THE UFAW HANDBOOK ON
The Care and Management of Laboratory and Other Research Animals

The Universities Federation for Animal Welfare

UFAW, founded in 1926, is an international independent, scientific and educational animal welfare charity and membership society. UFAW's vision is a world where the welfare of all animals affected by humans is maximised through a scientific understanding of their needs and how to meet them. UFAW aims to discover what matters to animals, develop scientific solutions to animal welfare problems and disseminate evidence-based animal welfare information by:

- Funding scientific research
- Supporting the careers of animal welfare scientists
- Disseminating animal welfare science knowledge both to experts and the wider public
- Providing expert advice to government departments and other bodies, helping to draft and amend laws and guidelines

You can help make even bigger strides in animal welfare science by donating, leaving a legacy or becoming a member of UFAW. For further information about UFAW and how you can help promote and support our work, please contact us at the following address:

Universities Federation for Animal Welfare
The Old School, Brewhouse Hill,
Wheathampstead, Herts AL4 8AN, United Kingdom
Phone: +44 (0) 1582 831818
Website: www.ufaw.org.uk
Email: ufaw@ufaw.org.uk

UFAW's aim with the UFAW/Wiley-Blackwell Animal Welfare book series is to promote interest and facilitate debate on the subject of animal welfare, while disseminating information relevant to improving the welfare of kept animals and those affected by human activities in the wild. The books in this series are the works of their authors, and the views they express do not necessarily reflect the views of UFAW.

THE UFAW HANDBOOK ON
The Care and Management of Laboratory and Other Research Animals

Ninth Edition

Edited by

Huw Golledge
Universities Federation Animal Welfare
UK

Claire Richardson
Universities Federation Animal Welfare
UK

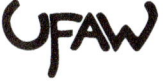

WILEY Blackwell

This edition first published 2024
© 2024 John Wiley & Sons Ltd

All rights reserved. No part of this publication may be reproduced, stored in a retrieval system, or transmitted, in any form or by any means, electronic, mechanical, photocopying, recording or otherwise, except as permitted by law. Advice on how to obtain permission to reuse material from this title is available at http://www.wiley.com/go/permissions.

The right of Huw Golledge and Claire Richardson to be identified as the authors of the editorial material in this work has been asserted in accordance with law.

Registered Offices
John Wiley & Sons, Inc., 111 River Street, Hoboken, NJ 07030, USA
John Wiley & Sons Ltd, The Atrium, Southern Gate, Chichester, West Sussex, PO19 8SQ, UK

For details of our global editorial offices, customer services, and more information about Wiley products visit us at www.wiley.com.

Wiley also publishes its books in a variety of electronic formats and by print-on-demand. Some content that appears in standard print versions of this book may not be available in other formats.

Trademarks: Wiley and the Wiley logo are trademarks or registered trademarks of John Wiley & Sons, Inc. and/or its affiliates in the United States and other countries and may not be used without written permission. All other trademarks are the property of their respective owners. John Wiley & Sons, Inc. is not associated with any product or vendor mentioned in this book.

Limit of Liability/Disclaimer of Warranty
The contents of this work are intended to further general scientific research, understanding, and discussion only and are not intended and should not be relied upon as recommending or promoting scientific method, diagnosis, or treatment by physicians for any particular patient. In view of ongoing research, equipment modifications, changes in governmental regulations, and the constant flow of information relating to the use of medicines, equipment, and devices, the reader is urged to review and evaluate the information provided in the package insert or instructions for each medicine, equipment, or device for, among other things, any changes in the instructions or indication of usage and for added warnings and precautions. While the publisher and authors have used their best efforts in preparing this work, they make no representations or warranties with respect to the accuracy or completeness of the contents of this work and specifically disclaim all warranties, including without limitation any implied warranties of merchantability or fitness for a particular purpose. No warranty may be created or extended by sales representatives, written sales materials or promotional statements for this work. This work is sold with the understanding that the publisher is not engaged in rendering professional services. The advice and strategies contained herein may not be suitable for your situation. You should consult with a specialist where appropriate. The fact that an organization, website, or product is referred to in this work as a citation and/or potential source of further information does not mean that the publisher and authors endorse the information or services the organization, website, or product may provide or recommendations it may make. Further, readers should be aware that websites listed in this work may have changed or disappeared between when this work was written and when it is read. Neither the publisher nor authors shall be liable for any loss of profit or any other commercial damages, including but not limited to special, incidental, consequential, or other damages.

Library of Congress Cataloging-in-Publication Data applied for:
[HB ISBN: 9781119555247]

Cover Design: Wiley
Cover Image: © tiripero/Getty Images

Set in 9/11pt Palatino by Straive, Pondicherry, India

Contents

List of contributors	vii
Foreword	xi

1. Introduction — Claire Richardson and Huw Golledge — 1

Part 1 Implementing the Three Rs in research using animals — 3

2. The Three Rs — Adrian Smith and Jon Richmond — 5

3. The design of animal experiments — Simon T. Bate and S. Clare Stanford — 23

4. An introduction to laboratory animal genetics — Michelle Stewart and Sara Wells — 40

5. Phenotyping of genetically modified mice — Jan-Bas Prins and Sara Wells — 54

6. Brief introduction to welfare assessment: a 'toolbox' of techniques — Jennifer Lofgren — 64

7. Welfare and 'best practice' in field studies of wildlife — Julie Lane and Robbie A. McDonald — 84

8. Legislation and oversight of the conduct of research using animals: a global overview — Kathryn Bayne, Javier Guillen, Malcolm P. France and Timothy H. Morris — 101

9. Planning, design and construction of the modern animal facility — Ken Applebee, Christopher Sear and Steven Cubitt — 122

10. Environmental enrichment: animal welfare and scientific validity — Hanno Würbel and Janja Novak — 137

11. Special housing arrangements — Mike Dennis — 150

12. Transportation of laboratory animals — Sonja T. Chou, Donna Clemons, Nicolas Dudoignon, Guy Mulder and Aleksandar Popovic — 171

13. Nutrition, feeding and animal welfare — Graham Tobin and Annette Schuhmacher — 191

14. Attaining competence in the care of animals used in research — Bryan Howard and Marcel Gyger — 220

15. The use of positive reinforcement training techniques to enhance the care and welfare of laboratory and research animals — Gail Laule — 236

16. 3Rs considerations when using ageing animals in science — J. Norman Flynn, Linda Horan, Carl S. Tucker, David Robb and Michael J.A. Wilkinson — 251

17. Euthanasia and other fates for laboratory animals — Huw Golledge — 268

18. Ethics review of animal research — I. Anna S. Olsson and Peter Sandøe — 281

Appendix — Penny Hawkins and Maggy Jennings — 294

Part 2 Species kept in the laboratory — 297

Mammals — 299

19. The laboratory opossum — John L. VandeBerg and Sarah Williams-Blangero — 301

20. Tree Shrews — Eberhard Fuchs — 324

Rodentia and Lagomorpha — 340

21. The laboratory mouse: Biology, behaviour, enrichment and welfare: first principles and real solutions for laboratory mice — Kathleen R. Pritchett-Corning and Joseph P. Garner — 340

22. The laboratory rat — Sietse F. de Boer and Jaap M. Koolhaas — 379

23. The laboratory gerbil — Elke Scheibler — 400

24. The Syrian hamster — Christina Winnicker and K.R. Pritchett-Corning — 419

25. Voles — Petra Kirsch — 430

26. The naked mole-rat (*Heterocephalus glaber*) — Chris G. Faulkes — 442

Appendix A — 459

27. The guinea pig — Sylvia Kaiser, Christine Krüger and Norbert Sachser — 465

28. The laboratory rabbit — Lena Lidfors and Therese Edström — 484

Carnivora	506
29 The ferret *Maggie Lloyd*	506
30 The laboratory dog *Laura Scullion Hall and Jackie Boxall*	518
31 The domestic cat *Emma Desforges*	546

Ungulates	570
32 Pigs and minipigs *Adrian Zeltner and Henrik Duelund Pedersen*	570
33 Cattle *Ute Weyer and Shellene Hurley*	596
34 Sheep and goats *Colin L. Gilbert and Cathy M. Dwyer*	609
35 The Horse *Heather Ewence and Fleur Whitlock*	628

Non-Human Primates	662
36 The mouse lemurs *Jennifer Wittkowski, Annette Klein, Annika Kollikowski, Marina Scheumann, Daniel Schmidtke, Elke Zimmermann and Ute Radespiel*	662
37 Marmosets and tamarins *Hannah M. Buchanan-Smith*	683
38 Capuchin monkeys *James R. Anderson, Elisabetta Visalberghi and Arianna Manciocco*	707
39 Old world monkeys *Jaco Bakker, Annet L. Louwerse, Marit K. Vernes and Jan A.M. Langermans*	721

Birds	**739**
40 The domestic fowl *Ian J.H. Duncan*	741
41 The Japanese quail *Rusty Lansford and Kimberly M. Cheng*	762
42 The zebra finch *Ruedi G. Nager, Michael J.A. Wilkinson and Graham Law*	787
43 Pigeons and doves *Stephen E.G. Lea, Anthony McGregor, Mark Haselgrove and Catriona M.E. Ryan*	807
44 The European starling *Melissa Bateson*	824
45 Corvids *Rachael Miller, Martina Schiestl and Nicola S. Clayton*	839

Reptiles and Amphibia	**853**
46 Terrestrial reptiles: lizards, snakes and tortoises *John E. Cooper*	855
47 An amphibian 'laboratory model', *Xenopus* *Richard Tinsley*	881

Fish	**905**
48 Fishes *Sonia Rey Planellas and Carlos Garcia de Leaniz*	907
49 Zebrafish *Carole Wilson*	933

Cephalopoda	**957**
50 Cephalopoda *Meghan Holst, Ryan B. Howard and Robyn J. Crook*	959

Decapoda	**991**
51 Decapod crustaceans *Robert W. Elwood and Ray W. Ingle*	993
Index	1012

List of contributors

†= have died before book was published

James R. Anderson
Department of Psychology, Graduate School of Letters,
Kyoto University
Kyoto, Japan

Kenneth A. Applebee
Applebee Advisory, Spectrum House
Hornchurch, Essex, UK

Jaco Bakker
Animal Science Department, Biomedical Primate
Research Centre
Rijswijk, The Netherlands

Simon T. Bate
CMC Statistics, GlaxoSmithKline Medicines Research Centre
Stevenage, UK

Melissa Bateson
Biosciences Institute, Newcastle University
Newcastle, UK

Kathryn Bayne
AAALAC International
Frederick MD, USA

Jackie Boxall
GSK, Stevenage, UK

Hannah M. Buchanan-Smith
Behaviour and Evolution Research Group, Psychology,
Faculty of Natural Sciences, University of Stirling
Scotland, UK

Kimberly M. Cheng
Avian Research Centre, University of British Columbia
Vancouver, Canada

Sonja T. Chou
Laboratory Animal Resources
NYU Shanghai, Shanghai, P. R. China

Nicola S. Clayton
Department of Psychology, University of Cambridge
Cambridge, UK

Donna Clemons
Comparative Medicine, AbbVie Inc.
North Chicago, IL, USA

John E. Cooper
Department of Veterinary Medicine, University of Cambridge
Cambridge, UK

Robyn J. Crook
Department of Biology, San Francisco State University
San Francisco, CA, USA

Steven J. Cubbitt
Cube Cleantech Limited, St John's Innovation Park
Cambridge, UK

Sietse F. de Boer
Behavioural Neuroscience group, GELIFES, University of
Groningen
Groningen, The Netherlands

Mike Dennis
Health Protection Agency
Porton Down, Salisbury, UK

Emma Desforges
Waltham Petcare Science Institute,
Waltham-on-the-Wolds, UK

Nicolas Dudoignon
Corporate Social Responsibility
Sanofi, Gentilly, France

Henrik Duelund Pedersen
Danish Medicines Agency, Regulatory & Clinical
Assessment
Copenhagen, Denmark

Ian J.H. Duncan
The Campbell Centre for the Study of Animal Welfare,
University of Guelph
Guelph, Canada

Cathy M. Dwyer
Animal Behaviour & Welfare, Animal & Veterinary Sciences,
Scottish Rural University College
Edinburgh, UK

Therese Edström
AstraZeneca R & D Mölndal
Mölndal, Sweden

Robert W. Elwood
Queen's University Belfast, School of Biological Sciences,
Belfast, UK

List of contributors

Heather Ewence
(formerly of) The Animal Health Trust
Suffolk, UK

Christopher G. Faulkes
School of Biological and Behavioural Sciences,
Queen Mary University of London
London, UK

J. Norman Flynn
Animals in Science Regulation Unit (ASRU),
Home Office Science, Security and Innovation, UK

Malcolm P. France
Consultant, Laboratory Animal Care and Management
NSW 2045, Australia

Eberhard Fuchs
Clinical Neurobiology Laboratory, German Primate Center,
Leibniz Institute for Primate Research
Göttingen, Germany

Carlos Garcia de Leaniz
Centre for Sustainable Aquatic Research, Swansea University
Wales, UK

Joseph Garner
Department of Comparative Medicine, Stanford University
Stanford, California, USA

Colin L. Gilbert
Babraham Institute
Babraham, Cambridge

Huw Golledge
UFAW
Wheathampstead, UK

Javier Guillen
AAALAC International
Pamplona, Spain

Marcel Gyger
Swiss Federal Institute of Technology, School of Life Sciences, Center of PhenogenomicsLausanne, Switzerland

Mark Haselgrove
University of Nottingham, School of Psychology
Nottingham, UK

Penny Hawkins
RSPCA, Animals in Science Department
Horsham, UK

Meghan Holst
Department of Biology, San Francisco State University
San Francisco, CA, USA

Linda Horan
University of Strathclyde, Strathclyde Institute of Pharmacy and Biomedical Sciences
Glasgow, UK

Ryan B. Howard
Department of Biology, San Francisco State University
San Francisco, CA, USA

Bryan Howard
(formerly of) University of Sheffield
Sheffield, UK

Shellene Hurley
Animal and Plant Health Agency, Pathology & Animal Sciences
Addlestone, Surrey, UK

Ray W. Ingle
Natural History Museum
London, UK

Maggy Jennings
RSPCA, Animals in Science Department
Horsham, UK

Sylvia Kaiser
University of Münster, Department of Behavioural Biology
Münster, Germany

Petra Kirsch
University Hospital Hamburg-Eppendorf
Hamburg, Germany

Annette Klein
Institute of Zoology, University of Veterinary Medicine Hannover
Hannover, Germany

Annika Kollikowski
Institute of Zoology, University of Veterinary Medicine Hannover
Hannover, Germany

Jaap M. Koolhaas
Behavioural Neuroscience group, GELIFES, University of Groningen
Groningen, The Netherlands

Christine Krüger
German Institute of Human Nutrition
Potsdam-Rehbruecke
Nuthetal, Germany

Julie M. Lane
The Food and Environment Research Agency
Sand Hutton, York, UK

Jan A.M. Langermans
Animal Science Department, Biomedical Primate Research Centre
Rijswijk, The Netherlands
Population Health Sciences, Unit Animals in Science and Society, Veterinary faculty
Utrecht University, The Netherlands

List of contributors ix

Rusty Lansford
Keck School of Medicine, University of Southern California
Los Angeles, USA

Gail Laule
Mandai Wildlife Group
Singapore

Graham Law†
University of Glasgow
Glasgow, UK

Stephen E. G. Lea
University of Exeter
Exeter, UK

Lena Lidfors
Department of Animal Environment and Health, Swedish University of Agricultural Sciences, Skara, Sweden

Maggie Lloyd
Red Kite Veterinary Consultants
Abingdon, UK

Jennifer Lofgren
Novartis Institutes for BioMedical Research Inc.
Cambridge, USA

Annet L. Louwerse
Animal Science Department, Biomedical Primate Research Centre
Rijswijk, The Netherlands

Arianna Manciocco
Istituto di Scienze e Tecnologie della Cognizione, Consiglio Nazionale delle Ricerche Rome, Italy

Robbie A. McDonald
The Food and Environment Research Agency
Sand Hutton, York, UK

Anthony McGregor
University of Durham, Department of Psychology
Durham, UK

Rachael Miller
Department of Psychology, University of Cambridge, Cambridge, UK
School of Life Sciences, Anglia Ruskin University, Cambridge, UK

Timothy H. Morris
The School of Veterinary Medicine and Science, The University of Nottingham
Sutton Bonington, UK

Guy Mulder
Research Models and Services, Charles River Laboratories, Inc.
Wilmington, MA, USA

Ruedi G. Nager
University of Glasgow, School of Biodiversity, One Health and Veterinary Medicine Glasgow, UK

Janja Novak
Division of Animal Welfare, Veterinary Public Health Institute, Vetsuisse Faculty, University of Bern
Bern, Switzerland

I. Anna S. Olsson
i3S - Instituto de Investigação e Inovação em Saúde and IBMC – Instituto de Biologia Molecular e Celular, Universidade do Porto
Porto, Portugal

Aleksandar Popovic
Research Models and Services, Charles River UK Ltd, Margate, UK

Kathleen R. Pritchett-Corning
Office of Animal Resources, Harvard University, Cambridge, MA, USA
Department of Comparative Medicine, University of Washington, Seattle, WA, USA

Jan-Bas Prins
The Francis Crick Institute, London, UK
Leiden University Medical Centre, The Netherlands

Ute Radespiel
Institute of Zoology, University of Veterinary Medicine Hannover
Hannover, Germany

Sonia Rey Planellas
Institute of Aquaculture, University of Stirling
Scotland, UK

Claire Richardson
UFAW
Wheathampstead, UK

Jon Richmond
Ethical Biomedical Research and Testing: Advice and Consultancy, UK

David Robb
Veterinary Services, Charles River Laboratories Edinburgh Ltd
Edinburgh, UK

Catriona M. E. Ryan
University of Exeter
Exeter, UK

Norbert Sachser
University of Münster, Department of Behavioural Biology
Münster, Germany

Peter Sandøe
Department of Food and Resource Economics, Science, Department of Veterinary and Animal Sciences, Health, University of Copenhagen
Denmark

Elke Scheibler
(formerly of) University of South Wales
UK

List of contributors

Marina Scheumann
Institute of Zoology
University of Veterinary Medicine Hannover
Hannover, Germany

Martina Schiestl
Faculty of Veterinary Medicine
University of Veterinary Sciences
Brno, Czech Republic

Daniel Schmidtke
Institute of Zoology
University of Veterinary Medicine Hannover
Hannover, Germany

Annette Schuhmacher
ssniff Spezialdiaeten
Soest, Germany

Laura Scullion Hall
(formerly of) University of Stirling
Stirling, UK

Christopher H.J. Sear
Cube Cleantech Limited
St John's Innovation Park
Cambridge, UK

Adrian Smith
Norecopa
Norwegian Veterinary Institute,
Norway

S. Clare Stanford
Department of Neuroscience, Physiology & Pharmacology
University College London
London, UK

Michelle Stewart
Mary Lyon Centre, MRC Harwell
Harwell Campus
Oxfordshire, UK

Richard Tinsley
School of Biological Sciences
University of Bristol
Bristol, UK

Graham Tobin
(formerly of) Harlan Teklad, Blackthorn
Bicester, UK

Carl S. Tucker
The QMRI (BVS) Aquatic Facilities, The Queen's Medical Research Institute
The University of Edinburgh
Edinburgh, UK

John L. VandeBerg
University of Texas Rio Grande Valley, Department of Human Genetics
South Texas Diabetes and Obesity Institute
Brownsville/Harlingen/Edinburg, Texas, USA

Marit K. Vernes
Animal Science Department
Biomedical Primate Research Centre
Rijswijk, The Netherlands

Elisabetta Visalberghi
Istituto di Scienze e Tecnologie della Cognizione
Consiglio Nazionale delle Ricerche Rome, Italy

Sara Wells
The Mary Lyon Centre at MRC Harwell
Harwell Science Campus
Oxfordshire, UK

Ute Weyer
Animal and Plant Health Agency
Pathology & Animal Sciences
Addlestone, Surrey, UK

Fleur Whitlock
(formerly of) The Animal Health Trust
Suffolk, UK

Michael J.A. Wilkinson
University of Glasgow, Biological Services, Veterinary Research Facility
Glasgow, UK

Sarah Williams-Blangero
University of Texas Rio Grande Valley, Department of Human Genetics
South Texas Diabetes and Obesity Institute
Brownsville/Harlingen/Edinburg, Texas, USA

Carole Wilson
University College London
London, UK

Christina Winnicker
Research Office of Animal Welfare Ethics Strategy and Risk
GlaxoSmithKline
Collegeville, Pennsylvania, USA

Jennifer Wittkowski
Institute of Zoology
University of Veterinary Medicine Hannover
Hannover, Germany

Hanno Würbel
Division of Animal Welfare, Veterinary Public Health Institute, Vetsuisse Faculty
University of Bern
Bern, Switzerland

Adrian Zeltner
Ellegaard Göttingen Minipigs A/S
Dalmose, Denmark

Elke Zimmermann[†]
Institute of Zoology
University of Veterinary Medicine Hannover
Hannover, Germany

Foreword

The use of animals in research is rightly a subject of a certain amount of public debate, but there is no doubt of the huge benefits to both human and animal health and well-being which has accrued as a result of highly regulated and scientifically based animal research. In this latest and impressive ninth edition, like its predecessors, this invaluable handbook from the Universities Federation for Animal Welfare (UFAW) continues to uphold the highest standards of animal welfare in research. It plays a crucial role in maintaining the social contract that allows for their ethical use.

The ninth edition comprehensively updates the eighth edition of 2010 and provides up-to-date, evidence-based information on the practical care and welfare of animals used in research to enable those who work with these animals to ensure the animals are cared for to the highest possible standard whilst also ensuring that they provide reliable research data.

Of 51 chapters, the first substantive one covers a priority issue, the Three Rs – *replacement*, *reduction* and *refinement* – which are a constant and continuing goal of all researchers. Very appropriately, the next chapter deals with the design experiments, which is critical to ensure statistically reliable results from as few animals as possible.

There follow a series of detailed chapters covering all the important general aspects of the care and use of laboratory animals, including welfare assessment, housing and the design of facilities, transport, nutrition and the legislation controlling the conduct of research. In addition to legislation, the use of animals now invariably requires ethical approval, the subject of another chapter. A further 33 authoritative chapters deal in depth with all types of animals used in research, including a major and brilliant chapter on laboratory mice. This makes the powerful point that providing enrichment and allowing animals control over their environments are critical to minimising their stress and maximising the biological relevance and predictive accuracy of any data derived from them. All of these chapters are written by experts in their fields from all over the world.

This superb handbook is of great value to researchers and to the welfare of the animals they use. Its authoritative and evidence-based exposition on such an important topic continues the exemplary contributions made by UFAW to the cause of animal welfare.

Emeritus Professor the Lord Trees, FRCVS,
FMedSci, HonFRSE
House of Lords,
London, SW1A 0PW,
United Kingdom
22 January 2024

1 Introduction

Claire Richardson and Huw Golledge

We are very pleased to introduce the 9th edition of *The UFAW Handbook on the Care and Management of Laboratory and Other Research Animals*. The first edition of this book, published in 1947, was the first ever laboratory animal handbook published with the aim of improving the welfare of animals used in research, and it continues to be a key reference for those in the field. Putting the latest animal welfare science into practice to improve animal welfare is central to the mission of Universities Federation for Animal Welfare (UFAW), and this handbook exemplifies this practical approach to improving the lives of animals.

The previous (8th) edition of the handbook was published in 2010. Chapters have been updated to reflect rapidly growing advances in the field, and new chapters have been added on nutrition, feeding and animal welfare (Chapter 14); 3Rs considerations when using ageing animals in science (Chapter 16); ethical review (Chapter 18); the naked mole rat (Chapter 26); corvids (Chapter 45); and zebrafish (Chapter 49).

Our thanks go to Dr. Robert Hubrecht, co-editor of the 8th edition of the handbook, who instigated this new edition before retiring as UFAW's chief executive in 2019. Although he retired before the project was complete, we are very grateful for his knowledge, insight and organisational skills, which were instrumental in initiating this project. We are also grateful for Dr. Hubrecht's longstanding commitment to promoting animal welfare and science. Our thanks also go to Dr. Birte Nielsen, Research Director of UFAW, for her editorial guidance, knowledge and encouragement in completing the handbook.

We are grateful to the Wiley publishing team, particularly Adalfin Jayasingh and Rathi Aravind, for their patience and professionalism throughout the production stage.

Our greatest thanks go to the members of the laboratory animal science and welfare community that came together to both write and peer-review the chapters of this handbook. Colleagues from around the world volunteered their time to provide their expertise and share their passion for animals and science to write the individual chapters. In addition, numerous anonymous referees generously volunteered their time and expertise to provide invaluable comments on draft chapters, which have significantly improved the contents of each.

It has not always been an easy journey, and progress was particularly difficult during the COVID pandemic, so we are grateful for the patience of the contributing authors who submitted chapters early in the production phase and to the resilience of the authors who submitted later on and endured our nagging emails. It has been our pleasure to learn from all those involved.

As a charity, UFAW relies on its members and donors to carry out its work, so we thank them as well as the UFAW staff and trustees, without whom we would not have been able to dedicate time and resources to produce this updated handbook.

As with previous editions, we have, as editors, aimed to ensure that the chapters reflect UFAW's approach to the care and husbandry of animals used in research; however, the chapters are the individual authors' work, and the views they have expressed should not be taken as UFAW's official opinions. Similarly, it is, of course, the responsibility of those working with animals to ensure that the practices they adopt comply with national legislation.

We hope that you find this handbook useful and that it helps to promote good welfare and good science.

The UFAW Handbook on the Care and Management of Laboratory and Other Research Animals, Ninth Edition.
Edited by Huw Golledge and Claire Richardson.
© 2024 John Wiley & Sons Ltd. Published 2024 by John Wiley & Sons Ltd.

PART 1
IMPLEMENTING THE THREE RS IN RESEARCH USING ANIMALS

2 The Three Rs

Adrian Smith and Jon Richmond

Opening remarks

The Universities Federation for Animal Welfare (UFAW) actively promotes the welfare of animals bred, kept and used for experimental and other scientific purposes by:

- championing a scientific approach to animal care and welfare, providing evidence-based insights into *'what is meaningful to the animal'*; and
- advocating that *'best welfare is indeed best science'* and that we must *'... aim at well-being rather than at mere absence of distress'* (Russell & Burch 1959).

In 1954, UFAW commissioned work by William Russell and Rex Burch which led to the publication in 1959 of *The Principles of Humane Experimental Technique* (Russell & Burch 1959). Russell and Burch reasoned that high standards of animal welfare facilitate better animal-based science. They concluded that *'... humanity can be promoted without prejudice to scientific and medical aims'* and *'... the humanest possible treatment of experimental animals ... is actually a prerequisite for successful animal experiments'*... *'If we are to use a criterion for choosing experiments to perform, the criterion of humanity is the best we could possibly invent ... The greatest scientific experiments have always been the most humane and most aesthetically attractive, conveying that sense of beauty and elegance which is the essence of science at its most successful'*.

They championed the principles of Replacement, Reduction and Refinement, now universally known as 'the Three Rs'. These principles, and an understanding that they must be embedded in the planning, conduct and review of animal-based research and testing, are now an integral part of mainstream biomedical science and form the basis of legislation on animal research and testing in many countries (Guillén 2017)[1].

This chapter provides a contemporary overview of the principles, art and practice of humane experimental technique as it has evolved since Russell and Burch's landmark publication. This chapter focuses on general principles as a prelude to the more detailed and context-specific material in later chapters.

Introduction

It is now accepted that some classes of animal, such as vertebrates, can experience negative welfare states such as pain, suffering and distress, and all of those involved in the production, care and use of live animals for scientific or other experimental purposes have a moral, and in many cases a legal, obligation to minimise any justifiable suffering caused.

It also generally accepted that animal studies should only be undertaken when all of the following conditions are met:

- the scientific objectives are timely, of sufficient importance, attainable, and that the scientific and societal benefits will be maximised;
- there is no non-sentient replacement alternative;
- all relevant and practical Reduction and Refinement strategies have been implemented; and
- the design and conduct of the study minimise the animal welfare cost in terms of the total pain, suffering and distress that may be produced, rather than simply minimising the number of animals used.

Implementing humane experimental technique to minimise animal welfare costs requires knowledge and understanding of:

- behaviours and clinical findings in normal, healthy animals;
- the impact of animal care systems and scientific procedures;
- how animal welfare can be evaluated; and
- the development and application of informed, practical solutions to identify, manage and minimise the animal welfare costs.

---

[1] See also https://en.wikipedia.org/wiki/Animal_testing_regulations (accessed 10 Jan 2022)

Simple words, complex meanings

The commonly used definitions of alternatives, Replacement, Reduction and Refinement, are deceptively simple. They conceal subtleties of meaning which must be fully understood in order to appreciate the power and relevance of the Three Rs.

The term 'alternatives', used by Smyth (1978) for the Three Rs, can mislead by creating the false impression that only Replacement is relevant, or that 'alternative' methods simply substitute for, but retain the scope and limitations of, the original animal models.

In reality, Replacement alternatives are not just substitutes for animal models: they are often better science, more powerful and versatile and the tools of choice. For example, the use of robotics and *in vitro* replacement systems for high-throughput screening of potential novel pharmaceuticals allows rates of progress not previously possible using animal models.

Reduction is better considered as optimisation of animal numbers. The intention is to minimise the number of animals required to provide suitably robust data. Using more is wasteful; using fewer at best requires that work is repeated and at worst results in misleading conclusions being drawn from the available data. There are occasions when the original estimates of the number of animals required prove on examination to be too few to meet the scientific objectives, and on these occasions properly applying the principles of Reduction will result in the justified use of more animals than originally estimated.

Reduction and Refinement are inseparable: the imperative is not to minimise the number of animals used, but to minimise the suffering that is caused.

The origin and evolution of the Three Rs

Early scientific use of animals was often curiosity-driven, and involved demonstrating biological phenomena, without necessarily having practical application (Barley 1999). A gradual shift then occurred towards understanding the underlying mechanisms and regulation of observed phenomena. This was, in turn, followed by a move to 'deductive science' – based on formulating and testing hypotheses, seeking results with practical applications, and publishing the results widely. These differing approaches to science are still reflected in the types of animal studies undertaken and animal models used (Festing 2011):

- exploratory models demonstrating biological phenomena or generating knowledge without necessarily being relevant to any immediate practical application;
- explanatory models elucidating the mechanisms;
- predictive models allowing problem solving and decision making.

The origins of the concepts of Replacement, Reduction and Refinement in relation to the use of animals in science date back to Victorian Britain (Richmond 2000). An editorial in the London Medical Gazette in 1839 advised that live animals should not be used

... till it is sufficiently clear that the fact pursued neither is, nor can be proved by any other evidence which is within reach, nor by any more mode of enquiry. (Anon. 1839)

Principles of humane experimental technique were set out in more detail in Marshall Hall's publications from the same period. In an article in the Lancet in 1847 he wrote:

We should never have recourse to experiment in cases which observation can afford us the information required; No experiment should be performed without a distinct and definite object and without the persuasion that the object will be attained and produce a real and uncomplicated result; We should not needlessly repeat experiments and cause the least possible suffering, using the lowest order of animals and avoiding the infliction of pain; We should try to secure due observation so as to avoid the necessity of repetition. (Hall 1847)

He composed the following seven principles (published posthumously by his widow in 1861)[2]

1. We should never have recourse to experiment in cases which observation can afford us the information required.
2. No experiment should be performed without a distinct and definite object, and without the persuasion, after the maturest consideration, that that object will be attained by that experiment, in the form of a real and uncomplicated result.
3. We should not needlessly repeat experiments which have already been performed by physiologists of reputation.
4. After due consideration that a given experiment is, at once, essential and adequate to the discovery of a truth, it should be instituted with the least possible infliction of suffering.
5. Every physiological experiment should be performed under such circumstances as will secure due observation and attestation of its results, and so obviate, as much as possible, the necessity for its repetition.
6. Facts should be laid before the public in the simplest, plainest terms. If there be a difference of opinion: '...add such views as may seem nearest the truth. These are neither wholly in accord with one opinion nor another, nor exceedingly at variance with both, ... a thing which may be observed in most controversies, when men seek impartially for truth'. (Celsus, translated from Latin)
7. In quoting the opinions of other authors, it should always be in their own words.

Russell and Burch originally defined:

- Replacement as '*any scientific method employing non-sentient material which may in the history of animal experimentation replace methods which use conscious living vertebrates*';
- Reduction as means of minimising, other than by Replacement, '*the number of animals used to obtain information of a given amount and precision*';

---

[2]https://www.ahajournals.org/doi/epdf/10.1161/01.CIR.48.3.651 (Accessed 12 Dec 2022)

- Refinement as measures leading to a *'decrease in the incidence or severity of inhumane procedures applied to those animals which have to be used'*.

The working definitions of the Three Rs commonly used today are often somewhat different to these originals (Buchanan-Smith *et al*. 2005; Tannenbaum and Bennett 2015; the NC3Rs web site[3]). More contemporary interpretations include:

- Replacement: methods which permit a given scientific objective to be achieved without conducting procedures on animals which impose any welfare cost;
- Reduction: methods for obtaining equivalent levels of information from the use of fewer animals in scientific procedures, or for obtaining more information from the same number of animals;
- Refinement: methods which alleviate or minimise potential pain, suffering or distress, and which enhance animal well-being.

The acceptance and application of the principles of humane experimental technique after Russell and Burch's book in 1959 was followed by a period of reduction in animal use and significant welfare gains, at a time of increasing investment and rapid advances in the biomedical sciences. The production and use of animals for experimental and other scientific purposes are, however, now increasing again, primarily due to the production and use of genetically altered animals[4,5]. Nevertheless, the principles of humane experimental technique, albeit with revised definitions, are proving to be sufficiently relevant and flexible to be applicable to areas of animal use not foreseen at the time of Russell and Burch's publication.

Progress with the Three Rs is not solely driven by a desire to improve animal welfare. Methodological improvements are required to overcome the limitations of existing animal models and open up new lines of scientific enquiry. In practice, 'alternative' methods based on the Three Rs are generally more technically advanced, cost effective, reliable, easily scalable and may be more scientifically valid than those traditionally used. The development and use of Adverse Outcome Pathways (AOP) to improve regulatory testing regimens is an example of these principles being applied in practice (Vinken 2013) to better protect the public and the environment.

Thus, the case for the Three Rs can be made simultaneously on three grounds:

- better animal welfare;
- better science in terms of quality and rate of progress; and
- logistics and economics.

Where implementation of the Three Rs is at times hampered by the lack of scientific evidence about, or a consensus on, what constitutes 'best practice', a useful approach to promoting the Three Rs and high-quality, humane animal-based research can be the Three Ss of good Sense, Sensibilities and Science (Rowsell 1977; Smith & Hawkins 2016).

---

[3]https://www.nc3rs.org.uk/the-3rs (accessed 10 Jan 2022)
[4]http://ec.europa.eu/environment/chemicals/lab_animals/reports_en.htm (accessed 10 Jan 2022)
[5]https://www.gov.uk/government/collections/animals-in-science-statistics (accessed 10 Jan 2022)

A holistic approach to the Three Rs

Russell and Burch recognised the need for a holistic, rather than sequential, approach to the Three Rs, particularly with respect to Reduction and Refinement. Tensions can exist, balances may have to be struck, and synergies exploited. Decisions must be made on a case-by-case basis in the context of the specific scientific objectives being pursued.

To minimise animal suffering, Reduction and Refinement must be considered concurrently. For example, there are technologies that involve initial surgical preparation but which then reduce the total number of animals required, minimise the stress animals subsequently experience and improve the quality of the findings. Implantable telemetry devices (Kramer & Kinter 2003) can allow the remote capture of intermittent or continuous streams of 'physiological data' while animals undertake normal activities unstressed by disturbances to the social group, sedation, handling or restraint. These technologies may permit the numbers of animals per study to be reduced by the capture of serial data and the re-use of telemetered animals. In such cases there are trade-offs to be made between the welfare costs of the initial surgical preparation, the reduction in the number of animals required to give meaningful results, the procedural stresses that can be avoided after recovery from surgery and the improved nature and quality of the data that can be gathered (Brockway *et al*. 1993; Schnell & Gerber 1997).

Serial diagnostic imaging can also reduce numbers, at the cost of the serial general anaesthetics that are normally required to restrain the animal during imaging.

These, and other, examples illustrate the need to take a holistic rather than a sequential approach when putting humane experimental technique into practice.

Replacement

Although we do not currently have the means to replace all forms of animal use without slowing scientific progress, Replacement is especially relevant to fundamental and applied biomedical research, regulatory testing and the use of animals in education and training. Replacement alternatives typically offer a range of benefits over the animal models they supersede, often allowing more rapid progress and in some cases providing scientific insights that were not possible using animal models.

Replacement alternatives must be based on sound science and produce responses that correlate with those of biological systems which they model. Their development requires an understanding of the underlying biological mechanisms and their responses, and is often dependent on the availability (or *de novo* generation) of reliable animal or human reference data, and new technologies.

Russell and Burch distinguished between 'absolute' Replacement, with no sentient animal use (for example, computer models), and 'relative' Replacement, using animals in procedures not causing pain, suffering or distress (for example, humane killing to obtain tissue, experiments under full terminal anaesthesia and the use of immature forms believed to be incapable of experiencing pain, suffering or distress).

Progress with Replacement has, to date, been largely with single-stage processes involving biological effects mediated by clearly understood single-event mechanisms, and for which there is high-quality human or relevant animal reference data. Devising non-animal models of dynamic and complex biological interactions is more difficult, but progress is being made, for example by producing so-called organs-on-chips (Marx *et al.* 2016; Trapecar 2021; Vulto & Joore 2021).

The range of Replacement options can be wide and varied, and may include:

- strategies avoiding the need to generate new animal-based data;
- systems allowing elements of evidence gathering, analysis or decision making to be undertaken without live animal use;
- animal-based methods and models providing the required insights without causing procedure-related pain, suffering or distress to sentient animals.

Replacement strategies

In some instances, new scientific objectives can be achieved without the need for animal use. Examples include:

- Rationalising and harmonising regulatory requirements and provisions to dispense with inessential tests. For example, the Abnormal Toxicity Test (Schwanig *et al.* 1997) is no longer required for the evaluation of a wide range of biologicals used in clinical practice.
- Harmonising international validation processes, regulatory testing requirements and decision making, to eliminate the need to use animals in different protocols to inform multiple regulators in different geographical regions about a single toxicological endpoint.
- Reformulating scientific objectives to allow relevant insights to be gained using existing data or new non-animal data.
- Reviewing published work to ensure that relevant existing data are not overlooked and animal experiments inadvertently replicated. There is, however, an important distinction to make between inadvertent, unnecessary duplication (the unintended repetition of studies that have already been completed and reported) and justified, intentional replication. The latter may be necessary to confirm findings, introduce new model systems, evaluate procedural changes, restart programmes of work after periods of inactivity, or when changing laboratories.
- Data sharing where previous relevant findings have not been published: for example, accessing data generated for in-house decision making or contained in regulatory submissions.
- Sharing tissues and samples from animals killed or used for scientific purposes.

Replacement methods

Where new data are required, a wide range of Replacement methods can be considered:

- The use of physico-chemical properties to predict biological effects to screen or fully evaluate test materials. Examples include the use of pH and buffer capacity to predict potential severe ocular irritation or corrosion (OECD, 2017); peptide reactivity assays to screen chemicals for skin sensitisation potential (Lalko *et al.* 2012); and the use of computer and mathematical models allowing molecular structure to be correlated with specific biological activities[6].
- The use of non-sentient organisms. Examples include the use of bacteria (Ames *et al.* 1973), roundworms (Leung *et al.* 2008) and fruit flies (Perrimon *et al.* 2016).
- The use of immature forms of sentient species incapable of experiencing pain, suffering or distress; for example, fish larvae to evaluate aquatic toxicity (Lilicrap *et al.* 2016).
- The use of *ex vivo* and *in vitro* systems, of animal or human origin, at the level of the organ, tissue slice, cell culture/suspension or sub-cellular component (Marx *et al.* 2016; Vulto & Joore 2021). These may be absolute replacements (for example, non-primary cell cultures that do not require to be maintained using foetal calf serum), or relative replacements (for example, animal primary cell cultures, or other cell culture systems requiring the use of serum).
- The collection of material shed by animals (e.g. their faeces, hair, saliva and urine) from which DNA can be retrieved, as an alternative to invasive capture and sampling methods (e.g. Bischof *et al.* 2020). The collection of environmental DNA is especially relevant in field research. Genotyping can be used to identify and track both individuals and populations.
- Human studies, subject to appropriate ethical safeguards. Data may be gathered in the course of volunteer, clinical-trial, post-marketing surveillance or epidemiological studies. New technologies (for example, improved methods of diagnostic imaging, and preclinical markers of biological effects) can offer new opportunities to work with ethically human subjects.

The pros and cons of animal use in education and training have been hotly debated for many years, both for ethical reasons and in the light of the Three Rs (Zemanova *et al.* 2021). A wide range of Replacement alternatives can be used in education and training, once the educational objectives have been clearly defined. These can be used to demonstrate biological phenomena, processes and interactions; train participants in manual skills and develop proficiency in problem solving. These 'alternatives' include models, films and videotapes of procedures, interactive software simulations and virtual reality systems. The NORINA database contains information on 3,000 alternatives and supplements to animal use in education and training, at all levels of academia and industry[7].

The high-fidelity fallacy

All model systems, whether they are animal or non-animal models, mimic only limited aspects of the human condition or other target system (Sams-Dodd 2006). This must be kept in

---

[6]https://echa.europa.eu/support/registration/how-to-avoid-unnecessary-testing-on-animals/qsar-models (accessed 10 Jan 2022)
[7]https://norecopa.no/NORINA (accessed 10 Jan 2022)

mind when the most appropriate model is selected, and findings analysed, interpreted, generalised and extrapolated. Scientists must be fully aware of the scope, and the limitations, of the models that they use (Pound & Ritskes-Hoitinga 2018).

Russell and Burch (1959) warned of the 'high-fidelity fallacy': the false assumption that high-fidelity (the closeness in biological terms of a model system to the actual system of interest) dictates the preferred model system. Non-human primates can be considered to be high-fidelity models of man as *'in their general physiological and pharmacological properties'* they are *'more consistently like us than are other organisms'*. However, any instinctive preference for high-fidelity models *'ignores all the advantages of correlation'*, whereby *'the responses of two utterly different systems may be correlated with perfect regularity'* (Russell and Burch (1959)).

High-fidelity models are generally not required in practice. What is essential is not that a model system 'looks like' the system of interest, but that it behaves like it. The essential quality of a good model system is high *discrimination*: its ability, in the context of a defined biological process or outcome, to produce responses which correlate with the response of the system which they model. Replacement alternatives (for example, isolated tissues, cell cultures and computer models) generally possess high discrimination but are, inevitably, low-fidelity. In the words of Russell and Burch, they *'reproduce one particular property of the original, in which we happen to be interested'*. This concept is partially fuelling a transition away from animal experimentation to studies of human cells, tissue or organs, particularly within the realm of toxicology where it is, at present, most feasible (Kimura *et al.* 2018).

Reduction

Reduction and Refinement must always be considered simultaneously. Focusing purely on decreasing numbers can lead to solutions that produce a disproportionate increase in the pain and distress caused to the animals that are used (Richmond 1999).

Reduction can be considered to comprise any strategy or method which:

- other than by Replacement reduces the need for animal studies; or
- minimises the number of animals required to achieve a defined scientific objective; or
- permits more data or product to be obtained from the animals that must still be used.

Experimental design

Elements of experimental design such as sample size, statistical power, variation, precision and the proper application of appropriate statistical methods are important means of determining the number of animals required and interpreting the data that is generated (see Festing & Altman 2002, and the Norecopa web site[8]). However, there are equally important non-statistical considerations. These include selection of suitable experimental subjects, husbandry and care systems, procedural details and other means of controlling and minimising unwanted stressors and unnecessary variables. See, among others, Chapter 15 (The use of positive reinforcement training techniques to enhance the care and welfare of laboratory and research animals).

Having exercised due diligence to ensure a new animal study is not unknowingly duplicating the work of others and that there are no suitable Replacement options, it is important to be aware of, and consider, the full range of Reduction options and opportunities.

The sequence in which a series of objectives are pursued and experiments are carried out is an important consideration. One of the most effective means of minimising the numbers of animals required for a programme of work is to apply tiered and hierarchical approaches to enable the early identification and discarding of models, materials and hypotheses not destined for further evaluation or development, thus avoiding the need for unnecessary animal studies. Using the assessment of the ocular safety of materials as an example (Gallegos Saliner & Worth 2007):

- consider a test material's structural and physicochemical properties;
- evaluate *in vitro* test results;
- conduct dermal safety tests; and
- identify strong skin irritants and corrosive materials.

These can combine to enable a reliable evaluation to be made of likely ocular safety without undertaking tests on live animals. When ocular safety tests on live animals are still required, testing first on a single animal can reduce the number of animals used, as materials giving strong positives in a single animal do not require confirmatory testing in more animals. This example also links to Refinement, by dispensing with the need to use animals to test the materials most likely to cause the greatest degrees of pain, suffering, distress and lasting harm.

Preliminary *in vitro* data can reduce the number of animals required for definitive studies. For example, cytotoxicity data is now used to reduce the number of animals used in acute toxicity studies by determining the appropriate doses of test materials to be used in the animal studies (ICCVAM 2001).

Small proof-of-concept studies, if they fail to demonstrate the expected outcomes, obviate the need for failed large-scale definitive studies.

Definitive studies can often only be planned in detail once preliminary animal data are available. Pilot experiments are useful: these are small-scale preliminary studies to examine and fully develop the working hypotheses and logistics of proposed definitive studies[9]. Even though in many cases the results will not be published, they will be used to design improved definitive studies by providing insights into:

- likely inter-individual variation and the number of animals required to obtain robust scientific results;
- the most appropriate dosing, and sampling routines;
- the nature, incidence, severity and timing of possible physiological, behavioural changes and adverse effects, and the required observation schedules;

---

[8]https://norecopa.no/prepare/4-experimental-design-and-statistical-analysis (accessed 10 Jan 2022)

[9]https://nc3rs.org.uk/conducting-pilot-study (accessed 10 Jan 2022)

- how adverse effects can best be avoided, elucidated or managed;
- importantly, they may identify and provide an opportunity to tackle unexpected, technical problems and extraneous experimental variables before larger-scale studies are undertaken.

The number of animals required to meet the scientific objectives reflects the required degree of precision and certainty. The number of animals required should be no more than is necessary to meet the scientific objective.

There may be opportunities for reducing the number of animals required by taking account of the prevalence of the outcome of interest (Hoffmann & Hartung 2006). It may require less data to identify candidate test materials with a common property, than with an uncommon property.

Where test materials are only to be assigned to general categories, requiring only an estimate of their biological properties, smaller numbers of animals may be sufficient, rather than the larger numbers required to calculate more precise or absolute values.

Control groups are in all other respects exposed to identical conditions, observations and investigations. They are used as standards for comparison, making conclusions about the relevance and significance of the results more robust by demonstrating that the test system is appropriately responsive and capable of correctly identifying biologically active and inactive test materials. They assist also in eliminating alternative explanations of experimental results: the possibility that the experimental subjects were prone to, or incapable of, giving appropriate positive or negative results. They may also be valuable in demonstrating other potential confounding variables within the test system, for example, the chance that some unrecognised, intercurrent problem influenced the responses observed.

When there is a need for control data, the number of animals can, in some circumstances, be minimised by the use of a single concurrent control to evaluate simultaneously a range of test materials for the same biological property, or by the use of historical controls, or when a number of test materials are tested in the same laboratory on the same day. The routine use of concurrent positive controls, to demonstrate that the test method as applied in a laboratory can produce an appropriate positive response, is generally unnecessary if the routine testing programme itself regularly produces both valid positive and negative results.

In some circumstances, a relatively large amount of extra information can be gained from the use of small additional satellite groups to pursue more than one scientific objective within a single experiment. For example, toxicokinetic data can be gathered in the course of single-dose toxicity studies (EMEA 1995).

The degree of uniformity (lack of variability) within and between experimental subjects is an important determinant of the number of experimental subjects required, and all reasonable efforts should be made to control relevant genetic and epigenetic factors. The use of purpose-bred animals permits varying degrees of control of genetic variability and microbiological status, and for many of the commonly used species the availability of inbred and isogenic strains allows the use of smaller group sizes than is possible with outbred or random-bred animals (see Chapter 4: An introduction to laboratory animal genetics). In some instances, it has been argued that the use of genetically identical animals allows scientific progress to be made that would otherwise be impossible (Festing & Fisher 2000). However, the relative merits of using inbred and outbred animals are still being debated (Tuttle et al. 2018).

Variability may be further reduced by providing a controlled and standardised environment, with the most uniform populations and results being produced when the environment is optimal for the animals' well-being (Chance 1957; Chance & Russell 1997). Whether or not research animals should be kept under controlled conditions is, however, currently the subject of debate (Würbel & Garner 2007; Karp 2018).

Stressed animals will inevitably have different baseline behaviours, physiological findings and range of responses to experimental interventions, from unstressed animals. Therefore, all reasonable efforts should be made to identify and remove or minimise unnecessary stressors (Poole 1997; Garner 2005).

Retrospective analyses of results may show that the number of animals needed could in future be reduced without loss of precision. This has been found to be the case with some vaccine potency assays (Hendriksen & Steen 2000).

Re-use of animals

Re-use may be defined as the second or subsequent scientific use of an animal that has already completed a series of procedures for a defined scientific purpose when the use of a naïve, unused animal would have also been scientifically satisfactory. While re-use may reduce the total of number of animals required for programmes of work, it has to be balanced against the increased, cumulative suffering experienced by the individual animal. Common examples include the re-use of animals as blood donors; and, subject to suitable recovery periods, the re-use of dogs or non-human primates in pharmacokinetic studies.

Re-use should only be considered when the following conditions are met:

- The first use has not compromised the suitability of the animal for the second or subsequent use (for example, animals which have been exposed to a pathogen or immunogen will not give a naïve response if subsequently re-exposed);
- Animals experienced only minimal pain, suffering and distress, and no lasting harm, from their earlier use;
- The animals have been shown on a case-by-case basis by a competent person, after completion of the first use, to have been restored to a normal state of well-being.

The re-use of animals is frequently regulated by legislation.

Optimising animal production

Matching the production of animals and the availability of animal tissues to known or likely demand avoids waste. Common examples include cryo preservation of genetically altered animal lines (Glenister & Rall 2000) rather than maintaining 'tick-over' colonies, preservation and archiving and sharing of other tissues and samples, and through tissue-sharing schemes such as AniMatch[10].

Refinement

Refinement improves the quality of life of every animal bred, kept and used for experimental and other scientific purposes, and potentially benefits every programme of work using live animals.

Animal welfare is a complex issue: it comprises not only the health of an animal, but also its state of well-being. It has both physical and psychological dimensions which can be compromised not only by unpleasant stimuli, but also by the denial of that which is pleasurable. It is important to be aware that there are many causes of suffering and distress other than pain. Refinement is not just a matter of minimising the incidence of adverse effects, or the number of animals used; it is about minimising the total, cumulative pain, suffering, distress and lasting harm that may be caused to animals bred, kept and used for scientific purposes. Thus, a higher incidence of findings not indicative of a high welfare cost, such as reduced weight gain, may be preferable in welfare terms to a lower incidence of endpoints clearly indicative of higher levels of suffering.

Consideration of Refinement starts the moment there is an intention to breed or keep an animal for experimental or other scientific purposes. It continues throughout the production and scientific use of the animal until it is humanely killed or otherwise disposed of; and, as in the case of Reduction, it does not end until the lessons learned are incorporated into future practice.

All reasonable efforts should be made to ensure that animals used for biomedical research and testing have normal baseline physiological parameters and behaviours, by refining systems for their care and use (Poole 1997; Bayne 2005).

Assessing animal well-being

To make proper provision for animal welfare it is essential to understand and recognise what is *'meaningful to the animal'* and to do *'what is right for the animals'* (Russell & Burch 1959). Recognition of an abnormal state depends on an awareness of, and familiarity with, normality in the species, strain and individual under observation.

The behavioural and physiological responses of animals to adverse effects are not uniform between species, strains, individuals of the same species and strain, or even in the same individual at different times (Scharmann 1999). Assessment of welfare must therefore take place at the level of the individual animal.

Welfare is assessed by taking into account behavioural, physiological, clinical and laboratory findings (see Chapter 6: Brief introduction to welfare assessment: A Toolbox of techniques). Of these, behavioural findings and changes are often the earliest, most sensitive and most meaningful indicators.

In the absence of evidence to the contrary, it should be assumed that any stimulus, experience or pathology that produces pain and discomfort in man, also does so in sentient animals (Home Office 1965; Smith & Hawkins 2016). Confidence in indices of welfare is best placed in findings which:

- occur in an appropriate context;
- progress with the nature and severity of the insult or pathology;
- are predictive of the ultimate welfare, clinical or pathological outcomes;
- can be controlled with appropriate specific, supportive or symptomatic treatment.

For example, signs considered to be indicative of pain should occur in contexts where there is reason to suspect or believe pain may be present, and should decline with prompt, effective analgesic administration.

However, it is important to recognise that:

- animals may be distressed, though not in pain, and therefore display signs which analgesics will not alleviate – this may be seen for example in animals with locomotor impairments due to neurological damage;
- analgesics can have direct pharmacological effects unrelated to pain relief producing behavioural and physiological changes, and altering clinical findings (Roughan & Flecknell 2000);
- identifying and managing chronic pain and distress, where the signs can be harder to detect, poses particular difficulties (Flecknell & Roughan 2004).

As the judgement of animal well-being ultimately rests with humans, a degree of critical anthropomorphism is perhaps inevitable. 'Critical' in this context implies empathy tempered with objective knowledge of the animal, its needs and normal behaviours, preceding events and the significance of any signs which may be seen.

Expert judgement can be required to understand the scope, limitations, possible interpretations and significance of even seemingly objective findings. Pitfalls to be borne in mind include the following:

- demonstrating behavioural or physiological differences may be contingent upon the animal's environment;
- preference testing (Kirkden & Pajor 2006) may only identify the least objectionable rather than the best option, and short-term preferences may not be indicative of long-term preferences, needs and benefits;
- although technology is improving, measuring even basic physiological phenomena and behaviours sometimes requires additional interventions that add welfare costs or influence the parameters being measured.

Severity scoring systems

A number of disturbance indices, pain, and severity scoring systems have been developed to assist with the assessment of the welfare of animals used for experimental purposes (for

---

[10]https://www.animatch.eu (accessed 10 Jan 2022)

example, Hendriksen & Morton 1999; Hawkins *et al.* 2011; Smith *et al.* 2018b; Zintzsch *et al.* 2017 and the Norecopa web site[11]). These can be used to identify protocols with high welfare costs where work on Replacement or Refinement might most usefully be commissioned, and to evaluate the impact of treatments and potential Refinement measures (see also Chapter 6: Brief introduction to welfare assessment: A 'toolbox' of techniques). They encourage the use of appropriate observation schedules, standard documentation and plain non-technical language with a limited range of keywords to identify, describe and record findings. These simplify staff training, provide a systematic approach to evaluating and documenting welfare and clinical findings, and facilitate communication within and between research groups.

Such systems are based upon indices of welfare, often with continuous variables categorised to reflect what we believe to be meaningful differences in levels of significance and suffering. Combinations of signs tend to be more significant than the occurrence of any sign in isolation. Although they must be adapted to reflect the research objectives, models and protocols, they should be valid whether impaired welfare is due to the immediate or delayed, local or systemic, or primary, secondary or tertiary effects of the procedures.

Observation schedules

Arrangements must be made to check animals under study at appropriate times to gather data and safeguard their welfare. All animals should be checked at least once a day by a competent person capable of recognising and arranging for welfare problems to be promptly remedied. The frequency of checks should be increased when problems are likely, or have already occurred. A policy for the availability of competent personnel seven days a week must be in place before the start of the experiment.

Findings of relevance to the animals' welfare, including normal findings, must be recorded, along with the action taken and the animal's response.

Contingent and direct harms

The welfare costs to animals bred, kept and used for experimental and other scientific purposes have two distinct components (Russell & Burch 1959):

- 'contingent' welfare costs (harms), comprising the welfare-negative aspects of animal production and care, whether caused deliberately or by omission;
- 'direct' costs (harms) resulting from the experimental procedures.

Animal facilities and care practices must facilitate high standards of animal welfare and high-quality research by eliminating, or identifying, controlling and minimising, unwanted variables. At the same time, the best possible, appropriate provision should be made for the physiological, social and behavioural needs of the animals (see later chapters such as Chapter 9: Planning, design and construction of efficient animal facilities and Chapter 10: Enrichment: animal welfare and scientific validity).

Contingent harms

Many elements of animal accommodation and care affect the welfare of animals and their response to experimental interventions (Poole 1997; Bayne 2005). These can affect the validity and reproducibility of findings to the extent that experimental results may only be valid for, and reproducible within, the specific conditions under which they were obtained. Key considerations are the animals' physical and behavioural needs, and how provision for these can best be made within the context of their production, care and use.

Ideally, the standards of animal care and accommodation provided would be based on objective evidence of what is required to make best provision for animal welfare. At present, much of the evidence required to derive and support such standards does not exist, with guidelines and regulations being based on a combination of empirical findings and what is believed to be existing good practice. These set only the minimum expected or acceptable standards of care and accommodation (see, for example, the EU legislation web site[12]).

Whenever possible, in order not to delay innovation and the introduction of better evidence-based care systems, standards should be written as performance standards (what outcomes they are intended to achieve) rather than as engineering standards (prescribing only the required inputs).

Pair- and group-housing

Animals, other than those that are naturally solitary, should be socially housed in stable groups of compatible individuals. It has been shown in many species that housing with one or more socially compatible conspecific significantly reduces stress, and that being kept singly in isolation compromises both an animal's welfare and its suitability as an experimental subject (Kappel *et al.* 2017). Care is required to ensure that pair- and group-housed animals are socially compatible, mindful that population density and group size influence the physiological and psychological state of the animal and affect experimental responses.

There will be some circumstances, for example the use of a single instrumented animal, when the companion animals will not be experimental subjects, yet will be exposed to any contingent harms.

Animals should only be singly housed on veterinary or other welfare grounds, or justified scientific need; in which case animal care and veterinary staff should be involved in the decision making, and additional measures taken to optimise animal welfare.

Space requirements and structure

Animals should be provided with a sufficiently spacious and complex environment to facilitate a wide range of normal activities and behaviours, taking account of their physiological and ethological needs. The preferred systems will vary

---

[11]https://norecopa.no/more-resources/severity-classification (accessed 10 Jan 2022)

[12]https://ec.europa.eu/environment/chemicals/lab_animals/legislation_en.htm (accessed 10 Jan 2022).

according to species, strain, age, physiological condition, stocking density and group size, and whether animals are kept as stock, for breeding or for experiments.

Basic physiological and ethological needs (such as freedom of movement, appropriate social contact and the ability to withdraw from social conflict; the performance of meaningful activities and access to food and water) should never be restricted without good cause, and then only to the justifiable minima.

Environmental enrichment

The laboratory environment can never reproduce the complexity of an animal's natural environment, nor adequately model human societal interactions. The intention is generally to mimic critical natural environmental factors so that normal, strongly motivated behaviours can be expressed, reinforced and maintained (Blanchard & Blanchard 2003). Not all natural behaviours are appropriate in the laboratory setting (Fraser 1993). They may represent what the animal needs or wants to, would not normally choose to do (for example, in response to environmental stressors), or will only choose to do when the need arises.

Environmental enrichment options can be categorised as:

- Social enrichment, generally characterised by housing with compatible conspecifics complemented by space of sufficient volume and complexity to permit an appropriate range of species-specific interactions and interaction with man. In many circumstances, social enrichment is both more effective than inanimate physical enrichment, and a prerequisite for the effectiveness of physical enrichment. Appropriate early social experience can be essential for the development of a normal behavioural repertoire. Conditions at breeding and rearing facilities play therefore a large part in determining the subsequent suitability of animals as experimental subjects or future breeding stock.
- Physical enrichment, including the provision of an adequate amount of suitably structured space, materials to manipulate, sensory stimuli and a varied diet. To prevent or reduce stress-induced behaviours, animals should be given a degree of control over their environment by encouraging species-appropriate physical exercise, foraging, manipulative and cognitive activities.

A creative and critical approach is required. Not all potential changes are beneficial; and if one form of enrichment is chosen others, which may be more effective, have to be rejected.

It is important that appropriate options are identified and critically evaluated in terms of their immediate and long-term impact on the animals' well-being and the research objectives (Bayne 2005; Benefiel *et al.* 2005). Assessing the impact of potential environmental enrichments depends on the ability of staff to evaluate the animal's state of mind and welfare state. It cannot be overemphasised that the most important resources required to devise and evaluate environmental enrichment opportunities are competent and caring staff.

Environmental enrichment is discussed in more detail in Chapter 10: Enrichment: animal welfare and scientific validity.

Restraint

During many husbandry and scientific procedures, animals may be restrained to minimise the risk of injury to the subject and handler, and facilitate the performance of the procedures. Restraint can be stressful, producing changes in physiological parameters and behaviours depending on the nature, duration and degree of restraint, particularly when the restrained animal is also removed from its enclosure or social group. Appropriate restraint will depend on the species and the nature and duration of the procedure for which the animal is being restrained, with the most refined method of restraint being that which causes the least stress to the animal and its social group.

Training of animals to accept reasonable restraint procedures is possible in a range of species, and has been shown to reduce the resulting physiological and behavioural changes (Wolfensohn & Honess 2005). Procedural training can in some circumstances encourage animals to allow the safe performance of routine procedures without the need for restraint (see Chapter 15: The use of positive reinforcement training techniques to enhance the care and welfare of laboratory and research animals).

Marking and identification of animals

Individual animals bred, kept and used for experimental and other scientific purposes need to be identified. This is generally achieved by marking individual animals, although biometric methods (identification based on an individual animal's natural physical characteristics) would be preferable. Faced with a choice of effective identification and marking methods, the preferred means is that which causes the least pain, suffering or distress to the animal. Many guidelines are available for marking[13] and identification[14] of research animals.

Transport of animals

The transport of animals, between or within establishments, can be stressful. All reasonable efforts must be made to avoid or minimise any stress that may be caused, and to ensure that animals are acclimatised to a new environment before being used for scientific purposes (see Chapter 12: Transportation of laboratory animals). Journey times should be minimised, the least stressful modes of transport used, and appropriate contingency plans should be in place.

The acclimatisation period will vary with the stresses imposed by transportation; the differences in the housing and care systems; and the species, strain and the condition of individual animals. It may be necessary to take expert advice to determine the appropriate minimum period for acclimatisation, and to confirm that animals have recovered before being used for scientific purposes.

In some cases, welfare costs can be minimised by transporting ova or embryos rather than live animals. This, and the resulting rederivation, is also a means of disease control when acquiring animals from facilities with different or unknown microbiological status.

---

[13] https://norecopa.no/search?q=guidelines%20marking&fq=db:%223r%22 (accessed 10 Jan 2022)

[14] https://norecopa.no/search?q=guidelines%20identification&fq=db:%223r%22 (accessed 10 Jan 2022)

Humane killing

The majority of animals produced and used for scientific purpose are humanely killed as part of, or at the end of, their scientific use; as are surplus stock animals.

Humane methods of killing, when properly applied, ensure rapid loss of consciousness without producing signs of pain or distress, result in the death of an animal with a minimum of physical and mental suffering, and should not interfere with any scientific data which is to be collected postmortem. They should also be aesthetically acceptable, and must incorporate careful and compassionate animal handling routines that avoid or minimise the stress due to any necessary restraint or the need to remove the animal from its enclosure or social group (see Chapter 17: Euthanasia and other fates for laboratory animals, and the Norecopa web site[15]). All require expertise which can only be developed by appropriate staff training, and the provision and maintenance of appropriate facilities and equipment.

After a humane killing method is applied, death must be confirmed in all cases before removing tissues or storing or disposing of cadavers.

Direct harms

A number of procedures applied to animals for experimental purposes impose welfare costs. The welfare costs tend to vary in proportion to:

- the degree of sentience and needs of the individual experimental subject;
- the nature, duration, intensity and frequency of the challenge;
- the biological systems and mechanisms involved;
- other factors which aggravate or ameliorate the suffering experienced by an individual experimental subject.

Choice of experimental subjects

Selection of appropriate experimental subjects requires understanding and control of factors including the animal's genotype; environmental conditions; other elements of animal husbandry, accommodation and care; and microbiological status.

The choice of species is relevant to refinement. Some species:

- are afforded specific legal protection;
- are believed to have a greater capacity to experience pain and distress (sometimes referred to as 'neurophysiological sensitivity'). Where there is flexibility in the interpretation and implementation of regulatory testing requirements, selection of the 'lowest' appropriate species should be on scientific considerations, not custom and practice or availability;
- have specific, complex husbandry requirements difficult to provide in the research context. Choosing the species whose needs can best be catered for in the laboratory setting may constitute Refinement.

Animal models of disease, animals expressing harmful natural genetic mutations and some lines of genetically altered animals (Wells *et al.* 2006) have specific problems and needs in addition to, or different from, those of normal animals of the same species. These special needs must be considered, identified and met when such animals are bred, kept or used for scientific purposes.

Wild-caught animals

The environmental, ethical, welfare and scientific benefits of using purpose-bred animals are so great that the use of non-purpose-bred, and in particular wild-caught, animals requires special justification. Where it can be justified, capture should be performed by competent persons using humane methods, minimising the impact of capture both on the captured animals and the remaining wildlife and habitat (see Chapter 7: Welfare and 'best practice' in field studies of wildlife). Arrangements should be in place for animals in poor health to be examined promptly by a competent person, and appropriate action taken.

Proper provision must be made for the transportation, acclimatisation, quarantine, housing, husbandry and care of wild-caught animals, mindful that their health status, behaviours and needs are likely to be different to those of animals bred in captivity. The eventual fate of wild-caught animals should be given due consideration before work begins.

Dosing

Research protocols commonly require that animals are dosed with test materials, and detailed advice on limit volumes and practical issues is available elsewhere (see Diehl *et al.* 2001 and the recommendations in the species-specific chapters in Part 2 of this book). In many cases, the most refined options to meet the scientific objective can only be determined by pilot studies. If the intention is to mimic natural exposure, to maintain a particular level at a target site, or to produce a specific effect (and not produce unwanted effects) pilot studies may be required to identify the appropriate dose or exposure.

Refinement is relevant to consideration of:

- The route of administration.
  - With oral administration, admixing the test material with food or water (providing stability and palatability are not problems) or administration in liquid, tablet or capsule form, may be more refined than gavage-dosing. The timing of the doses, and volumes administered, must neither compromise the animals' normal food and fluid intake, nor cause discomfort or other volume-related effects.
  - Test materials may be administered parenterally by injection or cannula. Other than administration directly into the circulation, this can lead to varying rates of uptake depending primarily on the injection site, the general condition of the animal and the volume and formulation used.
    - Administration by intraperitoneal injection is a special case: it results in the test material being partitioned and taken up simultaneously into the systemic circulation and hepatic portal circulation (where it may be metabolised by the liver before it enters the systemic circulation). How test materials partition between the portal and systemic circulations depends on the

---

[15]https://norecopa.no/more-resources/humane-killing (accessed 10 Jan 2022)

nature and volume of the test material, varies from subject to subject, and in the same subject from day to day.
    - Topical application of test materials to skin or mucous membranes may require some form of restraint, or other measures, to ensure the test material remains in place and is not ingested by the animal or its cage mates.
- The frequency and duration of dosing.
    - These are generally determined by the properties of the test material (for example, its bioavailability and biological effects), its interaction with the experimental subject (for example, its half-life, how it is metabolised, where it accumulates and how it is excreted) and the study objective.
- The equipment used.
    - For injection procedures, the smallest bore needle capable of delivering the volume required in an acceptable time should be used.
    - The need for multiple injections, and the associated restraint procedures, may be dispensed with by the placement and use of cannulae to permit repeated (or continuous) administration. To constitute Refinement, their use must be balanced against the welfare costs of the procedures to insert the cannulae, the restraint and other cannula-care procedures that may be required, and the possible cannula-related problems.
- The volumes to be administered.
    - For intravascular administration, the volume and the time over which materials are administered should avoid unwanted volume-related effects, and should not produce any biological changes due to the nature and volume of the vehicle used.
    - For injection into closed spaces (for example, intramuscular or intradermal injection), the volumes and rates of administration should avoid adverse effects due to pressure effects or over-stretching of tissues.
- The formulations to be administered.
    - The formulation and volume of test materials used are generally determined by the frequency of administration, the required accuracy of dosing, the nature and solubility of the test material, the required dose and preferred concentration.
    - In general, for parenteral administration the closer the osmolarity, pH, buffer capacity, viscosity and temperature of the test material are to normal body fluids, the greater the biocompatibility and the less discomfort and stress will be caused.

Non-invasive sampling

A range of biochemical parameters can be estimated or measured without the need to obtain blood samples. A number of hormones and metabolites can be measured in urine and faeces, allowing estimates to be made of recent circulating levels in unrestrained animals, mindful that there is a time lag between their production, release and excretion. In some cases, animals can be trained to deposit excreta in suitable receptacles without being restrained or removed from their social groups.

Although physiological responses to instantaneous stressors cannot be measured in urine or faeces, determination of salivary levels can provide a minimally invasive means for measurement of short-term responses for some materials, and for detecting and quantifying other metabolites and biomarkers (Chiappin et al. 2007).

Blood sampling

Blood sampling is one of the most common procedures used in animal research, and advice on volume limits (which should always be considered the justifiable maxima rather than the norm) and other practical issues is available elsewhere (e.g. Diehl et al. 2001 and the NC3Rs web site[16]), and in the species-specific chapters in Part 2 of this book.

Refinement is relevant to:

- The nature of the sample.
    - In many species, venous blood can be obtained from superficial veins by venepuncture or venesection.
    - Arterial blood is generally obtained by direct arterial puncture or closed cardiac puncture (the insertion of a needle directly through the chest wall into the left ventricle of the heart under general anaesthesia). Cardiac puncture is only appropriate for sampling under general anaesthesia from which the animals are not allowed to recover.
    - Blood obtained by retro-orbital puncture is not a physiological fluid: such samples comprise admixed capillary and venous blood, contaminated with other tissue fluids, in which a variety of clotting factors have been activated. Its haematological and biochemical parameters are neither physiological nor representative of blood anywhere in the systemic circulation. The technique is also likely to cause tissue damage and discomfort.
- The frequency of sampling and the volumes required.
    - The volumes, rates of withdrawal and frequency of sampling must be designed to prevent hypovolaemia and anaemia. Average blood volumes and limit sampling volumes are generally calculated on the basis of body weight (Joint Working Group on Refinement (JWGR) 1993; Wolfensohn & Lloyd 2003), but must be interpreted in the knowledge that the safe sampling limits are typically lower in animals whose welfare is already challenged. Microsampling is being used increasingly, particularly in the pharmaceutical and chemical industries[17].
    - If frequent samples are required, cannulation should be considered as a means of minimising the stress of sampling.

Reward or punishment?

Behavioural testing often requires that experimental subjects remain interested in performing prescribed tasks, and various means have been devised to motivate experimental subjects to undertake such tasks on demand or for longer periods.

---

[16]https://www.nc3rs.org.uk/3rs-resources/blood-sampling (accessed 10 Jan 2022)

[17]https://www.nc3rs.org.uk/microsampling (accessed 10 Jan 2022)

Methods of motivating test subjects may be based upon rewards/positive reinforcement (for example, access to a preferred food or drink as a reward for displaying the desired behaviours) or punishment/negative reinforcement (for example, exposure to an air-puff or mild electric shock to discourage other behaviours). In some cases, the reward may be made more desirable by a period of food or water deprivation (e.g. Prescott *et al.* 2010).

The most refined and ethically justifiable paradigms are those that rely solely on reward/positive reinforcement systems without prior deprivations. There are considerable opportunities to refine food deprivation in rodents[18]. Punishment/negative reinforcement regimens require specific justification.

Anaesthesia and analgesia

The informed and responsible use of anaesthetics and analgesics to prevent and manage pain is an essential component of contemporary animal research. A detailed review of current best practice in the use of anaesthetics and analgesics is beyond the scope of this chapter, and authoritative information can be found elsewhere (see, for example, Flecknell 2015, the Research Animal Training (RAT) web site[19], and the species-specific chapters in Part 2), but there are general principles particularly relevant to Refinement.

General anaesthetic agents affect many physiological mechanisms and parameters, and care must be taken to ensure this does not compromise experimental data or animal welfare. Appropriate steps should be taken to monitor and maintain the circulation, respiratory function, fluid balance, and the body temperature of the anaesthetised subject within normal physiological limits throughout surgery and until the effects of anaesthesia have worn off.

Recovery from general anaesthesia can be hazardous, and animals should not be left unattended until the effects have worn off, any necessary specific, symptomatic or supportive treatments have been given and their effectiveness determined. Consideration should be given to administering the first dose of analgesia, sometimes referred to as pre-emptive analgesia, before recovery from anaesthesia, since total post-operative analgesic requirements are reduced when the initial dose of analgesic precedes the animal's ability to feel pain.

Post-surgical analgesia must be the norm, and it should be administered as required to control pain and speed the restoration of normal behaviours, such as food and water intake, thus shortening the post-surgery catabolic phase and improving animal welfare. This requires appropriate observation schedules, with treatments based on the findings in, and needs of, individual animals.

Surgery

Surgical procedures must only be carried out by competent persons; using the best available surgical and animal care techniques; and the anaesthetic and analgesic regimens best suited to the species, the nature and duration of the procedure and the scientific objective. Surgery should be performed using aseptic technique in areas designed for, and dedicated to, this purpose.

The availability of trained, competent staff to take responsibility for the care of animals during the post-operative period must be confirmed before surgery is scheduled. To make best provision for post-operative care, it is recommended that complex surgical procedures are carried out as early in the working week, and working day, as possible.

Humane endpoints

Humane endpoints, minimising the direct welfare costs of justifiable animal-based research, are essential components of humane experimental technique, and a cornerstone of refinement (Richmond 1999)[20]. Humane endpoints incorporate all reasonable and practical steps that can be taken to minimise justifiable suffering by avoiding, or promptly recognising and remedying, unnecessary adverse effects arising during scientific procedures. Humane endpoints must be described in meaningful terms and be promptly recognised and acted on by those entrusted with the welfare of the animals.

To some, the term 'humane endpoint' mistakenly represents *'the earliest indicator in an animal experiment of severe pain, severe distress, suffering, or impending death'* (OECD 2000). That is a dangerous misconception.

Contrary to the narrow OECD definition, humane endpoints are often particularly appropriate when levels of pain and distress being experienced are not high and death is not imminent.

Humane endpoints in practice

Humane endpoints must be objective and evidence-based in order to:

- avoid the needless culling of animals whose welfare is less compromised than believed, or before the scientific objective has been achieved;
- prevent evidence indicative of significant suffering being missed;
- inform judgements about the severity of different procedures and models;
- evaluate potential refinements.

Although they must be designed within the context of the project, experiment and experimental group, they are best thought of as being applied to the individual animal: with early indicators often being the most meaningful, both with respect to welfare problems and to prevent scientific outcomes from being compromised by later undesirable changes, due to unnecessary and unwanted secondary or tertiary effects (Hendriksen *et al.* 2011).

Humane endpoints take account of legal, ethical, welfare and scientific considerations, and must cater for a number of eventualities, including the following:

- having achieved the experimental objective (or when it is recognised it cannot be achieved), even if there is no

---

[18] https://norecopa.no/3r-guide/fasting-in-rodents (accessed 10 Jan 2022)

[19] https://researchanimaltraining.com/elearning (accessed 10 Jan 2022)

[20] https://www.humane-endpoints.info/en (accessed 10 Jan 2022)

immediate welfare problem. Indeed, in some cases, preclinical endpoints can be set and implemented. For example, when intercurrent problems, such as a subclinical background infection, compromise the quality of the data or product, even when they may not have compromised the well-being of the animals – as is the case with mice found to be carrying the mouse hepatitis virus which, even in the absence of overt welfare problems, will result in atypical immune responses (e.g. Baker 1998; Hansen & Franklin 2019).
- experimental subjects experiencing pain, suffering, distress or lasting harm beyond that which is required or can be justified. Again, such endpoints are often invoked at low levels of suffering – for example, reduced weight gain can often be accepted as an early indication of overt toxicity.

When an endpoint is recognised, the action taken may take several forms including:

- the animal ceasing to be an experimental subject;
- adjusting the protocol to reduce or remove the immediate cause of the adverse effect to allow the animal to recover;
- the administration of specific, symptomatic or supportive treatments;
- humane killing.

Planning, implementing and reviewing humane endpoints

Before animal use begins, humane endpoints should be defined; minimum observation schedules determined; and arrangements for the provision or withholding of specific, symptomatic and supportive treatments, and other remedial measures, established. This requires an understanding and consideration of likely adverse effects (immediate and delayed: primary, secondary and tertiary), and how they will be avoided, recognised and remedied. The critical observation periods, training needs and resource implications should be identified and resolved before work starts. Thought must also be given to how unforeseen outcomes will be identified, interpreted, reported and managed. Particular care may be required both to predict and recognise transient pharmacological effects not indicative of true welfare problems. Pilot studies can inform the timing of observations and how the adverse effects should be identified and managed, minimising the welfare costs of definitive studies.

An understanding of relevant biological mechanisms and likely clinical findings allows appropriate symptomatic and supportive therapies to be delivered, permitting the processes of interest to continue while minimising or eliminating unnecessary suffering. In practice, primary changes are often subtle in nature and, even when symptomatic and supportive treatments are given, are overshadowed by less specific secondary (for example, anorexia) or tertiary (for example, weight loss or dehydration) changes. Untreated secondary and tertiary effects compromise both science and welfare: personnel do not need a reason to give supportive or symptomatic treatment, rather they need good reason not to do so.

It may well be possible to achieve the scientific objective using preclinical endpoints. The murine local lymph node assay for skin sensitisation (Kimber *et al.* 1990) is a case in point. It relies on subclinical changes caused by the induction phase of the sensitisation process; whereas its forerunner, the traditional guinea pig maximisation test, relied on the clinical changes and gross pathology of the acute dermatitis seen as a result of the subsequent full-blown allergic response.

In some cases, scientific judgements can be made on the basis of what might otherwise have been assumed to be general, non-specific changes (e.g. behaviour, appearance, body weight, food or water intake, or body temperature). Examples include the use of the HID_{50} (hypothermia-induced dose 50) as an indicator of impending overwhelming infection as an alternative to the significant morbidity and mortality associated with traditional LD_{50} or PD_{50} studies to establish bacteriological virulence (Soothill *et al.* 1992).

Death should seldom, if ever, be considered, set or accepted as a required scientific endpoint. As procedure-related death is often the result of secondary or tertiary changes, it may be that lethal endpoints are not consistent with good science and could be replaced by earlier humane killing and autopsy, or be avoided by improved observation schedules and supportive or symptomatic treatments. All instances where animals are killed *in extremis* or found dead should be reviewed and the endpoints and observational schedules revised as necessary. These events may indicate that opportunities for Refinement have been missed, data compromised and unnecessarily many animals used. This is a particular challenge in fish research.

The agreed humane endpoints and associated actions must be communicated to, and understood and implemented by the staff involved. The documentation and verbal descriptors should use plain language and be understood by the staff checking the animals; they should read across to other studies involving the same research team and establishment; and they should be meaningful to those working elsewhere in the same field of research to allow comparison with similar work performed by others, to define best practice and further raise standards.

Staff must be properly trained to recognise, and empowered to promptly implement, the endpoints. Welfare is not served by systems that demand that decisions and action require delayed or lengthy internal notifications, negotiations or consultations.

Once work is underway and insights are being gained into the likely welfare costs and scientific outcomes of procedures, those involved should again ask whether the specific experimental objective and findings to date justify the levels of suffering being produced, and whether the objective and/or methods can be adjusted to provide equally useful data at a lower welfare cost.

Completed studies should be reviewed to determine whether all of the likely clinical manifestations of the pathologies produced were detected, and if the scientific objectives could have been achieved if earlier endpoints were applied. This information should be taken into account when future studies are planned.

Published work should describe how endpoints were determined and implemented and summarise the welfare problems encountered. Russell and Burch offered sound advice in this area: the objective of publication is not just to enable others to '*do what you did*', but to allow them to '*see what you saw*'.

Responsibility for the Three Rs

The Three Rs of Replacement, Reduction and Refinement are now accepted and implemented at the level of individuals, their institutions, those who fund and publish research, and at national and international level.

Comprehensive guidelines for planning animal research and testing have been published (Smith *et al.* 2018a). These are entitled PREPARE (*Planning Research and Experimental Procedures on Animals: Recommendations for Excellence*) and consist of a 15-topic checklist, supported by a comprehensive website containing resources for each of the topics. The way forward for the Three Rs rests undoubtedly, to a large degree, on better awareness of such good practice resources, better planning to implement them (from day one when experiments which may involve animals or animal material are conceived) and better reporting.

The individual

There is no doubt that the most important factors promoting the development and application of humane experimental technique and the Three Rs are the expertise and culture of those responsible for the production, care and use of animals. Each individual involved must take responsibility for their own personal development and personal effectiveness, and must be given the necessary support by their institution (see below). This requires ensuring that individuals:

- obtain appropriate training and continued professional development (including periodic revalidation of existing skills), keep abreast of good practice by involvement with appropriate professional societies and scientific bodies, and seek opportunities to visit and benchmark against other establishments;
- make timely contributions to the planning and performance of animal production and use, and ensure that best practice is being followed;
- confirm that others with responsibility for the animal welfare are both competent and effective;
- make sure that only high-quality science is undertaken;
- require that outcomes are reviewed, lessons learned incorporated into future practice and technical improvements communicated to others;
- network with others, both to share their own expertise and capitalise on the knowledge and experience of others.

Scientific training and continuing professional development should instil and maintain the knowledge, mindset and practices that place the Three Rs at the heart of animal-based research and testing (see Chapter 14: Attaining competence in the care of animals used in research). The objective is not only to equip individuals with factual knowledge and technical skills relating to their immediate area of scientific interest, but also to develop the other competencies required to plan, conduct, assess and report high-quality, humane research and to keep abreast of technical progress.

Those who are responsible for animal production and use must have an awareness, acceptance and expectation that expert input from others is required, as it is no longer possible for any one person to have all of the necessary knowledge and skills; and even the largest and most successful research teams and organisations may at times have to seek expert advice. Accessing and assessing relevant information increasingly needs specialist training and skills, requiring either training scientists to do this better, or placing reliance on information specialists. Similarly, proper statistical design requires input from biostatisticians: it is no more reasonable to expect a short training course in statistics to turn a biological scientist into a competent statistician, than it would be to expect an equally short training in the biological sciences to turn a statistician into a competent biological scientist.

The institution

Institutions breeding, supplying and using animals for scientific purposes must display an appropriate 'culture of care'. The management culture and the attitudes and skills of those responsible for the care and use of animals used in research are important factors in achieving high welfare standards and conducting valid science. There is now an International Culture of Care Network to support these endeavours[21].

Institutional support extends far beyond simply providing suitable physical facilities and typically includes the provision of:

- expert advice on accommodation and care, statistics and other elements of experimental design, veterinary care and laboratory animal science;
- animal facilities and standards of accommodation which meet or surpass published minimum provisions and recommendations;
- systematic education, training and continued professional development to develop and maintain both the necessary technical competencies and the required culture of care;
- processes which encourage innovation and continuous improvement.

At the institutional level, the best and most refined use of animals in science requires an appropriate management culture, and a multidisciplinary-team approach. In partnership with scientists, laboratory animal veterinarians, laboratory animal scientists and animal care staff must play an active and expert part in refining animal care and use. Staff must be trained to recognise normal behaviours and signs of pain and distress, both to improve all aspects of animal care and facilitate the recognition of experimental effects (see also Chapter 14: Attaining competence in the care of animals used in research). Those responsible for assessing animal welfare must be empowered and resourced to make the best provision for their housing, care and use; and to take prompt action when scientific and welfare endpoints are approached or reached. They must be aware of contingency plans to deal promptly with unexpected adverse effects.

Funding bodies

Funding bodies should ensure that the Three Rs are given due consideration before programmes of work are funded, and that progress with the Three Rs made in the course of funded work is acknowledged and published.

---

[21] https://norecopa.no/coc (accessed 10 Jan 2022)

Scientific journals

The widespread adoption of new and improved technologies in animal research depends on the publication and acceptance of technical progress. However, in many cases little or no prominence is given to progress with the Three Rs in mainstream core-science journals. Although there are specialist publications and websites dedicated to the Three Rs, such as the journal *ATLA* (*Alternatives to Laboratory Animals*)[22] and Norecopa[23], this literature and these resources may be unfamiliar to many scientists.

Research journals should ensure that published work takes account of the Three Rs, and that progress with the Three Rs is published and is accessible to those who need to know. Scientists should also realise their responsibility for publishing techniques which advance the 3Rs in such a way that they are easily visible to others, for example, as separate methodological papers.

Despite the existence for over 30 years of reporting guidelines (a current example being the ARRIVE guidelines[24]) promoting more informative methods and findings sections, and their endorsement by funding bodies and journals, many scientific papers still include insufficient information (Avey *et al.* 2016; Leung *et al.* 2018), making it difficult to make informed judgements about the scientific validity of experiments and the degree to which the Three Rs were implemented.

International and national efforts

Science is a global activity, and international meetings focusing on the Three Rs such as the World Congresses on Alternatives and Animal Use in the Life Sciences[25], the annual meetings arranged by the European Society for Alternatives to Animal Testing (EUSAAT)[26], and laboratory animal science meetings held by Federation of European Laboratory Animal Science Associations (FELASA)[27], American Association for Laboratory Animal Science (AALAS) and others, provide opportunities to showcase progress with the Three Rs. These meetings are of high quality and well attended, but they tend mainly to attract those already active within the Three Rs.

In the case of regulatory testing, new and revised international regulatory requirements increasingly reflect the Three Rs. A large number of animals are used for regulatory testing, with test requirements generally determined at international level, but interpreted and implemented at regional or national level. There are a number of examples of how these test requirements take account of the Three Rs, but much remains to be done. There are still significant differences between, and in some cases within, economic regions in the legislative provision made for the protection of animals used for experimental and other scientific purposes. Regulatory requirements are still imperfectly harmonised and can be slow to adopt technical progress as scientific validation remains a time-consuming process and, despite the increasing co-operation between the validation centres, there is still the potential for different centres coming to different conclusions about the same data sets.

Despite numerous examples of animal studies showing poor reproducibility and translational failure when potential novel treatments are tried out in humans (Begley & Ellis 2012; Garner 2014), those promoting the Three Rs are generally expected to demonstrate that these more humane methods are scientifically as good or better than existing animal models and protocols even though the findings with these existing animal models are known to be imperfect.

Formal scientific validation of 'alternative' methods, with respect to their relevance and reliability for their stated purpose, is required if non-animal tests, and more refined animal tests, are to gain regulatory acceptance. Scientific validation addresses test optimisation and definition, within-laboratory variability, transferability between laboratories, between-laboratory variability, predictive capacity, applicability domain and minimum performance standards (Balls *et al.* 1995). These factors can either be addressed in a sequential process; or by '*modular*' approaches (Hartung *et al.* 2004) developed to take account the non-sequential development of alternatives; or by using '*weight-of-evidence*' (Balls *et al.* 2006) and '*catch-up*' schemes to cope more efficiently with variations on existing methods. The formal validation process is expensive and time consuming, and increasingly takes place at the international level in order to set agreed priorities, reduce the time required, pool available resources and ensure international acceptance of the outcomes.

Although at first sight the most appropriate means to assess the validity of any Replacement or more refined method would seem to be a direct comparison to reliable human (or other target species) data, this is seldom possible or appropriate. Available animal data tends to be of variable quality, and is generated using test systems that were not themselves fully standardised or scientifically validated, and which imperfectly reproduce the human response. There are also problems in finding reliable human data: the precise nature of the exposure to the material of interest is often unknown, and any non-symptomatic treatments given will interfere with the effects of the material.

An equally serious problem in practice is that an alternative test with greater specificity or sensitivity will produce different results in the established animal model. The inability to reproduce strictly the results obtained with imperfect but established test methods can delay the validation and acceptance of new and improved test systems.

National legislation for the protection of animals used for experimental and other scientific purposes is important to ensure that the Three Rs are given due consideration. Other support, such as government funding for work on the Three Rs, can be difficult to determine since funding primarily to improve methodologies is not necessarily based upon animal welfare considerations and may therefore not be readily identifiable as direct support for the Three Rs.

In recent years, there has been a steady increase in the number of national centres to champion the development and acceptance of alternative methods. These include the

---

[22] https://journals.sagepub.com/home/atl (accessed 10 Jan 2022)
[23] https://norecopa.no (accessed 10 Jan 2022)
[24] https://arriveguidelines.org (accessed 10 Jan 2022)
[25] http://alttox.org/10th-world-congress-going (accessed 10 Jan 2022)
[26] https://eusaat.eu (accessed 10 Jan 2022)
[27] https://felasa.eu (accessed 10 Jan 2022)

National Centre for the Three Rs (NC3Rs) in the UK[28], ZEBET in Germany[29], the Canadian Council on Animal Care (CCAC)[30], the Center for Alternatives to Animal Testing in the USA (CAAT)[31] and Europe (CAAT-Europe)[32], Denmark's 3R-Center[33], and Norecopa in Norway[34]. These act as focal points for the discussion and dissemination of good practice. An interactive global map of 3R centres and laboratory animal science associations is available on the Norecopa web site[35]. This site also contains a comprehensive listing of professional, industrial, academic and other non-governmental organisations specifically involved with developing and promoting alternative methods[36].

Concluding remarks

It is often difficult to trace the implementation and impact of the Three Rs at a national level, since the total number of animals used annually for experimental and other scientific purposes is determined by a range of factors. These include the level of spending on science, strategic funding priorities (for example, better understanding of gene function, interaction and control), the availability of new technologies (such as the ability to produce genetically altered animals) and changes in regulations to protect man and the environment (for example, the European Union REACH legislation[37]). Because of such drivers and the scientific activity they generate, progress with Replacement and Reduction cannot be judged simply on the basis of the total number of animals used for experimental and other scientific purposes. However, there are case studies of specific classes of animal use where Replacement and Reduction have had a demonstrable impact. For example, improved tissue culture systems have drastically reduced the use of animals to produce monoclonal antibodies by the ascites method, and the number of animals used in education and training has also declined.

The way forward for the Three Rs lies undoubtedly, in part, on better awareness, good practice resources and better planning, conduct, analysis and reporting of animal studies. Comprehensive Three R guidelines for planning animal research and testing such as PREPARE can help to guide scientists and animal facilities alike in these efforts (Smith *et al.* 2018a).

In addition to considering the principles set out in the preceding text, and applying the practices set out in later chapters and seeking further guidance as required, it is hoped that readers capitalise on, and communicate to others, their own successes, new insights and practical examples of how the principles of replacement, reduction and refinement can further contribute to both animal welfare and high-quality science.

References

Ames, B.N., Lee, F.D. and Durston, W.E. (1973) An improved bacterial test system for the detection and classification of mutagens and carcinogens. *Proceedings of the National Academy of Sciences USA*, **70**, 782–786.

Anon (1839) Editorial. *London Medical Gazette*, 24 May 1839, 212–215.

Avey, M.T., Moher, D., Sullivan, K.J. *et al.* (2016) The devil is in the details: Incomplete reporting in preclinical animal research. *PLoS One*, **11**. doi: 10.1371/journal.pone.0166733

Baker, D.G. (1998) Natural pathogens of laboratory mice, rats, and rabbits and their effects on research. *Clinical Microbiology Reviews*, **11**, 231–266.

Balls, M., Blaauboer, B.J., Fentem, J.H. *et al.* (1995) Practical aspects of the validation of toxicity test procedures. The report and recommendations of ECVAM workshop 5. *Alternatives to Laboratory Animals*, **23**, 129–147.

Balls, M., Amcof, P., Bremer, S. *et al.* (2006) The principles of weight of evidence validation of test methods and test strategies. *Alternatives to Laboratory Animals*, **34**, 603–620.

Barley, J.B. (1999) Animal experimentation, the scientist and ethics. *Animal Technology*, **50**, 1–10.

Bayne, K. (2005) Potential for unintended consequences of environmental enrichment for laboratory animals and research results. *Institute for Laboratory Animal Research Journal*, **46**, 129–139.

Begley, C.G. and Ellis, L.M. (2012) Drug development: Raise standards for preclinical cancer research. *Nature*, **483**, 531–533. doi: 10.1038/483531a

Benefiel, A.C., Dong, W.K. and Greenough, W.T. (2005) Mandatory 'enriched' housing of laboratory animals: the need for evidence-based evaluation. *Institute of Laboratory Animal Research Journal*, **46**, 95–105.

Bischof, R., Milleret, C., Dupont, P. *et al.* (2020) Estimating and forecasting spatial population dynamics of apex predators using transnational genetic monitoring. *Proceedings of the National Academy of Sciences*, 117, 30531–30538.

Blanchard, R.J. and Blanchard, D.C. (2003) Bringing natural behaviors into the laboratory: a tribute to Paul MacLean. *Physiology & Behaviour*, **79**, 515–524.

Brockway, B.P., Hassler, C.R. and Hicks, N. (1993) Minimizing stress during physiological monitoring. In: *Refinement and Reduction in Animal Testing*. Eds Niemi, S.M. and Willson, J.E., pp. 569. Scientists Center for Animal Welfare, Bethesda.

Buchanan-Smith, H.M., Rennie, A.E., Vitale, A. *et al.* (2005) Harmonising the definition of refinement. *Animal Welfare*, **14**, 379–384.

Chance, M.R.A. (1957) The contribution of environment to uniformity: variance control, refinement in pharmacology. *Laboratory Animals Bureau, Collected Papers*, **6**, 59–73.

Chance, M.R.A. and Russell, W.M.S. (1997) The benefits of giving experimental animals the best possible environment. In: *Comfortable Quarters for Laboratory Animals*, 8th edn. Ed. Reinhardt, V., pp. 12–14. Animal Welfare Institute, Washington, DC.

Chiappin, S., Antonelli, G., Gatti, R. *et al.* (2007) Saliva specimen: a new laboratory tool for diagnostic and basic investigation. *Clinica Chemica Acta*, **383**, 30–40.

Diehl, K.H., Hull, R., Morton, D. *et al.* (2001) A good practice guide to the administration of substances and removal of blood, including routes and volumes. *Journal of Applied Toxicology*, **21**, 15–23.

---

[28]https://nc3rs.org.uk (accessed 10 Jan 2022)
[29]https://www.bfr.bund.de/en/zebet-58194.html (accessed 10 Jan 2022)
[30]https://ccac.ca (accessed 10 Jan 2022)
[31]https://caat.jhsph.edu (accessed 10 Jan 2022)
[32]https://www.biologie.uni-konstanz.de/leist/caat-europe (accessed 10 Jan 2022)
[33]https://3rcenter.dk (accessed 10 Jan 2022)
[34]https://norecopa.no (accessed 10 Jan 2022)
[35]https://norecopa.no/global3R (accessed 10 Jan 202)
[36]https://norecopa.no/more-resources/organisations (accessed 10 Jan 2022)
[37]https://echa.europa.eu/regulations/reach/understanding-reach (accessed 10 Jan 2022)

EMEA (1995) Toxicokinetics: A Guidance for Assessing Systemic Exposure in Toxicity Studies, S3A. Available at: https://www.ema.europa.eu/en/documents/scientific-guideline/ich-s-3-toxicokinetics-guidance-assessing-systemic-exposure-toxicology-studies-step-5_en.pdf (accessed 10 Jan 2022).

Festing, M. (2011) How to Reduce the Number of Animals Used in Research by Improving Experimental Design and Statistics. *ANZCCART Fact Sheet T10.* https://anzccart.adelaide.edu.au/ua/media/553/reduce-numbers-in-animals.pdf (accessed 10 Jan 2022).

Festing, M.F.W. and Fisher, E.M.C. (2000) Mighty mice. *Nature*, **404**, 815.

Festing, M.F. and Altman, D.G. (2002) Guidelines for the design and statistical analysis of experiments using laboratory animals. *Institute for Laboratory Animal Research Journal*, **43**, 244–258.

Flecknell, P. (2015) *Laboratory Animal Anaesthesia*, 4th edn. Academic Press, London.

Flecknell, P.A. and Roughan, J.V. (2004) Assessing pain in animals – putting research into practice. *Animal Welfare*, **13**, S71–S75.

Fraser, D. (1993) Assessing animal well-being: common sense, uncommon science. Food Animal Well-Being 1993 – Conference Proceedings and Deliberations, Purdue University.

Gallegos Saliner, A. and Worth, A. (2007) Testing strategies for the prediction of skin and eye irritation and corrosion for regulatory purposes. EUR 22881 EN, JRC 37853 (available at http://publications.jrc.ec.europa.eu/repository/handle/JRC37853) (accessed 10 Jan 2022).

Garner, J.P. (2005) Stereotypies and other abnormal repetitive behaviors: potential impact on validity, reliability, and replicability of scientific outcomes. *ILAR Journal* **46**: 106–117.

Garner J.P. (2014) The significance of meaning: why do over 90% of behavioral neuroscience results fail to translate to humans, and what can we do to fix it? *ILAR journal*, **55**, 438–456. doi: 10.1093/ilar/ilu047

Glenister, P.H. and Rall, W.F. (2000) Cryopreservation and rederivation of embryos and gametes. In: *Mouse Genetics and Transgenics – a Practical Approach*. Eds Jackson, I.J. and Abbott, C.M., pp. 27–59. Oxford University Press, Oxford.

Guillén, J. (2017) *Laboratory Animals: Regulations and Recommendations for the Care and Use of Animals in Research*. Academic Press, Cambridge.

Hall, M. (1847) On experiments in physiology as a question of medical ethics. *The Lancet*, **1847**, 58–60.

Hansen, A.K. and Franklin, C. (2019) Microbiota, laboratory animals and research. *Laboratory Animals*, 53, 229–231.

Hartung, T., Bremer, S., Casati, S. et al. (2004) A modular approach to the ECVAM principles on test validity. *Alternatives to Laboratory Animals*, **32**, 467–472.

Hawkins, P., Dennison, N., Goodman, G. et al. (2011). Guidance on the severity classification of scientific procedures involving fish: Report of a Working Group appointed by the Norwegian Consensus-Platform for the Replacement, Reduction and Refinement of animal experiments (Norecopa). *Laboratory Animals*, **45**(4), 219–224. https://doi.org/10.1258/la.2011.010181 (accessed 10 Jan 2022).

Hendriksen, C.F.M. and Morton, D.B. (eds) (1999) *Humane Endpoints in Animal Experimentation for Biomedical Research*. In: Proceedings of the International Conference, 22–25 November 1998, Zeist, The Netherlands. The Royal Society of Medicine Press, London.

Hendriksen, C.F.M. and Steen, B. (2000) Humane endpoints for animals used in biomedical research and testing refinement of vaccine potency testing with the use of humane endpoints. *Institute for Laboratory Animal Research Journal*, V41, 105–113.

Hendriksen, C.F.M., Morton, D.B. and Cussler, K. (2011) Use of humane endpoints to minimise suffering. In: *The COST Manual of Laboratory Animal Care and Use: Refinement, Reduction and Research*. Eds Howard, B., Nevalainen, T. and Perretta, G., pp. 333–351. CRC Press: Boca Raton, FL.

Hoffmann, S. and Hartung, T. (2006) Toward an evidence-based toxicology. *Human & Experimental Toxicology*, **25**, 497–513.

Home Office (1965) *Report of the Departmental Committee on Experiments on Animals*. (The Littlewood Report). Her Majesty's Stationery Office, London.

Interagency Coordinating Committee on the Validation of Alternative Methods (ICCVAM) (2001) Guidance document on using in vitro data to estimate in vivo starting doses for acute toxicity. NIH publication no. 01-4500. https://ntp.niehs.nih.gov/iccvam/docs/acutetox_docs/guidance0801/iv_guide.pdf (accessed 10 Jan 2022).

Joint Working Group on Refinement (1993) Removal of blood from laboratory mammals and birds. First Report of the BVA/FRAME/RSPCA/UFAW Joint Working Group on Refinement. *Laboratory Animals*, **27**, 1–22.

Kappel, S., Hawkins, P. and Mendl, M. (2017) To group or not to group? Good practice for housing male laboratory mice. *Animals*, **7**, 88.

Karp, N.A. (2018) Reproducible preclinical research—Is embracing variability the answer? *PLoS Biology*, 16(3): e2005413. https://doi.org/10.1371/journal.pbio.2005413 (accessed 10 Jan 2022).

Kimber, I., Hilton, J. and Botham, P.A. (1990) Identification of contact allergens using the murine local lymph node assay. Comparisons with the Buehler Occluded Patch Test in Guinea Pigs. *Journal of Applied Toxicology*, **10**, 173–180.

Kimura, H., Sakai, Y. and Fujii, T. (2018) Organ/body-on-a-chip based on microfluidic technology for drug discovery. *Drug Metabolism and Pharmacokinetics*, **33**, 43–48.

Kirkden, R. and Pajor, E. (2006) Using preference, motivation and aversion tests to ask specific questions about animals' feelings. *Applied Animal Behaviour*, **100**, 29–47.

Kramer, K. and Kinter, L. (2003) Evaluation and applications of radiotelemetry in small laboratory animals. *Physiological Genomics*, **13**, 197–205.

Lalko, J.F., Kimber, I., Gerberick, G.F. et al. (2012) The direct peptide reactivity assay: Selectivity of chemical respiratory allergens. *Toxicological Sciences*, **129**, 421–431

Leung, M.C.K., Williams, P.L., Benedetto, A. et al. (2008) *Caenorhabditis elegans*: An emerging model in biomedical and environmental toxicology. *Toxicological Sciences*, **106**, 5–28.

Leung, V., Rousseau-Blass, F., Beauchamp, G. and Pang, D.S.J. (2018) ARRIVE has not ARRIVEd: Support for the ARRIVE (Animal Research: Reporting of in vivo Experiments) guidelines does not improve the reporting quality of papers in animal welfare, analgesia or anesthesia. *PLOS ONE* **13**, e0197882.

Lilicrap, A., Belanger, S., Burden, N. et al. (2016) Alternative approaches to vertebrate ecotoxicity tests in the 21st century: A review of developments over the last 2 decades and current status. *Environmental Toxicology and Chemistry*, **35**, 2637–2646. https://doi.org/10.1002/etc.3603 (accessed 10 Jan 2022).

Marx, U., Andersson, T., Bahinski, A. et al. (2016) Biology-inspired microphysiological system approaches to solve the prediction dilemma of substance testing. *ALTEX – Alternatives to animal experimentation*. 33, 272–321. doi:https://doi.org/10.14573/altex.1603161 (accessed 10 Jan 2022).

Organisation for Economic Co-operation and Development (OECD) (2000) *Guidance Document on the Recognition, Assessment, and Use of Clinical Signs as Humane Endpoints for Experimental Animals Used in Safety Evaluation*. Environmental Health and Safety Publications, Series on Testing and Assessment, No. 19 https://ntp.niehs.nih.gov/iccvam/suppdocs/feddocs/oecd/oecd_gd19.pdf (accessed 10 Jan 2022).

Organisation for Economic Co-operation and Development (OECD) (2017) Guideline for the testing of Chemicals: Acute Eye Irritation/Corrosion (TG405). https://www.oecd-ilibrary.org/docserver/9789264185333-en.pdf (accessed 10 Jan 2022).

Perrimon, N., Bonini, N.M. and Dhillon, P. (2016) Fruit flies on the front line: the translational impact of *Drosophila*. *Disease Models and Mechanisms*, **9**, 229–231.

Poole, T. (1997) Happy animals make good science. *Laboratory Animals*, **31**, 116–124.

Pound, P. and Ritskes-Hoitinga, M. (2018) Is it possible to overcome issues of external validity in preclinical animal research? Why most animal models are bound to fail. *Journal of Translational Medicine* **16**, 304.

Prescott, M.J., Brown, V.J., Flecknell, P.A. *et al.* (2010) Refinement of the use of food and fluid control as motivational tools for macaques used in behavioural neuroscience research: Report of a Working Group of the NC3Rs. *Journal of Neuroscience Methods*, **193**, 167–188.

Richmond, J. (1999) Criteria for humane endpoints. In: *Humane Endpoints in Animal Experiments for Biomedical Research: Proceedings of the International Conference*, 22–25 November 1998, Zeist, The Netherlands. Eds Hendriksen, C.F.M. and Morton, D.B., pp. 26–32. Royal Society of Medicine Press, London.

Richmond, J. (2000) The Three Rs: a journey or a destination? *Alternatives to Laboratory Animals*, **28**, 761–773.

Roughan, J.V. and Flecknell, P.A. (2000) Effects of surgery and analgesic administration on spontaneous behaviour in singly housed rats. *Research in Veterinary Science*, **69**, 283–288.

Rowsell, H.C. (1977) The ethics of biomedical experimentation. In *The Future of Animals, Cells, Models, and Systems in Research, Development, Education, and Testing*, pp. 267–281. National Academy of Sciences, Washington, D.C.

Russell, W.M.S. and Burch, R.L. (1959) *The Principles of Humane Experimental Technique*. Methuen and Co., London, England.

Sams-Dodd, F. (2006) Strategies to optimize the validity of disease models in the drug discovery process. *Drug Discovery Today*, **11**, 355–363.

Scharmann, W. (1999) Physiological and ethological aspects of the assessment of pain, distress and suffering. In: *Humane Endpoints in Animal Experiments for Biomedical Research: Proceedings of the International Conference*, 22–25 November 1998, Zeist, The Netherlands. Eds Hendriksen, C.F.M. and Morton, D.B., pp. 33–39. Royal Society of Medicine Press, London.

Schnell, C.R. and Gerber, P. (1997) Training and remote monitoring of cardiovascular parameters in non-human primates. *Primate Report*, **49**, 61–70.

Schwanig, M., Nagel, M., Duchow, K. *et al.* (1997) Elimination of abnormal toxicity test for sera and certain vaccines in the European Pharmacopoeia. *Vaccine*, **15**, 1047–1048.

Smith, A.J. and Hawkins, P. (2016) Good science, good sense and good sensibilities: The three Ss of Carol Newton. *Animals*, **6**, 70. doi:10.3390/ani6110070

Smith, A.J., Clutton, R.E., Lilley, E. *et al.* (2018a) PREPARE Guidelines for planning animal research and testing. *Laboratory Animals*, **52**(2) 135–141. doi:10.1177/0023677217724823

Smith, D., Anderson, D., Degryse, A.-D. *et al.* (2018b) Classification and reporting of severity experienced by animals used in scientific procedures: FELASA/ECLAM/ESLAV Working Group report. *Laboratory Animals*, **52**(1_suppl), 5–57. https://doi.org/10.1177/0023677217744587 (accessed 10 Jan 2022)

Smyth, D. (1978) *Alternatives to Animal Experiments*. Scolar Press, London.

Soothill, J.S., Morton, D.B. and Ahmad, A. (1992) The HID_{50} (hypothermia-inducing dose 50): an alternative to the LD_{50} for measurement of bacterial virulence. *International Journal of Experimental Pathology*, **73**, 95–98.

Tannenbaum, J. and Bennett, B.T. (2015) Russell and Burch's 3Rs then and now: The need for clarity in definition and purpose. *Journal of the American Association for Laboratory Animal Science*, **54**, 120–132.

Tuttle, A.H., Philip, V.M., Chesler, E.J. *et al.* (2018) Comparing phenotypic variation within inbred and outbred mice. *Nature Methods*, **15**, 994–996.

Trapecar, M. (2021) Multiorgan microphysiological systems as tools to interrogate interorgan crosstalk and complex diseases. *FEBS Letters*, Dec. 18. doi: 10.1002/1873-3468.14260.

Vinken, M. (2013) The adverse outcome pathway concept: a pragmatic tool in toxicology. *Toxicology*, **312**, 158–165.

Vulto, P. and Joore, J. (2021) Adoption of organ-on-chip platforms by the pharmaceutical industry. *Nature Reviews Drug Discovery*, **20**, 961–962.

Wells, D.J., Playle, L.C., Enser, W.E. *et al.* (2006) Assessing the welfare of genetically altered mice. *Laboratory Animals*, **40**, 111–114.

Wolfensohn, S. and Honess, P. (2005) *Handbook of Primate Husbandry and Welfare*. Blackwell Publishing, Oxford.

Wolfensohn, S. and Lloyd, M. (2003) *Handbook of Laboratory Animal Management and Welfare*, 3rd edn. Blackwell Publishing, Oxford.

Würbel, H. and Garner, J.P. (2007) Refinement of rodent research through environmental enrichment and systematic randomization. https://www.nc3rs.org.uk/sites/default/files/documents/Refinementenvironmentalenrichmentandsystematicrandomization.pdf (accessed 10 Jan 2022)

Zemanova, M., Knight, A. and Lybæk, S. (2021) Educational use of animals in Europe indicates reluctance to implement alternatives. *Alternatives to Animal Experimentation*, **38**, 490–506.

Zintzsch, A., Noe, E., Reißmann, M. *et al.* (2017) Guidelines on severity assessment and classification of genetically altered mouse and rat lines. *Laboratory Animals*, **51**, 573–582. https://doi.org/10.1177/0023677217718863 (accessed 10 Jan 2022).

3 The design of animal experiments

Simon T. Bate and S. Clare Stanford

Introduction

This chapter is aimed at anyone involved in research using laboratory animals, including: animal technicians and members of committees that focus on animal welfare and ethics ('Animal Welfare and Ethical Review Bodies' (AWERBs), in the UK; Institutional Animal Care and Use Committees (IACUCs) in the USA), as well as researchers. It covers the main principles of experimental design, but deliberately includes only a brief discussion of statistical analysis strategies.

Well-designed experiments not only improve the likelihood of achieving the scientific objectives of the study, but they can reduce the total number of animals used and so are more ethical, as well as saving money, time and effort. Such experiments will:
- Produce results that are less likely to be biased and/or misleading.
- Help to achieve accurate, consistent and reproducible results by addressing nuisance sources of variability.
- Have a suitable level of statistical power (the ability of the experiment to detect a biologically relevant response to an intervention). If experiments are too small, they will generate unreliable conclusions and so waste animals.
- Avoid running excessively large experiments that can either generate overly sensitive tests, or waste animals, time and other scientific resources.

Unfortunately, surveys of published papers suggest that there is scope for substantial improvement in both the design of animal experiments and their statistical analysis (Kilkenny et al. 2010; Leung et al. 2018; Hair et al. 2019). In many cases, fundamental principles, such as the need to control nuisance sources of variation, randomisation and blinding (whenever feasible), are either ignored or not reported (Macleod et al. 2009). Also, decisions on sample size often depend more on traditional, rather than scientific, principles (Festing et al. 2002).

To address these concerns, there are now several free tools available to animal researchers (see Box 3.1 below). For example, the National Centre for the 3Rs (NC3Rs) in the UK has developed a web-based tool (the 'Experimental Design Assistant' (EDA))[1] that enables users to generate well-designed experiments (du Sert et al. 2017).

The research strategy

Much animal research is aimed at curing or alleviating a specific human or animal disease. Careful thought needs to be given to developing a suitable research strategy to achieve this objective, which may involve a long series of experiments, ranging from *in vitro* studies, through experiments on animals, to clinical trials.

Choosing the animal and procedure

In vitro and animal experiments *in vivo* need to generate relevant and reliable results, and hence be capable of answering specific questions. It is highly unlikely that they will replicate all aspects of complex human disorders, which is what would be expected for a valid 'model', but they can still lead to a better understanding of the underlying disease process and its treatment (Sams-Dodd 2006).

There is surprisingly little literature on the theory of 'models' of human disorders in biomedical research. Russell and Burch (1959) recognised that there are at least two dimensions, *fidelity* and *discriminative ability*, which determine their use. They used the term 'fidelity' to describe the overall similarity of the experimental system to the target (say humans), with a high-fidelity system more likely to qualify as a 'model'.

---

[1]https://eda.nc3rs.org.uk/ (accessed 1 Jan 2022)

> **Box 3.1** Free tools available to life scientists
>
> *Experimental Design Assistant (EDA)*
> The National Centre for the 3Rs (NC3Rs) has developed a web-based tool (the 'Experimental Design Assistant' (EDA))[1] that enables users to generate robust experimental designs. Examples of EDA diagrams of some of the designs considered in this text are given in Karp and Fry (2021). Once a design has been defined within the EDA, it is then critiqued by the system using an automated algorithm so that any weaknesses can be identified and addressed. The system includes dedicated support for randomisation, blinding and statistical power calculation. The EDA website[1] also provides detailed information and advice to help researchers develop their experimental design. By using the EDA, researchers can build on the points covered in this chapter to ensure they optimise their experimental design and statistical analysis.
>
> *InVivoStat*
> Award winning statistical analysis software designed specifically for animal researchers who do not have access to a professional statistician. Alongside graphical tools and established techniques (such as regression, t-tests and ANOVA), it includes some more advanced statistical tools, such as mixed models and stepwise multiple comparison techniques. It also provides a description of the methods performed, advice on pitfalls to look out for and warnings to help the user perform more reliable analyses. Download from www.invivostat.co.uk
>
> *ARRIVE guidelines (Animal Research: Reporting of In Vivo Experiments)*
> These guidelines were developed by the NC3Rs in collaboration with a team of experts in biomedical research, experimental design and data analysis (Percie du Sert *et al.* 2020). They specify the topics that should be included in all reports of experiments that have used animals, although most of these topics (e.g. randomisation and blinding) apply to all types of biomedical research not just those involving animals. Originally published in PLoS Biol (Kilkenny *et al.* 2010), they have been translated into many different languages and officially endorsed by leading national and international journals and are available for free download from: https://www.nc3rs.org.uk/arrive-guidelines
>
> *PREPARE guideline (Planning Research and Experimental Procedures on Animals: Recommendations for Excellence)*
> These guidelines were designed to complement the ARRIVE guidelines and remind scientists of topics that should be considered when planning experiments, including those that affect health and safety of the experimenter and welfare of the animals, as well as regulatory matters. The guidelines are available (Open Access) from the journal, *Laboratory Animals* (Smith *et al.* 2018).
>
> [1]https://eda.nc3rs.org.uk/ (accessed 9 January 2022)

Thus, non-human primates would normally be considered high-fidelity because they resemble humans in many ways. In contrast, a cell-line would be low-fidelity. Fidelity influences the 'external validity' of an experiment, which is the extent to which results generated in an experiment can be reliably extrapolated to other settings, populations and species. See also Chapter 2: The Three Rs.

The second dimension defined by Russell and Burch is the 'discriminative ability' of the experimental system to distinguish between different experimental treatments and applies also to features of responses that could differ across species (see: Garner *et al.* 2017). This is not necessarily related to fidelity. For instance, a cell culture, which distinguishes the effects of carcinogens from other chemicals, would be a preferred experimental system in toxicity testing even though it is of low-fidelity.

Other attributes of 'models' are also important (Festing 2000). They must resemble the target, in ways that are relevant to the objectives of the experiment, but must differ from the target in other ways. For example, the mouse is widely used because it resembles humans in important respects, but differs from humans in being small, economical to maintain, easy to manipulate genetically and because experiments can be done using the mouse which could not be performed in humans due to ethical concerns.

It is important to bear in mind that the validity of an animal 'model' can depend on the objectives of the experiment. For instance, a procedure can have 'predictive' validity, when used as a drug screen, and yet have none of the underlying features of the disorder of interest, which would be required for a model to have 'construct validity' or 'face' validity (Willner 1984). It is now widely recognised that many different criteria need to be satisfied before abnormalities in animals' physiology or behaviour can be regarded as a valid model of the human disorder: these would include a wide range of different measures of pathology, including physiological, pharmacological, biochemical, behavioural and even genetic factors. It follows that, although the 'model' is chosen because the response of interest is thought to be relevant to humans, confirming that assumption is a multi-step process and is rarely achieved.

The first step in all animal research is to ensure the validity of the experimental system in the context of the objectives of the study. The next step is to design experiments that enable detection of relevant responses (e.g. in terms of the magnitude of the response, or dose of drug needed to evoke a response).

Defining the purpose of the experiment

Experiments should follow a planned strategy to address specific issues. There are at least three main types of experiment, each with a different purpose:

- *Pilot experiments* are studies carried out on small numbers of subjects, in order to gather preliminary information, before carrying out a full-scale experiment (if the pilot suggests this is justified). Such studies could consider, for example, the logistics of the procedure and whether or not the technology works, or the doses of the test drug are appropriate. These experiments might involve only a single animal, although performing such studies using small groups of animals can give useful information on inter-individual variation. In most cases, the results of these experiments will not be amenable to statistical analysis (or be published), but good use of pilot studies can lead to substantial improvements in the design of a subsequent full-scale study.

- *Exploratory experiments* are used to study the effect of an experimental intervention without having a clearly defined prediction for what will happen. They often involve measuring many different outcomes (e.g. genetic and behavioural abnormalities associated with a psychiatric disorder) and are used to generate hypotheses for further investigation. Data generated in such experiments can be subject to an appropriate statistical analysis, but any conclusion drawn from the analysis, and/or any hypothesis that emerges, will need to be confirmed in another independent experiment planned specifically to test it. Moreover, if many outcomes are assessed, there is a high risk of obtaining false positive results. As a consequence, the results of these experiments need to be interpreted with caution and further experiments must be carried out to confirm that the finding(s) can be replicated.

- *Confirmatory experiments* are used to test pre-planned hypotheses, often focusing on a single outcome. The sample size is determined by the predicted magnitude of a biologically relevant effect, the preferred statistical power and the variability of the response (which is estimated in the exploratory experiment). In animal experiments many additional outcomes may be measured during a confirmatory experiment, which can lead to the development of further hypotheses. Again, these need to be tested in follow-up experiments. Thus, confirmatory experiments often have a dual role: they are used primarily to test a planned hypothesis but can also incorporate exploratory analyses that lead to new hypotheses. It is important to acknowledge that confirmatory experiments test for a particular predicted outcome: the hypothesis should not be adjusted after the experimental results have been unblinded, a practice known as 'HARKing' (Hypothesising After the Results are Known; see: Munafo et al. 2017).

The purpose of each experiment needs to be clear because this will influence the choice of experimental design. For example, the design of an experiment that aims to explore the dose–response relationship for a novel drug will differ from one that aims to compare, say, the effect of three diets on body weight in both males and females. In all cases, the aim should be to design experiments that maximise the amount of information gathered, while using the minimum number of animals and other resources. For instance, the number of animals used in a study could be reduced by designing the experiment to test the effects of more than one experimental intervention in each animal. However, in so doing, the experimenter must consider the benefits of gathering more information from each animal *versus* the cumulative harm they experience (see also: the cross-over design in the following text).

The majority of experiments should include a control (no treatment) group of animals, but this is not invariably the case. For example, if a drug is predicted to cause hyperactivity, each animal can act as its own control (pre-treatment) because it is reasonable to assume that expression of hyperactivity, soon after the drug administration, was caused by the test treatment. Ideally, where ethical and scientific constraints allow, it is always best to let each animal act as its own control. Such designs allow treatments to be compared 'within animal', thus increasing both the reliability and probability of finding a true positive result (statistical power). This can dramatically reduce the total number of animals used. Even if this is not possible, a control group that has not been treated (even with vehicle) is always desirable, not least because the process of administering the drug or vehicle treatment (e.g. an intraperitoneal injection) can affect the response of interest (Stanford et al. 1984).

The decision-making process

When we conduct an experiment, regardless of its type, we make decisions based on the data generated: whether it be confirming a planned hypothesis (e.g. a novel drug is safe) or deciding which hypotheses to assess. Sometimes, estimating the intervention and control group means is the primary purpose of the experiment, but usually it is the difference between these means that is of interest.

When making a decision that is based on experimental data, the researcher needs to consider not only the biological relevance of the observed effects, but also the level of confidence they can place in that decision. Statistics provides a tool to quantify this. Generally, statistical approaches compare the size of the observed effect (the 'signal') to the background variability (the 'noise') of the system. This noise can be quantified, for example, by calculating the standard deviation of the responses. If the signal is large, compared with the background variability, then we can be more confident that the observed effect is real. Many statistics tests are based on evaluating this so-called '*signal-to-noise ratio*'. However, it should be noted that:

- In the statistical analysis, it is the amplitude of the signal-to-noise ratio that is important, not just the amplitude of the signal. To improve confidence in our decision (conclusion), we can either increase the amplitude of the signal, by changing the parameters of the experiment, or we can try to reduce the noise. We shall consider the latter in more detail in this chapter because the experimental design plays a key role in enabling the researcher to account for nuisance sources of variability in an experiment.

- Before drawing conclusions from the statistical analysis, the researcher should also consider the magnitude of the observed signal and decide whether or not it is of biological relevance. Observed effects that are small may well be statistically significant, if the noise is small, but might not be of any genuine biological or practical interest.

- In many experiments the variability of the response derives from multiple sources. A key part of any experimental process is to reduce extraneous sources of variability that could affect the results, such as differences in husbandry, research environment or experimenter. On the other hand, it is worth considering whether findings that are evident only in a highly controlled and constant environment are likely to be of biological importance, more generally, or relevant to the animals' response in their 'real world'. In animal experiments, it is often the pool of animals that will be the largest source of variability, as discussed in the next section, but this is not always the case. The experimental procedures themselves may be a considerable source of variability. For example, intraperitoneal injections are widely used in animal research, but they can occasionally be carried out incorrectly. This may introduce variability into the data set which, if not taken into account, could have a misleading effect on the conclusions drawn from the experiment (Das & North 2007).

Variation among the animals

To help minimise the noise in the signal-to-noise ratio, it is common practice to use animals that are as similar as possible. For instance, when using rodents, the experiment would aim to study animals of similar weight (and/or age). Note that it is sometimes desirable to use animals of a wider body weight or age range within an experiment. This strategy could increase the external validity of any conclusions drawn from the study, i.e. the extent to which the findings generalise to the whole population, (Voelkl & Würbel. 2021). However, any variability associated with body weight, which will have been amplified due to the wider range used in the study, must then be accounted for in the statistical analysis (see later in this chapter).

Animals used in experiments are also commonly Specific Pathogen-Free (SPF). Apart from any welfare considerations, illness in animals, whether caused by pathogens or other factors, not only increases variability, but also affect the results of the experiment. This is not least because diseased and healthy animals could respond differently to the treatment of interest. Most mice and rats supplied by commercial breeders are now of SPF quality and derive from colonies that are screened routinely for a wide range of pathogenic organisms. Animals that are bred in-house should similarly be screened regularly to ensure that they are pathogen-free. However, it should be borne in mind that there is now a great deal of evidence that naturalistic, non-pathogenic microbes (the microbiome) can influence the outcome of an experiment (e.g. Sherwin et al. 2018) and so it cannot be assumed that the results obtained using SPF animals are typical or would be replicated across all establishments.

Genetic heterogeneity is another factor that can increase phenotypic variability, but this is not invariably the case (Tuttle et al. 2018). Nevertheless, some researchers believe that an outbred stock of animals should always be used, on the grounds that humans are genetically diverse: see, for example, Martin et al. 2017. However, such genetic variation can result in a response to an experimental challenge being expressed in some, but not all subjects. If the treatment effect is assessed by estimating an overall shift in the mean response, then non-responders might mask a response in a subset of subjects, which reduces the power of the experiment and increases the risk of obtaining false negative results.

Another factor to consider is that experiments using outbred strains might be difficult to replicate because nothing is known about the genotypes of the individuals. Even the degree of genetic variability within an outbred colony is unclear because it depends on the previous history of the stock. For instance, there is a risk that each outbred colony has an element of inbreeding. Unless effective precautions are taken to prevent this, findings from experiments using outbred animals can differ from one outbred colony to another.

On the other hand, if a response is seen in an outbred strain, then it is likely to be an important finding because it either affects all subjects to some extent or indicates a large response in a subgroup of animals. The external validity of such an experiment will be strong because a similar 'stratification' of the response could also occur in humans. Moreover, such a finding could help to find ways of targeting treatments at those patients who are most likely to respond.

To avoid these potential confounders, some researchers recommend that (inbred or F1 hybrid) strains of rats and mice should always be used unless there is a compelling case for using outbred stocks (Festing 1999). Because inbred animals are more likely to be genetically identical, this could reduce the extraneous genetic 'noise' and potentially increase the power of the experiment, or enable the number of animals needed for the study to be reduced. Such an approach can reduce variability and so increase the internal validity of the experiment and strengthen the robustness of a study's findings, but this will also depend on factors such as how the experiment is designed and conducted (including the blinding of the experiment and the randomisation performed), as well as appropriate statistical analysis and reporting of the results. However, using inbred strains will almost certainly compromise external validity. For instance, a finding from a study of a particular inbred strain could be construed as a 'false positive' if it is assumed, incorrectly, to generalise to other inbred strains, or outbred animals.

For this reason, it is best to study the effects of the experimental challenge in at least two different inbred strains. 'Strain' can then be incorporated into the experiment as one factor in a factorial design (see later in this chapter). Although this strategy can increase the number of animals used (see: Martin et al. 2017 and Hsieh et al. 2017), in general such experiments are likely to be smaller, even after taking this duplication into account, than when using a single outbred strain. However, this approach assumes that at least one of the inbred strain(s) chosen for the study falls into the 'responder' category and so does not entirely remove the risk of obtaining a false positive or false negative result in respect of extrapolation to outbred animals.

If it is known that the variable of interest is abnormal (e.g. prominent or deficient), in a given inbred strain, then it can be justified to use only that strain to explore the mechanism(s) that underlie, or influence, that response. However, it would still be advisable to go on to confirm any inferences in a different strain. This is particularly important when studying genetically altered rodents because the effect of the mutation on the response to an experimental challenge can depend on the background strain of the animals (e.g. Jaramillo *et al*. 2018). However, such differences can be invaluable in providing clues to the underlying, biological factors that influence the response. More details of the origin, maintenance and characteristics of isogenic strains of rodents can be found at Jackson Laboratory[2] and the rat genome database[3].

Other factors should be considered as well as genetic variation and its effect on experimental results. For instance, an animal's response to an experimental challenge can depend on early life experience (e.g. maternal behaviour, which could be particularly important if the pups are cross-fostered), and/or interactions with littermates, or other environmental factors (e.g. Porter *et al*. 2015). The housing conditions of mice (e.g. individually ventilated cages *versus* standard, open-top cages and single *versus* group housed animals) can also have an appreciable effect on the physiology and behaviour of mice (Pasquarelli *et al*. 2017) and can increase the variability of experimental measures (Chvedoff *et al*. 1980). Other experimental factors that can affect variability include handling (see the preceding text) and environmental enrichment (see also, Chapter 10: Environmental enrichment: animal welfare and scientific validity).

There are other factors that can make the cage in which the animals are housed an important source of variation, but they can be difficult to deal with. For instance, the response to a given treatment could vary in different cages because the response of identically treated animals depends on social interactions within each cage. For this reason, an ideal design would fully randomise all the test treatment(s) and controls within all the cages. However, there may be situations where this is not feasible, such as when animals are to be given a drug in their drinking water or when the drug content in the faeces is to be measured for a pharmacokinetic study.

The position of the animals' cage in the animal facility can also be an important, but neglected, factor (Gore & Stanley 2005). For instance, animals housed on the top shelf of a rack are generally exposed to more light and possibly a warmer temperature than those on lower shelves. Ideally, the animals should either be randomly allocated to cages across all the shelves, or the shelf position should be included in the experimental design, using a complete block (by shelf) design (see later in this chapter). In such a design, each shelf has equal numbers of treated and control animals and any variability caused by differences between the shelves can be accounted for in the statistical analysis.

Steps in the design of an experiment

Defining which dependent variables to measure

The experimenter will usually measure one or more dependent variables (i.e. responses, also called 'outcome measures'), which are used to quantify the effect of the experimental intervention. Responses such as changes in body weight, haematology, clinical biochemistry, physiological variables (e.g. heart rate and blood pressure), behaviour and gene expression are all examples of 'outcomes', which could respond to the intervention and can be measured. Such measured variables can either be quantitative (i.e. consist of numerical levels), or qualitative (i.e. they consist of categorical levels, such as 'small', 'intermediate' and 'large'). As a rule of thumb, quantitative variables can be manipulated mathematically (i.e. added together, averaged, etc.) whereas qualitative variables cannot.

Quantitative dependent variables include:

- *Continuous*: Responses can be any numerical value.
- *Discrete*: Numeric responses that can be recorded only as fixed values, such as counts.

Qualitative dependent variables include:

- *Categorical*: Responses are non-numeric and can be either ordinal or nominal:
  - *Ordinal*: Levels of response are ordered, such as disease progression scores.
  - *Nominal*: Levels of response are not ordered, such as stress reaction behaviour.
- *Binary*: Response outcomes can be one of two values (i.e. yes/no, present/absent).

It should be noted that continuous responses contain the most information and binary responses have the least. As a consequence, more animals will generally be required to achieve the same level of statistical confidence in the experimental conclusions if the responses measured are not continuous.

Defining which effects to investigate

Researchers conduct experiments to investigate the effect of key variables (e.g. the effect of a test treatment, animal strain or set of equipment) on the outcome measure. These findings are then used to make predictions about what would happen in the 'real world'. The effects can be defined as either 'fixed' or 'random', depending on their influence on the outcome measure.

A 'fixed effect' has a consistent and reproducible effect on the response. Examples include: sex, strain, diet and housing condition. To assess the impact of a fixed effect, an experimental design is constructed which incorporates a 'fixed factor' (or 'independent variable') corresponding to the fixed effect. The levels of this fixed factor correspond to levels of the fixed effect that are of interest. For example, if the researcher wishes to investigate the effect of a drug treatment, over a specific range of doses, then a 'Treatment' factor is constructed at several levels (e.g. control, low, intermediate and high dose). Changes in the means for each test group, across the different levels of the Treatment factor (doses), will give an indication of the fixed effect of the treatment on the response.

In animal experiments, factors are usually considered to be 'categorical'. The levels of each factor are non-numeric, i.e. Sex has levels 'male' and 'female', Strain has levels 'wildtype' and 'transgenic', and Dose has levels 'control', 'low', 'intermediate' and 'high'. However, some factors can be considered 'continuous', where the levels of the factors are numeric

---

[2] http://www.jax.org/ (accessed 1 July 2019)
[3] http://rgd.mcw.edu (accessed 1 July 2019)

and hence the numerical difference between them can be taken into account in the statistical analysis. For example, the Dose factor, above, could alternatively be defined using numerical levels 0, 1, 5 and 10 (mg/kg) and in the statistical analysis a dose-response curve employed to model the dose effects, rather than fitting four individual means (corresponding to the four individual doses). Note that defining factors as continuous or categorical has implications for the choice of experimental design as well as the statistical analysis (see Bate & Clark (2014), Section 3.6.2).

By contrast, random effects introduce variability into the experimental results and include day-to-day variation, animal-to-animal variation, variation between rooms, cages, locations, researcher, sets of equipment and so on. The researcher often has little control, if any, over any of these sources of variation. To assess the influence of a random effect, a 'random factor' is incorporated into the experimental design. For example, in a dietary study, the weights of different animals, of the same age, will vary depending on the innate between-animal variability; this variability is captured by including an 'Animal' random factor in the experimental design. In the hyperactivity assessment, described above, where each animal acts as its own control, inclusion of the Animal factor in the analysis would enable the separation of the variability that is explained by baseline differences between the animals from the within-animal variability. The treatment effect can then be tested against the within-animal variability. The levels of such factors should be randomly sampled from a wider population: only then can the study conclusions be assumed to apply to this wider population. For instance, in the dietary study, if the levels of the Animal factor were selected at random from the male population, only, then any justifiable conclusion will be valid for males, but not necessarily for females.

The differences in the response across the different levels of the random factor will give an indication of the magnitude of the corresponding random effect. Generally, random effects should be controlled as much as possible, either by increased replication of the corresponding factor levels (i.e. the number of individual measurements) or by accounting for them in the experimental design (using, for example, a block design). These topics are discussed in detail in the following sections (see choice of sample size and block designs, respectively).

Some effects can be considered to be either fixed or random, depending on the purpose of the experiment. For example, if the test equipment itself affects the outcome measure, this is usually regarded as a fixed effect and it is assumed that, if different sets of equipment are used in the experiment, then each will introduce a different fixed amount of bias (i.e. each produces its own 'fixed' effect). However, if the aim of the experiment is to establish how much of the variability in the results can be attributed simply to the use of different sets of equipment, then each particular set used in the experiment would be regarded as a random sample from a wider population. In order to estimate this variability reliably, then many examples of the test equipment should be used (more than would be the case if the equipment effect is of no interest and is assumed to be a fixed effect). In this scenario, variation in the results when using different equipment reflects the underlying variability that can be attributed to this random effect.

Identifying the experimental unit

A fundamental principle when designing an experiment is to ensure that there is <u>independent</u> replication of the experimental interventions. The 'experimental unit' (sometimes called the 'unit of replication') is the unit of material that actually contributes $N=1$ to the experiment. The experimental unit can be defined as: *The unit (e.g. a tissue sample or animal) that independently receives a treatment such that the findings obtained from one experimental unit are unrelated to the findings obtained from any other.*

Properties of the experimental unit are that it:

- Is the smallest unit that independently receives one of the experimental interventions.
- Must not influence, or be influenced by, any of the other experimental units in the study (i.e. the response of one unit should not correlate with that of any other unit).
- Has an equal chance of receiving any of the interventions.

When making decisions about the experimental intervention, correct identification of the experimental unit is vital. This is because we need to compare the size of the response (signal) to the underlying variability of the units (noise) that receive the intervention. So, if animals receive either a treatment or no treatment (control), then the signal is the treated animals' mean response *versus* the control animals' mean response and this signal is assessed against the underlying animal-to-animal variability.

The experimental unit is often the animal, with animals being assigned to each of the interventions at random. However, if there are several animals in each cage and they all receive the same intervention, then it can be argued that it is the cage, not the individual animal, that is the experimental unit. In such cases, each cage should be assigned, at random, to one of the interventions and the statistical analysis should be performed on the mean outcome of <u>all</u> animals within each cage: i.e. if there are four animals in each cage, then the experimental unit is the mean of all four animals and $N=1$, not $N=4$, per cage. Incorrect definition of the experimental unit, in this case, leads to over-estimation of the number of experimental units (and hence 'total information' generated) in the study. This increases the risk of a false positive in the statistical analysis and, possibly, invalidates the conclusions of the whole study. Mistakes can also occur when multiple measurements are taken on each experimental unit but are not averaged before conducting the statistical analysis.

Another example where caution is necessary would be a teratology experiment in which a pregnant animal is treated with a test compound, but it is the abnormalities in each foetus that are counted. It is a common error to assume that each foetus is an experimental unit ('pseudo-replication'). However, the experimental unit is the mother, because it is the mother which was assigned to a specific treatment group, and each mother will have a score based on the average number of pup abnormalities in the litter. In this case, it may also be necessary to take account of litter size in the statistical analysis, as large litters will provide a better estimate of the susceptibility of the treated female than small litters. Additionally, it should be borne in mind that females with larger litters may respond differently from those with smaller ones.

Individual animals can sometimes provide multiple experimental units and it is possible to compare the response to different interventions within animal. For instance, if an animal is shaved, such that different treatments can be applied locally to individual patches of skin (e.g. in testing for an allergic skin reaction), then each patch can be regarded as an experimental unit because any two patches can receive a different treatment. Nevertheless, in such cases, the 'Animal' factor should still be included in the statistical analysis, potentially as a blocking factor (see the block design section).

Determining the sample size (replication of the experimental units)

As noted above, differences between the experimental units are usually the most important source of random variability, not least because the effects of the experimental intervention are compared with this variability. In general, random sources of variability are accounted for by increasing the replication of the corresponding factor in the experimental design (e.g. increasing the sample size). So, as the animals are a source of random variability and usually define the experimental unit, and ethical considerations mean that we should not use more animals than are necessary to reach a valid conclusion, we need to pay particular attention to the number of animals used.

Sample sizes that are based merely on traditional practice can lead to using either too many, or usually too few, animals and hence waste scientific resources. Two methods that are widely used and give a better estimate of the required sample size are 'power analysis' and the 'resource equation'. Both these methods have limitations but are substantially better than having an arbitrary, fixed number of replicates in each group.

The resource equation

The resource equation approach, in its simplest form, where there is only one treatment factor in the experimental design, involves considering E in the following equation:

$$E = N - T$$

where N is the number of experimental units (i.e. animals) and T is the number of treatments.

Mead (1988) suggests that E (the 'Error degrees of freedom') should be between 10 and 20. So if the number of treatments is 4 and the number of animals in each group is 5 then $E=20-4=16$. Note that in more general situations, E can be obtained from any analysis of variance (ANOVA) or analysis of covariance (ANCOVA) table (see following sections on analysis of variance and covariance, respectively).

The resource equation is useful when the researcher does not have an estimate of the variability of the response. However, its limitations are that it does not take into account the size of an effect that is biologically meaningful or indicate how that effect is related (in size) to the variability of the data. Additionally, this approach does not identify the probability of running a successful experiment. To investigate how these properties are influenced by replication of the design factors, a power analysis approach is required (and recommended).

Power analysis

Power analysis assesses the chance, for a given sample size, of achieving statistical significance when the impact of the intervention is of practical relevance. For example, if the aim of the experiment is to assess whether there is a difference between two treatment groups, then the following information is required:

- The type of *statistical test* which is to be used. This depends on the nature of the data/design. Quantitative data can normally be analysed using Student's t-test, ANOVA, or a non-parametric test. In the example described in Box 3.2, it is assumed that a quantitative variable is measured and that the group means are to be compared using a Student's t-test.
- An *estimate of the variability of the experimental units*. This information must be derived from an exploratory or pilot experiment, preferably from the same laboratory. Unfortunately, pilot studies are usually small, so any estimate of the variability is inevitably imprecise. This could result in an under- or over-estimate of the sample size required. This, and the fact that the variability cannot be assessed with confidence until the outcome has been measured, is a potential drawback.
- The *effect-size*. This is the minimum magnitude of the difference between the two groups in the experiment which would be of clinical or biological relevance. Clearly, a small difference would not be of great interest in most contexts, but it is important to be able to detect reliably a large difference.
- The *statistical power*. This is the probability, for a given biologically relevant difference between the two groups, of correctly rejecting the hypothesis that there is no effect. Somewhat arbitrarily, the power is usually set at 80–90%. A power of 80% implies that if there is a true effect as large, or larger, than that specified, then there will be an 80% chance of detecting it in the experiment. When choosing the desired level of power, the researcher should take into account the implications of incorrectly failing to detect an effect. If the consequences of a false negative are potentially serious, then a higher power should be specified.
- The *significance level*. This is the probability that the experiment generates a (false) positive conclusion when in reality there is no difference between the two groups (i.e. the probability of observing a 'sufficiently large' treatment effect purely due to chance). For the purposes of a power analysis, this is usually set at 0.05 (i.e. 5%), although this is entirely arbitrary and other levels may sometimes be selected instead. Using a significance level of 0.05 is well-established, although this may underestimate the false positive risk and so using a lower threshold is encouraged.
- The *'sidedness' of the test*. A two-sided test is used when it is not clear whether the effect of the intervention will be

> **Box 3.2**
>
> *The mean body weight of a group of F344 male rats in a growth trial is 259 g with a standard deviation of 11 g, which implies that the body weights among a group of 100 rats could be expected to range from about 230 to 290 g.*
>
> *Suppose a diet experiment is to be set up using these male F344 rats and that a 10 g difference in mean body weight between two groups of rats receiving two different diets is considered biologically important. It is assumed that the treatment does not alter the standard deviation. How many F344 rats will be needed to conclude there is an effect of the treatment, given that the true effect is 10 g?*
>
> If a Student's t-test is to be used to analyse the data, then to achieve a power of 90%, with a significance level of 0.05, InVivoStat's Power analysis suggests 27 rats per group will be required.
>
> However, if the weight range of the rats used in the study is restricted to 250–270 g, then applying this range would result in the standard deviation being reduced to about 5 g. This reduction in variability would mean that only 7, instead of 27 rats per group, would be required.
>
> Of course, this has the drawback that the conclusions of the experiment are now more limited as they would be valid only over a narrower range of body weights.
>
> An alternative strategy is to use a statistical procedure, known as ANCOVA, to account for the additional animal-to-animal variability associated with body weight (see ANCOVA section near end of the chapter), which can then be distinguished from the background variability that the treatment effect is compared to. When testing the effect of diet on body weight, this would be achieved by fitting each animal's baseline body weight as a covariate in the statistical analysis (Bate & Clark 2014). This approach has the advantage of allowing a wider range of animal body weights to be included in the experiment, and hence the conclusions are valid for a wider range, without necessarily requiring an increase in the sample size.

in a positive or negative direction. However, if the hypothesis is that the mean will change in a particular direction, then a one-sided test should be specified.

- The *sample size*. This is the number of experimental units needed for the experiment and is usually what is being estimated in the power analysis (see: Box 3.2). However, in some situations the sample size is fixed (by the availability of animals or limited equipment capacity, for instance). In such cases, the calculations can be used to determine the statistical power of the experiment.

Within InVivoStat[4] (Clark *et al.* 2012 and Bate *et al.* 2017), a free-to-use statistical software package aimed at animal researchers, there is a Power Analysis module that performs all the required calculations. The package generates plots, such as that given in Figure 3.1, so that the user can assess how changing the sample size, for difference biologically relevant effects, will influence the statistical power.

It is important to emphasise that when there is more than one response of interest, separate power calculations are needed for each of them and that their estimated sample sizes may differ. In such cases, it will be necessary to decide which response (or responses) is/are most important (known as the primary outcome(s)) and to ensure that the sample size selected is appropriate for them all.

Assessing the measurement and procedural variability

Increasing the number of replicates in an experiment enables the researcher to deal with the variability associated with the random effect. The previous section discussed the replication of the experimental units in order to account for individual differences between them. However, the variability of the experimental unit might not be the only source of variability in an experiment. There may be others we wish to investigate and take into account (Jeffery *et al.* 2018).

Some outcomes, such as measuring the activities of enzymes or gene expression, may involve multiple steps. Tissues may need to be removed, followed by extraction of a solute into a solution and an assay, using various types of apparatus. There may be variation in the calibration of the instruments, in the composition of the reagents, incubation

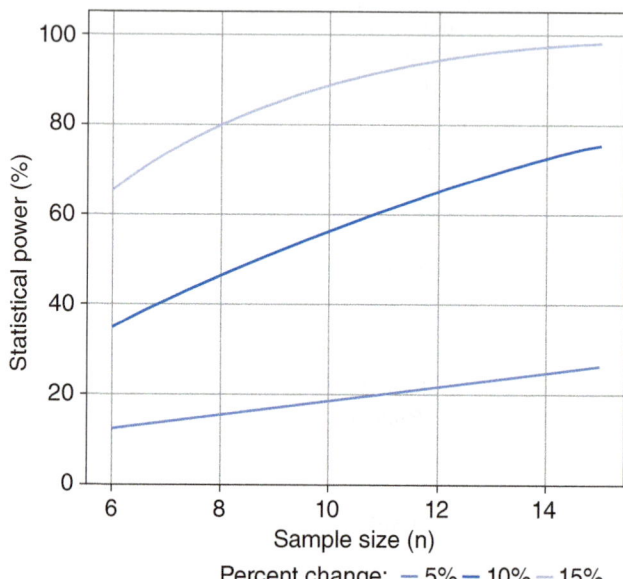

Figure 3.1 An InVivoStat power analysis plot for sample sizes ranging between 6 and 15. The lines show the percentage changes, above the control baseline, of 5, 10 and 15%, when the measure of variability (standard deviation) is equal to 1. To achieve 80% statistical power, when the true effect is a 15% change from control, a sample size of N=8 animals per group would be required.

---

[4] www.invivostat.co.uk (accessed 1 July 2019)

temperatures, pipetting errors, etc., leading to considerable measurement errors. In such situations, it can be advantageous to split the sample as soon as it is taken and run duplicate or triplicate determinations, which are then averaged for the formal statistical analysis. This is sometimes called 'technical replication' (or pseudo-replication), which is distinct from the 'biological replication' that is associated with differences between individuals (i.e. the experimental units). Note that technical replication does not increase the number of experimental units, but it does increase the precision with which each experimental unit is measured. This can then contribute to an increase in power and hence a reduction in sample size.

Behavioural observations provide another example. Different types of animal behaviour may be recorded for relatively brief periods. Although such observations may be adequate, they may not be a true reflection of the animals' typical behaviour. Modern apparatus is now available to record a wide range of behaviours automatically, over long periods of time, sometimes with several animals in their home cage (Redfern et al. 2017 and Bains et al. 2018). When using such approaches, measurement error in the assessment of behavioural phenotypes is likely to be reduced, by comparison with observations of individual animals for only brief periods of time. Nevertheless, technical limitations of such apparatus need to be taken into account and the data need to be interpreted with care, ideally with video confirmation.

All these experiments are examples of nested designs (Bate & Clark 2014), where multiple measurements must be taken at random within each experimental unit (typically, an animal): see Figure 3.2 for a diagrammatical representation of a nested design. With such designs, within-animal variability should be the only systematic difference between the within-animal measurements. There should be no trends across, or structure to, the within-animal responses that could be comparable across different animals: such cases could include, for example, time-dependent changes. Experiments in which repeated measurements are taken sequentially, and time-dependent changes are of interest, are not considered to be nested designs.

Effectively, applications of nested designs involve multiple (nested) random factors, where each factor corresponds to a source of variability. Because each random factor is nested within another, we can use statistical analysis to isolate, and hence estimate, the underlying sources of variability that correspond to the random factors in the design.

With nested designs, we can investigate whether there is any benefit in increasing the levels of replication of any of the multiple random factors. For example, by taking more measurements from each animal (thereby increasing the technical replication), can the number of animals per group be reduced without compromising the statistical power or causing appreciable more harm to the individual animal? The Nested Design Analysis module, within InVivoStat[4], allows researchers to answer such questions.

As well as investigating the known sources of variability, using a nested design, the researcher should always try to identify and record unexpected sources of variability when conducting the experiment (e.g. a change in the husbandry routine or the period of habituation to the laboratory environment). These can then be investigated, and/or taken into account in future experiments, thus allowing the researcher to construct more efficient designs, using fewer animals, next time.

Choosing an experimental design

So far, the choice of experimental design has not been considered, other than for determination of sample size. To comply with the obligation to reduce the number of experimental animals (and also to reduce the cost of the study), the sample size is usually kept as low as possible and yet must be large enough to reach a valid conclusion. When taken alongside the level of biological variability, this can be problematic for the statistical assessment. Nevertheless, the researcher has a good deal of control over the choice of experimental design, which can influence the number of animals required and so help to counterbalance the statistical issues of low sample size and high variability.

If we identify the largest sources of variability, then we can design our experiment to allow us to take these sources into account in the statistical analysis. This step is crucial. In the following section, we shall discuss some of these designs in more detail and show how they can be used to carry out more efficient experiments and to increase confidence in the conclusions.

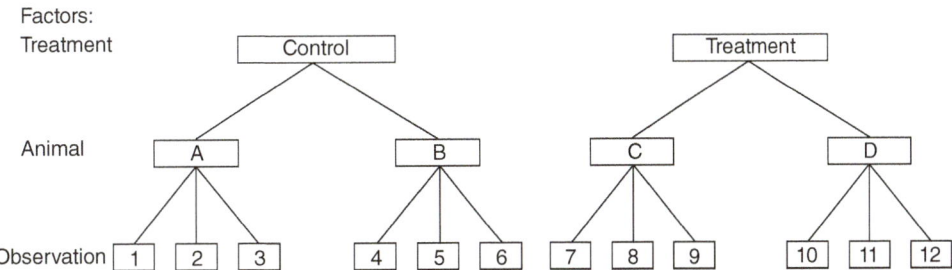

Figure 3.2 Schematic of a nested design involving two nested factors (Treatment and Animal). Two animals are randomly assigned to each of the two treatments and then three measurements are taken from each animal. In the nested design, the Animal factor (at four levels: A, B, C and D) is nested within the Treatment factor (two animals per treatment) and the Observation factor (12 levels: 1–12) is nested within the Animal factor (three observations taken per animal).

Randomising the experiment

Randomisation is of fundamental importance. Provided that it is maintained throughout the whole experiment, the aim of randomisation is to eliminate systematic differences between the experimental groups. For example, if all of the different drug treatments are assigned to every cage in a random order then it follows that we can assume that any observed differences in the outcome measure are due to either random inter-individual variation or the effect of the experimental intervention.

Randomisation also ensures that the variability estimate is itself unbiased. The aim of many statistical analyses is to quantify the extent to which group differences might have happened through chance. If the estimates of the intervention group means and the experimental unit variability are unbiased, then this assessment will be more reliable and reproducible.

Randomisation should be maintained throughout the whole experiment. To avoid any risk of introducing bias, interventions should be performed, and outcomes measured, in a random order. For instance, if all the controls are assessed first, followed by those receiving the experimental intervention, then extraneous time-related effects could introduce a bias that affects the difference in the outcome measures of the different groups.

Computer software is available to generate random sequences from a series of numbers (e.g. the Microsoft Excel function RAND). However, even randomisation by hand is simple and straightforward. For example, if the aim is to assign animals to five treatments (say a saline control and four levels for drug dose), with six animals per treatment group, the numbers 1, 2, 3, 4 and 5 could each be written six times on separate pieces of paper. These would then be shaken in a suitable receptacle. The first animal is then taken, and a piece of paper is withdrawn from the receptacle (and not replaced) to show the experimental group to which it should be assigned, and so on.

Blinding the experiment

Blinding of the conduct of the experiment ('allocation concealment') is another important way of avoiding bias because research workers cannot be regarded as unbiased. This leads to the problem that the expectations of an unblinded experimenter could affect the procedure, and even affect the animals, or influence the experimenter's observations of the animals' response. This is because, in most cases, researchers hope to see a 'positive' outcome. If there is any subjective element in assessing results, and the researcher knows which is the treatment group, then there is a high risk of subconscious bias when scoring the results. This can be avoided by blinding. However, blinding is not always possible because there can be obvious differences between groups: for example, the two strains of mice being compared may differ in coat colour, size or sex. If samples of tissue are taken from these animals, they should be coded so that any subsequent measurements can be done blind with respect to strain, sex or treatment.

The statistical analysis of the data should also be blinded to avoid any risk of bias, even at this final stage of the process. However, this should not be used as a replacement for blinding the experiment itself, as biases introduced when running the experiment cannot be removed by a blinded statistical analysis.

Performing the statistical analysis

When all the data have been collected, the statistical analysis can be performed. This analysis should match the experimental design and take into account all nuisance sources of variability that were included in the design. The analysis should be the most powerful available to the researcher: for example, parametric tests (rather than non-parametric tests) should be used whenever possible (Bate & Clark 2014). In the section below, we shall consider some of these tests in more detail.

Reporting the results of the experiment

When reporting the experiment, there should always be a statement to confirm whether or not randomisation and blinding were performed, together with the actual method of randomisation that was applied. Indeed, this is one of the points specified in the ARRIVE guidelines for reporting of animal experiments (Percie du Sert et al. 2020). Experiments which were not blinded and/or randomised are far more likely to have a 'positive' outcome than those which were (Bebarta et al. 2003), confirming that these precautions really do reduce bias.

Types of experimental designs

The completely randomised design

This is the simplest design with a single factor of interest: the number of factor levels corresponds to the number of different experimental interventions (i.e. treatments). One of the factor levels may be considered a 'control', or the aim may be to compare a set of qualitatively or quantitatively different interventions. The effects of many different interventions can be assessed and the number of experimental units receiving each intervention does not need to be the same (Bate & Karp 2014).

As explained above, the experimental units are assigned to intervention groups strictly at random: the order in which the interventions are given, the outcome measured and even the housing positions should all be randomised. The staff measuring the outcome should always be blinded with respect to the intervention group. Figure 3.3 is an example of a drug study where 16 animals are randomly assigned to four treatment groups with four animals per treatment.

Animal															
1	2	3	4	5	6	7	8	9	10	11	12	13	14	15	16
C	C	A	B	B	D	D	A	A	D	D	B	C	B	C	A

Figure 3.3 Example of the layout of a completely randomised design with four treatments (A, B, C and D) and four animals randomly assigned to each treatment. Thus, the first and second animals will be assigned to treatment C, the third to A, etc.

The randomised block design

Randomised block designs are an important class of designs as they enable the researcher to account for nuisance sources of variability. Researchers should consider using these designs routinely in all their experiments.

Consider, first, the drug study illustrated above in Figure 3.3. Assume that the singly housed animals were randomly assigned to cages on different shelves in a rack. If the responses to treatment are influenced by the shelf position (for example, the responses of animals housed on the top shelf are higher than those housed below), then shelf position will be a nuisance source of variability that is not accounted for by the randomisation.

If there is a nuisance source of variability, which is ignored, this could:

1. Increase the variability (or 'noise') of the responses, if not accounted for in the statistical analysis.
2. Bias the 'signal', if the intervention allocation leads to the random effect affecting the results for each intervention group in different ways.

A consequence of both of these issues is that the signal-to-noise ratio, as used in many statistical tests, may be unreliable. For example, in the drug study above, an unfortunate randomisation could lead to the control animals being housed mainly on the top shelf. The control group responses could therefore be higher than the treatment group responses, even before administration of the treatment, simply due to the shelf effect. This will result in a bias in any comparisons between the control and treatment groups.

However, we can accommodate any differences due to the influence of the shelf position by using a block design. This is a design that has been split up into several mini-experiments (or blocks), such that all the experimental units in a block share the same level of the nuisance effect. Every treatment should be replicated equally within each block, where possible, so that the nuisance effect does not bias any treatment comparisons. An example of a block design for the drug study (blocked by shelf position) is given in Figure 3.4.

Blocks can be separated in time so, for example, block 1 can be started in week 1, block 2 in week 2, etc. Blocks can also be separated in space, such as being on different shelves or in different rooms.

The results of these mini-experiments are then combined in a single statistical analysis so that any variability associated with the nuisance effect can be accounted for by including a 'blocking factor' in the statistical model. In this type of design, randomisation is done separately, within each block, as shown diagrammatically in Figure 3.4.

Some of the practical reasons for using a block design include:

- *To compensate for variation of the animals* in respect of some identifiable characteristic, such as weight, age, batch or source. Animals, which are similar for that characteristic, should be grouped in a 'block' and then assigned at random to the interventions. Typically, the number of experimental units in each block will be the same size as the number of interventions. So, if there are three treatments, then a block will consist of three animals that are as similar as possible for the measure of interest. The three animals within each block will be assigned at random to the three treatments. Alternatively, a block could consist of six animals with two assigned to each treatment, at random.
- *To enable the experiment to be carried out over a prolonged period.* For instance, if there are insufficient animals of the required specification to study all the blocks at the same time, then the experiment can be started with the first batch of animals as block 1, then other blocks can be added as the animals become available. As usual, the overall sample size for the experiment should be planned in advance.
- *To ensure that the results are repeatable over time.* This is common with *in vitro* studies, which are often repeated many times on different days. The researcher often considers these to be separate 'experiments' but, if they are pre-planned, then each 'experiment' qualifies as a block. This means that data from a series of experiments, split over a number of time-periods, can be combined and analysed as a randomised block design.

Note that the animals assigned to a block should be as similar as possible, but there can be multiple differences between blocks. Thus, block 1 might consist of uniformly heavy animals on the top shelf treated in week 1, with block 2 consisting of light animals on a lower shelf treated in week 2 and so on.

The Latin square design

If there are two or more sources of variability in the experiment, then a design can be constructed involving multiple blocking factors. When two blocking factors are required, a simple, if slightly constraining, way to do this is to base the experiment on a Latin square (see Figure 3.5). A Latin square is a matrix in which the rows of the square correspond to the levels of the first blocking factor and the columns correspond to the levels of the second blocking factor. The different levels of the intervention are arranged so that each one occurs only once in each row and once in each column of the square.

When using this design, the number of interventions must be the same as the number of rows and columns. For example, in testing the response to three different doses of a drug treatment (A, B and C), the rows might represent the shelf in a rack of cages and the columns represent their position from left to right. In Figure 3.5, every row and every column has

Block	Animal			
	1	2	3	4
I	B	C	A	D
II	D	A	B	C
III	A	B	D	C
IV	A	C	B	D
V	D	C	B	A

Figure 3.4 The plan for a randomised block design with four treatments (A, B, C and D) and sixteen animals, housed over four shelves/blocks. Note that the animals within each shelf/block are assigned at random to the four treatments.

A	B	C
C	A	B
B	C	A

Figure 3.5 A 3 × 3 Latin square design. There are three interventions A, B and C, three rows and three columns. Every row and column has only one of each of the interventions.

all three of the interventions A, B and C. By using this design, it is possible to account for the differences between both rows and columns and so the effects of the interventions can be assessed more accurately. Randomisation is achieved by first randomising the row order and then the column order.

When using a 3 × 3 Latin square, there will be only limited information to estimate the variability (if both blocking factors are included in the statistical model). However, this can be improved by replication of the Latin square.

The cross-over design

In many experiments, the largest source of variability is the animal. If each animal receives only one intervention, then this will be the variability that the intervention effects are assessed against. However, in certain situations it is possible to administer multiple interventions to each animal and hence block by animal. Consider a design in which each animal receives a series of different treatments over time, with one treatment per time-period. Such designs are defined as 'cross-over' designs and effectively involve blocking by both animal and treatment time-period. These designs are particularly powerful because they automatically control for much of the genetic and environmental variation. Such designs reduce considerably the number of animals needed to study the response to the treatment of interest but, unfortunately, cannot be used for experiments in which the intervention alters the animal permanently. Caution is also needed when using this design to study the response to test drugs: the researcher must ensure that each dose has been eliminated (undergone 'washout') before applying the next experimental intervention.

In cross-over designs, the experimental units are the combinations of animals and time-periods. For example, if the aim is to compare the effects of four anaesthetics on blood pressure in dogs, then all the anaesthetics might be administered to each dog sequentially with blood pressure being monitored each time. It is assumed that none of the treatments affect the dogs permanently and there is an adequate washout period between successive treatments. If necessary, this assumption can be tested in the statistical analysis (by comparing baseline measures between the different treatments, or at the end of the experiment). Although only 4 dogs were used in the trial, the total number of experimental units is 16 (4 dogs × 4 time-periods), but the sample size per group is $N=4$.

Cross-over experiments will usually involve several animals, determined by a power analysis (see the preceding text), with each receiving two or more interventions in a planned order. The sequence for administering the different interventions is usually defined using a Latin square, where columns of the square correspond to the animals, rows to the time-periods with animals being randomly assigned to the intervention sequences and each of the interventions being assigned randomly to the elements of the square.

Cross-over designs can be extremely powerful because the variation within an animal is usually much less than the variation between animals. However, a drawback of the cross-over design is that the animals will experience multiple procedures during the experiment and so the justification for the cumulative harm *versus* the reduction in the number of animals used in the study must be considered carefully in the harm-benefit analysis.

The factorial design

A design is defined as 'factorial' if there are two or more 'factors of interest' and some, or all, combinations of the levels of these factors are included in the design. The design is described as a 'full' factorial if all combinations are included. With such designs, it is possible to assess whether the effect of each factor influences ('interacts') with the others. For example, if interactions between two drugs are being studied, then one factor could be Drug A (at several dose levels) and another factor being Drug B (at several levels) and a two-factor full factorial design could be used to assess their effects. Statistical analysis of the results will indicate whether or not the actions of one drug affect the actions of the other, which is evidently important for predicting harmful or synergistic drug interactions in humans.

The factorial approach described in Box 3.3 has the added advantage that it is possible to assess, within a single

---

Box 3.3

Consider a drug trial with two factors of interest: Treatment (levels: control and test compound) and Mouse Strain (levels: C57BL/6 and BALB/c). A full factorial design based on these two factors would involve testing all the four combinations of the Treatment and Strain factors. If six mice are allocated to each combination, then 24 mice are needed in total.

It may also be desirable to know whether the response is the same in males and females. To do this, the experiment could be performed first in males and then repeated in females. This is known as the 'one factor at a time' approach and would involve using two batches of 24 mice in two separate experiments. Unfortunately, because the factor, Sex, would not be randomised across the two experiments, the response in males and females could not be compared directly and so there is no valid way of testing whether males and females responded in the same way.

A better approach would be to use a three-factor full factorial design. If three male and three female mice receive the test chemical and three male and three female mice receive the vehicle control (see Table 3.1), this would still give a total of six mice for each test factor (Treatment, Strain and Sex). This strategy would use only 24 mice to test the drug effects on the two sexes, rather than the 48 mice, which would be needed for two separate studies. This means that it is possible to study drug effects in both sexes, without any need to increase the total number of animals needed to answer the question of interest.

experiment, whether the treatment effect interacts with the sex of the animal: i.e. whether or not the treatment affects both sexes of mice in the same way. This is particularly important in light of the growing interest in sex differences in the response to experimental challenges. Moreover, more widespread adoption of factorial designs would help to alleviate the problem that female animals are often culled without being used for any research purpose.

If a significant interaction supports a conclusion that males and females respond to the treatment in different ways, there would be little point in considering the overall response to the treatment. In such cases, the treatment effect must be assessed separately for each sex. However, the noise estimate (in the signal-to-noise ratio) can still be estimated using all animals, and hence the statistical results will be more reliable as a result.

Factorial designs are often used in confirmatory experiments, where perhaps two or three factors of interest are assessed. It is usual practice to assess the difference between the means of pairs of factor levels using post-hoc tests, with suitable multiple comparison adjustment such as Bonferroni. This implies that an adequate sample size, for each combination of the levels of the factors, is required to achieve sufficient statistical power. Such designs are defined as 'small factorial designs' (Bate & Clark 2014) as they usually involve only two or three factors of interest. As the number of factors rises, so does the number of combinations of the factor levels and hence (with a suitable sample size at each combination of the levels of the factors) the total number of animals required can be impractically large.

While commonly used in confirmatory experiments, what is less well-known is that factorial designs can also be applied in exploratory studies. These designs, defined as 'large factorial designs' (Bate & Clark 2014), can have any number of factors, perhaps up to 10, and any number of levels of each factor (although it is often sensible to limit the number of levels of each factor to 2). The purpose of these studies is to screen the overall effect of the factors (and perhaps their interactions) rather than compare the mean of one combination of levels of the factors with another. Hence, the sample size per combination can be as low as $N=1$ or 2. These designs are employed in many fields of research, mainly using continuous rather than categorical factors. This strategy is known as Design of Experiments (or DoE).

Although large factorial designs are not suitable for confirmatory experiments, they have the advantage that they can be used to explore the relationships between many factors without using excessive numbers of experimental units and so the reduction in the number of animals needed for the study can be considerable. In practice, the analysis can be simplified by assuming that high-level interactions between the factors are negligible (i.e. interactions between three or more factors). This makes it possible to use as few as one or two animals per group in the large factorial designs and so this approach could play a useful role in optimising a screening programme for drug development (Shaw et al. 2002). More details are given by Montgomery (1997).

Another advantage of all factorial designs, whether large or small, is that they benefit from 'hidden replication'. In Table 3.1, there are only three mice for each of the eight combinations of treatments (i.e. a total of 24 mice). Assuming that

Table 3.1 Layout of a two (treatments) × two (sexes) × two (strains) factorial design. Although there are 12 mice in each 'intervention' group, only 3 are needed for each of combination of factors. For discussion, see text.

Strain	Treated		Control	
	Male	Female	Male	Female
C57BL/6	3	3	3	3
BALB/c	3	3	3	3

there is no interaction between any of the factors (Treatment, Sex and Strain), then for an overall comparison between the treated *versus* control mice there are actually 12 animals in both the treatment and control groups. This will also be the case when comparing the overall difference between males and females or between the two strains of mice. In short, the concept of group size needs to be modified when using factorial designs. Statisticians sometimes call this 'hidden replication', and it accounts for their higher efficiency. Note also that the noise in the signal-to-noise ratio can be estimated using all 24 animals, not just the 3 animals within each experimental group, and so the statistical analysis provides a potentially reliable estimate of the overall variability.

By contrast, should a researcher want to go on to carry out a pairwise comparison of the *mean* of one combination of the levels of the factors with another, a power analysis might decide that this would need as many as eight animals per combination.

In summary, a factorial design provides far more information than a single factor design, at no extra cost in terms of animals and scientific resources. The value of factorial designs has been recognised by statisticians for many years. According to R.A. Fisher:

> If the investigator ... confines his attention to any single factor we may infer either that he is the unfortunate victim of a doctrinaire theory as to how experimentation should proceed, or that the time, material or equipment at his disposal is too limited to allow him to give attention to more than one aspect of his problem. ... Indeed, in a wide class of cases (by using factorial designs), an experimental investigation, at the same time as it is made more comprehensive, may also be made more efficient if by more efficient we mean that more knowledge and a higher degree of precision are obtainable by the same number of observations. (Fisher 1960)

The repeated measures design

In many studies, the experimental units are measured sequentially over a period of time, as in monitoring the response to a drug treatment several times over several days. These samples will not be independent because, for example, if the animal (experimental unit) has a high count on day 1, it is also likely to have a high count on day 2. The samples are also not taken in a random order (day 1 must come before day 2!) and this structured sampling plan is the same for all the animals. Every animal has a 'day 1' result and a 'day 2' result and any systematic trends over time, across all animals, can be assessed.

In general, a repeated measures design consists of:

- A *core design*. This can be any experimental design and should incorporate randomisation, as described in the preceding text. The core design does not vary across repeated measurements.
- A *repeated factor*. Repeated measurements of the core design are taken in a fixed (non-random) order and the levels of these repeated measurements are indexed by the repeated factor.

One way of dealing with the non-random sampling is to use summaries of the repeated measurements: for example, the mean of the within-animal measurements, or the time to reach a certain value, or the area under the curve. An alternative approach, which enables a more detailed assessment of the response, at a given time point, is to use a repeated measures statistical analysis.

Consider an experiment to test the effect of a high fat diet on the body weight of a genetically-altered mouse, when compared to wildtype littermates. Male and female animals are assigned to either a high fat or normal diet and then measured repeatedly over several days. The core design is a 'factorial' design (see the preceding text), with two factors Sex and Diet (all four combinations of sex and diet are included in the experimental design). Day is a repeated factor as the levels of this factor index the days where the animals' body weight was recorded. The design is therefore an example of a repeated measures design. Because the levels of the repeated factor are not randomised, the results across this series of repeated measurements will be related, and this needs to be taken into account in the statistical analysis.

Bate and Clark (2014) describe seven types of design that involve taking multiple measurements of each animal, of which the repeated measures design is only one example. Other designs, such as cross-over and nested designs, discussed in the preceding text, involve taking multiple measurements of the animals but are not considered repeated measures designs. With cross-over designs, each animal receives a different treatment during each time-period. Hence, although animals are measured multiple times during the experiment, the design changes over time because a different treatment is administered to each animal in each time-period. Note that if, within each time-period, the animals are measured repeatedly in a non-random order (for example, at specific times within each time-period), then this would be defined as a 'repeated measures cross-over design'.

A special case of the repeated measures design is a 'before and after' experiment where an animal is used as its own control (and the repeated factor is equivalent to the treatment factor). Thus, the outcome of interest is first measured in the untreated animal (as a baseline measurement), then a treatment is applied, and the same outcome is again measured to assess the effect of the treatment. Data generated can be analysed using either a paired t-test or a within-subject mixed model. While this is a useful design in many cases, it suffers from the technical disadvantage that there is no randomisation. It is not possible to have an 'after' before the 'before' and hence any apparent treatment effects may be biased by time-related effects. The results therefore must be interpreted with caution.

Types of statistical analysis

Only a general description of some of the most useful statistical analysis techniques is given here. Detailed accounts, with worked numerical examples, are given in many textbooks (Bate & Clark 2014; Festing *et al*. 2002). All calculations described here can be performed using statistical packages such as InVivoStat[4] (Clark *et al*. 2012; Bate *et al*. 2017) or commercial software such as SPSS or MINITAB. The 'R' statistical software or 'language'[5] is widely used by professional statisticians and is free of charge, but it is command-driven, so initially may be difficult to learn.

The majority of experiments generate quantitative continuous numeric data, rather than discrete (e.g. binary) data. These experiments can usually be analysed using parametric tests, which involve assessing the model parameters (i.e. the mean and standard deviation); examples include the Student's t-test, ANOVA or ANCOVA. It follows that the valid use of these tests rests on making certain parametric assumptions, such as normality of the residuals (see the following text). However, in cases where the parametric assumptions do not hold, so-called 'non-parametric' methods may have to be used. As a first step in justifying this decision, it is important to examine the data graphically to gain a better understanding of the type and distribution of the observations.

The next step in any analysis is to screen the data for possible outliers. This is usually best done graphically. Although there are statistical tests that can be used to identify outliers, their use is not straightforward and can be misleading. Whichever technique is applied, the criteria for exclusion should be determined before starting the data analysis and the person performing the assessment should be blinded to treatment allocation when doing so. When potential outliers are detected, the records should be traced back to ensure that they are not explained by a potential problem with the experimental procedure (e.g. unexpected noise in the laboratory) or recording of the data. If the 'outlier' cannot be explained by any such practical issues, then it is best to perform the statistical analysis with and without this response in the dataset to assess its impact. If the exclusion of the 'outlier' does not affect the conclusions, then this provides reassurance of its relative importance and there is no need to consider any remedy. If excluding the outlier does have an impact, then the researcher should consider repeating the experiment to increase confidence in their conclusions. Whatever the case, the exclusion of outliers is not encouraged and should be reported, explicitly.

ANOVA and the t-test

The aims of ANOVA and the t-test are to compare the means of two groups (in the case of the t-test) or more than two groups (in the case of the ANOVA). Where there are three or more groups, the overall test in the ANOVA table does not indicate which specific groups differ from each other: the analysis merely indicates that it is unlikely that the group means are all the same. Further tests such as post-hoc

---

[5]http://www.r-project.org/ (accessed 1 July 2019)

comparisons or planned comparisons, described in most textbooks, are needed to determine which pairs of individual means differ from each other.

Randomised block designs are analysed using multi-way ANOVA with interactions between factors of interest (but not interactions between the factors of interest and the blocking factors), included in the analysis. Thus, ANOVA can deal with complex experimental designs. An excellent introduction to ANOVA is given by Roberts and Russo (1999).

ANOVA and the t-test, as implemented in most software packages, depend on three parametric assumptions:

1. The *residuals* (i.e. the deviation of each observation from its predicted mean) *are normally distributed*. Note that it is the residuals, not the observed responses themselves, that should follow a normal distribution.
2. The *variance is the same for all groups* (i.e. the data satisfy the assumption regarding homogeneity of sample variance).
3. The *observations are independent*. This depends on correct identification of the experimental unit and appropriate randomisation (see the preceding section on repeated measures and cross-over designs).

The first two of these assumptions can be examined using graphical plots of the residuals: a facility that is available in many statistics packages, such as InVivoStat[4]. For example, a normal probability plot of the residuals can be used to investigate assumption 1, and a plot of the residuals *versus* the predicted fits can be used to investigate assumption 2. However, the ANOVA is quite 'robust', even if there are deviations from these assumptions, especially assumption 1; only if they are seriously violated does the ANOVA give misleading answers. Unfortunately, it is not easy to give firm guidance on exactly when parametric methods should be abandoned in favour of non-parametric alternatives, and a statistician should be consulted if you are unsure. It is certainly important that the use of parametric *versus* non-parametric tests, or even the choice of parametric test is not based on finding an approach that supports the desired conclusion (P-hacking)!

When the assumptions are violated, for example, when there is a clear fanning effect observed on the residuals *versus* predicted plot (Bate & Clark 2014) then a transformation of the data to a different scale (e.g. $\log_{10}$ or square root), followed by a parametric analysis, should be attempted rather than using non-parametric methods. This is because when the assumptions hold, the parametric tests are more powerful than the non-parametric equivalents. For example, biological data often have a log-normal distribution (i.e. the distribution of the responses is skewed). Transforming the raw data for the observations into logarithms will usually result in the residuals from the analysis being normally distributed and hence the distribution of points on the predicted *versus* residuals plot looks like a random scatter (i.e. the fanning effect has been removed). In these cases, all the analyses should be carried out on the log-transformed data. The results can be presented either on the log scale, or back-transformed onto the original scale. Similar principles apply for responses that are expressed as ratios, which typically need a logit or arcsine transformation.

InVivoStat[4] has a module, the Single Measures Parametric Analysis module, which performs t-tests and ANOVA, produces diagnostic plots on the residuals and generates post-hoc tests on the group means. The module also enables the user to transform their data in several different ways (e.g. log, square root, arcsine) and, when data are log-transformed, it provides predictions on both the log-transformed scale and the back-transformed original scale.

Analysis of covariance

ANCOVA is similar to ANOVA in that it can be used when there are one or more factors in the experiment. ANCOVA is so-called because the statistical model includes covariates, which are continuous variables that could account for nuisance sources of variability. As with ANOVA, predicted group means from an ANCOVA analysis can be compared using planned comparisons.

In addition to the parametric assumptions described in the preceding text, ANCOVA relies on three additional assumptions:

- *The response variable and the covariate are related.* If the covariate does not account for variability in the response, then there is no benefit in including it in the statistical model.
- *The relationship between the response and the covariate should be the same for all interventions*, i.e. there is no 'intervention' by covariate interaction.
- *The covariate should not be influenced by the intervention.* For example, it can be assumed that baseline measurements of the response are not influenced by the intervention.

Covariates can be applied in many scenarios. For example, in a study of the effects of different diets on body weight, ANCOVA can be used to account for some of the variation in the body weight of the animals before the treatment is administered (Bate & Clark 2014). Covariate baselines can also enable a more reliable assessment of the response to the test treatment than can be achieved by the analysis of normalised data, such as the percentage change from baseline (Karp et al. 2012), which can distort the apparent magnitude of the response.

The chi-squared and Fisher's exact tests for discrete data (counts)

Discrete (often binary) data can be summarised as the proportion of animals in a group that has a particular attribute (e.g. the percentage of animals with a tumour). Such data can usually be analysed using a chi-squared test. Note that all calculations are performed using the actual number in each group rather than the percentages. The analysis assesses whether there is a difference in the proportions in the two (or more) groups. The main limitation of this test is that the expected numbers in all cells of the table should exceed five. If this is not the case, then it is necessary to use the more conservative (i.e. less powerful) Fisher's exact test. InVivoStat[4] has a module that performs both the chi-squared and Fisher's exact tests.

The non-parametric tests

Unlike parametric tests (see the preceding text), non-parametric tests tend to avoid investigating model parameters and focus instead on assessing the nature of the distribution. They do not depend on any assumptions about the distribution of the data and hence are used when the data are not normally distributed (to the extent that no transformation can be applied that would make it valid to use parametric analysis). As with parametric tests, non-parametric tests depend on the assumption that the measurements are all independent. However, non-parametric methods tend to lack statistical power, especially when compared to the equivalent parametric tests (when the parametric assumptions are satisfied) and so should not be used routinely.

The most commonly used tests include:

- The *Mann-Whitney* (or *Wilcoxon two sample rank sum*) test; the non-parametric equivalent of the t-test.
- The *Kruskal-Wallis* test; the non-parametric equivalent of one-way ANOVA.
- The *Friedman's* test; the non-parametric equivalent of two-way ANOVA without interaction, which can be used wheBln analysing randomised block designs.

Summary

Most textbooks include sections on these methods, and they are available in all good statistical software packages. For example, InVivoStat[4] has a dedicated non-parametric module that can perform these tests.

In these sections, we have explained how the statistical analysis should reflect the experimental design that was used in the study, which should be chosen to maximise the power of the analysis to be performed. This strategy will help to ensure that the impact of any sources of variability, which were identified when constructing the design, can be taken into account in the statistical analysis. The statistical test selected should be the most powerful available to the researcher. This will give more reliable/reproducible results, while allowing the researcher to reduce animal use. The analysis should also make use of all available information: for example, background information on the animals, to reduce the apparent between-animal variability and hence increase the sensitivity and reliability of the statistical tests.

Concluding remarks

In this chapter, we have highlighted seven criteria a researcher should aim to satisfy:

1. *Experiments should be simple to perform* so that the risk of making a mistake is minimised.
2. *Experiments should always be pre-planned*: additional treatment groups (or experimental units) should not be added later because randomisation will be compromised.
3. *The method of statistical analysis should be considered at the design stage* – not left until after the experiment is finished. Most importantly, there should be <u>independent</u> replication of the observations. This requires correct identification of the experimental unit, which may, for example, be all the animals in a single cage.
4. *The researcher should always aim to use block designs* to remove nuisance sources of variability.
5. *A factorial design should be used* if it is important to know whether the results depend on the strain, sex, diet or other factors, as is often the case. This approach will provide extra information at no additional cost (to the animals or researcher). Using such designs, it is possible to include both sexes and/or more than one inbred strain, in addition to a treatment, without increasing the total number of animals used in the study. However, when using these designs, it is essential to use the correct statistical analysis, otherwise all the advantages are lost.
6. *Experiments should have adequate power* to ensure that there will be a high probability of detecting a scientifically or clinically relevant intervention effect, when that is the true effect. This can be achieved by controlling the variation. For example, the animals could be the same age, weight, sex, health status and/or be housed in a controlled environment with similar prior experience or, if these effects are not controlled, they can be accounted for using covariates in the statistical analysis. Where there is detectable heterogeneity, or where there is some natural structure to the experimental material (e.g. the arrangements for housing the animals), then a randomised block design may be appropriate. Similarly, a cross-over design is often a powerful alternative because the variability of the responses for each animal is usually less than the variability between different animals. Once the variability has been assessed and controlled as much as possible, sample sizes can be determined (and minimised) using a power analysis.
7. *The experimental procedures should be unbiased*, with all treatment groups having the same environment (unless a study of the effect of 'environment' is an aim of the experiment). This is achieved by ensuring that the animals (or other experimental units) are randomised, both in respect of the allocation to a treatment and any subsequent steps throughout the experiment. The researcher should also perform the experiment blind, with respect to the assignment of treatments, the experimental measurement groups and the data analysis, so that no subjective bias is inadvertently introduced, favouring one particular group.

Acknowledgements

We would like to thank Michael Festing, the author of the first version of this chapter, upon which this updated version is based.

References

Bains, R.S., Wells, S., Sillito, R.R. *et al.* (2018) Assessing mouse behaviour throughout the light/dark cycle using automated in-cage analysis tools. *Journal of Neuroscience Methods*, **300**, 37–47.

Bate, S.T. and Clark, R.A. (2014) *The Design and Statistical Analysis of Animal Experiments*. Cambridge University Press, Cambridge.

Bate, S.T., Clark, R.A. and Stanford, S.C. (2017) Using InVivoStat to perform the statistical analysis of experiments. *Journal of Psychopharmacology*, **31**(6), 644–652.

Bebarta, V., Luyten, D. and Heard, K. (2003) Emergency medicine animal research: does use of randomization and blinding affect the results? *Academic Emergency Medicine*, **10**, 684–687.

Chvedoff, M., Clarke, M.R., Faccini, J.M. et al. (1980) Effects on mice of numbers of animal per cage: an 18-month study (preliminary results). *Archives of Toxicology*, Supplement 4, 435–438.

Clark, R.A., Shoaib, M., Hewitt, K.N. et al. (2012) A comparison of InVivoStat with other statistical software packages for analysis of data generated from animal experiments. *Journal of Psychopharmacology*, **26**(8), 1136–1142.

Das, R.G. and North, D. (2007) Implications of experimental technique for analysis and interpretation of data from animal experiments: outliers and increased variability resulting from failure of intraperitoneal injection procedures. *Laboratory Animals*, **41**, 312–320.

Percie du Sert, N., Ahluwalia, A., Alam, S. et al. (2020) Reporting animal research: explanation and elaboration for the ARRIVE guidelines 2.0. *PLoS Biology*, **18**(7), p.e3000411.

Festing, M.F.W. (2000) Reduction, model development and efficient experimental design. In: *Progress in the Reduction, Refinement and Replacement of Animal Experimentation*. Ed. Balls, M., pp. 721–727. Amsterdam, Elsevier Sciences BV.

Festing, M.F.W. (1999). Warning: the use of genetically heterogeneous mice may seriously damage your research. *Neurobiology of Aging*, 20, 237–244.

Festing, M.F.W., Overend, P., Gaines Das, R. et al. (2002) *The Design of Animal Experiments*. Laboratory Animals Ltd., London.

Fisher, R.A. (1960) *The Design of Experiments*. Hafner Publishing Company, Inc., New York.

Garner, J.P., Gaskill, B.N., Weber EM. et al. (2017) Introducing Therioepistemology: the study of how knowledge is gained from animal research. *Laboratory Animals*, **46**(4), 103–113.

Gore, K.H. and Stanley, P.J. (2005) An illustration that statistical design mitigates environmental variation and ensures unambiguous study conclusions. *Animal Welfare*, **14**(4), 361–365.

Hair, K., Macleod, M.R., Sena E.S. et al. (2019) A randomised controlled trial of an Intervention to Improve Compliance with the ARRIVE guidelines (IICARus). *Research Integrity and Peer Review*, Jun 12; **4**, 12. doi: 10.1186/s41073-019-0069-3: eCollection 2019.

Hsieh, L.S., Wen, J.H., Miyares, L. et al. (2017) Outbred CD1 mice are as suitable as inbred C57BL/6J mice in performing social tasks. *Neuroscience Letters*, 637, 142–147.

Jaramillo, T.C., Escamilla, C.O., Liu, S. et al. (2018). Genetic background effects in Neuroligin-3 mutant mice: Minimal behavioral abnormalities on C57 background. *Autism Research*, **11**, 234–244.

Jeffery, N.D., Bate, S.T., Safayi, S. et al. (2018) When neuroscience met clinical pathology: partitioning experimental variation to aid data interpretation in neuroscience. *European Journal of Neuroscience*, **47**(5), 371–379.

Karp, N.A. and Fry, D. (2021) What is the optimum design for my animal experiment? *BMJ Open Science*, **5**(1): e100126. doi: 10.1136/bmjos-2020-100126

Karp, N.A., Segonds-Pichon, A., Gerdin, A.K.B. et al. (2012) The fallacy of ratio correction to address confounding factors. *Laboratory Animals*, **46**(3), 245–252.

Kilkenny, C., Browne, W.J., Cuthill, I.C. et al. (2010) Improving bioscience research reporting: the ARRIVE guidelines for reporting animal research. *PLoS Biology*, **8**(6), e1000412.

Leung, V., Rousseau-Blass, F., Beauchamp, G. et al. (2018) ARRIVE has not ARRIVEd: Support for the ARRIVE (Animal Research: Reporting of in vivo Experiments) guidelines does not improve the reporting quality of papers in animal welfare, analgesia or anesthesia. *PLoS ONE*, **13**, e0197882.

Macleod, M.R., Fisher, M., O'collins, V. et al. (2009) Reprint: Good laboratory practice: preventing introduction of bias at the bench. *Journal of Cerebral Blood Flow & Metabolism*, **29**(2), 221–223.

Martin, M.D., Danahy, D.B., Hartwig, S.M. et al. (2017) Revealing the complexity in CD8 T cell responses to infection in inbred C57B/6 versus outbred Swiss mice. *Front Immunology*, 2017 Nov 22; **8**, 1527. doi: 10.3389/fimmu.2017.01527: eCollection 2017.

Mead, R. (1988) *The Design of Experiments*. Cambridge University Press, Cambridge.

Montgomery, D.C. (1997) *Design and Analysis of Experiments*. Wiley, New York.

Munafo, M., Nosek, B., Bishop, D.V.M. et al. (2017) A manifesto for reproducible science. *Nature Human Behaviour*, **1**, Article number: 0021.

Pasquarelli, N., Voehringer, P., Henke, J. et al. (2017) Effect of a change in housing conditions on body weight, behavior and brain neurotransmitters in male C57BL/6J mice. *Behavioral Brain Research*, **333**, 35–42.

Percie du Sert, N., Hurst, V., Ahluwalia, A. et al. (2020) The ARRIVE guidelines 2.0: Updated guidelines for reporting animal research. *PLoS Biology*, **18**(7): e3000410. https://doi.org/10.1371/journal.pbio.3000410

Percie du Sert, N., Bamsey, I., Bate, S.T. et al. (2017) The experimental design assistant. *PLoS Biology*, **15**(9), e2003779.

Porter, A.J., Pillidge, K., Tsai, Y.C. et al. (2015) A lack of functional NK1 receptors explains most, but not all, abnormal behaviours of NK1R-/- mice. *Genes Brain and Behavior*, **14**, 89–99.

Redfern, W.S., Tse, K., Grant, C. et al. (2017) Automated recording of home cage activity and temperature of individual rats housed in social groups: The Rodent Big Brother project. *PLoS One* **12**(9), e0181068.

Roberts, M.J. and Russo, R. (1999). *A Student's Guide to the Analysis of Variance*. Routledge, London.

Russell, W.M.S. and Burch, R.L. (1959) *The Principles of Humane Experimental Technique*. Potters Bar, Universities Federation for Animal Welfare.

Sams-Dodd, F. (2006) Strategies to optimize the validity of disease models in the drug discovery process. *Drug Discovery Today*, **11**, 355–363.

Shaw, R., Festing, M.F.W., Peers, I. et al. (2002) The use of factorial designs to optimise animal experiments and reduce animal use. *ILAR Journal*, **43**, 223–232.

Sherwin, E., Dinan, T.G. and Cryan, J.F. (2018) Recent developments in understanding the role of the gut microbiota in brain health and disease. *Annals of the N Y Academy of Science*, **1420**, 5–25.

Smith, A.J., Clutton, R.E. and Lilley, E. (2018) PREPARE: guidelines for planning animal research and testing. *Laboratory Animals*, **52**(2), 135–141.

Stanford, C., Fillenz, M. and Ryan, E. (1984). The effect of repeated mild stress on cerebral cortical adrenoceptors and noradrenaline synthesis in the rat. *Neuroscience Letters*, **45**(2), 163–167.

Tuttle, A.H., Philip, V.M., Chesler, E.J. et al. (2018). Comparing phenotypic variation between inbred and outbred mice. *Nature Methods*, **15**, 994–996.

Voelkl, B. and Würbel, H. (2021). A reaction norm perspective on reproducibility. *Theory in Biosciences*, **140**, 169–176.

Willner, P. (1984). The validity of animal models of depression. *Psychopharmacology*, **83**(1), 1–16.

4 An introduction to laboratory animal genetics

Michelle Stewart and Sara Wells

Introduction

The aim of this chapter is to introduce genetics to everyone using laboratory animals, both wild types and genetically altered (GA) strains. Even if gene studies are not the primary focus of a research project, the genome of the organism being used will be an influential context for most experiments. Most of the examples cited involve mice as they have been the most widely used and accessible model of mammalian genetic research over the last decade. However, the principles of inheritance are universal, with many genes being conserved during the evolution of different species. The principles of the technologies applied to mice are also similar in other organisms although important species differences do exist.

Since the initial publication of the human genome in 2001, biomedical science has been full of expectations. It was thought there would be an influx of ground-breaking discoveries into the function of human genes and their roles in disease. Furthermore, since the sequence was now available it was assumed that manipulating model organisms to recapitulate human genetic changes and disease would become more straightforward. The initial excitement has been followed by many years of technical developments which only now, nearly two decades later, place scientists in a position to be able to change genes in almost any organism. Being able to perform such genetic changes does not mean that ethically we always should. Indeed, concomitant with an increase in efficiency in targeting genes *in vivo* has been huge progress in achieving gene manipulations *in vitro*, including in-patient-derived cells as well as cell lines, providing an ever-increasing potential for replacement for whole animal experiments. It is also important to note at the very start of this chapter that much of the genome remains unexplored, with most research focusing on approximately 10% of human genes (Stoeger *et al.* 2018), and therefore the result of many of the genetic changes may be unpredictable. Ensuring that animal observation and care regimes are appropriate and stringent is central to any experimental design when generating novel GA animals.

This chapter will describe the journey from inbred strains of animals to genome editing, the importance of knowing and recording the genomic context of your experiments, and the benefits and limitations of the technologies which have been used to manipulate *in vivo* genomes.

Molecular genetics

DNA – the molecule of inheritance

There have been references to a 'heredity factor', something that passes from one generation to another, instilling a likeness between parents and offspring, since at least the times of Hippocrates and Aristotle. The work of Gregor Mendel (although largely overlooked for many decades) established that there were units of inheritance, later named *genes*, which were conferred in the germ cell (ova and sperm) from parents to offspring. However, it took until the 1940s and experiments from the biochemist Oswald Avery to prove that the genetic information being transferred was indeed the macro-molecule Deoxyribonucleic acid – DNA. Moreover, it took almost another decade for the molecular structure of DNA, to be elucidated by the much publicised work of Crick and Watson using data provided by Chargaff, Franklin and Wilkins (reviewed in Portin 2014).

Protein-coding DNA

A molecule conferring genetic information from one generation to another must have some key characteristics. The most important of which is that it must be able to tell cells how to put together the complex protein molecules, which are seminally responsible for directing almost all the body's physiological functions such as building cellular structures, catalysing chemical processes and even regulating genes themselves. Proteins contain many (usually hundreds of) subunits called *amino acids*, which come in 20 different forms. These are assembled in different numbers and combinations to make up the vast array of proteins needed for biological life.

DNA itself is composed of smaller subunits called *nucleotides*, which contain four different chemical bases: adenine (A), guanine (G), cytosine (C) and thymine (T). These collectively are arranged in different combinations to form a genetic code. However, as there are only four bases, any single nucleotide alone could not encode for 20 amino acids; indeed, any combination of 2 of them (for example, AA, AG, GC, TA) would only allow for 16 unique codes. In order to spell out a code for all 20 amino acids, groups of 3 nucleotides are needed. These triplets are called *codons*, and each of the 64 possible combinations instructs the cell to insert a particular amino acid into newly forming proteins or indeed to start or stop the process of protein synthesis (Figure 4.1). It is specific sequences of these nucleotides, coding for specific proteins, which form the heritable unit of a gene, with the entire genetic material of a cell being referred to as a *genome*.

The estimates in early 2019 of how many genes are in the human genome vary from 22,000 to 25,000. The precise number is subject to change as genomic sequences from different human populations are explored, more functional interrogation of potential genes occurs and new bioinformatics technologies improve the capacity for predicting the location of genes.

Gene structure

The vast lengths of DNA sequences contained within the chromosomes are not simply arrays of genes but include many sequences called *non-coding DNA*. The majority of genes are split into smaller entities, called *exons*, which are interspersed by non-coding sequences called *introns*. For example, the gene for growth hormone, which is largely responsible for pubescent growth, is split into 5 exons with 4 introns in between.

Chromosomes

Sequences for protein-coding genes are not arranged individually on pieces of DNA within the cell nucleus but rather strung together on extremely long DNA molecules which themselves are organised into a double helix. This structure can be formed because of the creation of base pairs, that is the very organised and specific binding between A and T or G and C bases. Every molecule of DNA has two strands, running in opposite directions to each other (Figure 4.2) and held together by these bonds between complementary base pairs (for A, it is always T and for G, it is always C and vice versa).

The human genome for example has over 3 billion bases, which are divided over 23 different structures called *chromosomes*, each of which has many millions of base pairs of DNA twisted and bound to proteins called *histones*, which protect, regulate and pack the DNA sequences. The DNA in a human cell, if stretched out, would be 2 metres long, and this has to be packed into the nucleus of a cell, which is about a million times smaller. Chromosomes are such large and complex structures that they can be viewed under a light microscope. Interestingly, the number of chromosomes varies widely between species, with the mouse having 20, zebrafish 25 and guinea pigs an amazing 64! This does not mean the guinea pig has three times the number of genes than the mouse, merely that evolutionary changes in the organisation of the DNA molecules have led to them being arranged in smaller groupings.

Genes and alleles

Although each germ cell organism contains a set of chromosomes, this in fact is only half the story, as chromosomes exist in most cells as pairs, one inherited from each parent. The somatic cells (non-germ cells) of humans are described as diploid as there are 46 chromosomes. Twenty-two pairs of which are called *autosomes*, found in both males and females, while the final pair are the sex chromosomes, in humans known as the X and Y chromosomes. Females (XX) are different from males (XY) who have one X chromosome and one male-specific Y chromosome. So, in total, we have inherited 23 chromosomes from our mother and 23 from our father. If you are female, you inherited an X chromosome from your father; if you are male, a Y chromosome. Although the corresponding genes within each chromosome pair code for the same proteins,

		Second letter				
		T	C	A	G	
First letter	T	TTT TTC Phe TTA TTG Leu	TCT TCC TCA TCG Ser	TAT TAC Tyr TAA TAG Stop	TGT TGC Cys TGA Stop TGG Trp	T C A G
	C	CTT CTC CTA CTG Leu	CCT CCC CCA CCG Pro	CAT CAC His CAA CAG Gln	CGT CGC CGA CGG Arg	T C A G
	A	ATT ATC Ile ATA ATG Met	ACT ACC ACA ACG Thr	AAT AAC Asn AAA AAG Lys	AGT AGC Ser AGA AGG Arg	T C A G
	G	GTT GTC GTA GTG Val	GCT GCC GCA GCG Ala	GAT GAC Asp GAA GAG Glu	GGT GGC GGA GGG Gly	T C A G

Third letter

Figure 4.1 All possible combinations of nucleic acid codons and the amino acids they encode for.

42 An introduction to laboratory animal genetics

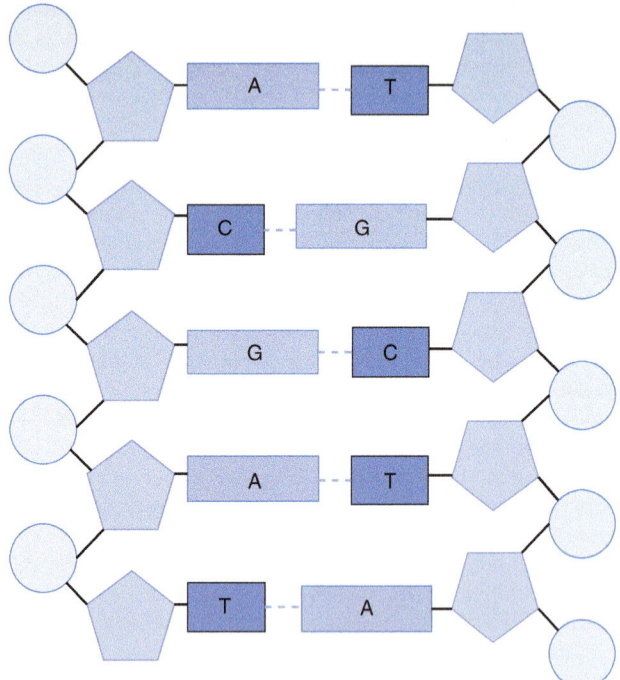

Figure 4.2 A schematic representation of the structure of DNA. The green pentagons represent the deoxyribose sugar, the yellow circles a phosphate backbone and the individual bases with their specific pairings (A=adenine, T= Thymine, C=cytosine and G=guanine).

the version of the gene inherited from each parent may be different. Alleles are variant forms of the same gene, which code for the diversity we see between individuals such as different blood groups or hair colours or enzymatic function.

During a specialised type of cell division called *meiosis*, which results in the formation of germ cells in the testis and in the ovary, chromosome pairs are separated to produce sperm or ova with only one copy of each pair (a state called *haploid*). The joining of these chromosomes at fertilisation recreates the diploid state and forms an organism with a different combination of alleles from either of the parents.

Protein synthesis

During protein synthesis, another nucleic acid, called *messenger RNA* (mRNA), acts as an intermediary molecule, carrying a representation of the sequence of the DNA bases from the nucleus of the cell, out into the cytoplasm, where the proteins are synthesised. Messenger RNA is assembled only when a gene is being 'expressed', a term used when a gene is turned on and actively directing protein synthesis. RNA shares many chemical characteristics with DNA and although it is only a single-stranded molecule which does not form a double helix, it does contain bases. The only difference between the bases of RNA and DNA is that thymine in DNA is substituted for a base called *Uracil* (U) in RNA. The complementary bases of the RNA molecule bind to the DNA sequence and produce an mRNA molecule which faithfully represents the sequence of the gene as dictated by the DNA. For example, the mRNA sequence for a DNA code of AAGTCCT would be UUCAGGA. The process of generating the mRNA molecule is called *transcription* after which the exonic sequences of mRNA that code for the protein itself get spliced together to remove intronic sequences. The spliced mRNA is then transported to the cytoplasm.

In the cytoplasm, cellular machinery, coordinated around a structure also made of protein and RNA called the *ribosome*, directs a third type of RNA – transfer RNA (tRNA) – to bring the correct amino acid to join the protein being assembled. This process is called *translation* with each codon binding to a specific tRNA molecule which is physically attached to the corresponding amino acid. The sequence of this biological process, DNA being transcribed into RNA, RNA then being translated into protein is often called the *central dogma of biology*, a term coined by Francis Crick in 1957 (Figure 4.3). Although Crick used this term initially as 'dogma', he represented an idea for which there was no reasonable evidence.

Regulatory DNA and cell-specificity

In addition to introns, there are other non-coding sequences surrounding the gene. This actually constitutes the majority of the genome (estimated at over 95%), which include intronic sequences within the gene as well intergenic DNA. Interestingly, there are some extraordinary species differences in the amount of non-coding DNA that individual genomes have, including those of the smooth pufferfish (Tetraodontidae) which have the smallest vertebrate genome at eight times smaller than the human genome, largely due to the reduction in non-coding DNA (Neafsey & Palumbi 2003). Some of these stretches of nucleotides function to direct the cell to turn a gene on or off. Such regions of DNA are called *regulatory sequences*; these are often before the start of a specific gene and are called *promoters*. However, sequences regulating an individual gene can be many base pairs away – both before (upstream), after (downstream) or in the intronic sequence of a gene, these are called *enhancers*.

These sequences direct the biological basis of complex organisms; if every protein was made in every cell of the body, all cells would be identical. Clearly, this is not the case in multicellular complex organisms like humans. Cells in our liver make enzymes specific for the function of the liver, whereas

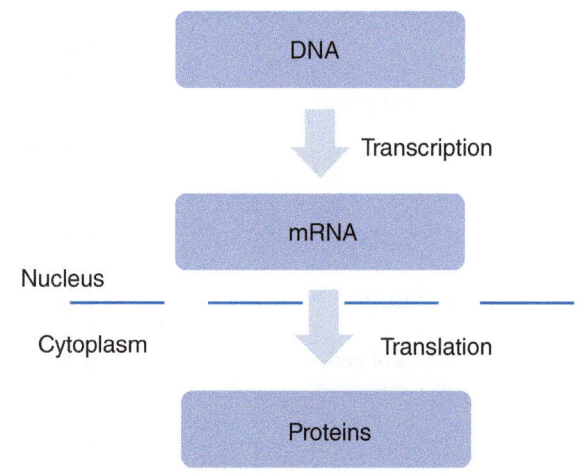

Figure 4.3 The central dogma of molecular genetics.

neurons make the neurotransmitters necessary for signal transmission in the brain. Cell-specificity of protein production is the direct function of the regulatory sequences of the gene. For example, in a liver cell these regulatory sequences bind to particular proteins, only present in specific combinations in those cells and which only enable the gene to be expressed in the liver. In the brain, these proteins would not be there and therefore do not bind to the enhancer and do not turn on the liver-specific genes. The specificity of gene regulation also occurs at different times as well as in different cells. The proteins required for the development of an embryo would need to be active during gestation and may have a different or limited function in the adult. By carefully controlling and orchestrating when and where genes are expressed, regulatory sequences ensure that proteins are only made in places and times where they are needed.

Other non-coding DNA

The complexity of genome structure does not end with genes, introns and regulatory sequences. Indeed nearly 50% of the human genome is made up of repetitive DNA sequences (Richard *et al.* 2008). Chromosomes also include sequences which direct the production of RNA molecules not destined to be exported to the cytoplasm or to make proteins. These molecules have key functions in protein synthesis or can be involved in gene regulation, for example microRNAs are small (20-25 bases) RNA molecules, encoded by genomic DNA, that play an active role in suppressing and modulating gene expression. Other chromosomal regions contain sequences essential for replicating DNA, or are involved in maintaining the structure of the chromosome itself.

Mutations and variation

DNA replicates during cell division in order to produce a faithful copy of the genome for all daughter cells. During this process of assembling billions of bases, errors occur which change the sequence of the nucleotides. These changes are called *mutations* and can occur with no consequence at all, can alter gene sequences and thereby change the protein which is being encoded for or can indeed alter chromosomal number or structures. In such ways, mutations in genes are responsible for the huge variations in appearance, physiological processes and potential disease states that are apparent in all species.

Genetics and the laboratory animal

Gene nomenclature

As many thousands of genes in many hundreds of organisms have now been sequenced, it is imperative that there are rules used to name genes so that researchers across the world are referring to the same genetic locus when they report their studies. The gene nomenclature for each species is controlled by specialist groups of experts including the HUGO gene nomenclature committee[1] for human genes, the International Committee for Standardized Genetic Nomenclature for mice and rats[2] and the Zebrafish Nomenclature Committee[3].

As a general rule, gene symbols are italicised with the allele being represented as a superscript. There are some variations between organisms in terms of gene symbols. For example, humans, non-human primates and most domestic species use a 3- to 6-letter symbol in capitals, mouse and rat genes are written with only the first letter in uppercase and fish genes are displayed entirely in lower case. For example, insulin-like growth factor 1 gene in humans is represented as *IGF1*, in mice as *Igf1* and in zebrafish as *igf1*.

Not only is it important to be specific as to which gene is being referred to, it is also necessary to be consistent and correct with the naming of each allele of each gene; that is the symbol in superscript next to the corresponding gene name. It is conventional for the allele which is present in a normal population to be referred by '+' symbol and be termed *wild type*, whereas alleles which arose as a process of mutation are allocated symbols by the committees for the respective organism, as we will discuss later. Usually for genetically engineered animals (especially, mice), these symbols reflect either the mechanism by which the mutation was introduced or the historical naming of the mutant strain.

Inbred strains

The beginning of any discussion on the use of laboratory animals in genetic research will inevitably focus on the generation of inbred strains, particularly for mice. It is very obvious from the diversity of the human population alone that we all contain many different combinations of many gene alleles. That is as humans we are heterozygotes for many genes and carry two different alleles, with a number of different alleles for each gene being present in any population. With the exception of monozygotic (identical) twins, siblings inherit different combinations of genes from each parent and therefore often exhibit many diverse characteristics (called *phenotypes*). The scale of differences between individuals means that trying to find the specific change in a gene(s) that results in a different phenotype, whether it is hair colour or symptoms of a disease, is very complicated. Hunting for the one or two specific nucleotide changes in the millions that differ between two individuals is still a daunting and sometimes insurmountable task.

Although Lucien Cuénot (a French scientist largely forgotten for this contribution to genetics) had used mice to investigate Mendel's theories of inheritance, it was North American scientists such as William Castle and Clarence C. Little who realised the potential of mice for inheritance studies[4]. Specifically, Little exploited the potential to be able to circumvent the genetic heterogeneity hindering genetic studies

---

[1] https://www.genenames.org/about/guidelines/ (accessed 19 February 2020)

[2] http://www.informatics.jax.org/mgihome/nomen/gene.shtml (accessed 19 February 2020)

[3] https://wiki.zfin.org/display/general/ZFIN+Zebrafish+Nomenclature+Conventions (accessed 19 February 2020)

[4] http://www.informatics.jax.org/morsebook/contents.shtml (accessed 19 February 2020)

by adopting inbreeding mating schemes in an attempt to limit the diversity between individuals of the same strain.

By mating brother and sister mice from the same litter, through many generations (over 20), the ancestry of the *inbred* mouse strains we are so familiar with today such as DBA/2, C57BL/6 and 129 was established. However, this was not a trivial breeding exercise, as in the 1900s and still today, generating new inbred lines requires a significant effort (Bogue *et al.* 2015). This is due to the increasing number of genes that become homozygous, with individuals inheriting identical alleles from both parents, during the inbreeding process. Any deleterious alleles (or combinations of alleles) or those responsible for infertility will cause significant losses and/or breeding issues leading to the abandonment of many lines during the progress to 20 or more generations. The process of inbreeding to create new lines therefore has significant potential welfare and ethical issues and should not be embarked upon unless these are scientifically justified. During the collaborative cross, a recent breeding effort to produce more genetically varied inbred lines, more than 70% of lines were not fecund or healthy enough to reach 20 generations (Shorter *et al.* 2017).

This withstanding, hundreds of inbred strains are described in the Mouse Genome Informatics resource[5]. In these colonies of mice, each individual contains two identical alleles at every gene locus, termed *homozygous*, always inheriting the same allele from both parents. Therefore, a phenotype, resulting from the alteration of a single gene in an inbred strain, can only be caused by that difference in sequence between the mutant and the non-mutant as there are no other genetic differences.

The power of genetic homogeneity in mice and other species has greatly assisted the discovery of many genes and many gene variants over the last century. The most widely used of the many hundreds of inbred strains of mouse is undoubtedly the C57BL/6 strains. The ancestral strain for many other substrains (see the following text) was bred by Clarence C. Little, from the mating of female 57 of a nonagouti (the official name for a black coat colour) strain to male 52. As with all genetically distinct colonies, inbred lines have a very tightly regulated nomenclature which is often overlooked in many scientific publications (Figure 4.4).

Genetic drift

As described in the preceding text, the replication of DNA during gametogenesis introduces a number of errors in the billions of base pairs that are being copied each time a germ cell is produced. This constant tendency for genes to evolve is termed as *genetic drift*. The chance of any individual DNA residue mutating probably varies according to its genomic context, for example, what sequences surround it or whether it is bound to proteins or other factors. Some estimates put the rate of genetic drift between each generation at around one single nucleotide change per 26Mb (megabases). This

---

[5] http://www.informatics.jax.org (accessed 19 February 2020)

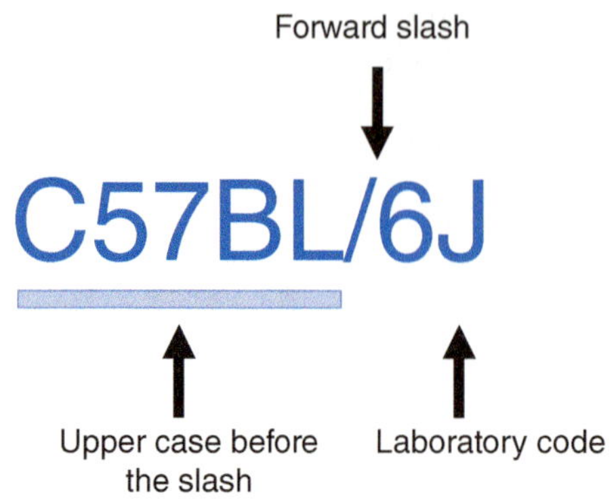

Figure 4.4 The nomenclature of an inbred mouse strain.

equates to the introduction of approximately 100 new single nucleotide polymorphisms (SNPs) every generation (Lynch 2011). Others, using whole genome sequencing, put the rate of single base changes in C57BL/6 mice five-fold lower (Uchimura *et al.* 2015). Of course, many of these changes will not have an impact on the phenotype of the strain being examined; however, over many generations as these changes accumulate so does the risk that they will affect experimental data and/or comparisons with previous research findings. Next-generation sequencing and advanced whole genome analysis – that is, very rapid sequencing of the entire genome of individual mouse strains and the subsequent comparison of these sequences – has provided much molecular information on the specific alleles carried by the most commonly used inbred strains (Doran *et al.* 2016; Lilue *et al.* 2018). In mice, it is therefore possible to examine genome sequence and alleles of individual inbred strains and use this information to select the most appropriate strain for your experiments.

Substrains

Any mouse breeding line which has been continued for more than 10 generations from the original breeding colony is called a *substrain* and must be differentiated from the parental strain by nomenclature. An example of this, which will be pertinent for many mouse genetic projects, is the development of the C57BL/6N substrain from its parental strain C57BL/6J. In 1948, the C57BL/6J strain was established at the Jackson Laboratory, Maine USA. Several years later in 1951, when the colony had reached the 32nd generation of inbreeding, some breeding stock was sent to the National Institutes of Health (NIH), leading to the C57BL/6N line. Therefore, these two strains have been bred separately for upward of 220 generations. An in-depth comparison of both genotypes and phenotypes has revealed many differences including a significant number of SNPs, structural variants (parts of the genome deleted, inserted or rearranged) but most importantly, a number of changes to the phenotypes of the strains (Simon *et al.* 2015). These include behavioural, metabolic and sensory differences such as the observation of the *rd8* mutations in the *Crb1* gene in C57BL/6N which causes white flecking on the retina

(Mattapallil *et al.* 2012) and a deletion which includes the *Nnt* locus in C57BL/6J causing impaired glucose tolerance (Freeman *et al.* 2006).

The differences are very important if you are comparing data between two different inbred lines. For example, as large international consortium efforts such as the International Mouse Phenotyping Consortium[6] (IMPC) use C57BL/6N as the background strain for all gene modifications, data produced from these strains cannot be directly compared to previous data gathered from other background strains without an appreciation of the genomic differences. The 129 strains which are of historical importance in genetic research, especially with respect to gene modification, have a remarkable pedigree. The original 129 strain was bred in 1928 and since then has been exported to many different laboratories and crossed to many different strains including C3H/Hu, 101, WCB6F1 and even strains of unknown origin (Simpson *et al.* 1997; Threadgill *et al.* 1997). This has resulted in a collection of strains with widely varying phenotypic and genotypic differences, so much so that the nomenclature of all 129 substrains was revised to reflect their origins and phenotypes[7].

Maintaining inbred strains

The history of many inbred strains is a reflection of the history of breeding practices (good and bad) over many generations (Beck *et al.* 2000) and includes incidence of stock contamination and poor record-keeping. Today, there are clear standards (Table 4.1) for maintaining inbred strains which are adhered to by breeders and should be reflected also in the management of any local inbred colonies at research institutions. These rules are in place to reduce the incidence of genetic drift and ensure the traceability of any individual animal to deliver the genetic integrity required for modern genetic studies. It is noteworthy that these rules are not specific for mice and can be applied to any inbred strain in any species.

Characteristics of an inbred line

Inbred lines of any species have a number of characteristics that enable and facilitate genetic research. For a start they are isogenic, that is they are genetically identical to one another. Inbred strains display similar phenotypes although it is noteworthy that the word 'similar' is used here as the phenotype of an animal is a combination of both genetics and environment, plus variation in the phenotypic assay. Therefore, no two C57BL/6J mice are likely to produce exactly the same values in assays. However, all inbred animals of a single strain would present a phenotype within a specific range and the ranges for many characteristics from growth curves to

Table 4.1 Standards and good practice for breeding inbred strains.

Establishment	• Inbred strains come from at least 20 consecutive sibling matings (brother–sister) arising from a single pair mating
	• Inbred strains are always bred by brother–sister mating schemes
	• Inbred strains have distinct nomenclature
Supply	• Always source new strains from a reputable supplier adhering to strict mating regimes
	• Ensure that you are consistently ordering the same substrain. Different suppliers are likely to issue different substrains
Husbandry practices	• All animals within a colony must be traceable (i.e. their pedigree must be recorded) to assist with tracking any phenotypic changes observed. To assist with traceability, excellent breeding records and clear, consistent processes of identifying individuals is essential
	• It is preferable to house strains of the same coat colour in different locations (racks or rooms) and handle at different times
	• Husbandry standard operating procedures (SOPs) should include protocols for the careful observation of individuals, detection of any *phenodeviants* and clear reporting and recording instructions. This allows for any changes exhibited by individuals within an inbred colony to be managed
Genetic quality	• If housing many similar-looking strains (such as C57BL/6J and C57BL/6N), it may be beneficial to periodically genotype a proportion of the colony (for example, the breeders) for sequences specific to each strain
	• Restock the breeding stock of inbred colonies every 5–10 generations from either the original source or from an archive of cryopreserved embryos, this will limit the genetic drift

more involved phenotypic assessments are available in public databases[8,9]. See also Chapter 5: Phenotyping of genetically modified mice.

Importantly, all inbred strains have specific alleles fixed in their genome and due to many years of selective breeding, these alleles encode for very specific biological characteristics (Table 4.2). The most obvious variants are those genes which govern coat colours producing non-agouti mice such as C57BL/6 strains and/or albinism in BALB/c strains. However, there is much variation in many other alleles which will only become obvious during specific tests and in some cases conferring detrimental phenotypes. These allelic variants which have become fixed in the genetic background of laboratory strains are both a research resource and also a hurdle if they conflict or interfere with experimental results.

---

[6] http://www.mousephenotype.org/ (accessed 19 February 2020)
[7] http://www.informatics.jax.org/mgihome/nomen/strain_129.shtml (accessed 19 February 2020)
[8] https://phenome.jax.org/ (accessed 19 February 2020)
[9] http://www.mousephenotype.org/ (accessed 19 February 2020)

Table 4.2 Gene variants in common inbred mouse strains.

Inbred strain(s)	Phenotype	Gene mutated	Allele symbol
BALB/c – all substrains	Albinism	Tyrosinase	Tyr^c
C57BL/6JOlaHsd	Behavioural deficits	Alpha-synuclein	$Del(6Snca)1Slab$
C57BL/6J	Reduced insulin secretion	Nicotinamide nucleotide transhydrogenase	$Nnt^{C57BL/6J}$
129 – all substrains	Impaired memory	Disrupted in schizophrenia-1	$Disc1^{del}$
C3H – all substrains	Retinal degeneration	Phosphodiesterase 6B	$Pde6b^{rd1}$

Selecting an appropriate inbred strain

A multitude of publications describe the phenotypic differences between inbred strains (for examples, see Table 4.3). The most relevant and appropriate strain for experimental studies is dependent upon many factors. Obvious reasons for selecting a strain include the ability to measure specific parameters and physiological traits. For example, the sensory phenotypes of hearing and sight are compromised in two of the most common inbred strains, with C57BL/6 strains carrying a mutation in *Cdh23* causing hearing loss as the mice mature (Noben-Trauth *et al.* 2003) and C3H carrying the *Pde6b*^{rd1} mutation causing sight-loss by three weeks of age (Hart *et al.* 2005). Therefore, neither of these strains would be appropriate for research in hearing or vision respectively. However, there are also some more subtle considerations in terms of strain selection; these will be different for each study but include the availability of wild-type stock for ongoing breeding programmes, the strains used in historical data on which hypotheses are based and technical issues around modifying that particular strain or allele.

Inbred strains of other species

The ease, speed and relatively low-cost of mouse breeding has led to the proliferation of many inbred mouse strains as described above. However, the desire for genetic homogeneity has not only been confined to laboratories using mice. Inbred strains of rats have been developed concurrently with mouse inbred strains since the early part of the twentieth century. Strains such as Fischer 344, Lewis, Brown Norway and the SHR (spontaneously hypertensive rat) have been widely used to characterise and explore pathophysiological traits including their wide-spread use in cardiovascular and neurological (Gulley *et al.* 2007) studies. Although their size, blood volume and cognitive abilities make rats suitable for many *in vivo* studies, they have been less widely exploited in genetic engineering efforts (see the following text) and analyses of their genomic sequences have attracted less attention (Aitman *et al.* 2008) until relatively recently (Hermsen *et al.* 2015). Previous technical constraints with respect to changing genes in rat embryos and the significantly higher costs of housing and maintenance mean that there are fewer rat strains compared with mice; however, new technologies are likely to address this (Meek *et al.* 2017).

There have of course been efforts to generate inbred strains of other species including Zebra fish (Shinya & Sakai 2011) and pigs (Nicholls *et al.* 2016). The degree of homogeneity for both of these examples is reported at a far lower level than the mouse strains. This is likely to be largely the result of residual heterozygosity from the parental strains due to the limited number of sibling crosses (20 generations as compared to over 200 for many mouse strains). The principle of using genetic homogeneity in order to identify discrete, individual genetic changes or to reduce potential variation in an experimental group remains the same regardless of species.

Outbred strains

As opposed to the genetic homogeneity of inbred strains, colonies of outbred animals are specifically maintained to retain a high level of genetic heterogeneity. By using schemes which limit breeding between closely related individuals, outbred strains have a number of genetic loci which carry different alleles in different individuals. The characteristics of outbred stocks include high fecundity and characteristics which may change over generations and introduce a higher level of variability into an experimental paradigm, although this is disputed for some research outcomes (Tuttle *et al.* 2018).

Outbred rodents are routinely used in toxicology and other fields where genetic and, therefore, potential phenotypic variability might be thought to more closely reflect the genetic diversity of the human population and be more translational. However, this is still a subject of some controversy with some claiming that this selection is not based on scientific evidence (Festing 2010) and that the most commonly used laboratory strains of outbred mice lack significant genetic heterogeneity to be a useful comparison to the human population (Yalcin *et al.* 2010).

GA laboratory animals

The most logical way of examining how any component in a biological system works (or any system actually) is to change it or take it away. Therefore, in order to study the function of

Table 4.3 References describing differences in phenotypes between inbred strains

Phenotype category	References
Behaviour	Different levels of anxiety (Võikar *et al.* 2001)
Metabolism	Variable insulin resistance (Berglund *et al.* 2008)
Infection	**Variable resistance to Salmonella *typhimurim* by some inbred strains (Hormaeche 1979)**
Cardiac	Differential heart growth (Kiper *et al.* 2013)
Sensory	Variable nociception response (Tsuda *et al.* 2002)

any singular gene, biologists have been striving to change the DNA of laboratory animals in order to gain information on the function of that specific DNA sequence. This began before the development of molecular technologies and indeed many years before DNA was known to be the molecule conferring inheritance. In this section, we will discuss the means by which these genetic changes have been introduced and how the protocols of care, welfare assessment and breeding of these stocks need adapting from wild-type colonies.

Terminology

Over several decades, the terminology used to describe laboratory strains carrying a genetic difference from the equivalent wild-type strain has evolved and changed concurrently with the establishment of new technologies. There are many acronyms and names for GA animals including GMO (genetically modified organism), GEMM (genetically engineered mouse mutants), harmful and non-harmful mutants and genetic variants (Wells & Stéphane 2017). For the purpose of this chapter, we will use the term *genetically altered* (GA) to cover any change from the wild-type sequence made to the germ-line DNA (that is, DNA that is passed on from generation to generation) in a strain of laboratory animal. Much of the work discussed below will concentrate on the use of mice in genetic research, however with emerging technologies, the possibilities of genetically altering every single species (including human) becomes a relative and an ethical quandary we must all consider.

Spontaneous mutations

As already alluded to, many strains of laboratory inbred animals carry mutations which have arisen during selective breeding due to errors in DNA replication when forming gametes (oocytes and sperm). Following the establishment of some of our classical inbred mouse strains in the first half of the twentieth century, many breeding programs have detected deviants from the normal in terms of the appearance of the animal or the animal's behaviour. Indeed, it is an essential aspect of the role of an animal care worker to be so familiar with the normal characteristics of the animals they are looking after, that they can detect any subtle changes as well as obvious deviations such as coat colours. Many valuable biological discoveries have been made as a consequence of observant researchers and technicians identifying oddities in their colonies. One such example is the identification of mice in a BALB/c colony exhibiting nervous head movements and circling, which upon investigation were found to be deaf (Lord 1929). This led to the cloning of the *Myo7a* gene (Gibson *et al*. 1995) and the establishment of its role in a number of sensory and physiological functions such as hearing and vision (Self *et al*. 1998).

It is worth remembering that spontaneous mutations can occur in any animal including those already carrying mutations introduced by other methods such as chemical mutagenesis (Oliver *et al*. 2011) or gene targeting efforts (Westrick *et al*. 2010). In both cases noted here, the research groups were involved in projects using technical interventions to produce mutant alleles; however, molecular analysis uncovered that the mutation responsible for the observed phenotypes was indeed spontaneous and not deliberately induced or introduced in any way. The obvious lessons learnt from such an experience are that keen observations of the animals and consideration of the possibility of new mutations in every generation is key to good genetic research.

Inducing mutations in laboratory animals

Although spontaneous mutations have and will continue to be very important in genetic research, their generation is serendipitous and uncontrolled. In addition, gene mutations manifesting themselves as physical or behavioural anomalies will only ever reveal the function of a subset of the genome. Those involved in biological systems less easy to identify at cage-side or those genes involved when the body is challenged (for example, by infection or an environmental challenge) will be recognised at a much lower frequency. The induction of mutants at higher rates of incidence, by a variety of interventions, in combination with increasingly more sensitive phenotyping screens have delivered the plethora of mouse mutant strains now available.

The rate of mutagenesis has been increased by different physical, chemical and genetic methods, and concomitantly the chances of revealing the genetic causes of diseases have increased.

Radiation-induced germ-line mutagenesis

Following the atomic bombs which heralded the end of the Second World War, the mouse genetic programs at Oak Ridge, Tennessee, US (Russell 2013) and MRC Radiobiology Unit in Edinburgh, UK (de Chadarevian 2006) were initiated. The broad objectives of these projects were to mimic and explore the effects of radiation on genetic changes to mammalian germ cells. The application of radiation either in acute doses or chronically over longer periods of time resulted in a much higher yield of mouse mutations, many fold higher than those occurring spontaneously. These rates are largely dependent upon sex, test system, radiation quality, dose rates and other variables[10]. Radiation not only increases the frequency of changes in individual genes but also creates large chromosomal changes. These include deletions of regions of chromosomes, inversions (where a portion of the chromosome breaks off and joins the chromosome again in the opposite orientation) and translocations (where the broken-off portion joins another chromosome). These large chromosomal rearrangements provided the mouse strains for many seminal biological research projects, including the field of imprinting (Tucci *et al*. 2019) and facilitated efforts to discover the positions of genes relative to each other on individual chromosomes (called *linkage*).

Chemical-induced mutagenesis

In order to monitor how mutagenic a treatment was, specific strains of mice were bred which carried a collection of recessive mutations. These were largely coat and eye colour, hair

---

[10] http://informatics.jax.org/greenbook/chapters/chapter10.shtml

texture and ear abnormalities. By scoring any change to these characteristics, a rate for mutational changes could be estimated. This was called the *specific-locus test* and was not only used in radiation studies but also to assess the mutagenic effect of chemical treatments. The specific-locus test revealed a chemical called *N-ethyl-N-nitrosourea* (ENU) as a powerful super-mutagen of germ-line DNA (Russell *et al.* 1979).

Common ENU mutagenesis protocols involve male mice being given several intraperitoneal injections of doses of the chemical (Russell *et al.* 1982). The impact of this aggressive mutagen is to render the mice sterile for several months due to a depletion of their germ cells. Once fertility is regained, the sperm produced contain many unique mutations which are apparent in the phenotypes of their offspring. Unlike radiation, most of the mutations caused by ENU are single base-pair substitutions (e.g. A/T to T/A transversions (44%) or A/T to G/C transitions (38%) (Barbaric *et al.* 2007)).

ENU mutagenesis has been used to generate large numbers of potential mutants, which have been screened for many different phenotypes, and subsequently the causative genes were mapped and identified. This method has been instrumental in identifying the difficult-to-predict function of unknown genes and was really gathering pace by the 1990s. The limitation to discovering new gene functions no longer rested with the frequency of occurrence of genetic changes but with the sensitivity and logistics of phenotyping screens. Large-scale mouse chemical mutagenesis programmes were launched (Nolan *et al.* 2000; Arnold *et al.* 2012; Oliver & Davies 2012) and over many years this so-called *forward genetics* approach (from phenotype to gene) revealed the function of many mammalian genes and produced many models of human disease which are still used in research today. Chemical mutagenesis is not just restricted to mice and has been used in other species namely rats (Smits *et al.* 2006), zebrafish (Solnica-Krezel *et al.* 1994) and pigs (Hai *et al.* 2017) with the goal of discovering novel genes relating to observed phenotypes.

Creating many new mouse strains may have advantages in terms of seeking genetic knowledge; however, the impact on individual animals can be significant. Applying radiation or chemicals to animals often results in side-effects including tumours such as lymphomas (Smith *et al.* 2009). Careful and precise monitoring of mutagenised animals is required in all cases to observe early signs of ill health and distress.

Transgenesis – the new era of genetic engineering

Spontaneous, radiation and chemical mutants have inevitably led to the uncovering of the function of many genes. However, these techniques are limited by the untargeted nature of how they occur. Using these methods, it is not possible to direct changes to a specific region or gene within an organism's genome. Moreover, once a deviant phenotype is revealed, complex molecular mapping and/or genome sequencing and further breeding are required to first detect possible causative changes in the DNA and secondly, to prove without a doubt that these changes are responsible for the characteristics observed.

In the early 1980s, the field of molecular biology was expanding dramatically. New laboratory techniques allowed for the isolation of DNA and the identification of specific sequences within genomes. Importantly, these new molecular biology techniques facilitated the ability to combine different pieces of DNA together to form artificial sequences (so-called *constructs*) which potentially could combine any gene from any organism with regulatory sequences from any other. This laid the foundation for transgenesis in mammals; that is the introduction of DNA from one organism into another, creating a transgenic mouse. Foreign DNA had been delivered into an embryo of a mouse oocyte in the 1970s (Jaenisch & Mintzt 1974); however, the introduced sequence was not transmitted to subsequent generations. This discussion will concentrate on the generation of GA strains (also called *transgenic strains*), this being those strains in which the alteration is integrated into the genome to be inherited by subsequent progeny.

Integrational transgenesis

Integrational transgenesis is the term given to an additive process of delivering DNA, usually to an early-stage embryo, which then becomes integrated into the host genome at a random locus. The most commonly used method to introduce exogenous DNA into a whole organism, such as a mouse, is microinjection. A fine glass capillary is filled with the multiple copies of the sequence to be introduced (the transgene) and under high-powered microscopes, the DNA is injected into one of two pronuclei of a one-celled fertilised embryo. Each pronucleus contains the haploid genetic material of either the sperm or the oocyte before the nuclei fuse. In the mouse, this was first performed by injecting a construct which combined the promoter of the mouse metallothionein-I gene fused to the structural gene of rat growth hormone (Palmiter *et al.* 1982). The resulting lines gave rise to significantly larger mice, thus demonstrating the possibility of manipulating the mammalian genome.

Since these early experiments in the 1980s, constructs have been developed and refined in order to enable many foreign proteins to be expressed in not only mice but rats (Bachmann *et al.* 1992), farm animals (Wolf *et al.* 2000), fish (Tonelli *et al.* 2017) and primates (Sasaki *et al.* 2009). Some species require modification to this technique and the use of a specialised virus to deliver the DNA. These genetic alterations have been used widely for a number of purposes (Table 4.4).

Although the sequence of the DNA being introduced is carefully controlled in a laboratory, the place where it inserts into the genome is uncontrolled and this can impact on the subsequent phenotype of the animal. Indeed, a large-scale project to identify the sites of integration of a large number of widely used transgenic mouse lines has revealed disruption in endogenous coding sequences in half of the lines, some of these accompanied by notable deletions and structural variations at the site of integration (Goodwin *et al.* 2019). In these cases, it is possible that disruption of the gene at the integration site may be responsible for the phenotype, rather than the transgene itself.

In addition to introducing DNA fragments by microinjection, other methods to add sequences to a host genome have been used especially for some large-scale mutagenesis projects which includes the use of transposons (Takeda *et al.* 2007). These are DNA sequences that change their positions in the genome by either duplicating themselves with

Table 4.4 Uses of different types of integrational transgenic animals.

Type	Description	Use
Disease models	Animals carrying an allele which confers a disease in another species or individual	In studies of disease progression such as Huntington's disease where transgenic models carry the expanded nucleotide repeat present in human sufferers (Li et al. 2005)
Overexpression models	Animals carrying multiple copies of a protein-coding gene or a gene under the control of a very strong promoter producing much more protein than in the wild type	For disease models where protein over-production is a problem and analysis of gene function (Cheng et al. 2016) Also for the production of recombinant therapeutic proteins (Wang et al. 2013)
Reporter gene	Animals bearing transgenes which code for proteins which can easily be detected by microscopy or laboratory techniques such as fluorescent proteins or enzymes	Labelling of a specific cell type often for visualisation, cell-sorting or cell lineage tracking (Li et al. 2018)
Promoter sequence analysis	Animals produced carrying specific fragments of regulatory regions, often linked to a reporter gene	For investigating DNA elements controlling gene regulation

the copy being inserted elsewhere or a sequence excising from their existing position and recombining back into the chromosomes somewhere else. Often, they result in gene disruption and are useful in analysing gene function.

Targeted transgenesis

Additive transgenesis gave scientists the ability to insert DNA constructs they had designed in order to answer specific scientific questions, into the genomes of mammals. Nevertheless, it did not permit the specific targeting of endogenous loci hence accessing an individual gene and altering its sequence still remained elusive. However, *in vitro* studies using cell lines were increasingly recognising a process called *homologous recombination* as a mechanism for replacing existing gene sequences with those designed in the laboratory. This involved the production of a DNA construct which contained the altered sequence flanked by regions that were the same (homologous) to the endogenous genome, called *homology arms*. Inside certain cells, these regions of homology would recombine with the homologous sequence in the genome (Figure 4.5). This results in the transgene being precisely inserted in replacement for the endogenous sequence (Folger *et al.* 1982).

At the same time, embryonic stem (ES) cell lines were being developed for the mouse (Evans & Kaufman 1981). These specialist cells, derived from the inner cell mass of blastocyst-stage embryos, remain pluripotent when cultured under specific conditions. That is, they retain the ability to differentiate into any cell type. By combining both the process of homologous recombination and the ability to culture embryonic stem cells, it became possible to engineer ES cells with specific parts of their genomes replaced with transgenes.

When introduced back into an early-stage blastocyst embryo by microinjection, these engineered ES cells could colonise parts of the embryo generating chimaeric mice, containing a mixture of cells derived from both the injected embryo and ES cells. These chimaeras, which contain the genetic information of four parents, could potentially transmit the altered gene to the next generation (Koller *et al.* 1989). At last, it seemed possible to be able to precisely and accurately target any place in the genome. For mouse genetic research, this truly was a turning point, with ES cell technologies being used prolifically to disrupt genes and produce knockout mice, missing individual genes and their respective proteins. Manipulating ES cells has become the basis for generating a huge array of new mouse strains with increasing molecular sophistication. As well as knockout mice where specific genes are inactivated, many

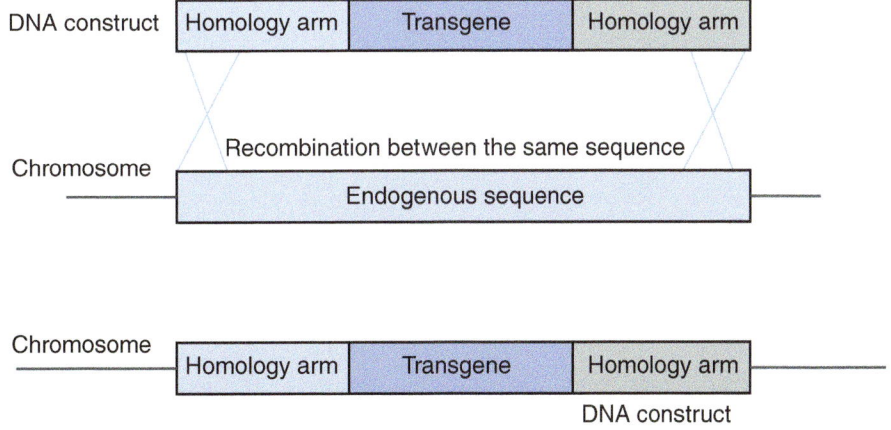

Figure 4.5 Homologous recombination resulting in the targeted insertion of a transgene.

knockin strains are now available. By replacing the mouse sequence with specific engineered sequences, it is now possible to turn genes on and off in both specific tissues and at specific times, so-called *conditional transgenesis*.

ES cells have also been developed for other species such as the rat (Buehr *et al.* 2008). However, species-specific differences and technical issues relating to their culture and targeting have limited their use. For the mouse, there are some significant differences between the ability of ES cells from different background strains to transmit gene alterations. Initially, all experiments were performed using ES cells from 129 strains. Although efficient in the production of GA mice, the 129 background is not optimal for many types of phenotyping (especially, neuroscience where the 129 strains have vastly different behavioural profiles than C57BL/6 strains). Moreover, although the technology allowed specific genes to be targeted, the process of construct preparation, ES cell targeting, chimaera generation and breeding for germ-line transmission was laborious, fraught with technical issues and often takes several years.

To facilitate the issues around the restrictive background of the 129 ES cells and the time taken for targeting and ES culture, an international effort was established in the early 2000s. The International Knockout Mouse Consortium[11] now provides targeted ES cells for many of the genes in the mouse genome on a C57BL/6N background (Skarnes *et al.* 2011). However, three major problems remained in terms of targeting genomic sequences, firstly for most species and including most strains of mice, ES cells are not available. Secondly, the efficiency of generating new animal models using ES technologies can be low, as not all ES cell clones retain pluripotency and lead to germ-line transmission of a genetic alteration. Lastly, ES cell work is costly, time-consuming and restrictive for most PhD students or post-doctoral researchers on time-limited research programmes.

Gene editing – a revolution for the generation of GA animal models

In an ideal situation, the generation of GA animals would not be hampered by long cell culture protocols or the efficiency of transgene transmission. It would be applicable to any species and any strain, be rapid and cost less than previous methods. The development of RGEN (RNA-guided endonucleases) addresses all of these issues and has set alight the world of mammalian genetics (Hsu *et al.* 2014).

This technology comes with the promise that the genome of potentially any organism could be changed easily and efficiently. In rodents, for example, this can be done by simply injecting one-cell fertilised embryos with a prokaryote-derived nuclease and one or more 'guide' RNAs which direct the precise alteration of single or multiple genes (Sander & Joung 2014). Although other genome editing technologies such as zinc-finger nucleases (ZFNs) and transcription activator-like effector nucleases are available, this discussion will concentrate on the most prolific of these technologies, CRISPR/Cas9.

[11] https://www.mousephenotype.org/about-impc/about-ikmc/ (accessed 19 February 2020)

CRISPR/Cas9

Viruses that infect bacteria (called *bacteriophages*) do so by injecting their own genomes inside bacterial cells. These nucleic acids that make up the viral genome are then incorporated into the bacterial genome and transcribed as if they were endogenous genes, generating new viral particles and completing the infectious cycle. *CRISPR* stands for Clustered Regularly Interspaced Short Palindromic Repeats, which are short sequences within the bacterial genome representing remnants of previous viral infections. These form a store of DNA sequences which can be recognised during future infections. Bacteria use this library of viral DNA to synthesise RNA molecules, which then guide a nuclease called *Cas9* to the complementary sequences of invading viruses, cleaving them and rendering them inactive. In recent years, this system has been adapted for use in eukaryotes (Jinek *et al.* 2012) and has allowed prolific targeting and cleaving of almost any sequence in any organism so far attempted.

In more detail, Cas9 has the ability to cut genomic DNA in a specific place when bound by a guide RNA molecule (gRNA). Therefore, we now have the ability to design a gRNA with a sequence complementary to almost any region of the genome we need to target. This RNA molecule, along with Cas9, can be microinjected or electroporated straight into pre-implantation-stage embryos, without any prior cell culture. When the gRNA binds to its complementary sequence in the genome of the organism being targeted (Figure 4.6) the Cas9 protein cleaves both strands of the DNA. This double-stranded breaking of the DNA initiates two main cellular DNA repair processes. In non-homologous end-joining (NHEJ), the two cut ends of the DNA are forced back together, during which time it is likely that some nucleotides are deleted or inserted. Often small insertions or deletions are enough to render a gene inactive, thereby creating a knockout allele. The second process is called *homology-directed repair* (HDR) (Figure 4.7). In this case, rather than forcing the ends together, the cell attempts to fix the DNA by replicating the broken sequence from a template. By providing a third element, an artificial template or 'donor' (usually, DNA), which contains the complementary sequence to either side of the cut site, incorporation of a multitude of different sequences will result in knockin alleles.

CRISPR/Cas9 technologies work in every mammalian species so far attempted including humans, mice and macaques (Chen *et al.* 2015), but there are limitations. Technically, there are some sequence constraints as Cas9 does not cut everywhere in the genome. Often the genomic alterations do not occur until the embryonic DNA has replicated, leading to the generation of a *mosaic* animal that carries cells of differing genotypes. It is also currently difficult to insert larger fragments of DNA directly into the genomes via the embryo. Therefore, for complex allelic changes, ES cell technologies (sometimes in combination with CRISPR/Cas9) are still widely utilised. Lastly, there are widely reported issues of genetic integrity in terms of the quality of the strains generated. Anxiety about off-target effects (where the Cas9 generates alterations at sites other than the target locus) and concerns about the allelic

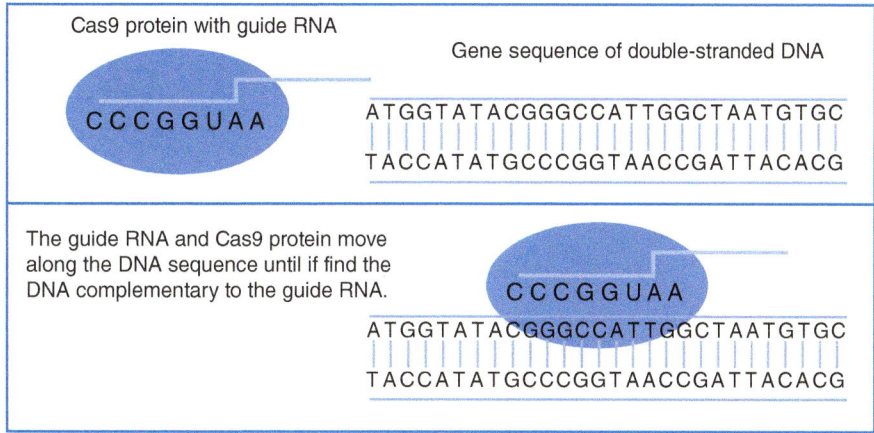

Figure 4.6 The binding of guide RNA molecules to their complementary genomic sequences.

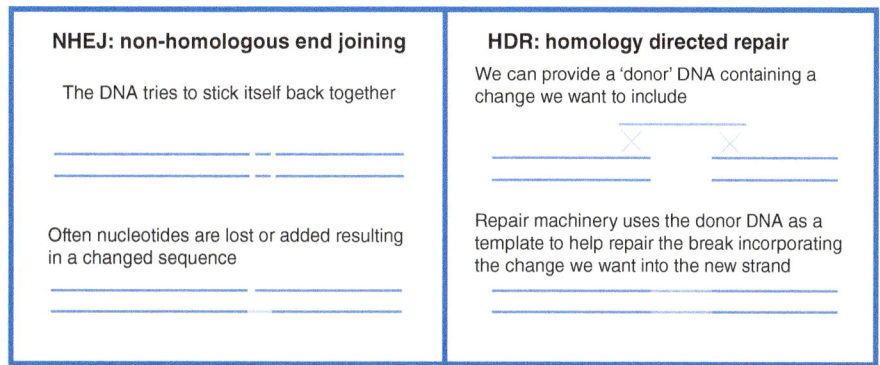

Figure 4.7 The two main mechanisms of double-stranded DNA repair, non-homologous end-joining and homology-directed repair.

changes (Kosicki *et al.* 2018) need to be addressed by rigorous quality control processes. However, we should not underestimate the importance of this technology and/or the potential that newer versions of similar systems will improve on all the drawbacks listed above. There is no doubt that genome editing will form the basis of GA laboratory animals for some time to come.

Concluding remarks

As a scientific community, we have striven to alter the genetic composition of the laboratory animals we use in research over many decades. Initially by breeding methods and latterly by molecular technologies, we have generated animals carrying mutations and expressing modified proteins in order to elucidate gene function and disease mechanisms. This has rapidly accelerated with the establishment of genome editing tools throughout the globe, allowing any genomic change to be made, in any genome and any species. We are now in a position to refine previous animal models and generate new strains, with high relevance to disease and potentially invaluable to translational research. This is indeed exciting in a time when many human genome projects are revealing the true diversity and number of genetic variations in the human genome. Understanding the function of many of these genetic variations may require the production of novel GA animal strains.

Technologies old and new do not come without responsibilities, challenges and costs. It is worth remembering in one of the opening statements of this chapter that being able to perform such genetic changes does not mean that ethically we always should. The cost to animals in terms of numbers used in the production and breeding of new strains as well as the cost to the individual animal bearing a debilitating mutation need constantly reviewing. Methods that are more efficient should not assuage the need for a scientific and medical need that outweighs the burden on the laboratory animal.

Acknowledgements

We thank the staff of MRC Harwell, especially Dona Reddiar, for their encouragement and support while writing this chapter. We are also grateful to Michael Festing and Cathleen Lutz, authors of this chapter in previous editions, for their inspiration and knowledge.

References

Aitman, T.J., Critser, J., Cuppen, E. et al. (2008) Progress and prospects in rat genetics: A community view. *Nature Genetics*, **40**(5), 516–522. doi: 10.1038/ng.147.

Arnold, C.N., Barnes, M., Berger, M. et al. (2012) ENU-induced phenovariance in mice: inferences from 587 mutations. *BMC Res Notes*, **5**, 577. doi: 10.1186/1756-0500-5-577.

Bachmann, S., Peters, J., Engler, E. et al. (1992) Transgenic rats carrying the mouse renin gene – morphological characterization of a low-renin hypertension model. *Kidney International*, **41**(1), 24–36. doi: 10.1038/ki.1992.4.

Barbaric, I., Wells, S., Russ, A. and Dear T.N. et al. (2007) Spectrum of ENU-induced mutations in phenotype-driven and gene-driven screens in the mouse. *Environmental and Molecular Mutagenesis*, **48**(2), 124–142. doi: 10.1002/em.20286.

Beck, J.A., Lloyd, S., Hafezparast, M. et al. (2000) Genealogies of mouse inbred strains. Nature Genetics, 24, 23–25. doi: 10.1038/71641.

Berglund, E.D., Li, C., Poffenberger, G. et al. (2008) Glucose metabolism in vivo in four commonly used inbred mouse strains. *Diabetes*, **57**(7), 1790–1799. doi: 10.2337/db07-1615.

Bogue, M.A., Churchill, G.A. and Chesler, E.J. (2015) Collaborative cross and diversity outbred data resources in the mouse phenome database. *Mammalian Genome*, Springer US, **26**(9–10), 511–520. doi: 10.1007/s00335-015-9595-6.

Buehr, M., Meek, S., Blair, K. et al. (2008) Capture of authentic embryonic stem cells from rat blastocysts. *Cell*. **135**(7), 1287–1298. doi: 10.1016/j.cell.2008.12.007.

Chen, Y., Zheng, Y., Kang, K. et al. (2015) Functional disruption of the dystrophin gene in rhesus monkey using CRISPR/Cas9. *Human Molecular Genetics*, **24**(13), 3764–3774. doi: 10.1093/hmg/ddv120.

Cheng, N., Jiao, S., Gumaste, A. et al. (2016) APP overexpression causes Aβ-independent neuronal death through intrinsic apoptosis pathway. *eNeuro*, **3**(4), 208–245. doi: 10.1523/ENEURO.0150-16.2016.

de Chadarevian, S. (2006) Mice and the reactor: The "genetics experiment" in 1950s Britain. *Journal of the History of Biology*, **39**, 707–735. https://doi.org/10.1007/s10739-006-9110-8.

Doran, A.G., Wong, K., Flint, J. et al. (2016) Deep genome sequencing and variation analysis of 13 inbred mouse strains defines candidate phenotypic alleles, private variation and homozygous truncating mutations. *Genome Biology*, **17**(1), 167. doi: 10.1186/s13059-016-1024-y.

Evans, M.J. and Kaufman, M.H. (1981) Establishment in culture of pluripotential cells from mouse embryos. *Nature*, **292**, 154–156. https://doi.org/10.1038/292154a0.

Festing, M. (2010) Inbred strains should replace outbred stocks in toxicology, safety testing, and drug development. *Toxicologic Pathology*, 681–690. doi: 10.1177/0192623310373776.

Folger, K.R., Wong, E., Wahl, G. et al. (1982) Patterns of integration of DNA microinjected into cultured mammalian cells: evidence for homologous recombination between injected plasmid DNA molecules. *Molecular and Cellular Biology*, **2**(11), 1372–1387. doi: 10.1128/mcb.2.11.1372.

Freeman, H.C., Hugill, A., Dear, N. et al. (2006) Deletion of nicotinamide nucleotide transhydrogenase: A new quantitive trait locus accounting for glucose intolerance in C57BL/6J mice. *Diabetes*, **55**(7), 2153–2156. doi: 10.2337/db06-0358.

Gibson, F., Walsh, J., Mburu, P. et al. (1995) A type VII myosin encoded by the mouse deafness gene shaker-1. *Nature*, **374**(6517), 62–64. doi: 10.1038/374062a0.

Goodwin, L.O., Splinter, E., Davis, T. et al. (2019) Large-scale discovery of mouse transgenic integration sites reveals frequent structural variation and insertional mutagenesis. *Genome Research*, **29**(3), 494–505. doi: 10.1101/gr.233866.117.

Gulley, J.M., Everett, C.V. and Zahniser, N.R. (2007) Inbred Lewis and Fischer 344 rat strains differ not only in novelty and amphetamine-induced behaviors, but also in dopamine transporter activity in vivo. *Brain Research*, **2**(1151), 32–45. doi: 10.1016/j.brainres.2007.03.009.

Hai, T., Cao, C., Shang, H. et al. (2017) Pilot study of large-scale production of mutant pigs by ENU mutagenesis. *eLife*, **6**, 1–21. doi: 10.7554/eLife.26248.

Hart, A.W., McKie, L., Morgan, J. et al. (2005) Genotype-phenotype correlation of mouse Pde6b mutations. *Investigative Ophthalmology and Visual Science*, **46**(9), 3443–3450. doi: 10.1167/iovs.05-0254.

Hermsen, R. De Ligt, J., Spee, W. et al. (2015) Genomic landscape of rat strain and substrain variation. *BMC Genomics*, **16**(1). doi: 10.1186/s12864-015-1594-1.

Hormaeche, C.E. (1979) Natural resistance to Salmonella typhimurium in different inbred mouse strains. *Immunology*, **37**(2), 311–318.

Hsu, P.D., Lander, E.S. and Zhang, F. (2014) Development and applications of CRISPR-Cas9 for genome engineering. *Cell*, **157**(6), 1262–1278. doi: 10.1016/j.cell.2014.05.010.

Jaenisch, R. and Mintzt, B. (1974) Simian virus 40 DNA sequences in DNA of healthy adult mice derived from preimplantation blastocysts injected with viral DNA. *Proceedings of the National Academy of Sciences of the United States of America*, **71**(4), 1250–1254.

Jinek, M., Chylinski, K., Fonfara, I. et al. (2012) A programmable dual-RNA-guided DNA endonuclease in adaptive bacterial immunity. *Science*, **337**(6096), 816–821. doi: 10.1126/science.1225829.

Kiper, C., Grimes, B., Zant, G., et al. (2013) Mouse strain determines cardiac growth potential. *PLoS ONE*, **8**(8), 1–13. doi: 10.1371/journal.pone.0070512.

Koller, B.H., Hagemann, L.J., Doestschman, T. et al. (1989) Germ-line transmission of a planned alteration made in a hypoxanthine phosphoribosyltransferase gene by homologous recombination in embryonic stem cells. *Proceedings of the National Academy of Sciences of the United States of America*, **86**(22), 8927–8931. doi: 10.1073/pnas.86.22.8927.

Kosicki, M., Tomberg, K. and Bradley, A. (2018) Repair of double-strand breaks induced by CRISPR–Cas9 leads to large deletions and complex rearrangements. *Nature Biotechnology*, **36**(8). doi: 10.1038/nbt.4192.

Li, J.Y., Popovic, N. and Brundin, P. (2005) The use of the R6 transgenic mouse models of Huntington's disease in attempts to develop novel therapeutic strategies. *NeuroRx*, **2**(3), 447–464. doi: 10.1602/neurorx.2.3.447.

Li, S., Chen, L., Peng, X. et al. (2018) Overview of the reporter genes and reporter mouse models. *Animal Models and Experimental Medicine*, **1**(1), 29–35. doi: 10.1002/ame2.12008.

Lilue, J., Dorna, A., Fiddes, I. et al. (2018) Sixteen diverse laboratory mouse reference genomes define strain-specific haplotypes and novel functional loci. *Nature Genetics*, **50**(11), 1574–1583. doi: 10.1038/s41588-018-0223-8.

Lord, E.M. (1929) Shaker, a new mutation of the house mouse (Mus musculus). *The American Naturalist*, **63**(688), 435–442. doi: 10.1086/280276.

Lynch, M. (2011) Evolution of the mutation rate. *Trends in Genetics*, **26**(8), 345–352. doi: 10.1016/j.tig.2010.05.003.

Mattapallil, M.J., Wawrousek, E., Chan, C. et al. (2012) The Rd8 mutation of the Crb1 gene is present in vendor lines of C57BL/6N mice and embryonic stem cells, and confounds ocular induced mutant phenotypes. *Investigative Ophthalmology & Visual Science*, **53**(6), 2921–2927. doi: 10.1167/iovs.12-9662.

Meek, S., Mashimo, T. and Burdon, T. (2017) From engineering to editing the rat genome. *Mammalian Genome*, **28**(7), 302–314. doi: 10.1007/s00335-017-9705-8.

Neafsey, D.E. and Palumbi, S.R. (2003) Genome size evolution in pufferfish: A comparative analysis of diodontid and tetraodontid pufferfish genomes. *Genome Research*, **13**(5), 821–830. doi: 10.1101/gr.841703.

Nicholls, S., Pong-Wong, R., Mitchard, L. *et al.* (2016) Genome-wide analysis in swine associates corneal graft rejection with donor-recipient mismatches in three novel histocompatibility regions and one locus homologous to the mouse H-3 locus. *PLoS ONE*, **11**(3), 1–12. doi: 10.1371/journal.pone.0152155.

Noben-Trauth, K., Zheng, Q.Y. and Johnson, K.R. (2003) Association of cadherin 23 with polygenic inheritance and genetic modification of sensorineural hearing loss. *Nature Genetics*, **35**(1), 21–23. doi: 10.1038/ng1226.

Nolan, P.M., Peters, J., Strivens, M. *et al.* (2000) A systematic, genome-wide, phenotype-driven mutagenesis programme for gene function studies in the mouse. *Nature Genetics*, **25**(4), 440–443. doi: 10.1038/78140.

Oliver, P.L. and Davies, K.E. (2012) New insights into behaviour using mouse ENU mutagenesis. *Human Molecular Genetics*, **21**(R1), 72–81. doi: 10.1093/hmg/dds318.

Oliver, P.L., Finelli, M.J., Edwards, B. *et al.* Oxr1 is essential for protection against oxidative stress-induced neurodegeneration. *PLOS Genetics*, **7**(10), e1002338. https://doi.org/10.1371/journal.pgen.1002338.

Palmiter, R.D., Brinster, R., Hammer, R. *et al.* (1982) Dramatic growth of mice that develop from eggs microinjected with metallothionein–growth hormone fusion genes. *Nature*, **300**(5893), 611–615.

Portin, P. (2014) The birth and development of the DNA theory of inheritance: Sixty years since the discovery of the structure of DNA. *Journal of Genetics*, **93**(1), 293–302. doi: 10.1007/s12041-014-0337-4.

Richard, G.-F., Kerrest, A. and Duion, B. (2008) Comparative genomics and molecular dynamics of DNA repeats in eukaryotes. *Microbiology and Molecular Biology Reviews*, **72**(4), 686–727. doi: 10.1128/MMBR.00011-08

Russell, L. B. (2013) The Mouse House: A brief history of the ORNL mouse-genetics program, 1947-2009. *Mutation Research – Reviews in Mutation Research*, **753**(2), 69–90. doi: 10.1016/j.mrrev.2013.08.003.

Russell, W.L., Hunsicker, P., Carpenter, D. *et al.* (1982) Effect of dose fractionation on the ethylnitrosourea induction of specific-locus mutations in mouse spermatogonia. *Proceedings of the National Academy of Sciences of the United States of America*, **79**(11), 3592–3593. doi: 10.1073/pnas.79.11.3592.

Russell, W.L., Kelly, E., Hunsicker, P. *et al.* (1979) Specific-locus test shows ethylnitrosourea to be the most potent mutagen in the mouse. *Proceedings of the National Academy of Sciences*, **76**(11), 5818–5819. doi: 10.1073/pnas.76.11.5818.

Sander, J.D. and Joung, J.K. (2014) CRISPR-Cas systems for genome editing, regulation and targeting, *Nature Biotechnology*, **32**(4), 347–355. doi: 10.1038/nbt.2842.

Sasaki, E., Suemizu, H., Shimada, A. *et al.* (2009) Generation of transgenic non-human primates with germline transmission. *Nature*, **459**(7246), 523–527. doi: 10.1038/nature08090.

Self, T., Mahony, M., Fleming, J. *et al.* (1998) Shaker-1 mutations reveal roles for myosin VIIA in both development and function of cochlear hair cells. *Development*, **125**(4), 557–566.

Shinya, M. and Sakai, N. (2011) Generation of highly homogeneous strains of zebrafish through full sib-pair mating. *G3: Genes, Genomes, Genetics*, **1**(5), 377–386. doi: 10.1534/g3.111.000851.

Shorter, J.R. (2017) Male infertility is responsible for nearly half of the extinction observed in the mouse collaborative cross. *Genetics*, **206**, 557–572. doi: 10.1534/genetics.116.199596.

Simon, M.M., Greenaway, S., White, J. *et al.* (2015) Current strategies for mutation detection in phenotype-driven screens utilising next generation sequencing. *Mammalian Genome*. **26**(9–10), 486–500. doi: 10.1007/s00335-015-9603-x.

Simpson, E.M., Carbonetto, P., Engle, K. *et al.* (1997) Genetic variation among 129 substrains and its importance for targeted mutagenesis in mice. *Nature Genetics*, **16**, 19–27.

Skarnes, W.C., Rosen, B., West, A. *et al.* (2011) A conditional knockout resource for the genome-wide study of mouse gene function. *Nature*. **474**(7351), 337–344. doi: 10.1038/nature10163.

Smith, A.P.L., Polley, S., Wells, S. *et al.* (2009) Analysis of breeding and pathology helps refine management practices of a large-scale N'-ethyl-N'-nitrosourea mouse mutagenesis programme. *Laboratory Animals*, **43**(1), 1–10. doi: 10.1258/la.2008.007072.

Smits, B.M.G., Muddle, J., Van De Belt, J. *et al.* (2006) Generation of gene knockouts and mutant models in the laboratory rat by ENU-driven target-selected mutagenesis. *Pharmacogenetics and Genomics*, **16**(3),159–169. doi: 10.1097/01.fpc.0000184960.8290.8f.

Solnica-Krezel, L., Schier, A.F. and Driever, W. (1994) Efficient recovery of ENU-induced mutations from the zebrafish germline. *Genetics*, **136**(4), 1401–1420. Available at: http://www.genetics.org/cgi/reprint/136/4/1401.

Stoeger, T. Gerlach, M., Morimoto, R. *et al.* (2018) Large-scale investigation of the reasons why potentially important genes are ignored. *PLoS Biology*, **16**(9), 1–25. doi: 10.1371/journal.pbio.2006643.

Takeda, J., Keng, V.W. and Horie, K. (2007) Germline mutagenesis mediated by Sleeping Beauty transposon system in mice. *Genome Biology*, **8**(Suppl. 1), S14. doi: 10.1186/gb-2007-8-s1-s14.

Threadgill, D.W., Yee, D., Matin, A. *et al.* (1997) Genealogy of the 129 inbred strains: 129/SvJ is a contaminated inbred strain. *Mammalian Genome*, **8**(6), 390–393. doi: 10.1007/s003359900453.

Tonelli, F.M.P., Lacaerda, S., Toneli, F.C.P. *et al.* (2017) Progress and biotechnological prospects in fish transgenesis, *Biotechnology Advances*, **35**(6), 832–844. doi: 10.1016/j.biotechadv.2017.06.002.

Tsuda, M. Shigemoto-mogami, Y., Ueno, S. *et al.* (2002) Downregulation of P2X 3 receptor-dependent sensory functions in A / J inbred mouse strain. *European Journal of Neuroscience*, **15**(9), 1444–1450. doi: 10.1046/j.1460-9568.2002.01982.x.

Tucci, V., Isles, A., Kelsey, G. *et al.* (2019) Genomic imprinting and physiological processes in mammals. *Cell*, **7**. doi: 10.1016/j.cell.2019.01.043.

Tuttle, A.H., Philip, V., Chesler, E. *et al.* (2018) Comparing phenotypic variation between inbred and outbred mice. *Nature Methods*, **15**(12), 994–996. doi: 10.1038/s41592-018-0224-7.

Uchimura, A., Higuchi, M., Minakuchi, Y., *et al.* (2015) Germline mutation rates and the long-term phenotypic effects of mutation accumulation in wild-type laboratory mice and mutator mice'. *Genome Research*, **25**, 1125–1134. doi: 10.1101/gr.186148.114.25.

Võikar, V. Kõks, S., Vasar, E. *et al.* (2001) Strain and gender differences in the behavior of mouse lines commonly used in transgenic studies. *Physiology and Behavior*, **72**(1–2), 271–281. doi: 10.1016/S0031-9384(00)00405-4.

Wang, Y., Zhao, S., Bai, L. *et al.* (2013) Expression systems and species used for transgenic animal bioreactors. *BioMed Research International*, 580463. doi: 10.1155/2013/580463.

Wells, S. and Stéphane, J. (2017) The trouble with collective nouns for genome editing. *Mammalian Genome*, **28**(7), 365–366. doi: 10.1002/jsfa.7523.

Westrick, R.J., Mohlke, K.L., Yang, A.Y. *et al.* (2010) Spontaneous Irs1 passenger mutation linked to a gene-targeted SerpinB2 allele. *Proceedings of the National Academy of Sciences of the United States of America*, **107**(39), 16904–16909. doi: 10.1073/pnas.1012050107.

Wolf, E. Schernthaner, W., Zakhartchenko, V. *et al.* (2000) Transgenic technology in farm animals – Progress and perspectives. *Experimental Physiology*, **85**, 615–625.

Yalcin, B., Nicod, J., Bhomra, A. *et al.* (2010) Commercially available outbred mice for genome-wide association studies. *PLoS Genetics*, **6**(9). doi: 10.1371/journal.pgen.1001085.

5 Phenotyping of genetically modified mice

Jan-Bas Prins and Sara Wells

Introduction

The development of techniques to create genetically modified (GM) mice has allowed tremendous progress in biomedical research and the life sciences during the last decades. GM animals have been used to provide a multitude of animal models for human conditions and their use has increased dramatically.

Each new GM mouse generated transmitting the genetic modification to the next generation is a founder of a new line. A GM animal may or may not show altered characteristics (phenotypic changes) compared to the wild-type, non-modified, counterpart. The phenotype of a GM mouse is the sum of observable characteristics of an induced or spontaneous mutation and the impact of its environment which includes housing, diet and pathogen. See also Chapter 4: An introduction to laboratory animal genetics.

The phenotypic consequences of a genetic modification cannot always be predicted and, consequently, it is essential to characterise each new GM line's phenotype. Phenotypic characterisation, or phenotyping, is the discipline of identifying and describing new characteristics as compared to the non-mutated wild type. Ideally, phenotyping should uncover any new trait. A vast number of tests could be applied to a mouse strain in order to reveal the full extent of the impact of the genetic change. Phenotyping is essential to know the characteristics of a GM line so that decisions can be made as to whether the line will be suitable as model system for a particular area of research and whether there are any co-occurring phenotypes which may interfere with subsequent testing. For example, if it has become clear though phenotyping that a GM line is deaf, the acoustic startle response test is an inappropriate test to use for this line. Knowing a strain's phenotype will also help in making welfare decisions for these animals.

The resultant phenotype of a genetic modification is dependent on the role of the gene(s) in normal development, the functioning of the organism and on the type of the modification. To date, however, the function of many genes is still unknown, let alone much of the function of DNA sequences labelled as non-coding. The scale at which GM mutants, which are generated to address a specific research question, are phenotyped is very often limited by the expertise, interest and resources available to the individual investigator. However, the systematic broad-based phenotypic screens by consortia of mouse clinics complements these efforts with phenotyping of large numbers of different GM mutant strains. These efforts provide a basis for the characterisation of relationships between gene and function, i.e. associated phenotype. At the same time the phenotyping data coming from these consortia allow an assessment to be made of the scale of potential welfare issues accompanying the widespread generation of GM animals (Osborne *et al*. 2018).

The welfare of GM animals

There has been a focus on animal welfare since the beginning of the era of genetic modification as demonstrated by the inception of an EU workshop in 1995 named Welfare Aspects of Transgenic Animals (Van Zutphen & Van Der Meer 1997). Since then, the topic has been addressed in multiple articles and reports. This literature is summarised and discussed in a recent review (Osborne *et al*. 2018).

Phenotyping is important for keeping and breeding GM animals. It should provide information about any specific problems of a particular strain, thereby allowing the animal care staff to act and improve the conditions of the animals, such as: providing a special diet, special housing or medication. In this context the use of a common language is essential (Bussell & Wells 2015). Ultimately, this will improve animal welfare and the quality of science at the same time (Prescott & Lidster 2017). In addition, the assessment of harm and distress and the setting of humane endpoints can be better informed.

Welfare assessment

In the proceedings of the above-mentioned 1995 EU workshop, indices of good and bad welfare were defined (Broom 1995). Those relating to the former were listed as: changes to normal behaviours; changes to the ability of the animal to perform strongly preferred behaviours and changes to physiological and behavioural indicators of pleasure. The list of indices reflecting poor welfare was much longer and included: reduced life expectancy; reduced ability to grow or breed; body damage; disease; immunosuppression; impairment of physiological and behavioural attempts to cope; behavioural pathology; self-narcotisation when given the opportunity; changes to behavioural aversions; changes to normal behaviour and changes to normal physiological processes and anatomical development.

The relevant tests for assessing the above-mentioned indices can be roughly grouped into: (1) behavioural tests; (2) measurement of production parameters and (3) physiological tests. Most often a combination of indices will have to be studied in order to comprehensively assess the well-being of individual animals or assess the welfare impact of a (combination of) genetic modification.

In 2011, the BVAAWF/FRAME/RSPCA/UFAW Joint Working Group on Refinement[1] published a practical guidance on setting up and operating effective protocols for the welfare assessment of animals used in research and testing (Hawkins et al. 2011). It sets out general principles for more objective observation of animals, recognising and assessing indicators of pain or distress and tailoring these to individual projects. Systems for recording indicators, including score sheets, are reviewed. Guidance is set out on determining practical monitoring regimes that are more likely to detect any signs of suffering. See also Chapter 6: Brief Introduction to welfare assessment: A toolbox of techniques. This practical guidance is equally applicable to the more specific category of GM mice.

The accumulation of data concerning GM mouse lines and their sharing has fuelled discussions on the most appropriate means of making the data available and accessible. The concept of a mouse passport or certificate has been suggested (Jegstrup et al. 2003; Wells et al. 2006). However, with the availability of resources on the web such as Mouse Genome Informatics[2], the Mouse Phenome Database[3] and the International Mouse Phenotyping Consortium[4] the scientific community has access to relevant genome and phenotypic information. It could be argued that putting all that information in one location would be beneficial and reduce the risk of duplication (Osborne et al. 2013).

---

[1] The UK Joint Working Group on Refinement (JWGR) was established in 1989 by the British Veterinary Association Animal Welfare Foundation (BVAAWF), the Fund for the Replacement of Animals in Medical Experiments (FRAME), the Royal Society for the Prevention of Cruelty to Animals (RSPCA) and the Universities Federation for Animal Welfare (UFAW).
[2] http://www.informatics.jax.org (accessed 25 February 2020)
[3] http://phenome.jax.org (accessed 25 February 2020)
[4] https://www.mousephenotype.org/ (accessed 25 February 2020)

Phenotypic characterisation

Phenotyping is essential to establish the relationship between genes and phenotype and to characterise a GM animal. The benefits of a better understanding of the welfare impacts of a genetic modification are also that it contributes to an improved description of the model, which is important for the science in assessing the validity of the animal model.

Forward genetics, an approach used to identify genes responsible for a particular phenotype, is totally dependent on effective phenotyping. ENU (N-ethyl-N-nitrosourea) mutagenesis is aimed at introducing random and mainly point mutations in the genes of premeiotic spermatogonia. See also Chapter 4: An introduction to laboratory animal genetics. After breeding, successful mutations are identified through thorough phenotyping of every animal. This way, any new trait that has arisen as a consequence of the ENU treatment can be discovered (phenotype-driven approach) (Justice et al. 1999).

This broad-based phenotyping strategy should optimise the chance of detecting unexpected effects of any mutation as well (Brown et al. 2006). The phenotype of any genetic modification is a complex interaction between gene allele and genetic background, among other factors. Therefore, the successful targeted mutation of a particular gene may not necessarily result in the expected phenotype (of that gene) or be the only phenotypical change.

For decades, it has been accepted that microbiological and genetic standardisation and quality control of laboratory animals are essential to reduce variability and increase replicability of studies. The same is true for phenotypic characterisation of GM animals. Lack of phenotypic characterisation increases the risk that unidentified traits can cause extraneous variability, as they are not considered when designing the experiment. This could increase the risk of systematic errors which might intervene and confound results leading to false conclusions. See also Chapter 3: The design of animal experiments. Phenotyping the mutant model before setting up the experiment will provide the user with scientifically important information about the animal and allow him/her to implement a better design of the experiment leading to more valid results. Furthermore, new and unexpected traits may be detected that could be of scientific interest to other areas of research. Therefore, accurate characterisation must be considered as an essential aid in defining and selecting the best model and designing the best experiment possible (Barthold 2004).

Systematic, broad-based phenotyping

Early phenotyping protocols

As long ago as 1968, Irvin introduced protocols for systematic identification of behavioural and physiological phenotypes of mice (Irwin 1968). These protocols were designed primarily for pharmacology and toxicology. They have served as an inspiration for protocols such as the SHIRPA protocols[5] (Rogers et al. 1997), which was initially developed for

---

[5] **S**mithKline Beecham, **H**arwell MRC, **I**mperial College School of Medicine at St Mary's, **R**oyal London Hospital **P**henotype **A**ssessment

characterisation of neurological models and based on the principle of a broad primary test battery followed by more specialised secondary and tertiary tests. The SHIRPA protocols have been in use since their introduction, sometimes in a modified form. They have had a profound influence on more recent comprehensive phenotyping protocols.

In 1997, Crawley and Paylor published a series of neurological and neuropsychological tests and a series of specific behavioural paradigms clustered by category, including learning and memory, feeding, analgesia, aggression, anxiety, depression, schizophrenia and drug abuse models, to investigate behavioural phenotypes of transgenic and knockout mice (Crawley & Paylor 1997).

The Mouse Phenome Project

The Mouse Phenome Project[6] was initiated in 2000 by the Jackson Laboratories to develop a comprehensive database encompassing phenotypes of inbred mouse strains and those of GM mice. Data sets are voluntarily contributed by researchers from a variety of institutions and settings, or in some cases, retrieved by the Mouse Phenome Database (MPD) staff from public sources. The MPD maintains a growing collection of standardised reference data that assists investigators in selecting mouse strains for research applications; it houses treatment and control data for drug studies and other interventions; offers a standardised platform for discovering genotype–phenotype relationships and provides tools for hypothesis testing (Maddatu et al. 2012). The MPD also holds phenotyping data on the recently introduced Collaborative Cross and Diversity Outbred mice, which share an extensive pool of genetic variation from eight founder inbred strains (Bogue et al. 2015). The MPD provides several tools for downloading and viewing the phenome data. The tools can be used in combination to enable the scientist to mine the biological information for relevant patterns and correlations (Grubb et al. 2014; Bogue et al. 2018; Bogue et al. 2020).

Eumorphia

Eumorphia (European Union Mouse Research for Public Health and Industrial Applications) was an integrated research programme funded by the European Commission. It was involved in the development of new approaches in phenotyping, mutagenesis and informatics leading to improved characterisation of mouse models for the understanding of human physiology and disease. Eighteen laboratories from eight European countries formed the consortium, which developed over 150 Standard Operating Procedures (SOPs) for phenotyping from 2002 to 2006. These were collected in a database called EMPReSS (European Mouse Phenotyping Resource for Standardised Screens), now called IMPReSS (see the following text). This was the start of a cross-centre comparison of phenotypic data. Across the participating laboratories, SOPs were standardised and validated by using four phenotypically distinct inbred strains (Mandillo et al. 2008).

From EUMODIC to IMPC

Two large-scale phenotyping efforts, the European Mouse Disease Clinic (EUMODIC) and the Wellcome Trust Sanger Institute Mouse Genetics Project (SANGER-MGP), started during the late 2000s with the aim to deliver a comprehensive assessment of phenotypes or to screen for robust indicators of diseases in mouse mutants. They both took advantage of available mouse mutant lines but predominantly of the embryonic stem (ES) cells resources derived from the European Conditional Mouse Mutagenesis programme (EUCOMM) and the Knockout Mouse Project (KOMP) to produce and study 799 mouse models that were systematically analysed with a comprehensive set of physiological and behavioural paradigms (Ayadi et al. 2012).

The EUMODIC consortium captured data from over 27,000 mice and found that 83% of the mutant lines were phenodeviant with, in 65% of the cases, one gene influencing two or more apparently unrelated phenotypes. Furthermore, there were significant differences in phenotype annotations according to the degree of similarity between alleles for each trait (de Angelis et al. 2015).

All lines from the EUMODIC consortium were stored in the European Mouse Mutant Archive (EMMA) repository[7]. EMMA has merged with the wider INFRAFRONTIER project[8] and supports standardised mouse phenotyping services in Europe to ensure results are robust and reproducible. The merger of the two projects has the expanded goals of: Providing access to mouse models, data and scientific platforms and services; Determining genotype–phenotype interactions through cutting-edge analytical and diagnostic methodology in the INFRAFRONTIER mouse clinics[9], one of which is the German Mouse Clinic (Fuchs et al. 2018); Archiving and distribution of mouse strains (Consortium 2015). INFRAFRONTIER closely collaborates with and contributes to the International Mouse Phenotyping Consortium (IMPC)[10].

IMPC was established in 2010 with the aim of completing a catalogue of gene function by deleting and phenotyping all the protein-coding genes in the mouse genome. This project produces knockout mice and carries out high-throughput phenotyping of each line in order to determine the gene function. These mice are preserved in repositories and made available to the scientific community, representing a valuable resource for basic scientific research as well as generating new models for human diseases. IMPC takes every newly generated knockout line through standardised embryo and adult mouse phenotyping protocols.

The IMPC adult phenotyping pipeline involves the analysis of cohorts of at least seven male and seven female mice with a broad spectrum of in-life tests between the ages of 9 and 15 weeks, followed by various terminal tests at 16 weeks. The IMPC pipeline incorporates 20 phenotyping platforms, encompassing diverse biological systems such as

---

[6] https://phenome.jax.org/ (accessed 25 February 2020)

[7] https://www.infrafrontier.eu/infrafrontier-research-infrastructure/organisation/european-mouse-mutant-archive (accessed 25 February 2020)

[8] https://www.infrafrontier.eu/ (accessed 25 February 2020)

[9] https://www.infrafrontier.eu/procedures/animal-welfare-and-ethics/mouse-clinics (accessed 1 May 2020).

[10] http://www.mousephenotype.org (accessed 25 February 2020)

neurological and neuromuscular, sensory, behavioural, cardiovascular, metabolic, respiratory, bone, haematological and clinical chemistry, among others (Brown & Moore 2012). The embryonic pipeline encompasses histopathology and gross morphology of the embryo at defined days *post coitum* and of the placenta.

A wide range of *in vivo* imaging modalities have become available for small animals, some of which are included in the IMPC phenotyping pipeline. Research applications of positron emission tomography (PET), single-photon emission computed tomography (SPECT), computed tomography (CT) and magnetic resonance imaging (MRI) in small animals have been reviewed (Fine et al. 2014).

The phenotype pipeline is available through the International Mouse Phenotyping Resource of Standardised Screens (IMPReSS)[11] (Koscielny et al. 2014). IMPReSS contains definitions of the phenotyping pipelines and mandatory and optional procedures and parameters carried out and data collected by international mouse clinics following the protocols defined. This allows data to be comparable and shareable and ontological annotations permit inter-species comparison which may help in the identification of phenotypic mouse models of human diseases. The IMPReSS protocols do not include welfare assessment.

IMPC has created over 9,000 new knockout lines. The consortium identified 410 lethal genes during the production of the first 1,751 unique gene knockouts, which amounts to about 23% of the genes targeted so far. Furthermore, they observed instances of phenotypes that displayed incomplete penetrance, including variable lethality (sub-viability) (Dickinson et al. 2016).

These efforts to generate a genome-wide catalogue of gene function, taken together with the type of genetic modification technique used, will aid efforts to make a more informed prospective welfare assessment possible and to narrow the attention to specific phenotypes that arise based on the known function(s) of the modified gene(s) (Osborne et al. 2018).

Hypothesis-driven phenotyping

The systematic approach of phenotyping consortia is not common in the more general practice of genetic modification by individual researchers. With gene editing technologies (Certo & Morgan 2016) becoming increasingly commonly used, most GM animals will be generated without the systematic approach of phenotyping. Hence, phenotypes may go undetected, effects on animal welfare may go unnoticed and the effects of confounding and bias may be underestimated.

Before phenotyping – search for information

It is advisable to carry out a thorough (systematic) literature/database review to obtain information about the gene(s) to be modified or the already modified genes of a GM mouse line new to the researcher and/or the institute (Bult 2012). This way, potential phenotypic deviations can be anticipated and acted upon at an early stage. Results from animals with similar mutations and/or mutations in the same area of the genome can also be of great value when gathering information about a particular genetic mutation.

Although a comprehensive database of results from all GM lines does not exist to date, only a limited number of websites need to be searched. The most prominent ones are listed in this chapter.

The MPD[12] (Grubb et al. 2004) and the IMPC consortium website[13] are central databases holding substantial information about phenotypes. Both are annotated according to the Mammalian Phenotype (MP) Ontology (Gkoutos et al. 2005; Smith et al. 2005) and have tools for browsing and searching for phenotypes.

Testing for new traits – the hierarchical approach

In principle, any clinical test could be used to uncover phenotypic details about a specific GM mouse and a variety of SOPs for these tests can be found in published protocols. In view of the huge number of possible tests, it is worth prioritising these to obtain relevant results as quickly and efficiently as possible while also acknowledging the value of negative results. A practical approach to gaining useful information about a mouse strain is to first apply a battery of relatively unsophisticated tests or primary screens such as those of the SHIRPA test (Rogers et al. 1997). These provide a superficial but broad assessment of a mouse phenotype. Various protocols have been proposed which employ this hierarchical approach, focusing either on specific functional domains such as behaviour (Crawley & Paylor 1997; Crawley 2003) or employing a wider selection of screens (Rogers et al. 1997; Murray 2002). Results from these primary screens should point the way to more detailed tests. For example, if a mouse shows a hearing deficiency in the auditory startle test during the primary phenotyping screen, a comprehensive examination of the auditory tract should follow. In this way, phenotypes of interest identified by the primary screen are followed up by more time-consuming, detailed secondary screens.

Phenotyping - how far do you take it?

When phenotyping a mouse strain, difficulties may be encountered in deciding how comprehensive the phenotyping project should be. How many and which tests should be included? Looking at the protocols for phenotyping published in the literature and on the internet, it is obvious that no working procedure is unanimously recommended. As pointed out earlier, GM mice can be very different and are used in so many ways that specific phenotyping needs often arise. However, it is important to avoid approaches that are non-systematic and subjectively biased. It is advised to carry out a systematic investigation into the need for phenotyping and the contribution that the individual protocols can yield in

---

[11] https://www.mousephenotype.org/impress/ (accessed 25 February 2020)

[12] http://phenome.jax.org (accessed 25 February 2020)
[13] http://www.mousephenotype.org (accessed 25 February 2020)

every case of phenotyping, before the project is started. The question of how wide-ranging a basic phenotyping protocol should be – or what the minimum requirements for phenotyping are to obtain meaningful results from the GM line(s) in question – needs to be answered for every single GM line and purpose.

Issues with conventional phenotyping in mice

In our eagerness to find mechanisms and possible cures for human diseases, we should not forget that mice are not small humans. There are a number of fundamental biological differences including the fact they are nocturnal, although we largely phenotype them during daylight hours (Hawkins & Golledge 2018). In addition, our housing conditions may be challenging in terms of inter-species comparisons. The constant need to expend energy for thermoregulation at our laboratory temperatures and constant access to food are not environmental conditions which mirror that experienced by humans.

As new technologies are being developed, progress towards collecting data under more relevant conditions should be a priority.

Automated in-cage behavioural phenotyping

Developments in in-cage automated phenotyping as a complement and potentially a replacement to conventional out-of-cage phenotyping have been reviewed recently (Bains et al. 2018). 'In cage' is the more neutral, precise term, but often the term 'home-cage monitoring' is used. Typically, in-cage monitoring installations make use of different technologies in different combinations, among others: (Infra-Red) video cameras, electromagnetic field sensors, radio-frequency identification (RFID) tags (which requires an intervention to introduce the tag) and ultrasound monitors.

Automated in-cage behavioural phenotyping allows for the non-invasive monitoring of animal behaviours 24 hours a day, 7 days a week (24/7). With this technology, one is less dependent on the availability of reverse daylight suites to study nocturnal animals during their active phase unless one is prepared to work night shifts under more normal light-regimes.

In particular, the non-invasive nature of the continuous monitoring of individual and group-housed mice has proven to be beneficial. This can be carried out in an experimental setting or truly in a home-cage situation, i.e. the cage in which the animals are normally housed in an animal facility. The latter has allowed for the detection of hitherto unobserved activity i.e. locomotion phenotypes in particular mouse models during the dark phase (Richardson 2015). In combination with regular monitoring by experienced staff, continuous monitoring can greatly refine the welfare monitoring of mice (Bains et al. 2018).

After Bains' comparison of home-cage monitoring systems, the digital individually ventilated cage system (DVC™, Tecniplast Spa) has been introduced (Iannello 2019; Pernold et al. 2019). The system's activity metrics represents the overall in-cage activity generated by all mice in a cage, it does not track activity of individual group-housed animals.

Also, a fully automated, high-throughput system for self-initiated conditioning of up to 25 group-housed, RFID-tagged mice was published recently (Erskine et al. 2019). The system can train large cohorts of mice, producing thousands of trials per day across these animals and motivating them to perform without resorting to methods such as severe water restriction. The automated nature of the system largely eliminates the need for experimenter presence and intervention during behavioural tasks.

Phenotyping challenges – the environment

The results of phenotyping not only depend on the genetic make-up of the mutant but can also be influenced by environmental factors, such as cage environment, diet and the microbiological status of the animals (Barthold 2004; Balcombe 2006). Some phenotypes are not expressed until provoked by the environment; for example, diabetes may not develop until the animals are fed a high-fat diet. There is increasing evidence supporting a role of the gut microbiome in behavioural responses associated with pain, emotion, social interactions, food intake (Martin & Mayer 2017; Scheepers et al. 2020). Therefore, the microbiological quality is likely to influence the outcome of behavioural phenotyping tests.

Also, common husbandry practices and experimental procedures significantly influence mouse physiology and behaviour (Gerdin et al. 2012). For example, it has been shown that non-aversive tunnel handling substantially improved mouse performance in behavioural tests compared to traditional tail handling (Gouveia & Hurst 2017)[14]. The procedure whereby an animal is removed from its cage, immobilised and a blood sample taken by puncturing a vein will lead to some level of anxiety, which can significantly influence results obtained.

It is generally thought that when behavioural phenotyping results need to be comparable and replicable it is recommended that environmental conditions are standardised as much as possible and that the conditions under which the results are obtained are documented (Brown et al. 2006). Different environmental factors influence phenotyping results to different degrees and the results of behavioural tests are prone to being very sensitive to variation in environmental factors. However, despite attempts to standardise six behavioural testing modalities between three laboratories, systematic differences in behavioural test outcomes across the three laboratories were detected (Crabbe et al. 1999). This has led others to argue that systematic variation of genetic background and environmental conditions, instead of excessive standardisation, is needed to control the robustness of the results and to detect biologically relevant interactions between the mutation and the genetic background and environmental conditions of the animals (Voelkl et al. 2018). However, changes in environmental enrichment do not appear to lead to increased variation in experimental results (Andre et al. 2018; Bailoo et al. 2018).

---

[14]https://www.nc3rs.org.uk/how-to-pick-up-a-mouse (accessed 3 May 2020)

Another important environmental factor is the phenotyping test itself, and the aspect that different equipment may have different detection sensitivities. Also, the order in which the individual tests are performed can influence the results. This has been investigated in behavioural tests and it has been reported that certain test variables are sensitive to the test order while others are resistant (McIlwain *et al.* 2001). Mice that have become experienced through their participation in some tests change their behaviour significantly in subsequent tests compared with naïve mice (Voikar *et al.* 2004). For this reason, it is best to start with tests that assess anxiety and exploratory activity and to perform the cognitive tests at a later stage.

Phenotyping challenges – other issues

Age and sex

As with comprehensive phenotyping by consortia like IMPC, everyone embarking on phenotyping GM mouse lines should test and characterise animals at different stages of their lives. It has been suggested that animals should be tested at three ages: young, adult and geriatric (Wells *et al.* 2006). Testing takes place at different life stages, because some phenotypic changes are subtle and can be compensated for by other mechanisms. Some may not be apparent in the young animal, but may become apparent at a later stage of life. Some phenotypes are seen only at a specific developmental stage and some in connection with specific physiological conditions such as pregnancy. For those reasons, animals should be characterised at different stages of their lives. Some new traits have been shown not to reveal themselves until after a couple of generations (Van Hoosier 1999). Therefore, consideration should be given to phenotyping strains for several generations.

Also, one should be aware that a phenotype could vary between sexes and so both male and female animals should be tested (Karp *et al.* 2017). Sex is a biological variable, which should be included into the research design and analysis of data (Clayton & Collins 2014; Clayton 2018). Oestrous cycle effects on behaviour have been reported in C57BL/6J and BALB/cByJ female mice (Meziane *et al.* 2007). However, in a meta-analysis of 293 articles, behavioural, morphological, physiological and molecular traits were monitored in male mice and females tested without regard to estrous cycle stage; variability was not significantly greater in females than males for any endpoint and was substantially greater in males for several traits (Prendergast *et al.* 2014).

Genetics

Phenotypic characterisation of a GM line will lead to more reliable results only after reaching genetic stability. Depending on the method of modification, genetic stability may only occur after breeding for some generations (Mertens & Rülicke 2002; Benavides *et al.* 2020). Genetic stability includes a stable mode of transmission of the modification as well as a non-segregating genetic background. Each GM animal created by a gene editing method, such as CRISPR/Cas9, is unique and needs to be analysed for the presence of the correct modification while also identifying mosaic founders. Once identified, the selected founder should be bred with wild-type animals of the same genetic background to evaluate stable transmission of the mutation (Benavides *et al.* 2020). GM animals created by more traditional modification methods may still have a mixed genetic background. This means that the genetic background is a mixture of the strains used in the generation of the mutant (for example: 129 and C57BL/6). The genetic background could contain modifier genes affecting the phenotypic expression of the mutation; hence the 'mixed background' will give variations in the phenotype of these animals – even among siblings. Therefore, ideally phenotyping should not be undertaken until the line is truly congenic (Silva *et al.* 1997; Wakeland *et al.* 1997), and both age-matched homo- and heterozygous animals are tested. Phenotyping of earlier generations of congenic breeding is acceptable when the mixed background status is accurately determined and reported together with the phenotyping results.

The importance of assigning the correct name to a GM line cannot be underestimated. A name designed to according to the international nomenclature rules[15] is the only means to unambiguously distinguish strains from each other (Benavides *et al.* 2020).

Situations might occur where animals are not completely backcrossed to a congenic state before they are used. In that case, it is best to use a larger number of animals for the tests to compensate for the variation in the genetic background. However, establishing this point by breeding or backcrossing several generations can be difficult and also contradictory to welfare considerations in case the strain has a phenotype with a negative impact on the welfare of the animal.

Furthermore, in order to prevent the mutant strain from accumulating genetic changes as a result of genetic drift over time, it is recommended that the strain is maintained by backcrossing to the parental wild-type colony. Also, the wild-type colony should be controlled for genetic drift.

Controls

Colonies shouldn't be kept as homozygous colonies at least for the purpose of phenotyping. The proper controls are age- and sex-matched wild-type siblings from the same breed and parental genotype.

Number of animals

The aim of phenotyping is to find new traits that affect the scientific use of the strain and that may be pertinent in welfare assessment. In order to optimise the chance of detecting these, a sufficient number of animals will have to be tested. As outlined earlier, traits might be subtle or only identifiable under certain conditions (e.g. with age, stress or feeding a specific diet) (Fitzgerald *et al.* 2003). Also, the level

---

[15] https://www.jax.org/jax-mice-and-services/customer-support/technical-support/genetics-and-nomenclature (accessed 3 May 2020)

of intra-strain variability of response will affect the number of mice recommended for a particular test, as the 'background noise' might mask potential phenotypic differences. Furthermore, different test methods have different levels of sensitivity. Such factors make it difficult to estimate how many animals should be used for phenotyping a particular strain. A pilot study should be carried out or previous experimental data referred to in order to establish the values of the above parameters and calculate sample sizes accordingly (Meyer et al. 2007).

Mertens and Rülicke (2002) concluded that for animal welfare, time and expense reasons, it is important to consider the number of animals thoroughly. They have stated that it is not feasible to make a clear-cut recommendation as many factors, such as genetic background, penetration and expression of the mutation and welfare implications, would influence the size of the group necessary. However, they recommended starting with approximately 10 wild-type, 10 hemi- or hetero- and 10 homozygous animals (50% males and 50% females). This would allow statistical calculations and should be regarded as the minimal number of animals for testing. Depending on the results, more animals could be included (Mertens & Rülicke 2002; Bailey et al. 2006). As more results accumulate, one should make a more informed decision on the minimum number of animals that should be included (Festing 2018; Lazic 2018).

It is clear that different GM lines will require different numbers depending also on the effect size. One could use the NC3Rs Experimental Design Assistant as an aid to determine appropriate group sizes (Percie du Sert et al. 2017); see also Chapter 3: The design of animal experiments.

A different, but often very troublesome issue that can affect the number of animals available for phenotyping is the breeding capability of the GM lines. However, if homozygous breeding is avoided, reduced reproductive performance is not much of an issue.

Scientific reporting

While the PREPARE guidelines and checklist cover the three broad areas which determine the quality of the preparation for animal studies (Smith et al. 2018), the implementation of the ARRIVE guidelines and checklist lead to transparent and comprehensive scientific reporting which is essential for the phenotyping methods and results to be scrutinised, evaluated for their methodological rigour, and reproducible (Kilkenny et al. 2010; Percie du Sert et al. 2019).

Summary

In this chapter, we have addressed many aspects of phenotyping. Bearing in mind the many reasons for using GM mice, we shall not attempt to suggest which set of tests to use. Rather, we urge the scientist responsible for the characterisation of the animal to give the issue careful consideration based on the information provided in this chapter. Comprehensive phenotyping may be contracted out to expert centres and networks (Gulinello et al. 2019; Bikovski et al. 2020). However,

the same principles put in place by the expert centres apply to the smaller scale i.e. 'in-house' phenotyping exercises:

1. Search for existing information;
2. Conduct a welfare assessment;
3. Investigate the basic functions of the animal, e.g.:
   a. growth and development of the animal,
   b. lifespan and age-specific mortality,
   c. fertility,
   d. physical examination,
   e. clinical chemistry and haematology,
   f. behaviour;
4. Conduct necropsies (Adissu et al. 2014).

We recommend testing every new strain at three stages: young, adult and geriatric. The mice in each group should be approximately the same age. Homo-, heterozygous and wild-type mice should be tested in both sexes. The line should be backcrossed to full congenicity (more than 10 generations, maybe less when a marker-assisted backcrossing or speed-congenics approach is used) before phenotyping. The order of tests should be considered to minimise one test affecting the result of the next.

It is worth considering testing the strain for several generations and investigating the mutation on different genetic backgrounds. The number of animals in every test group should be at least 10 for the initial testing. Pilot studies for the identification of the optimal number of animals should be carried out.

Concluding remarks

Only very few GM mice are systematically phenotyped – often the process involves no more than daily observation by animal technicians. The widespread use of such observation for the detection of welfare impingement and new phenotypic traits is in many cases regarded as sufficient. There is no doubt that a talented and experienced animal technician is likely to discover even subtle deviations in a GM mouse. Nevertheless, there are traits that produce no immediately observable symptoms. Systematic testing using phenotyping protocols increases the chance of identifying traits, and should be carried out.

For welfare assessment, observation is an excellent tool, as much welfare assessment is based on behavioural studies. However, observation of behaviour alone is not sufficient to evaluate welfare. Furthermore, observations should always be recorded for later reference.

Phenotyping takes time and requires an investment in resources. Testing requires a certain number of age-matched pups. Producing these from a founder animal is a laborious and time-consuming task. Carrying out the actual phenotyping tests can take months and if the mouse is tested at different ages the required time investment increases. However, the advantages of thoroughly phenotyping before using an animal for scientific purposes are obvious and the time for phenotyping should be allocated to any project including GM rodents.

Phenotyping requires expertise. The tests that are used to identify new traits are often complicated and demanding to perform. Behavioural testing is the classic example of a task which requires special skills. The histo-pathological analysis should be performed by a trained and qualified laboratory animal histo-pathologist. The tendency of phenotyping protocols to grow both in size (by adding more tests) and in complexity (by developing more sophisticated methods) leads to increasing demand for specific expertise and resources. However, adequate phenotyping of GM lines is an essential contribution to establishing the validity and reliability of an animal model hence to the quality of the science based on these models and to their welfare assessment.

Acknowledgement

Revised from 'Phenotyping of genetically modified mice' by Rikke Westh Thon, Merel Ritskes-Hoitinga, Hillary Gates and Jan-Bas Prins in *The UFAW Handbook on The Care and Management of Laboratory and Other Research Animals*, eighth edition, Wiley-Blackwell, 2010.

References

Adissu, H.A., Estabel, J., Sunter, D. *et al.* (2014) Histopathology reveals correlative and unique phenotypes in a high-throughput mouse phenotyping screen. *Disease Models & Mechanisms*, **7**, 515–524. doi: 10.1242/dmm.015263.

Andre, V., Gau, C., Scheideler, A. *et al.* (2018) Laboratory mouse housing conditions can be improved using common environmental enrichment without compromising data. *PLoS Biology*, **16**, e2005019. doi: 10.1371/journal.pbio.2005019.

Ayadi, A., Birling, M.C., Bottomley, J. *et al.* (2012) Mouse large-scale phenotyping initiatives: overview of the European Mouse Disease Clinic (EUMODIC) and of the Wellcome Trust Sanger Institute Mouse Genetics Project. *Mamm Genome*, **23**, 600–610. doi: 10.1007/s00335-012-9418-y.

Bailey, K.R., Rustay, N.R. and Crawley, J.N. (2006) Behavioral phenotyping of transgenic and knockout mice: practical concerns and potential pitfalls. *ILAR Journal*, **47**, 124–131. doi: 10.1093/ilar.47.2.124.

Bailoo, J.D., Murphy, E., Boada-Sana, M. *et al.* (2018) Effects of cage enrichment on behavior, welfare and outcome variability in female mice. *Front Behav Neurosci*, **12**, 232. doi: 10.3389/fnbeh.2018.00232.

Bains, R.S., Wells, S., Sillito, R.R. *et al.* (2018) Assessing mouse behaviour throughout the light/dark cycle using automated in-cage analysis tools. *Journal of Neuroscience Methods*, **300**, 37–47. doi: 10.1016/j.jneumeth.2017.04.014.

Balcombe, J.P. (2006) Laboratory environments and rodents' behavioural needs: a review. *Laboratory Animals*, **40**, 217–235. doi: 10.1258/002367706777611488.

Barthold, S.W. (2004) Genetically altered mice: phenotypes, no phenotypes, and Faux phenotypes. *Genetica*, **122**, 75–88.

Benavides, F., Rulicke, T., Prins, J.B. *et al.* (2020) Genetic quality assurance and genetic monitoring of laboratory mice and rats: FELASA Working Group Report. *Laboratory Animals*, **54**, 135–148. doi: 10.1177/0023677219867719.

Bikovski, L., Robinson, L., Konradsson-Geuken, A. *et al.* (2020) Lessons, insights and newly developed tools emerging from behavioral phenotyping core facilities. *Journal of Neuroscience Methods*, **334**, 108597. doi: 10.1016/j.jneumeth.2020.108597.

Bogue, M.A., Churchill, G.A. and Chesler, E.J. (2015) Collaborative cross and diversity outbred data resources in the Mouse Phenome Database. *Mammalian Genome*, **26**, 511–520. doi: 10.1007/s00335-015-9595-6.

Bogue, M.A., Grubb, S.C., Walton, D.O. *et al.* (2018) Mouse Phenome Database: an integrative database and analysis suite for curated empirical phenotype data from laboratory mice. *Nucleic Acids Research*, **46**, D843–D850. doi: 10.1093/nar/gkx1082.

Bogue, M.A., Philip, V.M., Walton, D.O. *et al.* (2020) Mouse Phenome Database: a data repository and analysis suite for curated primary mouse phenotype data. *Nucleic Acids Research*, **48**, D716–D723. doi: 10.1093/nar/gkz1032.

Broom, D.M. (1995) Assessing the welfare of transgenic animals. In *Welfare Aspects of Transgenic Animals. Proceedings EC-Workshop*. Eds Van Zutphen, L.F.M. and Van Der Meer, M. Springer.

Brown, S.D., Hancock, J.M. and Gates, H. (2006) Understanding mammalian genetic systems: the challenge of phenotyping in the mouse. *PLoS Genetics*, **2**, e118. doi: 10.1371/journal.pgen.0020118.

Brown, S.D. and Moore, M.W. (2012) Towards an encyclopaedia of mammalian gene function: the International Mouse Phenotyping Consortium. *Disease Models & Mechanisms*, **5**, 289–292. doi: 10.1242/dmm.009878.

Bult, C.J. (2012) Bioinformatics resources for behavior studies in the laboratory mouse. *International Review of Neurobiology*, **104**, 71–90. doi: 10.1016/B978-0-12-398323-7.00004-5.

Bussell, J. and Wells, S.E. (2015) Talking welfare: the importance of a common language. *Mammalian Genome*, **26**, 482–485. doi: 10.1007/s00335-015-9591-x.

Certo, M.T. and Morgan, R.A. (2016) Salient features of endonuclease platforms for therapeutic genome editing. *Molecular Therapy*, **24**, 422–429. doi: 10.1038/mt.2016.21.

Clayton, J.A. (2018) Applying the new SABV (sex as a biological variable) policy to research and clinical care. *Physiology & Behavior*, **187**, 2–5. doi: 10.1016/j.physbeh.2017.08.012.

Clayton, J.A. and Collins, F.S. (2014) Policy: NIH to balance sex in cell and animal studies. *Nature*, **509**, 282–283.

Consortium, I. (2015) INFRAFRONTIER – providing mutant mouse resources as research tools for the international scientific community. *Nucleic Acids Research*, **43**, D1171–1175. doi: 10.1093/nar/gku1193.

Crabbe, J.C., Wahlsten, D. and Dudek, B.C. (1999) Genetics of mouse behavior: interactions with laboratory environment. *Science*, **284**, 1670–1672.

Crawley, J.N. (2003) Behavioral phenotyping of rodents. *Comparative Medicine*, **53**, 140–146.

Crawley, J.N. and Paylor, R. (1997) A proposed test battery and constellations of specific behavioral paradigms to investigate the behavioral phenotypes of transgenic and knockout mice. *Hormones and Behavior*, **31**, 197–211. doi: 10.1006/hbeh.1997.1382.

de Angelis, M.H., Nicholson, G., Selloum, M. *et al.* (2015) Analysis of mammalian gene function through broad-based phenotypic screens across a consortium of mouse clinics. *Nature Genetics*, **47**, 969–978. doi: 10.1038/ng.3360.

Dickinson, M.E., Flenniken, A.M., Ji, X. *et al.* (2016) High-throughput discovery of novel developmental phenotypes. *Nature*, **537**, 508–514. doi: 10.1038/nature19356.

Erskine, A., Bus, T., Herb, J.T. and Schaefer, A.T. (2019) AutonoMouse: high throughput operant conditioning reveals progressive impairment with graded olfactory bulb lesions. *PLoS One*, **14**, e0211571. doi: 10.1371/journal.pone.0211571.

Festing, M.F. (2018) On determining sample size in experiments involving laboratory animals. *Laboratory Animals*, 002367721773826. doi: 10.1177/0023677217738268.

Fine, E.J., Herbst, L., Jelicks, L.A. *et al.* (2014) Small-animal research imaging devices. *Seminars in Nuclear Medicine*, **44**, 57–65. doi: 10.1053/j.semnuclmed.2013.08.006.

Fitzgerald, S.M., Gan, L., Wickman, A. and Bergstrom, G. (2003) Cardiovascular and renal phenotyping of genetically modified mice: a challenge for traditional physiology. *Clinical and Experimental Pharmacology and Physiology*, **30**, 207–216. doi: 10.1046/j.1440-1681.2003.03818.x.

Fuchs, H., Aguilar-Pimentel, J.A., Amarie, O.V. *et al.* (2018) Understanding gene functions and disease mechanisms: phenotyping pipelines in the German Mouse Clinic. *Behavioural Brain Research*, **352**, 187–196. doi: 10.1016/j.bbr.2017.09.048.

Gerdin, A.K., Igosheva, N., Roberson, L.A. et al. (2012) Experimental and husbandry procedures as potential modifiers of the results of phenotyping tests. *Physiology & Behavior*, **106**, 602–611. doi: 10.1016/j.physbeh.2012.03.026.

Gkoutos, G.V., Green, E.C., Mallon, A.M. et al. (2005) Using ontologies to describe mouse phenotypes. *Genome Biology*, **6**, R8. doi: 10.1186/gb-2004-6-1-r8.

Gouveia, K. and Hurst, J.L. (2017) Optimising reliability of mouse performance in behavioural testing: the major role of non-aversive handling. *Scientific Reports*, **7**, 44999. doi: 10.1038/srep44999.

Grubb, S.C., Bult, C.J. and Bogue, M.A. (2014) Mouse phenome database. *Nucleic Acids Research*, **42**, D825–834. doi: 10.1093/nar/gkt1159.

Grubb, S.C., Churchill, G.A. and Bogue, M.A. (2004) A collaborative database of inbred mouse strain characteristics. *Bioinformatics*, **20**, 2857–2859. doi: 10.1093/bioinformatics/bth299.

Gulinello, M., Mitchell, H.A., Chang, Q. et al. (2019) Rigor and reproducibility in rodent behavioral research. *Neurobiology of Learning and Memory*, **165**, 106780. doi: 10.1016/j.nlm.2018.01.001.

Hawkins, P. and Golledge, H.D.R. (2018) The 9 to 5 Rodent – Time for change? Scientific and animal welfare implications of circadian and light effects on laboratory mice and rats. *Journal of Neuroscience Methods*, **300**, 20–25. doi: 10.1016/j.jneumeth.2017.05.014.

Hawkins, P., Morton, D.B., Burman, O. et al. (2011) A guide to defining and implementing protocols for the welfare assessment of laboratory animals: eleventh report of the BVAAWF/FRAME/RSPCA/UFAW Joint Working Group on Refinement. *Laboratory Animals*, **45**, 1–13. doi: 10.1258/la.2010.010031.

Iannello, F. (2019) Non-intrusive high throughput automated data collection from the home cage. *Heliyon*, **5**, e01454. doi: 10.1016/j.heliyon.2019.e01454.

Irwin, S. (1968) Comprehensive observational assessment: Ia. A systematic, quantitative procedure for assessing the behavioral and physiologic state of the mouse. *Psychopharmacologia*, **13**, 222–257.

Jegstrup, I., Thon, R., Hansen, A.K. and Hoitinga, M.R. (2003) Characterization of transgenic mice – a comparison of protocols for welfare evaluation and phenotype characterization of mice with a suggestion on a future certificate of instruction. *Laboratory Animals*, **37**, 1–9. doi: 10.1258/002367703762226647.

Justice, M.J., Noveroske, J.K., Weber, J.S. et al. (1999) Mouse ENU mutagenesis. *Human Molecular Genetics*, **8**, 1955–1963. doi: 10.1093/hmg/8.10.1955.

Karp, N.A., Mason, J., Beaudet, A.L. et al. (2017) Prevalence of sexual dimorphism in mammalian phenotypic traits. *Nature Communications*, **8**, 15475. doi: 10.1038/ncomms15475.

Kilkenny, C., Browne, W.J., Cuthill, I.C. et al. (2010) Improving bioscience research reporting: the ARRIVE guidelines for reporting animal research. *PLoS Biology*, **8**, e1000412.

Koscielny, G., Yaikhom, G., Iyer, V. et al. (2014) The International Mouse Phenotyping Consortium Web Portal, a unified point of access for knockout mice and related phenotyping data. *Nucleic Acids Research*, **42**, D802–809. doi: 10.1093/nar/gkt977.

Lazic, S.E. (2018) Four simple ways to increase power without increasing the sample size. *Laboratory Animals*, **52**, 621–629. doi: 10.1177/0023677218767478.

Maddatu, T.P., Grubb, S.C., Bult, C.J. and Bogue, M.A. (2012) Mouse Phenome Database (MPD). *Nucleic Acids Research*, **40**, D887–894. doi: 10.1093/nar/gkr1061.

Mandillo, S., Tucci, V., Holter, S.M. et al. (2008) Reliability, robustness, and reproducibility in mouse behavioral phenotyping: a cross-laboratory study. *Physiol Genomics*, **34**, 243–255. doi: 10.1152/physiolgenomics.90207.2008.

Martin, C.R. and Mayer, E.A. (2017) Gut-brain axis and behavior. *Nestle Nutrition Institute Workshop Series*, **88**, 45–53. doi: 10.1159/000461732.

McIlwain, K.L., Merriweather, M.Y., Yuva-Paylor, L.A. and Paylor, R. (2001) The use of behavioral test batteries: effects of training history. *Physiology & Behavior*, **73**, 705–717. doi: 10.1016/s0031-9384(01)00528-5.

Mertens, C. and Rülicke, T. (2002) Phenotype Characterisation and Welfare Assessment of Transgenic Mice. 3R-Info-Bulletin. from http://www.forschung3r.ch/index.html.

Meyer, C.W., Elvert, R., Scherag, A. et al. (2007) Power matters in closing the phenotyping gap. *Naturwissenschaften*, **94**, 401–406. doi: 10.1007/s00114-006-0203-1.

Meziane, H., Ouagazzal, A.M., Aubert, L. et al. (2007) Estrous cycle effects on behavior of C57BL/6J and BALB/cByJ female mice: implications for phenotyping strategies. *Genes Brain Behav*, **6**, 192–200. doi: 10.1111/j.1601-183X.2006.00249.x.

Murray, K.A. (2002) Issues to consider when phenotyping mutant mouse models. *Laboratory Animals (NY)*, **31**, 25–29. doi: 10.1038/5000123.

Osborne, N., Chadwick, C., Haskings, M.-A. et al. (2013) GA passports workshop report - IAT/LAVA congress 2013. *Animal Technology and Welfare*, **12**, 105–109.

Osborne, N., Morton, D. and Prins, J.B. (2018) Welfare concerns in genetically modified laboratory mice and rats. In *Are We Pushing Animals to Their Biological Limits? Welfare and Ethical Implications*, Eds Grandin, T. and Whiting, M., pp. 122–140, CABI, Wallingford, Oxfordshire OX10 8DE, United Kingdom.

Percie du Sert, N., Bamsey, I., Bate, S.T. et al. (2017) The experimental design assistant. *PLoS Biology*, **15**, e2003779. doi: 10.1371/journal.pbio.2003779.

Percie du Sert, N., Hurst, V., Ahluwalia, A. et al. (2019) The ARRIVE guidelines 2019: updated guidelines for reporting animal research. doi: 10.1101/703181.

Pernold, K., Iannello, F., Low, B.E. et al. (2019) Towards large scale automated cage monitoring – Diurnal rhythm and impact of interventions on in-cage activity of C57BL/6J mice recorded 24/7 with a non-disrupting capacitive-based technique. *PLoS One*, **14**, e0211063. doi: 10.1371/journal.pone.0211063.

Prendergast, B.J., Onishi, K.G. and Zucker, I. (2014) Female mice liberated for inclusion in neuroscience and biomedical research. *Neuroscience & Biobehavioral Reviews*, **40**, 1–5. doi: 10.1016/j.neubiorev.2014.01.001.

Prescott, M.J. and Lidster, K. (2017) Improving quality of science through better animal welfare: the NC3Rs strategy. *Laboratory Animals (NY)*, **46**, 152–156. doi: 10.1038/laban.1217.

Richardson, C.A. (2015) The power of automated behavioural homecage technologies in characterizing disease progression in laboratory mice. *Applied Animal Behaviour Science*, **163**, 9.

Rogers, D.C., Fisher, E.M., Brown, S.D. et al. (1997) Behavioral and functional analysis of mouse phenotype: SHIRPA, a proposed protocol for comprehensive phenotype assessment. *Mammalian Genome*, **8**, 711–713. doi: 10.1007/s003359900551.

Scheepers, I.M., Cryan, J.F., Bastiaanssen, T.F.S. et al. (2020) Natural compulsive-like behaviour in the deer mouse (*Peromyscus maniculatus bairdii*) is associated with altered gut microbiota composition. *European Journal of Neuroscience*, **51**, 1419–1427. doi: 10.1111/ejn.14610.

Silva, A.J., Simpson, E.M., Takahashi, J.S. et al. (1997) Mutant mice and neuroscience: recommendations concerning genetic background. *Neuron*, **19**, 755–759. doi: 10.1016/s0896-6273(00)80958-7.

Smith, A.J., Clutton, R.E., Lilley, E. et al. (2018) PREPARE: guidelines for planning animal research and testing. *Laboratory Animals*, **52**, 135–141. doi: 10.1177/0023677217724823.

Smith, C.L., Goldsmith, C.A. and Eppig, J.T. (2005) The Mammalian Phenotype Ontology as a tool for annotating, analyzing and comparing phenotypic information. *Genome Biology*, **6**, R7. doi: 10.1186/gb-2004-6-1-r7.

Van Hoosier, G.L. (1999) The age of biology: opportunities and challenges for laboratory animal medicine. *Scandinavian Journal of Laboratory Animal Science*, **26**, 181–192.

Van Zutphen, L.F.M. and Van Der Meer, M. (1997) *Welfare Aspects of Trangenic Animals*. Springer, Berlin, Germany.

Voelkl, B., Vogt, L., Sena, E.S. and Wurbel, H. (2018) Reproducibility of preclinical animal research improves with heterogeneity of study samples. *PLoS Biology*, **16**, e2003693. doi: 10.1371/journal.pbio.2003693.

Voikar, V., Vasar, E. and Rauvala, H. (2004) Behavioral alterations induced by repeated testing in C57BL/6J and 129S2/Sv mice: implications for phenotyping screens. *Genes, Brain and Behavior*, **3**, 27–38. doi: 10.1046/j.1601-183x.2003.0044.x.

Wakeland, E., Morel, L., Achey, K. *et al.* (1997) Speed congenics: a classic technique in the fast lane (relatively speaking). *Immunol Today*, **18**, 472–477. doi: 10.1016/s0167-5699(97)01126-2.

Wells, D.J., Playle, L.C., Enser, W.E. *et al.* (2006). Assessing the welfare of genetically altered mice. *Laboratory Animals*, **40**, 111–114. doi: 10.1258/002367706776318971.

6 Brief introduction to welfare assessment: a 'toolbox' of techniques

Jennifer Lofgren

Introduction

It is critical both for the direct benefit to the animals and the resulting science that those responsible for the care and engagement of animals in research be able to accurately assess their welfare. As better tools for welfare assessments are developed and validated, a better understanding of how to not only minimise negative welfare states but build positive welfare states can be achieved. Welfare assessments are at the heart of one of the 3Rs, refinement, as one can only improve the animal's experience in research if one first understands how to accurately measure current welfare state and identify an improvement through the proposed refinement. This chapter will explore the basic principles of a welfare assessment and provide species-specific examples of commonly used welfare assessments to form a welfare assessment 'toolbox'.

Basic principles of welfare assessment

Unlike adult humans, the welfare of animals cannot be assessed by asking for a direct verbal indication of their subjective state (which is generally accepted as the 'gold standard' indicator of subjective experiences) (Paul et al. 2005). Instead, there is a range – a 'toolbox' – of indirect measures of the clinical, physiological and neurophysiological/chemical, and behavioural components that reflect the welfare of non-human animals. These tools can be used to ask two questions that, between them, capture both the physical and mental aspects of animal welfare: 'are animals healthy?' and 'can they engage in their telos?' (Dawkins 2004; Rollins 2015). By this, it is meant that not only is their body sound and free of physical harm but that they are able to express the species-typical behaviours that allow them to fulfil their natural drivers (Christiansen & Forkman 2007). Since these tools only provide an indirect indication of an animal's health or its subjective state, it is necessary to use multiple welfare assessments to triangulate their welfare state.

Considerations when assessing welfare

What is normal?

When developing new or choosing established welfare assessments, one must ensure that the background or normal state for a given species for a given parameter is known, and the assessment must be evidence based. Even within a particular species, *Mus musculus* for example, significant diversity in normal behaviours has been demonstrated in males versus females, young versus old, and between strains (Chesler et al. 2002; Sternberg et al. 2004; Rosen et al. 2017; Lariviere & Mogil 2010; Mogil et al. 2020). Therefore, whether developing an entirely new welfare assessment or applying a validated assessment to new conditions or patient population, it is important to first become familiar with what is normal for a given parameter in the animals to be evaluated (Table 6.1).

In addition to the signalment of the animal, one must consider potential influence of other variables to common welfare assessments. What is normal for the animal may change significantly throughout a light/dark cycle, as well as throughout the seasons in the year. Even in a controlled laboratory environment, animals practice a circadian rhythm of activity and respond to subtle changes in humidity and temperature throughout the year (Chelser et al. 2002). For example, nocturnal animals have higher thresholds for mechanical and thermal stimuli at night when they are more active and lower thresholds during the day when they are at rest (Christina et al. 2004). So, it is helpful to understand these normal fluctuations in baseline welfare assessments to both understand when the measures may be most accurate for the assessment being made and to keep measurement times consistent to help control for these changes.

The UFAW Handbook on the Care and Management of Laboratory and Other Research Animals, Ninth Edition.
Edited by Huw Golledge and Claire Richardson.
© 2024 John Wiley & Sons Ltd. Published 2024 by John Wiley & Sons Ltd.

Table 6.1 Key references providing information about the natural biology and behaviour of mice and rats (see also the species-specific chapters in this handbook for information about these and other laboratory animals).

Species	Relevant publications
Rodents	Würbel, H., Burn, C. and Latham, N. (2015). The behaviour of laboratory mice and rats. In: *The Ethology of Domestic Animals: An Introductory Text*, 3rd edition (ed. P. Jensen), 272–284. Boston: CABI.
Mouse (*Mus musculus*)	• See the website Mousebehavior.org for behaviour definitions, including video examples, by Dr. Joseph Garner and colleagues (2002) at the Stanford School of Medicine and Garner (2006). • Latham and Mason (2004) From house mouse to mouse house: the behavioural biology of free-living *Mus musculus* and its implications in the laboratory. *Applied Animal Behaviour Science*, **86**, 261–289. • Olsson *et al*. (2003) Understanding behaviour: the relevance of ethological approaches in animal welfare science. *Applied Animal Behaviour Science*, **81**, 245–264.
Rat (*Rattus norvegicus*)	• Burn (2008) What is it like to be a rat? Rat sensory perception and its implications for experimental design and animal welfare. *Applied Animal Behaviour Science*, **112**, 1–32. • Whishaw and Kolb (Eds) (2004) *The Behavior of the Laboratory Rat*. Oxford University Press, New York.

The 'welfare assessment toolbox'

Now that we have reviewed what considerations must be made to maximise the potential for accurately assessing welfare, a welfare assessment can be selected. There are several different reasons for assessing welfare, and these influence which tool may be right for the job.

For example, the method will depend upon factors such as:

1. assessing day-to-day welfare;
2. assessing positive, negative or neutral change to welfare following an environmental manipulation (e.g., the provision of a potential environmental enrichment);
3. assessing preference or strength of motivation for particular resources (e.g., social access, food, etc.);
4. assessing for the presence of negative welfare (specifically unalleviated pain) following an experimental procedure.

The next sections describe the tools available to those wishing to assess welfare in relation to the conditions in which they might be useful. However, note that this is only intended as a brief introduction to each of these methods. Many of the welfare assessment techniques described below could fill an entire chapter or article in themselves (and indeed do in other publications, e.g., Hawkins *et al*. 2011; Mellor 2017; Appleby *et al*. 2018). Thus, those wishing to use any of the following methods are encouraged to familiarise themselves more fully with the literature about their chosen method(s) – particularly in relation to their subject animal of interest.

Routine welfare monitoring

Cage observations

Particularly for prey and non-diurnal species, direct observation of the animal for evidence of poor welfare can be limited; thus, careful evaluation of the home-cage environment may provide more obvious and sensitive indicators of the animal's health and well-being. Where direct observation of the animal may allow for the identification of new behaviours indicative of poor welfare, such as limping, cage observation typically yields evidence of a lack of normal behaviours, such as unused nesting material. These types of measures have been termed '*resource input*' measures of welfare assessment (Leach *et al*. 2008) or '*proxy indicators*' of welfare (Dunbar *et al*. 2016). Interestingly, these kinds of assessments can be more sensitive indicators of welfare than other more traditional measures of welfare such as weight loss (Oliver *et al*. 2018) allowing for earlier identification of declining welfare and, therefore, more timely interventions. This may be because engagement in these kinds of behaviours, such as nest building, is more optional for maintaining homeostasis, and therefore, they are discontinued more easily and earlier than more requisite behaviours, such as eating or drinking. Examples of this kind of approach can be found in Table 6.2. While the assessments described in this table are rodent focused, similar types of assessments could be made for any species. As discussed in the above section, once a normal repertoire of behaviour is known, visual evidence that those normal behaviours occurred in the home cage can be identified. This may be disappearance (consumption or hoarding) of favourite treats, a well-formed resting space or manipulation of a toy, shelter or other environmental enrichment. If that visual cue is not present, the animal is likely not engaging in that normal behaviour. For an example that takes advantage of the average home-cage set-up, see Arras *et al*. 2017. For examples that include an addition of a research intervention, i.e., burrowing (Jirkof *et al*. 2010) or grooming assessments, see Figure 6.1. Note that the home environment must be furnished with valued, interactive structural and non-structural enrichments to help facilitate expression of species-typical behaviours. A barren home environment leaves little opportunity for the expression or assessment of normal behaviours. See also Chapter 10: Enrichment: animal welfare and scientific validity. Additionally, the strength of the motivation to engage in particular behaviour must be considered. If the motivation is extremely high, as was the case with guinea pigs and the consumption of parsley,

Table 6.2 Examples of home-cage assessments that may indicate health and/or welfare problems in laboratory animals.

Assessment	Reference
Nest consolidation	Rock *et al*. 2014; Negus *et al*. 2015; Oliver *et al*. 2018
Nest score	Gaskill *et al*. 2013a; Jirkof *et al*. 2013
Cage organisation	Arras *et al*. 2007
Grooming efficacy	Oliver *et al*. 2018
Burrowing	Deacon 2006; Jirkof *et al*. 2010
Wheel running	Häger *et al*. 2018

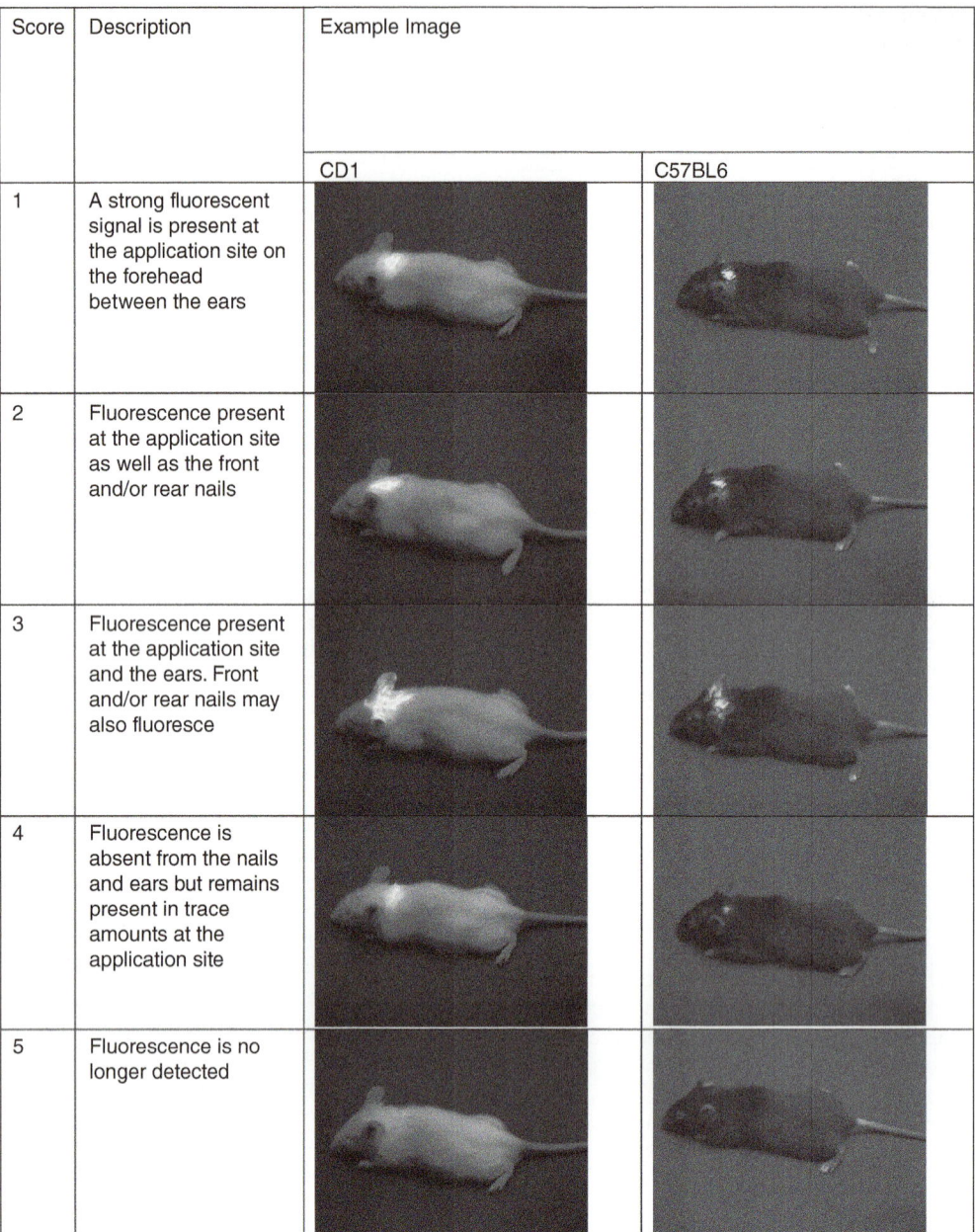

Figure 6.1 Grooming transfer test: as the mice engage in normal grooming behaviour, they transfer an inert pigment suspended in mineral oil from the site of application on the top of their head to their paws and ears before they begin to effectively groom it completely away. The time course required for this sequence of events is delayed if the animals have a disruption to their normal grooming behaviours, such as after a surgery (Oliver *et al*. 2018 / with permission form AALAS).

the animal may choose to engage in that behaviour in conditions of positive or negative welfare (Dunbar *et al*. 2016). Thus, pilot assessments and validation of new measures are recommended prior to reliance on a novel proxy indicator for welfare assessment.

Other cage assessments can include evidence of unconsumed food or water, presence of diarrhoea, urine, blood or other secretions around the cage walls or bedding should lead to a closer examination of animals within (and possibly also within neighbouring cages) to check for physical signs that may identify the affected individual(s), e.g., matted fur around the anogenital area, signs of dehydration (e.g., as assessed by the skin tent test) (Thurman *et al*. 1999). The number of fecal boli produced in a new space or after an acute stressor, such as after placement in a clean cage or exposure to predator scent, has been used as an indicator of stress in rats (Ennaceur *et al*. 2006; Bowen *et al*. 2012; Franks *et al*. 2014).

Physical condition

Monitoring the physical appearance of animals can be a quick and non-invasive method of assessing welfare and the one that can easily be incorporated into routine daily or weekly checks

(Leach *et al.* 2008; Campos-Luna *et al.* 2019). Examples of some of the parameters that can be assessed are given in Table 6.3.

Table 6.3 Examples of routine observations of physical appearance (note that some of these are specific to certain species).

Body area	Observations
Head	Is the head consistently being tilted to one side?
Ears	Are ears upright and alert or rotated down or to the side of the head?
Eyes	Is there evidence of orbital tightening or are eyes fully open?
	Are the eyes sunken or bulging?
	Are the pupils constricted or dilated?
	Are there signs of opacity in the eyes?
	Are there abnormal secretions, crusting or signs of inflammation of the mucous membranes?
Nose	Are there signs of chromodacryorrhoea[a]?
	Is the skin over bridge of the nose contracted resulting in cheek bulging or a V shaped nasal planum?
	Are there abnormal secretions or crusting?
Teeth	Are the teeth overgrown or damaged? Is the fur on the chin wet or matted?
Whiskers	Are there any signs of damage to the whiskers (possibly due to barbering) (Figure 6.2)?
	Are whiskers relaxed and cascading in an arch from the cheek or are they extending rigidly straight and perpendicular from the head?
Body	What is the body condition of the animal (e.g., emaciated, obese, etc.)?
	Are there any obvious lumps?
	Is the body shape asymmetrical?
	Are there any wounds from fighting?
	Is the curve of the back gentle and relaxed or is it arched with the feet tucked under the abdomen?
Fur	Is the fur dull and unkept?
	Are there signs of piloerection (raised fur)?
	Is there any hair loss?
Anogenital area	Are there signs of rectal or vaginal prolapse? Urine or fecal staining?
Breathing	Is the animal's breathing noisy or laboured?
	Is there an abdominal component to the breathing?

[a] discussed in detail in Assessing welfare: physical and physiological measures section.

Physical condition measures such as these are often incorporated into distress scoring systems (e.g., the scoring sheets as displayed in Committee on Recognition and Alleviation of Distress in Laboratory Animals 2008, p. 109–110), body condition scoring assessments in mammals (Ullman-Cullere & Foltz 1999; Clingerman & Summers 2005) and zebra fish (Clark *et al.* 2018) and guidelines for assessing health and physical condition in laboratory animals (e.g., Foltz & Ullman-Cullere 1999; Campos-Luna *et al.* 2019). A review of score sheets ranging from osteotomy models and abdominal surgery to neurosurgical models and experimental autoimmune encephalomyelitis can be found in a special issue of *Laboratory Animals* (Golledge & Jirkof 2016; Lang *et al.* 2016; Graf *et al.* 2016; Pinkernell *et al.* 2016; Palle *et al.* 2016). In non-human primates (NHPs), alopecia scoring is commonly used as a welfare indicator (Luchins *et al.* 2011). Many of these physical signs are vague in nature and do not indicate a specific underlying problem or aetiology. Thus, animals exhibiting signs of poor physical condition (particularly multiple signs, or physical *and* behavioural signs [see earlier in this chapter]) should be assessed by veterinary staff. The assessment of such parameters is somewhat more qualitative (and hence can be more susceptible to between-observer variability; see, e.g., Beynen *et al.* 1987 and Campos-Luna *et al.* 2019) than some other measures of physical condition, e.g., body weight (which will be discussed later on). However, the assessment of physical appearance can have benefits over other more quantifiable measures in certain situations. For example, physical appearance can be assessed non-intrusively (i.e., the animals can be assessed visually and do not need to be removed from the home cage) (Ullman-Cullere & Foltz 1999). In certain situations, though, it may be beneficial to supplement visual examinations of an animal's condition with a physical examination. For example, Beynen *et al.* (1987) found that gallstone-bearing mice did not differ in physical appearance from non-gallstone-bearing individuals but did differ by exhibiting signs of discomfort during abdominal palpation. Additionally, body condition scoring is often more accurate when it includes palpation of the animal, such as in the case of tumour growth or ascites, which can mimic a higher body condition score due to masking of loss of muscle or fat stores.

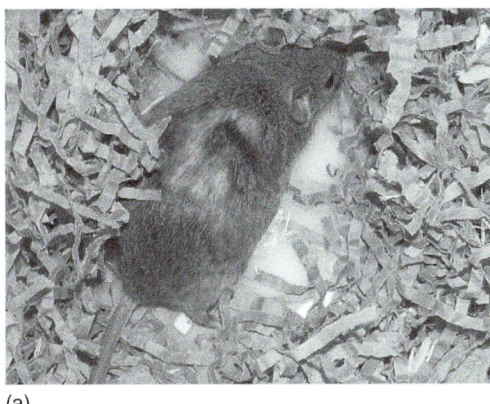
(a)

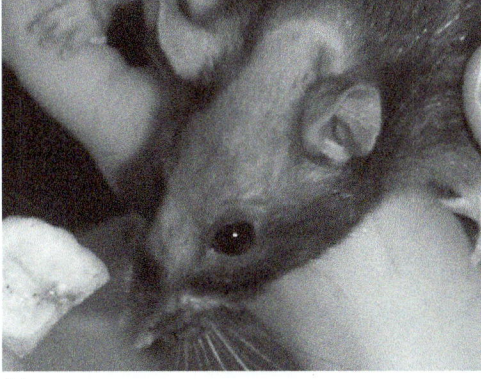
(b)

Figure 6.2 (a) A mouse that has been barbered on its head and whiskers and on its back respectively. (b) A rat that has been barbered on its head. (Pictures: N. Latham.)

Chromodacryorrhoea

Chromodacryorrhoea (also sometimes known as 'red tears' or 'bloody tears') is the name for red staining around the eyes and nose that occurs when the Harderian glands over-secrete porphyrin. This is commonly used as a welfare indicator in rats, with chromodacryorrhoea occurring (or becoming more severe) following 'stressors' such as cage-cleaning, visits by unfamiliar people, handling or restraint, and animal facility maintenance (Harkness & Ridgway 1980; Mason *et al.* 2004; Abou-Ismail *et al.* 2008; Burn *et al.* 2008), but has also been used as a welfare indicator in pigs (Telkänranta *et al.* 2016). Chromodacryorrhoea has also been used (in rats and other species) to assess the effects of certain pharmacological manipulations (Burgen 1949; Harkness & Ridgway 1980; Rupniak & Williams 1994), including the pharmacological induction of acute inflammation (Harper *et al.* 2001). Chromodacryorrhoea has a number of advantages over other physiological measures of 'stress'. For example, it can be assessed non-invasively and relatively non-intrusively, and unlike other physiological stress responses (e.g., hypothalamic–pituitary–adrenal (HPA) axis activity), it has not yet been reported to be increased by physical activity *per se* or 'excitement' (Burn *et al.* 2006). However, this measure has the disadvantage that it is of limited use in species other than rats (since many other laboratory species do not exhibit chromodacryorrhoea), and it is a product of parasympathetic activity, which is not well understood in terms of welfare.

The onset of chromodacryorrhoea is relatively quick. For example, chromodacryorrhoea has been reported to occur within 10 minutes of handling or 20 minutes of restraint (although onset can vary according to the size of the individual) and ceases after approximately 2 hours (Harkness & Ridgway 1980; Burn 2005). Since grooming (which can also be elicited by 'stressors') removes evidence of chromodacryorrhoea, observations must be made within the initial time period during which chromodacryorrhoea occurs (Burn *et al.* 2006). Several numerical scoring systems are published for grading the severity of chromodacryorrhoea; for examples of a scoring system, see Telkänranta *et al.* 2016 for pigs and Figure 6.3 for rats.

Body weight

Body weight is commonly used as an indicator of health and/or welfare in research animals. Body weight is often measured repeatedly during a study, in order to allow the ongoing assessment of this measure as well as comparison between treatments (Spangenberg *et al.* 2006; Abou-Ismail *et al.* 2008; Simone *et al.* 2008; Brenneis *et al.* 2017). However, a number of other factors may also influence this measure, including age, activity levels and reproductive cycling (Spangenberg *et al.* 2005; CRADLA 2008, p. 34), as well as tumours and fluid accumulation (as discussed above). Body weight can also be significantly influenced by anaesthetic and analgesics, opiates in particular as they suppress consumptive behaviour in mice and guinea pigs (Oliver *et al.* 2017, 2018) and can, at high doses, induce pica in rats (Schaap *et al.* 2012; Nunamaker *et al.* 2018). Thus, assessments of body weight should ideally include comparisons with appropriate (e.g., age- and sex-matched) controls and, where possible, after first quantifying the impact of confounders, such as anaesthetics or analgesics, that may mask benefits or harms of an intervention or procedure. Body weight may also be used as a criterion for humane end points in studies, as the rapid loss of a certain percentage of weight can be considered one criterion for euthanasia; while 20% body weight

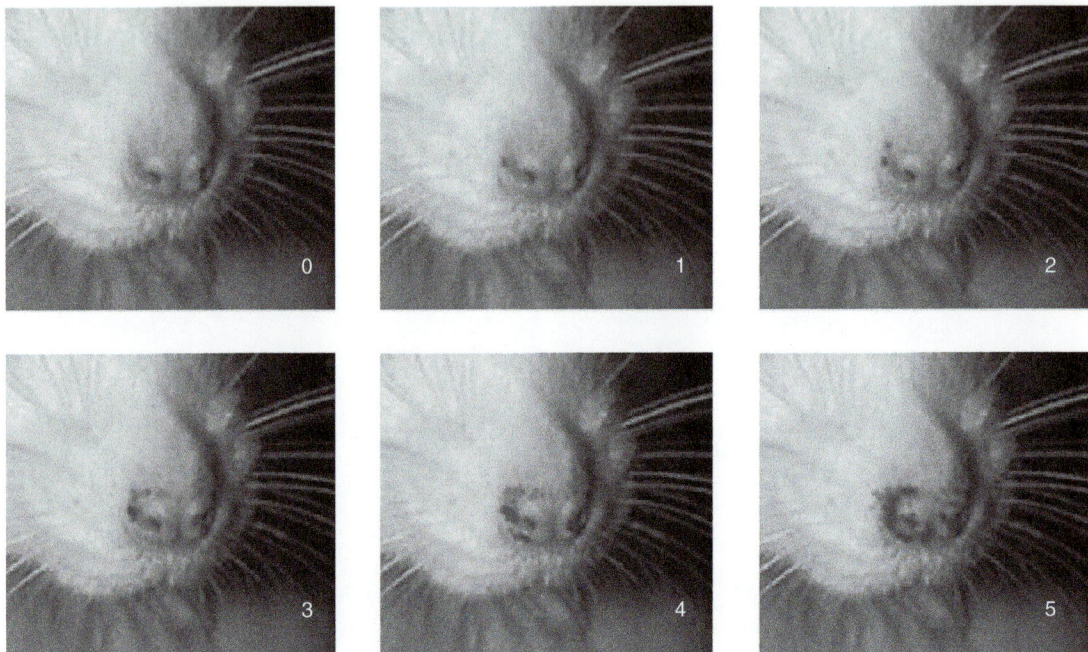

Figure 6.3 Scoring system for assessing the severity of chromodacryorrhoea in rats. Note that the pictures are not actual photographs of chromodacryorrhoea of differing severities. The pictures have been digitally altered to illustrate the severity of chromodacryorrhoea required for each of the scoring grades. (Picture: Charlotte Burn.)

loss is often used in rodents (Ullman-Cullere & Foltz 1999), the exact percentage should be selected with consideration to the specific model and experimental procedures (Talbot et al. 2020).

Assessing welfare and changes in welfare: physiological measures

HPA axis activity

HPA axis activity culminates in the release of glucocorticoids – usually corticosterone in rodents and cortisol in other animals – from the adrenal cortex. This release of glucocorticoids functions to mobilise energy stores (CRADLA 2008, p. 37), and therefore, HPA axis activity often increases in conditions where an increase in activity may be appropriate. Increases in HPA axis activity then additionally occur during flight/fight responses in aversive situations, but they also occur during other heightened states of arousal, including during coitus and hunting prey (Szechtman et al. 1974; Rushen 1991; Walker et al. 1992; Toates 1995) and, therefore, have frequently been used as indicators of welfare. Increases are measurable after common laboratory animal experiences, such as transportation or cage change (Fernstrom et al. 2008; Ochi et al. 2016). There are a number of variables that significantly impact HPA axis independent of changes in welfare. For example, glucocorticoid levels exhibit circadian variation, with peak levels occurring prior to the onset of the active phase (Terlouw et al. 1995) necessitating taking samples at the same time of day or samples that are averaged over a 24-hour period; additionally, the provision of anaesthetics, frequently needed to collect blood samples, can also increase glucocorticoid levels (Crockett et al. 2000; Hohlbaum et al. 2018). Thus, although HPA axis activity is commonly referred to as the 'physiological stress response', it is necessary to remember that increases in glucocorticoids are not restricted to aversive situations. Additionally, chronic stress may actually result in a dulled and ineffective HPA axis, decreasing stress hormone release (Novak et al. 2013). Hence, measures of HPA axis activation must be interpreted cautiously (and, preferably, in combination with other indices of welfare). A thorough review of how and when HPA axis assessments is *Limits to using HPA axis activity as an indication of animal welfare* by Otovic and Hutchinson (2015).

Glucocorticoids, or their metabolites, can be assessed in blood (Vahl et al. 2005), saliva (Lutz et al. 2000), urine (Touma et al. 2003), faeces (Lepschy et al. 2007) or even hair samples (Davenport et al. 2006), and the timescales differ for each of these sampling methods. Thus, glucocorticoids are released into the blood within a few minutes; they appear in the saliva a few minutes later (Kirschbaum & Hellhammer 2000); their metabolites appear in urine and faeces roughly 1–2 hours and 9–10 hours later, respectively, although this varies according to species, sex and the time of glucocorticoid release (Touma et al. 2003; Lepschy et al. 2007); and changes in glucocorticoid levels can be measured in hair samples some weeks later (Davenport et al. 2006). Due to the differences involved in sample collection and the timescales over which the responses appear, there are pros and cons to each of the sampling techniques listed above, and these are detailed briefly in Table 6.4.

Table 6.4 Pros and cons of the different methods of glucocorticoid analysis.

Sample type	Pros	Cons
Blood	Allows accurate assessment of acute glucocorticoid responses	Sample collection is invasive Potential risk of sampling procedure influencing sample levels (if sample is not collected quickly enough) Provides information about levels at one moment in time ('point sample'[a]) Low sample stability[d] Vulnerable to circadian variation[b,d]
Saliva	Allows accurate assessment of acute glucocorticoid responses Non-invasive sampling method	Only non-invasive in species that can be trained to provide samples or that readily chew the collection device Training may be lengthy and not always successful[c] Provides information about levels at one moment in time ('point sample'[a]) Vulnerable to circadian variation[b,d]
Urine/faeces	Sampling can be non-invasive Less vulnerable (but not invulnerable) to circadian variation Provides an assessment of glucocorticoid levels over several hours ('steady-state' sample[a])	Assessment of acute responses may require repeated sampling during the time period at which responses typically appear in the urine/faeces Represents stress incurred over hours to a day rather than in previous minutes before sampling[d]
Hair	Non-invasive sampling method Not vulnerable to circadian variation[d] The most stable sample[d]	Provides only a chronic index on the order of months of glucocorticoid responses

[a] CRADLA (2008).
[b] samples must be collected at the same time of day.
[c] Lutz et al. (2000).
[d] Novak et al. (2013).

Other 'stress' hormones

Although HPA axis activity is the most commonly assessed hormonal 'stress' response, plasma levels of various other hormones are also sometimes monitored. These include catecholamines, such as adrenaline (epinephrine), prolactin, growth hormone, luteinising hormone and oxytocin (Manteca 1998; Paul et al. 2005; CRADLA 2008). Similar caveats to those that apply to HPA axis activity also apply to many of these measures in terms of the influence of circadian variation, invasive sampling techniques and the fact that these hormones are also released in response to neutral or even pleasurable stimuli. Indeed, oxytocin release (in contrast to many physiological measures) often occurs during bonding experiences, such as suckling and maternal care as well as social bonding, and, therefore, tends to be interpreted as indicating positive affective responses (Carter 2001; Rault et al. 2017). Vasopressin has also been indicated in the reward and social bonding neural networks in a variety of species (Albers 2015). Hence, this may be a potential measure if we consider welfare to be not only about the reduction of negative feelings but also the promotion of positive feelings (Paul et al. 2005; Boissy et al. 2007; Yeates & Main 2008).

Immune response

There is an important intersection between stress hormones, the HPA axis, and immune system function. Acute and chronic stress can induce changes in the white blood cell populations, sometimes referred to as a stress leukogram characterised by a neutrophilia and lymphopenia, resulting in a decreased lymphocyte:neutrophil ratio (Jain 2005; Moroni et al. 2011). This has been demonstrated in a wide range of laboratory animals, including fish (Fuentes & Newgren 2008; Swan & Hickman 2014; Grzelak et al. 2017; Hickman 2017). In addition, increased stress hormones can result in decreased immune system effectiveness, resulting in changes in thymocytes, increased tumour growth and metastasis (Franchi et al. 2007; Benish & Ben-Eliyahu 2010; Hutchinson et al. 2012; Peterson et al. 2017; Jirkof 2017; Lofgren et al. 2018). Natural Killer cell activity is known to become suppressed by increasing corticosterone and other stress hormones (Gaspani et al. 2002; Franchi et al. 2007). Leukocyte coping, as measured by oxygen radical production, is a more recent welfare assessment tool demonstrated to be negatively impacted by increasing stress (Gelling et al. 2010; Gaudio et al. 2018; Huber et al. 2019).

Autonomic responses

Autonomic responses, such as heart rate (particularly 'stress-induced' elevations from baseline levels), heart rate variability, blood pressure, respiratory rate and body temperature, are frequently used to assess welfare animals (Duke et al. 2001; Boissy et al. 2007; von Borell et al. 2007; Arras et al. 2007; Taitt & Kendall 2019). Autonomic responses are also commonly used to monitor physiological functioning in biomedical research and to monitor general activity levels (Irvine et al. 1997; Gross et al. 2008). However, these measures seem to be less commonly used, at present at least, to assess welfare in research animals (although some examples include Beerda et al. 1998; Duke et al. 2001; Sharp et al. 2002; Arras et al. 2007). Autonomic responses may be less commonly used here because monitoring them often requires the use of telemetry devices that: (i) must be surgically implanted into the research subjects; and (ii) are still relatively large and heavy compared to the body size of most research animals (the vast majority of which are mice and rats). Thus, although some researchers report that telemetric assessment of autonomic responses provides information about welfare that otherwise may not have been observed (Arras et al. 2007), the low popularity of this method may stem from the desire to avoid using a method that requires surgical implantation of a device that may cause discomfort once implanted. Nonetheless, where animals are telemeterised for the purposes of research, there is an opportunity to use the data for assessing welfare. Recent developments in automated, non-invasive assessments including for respiratory rate that can be paired with general activity measures, wheel running, and even automated ethogram scoring may provide new opportunities to assess some physiological parameters without requiring surgery (Rasid et al. 2012; Lim et al. 2019; Baran et al. 2020; Baran et al. 2021). A drawback to this technology is that it may require single housing, thus incurring welfare costs of its own. New commercially available jacket telemetry is now available not only for larger species like NHPs and dogs but also rats. These may more easily facilitate social housing during data collection. Another approach is to co-house an animal with a telemeter with a non-telemeterised animal to ensure a clear individual signal while also providing social housing.

Assessing welfare and changes in welfare: behavioural measures

Behavioural signs associated with reduced welfare range from gross changes in the home-cage behaviour of animals to subtle (but significant) changes in cognitive testing paradigms. As alluded to earlier, the ability to identify changes, particularly in spontaneous home-cage behaviour, that (are likely to) indicate reduced welfare requires an understanding of the species' natural behaviour and the animals' normal behaviour under captive conditions. Thus, researchers assessing behavioural measures of welfare should ensure that they are familiar with both of these aspects of their subject animals' behaviour.

Monitoring routine behaviour

Routine checks of home-cage behaviour can also be used to monitor welfare in laboratory animals (Leach et al. 2008) and, like physical parameters, behaviour is often incorporated into distress scoring systems (CRADLA 2008, p. 109–110) and guidelines on assessing health and welfare (Foltz & Ullman-Cullere 1999; Campos-Luna et al. 2019). General activity in the home cage can be helpful indices of welfare, and new automated systems are making this far easier and more powerful (Brenneis et al. 2017; Lim et al. 2019).

If the animals are inquisitive about human observers, expressed by approaching or staying oriented and alert to the observer, rearing, sniffing or vocalising when the observer

Table 6.5 Examples of home-cage behaviours that may indicate health and/or welfare problems in laboratory animals.

Inactivity or lethargy
Hyperactivity
Aggression
Abnormal gait
Reduced exploratory behaviour
Social isolation
Hunched or abnormal posture
Huddling
Ataxia (lack of coordination)
Signs of paresis or paralysis
Writhe
Twitch
Back arch
Weight shifting

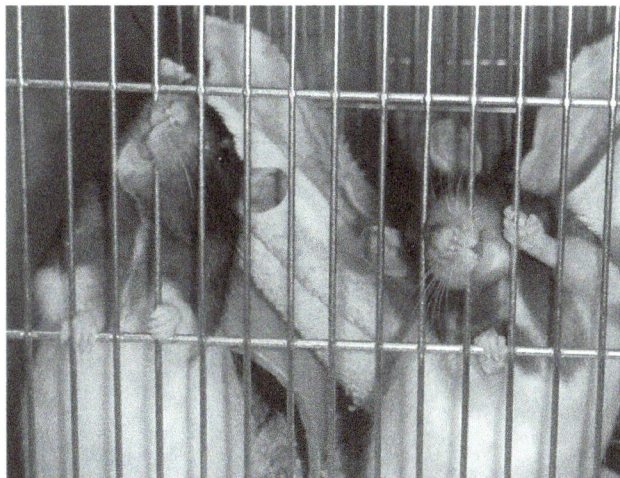

Figure 6.4 Bar-biting in rats. (Picture: Charlotte Burn.)

is cageside, this may also serve as a normal behaviour to assess. Routine positive interactions with care or research staff not only help build human–animal bonds and acclimation to people but can also facilitate this kind of interactive behaviour as a simple animal welfare screening tool. An example from one facility was a care technician who hand fed each rabbit in their room a Cheerio (a small whole grain cereal) during morning rounds. When a rabbit did not hop to the front of their pen to take their morning treat, the technician knew the rabbit required additional welfare assessments. More quantitative approaches can be used, as well. Similar approaches are well described for many large animal species such as cats (Stella & Croney 2019), dogs and NHPs (Bloomsmith et al. 2018). A more detailed overview of behavioural assessment methods that can be used cageside or when reviewing remotely recorded video can be found in Bateson and Martin (2021). Examples of home-cage behaviours that might indicate health and/or welfare problems are given in Table 6.5 (note that this table deals primarily with those behaviours that might be observed in quick, routine checks on animals – it does not include those behaviours that must be assessed over longer time periods, such as stereotypic behaviour, as these will be addressed later in the chapter). Observations of home-cage behaviour (e.g., the frequency of twitching, writhing and rearing behaviour) can also be useful in assessing pain following experimental procedures (see section on assessing pain) but may require remote video if animals suppress pain-associated behaviours in the presence of an observer (Oliver et al. 2017). Automated ethogram scoring is possible in several behavioural assessment platforms (Flecknell & Roughan 2004; Roughan & Flecknell 2006), though only recently have these been developed to include assessments in the home cage, even when animals are socially housed (Bains et al. 2016, 2018; Redfern et al. 2017).

Stereotypic behaviour

Stereotypic behaviours are highly repetitive behaviours that do not have a readily apparent function caused by myriad of drivers that may or may not correlate to poor welfare (Poirier & Bateson 2017; Cabib 2006). When developing a welfare assessment toolbox, it is important to be able to recognise stereotypies when they arise, as in some circumstances they can be symptoms of an animal's unmet social, environmental or medical need. Common examples of stereotypic behaviour in laboratory rodents include bar-biting (Figure 6.4), somersaulting ('back-flipping') and jumping (Würbel 2006), while examples in research primates include pacing, rocking and digit-sucking (Novak et al. 2006). There is also an enormous diversity in the prevalence and severity of stereotypic behaviour observed in different laboratory species. For example, stereotypic behaviours have been estimated to develop in approximately 50% of mice in standard laboratory cages, but they appear to be much less common in rats and possibly even absent in guinea pigs (Würbel 2006, p. 88); lower prevalence of stereotypic behaviour has been reported more recently in mice, but behavioural observations were made during the light portion of the light cycle, when mice are typically less active (Leach & Main 2008). However, species differences may be due, in part, to inconsistencies in whether or not comparable behaviours are defined as stereotypic in different studies (see the example of bar-biting in rats cited by Würbel (2006) and discussed later in this section).

Stereotypic behaviour is the most commonly used behavioural measure of welfare, but the relationship between stereotypic behaviour and welfare is somewhat complex. The diversity of stereotypic behaviours performed by animals may reflect the diversity of underlying mechanisms that can cause their performance. Some stereotypic behaviours may indeed stem from repeated, frustrated attempts to perform motivated behaviours. Indeed, although stereotypic behaviours often superficially appear to be functionless, a number of studies have elegantly demonstrated the underlying motivation and affective states leading to the behaviour (Dallaire et al. 2011; Pomerantz et al. 2012a,b; Novak et al. 2016; Poirier & Bateson 2017). For example, bar-biting in mice stems from attempts to escape from the cage (Nevison et al. 1999b), and stereotypic digging in gerbils stems from the desire for a naturalistic burrow (Wiedenmayer 1997). However, in some cases, the performance of the stereotypic behaviour itself may be rewarding, acting as a substitute behaviour for motivated behaviours (termed 'DIY enrichments'). In other cases, the stereotypic behaviour may reflect environmentally induced changes in behavioural control processes that cause animals to be unable to inhibit behavioural responses to environmental stimuli ('perseverative' behaviour) (Mason & Latham 2004). Stereotypic behaviours may also, through frequent repetition, become performed out of habit (and shifted into an automatic form of processing known as 'central control'). As a result, different types of stereotypic behaviour (within the same species, and even within individuals) should not necessarily be considered directly comparable in their implications for welfare. Hence, while it is generally accepted that environments that increase stereotypic behaviour are associated with decreased welfare, those individuals exhibiting the most stereotypic behaviour within stereotypy-inducing environments may not have the worst welfare (as assessed by other welfare measures) – perhaps because they have found a stereotypic behaviour that helps them to 'cope' with their poor environment, or because their stereotypic behaviour reflects changes in behavioural control processes (Mason & Latham 2004).

Vocalisations

Vocalisations, including ultrasonic vocalisations that are outside the range audible to humans, have been well studied in research animals for many years. Vocalisations are increasingly being used as a tool to assess both positive and negative welfare in a variety of species. There is a large body of work utilising vocalisations as welfare indicators in rodents (mice (Weiner et al. 2016); rats (Brudzynski & Ociepa 1992; Burman et al. 2007; Mällo et al. 2007; Cloutier & Newberry 2008; Chisholm et al. 2013; Cloutier et al. 2014). Vocalisations have also been used as a method of welfare assessment in primates (olive baboons, Crowell Comuzzi 1993; marmosets, Cross & Rogers 2006; Bakker et al. 2014), companion species (dogs, Gazzano et al. 2008) and even agricultural species (pig, Maigrot 2018; Viscardi & Turner 2018; Laurijs et al. 2021 and cattle, Green et al. 2018). Most attention has been paid to vocalisations associated with negative subjective states, such as ultrasonic alarm calls (22 kHz) (Cuomo et al. 1992; Litvin et al. 2007; Chisholm et al. 2013) or audible vocalisations (Burman et al. 2008a) in rats. Indeed, questions concerning the welfare of animals within auditory range of conspecifics producing such vocalisations have also been raised (Burman et al. 2007). Since welfare researchers are increasingly acknowledging the importance of positive subjective states for good welfare (Paul et al. 2005; Boissy et al. 2007; Yeates & Main 2008), there is an increasing focus upon vocalisations that indicate positive feelings. The best known and most commonly studied of these is the 50-kHz call in rats – the so-called rat 'laughter', which can be elicited by tickling rats and mimicking play behaviour (Panksepp & Burgdorf 2000, 2003; Rygula et al. 2012; LaFollette et al. 2017) or which increase during food consumption, mating, electrical self-stimulation of the brain or the use of addictive drugs (Wöhr et al. 2008). However, some researchers have recently suggested that experience, context and individual differences can influence 50-kHz calls, and that some caution is required when interpreting these calls with respect to their welfare implications (Wöhr et al. 2008; Webber et al. 2012; Schwarting 2018).

Anticipatory behaviour

Anticipatory behaviour is the behavioural response that is *'elicited by rewarding stimuli that lead to and facilitate consummatory behaviour'* (Spruijt et al. 2001). Anticipatory behaviour is associated with feelings of 'wanting'; this is termed 'incentive salience' and is different to 'liking', which is the hedonic pleasure associated with consummatory behaviour (Berridge & Robinson 1998). Anticipatory behaviour has mainly been investigated in rats using classical Pavlovian training tasks, whereby a 'reward' (such as a sugary food, the opportunity to mate or interact with others) is announced by a 'conditioned stimulus', e.g., the sound of a bell. The amount of active behaviour performed by the animal(s) is then scored during the intervening period between the animal hearing the bell and the presentation of the reward (Van den Berg et al. 1999, 2000; Von Frijtag et al. 2000, 2001). This activity score is then compared with that of control animals that heard the bell but did not receive the reward. However, anticipatory activity is not expressed in the same way in different species and is not universally associated with negative affective state, anxiety or frustration (Makowska & Weary 2016; Krebs et al. 2017; Riemer et al. 2018; Chincarini et al. 2019). For example, rats exhibit an increase in anticipatory activity in the period between the conditioned stimulus and the arrival of the reward, while domestic cats exhibit a decrease in the number of behavioural transitions during this time. It has been suggested that this may reflect species differences in food-acquisition behaviour: for example, rats actively explore for food while cats often employ a 'sit-and-wait' strategy when close to prey (Van den Bos et al. 2003). Anticipatory behaviour can be used to assess sensitivity (incentive salience) to different types of rewarding stimuli (Van Der Harst et al. 2003b, 2005), or to assess (poor) housing-induced sensitisation of the mesolimbic dopaminergic system (Van Der Harst et al. 2003a). Caution should be used when interpreting the underlying mechanisms driving a change in anticipatory behaviour. For example, while a more barren housing condition increases anticipatory behaviour in rats, medications that treat anxiety and depression were ineffective in lessening this change (Makowska & Weary 2016).

Affect-driven attention biases including cognitive biases

Tasks assessing affect-driven attention biases (ADABs) are one of the most recently developed tools in the welfare assessor's toolbox and are nicely reviewed in detail by Crump et al. (2018). One of the simplest methods available is looking time, which refers both to how quickly and how long the subject looks at a cue and benefits from technical advances in automated eye tracking. This technique has been used to assess welfare in a wide variety of species including sheep, cattle, dogs, birds and NHPs (Brilot et al. 2009; Bethell et al. 2012; Lee et al. 2016; Monk et al. 2018; Lee et al. 2018). Look time at a cue associated with stress can decrease with anxiolytics and enriched environments (Vögeli et al. 2014; Lee et al. 2016; Monk et al. 2018). Importantly, look time must be considered in the context of the species' natural behaviours. For example, while typically cues perceived as threats are looked at for longer periods of time, stressed rhesus macaques decrease their look time at images of other rhesus demonstrating threatening faces (Bethell et al. 2012).

More advanced ADABs include cognitive bias. Cognitive bias methods of animal welfare assessment were proposed by Mendl, Paul and colleagues (Mendl & Paul 2004; Harding et al. 2004; Paul et al. 2005) and are based on the wealth of evidence from the human literature that people who report negative feelings tend to make negative judgements about ambiguous stimuli or anticipated events, while those reporting positive feelings tend to make more optimistic judgements (Paul et al. 2005). Recently, these tasks have been modified for use in animals (Roelofs et al. 2016; Crump et al. 2018). For example, Harding et al. (2004) trained rats to perform a lever press to one auditory stimulus (a tone) in order to receive a food reward and to refrain from pressing the lever following a different tone in order to avoid 30 seconds of loud white noise. The rats were then housed in different types of housing and subsequently tested with the training tones and three intermediate (ambiguous) tones. Harding and colleagues found that rats housed in 'unpredictable' housing made fewer and slower responses to the tone associated with food and the ambiguous tones that were closer to it – findings that are comparable with those in anxious or depressed humans. Similar techniques and results indicating 'pessimistic' and 'optimistic' behaviour have subsequently been published in further studies in a wide variety of species (Mendl et al. 2009; Bateson & Matheson 2007; Matheson et al. 2008; Burman et al. 2008b). Given the increased emphasis on positive subjective feelings in welfare research (Boissy et al. 2007; Yeates & Main 2008), tasks that enable us to assess positive feelings (such as optimism) are, thus, an important addition to the welfare assessment toolbox. A caution regarding cognitive bias studies in animals was published: in exposing animals to the ambiguous probe, the study design must be careful not to inadvertently extinguish response behaviours to the positive and negative options (Barker et al. 2018). This inadvertent study design confounder can be avoided by including both choice and latency measures (Crump et al. 2018).

Assessing welfare and changes in welfare: brain measures

The processes that lead to affective states and the physiological and behavioural indicators of welfare that we assess are regulated by the brain. Thus, affective states are elicited by neural processing (e.g., in the amygdala and limbic regions) of the rewarding and punishing properties of sensory stimuli (Rolls 1999; Panksepp 2003; Burgdorf & Panksepp 2006). Stimuli then elicit physiological responses by additional processing through regions including the hypothalamus, pituitary and brainstem, and behavioural responses by additional processing through the basal ganglia, ventral tegmental area, motor cortical areas and cerebellum (Sapolsky 1992; Toates 2004). Thus, welfare can be assessed by monitoring activity or changes in these regions: for example, by assessing glucocorticoid activity or receptor levels or neurotransmitter functioning (e.g., dopaminergic functioning) (Broom & Zanella 2004). Indeed, a number of aspects of brain functioning have been correlated with physiological or behavioural indicators of welfare: for example, numerous studies have found a correlation between aspects of dopaminergic functioning (particularly dopamine receptor levels) and stereotypic behaviour (McBride & Hemmings 2005; Lewis et al. 2006; Wilkes et al. 2020). Cytochrome oxidase, reflective of neuronal metabolic activity, in the basal ganglia has been used to assess the potential impact of either standard or super-enriched environments on the welfare of deer mice (Bechard et al. 2017). One disadvantage of assessing brain function is that it can be invasive, such as requiring surgical electrode implants or requiring post-mortem brain analysis, and in some cases, the most humane killing methods cannot be used because they disrupt the brain regions of interest. While previously limited to human emotional states, new technological advances with functional magnetic resonance imaging (fMRI), positron emission tomography (PET) and two-photon microscopy, it is now possible to assess brain activity non-invasively in conscious animals (Phan et al. 2004; Harris et al. 2015; Dopfel & Zhang 2018; Sugita et al. 2018). However, refinements may still be necessary to effectively utilise these methods to evaluate animal welfare as the restraint training required for imaging of awake animals can, in and of itself, impact the animal's welfare (Jennings et al. 2014; Low et al. 2016).

Assessing animals' preferences and motivation for resources

In addition to assessing welfare itself, the welfare researchers' toolbox also includes tools for identifying potential methods of improving welfare. Thus, we can assess animals' preferences and motivation for resources by asking animals to 'vote with their feet' (or fins in the case of fish) and tell us how they feel about their environment and choices that we offer them (Dawkins 1980; Held et al. 1995; Kirkden & Pajor 2006; Krueger et al. 2020). A thorough review on the various published approaches to assessing preference and motivation can be found in (Franks 2019). These assessments are often used as a way of identifying potential refinements to laboratory housing (e.g., environmental enrichments), and the two most commonly used methods (and hence those that will be discussed here) are preference tests and consumer demand studies. However, while these tools enable us to identify potential refinements, the long-term effects of these refinements should then be double-checked using the tools described in previous sections. This additional assessment is necessary because, for example, defendable resources may elicit undesirable behaviours such as territorial behaviour in group-housed animals, and animals (like humans) do not always make choices or behave in ways that maximise their long-term welfare (Silverman 1978; Rutherford 2002).

Preference tests

Preference tests (as their name implies) investigate the preference of animals for particular resources when given a choice, and they have been a popular tool in welfare research for many years (Amdam & Hovland 2011; Bateson 2004). Preference tests can be used to assess animals' preferences for different environmental characteristics such as: cage cleanliness (Godbey et al. 2011), cage height and light intensity (Blom et al. 1992; Colson et al. 2021); cage temperature (Gaskill et al. 2012), different substrates (Kirchner et al. 2012); nesting surface (Hunniford et al. 2017; running wheels (Walker & Mason 2018); social contact (Sørensen et al. 2010); climbing structure orientation, e.g., with marmosets (Pines et al. 2005); and environmental enrichment options, e.g., with singly housed fish (Krueger et al. 2020). Preference for the resources is usually measured by time spent with (using) the resources (whereby most time = most preferred). Automated systems are now available to automatically score time spent in various chamber choices (Tsai et al. 2021).

However, there are a number of criticisms that have been levelled at preference tests and *caveats* that should be borne in mind when using them. These have been addressed in detail in a number of places (Kirkden & Pajor 2006; Franks 2019), so the main criticisms detailed in these other reviews will only be briefly discussed here. The first of these is that preference tests only tell you about the relative preference for different resources, not the absolute strength of motivation for any of the resources. Thus, a preferred resource may only be weakly more reinforcing – e.g., a preference for strawberries over blackberries – or alternatively it may be much more reinforcing – e.g., copulatory rather than exploratory behaviour.

Second, short-term and long-term welfare are not necessarily always compatible. Hence, animals may exhibit preferences for resources that maximise their immediate welfare, but welfare but may adversely affect their longer-term welfare. For example, rodents develop qualities of addiction when able to self-administer substances in their home cage, later developing qualities of alcohol and opiate abuse (Green & Grahame 2008; Monroe & Radke 2021). A further interesting example is provided by Buttigieg et al. (2014) who found that after a short-term feeding of either high-fat diet or regular diet, those mice in the high-fat diet group subsequently preferred the high-fat diet when given a subsequent choice, whereas those in the regular diet group continued to have no preference. If the mice continue on the high-fat diet, they can develop negative metabolic effects.

Third, behaviour in preference tests may be confounded by differential use of the resources, for example, due to time of day effects (Van de Weerd et al. 1998), or strong but periodic motivation to use resources that provide opportunities for motivated behaviours (such as an enhanced motivation for nesting material in pre-parturient animals, or access to a potential mate when females are in oestrus). Fourth, preferences can be influenced by the prior experience of the animals. Thus, for example, animals that are used to living in cages may initially show a preference for cages rather than an outdoor pen (Fraser & Matthews 1995). Deer may also demonstrate a significant preference for familiar feeding sites, even when new comparable feeding sites become available (Ranc et al. 2020).

Finally, preference tests are designed to test preference between two substitutable resources (i.e., two resources that satisfy the same motivation). Kirkden and Pajor (2006) (see also Fraser & Matthews 1995) suggest that a preference test between non-substitutes (e.g., food versus litter) would have little meaning from the animals' point of view since the comparison would not be between the resources but between the strengths of the different motivations. Thus, preference tests can provide useful information about environmental features that may enhance animals' welfare. However, preference tests must be carefully designed so that the link between an animal's preferences and their welfare is valid and reliable.

Consumer demand

Consumer demand tasks were introduced into animal welfare research in the 1980s, and they are based on ideas traditionally used by economists studying the spending patterns of humans faced with a choice of products and limited income (Dawkins 1983). The basic premise behind consumer demand tasks is that there is an inverse relationship between the price of a resource and the amount that a consumer will buy. By increasing the price of the resource, the researcher can then quantify the value that the consumer places on the resource, measuring one or more of the following: (1) the top price that the consumer is willing to pay ('reservation price'); (2) the total amount of income spent on the resource ('consumer surplus'); and (3) the willingness of the consumer to keep on paying for the resource as the price increases ('elasticity of demand') (Varian 1993; Gwartney et al. 2005, pp. 56–82). The advantages and limitations of these methods in animal welfare research are addressed in detail by Kirkden and Pajor (2006) (see also Jensen et al. 2004).

Consumer demand studies have an advantage over preference tests in that they can tell us about the strength of motivation for different resources; we can even determine the absolute strength of this motivation if we 'titrate' it against motivation for essential resources, such as food (termed '*yardstick*' resources, Dawkins 1983; see also Warburton & Mason 2003). In animal welfare studies, consumer demand tasks require animals to 'pay' to gain access to resources, either by performing an operant task (e.g., lever pressing – termed fixed ratio (FR) schedules) (e.g., Sherwin 2004b, 2007) or by increasing the effort required (e.g., pushing weighted doors or traversing water) to achieve access to various resources such as food or a conspecific (Sherwin & Nicol 1995, 1996; Seaman et al. 2008). These can be powerful tools for questioning assumptions about the animal's relative priorities. For example, female New Zealand White (NZW) rabbits worked just as hard for access to food as they did for access to a conspecific, countering the assumption that NZW rabbits are not a social species and underscoring the need to provide social housing to this common laboratory animal (Seaman et al. 2008). Consumer demand tasks can, thus, be used to assess (quantitatively) motivation for different environmental characteristics in laboratory animals (Manser et al. 1996; Sherwin 1998; Seaman et al. 2008), farmed animals, where consumer demand techniques are probably even more extensively utilised (Gunnarsson et al. 2000; Mason et al. 2001; Jensen et al. 2004; Dixon et al. 2014), and even fish (Sullivan et al. 2016).

However, like preference tests, there are a number of factors that must be borne in mind when designing consumer demand tasks; these are also reviewed in more detail by Kirkden and Pajor (2006). For example, motivation for some resources may be influenced by whether or not the resource can be seen (i.e., for some resources *'out of sight = out of mind'*) (Warburton & Mason 2003), and where the cost of accessing the resource must be *'paid'*, e.g., whether the cost is paid on entry or exit from the resource (Warburton & Nicol 1998). Furthermore, many consumer demand tasks use animals that are individually housed, yet individual housing may affect motivation for resources (Sherwin 2003; Cooper 2004); see also the Anticipatory Behaviour section). Thus, finding methods of assessing motivation in group-housed animals (Sherwin 2004b, 2007) may be more complex, but ultimately more appropriate where animals are typically group housed (as most laboratory animals are).

Assessing pain

Animals' experience of pain has been the centre of as much debate as animals' experience of affective states ('emotions') such as pleasure or suffering. Pain is defined as *'An unpleasant sensory and emotional experience associated with, or resembling that associated with, actual or potential tissue damage'* (Raja et al. 2020). In addition to the physical components of pain in animals, it is known that psychological stress can exacerbate pain in animals (Low et al. 2016). Common regulations governing education and research with animals require the assumption that animals can experience pain. For example, the U.S. Government Principles for the Utilization and Care of Vertebrate Animals Used in Testing, Research, and Training state that 'Unless the contrary is established, investigators should consider that procedures that cause pain or distress in human beings may cause pain or distress in other animals'[1].

As in general welfare assessment, the ability to assess pain is greatly enhanced by understanding animals' normal appearance and behaviour and species-typical pain responses (Flecknell & Thomas 2015 Flecknell 2018; American College of Laboratory Animal Medicine (ACLAM) 2007; Turner et al. 2019). Without a clear understanding of these differences, one may misinterpret a post-procedural welfare assessment as negative when it may be reflective of a normal state, or vice versa. For example, C3H strain male mice have a significantly higher mouse grimace score than their female counterparts, as well as several other strains, even in the absence of any painful procedure (Miller & Leach 2015; Miller et al. 2015). Without first understanding their baseline, a high grimace score for these mice after surgery may result in a false positive score for pain when in fact, if there is no difference in the pre to post-procedural score, appropriate analgesia has been achieved. The converse can also be true. Guinea pigs can be highly treat motivated. Without appropriate understanding of this significant behavioural driver, one might assume that a guinea pig that quickly consumes a treat, such as parsley, after surgery indicates they are comfortable and have effective analgesia. However, when paired with a remotely scored ethogram and mechanical nociceptive assay, it was identified that the guinea pigs were actually demonstrating significant behavioural signs of unalleviated pain, even while also quickly consuming their parsley treat (Dunbar et al. 2016).

The presence of anaesthetics and analgesics can have direct drug effects on pain assessments, even in the absence of pain. Without understanding the expected effect size and duration of a drug on a pain measurement, one might over or under interpret the presence of unalleviated pain. For example, opiate analgesia given in the absence of a painful procedure may suppress consumptive behaviours in rodents resulting in weight loss similar to what is measured in post-surgical rodents for which no analgesia was given (Olivier et al. 2017, 2018). If weight loss alone is used as a measure of pain, the presence of opiates may result in a false positive indication of poor welfare. Buprenorphine can also significantly increase ambulatory behaviours in mice, confounding the ability to use distance travelled or ambulatory activity as a welfare measurement (Miller et al. 2015; Olivier et al. 2018; Lofgren et al. 2018). Isoflurane, in the absence of any other stimuli, can significantly delay nesting consolidation behaviour and grooming in mice as well as suppress grimace scores (Miller et al. 2015; Miller et al. 2016; Olivier et al. 2018). However, application of anaesthetics and analgesics is a necessary and important component of assuring appropriate animal welfare and should not be avoided simply to reduce confounders to welfare assessments. Rather, understanding the potential impact of a given drug on the welfare assessment is important to allow for the estimation of the 'drug effect' and allows for the isolation of a 'pain effect' in the post-procedural setting. For example, in analgesia efficacy studies, it is valuable to have animals serve as their own controls with assessments at baseline, after drugs in the absence of the potentially painful procedure, and again after an appropriate washout period, with the same drugs are provided in combination with the potentially painful procedure. Not only does this allow for fewer animals to be used for the study, but it provides better control of inter-animal variation and quantifies the impact of the drugs on the assessments such that they can be controlled for and a true assessment for the presence of unalleviated pain can be made. It is equally important to note that despite potential negative impacts of anaesthetics and analgesics on either the animals themselves, such as weight loss, or on the resulting research, unalleviated pain can have significant and negative impacts that in some research models may be a greater variable posed by than the analgesic (Franchi et al. 2007; Lofgren et al. 2018).

The research environment itself can mask or exacerbate the outcome of a welfare assessment. Therefore, careful acclimation of the animal patient to the environment in which the assessments will occur and the staff that will be involved in the assessments present, prior to a potentially painful development, is key for facilitating baseline, as well as unmodulated post-procedural response. Where possible, the same person should take serial measurements throughout the study period to reduce inter-observer variation and reduce stress on the animals. It can take up to a week for mice to acclimate after shipping and the presence of new or unfamiliar animals, sounds, smells, or sights can result in a similar stress, potentially altering the welfare measurement. So, provision of an appropriate acclimation and conditioning period is always advisable. This includes acclimation to their cagemates, as the presence of unfamiliar cagemates,

---

[1] https://olaw.nih.gov/policies-laws/phs-policy.htm (Accessed December 5, 2022)

particularly among males, can result in suppression of pain behaviour expression (Langford *et al.* 2006; Mogil & Bailey 2010). Who is doing the measuring and how they are taking the measurement can also significantly impact welfare assessments (Mogil 2017). One study evaluating the potential impact of a variety of environmental factors on mouse nociceptive assays identified the experimenter performing the test as the most important factor, more so than the animal's sex, time of day or cage density (Chesler *et al.* 2002). Therefore, it is important that the same person perform pain assessments for longitudinal evaluations of an animal's pain state. The sex of the human conducting the welfare assessment, if conducted in the presence of the animals, has been shown to significantly alter the animal's response. The presence of a human male has been shown to result in suppression of some pain behaviours in mice; interestingly, this suppression was prevented if human female pheromones were also present (Sorge *et al.* 2014). However, even female handlers, simply by being present cageside, can result in significant suppression of pain behaviours such as the mouse grimace score and behavioural ethogram in guinea pigs (Miller & Leach 2015; Olivier *et al.* 2017). Handling and restraint have also been shown to layer on a level of stress that can significantly modulate response, whether physiological or behavioural, to painful stimuli (Mogil 2017). For both of these reasons, remote evaluation through technologies like telemetry, video and smart caging can be advantageous for identifying authentic responses to a potentially painful or distressing aspect of a study.

Thorough reviews of clinically relevant pain assessments in rodents can be found in (Tappe-Theodor *et al.* 2019) and (Negus 2019). Indeed, training in pain assessment techniques ranging from recognition of new, pain-specific behaviours including use of a behavioural ethogram featuring behaviours such as writhing or twitching, scoring pain faces (i.e., grimace scale scores, to assessing for loss of normal behaviours such as reduced use of environmental enrichments or grooming (see earlier in the chapter for examples) may help researchers to identify and score pain more accurately and sensitively (Flecknell & Roughan 2004, Flecknell 2018). Like welfare, pain is often assessed by monitoring general measures of body functioning, such as changes in body weight, reduced feeding and drinking (Weary *et al.* 2006), physiological responses, including HPA axis activity (Wright-Williams *et al.* 2007) and behaviour, including pain-related behaviour, vocalisations and loss of normal behaviours (Cooper & Vierck 1986; Jourdan *et al.* 1998); see also ACLAM (2007).

Concluding remarks

Laboratory animal welfare is critical, not only for ethical reasons but also because of its often under-appreciated impact on scientific validity (Gaskill & Garner 2017; Garner *et al.* 2017). Although animals cannot be asked about their feelings directly, there is a broad (and increasing) range of tools available, which can be used to provide an indirect indication of animals' subjective states. Many of these tools have been described in this chapter. The diversity of tools in the welfare assessor's toolbox means that different methods are available for the different types of welfare assessment that might be necessary during the course of a research animal's life. Thus, the physical appearance and home-cage behaviour of animals can be used to monitor their welfare on a day-to-day basis, while longer-term or treatment effects on welfare can be assessed by measuring physiological responses (e.g., HPA axis activity – the physiological 'stress response'), immune function, brain function, home-cage behaviour (e.g., stereotypic behaviour), vocalisations and performance in behavioural paradigms that reveal sensitivity to rewarding stimuli and cognitive states, such as optimism.

Tools are also available (tasks designed to assess preference and motivation for resources) that enable potential refinements and the building of positive welfare to laboratory housing to be identified – techniques that are regularly used in the growing field of refinement research. When used, and appropriately analysed, these techniques can help the identification and assessment of animals' negative and positive subjective states and find techniques of refining housing and husbandry practices and experimental procedures that make a genuine and meaningful difference to the welfare of research animals. Thus, for example, such research has shown that laboratory mice prefer environments that contain nesting material and indeed will work to get nesting material (Roper 1975; Van de Weerd *et al.* 1998), and that providing nesting material can help to reduce behavioural problems such as aggression (Van Loo *et al.* 2002) as well as reduce the significant variable of cold stress (David *et al.* 2013; Ganeshan & Chwala 2017). Hence, the provision of nesting material is now widely recommended for laboratory mice (Jennings *et al.* 1998; Gaskill *et al* 2013b and c), and its presence in mouse cages is used as a 'resource input' measure of welfare by animal care staff and researchers (Leach *et al.* 2008; Gaskill *et al.* 2013a; Jirkof *et al.*, 2013; Rock *et al.* 2014; Oliver *et al.* 2017).

Finally, for many years (even dating back to the thoughts of Jeremy Bentham 1789), questions about welfare have focused upon animal suffering. Therefore, it is encouraging that the increased interest in finding tools that enable us to assess positive subjective states reflects the increasing emphasis on the importance of ensuring that research animals do not suffer more than is necessary, and that they experience positive subjective states, such as pleasure, and hence actually have good (and not just the absence of poor) welfare.

Acknowledgements

I would like to thank Dr Naomi Latham, the author of the first version of this chapter which I have updated.

References

Abou-Ismail, U., Burman, O., Nicol, C. *et al.* (2008) Let sleeping rats lie: does the timing of husbandry procedures affect laboratory rat behaviour, physiology and welfare? *Applied Animal Behaviour Science*, **111**, 329–341.

Albers, H.E. (2015) Species, sex and individual differences in the vasotocin/vasopressin system: relationship to neurochemical signaling in the social behavior neural network. *Frontiers in Neuroendocrinology*, **36**, 49–71.

American College of Laboratory Animal Medicine (2007) Guidelines for the assessment and management of pain in rodents and rabbits. *Journal for the American Association of Laboratory Animal Science*, **46**, 97–108.

Amdam, G.V. and Hovland, A.L. (2011) Measuring animal preferences and choice behavior. *Nature Education Knowledge*, **3**(10), 74.

Appleby, M.C., Olsson, A.S. and Galindo, F. (Eds) (2018) *Animal Welfare*, 3rd edn. CABI, Wallingford, UK.

Arras, M., Rettich, A., Cinelli, P. *et al.* (2007) Assessment of post-laparotomy pain in laboratory mice by telemetric recording of heart rate and heart rate variability. *BMC Veterinary Research*, 2; 3, 16.

Bains, R.S., Cater, H.L., Sillito, R.R. *et al.* (2016) Analysis of individual mouse activity in group housed animals of different inbred strains using a novel automated home cage analysis system. *Frontiers in Behavioral Neuroscience*, **10**, 106.

Bains, R.S., Wells, S., Sillito, R.R. *et al.* (2018) Assessing mouse behaviour throughout the light/dark cycle using automated in-cage analysis tools. *Journal of Neuroscience Methods*, **300**, 37–47.

Bakker, J., Van Nijnatten, T.J., Louwerse, A.L. *et al.* (2014) Evaluation of ultrasonic vocalizations in common marmosets (Callithrix jacchus) as a potential indicator of welfare. *Lab Animal*, **43**(9), 313–320.

Baran, S.W., Gupta, A.D., Lim, M.A. *et al.* (2020) Continuous, automated breathing rate and body motion monitoring of rats with paraquat-induced progressive lung injury. *Frontiers in Physiology*, **11**, 569001.

Baran, S.W., Lim, M.A., Do, J.P. *et al.* (2021) Digital biomarkers enable automated, longitudinal monitoring in a mouse model of aging. *The Journals of Gerontology: Series A*, **76**(7), 1206–1213.

Barker, T.H., Howarth, G.S. and Whittaker, A.L. (2018) Increased latencies to respond in a judgment bias test are not associated with pessimistic biases in rats. *Behavioural Processes*, **146**, 64–66.

Bateson, M. and Martin, P. (2021) *Measuring Behaviour: An Introductory Guide*. New York, NY: Cambridge University Press.

Bateson, M. (2004) Mechanisms of decision-making and the interpretation of choice tests. *Animal Welfare*, **13**, S115–120.

Bateson, M. and Matheson, S. (2007) Performance on categorisation tasks suggests that removal of environmental enrichment induces 'pessimism' in captive European starlings (Sturnus vulgaris). *Animal Welfare*, **16**(S), 33–36.

Bechard, A.R., Bliznyuk, N. and Lewis, M.H. (2017) The development of repetitive motor behaviors in deer mice: effects of environmental enrichment, repeated testing, and differential mediation by indirect basal ganglia pathway activation. *Developmental Psychobiology*, **59**(3), 390–399.

Beerda, B., Schilder, M., van Hooff, J. *et al.* (1998) Behavioural, saliva cortisol and heart rate responses to different types of stimuli in dogs. *Applied Animal Behaviour Science*, **58**, 365–381.

Benish, M. and Ben-Eliyahu, S. (2010) Surgery as a double-edged sword: a clinically feasible approach to overcome the metastasis-promoting effects of surgery by blunting stress and prostaglandin responses. *Cancers*, **2**(4), 1929–1951.

Bentham, J. (1789) *Introduction to the Principles of Morals and Legislation*. Clarendon Press, Oxford.

Berridge, K. and Robinson, T. (1998) What is the role of dopamine in reward: hedonic impact, reward learning or incentive salience? *Brain Research Reviews*, **28**, 309–369.

Bethell, E.J., Holmes, A., MacLarnon, A. and Semple, S. (2012) Evidence that emotion mediates social attention in rhesus macaques. *PLoS One*, **7**(8), e44387.

Beynen, A., Baumans, V., Bertens, P. *et al.* (1987) Assessment of discomfort in gallstone-bearing mice: a practical example of the problems encountered in an attempt to recognize discomfort in laboratory animals. *Laboratory Animals*, **21**, 35–42.

Blom, H., Van Vorstenbosch, C., Baumans, V. *et al.* (1992) Description and validation of a preference test system to evaluate housing conditions for laboratory mice. *Applied Animal Behaviour Science*, **35**, 67–82.

Bloomsmith, M.A., Perlman, J.E., Hutchinson, E. *et al.* Behavioral management programs to promote laboratory animal welfare. In: *Management of Animal Care and Use Programs in Research, Education, and Testing*, 2nd edn. Eds Weichbrod, R.H., Thompson, G.A.H. and Norton, J.N. CRC Press/Taylor & Francis, Boca Raton (FL); 2018. Chapter 5. Available from: https://www.ncbi.nlm.nih.gov/books/NBK500424/ doi: 10.1201/9781315152189-5

Boissy, A., Manteuffel, G., Jensen, M. *et al.* (2007) Assessment of positive emotions in animals to improve their welfare. *Physiology and Behavior*, **92**, 375–397.

Bowen, M.T., Keats, K., Kendig, M.D. *et al.* (2012) Aggregation in quads but not pairs of rats exposed to cat odor or bright light. *Behavioural Processes*, **90**, 331–336.

Brenneis, C., Westhof, A., Holschbach, J. *et al.* (2017) Automated tracking of motion and body weight for objective monitoring of rats in colony housing. *Journal of the American Association for Laboratory Animal Science*, **56**(1), 18–31.

Brilot, B.O., Normandale, C.L., Parkin, A. and Bateson, M. (2009) Can we use starlings' aversion to eyespots as the basis for a novel 'cognitive bias' task?. *Applied Animal Behaviour Science*, **118**(3–4), 182–190.

Broom, D. and Zanella, A. (2004) Brain measures which tell us about animal welfare. *Animal Welfare*, **13**, S41–45.

Brudzynski, S. and Ociepa, D. (1992) Ultrasonic vocalization of laboratory rats in response to handling and touch. *Physiology and Behavior*, **52**, 655–660.

Burgdorf, J. and Panksepp, J. (2006) The neurobiology of positive emotions. *Neuroscience and Biobehavioral Reviews*, **30**, 173–187.

Burgen, A. (1949) The assay of anticholinesterase drugs by the chromodacryorrhoea response in rats. *British Journal of Pharmacology*, **4**, 185–189.

Burman, O., Ilyat, A., Jones, G. *et al.* (2007) Ultrasonic vocalizations as indicators of welfare for laboratory rats (Rattus norvegicus). *Applied Animal Behaviour Science*, **104**, 116–129.

Burman, O., Owen, D., Abou-Ismail, U. *et al.* (2008a) Removing individual rats affects indicators of welfare in the remaining group members. *Physiology and Behavior*, **93**, 89–96.

Burman, O.H.P., Parker, R.M.A., Paul, E.S. and Mendl, M.T. (2008b) A spatial judgement task to determine background emotional state in laboratory rats, Rattus norvegicus. *Animal Behaviour*, **76**, 801–809.

Burn, C. (2005) Effects of husbandry and the laboratory environment on rat welfare. In: *Zoology*. University of Oxford, Oxford.

Burn, C. (2008) What is it like to be a rat? Rat sensory perception and its implications for experimental design and rat welfare. *Applied Animal Behaviour Science*, **112**, 1–32.

Burn, C., Deacon, R. and Mason, G. (2008) Marked for life? Effects of early cage cleaning frequency, delivery batch and identification tail-marking on adult rat anxiety profiles. *Developmental Psychobiology*, **50**, 266–277.

Burn, C., Peters, A. and Mason, G. (2006) Acute effects of cage-cleaning at different frequencies on laboratory rat behaviour and welfare. *Animal Welfare*, **15**, 161–172.

Buttigieg, A., Flores, O., Hernández, A. *et al.* (2014) Preference for high-fat diet is developed by young Swiss CD1 mice after short-term feeding and is prevented by NMDA receptor antagonists. *Neurobiology of Learning and Memory*, **107**, 13–18.

Cabib, S. (2006) The neurophysiology of stereotypies II: The role of stress. In: *Stereotypic Behaviour: Fundamentals and Applications to Welfare*. Ed. Mason, G., pp. 227–255. CAB International, Wallingford.

Campos-Luna, I., Miller, A., Beard, A. and Leach, M. (2019) Validation of mouse welfare indicators: a Delphi consultation survey. *Scientific Reports*, **9(1)**, 10249.

Carter, C. (2001) Is there a neurobiology of good welfare? In: *Coping with Challenge. Welfare in Animals Including Humans*. Ed. Broom, D., pp. 11–30. Dahlem University Press, Berlin.

Chesler, E.J., Wilson, S.G., Lariviere, W.R. et al. (2002) Identification and ranking of genetic and laboratory environment factors influencing a behavioral trait, thermal nociception, via computational analysis of a large data archive. *Neuroscience and Biobehavioral Reviews*, **26(8)**, 907–923.

Chincarini, M., Qiu, L., Spinelli, L. et al. (2019) Evaluation of sheep anticipatory response to a food reward by means of functional near-infrared spectroscopy. *Animals*, **9(1)**, 11.

Chisholm, J., De Rantere D., Fernandez, N.J. et al. (2013) Carbon dioxide, but not isoflurane, elicits ultrasonic vocalizations in female rats. *Laboratory Animals*, **47(4)**, 324–327.

Christiansen, S. and Forkman, B. (2007) Assessment of animal welfare in a veterinary context – a call for ethologists. *Applied Animal Behaviour Science*, **106**, 203–220.

Christina, A., Merlin, N., Vijaya, C. et al. (2004) Daily rhythm of nociception in rats. *Journal of Circadian Rhythms*, **2(1)**, 2.

Clark, T.S., Pandolfo, L.M., Marshall, C.M. et al. (2018) Body condition scoring for adult zebrafish (Danio rerio). *Journal of the American Association for Laboratory Animal Science*, **57(6)**, 698–702.

Clingerman, K. and Summers, L. (2005) Development of a body scoring system for nonhuman primates using *Macaca mulatta* as a model. *Laboratory Animals*, **34**, 31–36.

Cloutier, S. and Newberry, R. (2008) Use of a conditioning technique to reduce stress associated with repeated intra-peritoneal injections in laboratory rats. *Applied Animal Behaviour Science*, **112**, 158–173.

Cloutier, S., Wahl, K., Baker, C. and Newberry, R.C. (2014) The social buffering effect of playful handling on responses to repeated intra-peritoneal injections in laboratory rats. *Journal of the American Association for Laboratory Animal Science*, **53(2)**, 168–173.

Colson, V., Ferreira, V.H.B., Luchiari, A.C. et al. (2021) Loss of light colour preference after chronic embryonic stress in rainbow trout fry: A novel and potential indicator of fish welfare?. *Applied Animal Behaviour Science*, **239**, 105335.

Cooper, B. and Vierck, C. (1986) Vocalizations as measures of pain in monkeys. *Pain*, **26**, 393–407.

Cooper, J. (2004) Consumer demand under commercial husbandry conditions: practical advice on measuring behavioural priorities in captive animals. *Animal Welfare*, **13**, S47–56.

Crockett, C.M., Shimoji, M. and Bowden, D.M. (2000) Behavior, appetite, and urinary cortisol responses by adult female pigtailed macaques to cage size, cage level, room change, and ketamine sedation. *American Journal of Primatology*, **52(2)**, 63–80.

Committee on Recognition and Alleviation of Distress in Laboratory Animals (CRADLA) (2008) *Recognition and Alleviation of Distress in Laboratory Animals*. National Academies Press, Washington.

Cross, N. and Rogers, L. (2006) Mobbing vocalizations as a coping response in the common marmoset. *Hormones and Behavior*, **49**, 237–245.

Crowell Comuzzi, D. (1993) Baboon vocalizations as measures of psychological well-being. *Laboratory Primate Newsletter*, **21**, 5–6.

Crump, A., Arnott, G. and Bethell, E.J. (2018) Affect-driven attention biases as animal welfare indicators: review and methods. *Animals*, **8(8)**, 136.

Cuomo, V., Cagiano, R., De Salvia, M. et al. (1992) Ultrasonic vocalization as an indicator of emotional state during active avoidance learning in rats. *Life Sciences*, **50**, 1049–1055.

Dallaire, J.A., Meagher, R.K., Díez-león, M. et al. (2011) Recurrent perseveration correlates with abnormal repetitive locomotion in adult mink but is not reduced by environmental enrichment. *Behavioural Brain Research*, **224**, 213–222.

Davenport, M., Tiefenbacher, S., Lutz, C. et al. (2006) Analysis of endogenous cortisol concentrations in the hair of rhesus macaques. *General and Comparative Endocrinology*, **147**, 255–261.

David, J.M., Knowles, S., Lamkin, D.M. and Stout, D.B. (2013) Individually ventilated cages impose cold stress on laboratory mice: a source of systemic experimental variability. *Journal of the American Association for Laboratory Animal Science*, **52(6)**, 738–744.

Dawkins, M. (1980) *Animal Suffering: The Science of Animal Welfare*. Chapman and Hall, London.

Dawkins, M. (1983) Battery hens name their price: consumer demand theory and the measurement of ethological needs. *Animal Behaviour*, **31**, 1195–1205.

Dawkins, M. (2004) Using behaviour to assess animal welfare. *Animal Welfare*, **13**, S3–7.

Deacon, R.M. (2006) Burrowing in rodents: a sensitive method for detecting behavioral dysfunction. *Nature Protocols*, **1**, 118–121.

Dixon, L.M, Brocklehurst, S., Sandilands, V. et al. (2014) Measuring motivation for appetitive behaviour: food-restricted broiler breeder chickens cross a water barrier to forage in an area of wood shavings without food. *PLoS One*, **9(7)**, e102322.

Dopfel, D. and Zhang, N. (2018) Mapping stress networks using functional magnetic resonance imaging in awake animals. *Neurobiology of Stress*, **9**, 251–263.

Duke, J., Zammit, T. and Lawson, D. (2001) The effects of routine cage-cleaning on cardiovascular and behavioral parameters in male Sprague-Dawley rats. *Contemporary Topics in Laboratory Animal Science*, **40**, 17–20.

Dunbar, M.L., David, E.M., Aline, M.R. and Lofgren, J.L. (2016) Validation of a behavioral ethogram for assessing postoperative pain in guinea pigs (*Cavia Porcellus*). *Journal of the American Association for Laboratory Animal Science*, **55(1)**, 29–34.

Duke, J.L., Zammit, T.G. and Lawson, D.M. (2001) The effects of routine cage-changing on cardiovascular and behavioral parameters in male Sprague-Dawley rats. *Contemporary Topics in Laboratory Animal Science*, **40(1)**, 17–20.

Ennaceur, A., Michalikova, S. and Chazot, P.L. (2006) Models of anxiety: Responses of rats to novelty in an open space and an enclosed space. *Behavioural Brain Research*, **171**, 26–49.

Fernström, A.L., Sutian, W., Royo, F. et al. (2008) Stress in cynomolgus monkeys (*Macaca fascicularis*) subjected to long-distance transport and simulated transport housing conditions, *Stress*, 11: 6, 467–476.

Flecknell, P. and Molony, V. (1997) Pain and injury. In: *Animal Welfare*. Eds Appleby, M. and Hughes, B., pp. 63–73. CAB International, Wallingford.

Flecknell, P. and Roughan, J. (2004) Assessing pain in animals – putting research into practice. *Animal Welfare*, **13**, S71–76.

Flecknell, P.A. and Thomas, A.A. (2015) Chapter 39: Comparative anesthesia and analgesia of laboratory animals. In: *Veterinary Anesthesia and Analgesia*. Eds Grimm, K.A., Lamont, W.J., Greene, S. and Robertson, S.A., pp. 754–763. Wiley. DOI:10.1002/9781119421375

Flecknell, P. (2018) Rodent analgesia: Assessment and therapeutics. *The Veterinary Journal*, **232**, 70–77.

Foltz, C. and Ullman-Cullere, M. (1999) Guidelines for assessing the health and condition of mice. *Laboratory Animal*, **28**, 28–32.

Franchi, S., Panerai, A.E. and Sacerdote, P. (2007) Buprenorphine ameliorates the effect of surgery on hypothalamus-pituitary-adrenal axis, natural killer cell activity and metastatic colonization in rats in comparison with morphine or fentanyl treatment. *Brain, Behavior, and Immunity*, **21**, 767–774.

Franks, B., Higgins, E.T. and Champagne, F.A. (2014) A theoretically based model of rat personality with implications for welfare. *PLoS One*, **9(4)**, e95135.

Franks, B. (2019) What do animals want. *Animal Welfare*, **28**, 1–10.

Fraser, D. and Matthews, L. (1995) Preference and motivation testing. In: *Animal Welfare*. Eds Appleby, M. and Hughes, B., pp. 159–174. CAB International, Wallingford.

Fuentes, G.C. and Newgren, J. (2008) Physiology and clinical pathology of laboratory New Zealand white rabbits housed individually and in groups. *Journal of the American Association for Laboratory Animal Science.* **47**(2), 35–38.

Ganeshan, K. and Chawla, A. (2017) Warming the mouse to model human diseases. *Nature Reviews Endocrinology*, **13**(8), 458–465.

Garner, J. (2006) Perseveration and stereotypy – systems-level insights from clinical psychology. In: *Stereotypic Animal Behaviour: Fundamentals and Applications to Welfare.* Eds Rushen, J. and Mason, G., pp. 121–152. CAB International, Wallingford.

Garner, J. and Mason, G. (2002) Evidence for a relationship between cage stereotypies and behavioural disinhibition in laboratory rodents. *Behavioural Brain Research*, **136**, 83–92.

Garner, J.P., Gaskill, B.N., Weber, E.M. *et al.* (2017) Introducing Therioepistemology: the study of how knowledge is gained from animal research. *Lab Animal*, **46**(4), 103–113.

Gaskill, B.N., Gordon, C.J., Pajor, E.A. *et al.* (2012) Heat or insulation: behavioral titration of mouse preference for warmth or access to a nest. *PLoS One*, **7**(3), p.e32799.

Gaskill, B.N., Karas, A.Z., Garner, J.P. and Pritchett-Corning, K.R. (2013a) Nest building as an indicator of health and welfare in laboratory mice. *Journal of Visualized Experiments: JoVE*, **82**, 51012.

Gaskill, B.N., Gordon, C.J., Pajor, E.A. *et al.* (2013b) Impact of nesting material on mouse body temperature and physiology. *Physiology & Behavior*, **110**, 87–95.

Gaskill, B.N. and Garner, J.P. (2017) Stressed out: providing laboratory animals with behavioral control to reduce the physiological effects of stress. *Lab Animal*, **46**(4), 142–145.

Gaskill, B.N., Pritchett-Corning, K.R., Gordon, C.J. *et al.* (2013c) Energy reallocation to breeding performance through improved nest building in laboratory mice. *PLoS One*, **8**(9), p.e74153.

Gaspani, L., Bianchi, M., Limiroli, E. *et al.* (2002) The analgesic drug tramadol prevents the effect of surgery on natural killer cell activity and metastatic colonization in rats. *Journal of Neuroimmunology*, **129**(1–2), 18–24.

Gaudio, E., Bordin, S., Lora, I. *et al.* (2018) Leukocyte coping capacity chemiluminescence as an innovative tool for stress and pain assessment in calves undergoing ring castration, *Journal of Animal Science*, **96**(11), 4579–4589.

Gazzano, A., Mariti, C., Notari, L. *et al.* (2008) Effects of early gentling and early environment on emotional development of puppies. *Applied Animal Behaviour Science*, **110**, 294–304.

Gelling, M., Montes, I., Moorhouse, T.P. and Macdonald, D.W. (2010) Captive housing during water vole (*Arvicola terrestris*) reintroduction: does short-term social stress impact on animal welfare?. *PLoS One*, **5**(3), e9791.

Godbey, T., Gray, G. and Jeffery, D. (2011) Cage-change interval preference in mice. *Lab Animal*, **40**(7), 225–230.

Golledge, H. and Jirkof, P. (2016) Score sheets and analgesia. *Laboratory Animals*, **50**(6), 411–413.

Graf, R, Cinelli, P, Arras, M. (2016) Morbidity scoring after abdominal surgery. *Laboratory Animals*, **50**, 453–458.

Grzelak, A.K., Davis, D.J., Caraker, S.M. *et al.* (2017) Stress leukogram induced by acute and chronic stress in zebrafish (*Danio rerio*). *Comparative Medicine*, **67**(3), 263–269.

Green, A.S. and Grahame, N.J. (2008) Ethanol drinking in rodents: is free-choice related to the reinforcing effects of ethanol? *Alcohol*, **42**, 1–11.

Green, A.C., Johnston, I.N. and Clark, C.E.F. (2018) Invited review: the evolution of cattle bioacoustics and application for advanced dairy systems. *Animal.* 12(6): 1250–1259.

Gross, V., Tank, J., Partke, H.-J. *et al.* (2008) Cardiovascular autonomic regulation in non-obese diabetic (NOD) mice. *Autonomic Neuroscience: Basic and Clinical*, **138**, 108–113.

Gunnarsson, S., Matthews, L., Foster, T. *et al.* (2000) The demand for straw and feathers as litter substrates by laying hens. *Applied Animal Behaviour Science*, **65**, 321–330.

Gwartney, J., Stroup, R., Sobel, R. and Macpherson, D. (2005) *Economics. Private and Public Choice.* Thomson South-Western, Mason.

Häger, C., Keubler, L.M., Talbot, S.R. *et al.* (2018) Running in the wheel: Defining individual severity levels in mice. *PLoS Biology*, **16**(10), e2006159.

Harding, E., Paul, E. and Mendl, M. (2004) Animal behaviour – cognitive bias and affective state. *Nature*, **427**, 312.

Harkness, J. and Ridgway, M. (1980) Chromodacryorrhea in laboratory rats (*Rattus norvegicus*): etiologic considerations. *Laboratory Animal Science*, **30**, 841–844.

Harper, R., Kerins, C., McIntosh, J. *et al.* (2001) Modulation of the inflammatory response in the rat TMJ with increasing doses of complete Freund's adjuvant. *Osteoarthritis and Cartilage*, **9**, 619–624.

Harris, A.P., Lennen, R.J., Marshall, I. *et al.* (2015) Imaging learned fear circuitry in awake mice using fMRI. *European Journal of Neuroscience*, **42**(5), 2125–2134.

Hawkins, P., Morton, D.B., Burman, O. *et al.* (2011) A guide to defining and implementing protocols for the welfare assessment of laboratory animals: eleventh report of the BVAAWF/FRAME/RSPCA/UFAW Joint Working Group on Refinement. *Laboratory Animals*, **45**(1), 1–13.

Held, S., Turner, R. and Wootton, R. (1995) Choices of laboratory rabbits for individual or group-housing. *Applied Animal Behaviour Science*, **46**, 81–91.

Hickman, D.L. (2017) Evaluation of the neutrophil:lymphocyte ratio as an indicator of chronic distress in the laboratory mouse. *Lab Animal (NY)*, **46**(7), 303–307.

Hohlbaum, K., Bert, B., Dietze, S. *et al.* (2018) Impact of repeated anesthesia with ketamine and xylazine on the well-being of C57BL/6JRj mice. *PLoS One*, **13**(9), e0203559.

Huber, N., Marasco, V., Painer, J. *et al.* (2019) Leukocyte coping capacity: An integrative parameter for wildlife welfare within conservation interventions. *Frontiers in Veterinary Science*, **6**, 105.

Hunniford, M.E., Woolcott, C., Siegford, J. and Widowski, TM. (2017) Nesting behavior of Hy-Line hens in modified enriched colony cages. *Poultry Science*, **96**(6), 1515–1523.

Hutchinson, E.K., Avery, A.C. and Vandewoude, S. (2012) Environmental enrichment during rearing alters corticosterone levels, thymocyte numbers, and aggression in female BALB/c mice. *Journal of the American Association for Laboratory Animal Science: JAALAS*, **51**(1), 18–24.

Irvine, R., White, J. and Chan, R. (1997) The influence of restraint on blood pressure in the rat. *Journal of Pharmacological and Toxicological Methods*, **38**, 157–162.

Jain, N.C. (2005) Leukocytic disorders. In: *The Merck Veterinary Manual*, 9th edn. Ed. Kahn C.M., pp. 46–52. Merck and Company, Whitehouse Station (NJ).

Jennings, E.M., Okine, B.N., Roche, M. and Finn, D.P. (2014) Stress-induced hyperalgesia. *Progress in Neurobiology*, **121**, 1–18.

Jennings, M., Batchelor, G., Brain, P. *et al.* (1998) Refining rodent husbandry: the mouse. *Laboratory Animals*, **32**, 233–259.

Jensen, M., Pedersen, L. and Ladewig, J. (2004) The use of demand functions to assess behavioural priorities in farm animals. *Animal Welfare*, **13**, S27–32.

Jirkof, P. (2017) Side effects of pain and analgesia in animal experimentation. *Lab Animal (NY).* 22; **46**(4), 123–128.

Jirkof, P., Cesarovic, N., Rettich, A. *et al.* (2010) Burrowing behavior as an indicator of post-laparotomy pain in mice. *Frontiers in Behavioral Neuroscience*, **4**, 165.

Jirkof, P., Fleischmann, T., Cesarovic, N. *et al.* (2013) Assessment of postsurgical distress and pain in laboratory mice by nest complexity scoring. *Lab Animal*, **47**(3), 153–161.

Jourdan, D., Ardid, D., Chapuy, E. *et al.* (1998) Effect of analgesics on audible and ultrasonic pain-induced vocalisation in the rat. *Life Sciences*, **63**, 1761–1768.

Kirchner, J., Hackbarth, H., Stelzer, H.D. and Tsai, P.P. (2012) Preferences of group-housed female mice regarding structure of softwood bedding. *Laboratory Animals*, **46(2)**, 95–100.

Kirkden, R. and Pajor, E. (2006) Using preference, motivation and aversion tests to ask scientific questions about animals' feelings. *Applied Animal Behaviour Science*, **100**, 29–47.

Kirschbaum, C. and Hellhammer, D. (2000) Salivary cortisol. In: *Encyclopedia of Stress*. Ed. Fink, G., pp. 379–383. Academic Press, Boston.

Krebs, B.L., Torres, E., Chesney, C. et al. (2017) Applying behavioral conditioning to identify anticipatory behaviors. *Journal of Applied Animal Welfare Science*, **20(2)**, 155–175.

Krueger, L.D., Thurston, S.E., Kirk, J. et al. (2020) Enrichment preferences of singly housed zebrafish (Danio rerio). *Journal of the American Association for Laboratory Animal Science*, **59(2)**, 148–155.

LaFollette, M.R., O'Haire, M.E., Cloutier, S. et al. (2017) Rat tickling: a systematic review of applications, outcomes, and moderators. *PLoS One*, **12(4)**, e0175320.

Lang, A., Schulz, A., Ellinghaus, A. and Schmidt-Bleek, K. (2016) Osteotomy models – the current status on pain scoring and management in small rodents. *Lab Animal*, **50**, 433–441.

Langford, D.J., Crager, S.E., Shehzad, Z. et al. (2006) Social modulation of pain as evidence for empathy in mice. *Science*, **312(5782)**, 1967–1970.

Latham, N. and Mason, G. (2004) From house mouse to mouse house: the behavioural biology of free-living *Mus musculus* and its implications in the laboratory. *Applied Animal Behaviour Science*, **86**, 261–289.

Lariviere, W.R. and Mogil, J.S. (2010) The genetics of pain and analgesia in laboratory animals. *Methods in Molecular Biology*, **617**, 261–278.

Laurijs, K.A., Briefer, E.F., Reimert, I. and Webb, L.E. (2021) Vocalisations in farm animals: A step towards positive welfare assessment. *Applied Animal Behaviour Science*, **236**, 105264.

Leach, M. and Main, D. (2008) An assessment of laboratory mouse welfare in UK animal units. *Animal Welfare*, **17**, 171–187.

Leach, M., Thornton, P. and Main, D. (2008) Identification of appropriate measures for the assessment of laboratory mouse welfare. *Animal Welfare*, **17**, 161–170.

Lee, C., Verbeek, E., Doyle, R. and Bateson, M. (2016) Attention bias to threat indicates anxiety differences in sheep. *Biology Letters*, **12(6)**, 20150977.

Lee, C., Cafe, L.M., Robinson, S.L. et al. (2018) Anxiety influences attention bias but not flight speed and crush score in beef cattle. *Applied Animal Behaviour Science*, **205**, 210–215.

Lepschy, M., Touma, C., Hruby, R. et al. (2007) Non-invasive measurement of adrenocortical activity in male and female rats. *Laboratory Animals*, **41**, 372–387.

Lewis, M., Presti, M., Lewis, J. et al. (2006) The neurobiology of stereotypy 1: environmental complexity. In: *Stereotypic Animal Behaviour: Fundamentals and Applications to Welfare*. Eds Rushen, J. and Mason, G., pp. 190–226. CAB International, Wallingford.

Lim, M.A., Defensor, E.B., Mechanic, J.A. et al. (2019) Retrospective analysis of the effects of identification procedures and cage changing by using data from automated, continuous monitoring. *Journal of the American Association for Laboratory Animal Science*, **58(2)**, 126–141.

Litvin, Y., Blanchard, D. and Blanchard, R. (2007) Rat 22 kHz ultrasonic vocalizations as alarm cries. *Behavioural Brain Research*, **182**, 166–172.

Lofgren, J., Miller, A.L., Lee, C. et al. (2018) Analgesics promote welfare and sustain tumour growth in orthotopic 4T1 and B16 mouse cancer models. *Laboratory Animals*, **52(4)**, 351–364.

Low, L.A., Bauer, L.C., Pitcher, M.H. and Bushnell, M.C. (2016) Restraint training for awake functional brain scanning of rodents can cause long-lasting changes in pain and stress responses. *Pain*, **157(8)**, 1761.

Luchins, K.R. Baker, K.C., Gilbert, M.H. et al. (2011) Application of the diagnostic evaluation for alopecia in traditional veterinary species to laboratory rhesus macaques (*Macaca mulatta*). *Journal of the American Association for Laboratory Animal Science*, **50(6)**, 926–938.

Lutz, C., Tiefenbacher, S., Jorgensen, M. et al. (2000) Techniques for collecting saliva from awake, unrestrained, adult monkeys for cortisol assay. *American Journal of Primatology*, **52**, 93–99.

Maigrot, A.L., Hillmann, E. and Briefer, E.F. (2018) Encoding of emotional valence in wild boar (Sus sucrofa) calls. *Animals*, **8(6)**. Pii: E85.

Makowska, I.J. and Weary, D.M. (2016) Differences in anticipatory behaviour between rats (Rattus norvegicus) housed in standard versus semi-naturalistic laboratory environments. *PLoS One*, **11(1)**, e0147595.

Mällo, T., Matrov, D., Herm, L. et al. (2007) Tickling-induced 50 kHz ultrasonic vocalization is individually stable and predicts behaviour in tests of anxiety and depression in rats. *Behavioural Brain Research*, **184**, 57–71.

Manser, C., Elliott, H., Morris, T. et al. (1996) The use of a novel operant test to determine the strength of preference for flooring in laboratory rats. *Laboratory Animals*, **30**, 1–6.

Manteca, X. (1998) Neurophysiology and assessment of welfare. *Meat Science*, **49**, S205–218.

Mason, G. (1991) Stereotypies: a critical review. *Animal Behaviour*, **41**, 1015–1037.

Mason, G. (2006) Stereotypic behaviour in captive animals: fundamentals, and implications for welfare and beyond. In: *Stereotypic Animal Behaviour: Fundamentals and Applications to Welfare*. Eds Rushen, J. and Mason, G., pp. 325–326. CAB International, Wallingford.

Mason, G., Cooper, J. and Clarebrough, C. (2001) Frustrations of fur-farmed mink. *Nature*, **410**, 35–36.

Mason, G. and Latham, N. (2004) Can't stop, won't stop: is stereotypy a reliable animal welfare indicator? *Animal Welfare*, **13S**, S57–S69.

Mason, G., Wilson, D., Hampton, C. et al. (2004) Non-invasively assessing disturbance and stress in laboratory rats by scoring chromodacryorrhoea. *ATLA, Alternatives to Laboratory Animals*, **32(1A)**, 153–159.

Matheson, S., Asher, L. and Bateson, M. (2008) Larger, enriched cages are associated with 'optimistic' response biases in captive European starlings (*Sturnus vulgaris*). *Applied Animal Behaviour Science*, **109**, 374–383.

McBride, S. and Hemmings, A. (2005) Altered mesoaccumbens and nigro-striatal dopamine physiology is associated with stereotypy development in a non-rodent species. *Behavioural Brain Research*, **159**, 113–118.

Mellor, D. (2017) Operational details of the five domains model and its key applications to the assessment and management of animal welfare. *Animals*, **7**, 60; doi:10.3390/ani7080060

Mendl, M. and Paul, E. (2004) Consciousness, emotion and animal welfare: insights from cognitive science. *Animal Welfare*, **13**, S17–25.

Mendl, M., Burman, O.H., Parker, R.M. and Paul, E.S. (2009) Cognitive bias as an indicator of animal emotion and welfare: Emerging evidence and underlying mechanisms. *Applied Animal Behaviour Science*, **118(3–4)**, 161–181.

Miller, A.L. and Leach, M.C. (2015) The mouse grimace scale: a clinically useful tool? *PLoS One*, **10(9)**, p.e0136000.

Miller, A., Kitson, G., Skalkoyannis, B. and Leach, M. (2015) The effect of isoflurane anaesthesia and buprenorphine on the mouse grimace scale and behaviour in CBA and DBA/2 mice. *Applied Animal Behaviour Science*, **172**, 58–62.

Miller, A.L., Golledge, H.D. and Leach, M.C. (2016) The influence of isoflurane anaesthesia on the rat grimace scale. *PLoS One*, **11(11)**, p.e0166652.

Mogil, J.S. and Bailey, A.L. (2010) Sex and gender differences in pain and analgesia. *Progress in Brain Research*, **186**, 140–157.

Mogil, J.S. (2017) Laboratory environmental factors and pain behavior: the relevance of unknown unknowns to reproducibility and translation. *Lab Animal*, **46(4)**, 136–141.

Mogil, J.S., Pang, D.S.J., Silva Dutra, G.G. and Chambers, C.T. (2020) The development and use of facial grimace scales for pain measurement in animals. *Neuroscience & Biobehavioral Reviews*, **116**, 480–493.

Monk, J.E., Doyle, R.E., Colditz, I.G. et al. (2018) Towards a more practical attention bias test to assess affective state in sheep. *PLoS One*, **13(1)**, p.e0190404.

Monroe, S.C. and Radke, A.K. (2021) Aversion-resistant fentanyl self-administration in mice. *Psychopharmacology*, **238(3)**, 699–710.

Moroni, M., Coolbaugh, T.V., Mitchell, J.M. et al. (2011) Vascular access port implantation and serial blood sampling in a Gottingen minipig (Sus scrofa domestica) model of acute radiation injury. *Journal of the American Association for Laboratory Animal Science*, **50(1)**, 65–72.

Negus, S.S. (2019) Core outcome measures in preclinical assessment of candidate analgesics. *Pharmacological Reviews*, **71(2)**, 225–266.

Negus, S.S., Neddenriep, B., Altarifi, A.A. et al. (2015) Effects of ketoprofen, morphine, and kappa opioids on pain-related depression of nesting in mice. *Pain*, **156(6)**, 1153–1160.

Nevison, C., Hurst, J. and Barnard, C. (1999b) Why do male ICR(CD-1) mice perform bar-related (stereotypic) behaviour? *Behavioural Processes*, **47**, 95–111.

Novak, M.A., Hamel, A.F., Kelly, B.J. et al. (2013) Stress, the HPA axis, and nonhuman primate well-being: a review. *Applied Animal Behaviour Science*, **143(2–4)**, 135–149.

Novak, M., Meyer, J., Lutz, C. et al. (2006) Deprived environments: developmental insights from primatology. In: *Stereotypic Animal Behaviour: Fundamentals and Applications to Welfare*. Eds Rushen, J. and Mason, G., pp. 86–120. CAB International, Wallingford.

Novak, J., Bailoo, J.D., Melotti, L. and Würbel, H. (2016) Effect of cage-induced stereotypies on measures of affective state and recurrent perseveration in CD-1 and C57BL/6 mice. *PLoS One*, **11**, e0153203.

Nunamaker, E.A., Goldman, J.L., Adams, C.R. and Fortman, J.D. (2018) Evaluation of analgesic efficacy of Meloxicam and 2 formulations of buprenorphine after laparotomy in female Sprague-Dawley Rats. *Journal of the American Association for Laboratory Animal Science*, **57(5)**, 498–507.

Ochi, T., Yamada, A., Naganuma, Y. et al. (2016) Effect of road transportation on the serum biochemical parameters of cynomolgus monkeys and beagle dogs. *The Journal of Veterinary Medical Science*, **78(5)**, 889–893.

Oliver, V.L., Athavale, S., Simon, K.E. et al. (2017) Evaluation of pain assessment techniques and analgesia efficacy in a female guinea pig (Cavia porcellus) model of surgical pain. *Journal of the American Association for Laboratory Animal Science*, **56(4)**, 425–435.

Oliver, V.L., Thurston, S.E. and Lofgren, J.L. (2018) Using cageside measures to evaluate analgesic efficacy in mice (Mus musculus) after surgery. *Journal of the American Association for Laboratory Animal Science*, **57(2)**, 186–201.

Olsson, I., Nevison, C., Patterson-Kane, E. et al. (2003) Understanding behaviour: the relevance of ethological approaches in laboratory animal science. *Applied Animal Behaviour Science*, **81**, 245–264.

Otovic, P. and Hutchinson, E. (2015) Limits to using HPA axis activity as an indication of animal welfare. *ALTEX*, **32(1)**, 41–50.

Palle, P., Ferreira, F.M., Methner, A. and Buch, T. (2016) The more the merrier? Scoring, statistics and animal welfare in experimental autoimmune encephalomyelitis. *Laboratory Animals*, **50**, 427–432.

Panksepp, J. (2003) At the interface of the affective, behavioral, and cognitive neurosciences: decoding the emotional feelings of the brain. *Brain and Cognition*, **52**, 4–14.

Panksepp, J. and Burgdorf, J. (2000) 50-kHz chirping (laughter?) in response to conditioned and unconditioned tickle-induced reward in rats: effects of social housing and genetic variables. *Behavioural Brain Research*, **115**, 25–38.

Panksepp, J. and Burgdorf, J. (2003) 'Laughing' rats and the evolutionary antecedents of human joy? *Physiology and Behavior*, **79**, 533–547.

Paul, E., Harding, E. and Mendl, M. (2005) Measuring emotional processes in animals: the utility of a cognitive approach. *Neuroscience and Biobehavioral Reviews*, **29**, 469–491.

Peterson, N.C., Nunamaker, E.A. and Turner, P.V. (2017) To treat or not to treat: the effects of pain on experimental parameters. *Comparative Medicine*, **67(6)**, 469–482.

Phan, K., Wager, T., Taylor, S. et al. (2004) Functional neuroimaging studies of human emotions. *CNS Spectrums*, **9**, 258–266.

Pines, M., Kaplan, G. and Rogers, L. (2005) Use of horizontal and vertical climbing structures by captive common marmosets (Callithrix jacchus). *Applied Animal Behaviour Science*, **91**, 311–319.

Pinkernell, S, Becker, K, Lindauer, U. (2016) Severity assessment and scoring for neurosurgical models in rodents. *Lab Animal*, **50**, 442–452.

Poirier, C. and Bateson, M. (2017) Pacing stereotypies in laboratory rhesus macaques: Implications for animal welfare and the validity of neuroscientific findings. *Neuroscience and Biobehavioral Reviews*, **83**, 508–515.

Pomerantz, O., Paukner, A. and Terkel, J. (2012a) Some stereotypic behaviors in rhesus macaques (Macaca mulatta) are correlated with both perseveration and the ability to cope with acute stressors. *Behavioural Brain Research*, **230**, 274–280.

Pomerantz, O., Terkel, J., Suomi, S.J. and Paukner, A. (2012b) Stereotypic head twirls, but not pacing, are related to a pessimistic-like judgment bias among captive tufted capuchins (Cebus apella). *Animal Cognition*, **15**, 689–698.

Raja, S.N., Carr, D.B., Cohen, M. et al. (2020) The revised IASP definition of pain: concepts, challenges, and compromises. *Pain*, **161(9)**, 1976.

Ranc, N., Moorcroft, P.R., Hansen, K.W. et al. (2020) Preference and familiarity mediate spatial responses of a large herbivore to experimental manipulation of resource availability. *Scientific Reports*, **10(1)**, 1–11.

Raşid, O., Chirita, D., Iancu, A.D. et al. (2012) Assessment of routine procedure effect on breathing parameters in mice by using whole-body plethysmography. *Journal of the American Association for Laboratory Animal Science*, **51(4)**, 469–474.

Rault, J.L., van den Munkhof, M. and Buisman-Pijlman, F. (2017) Oxytocin as an indicator of psychological and social well-being in domesticated animals: a critical review. *Frontiers in Psychology*, **8**, 1521.

Redfern, W.S., Tse, K., Grant, C. et al. (2017) Automated recording of home cage activity and temperature of individual rats housed in social groups: The Rodent Big Brother project. *PLoS One*, **12(9)**, e0181068.

Riemer, S., Thompson, H. and Burman, O.H. (2018) Behavioural responses to unexpected changes in reward quality. *Scientific Reports*, **8(1)**, 1–11.

Rock, M.L., Karas, A.Z., Rodriguez, K.B. et al. (2014) The time-to-integrate-to-nest test as an indicator of wellbeing in laboratory mice. *Journal of the American Association for Laboratory Animal Science*, **53(1)**, 24–28.

Roelofs, S., Boleij, H., Nordquist, R.E. and van der Staay, F.J. (2016) Making decisions under ambiguity: judgment bias tasks for assessing emotional state in animals. *Frontiers in Behavioral Neuroscience*, **10**, 119.

Rollins, B. (2015) Telos, conservation of welfare, and ethical issues in genetic engineering of animals. *Current Topics in Behavioral Neurosciences*, **19**, 99–116.

Rolls, E. (1999) *The Brain and Emotion*. Oxford University Press, Oxford.

Roper, T. (1975) Self-sustaining activities and reinforcement in the nest building behaviour of mice. *Behaviour*, **59**, 40–57.

Rosen, S., Ham, B. and Mogil, J.S. (2017) Sex differences in neuroimmunity and pain. *Journal of Neuroscience Research*, **95**(1–2), 500–508.

Roughan, J. and Flecknell, P. (2001) Behavioural effects of laparotomy and analgesic effects of ketoprofen

Roughan, J. and Flecknell, P. (2006) Training in behaviour-based post-operative pain scoring in rats – an evaluation based on improved recognition of analgesic requirements. *Applied Animal Behaviour Science*, **96**, 327–342.

Rupniak, N. and Williams, A. (1994) Differential inhibition of foot tapping and chromodacryorrhoea in gerbils by CNS penetrant and non-penetrant tachykinin NK1 receptor antagonists. *European Journal of Pharmacology*, **265**, 179–183.

Rushen, J. (1991) Problems associated with the interpretation of physiological data in the assessment of animal welfare. *Applied Animal Behaviour Science*, **28**, 381–386.

Rutherford, K. (2002) Assessing pain in animals. *Animal Welfare*, **11**, 31–53.

Rygula, R., Pluta, H. and Popik, P. (2012) Laughing rats are optimistic. *PLoS One*, **7**(12), e51959.

Sapolsky, R. (1992) Neuroendocrinology of the stress-response. In: *Behavioral Endocrinology*. Eds Becker, J., Breedlove, S. and Crews, D., pp. 287–324. Massachusetts Institute of Technology, Cambridge, Massachusetts

Schaap, M.W.H., Uilenreef, J.J., Mitsogiannis, M.D. *et al.* (2012) Optimizing the dosing interval of buprenorphine in a multimodal postoperative analgesic strategy in the rat: minimizing side-effects without affecting weight gain and food intake. *Laboratory Animals*, **46**(4), 287–292.

Schwarting, R.K.W. (2018) Ultrasonic vocalization in female rats: A comparison among three outbred stocks from pups to adults. *Physiology & Behavior*, **196**, 59–66.

Seaman, S., Waran, N., Mason, G. *et al.* (2008) Animal economics: assessing the motivation of female laboratory rabbits to reach a platform, social contact and food. *Animal Behaviour*, **75**, 31–42.

Sharp, J., Zammit, T., Azar, T. *et al.* (2002) Does witnessing experimental procedures produce stress in male rats? *Contemporary Topics in Laboratory Animal Science*, **41**, 8–12.

Sherwin, C. (1998) The use and perceived importance of three resources which provide caged laboratory mice the opportunity for extended locomotion. *Applied Animal Behaviour Science*, **55**, 353–367.

Sherwin, C. (2003) Social context affects the motivation of laboratory mice, *Mus musculus*, to gain access to resources. *Animal Behaviour*, **66**, 649–655.

Sherwin, C. (2004b) The motivation of group-housed laboratory mice, *Mus musculus*, for additional space. *Animal Behaviour*, **67**, 711–717.

Sherwin, C. (2007) The motivation of group-housed laboratory mice to leave an enriched laboratory cage. *Animal Behaviour*, **72**, 29–35.

Sherwin, C. and Nicol, C. (1995) Changes in meal patterning by mice measure the cost imposed by natural obstacles. *Applied Animal Behaviour Science*, **43**, 291–300.

Sherwin, C. and Nicol, C. (1996) Reorganisation of behaviour in laboratory mice, *Mus musculus*, with varying cost of access to resources. *Animal Behaviour*, **51**, 1087–1093.

Silverman, A. (1978) Rodents' defence against cigarette smoke. *Animal Behaviour*, **26**, 1279–1281.

Simone, L., Bartolomucci, A., Palanza, P. *et al.* (2008) On-ground housing in 'Mice Drawer System' (MDS) cage affects locomotor behaviour but not anxiety in male mice. *Acta Astronautica*, **62**, 453–461.

Sørensen, D., Hanse, H., Krohn, T. and Bertelsen, T. (2010) Preferences for limited versus no contact in SD rats. *Laboratory Animals*, **44**(3), 274–277.

Sorge, R.E., Martin, L.J., Isbester, K.A. *et al.* (2014) Olfactory exposure to males, including men, causes stress and related analgesia in rodents. *Nature Methods*, **11**(6), 629–632.

Spangenberg, E., Augustsson, H., Dahlborn, K. *et al.* (2005) Housing-related activity in rats: effects on body weight, urinary corticosterone levels, muscle properties and performance. *Laboratory Animals*, **39**, 45–57.

Spangenberg, E., Bjorklund, L. and Dahlborn, K. (2006) Outdoor housing of laboratory dogs: effects on activity, behaviour and physiology. *Applied Animal Behaviour Science*, **98**, 260–276.

Spruijt, B., van den Bos, R. and Pijlman, T. (2001) A concept of welfare based on reward evaluating mechanisms in the brain: anticipatory behaviour as an indicator for the state of reward systems. *Applied Animal Behaviour Science*, **72**, 145–171.

Stella, J. and Croney, C. (2019) Coping styles in the domestic cat (*Felis silvestris catus*) and implications for cat welfare. *Animals*, **9**(6), 370.

Sternberg, W.F., Ritchie, J. and Mogil, J.S. (2004) Qualitative sex differences in kappa-opioid analgesia in mice are dependent on age. *Neuroscience Letters*, **363**(2), 178–181.

Sugita, T., Kondo, Y., Ishino, S. *et al.* (2018) Evaluation of drug effects on cerebral blood flow and glucose uptake in un-anesthetized and un-stimulated rats: application of free-moving apparatus enabling to keep rats free during PET/SPECT tracer injection and uptake. *Nuclear Medicine Communications*, **39**(8), 753.

Sullivan, M., Lawrence, C. and Blache, D. (2016) Why did the fish cross the tank? Objectively measuring the value of enrichment for captive fish. *Applied Animal Behaviour Science*, **174**, 181–188.

Swan, M.P. and Hickman, D.L. (2014) Evaluation of the neutrophil-lymphocyte ratio as a measure of distress in rats. *Lab Animal (NY)*, **43**(8), 276–282.

Szechtman, H., Lambrou, P., Caggiula, A. *et al.* (1974) Plasma corticosterone levels during sexual behaviour in male rats. *Hormones and Behaviour*, **5**, 191–200.

Taitt, K.T. and Kendall, L.V. (2019) Physiologic stress of ear punch identification compared with restraint only in mice. *Journal of the American Association for Laboratory Animal Science*, **58**(4), 438–442.

Talbot, S.R., Biernot, S., Bleich, A. *et al.* (2020) Defining body-weight reduction as a humane endpoint: a critical appraisal. *Laboratory Animals*, **54**(1), 99–110.

Tappe-Theodor, A., King, T. and Morgan, M.M. (2019) Pros and cons of clinically relevant methods to assess pain in rodents. *Neuroscience & Biobehavioral Reviews*, **100**, 335–343.

Telkänranta, H., Marchant-Forde, J.N. and Valros, A. (2016) Tear staining in pigs: a potential tool for welfare assessment on commercial farms. *Animal*, **10**(2), 318–325.

Terlouw, E., Schouten, W. and Ladewig, J. (1995) Physiology. In: *Animal Welfare*. Eds Appleby, M. and Hughes, B., pp. 143–158. CAB International, Wallingford.

Thurman, J., Tranquilli, W. and Benson, G. (1999) *Essentials of Small Animal Anaesthesia and Analgesia: Small Animal Practice*. Blackwell Publishing, Oxford.

Toates, F. (1995) *Stress: Conceptual and Biological Aspects*. John Wiley & Sons, Chichester.

Toates, F. (2004) Cognition, motivation, emotion and action: a dynamic and vulnerable interdependence. *Applied Animal Behaviour Science*, **86**, 173–204.

Touma, C., Sachser, N., Mostl, E. *et al.* (2003) Effects of sex and time of day on metabolism and excretion fo corticosterone in urine and feces of mice. *General and Comparative Endocrinology*, **130**, 267–278.

Tsai, P.P., Nagelschmidt, N., Kirchner, J. *et al.* (2012) Validation of an automatic system (DoubleCage) for detecting the location of animals during preference tests. *Laboratory Animals*, **46**(1), 81–84.

Turner, P.V., Pang, D.S. and Lofgren, J.L. (2019) A review of pain assessment methods in laboratory rodents. *Comparative Medicine*, **69**(6), 451–467.

Ullman-Cullere, M. and Foltz, C. (1999) Body condition scoring: a rapid and accurate method for assessing health status in mice. *Laboratory Animal Science*, **49**, 319–323.

Vahl, T., Ulrich-Lai, Y., Ostrander, M. et al. (2005) Comparative analysis of ACTH and corticosterone sampling methods in rats. *American Journal of Physiology and Endocrinology Metabolism*, **289**, E823–828.

Van de Weerd, H., Van Loo, P., Van Zutphen, L. et al. (1998) Strength of preference for nesting material as environmental enrichment for laboratory mice. *Applied Animal Behaviour Science*, **55**, 369–382.

Van den Berg, C., Pijlman, T., Koning, H. et al. (1999) Isolation changes the incentive value of sucrose and social behaviour in juvenile and adult rats. *Behavioural Brain Research*, **106**, 133–142.

Van den Berg, C., Van Ree, J. and Spruijt, B. (2000) Morphine attenuates the effects of juvenile isolation in rats. *Neuropharmacology*, **39**, 969–976.

Van den Bos, R., Meijer, M., van Renselaar, J. et al. (2003) Anticipation is differently expressed in rats (*Rattus norvegicus*) and domestic cats (*Felis silvestris catus*) in the same Pavlovian conditioning paradigm. *Behavioural Brain Research*, **141**, 83–89.

Van Der Harst, J., Baars, A. and Spruijt, B. (2003a) Standard housed rats are more sensitive to rewards than enriched housed rats as reflected by their anticipatory behaviour. *Behavioural Brain Research*, **142**, 151–156.

Van Der Harst, J., Baars, A. and Spruijt, B. (2005) Announced rewards counteract the impairment of anticipatory behaviour in socially stressed rats. *Behavioural Brain Research*, **161**, 183–189.

Van Der Harst, J., Fermont, P., Bilstra, A. et al. (2003b) Access to enriched housing is rewarding to rats as reflected by their anticipatory behaviour. *Animal Behaviour*, **66**, 493–504.

Van Loo, P., Kruitwagen, C., Koolhaas, J. et al. (2002) Influence of cage enrichment on aggressive behaviour and physiological parameters in male mice. *Applied Animal Behaviour Science*, **76**, 65–81.

Varian, H. (1993) *Intermediate Microeconomics: A Modern Approach*. WW Norton, London.

Viscardi, A.V. and Turner, P.V. (2018) Efficacy of buprenorphine for management of surgical castration pain in piglets. *BMC Veterinary Research*, **14**(1), 318.

Vögeli, S., Lutz, J., Wolf, M. et al. (2014) Valence of physical stimuli, not housing conditions, affects behaviour and frontal cortical brain activity in sheep. *Behavioural Brain Research*, **267**, 144–155.

von Borell, E., Langbein, J., Despres, G. et al. (2007) Heart rate variability as a measure of autonomic regulation of cardiac activity for assessing stress and welfare in farm animals – a review. *Physiology and Behavior*, **92**, 293–316.

Von Frijtag, J., Reijmers, L., Van Der Harst, J. et al. (2000) Defeat followed by individual housing results in long-term impaired reward- and cognition-related behaviours in rats. *Behavioural Brain Research*, **117**, 137–146.

Von Frijtag, J., Van den Bos, R. and Spruijt, B. (2001) Imipramine restores the long-term impairment of appetitive behaviour in socially stressed rats. *Psychopharmacology*, **162**, 232–238.

Walker, C., Lightman, S., Steele, M. et al. (1992) Suckling is a persistent stimulus to the adreno-cortical system of the rat. *Endocrinology*, **130**, 115–125.

Walker, M. and Mason, G. (2018) A comparison of two types of running wheel in terms of mouse preference, health, and welfare. *Physiology & Behavior*, **191**(1), 82–90.

Warburton, H. and Mason, G. (2003) Is out of sight out of mind? The effects of resource cues on motivation in mink, *Mustela vison*. *Animal Behaviour*, **65**, 755–762.

Warburton, H. and Nicol, C. (1998) Position of operant costs affects visits to resources by laboratory mice, *Mus musculus*. *Animal Behaviour*, **55**, 1325–1333.

Weary, D., Niel, L., Flower, F. et al. (2006) Identifying and preventing pain in animals. *Applied Animal Behaviour Science*, **100**, 64–76.

Webber, E.S., Harmon, K.M., Beckwith, T.J. et al. (2012) Selective breeding for 50 kHz ultrasonic vocalization emission produces alterations in the ontogeny and regulation of rough-and-tumble play. *Behavioural Brain Research*, **229**(1), 138–144.

Weiner, B., Hertz, S., Perets, N. and London, M. (2016) Social ultrasonic vocalizations in awake head-restrained mouse. *Frontiers in Behavioral Neuroscience*, **10**, 236.

Whishaw, I. and Kolb, B. (2004) *The Behavior of the Laboratory Rat*. New York: Oxford University Press.

Wiedenmayer, C. (1997) Causation of the ontogenic development of stereotypic digging in gerbils. *Animal Behaviour*, **53**, 461–470.

Wilkes, B.J., Bass, C., Korah, H. et al. (2020) Volumetric magnetic resonance and diffusion tensor imaging of C58/J mice: neural correlates of repetitive behavior. *Brain Imaging and Behavior*, **14**(6), 2084–2096.

Wöhr, M., Houx, B., Schwarting, R. et al. (2008) Effects of experience and context of 50-kHz vocalizations in rats. *Physiology and Behavior*, **93**, 766–776.

Wright-Williams, S., Courade, J.-P., Richardson, C. et al. (2007) Effects of vasectomy surgery and meloxicam treatment on faecal corticosterone levels and behaviour in two strains of laboratory mouse. *Pain*, **130**, 108–118.

Würbel, H. (2006) The motivational basis of caged rodents' stereotypies. In: *Stereotypic Animal Behaviour: Fundamentals and Applications to Welfare*. Eds Rushen, J. and Mason, G., pp. 86–120. CAB International, Wallingford.

Würbel, H., Burn, C. and Latham, N. (2015). The behaviour of laboratory mice and rats. In: *The Ethology of Domestic Animals: An Introductory Text*, 3rd edition (ed. P. Jensen), 272–284. Boston: CABI.

Yeates, J. and Main, D. (2008) Assessment of positive welfare: a review. *The Veterinary Journal*, **175**, 293–300.

7 Welfare and 'best practice' in field studies of wildlife

Julie Lane and Robbie A. McDonald

Introduction

Wildlife research is exciting and is an appealing career for many aspiring scientists. The life of the wildlife biologist or vet and the thrill of capturing and handling wild animals are glamorised by the media, and the professions are often treated as being synonymous with working to promote animal welfare and conservation. However, field studies of wild animals carry with them multiple risks for the animal subjects. Unfortunately, these risks and problems are sometimes given scant consideration by practitioners, often because they are judged relative to natural processes or are incurred 'for the good of the species' or population. Wild animals undoubtedly suffer a range of markedly inhumane fates in the wild, and some are in grave need of intervention for conservation and management reasons. The ethical/moral absolute of the welfare of the individual animal and the corresponding deep concern felt by society mean that field research on wild animals requires an approach to ethical issues and the implementation of the three Rs that is as rigorous as for other areas of research using animals.

For a range of historical and subjective reasons, 'wildlife' is most commonly construed as naturally free-living vertebrates, most commonly mammals and birds, and to a slightly lesser extent, reptiles, amphibians and 'fish'. The huge diversity within and among these taxa means that there is little consistency in their physiology, let alone their behaviour. Even within species, individuals and populations are likely to be behaviourally distinct; indeed, this fine-scale variation is itself often the focus of field investigation. Generalising the needs and responses of individuals of particular populations and species is, therefore, an ambitious and probably unrealistic endeavour. Investigators and regulators must view field studies on a case-by-case basis, bringing relevant experience to bear where possible, but being prepared for exception and novelty due to the unexpected events that can occur in a natural situation. Since much of the legislation dealing with scientific procedures on animals is restricted to vertebrates (see Chapter 8: Legislation and oversight of the conduct of research using animals: a global overview), we will not consider invertebrates in this chapter. *Octopus vulgaris*, for example, is covered by legislation in the UK and, at a European level, protection may be extended to all cephalopods and decapod crustaceans. We do not consider kept animals, such as companion animals and farm livestock. However, cats *Felis catus*, dogs *Canis familiaris*, pigs/boar *Sus scrofa*, goats *Capra aegagrus hircus*, horses *Equus caballus* and other kept animals, such as ferrets *Mustela furo* mink *Neovison vison*, often return to a free-living state, sometimes outside of their native range, where they can revert to wild-type appearance and behaviour. Such feral animals are, to all intents and purposes, wild and so they fall within our scope.

The object of field studies is to examine how wild animals behave in the wild or in as natural a situation and habitat as possible. Observations in the field might require little direct intervention and be as apparently straightforward as observing animals from a distance, comparable to a birdwatcher's hobby. However, interventions might involve animals being filmed or camera-trapped, or physically trapped, potentially anaesthetised, and equipped with tags or telemetry devices and less conspicuously if they are treated with internal markers, drugs or if their social or physical environment is manipulated around them. Other treatments, procedures and observations might take place in the laboratory or in other situations where wild animals are trapped and held captive for periods of time. Therefore, our review extends to any interaction with wild animals in the field, the taking of animals from the wild and includes making observations or applying treatments in captivity, where captivity is temporary and takes place in the field or requires holding animals for periods for up to a few days. We do not dwell on the use of wild-caught animals in prolonged or terminal laboratory work, but focus on cases where animals are subsequently released back to the wild.

By studying animals in the wild and capturing the natural variability of their environment and behaviour, investigators are by definition and intent exposing the animals in the study environment to uncertainty and unpredictability. It is never certain, for example, how many animals might be caught in a trap round or cannon net or how individuals might behave or

---

The UFAW Handbook on the Care and Management of Laboratory and Other Research Animals, Ninth Edition.
Edited by Huw Golledge and Claire Richardson.
© 2024 John Wiley & Sons Ltd. Published 2024 by John Wiley & Sons Ltd.

respond to capture or interventions. With experience, many of these risks can be identified or predicted and mitigated. Expecting the unexpected and building appropriate contingency plans and budgets carries financial costs, but these are usually minor relative to the cost of mistakes and misjudgement, which may lead to a project being abandoned because of failures to comply with legislation and/or public opposition.

Reasons for wildlife research

The management of wild animals is an intrinsic part of land management. Often these practices have developed over centuries of common practice and form part of routine pest management for disease control and crop protection, as well as for food and sport. More recently, as the awareness of the threats to biodiversity conservation has increased, management is frequently undertaken to enhance the status of endangered or threatened species. As society and the environment changes, it is becoming much more important that we understand how wild animals respond to management actions. Regulatory authorities and private sector interests can intervene in management, by requiring evidence of humane treatment, efficacy or cost-effectiveness.

Studies may be carried out to examine wild animal biology, including population dynamics and individual behaviour and welfare. Wild animals are also used as indicators of environmental health. For these studies, the benefits in terms of knowledge, understanding and the conservation of the species are usually clearly articulated; however, the costs incurred to the welfare of the individual animals are often not as well understood.

One critical difference between wild animal studies and the use of laboratory animals in research is that with wild animals, the subject of interest and focus of investigation is the subject animal in its own right rather than as a model for the human condition or some other living system, as with many laboratory studies. For this reason, the total replacement of animals in wildlife research (unlike, for example, clinical studies) will never be a feasible option (see Cuthill 2007 and Barnard 2007 for fuller discussions on this topic), and for many wildlife studies, captive or captive-bred animals will never be a substitute for free-living animals. Nonetheless, due consideration should always be given to seeking alternatives where possible, in order to reduce the number of animals impacted.

Welfare impacts of wildlife studies

Effects of stress

All interactions between humans and animals have the potential to cause stress and behavioural or physiological changes, and this is particularly likely with wild animals, where any kind of direct interaction is usually perceived as a threat. Stress is an integral part of all animals' lives, and the body has developed many mechanisms for coping with both psychological and physical stressors (see (Broom & Johnson 1993) for review). However, acute or prolonged stress can have diverse, profound and deleterious effects on the psychological and physiological health of animals, and it is usually in the latter case that animals are said to be 'suffering from distress'. In wildlife studies, the onset of these stress-related effects is of particular importance; they may be difficult if not impossible to identify as animals are normally released into the wild and any symptoms may not be observed. And, unlike laboratory subjects, wild animals are not constantly provided with the essentials of life (such as food, water and shelter) and so their survival is routinely challenged on a range of fronts.

In severe cases, acute stress can cause death from cardiac failure, but in the majority of cases the effects will be more long term and harder to define. Physiological indicators of stress that may be observed during capture include shortness of breath (panting) and tachycardia (racing heart). However, from a behavioural point of view, stress reactions are more difficult to ascertain and very much rely on having detailed knowledge of the biology of the study animals. For example, some animals become motionless (e.g., rabbits *Oryctolagus cuniculus*) or may appear relaxed (e.g., badgers *Meles meles*) when confronted with a stressor, whereas other animals will be hyperactive and spend a great deal of time in escape behaviours (e.g., rats *Rattus* spp.). In addition, response to stressors can vary within a species, with differences apparent between dominant and subordinate individuals and between genders (Overli *et al*. 2006).

The long-term physiological components of stress can affect most aspects of an animal's biology. High levels of stress hormones (such as glucocorticoids) are linked to poor reproductive success in males and females (Rivier & Vale 1984; Sapolsky *et al*. 2000) and reduced immunity from disease (Munck *et al*. 1984), both of which have the potential for significant impact on a wild animal's life and fitness. See also Chapter 6: Brief introduction to welfare assessment: a 'toolbox' of techniques.

Injuries

Apart from physiological effects, there are also adverse physical consequences of field studies, primarily arising from capture and captivity. These range from minor injuries such as skin abrasions and tooth and claw damage in animals attempting to escape from cage or box traps and abrasions from external devices (e.g., radio/GPS collars) up to more severe injuries such as broken limbs (e.g., birds in mist nets, 'foul' captures in traps), adverse reactions to drugs, predator attacks or death (e.g., fish in gill nets) (Powell & Proulx 2003).

One particularly serious problem associated with capture of wild animals is myopathy. This occurs when an animal is subjected to stress and intense physical exertion. It is unusual with cage trapping but can be found with netting or prolonged pursuit and handling of large mammals, particularly deer (Haulton *et al*. 2001). The condition is caused by a build-up of lactic acid in muscles leading to stiffness, paralysis and, in extreme cases, death (Breed *et al*. 2019; Conner *et al*. 1987). Symptoms normally have a delayed onset (sometimes over one week) and, hence, are rarely identified during capture, instead occurring after the animal has been released and usually no longer under observation. Hence, it is imperative that stress levels are minimised by ensuring confident and effective handling and brief periods of pursuit and capture.

Other welfare effects

If the welfare status of an animal is unduly compromised, this is not only of ethical significance but also impacts the validity and rigour of the scientific study itself. The stress associated with capture (and particularly when associated with anaesthesia) can have wide-ranging effects on an animal's biology, behaviour and ecology, and these must be taken into account. Poor welfare arising from studies can have effects on the following:

i) Social structure and behaviour

The establishment and maintenance of social status within animal groups is complex and varies greatly with taxonomy, environment and among individuals. Social rank in a group is determined by many factors, but higher rank is often gained through aggressive behaviour linked to levels of the male hormone testosterone (Abbott *et al*. 2003; Schaffner & French 2004). Stress can alter testosterone levels and may, therefore, compromise dominance hierarchies within a population, particularly in group-living animals such as wolves. In addition, even the temporary removal of an animal from its social group (especially the dominant male and female) may affect its subsequent position and the relative status of several others, and this may cause unrest and heightened aggression in the group. The effect of large-scale permanent removal of individuals on social structure has been well documented in badgers. Badger culling employed for the control of tuberculosis (TB) has resulted in disruption of territoriality, increased ranging behaviour and mixing between social groups (Carter *et al*. 2007).

ii) Reproductive behaviour

The effect of stress on levels of reproductive hormones is well documented and could have wide-ranging effects for males and females, with respect to their reproductive investment and success. Anaesthesia has the potential to cause abortion in the early part of gestation and premature birth in late pregnancy. It has also been shown that handling young can cause the mother to kill or abandon them. Therefore, where reproduction is not a focus of the research, studies should, where possible, be carried out outside sensitive times during the breeding seasons. There are also instances where the procedure itself can influence mating behaviour. This has been demonstrated in bird species that use 'badges of status' where ringing these birds can have an impact on mate choice (Burley 1986; Song *et al*. 2017).

iii) Foraging behaviour

Anaesthesia and stress can affect the metabolic condition (Smith 1993) and cognitive ability of an animal in the short term rendering it less able to forage. Alternatively, periods of captivity in the absence of preferred food may affect an animal's nutritional status and foraging choices upon release. This problem can be minimised if studies are conducted at times when there are fewer external pressures such as low food availability.

iv) Spatial behaviour

Some animals have been shown to move away from an area from where they have experienced capture and anaesthesia presumably as the stress of this experience is associated with this geographical area (Teixeira *et al*. 2007). Others tend to be more sedentary than normal after capture and release. This has, potentially, wide-ranging effects on the population dynamics of group living animals and also on the survival of individual animals that forsake their known home ranges and food sources. While such changes may be temporary, scientific measurements made during the affected period may give a misleading impression of typical ranging behaviour. Where observation periods are brief, these measures will be even more prone to bias.

v) Survival and mortality rates

Even the ringing of birds can have an effect on mortality in a population (Recher *et al*. 1985; Inglis *et al*. 1997). The procedure itself can directly affect the probability of survival due to impact of stress, and in addition, wild animals often carry underlying latent infections such as toxoplasmosis (e.g., in sparrows) that may, as a result of lowered immunity due to stress, develop into clinical disease (Bermúdez *et al*. 2009).

vi) Population dynamics

There is always the potential that the study itself might have a direct effect on the results obtained. Increased mortality and disease are both possibilities, but more subtle effects may be more difficult to determine. Moorhouse and Macdonald (2005) demonstrated that the sex ratio of a population of water voles was affected by a trapping and radio-tracking programme over a three-year period. Over this time, one discrete population of the water voles was regularly trapped and anaesthetised, whereas a separate population was left undisturbed. After three years, both populations were trapped and the numbers estimated. It was found that the first population had a significantly higher ratio of males to females than the undisturbed voles. The authors concluded that the stress of capture and tracking had caused the mothers to produce higher levels of testosterone leading to an increase in male births.

vii) Effects on others

One of the main differences in welfare terms between laboratory and wildlife studies is the fact that the latter has the potential to affect not only the study animals but also many other individuals in the surrounding area. Although this may not be avoidable, it is always important to be aware of the consequences of any study and factor it into the ethical assessment:

a) Conspecifics

The effect of a study on an individual also has potential repercussions for conspecifics especially with respect to group living animals. This includes changes in dominance hierarchies and the onset of disease (see section on *Survival and mortality rates* above).

b) Dependents

Removing parent animals from their dependents may cause malnutrition and, in severe cases, death of the young, particularly among animals with altricial young and those in the earliest stages of life. Treatment with drugs, including anaesthesia, has the potential to affect lactation (Yokoyama 1965), potentially exacerbating nutritional problems. Where breeding is not itself the focus of the study, trapping when young are dependent is a risk that should be avoided where possible or mitigated. If there are obvious signs that the animals caught have dependent young (e.g., lactation and brood patches), then it is advisable to release them as soon as possible, which may involve a judgement as to whether to carry out all of the intended procedures.

c) Non-targets

Capturing non-target species or individuals is almost unavoidable in wildlife studies, but the consequences can be more severe than those for the intended subject, and selective traps should be used wherever possible (Virgós *et al.* 2016). For example, it may be the breeding season of the non-target but not of the target, or the trap though suitable for the target may not be appropriate for non-target species (e.g., weasels *Mustela* spp. caught in uncovered cage traps can die through hypothermia).

The three Rs and welfare

Exact numbers of wild animals used in procedures regulated under the Animals (Scientific Procedures) 1986 Act are difficult to ascertain and are not often specifically quoted for wildlife species. In the UK, Home Office statistics[1] provide numbers of each species used in a range of subjects, but it is not clear how many wild animals are studied in the field. For example, there were 5451 procedures carried out in the category of protection of the natural environment in 2020, which would presumably include wild animal research. The majority of these were fish (4158), many of which were tagged and released as part of fisheries research, though others were captive animals used in behavioural ecology research in the laboratory. The remaining individuals largely fell into the categories: Other rodent, Other carnivore, Other mammal (180) and Other bird (2) with no amphibian or reptile use recorded in this year for this purpose. In addition, wild species are also likely to have been used in other fields of study (e.g., basic research where 202 Other amphibians were used). Many wildlife studies, including observational studies or minor interventions such as bird ringing, may not involve regulated procedures but nonetheless could affect the welfare of the subject animal. Although the three Rs concept (Replacement, Reduction and Refinement) was originally developed with laboratory studies in mind, the same principles and philosophy can be extended to many other areas in which there are human–animal interactions, as a means of ensuring the highest standards of welfare (see Cuthill 2007). See also Chapter 2: The three Rs. Unfortunately, most of the information readily available with respect to the three Rs tends to be aimed at their implementation in laboratory studies, and many examples are not applicable to wildlife research (e.g., cell culture and refinement of housing). This, however, should not lead to the conclusion that the three Rs are not relevant to wildlife research. Here, we provide a number of practical examples of how the three Rs can be incorporated into field studies.

Replacement

Replacement is often not considered a valid concept in studies of the behaviour and ecology of wildlife species, where the specific animals and their natural behaviour are intrinsic to the study (see section *Reasons for wildlife research* above). However, sometimes alternative techniques can give us a greater understanding of these topics without the use of animals themselves.

i) *In silico* studies (i.e., computer modelling)

This approach can be used to generate predictions of treatment effects, often taking into account uncertainty associated with observations and outcomes. In this way, the results of modelling can be more general than those of specific or localised observational studies. While such modelling requires understanding of the quality and representative nature of input data, modelling can also help evaluate the most important avenues of investigation allowing the field study to be refined. This approach has proven particularly effective in estimating population changes and for evaluating methods of management and disease control (Wilkinson *et al.* 2004).

ii) Use of less sentient species

The substitution of a less sentient and/or non-protected species is usually classed as a form of replacement but is often not appropriate for the majority of wildlife studies, where the species itself is the subject of investigation. However, there is potential for using this type of replacement in ecotoxicology studies, where invertebrate models (e.g., the shrimp *Gammarus*) can be used to assess levels of pollutants (Ashauer *et al.* 2007).

iii) Read-across approach

This approach is more commonly associated with pharmaceutical and toxicity testing, usually in combination with computer modelling (Schultz *et al.* 2009). At a basic level, it involves using data from one species to predict outcomes in others. Although this may not be appropriate for many field studies, it may be useful in more heavily regulated areas

---

[1] https://www.gov.uk/government/statistics/statistics-of-scientific-procedures-on-living-animals-great-britain-2020 (Accessed March 16, 2023)

such as ecotoxicology and developing population control methods. For example, if determining the effect of pesticides on non-target species, data from wood mice (*Apodemus sylvaticus*) may be used to extrapolate to other small rodents such as harvest mice (*Micromys minutes*).

Reduction

Most of the principles and techniques of minimising animal use in the laboratory are also applicable to studies in the field:

i) Statistical design

The use of robust statistical approaches before, during and after the study can help ensure an efficient study where minimum numbers of animals are used and resources are deployed to best effect. Power analysis, where the project scale and sampling techniques are evaluated with respect to a range of probable effect sizes, is particularly important in planning investigations. See also Chapter 3: The design of animal experiments. It can now be applied to a range of complex analytical approaches, though often requiring repeated simulations of statistical outcomes rather than the off-the-peg power analyses available in standard packages (see Dytham 2003).

As with laboratory studies, the precision and accuracy of observations in relation to the magnitude of any effect size are vital in considering the required sample size. Similarly, variance in outcomes can be inflated by sampling across outwardly similar groups or environments, potentially masking treatment effects. Sampling design may need to be modified to account for, or avoid, these sources of potential variance. However, sample size and sampling design cannot be easily controlled in the field, and natural error variance and sampling error, if anything, tend to be more pronounced (see Feinsinger 2001). The following factors often confound field investigations and should be taken into account in developing the study design:

- Species, sex and age
- Weather conditions
- Presence and number of non-targets
- Interference by others (e.g., members of the public)

The other factor to consider is that if the sample size is too small, repeating studies to gain the data required is more difficult than in the laboratory, due to the inability to mimic the exact conditions used in previous trials.

ii) Sequential testing

Sequential testing (or phasing) is where the sample size is not fixed in advance. Instead, data are evaluated as these are collected and further sampling is stopped in accordance with a pre-defined stopping rule as soon as significant results are observed. Thus, a conclusion may sometimes be reached at a much earlier stage than would be possible with more classical hypothesis testing or estimation, with the potential to use fewer animals. With these techniques, as the study progresses, the design can be refined or the study halted as appropriate

iii) Using published or available data

Literature and other resources should be used to inform experimental design, perhaps in a power analysis, and hence reduce the number of animals or trials needed. It is important to note that the read-across approach works in this instance as well (i.e., if no data are available for a particular species, searches should be made for data on related animals).

iv) Sharing data

Data sharing is an important method for reducing animal use across the whole spectrum of animal related studies. Data are normally shared within a scientific discipline via publications or presentations at conferences, but this tends to focus only on positive results and finalised studies. It is as important, if not more so, that negative results and potential pitfalls of animal work are highlighted, and a particularly good way of achieving this is by the use of specialist user groups on the web. These can provide an easily accessible and low-cost method to exchange data and ideas.

Samples can be shared as well as information. If different research teams (especially in the same geographical area) all require samples (e.g., blood, hair and swabs) from the same species, then it may be possible to work together so that the animals only need to be caught and sampled once. This needs to carry the caveat that the numbers, quantities and types of samples taken from an individual must remain within the best practice guidelines (see below) and have the appropriate licensing authority.

v) Multi-use technique

This technique is particularly applicable to field use. It is a method of minimising the overall number of animals used by gaining data from one event that may be required for different parts of the study or for a completely separate study (e.g., trapping animals for marking for ecological study and taking blood samples for a disease monitoring programme). A good degree of forethought needs to be exercised when undertaking multi-use studies so that appropriate permissions are in place for all uses and any caveats observed before the studies are initiated.

The PREPARE and ARRIVE guidelines, although designed for laboratory studies, can also be useful in guiding the design and subsequent reporting of studies involving wildlife.

Refinement

The main way of addressing refinement with respect to wildlife studies is through opting for the least invasive techniques and always referring to 'best practice' guidelines and recent experience for capture, handling, marking and sampling appropriate for the species (see section *Capture, handling, release* below)

More specific, less-invasive methods include:

i) Remote cameras

This method involves using remotely triggered cameras to gain information without any capture or manipulation of an animal. With digital technology, these cameras are more

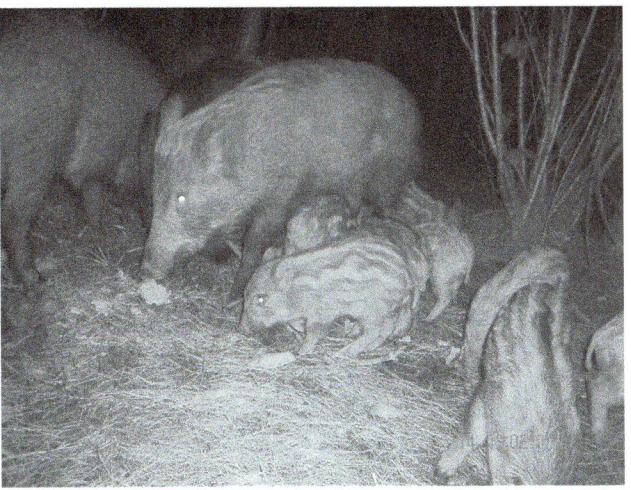

Figure 7.1 Image of wild boar using an infrared camera trap.

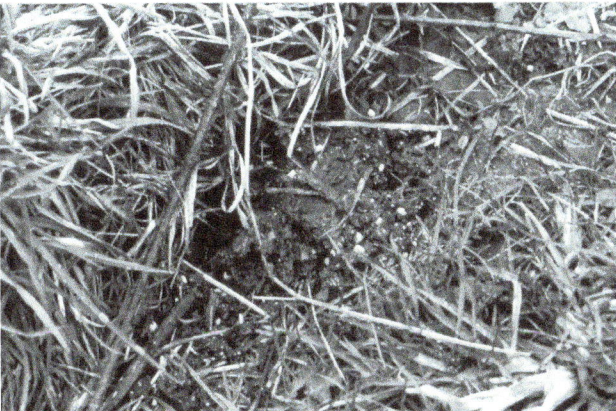

Figure 7.2 Coloured beads as bait markers in badger latrine. A non-invasive and effective method to monitor bait uptake is to add coloured beads to baits which can then be detected in the faeces negating the need for any procedure or capture of the animal.

sophisticated and can create photographs in various formats, use time lapse technology, motion-sensitive, and can operate at night using infrared (see Figure 7.1). In addition, there are now cameras that allow video and photographs to be sent via 4G over the GSM network to a smart phone or computer. Using video recording and/or still photographs has the advantage over direct observations in that there is less disturbance (and hence less stress imposed) on the animal, and it requires less input from the investigator. This technique sometimes requires prior catching for marking (depending on the type of study) but still has the benefit of reducing capture and handling.

ii) Non-invasive sampling methods

Many field studies involve the taking of samples to measure physiological parameters or pathological indicators. Although most of these factors have been traditionally measured in the blood, other less invasive approaches to sampling (e.g., saliva and faeces) can be used in many instances to gain the same data. Faecal sampling is of particular interest as it can be used easily without disturbing the subject and without interfering with other welfare measures running in parallel, such as behavioural assessment (Lane 2006). Faecal sampling can be used to investigate hormonal levels (e.g., cortisol and testosterone), conduct DNA analyses and for bait marking purposes (see Figure 7.2). For some species, natural markings can be used as a completely non-invasive method of identification (see section *Marking* below).

iii) Smart traps

There have been a number of very recent advances in 'smart trapping' enabling the capture of non-targets to be eliminated and the time of capture of target animals to be significantly reduced, thereby improving animal welfare on a number of fronts. Some traps can select animals which are over a specific weight ensuring no juveniles or other similar smaller species are caught or they can only be accessed by animals already with a passive integrated transponder (PIT) tag[2]. In addition, some smart traps can release the door after a set amount of time that can be useful for collecting faecal samples without human interference or can ensure that animals not processed within the maximum amount of time (e.g., through human error) will be automatically released. Other electronic monitoring devices (e.g., MINKPOLICE™) can send text messages once activated, thereby reducing the amount of time the animal needs to spend in captivity. There are also instances where camera identification can be used to allow only certain species to access the trap. However, this technology is still in its infancy and is very expensive and currently only be bespoke made for particularly high-profile work (e.g., snow leopards).

It is also important to be aware of outdated techniques that should not be used in most circumstances due to the availability of more refined alternatives. A good example of this is the use of toe-clipping to permanently mark small mammals and amphibians. This invasive technique permanently removes part of an animal's toe, causing tissue damage (Golay & Durrer 1994; Reaser 1995) and affecting survival (Clarke 1972), and it has been demonstrated to cause pain and suffering (May 2004). For these reasons, it should, wherever possible, be replaced by a non-invasive technique such as using natural markings or if not possible a less damaging technique such as microchipping.

With respect to refinement, it is also important to always consider the fate of non-targets as well as study animals. Non-targets may encounter the same potential costs to welfare as the target animals such as stress and injury caused by cage trapping or mist netting or in some cases (due to the trap not being designed for that species), the impact on non-targets can be even more sever and occasionally fatal. Hence, it is vitally important that best practice methods of capture are employed to reduce the incidence of non-target captures (see below).

---

[2] www.knowleslab.com/research/new-technology-for-wildlife-monitoring (Accessed September 19, 2022)

Capture, handling, release

Most wildlife studies in the field include the use of capture, mark and release programmes. The techniques adopted in these programmes can have far-reaching welfare consequences, and therefore, it is important to be aware of, and where possible, minimising the potential adverse effects not only on the study animals but also on the other animals in the environment.

General welfare issues

i) Time of year

Research may lead to disruption of normal animal activities, whether as part of the study procedure or incidental to it (directly or indirectly) Disturbance of breeding individuals and dependent juveniles is of particular concern. Investigators should be aware of the breeding seasons of the species that they propose to study and ensure that there are no significant welfare implications associated with the timing of their research.

ii) Time of day

An awareness of an animal's circadian activities is essential for appropriate capture and handling, or for making observations. Nocturnal animals should be kept in darkness when held in traps, as being away from cover during daylight hours will cause them further stress. Animals that are caught without the use of food baits (e.g., mist netting of birds and bats) should be released with enough time to forage before they return to burrows or roost. If this is not possible, consideration should be given to provision of supplementary food and water or a glucose solution before release.

iii) Extreme weather conditions (heat or cold)

Checking weather forecasts should always be a priority when carrying out field work. In the UK, the Met Office provide a paid service in which detailed, tailored forecasts can be sent directly to your email account, and there are a number of phone apps that also give reasonably accurate forecasts (although not in the detail that the Met Office provide). Trapping should be avoided during extreme weather conditions to reduce the possibility of hyper- or hypothermia. Shelter and extra warmth should be considered especially when anaesthetising animals in cold conditions (e.g., heat pads, blankets and bubble wrap).

iv) Non-targets

The capture of non-targets is always a possibility with trapping, so, where possible, use selective methods that maximise the capture of the intended target and reduce the capture of other species (e.g., son a run, or use smart traps; see above). However, always be prepared to deal with non-targets if the need arises. In some cases, certain non-target species, usually invasive non-native species (e.g., grey squirrel, mink in the UK), may not be released back to the wild under conservation legislation

Capture

The choice of capture method should be made according to the species involved and availability of technology and personnel, potentially including veterinary cover. Methods of capture may be physical, such as the use of traps and nets. Small–medium mammals and birds are often caught in live traps and netting tends to be the most common method for catching small birds and bats. Larger mammals may be trapped by a variety of methods (live trapping and netting) and may also be chemically sedated using darts. Capture efficiency and capture-related mortality rates have been found to differ considerably between methods and operators, and this should be considered before a decision is made.

i) Live trapping

It is vitally important that you only catch as many animals that you can effectively and safely deal with in the time period available. With cage traps, only set the number that you can check and process within the allocated time (usually a maximum of 24 hours, though note that traps checked every 24 hours could hold animals captive for nearly 48 hours). It is also beneficial to have a good idea of variation in trap efficiency in your study system (e.g., number of captures/100 trap night) so that you can check your plan is achievable. Traps should always be shut or wired open if you are unable to check with the required frequency.

Being caught and held in a trap can be a very stressful experience for an animal, but the trauma can be minimised by:

- Avoiding exposed areas (so they are less likely to be bothered by cold, predators, noise, etc.)
- Providing shade/cover and bedding or similar material where applicable – apart from calming the animal this can also reducing biting and scratching (see Figures 7.3 and 7.4)

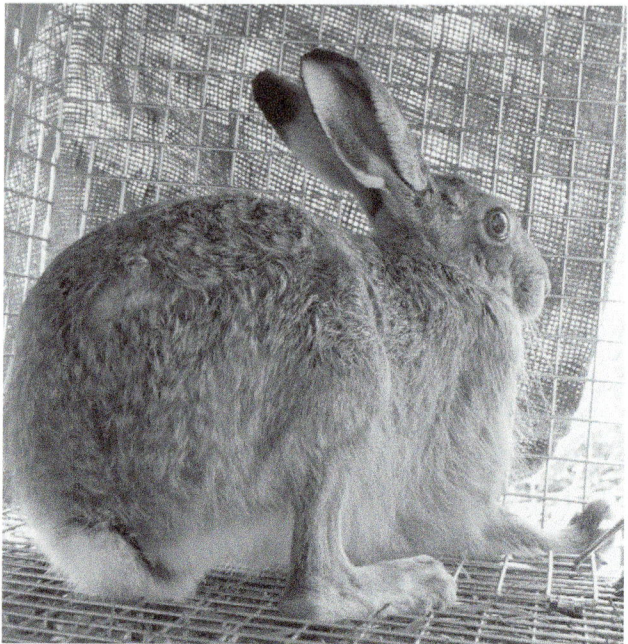

Figure 7.3 Hare in cage trap. Covering traps prevents exposure to the elements and predators and has a calming effect on most species.

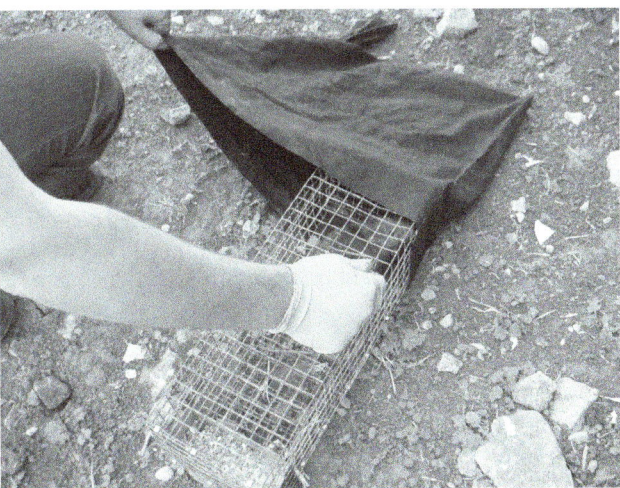

Figure 7.4 Transferring wild rat from cage trap. When dealing with wild animals, it is always beneficial if they can be studied with minimal handling. A simple black bag provides a device to extricate wild rats simply and safely from a cage trap. The rats seeking solace in the darkness will run directly into the bag precluding the need for direct handling.

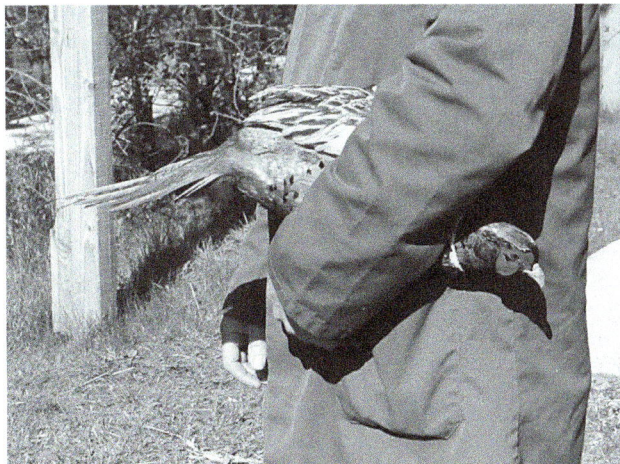

Figure 7.5 Correct handling of a pheasant. Wings and feet are safely secured so that the bird cannot damage itself or the handler.

- Ensuring traps (and animals) are clearly labelled, particularly if the animals are being moved for processing so that you know exactly where to return them for release
- Checking frequently – especially with small animals such as shrews (preferably at least twice a day)
- With netting, it is important to be able to close down the nets as you approach your handling capacity in the specified time period. Small animals have high metabolic rates and can quickly lose condition, so efficiency is of the essence.

Most cage traps rely on a baiting system, so food is usually available, but it is also recommended that water or food with high water content is provided. In addition, if using live traps for small mammals, food should be provided for shrews (e.g., fly pupae) even if they are not the target.

Handling

Wild animals should not be handled unless necessary for the procedure. If handling is required, the amount of contact should be kept to a minimum and the safety of the handler and of the animal needs to be considered (see Figure 7.4). Wild animals are likely to bite or peck and scratch and are carriers of many zoonotic diseases (e.g., *Leptospira*, Cryptosporidium) and so caution needs to be exercised at all times and risk assessments carried out before handling any wild animal. The method of handling will depend on the species of the animal and on the procedure to be carried out. However, there are key rules that should be followed:

- Handling should be kept to a minimum
- Most animals like to be covered as it produces a calming effect–this is NOT the case for some species of deer (e.g., muntjac), which find being covered more stressful
- Handlers need to be confident and competent at dealing with the appropriate species
- Rodents should never be lifted by the end of their tail
- With birds the hold must include the wings and legs in order to prevent damage to these appendages. Certain species may have specific requirements for physical restraint, including those with long legs and necks (see Figure 7.5). Birds breathe by a bellows-like action of the ribs and sternum. Therefore, care should be taken so that the method of restraint does not interfere with the ventilatory movements of the sternum or impede the respiratory air flow.

Anaesthesia

In the UK, under Schedule 2(A) of Animal Scientific Procedures Act, anaesthesia should be used for all regulated procedures unless the use of these compounds is likely to cause more harm and distress. For wild animals, it may be that some procedures that are not inherently painful (e.g., fitting a radio GPS collar) may still require sedation and/or anaesthesia, even if brief, for the handler's safety and the animal's welfare.

With all wild animal anaesthesia, veterinary input and advice should be sought from the outset. Doses, routes and recovery should be discussed fully with a veterinary surgeon before embarking on anaesthetising any wild animal. The following information is for guidance only.

After administering an anaesthetic, the animal must be monitored to check that they are at the required depth of anaesthesia and that their vital body functions have not become dangerously depressed. Respiratory and cardiac function must both be monitored closely. When anaesthetising wild animals in the field, inhalation or injectable anaesthetics may be used (see Hall *et al.* 2000 for overview).

i) Inhalation anaesthetics

These types of anaesthetics tend to be used for small mammals and birds. There are portable versions of gaseous anaesthetic machines (see Figure 7.6) or anaesthetics can be delivered in a

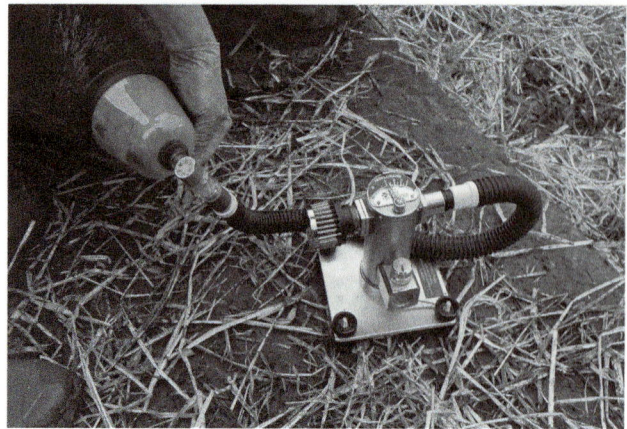

Figure 7.6 Anaesthesia of a wild boar. Portable gaseous anaesthetic machines are an effective and safe way of maintaining anaesthesia (after initial darting or injection) in medium- and large-sized mammals in field situations.

chamber in which the liquid compound is poured onto a gauze or cotton wool pad. The former set-up is preferable is it allows much more control of the depth and recovery from anaesthesia and, hence, should be used whenever possible and practical to do so. In the latter device, the concentration is dependent on the temperature, and in cold winter weather, it may be difficult to ensure that the anaesthetic agent actually vaporises and does so sufficiently quickly. All volatile anaesthetics are irritant when in their liquid state, so the chamber must be designed to separate the anaesthetic-soaked gauze or cotton wool from the animal. It can be more difficult to safely judge the correct depth of anaesthesia for birds. The avian respiratory system, which consists of a pair of relatively fixed lungs and a group of mobile air sacs, is more efficient at gas exchange than mammals, and therefore, birds will often demonstrate a more rapid response to the effects of inhaled anaesthetics. In addition, due to the large volume of stored gases in air sacs, birds can be slow to eliminate the anaesthetics. Recovery from anaesthesia can be facilitated by maintaining the bird in lateral recumbency and turning it from one side to the other every few minutes.

ii) Injectable anaesthetics

These are commonly used for larger mammals delivered through a hypodermic needle and syringe to a trapped or caged animal (e.g., badgers and wild boar) or from a distance via a dart (e.g., wild boar, deer) and will usually be delivered intramuscularly.

Injectable anaesthetics may be used to induce anaesthesia, which is then maintained with a gaseous anaesthetic. In some instances, particularly with small animals that are highly active, such as weasels (*Mustela nivalis*), the opposite may apply, with short-term anaesthesia induced by inhalation and maintained by injection. It should also be noted that the injectable agent ketamine (when used in isolation) has been shown to cause psychosis in humans particularly with repeated use and, hence, should be avoided for wild animal anaesthesia unless used in a cocktail with other drugs (such as medetomidine) (de Leeuw *et al.* 2004).

Darting: Use of a dart-gun to dart wild animals is a specialist skill and may be subject to a number of restrictions. In the UK, dart rifles and blow pipes are classified as Section 5 prohibited weapons under the Firearms Act 1968 and its subsequent amendments. Exemptions for tranquilising and treating animals are available and require both a permit from the Home Office and permission from the statutory authority before use including suitable secure storage facilities. Furthermore, there are restrictions on the number of darts that may be held by one individual. Details may vary between authorities, and advice should always be sought. When firing a dart, the aim is for the dart to hit the animal at right angles, ensuring that the needle penetrates the subcutaneous fat and enters the muscle. The propellant pressure of the rifle should be adjusted depending upon the distance between the operator and the animal to ensure that the dart has sufficient velocity to penetrate to the muscle, but not so much that it enters the body cavity. It is essential to practice thoroughly and regularly before using this equipment on animals.

Recovery from anaesthesia

It is vitally important that all animals are monitored in the recovery phase of anaesthesia. Reflexes such as the swallowing and cough reflexes are usually suppressed during anaesthesia, and although reasonably rare there is a risk of choking and struggling to breathe. Operators should be prepared to handle the animal (e.g., lightly swinging the individual) to get more air into the lungs to enable the animal to breathe properly if this occurs. These reflexes will gradually return as the animal recovers consciousness. Anaesthetics also cause hypothermia, so keeping the animal warm and away from wind and rain is important both pre, during and post-anaesthesia.

With injectable anaesthetics, it is always useful to use a reversing agent where possible. For example, Antisedan will rapidly reverse the sedative effect of medetomidine).

All animals should be fully conscious before release back into the wild, and if the animal is still experiencing effects of the anaesthetic (such as unsteadiness on their feet), they should be kept quiet and warm whilst they fully recover.

Sampling

Methods and volumes for blood sampling of wild species are similar to those for laboratory species[3] (see JWGR 1993) in many instances, although sedation or anaesthesia may be needed for restraint. Due consideration should be given to the health and physiological status of the animal as this can affect the level of handling or the amount of blood that can be safely withdrawn without causing the animal to go into hypovolaemic shock. As with laboratory animals, no more blood should be taken than is necessary, and where alternative less-invasive sampling methods are available (eg use of saliva (see Figure 7.7) or faeces), these should be chosen.

---

[3]https://www.nc3rs.org.uk/3rs-resources/blood-sampling (Accessed 19 September, 2022)

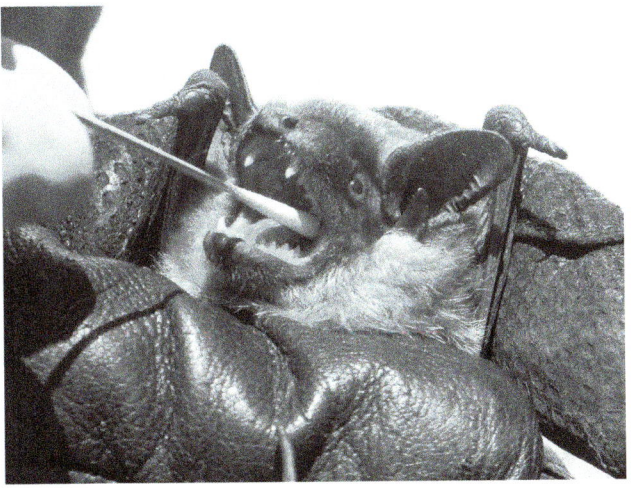

Figure 7.7 Salivary sampling of a serotine bat. Saliva can be collected without anaesthesia in many species and used instead of blood for a variety of physiological measures (e.g., immunoglobulins, stress and reproductive hormones).

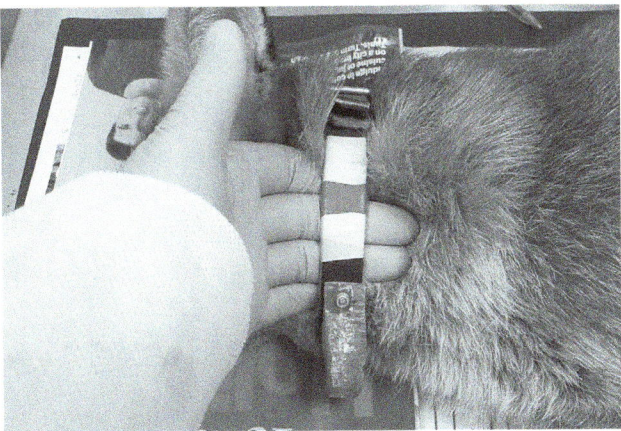

Figure 7.8 Fitting a radio collar to a red fox. It is essential that fitting of the collar is comfortable and allows for growth.

If hair and/or whiskers (vibrissae) are to be taken, cutting/shaving rather than plucking is preferable if the follicles are not required. Whiskers should be taken equally from both sides of the face, and only a small percentage of the total numbers of whiskers should be removed at any one time (e.g., three or four whiskers from each side). Feathers should be taken from less essential areas of birds (e.g., from the back rather than the wings). For stable isotope sampling of tissues, it is important to consider the time at which tissues were formed.

Risk of infection is high in wild animals (perhaps particularly in fossorial species), and hence, the use of antibacterial sprays and/or use of surgical glue is recommended for skin protection following invasive sampling.

Marking

Recognition of individual animals plays an important part in most wildlife research. Marking can provide information about survival, site fidelity, population dynamics, social behaviour, feeding ecology and almost every facet of an animal's ecology. Several techniques are available, such as:

- Telemetry: External and internal, VHF, GPS and proximity transmitters
- External ringing and tagging (bird and bat banding, mammal ear-tags, wing tags)
- Physical marking (tattooing, fur-clipping and scale marking)
- Internal marking (microchips and fish wire-tags)
- Natural markings

i) Telemetric/GPS devices

A wide variety of attachment methods for both types of transmitters exist (collars, tags and implants). External devices should be as light in weight as possible and should not exceed 5% of the body mass of the animal (<3% is recommended).

In many species (especially those that swim or fly), it is not just the weight of the tag that is important but also the shape that can affect the impact of the device. Birds that are subject to high G forces are particularly affected by tags, and care must be taken when using these species. There are some areas in which species specific information on tag weights and design are available[4].

Devices that break away after sampling at the end of the useful life of the transmitter or those with a remote release are preferable. Collars/harnesses should always be fitted to allow room for growth and natural variation in body mass, which can be pronounced in some species. For example, when fitting collars on small–medium mammals, insert fingers between the neck and the collar to judge the appropriate fit (see Figure 7.8).

ii) Ringing

This is the most accepted method of marking birds. In the UK, ringing is not regulated under legislation relating to animals used in research, but attachment of any marks or tags to wild birds requires formal training and a permit from the British Trust for Ornithology[5]. Scientists can obtain scientific permits that are more restricted in their scope, but may require less diverse training and accreditation.

iii) Tagging

When tagging animals, bright colours should be used with caution as they may affect camouflage and act as an attractant for predators – they also make the animals visible to members of the public. In addition, tags should be thoughtfully placed so that they are not likely to snag or get caught on vegetation, potentially leading to tissue damage; this is of particular relevance for animals that squeeze through crevices or holes (e.g., bats and rats).

---

[4] https://www.swansea.ac.uk/staff/science/biosciences/wilson-r-p/#publications=is-expandedhttps://royalsocietypublishing.org/doi/10.1098/rspb.2021.2005 (Accessed 19 September, 2022)

[5] www.bto.org/ringing (Accessed 19 September, 2022)

iv) Physical marking

The type of physical marking chosen will depend on whether the study requires the animal to be identified remotely (e.g., by camera or binoculars) or after re-capture. Fur-clipping is good non-invasive method of temporary marking (as long as the fur removed does not affect thermo-regulation) an individual, but its use is limited in most studies due to its short duration. In contrast, tattooing is a permanent mark and of great benefit in long-term population studies. However, it should be noted that it always requires anaesthesia and does pose a risk of infection (especially for fossorial animals), and hence, the use of antiseptic sprays or creams on the tattooed area is recommended.

v) Microchipping

Microchipping or the use of PIT tags are often the most popular method of choice with many small mammals and amphibia. These devices are commonly used in pets such as cats and dogs. The tag itself is a small cylinder (approximately 7–12 mm or 7 mm in length), and it is usually injected subcutaneously in the scruff of the neck or can be implanted in the lymphatic cavity (particularly in amphibians or reptiles). Although available data suggest no strong evidence for lasting detrimental effects of these tags (Brown 1997), most studies concentrate on efficacy and cost rather than welfare, behaviour, growth and survival. There is anecdotal evidence suggesting that subcutaneous PIT tags can occasionally migrate, potentially leading to problems with the tag moving around the scapular region or even being expelled from the body. There is also some concern that implanting tags into the abdomen through the muscle is a relatively invasive procedure and has the potential to cause pain, necrosis of tissue and/or inflammation around the site. In addition, in some cases, PIT tags are not retained as reliably as other marking techniques (Ott & Scott 1999), but in some species, this method can be very reliable with up to 99% retention recorded (D'Arcy et al. 2020).

vi) Natural marking

Individual-identification-based upon natural markings is an underutilised refinement method. The theory behind individual identification involves the use of physical markings, patterns or colouration, or old injuries such as scars or torn ears to distinguish between conspecifics. The advantage of this method is that it enables identification without the need for handling, therefore minimising disturbance to the animal. It also has low cost compared to other methods (Doody 1995). The age of digital photography has also provided a method of storing a large number of pictures, which can be viewed easily and transferred between facilities. The method has now been used for range of different species including many types of amphibian (Loafman, 1991; Doody 1995), cetaceans (Rugh et al. 1992; Neumann et al. 2002), birds, (Bretagnolle et al. 1994), cheetahs (Kelly 2001), whale sharks (Arzoumanian et al. 2005) and zebras (Briand Peterson 2008).

vii) Invasive tissue marking

Marking techniques that cause significant tissue injury, such as branding and toe, ear and tail clipping (normally used for amphibians or mice), should be avoided. If no alternative methods can achieve the desired results, then researchers need to ensure that the marking process does not cause unnecessary tissue damage, pain, and/or severe blood loss. Adequate pain and infection control is a necessity when undertaking such procedures.

The method used will depend on the species and type of study. When choosing a marking technique, primary consideration should be given to methodologies that are the least invasive, do not require recapture for identification and will remain visible for the duration of the study. In addition, marks should:

- be quick and easy to apply;
- be readily visible and distinguishable;
- persist on animals until all research objectives are fulfilled;
- not introduce bias by having variable tag retention rates;
- not cause long-term adverse effects on health, behaviour, longevity or social life;
- comply with any legal restrictions or regulations;
- allow for seasonal changes in mass and growth of juvenile animals.

Release

Animals should be released back to the point of capture when fully recovered from the procedures performed. If an animal is injured or showing signs of illness, euthanasia may be required. The most humane method of despatch in the field will depend on the species and the experience of the investigator. Table 7.1 lists some suggested methods, but see also Chapter 17: Euthanasia and other fates for laboratory animals, AAZV guidelines[6] and the AVMA 2020 guidelines[7].

Table 7.1 Methods of dispatch. Please note that these methods are not the only, or necessarily the most, appropriate methods to be used in all situations. The method of dispatch used should always be decided on the health status of the individual, the situation, the setting and the competence of the personnel. In addition, confirmation of death by a secondary method (such as onset of rigor mortis) must always be undertaken.

Animal	Suggested method of dispatch
Small rodents Rats Birds	Dislocation of neck or overdose of gaseous anaesthesia
Rabbit	Dislocation of neck (requires highly skilled operator)
Hedgehog	Overdose of gaseous anaesthesia
Badger	Overdose of anaesthesia (injectable)
Bats	Overdose of gaseous anaesthesia
Fox Deer Wild boar	Overdose of anaesthesia (injectable) or Shooting

[6] https://www.avma.org/sites/default/files/2020-02/Guidelines-on-Euthanasia-2020.pdf (Accessed 20 September, 2022)
[7] https://www.avma.org/sites/default/files/2020-02/Guidelines-on-Euthanasia-2020.pdf (Accessed 20 September, 2022)

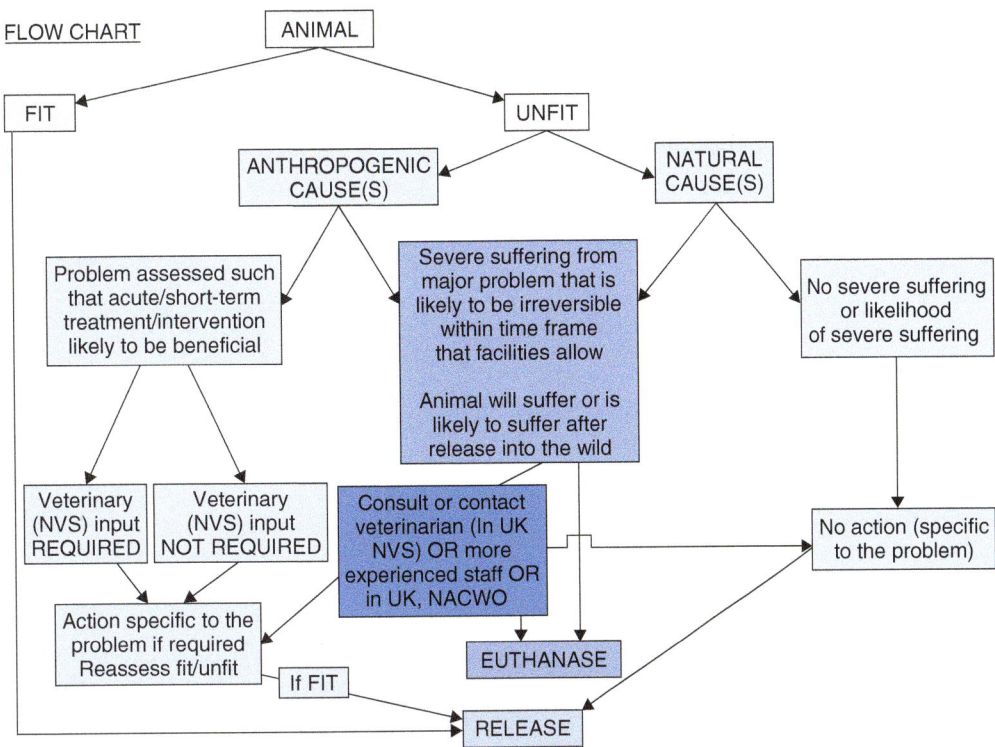

Figure 7.9 Example flow chart on dealing with injured animals in the field. It is vital that all field workers are aware of how to deal with injured target and non-target animals. This flow chart shows an example of strategies for dealing with injuries that are due to the procedure (iatrogenic) or which the animal sustained prior to capture.

The investigator should always have the necessary equipment to euthanise target or non-target animals where appropriate (e.g., anaesthetics for overdose) or in the case of larger animals where veterinary advice may need to be sought contact numbers for 24-hour cover. The type of euthanasia to be used where necessary should be discussed with your Named Veterinary Surgeon prior to commencing studies in the field.

To treat or not to treat?

There are often ethical and moral dilemmas to be faced in the treatment of wild animals. Interference with a natural process could lead to perturbation of the ecological balance, and this must be considered when deciding whether or not to treat a wild animal. As a general guideline, it is accepted that injuries and illnesses that have anthropogenic causes, for example, trap injuries, should be treated (see Figure 7.9 for an example flow chart). In many other cases, the researcher must make an informed choice based upon his/her knowledge of the animal, the injury (or illness) and the situation. The final decision should be one that the researcher has the ability and confidence to defend.

Legislation appropriate to wildlife studies

Anyone proposing to conduct research on, study, capture, hold or release wildlife should be familiar with, and comply with, the relevant legislation governing their use. In many cases, licences or permits are required to conduct work with wildlife. As an example, the paragraphs below list some of the provisions pertaining to wildlife research in the UK.

Legislation relating to the use of animals in research

Animal research in the European Union (EU) is regulated under Directive 2010/63/EU on the protection of animals used for scientific purposes.

In the UK, the ability to perform animal experiments is regulated by the Animals (Scientific Procedures) Act 1986 (ASPA 1986). ASPA has been revised to transpose European Directive 2010/63/EU on the protection of animals used for scientific purposes into UK law. The revised legislation came into force in 2013. The basic relationship between these two pieces of legislation is that ASPA 1986 defines the regulations and 2013/63 provides harmonisation with other EU member states. The European legislation has made very few changes to the UK apart from increases in number and type of records required. In the UK, the Animals (Scientific procedures) Act 1986 A(SP)A states that all regulated work must be carried out at a Licensed Establishment (LE) unless the work requires:

- Wild animals or farm species at sites that could not be reasonably part of an LE.
- Studies that depend upon access to the wild environment or commercial husbandry standards.

When regulated work under A(SP)A is carried out at field sites, these are classed as Places Other than Licensed

Establishments (POLEs). At POLEs, procedures must be conducted and welfare standards maintained as near as practicable to those achievable in LEs. Additional controls also apply to POLEs to enable appropriate controls to be applied, such as notification conditions (i.e., usually the Inspector is required to be notified of all POLE sites at least seven days before the onset of a regulated study). Landowners' consent, where appropriate, must be obtained prior to applying for a licence under ASPA, and provision must be made to allow Inspectors onto all POLE sites.

Wildlife studies and/or techniques that are not regulated under A(SP)A include the following:

- The ringing, tagging or marking of an animal or the use of any other humane procedure for the *primary* purpose of enabling an animal to be identified is not a regulated procedure under A(SP)A if it causes only momentary pain or distress and no lasting harm.
- Humane killing by a recognised method.
- Procedures applied in the course of recognised veterinary practice.
- Capture and release of wild animals unless the method of capture itself is being studied (as long as the capture method does not cause 'avoidable pain, suffering, distress or lasting harm').

However, it should be noted that any of the above do become regulated if anaesthesia is used. Advice should always be sought from the ASRU in case of any doubt as to whether a procedure is regulated or not.

Certain species (known as Schedule 2 animals) to be used in research may be obtained only from a designated breeding establishment, unless an official exemption is granted. Therefore, it is also illegal to trap these animals in the wild without an exemption granted by the Home Office. The animals on this list include mouse, rat, rabbit, ferret and quail. Moreover, release of animals back to the wild will only be authorised if:

- the maximum possible care has been taken to safeguard the animal's well-being;
- the animal's state of health allows it to be set free;
- setting the animal free poses no danger to public health and the environment.

A(SP)A licences do not absolve the licensee from their duties under other wildlife legislation. Hence, all work must comply with other appropriate legislation, and other applicable licences must be in place before any studies commence.

The Habitats Directive

The Habitats Directive[8] is the short name for European Union Council Directive 92/43/EEC on the conservation of natural habitats and of wild fauna and flora. The Directive led to the establishing of European sites and setting out how they should be protected; it also extends to other topics such as European protected species. Most member states then have legislation that they enact that sits under this act and performs the protection needed.

i) The Conservation (Natural Habitats, &c.) Regulations 1994

This implements the EC Directive 92/43/EEC in the UK under which it is an offence, with certain exceptions, to:

- deliberately capture or kill any wild animal of a European protected species;
- deliberately disturb any such animal;
- deliberately take or destroy eggs of any such wild animal;
- damage or destroy a breeding site or resting place of such a wild animal;
- deliberately pick, collect, cut, uproot or destroy a wild plant of a European protected species;
- keep, transport, sell or exchange, or offer for sale or exchange, any live or dead wild animal or plant of a European protected species, or any part of, or anything derived from such a wild animal or plant.

Wildlife and Countryside Acts

The Wildlife and Countryside Act (WCA) 1981 is the principle mechanism for the legislative protection of wildlife in Great Britain but does not extend to Northern Ireland (where the wildlife (NI) order is equivalent in many respects, the Channel Islands or the Isle of Man) but most countries have similar legislation particularly in the EU. This legislation is the means by which the Convention on the Conservation of European Wildlife and Natural Habitats (the 'Bern Convention') and the European Union Directives on the Conservation of Wild Birds (79/409/EEC) and Natural Habitats and Wild Fauna and Flora (92/43/EEC) are implemented in Great Britain. Similar legislation is enacted to fulfil these obligations elsewhere in the UK. The WCA is divided into four parts with Part I being concerned with the protection of wildlife.

Part I of the WCA protects all wild birds and protected animals (includes some mammals, all species of bat; species of dolphin; amphibians, reptiles; porpoise; otter; and many species of insects). A wild bird is defined as any bird of a species that is resident in or is a visitor to the European Territory of any member state in a wild state. Under the WCA, it is an offence to:

- take, injure, kill or sell a protected species;
- disturb a protected species in its nest or place of shelter;
- possess a protected species.

There are additional clauses and various additional forms of protection.

However, many activities prohibited under the WCA can be carried out after acquiring a licence issued by the appropriate authority to avoid committing an offence. For example, scientific study that requires capturing protected animals (under schedule 5 of the Act) can be allowed by obtaining a licence.

Since the passing of the WCA in 1981, there have been various amendments to the Act, through the Countryside and Rights of Way (CRoW) Act 2000 (in England and Wales) and the Nature Conservation (Scotland) Act 2004 (in Scotland), but also through other legislation including the

---

[8] https://ec.europa.eu/environment/nature/legislation/habitatsdirective/index_en.htm (Accessed 20 September, 2022)

Environmental Protection Act 1990. There have also been many changes to the species listed in the schedules through Variations to the Schedules Orders. There is a statutory five-yearly review of Schedules 5 (protected wild animals) undertaken by the statutory conservation agencies but changes to the schedules can be made by the Secretary of State at any time, if it is considered necessary because of a threat of extinction or in response to international obligations. Hence, it is always worth checking whether a species does fall under any of the schedules under the WCA before commencing work (even if this has not been the case previously).

Other wildlife legislation

i) Wild Mammals (Protection) Act 1996

This Act covers unprotected mammals to prevent unnecessary suffering by certain methods such as self-locking snares, explosives, drowning, asphyxiation and use of live decoys. The Wild Mammals (Protection) Act 1996 does not apply in legal pest control or in the humane killing of an injured animal.

ii) The Destructive Imported Animals Act (1932)

This Act restricts the import and keeping of certain destructive non-indigenous animals including Muskrat *Ondata zibethicus*, Coypu *Myocastor coypus*, Grey Squirrel *Sciurus carolinensis*, Mink *Mustela vison* and 'non-indigenous' rabbits. The appropriate licensing authority (Natural England Natural Resources Body for Wales in Wales) may licence imports for research or exhibition purposes.

iii) Animal Welfare Act 2006

This Act ensures that it is not only against the law to be cruel to an animal, but also the welfare needs of the animals must be met. A 'protected animal' under this Act is a non-human vertebrate that is domesticated, not living in a wild state, or under control of man (either permanently or temporarily). The latter does include wild animals captured even for a short period. An offence is caused when an 'act of a responsible person causes an animal to suffer … and suffering is unnecessary'. 'Suffering for a legitimate purpose', e.g., research is permissible but only if; suffering is proportionate to the purpose of the conduct, and could not have been avoided or reduced, and conduct concerned was that of a reasonably competent and humane person.

Further information on how this Act implies to wildlife work can be gained from Natural England Natural England. 2010[9].

iii) The Agreement on International Humane Trapping Standards (AIHTS)

The Agreement on International Humane Trapping Standards (AIHTS) was reached with the EU, Canada and Russia with a separate agreement reached between the EU and United States[10]. Both Agreements incorporate the same standards. The AIHTS establishes criteria for rating traps by species and by method of use. Killing traps are rated according to the time to loss of consciousness. Restraining traps are rated according to injuries indicative of poor welfare. Ratings form part of the trap approval process.

The Agreement prohibits the use of restraining and killing traps that are not certified in accordance with the Standards. However, it does not prevent individuals from constructing and using traps that comply with designs approved by the competent authorities. (Competent authorities are legal bodies that regulate trapping, including governments, government mandated agencies and those Aboriginal groups with authority to regulate wildlife management activities.) Traps not meeting the Agreement Standards must be phased out by the signatories. If there are no traps certified for a particular species, all traps legal for use for that species can continue to be used until certified traps become available and provided research continues to search for traps that meet the Agreement Standards

This agreement is also implemented in the UK via the Humane Trapping Standards Regulations 2019. This seeks to improve the welfare of fur-bearing animals trapped for their pelts as well as for conservation and pest control purposes. It does this by providing minimum humaneness standards for most killing and restraining traps as well as trap testing procedures.

In the UK a licence from Natural England is currently required to trap (both restraining and kill traps):

- Otter (*Lutra lutra*)
- Badger (*Meles meles*)
- Beaver (*Castor fiber*)
- Pine marten (*Martes martes*)
- Stoat (*Mustela erminea*)

Any trap used under the authority of a licence must be certified as meeting the AIHTS and suitable for the humane live capture of the above species.

However, if you want to use a live capture trap that has not yet been considered for certification in England, the use of the trap may be permitted under individual licence, subject to a trap humaneness assessment being undertaken, recorded and reported to the relevant authority (e.g., Natural England in England).

iv) Invasive Alien Species Order

The EU Regulation (1143/2014) on invasive alien (non-native) species entered into force on 1 January 2015. The Regulation imposes restrictions on a list of species known as 'species of Union concern' (see Table 7.2). These are species whose potential adverse impacts across the EU are such that concerted action across Europe is required. This list is drawn up by the European Commission and managed with Member States using risk assessments and scientific evidence.

---

[9]http://www.adlib.ac.uk/resources/000/263/401/TIN072.pdf (Accessed 22 September, 2022)

[10]https://www.face.eu/international-agreements/aihts/ (Accessed 22 September, 2022)

Table 7.2 EU list of invasive non-native species of concern, invasion status in England and organisation responsible for response.

Species	Species	Group
Acridotheres tristis	Common myna	Bird
Alopochen aegyptiacus	Egyptian goose	Bird
Corvus splendens	Indian house crow	Bird
Oxyura jamaicensis	Ruddy duck	Bird
Threskiornis aethiopicus	Sacred ibis	Bird
Callosciurus erythraeus	Pallas' squirrel	Mammal
Herpestes javanicus	Small Asian mongoose	Mammal
Muntiacus reevesi	Muntjac deer	Mammal
Myocastor coypus	Coypu	Mammal
Nasua nasua	Coati	Mammal
Nyctereutes procyonoides	Raccoon dog	Mammal
Ondatra zibethicus	Muskrat	Mammal
Procyon lotor	Raccoon	Mammal
Sciurus carolinensis	Grey squirrel	Mammal
Sciurus niger	Fox squirrel	Mammal
Tamias sibiricus	Siberian chipmunk	Mammal
Vespa velutina nigrithorax	Asian hornet	Invert - insect
Lithobates catesbeianus	American bullfrog	Amphibian
Trachemys scripta	Red-eared, yellow-bellied, Cumberland sliders	Reptile
Arthurdendyus triangulates	New Zealand flatworm	Invert - worm
Lepomis gibbosus	Pumpkinseed	Fish
Percottus glenii	Amur sleeper	Fish
Plotosus lineatus	Striped eel catfish	Fish
Pseudorasbora parva	Stone moroko	Fish
Eriocheir sinensis	Chinese mittencrab	Crustacean
Orconectes limosus	Spiny-cheek crayfish	Crustacean
Orconectes virilis	Virile crayfish	Crustacean
Pacifastacus leniusculus	Signal crayfish	Crustacean
Procambarus clarkii	Red swamp crayfish	Crustacean
Procambarus fallax virginalis	Marbled crayfish	Crustacean

Under Article 8 of the EU IAS Regulation, the UK issues permits to carry out research on, or ex-situ conservation of, invasive alien species of Union concern. Permits are issued by the Animal and Plant Health Agency (APHA) on behalf of Defra and the devolved administrations. Other countries in the EU will have a different licensing system for this regulation[11].

iv) Convention on International Trade of Endangered Species

The Convention on International Trade of Endangered Species (CITES)[12] provides protection to specified endangered species and controls the taking, handling and transport of samples taken or collected from them. This can constrain the international movement of samples collected for scientific purposes, so advice should always be sought about the application of CITES regulations in research on CITES listed species.

v) Other examples of legislation include Acts that are designed for the protection of specific groups of wildlife. In the UK, this includes Acts such as:

The Protection of Badgers Act 1992
The Deer Act 1991,
The Ground Game Act 1880,
The Whaling Industry (Regulation) Act 1934,
The Conservation of Seals Act 1970,
The Salmon and Freshwater Fisheries Act 1975,
The Dangerous Wild Animals Act 1976,

(some of these Acts have parallel legislation in Scotland and Northern Ireland).

Licences

There are different bodies across the UK that are responsible for issuing licences and permits through their Wildlife Management and Licensing Service under a range of wildlife legislation for activities that would otherwise be illegal but where a valid justification exists. These are:

Natural England: England
NatureScot: Scotland

---

[11] https://ec.europa.eu/environment/nature/invasivealien/index_en.htm (Accessed September 22, 2022)
[12] https://cites.org/eng/disc/what.php (Accessed 22 September, 2022)

Natural Resource Wales: Wales

Department of Agriculture, Environment and Rural Affairs (DAERA): Northern Ireland

The Joint Nature Conservation Committee (JNCC) is the advisor on nature conservation to the government across the whole of the UK.

International legislation

Many countries have their own guidance and legislation regarding the use of animals in research and the protection of animals in the wild. It is important that researchers are aware of the local regulations in different countries and abide by these and the 'best practice' guidelines (see below).

Best practice' guidelines

The key to carrying out wildlife studies in the field to the highest standards is to follow best practice guidelines wherever possible. Below is a selection of relevant websites, most of which have links to further resources.

UK

i) National Centre for 3Rs (NC3Rs)
    Microsites on a number of topics with relevance to field studies; of particular interest is their site on 3Rs and wildlife research, but also there are sites on dosing and sampling and anaesthesia that include information appropriate to studying animals in the field
    www.nc3rs.org.uk

ii) Association for the Study of Animal Behaviour (ASAB)
    Guidelines relating to conducting animal research with some areas particularly associated with field studies (e.g., marking) and also have links with other websites that contain information with respect to welfare and ethical treatment of animals
    https://www.asab.org/

iii) British Association for Shooting and Conservation (BASC)
    Although not a welfare organisation BASC has Codes of Practice on the Trapping of Pest Mammals and Pest Birds which include information on the different legislations, and practical tips on topics such as how to reduce non-target capture and the appropriate setting and positioning of traps which may be of help in conducting field studies of these species.
    www.basc.org.uk

Worldwide

i) Norwegian Consensus-platform for Replacement, Reduction and Refinement (norecopa)
    Guidelines for wildlife research particularly relating to the 3Rs
    www.norecopa.no

ii) Canadian Council for Animal Care (CCAC)
    3Rs microsite with a special section on its implementation on wildlife research and refinement alternatives for marking and tagging
    www.ccac.ca

Summary

This chapter is intended as a signpost to the issues that a potential researcher should be considering but does not cover all possible issues that are important in an ever-changing environment. Before embarking on a field study, preparation is key. A checklist of considerations can be of great benefit, an example of which is given below:

- Do you need to use animals to achieve your aims?
- Are you using the lowest number of animals to achieve your aims?
- Are you using the least invasive but effective methods?
- Have you checked 'best practice' guidelines?
- Have you got the appropriate legal authorities (e.g., licences)?
- Have you got the necessary Home Office license (in the UK) or other ethical permissions?
- Is your planned research otherwise within the wildlife law of the country concerned?
- Have you sought advice from others (e.g., veterinary surgeon)?
- Have you checked the weather forecast?
- Have you checked breeding seasons?
- Have you checked your field equipment is the most appropriate for your target species and is fully functional?
- Have you minimised non-target risk?
- Do you know how to treat/despatch injured animals?
- Do you know how to check and ensure the welfare of the animals before discharging from your care?

The wildlife researcher has to be prepared for any eventuality and ensure that the welfare of the animals within their care is maintained at the highest possible level. This is best achieved by always considering the three Rs, being aware of best practice guidelines and taking advice from colleagues and other experts in the relevant scientific fields.

References

Abbott, D.H., Keverne, E.B., Bercovitch, F.B. *et al.* (2003) Are subordinates always stressed? A comparative analysis of rank differences in cortisol levels among primates. *Hormones and Behavior*, **43**, 67–82.

Ashauer, R., Boxall, A.B. and Brown, C.D. (2007) New ecotoxicological model to simulate survival of aquatic invertebrates after exposure to fluctuations and sequential pulses of pesticides. *Environmental Science and Technology*, **41**, 1480–1486.

Arzoumanian, Z., Holmberg, J. and Norman, B. (2005) An astronomical pattern matching algorithm for computer-aided identification of whalesharks Rhincondon type. *Journal of Applied Ecology*, **42**, 999–1011.

Barnard, C. (2007) Ethical regulation and animal science: why animal behaviour is special. *Animal Behaviour*, **74**, 5–13.

Bermúdez, R., Faílde, L.D., Losadab, A.P. et al. (2009) Toxoplasmosis in Bennett's wallabies (*Macropus rufogriseus*) in Spain. *Veterinary Parasitology*, **160**, 155–158.

Breed, D., Meyer, L.C.R., Steyl, J.C.A. et al. (2019). Conserving wildlife in a changing world: Understanding capture myopathy – a malignant outcome of stress during capture and translocation. *Conservation Physiology*, **7** issue 1

Bretagnolle, V., Thibault, J. and Dominici, J. (1994) Field identification of individual osprey using head marking pattern. *Journal of Wildlife Management*, **58**, 175–178.

Briand Peterson, J.C. (2008) An idneitfication system for zebra (Equus burchelli, Gray). *African Journal of Ecology* **10**, 59–63.

Broom, D.M. and Johnson, K. (1993) *Stress and Animal Welfare*. Blackwell Science, Oxford, UK.

Brown, L.J. (1997) An evaluation of some marking and trapping techniques currently used in the study of anuran population dynamics. *Journal of Herpetology*, **31**, 410–419.

Burley, N. (1986) Sexual selection for aesthetic traits in species with biparental care. *American Naturalist*, **127**, 415–445.

Carter, S.P., Delahay, R.J., Smith, G.C. et al. (2007) Culling-induced social perturbation in Eurasian badger *Meles meles* and management of TB in cattle: an analysis of a critical problem in applied ecology. *Proceedings of The Royal Society of London B*, **274**, 2769–2777.

Clarke, R.D. (1972) The effect of toe clipping on survival in fowlers toad (*Bufo woodhousei fowleri*). *Copeia*, **1**, 182–185.

Conner, M.C., Soutiere, E.C. and Lancia, R.A. (1987) Drop-netting deer: costs and incidence of capture myopathy. *Wildlife Society Bulletin*, **15**, 434–438.

Cuthill, I.C. (2007) Ethical regulation and animal science: why animal behaviour is not so special. *Animal Behaviour*, **74**, 15–22.

D'Arcy, J., Kelly, S., McDermott, T. et al. (2020) Assessment of PIT tag retention, growth and post-tagging survival in juvenile lumpfish, *Cyclopterus lumpus*. *Animal Biotelemetry* **8** Article number 1.

Doody, J.S. (1995) A photographic mark-recapture method for patterned amphibians. *Herpetological Review*, **26**, 19–21.

Dytham, C. (2003) *Choosing and Using Statistics. A Biologists Guide*. Blackwell Science, Oxford, UK.

Feinsinger, P. (2001) *Designing Field Studies for Biodiversity and Conservation*. Island Press, Washington DC, USA.

Golay, N. and Durrer, H. (1994) Inflamation due to toe clipping in natterjack toads (Bufo calamita). *Amphibia-Reptilia*, **15**, 81–83.

Hall, L.W., Clarke, K.W. and Trim, C.M. (2000) Chapter 17: Anaesthesia of birds, laboratory animals and wild animals. In: *Veterinary Anaesthesia*, 10th edn, pp. 463–478. Elsevier Press Ltd, UK.

Haulton, S.M., Porter, W.F. and Rudolph, B.A. (2001).Evaluating 4 methods to capture white-tailed deer. *Wildlife Society Bulletin*, **29**, 255–264.

Inglis, I.R., Isaacson, A.J., Smith, G.C. et al. (1997) The effect on the woodpigeon (*Columba palumbus*) of the introduction of oilseed rape into Britain. *Agriculture Ecosystems & Environment*, **61**, 113–121.

JWGR (1993) Removal of blood from laboratory mammals and birds. First Report of the BVA/FRAME/RSPCA/UFAW Joint Working Group on Refinement. *Laboratory Animals*, **27**, 1–22.

Kelly, M.J. (2001) Computer-aided photograph matching in studies using individual identification: and example from Serengeti cheetahs. *Journal of Mammology*, **82**, 440–449.

Lane, J. (2006) Can non-invasive glucocorticoid measures be used as reliable indicators of stress in animals? *Animal Welfare*, **15**, 331–342.

de Leeuw, A.N.S., Forrester, G.J. and Spyvee, P.D. (2004) Experimental comparison of ketamine with a combination of ketamine, butorphanol and medetomidine for general anaesthesia of the Eurasian badger (Meles meles L.). *Veterinary Journal*, **167**, 186–193.

Loafman, R. (1991) Identifying individual spotted salamanders by spot pattern. *Herpetologica Review*, **22**, 91–92.

May, R. (2004) Ecology: Ethics and amphibians. *Nature*, **431**, 403.Moorhouse, T.P. and Macdonald, D.W. (2005) Indirect negative impacts of radio-collaring: sex ratio variation in water voles. *Journal of Applied Ecology*, **42**, 91–98.

Munck, A., Guyre, P.M. and Holbrook, N.J. (1984) Physioloigical functions of glucocrticoids in stress and their relation to pharmacological actions. *Endocrine Review*, **5**, 25–41.

Neumann, D.R., Leitenberger, A. & Orams, M.B. (2002) Photo identification of short beaked common dolphins (*Delphinus delphis*) in north east New Zealand: a photo catalogue of recognisable individuals. *New Zealand Journal of Marine and Freshwater Research*, **36**, 593–604.

Ott, J.A. and Scott, D.E. (1999) Effects of toe clipping and PIT-tagging on growth and survival in metamorphic Ambystomaopacum. *Journal of Herpetology*, **33**, 344–348.

Overli, O., Sorensen, C. and Nilsson, G.E. (2006) Behavioral indicators of stress-coping style in rainbow trout: do males and females react differently to novelty? *Physiology & Behavior*, **87**, 506–512

Powell, R.A. and Proulx, G. (2003) Trapping and marking terrestrial mammals for research: Integrating ethics, performance criteria, techniques, and common sense. *ILAR Journal*, **44**, 259–276.

Reaser, J. (1995) Marking amphibians by toe-clipping; a response to Halliday. *FROGLOG*, **12**, 1–2.

Recher, H., Gowing, G. and Armstrong, T. (1985) Causes and frequency of deaths among birds mist-netted for banding studies at 2 localities. *Australian Wildlife Research*, **12**, 321–326.Rivier, C. and Vale, W. (1984) Influence of CRF on reproductive functions in the rat. *Endocrinology*, **114**, 914–921.

Rugh, D.J., Braham, H.W. and Miller, G.L. (1992) Method of photographic identification of bowhead whales, Balaena mysticetus. *Canadian Journal of Zoology*, **70**, 617–624.

Sapolsky, R.M., Romero, L.M. and Munck, A.U. (2000) How do glucocorticoids influence stress responses? Integrating Permissive, suppressive, stimulatory and preparative actions. *Endocrine Reviews*, **21**, 55–89.

Schaffner, C.M. and French, J.A. (2004) Behavioral and endocrine responses in male marmosets to the establishment of multi-male breeding groups: Evidence for non-monopolizing facultative polyandry. *International Journal of Primatology*, **25**, 709–732.

Schultz, T.W., Rogers, K. and Aptula, A.O. (2009) Read-across to rank skin sensitization potential: subcategories for the Michael acceptor domain. *Contact Dermatitis*, **60**, 21–31.

Smith, W. (1993) Responses of laboratory animals to some injectable anaesthetics. *Laboratory Animals*, **27**, 30–39.

Song, Z., Liu, Y., Booksmthe, I. and Ding, C. (2017) Effects of individual-based preferences for colour banded mates on sex allocation in zebra finches. *Behavioural Ecology* **28**, 1228–1235.

Teixeira, C.P., De Azevedo, C.S. and Mendl, M. (2007) Revisiting translocation and reintroduction programmes: the importance of considering stress. *Animal Behaviour*, **73**, 1–13.

Virgós, E., Lozano, J., Cabezas-Díaz, S. et al. (2016) A poor international standard for trap selectivity threatens carnivore conservation. *Biodiversity and Conservation*, **25**, 1409–1419.

Wilkinson, D., Smith, G.C. and Delahay, R.J. (2004) A model of bovine tuberculosis in the badger *Meles meles*: an evaluation of different vaccination strategies. *Journal of Applied Ecology*, **41**, 492–501.

Yokoyama, A.K. (1965) The effect of anaesthesia on milk yield and maintenance of lactation in the goat and rat. *Journal of Endocrinology*, **33**, 341–351.

8 Legislation and oversight of the conduct of research using animals: a global overview

Kathryn Bayne, Javier Guillen, Malcolm P. France and Timothy H. Morris

Introduction

This chapter serves to highlight key aspects of laws, regulations, policies and/or codes that apply to the use of animals in biomedical research and testing. An exhaustive review of all relevant, but adjunct regulations (e.g. pertaining to animal transportation both domestically and internationally; occupational health and safety; importation/exportation) is beyond the scope of this chapter. In addition, in some jurisdictions the conduct of veterinary clinical research and veterinary clinical trials of new devices, vaccines and pharmaceuticals may be covered by separate mechanisms of oversight. However, as these subjects can have a significant role in the operation of an animal facility, readers are encouraged to review applicable standards in these areas.

Many, but not all, countries and jurisdictions around the world have laws, regulations, policies and other systems of oversight relating to the use of animals in science. There are variations in scope, scale, approach; in legal basis; in social and cultural perspectives; and in implementation. Variability in regulatory delivery and application of such oversight is likely to continue, but there is increasing convergence of the outputs of this oversight. In particular, there is increased emphasis on a wider scope of oversight to include all facets of animal use, in particular on ethical aspects, and on standards and approaches to animal care and welfare.

The regulatory environment for animals in biomedical research and testing is, therefore, both variable across countries, and also in many parts of the world is in a state of evolution. Different approaches have been taken by various countries to improve the welfare of animals used in research, to develop and maintain high-quality science and to address ethical issues. In some countries, the individual scientist is licensed to conduct research, while elsewhere the institution (e.g. university or pharmaceutical company) may hold the licence to do animal-based research. In some countries, a wide range of animals (vertebrate and invertebrate, warm and cold blooded) is covered by government standards, while in other countries there are no government regulations, or government standards cover select species of animals. Some countries require ethical review of proposed research, while in others no institutional or governmental review of the proposed study is necessary before work can begin. Similarly, some countries require researchers to have appropriate training and qualifications while others do not. Voluntary oversight schemes are of importance in numerous countries. This chapter describes some of the similarities and distinctions between countries/regions where biomedical research is conducted by describing the regulatory climate and systems of oversight in several countries. Its purpose is to provide an introduction to the range of legislative approaches, and it is neither a summary of all national regulations nor a critical review.

The increasing availability of laws and regulations in an electronic format has enhanced access to this information by countries that are in the process of developing their own standards. Some countries (e.g. Singapore) have assessed the regulations of many different countries and selected those that apply best for their cultural and scientific environment. In addition, countries that are members of the World Organisation for Animal Health (the OIE), by virtue of their membership, are encouraged to implement normative documents regarding animal health and welfare, including in the field of animal use in research and education[1] as the OIE is the only international reference organisation for animal health. Such actions can lead to a convergence of approaches in providing animal research oversight, as oversight systems viewed as useful are used as resources for developing a customised regulatory framework. In general, such increased availability of information has increased harmonisation in approaches to ensuring research animal welfare.

The growing internationalisation of research has led to greater interest in systems of accreditation, both for

---

[1] http://www.oie.int/index.php?id=169&L=0&htmfile=chapitre_aw_research_education.htm (accessed 24 June 2021)

The UFAW Handbook on the Care and Management of Laboratory and Other Research Animals, Ninth Edition.
Edited by Huw Golledge and Claire Richardson.
© 2024 John Wiley & Sons Ltd. Published 2024 by John Wiley & Sons Ltd.

institutions in emerging scientific locations to demonstrate their standards and for institutions in established scientific areas to assure standards. Non-governmental oversight bodies (e.g. AAALAC International) have a key role, and in some cases the primary role, in harmonising standards for animal care and use around the world, for example, by requiring committee review of proposed research at institutions in countries where there is no such requirement. Thus, while approaches may differ among countries, the goals of good animal welfare, attention to ethics and high-quality science are the same (Guillen & Vergara 2018). Nonetheless, differences remain in the standards required by different nations. Therefore, there is an ongoing imperative, for animal welfare reasons, and to promote good science and a level economic playing field, that regulations and other means of oversight should reflect current knowledge of animal welfare science.

History

Animals have been used in science for centuries (Dunlop & Williams 1996), but formal oversight of such animal use developed during the eighteenth century. This was the period when the study of animals was revived on a larger scale in European and North American universities, having fallen into disuse after earlier extensive use by Greek and Arab societies. As this use grew, so too did concern, both for the animals themselves, and also about how lack of respect for animals and how they were used would *'corrupt'* humans. Even before laws were proposed in the nineteenth century in the UK to regulate research using animals, the tensions between the need for such research and animal welfare were present. There was both support for animal use as well as concern for their *'pain and suffering'* (Dunlop & Williams 1996). It is interesting that one prescient set of principles for research laid out at that time was that there should be: (1) no alternative; (2) a clear objective; (3) avoidance of repetition of work; (4) minimisation of suffering; and (5) full and detailed publication (Rupke 1987). See also the discussion of early proposals similar to the Three Rs in Chapter 2.

A general trend in oversight has been to move the focus from avoiding 'cruelty' and on sanitary aspects, to a wider perspective on experimental animal health, welfare and ethics. Early laws and guidelines gave fellow scientists control over other scientists' specified use of animals (Select Committee on Animals in Scientific Procedures 2002) and were aimed at controlling and excluding diseases that clearly confounded early animal experimentation (Walker & Poppleton 1967).

It is important to note that while oversight is anchored on legal requirements, this baseline may be buttressed by voluntary adherence to additional standards. This approach results in broader attention to animal welfare and ethical issues (Orlans 2001). For example, initially the Russian law on animal experimentation (Russian Ministry of Health 1973) focused on hygiene, husbandry and facilities but a more recent law, 'Protection of Animals Against Ill Treatment', adopted by the Duma in 1999, addresses in general terms the need to reduce the suffering of animals used in research, testing and education. However, Russian establishments are becoming increasingly aware of broader issues, and some are voluntarily following the European Directive 2010/63/EU. Key guidance documents have been translated into many languages, including Russian (e.g. National Research Council 2011). Some countries have based their guidance documents on those developed in other countries. For example, the 2018 Taiwan 'Guidelines for Laboratory Animal Use and Care'[2] references the *Guide for the Care and Use of Laboratory Animals* (*Guide*, National Research Council 2011), the *Guide for the Care and Use of Agricultural Animals in Research and Teaching* (FASS 2010) and the Euroguide (FELASA 2007), and addresses topics such as semi-annual programme reviews/facility inspections, as well as animal reuse, retirement, rehabilitation and rehoming. A recent example of new regulatory requirements is the 2015 Thai Animals for Scientific Procedures Act[3] which incorporates several principles in the *Guide*.

Principles

The Three Rs

The principles of the Three Rs, consisting of replacement, reduction and refinement (see Chapter 2), were developed by the UFAW scholars Professors William MS Russell and Rex Burch. The Three Rs were first presented at a UFAW symposium in 1957 entitled *'Humane Techniques in the Laboratory'* and published as *'The Principles of Humane Experimental Technique'* in 1959 (Russell & Burch 1959). The term *alternatives*, while sometimes confused with replacement is commonly used to refer to all Three Rs. Definitions of the Three Rs have evolved over the last half century (Buchanan-Smith *et al.* 2005), but the original text (Russell & Burch 1959) remains valid and important:

> We shall use the term 'replacement technique' for any scientific method employing non-sentient material which may in the history of experimentation replace methods which use conscious living vertebrates.
>
> Reduction means reduction in the numbers of animals used to obtain information of a given amount and precision.
>
> Suppose, for a particular purpose, we cannot use replacing techniques. Suppose it is agreed that we shall be using every device of theory and practice to reduce to a minimum the number of animals we have to employ. It is at this point that refinement starts, and its object is simply to reduce to an absolute minimum the amount of distress imposed on those animals that are still used.

Since 1957, and in particular over the last 20 years, the Three Rs have increasingly become, either explicitly (e.g. CIOMS/ICLAS 2012, European Parliament and Council of European Union 2010) or implicitly (e.g. Interagency Research Animal Committee (IRAC) 1985), a key, if not the leading, ethical principle for the care and use of animals used in science worldwide.

---

[2]https://www.aaalac.org/resources/Taiwan%20ROC%20Guideline%20for%20the%20Care%20and%20Use%20of%20Laboratory%20Animals.pdf) (accessed 24 June 2021)

[3]Thai Animals for Scientific Purposes Act English Translated version (aaalac.org)

International Guiding Principles for Biomedical Research Involving Animals

The International Guiding Principles for Biomedical Research Involving Animals were developed by the Council for International Organizations of Medical Sciences (CIOMS) and, in collaboration with the International Council for Laboratory Animal Science (ICLAS) were revised (CIOMS/ICLAS 2012) to reflect contemporary principles. CIOMS is an international, non-governmental, non-profit organisation established jointly by the World Health Organization and the United Nations in 1949 and is representative of a substantial proportion of the biomedical scientific community. ICLAS is 'an international scientific organization dedicated to advancing human and animal health by promoting the ethical care and use of laboratory animals worldwide'. These principles for animal experimentation were, in part, created because national and international ethical codes and laws for human experimentation mandate that new substances or devices should not be used for the first time on human beings unless previous tests on animals have provided a reasonable presumption of their safety. The principles provide a framework for ethical animal use (Box 8.1). Other areas covered include animal acquisition, transportation, housing, environmental conditions, nutrition, the provision of veterinary care, the maintenance of records, euthanasia, the monitoring of animal care and use, the implementation of the Three Rs, and the training of investigators and others in animal care and use.

The World Organisation for Animal Health (OIE)

In recent years, the OIE has taken an interest in the use of animals in research. Principle-based standards have been published for OIE members to follow when formulating regulatory requirements for the use of live animals in research, testing or teaching, as described in Chapter 7.8 of the Terrestrial Animal Health Code (World Organisation for Animal Health 2013). The standards give prominence to the Three Rs, protocol and programme review, training of those involved in veterinary care, the animal facilities, as well as animal health control.

Engineering versus performance standards

Standards can be performance based, specifying the outcomes but not the methods to achieve outcomes, or engineering based, specifying measurements, activities or processes (National Research Council 2011). Performance standards have the advantage of flexibility, which may be useful where

---

Box 8.1 CIOMS/ICLAS International Guiding Principles for Biomedical Research Involving Animals (2012)

I. The advancement of scientific knowledge is important for improvement of human and animal health and welfare, conservation of the environment, and the good of society. Animals play a vital role in these scientific activities and good animal welfare is integral to achieving scientific and educational goals. Decisions regarding the welfare, care, and use of animals should be guided by scientific knowledge and professional judgment, reflect ethical and societal values, and consider the potential benefits and the impact on the well-being of the animals involved.

II. The use of animals for scientific and/or educational purposes is a privilege that carries with it moral obligations and responsibilities for institutions and individuals to ensure the welfare of these animals to the greatest extent possible. This is best achieved in an institution with a culture of care and conscience in which individuals working with animals willingly, deliberately, and consistently act in an ethical, humane and compliant way. Institutions and individuals using animals have an obligation to demonstrate respect for animals, to be responsible and accountable for their decisions and actions pertaining to animal welfare, care and use, and to ensure that the highest standards of scientific integrity prevail.

III. Animals should be used only when necessary and only when their use is scientifically and ethically justified. The principles of the Three Rs – Replacement, Reduction and Refinement – should be incorporated into the design and conduct of scientific and/or educational activities that involve animals. Scientifically sound results and avoidance of unnecessary duplication of animal-based activities are achieved through study and understanding of the scientific literature and proper experimental design. When no alternative methods, such as mathematical models, computer simulation, *in vitro* biological systems, or other non-animal (adjunct) approaches, are available to replace the use of live animals, the minimum number of animals should be used to achieve the scientific or educational goals. Cost and convenience must not take precedence over these principles.

IV. Animals selected for the activity should be suitable for the purpose and of an appropriate species and genetic background to ensure scientific validity and reproducibility. The nutritional, microbiological, and general health status as well as the physiological and behavioral characteristics of the animals should be appropriate to the planned use as determined by scientific and veterinary medical experts and/or the scientific literature.

V. The health and welfare of animals should be primary considerations in decisions regarding the program of veterinary medical care to include animal acquisition and/or production, transportation, husbandry and management, housing, restraint, and final disposition of animals, whether euthanasia, rehoming, or release. Measures should be taken to

(Continued)

Box 8.1 (Continued)

ensure that the animals' environment and management are appropriate for the species and contribute to the animals' well-being.

VI. The welfare, care, and use of animals should be under the supervision of a veterinarian or scientist trained and experienced in the health, welfare, proper handling, and use of the species being maintained or studied. The individual or team responsible for animal welfare, care and use should be involved in the development and maintenance of all aspects of the program. Animal health and welfare should be continuously monitored and assessed with measures to ensure that indicators of potential suffering are promptly detected and managed. Appropriate veterinary care should always be available and provided as necessary by a veterinarian.

VII. Investigators should assume that procedures that would cause pain or distress in human beings cause pain or distress in animals, unless there is e evidence to the contrary. Thus, there is a moral imperative to prevent or minimize stress, distress, discomfort, and pain in animals, consistent with sound scientific or veterinary medical practice. Taking into account the research and educational goals, more than momentary or minimal pain and/or distress in animals should be managed and mitigated by refinement of experimental techniques and/or appropriate sedation, analgesia, anesthesia, non-pharmacological interventions, and/or other palliative measures developed in consultation with a qualified veterinarian or scientist. Surgical or other painful procedures should not be performed on unanesthetized animals.

VIII. Endpoints and timely interventions should be established for both humane and experimental reasons. Humane endpoints and/or interventions should be established before animal use begins, should be assessed throughout the course of the study, and should be applied as early as possible to prevent, ameliorate, or minimize unnecessary and/or unintended pain and/or distress. Animals that would otherwise suffer severe or chronic pain, distress, or discomfort that cannot be relieved and is not part of the experimental design, should be removed from the study and/or euthanized using a procedure appropriate for the species and condition of the animal.

IX. It is the responsibility of the institution to ensure that personnel responsible for the welfare, care, and use of animals are appropriately qualified and competent through training and experience for the procedures they perform. Adequate opportunities should be provided for on-going training and education in the humane and responsible treatment of animals. Institutions also are responsible for supervision of personnel to ensure proficiency and the use of appropriate procedures.

X. While implementation of these Principles may vary from country to country according to cultural, economic, religious, and social factors, a system of animal use oversight that verifies commitment to the Principles should be implemented in each country. This system should include a mechanism for authorization (such as licensing or registering of institutions, scientist, and/or projects) and oversight which may be assessed at the institutional, regional, and/or national level. The oversight framework should encompass both ethical review of animal use as well as considerations related to animal welfare and care. It should promote a harm-benefit analysis for animal use, balancing the benefits derived from the research or educational activity with the potential for pain and/or distress experienced by the animal. Accurate records should be maintained to document a system of sound program management, research oversight, and adequate veterinary medical care.

species, previous history of the animals, facilities, expertise of the people and research goals need to be taken into account, but are open to more variability. The performance approach requires professional input and judgement to achieve outcome goals. Engineering standards are useful to establish a baseline, but are not as useful when a goal or outcome, such as well-being, sanitation or personnel safety, needs to be specified. Moreover, they may not encourage the development of higher standards. Optimally, engineering and performance standards should be used in tandem, thereby providing baseline standards while allowing flexibility and the application of informed professional judgement.

Adequate veterinary care

Veterinary care by trained and experienced specialists is fundamentally important to the delivery of a programme of humane and scientifically valid animal care and use. This is reflected in many countries' provisions for regulation or oversight.

The United States Department of Agriculture's (USDA) Animal Welfare Regulations (US Department of Agriculture 2017) and the Public Health Service (PHS) Policy on Humane Care and Use of Laboratory Animals (Policy) (Office of Laboratory Animal Welfare (OLAW) 2015) stipulate that the veterinarian has the authority to oversee several key components of the animal care and use programme, including: animal procurement and transportation; quarantine, stabilisation and separation of animals; surveillance, diagnosis, treatment and control of disease; surgery; the selection of analgesic and anaesthetic agents; method of euthanasia; animal husbandry and nutrition; sanitation practices; zoonosis control; and hazard containment. The veterinarian must be qualified through either experience or training in laboratory animal medicine or in the species being used. The veterinarian brings a specific perspective to the deliberations of the Institutional Animal Care and Use

Committee (IACUC), and is a voting member of the IACUC. The Animal Welfare Regulations describe the programme of adequate veterinary care as including:

- the availability of appropriate facilities, personnel, equipment and services;
- the use of appropriate methods to prevent, control, diagnose and treat diseases and injuries, inclusive of the availability of emergency, weekend and holiday care;
- daily observation of all animals to assess their health and well-being;
- guidance to researchers regarding handling, immobilisation, anaesthesia, analgesia, tranquillisation and euthanasia;
- nutrition;
- pest and parasite control; and
- adequate pre-procedural and post-procedural care in accordance with current professional standards.

The *ACLAM Position Statement on Adequate Veterinary Care* (American College of Laboratory Animal Medicine 2016) describes a program of adequate veterinary care as including:

- disease detection and surveillance, prevention, diagnosis, treatment and resolution;
- provision of guidance on anaesthetics, analgesics, tranquilliser drugs and methods of euthanasia;
- the review and approval of all pre-operative, surgical and post-operative procedures;
- the promotion and monitoring of an animal's well-being before, during and after its use; and
- involvement in the review and approval of all animal care and use at the institution.

This report is used by AAALAC International (see later in this chapter) as a reference standard in its assessments of animal care and use programmes. Also, AAALAC International has established a Position Statement on 'The Attending Veterinarian and Veterinary Care' which describes clinical and IACUC responsibilities of this individual.[4]

The Federation of European Laboratory Animal Science Associations (FELASA), the European Society of Laboratory Animal Veterinarians (ESLAV) and the European College of Laboratory Animal Medicine (ECLAM) produced European Guidelines for the Veterinary Care of Laboratory Animals (Joint Working Group on Veterinary Care 2008). Core veterinary roles described in the guidelines include:

- all activities directly related to the animals to promote their welfare, such as during transportation, health monitoring and health management, husbandry, selection of environmental enrichment, surgery, anaesthesia, analgesia and euthanasia;
- scientific activities, often as a scientific collaborator and adviser in laboratory animal science;
- activities related to regulatory and administrative compliance; the veterinarian must be knowledgeable about relevant legislation, including any appropriate ethical review process;

- education and training of personnel and guidance of administrative staff, animal care staff and scientists to the benefit of the animals, the science and the institution.

The guidelines also emphasise the need for appropriate training and continuing professional development to ensure competence is established and maintained. Subsequently, ESLAV, ECLAM, the Laboratory Animal Veterinary Association (LAVA) and the Association for European Veterinarians in Education, Research and Industry (EVERI) published recommendations for the roles, responsibilities and training of the laboratory animal veterinarian and the designated veterinarian under Directive 2010/63/EU (Poirier *et al.* 2015), the European Directive controlling animal experimentation (European Parliament and Council of European Union 2010). This document reviews the references to the designated veterinarian across the Directive and recommends how the veterinary input should be organised in all these cases (e.g. input to the Animal Welfare Body and the project evaluation), and offer guidance on how to achieve training and continuing education.

Training and competence

The importance of adequate training and competence for all those involved in the animal care and use programme is underscored by the emphasis it receives in regulation and policy such as the US Animal Welfare Regulations, PHS Policy on Humane Care and Use of Laboratory Animals (PHS Policy), the *Guide* (National Research Council 2011), Directive 2010/63/EU; the ETS Resolution on education and training (Council of Europe 1993); the working document on the development of a common education and training framework to fulfil the requirements under the Directive (National Competent Authorities 2014), an emphasis also reflected in other jurisdictions such as Canada (Canadian Council on Animal Care 2015) and Australia (Australian Government *et al* 2013). These modern guidance documents highlight the importance not only of training, but also of demonstrating the necessary competency, after a period of supervision, to perform animal care and use practices.

The US Animal Welfare Regulations and PHS Policy require institutions to ensure that people caring for or using animals are qualified to do so. The Animal Welfare Regulations stipulate that several key topics be included in the institution's training programme. They are:

- humane methods of animal maintenance and experimentation, including the basic needs of each species of animal, proper handling and care for the various species of animals used by the institution, proper pre-procedural and post-procedural care of animals, and aseptic surgical methods and procedures;
- the concept, availability and use of research or testing methods that limit the use of animals or minimise animal distress;
- proper use of anaesthetics, analgesics and tranquillisers for any species of animal at the institution;
- methods to report any deficiencies in animal care and treatment;

---

[4]https://www.aaalac.org/accreditation/positionstatements.cfm#vetcare (accessed 24 June 2021)

- use of the services at the National Agricultural Library, such as appropriate methods of animal care and use, alternatives to the use of live animals in research, prevention of unintended and unnecessary duplication of research involving animals, information regarding the intent and requirements of the Animal Welfare Act.

The *Guide* urges that adequate training should be provided to members serving on the IACUC so that they can appropriately discharge their responsibilities. In addition, the *Guide* recommends that the professional and technical personnel caring for animals should be trained, as should investigators, research technicians, trainees (including students) and visiting scientists. The *Guide* also endorses training in occupational health and safety, in procedures that are specific to an employee's job, and in procedures specific to research (e.g. anaesthesia, surgery, euthanasia, recognition of the signs of pain and/or distress).

Over the last several years, there has been regionalisation and internationalisation of training standards. A particularly strong example was the development of training guidelines across Europe which defined four categories of persons working with laboratory animals and their training needs:

- Category A: persons taking care of animals;
- Category B: persons carrying out procedures;
- Category C: persons responsible for directing or designing procedures;
- Category D: laboratory animal science specialists.

FELASA elaborated these training requirements for each of these categories into training guidelines (Federation of European Laboratory Animal Science Associations 2000, Federation of European Laboratory Animal Science Associations 2010a, Federation of European Laboratory Animal Science Associations 2010b) and an accreditation scheme for provision of this training (Federation of European Laboratory Animal Science Associations 2018). These guidelines became the *de facto* requirement for training and education across Europe for several years, and have been and still are also being used elsewhere in the world. In the European Union, these FELASA Categories have been surpassed by the functions defined in Directive 2010/63/EU, which require personnel must be educated and trained before:

- Carrying out procedures on animals
- Designing procedures and projects
- Taking care of animals
- Killing animals

In addition to this training, the Directive also requires the participation of the designated veterinarian, and one or several persons responsible for overseeing the welfare and care of the animals in the establishment.

This trend to wider application of guidelines is seen in other areas. Animal technology certification is heavily influenced by the certification programmes of the American Association for Laboratory Animal Science across the Americas, while in Europe and beyond, FELASA has adapted its accreditation programme to the new legal requirements and the European Federation of Animal Technicians is increasingly influenced by the programmes from the UK Institute of Animal Technology. More recently, there have been moves to share standards for certification of specialists in Laboratory Animal Medicine by the formation of an International Association of Colleges of Laboratory Animal Medicine[5].

Institutional and governmental review, oversight and authorisation of animal activities

An institution-based process is the commonest method of animal activity evaluation and authorisation around the world. While there may be oversight of these activities by a national authority, often this is the sole layer of authorisation.

The committee or process that is designated to review proposed uses of animals has been variously called the Animal Care Committee (Canada), Ethics Committee or Animal Welfare Body (Europe) and the IACUC (US and several countries in Asia). This group of individuals, operating as a committee or process, representing institutional and public interests, has the responsibility for oversight and evaluation of the entire animal care and use programme and facilities. Because they act on behalf of the institution, their role is pivotal to engendering a humane and progressive animal care and use programme. The term programme is used to describe all aspects of animal care and use. The successful programme is overseen by a committee that is engaged, knowledgeable and receives strong administrative support. As the committee is responsible for investigating reports of concern regarding animal welfare, the committee's functions must be well known throughout the institution and there must be ready (and confidential) access to the committee.

In many countries, the institutional committee is the main body responsible for not only the protocol or project evaluation, but also for other oversight activities. This is the case, for example, with the IACUCs in the US. In countries lacking specific legislation, some institutions establish institutional committees on their own initiative to improve animal oversight and satisfy researchers' needs in terms of protocol evaluation for publication of research, international collaborations or conditions of funding and/or accreditation.

In the European Union, following implementation of Directive 2010/63/EU, three levels of review, oversight and authorisation may be observed. All establishments must have an Animal Welfare Body with several advisory duties, especially in the Three Rs domain. Although the project evaluation is assigned to the (public) competent authority, some functions (including project evaluation) can be delegated to other bodies that are considered competent authorities. This has resulted in some countries allowing institutional Animal Welfare Bodies or Ethics Committees to perform the evaluation, others allowing also external bodies (neither institutional nor public) to do it, and some to retain the process at public Competent Authorities level (Guillen *et al.* 2015). However, regardless of the process in place, final authorisation must be issued by the public competent authority except in Belgium, where the institutional bodies can perform both evaluation and authorisation.

---

[5] http://www.iaclam.org (accessed 24 June 2021)

An ethical component of the review process may be explicit or implicit, depending on regulatory requirements, but especially on the cultural norms in each jurisdiction. In the European Union, the evaluation process refers to 'project evaluation' due to concerns expressed by some countries regarding the term, although in Art. 38(2) d, the harm-benefit analysis expected in the evaluation process has to take into account 'ethical considerations'. In Asia, the review process may be less explicit in terms of 'ethical review'; but ethics is implicit in approaches such as memorials to animals used in research which encourage reflection on ethical aspects of such animal use (Slaughter 2002) and reference to adherence to the Three Rs (e.g. Science Council of Japan 2006; Korea Animal Protection Act 2017).

Inspection and compliance

Systems of inspection, with consequences for non-compliance, are operated in some jurisdictions. The scope of these systems is highly variable across the globe, but can include evaluation of animal health, facility inspections, assessment of the IACUC's/comparable oversight body's functions, husbandry, animal housing, veterinary authority over animal welfare and other programme elements. The inspection system is usually government controlled but there may also be other means of oversight, such as the peer-review system used by AAALAC International. Sanctions for non-compliance are highly varied and may include fines, imprisonment, denial of authority to conduct research or withdrawal of accreditation.

In the European Union, Directive 2010/63/EU defines the minimum requirements for inspections, which have to be carried out on at least one-third of the users each year with the exception of institutions housing nonhuman primates, which must be inspected once a year. The systems is based on a risk analysis to determine the frequency of inspections.

International accreditation of animal care and use programmes

There are two systems of accreditation that occur around the globe: domestic or international. Programmes of accreditation with a domestic (i.e. in-country) scope are found in Canada, Japan and the People's Republic of China. An accreditation system that is international in scope is offered by AAALAC International. AAALAC International is a non-profit organisation that was formed in 1965. AAALAC's mission is to promote the humane treatment of animals in science through confidential, voluntary accreditation of animal care and use programmes. International accreditation promotes scientific validity across country borders. Institutions also seek international accreditation to facilitate academic collaborations, to promote the biomedical research enterprise in their country, to assist in the recruitment of high-calibre scientists from around the world and, importantly, to assure stakeholders and the general public that a global standard of animal welfare is in place for animals used in science. Institutions in countries without either a regulatory framework or a domestic accreditation programme validate the quality of their animal research programmes by achieving international accreditation.

AAALAC does not establish policies to which institutions must conform. Rather, AAALAC International relies principally on the *Guide*, the *Guide for the Care and Use of Agricultural Animals in Research and Teaching* (*Ag Guide*, American Dairy Science Association®, the American Society of Animal Science, and the Poultry Science Association 2020) and ETS 123 (including Appendix A and Appendix B), collectively referred to as AAALAC's 'Three Primary Standards'. The Three Primary Standards are used in conjunction with national laws, regulations and policies, and numerous scientifically based standards, referred to as '*reference resources*', which address specific subject areas (e.g. recombinant DNA, surgery, euthanasia), for evaluation of animal care and use programmes around the world (Bayne & Martin 1998; Bayne & Miller 2000). AAALAC has developed several 'Position Statements' that fill in gaps in the Three Primary Resources, and these are considered mandatory requirements for institutions seeking accreditation. In addition, AAALAC's Council on Accreditation has crafted numerous responses to 'frequently asked questions'. The topics addressed include: institutional responsibilities; animal environment, housing and management; veterinary medical care; physical plant; and some administrative points related to the accreditation process.

The accreditation process includes an extensive internal review conducted by the institution, which is summarised in an animal care and use programme description based on a template questionnaire provided by AAALAC. On-site visits are announced and conducted every 3 years, though interim 'drop-in' visits may be conducted '*for cause*'. These visits are led by one or more members of the Council on Accreditation with the assistance of *ad hoc* consultants or specialists. At the time of this writing, the Council functions in geographically based sections: Europe, North America and the Pacific Rim. Significant effort is invested in ensuring consistency in the application of accreditation standards across the globe. The standards and process for accreditation are described in the Association's Rules of Accreditation. Non-conformance with AAALAC International standards results in formal notification that full accreditation has not been granted and provision of a timeline for correcting identified deficiencies. Sustained or serious non-conformance can result in revocation of accreditation. Accredited institutions are required to submit an annual report and to promptly report adverse events.

Regional and international harmonisation of guidelines

Regionally or internationally, some organisations promote harmonisation of standards. As examples, FELASA has issued guidelines that include health monitoring, control of pain and distress and use of transgenic animals, and ICLAS has a programme of producing harmonised guidance that includes euthanasia and humane endpoints. Also, FELASA has collaborated with AALAS to develop a two-part report (Brønstad *et al*. 2016; Laber *et al*. 2016) containing recommendations for conducting a harm-benefit analysis of animal experiments and how to implement this as part of the ethical review.

Europe

Harmonisation in the region

Very important harmonisation initiatives have been implemented at the European level when in 1876 the UK passed the Cruelty to Animals Act, the first legislation in the world to regulate animal research, which made provision to permit experiments on live animals under certain conditions (United Kingdom Parliament 1876). The main harmonisation initiatives were promoted by the Council of Europe and the European Union in 1986 through, respectively, the Convention for the Protection of Vertebrate Animals used for Experimental and other Scientific Purposes (ETS 123) (Council of Europe 1986), and the European Union's Council Directive on the approximation of laws, regulations and administrative provisions of the Member States regarding the protection of animals used for experimental and other scientific purposes (European Council 1986). The 1986 Directive was later replaced by Directive 2010/63/EU of the European Parliament and of the Council of 22 September 2010 on the Protection of Animals used for Scientific Purposes (European Parliament and Council of the European Union 2010).

Theoretically, the provisions of the ETS 123 could impact more countries, as the Council of Europe includes 47 European countries, as compared to the 27 European Union Member States. However, there are some very important differences between the legal power of the Council of Europe and the European Union that affect the way the provisions of their respective documents are implemented in practice. The Council of Europe is an inter-governmental organisation, has no legislative power but seeks voluntary cooperation by means of Recommendation, Agreements and Conventions. Conventions such as the ETS 123 have to be voluntarily signed and ratified by the members of the Council of Europe, who by these actions commit to enforce the provisions of the Convention. At the time of this writing, 21 out of the 47 members, and also the European Union, have signed and ratified the ETS 123.

On the other hand, the European Union is a supra-national entity with policy-making and legislative powers delegated by the Member States, and can pass Regulations, which become enforceable as law in all Member States simultaneously without modification, and Directives, which will be transposed by Member States into national legislation in a given period of time. The transposition process of Directives gives Member States some flexibility in the way provisions can be implemented, therefore, creating some practical differences on the ground at the national level, while trying to ensure the same outcome.

The importance of ETS 123 is that it established a common European framework for the protection of animals used in research that has been the basis for subsequent legislation throughout the continent. Due to progress in knowledge about sentience, animal welfare and societal concerns, Directive 2010/63/EU (Directive), published more than 20 years later, has some more advanced requirements and builds on the primary and fundamental principles of ETS 123. Unfortunately, there is no plan for the Council of Europe to update ETS 123. The Directive was published taking into account the objectives of improving animal welfare through implementation of the Three Rs, establishing a level framework for research across the European Union, and promoting transparency on animal research matters. The UK continues to apply Directive 2010/63/EU after leaving the EU.

From ETS 123 to Directive 2010/63/EU

In the 'General Principles' section (Part II), ETS 123 describes terms such as 'animal', 'procedure' and 'competent person' (a term widely used in the Directive), and lists the only purposes for which procedures may be performed. Vertebrates, including free-living and/or reproducing larval forms but excluding foetal or embryonic forms, are considered animals, while in the Directive, foetal forms of mammals from the last third of their development, and live cephalopods are also covered, which is one of the differences between both documents. The original list of eight species to be purpose bred has been extended in the Directive to include the Chinese hamster, the Mongolian gerbil, all species of nonhuman primates, frogs and zebrafish, while the quail has been removed. The original definition of 'procedure' in ETS 123 referred to actions that could cause pain, suffering, distress or lasting harm, but this has been further defined in the Directive to specify that any level of activity equivalent to, or higher than, that caused by the introduction of a needle is considered a procedure. An important step taken in the Directive has been the classification of the severity of procedures, which can be 'non-recovery', 'mild', 'moderate' or 'severe'.

The scope of purposes of procedures is very similar between the Directive and ETS 123. The Directive has somewhat refined the list in ETS 123 based on research purposes (which in the Directive has been more explicitly defined as basic, translational or applied), protection of the environment, education and training (which in the Directive has been enhanced to 'higher education, or training for the acquisition, maintenance or improvement of vocational skills'), and forensic enquiries. Specific restrictions are included in the Directive concerning the use of nonhuman primates, and the use of great apes is forbidden. However, for this particular point and others (i.e. procedures involving long-lasting harm), a safeguard clause could allow their use in exceptional circumstances.

ETS 123 refers implicitly to the principles of the Three Rs in several articles of Part III (Conduct of Procedure) indicating that procedures shall not be performed if other methods are available, that minimum numbers shall be used, and that procedures shall cause the least pain suffering, distress or lasting harm. The Directive is much more explicit, with multiple references to the Three Rs and even a specific article (Article 4) dedicated to them.

The most tangible connection between ETS 123 and the Directive relates to the care and accommodation of animals. In ETS 123, Appendix A addresses this topic. The Appendix was revised in 2006 (Council of Europe 2006), and the European Union subsequently recommended Member States consider the guidelines set out in the document (European Commission 2007). Appendix A contains detailed recommendations on the housing, environment and care of the most commonly used species, as well as birds, fish, reptiles and amphibians. Appendix A is particularly important because part of it, including recommended minimum cage sizes, was incorporated to the Directive and therefore considered legal requirements. Therefore, what was a 'should' in ETS 123 became more mandatory with the 'shall' in the Directive. Initially, this had a significant impact on animal facilities because some of the minimum cage/enclosure sizes in the revised Appendix A, and therefore in the 2010 Directive, were significantly larger than those in the original Appendix A and the 1986 Directive. Currently, all animals in the European Union must be housed under these standards. A positive result of the evolution of standards from ETS 123, Appendix A to the Directive is that the Directive not only enforces engineering standards such as cage sizes, but also applies performance standards. For example, the Directive does not require specific ranges for ventilation, temperature or relative humidity, but rather requires that these are appropriate for the species and do not adversely affect welfare.

Levels of authorisation to work with animals

An important recommendation in ETS 123 that is maintained and further developed in the Directive is the need for breeder, supplier and user establishments to be registered and authorised. It can be said that, in general, there are three levels of authorisation: the establishment, the personnel and the research project. Establishments can belong to either breeders, suppliers or users, who have to be authorised by, and registered with, the competent authority.

With regard to personnel, ETS 123 states that 'Persons who carry out procedures, or take part in procedures, or take care of animals used in procedures, including supervision, shall have had appropriate education and training', and that 'Authorisation (for persons carrying out procedures) shall be granted only to persons deemed to be competent by the responsible authority'. The Directive describes four functions for which personnel shall be adequately trained: (a) carrying out procedures on animals; (b) designing procedures and projects; (c) taking care of animals and (d) killing animals. Also, it requires the participation of a designated veterinarian with expertise in laboratory animal medicine or a suitable qualified expert where more appropriate; person(s) for overseeing the welfare and care of the animals in the establishment, person(s) who ensure that staff dealing with animals have access to the necessary information, and person(s) responsible for ensuring training and competence of personnel. The concept of 'competence' has been further developed in the Directive with a requirement that personnel carrying out functions referred to above in points (a), (c) or (d) shall be supervised in the performance of their tasks until they have demonstrated the requisite competence. However, the European Commission (the European Union 'Government') has no legal authority over educational matters, which are under the purview of Member States. Thus, the Directive requires Member States to ensure that this is achieved without defining specific requirements on how to do it. To promote harmonisation, 'Guidance on the development of a common education and training framework to fulfil the requirements under the Directive' has been produced by an Expert Working Group organised by the European Commission, endorsed by Member States, and is available online.[6] In addition, the European Commission promoted the establishment of the Education and Training Platform for Laboratory Animal Science (ETPLAS), as an information portal to enable information sharing and communication among training providers, approval/accrediting bodies, employers and Member-State authorities.[7]

Projects must be authorised by the competent authority after a favourable (ethical) project evaluation before work can commence. ETS 123 does not specifically require the procedure or project evaluation, although this process is well described as one of the most important requirements in the Directive.

Initially, the evaluation and authorisation process occurs at the level of a project, defined as a programme of work having a defined scientific objective and involving one or more procedures. According to the Directive, a procedure means any use, invasive or non-invasive, of an animal for experimental or other scientific purposes, with known or unknown outcome, or educational purposes, which may cause the animal a level of pain, suffering, distress or lasting harm equivalent to, or higher than, that caused by the introduction of a needle in accordance with good veterinary practice. This includes any course of action intended, or liable, to result in the birth or hatching of an animal or the creation and maintenance of a genetically modified animal line in any such condition, but excludes the killing of animals solely for the use of their organs or tissues. A project means a programme of work having a defined scientific objective and involving one or more procedures. Projects will be authorised only if a favourable project evaluation by the competent authority has been received.

In addition to the typical elements of a research project to be evaluated, the application must include a non-technical project summary (NTS). The NTS is one means of providing evidence of transparency, one of the main aims of the current European legislation, and is made available to the public by the Member States.

As previously noted, transposition of Directives into Member States legislation provides some flexibility, and the project evaluation is the best example of how the same process is being implemented in different ways across the European Union. Although the project evaluation function is assigned to the (public) competent authority, Article 59 of the Directive indicates that Member States may designate bodies other than public authorities for the implementation of specific tasks laid down in the Directive if there is proof that the body: (a) has the expertise and infrastructure required to carry out the tasks; and (b) is free of any conflict of interests with regard to the performance of the tasks. Bodies thus designated shall be considered competent authorities for the purposes of the Directive. Based upon this Article, a number of Member States have chosen to delegate the project evaluation to other bodies, either external to government and institutions, or directly to institutional bodies. Therefore, there are countries where the evaluation is performed by the public competent authority, others by external bodies, others by

---

[6]http://ec.europa.eu/environment/chemicals/lab_animals/pdf/Endorsed_E-T.pdf (accessed 24 June 2021)
[7]Home - Education and Training Platform for Laboratory Animal Science (etplas.eu) (accessed 24 January 2022)

institutional bodies (e.g. an Ethics Committee) or even by a combination of any of these options (Guillén et al. 2015). Despite the differences, the important common element is that animal use must be subjected to a previous ethical evaluation, which must also include retrospective assessment for, at least, projects categorised as severe and/or involving the use of nonhuman primates.

Other important aspects of the European framework

The Animal Welfare Body (AWB), required by the Directive in all establishments, play an important role in oversight activities of the programme. The AWB is assigned mainly advisory roles in terms of the Three Rs and animal welfare, but also is responsible for monitoring the development and outcome of projects and advising on rehoming schemes. Although the minimum composition of the AWB (person or persons responsible for the welfare and care of the animals and, in the case of a user, a scientific member) may be considered too limited, most institutions extend the composition to reflect the complexity of the institution. It is the key body responsible for implementing a culture of care, as in the United Kingdom, for example, where it is called Animal Welfare and Ethical Review Body (AWERB). In certain countries, the AWB performs an internal review of the projects before they are submitted to the competent authority. In others (e.g. France), this function is performed by another independent institutional body, the Ethics Committee.

While both ETS 123 and the Directive require arrangements for the provision of veterinary advice and treatment, the veterinarian is assigned only an advisory role, including provision of input to the AWB (some Member States have included the designated veterinarian in the AWB in the national legislation), with little definition of authority over or details regarding the veterinary care programme. This has prompted professional organisations to publish recommendations on the role of the designated veterinarian under the Directive, highlighting all the potential activities where veterinarians have an important role (Poirier et al. 2015). One aspect of the veterinary medical programme addressed in more detail in the Directive are methods of euthanasia. Annex IV lists the authorised killing methods by species.

As previously noted, transparency is key in the Directive, which requires including in the statistical reports information on the actual severity of the procedures and on the origin and species of nonhuman primates used in procedures. To make this possible, recently the European Commission has developed the 'ALURES' database to facilitate the sharing of all statistical information by the Member States, which is accessible to the public.[8] Also, as noted in the preceding text, the NTS have to be made publicly available by Member States.

Member States are not allowed to implement stricter measures than those in the Directive, but are allowed to maintain provisions in force before the Directive. Transposition of the Directive into national legislation has led to a certain level of diversity in practice. To harmonise the implementation of the Directive across the European Union, the European Commission has been establishing numerous Expert Working Groups, where representatives of the national competent authorities (National Contact Points) and representatives of expert stakeholder organisations have developed guidance intended to assist Member States and others affected by the Directive to arrive at a common understanding of the provisions contained in the Directive and promote uniform implementation and application. The documents produced have been endorsed by the National Contact Points. They refer to: Animal Welfare Bodies and National Committees; Education and Training; Genetically Altered Animals; Inspections and Enforcement; Non-Technical Project Summaries; Project Evaluation/Retrospective Assessment; Severity Assessment; and Severity Assessment – Illustrative Examples. Another document prepared by the European Commission and the National Contact Points relates to interpretation of various specific articles of the Directive. All these articles are available online.[9] Additional Expert Working Groups are in the process of preparing reports, which represent additional evidence of the efforts taken at European level to harmonise the protection, care and use of animals in research.

North America

Canada

The Canadian Constitution precludes federal legislation pertaining to the use of animals in research, testing or education, and as a result such use is under provincial jurisdiction. All provinces have established animal protection Acts and regulations, and Ontario has an Act specific to research animals. Five provinces have legislation and/or regulations that directly reference the standards of the national accreditation body, the Canadian Council on Animal Care (CCAC). Although there is no federal requirement to participate in the CCAC assessment programme, the two principal funding agencies (Canadian Institutes for Health Research (CIHR) and the Natural Sciences and Engineering Research Council (NSERC)) require grantee institutions to have a Certificate of GAP – Good Animal Practice® and to comply with CCAC guidelines and policies for continued funding of animal-based projects. Contractors performing work for the federal government are required to adhere to CCAC guidelines, as specified in the Public Works and Government Services Canada Standard Acquisition Clauses and Conditions Manual, Section 5, Subsection A, Clause A9015C: Experimental Animals. Also, the Canadian Food Inspection Agency imposes conformance with CCAC standards as part of the agency's requirements for importation of nonhuman primates into Canada and veterinary biologics guidelines.

The CCAC, founded in 1968, places responsibility for humane animal care and use with the Animal Care

---

[8] https://ec.europa.eu/environment/chemicals/lab_animals/alures_en.htm (accessed 24 January 2022)

[9] http://ec.europa.eu/environment/chemicals/lab_animals/interpretation_en.htm (accessed 24 June 2021)

Committee (ACC) at each institution. The ACCs are granted specific authority and provided with terms of reference under which they operate (e.g. membership, authority, responsibilities and functioning). The CCAC's mission is:

> 'ensure that animal-based science in Canada takes place only when necessary and that the animals in the studies receive optimal care according to high-quality, research-informed standards'.

The CCAC has three principal functions: (1) the development of guidelines and policies to govern experimental animal care and use; (2) to monitor compliance with those guidelines and policies and confer a certification to that effect and (3) to provide education, training and networking opportunities in implementing the CCAC standards. The CCAC is an independent organisation and receives funding from CIHR and NSERC as well as federal science-based departments and agencies.

The CCAC establishes guidelines and policies for its certified institutions to follow, available on the CCAC website and categorised as General Guidelines[10] (e.g. antibody production, endpoints, euthanasia, husbandry) and Types of Animals (e.g. amphibians, cats, dogs, various rodent, nonhuman primates). All CCAC guidelines are based on fundamental principles[11] contained in three policies: (1) ethics of animal investigation; (2) social and behavioural requirements of experimental animals and (3) categories of invasiveness in animal experiments. The CCAC also has established several policies[12] relevant to the assessment and certification programme that address a variety of topics such as animal-based projects involving two or more institutions and pedagogical merit of live animal-based teaching and training.

Regular on-site assessments using panels of experts from the animal care and use community and a representative normally nominated by the Canadian Federation of Humane Societies are conducted every six years, though interim visits are conducted mid-cycle (at three years) by a smaller review panel. An institution is deemed to be in compliance if the CCAC report prepared by the assessment panel and Secretariat, and approved by the Assessment and Certification Committee (a standing committee composed of a chairperson and at least 11 other members) contains no recommendations, or the CCAC report contains 'Major' recommendations that the institution has corrected immediately and appropriately, or 'Serious' or 'Regular' recommendations for which the institution has provided corrective action implementation reports. These institutions will receive a CCAC Certificate of GAP - Good Animal Practice®. The institution may receive a CCAC Probationary Certificate of GAP - Good Animal Practice® if the institution has serious and as yet unresolved deficiencies in the animal care and use programme. All relevant funding agencies and government ministries and departments are notified when there is a change in the institution's category of certification (CCAC 2016). Sustained non-compliance with CCAC guidelines and policies can ultimately result in withdrawal of all animal-based research funding to the institution.

The United States

In the US, oversight of animal care and use for research, testing and teaching is achieved by a matrix of federal and state laws, regulations, policies and guidelines from two principal government organisations: the USDA and the PHS. Other guidance may be derived from scientific panels or professional societies and endorsed by the government as required standards. Federal laws are annually compiled and categorised into their respective subjects (e.g. agriculture) and published as the United States Code (USC). The USC includes a discussion of the intent of Congress for establishing the law and any interpretations from the courts. Regulations are promulgated to enforce the corresponding law. Proposed regulations are published in the Federal Register for public comment. After the responsible agency reviews and addresses the public comments, the regulations are again published in the Federal Register in final format and then incorporated into the Code of Federal Regulations (e.g. 9 CFR) (Bayne & Morris 2012, Bayne & Anderson 2015). In general, laws address two specific areas: animal welfare and procurement, and animal importation and shipment.

US Department of Agriculture

Federal laws for the humane treatment of animals have been in place since 1873. The first federal law to protect non-farm animals was not passed until 1966 and was called the Laboratory Animal Welfare Act, administered by APHIS, USDA. The Laboratory Animal Welfare Act of 1966 was amended in 1970, 1976, 1985, 1990, 2002, 2007 and 2014 to broaden coverage of the law. Public Law 91-579, the Animal Welfare Act of 1970, increased the species of animals covered under the law to include all warm-blooded animals and increased the scope of applicability of the law to include the time animals were held in the facility. Specifically, exempted were horses not used in research and agricultural animals used in food and fibre research, retail pet stores, state and county fairs, rodeos, purebred cat and dog shows, and agricultural exhibitions. Public Law 94-279, the Animal Welfare Act Amendments of 1976, included common commercial carriers, such as airlines, and this subsequently led to standards being developed for shipping containers and conditions of shipment. Public Law 99-198, the Improved Standards for Laboratory Animals Act (1985), added several new provisions to the law including: minimisation of animal pain and distress and consideration of alternatives to painful procedures; consultation with a doctor of veterinary medicine for any practice which could cause pain to animals; limitation on conducting more than one major survival surgery on an animal (i.e. multiple major survival surgical procedures may be permitted if they are interrelated to the scientific goal of the study); establishment of an IACUC to provide oversight of the animal care and use programme and facilities; provision of

---

[10]https://www.ccac.ca/en/standards/guidelines/ (accessed 24 June 2021)

[11]https://www.ccac.ca/en/standards/fundamental-principles.html (accessed 24 June 2021)

[12]https://www.ccac.ca/en/certification/about-certification/policies-and-prerequisites.html (accessed 24 June 2021)

specific training to personnel; provision of exercise to dogs; and a stipulation to promote the psychological well-being of nonhuman primates. The 1990 amendment to the Animal Welfare Act, Public Law 101-624, Food, Agriculture, Conservation, and Trade Act of 1990, Section 2503, Protection of Pets, established a holding period for dogs and cats at shelters and other holding facilities prior to sale. The goal of the amendment was to allow owners or prospective owners to claim or adopt the animal, and the added documentation requirement ensured the animals were legally obtained as the law also required dealers to provide written certification to the recipient regarding the background of each animal. The Act was further amended in 2014 to establish thresholds for *de minimis* activity and exemptions from licensing under the Act. Accompanying regulations were issued in 2018. Changes in required administrative processes were adopted by the USDA in accordance with the 21st Century Cures Act.[13]

The 1970 amendment to the Animal Welfare Act defined an animal as: *'any live or dead dog, cat, monkey (nonhuman primate animal), guinea pig, hamster, rabbit, or other such warm-blooded animal as the Secretary may determine is being used, or is intended for use, for research, testing, experimentation, or exhibition purposes, or as a pet'*. In this way, the Secretary of the Department of Agriculture was provided the authority to determine which animals would be covered by the Act. In 1977, the USDA promulgated regulations that specifically excluded rats, mice and birds from the definition of 'animal'. The Helms amendment to the 2002 Farm Bill explicitly excluded rats, mice and birds used for research from the Act. As the USDA regulates only those species covered by the Animal Welfare Act, the passage of this bill into law removed USDA oversight of these species. Rationale for Congress to accept their exclusion from the Act was based in large part on the fact that these species are covered by other federal (e.g. PHS Policy) and private (e.g. AAALAC International) systems of oversight.

Since the 1966 Act, the USDA has been vested by Congress with both promulgation and enforcement authority. The USDA is required to conduct unannounced annual inspections of research facilities, with follow-up inspections until any cited deficiency has been corrected. Exempt from this provision are federal research facilities. Research institutions, intermediate handlers and common carriers are required to register with the USDA, while animal dealers and exhibitors must be licensed. Research facilities and US government agencies are required to purchase animals only from licensed sources, unless the source is exempted from obtaining a licence. Failure to comply with regulatory requirements, despite formal notification of an item(s) of non-compliance and an opportunity to effect a correction, can result in fines levied on the facility, suspension of authority to operate and even permanent revocation of the facility's licence to operate. Thus, the enforcement arm of the USDA's oversight responsibility is strong, and has been used over the years to improve animal welfare at dealers, exhibits and research facilities.

Public Health Service Policy

The other federal agency charged with oversight of research animal care and use is the PHS. The PHS Policy was implemented in 1973 and has been revised periodically, with the most recent revision in 2015. The PHS Policy covers all vertebrate animals used in research, testing or education. The PHS's authority is derived from Public Law 99-158, the Health Research Extension Act of 1985, Section 495, Animals in Research. Under this Act, institutions conducting animal research using PHS funding, such as through the National Institutes of Health (NIH), must comply with the PHS Policy (Office of Laboratory Animal Welfare 2015). The PHS Policy requires the funding recipient (referred to as an '*awardee institution*') to submit an Animal Welfare Assurance statement. This Animal Welfare Assurance statement must be approved by the PHS's OLAW, a component of the NIH. It commits the institution to following the US Government Principles for the Utilization and Care of Vertebrate Animals Used in Testing, Research, and Training (Interagency Research Advisory Committee 1985). In addition to stating a commitment to animal welfare, the Assurance must designate clear lines of authority and responsibility for institutional oversight of the work, inclusive of a designated '*Institutional Official*' who is ultimately responsible for the animal care and use programme; identify a qualified veterinarian who is involved in the programme; provide a description of the occupational health and safety programme for relevant personnel in the programme; describe mandated training and describe the facility. The Assurance is renegotiated with OLAW every 5 years. OLAW can approve, disapprove, restrict or withdraw approval of the Assurance.

PHS awarding agencies, such as the NIH, may not make an award for an activity involving live vertebrate animals unless the prospective awardee institution and all other institutions participating in the animal activity have an approved Assurance with OLAW and provide verification that the IACUC has reviewed and approved those sections of the grant application that involve the use of animals. Applications from organisations with approved Assurances must address five specific points pertaining to the use of animals:

- a detailed description of the proposed work, including species, strain, sex, age and number of animals to be used in the proposed work;
- a justification of the use of animals, species and number of animals;
- information regarding the veterinary care for the animals;
- a description of the procedures for ensuring that discomfort, distress, pain and injury will be minimised;
- a description of the method of euthanasia and the reason for the selection of that method, including a justification for any method that does not conform with the American Veterinary Medical Association's (AVMA) Euthanasia Guidelines (2020).

Awardee institutions that do not comply with the standards of the *Guide*, the USDA Animal Welfare Regulations and other standards referenced in the PHS Policy (e.g. the AVMA's Euthanasia Guidelines (American Veterinary Medical Association 2020)), may have their Assurance

---

[13] USDA APHIS | APHIS Announces Changes to Requirements for Research Facilities to Implement the 21st Century Cures Act

restricted, which in turn can limit access to PHS funding for research. Sustained non-compliance with the PHS Policy can result in withdrawing the approval of the Assurance and cessation of all PHS funding for animal-based activities.

The awardee institution must also submit an annual report. Institutions that are reviewed by an outside accrediting body, and AAALAC International is the sole accrediting body recognised by the PHS (Category 1 institutions), must indicate in the annual report if that accreditation status has been removed. Institutions that are not accredited by an external review group (Category 2) must provide the most recent copy of their IACUC's semi-annual programme review and facility inspection with the Assurance. The role of the IACUC in providing local oversight of animal care and use is a key element of the PHS Policy. Although the required composition of the IACUC for the PHS differs slightly from USDA requirements, due to a Memorandum of Understanding concerning laboratory animal welfare among APHIS/USDA, the Food and Drug Administration (FDA) and the NIH that sets forth procedures for cooperation among the three agencies in their oversight of animal care and use programmes, the general functions and responsibilities of the IACUC are similar.

OLAW conducts site visits of awardee institutions both *'for cause'* and *'not for cause'*. In addition, an ongoing significant mission of OLAW is the educational outreach it performs in collaboration with awardee institutions and various associations (e.g. IACUC 101/201/301 series, Public Responsibility in Medicine and Research, IACUC Administrators Association, Scientists Center for Animal Welfare). Jointly sponsored workshops focus on information of value to Institutional Officials and IACUCs to provide appropriate oversight of animal care and use. OLAW also provides guidance through articles in journals, commentary on other articles, NIH Guide Notices and a listserve[14].

Other laws and regulations with international scope

In 1978, the FDA initially promulgated regulations for the conduct of animal research on new or existing pharmaceutical agents, food additives or other chemicals. These regulations, known as the Good Laboratory Practice (GLP) regulations (which have been subsequently revised), specify appropriate diagnosis, treatment and control of disease in animals used in the work (see 21 CFR Part 58[15] (Code of Federal Regulations 1998)). The Environmental Protection Agency (EPA) has issued companion regulations (Code of Federal Regulations 1997) for conducting research pertaining to health effects, environmental effects and chemical fate testing in a separate set of GLP regulations[16]. Both the FDA and EPA GLP regulations rely heavily on detailed record keeping. Records must include standard operating procedures, animal identification, food and water analysis, documentation that any pesticides or chemicals used near the animals do not interfere with the study, and documentation of any disease and treatments animals experience. On-site inspections are conducted to ensure compliance with GLP standards.

The Department of Defense (DoD) developed a 'Policy on Experimental Animals' in 1961 to ensure that all research at DoD facilities involving animals was conducted in accordance with certain principles of animal care. Later versions of this Policy included overseas sites. Subsequently, a joint regulation, entitled 'The Use of Animals in DoD Program', from the Army, Navy, Air Force, Defense Nuclear Agency, and Uniformed Services University required all DoD facilities to 'attain and maintain' AAALAC accreditation and consider accreditation of vendors supplying animals for DoD sponsored research and training. Exemptions to this requirement may be allowed if deemed appropriate. This DoD Instruction also frames the approval and oversight responsibilities of local institutional animal care and use committees (Department of Defense 2010, most recently revised 2019).

Asia

Japan

The Act on Welfare and Management of Animals was enacted in 1973 (the name was changed to this in 2009), with the most recent revision made in 2017. The Act covers most vertebrate animals, with the exception of amphibians and fish. It is the main law that governs the use of animals in research, and is supplemented by various guidelines. Self-regulation characterises the oversight system. Before the 2017 revision of the Act, Refinement was the only 'R' of the Three Rs that was directly included (Bayne *et al.* 2019). The principles of Reduction and Replacement were subsequently added to the Act. More specific to laboratory animals, the 'Standards Relating to the Care and Keeping of Laboratory Animals' were implemented in 1980 and revised in 2013 by the Ministry of Environment. At this time, the name was changed to 'Standards Relating to the Care and Keeping and Reducing Pain of Laboratory Animals' (Notice of the Ministry of the Environment No. 84 of 2013). Guidelines for this standard were published by the Ministry of Environment in 2017. The guidelines provide an explanation of the standard and resemble the *Guide* (National Research Council 2011) quite closely.

With effect from 1 June 2006, the Science Council of Japan (SCJ) issued 'Guidelines for Proper Conduct of Animal Experiments' as a result of the amended Law for the Humane Treatment and Management of Animals (amended 2005) and at the request of the Ministry of Education, Culture, Sports, Science and Technology (MEXT) and the Ministry of Health, Labour and Welfare (MHLW, Science Council of Japan 2006). The SCJ guidelines place ultimate responsibility for all experiments with the director of the institution, but also encourage the formation of an IACUC. Therefore, the IACUC's role is to provide the institutional director with a report on the committee's deliberations regarding a proposed study, and then the director approves or disapproves the protocol. Of particular note, the amended law and SCJ Guidelines require attention to the Three Rs in the planning and conduct of

---

[14]https://olaw.nih.gov/resources/list.htm (accessed 24 June 2021)

[15]https://www.accessdata.fda.gov/scripts/cdrh/cfdocs/cfcfr/CFRSearch.cfm?CFRPart=58 (accessed 24 June 2021)

[16]https://ntp.niehs.nih.gov/iccvam/suppdocs/feddocs/epa/epa_glp40_160.pdf (accessed 24 June 2021)

research activities, though in practice, particular emphasis is placed on refinement. The detailed guidelines promulgated by the SCJ build upon the more basic guidelines, 'Fundamental guidelines for proper conduct of animal experiment and related activities in academic research institutions under the jurisdiction of the Ministry of Education, Culture, Sports, Science and Technology', 'Basic policies for the conduct of animal experimentation in the Ministry of Health, Labour and Welfare' and 'Standards Relating to the Care and Management of Laboratory Animals and Relief of Pain' (Ministry of Environment 2006).

The SCJ Guidelines encourage each institution to develop and implement its own policies for the conduct of animal-based research, typically through the IACUC. The number of IACUC members may vary with the size and complexity of the institution, but the committee should include researchers who conduct animal experiments, laboratory animal specialists and *'other persons of knowledge and experience'* (Science Council of Japan 2006). The primary role of the IACUC is to evaluate the scientific merit of the proposed study, taking into consideration the aforementioned law, standards and policies. The IACUC is also charged with reviewing the education and training of the investigator and to make recommendations to the director of the institution as necessary.

The SCJ Guidelines provide general recommendations regarding items for the IACUC to consider when reviewing a protocol, items that should be contained on the protocol form, facility and equipment considerations, animal restraint, food and water restriction, surgical procedures, analgesics and anaesthetics, humane endpoints, euthanasia, safety considerations and reporting of experimental results. This latter item suggests that the investigator report to the director of the institution the number of animals used, whether any changes were made to the protocol and the results of the experiment. Other topics covered include laboratory animal selection and receipt, the care and management of laboratory animals, laboratory animal health management, as well as education and training. Under the topic of laboratory animal care and management, cage space is discussed. The SCJ Guidelines recommend considering the animal's characteristics (e.g. species, age) and its behaviour when determining appropriate cage size, or alternatively to use the *Guide* (National Research Council 1996). The SCJ Guidelines provide additional recommendations on environmental conditions and other related animal care and use programme information. Although a government inspection system does not validate conformity with these standards and guidelines, a third-party audit system is encouraged, which may be met by the national audit system or through assessments and accreditation provided by AAALAC International. As noted previously, Japan not only participates in the international accreditation program offered by AAALAC International, but two domestic accreditation programs exist (Ogden *et al*. 2016). The Center for Accreditation of Laboratory Animal Care and Use was established by the Japan Health Science Foundation, under the jurisdiction of the Ministry of Health, Labor and Welfare (for government, pharmaceutical and contract research organizations). In 2009, the Japanese Association of Laboratory Animal Facilities of National University Corporations, under the Ministry of Education, Culture, Sport, Science Technology, launched its accreditation program for Japanese universities.

Republic of Korea

The first Korean Animal Protection Law (Ministry of Agriculture Food and Rural Affairs) was passed in 1991, but primarily addressed preventing abuse of companion animals (Ogden *et al*. 2016). The law did formally allow the use of animals for teaching, research, *'or other scientific study'* and specified reduction of pain and humane euthanasia. It did not contain any enforcement language, and thus was subsequently determined to be inadequate. As a result, a revised law was promulgated in 2007. The amended law addressed several key principles, including consideration of harm/benefit, alternatives, using the minimum number of animals necessary to achieve the scientific goal, ensuring appropriate training and experience of the investigator, pain mitigation and euthanasia. Importantly, the amended law requires the establishment of an Animal Experimentation Ethics Committee to *'oversee the protection and ethical treatment'* of research animals. Around the same timeframe (2008), a separate law specific to research animals (Laboratory Animal Act) was issued by the Ministry of Food and Drug Safety (MFDS). The two laws had different requirements for the composition of the IACUC, which were later resolved by the publication of IACUC Standard Operating Guidelines, prepared by the MFDS and the Animal and Plant Quarantine Agency and which have been formally recognised by both ministries (Ogden *et al*. 2016). A fine may be levied against the head of an animal facility who has not appointed an Animal Experimentation Ethics Committee. Under the terms of the amended law, an annual report must be submitted to the Minister of Agriculture and Forestry regarding animal experimentation activities. In addition, other guidelines have been published to assist the IACUC in its review of protocols (e.g. pain classification).

People's Republic of China

There is a tiered system of oversight of research animal use in China (Ogden *et al*. 2016; Bayne *et al*. 2019). The 'Regulations for the Administration of Affairs Concerning Experimental Animals' was approved by the State Council in 1988 (State Science and Technology Commission 1988). The Ministry of Health subsequently published 'Implementing Detailed Rules of Medical Laboratory Animal Administration'. In general, these regulations are designed to ensure high-quality animals for research. The standards, 'Laboratory animal – Requirements of environment and housing facilities' (GB 14925-2001) were revised in 2001. Standards are described regarding construction of the animal housing areas; separation of animals by source, species, strain, experiment and pathogen status; quality of food, water and bedding provided to the animals; quarantine procedures; preventive medicine and animal transportation. In 2006, the Ministry of Science and Technology (MOST) issued guidelines for the humane treatment of laboratory animals. This was the first state policy-related document which directs administrators and technicians to attend to the welfare of laboratory animals. In this manner, concepts such as the Three Rs and scientific merit have begun to be included in Chinese regulations. In 2018, China issued two national standards, 'Laboratory Animals-General requirements for animal experiment' (GB/T 35823-2018) and 'Laboratory Animal-Guideline for the ethical review of animal welfare' (GB/T 35892-2018). An English translation is available (MacArthur Clark and Sun 2020); in general, the new standards are an amalgamation of the recommendations of the *Guide* (National Research Council 2011) and elements of ETS 123, while being context specific to the Chinese culture.

The Beijing Municipality requires licensure of organisations or individuals engaged in the production, supply or operation of laboratory animals and in Article 8 stipulate 'having animal welfare and animal experiment ethics review systems' (Beijing Bureau of Municipal Science and Technology 2005). The municipal regulations require personnel training, and technical staff must complete a technical competency assessment. Proper care, handling and treatment of the animals are emphasised throughout the regulations. The province also has established guidelines for the care of laboratory animals (Beijing Administrative Office of Lab Animal 2006). Similar approaches are established in other cities where scientific research is important, such as Shanghai.

Taiwan, ROC

In Taiwan, the Animal Protection Law (Taiwan Animal Protection Law 1998 and as amended in 2021 to become the Animal Protection Act), under the auspices of the Council of Agriculture (COA), has provisions that address animals used for commercial purposes (e.g. meat, milk, fur), science (teaching and research) and animals kept as pets. Chapter II, Article 12 of the Animal Protection Law precludes the killing of animals, with certain exceptions such as killing for scientific purposes. Chapter III, Articles 15–18 specify the conditions for the '*scientific application of animals*'. Included in this chapter is the mandate that the minimum number of animals necessary will be used in ways that cause the minimum amount of pain or injury. Article 16 requires that the institution that is using animals form a '*panel*' to oversee the scientific utilisation of the laboratory animals. In addition, Article 16 states the central competent authority 'shall invite scholars, experts, officials from related agencies and registered civic animal welfare groups to regularly supervise and manage the scientific application of animals. There should be at least one veterinarian and one representative from a civil group on this list'.

More recently, the COA Executive Yuan published the 'Guidelines for Laboratory Animal Use and Care'[17] which became effective in June 2018. An English translation is not available. The guidelines address a variety of species (rodents, dogs, cats, nonhuman primates, aquatic species) and farm animals used in research (pigs, sheep, cattle, poultry). The four chapters of the Guidelines address: institutional policy and responsibility; veterinary care and management; animal room and supportive area and functional facility and management. Most of the recommendations, including minimum space for animals, are consistent with the *Guide* (National Research Council 2011). A difference between the Guidelines and the *Guide* is that the Guidelines require that the IACUC have an Executive Secretary position and that the Secretary must have received a minimum of 12 hours of IACUC training recognised by the Central Authority of Taiwan. The Secretary can be a member of the IACUC or hold a separate position. Also, if the institution uses dogs, cats or nonhuman primates or reuses animals, the IAUC must establish an animal reuse policy or a retirement, rehabilitation and rehoming policy. The Guidelines require semi-annual programme reviews and facility inspections. The Guidelines reference the 2013 version of the AVMA Guidelines for the Euthanasia of Animals, but allow the use of non-pharmaceutical-grade chemicals for the euthanasia of animals.

India

The Animal Welfare Board of India was set up in accordance with Chapter II of The Prevention of Cruelty to Animals Act 1960 (No. 59 of 1960), the first law to govern animal welfare in the country. The scope of the law includes 'any living creature other than a human being' and thus takes invertebrate species into consideration. The Ministry of Food and Agriculture constituted the Animal Welfare Board of India in 1962. Since 1998, oversight of the Animal Welfare Board is the purview of the Ministry of Social Justice and Empowerment. Among the functions of the Board are: to advise the government on promulgating rules with a view to preventing unnecessary pain or suffering of captive animals and on potential amendments to the law. Chapter IV of the Prevention of Cruelty to Animals Act addresses experimentation on animals. Included in the act is the authority for the government to appoint a Committee for the Purpose of Control and Supervision of Experiments on Animals (CPCSEA). The committee must ensure that animals are not subjected to unnecessary pain or suffering before, during or after the performance of experiments on them. To achieve this, the committee may, subsequent to notification in the Gazette of India, develop rules regarding the conduct of experiments. In general, the rules for animal experimentation pertain to appropriate qualifications of individuals conducting the experiment, minimisation of animal pain by the use of anaesthetics, euthanasia, consideration of alternatives to animal experimentation, that pre- and post-procedural care be provided to the animal, and that suitable records are maintained. The committee can authorise inspection of the location of the experiment and can suspend animal work by an individual or an institution.

The Indian National Science Academy is responsible for the development of guidelines for the operation of the Institutional Animal Ethics Committees (IAEC). For example, protocols must be provided to the IAEC 30 days in advance of the committee meeting. The IAEC's principal responsibility is the review and authorisation of proposed

---

[17]https://www.animallaw.info/statute/taiwan-cruelty-taiwan-animal-protection-law

animal experimentation, with due regard for the Three Rs. In addition, the CPCSEA requires consideration of a Fourth R, rehabilitation for experiments using any large animal. The CPCSEA policy (2004) states:

> 'the aftercare rendered to animals that have been (i) bred for the purpose of experimentation; (ii) subject to any form of experimentation; (iii) retained in laboratory animal houses or breeding houses for the purpose of experimentation, both for education and research, with the sole intention of alleviating the pain/distress or suffering due to the physical, physiological and psychological trauma that the animals have been exposed to and to provide the animal a life distinctly different from laboratory housing and care, until the point of natural death'.

Implementation of the Fourth R has been challenging and is still under development (Qadri & Ramachandra 2018).

The IAEC is also responsible for inspecting the animal facility at least twice annually. A copy of the inspection report must be provided to the CPCSEA. Each IAEC includes a member of the CPCSEA. Most experimentation is conducted on small laboratory animals (e.g. mice, rats, guinea pigs, rabbits); permission must be obtained from a subcommittee of the CPCSEA to conduct research on larger animals.

Singapore

The National Advisory Committee for Laboratory Animal Research (NACLAR) Guidelines on the Care and Use of Animals for Scientific Purposes were published in 2004 (National Advisory Committee for Laboratory Animal Research 2004). They draw heavily on US, Australian and Canadian standards for husbandry, care and protocol authorisation, and on European standards for training guidelines. The guidelines are comprised of three main sections: (1) Guiding principles for the Care and Use of Animals for Scientific Purposes; (2) Guidelines for Institutional Animal Care and Use Committee and (3) Training. Retnam et al. (2016) provide an excellent overview of the content of the Guidelines. The Animal & Veterinary Service (AVS), the government authority that issues licences to research institutions, requires institutional compliance with the NACLAR Guidelines for its animal research programme for that facility to be licensed. While enforcement of compliance occurs at the institutional level through self-regulation by the IACUC, the AVS audits the IACUCs to ensure appropriate self-regulation.

Australia and New Zealand

Australia

Animal research in Australia is regulated at the state or territory level rather than at the national level. In most of these jurisdictions, the regulatory framework for animal research lies within broader animal welfare legislation. The only exception is the state of New South Wales although it is expected that animal research in this jurisdiction will also be amalgamated into a broader animal welfare legislation following a review due for completion in 2022.

The core principles and objectives of the regulations are similar in each Australian jurisdiction although minor operational differences exist. These include differences in licensing procedures, coverage of non-vertebrate species and reporting of animal use numbers, all of which may have implications for projects being conducted in more than one jurisdiction (Bain & Debono 2013; Zrna 2017).

Despite these differences, the regulation of animal research is united by a national standard which is legally binding by virtue of its incorporation into state and territory laws. Now in its eighth edition, this standard is known as The Australian Code for the Care and Use of Animals for Scientific Purposes (National Health and Medical Research Council 2013) ('the Code' not to be confused with the US 'Code').

The first edition of the Code was published in 1969 as an initiative of the scientific community. Later editions, however, have been prepared by broad-based working parties with representatives from animal welfare organisations, state and territory regulators, federal government departments, funding bodies and the research community. Input from the broader community is sought through public consultation phases involving the release of a draft for comment.

The scope of the Code has expanded considerably through the course of its revisions (Rose and Grant 2013). Beginning with a focus on the nexus between animal welfare and scientific outcomes in its first edition, it now encompasses consideration of ethical justification, the 3Rs, lines of responsibility, scientific integrity, competency assessment and wildlife research. The latest edition articulates these in a set of Governing Principles linked to an opening declaration that states 'Respect for animals must underpin all decisions and actions involving the care and use of animals for scientific purposes'. Rather than being prescriptive, the Code provides an ethical framework to guide the decisions of all those involved in the care and use of animals. This allows a common set of principles to be applied on a case-by-case basis in a wide range of circumstances. In 2021, the Code was amended to include a new section which bans the use of animals for testing of chemical ingredients in cosmetics and for testing of finished cosmetic products.

At the core of both the Code and the state and territory legislation is the role played by Animal Ethics Committees (AECs). Constituted locally by research institutions, AECs operate under the oversight of their state or territory regulator and so form part of a system of enforced self-regulation. A key responsibility of AECs is the assessment and approval of applications to use animals in research (whether biomedical or field research) based on whether the proposed use is judged to be ethically acceptable after balancing the potential effects on the well-being of the animals against the potential benefits of the research. AECs also play a formal role in monitoring of research activities and review of research outcomes at the end of a project. Committee membership must include a veterinarian with relevant expertise, a scientist with experience in animal-based research, a person with a demonstrable commitment to animal welfare and a person who has never been involved in animal research and who should be viewed by the wider community as bringing a completely independent view. Members in the latter two categories must be external to the institution and must comprise at least one-third of those present for a meeting to be deemed quorate. Individuals with relevant expertise in other areas such as a representative of the institution's animal facilities or a statistician may also be part of the committee although they do not usually form part of the decision-making quorum. To support the aims of the Code, some jurisdictions also publish guidelines which may not be mandatory but are still expected to be considered carefully during the approval process for animal research projects. One such example is the Best Practice Methodology in the Use of Animals for Scientific Purposes which was developed in response to concerns over reproducibility in animal research (National Health and Medical Research Council 2018).

An important element in supporting regulatory compliance is the requirement for all institutions and their AECs to undergo an independent external review at least once every four years. These reviews must be conducted by a panel whose members have relevant expertise and who are independent of the institution. Panels are usually constituted on an ad hoc basis and so may include representatives from the regulatory body, specialist consultants, community members with animal welfare credentials or a combination of these. The panel must evaluate all aspects of the animal research programme including researcher compliance, standards of animal care, institutional support and the effectiveness of AEC operations.

As is the case in many other countries, the regulation of animal research in Australia is also subject to a range of other laws applicable in specific cases. These include state and federal laws relating to quarantine, wildlife management, genetic manipulation and work health and safety.

New Zealand

The principal legislation regulating animal research in New Zealand lies within the Animal Welfare Act 1999. This reformed earlier animal welfare legislation promulgated in 1960 and marked a change in emphasis from punishment for cruelty to preventing undue pain or distress (Ministry of Agriculture and Forestry 2000). Provisions relating specifically to animal research (which in New Zealand's regulatory system is routinely designated 'research, testing and teaching' or RTT) are found in Part 6 of the Act.

The Act explicitly promotes efforts to support the 3Rs and was one of the first pieces of legislation worldwide to prohibit research involving gorillas, chimpanzees, bonobos or orangutans ('great apes') unless it is in the best interests of the individual animal or the species to which that animal belongs; a special evaluation process is also required for such research. In addition to all nonhuman vertebrates, the definition of 'animal' under the Act extends to octopus, squid, crab, lobster, crayfish and vertebrate foetuses in the second half of gestation or development.

Institutions conducting animal research must hold an accreditation known as a Code of Ethical Conduct (CEC). CECs are issued by New Zealand's Ministry for Primary Industries (MPI; Māori: Manatū Ahu Matua) upon approval of an application demonstrating that the institution has the capacity to meet its obligations under the Act; institutional policies, staff skills, experience and institutional history are among the factors taken into account. Periodic review of the CEC is enforced by an approval limit of 5 years with renewal being subject to satisfactory review by an independent, government-accredited reviewer.

Every Code-holder must establish an AEC whose roles include review of animal research applications and monitoring compliance. AECs may only approve applications if there is good reason to believe that the direct or indirect benefits of using animals will not be outweighed by the likely harm to the animals. AECs must have at least four members, three of whom must be external to the institution: a veterinarian nominated by the New Zealand Veterinary Association, a nominee from an approved animal welfare organisation and a person nominated by a local government who is not associated with research or an animal welfare agency. New Zealand is one of very few countries where membership of animal ethics review bodies must include a person with a demonstrable commitment to animal welfare in addition to a veterinarian. The fourth category of membership comprises a senior person from the institution with the capability to evaluate the scientific merits of an application.

A National Animal Ethics Advisory Committee (NAEAC) was established under the Act although its origins date back to a 1983 amendment of the previous legislation. The NAEAC provides independent advice and recommendations to the Minister, the MPI and AECs on policies and implementation of the Act. Membership is by ministerial appointment and must ensure a balance of expertise across relevant sciences, animal use, ethics and animal welfare advocacy. Within the constraints referred to earlier, the NAEAC must also be consulted by the Director-General of the MPI as part of the review process should an application be made to conduct research involving great apes. A prominent publication supported by NAEAC is a best practice guide for the use of animals in research, teaching and field trials which provides guidance on animal care, animal supply, ethical oversight and responsibilities (Ministry for Primary Industries 2010; Noonan and Williams 2017).

A number of revisions to the Act were introduced with the Animal Welfare Amendment Act (No. 2) 2015. These included formal recognition of animal sentience and a prohibition on the use of animals for testing cosmetics or ingredients intended exclusively for use in cosmetics. A broadening of definitions under the Act also meant that the breeding of research animals or the killing of animals for tissue collection must now be approved by an AEC and the number of such animals included in the institution's mandatory reporting of animal use data. Prior to this, and subject to certain safeguards relating to avoidance of pain or distress, AECs were not formally required to include loss of animal life in harm-benefit analyses.

Although animal-based toxicology is only conducted on a small scale in New Zealand, specific legislation with the potential to require animal testing of psychoactive substances for recreational use has prompted controversy (Brown 2014). Animal research activities in New Zealand may also be subject to other regulatory frameworks in areas such as occupational health and safety and genetic modification depending on the nature of the project (Schofield et al. 2014).

Examples of oversight elsewhere in the world

Latin America

Animal-based research is conducted throughout most of Latin America. However, the legislative framework governing such use is highly variable across the region. Some countries (e.g. Brazil, Chile, Costa Rica, Cuba) have laws specific to the welfare of research animals, while other countries have only general animal protection laws in place. For example, in Peru, the protection of Domestic Animals Law (2000) covers the use of cats and dogs used in research. In Costa Rica, the law references the ethical principles of the Three Rs. Of note, Mexico was the first country in Latin America to implement a law regarding research animals, NOM-062-ZOO-1999. The national or local governments of, and professional societies in, several countries have buttressed the legal framework though the publication of guidance documents (e.g. Cuba's Regulation 64/12 (Ministerio de Salud Pública 2013), the 'Guide for Determination of Humane Final Endpoint in Animals Used in Biomedical Research'). In Brazil, animal welfare is encompassed in the Constitution (Article 225) and the Federal Decree on Anti-Cruelty (1934). However, the Brazilian Environmental Crimes Law (1998) supplements the Constitution to include cruelty crimes against animals. Article 32 of the Environmental Crimes Law specifically addresses the use of animals in research. This Article encourages the use of alternatives and requires the use of anaesthesia for painful procedures. In addition, in Brazil, various states and municipalities have additional animal laws in place.

Russian Federation

There is no specific law in Russia on the protection of research animals that is similar to the ones existing in other European countries. However, the Russian Association for Laboratory Animal Science (Rus-LASA) developed 'Guidelines for the Care and Use of Laboratory Animals based on ETS 123 Appendix A', and they have been officially accepted as terms of reference by the Federal Agency on Standardization (Federal Agency on Technical Regulating and Metrology 2014, 2017). Rus-LASA has also translated into Russian and distributed the *Guide* (National Research Council 2011) to promote implementation of international standards.

Israel

The Israeli Animal Welfare Law (Experiments with Animals) 1994 establishes a review system and standards that are very similar to the US system based on the IACUC, the Attending Veterinarian, and the animal care and use programme (Israel Ministry of Public Health 1994). The Law established a National Council for Experiments on Animal Subjects that authorises institutions to perform animal research, and also authorises IACUCs. For institutions not having authorised IACUCs, a National Permit Committee with members of the National Council will authorise the animal research projects. In addition to the Animal Welfare Law, the Animal Welfare Rules (Israel Ministry of Public Health 2001) give legal status to the latest edition of the *Guide* (National Research Council 2011). Therefore, institutions in Israel currently follow the standards of the 2011 *Guide*.

South Africa

The South African National Standard, 'The care and use of animals for scientific purposes' (SANS 10386:2008 (South African Bureau of Standards 2008)) encompasses all aspects of the care and use of animals for medicine, biology, agriculture, veterinary and other animal science, as well as industry and teaching. These standards define an animal as *'live, sentient nonhuman vertebrate, including eggs, foetuses and embryos, that is fish, amphibians, reptiles, birds and mammals ... and higher invertebrates such as the advanced members from the Cephalopoda and Decapoda'*. The SANS 10386 requires approval of animal activities by an AEC, using the tenets of the Three Rs.[18] Competency of those involved in animal research is regulated by the South African Veterinary Council. Some institutions have supplemented the national standards with their own guidelines. For example, the University of the Free State, Faculty of the Health Sciences has published the 'Guide to the Care and Use of Animals in Research and Teaching' (Faculty of Health Sciences 2016). This document includes a Fourth R, 'Responsibility' whereby the *'reduction of the sum total of discomfort and pain... is the Responsibility of the user for the care and welfare of the animals under his/her control'*.

References

American College of Laboratory Animal Medicine (2016) ACLAM position statement on adequate veterinary care. *JAALAS*, **55**, 826–828.

American Dairy Science Association®, the American Society of Animal Science, and the Poultry Science Association (2020) *Guide for the Care and Use of Agricultural Animals in Research and Teaching, Fourth edition*. Ag Guide 2020 4th Edition (aaalac.org) (accessed 20 January 2022).

American Veterinary Medical Association (2020) *AVMA Guidelines for the Euthanasia of Animals: 2020 Edition*. Schaumburg, IL. 2020-Euthanasia-Final-1-17-20.pdf (avma.org) (accessed 21 January 2022).

Australian Government, National Health and Medical Research Council, Australian Research Council (2013). *Australian Code for the Care and Use of Animals for Scientific Purposes*, 8th edn. Commonwealth of Australia. ISBN Online: 1864965975. https://www.nhmrc.gov.au/about-us/publications/australian-code-care-and-use-animals-scientific-purposes (accessed 3 July 2019).

Bain, S. and Debono, K. (2013) *Australian Scientific Animal Use Statistics: A History of Fragmentation, a Future of Hope*. In: Australian and New Zealand Council for the Care of Animals in Research and Teaching, 2013 Annual Conference Proceedings, pp. 22–26.

Bayne, K. and Martin, D. (1998) AAALAC International: Using performance standards to evaluate an animal care and use program. *Laboratory Animals*, **27**, 32–35.

Bayne, K. and Miller, J. (2000) Assessing animal care and use programs internationally. *Lab Animal*, **29**, 27–29.

---

[18] https://www.sun.ac.za/english/research-innovation/Research-Development/Documents/Animal%20Ethics/ENGLISH/SANS10386.pdf (accessed 24 June 2021)

Bayne, K. and Morris, T.H. (2012) Laws, regulations and policies relating to the care and use of nonhuman primates in biomedical research. In: *Nonhuman Primates in Biomedical Research: Biology and Management, Volume 1*. Eds Abee, C., Mansfield, K., Tardiff, S. and Morris, R., pp. 35–56. Elsevier Inc., New York.

Bayne, K. and Anderson, L.C. (2015) Laws, regulations, and policies affecting the use of laboratory animals. In: *Laboratory Animal Medicine*, 3rd edn. Eds Fox, J.G., Anderson, L.C., Otto, G. et al., pp. 23–42. Elsevier/Academic Press, New York.

Bayne, K., Howard, B.R., Kurosawa, T.M., and Najera, M.E.A. (2019) An overview of global legislation, regulation and policies. In: *Handbook of Laboratory Animal Science*, 4th edn. Eds Hau, J. and Shapiro, S., pp. 899–922. CRC Press LLC, New York.

Beijing Bureau of Municipal Science and Technology (2005) *Beijing Laboratory Animal License Management Measures*. https://www.lascn.net/Item/11982.aspx (accessed 16 January 2019).

Beijing Administrative Office of Lab Animal (2006) *Guide of the Beijing Municipalities for the Review of Laboratory Animal Welfare and Ethics*. http://www.nicpbp.org.cn/sydw/CL0251/1377.html (accessed 16 January 2019).

Brønstad, A., Newcomer, C.E., Decelle, T. et al. (2016) Current concepts of Harm-Benefit Analysis of animal experiments – Report from the AALAS-FELASA Working Group on Harm-Benefit Analysis – Part 1. *Laboratory Animals* **50**, 1–20.

Brown, R. (2014) Our 'psycho' psychoactive substances legislation. *Matters of Substance* **25**(4) November 2014. NZ Drug Foundation. Te Tūāpapa Tarukino o Aotearoa.

Buchanan-Smith, H.M., Rennie, A.E., Vitale, A. et al. (2005) Harmonising the definition of refinement. *Animal Welfare*, **14**, 379–384.

Canadian Council on Animal Care (2015) CCAC guidelines on: training of personnel working with animals in science. ISBN: 978-0-919087-59-0. https://www.ccac.ca/Documents/Standards/Guidelines/CCAC_Guidelines_on_Training_of_Personnel_Working_With_Animals_in_Science.pdf (accessed 3 July 2019).

Canadian Council on Animal Care (2016) *CCAC Policy Statement on: The Certification of Animal Ethics and Care Programs*. https://www.ccac.ca/Documents/Standards/Policies/Certification-of-animal-ethics-and-care-programs.pdf (accessed 15 January 2019).

Code of Federal Regulations (1998) *Title 21: Food and Drugs*; Chapter 1: Feed and Drug Administration, Department of Health and Human Services; Subchapter A: General; Part 58: Good Laboratory Practice for Nonclinical Laboratory Studies, Office of the Federal Register, Washington, DC.

Code of Federal Regulations (1997) *Title 40: Protection of the Environment*; Chapter 1: Environmental Protection Agency; Subchapter E: Pesticide Programs; Part 160: Good Laboratory Practice Standard, Office of the Federal Register, Washington, DC.

Council for International Medical Sciences/International Council for Laboratory Animal Science (CIOMS/ICLAS)_(2012) *International Guiding Principles for Biomedical Research Involving Animals*. https://olaw.nih.gov/sites/default/files/Guiding_Principles_2012.pdf (accessed 30 December 2018).

Council of Europe (1986) *Convention for the Protection of Vertebrate Animals used for Experimental and other Scientific Purposes* (ETS 123). Strasbourg. https://rm.coe.int/168007a67b (accessed 31 December 2018).

Council of Europe (2006). *Appendix A of the European Convention for the Protection of Vertebrate Animals Used for Experimental and Other Scientific Purposes (ETS No. 123)*. Guidelines for accommodation and care of animals (Article 5 of the convention). Approved by the multilateral consultation. Cons 2006;123:3. https://rm.coe.int/CoERMPublicCommonSearchServices/DisplayDCTMContent?documentId=090000168007a445 (accessed 2 January 2019).

CPCSEA (2004) *Report of the Consultative Group on Review of the Norms and Practices for Regulation of Animal Experimentation*. (https://www.aaalac.org/resources/CPCSEA_Conference_Rehabilitation.pdf (accessed 16 January 2019).

Department of Defense. (2019) DoD Instruction 3216.01, *Use of Animals in DoD Conducted and Supported Research and Training*, DoDI 3216.01, March 20, 2019 (whs.mil) (accessed 21 January 2022).

Dunlop, R. and Williams, D. (1996) Bioethics, Animal experimentation and sentience. In: *Veterinary Medicine: An Illustrated History*. pp. 619–642. Mosby, Philadelphia.

European Commission (2007) *Commission Recommendations of 18 June 2007 on Guidelines for the Accommodation and Care of Animals Used for Experimental and Other Scientific Purposes*. https://eur-lex.europa.eu/legal-content/EN/TXT/PDF/?uri=CELEX:32007H0526&from=EN (accessed 2 January 2019).

European Council (1986) Council Directive 86/609/EEC of 24 November 1986 on the approximation of laws, regulations and administrative provisions of the Member States regarding the protection of animals used for experimental and other scientific purposes. *Official Journal of the European Communities* L 358, 1–29. https://eur-lex.europa.eu/legal-content/EN/TXT/PDF/?uri=CELEX:31986L0609&from=EN (accessed 31 December 2018).

European Parliament and Council (2010) Directive 2010/63/EU of the European Parliament and of the Council of 22 September 2010 on the Protection of Animals Used for Scientific Purposes. *Off J Eur Union* 2010; L 276/33–79. https://eur-lex.europa.eu/LexUriServ/LexUriServ.do?uri=OJ:L:2010:276:0033:0079:EN:PDF (accessed 31 December 2018).

Faculty of Health Sciences, University of the Free State (2016) *Guide to the Care and Use of Animals in Research and Teaching (Version 1)*. https://www.ufs.ac.za/docs/librariesprovider25/ethics-documents/animal_ethics_guide_ufs_may16_aec_accepted.pdf?status=Temp&sfvrsn=0.2821812948629828 (accessed 16 January 2019).

Federal Agency on Technical Regulating and Metrology (2014) *Standard GOST 33215-2014 Guidelines for Accommodation and Care of Animals: Environment, Housing and Management*. https://docs.cntd.ru/document/1200127789 (accessed 24 January 2022).

Federal Agency on Technical Regulating and Metrology (2017) Standard GOST 34088-2017 *Guidelines for Accommodation and Care of Laboratory Animals. Guidelines for the Maintenance and Care of Laboratory Animals. Rules for Keeping and Caring for Farm Animals* (internet--law-ru.translate.goog) (accessed 21 January 2022).

Federal Service for Supervision of Consumer Rights Protection and Human Well-Being (2014) *Sanitary Rules for Organization and Managing Vivariums* SP 2.2.1.3218-14 from 29.08.2014.

Federation of European Laboratory Animal Science Associations (2000) Recommendations for education and training: Category B. *Laboratory Animals*, **34**, 229–235. http://www.felasa.eu/recommendations/recommendation/recommendations-on-education-and-training-categories-b/ (accessed 3 January 2019).

Federation of European Laboratory Animal Science Associations (FELASA) (2007) *Euroguide: On the Accommodation and Care of Animals Used for Experimental and Other Scientific Purposes*. Royal Society of Medicine Press, London. http://www.felasa.eu/about-us/library/ (accessed 11 January 2019).

Federation of European Laboratory Animal Science Associations (2010a) Recommendations for education and training: Category A. *Laboratory Animals*, **44**, 163–169. http://www.felasa.eu/recommendations/recommendation/recommendations-for-education-and-training-category-a-revision/ (accessed 3 January 2019)

Federation of European Laboratory Animal Science Associations (2010b) *Guidelines for Continuing Education for Persons Involved in Animal Experiments*. http://www.felasa.eu/recommendations/guidelines/guidelines-for-continuing-education-for-persons-involved-in-animal-experime/ (accessed 4 January 2019)

Federation of European Laboratory Animal Science Associations (2018) FELASA accreditation of education and training courses in laboratory animal science according to the Directive 2010/63/EU. *Laboratory Animals*, Jul 24: 23677218788105. doi: 10.1177/0023677218788105.

[Epub ahead of print]. https://journals.sagepub.com/doi/pdf/10.1177/0023677218788105 (accessed 3 January 2019)

Guillén, J. and Vergara, P. (2018). Global Guiding Principles: A Tool for Harmonization In: *Laboratory Animals: Regulations and Recommendations for the Care and Use of Animals in Research*, 2nd edn. Ed. Guillén, J. pp. 1–13. Academic Press, London.

Guillén, J., Robinson, S., Decelle, T. *et al.* (2015) Approaches to animal research project evaluation in Europe after implementation of Directive 2010/63/EU. *Lab Animal Europe* **44**, 23–31.

Interagency Research Advisory Committee (1985) US Government Principles for the Utilization and Care of Vertebrate Animals Used in Testing, Research, and Training. *Federal Register*, May 20, **50**. https://www.ncbi.nlm.nih.gov/books/NBK54048/ (accessed 28 December 2018).

Israel Ministry of Public Health (1994) *Animal Welfare Law – Prevention of Cruelty to Animals Law* (experiments on animals) 5754, 1994. https://www.aaalac.org/intlRefs/Israel/Israel-Law.pdf (accessed 10 January 2019).

Israel Ministry of Public Health (2001) *Animal Welfare Rules – Prevention of Cruelty to Animals Rules (Experiments on Animals)* 5761. https://www.aaalac.org/intlRefs/Israel/Israel-Law.pdf (accessed 10 January 2019).

Joint Working Group on Veterinary Care: Voipio, H-M., Baneux, P., Gomez de Segura, I.A. *et al.* (2008) Guidelines for the veterinary care of laboratory animals: report of the FELASA/ECLAM/ESLAV Joint Working Group on Veterinary Care. *Laboratory Animals*, **42**, 1–11.

Korea Animal Protection Act. (2017) http://law.go.kr/LSW/eng/engLsSc.do?menuId=2&query=#liBgcolor12 (accessed 28 December 2018).

Laber, K., Newcomer, C.E., Decelle, T. *et al.* (2016) Recommendations for addressing Harm-Benefit Analysis and implementation in ethical evaluation – Report from the AALAS-FELASA Working Group on Harm-Benefit Analysis – Part 2. *Laboratory Animals*, **50**, 21–42.

MacArthur Clark, J., Sun, D. (2020) Guidelines for the ethical review of laboratory animal welfare, People's Republic of China National Standard GB/T 35892-2018 (issued 6 February 2018, effective from 1 September 2018). Guidelines for the ethical review of laboratory animal welfare People's Republic of China National Standard GB/T 35892-2018 (aaalac.org) (accessed 21 January 2022).

Ministerio de Salud Pública. Cuba. Regulación 64/12, Lineamiento para la Constitución y Funcionamiento de los Comités Institucionales para el Cuidado y Uso de los Animales de Laboratorio. Cuba. 2013.

Ministry for Primary Industries (2010) *Good Practice Guide for the Use of Animals in Research, Testing and Teaching*. https://www.mpi.govt.nz/protection-and-response/animal-welfare/national-animal-ethics-advisory-committee/naeac-publications/ (accessed 22 January 2019)

Ministry of Agriculture and Forestry (2000) *The Use of Animals in Research Testing and Teaching. Users Guide to Part 6 of the Animal Research Act 1999*. MAF Policy Information Paper 33, May 2000.

Ministry of Environment, Japan (2006) *Standards Relating to the Care and Management of Laboratory Animals Reducing Pain of Laboratory Animals* (Notice No. 88); Latest revision: Notice of the Ministry of the Environment No. 84 (2013). https://www.env.go.jp/nature/dobutsu/aigo/2_data/laws/nt_h25_84_en.pdf (accessed 15 January 2019)

National Advisory Committee for Laboratory Animal Research (2004) *Guidelines on the Care and Use of Animals for Scientific Purposes*. Singapore. https://www.ava.gov.sg/docs/default-source/tools-and-resources/resources-for-businesses/attach3_animalsforscientificpurposes (accessed 16 January 2019).

National Competent Authorities for the implementation of Directive 2010/63/EU on the protection of animals used for scientific purposes (2014). A working document on the development of a common education and training framework to fulfil the requirements under the Directive – Replacing consensus document of 18–19 September 2013 – http://ec.europa.eu/environment/chemicals/lab_animals/pdf/Endorsed_E-T.pdf (accessed 3 July 2019).

National Health and Medical Research Council (2013) *Australian Code for the Care and Use of Animals for Scientific Purposes*, 8th edn. Canberra, ACT, Australia: National Health and Medical Research Council.

National Research Council (1996) *Guide for the Care and Use of Laboratory Animals*. National Academies Press, Washington DC. https://www.cpp.edu/~research/acuc/doc/guide%20to%20use%20lab%20animals.pdf (accessed 7 January 2019).

National Research Council (2011) *Guide for the Care and Use of Laboratory Animals*. National Academies Press, Washington DC. https://www.aaalac.org/resources/theguide.cfm (accessed 7 January 2019).

Noonan, D and Williams, V (2017) Chapter 12, Laboratory Animals Regulations and Recommendations: Australia and New Zealand. In *Laboratory Animals: Regulations and Recommendations for the Care and Use of Animals in Research*, 2nd edn. Ed. J. Guillen, pp. 375–419. San Diego: Academic Press.

Office of Laboratory Animal Welfare, National Institutes of Health (2015) *Public Health Service Policy on Humane Care and Use of Laboratory Animals*. Bethesda, MD.

Ogden, B., Pang, W., Agui, T. and Lee, B.H. (2016) Laboratory animal laws, regulations, guidelines and standards in China Mainland, Japan, and Korea. *ILAR Journal* **57**, 301–311

Orlans, B. (2001) Ethical themes of national regulations governing animal experiments: An international perspective. In: *Applied Ethics in Animal Research. Philosophy, Regulation, and Laboratory Applications*. Eds Gluck, J., DiPasquale, T. and Orlans, B., pp. 131–147. Purdue University Press, West Lafayette.

Poirier, G.M., Bergmann, C., Denais-Lalieve, D.G. *et al.* (2015) ESLAV/ECLAM/LAVA/EVERI recommendations for the roles, responsibilities and training of the laboratory animal veterinarian and the designated veterinarian under Directive 2010/63/EU. 2015. *Laboratory Animals* **49**, 89–99.

Qadri, S.S.Y.H. and Ramachandra, S.G. (2018) Laws, regulations, and guidelines governing research animal care and use in India. In: *Laboratory Animals: Regulations and Recommendations for the Care and Use of Animals in Research*, 2nd edn. Ed. Guillen, J., pp. 237–261. Academic Press, Elsevier Inc., London.

Retnam, L., Chatikavanij, P., Kunjara, P. *et al.* (2016) Laws, regulations, guidelines and standards for animal care and use for scientific purposes in the countries of Singapore, Thailand, Indonesia, Malaysia, and India. *ILAR Journal* **57**, 312–323

Rose, M. and Grant, E. (2013) Australia's ethical framework for when animals are used for scientific purpose. *Animal Welfare*, **22**, 315–322.

Rupke, N. (1987) *Vivisection in Historical Perspective*. Croon-Helm, London.

Russell, W. and Burch, R. (1959) *The Principles of Humane Experimental Technique*. Methuen, London (2nd edn. 1992, UFAW). http://altweb.jhsph.edu/pubs/books/humane_exp/het-toc (accessed 11 January 2019).

Schofield, J., Noonan, D., Chen, Y. and Penson, P. (2014) Laboratory Animal Regulations and Recommendations for Global Collaborative Research: Australia and New Zealand. In *Laboratory Animals: Regulations and Recommendations for Global Collaborative Research*, Ed. Guillen, J., pp. 333–376. San Diego: Academic Press/Elsevier.

Science Council of Japan (2006) *Guidelines for Proper Conduct of Animal Experiments*. Tokyo, Japan. http://www.scj.go.jp/ja/info/kohyo/pdf/kohyo-20-k16-2e.pdf (accessed 17 January 2019).

Select Committee on Animals in Scientific Procedures (2002) *Memorandum by the Chief Inspector*, **III** 179, (HL paper 150-III). House of Lords, London.

Slaughter, B. (2002). Animal use in biomedicine: an annotated bibliography of Buddhist and related perspectives. *Journal of Buddhist*

Ethics, **9**, 149–158. http://blogs.dickinson.edu/buddhistethics/files/2010/04/slaug021.pdf (accessed 17 January 2019).

South African Bureau of Standards (2008) The care and use of animals for scientific purposes. *Standards Bulletin*, September 2008. https://www.sun.ac.za/english/research-innovation/Research-Development/Documents/Animal%20Ethics/ENGLISH/SANS10386.pdf (accessed 16 January 2019).

State Science and Technology Commission (1988) *Regulations of People's Republic of China for the Administration of Affairs Concerning Experimental Animals*. http://en.pkulaw.cn/display.aspx?cgid=3f3dc921e8e837aebdfb&lib=law (accessed 16 January 2019).

Taiwan Animal Protection Law. 4 November 1998. https://www.animallaw.info/statute/taiwan-cruelty-taiwan-animal-protection-law (accessed 16 January 2019).

The Prevention of Cruelty to Animals Act 1960 (No. 59 of 1960), Amended by Central Act 26 of 1962, Republic of India. http://www.envfor.nic.in/legis/awbi/awbi01.pdf (accessed 16 January 2019).

United Kingdom Parliament (1876) 39 & 40 Vict, Public Acts, c. 77. An Act to amend the Law relating to Cruelty to Animals. https://web.archive.org/web/20061214034848/http://homepage.tinet.ie/~pnowlan/Chapter-77.htm (accessed 31 December 2018).

US Department of Agriculture (2017) Animal Welfare Regulations. Code of Federal Regulations, Title 9, Animals and Animal Products, Chapter 1, Subchapter A https://www.aphis.usda.gov/animal_welfare/downloads/AC_BlueBook_AWA_FINAL_2017_508comp.pdf (accessed 11 January 2019).

Walker, A. and Poppleton, W. (1967) The establishment of a specific pathogen-free (SPF) rat and mouse breeding unit. *Laboratory Animals*, **1**, 1–5.

World Organisation for Animal Health (2013) *Use of Animals in Research and Education*. Chapter 7.8, Terrestrial Animal Health Code. http://www.oie.int/index.php?id=169&L=0&htmfile=chapitre_aw_research_education.htm (accessed 11 January 2019).

Zrna, S. (2017) *Operating a National Animal Ethics Committee under State Based Licences*. In: Australian and New Zealand Council for the Care of Animals in Research and Teaching, 2017 Annual Conference Proceedings, pp. 53–59.

9 Planning, design and construction of the modern animal facility

Ken Applebee, Christopher Sear and Steven Cubitt

Introduction

The purpose of this chapter is to inform those who rarely get called upon to participate in the design of a new research animal facility; but who have to come forward when requested and, with very little preparation, contribute their experience, expertise and aspirations within the context of a new facility design process. These individuals are usually the existing facility management and their senior team. This chapter is for their benefit, and will explain how a vivarium building project evolves, when they should expect to be involved and what types of roles they can be asked to fulfil in order to ensure the project's success.

The chapter does not provide an exhaustive discussion of the different rooms, services and functions that make up the new facility. Facility managers usually have a clear idea of what they need to support their scientists and provide for the animals in their care, but if required, these can be found in excellent treatises such as 'Guidelines on laboratory animal facilities – characteristics, design and development'[1]. Rather, our intention is to provide guidance on how the design and construction processes work, and how they should be co-ordinated to ensure that the new facility functions as designed, specifically to meet scientific needs and comply with the local regulations.

The purpose and function of a research animal facility is to effectively support an institution's biomedical research goals by providing appropriate laboratory space and services, plus promoting the health and welfare of the housed animals and its staff. When contemplating a new facility or a major refurbishment, creating and maintaining these functions requires carefully detailed and co-ordinated up-front and follow-through planning.

We stress at the outset that adequate budgetary planning is a crucial pre-requisite. Animal research facilities, also known as 'vivaria' or some other less 'direct' terminology, are a specially designed building type that provide accurately controlled environments for the care and maintenance of animals bred and used in research, and the procedures that researchers require them to undergo. Animal research facilities are thus a distinct subset of research laboratories whose integrated functions require the buildings to be necessarily complex and expensive to construct and to operate. Their value is immense and lies in their specific utility for biomedical research. They provide the safe and humane environments for both animals and the researchers that work with them: the vital infrastructure supporting high-quality ethical pre-clinical science.

In addition to the immediate management team, the key groups that will be involved in the planning and construction stages of a new facility include:

- The institution's management who control the budgets for design-and-build expenditure. Throughout this chapter, we refer to the institution as the 'client', as represented by its management and those staff designated to work with third-party contractors as employers.
- Scientists, sometimes referred to as researchers who will plan and conduct studies within the facility.
- Animal technicians who will service the facility and care for the animals held within it.
- Veterinarians who will have specific responsibilities for maintaining defined animal health and overseeing animal welfare.
- Engineers and other support staff who will maintain the fabric of the building and its plant in working order.
- Institutional health and safety advisors.
- Regulators and those with specific responsibilities for ensuring compliance with regulations.
- The design team comprising architects, space planners and engineers.
- Contractors who build, fit out, commission and validate the new facility.

---

[1] https://ccac.ca/Documents/Standards/Guidelines/Facilities.pdf?msclkid=250b7a33cfa711ecb4e748be2803f7e9 (Accessed 31 May 2022)

Overriding requirements for all research animal facilities

An animal facility must:

- Satisfy the needs of the animals in that they should be free of disease, stress and injury; and occupy a safe, comfortable and enriched environment.
- Meet the needs of the research and the researchers.
- Satisfy the needs of the facility staff, and the health and safety of all personnel.
- Meet the facility operational needs of stability, efficiency and durability.
- Comply with regulatory requirements that can influence the design, construction, operational model and the overall philosophy.
- Provide environmental stability that should include uninterrupted maintenance of the animals' physical environment necessitating the provision of redundancy for several critical components of the heating, ventilation and air conditioning system (normally abbreviated to HVAC).
- Maintain bioexclusion barriers and biocontainment facilities by physical separation and directional airflow created by differential air pressures between defined spaces.

Project brief

A project brief summarises what the client desires to achieve in the new or refurbished facility, where they hope to achieve it, and at what scale and cost.

The project brief for an animal research building project is informed by seven factors:

1. Institutional/governmental/geographical factors:
    Careful, detailed planning encompassing all phases of facility programming, planning, design, construction and commissioning should be based around local institutional, governmental and geographic requirements, to ensure that the facility will function effectively and efficiently support the institution's research programmes.
    Different funding-providers, whether public, private or charity-based, can have a strong influence on the design and function of animal research facilities and should be consulted well in advance of the design and build.
    Facilities with similar functions may differ in detail locally, due to different regulations and design approaches in different countries.
2. Environmental/sustainability factors:
    Those responsible for managing and designing laboratory animal facilities need to make carefully co-ordinated and well-considered choices in design, equipment and working practices to create working environments that support animal and staff welfare in a sustainable fashion. It is important that any new or refurbishment project provides high-quality barriered facilities meeting the needs of science while housing a sufficiently large number of animals under welfare-focused conditions.
    There are many synergies between sustainability and good working conditions for both staff and animals. Natural daylight and ventilation, especially in staff rest and office areas, associated with increased productivity and reduced absenteeism.
    There is a growing recognition of the need to make laboratories more sustainable. The International Institute for Sustainable Laboratories[2] (I²SL) has developed and published much guidance material and is now having a major influence on laboratory design in North America. A number of such laboratories are using their achievements of legal compliance plus the former Labs 21 guidance (adopted by I²SL) to emphasise their environmental commitment and bolster their world class status. These initiatives are enabling such organisations to minimise their operating costs while maintaining their animal and human welfare responsibilities, enhancing their facility's attractiveness to staff, and thereby enhancing productivity, recruitment and retention.
    A UK initiative called 'S-labs' has also been established and is developing similar guidance for the UK[3]. It is also working with those promoting equivalent guidance in other countries, such as the German Laboratory 2020 programme, to develop a European initiative. S-Labs UK aims to reduce the environmental impact of laboratories and move towards net zero carbon emissions. Although this may not be achievable for animal research facilities, they are one of the biggest users of energy on research campuses, and therefore, a reduction in energy usage of, for example 30%, would still have a major impact. The authors believe that such significant energy reductions are possible, but to achieve them will require a focus on the primary animal environment, rather than the conditioning of the whole facility environment. The UK initiative is building on the former US Labs 21 programme and promoting new approaches to design and operation which should result in significant environmental, financial and other benefits.
3. Specialist scientific factors:
    Animal research facilities often contain a number of specialised local environments that are designed to support a range of diverse specific functions, and these need to be defined at the start of the design process (e.g. quarantine, live imaging, biocontainment and cage washing).
    A potential downside to specialisation of space for specific functions is that it can add cost and reduce future flexibility, which should also be recognised at the project brief stage.
4. Regulatory factors:
    Design, construction and the operating model should be integrated to meet all applicable codes and regulations governing animal care and use, as well as human health and safety.
5. Animal welfare factors:
    Modern laboratory animal facilities should meet the needs of the animals and provide a safe, comfortable and enriched environment that is free of disease, stress and injury.
    It is now accepted that animal welfare can be greatly impacted by poor environmental conditions. An

---

[2] https://www.i2sl.org/index.html (Accessed 31 May 2022)
[3] http://www.effectivelab.org.uk/about-s-lab.html (Accessed 31 May 2022)

extreme example is ringtail in rats, also known as tail necrosis, and is attributed to low environmental humidity and high temperatures. Other examples of poor environmental factors include high frequency ultrasound, vibration emanating from mechanical components of equipment (e.g., HVAC system, cage washers, autoclaves) and high-lux lighting levels which can all have negative impacts on animals' well-being and behaviours. See also Chapter 10: Enrichment: animal welfare and scientific validity. These and many other potentially adverse environmental conditions must be carefully considered when building the animal facility.

Simple measures such as automatic opening doors with soft closures, swipe access, all of which lessen sudden noise, light-tight doors eliminating extraneous light into animal rooms during dark periods, dusk and dawn lighting cycles, plus many other design initiatives can all help to reduce stress levels in animals.

There will also be species-specific considerations that need to be considered and factored into the design and build, which will ensure the optimum levels of animal welfare and, therefore, the quality of the scientific outcomes (e.g. the provisions of floor pens for intermediate-sized animals, such as rabbits).

Continuous monitoring and control of temperature, humidity, sound, light, etc. provide environmental stability, essential for the animals' physical well-being, as well as for scientific reproducibility.

Maintenance of differential air pressures in barrier and containment facilities is a critical factor in maintaining biosecurity and protecting staff from biological hazards.

To ensure that such welfare-centric requirements are met, the design and construction of the facility should follow an evidence-based approach to meeting the needs of species, strain, sex, age, health status and experimental conditions, rather than a rules-based approach. An evidence-based study and report, that documents how the facility will achieve its animal and human welfare objectives, should, therefore, be used right from the start of the project, to inform and direct the design and construction processes. Regulators can be given access to this report, so that, when auditing the finished facility, they can be directed to the evidence that demonstrates the compliance they expect to see.

6. Benchmarking factors:

The project brief should provide comparisons with some examples of similar facilities. Such benchmarking can assist with the selection, sizing and adjacencies of spaces and equipment; how animal care and welfare requirements can be met; and environmental footprints minimised. Benchmarking can also help to establish a realistic budget.

7. Contract/procurement factors:

Forms of contract and different types of procurement influence the staging of the project programme and the milestones that lead to completion. The way that users, veterinarians and technicians input their requirements, and the timing of such inputs, will vary according to contract type and procurement process. Specialist areas such as surgical, imaging and behavioural suites and specific/unique equipment should be closely specified by experts in their field to prevent misunderstandings by the design team. It is essential that clients have a good understanding about this, so that the vital information is not provided too late in the design process and thus be unable to influence it, potentially attracting extra design and construction costs.

Types of animal research facility

Animal research facilities may be operated for different purposes by several different types of organisations:

- University (e.g. academic multi-purpose research);
- Government (e.g. containment facilities for research of national health interest);
- Hospital/NHS (e.g. infection control; personalised medicine);
- Pharmaceutical R&D (e.g. new drug development);
- Contract Research Organisation (CROs) (e.g. drug safety and efficacy testing);
- Biotech/start-up companies (e.g. application of new bio-technologies);
- Commercial breeders (e.g. breed and supply of highly defined animals for research).

The type of facility and how it is funded, designed and built will vary according to the organisation that owns/operates the animal research laboratories. For example, government-funded projects have very different procurement processes when compared with the pharmaceutical industry, as they have different financing, tendering and legal obligations.

Facility accommodation factors

Animal facilities comprise a variety of different workspaces designed to meet the needs of the users' particular research foci, species requirements, local legislation and *raison d'être*. Below is a list of workspaces commonly found in modern research animal facilities, although the list should not be regarded as exclusive or mandatory:

- Animal holding (e.g. breeding/ageing);
- Staff services (e.g. clothes changing/showering/training/office/break);
- Support services (e.g. cage cleaning and sterilisation for reuse/storage);
- Surgery (with separate preparation, surgical procedure and post-operative provisions);
- Procedural (general or specialised, with all support equipment);
- Imaging (with provisions for several modalities and short-term and longitudinal studies);
- Specialist scientific equipment that must be located adjacent to animal holding;
- Behavioural (with provisions for several test modalities and adjacencies to related functions);
- Areas meeting the requirements of GLP (e.g. pre-clinical toxicology and efficacy studies);
- Clinical support (e.g. xenotransplantation);

- Containment (CL2, CL3, CAT2, CAT3, SAPO, BS, etc.);
- Bioexclusion (to maintain animals of a defined health status such as SPF, SOPF or Germ-Free).

Legislation

Legislation has become increasingly harmonised, globally, with the UK, European Union, USA, Canada and Australia influencing the wider geopolitical regulatory frameworks. It is covered in detail in Chapter 8: Legislation and oversight of the conduct of research using animals: a global overview.

Legislation impacts the design of research animal facilities through the type of approach to approval/certification/licensure of the new facility taken by the specific regulatory authority. The main differences in approach can be summarised as 'rules-based' in which the regulatory requirements must be followed exactly as described in legal documentation or 'evidence-based' in which the performance of the new facility must be shown to be appropriate for the animals housed and the experimental work to be performed. The 'evidence-based' approach is becoming increasingly used for facilities that must cater for animal welfare and human health and safety.

The facility client will know which legislative framework the new facility and its design must comply with, and it is their responsibility to ensure that the necessary requirements are understood by the design team and contractors. There will be differences between different countries and different regulatory authorities, and these differences are outside the scope of this chapter.

The main types of legislation that always apply to animal research laboratories in the UK are listed below.

- Animal Welfare (e.g. UK: Animals (Scientific Procedures) Act 1986[4] and related Code of Practice for the Housing and Care of Animals Bred, Supplied or Used for Scientific Purposes 2014[5]);
- Human Safety (e.g. UK: Health and Safety at Work etc. Act, 1974[6]; Control of Substances Hazardous to Health (COSHH) Regulations 2002[7]);
- Biocontainment (e.g. HSE Sealability of Microbiological Containment Level 3 and 4 Facilities[8]; HSE Management and operation of microbiological containment laboratories ACDP 2019[9]);
- BS 5726: 2005 Microbiological safety cabinets – siting and use of cabinets[10].
- BS EN12469: 2000 Performance criteria for microbiological safety cabinets[11]);
- Bioexclusion (No legislative standards);
- Biosecurity (No legislative standards);
- Good manufacturing processes (GMP) (e.g. UK: MHRA Orange Guide 2017[12]);
- Genetic Modification (e.g. UK: Genetically Modified Organisms (Contained Use) Regulations 2014[13]).

Specialist regulations may also apply to animal research laboratories, and these should be consulted during the design of a new facility. Those that apply in the UK shall serve as examples here:

- Veterinary Medicines Regulations 2013[14];
- Anti-terrorism, Crime and Security Act 2001[15];
- BS2646: 2021 Autoclaves for sterilisation in laboratories Part 5[16];

There may also be official documentation that provides useful guidance on design considerations, such as the following current in the UK:

- Higher Education Safety and Health Forum (HESH)[17];
- Working safely with research animals: Management of infection risks Guidance HSE[18];
- Scientific Advisory Committee on Genetic Modification Section 5 (SACGM)[19];
- HSE Guidance note EH76 – Control of laboratory animal allergy[20];
- HSE Guide paper HSG 258 – Controlling airborne contaminants at work[21];
- Royal Institute of British Architects (RIBA) Workplan (2020)[22].

---

[4] https://www.legislation.gov.uk/ukpga/1986/14/introduction (Accessed 31 May 2022)

[5] https://assets.publishing.service.gov.uk/government/uploads/system/uploads/attachment_data/file/388895/COPAnimalsFullPrint.pdf (Accessed 31 May 2022)

[6] https://www.legislation.gov.uk/ukpga/1974/37/contents?msclkid=d6647c21cfa811eca9b1c5d97d116c69 (Accessed 31 May 2022)

[7] https://www.hse.gov.uk/coshh/index.htm (Accessed 31 May 2022)

[8] https://www.hse.gov.uk/biosafety/gmo/guidance/sealability.pdf?msclkid=7ba83b62cfa911ec8c816d5caa15b9dd (Accessed 31 May 2022)

[9] https://www.hse.gov.uk/biosafety/management-containment-labs.pdf?msclkid=c4bde91ccfa911eca2ce707e2e57718e (Accessed 31 May 2022)

[10] https://www.standardsuk.com/products/BS-5726-2005?msclkid=f3d6f99fcfa911ec8c7953fd51536add (Accessed 31 May 2022)

[11] https://www.en-standard.eu/bs-en-12469-2000-biotechnology-performance-criteria-for-microbiological-safety-cabinets/?msclkid=9ea208abcfaa11ecab8408b05dbfaf80 (Accessed 31 May 2022)

[12] https://mhrainspectorate.blog.gov.uk/2016/12/02/the-2017-orange-and-green-guides/?msclkid=d33af6cacfaa11ec819244697dbde60f (Accessed 31 May 2022)

[13] https://www.legislation.gov.uk/uksi/2014/1663/contents?msclkid=246a8672cfac11ecac91984582793be3 (Accessed 31 May 2022)

[14] https://www.legislation.gov.uk/uksi/2013/2033/contents (Accessed 31 May 2022)

[15] https://www.legislation.gov.uk/ukpga/2001/24/contents?msclkid=ce10df21cfad11ecb887ea730f08e349 (Accessed 8 June 2022)

[16] https://www.bsigroup.com/en-GB/standards/bs-2646-12021/?msclkid=fe6ed657cfad11ec9b0cda7f4e45afed (Accessed 8 June 2022)

[17] https://www.hse.gov.uk/services/education/hesh.htm (Accessed 8 June 2022)

[18] https://www.hse.gov.uk/pubns//priced/animal-research.pdf (Accessed 8 June 2022)

[19] https://www.hse.gov.uk/biosafety/gmo/acgm/acgmcomp/?msclkid=b3080839cfb211ecbfa4752a4c19b027 (Accessed 8 June 2022)

[20] https://www.hse.gov.uk/pubns/eh76.pdf?msclkid=38b23041cfb311ecb3c14ef4c94025a9 (Accessed 8 June 2022)

[21] https://www.hse.gov.uk/pubns/priced/hsg258.pdf (Accessed 8 June 2022)

[22] https://www.architecture.com/knowledge-and-resources/resources-landing-page/riba-plan-of-work (Accessed 8 June 2022)

Biocontainment and GMP are, in general, more strictly regulated, with GMP requiring defined, controlled and recorded processes during design, construction, commissioning and pre-operational activities.

To ensure that the current legislation is adopted and followed, it may be appropriate for the client to appoint, early in the design process, specialist consultants who will be able to advise the design team on the appropriate actions to be taken under the subject headers above, including how and when to liaise with the regulators, how to propose and justify the most appropriate approaches for compliance, and how to document and co-ordinate all the necessary interactions in a timely manner.

Procurement models

Project procurement strategy

Procurement is the process of purchasing goods or services. There are many different routes by which the design, construction and equipping of a building can be procured. The selected procurement route should follow a strategy which fits the long-term objectives of the client's business plan and for many institutions, is a legally prescribed process. Considerations are likely to include:

- Speed;
- Cost;
- Quality;
- Specific project requirements and/or constraints;
- Risk;
- Asset ownership;
- Financing.

The client should develop the procurement strategy for the project in its very early stages, in consultation with the project manager and the design team. This preliminary process should be based upon the overall objectives of the project and will vary from project to project.

Contractor procurement models

The contractor procurement models commonly used are as follows:

1. **Traditional model**
   The traditional model affords the client a great deal of control over the project quality, specification and cost, by having the design completed in detail before the contractor tender process commences.

   The timescale is, therefore, lengthened in order to complete the concept and detailed design with all specifications included.

   The client assumes all the risks associated with the consultants' design and the consequences of any unforeseen items (e.g. changes in ground conditions). The client also fails to benefit from the buildability input that can be provided by a contractor when appointed before the design is complete (see below).

   As the contractor has no responsibility for the design, the client is responsible for any design mistakes or omissions that might become apparent during the construction process. Although some risk can be shared with the contractor, the MAJORITY of the development liability is assumed by the client, who is totally dependent on the design team for successfully interpreting his requirements.

   Good for: Client maintaining control of quality and specifications, and some cost certainty at the point of accepting the successful contractor's tender.

   Bad for: Client assuming almost 100% of the risks associated with the tender design and can, therefore, exert limited impact on the contractors' cost control during the construction works.

2. **Single- and two-stage design-and-build models**
   These models transfer the majority of the risk to the contractor at a relatively early stage in the project. There are various sub-types of the design-and-build model; however, the basic parameters remain the same: at a certain point in time, the contractor becomes responsible for completing the design and construction of the project for an agreed fixed sum. A fixed price is, therefore, achieved prior to construction, and offers the client a high level of cost certainty.

   For building projects in the UK, the RIBA have provided direction that the client must initially complete a formal document that describes the user's requirements, which can range from a simple accommodation schedule (for a very basic project) to an almost fully worked-out design. Regardless of the size and complexity of the project, the authors' recommendation is that the client creates a team that prepares a User Requirement Specification (URS) as described below. This will comprise the sections of the client's/employer's Requirements Document that describes all the necessary specifications related to the animal research facility, as required by RIBA. Adequate time must be allowed for the client's requirements and proposals to be properly prepared, including the completion of floor layouts and room data sheets, and taking the project to the end of RIBA Stage 3 (described later in this chapter under 'The design process' and 'Project stages as defined by RIBA'). At this point, the project goes out to tender, either via a single or a two-stage process, and upon completion of the tender process, the successful contractor becomes responsible for the completion of the design, fulfilling the client's documented requirements, and assuming all the construction risks (RIBA 2020).

   The design team may be novated to (i.e. re-hired by) the contractor and is then no longer controlled by the client. However, most clients choose to retain the services of the quantity surveyor, so that some control can be maintained over costs. If the client requires any changes during the construction works, they are controlled by the contractor, but all the additional costs are the responsibility of the client as variation orders. The design team will work closely with the client to ensure that his requirements are fully described in the scope of the works presented in the tender documents, and thereby endeavour to avoid the need for any changes during the construction stage.

The two main variants of this model are:

Single-stage, where the client's requirements are well-established and described, and potential contractors can be expected to price for the entire project, comprising several work packages, as a one-step process.

Two-stage, where the contractor is chosen, based on a preliminary tender which includes only certain criteria: normally, site management costs plus a percentage for profit and overheads. The contractor, having been chosen on the basis of this limited information, then works with the client and principal suppliers to provide each work package on an individual basis. This two-stage approach normally allows the contractor to commence works sooner on site, but at a risk to the client, as some packages will not be fully priced at that stage.

The advantages and disadvantages of the two main facility procurement methods are summarised in Table 9.1.

Table 9.1 The advantages and disadvantages of the two main facility procurement methods.

Procurement route	Advantages	Disadvantages
Traditional contract	Control over design process and quality.	Design must be fully developed before tender procedure. Longer timescale.
	Cost certainty at point of appointing the contractor.	
	Client retains direct contractual relationship with consultants and main contractor.	Low risk to contractors. Client must have the resources and expertise to administer the contracts of the design team and main contractor.
Design and build	Transfers risk to contractor for construction, delivery and design development.	Client has less control over design quality and this creates cost risks.
	Cost certainty.	Changes by client are unadvisable – heavy cost penalties.
	Shorter programme.	Client's requirements must be fully detailed before signing contract.
	Single point of responsibility for design and cost risks. Early contractor involvement assists with buildability.	

The client team

The role of user advisors

It is important that the client institution establishes a clear governance process for the new facility development before professional designers are appointed, and that time is properly allocated for those individuals who need to interface with the users: the design team and the construction team. This is the role of the user advisor.

It is important on all projects that there are designated user advisors, '…to take responsibility for design quality throughout the project. This may be a departmental user advisor with a responsibility for all the organisation's construction projects or an individual assigned the role, specifically for the (current) project' (RIBA 2020).

Normally, for an animal facility project, the user advisor is selected directly from within the client's organisation and takes responsibility for that particular project only, and is often the facility manager.

Sometimes, it is appropriate to appoint a number of user advisors if, for example, the project is large and/or comprises a number of specialist areas; but in this instance, one user advisor must then be appointed as the lead, and assumes the responsibility for interfacing effectively and directly between all user groups and the project team. The communication routes will vary depending on the size of the project and its participants.

The role of the user advisor is to harness information from all those who will use and maintain the new facility, and to present that information to the project team, in such a way that the functional requirements intended for the facility are comprehensively understood and translated into effective design features by the project designers. This is what is meant by achieving 'design quality'.

A representative from the client's facility management (FM) team should adopt the role of Soft Landings user advisor, to ensure the design is capable of optimising the facility's operational performance and that there is a smooth transition from construction to occupation with appropriate aftercare. 'Soft Landings' is explained in a later section.

The role of user advisor might include:

- Articulating the vision for the project
- Ensuring that design objectives are clearly described in briefing documents and the URS
- Articulating the client's aspirations for the design quality – what he wants the project to achieve in a descriptive, practical sense
- Evaluating design quality throughout the design process
- Chairing user groups relevant to their particular area of responsibility so that information contributing to the above can be collected and documented
- Determining the appointment, of (other) appropriately skilled and experienced user advisors

It is important that user advisors are appointed as soon as possible, at the commencement of a new project, so that they fulfil their important role in establishing and communicating the vision for the project and in practical detail. User advisors do not need to have experience of construction projects. It is more important that their role is clearly focused around their area of expertise and experience within the institutional context, and that they are given the authority, time and support to effectively describe and justify the project.

Documentation of the User Requirement Specification (URS)

User advisors are critically engaged in this process which follows the development of the project brief.

The User Requirement Specification is a formal document approved by the institution's management that defines the client's intended usage of the new facility, and translates that into the structural, functional and legislative requirements of the new building. This ensures that the effective transfer of critical knowledge from the client's users to the design team.

The URS defines the characteristics of the facility spaces, important functional adjacencies, the research process systems the rooms contain, and the plant and equipment that supports them. The significance of the URS lies in its structure that lays down precisely the basic elements of the quality requirements and thus reduces the client's risks to an acceptable level. The URS should be a point of reference throughout the design and construction periods.

The URS will also define the environmental conditions required and how they are controlled to meet the needs of animal species, strain, sex, age and experimental usage anticipated in the new facility. This must be in accord with legislative requirements and guidance and should be documented and shared with the licensing body before the design team is appointed.

Figure 9.1 summarises the processes involved in developing the URS, where all the relevant data is collated using the client's internal staff and/or by employing an external industry specialist. The independent nature of the latter may carry advantages for the institution.

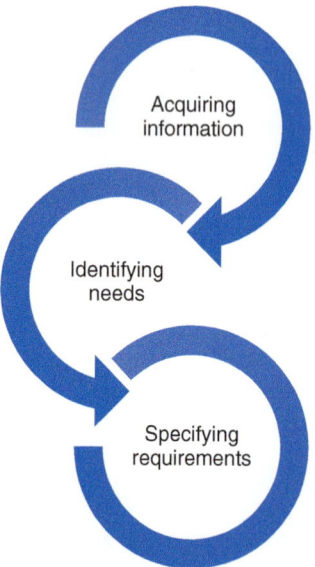

Figure 9.1 The process flow of client information that facilitates the description of the User Requirement Specification for a research animal facility.

Cost consultants

A quantity surveyor (QS) is primarily concerned with providing cost analysis and related financial advice to the client throughout all stages of the project.

During the preliminary stages, the QS may provide early cost estimates for the project brief, which might be modified upon completion of the URS. These cost estimates are then refined as the project evolves through concept, developed and technical design stages.

During the design stages, the QS will assist the project manager in providing advice on procurement routes for the main contractor, preparing the tender documentation, receiving and analysing tenders and preparing the tender report for the client and recommendations for approval. The QS will prepare the contract documentation on behalf of the client. Where the client has a procurement department, it is essential the QS liaise with them throughout the procurement process to ensure adherence with institutional financial policies.

During the contract period, the QS monitors the project spend, providing regular reports to the client. The QS will also receive monthly valuations for work done from the main contractor and will check these, before authorising the architect to approve payment in the form of an architect's certificate.

The QS will also assist with negotiations between the client and the contractor if any variations (changes) having a financial impact occur during the construction phase.

Following completion of the construction works, the QS will liaise with the contractor in agreeing the final account. It is normal for this to take several months after completion, but it can take much longer if the project is complex and there are many variations to account for.

Budget

The most important cost consideration is to correctly set the budget around a design brief that has been informed from a properly developed URS.

If the budget does not match the URS, then the scope of the project should be reduced to ensure that construction quality is not impacted.

If this process is not followed, the usual result is a building that neither meets the URS specifications, nor the scientific needs of the client users.

Value engineering (VE)

VE is used to solve problems and identify and eliminate unwanted costs, while improving function and quality. The aim is to increase the value of a product or system by studying and satisfying the clients' requirements for the product's or system's performance and achieving this at the lowest possible cost.

In construction, VE involves considering the availability of materials, construction methods, transportation issues, site limitations or restrictions, planning and organisation, costs to instal and operate, etc. Benefits that can be delivered by VE include a reduction in life cycle costs, improvement in quality, reduction of environmental impacts, etc.

VE should be considered at project inception when the benefits can be greatest. However, when the contractor is appointed, they may also offer a significant contribution via

VE, but such offers must be analysed and only taken up if the proposed changes to the contract do not affect the project timescales, completion dates or incur additional costs that outweigh the savings on offer.

If a URS has been prepared for the new facility, then VE should always respect the specifications defined for the project components and systems. The URS should, therefore, be prepared with a full understanding of the VE process in mind, thus preventing the misapplication of VE in critical areas that effect lower operational costs/energy, functionality, performance, research and most importantly animal and human welfare.

The design process

Broadly speaking, design is the process of translating the description of a new facility, incorporating the client's requirements, into detailed plans and specifications.

Construction planning is the process of identifying activities and resources required to make the final design a physical reality. The steps involved are influenced by contract and procurement methods but broadly follow the stages, described below, from the RIBA Workplan (2020).

The client should organise his user advisors to deliver and discuss the institutional inputs at the key points of influence provided by RIBA Stages 0–3 below, and at commissioning and handover (Stages 5 and 6).

Project stages as defined by RIBA

0. **Strategic definition** – The proposed new project is strategically appraised by senior client management and defined in principle before a detailed brief is created. Typical issues to address at this stage are: What does the institution desire that the project achieves and is it sustainable? Can there be reuse of existing facilities, components or materials? What skills/expertise will be needed to realise the project? Some institutions employ external specialists to assist them explore realistic options based on their scientific strengths and aspirations.
1. **Development of the brief** – The project brief is a comprehensive word description of the project and must consider the desired research and operational outcomes, the project's spatial requirements, the location site or context, and an estimation of the budget.

    To provide the necessary detail, a third-party specialist may be employed to define a URS (see Figure 9.1) or, if the project is complex with several options to consider, a third party may be required to conduct a feasibility study which may incorporate a comparative risk assessment to define the risks of doing nothing or of adopting one of the several options. The feasibility study can also be used to estimate a project programme (a timeline of the works required) and a procurement strategy.

    The project brief, URS and/or feasibility study should be signed off by the client before the project proceeds to the design stage.
2. **Concept design** – The initial concept design is drawn up to faithfully accommodate and realise the requirements of the project brief and/or URS. The concept design takes into account proposals for floor and room layouts, structural components, cost information and building services systems as well as preliminary work on a number of relevant project inputs, such as planning applications, health and safety, construction type, handover, sustainability, SOPs, operational flows and choice and maintenance of plant and equipment. The project programme is reviewed and procurement activities started with potential suppliers.

    The concept design should be signed off, signifying acceptance by the client, before the project proceeds to the detailed design stage.
3. **Detailed design** – This stage creates more detail and also takes into account updated proposals for structure and layout, building services, cost information and project strategies, which were initially defined in Stage 2. A full sustainability assessment is carried out. Project strategies and risk assessments are reviewed and updated, and procurement activities continue. Owing to facility complexity and the consequential number of considerations requiring exchange of information, the developed design may be amended several times.

    The detailed design should be signed off, signifying acceptance by the client, before the project proceeds to the technical design stage.
4. **Technical design** – The architectural, building services and structural engineering designs are now further refined to provide full technical definition to the project. The design work of specialist sub-contractors is often a necessary component of this stage (e.g. mechanical, electrical and plumbing (MEP) engineers; and commissioning agents).

    The technical design should be signed off to signify acceptance by the client before the project proceeds to the contractor procurement stage, which usually involves publishing the technical design and inviting potential contractors to bid for the contract. After a tender evaluation process, the contractor is chosen for a traditional contractor procurement.
5. **Construction** – Building work starts. The building contract will include the requirement for regular site inspections, reviews of progress and resolution of any design/construction queries as they arise. Supporting tasks are focused on on-site health and safety, and on-site security. Information is acquired and plans implemented when appropriate for plant and equipment commissioning, training in the use of equipment and plant, handover, asset management, future monitoring and maintenance. Reviews and updates to the sustainability strategy may be necessary. Some plant and equipment may require the production of non-technical user guides or SOPs where required for everyday use by laboratory staff (e.g. robotic cage processors) and the organisation of aftercare service, where it interferes with normal operations.
6. **Handover** and **close-out** – Handover of building and conclusion of building contract. Carry out handover activities listed in the handover strategy, including client's feedback on the project, which can be used to support and develop future projects. A defect liability

period is usually started after handover. It is important to note that this is a period during which the contractor may be recalled to rectify defects which appear after operations commence, and is not a chance for the contractor to correct problems that were apparent at practical completion. If there are defects apparent before practical completion, then these should be rectified before the certificate of practical completion is issued.
7. **In-Use** – Concludes the activities listed in the handover strategy and implement. In-Use services such as plant and equipment maintenance. Post-occupancy evaluation and a review of project performance are completed. Feedback processes which will continue until the end of the building's life are implemented (see Soft Landings section later in this chapter).

The project team

Projects intended to design and construct buildings can involve large numbers of people, and on major projects many thousands of people. The structure and composition of the project team tends to change through the duration of the project. Some team members might only have a very brief involvement, bringing specialist knowledge and advice about specific components or the intended scientific process during a particular phase, while others, such as client managers and user advisors, project managers or lead consultants may be involved for the duration of the project, possibly a number of years.

Project manager (PM)

The PM is responsible for directing and co-ordinating the entire scope of the project components and staff from commencement to handover. The person appointed has considerable experience and knowledge of similar animal facility projects and acts as the most senior project-related manager on behalf of the client to direct the design team and contractor(s), ensuring that they have the appropriate information and understanding to effectively plan and complete the project. The scope of works under the purview of the PM will depend on the size and complexity of the project. The client's responsibility to the PM is to clearly define the scope of their role, within the context of the client's requirements, from the outset. This emphasises the crucial role of the user advisor who shall need to work closely with the PM. The PM has an obligation to recognise and respect the client's team and also the professional knowledge and skills of the various disciplines (architectural and engineering) that make up the project team.

Dependent on the size of the project and the availability of appropriate internal resources, the client institution may decide to either appoint a PM from its own staff, possibly a senior member of their estates team, or to appoint an external manager. However, the full-time nature of the job demands considerable commitment and should not be seen as an easy add-on to existing duties. Depending upon the scope of the project, the institutional resources and where such projects are resource-intensive, it may be appropriate to appoint two PMs: one being an external professional and the other a senior individual from within the client's staff. The appointment of the PM is normally made before the design team is appointed. The PM will then work with the client institution to assist with the appointment of the other design team members.

The PM's main responsibility is, therefore, to the client institution, acting as the interface between the client team, the design team and the contractor(s), and guiding them through the project to completion. An important early part of the role is ensuring that a comprehensive project brief and/or URS is prepared, ensuring that comprehensive but concise information about functionality, specifications, timescale and cost estimates are documented. The PM will also provide management of all the other key actions required to deliver the project, from advising on the types of contractor procurement options, managing risk, monitoring and reporting on the design and construction works as they proceed on site, assisting with the procurement and management of equipment and fit-out systems, plant and equipment commissioning and facility validation, and making arrangements for planning permission, demolitions and removals.

Design team

The PM works with the client to appoint a design team having the necessary disciplines to adequately service the project. Once appointed, the design team can proceed to work through the various stages of the design process with the client.

The PM will co-ordinate the information gathering activities, using source material from the project brief, the URS and user advisor(s) and, with the design team, translate the whole into concise descriptions of design specifications that meet functional needs, cost implications and options, and a project timescale. The quality and accuracy of this briefing process will greatly influence the success or otherwise of the project. Sufficient time must be committed to completing these stages in an organised way, so that the client can comprehensively consider, decide, then authorise the design implications by 'signing off' the documentation and thereby 'freezing' the project parameters. There are practical and financial reasons for ensuring that no changes are made to the design specifications once it has been signed off at the end of RIBA Stage 3; principally this reduces the risk of introducing variations (changes) that create delay and additional design and/or construction costs if requested during the later stages of the project.

A well-prepared project brief and URS will form the basis of all the subsequent project actions including design detailing, contractor tenders, service, plant and equipment choice and construction works. At the end of each RIBA stage, the design team usually produces a co-ordinated report, which will confirm all the relevant project information accumulated to date, with relevant design implications. It is essential that the client reviews the reports, consulting with all relevant in-house colleagues, and providing any necessary feedback to the design team, who will action changes and update the reports accordingly. Updated reports should be checked and 'signed off' by the appropriate senior officers of the client organisation, to confirm their agreement with the documented specifications, including any potential changes and subsequent implications, including potential cost increases.

The client must understand that their involvement in and contribution to the design process effectively concludes at the end of RIBA Stage 3. To engage again with changes after that will very likely incur delays and additional charges.

Architect

The architect's responsibility is to interpret and develop the project brief into design plans and construction specifications at appropriate stages of the project, and to co-ordinate the inputs of the various specialist disciplines with their own. The architect will define and refine the client's requirements as construction drawings and specifications, identifying constraints, advising on the usefulness of any feasibility studies and options appraisals, arrange site investigations, establish the preferred solutions when options have been studied, advise on sustainability, manage health and safety issues, prepare room data sheets, obtain client input and 'sign-off' of the design at appropriate stages, advise on the selection of materials, furniture and equipment, provide space planning services and, recognising every detail of the project brief, prepare a design which meets all the client requirements, including an outline budget and timescale.

The architect will prepare and lodge the planning application and building warrants sometimes with the assistance of a local planning specialist. During the construction phase, the architect will assist the Clerk of Works in monitoring build quality on site. At handover the architect will assist in ensuring that the works are complete, that the client's needs as described in the project brief and URS have been met and will continue their involvement through the defect liability period assuring the final resolution of any new defects.

After novation (in the case of a design-and-build contract), the architect will work for the main contractor and will no longer be in the direct employment or control of the client.

Services engineer (mechanical, electrical and plumbing services – MEP)

The services engineer has the responsibility to design and specify all the MEP services for the building to meet the needs of the client's functional requirements, bearing in mind any additional needs to achieve high environmental impact standards (e.g. BREEAM 'excellent' in the UK, 'CASBEE' in Japan, 'LEED' in the USA and 'Green Star' in Australia) and to minimise long-term building running costs.

The services engineer will co-ordinate their work with that of the architect and the structural engineer, providing appropriate cost advice to the QS to allow for the necessary cost planning and monitoring. The services engineer provides the requisite advice to the client in order to allow them to make the best decisions in terms of sustainability, energy use, life cycle costs and relevant 'Green Issues'.

After novation (in the case of a design-and-build contract), the services engineer will work for the main contractor and will no longer be in the direct employ or control of the client.

Fire protection engineer (FP)

The FP engineer is a specialist services engineer who works closely with the design team and the institutional fire safety officer to study, propose and deliver a design for the fire prevention and protection features of the new building, having due regard for the purpose of the facilities and their operability. For research animal facilities, this entails an appreciation of the requirements for animal welfare, and how they may impact the emergency exit routes, the conduct of the fire drills and the types of fire detectors, alarm sounders and sprinkler systems that may be deployed as part of the fire safety management plan.

Structural engineer (SE)

The SE has the responsibility to design the structural fabric and method of construction of the new building, including drainage installations; and must ensure that their designs are co-ordinated with the layouts and specifications created by the architect and the services engineer. The SE will advise the client on the most appropriate form of structure for the building, taking into account its future functionality, and will also provide cost advice to the QS in relation to all aspects of the building structure.

Building information modelling (BIM), the design of complex buildings that must simultaneously satisfy a variety of functional and regulatory requirements, is dependent on electronic methods of drafting that establish the appropriate locations and adjacencies of structural elements, plant and equipment.

Two-dimensional drafting was the mainstay architectural tool, but computer-aided design (CAD) has provided the means to integrate designs from different sources and manipulate them to optimise location and functionality.

Building information modelling (BIM) is a very broad term that describes the relatively new process of creating a comprehensive digital model of all the constituent components of a building or proposed refurbishment.

In addition to providing a 3D visualisation of the building and services (which can assist with detailed planning and the potential for accommodating 'late' changes), the adoption of BIM can provide a design tool that allows more work to be done by a smaller team. This can lower costs and lessen the impacts of miscommunications, as less time and money are spent in design processes and administration because of better visualisation and document quality: hence more efficient pre-construction planning. One of the biggest benefits in using BIM is the additional efficiency that can be brought to the design development and co-ordination of the MEP and FP systems. For animal facilities, this can represent a large cost saving, as the MEP and FP services are complex systems to co-ordinate.

In the UK, the Government Construction Strategy: 2016-2020 published in 2016 stated that the UK Government '….supports the digitisation of construction and uses information relating to the asset to build a three dimensional model' (Infrastructure and Projects Authority 2016). In most developed countries, all large construction projects are now carried out using BIM and it is becoming equally important for the supply chain, including equipment suppliers, to also work in BIM.

The range of levels that this form of modelling can take are described as 'maturity levels' and are described below.

Level 0 BIM

Unmanaged CAD including 2D drawings, and text with paper-based or electronic exchange of information but without common standards and processes. Essentially, this is a digital drawing board.

Level 1 BIM

Managed CAD, with the increasing introduction of spatial co-ordination, standardised structures and formats as it moves towards Level 2 BIM. This may include 2D information and 3D information such as visualisations or concept development models. Level 1 can be described as 'Lonely BIM' as models are not shared between project team members.

Level 2 BIM

Managed 3D environment with data attached, but created in separate discipline-based models. These separate models are assembled to form a federated model, but do not lose their identity or integrity. Data may include construction sequencing (4D) and cost (5D) information. This is sometimes referred to as 'pBIM' (proprietary BIM).

Level 3 BIM

A single collaborative, online, project model with construction sequencing (4D), cost (5D) and project life cycle information (6D). This is sometimes referred to as 'iBIM' (integrated BIM) and is intended to deliver better business outcomes.

Level 4 BIM

Level 4 introduces the concepts of improved social outcomes and well-being.

ISO 19650

The ISO 19650 standard[23] is an international standard for managing information over the whole life cycle of a built asset, using BIM. It contains all the same principles and high-level requirements as the UK BIM Framework and is closely aligned with the current UK 1192 standards.

Construction team

Main contractor

The construction team is led by the main contractor, whose responsibility it is to deliver the entire building project in accordance with the client's requirements, as expressed in the project brief and URS, to budget and within the projected completion time. The main contractor will sub-contract various parts of the construction works to specialist sub-contractors, but will be responsible for the overall project performance, co-ordinating all sub-contractor works accordingly. The main contractor is also responsible for on-site health and safety and for ensuring that all persons working on or visiting the building site are aware of their responsibilities.

The sub-contractors

Sub-contractors deliver their specialist work packages in close co-ordination with the work of the main contractor and other sub-contractors. Nowhere is this co-ordination more important than with the MEP sub-contractors whose work is always closely integrated with construction activities.

The suppliers

The suppliers of building materials, plant and equipment have the responsibility to provide goods and/or services to the project as per the requirements, timescale and budget. Suppliers include manufacturers and installers of cages, cage racks, autoclaves and cage-cleaning systems, etc.

Heating, ventilation and air conditioning (HVAC)

HVAC is the technology that provides indoor environmental comfort. Its goal is to provide acceptable indoor air quality (as determined by temperature, humidity and airflow) suitable for the purposes served: in this case the housing and husbandry of laboratory animals by animal care staff, and the provisions for surgery and experimentation in purpose-designed procedure rooms.

HVAC system design is an important sub-discipline of mechanical engineering, based on the principles of thermodynamics, fluid mechanics and heat transfer.

Building management system (BMS)

A building management system is an electronic control system that is used to monitor, control and thereby manage the MEP services in a research animal facility. All such systems are reliant on their connections, hard-wired for BMS and/or via wi-fi for EMS, to a network of sensors appropriately calibrated and positioned in the locations of interest. It is a crucially important component of the facility systems that operate 24/7 in order to maintain the various environmental conditions and ensure that back-up systems come online when required.

The BMS is also often used to monitor and record the environmental conditions within specific animal housing rooms, thus providing evidence of stability and demonstrating compliance with animal welfare legislation. The need to provide independent environmental records that demonstrate GLP/GMP compliance requires an environment monitoring system (EMS) completely separate from the BMS.

---

[23] https://ukbimframework.org/wp-content/uploads/2019/11/ISO-19650-Guidance-Part-2-Single-Page-Print.pdf (Accessed 8 June 2022)

Specifications

Specifications are written documents that describe the materials and workmanship required for a development. They do not include cost, quantity or drawing information but should be read alongside other contract documentation such as quantities, schedules and drawings.

There are two main types of specifications that define and shape a laboratory building project: prescriptive specifications and performance specifications. Prescriptive specifications are detailed descriptions, giving the client more certainty about the end product, and thus defining more precisely the final investment decision (i.e. when the client appoints the main contractor). The alternative, the performance specification is 'more simple' in that it focuses on a description of the end product – the performance expected of the finished building. This gives the main contractor and suppliers more scope to innovate and adopt cost effective methods of work: potentially offering better value for money. However, a possible downside is that the main contractor may sacrifice quality to cut costs, thus compromising build finish and long-term serviceability of equipment.

Prescriptive specifications

Prescriptive specifications typically contain precise detailed descriptions of the following components:

- The location, compartmentalisation and shape of the whole building;
- General requirements relating to functionality, regulations and standards;
- The type of materials, services and plant products required;
- The build execution and installation methods required.

Prescriptive specifications place a greater burden on the design team to ensure proper construction and installation, rather than the main contractor. Typically, prescriptive specifications are usually written for more complex buildings, or buildings where the client has specific requirements that might not be familiar to contractors or suppliers, where the exact nature of the completed development is very specific to the client's requirements, e.g. category 3 and 4 containment facilities; *in vivo* imaging etc.

Performance specifications

Performance (open) specifications describe what the finished building and equipment are needed to do – which means that the main contractor and his suppliers have a responsibility to satisfy those requirements, which in effect requires the main contractor to complete the design with considerable input from the plant and equipment suppliers. The nature of the performance required may be defined by listing and describing the desired outcomes, and/or by reference to standards. In the latter case, it is important to ensure that the standards referred to are 'current' and not 'obsolete'.

Commissioning

Commissioning is the systematic process of inspecting, testing and documenting the operation of the facility's plant systems and equipment to verify that their installation and performance comply with the manufacturers' specifications and the requirements of the project brief, as defined in the URS.

A commissioning manager is appointed by the client or PM to lead the commissioning activities which are conducted by the commissioning team, comprising members from the main contractor, the engineers, and the client teams. The client or PM may also choose to employ an independent commissioning manager and team from outside of the project. The commissioning manager is responsible for planning and implementing the commissioning programme, and writes and manages the commissioning plan.

The purpose of the commissioning plan is to verify that the performance of the plant and equipment that create and control the environment, and executes the client's stated processes, do so in compliance with the requirements of the URS. On a practical level, the commissioning plan also provides direction for the execution of the commissioning processes, with particular attention to the complexity of processes and procedures adopted in a laboratory animal science facility, and those aspects that could not be fully developed during the design stage. These include all necessary activities such as scheduling of observations and tests, roles and responsibilities of the various project team members, communications, co-ordination, workflow and subsequent resolution of any identified issues.

The commissioning plan is intended to achieve the following specific objectives:

- Ensure that all applicable equipment and systems are installed according to the manufacturers recommendations and to industry-acceptable standards, and that they receive adequate and certified inspections by the installation engineers during normal operation and simulated failure modes
- Verify and document the proper performance of equipment and systems within the context of the client's requirements
- Identify and track through to resolution all issues related to improper equipment and systems installation, performance and maintenance-related conditions

Pre-handover demonstration of facility reliability

Verification, validation, stability, reliability

Verification is intended to demonstrate that a product, service or system meets a defined set of design specifications. Verification procedures involve normal operation at partial and complete capacity, and performing special stress tests to simulate and model failure of all or part of the entire system.

Validation is a process intended to demonstrate that the operation of a system, or combination of systems, such as a fully functional vivarium, results in environments and facility conditions that meet the requirements of the client. The qualification requirements used as the basis of the validation process are defined by the client as the operational specifications and regulations defined in the project brief and URS.

A research animal facility is a complex capital-intensive building that requires meticulous attention to operational detail if it is to realise the research aspirations of the client institution and their scientific potential; and protect the welfare of its animals and staff. It is, therefore, essential that its preparation for use includes a period of operation and technical scrutiny before it is handed over to the client team. This period is known by several different names in different locations, but all apply similar assessment principles: Facility Reliability Test (FRT), Pre-handover Compliance Test, Stability Test, Shake-down and Burn-in. We shall use FRT.

Facility Reliability Test (FRT)

The purpose of FRT is to ensure that the new building, its plant and equipment, are capable of working together for an extended period in real time (typically, 30 days), under the full range of light to heavy loading, and in normal and fault-stressed scenarios, performing in all circumstances to the user's specifications.

The primary objective is to demonstrate that the new building is capable of continuously supporting the processes and plant that create and deliver stable environments for staff and animals, as defined in the project brief. The parameters of interest shall be scrutinised at audit by the regulatory authorities when they inspect to award facility licensure or certification and are listed below (under Environment).

Secondary objectives include the completion of performance qualifications for some equipment (e.g. autoclaves which must be adjusted to deliver several different sterile load types), the training of scientific and maintenance staff in the use and servicing of new equipment, and the completion of process SOPs that were drafted during the design stage.

Prerequisites

Prior to commencement of the FRT, completion and approval of the commissioning report is absolutely essential. This provides the necessary assurance that the individual items of plant and equipment are verified as working in accordance with their manufacturers' specifications, within the new facility.

In addition, it is essential that the building is cleaned, so that all the building service systems, such as the HVAC, are operating at optimal efficiency and reliability, as previously demonstrated during the commissioning period.

To ensure that unnecessary and costly interruptions are avoided, rooms undergoing stability testing are subject to restricted access during the period of the FRT.

The BMS is the central instrument for monitoring and controlling the animal room environments in a research animal facility. It is, therefore, essential that the BMS is fully commissioned prior to the facility testing, and operated and monitored by competent, trained staff during the FRT period.

The BMS's record of the critical environmental parameters will be examined every day and compared with the data collected from independent measuring devices deployed throughout the facility (e.g. temperature and relative humidity data loggers, thermo-hygrographs, etc.). Procedures should be put in place and training provided to ensure that any BMS alarms detected during the FRT are reacted to promptly and appropriately, including the recording of any remedial actions undertaken.

Maintenance

The client's facility maintenance staff should inspect the plant and services regularly (at least daily including weekends) throughout the FRT, following their SOPs. Maintenance procedures should be performed and recorded as necessary, again following the planned servicing protocols.

FRT process

First two weeks

The first two-week period of the FRT will be used to establish stability by fine-tuning the control of systems and equipment operating together for the first time and correcting any faults or failures that may occur (see below).

The secondary objectives will also be commenced during the first two weeks.

Second two weeks

The second period of two weeks will specifically simulate 'normal operations' and focus on the demonstration of stable and reliable operation and the collection of data as evidence for compliance purposes.

Operational problems, how they were resolved and how timely the resolutions were made should be documented according to the relevant SOPs, discussed as soon as possible after the event, and certainly at the FRT daily briefing, by all interested parties. Problems and their resolution can be categorised as follows:

- Minor issues and faults should be considered part of the learning process involved in operating and delivering a new building (e.g. recalibration or replacement of a room temperature probe which persistently produces BMS data deviating from the independent measurements taken in that room).
- Major issues and faults should be responded to as if the building were live, and fully documented by the facility maintenance staff (e.g. a plant failure which affects its ability to maintain the required pressure differentials in the animal rooms should be rectified immediately, irrespective of the time of day or night).

System/Equipment failure

If during the 30-day period there is a failure of a significant piece of equipment or building system, the FRT should be put 'on hold', and only recommenced when the faulty equipment or system has been rectified. The other equipment and systems in the building that have remained working properly should continue to function to the original test schedule, as far as it is possible. All failures should be documented according to the relevant SOPs, recording the nature of the fault, the necessary root cause analysis and the steps taken to rectify the issue in order to prevent a recurrence.

A 'failure condition' is where an entire piece of equipment or system, or a major constituent component, malfunctions and requires replacement. For clarification, this is any situation where the client users, or their intended processes operating within the compliance framework, would be adversely affected if the aberrant condition of the equipment or system were allowed to continue.

A 'termination and restart' condition causes the whole or a significant part of the facility to be shut down. The FRT is then terminated and only restarted when the rectification is completed and shown to reinstate stable operating conditions. The decision whether to resume from the day of the shut-down, or whether to start again from a new Day 0, or a later time, shall be determined by discussion between the FRT manager, the main contractor and the client. Note that for the unambiguous demonstration of compliance with the appropriate regulations (e.g. the Home Office ASPA Code of Practice in the UK[24]), the final 14-day continuous period cannot be interrupted and restarted mid-period, and must, therefore, always be started again from Day 0 under these circumstances.

Special requirements for research animal facilities

Because animal research facilities must support live animals under optimal conditions of care and welfare, they are subjected to more stringent stability testing than a standard wet laboratory. Selected animal rooms will be heat loaded (typically using convector heaters) to simulate the heat loads generated by the intended animal occupants in their cages. It is recommended that this heat stress period is maintained for 48 hours and is closely monitored by the BMS and the independent room data loggers/thermo-hygrographs. Failure of the critical room parameters to remain stable, within the specified ranges, will require investigation and subsequent adjustment of one or more of the BMS, the environmental sensors or the HVAC system controls, followed by a period of re-testing.

The below list summarises the test parameters that should be monitored in the rooms and facilities intended to hold research animals, before and/or during the FRT:

Environment

- Temperature;
- Relative humidity;
- Light levels;
- Noise pressure levels, audible and ultrasound;

- Air change rates;
- Differential pressures between rooms, groups of rooms and corridors;
- Vibration (for specific equipment known to generate it).

Barrier integrity

- HEPA (or other) filter integrity checks;
- Directional airflow patterns deduced from smoke visualisation;
- BMS operation and calibration of all probes, with cause-and-effect analysis;
- HVAC system performance monitoring by BMS or EMS, plus alarm functions;
- Microbiological challenge of sanitising and sterilising equipment to verify performance *in situ*;
- Microbiological (settle plate) monitoring of surface environments after fumigation.

Acceptance of FRT data

Recommendations for acceptance are based on conclusive tests and verifications of performance, including certifications where necessary. The items subject to test include but are not limited to:

- Animal holding systems – equipment and processes;
- Primary biocontainment device effectiveness (e.g. microbiological safety cabinets);
- Scientific equipment (e.g. electrophysiology rigs);
- Imaging equipment and processes;
- Aseptic surgery processes, including separation of preparation, surgical procedure and recovery;
- Facility and room decontamination systems, and their integration with facility functions;
- Decontamination chamber cycles;
- Robotic cage processing systems;
- Cage washer cycles;
- Autoclave cycles;
- Animal watering systems (e.g. reverse osmosis systems);
- Waste handling systems (for liquids and solids);
- Redundancy tests on mission-critical equipment (including response time from standby mode);
- Procedures for failure analysis of primary systems (fans, pumps, etc.);
- Standby or emergency power tests.

Soft Landings

There is a broad consensus that buildings in operation, particularly new or refurbished ones, do not perform as well as they should. There is frequently a significant gap between a facility's expected performance and what is achieved in practice, often resulting from one or more contributory factors. These include short-comings in briefing, design and construction and subsequently from poor operability or inadequate post-completion maintenance. Such problems are often caused by or exacerbated when

---

[24] https://assets.publishing.service.gov.uk/government/uploads/system/uploads/attachment_data/file/388895/COPAnimalsFullPrint.pdf (Accessed 8 June 2022)

there is a separation of operational comment and influences before and during the construction phase. A well-executed URS can correct this by specifying weekly meetings of contractors with PM, user advisor and other project team members as necessary throughout the construction and commissioning phases.

The Soft Landings Framework is a joint initiative between the Building Services Research and Information Association (BSRIA) and the Usable Buildings Trust (UBT). It is an open-source informational framework available on the BSRIA website that is intended to '. . .smooth the transition into use and to address problems that post-occupancy evaluations (POEs) show to be widespread' (BSRIA 2018). It was first published in 2009 and was updated in 2014 to align with the RIBA 2013 design stages described earlier. The Soft Landings Framework is now promoted and developed by the BSRIA Soft Landings Group (see *BSRIA Soft Landings Core Principles* 2018).

The term 'Soft Landings' refers to a strategy that is adopted by the client team, notably involving the facility manager, to ensure the transition from construction to occupation is 'bump-free' and that subsequent operational performance is optimised in line with the client's expectations.

This transition needs to be considered throughout the development of a project, not just at the point of handover. Ideally, the client should commit to adopting a Soft Landings strategy in the very early stages so that an appropriate budget can be allocated to appoint those who will be involved, and to ensure that the project brief includes the relevant requirements. This should include agreements from designers, service engineers, main and sub-contractors and suppliers to provide the necessary dossiers of information required for the management of commissioning, training in the use of plant and equipment, facility service and maintenance of plant and equipment, and increasingly will include the output from the BIM analysis (see section earlier in this chapter).

To ensure that a Soft Landings strategy is implemented properly from the outset, it may be appropriate to appoint an experienced and independent Soft Landings champion or manager to oversee the whole process and train the estates team in this relatively new approach to buildings handover.

The key stages of the Soft Landings approach may be summarised as:

- Project inception/briefing – an early understanding of the project purpose;
- Ensuring that the client's needs and required outcomes are clearly defined (e.g. in an URS);
- Design development and review;
- Reviewing comparable projects and assessing proposals about facility management and use of the building by scientific staff;
- Pre-handover requirements and evaluation;
- Ensuring that operators properly understand all systems before occupation;
- Initial post-handover aftercare requirements and evaluation;
- Extended aftercare and POE (e.g. defect liability periods of 2–3 years).

Conclusions

The purpose of this chapter has been to educate and inform all those who may be asked to participate in the design and construction of a new research animal facility, whether they be research animal users or facility managers and engineers: they all need to have a comprehensive understanding of the process and how their individual efforts combine to realise the new facility.

The design and construction framework we have described above is based upon our varied experience and roles in the UK and overseas, which may not correspond with the precise requirements in every country. If readers find apparent contradictions with their national process guidelines, then we hope that this framework can be used early in their project to define and resolve differences and create an effective design and build process.

The design and build of a research animal facility is a complex matter, involving the co-ordination and integration of biomedical, operational, infrastructural and regulatory factors. At the outset, it can seem to be a daunting task, and we recommend that new participants avail themselves of relevant information from this chapter and consult with industry experts who can provide specialist advice, even manage the project if so desired, so that risks are reduced and budgets conserved.

Our experience of such projects over the past 30 years has highlighted two critically important factors for success: firstly, early involvement of the client institution and its end-users to establish their requirements in detail and ensure the design meets all experimental and animal welfare needs; and secondly, strong, knowledgeable project management that motivates, organises and co-ordinates the diverse teams of expert professionals whose combined efforts shall bring the enterprise to a successful completion.

Acknowledgement

The authors wish to thank the College of Laboratory Animal Science and Technology www.clast.org.uk and Level 6 tutor Auriol Lamb Cubitt for information accessed from the Level 6 Unit in Animal Facility Management and Design.

References

BSRIA. (2018) *Soft Landings Core Principles*, 2nd edn (BG38/2018). BSRIA. https://www.bsria.com/uk/product/BxP8EB/soft_landings_core_principles_2nd_edition_a15d25e1/?msclkid=5e7562b9cfb611ec808501f572a919ae

Infrastructure and Projects Authority. (2016) *Government Construction Strategy: (2016–2020)*. UK Government Infrastructure and Projects Authority. https://www.gov.uk/government/publications/government-construction-strategy-2016-2020 (Accessed 8 June 2022).

Royal Institute of British Architects (RIBA) Workplan. (2020) *The RIBA Plan of Work*. https://www.architecture.com/knowledge-and-resources/resources-landing-page/riba-plan-of-work (Accessed 8 June 2022).

10 Environmental enrichment: animal welfare and scientific validity

Hanno Würbel and Janja Novak

'The need for designing animal facilities that provide the basic needs of shelter, food, water and a degree of environmental stability has long been appreciated. Currently, however, it is recognised that science also has an ethical responsibility to house animals according to their species-specific needs, and that responsibility invokes the concept of behavioural and environmental enrichment'. (Wolfle 2005)

Introduction

It is now over 60 years since Russell and Burch pointed to the need to refine animal experiments by reducing *'to an absolute minimum the amount of stress imposed on those animals that are still used'* (Russell & Burch 1959, reprinted 1992). More recently, Buchanan-Smith *et al.* (2005) specified the definition of refinement as: *'any approach which avoids or minimises the actual or potential pain, distress and other adverse effects experienced at any time during the life of the animals involved, and which enhances their well-being'*. However, it is only more recently that the focus has started to shift from merely minimising adverse effects to enhancing animal well-being (Mellor 2016). Environmental enrichment having any of these effects – minimising actual or potential harms and enhancing animal well-being – can thus be considered as refinement, which according to the Three Rs' principle must be implemented wherever possible.

For a long time, barren housing conditions were the norm, but over the last 30 years there has been a remarkable growth in the provision of environmental enrichment for animals used in research. Several factors have likely contributed to this change, not least the development of enriched housing conditions in other areas of animal use. Zoos were relatively early adopters of enrichment in the 1970s (Markowitz 1982), based on concerns about the occurrence of abnormal behaviour (e.g. Hediger 1950) and a better understanding of animal behaviour and of the effects of sensory and motor deprivation on the behaviour and physiology of captive animals (Shepherdson 1998, 2003; Würbel 2006). Within agricultural practice, the Brambell report on farm animal welfare of 1965 stimulated welfare research, calling for studies in the fields of veterinary medicine, stress physiology, animal science and animal behaviour (Fraser 2008). Already then, it was suggested that animal welfare might be advanced by studies of motivation and preference: an early call for studies that have since become a major component of animal welfare research (Fraser & Nicol 2018; Franks 2019).

Since these early days, animal welfare science has developed rapidly, and its research has influenced legal regulations and codes of practice governing the care and use of laboratory animals, including environmental enrichment in laboratory animal housing (EU Directive 2010/63/EU; FELASA 2006; see Chapter 8: Legislation and oversight of the conduct of research using animals: a global overview). However, it is important to recognise that the impetus for improvements in housing and husbandry has not just come from legislators and animal welfare researchers but also from those directly involved in using and caring for animals in research. Many institutions, even facilities carrying out regulatory work, have developed innovative enrichment strategies as a means to achieving high welfare standards (Dean 1999; Johnson *et al.* 2003; Winnicker *et al.* 2012).

Nonetheless, experience shows that implementation of enrichment varies between institutions and countries and that some species (e.g. primates, dogs) are more likely to be provided with enrichment, and are provided with more extensive enrichment than others. In the past, many researchers have been very critical of enrichment (e.g. Benefiel *et al.* 2005; Toth *et al.* 2011) or even resisted the use of enrichment for various reasons discussed below. Since the incorporation of the 3Rs into legislation (EU Directive 2010/63/EU), refinement, including enrichment, has been receiving more attention by the laboratory animal research community (Franco *et al.* 2018). However, differences in implementation remain and reasons may include concerns about labour, cost, altered experimental outcomes, increased variation in results, potential risks to the animals or a lack of understanding of the welfare impact of enrichment. In order to mitigate these

The UFAW Handbook on the Care and Management of Laboratory and Other Research Animals, Ninth Edition.
Edited by Huw Golledge and Claire Richardson.
© 2024 John Wiley & Sons Ltd. Published 2024 by John Wiley & Sons Ltd.

concerns, it is important that animal care staff understand the implications of enrichment for both animal welfare and experimental outcomes. The aim of this chapter is to provide a short introduction to the subject by discussing what enrichment is, why and when it is needed, how it might interact with research requirements, and the practicalities of providing environmental conditions that meet the animals' needs.

Terminology

As others have noted, the term environmental enrichment has been used inconsistently in the scientific literature (Bayne 2005; Benefiel et al. 2005; Würbel & Garner 2007). In neurobiology research, where enrichment serves as a paradigm to investigate neural plasticity, it has been defined as *'a combination of complex inanimate and social stimulation'* (Rosenzweig et al. 1978, cited in van Praag et al. 2000). These studies use enrichment to stimulate sensory and motor systems, regardless of the consequences for the animals' well-being. Thus, the animals may be housed in bigger cages and in large social groups with various enrichment items (e.g. tunnels, shelters, running wheels, and toys) that may be changed regularly to induce novelty (van Praag et al. 2000).

Such conditions need not be beneficial for the animals' well-being, as stressful conditions may also enhance sensory and motor stimulation. Therefore, enrichment as found in the scientific literature should not be mistaken for refinement, and Würbel & Garner (2007) proposed to distinguish between adverse, neutral and beneficial enrichment. However, for those concerned about animal husbandry, the sole purpose of enrichment is that it should be beneficial to the animals. Hence, Newberry (1995) defined environmental enrichment as *'an improvement in the biological functioning of captive animals resulting from modifications in their environment'*, and Shepherdson (1998) as a *'husbandry principle that seeks to enhance the quality of captive animal care by identifying and providing the environmental stimuli necessary for optimal psychological and physiological well-being'*. Olsson & Dahlborn (2002) further suggested that changes to the environment should be considered as enrichment only if their use results in an improvement in animal welfare.

Welfare legislation and codes of practice for animals have adopted these latter definitions of enrichment, implying beneficial effects on animal welfare. Moreover, with a better understanding of the relationship between behaviour and welfare, special emphasis was also placed on the expression of the animals' species-typical behaviour. Thus, the 'Guide for the care and use of laboratory animals' states *'the aim of environmental enrichment is to enhance animal well-being by providing animals with sensory and motor stimulation, through structures and resources that facilitate the expression of species-typical behaviors and promote psychological well-being'* (NRC 2011). Similarly, the 'EU Directive on the protection of animals used for scientific purposes' (EU Directive 2010/63/EU, Annex III) states *'all animals shall be provided with space of sufficient complexity to allow expression of a wide range of normal behaviour'*. As there is no single common currency for the assessment of animal welfare, legal regulations and codes of practice (implicitly or explicitly) refer to three separate, though overlapping, aspects of animal welfare; namely, health and biological function, species-typical behaviour and subjective well-being. This is often referred to as the Three Circles model of animal welfare, originally framed by Fraser et al. (1997).

Approaches to enrichment

There is a wide variety of approaches to the refinement of laboratory animal housing conditions through the implementation of environmental enrichment. Initially, enrichment merely meant a change from traditional single housing to group housing, and the addition of simple objects to an otherwise barren environment to enhance sensory and motor stimulation and occupy the animals. Over time, attention has shifted to species-specific resources (e.g. nesting material, burrowing substrate, and feeding and foraging options) to meet the animals' most essential behavioural and physiological needs (Bloomsmith et al. 1991; Young 2003; Winnicker et al. 2012; Baumans & van Loo 2013). More recently, attention is also given to structural aspects of cage or pen design, such as visual barriers (Tallent et al. 2018; Mertens et al. 2020) or spatial segregation, which also promotes the expression of species-typical behaviour (Makowska et al. 2019; Makowska & Weary 2016). Researchers have further emphasised the importance of behavioural choices and control over the environment for animals to be able to cope successfully with the challenges of confinement (Carlstead & Shepherdson 2000; Young 2003, Makowska & Weary 2019). This is reflected in the EU Directive stating that animals *'shall be given a degree of control and choice over their environment to reduce stress-induced behaviour'* and that *'establishments shall have appropriate enrichment techniques in place, to extend the range of activities available to the animals and increase their coping activities'* (EU Directive 2010/63/EU, Annex III). Despite these advances in both conceptualisation and regulation of enrichment, implementation is lagging behind. This is only partly due to resistance to change practice in housing and husbandry procedures in animal facilities. For most species, including mice (e.g. Bailoo et al. 2018), we still lack well validated examples of practicable enrichments with proven beneficial effects.

Why is enrichment needed?

Animal behaviour and enrichment in captive environments

Conventional standard laboratory housing provides a highly restricted and barren environment compared to the natural habitats in which animals evolved; these natural environments contain all essential resources, are usually complex, rich in stimuli and much less predictable. Therefore, enrichment should be considered more of a reversal of the impoverished laboratory setting than an enrichment of a natural setting (van Praag et al. 2000). As will be discussed in the following sections, there is a considerable body of evidence from both deprivation studies and studies of environmental enrichment (which are fundamentally similar except for the reversal of the experimental and control groups

(Fuller 1967)), that barren environments, or housing conditions designed without taking into account the natural history of the animal, can result in impaired functioning, abnormal behaviour and compromised health (Würbel 2001; Cait *et al*. 2022).

Animals are complex organisms with behaviour and physiology adapted to their natural habitats. Evolution has shaped organisms to function and behave in ways that maximise their chances of reproduction and minimise their risk of harm. This, of course, does not mean that animals in their natural environments always experience good welfare. Life in all environments, including natural habitats, likely includes stressors (defined as real or perceived perturbations to an organism's physiological homeostasis or psychological well-being) (NRC 2008). However, animals have evolved to respond to natural stressors using species-specific decision rules and appropriate response patterns (Barnard & Hurst 1996). This armoury of coping mechanisms may include behavioural, hormonal and immune function changes. In captivity, welfare problems may thus arise when the conditions do not allow the expression of appropriate coping responses, when stressors occur for which animals do not have appropriate coping responses or when the animals' coping capacity is overtaxed, leading to a chronic state of distress and a higher susceptibility to disease (Mason 2010; Mason *et al*. 2013; Cait *et al*. 2022).

Control over the environment requires that the environment offers certain choices, and some degree of predictability and control over the environment are important in reducing the likelihood that stress will tip into distress (Wiepkema & Koolhaas 1993; Rennie & Buchanan-Smith 2006; NRC 2008). Making choices not only matters in terms of coping with stress, it is also inherently rewarding (Leotti & Delgado 2011; Špinka 2019). There is, however, a balance to be struck between too much predictability, which may result in boredom (Burn 2017), and too little, which can lead to prolonged arousal of HPA axis activation (Sambrook & Buchanan-Smith 1997; Bassett & Buchanan-Smith 2007).

Enrichment can offer opportunities for animals to make choices that allow them to cope with their environment successfully. For example, mice are commonly housed at 20–24 °C, which is outside their thermoneutral zone of 26–34 °C, and when given the choice they prefer warmer temperatures, especially during resting (Gaskill *et al*. 2009; Gaskill *et al*. 2012; Gordon 2012). Adequate nesting material allows them to express such choices by creating a resting area with the preferred microclimate. Similarly, a well-structured cage design, which allows animals to move out of sight of other animals, may allow them to better cope with the challenges of social life, which in male mice may reduce escalating aggression (Tallent *et al*. 2018; but see Mertens *et al*. 2020). It may also give mice a choice to segregate nesting and elimination areas (Makowska *et al*. 2019).

Barren housing conditions that are detrimental to animal health and functioning or compromise the expression of highly motivated behaviour are likely also associated with negative affective states, as these three domains of animal welfare are highly interconnected and largely overlapping Fraser 2008, Würbel 2009). Thus, by reducing abnormal behaviour, enrichment may at the same time stimulate species-typical behaviour, allow animals to better cope with stressors, as well as improve the animals' subjective well-being (also referred to as affective states, emotions or feelings). Moreover, it is becoming increasingly accepted that we should not merely be concerned about negative affective states but should also promote positive ones, which over an animal's lifespan will lead to 'a life worth living' (Yeates 2012; Green & Mellor 2012). As discussed in the sections below, there is a growing body of research indicating that animals' affective states can be adversely affected by conventional housing conditions. Under such conditions, animals exhibit a strong motivation to attain certain types of environmental enrichment. Providing adequate environmental enrichment may thus be crucial, if our aim is to provide animals a life worth living.

Behaviour in captivity associated with poor welfare

Barren housing conditions are associated with signs of stress and anxiety and can cause a variety of abnormal behaviours (Würbel 2001). Stereotypic behaviour has received most attention in the captive animal behaviour literature (Mason 1991a; Würbel 2006), and was one of the earliest indicators used in the evaluation of environmental enrichment effects on animal welfare (Hediger 1950; Meyer-Holzapfel 1968; Young 2003). Stereotypies are defined as repetitive, invariant behaviour patterns without obvious goal or function (Ödberg 1978). They reflect impaired welfare (Mason & Latham 2004) and are considered a sign that, at some point, conditions for the animal have not been adequate (reminiscent of a 'scar': Mason 1991b). Stereotypies are relatively common in some species used in research. In particular, some strains of laboratory mice show a high prevalence and may spend a large part of their active time performing stereotypies, such as bar-chewing, jumping, route-tracing and somersaulting, when raised in barren laboratory cages (Würbel & Stauffacher 1994, reported in Würbel 2006; Gross *et al*. 2011; Novak *et al*. 2016). The extent of the behaviour may come as a surprise to some animal care staff, but this is because much of the active behaviour occurs during the dark phase, which in most laboratories is at night, when the animal care staff is not there.

Gerbils are also prone to develop stereotypies under standard laboratory housing conditions (Wiedenmayer 1997). Similarly, for primates, up to 89% of individually housed and 48% of group-housed rhesus monkeys at a research centre showed abnormal behaviour, with pacing occurring in 78% and self-injurious behaviour in 11% of the monkeys (Novak *et al*. 2006; Lutz *et al*. 2003). In carnivores, home range size is linked to their propensity to develop stereotypies (Clubb & Mason 2007), and up to 90% of mink can develop stereotypies in captivity (Meagher *et al*. 2014). As dogs can range over substantial areas (Hubrecht 1995) it is, perhaps, not surprising that they also develop stereotypies when kept in restricted social or environmental conditions. In one study, 13% of single-housed laboratory dogs spent more than 10% of their time in repetitive behaviour patterns (Hubrecht *et al*. 1992), and some dogs spent up to 51% of their time performing such behaviours.

Stereotypies have been considered as indicator of poor welfare mainly because they develop from thwarted motivations to express highly motivated behaviours (Ödberg 1978;

Mason 1991b; Nevison *et al.* 1999a; Würbel 2006). However, they vary in their associations with other welfare indicators, with some studies reporting associations with measures of negative affective states (Pomerantz *et al.* 2012; Novak *et al.* 2016), while others found no associations with HPA axis activation (Nevison *et al.* 1999b).

Barren housing conditions can also increase inactivity, reflecting boredom, fear or apathy, as reported for mink (Meagher *et al.* 2017), rhesus monkeys (Hennessy *et al.* 2014) and laboratory mice (Fureix *et al.* 2016). Inactivity appears to be an alternative response to barren housing conditions. It may reflect thwarted motivation for general stimulation (Burn 2017) and possibly indicate a state of depression (Fureix *et al.* 2016).

It has long been known that inadequate social environment during development can lead to abnormal behaviour in the adult. Harlow and his followers in the 1960s demonstrated the importance of a normal social environment for macaques during their development (Novak *et al.* 2006; NRC 2008). Similarly, Fuller (1967) showed that dogs reared under a partial social isolation regimen became less social and interacted less with their environment; early weaning of mice can lead to increased anxiety, as tested in an elevated plus maze (Berry *et al.* 2012), and poorer maternal behaviour (Kikusui *et al.* 2005). Separation of animals after they have developed social ties can also cause stress (Taylor *et al.* 2014). Self-injurious behaviour is much more common in individually housed than socially housed rhesus macaques (Novak *et al.* 2006), while Fox and Stelzner (1966, 1967) found that isolating dogs from conspecifics led to later deficits even if human social contact was provided.

Barren housing conditions also increase agonistic behaviour and aggression in rats (Abou-Ismail 2011) and mice (Hutchinson *et al.* 2012; Nip *et al.* 2019). Behavioural signs of fear and anxiety, which are often increased in barren environments, may reflect negative affective states and indicate poor welfare (Olsson & Dahlborn 2002). In contrast, environmental enrichment may decrease fear responses (Meagher *et al.* 2014; Ross *et al.* 2019) and anxiety (Lambert *et al.* 2016).

Behaviour in captivity associated with good welfare

Similar to indicators of poor welfare, positive welfare can also be assessed from behavioural responses and cognitive processes (Yeates & Main 2008). Provision of environmental enrichment stimulates exploration and interactions with the environment (Freund *et al.* 2015; Hendershott *et al.* 2016; Bailoo *et al.* 2018) and enables animals to express behaviours which are related to positive affect. For example, young rats in naturalistic environments were reported to burrow 30 times per day (Makowska & Weary 2016) and emit more 50-kHz vocalisations (Hinchcliffe *et al.* 2022). Affiliative behaviours, such as grooming and play also increased in enriched environments (Bortolini & Bicca-Marques 2011; Reinhold *et al.* 2019; Pietropaolo *et al.* 2004).

Animals housed with enrichment also display a positive cognitive bias (Brydges *et al.* 2011; Richter *et al.* 2012; Bethell *et al.* 2015; Douglas *et al.* 2012), suggesting that enrichment can induce positive affective states in many species (Mendl *et al.* 2009).

Effect of environmental enrichment on behaviour and welfare

Adequate environmental enrichment facilitates the expression of species-typical behaviour and stimulates interactions with the environment. Young (2003) reviewed the literature for this on farm, zoo and laboratory animals. Lutz and Novak (2005) and Honess and Marin (2006) provide extensive reviews of positive effects of various types of enrichment on non-human primate behaviour. However, it is important to take into account the full spectrum of behaviour elicited by a particular form of enrichment to identify potential adverse effects. For example, Marashi *et al.* (2003) found that their enrichment of cages for male mice increased play behaviour (an indicator of good welfare), but also aggression, possibly because of the presence of defendable resources.

Enrichment can not only promote normal behaviour, but also reduce abnormal behaviour (Mason *et al.* 2007). In most studies, the expression of stereotypic behaviour in enriched environments was, to variable extents, lower compared to standard cages, but was not completely prevented. For example, up to 20% of mice reared in enriched laboratory cages still displayed stereotypic behaviour (Gross *et al.* 2011; Bailoo *et al.* 2018) and in mink, enrichment reduced the prevalence and level of stereotypic behaviour by 50% or less (Dallaire *et al.* 2012; Buob *et al.* 2013; Polanco *et al.* 2018). This does not mean that enrichment cannot be fully effective, but that the enrichments used in these studies were not. This is supported by a study in mice showing that only the most extensively enriched housing conditions ('super-enriched') completely prevented stereotypies in mice (Bailoo *et al.* 2018). Shyne (2006) carried out a meta-analysis of zoo animal enrichment studies, showing that attempts to enrich housing have generally been effective in reducing stereotypies, but to have their best effect, animals should be exposed to an enriched social and physical environment throughout their development. Similarly in mice, effects of environmental enrichment on stereotypy are greater when provided at a young age (Tilly *et al.* 2010). Enrichment later in the animal's life can still be beneficial, but may not undo the damage caused by an inadequate environment during development (squirrel monkeys: Fekete *et al.* 2000; deer mice: Hadley *et al.* 2006).

Different types of enrichment might also have different effects on behaviour: social enrichment, rather than physical items such as toys or foraging devices, seems to be more likely to result in improvements for non-human primates (Lutz & Novak 2005). Nonetheless, some improvement can occur; for example, mealworm feeders decreased marmoset stereotyped pacing (Vignes *et al.* 2001), and Würbel *et al.* (1998) showed that the provision of a simple tube reduced bar-chewing in mice by 40%. Similarly, scrabbling in mink can be reduced by removing neighbours, while physical enrichment is a better treatment for head-only and whole-body stereotypies (Polanco *et al.* 2018). Therefore, provision of enrichment should be tailored to address specific behavioural problems or needs.

It has been asserted that because enrichment of rodent laboratory cages does not completely abolish abnormal behaviour, it has no effect on their well-being (Benefiel & Greenough 1998). However, stereotypies resulting from chronic exposure to a sub-optimal environment can be thought of as a behavioural scar (Mason 1991b). Hence, stereotypies are not necessarily a good indicator of current welfare status (Mason & Latham 2004; see also Chapter 6: Brief introduction to welfare assessment: A toolbox of techniques) and they can be resistant to improvements in housing condition. Failure to eradicate established stereotypies, therefore, does not necessarily indicate that the enrichment is a failure.

Animals used in research are inevitably exposed to stressors during both husbandry and experimental procedures. Enrichment that improves their ability to cope with such stressors will improve their welfare. There is evidence for a range of species that enrichment can produce less fearful, more confident and adaptable animals than those kept in barren conditions (Chamove 1989; Prior & Sachser 1994; Larsson et al. 2002; van de Weerd et al. 2002; Young 2003; van Loo et al. 2004; Friske & Gammie 2005; Meagher et al. 2014; Ross et al. 2019). A study carried out by Sherwin and Olsson (2004), in which mice were allowed to self-dose with an anxiolytic, indicated that mice housed in enriched cages may be less anxious than those housed in barren cages. Environmental enrichment can decrease stress reactivity as shown by behaviour in the elevated plus maze, defaecation in a novel environment, defensive responses to a predator and open-field exploration (Lewis 2004; Urakawa et al. 2013; Lambert et al. 2016). Other examples include the study by Benaroya-Milshtein et al. (2004), in which enrichment attenuated behavioural and physiological responses to an electrical shock, and that by van Loo et al. (2004), who showed that provision of nesting material reduced corticosterone levels in male Balb/c and CD-1 mice.

For laboratory mice, nesting material is nowadays found throughout European animal facilities, as its provision is required by law. Studies have reported that neither complexity nor novelty have additional effects on stereotypic and anxiety-related behaviour beyond those of nesting material (Gross et al. 2011). However, this might be different if more extensive forms of complexity and novelty were used. In line with this, a recent study comparing female C57BL/6 and SWISS mice found that only extensively enriched ('super-enriched') housing conditions (including more space, complexity, resources and novelty compared to more conventionally enriched laboratory conditions) reduced stereotypic behaviour, anxiety and stress in a manner consistent with improved animal welfare compared to the other housing conditions with less enrichment (Bailoo et al. 2018).

Reductions in stress responses suggest that enrichment not only has the potential to improve the animals' welfare during husbandry but could also help to refine procedures. For example, Meijer et al. (2006) found that enrichment and frequent handling of mice reduced their temperature and heart rate following procedures such as injection or restraint. Environmental enrichment can also facilitate recovery from physical injury or illness (Jirkof 2015).

Those implementing enrichment programmes should be aware that some common forms of enrichment may not work for a specific sex or strain, resulting in increased stress rather than a reduction. Enrichment can increase aggression in some mouse strains in both male and female mice (McQuaid et al. 2012; Mesa-Gresa et al. 2013). In males of some strains of mice, the provision of shelter has been associated with increases in testosterone, and corticosterone that may be linked to territoriality (Howerton et al. 2008; Haemisch et al. 1994; Haemisch & Gärtner 1994; Nevison et al. 1999b; van Loo et al. 2002). In contrast, some studies found that mice in enriched environments had fewer tail wounds (Hutchinson et al. 2012) and displayed less agonistic behaviour (Harper et al. 2015; Clipperton-Allen et al. 2015; Nip et al. 2018). However, not all enrichment items have the same effect on aggression: male mice with cage partitions (Tallent et al. 2018), and female mice with dispersed enrichment items (Akre et al. 2011) show less aggression. Thus, effects of enrichment on aggression may vary not only with strain and sex, but also with enrichment type.

Effects of enrichment on experimental outcomes

Researchers have been concerned that enrichment could affect experimental results in ways that are detrimental to their scientific validity (Benefiel et al. 2005; Toth et al. 2011). There are three separate potential issues wrapped up in this concern that are often confounded. These are: that enrichment might bias the results by altering the animals' responses to experimental treatments; that it might decrease precision of the results by increasing variation in the data thus reducing test sensitivity; and that it might decrease replicability of the results by increasing between-laboratory variation (Würbel 2000; Garner 2005; Würbel & Garner 2007). These issues are addressed in the following sections.

Bias and internal validity

Enrichment (as defined by Rosenzweig et al. 1978) certainly does have the potential to alter experimental outcomes (Federation of European Laboratory Animal Science Associations (FELASA) 2006). For example, enrichment has been found to promote wound healing in rodents (Bice et al. 2017; Vitalo et al. 2012) and increase lifespan (Arranz et al. 2010; Bice et al. 2017). These benefits may be mediated by effects of enrichment on immune system function, including increased natural killer cell activity (Arranz et al. 2010; Benaroya-Milshtein et al. 2004), increased wound-site plasma secretions of IgA antibodies (Bice et al. 2017) and increased lymphocyte proliferation (Arranz et al. 2010). Furthermore, enrichment was found to result in increased neurogenesis, gliogenesis, capillary development and synaptogenesis (Kempermann 2019; Nithianantharajah et al. 2004), as well as changes in neurotransmitter activity (Varman & Rajan 2015), hormone levels (Sztainberg et al. 2010), gene expression in many cells and tissues (Rattazzi et al. 2016; Zhang et al. 2018), and changes in protein production (Zhang et al. 2016). Similar effects have been found for other mammalian and avian species, including cats, monkeys and even humans (Healy & Tovée 1999).

These structural changes in animals kept in enriched environments are associated with functional changes, including improved learning, memory and behavioural plasticity (Zimmermann et al. 2001; Schrijver et al. 2002; Lewis 2004; Garthe et al. 2016), as well as sensory functions. For example, visual acuity of enriched mice was 18% greater than those of mice kept in standard conditions (Prusky et al. 2000), and the cortical representations of the rats' sensory whiskers became refined and more focused, contracting by up to 46%, compared to rats housed in standard cages (Polley et al. 2004). Moreover, improved immune system and decreased oxidative-inflammatory stress have been reported in animals housed with enrichment (Arranz et al. 2010; Singhal et al. 2014).

So, does enrichment bias experimental outcomes? If it does, it would seem that it does so for the better. The findings summarised in the preceding text indicate that animals reared under non-enriched conditions exhibit structural and functional deficiencies that may negatively affect experimental outcomes (Würbel 2001; Garner 2005). This is further supported by findings indicating that non-enriched housing conditions are associated with signs of impaired welfare, including increased morbidity, abnormal repetitive behaviour, stress and fearfulness (Chapillon et al. 1999; Würbel 2001; Garner 2005; Würbel 2006; Bailoo et al. 2018; Cait et al. 2022).

Conversely, beneficial enrichment should result in animals that are more 'normal' and thereby increase the validity of experimental results by normalising brain function, physiology and behaviour (Würbel 2001; Garner 2005). Thus, beneficial enrichment should help to avoid bias caused by housing conditions rather than create it.

Despite the arguments outlined in the preceding text, enrichment may or may not alter the results of any given study. Not all experimental outcomes are sensitive to environmental effects on the animals' phenotype. However, if an experimental outcome does vary depending on the animals' housing conditions, the question is no longer just what housing condition to choose, but how many. Housing-dependent variation in an outcome measure indicates that the outcome is sensitive to phenotypic plasticity (Voelkl & Würbel 2016). In that case, it is important to vary conditions to assess whether a finding is robust against some environmental variation or is valid only under highly specific environmental conditions (Würbel 2000; Richter et al. 2009). In the latter case, a finding may show poor replicability and may not be as important a finding as one that generalises across a wider range of conditions (Bailoo et al. 2014; Würbel 2017). This will be discussed further in the following text (cf. external validity and replicability).

Precision and test sensitivity

Researchers may be concerned that enrichment will compromise standardisation of experiments leading to less precise (i.e. more variable) results, which will also compromise test sensitivity. Because higher test sensitivity (i.e. less variation) allows a reduction of sample size, standardisation is sometimes promoted for ethical as a means of reducing animal use (Festing 2004a,b).

These concerns seem to be based on the fact that environmental enrichment renders the animals' environment more complex. Given that a more complex environment offers animals more choices, concerns were raised that this could lead to higher variability in experimental results. However, empirical evidence does not support these concerns (van de Weerd et al. 2002; Augustsson et al. 2003; Wolfer et al. 2004;

Baumans et al. 2010; André et al. 2018; Bailoo et al. 2018). As long as enrichment is beneficial as outlined in the preceding text, there seems to be no reason for concerns of increased variation in experimental results.

External validity and replicability

Researchers may further be concerned that variable implementation of enrichment will compromise standardisation between sites, leading to poor replicability (e.g. Benefiel et al. 2005; Toth et al. 2011). However, this concern seems to be based on two logical fallacies. First, so-called standard housing is, itself, not particularly well standardised across animal facilities, with variation in hygiene levels, macro-environment, cage design, materials, feed and husbandry, including human-animal interaction (e.g. handling procedures). Variation in any of these factors can induce variation in experimental results between replicate studies conducted independently by different laboratories. There is no good reason why enrichment should be special in this respect.

Secondly, even when conditions between laboratories are rigorously standardised, systematic differences between them still remain (Crabbe et al. 1999). Conflicting findings even between rigorously standardised replicate studies indicate that standardisation itself may be the cause of this problem. Because many environmental factors resist standardisation between laboratories (e.g. microbiome, experimenter, noises, odours; Richter et al. 2009; Voelkl & Würbel 2016), animals within laboratories will be more homogenous than animals between laboratories when environmental conditions are standardised. Therefore, increasingly rigorous environmental standardisation produces results that are increasingly distinct between laboratories and hence less reproducible. This has been referred to as the 'standardisation fallacy' (Würbel 2000). Environmental standardisation could therefore be a major cause of, rather than a cure for, spurious results and conflicting findings in the scientific literature (Richter et al. 2009). Instead of environmental standardisation, these researchers thus proposed systematic environmental variation (i.e. heterogenisation) to improve the external validity and thus the reproducibility of results from animal experiments. Different types of environmental enrichment might serve to introduce systematic environmental variation.

Conclusions

Taken together, current evidence suggests that environmental enrichment improves the well-being of laboratory animals without reducing the precision and replicability of experimental results, while at the same time 'attenuating abnormal brain function and anxiety – both of which are possible confounds in animal experiments' (Wolfer et al. 2004).

Finally, while there is a growing body of literature on the value of many types of enrichment, which has helped to inform guidance given in this volume and elsewhere, it remains true that further work is needed to develop practicable and effective ways of improving the housing conditions of laboratory animals in ways that promote both the well-being of the animals and the scientific validity of the research.

Factors to consider when choosing enrichment

What are the benefits of the proposed enrichment?

The aim of enrichment in laboratory animal husbandry is to improve welfare. However, what does this mean in practice? Young (2003) provides the following list of goals, which should help to focus planning and to assess success: Goals of enrichment are to:

1. increase behavioural diversity;
2. reduce the frequencies of abnormal behaviour;
3. increase the range or number of normal behaviour patterns;
4. increase positive utilisation of the environment;
5. increase the ability to cope with challenges in a more normal way.

As discussed earlier, some so-called enrichments may turn out to have no effect or even negative effects on the animals' welfare. Therefore, it is important to avoid filling the animals' enclosure with a random selection of items in the hope that the animal will make use of them. Instead, enrichment choices should be based on a sound understanding of the animal's biology and preferably on experimental research. A good example of enrichment that combines these features is the provision of refuges with tunnels for gerbils. Gerbils commonly develop stereotypic behaviour in laboratory cages. See also Chapter 23: The laboratory gerbil. The reason for this was not understood until Wiedenmayer (1997) showed that gerbils not only need a refuge, but also a tunnel of a certain length leading to that refuge to avoid the development of stereotypic digging behaviour. It is likely that this is because gerbils, in the wild, dig burrows that are connected to the surface by tunnels of a sufficient length to reduce the risk of predation and to protect them from other hazards. As a result, it seems that they are strongly motivated to keep digging if they are not able to achieve this goal in captivity. Those implementing behavioural strategies should therefore review the literature to familiarise themselves with the natural history of the species and to identify any proven beneficial enrichments.

While enrichment should be biologically relevant (Garner 2005), it need not be naturalistic (i.e. designed to mimic features of the wild environment). Some findings indicate that to rats, for example, natural-like enrichment items (wooden sticks, stones) may be more relevant than artificial (plastic) (Lambert et al. 2016; Stevens et al. 2018). However, non-naturalistic objects such as bells, marbles, metal manipulanda should be evaluated to ensure that they really are beneficial and that they are not harmful or distressing to the animals. Even if animals do make use of, or manipulate, items placed in their cage as enrichment, it is important to consider whether they are doing so for positive reasons, and not perhaps just trying to remove them from their living areas. The answers to these questions lie in carefully designed behavioural experiments, which, if the enrichment is a commercially marketed one, should be the responsibility of the manufacturer. To help encourage manufacturers to carry out this research, customers of companies selling enrichment should ask to see the scientific data that support their claims.

Enrichment and animal safety

As the aim of enrichment in laboratory animal husbandry is to improve animal welfare, only beneficial, or conditionally beneficial, items should be used. However, the addition of any novel item to an animal's environment carries some risks. It is therefore necessary to attempt to identify these and to weigh them against the likely benefits arising from the items before using a new enrichment. This assessment is likely to require considerable input from care staff, which includes veterinary care staff (Nelson & Mandrell 2005).

Physical items can result in injury, either directly, or by increasing aggression. Bayne (2005) reviews harms (as well as benefits) arising from attempts to provide enrichment for non-human primates as well as rodents and rabbits. Animals can become entangled in objects. Murchison (1993), for example, described a case of a pig-tailed macaque becoming entangled in a ring toy. Items placed into a cage may be ingested, even if that is not the specific aim of the enrichment, so there may be risks of choking or obstruction. It is possible that certain types of food enrichment, if not properly controlled, may lead to obesity or tooth decay. Moreover, commonly used enrichments may result in problems for particular strains, e.g. particular nesting material for nude mice (Bazille et al. 2001). Enrichment may result in increased aggression, either because the items may be desirable resources in themselves or because they allow the animals to divide the enclosure into territorial units as previously described for mice. Enrichment within the animals' environment can make cleaning more difficult, and the enrichment items themselves could act as fomites (Bayne et al. 1993). To help put these risks into context, it is worth considering that no environment is entirely safe, that incidences of disease related to enrichment items seem to be very rare, that enrichment can also reduce aggression (Honess & Marin 2006) and that injuries (and other deleterious health effects) can occur even in an unenriched environment. Marmosets have been known to entangle their arms in the mesh of their cages; dogs without chews may chew through the steel cable holding up pop holes or even at the walls, with consequent tooth damage. The increased risk of injury from most physical enrichment options is likely to be small, and there are few published reports of enrichment devices resulting in injury (Young 2003; Nelson & Mandrell 2005). This lack of data may not be surprising, given its sensitive nature, but there are obvious benefits that could arise if both failures and successes were published. While the increased risk of injury or disease when using well-established enrichment items is small, it is best to avoid problems. The checklist of safety considerations provided by Young (2003) is a useful starting point in carrying out a risk assessment. As Young points out, safety assessment should be an ongoing process, as animals may use enrichment in new and unexpected ways.

Enrichment and human safety

Enrichment strategies must meet the needs of staff and researchers as well as the animals. Clearly, any enrichment must be practical and cost effective, and any health and safety issues for the staff must also be addressed. Concerns may include trip hazards, increased weight of enclosures, increased exposure to allergens, exposure to sharp objects (e.g. after animals have gnawed or broken them). Some species such as primates or apes may cause injury by throwing enrichment items. Excessive enrichment might also compromise the ability of staff to avoid potentially dangerous animals. Again, an attempt should be made to identify risks to human safety before introducing the enrichment and to find ways of ameliorating these by reconsidering housing and management regimens.

Enrichment and the experiment

Previous sections have discussed the issues of enrichment and experimental outcomes, but it goes without saying that before introducing enrichment both scientists and care staff must be content that it will not adversely affect the outcomes of experiments in which the animals or their offspring might be used. Where there are concerns that a proposed enrichment might have such effects, it is important to carefully assess the validity of these concerns, bearing in mind that enrichment programmes have been successfully adopted in many experimental protocols. It is also important to consider whether the procedures carried out on the animals might impact on the way in which they interact with the enrichment. If, for example, the research involves damage to the animals' motor or sensory function, then this might necessitate changes to enrichment regimens to avoid safety issues.

Validating new enrichment

The Directive 2010/63/EU mandates the implementation of enrichment programmes appropriate to the species, and ensuring that enrichment is beneficial is an important component of any programme. This issue is discussed in detail in a FELASA working group document (FELASA 2006), which points out that the techniques used to demonstrate a welfare benefit (e.g. preference/choice tests, demand studies, physiological measurements) can be difficult to use and to interpret.

Most commonly, efficacy for improving welfare is inferred from the degree to which enrichment is used (Hoy et al. 2010; Meagher et al. 2014; Bailoo et al. 2018; Ratuski et al. 2021). Active use is the most obvious method to evaluate the underlying motivation to use resources (e.g. interaction with balls or toys by mink (Meagher et al. 2014)); however, it may not always accurately represent the resource's value. Inactive use of enrichments, which provide tactile comfort or thermoregulation could also be rewarding. For example, when given access to an enriched environment, some mink spent most of their inactive time on elevated platforms and spent little time actively interacting with other enrichment items. These individuals also showed most reduction in stereotypy levels (Dallaire et al. 2012).

As previously discussed, rate of interaction, choice or preference tests, for example, can provide some indication of the relative value that an animal attaches to a resource, but they do not tell how much an animal either likes or dislikes a resource, or why the animal has made the choice. The test might therefore reflect the animal's motivation to minimise deprivation, maximise pleasure or monitor unwanted problems; and the value of the enrichment in question would be very dependent on which of these was the underlying motivation. Past experience, familiarity with the item, reproductive status of the animal, season or time of day can also strongly affect preference test outcomes. For example, individual differences in enrichment use may be attributed to differences in neophobia (Walker & Mason 2011), among others. In some cases, animals may make short-term choices that result in a long-term reduction in welfare or health, such as through diet choices that ultimately result in obesity or dental caries. Finally, the enrichment needs of animals can vary between strain, by sex and with age.

Some studies have applied a cost with incremental increases (push-door with increasing weight, grids with electric shocks) on accessing enrichment, to quantify the rewarding property of enrichment and to see which resources are most valued (Spangenberg & Wichman 2018; Kirkden & Pajor 2006; Tilly et al. 2010; Walker & Mason 2018). Enriched environments are generally preferred by animals: they voluntarily interact with them, and may even work to access them, indicating high motivation (Dallaire et al. 2012; Elmore et al. 2011; Tilly et al. 2010).

For the reasons outlined in the preceding text, the initial determination of the types of enrichment required by a species will normally best be carried out either by, or in collaboration with, specialist animal welfare scientists who will be aware of the pitfalls of these studies and will have the necessary experience to choose appropriate measures and study designs.

Once an enrichment has been validated as beneficial, it would normally be a waste of time and resources for individual laboratories to repeat this process. For example, it is well known that foraging enrichment is beneficial for primates and further research to corroborate this is unnecessary. Nonetheless, there may be local variations in the implementation of categories of enrichment, and these details may need to be evaluated to ensure that they function as expected, that there are no safety concerns and that the enrichment will not compromise the study.

Managing an enrichment programme

Successful enrichment strategies depend on good communication and management. Research institutions should be committed to providing a high quality of housing for their animals; and animal care staff, veterinarians and research scientists should receive sufficient training to understand this concept. Enrichment should not be introduced piece-meal, but should be properly planned and discussed, particularly with the scientists who will be using the animals.

Ideally, the effect of enrichment items on welfare should be evaluated by well-designed experiments and published in peer-reviewed journals. However, new items are often assessed by animal care staff, who make informal observations of enrichment use during routine husbandry. Many facilities use a more formal process of assessing novel enrichment by having a committee charged with developing, assessing and implementing the programme (Schaller 2014; Schimmel & Hlavka 2014). For some research programmes, the normal enrichment and housing conditions may not be compatible with the aims of the research, but requests to keep animals without enrichment should always be carefully examined to determine whether an alternative enrichment programme, perhaps using different materials, is possible.

Management should ensure that there is a reasonable and sufficient budget to meet enrichment needs and to fund any research necessary to validate the programme. However, simple enrichments can be as effective as more complex and expensive options (Schapiro *et al*. 1997). Enrichment items need not be expensive, and can be made from everyday items such as old water bottles, cardboard rolls. Nonetheless, such items should be used with care as they may contain undesirable substances, and their composition may not remain consistent. Commercial enrichment products have the advantage that they can often be obtained with a certificate of analysis, which is necessary for regulatory studies. Further advice on implementing enrichment within a Good Laboratory Practice (GLP) framework is available from FELASA (2006).

The extra costs arising from an enrichment programme should not impact adversely on research. For commercial establishments, the costs of enrichment are usually trivial compared to overall budgets. Moreover, as enrichment becomes more widely accepted, competitive disadvantages between commercial organisations adopting enrichment should decrease. Moreover, within the UK, the major funding bodies emphasise the importance of the Three Rs, and of housing animals in a complex and varied physical environment in appropriate social groupings, with the aim of promoting exercise and performance of species-typical behaviours. This is reflected by their support for the National Centre for the Replacement, Refinement & Reduction of Animals in Research (NC3Rs). Similar developments supported by national 3Rs centres are currently observed worldwide. Therefore, it should no longer be a problem for academic researchers to obtain the funds that are necessary to provide appropriate enrichment.

Within the animal house, records should be kept of the enrichment used and of any rotation of enrichment items. As part of continuing professional development, staff should be given access to current literature to keep up-to-date with the literature on enrichment, should visit other research sites and attend conferences at which enrichment is discussed. It is also useful to invite experts on various species to visit and comment on the enrichment programmes in place. When animals are obtained from outside institutions, it is important to determine the husbandry and enrichment systems of the supplying institution. This is partly to minimise adverse effects resulting from a change of husbandry, and also to encourage the worldwide spread of high standards. Finally, institutions should make efforts to disseminate information on the successes or failures of their enrichment programmes.

Acknowledgement

This chapter was originally written by Robert Hubrecht for the 8th edition of the UFAW Handbook and has now been updated by us. It still contains a lot of Robert's original content, and we hope that we could also preserve a sense of his deep commitment to promoting good welfare and good science.

References

Abou-Ismail, U.A. (2011) The effects of cage enrichment on agonistic behaviour and dominance in male laboratory rats (Rattus norvegicus). *Research in Veterinary Science*, **90**, 346–351.

Akre, A.K., Bakken, M., Hovland, A.L. *et al*. (2011) Clustered environmental enrichments induce more aggression and stereotypic behaviour than do dispersed enrichments in female mice. *Applied Animal Behaviour Science*, **131**, 145–152.

André, V., Gau, C., Scheideler, A. *et al*. (2018) Laboratory mouse housing conditions can be improved using common environmental enrichment without compromising data. *PLoS biology*, **16**(4), e2005019.

Arranz, L., De Castro, N.M., Baeza, I. *et al*. (2010) Environmental enrichment improves age-related immune system impairment: long-term exposure since adulthood increases life span in mice. *Rejuvenation Research*, **13**, 415–428.

Augustsson, H., van de Weerd, H.A., Kruitwagen, C.L.J.J. and Baumans, V. (2003) Effect of enrichment on variation and results in the light/dark test. *Laboratory Animals*, **37**, 328–340.

Bailoo, J.D., Murphy, E.M., Boada-Saña, M. *et al*. (2018) Effects of cage enrichment on behavior, welfare and outcome variability in female mice. *Frontiers in Behavioral Neuroscience*, **12**, 232.

Bailoo, J.D., Reichlin, T.S. and Würbel, H. (2014) Refinement of experimental design and conduct in laboratory animal research. *ILAR Journal*, **55**, 383–391.

Barnard, C.J. and Hurst, J.L. (1996) Welfare by design: the natural selection of welfare criteria. *Animal Welfare*, **5**, 405–433.

Bassett, L. and Buchanan-Smith, H.M. (2007) Effects of predictability on the welfare of captive animals. *Applied Animal Behaviour Science*, **102**(3–4), 223–245.

Baumans, V. and Van Loo, P.L.P. (2013) How to improve housing conditions of laboratory animals: The possibilities of environmental refinement. *The Veterinary Journal*, **195**, 24–32.

Baumans, V., Van Loo, P.L.P. and Pham, T.M. (2010) Standardisation of environmental enrichment for laboratory mice and rats: utilisation, practicality and variation in experimental results. *Scandinavian Journal of Laboratory Animal Sciences*, **37**, 101–114.

Bayne, K. (2005) Potential for unintended consequences of environmental enrichment for laboratory animals and research results. *ILAR Journal*, **46**, 129–139.

Bayne, K.A.L., Dexter, S.L., Hurst, J.K. *et al*. (1993) Kong® Toys for laboratory primates: are they really an enrichment or just fomites? *Laboratory Animal Science*, **43**, 78–85.

Bazille, P.G., Walden, S.D., Koniar, B.L. *et al*. (2001) Commercial cotton nesting material as a predisposing factor for conjunctivitis in athymic nude mice. *Laboratory Animal*, **30**, 40–42.

Benaroya-Milshtein, N., Hollander, N., Apter, A. *et al*. (2004) Environmental enrichment in mice decreases anxiety, attenuates stress responses and enhances natural killer cell activity. *European Journal of Neuroscience*, **20**, 1341–1347.

Benefiel, A.C., Dong, W.K. and Greenough, W.T. (2005) Mandatory 'enriched' housing of laboratory animals: the need for evidence based evaluation. *ILAR Journal*, **46**, 95–105.

Benefiel, A.C. and Greenough, W.T. (1998) Effects of experience and environment on the developing and mature brain: implications for laboratory animal housing. *ILAR Journal*, **39**, 5–11.

Berry, A., Bellisario, V., Capoccia, S. *et al*. (2012) Social deprivation stress is a triggering factor for the emergence of anxiety- and depression-like behaviours and leads to reduced brain BDNF levels in C57BL/6J mice. *Psychoneuroendocrinology*, **37**, 762–772.

Bethell, E.J. and Koyama, N.F. (2015) Happy hamsters? Enrichment induces positive judgement bias for mildly (but not truly) ambiguous cues to reward and punishment in Mesocricetus auratus. *Royal Society Open Science*, **2**, 140399.

Bice, B.D., Stephens, M.R., Georges, S.J. *et al*. (2017) Environmental enrichment induces pericyte and IgA-dependent wound repair and lifespan extension in a Colon Tumor Model. *Cell Reports*, **19**, 760–773.

Bloomsmith, M.A., Brent, L.Y. and Schapiro, S.J. (1991) Guidelines for developing and managing an environmental enrichment program for nonhuman primates. *Laboratory Animal Science*, **41**, 372–377.

Bortolini, T.S. and Bicca-Marques, J.C. (2011) The effect of environmental enrichment and visitors on the behaviour and welfare of two captive hamadryas baboons (*Papio hamadryas*). *Animal Welfare–The UFAW Journal*, **20(4)**, 573.

Brydges, N.M., Leach, M., Nicol, K. et al. (2011) Environmental enrichment induces optimistic cognitive bias in rats. *Animal Behaviour*, **81**, 169–175.

Buchanan-Smith, H.M., Rennie, A.E., Vitale, A. et al. (2005) Harmonising the definition of refinement. *Animal Welfare*, **14**, 379–384.

Buob, M., Meagher, R., Dawson, L. et al. (2013) Providing 'get-away bunks' and other enrichments to primiparous adult female mink improves their reproductive productivity. *Applied Animal Behaviour Science*, **147**, 194–204.

Burn, C.C. (2017) Bestial boredom: A biological perspective on animal boredom and suggestions for its scientific investigation. *Animal Behaviour*, **130**, 141–151.

Cait, J., Cait, A., Scott, R. W., et al. (2022) Conventional laboratory housing increases morbidity and mortality in research rodents: results of a meta-analysis. *BMC biology*, 20(1), 1–22.

Carlstead, K. and Shepherdson, D. (2000) Alleviating stress in zoo animals with environmental enrichment. In: *The Biology of Animal Stress: Basic Principles and Implications for Animal Welfare*. Eds Moberg, G.P. and Mench, J.A., pp. 337–354. CABI Publishing, Wallingford, UK.

Chamove, A.S. (1989) Cage design reduces emotionality in mice. *Laboratory Animal*, **23**, 215–219.

Chapillon, P., Manneche, C., Belzung, C. and Caston, J. (1999) Rearing environmental enrichment in two inbred strains of mice: 1. Effects on emotional reactivity. *Behavior Genetics*, **29**, 41–46.

Clipperton-Allen, A.E., Ingrao, J.C., Ruggiero, L. et al. (2015) Long-term provision of environmental resources alters behavior but not physiology or neuroanatomy of male and female BALB/c and C57BL/6 mice. *Journal of the American Association for Laboratory Animal Science*, **54**, 718–730.

Clubb, R. and Mason, G.J. (2007) Natural behavioural biology as a risk factor in carnivore welfare: How analysing species differences could help zoos improve enclosures. *Applied Animal Behaviour Science*, **102**, 303–328.

Crabbe, J.C., Wahlsten, D. and Dudek, B.C. (1999) Genetics of mouse behavior: interactions with laboratory environment. *Science*, **284**, 1670–1672.

Dallaire, J.A., Meagher, R.K. and Mason, G.J. (2012) Individual differences in stereotypic behaviour predict individual differences in the nature and degree of enrichment use in caged American mink. *Applied Animal Behaviour Science*, **142**, 98–108.

Dean, S.W. (1999) Environmental enrichment of laboratory animals used in regulatory toxicology studies. *Laboratory Animals*, **33**, 309–327.

Douglas, C., Bateson, M., Walsh, C. et al. (2012) Environmental enrichment induces optimistic cognitive biases in pigs. *Applied Animal Behaviour Science*, **139**, 65–73.

Elmore, M.R.P., Garner, J.P., Johnson, A.K. et al. (2011) Getting around social status: Motivation and enrichment use of dominant and subordinate sows in a group setting. *Applied Animal Behaviour Science*, **133**, 154–163.

EU Directive 2010/63/EU of the European Parliament and of the Council on the protection of animals used for scientific purposes. https://eur-lex.europa.eu/LexUriServ/LexUriServ.do?uri=OJ:L:2010:276:0033:0079:EN:PDF (accessed 28 March 2020).

Federation of European Laboratory Animal Science Associations (2006) *FELASA Working Group Standardization of Enrichment, Working Group Report*. http://www.felasa.eu/working-groups/reports/standardization-of-enrichment/ (accessed 3 April 2020).

Fekete, J.M., Norcross, J.L. and Newman, J.D. (2000) Artificial turf foraging boards as environmental enrichment for pair-housed female squirrel monkeys. *Contemporary Topics in Laboratory Animal Science*, **39**, 22–26.

Festing, M. F. (2004a). Refinement and reduction through the control of variation. *Alternatives to Laboratory Animals*, **32** (Suppl. 1), 259–263.

Festing, M.F. (2004b). The choice of animal model and reduction. *Alternatives to Laboratory Animals*, **32** (Suppl. 2), 59–64.

Fox, M.W. and Stelzner, D. (1966) Behavioural effects of differential early experience in the dog. *Animal Behaviour*, **14**, 273–281.

Fox, M.W. and Stelzner, D. (1967) The effects of early experience on the development of inter and intraspecies social relationships in the dog. *Animal Behaviour*, **15**, 377–386.

Franco, N.H., Sandøe, P. and Olsson, I.A.S. (2018) Researchers' attitudes to the 3Rs – An upturned hierarchy? *PLOS One*, **13**, e0200895.

Franks, B. (2019) What do animals want? *Animal Welfare*, **28**, 1–10.

Fraser, D. (2008) *Understanding Animal Welfare: The Science in its Cultural Context*. John Wiley & Sons, Chichester, UK.

Fraser, D. and Nicol, C.J. (2018) Preference and motivation research. In: *Animal Welfare*, 3rd edn. Eds Appleby, M.C. et al., pp. 213–231. CABI, Cambridge, MA, USA.

Fraser, D., Weary, D.M., Pajor, E.A. et al. (1997) A scientific conception of animal welfare that reflects ethical concerns. *Animal Welfare*, **6**, 187–205.

Freund, J., Brandmaier, A.M., Lewejohann, L. et al. (2015) Association between exploratory activity and social individuality in genetically identical mice living in the same enriched environment. *Neuroscience*, **309**, 140–152.

Friske, J.E. and Gammie, S.C. (2005) Environmental enrichment alters plus maze, but not maternal defense performance in mice. *Physiology & Behavior*, **85**, 187–194.

Fuller, J.L. (1967) Experiential deprivation and later behaviour. *Science*, **158**, 1645–1652.

Fureix, C., Walker, M., Harper, L. et al. (2016) Stereotypic behaviour in standard non-enriched cages is an alternative to depression-like responses in C57BL/6 mice. *Behavioural Brain Research*, **305**, 186–190.

Garner, J.P. (2005) Stereotypies and other abnormal repetitive behaviors: potential impact on validity, reliability, and replicability of scientific outcomes. *ILAR Journal*, **46**, 106–117.

Garthe, A., Roeder, I. and Kempermann, G. (2016) Mice in an enriched environment learn more flexibly because of adult hippocampal neurogenesis. *Hippocampus*, **26**, 261–271.

Gaskill, B.N., Gordon, C.J., Pajor, E.A. et al. (2012) Heat or insulation: behavioral titration of mouse preference for warmth or access to a nest. *PLOS One*, **7**, e32799.

Gaskill, B.N., Rohr, S.A., Pajor, E.A. et al. (2009) Some like it hot: mouse temperature preferences in laboratory housing. *Applied Animal Behaviour Science*, **116**, 279–285.

Gordon, C.J. (2012) Thermal physiology of laboratory mice: defining thermoneutrality. *Journal of Thermal Biology*, **37**, 654–685.

Green, T.C. and Mellor, D.J. (2011) Extending ideas about animal welfare assessment to include 'quality of life' and related concepts. *New Zealand Veterinary Journal*, **59**, 263–271.

Gross, A.N.M., Engel, A.K.J. and Würbel, H. (2011) Simply a nest? Effects of different enrichments on stereotypic and anxiety-related behaviour in mice. *Applied Animal Behaviour Science*, **134**, 239–245.

Hadley, C., Hadley, B., Ephraim, S. et al. (2006) Spontaneous stereotypy and environmental enrichment in deer mice (*Peromyscus maniculatus*): reversibility of experience. *Applied Animal Behaviour Science*, **97**, 312–322.

Haemisch, A. and Gärtner, K. (1994) The cage design affects intermale aggression in small groups of male laboratory mice: strain specific consequences on social organization, and endocrine activations in two inbred strains (DBA/2J and CBA/J). *Journal of Experimental Animal Science*, **36**, 101–116.

Haemisch, A., Voss, T. and Gärtner, K. (1994) Effects of environmental enrichment on aggressive behavior, dominance hierarchies, and endocrine states in male DBA/2J Mice. *Physiology & Behavior*, **56**, 1041–1048.

Harper, L., Choleris, E., Ervin, K. et al. (2015) Stereotypic mice are aggressed by their cage-mates, and tend to be poor demonstrators in social learning tasks. *Animal Welfare*, **24**, 463–473.

Healy, S.D. and Tovée, M.J. (1999) Environmental enrichment and impoverishment: neurophysiological effects. In: *Attitudes to Animals Views in Animal Welfare*. Ed. Dolins, F.L., pp. 54–76. Cambridge University Press, Cambridge.

Hediger, H. (1950) *Wild Animals in Captivity*. Butterworths, London.

Hendershott, T.R., Cronin, M.E., Langella, S. et al. (2016) Effects of environmental enrichment on anxiety-like behavior, sociability, sensory gating, and spatial learning in male and female C57BL/6J mice. *Behavioural Brain Research*, **314**, 215–225.

Hennessy, M.B., McCowan, B., Jiang, J. and Capitanio, J.P. (2014) Depressive-like behavioral response of adult male rhesus monkeys during routine animal husbandry procedure. *Frontiers in Behavioral Neuroscience*, **8**, 309.

Hinchcliffe, J.K., Jackson, M.G. and Robinson, E. S. (2022) The use of ball pits and playpens in laboratory Lister Hooded male rats induces ultrasonic vocalisations indicating a more positive affective state and can reduce the welfare impacts of aversive procedures. *Laboratory Animals*, 00236772211065920 [online].

Honess, P.E. and Marin, C.M. (2006) Enrichment and aggression in primates. *Neuroscience and Biobehavioral Reviews*, **30**, 413–436.

Howerton, C.L., Garner, J.P. and Mench, J.A. (2008) Effects of a running wheel-igloo enrichment on aggression, hierarchy linearity, and stereotypy in group-housed male CD-1 (ICR) mice. *Applied Animal Behaviour Science*, **115**, 90–103.

Hoy, J.M., Murray, P.J. and Tribe, A. (2010) Thirty years later: Enrichment practices for captive mammals. *Zoo Biology*, **29**, 303–316.

Hubrecht, R.C. (1995) Dog welfare. In: *The Domestic Dog: Evolution, Behaviour, and Interactions with People*. Ed. Serpell, J., pp. 179–198. Cambridge University Press, Cambridge.

Hubrecht, R.C., Serpell, J.A. and Poole, T.B. (1992) Correlates of pen size and housing conditions on the behaviour of kennelled dogs. *Applied Animal Behaviour Science*, **34**, 365–383.

Hutchinson, E.K., Avery, A.C. and Vandewoude, S. (2012) Environmental enrichment during rearing alters corticosterone levels, thymocyte numbers, and aggression in female BALB/c mice. *Journal of the American Association for Laboratory Animal Science*, **51**, 18–24.

Jirkof, P. (2015) Effects of experimental housing conditions on recovery of laboratory mice. *Lab Animal*, **44**, 65–70.

Johnson, C.A., Pallozzi, W.A., Geiger, L. et al. (2003) The effect of an environmental enrichment device on individually caged rabbits in a safety assessment facility. *Contemporary Topics in Laboratory Animal Science*, **42**, 27–30.

Kempermann, G. (2019) Environmental enrichment, new neurons and the neurobiology of individuality. *Nature Reviews Neuroscience*, **20**, 235–245.

Kikusui, T., Isaka, Y. and Mori, Y. (2005) Early weaning deprives mouse pups of maternal care and decreases their maternal behavior in adulthood. *Behavioural Brain Research*, **162**, 200–206.

Kirkden, R. and Pajor, E. (2006) Using preference, motivation and aversion tests to ask scientific questions about animals' feelings. *Applied Animal Behaviour Science*, **100**, 29–47.

Lambert, K., Hyer, M., Bardi, M. et al. (2016) Natural-enriched environments lead to enhanced environmental engagement and altered neurobiological resilience. *Neuroscience*, **330**, 386–394.

Larsson, F., Winblad, B. and Mohammed, A.H. (2002) Psychological stress and environmental adaptation in enriched vs. impoverished housed rats. *Pharmacology, Biochemistry and Behavior*, **73**, 193–207.

Leotti, L.A. and Delgado, M.R. (2011) The inherent reward of choice. *Psychological Science*, **22**, 1310–1318.

Lewis, M.H. (2004) Environmental complexity and central nervous system development and function. *Mental Retardation and Developmental Disabilities Research Reviews*, **10**, 91–95.

Lutz, C.K. and Novak, M.A. (2005) Environmental enrichment for non-human primates: theory and application. *ILAR Journal*, **46**, 178–191.

Lutz, C., Well, A. and Novak, M. (2003) Stereotypic and self-injurious behavior in rhesus macaques: a survey and retrospective analysis of environment and early experience. *American Journal of Primatology*, **60**, 1–15.

Makowska, I.J., Franks, B., El-Hinn, C. et al. (2019) Standard laboratory housing for mice restricts their ability to segregate space into clean and dirty areas. *Scientific Reports*, **9**, 1–10.

Makowska, I.J. and Weary, D.M. (2016) The importance of burrowing, climbing and standing upright for laboratory rats. *Royal Society Open Science*, **3**, 160136.

Makowska, I.J. and Weary, D.M. (2019) A good life for laboratory rodents? *ILAR Journal*, **60(3)**, 373–388.

Marashi, V., Barnekow, A., Ossendorf, E. et al. (2003) Effects of different forms of environmental enrichment on behavioral, endocrinological, and immunological parameters in male mice. *Hormones and Behavior*, **43**, 281–292.

Markowitz, H. (1982) *Behavioural Enrichment in the Zoo*. Van Nostrand Reinhold, New York.

Mason, G.J. (1991a) Stereotypies: a critical review. *Animal Behaviour*, **41**, 1015–1037.

Mason, G.J. (1991b) Stereotypies and suffering. *Behavioural Processes*, **25**, 103–115.

Mason, G.J. (2010) Species differences in responses to captivity: stress, welfare and the comparative method. *Trends in Ecology & Evolution*, **25**, 713–721.

Mason, G., Burn, C.C., Dallaire, J.A. et al. (2013) Plastic animals in cages: behavioural flexibility and responses to captivity. *Animal Behaviour*, **85**, 1113–1126.

Mason, G., Clubb, R., Latham, N. and Vickery, S. (2007) Why and how should we use environmental enrichment to tackle stereotypic behaviour? *Applied Animal Behaviour Science*, **102**, 163–188.

Mason, G.J. and Latham, N.R. (2004) Can't stop, won't stop: is stereotypy a reliable animal welfare indicator? *Animal Welfare*, **13**, S57–S69.

McQuaid, R.J., Audet, M.C. and Anisman, H. (2012) Environmental enrichment in male CD-1 mice promotes aggressive behaviors and elevated corticosterone and brain norepinephrine activity in response to a mild stressor. *Stress*, **15**, 354–360.

Meagher, R.K., Dallaire, J.A., Campbell, D.L. et al. (2014) Benefits of a ball and chain: Simple environmental enrichments improve welfare and reproductive success in farmed American mink (*Neovison vison*). *PLOS One*, **9**, e110589.

Meagher, R.K., Campbell, D.L. and Mason, G.J. (2017) Boredom-like states in mink and their behavioural correlates: a replicate study. *Applied Animal Behaviour Science*, **197**, 112–119.

Meijer, M.K., Kramer, K., Remie, R. et al. (2006) The effect of routine experimental procedures on physiological parameters in mice kept under different husbandry conditions. *Animal Welfare*, **15**, 31–38.

Mellor, D.J. (2016) Updating animal welfare thinking: moving beyond the "Five Freedoms" towards "a Life Worth Living". *Animals*, **6**, 21.

Mendl, M., Burman, O.H., Parker, R.M. and Paul, E.S. (2009) Cognitive bias as an indicator of animal emotion and welfare: Emerging evidence and underlying mechanisms. *Applied Animal Behaviour Science*, **118**, 161–181.

Mertens, S., Gass, P., Palme, R. et al. (2020) Effect of a partial cage dividing enrichment on aggression-associated parameters in group-housed male C57BL/6NCrl mice. *Applied Animal Behaviour Science*, 104939.

Mesa-Gresa, P., Pérez-Martinez, A. and Redolat, R. (2013) Environmental enrichment improves novel object recognition and enhances agonistic behavior in male mice. *Aggressive Behavior*, **39**, 269–279.

Meyer-Holzapfel, M. (1968) Abnormal behavior in zoo animals. In: *Abnormal Behavior in Animals*. Ed. Fox, M.W., pp. 476–503. Saunders, Philadelphia.

Murchison, M.A. (1993) Potential animal hazard with ring toys. *Laboratory Primate Newsletter*, **32**, 7.

Nelson, R.J. and Mandrell, T.D. (2005) Enrichment and nonhuman primates: 'First, Do No Harm'. *ILAR Journal*, **46**, 171–177.

Nevison, C.M., Hurst, J.L. and Barnard, C.J. (1999a). Why do male ICR (CD-1) mice perform bar-related (stereotypic) behaviour? *Behavioural Processes*, **47(2)**, 95–111.

Nevison, C.M., Hurst, J.L. and Barnard, C.J. (1999b) Strain-specific effects of cage enrichment in male laboratory mice (*Mus musculus*). *Animal Welfare*, **8**, 361–379.

Newberry, R.C. (1995) Environmental enrichment: increasing the biological relevance of captive environments. *Applied Animal Behaviour Science*, **44**, 229–243.

Nip, E., Adcock, A., Nazal, B. et al. (2019) Why are Enriched Mice Nice? Investigating how environmental enrichment reduces agonism in female C57BL/6, DBA/2, and BALB/c Mice. *Applied Animal Behaviour Science*, **217**, 73–82.

Nithianantharajah, J., Levis, H. and Murphy, M. (2004) Environmental enrichment results in cortical and subcortical changes in levels of synaptophysin and PSD-95 proteins. *Neurobiology of Learning and Memory*, **81**, 200–210.

Novak, J., Stojanovski, K., Melotti, L. et al. (2016) Effects of stereotypic behaviour and chronic mild stress on judgement bias in laboratory mice. *Applied Animal Behaviour Science*, **174**, 162–172.

Novak, M.A., Meyer, J.S., Lutz, C. et al. (2006) Deprived environments: developmental insights from primatology. In: *Stereotypic Animal behaviour: Fundamentals and Applications to Welfare*. Eds. Mason, G. and Rushen, J., pp. 19–57. CAB International, Wallingford.

National Research Council (2008) *Recognition and Alleviation of Distress in Laboratory Animals*. Committee on Recognition and Alleviation of Distress in Laboratory Animals. National Research Council, National Academy Press, Washington, DC.

National Research Council NRC (2011) Guide for the Care and Use of Laboratory Animals. Washington, DC: Committee for the Update of the Guide for the Care and Use of Laboratory Animals. *Institute for Laboratory Animal Research, Division on Earth and Life Studies, National Research Council*.

Ödberg, F.O. (1978) Abnormal behaviours: stereotypies. In: *Proceedings of the First World Congress on Ethology Applied to Zootechnics*, pp. 475–480. Industrias Graficas Espana, Madrid.

Olsson, I.A.S. and Dahlborn, K. (2002) Improving housing conditions for laboratory mice: a review of environmental enrichment. *Laboratory Animals*, **36**, 243–270.

Pietropaolo, S., Branchi, I., Cirulli, F. et al. (2004) Long-term effects of the periadolescent environment on exploratory activity and aggressive behaviour in mice: social versus physical enrichment. *Physiology & Behavior*, **81(3)**, 443–453.

Polanco, A., Díez-León, M. and Mason, G. (2018) Stereotypic behaviours are heterogeneous in their triggers and treatments in the American mink, *Neovison vison*, a model carnivore. *Animal Behaviour*, **141**, 105–114.

Polley, D.B., Kvasnák, E. and Frostig, R.D. (2004) Naturalistic experience transforms sensory maps in the adult cortex of caged animals. *Nature*, **429**, 67–71.

Pomerantz, O., Terkel, J., Suomi, S.J. and Paukner, A. (2012) Stereotypic head twirls, but not pacing, are related to a 'pessimistic'-like judgment bias among captive tufted capuchins (*Cebus apella*). *Animal Cognition*, **15**, 689–698.

Prior, H. and Sachser, N. (1994) Effects of enriched housing environment on the behaviour of young male and female mice in four exploratory tasks. *Journal of Experimental Animal Science*, **37**, 57–68.

Prusky, G.T., Reidel, C. and Douglas, R.M. (2000) Environmental enrichment from birth enhances visual acuity but not place learning in mice. *Behavioural Brain Research*, **114**, 11–15.

Rattazzi, L., Piras, G., Brod, S. et al. (2016) Impact of enriched environment on murine T cell differentiation and gene expression profile. *Frontiers in Immunology*, **7**, 381.

Ratuski, A.S., Makowska, I.J., Dvorack, K.R. and Weary, D.M. (2021) Using approach latency and anticipatory behaviour to assess whether voluntary playpen access is rewarding to laboratory mice. *Scientific Reports*, **11(1)**, 1–13.

Reinhold, A.S., Sanguinetti-Scheck, J.I., Hartmann, K. and Brecht, M. (2019) Behavioral and neural correlates of hide-and-seek in rats. *Science*, **365**, 1180–1183.

Rennie, A.E. and Buchanan-Smith, H.M. (2006) Refinement of the use of non-human primates in scientific research. Part II: housing, husbandry and acquisition. *Animal Welfare*, **15**, 215–238.

Richter, S.H., Garner, J.P. and Würbel, H. (2009) Environmental standardization: cure or cause of poor reproducibility in animal experiments? *Nature Methods*, **6**, 257–261.

Richter, S.H., Schick, A., Hoyer, C. et al. (2012) A glass full of optimism: enrichment effects on cognitive bias in a rat model of depression. *Cognitive Affective & Behavioral Neuroscience*, **12**, 527–542.

Rosenzweig, M.R., Bennett, E.L., Hebert, M. et al. (1978) Social grouping cannot account for cerebral effects of enriched environments. *Brain Research*, **153**, 563–576.

Ross, M., Garland, A., Harlander-Matauschek, A. et al. (2019) Welfare-improving enrichments greatly reduce hens' startle responses, despite little change in judgment bias. *Scientific Reports*, **9**, 1–14.

Russell, W.M.S. and Burch, R.L. (1959) *The Principles of Humane Experimental Technique*. Methuen & Co Ltd, London, reprinted UFAW 1992, Potters Bar.

Sambrook, T.D. and Buchanan-Smith, H.M. (1997) Control and complexity in novel object enrichment. *Animal Welfare*, **6**, 207–216.

Schaller, T.L. (2014) A committee approach to environmental enrichment. American Association for Laboratory Animal Science [AALAS] Meeting Official Program, 534 (Abstract #PS35).

Schapiro, S.J., Bloomsmith, M.A., Suarez, S.A. et al. (1997) A comparison of the effects of simple versus complex environmental enrichment on the behaviour of group-housed, subadult rhesus macaques. *Animal Welfare*, **6**, 17–28.

Schimmel, A. and Hlavka, R. (2014) Enhancing environmental enrichment without breaking the bank. American Association for Laboratory Animal Science [AALAS] Meeting Official Program, 562–563 (Abstract #P51).

Schrijver, N.C.A., Bahr, N.I., Weiss, I.C. and Würbel, H. (2002) Dissociable effects of isolation rearing and environmental enrichment on exploration, spatial learning and HPA activity in adult rats. *Pharmacology Biochemistry and Behavior*, **73**, 209–224.

Shepherdson, D.J. (1998) Tracing the path of environmental enrichment in zoos. In: *Second Nature: Environmental Enrichment for Captive Animals*. Eds Shepherdson, D.J., Mellen, J.D. and Hutchins, M., pp. 1–12. Smithsonian Institution, Washington, DC.

Shepherdson, D.J. (2003) Environmental enrichment: past, present and future. *International Zoo Yearbook*, **38**, 118–124.

Sherwin, C.M. and Olsson, I.A.S. (2004) Housing conditions affect self-administration of anxiolytic by laboratory mice. *Animal Welfare*, **13**, 33–38.

Shyne, A. (2006) Meta-analytic review of the effects of enrichment on stereotypic behavior in zoo mammals. *Zoo Biology*, **25**, 317–337.

Singhal, G., Jaehne, E.J., Corrigan, F. and Baune, B.T. (2014) Cellular and molecular mechanisms of immunomodulation in the brain through environmental enrichment. *Frontiers in Cellular Neuroscience*, **8**, 97.

Spangenberg, E.M. and Wichman, A. (2018) Methods for investigating the motivation of mice to explore and access food rewards. *Journal of the American Association for Laboratory Animal Science*, **57**, 244–252.

Špinka, M. (2019) Animal agency, animal awareness and animal welfare. *Animal Welfare*, **28**(1), 11–20.

Stevens, C., Hawkins, P., Lovell-Badge, R. et al. (2018) Report of the 2016 RSPCA/UFAW Rodent and Rabbit Welfare Group meeting. Animal Technology & Welfare.

Sztainberg, Y., Kuperman, Y., Tsoory, M. et al. (2010) The anxiolytic effect of environmental enrichment is mediated via amygdalar CRF receptor type 1. *Molecular Psychiatry*, **15**, 905–917.

Tallent, B.R., Law, L.M., Rowe, R.K. and Lifshitz, J. (2018) Partial cage division significantly reduces aggressive behavior in male laboratory mice. *Laboratory Animals*, **52**, 384–393.

Taylor, J.H., Mustoe, A.C. and French, J.A. (2014) Behavioral responses to social separation stressor change across development and are dynamically related to HPA activity in marmosets. *American Journal of Primatology*, **76**(3), 239–248.

Tilly, S.L.C., Dallaire, J. and Mason, G.J. (2010) Middle-aged mice with enrichment-resistant stereotypic behaviour show reduced motivation for enrichment. *Animal Behaviour*, **80**, 363–373.

Toth, L.A., Kregel, K., Leon, L. and Musch, T.I. (2011) Environmental enrichment of laboratory rodents: the answer depends on the question. *Comparative Medicine*, **61**, 314–321.

Urakawa, S., Takamoto, K., Hori, E. et al. (2013) Rearing in enriched environment increases parvalbumin-positive small neurons in the amygdala and decreases anxiety-like behavior of male rats. *BMC Neuroscience*, **14**, 13.

Van de Weerd, H.A., Aarsen, E.L., Mulder, A. et al. (2002) Effects of environmental enrichment for mice: variation in experimental results. *Journal of Applied Animal Welfare Science*, **5**, 87–109.

Van Loo, P.L.P., Kruitwagen, C.L.J.J., Koolhaas, J.M. et al. (2002) Influence of cage enrichment on aggressive behaviour and physiological parameters in male mice. *Applied Animal Behaviour Science*, **76**, 65–81.

Van Loo, P.L.P., van der Meer, E., Kruitwagen, C.L.J.J. et al. (2004) Long-term effects of husbandry procedures on stress-related parameters in male mice of two strains. *Laboratory Animals*, **38**, 169–177.

van Praag, H., Kempermann, G. and Gage, F.H. (2000) Neural consequences of environmental enrichment. *Nature Reviews: Neuroscience*, **1**, 191–198.

Varman, D.R. and Rajan, K.E. (2015) Environmental enrichment reduces anxiety by differentially activating serotonergic and neuropeptide Y (NPY)-ergic system in Indian field mouse (*Mus booduga*): an animal model of post-traumatic stress disorder. *PLOS One*, **10**, e0127945.

Vignes, S., Newman, J.D. and Roberts, R.L. (2001) Mealworm feeders as environmental enrichment for common marmosets. *Contemporary Topics in Laboratory Animal Science*, **40**, 26–29.

Vitalo, A.G., Gorantla, S., Fricchione, J.G. et al. (2012) Environmental enrichment with nesting material accelerates wound healing in isolation-reared rats. *Behavioural Brain Research*, **226**(2), 606–612.

Voelkl, B. and Würbel, H. (2016) Reproducibility crisis: are we ignoring reaction norms? *Trends in Pharmacological Sciences*, **37**, 509–510.

Walker, M.D. and Mason, G. (2011) Female C57BL/6 mice show consistent individual differences in spontaneous interaction with environmental enrichment that are predicted by neophobia. *Behavioural Brain Research*, **224**, 207–212.

Walker, M. and Mason, G. (2018) Using mildly electrified grids to impose costs on resource access: A potential tool for assessing motivation in laboratory mice. *Applied Animal Behaviour Science*, **198**, 101–108.

Wiedenmayer, C. (1997) Causation of the ontogenetic development of stereotypic digging in gerbils. *Animal Behaviour*, **53**, 461–470.

Wiepkema, P.R. and Koolhaas, J.M. (1993) Stress and animal welfare. *Animal Welfare*, **2**, 195–218.

Winnicker, C., Gaskill, B., Garner, J. and Prichett-Corning, K.R. (2012) *A Guide to the behavior & Enrichment of Laboratory Rodents*. Charles River Laboratories.

Wolfer, D.P., Litvin, O., Morf, S. et al. (2004) Laboratory animal welfare. Cage enrichment and mouse behaviour. *Nature*, **432**, 821–822.

Wolfle, T.L. (2005) Environmental enrichment. *ILAR Journal*, **46**, 79–82.

Würbel, H. (2000) Behaviour and the standardization fallacy. *Nature Genetics*, **26**, 263.

Würbel, H. (2001) Ideal homes? Housing effects on rodent brain and behaviour. *Trends in Neurosciences*, **24**, 207–211.

Würbel, H. (2006) The motivational basis of caged rodents' stereotypies. In: *Stereotypic Animal Behaviour: Fundamentals and Applications to Welfare*. Eds Mason, G. and Rushen, J., pp. 19–57. CABI, Wallingford.

Würbel, H. (2009) Ethology applied to animal ethics. *Applied Animal Behaviour Science*, **118**, 118–127.

Würbel, H. (2017) More than 3Rs: the importance of scientific validity for harm-benefit analysis of animal research. *Laboratory Animal*, **46**, 164–166.

Würbel, H., Chapman, R. and Rutland, C. (1998) Effect of feed and environmental enrichment on development of stereotypic wire-gnawing in laboratory mice. *Applied Animal Behaviour Science*, **60**, 69–81.

Würbel, H. and Garner, J.P. (2007) Refinement of rodent research through environmental enrichment and systematic randomization. NC3Rs Article #9.

Würbel, H. and Stauffacher M. (1994) Standardhaltung für Labormäuse – Probleme und Lösungsasätze. *Tierlaboratorium*, **17**, 109–118. https://www.nc3rs.org.uk/sites/default/files/documents/Refinementenvironmentalenrichmentandsystematicrandomization.pdf (accessed 3 April 2020).

Yeates, J.W. and Main, D.C. (2008) Assessment of positive welfare: a review. *The Veterinary Journal*, **175**, 293–300.

Yeates, J. (2012) Quality time: Temporal and other aspects of ethical principles based on a "life worth living". *Journal of Agricultural and Environmental Ethics*, **25**, 607–624.

Young, R.J. (2003) *Environmental Enrichment for Captive Animals*. Blackwell Publishing, Oxford.

Zhang, Y., Crofton, E.J., Fan, X. et al. (2016) Convergent transcriptomics and proteomics of environmental enrichment and cocaine identifies novel therapeutic strategies for addiction. *Neuroscience*, **339**, 254–266.

Zhang, T.Y., Keown, C.L., Wen, X. et al. (2018) Environmental enrichment increases transcriptional and epigenetic differentiation between mouse dorsal and ventral dentate gyrus. *Nature Communications*, **9**, 1–11.

Zimmermann, A., Stauffacher, M., Langhans, W. and Würbel, H. (2001) Enrichment-dependent differences in novelty exploration in rats can be explained by habituation. *Behavioural Brain Research*, **121**, 11–20.

11 Special housing arrangements

Mike Dennis

Introduction

While it is desirable to maintain laboratory animals in accommodation that is as close as possible (excluding harmful aspects) to their natural habitats, there are several reasons why special housing arrangements are required in some cases, in order to meet more exacting experimental requirements than are provided by conventional caging or penning systems.

Special housing arrangements may be required to achieve any of the following:

- to prevent contamination of germ-free animals.
- to protect animals that are particularly sensitive to infection, for example, genetically immunocompromised animals such as severe combined immunodeficient (SCID) or nude (athymic) mice.
- to protect animal handlers from allergens or infections that are deemed to be a potential risk (e.g., from animals of unknown health provenance or that have been administered an infectious agent).
- to isolate (quarantine) animals of unknown microbiological status that might pose an infection risk to other animals within a facility.

Many approaches and systems have been developed over the years to address these issues, but the main principles involve a physical barrier, a directional/laminar airflow or a combination of both.

Physical barriers may be provided by:

- protective clothing;
- animal rooms;
- flexible film or rigid isolators;
- filter-top boxes;
- independently ventilated cages;
- laminar flow hoods;
- isolation booths;
- rigid cabinets.

Although all barriers, even one as simple as the handler wearing protective clothing, can have an impact upon the welfare of the animals, there is still an obligation to ensure that the mental and physical needs of animals in our care are met wherever possible by addressing what are frequently referred to as the 'Five Freedoms': Freedom from Hunger and Thirst, Discomfort, Pain, Injury or Disease, Fear and Distress and freedom to express normal behaviours (Webster 2005) or the more recent framework suggested by Mellor (2016) of 'a life worth living'. Addressing these issues may, of course, be somewhat limited by enrolment of animals in scientific procedures.

This chapter will not detail legislative requirements but will address the practical aspects affecting the welfare of animals held in special housing. It will first describe the types of containment systems currently in use and then address their use with individual species together with suggested methods for optimising welfare. It will not cover highly specialised housing situations such as metabolic cages, isolation chambers for determining methane production (Llonch *et al.* 2016) or harnessing for periods of microdialysis (Lanni *et al.* 2021). While the welfare concerns associated with their use are in many ways similar to those associated with those described in this chapter, there may be additional factors such as single housing that increase the severity rating and require specific permission/justification from the relevant licencing authorities.

In addition, it must be considered that the majority of special housing environments and strategies described here have been put in place to provide protection to staff or the environment from infectious agents in line with legislation. Biocontainment strategies are required by national regulatory bodies such as the Health and Safety Executive (HSE) in the UK and meeting these safety imperatives can often conflict with legislation covering the scientific use of animals that demands optimisation of welfare for animals involved in experiments. Staff familiar with individual animals and species biology should be those that assess clinical or behavioural signs. Humane endpoints with clear definition of criteria that are unambiguous and easy to evaluate should be used. Animals should be acclimatised to the containment system or to protective clothing, using staff who are familiar to the animals.

Enrichment should be designed to increase an animal's number and range of normal behaviours, decrease abnormal behaviours, increase interaction with the environment and enhance its ability to cope with behavioural and physiological challenges imposed by housing within specialised environments.

The UFAW Handbook on the Care and Management of Laboratory and Other Research Animals, Ninth Edition.
Edited by Huw Golledge and Claire Richardson.
© 2024 John Wiley & Sons Ltd. Published 2024 by John Wiley & Sons Ltd.

Types of containment

Protective clothing

This is probably the most common physical barrier used in animal facilities. Personal protective equipment (PPE) may be as simple as a gown over normal clothing and a pair of gloves but may also include hats and masks. For higher levels of operator protection, it may be necessary to undertake a complete change of clothes and to use respiratory protective equipment (RPE) (Figure 11.1). Other protection strategies may require the use of powered respirators or suits with their own integral air supplies, depending on the danger presented by the infectious or chemical agent that is being used (Figures 11.2 and 11.3).

Welfare considerations

Protective clothing may impact on animal welfare in a number of ways. This impact may be accentuated if a sudden change in regime is adopted, for example after an experimental challenge with an infectious agent (i.e., a sudden change in appearance and practices may well have an influence on the dynamics of the relationship between the animal, its handler and even its cage mates). Animals that have become habituated to their care staff may be affected by any of the following changes:

- Odours: the use of PPE may remove smells that have become familiar to the animals; or PPE equipment may have a distinctive odour of its own that is unfamiliar and may be aversive to the animals.
- Colours: a change in the colour of protective apparel from the previous everyday laboratory gown can affect some species.
- Noise from powered air supplies: these can disturb animals and even if they may seem quiet to the wearer, there can be sub- or super-sonic noise that certain species find disturbing.

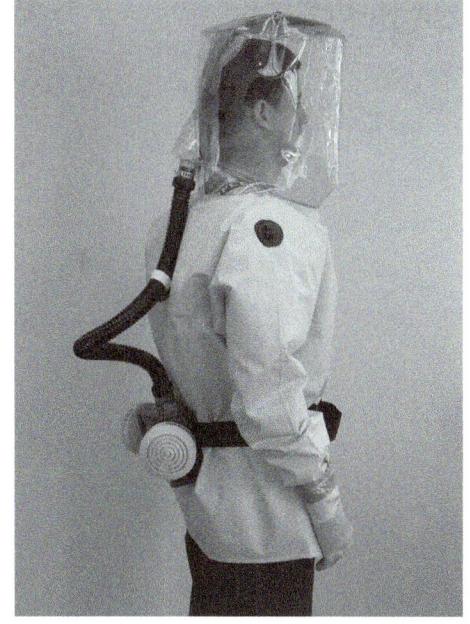

Figure 11.2 A Martindale-type suit with a filtered, powered air supply. Source: Courtesy of UK Health Security Agency.

- Visibility:
  - the profile of an individual may be changed by protective wear such that they can no longer be recognised. Face masks or other RPE hide usual visual signals that are used by some species for recognition and to assess intent.
  - the vision of the operator may be restricted either directly or by reduction of peripheral awareness such that observation of subtle changes in appearance or behaviour are impaired.
- The complex configuration of a high containment suite may result in startling by sudden appearance without the usual clues of approach (e.g., if emerging from a

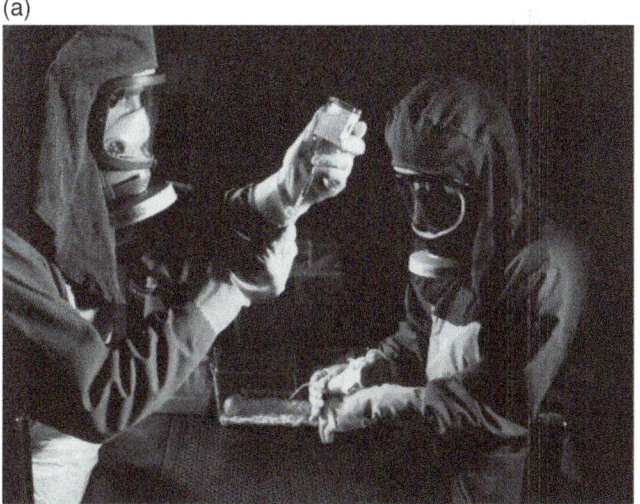
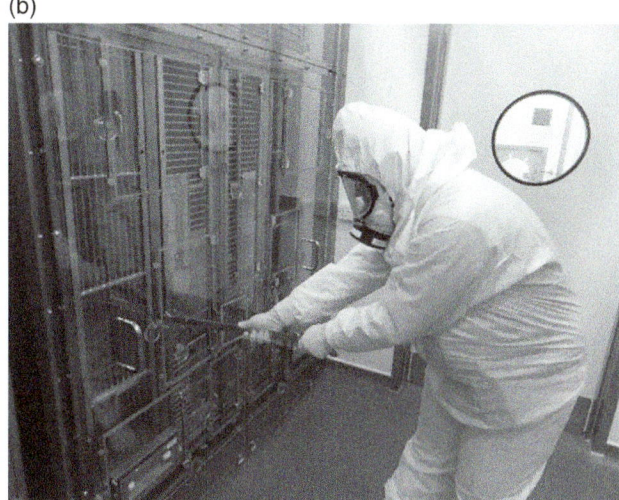

Figure 11.1 (a) The use of RPE plus down-draught table and RPE plus protective Tyvek suit to protect the operators during procedures or husbandry tasks on infected animals. Source: Courtesy of UK Health Security Agency.

152 Special housing arrangements

Welfare aspects of higher levels of PPE (e.g., suits, half suits, powered RPE with full clothing change)

The use of specialised apparel with higher levels of PPE usually involves strict changing and showering regimes that are time-consuming and reduce the number of visits that can be made per day. Copps (2005) in a review of the issues related to the use of animals in containment facilities pointed out that the higher the level of biocontainment, the longer it took to conduct a simple procedure such as taking a blood sample due to the length of time required to put on and remove protective clothing and to undergo decontamination procedures. The example given was that removing a blood sample from a pig took 15 minutes at biocontainment level (BCL) 2, 30 minutes at BCL3 and an hour at BCL4. This would also apply to the ability to respond in a timely manner to any welfare issue that may arise. In addition, protective equipment can restrict movement, hearing and dexterity, and its use has an inherent level of discomfort that reduces the amount of time that can be safely spent on any one visit. A further problem with this equipment is the lack of facial signals to animals because of reduced clarity or reflectivity of visors or other headgear. While some protective clothing may be considered to provide more facial visibility (e.g. Martindale-type suits) other considerations such as dexterity, ergonomics and verbal communication might indicate the use of other strategies at high biocontainment levels.

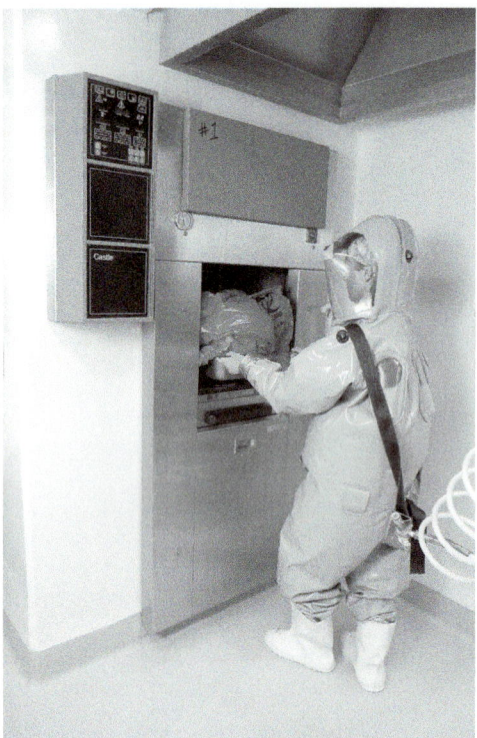

Figure 11.3 A one-piece full suit that might be required for work with dangerous pathogens. Source: Courtesy of the Canadian Science Centre for Human & Animal Health.

The animal room

In some cases, the boundaries of the animal room itself may be considered as the primary barrier between the animals and the rest of the facility. This type of barrier system is likely to be required where the work involves species that cannot be housed with any degree of practicability in other containment systems. Examples may include juvenile or adult farm animals such as cattle, pigs, or sheep or other species such as cervids (Figure 11.4). In such cases and where high-level

changing room, rather than directly from a corridor). Wherever possible, this effect can be minimised by the strategic placement of windows in doors to increase visibility while giving due regard for modesty during changes of clothing or showering.
- Gloves: the wearing of gloves has been shown to affect dexterity and this may result in clumsier, more stressful handling of smaller species.

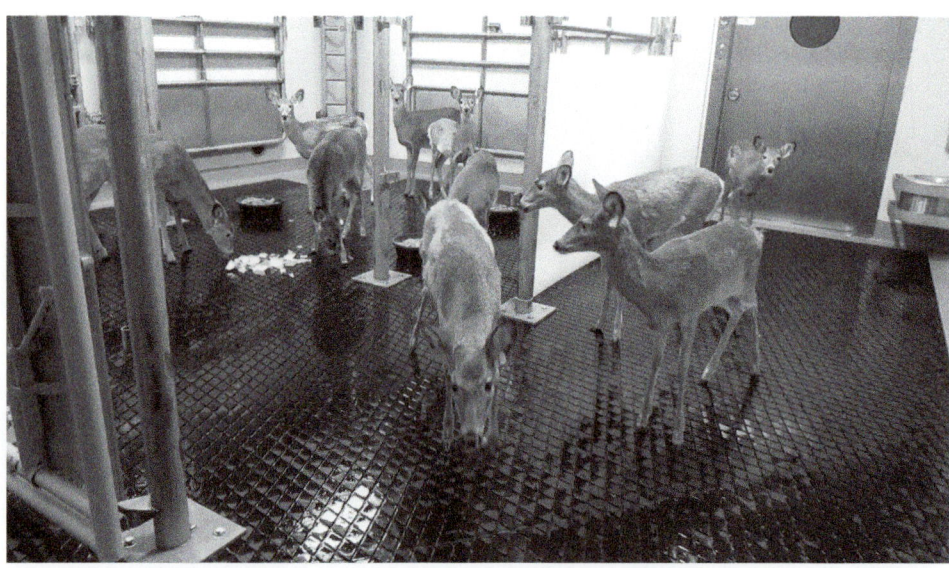

Figure 11.4 White-tailed deer in biocontainment (Source: Courtesy of VIDO-intervac, Saskatoon, Canada).

biocontainment is required, the room might need to be modified and this may impact upon animal welfare in ways that are not immediately obvious. Containment of pathogens dangerous to humans or to other animals may require the provision of en suite changing rooms, showers, fumigation chambers and autoclaves. The supply air, extracted air – or both – may require high-efficiency particulate air (HEPA) filtration, and the room may need to be maintained at negative pressure, depending on the defined biosafety level.

Welfare considerations

Safety and biocontainment legislation such as those relating to high consequence animal or human pathogens and genetically manipulated organisms (GMOs) will inevitably drive the design of facilities and the practices within a particular room: for example, if effluent treatment is part of the containment strategy, then the use of water for cleaning may be restricted. In addition, the type of bedding that can be used may have to be modified to avoid blocking the drains that lead to the treatment plant. Due consideration needs to be given to where procedures and necropsies are to be performed, bearing in mind both the welfare of other animals and any safety requirement to prevent release of pathogens. It is highly likely, where the confines of the room itself are used as the primary barrier, that protocols will also prescribe some level of protective clothing for animal care and scientific staff, as described in the section on clothing in the preceding text. The needs of high-level biocontainment may dictate the use of sealable submarine-type doors to prevent escape of pathogens, to enhance air pressure cascades and to allow regular fumigation. Current biosecurity and health and safety requirements are often stringent in demanding that facilities using certain infectious agents should have robust physical security, such as coded locks or swipe access, to limit access. As these layers of mechanical or procedural strategies are built up to address safety issues or to ensure the integrity of the experiment, then more attention needs to be paid to the impact upon the welfare of the animals and adherence to any welfare legislation, as they become more isolated from the rest of the facility and its day-to-day activities. Table 11.1 provides a summary of potential welfare issues and solutions relating to using rooms as a barrier.

Staff training

Use of the highly specialised systems and strategies described here requires a high level of staff training and competence in order to ensure staff safety and animal welfare. It is essential, therefore, to have in place a rigorous competency framework with sufficient staff to provide resilience to meet the needs of such demanding work. It is essential that staff are fully trained to understand animals' behaviour and the impact of their own behaviour so as to minimise stress or aggression.

Flexible film isolators

Flexible film isolators are used extensively for the microbial isolation of experimental animals. The original flexible film isolators were developed by Trexler and Reynolds (1957), and designed specifically to maintain germ-free (animals with no detectable microbial flora) or gnotobiotic animals (derived germ-free but having a defined, given microbial agent) and to prevent contamination of these animals by environmental microbes. Germ-free animals are derived free of microbial contamination by removal directly from the uterus under sterile conditions either by hysterotomy or hysterectomy in the case of mammals (decontamination of newborn has also been reported) or by decontamination of eggs in the case of birds.

Flexible film technology has proved to be extremely effective and adaptable as a microbiological barrier and a wide range of species, from rodents to farm animals such as pigs, sheep and calves, have been maintained under germ-free or gnotobiotic conditions (Tavernor et al. 1971; Alexander et al. 1973; Dennis et al. 1976). Microbial isolation is achieved by the physical barrier of the flexible film canopy, enhanced by positive pressure and HEPA filtration of both incoming and outgoing air.

Germ-free or gnotobiotic animals have become a powerful tool for investigating the functional effects of the microbiome on a range of human disorders (Basic & Bleich 2019) and interaction with pathogens (Kim et al. 2020). They are used to investigate the development of the immune system (Butler et al. 2005; Hope et al. 2005); the influence of microbiota on the brain and behaviour (Luczynski et al. 2016) in studies of gene expression (Chowdhury et al. 2007) or to provide an insight into diseases of unknown aetiology (Wyatt et al. 1979; Bridger et al. 1984). Mobile versions of plastic film isolators have recently been developed to enable medical imaging of infected animals using mobile scanners (Dennis et al. 2015).

Welfare and handling considerations

The use of isolators can impact upon animal handling with potential knock-on welfare consequences in various ways:

- If the operator's vision is reduced or restricted, this may impact upon animal observations and checks on wellbeing. Plastic canopies, even if of clear PVC, will reduce optical clarity, although clearer panels can be introduced to enhance visibility in key areas of the canopy.
- Reduced dexterity may affect the handling of smaller species and hinder sampling or administration procedures. Access to cages and to the animals will be via glove sleeves built into the walls of the isolator (Figure 11.5) or by the use of integral half suits (Figure 11.6). These gloves will normally be fixed in place and will thus have to be of a size to accommodate all users.
- The length and position of glove sleeves may mean that there are certain areas within the isolator that cannot be reached. There needs to be a contingency plan in place to deal with animals that have escaped from cages within the isolator so that this will not compromise the experiment (e.g., by chewing through the isolator wall or a glove) or stress the animals during attempts at recapture.
- While not a direct effect of the use of isolators, the reason for their use should be considered in the context of good practice to ensure animal welfare: For example, the reduced or absent gut microflora of gnotobiotic animals

Special housing arrangements

Table 11.1 Potential welfare issues of the room as a containment barrier.

Parameter	Potential welfare issues	Solution
HEPA filtration	Room reliant on air-handling system for adequate ventilation/environmental control. Failure of fans could lead to inability to control temperature, humidity and build-up of waste gases	Build in redundancy on air handling equipment and have reliable emergency power with automatic cut in
Negative (or positive) air pressure	Pressure differentials need to be well controlled, such that sudden changes in pressure are avoided, as these can be distressing	Have reliable feedback linkage between supply and extract, build in a delay in variable fan speed to allow for door opening between rooms or changing areas
Limited access due to time-consuming changing and showering regimes	Reduced time and frequency of observation and interaction with animals	Consider CCTV and environmental enrichment appropriate for species such as TVs on timers. Consider practices that reduce the time taken to enter/exit (e.g., is showering necessary? Could air showers be used to speed up the process?)
En suite autoclave/fumigation chamber	Exposure to noise, heat, noxious fumes	Ensure good sound and heat insulation, use an ante-room if possible, have local ventilation that will cope with steam or leakage of fumigant. Ensure compliance with national safety regulations by regular testing of door seals or other areas of potential egress
Procedures and necropsies	Requirement for biocontainment may limit separate procedures room or use of a shared remote post-mortem room. Animals will potentially become distressed if their cage mates are killed within sight, sound or smell so this should be considered as appropriate the species concerned	Animals should be removed from any husbandry room to an area that prevents sight, sound and smell so a separate procedures/necropsy area should be designed with this in mind and include cascade pressure regime away from the animal accommodation to the procedures area
Effluent treatment	Capacity issues or fear of blockage may restrict use of water and certain types of bedding. This may impact on natural behaviours such as foraging for food and may lead to a build-up of faeces or urine if wash-down restricted	Consider using a system of screen filters for the drains and have separated areas where deep litter can be used and then bagged for disposal
Use of PPE/RPE	1. Stress may be caused by unfamiliar suits/respirators and lack of usual facial and olfactory signals 2. Time taken to respond to a welfare issue will increase at higher levels of biocontainment due to the lengthy time it takes to change into the equipment and enter the unit	1. Acclimatise animals by wearing apparel on occasions before study start or by hanging suits in room 2. Consider use of CCTV and refinement of welfare monitoring strategies to allow early humane intervention. This would involve the evolution of stringent clinical scoring systems based on experience with a particular pathogen, and protocols that trigger prompt progression from CCTV observation to physical intervention
Requirements of disease hygiene/biosecurity	The need to keep rooms clean/disinfected for biosecurity reasons may lead to creation of a barren environment	Creative use of space, use of cleanable/disposable items for enrichment

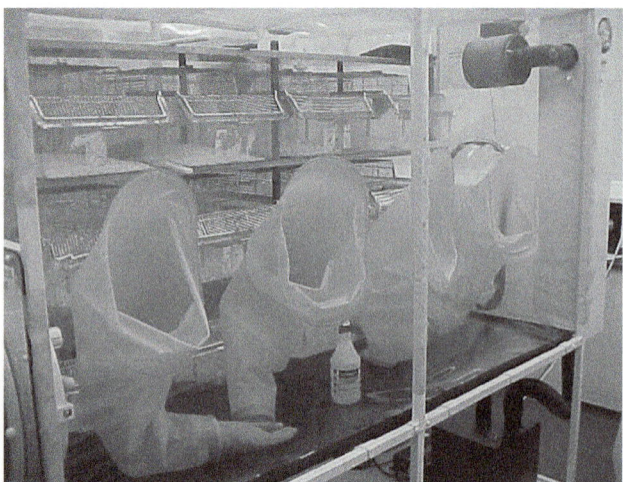

Figure 11.5 A flexible film isolator used to house infected mice or guinea pigs. Source: Courtesy of UK Health Security Agency.

may affect their digestion or utilisation of nutrients that are usually made available by commensal organisms. In addition, the normal microflora may act as a barrier to pathogenic or opportunist organisms, and animals in which this flora is absent or restricted may be more susceptible to infection.

- Some species may be colostrum-deprived in order to maintain naïve immune status and so be deficient in protective maternal antibodies, resulting in greater susceptibility to disease by opportunist organisms, or to any pathogens given experimentally.

The environment within isolators is dependent upon a constant adequate airflow through the isolator to prevent high temperature, high humidity or excesses of gases such as of ammonia and carbon dioxide and welfare will be at risk if these systems should fail. However, with the latest technology, the smaller air spaces involved provide the opportunity to control temperature and humidity within much tighter ranges.

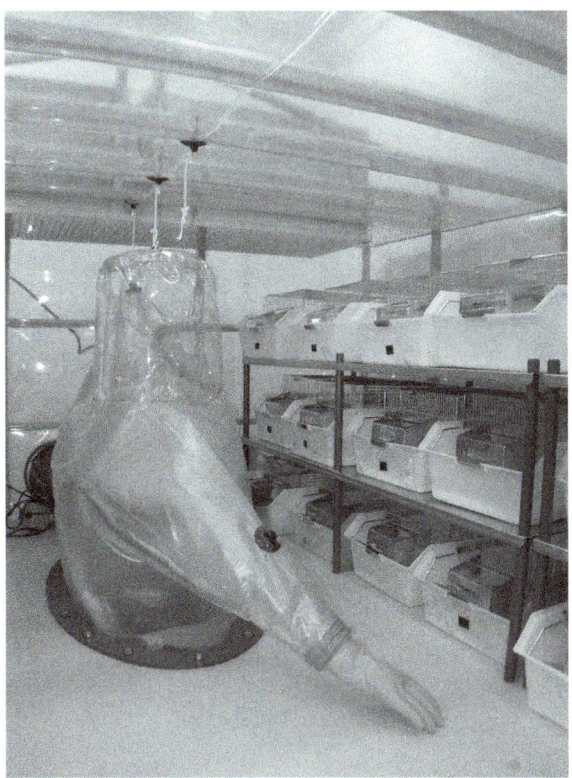

Figure 11.6 The interior of a half-suit isolator used to house infected guinea pigs. Source: Courtesy of UK Health Security Agency.

Activities such as the removal of waste and introduction of food, water, bedding and other materials into isolators pose risks to the integrity of the system and require strict decontamination protocols. Usually, these materials are pre-sterilised by autoclaving, filtration or irradiation and sealed into plastic bags or other containers that can then be introduced to the isolator via a transfer port after surface decontamination. It is important to check that treating food by autoclaving or irradiation will not result in loss of essential trace elements or nutritional value. Wherever possible, such diet should be obtained from commercial suppliers who can provide a certificate of analysis of nutritional content.

The use of chemical disinfection may potentially expose animals to unpleasant or toxic fumes. It is important to select non-toxic disinfectants, those that break down rapidly to non-toxic components (e.g., peracetic acid breaks down to water, carbon dioxide and oxygen) or to design isolators to have some sort of ventilation system to remove unpleasant or toxic fumes.

More recently, isolator technology has been adapted as a strategy for primary containment of infected animals and, in this scenario, the isolator is maintained under negative pressure to enhance operator protection (Figures 11.5 and 11.6). The same points listed apply regarding potential impact on animal welfare. Flexible canopies need robust support to prevent collapse on to the animals' cages due to the negative pressure (UK Health and Safety Executive guidelines (Guidance on the use, testing and maintenance of laboratory and animal isolators for the containment of biological agents[1]) recommend a minimum operating pressure of 30 Pa below laboratory pressure). In order to safeguard animals' welfare, isolators need to be equipped with alarms that indicate out-of-range pressure changes and air supply failure. They also need to be linked to standby generators and to emergency battery back-up that will cut in to maintain the air supply, allowing sufficient operating time to allow any remedial action to be completed. Isolators are now used to house a number of species such as mice, guinea pigs and ferrets at the highest level of biocontainment (BCL4), and the added complexity required to address safety issues demands highly trained and experienced staff to operate safely and to monitor animal welfare (Figure 11.7; Advisory Committee on Dangerous Pathogens Management of hazard Group 4 viral haemorrhagic fevers and similar human infectious diseases of high consequence 2015).

Rigid isolators

Rigid isolators operate in the same way as flexible film isolators, but their walls are made of rigid plastic. This makes them more resistant to physical damage, but the rigid nature of the walls limits the access reach of glove sleeves; this normally necessitates the use of integral half suits to improve access and user ergonomics. The other disadvantage of these isolators is that they are less able to absorb sudden pressure fluctuations such as those that occur when entering the glove sleeves or half suit and this could potentially compromise the protective efficacy of a negative- or positive-pressure regime unless carefully managed. Rigid isolators have been used where a more robust structure is required such as for housing infected marmosets (Brown & Hearson 2008) or poultry (Timms et al. 1979). Table 11.2 provides a summary of potential welfare issues and solutions relating to using isolators.

Individually ventilated cages

The principle of the individually ventilated cage (IVC) is for each to be a mini containment system (Figure 11.8), mostly to house small rodents. Each cage has a removable lid that, for effective containment purposes, is clamped and sealed to the top rim of the cage. Ventilation for the occupants is provided by plugging each cage into a dedicated rack system that has either an integrated air supply/extract or which, less frequently, plumbs into the room air-handling system in some way. The supply and extract air can be balanced to provide either positive or negative pressure within the cage, depending upon the experimental requirements. For effective high-level biocontainment, the integrity of these air penetrations is managed by use of small in-line HEPA filters or by snap-shut valve systems or a combination of both. IVCs are often used as the preferred option for protecting staff from exposure to animal allergens (Renström et al. 2001; Feistenauer et al. 2014) or, in older facilities, as a less expensive method of meeting recommended air change rates, in place of total

---

[1] https://www.hse.gov.uk/biosafety/isolators.pdf (Accessed 21 February 2022)

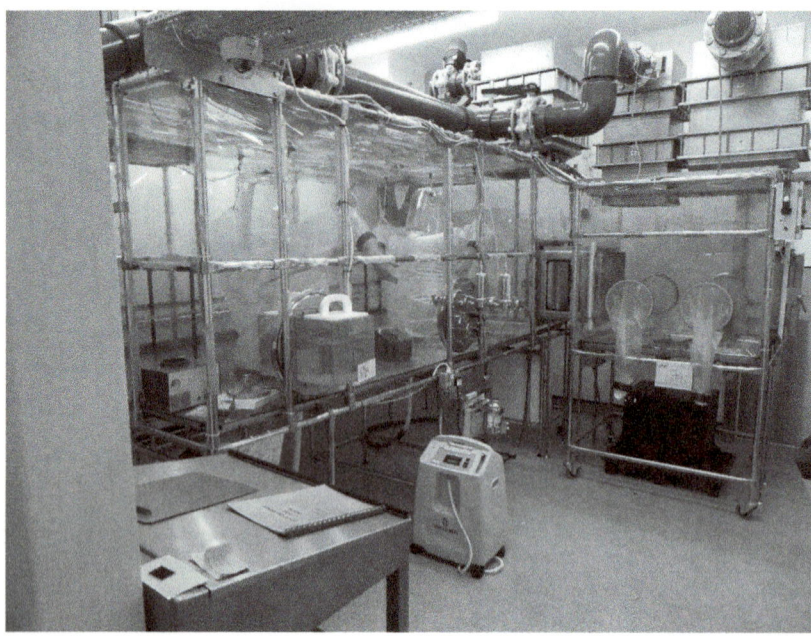

Figure 11.7 The added complexities of operating at BCL4. Source: Courtesy of UK Health Security Agency.

Table 11.2 Potential welfare issues of isolators.

Parameter	Potential welfare issues	Solution
Air supply	Restricted space requires constant airflow to be maintained to provide oxygen and avoid unsuitably high humidity, temperature fluctuations or build-up of waste gases (e.g., ammonia). Failure of power or fans will rapidly cause problems. Air supply and extract fans may provide vibration that may disturb certain species	Have over-capacity for fans. Have reserve fan or twin-motored fan. Emergency generator is essential and battery back-up to power fans is recommended. Alarms and out-of-hours response to alarms. Minimise vibration by use of remote fans and sound insulated ducting
Use of supply ports	Potential route for contamination. Potential for exposure to chemical disinfectants	Minimise frequency of use of entry ports by use of supply isolators and/or extended waste bags. Choose disinfectants that will decompose into non-toxic components or ventilate the port
Sterilisation of food	This may affect nutritional value	Select least drastic sterilisation technique. When specifying diet composition, allow for decay of essential vitamins or trace elements. This assessment should be species-specific
Interaction with staff	Reduced visibility, dexterity and ergonomics may limit observation of animals, precision for handling or procedures and may reduce the time staff can spend at one session	Consider lighting levels, glove positions, number of cages per isolator and positioning. Consider integral half suits for improved ergonomics. Environmental enrichment and group housing can be the same as for conventional rooms
Reduced social interaction	Limited space within isolators may induce social isolation in some species	House in compatible groups wherever possible and consider caging that provides visual, aural and olfactory contact. Provide increased bedding and enrichment as appropriate for species
Procedures and necropsies	Confined space and biosafety requirements may lead to procedures and necropsies being performed in close proximity to other animals	Where possible have a separate isolator or cabinet attached for conduct of procedures/necropsies. For more intricate procedures, removal to a downdraught table may be required to improve dexterity and duration of procedure
Absence of natural microflora	Germ-free or gnotobiotic state may affect ability to utilise food	Consider supplementation of diet or possibility of introducing a balanced microflora
Escape from cage	Escaped animals may damage canopy or sleeves and this may compromise the experiment	A strict regime of checking cage security is required. Caps can be used to prevent access to glove sleeves
General ergonomics	There may be areas in the isolator that cannot be reached due to restrictions of glove sleeves	Design out any dead spaces or ensure that some form of humane capture such as netting can be used successfully
Staff competence	These systems are highly specialised and demand complex protocols for effective operation	Have in place a rigorous competency framework that includes training and onward mentoring of an adequately sized team to allow for staff absence/leave

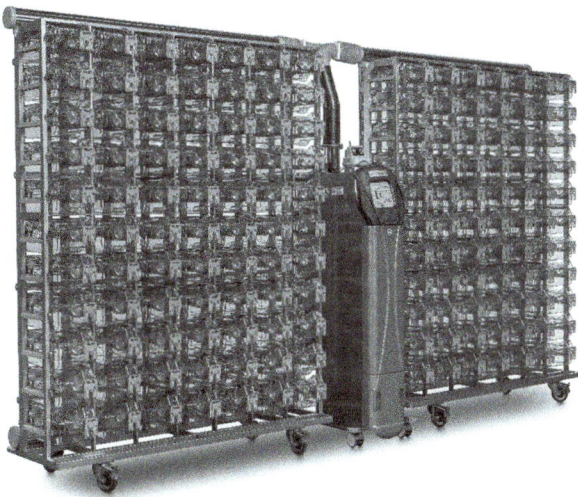

Figure 11.8 A rack of IVCs used to house mice (Source: Courtesy of Tecniplast UK).

refurbishment. Studies have been reported comparing the efficacy of IVCs to isolators in maintaining microbiological status (Lundberg 2017) and one group has reported using a combination of IVCs and Biobubble technology as a less technically demanding method of conducting microbiome research (Ka et al. 2021).

Welfare considerations in the use of IVCs

Individually ventilated cages are capable of providing good air change rates and environmental conditions when working well (Clough et al. 1995; Teixeira et al. 2006). However, dust clogging of filters may affect performance (Höglund & Renström 2001). They can provide protection from external disease or cross-contamination from experimental infection (Lipman et al. 1993; Morrell 1997), but there is reduced visibility of the occupants. To improve visibility, the food hopper can be moved to the rear of the cage.

Kallnik et al. (2007) found that, for some inbred mouse strains, housing in IVCs reduced activity and increased anxiety-related behaviour, and Logge et al. (2014) reported that IVC housing affected the behaviour of mutant or genetically modified mice and recommended that publications, particularly in the field of behavioural studies, should provide more detail on the cage systems used.

David et al. (2013) reported that the use of IVCs can induce cold stress in mice and that this can introduce experimental variability in a tumour growth model compared to conventional housing but that this could be avoided by the provision of shelters and nesting material. Spangenberg et al. (2014) reported differences in maternal performance and pup development in different types of IVC and attributed this mainly to the physical construction of the cage and position of air inlet and outlets.

IVC cages are labour-intensive to service: a change of bedding requires transfer of each cage to cabinet prior to removal of lid and strict disinfection regimes to prevent cross-contamination (Figure 11.9) (Höglund & Renström 2001). There is a risk of uneven distribution of air throughout cages

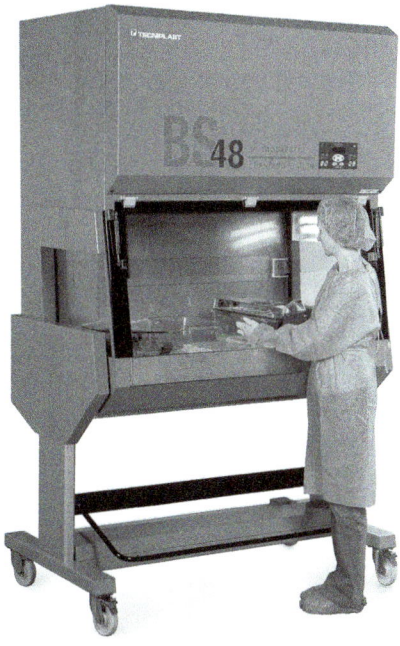

Figure 11.9 An IVC being serviced in a Class-II-type cabinet (Source: Courtesy of Tecniplast UK).

depending on their position on the rack but more recently the majority of commercially available systems have improved airflow technology to avoid this issue. Other potential disadvantages or problems include:

- There is a risk of suffocation if the air supply fails (therefore, they need good back-up support and visible evidence of airflows for each cage on the rack, plus good alarm systems) (Krohn & Hansen 2002). An uninterruptible power supply (UPS) is essential to guarantee the well-being of the occupants.
- Care must be taken that the noise and vibration of air handling units is not transferred to the cages. This should include any frequencies beyond the normal human range. Noise-level considerations should also extend to the cabinet where cage changes or procedures may be conducted.
- Disturbance during cage changes may affect breeding performance (Reeb-Whitaker et al. 2001). In the most recent systems, the improved level of ventilation means that cages need cleaning out at fortnightly rather than weekly intervals.
- Reduced frequency of cleaning may mean that welfare problems may go unnoticed unless a strict discipline of observation by animal care staff is enforced. This practice may also require the use of large food hoppers and drinking bottles that may intrude upon and reduce the amount of three-dimensional cage space available to the occupants.

A drive towards more efficient use of room space may lead to the deployment of cage racks that are too tall for direct observation of all animals. Similarly, library racking systems may present a tempting economy of room usage but working practices must be in place to ensure that cages are observed at least once per day by a competent individual.

158 Special housing arrangements

The environment in which a laboratory animal is housed can significantly influence its behaviour and welfare, acting as a potential confounding factor for those studies in which it is utilised. Burman *et al.* (2014) investigated the impact of two Individually Ventilated Cage (IVC) housing systems on anxiety-related behaviour and welfare indicators in two common strains of laboratory mice and showed significant differences between strains and housing systems. Increased anxiety and aggression have been reported in highly ventilated cages due to odours related to maintenance of the social dominance hierarchy being constantly removed (Logge *et al.* 2013).

Table 11.3 provides a summary of potential welfare issues and solutions relating to using IVCs.

Filter-top cages

Filter-top cages provide a simple method of preventing cross-contamination between cages by providing a physical barrier to larger particles (Figure 11.10). Typically, they consist of a

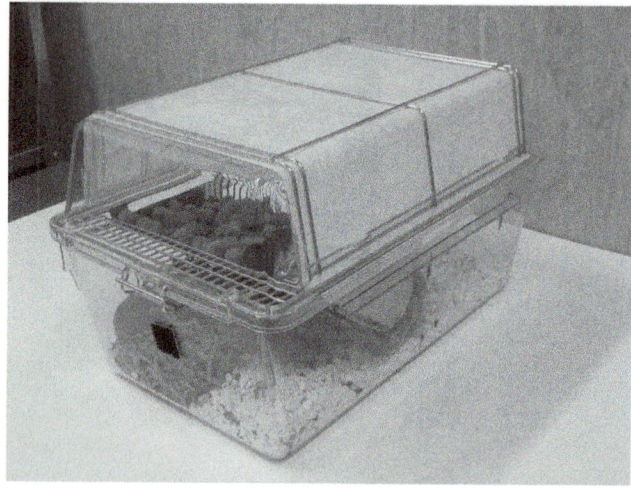

Figure 11.10 A filter-top box housing hamsters infected with *Clostridium difficile*. Source: Courtesy of UK Health Security Agency.

Table 11.3 Potential welfare issues of IVCs.

Parameter	Potential welfare issues	Solution
Air supply	Sealed lids and small volume of airspace require constant airflow to be maintained to provide oxygen and avoid build-up of humidity, temperature or waste gases (e.g., ammonia) Failure of power or fans will rapidly cause problems and may lead to suffocation if prolonged	Have a system that ensures even distribution of air to all cages. Have reserve fan or twin-motored fan. Emergency generator is essential and battery back-up to power fans is recommended (UPS). A schedule of regular servicing should be in place to ensure optimum performance
Filtration	Effective biocontainment will involve filtration of air. Filters will become clogged with dust and dander and this will affect performance	Either change filters frequently (expensive) or have a disposable pre-filter that can be discarded Have a monitoring system that will warn of reduction in performance (preferably for each cage)
Cage cleaning/ changing	Complete change of bedding has been shown to increase aggression	Consider revising bedding change regimes while retaining ability to provide adequate food and water and welfare/clinical observation
Interaction with staff	Reduced visibility and ergonomics may limit observation of animals	Organise cages to allow maximum visibility of occupants and food hopper (e.g., move food hopper from front of cage)
	Requirement to move to cabinet before removing lid may reduce the time staff can spend at one session	Have strict daily observation regime in place Mobile transportation units are available to move batches of cages while maintaining air supply
Procedures	Cages need to be transferred to a cabinet or downdraught table to conduct experimental procedures. This will be time-consuming and may lead to fatigue Incorrect replacement of cage could prevent adequate air supply	Design experiments so that groups of animals can be dealt with in a tolerable time-period. Do not be over-ambitious with the types of procedures that can be conducted, bearing in mind group sizes and the limitations of cabinet work Use IVCs with added filters to allow passive air transfer and mechanisms that ensure correct placement on rack
Cross-contamination	The use of a cabinet for husbandry or procedures means that there is a risk of cross-contamination between groups of animals	Strict operating procedures are required to schedule the order in which groups of cages are opened and to define disinfection regimes for exposed surfaces
Size constraints for practical or ergonomic reasons	Could tend towards a barren environment and social isolation	Consider latest enrichment provisions for IVC cages such as play wheels, shelters, platforms
Health monitoring	Changes in health screening regime (e.g. use of sentinel animals) could lead to biosafety breakdown	The development of sampling techniques allowing detection of microbes from live animals (e.g. for blood samples, swabs and faecal pellets)

shoebox-type cage with a lid consisting of a polycarbonate frame fitted with a piece of filter media. Such systems have been shown to protect the cage occupants from exposure to pathogens in adjacent cages (Lipman et al. 1993). While they can be used successfully to prevent cross-contamination between groups of infected animals such as hamsters infected with *Clostridium difficile* (Roberts et al. 2012), they are not recommended for use with pathogens dangerous to humans without the additional use of some other, more robust form of containment.

Welfare considerations in the use of filter-top cages

The presence of a filter lid reduces visibility of the occupants and of food and water levels. Also, the presence of a filter without a forced air supply reduces ventilation and can lead to a build-up of waste gases. Reviews of the environmental conditions within such cages indicate that the reduced airflow observed within these cages could lead to a build-up of gaseous pollutants that may adversely affect the animals' health (Keller et al. 1989) and that the high relative humidity, ammonia and carbon dioxide levels result in lower body weight gain and lower water consumption (Corning & Lipman 1991; Memarzadeh et al. 2004).

However, if due consideration is given to the number of animals housed per cage, the provision of bedding that will absorb waste effectively and to the frequency of bedding change (Reeb et al. 1998), then these cages provide a simple and effective means of preventing cross-contamination.

The filter lid should only be removed in a contained environment such as a safety cabinet, otherwise the benefits of using the lid will be lost and the resultant cross-contamination may invalidate the experiment. A strict working practice regime, including disinfection, placing only similarly infected groups of cages in the cabinet at the same time, and working from the lowest dose upwards, is required for this system to work effectively.

Ventilated cabinets

Ventilated cabinets are cabinets with sets of shelves on which the animal cages are placed. They can provide low-grade protection or isolation (Figure 11.11a). There are usually one or two doors at the front to allow access to the cages, and air is supplied either by an integral air-handling system or by plumbing into the room air system. The air handling can usually be switched between supply or extraction so that the cabinet can be operated at either negative or positive pressure. The shelves may be perforated to allow better distribution of air. Ventilated cabinets are frequently used in combination with filter-top cages, as any protective efficacy is lost as soon as a cabinet door is opened. Ventilated cabinets can be fitted with a range of optional extras to suit user requirements, such as building in a variable circadian rhythm with light/dark time control or fitting temperature control to allow post-operative recovery (Figure 11.11b).

Welfare considerations in the use of ventilated cabinets

Ventilated cabinets limit the observation of occupants, especially if used in combination with filter-top boxes. Ventilation is limited in the event of a power failure. As with other ventilated systems, due consideration should be given to the

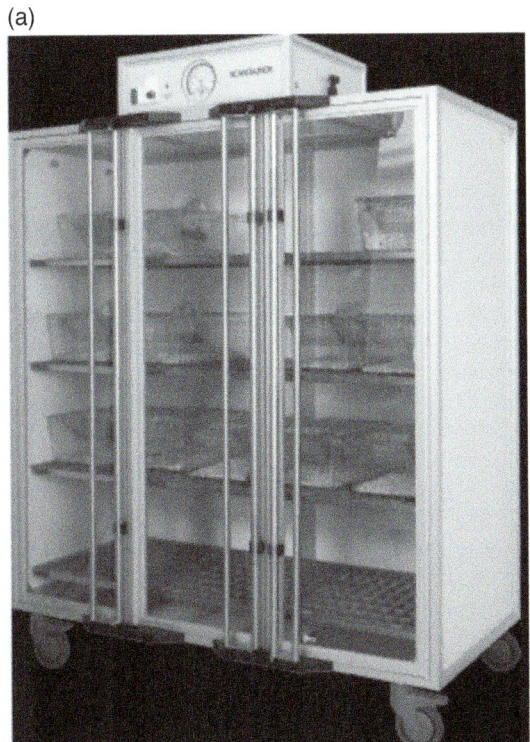
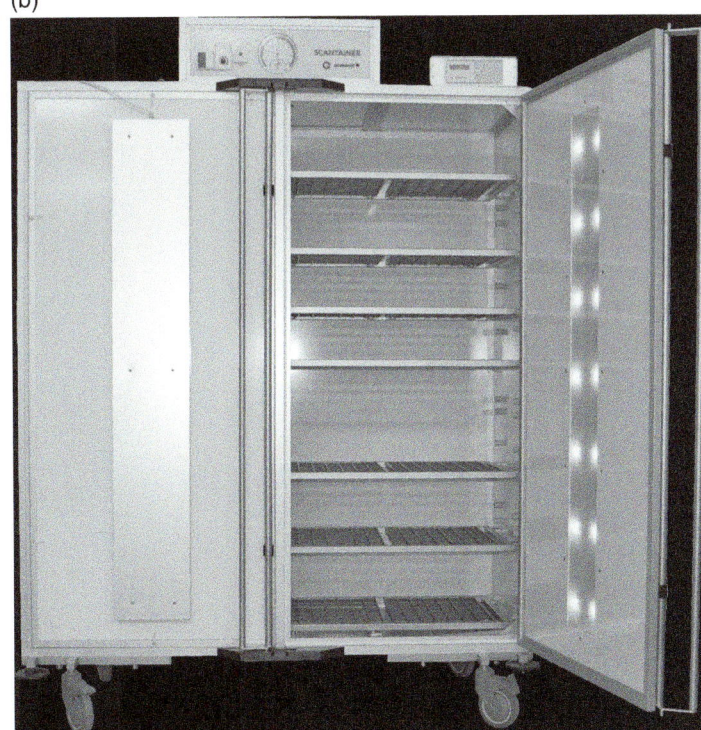

Figure 11.11 (a) A typical ventilated cabinet containing mouse cages. (b) Light cycles can be programmed (Source: Courtesy of Scanbur UK).

transfer of noise and vibration from air handling systems. There may be a temptation to conduct more than one experiment in a room as the cabinets appear very self-contained. For such a strategy to succeed, there need to be strict protocols in place for removal of cages for husbandry or experimental procedures. The latest versions of ventilated cabinets have improved control over ventilation and humidity +/- 3% RH (Leonhardt & Domone 2015).

Laminar flow booths or cubicles

Laminar flow booths are essentially miniature rooms with their own air handling systems, and they are used to subdivide an animal room into several independent units. Their main advantage is that this subdivision of a room enables more efficient use of space, where this is at a premium, by allowing several different experiments to be conducted simultaneously (Figure 11.12).

Typical isolation booths include: a wall system, a ceiling containing controls and an air handling system and a vertically telescoping front access door with transparent windows. They can be operated at either positive pressure, to protect the occupants, or at negative pressure, to protect staff. They can be custom-built to fit any particular space and are usually accessed from the front by upward-opening sectioned doors. As with ventilated cabinets, any protective efficacy afforded by the pressure differential or direction of airflow is considerably reduced when the doors are opened to access the occupants of the booth. The use of upwardly telescoping, rather than outward-opening doors reduces this effect and allows the air handling system to cope more efficiently with the breach in the barrier that is created. The vulnerability of the occupants of such systems to power or fan failure is very much dependent on the size of the booth.

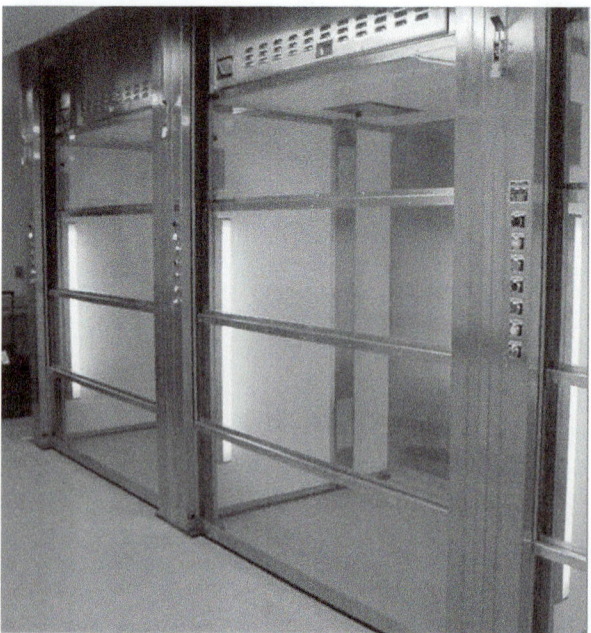

Figure 11.12 A typical containment booth with upwardly telescoping sectioned doors. Source: Courtesy of Britz & Co., USA.

For smaller booths, animals will need to be removed to a separate area or cabinet to perform daily husbandry or procedures, but larger booths can incorporate a section to allow such functions.

Welfare considerations in the use of laminar flow booths

These booths can provide a degree of microbiological separation, but they permit only poor observation of occupants from outside the booth and the potential for social isolation of the occupants. Other potential problems include:

- limited ventilation in the event of power failure;
- as with other ventilated systems, there is the potential for transfer of noise from air handling equipment or generated by the flow of air.

The environment of a booth can be easier to control in terms of air changes, temperature and humidity than that of an entire room. A controlled light–dark system can also be incorporated if required. A strict regime of daily practice is required for staff to prevent cross-contamination between booths and where smaller booths are sharing an area or cabinet for procedures, robust protocols must be in place to prevent cross-contamination between separate experiments. As with any enclosed system, a reliable UPS is essential.

Bespoke systems

For some species, no systems that offer acceptable levels of operator protection are commercially available and bespoke systems have to be developed according to need. An example of this is the directional flow containment system developed at UK Health Security Agency, to enable group housing of macaques that have been challenged with infectious agents (Figure 11.13a,b). Here, operator protection depends upon a directional flow of air that is maintained to a minimum velocity of 0.7 m/s at all times, even when accessing the animals. The room air-handling system is used to provide the ventilation for the system. The primates are physically isolated from the general room area by a solid transparent plastic barrier fixed to the front of the cage system. This barrier serves to enhance the directional airflow and to provide a physical barrier to potentially contaminated material generated by coughing, urination or defecation. The flexibility of such a system has been demonstrated by using them for other species such as rabbits and ferrets where high levels of biocontainment are required.

The risks associated with the husbandry of infected primates are controlled by strict discipline with regard to feeding, watering and waste removal regimes. The risks associated with handling of the primates are controlled by a strict regime whereby animals are sedated by injection before any handling or removal from the cage. Injection for sedation is accomplished by the use of a winding mechanism that gently brings the animal to the front of the cage and a strategically placed access door to allow injection. Sedated animals are removed from the cage into a carrying box that will be used at all times for transportation to and from a separate procedures area. All procedures are conducted on validated downdraught tables.

(a) 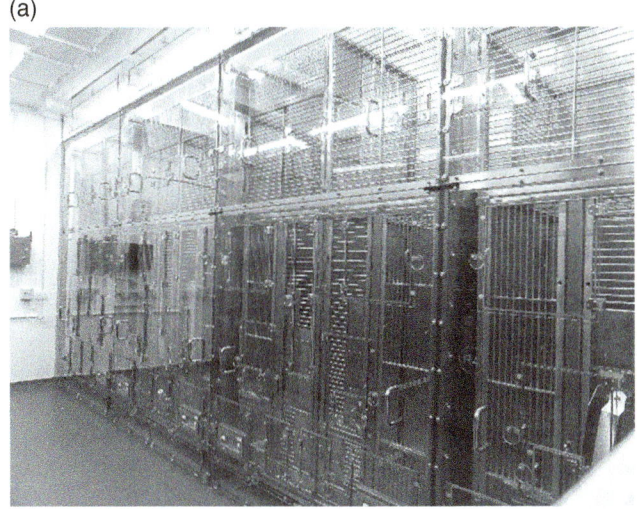 (b)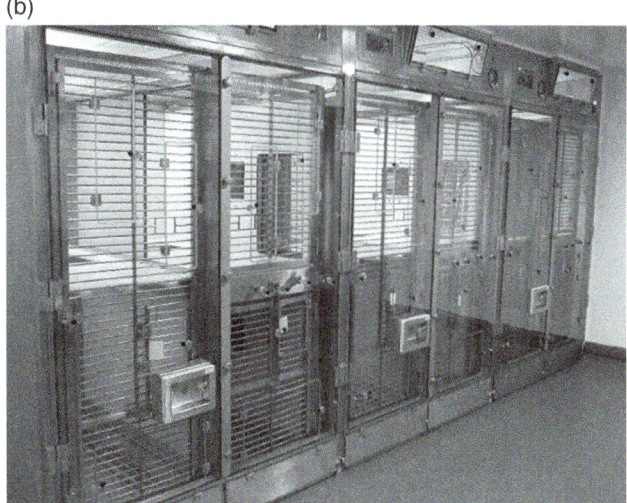

Figure 11.13 Two versions of directional flow containment systems that can house social groups of macaques infected with level 3 pathogens. Note in (a) floor to ceiling height and use of full length of room to maximise available space beyond ETS 123 housing standards and in (b) use of non-metal materials such as Trespa. Source: Courtesy of UK Health Security Agency.

Welfare considerations of bespoke systems

Access to the animals is restricted compared to the situation when using an open cage system. It is essential that all systems are designed so that animals can be accessed and isolated without causing undue stress for sedation or for remedial treatment in case of injury. In these systems, observations of animals can be limited by reflection of the plastic barrier. Overhead lighting needs to be positioned carefully to avoid this. Observation periods are also limited due to the demanding entry and exit procedures that require the use of protective clothing and strict disinfection regimes. Solid barriers inevitably alter the relationship between the care staff and the animals. This is no great problem if the animals are housed in social groups. Such systems can change the ergonomics of husbandry procedures and consideration needs to be given at the design stage to the potential for fatigue or strain in staff conducting day-to-day husbandry procedures. It is good practice to take any opportunity for positive enforcement training, such as presenting for injection or entering sedation boxes, while animals are housed at lower containment levels, such as BCL2, as this has the potential to provide better welfare once transferred to higher containment (see Chapter 15: Attaining competence in the care of animals used in research).

Species

Mice

IVCs are now in common usage for mice for containment of infection, for reduction of animal allergens or to protect susceptible animals from outside contamination. The ability to 'quarantine' animals of unknown health status in such systems has led to increased usage linked to the increasing traffic of transgenic strains of mice between research groups in different countries.

The other obvious attraction of these systems is that more efficient use can be made of animal accommodation, while not compromising health status (increases in stocking density per room of up to 50% are claimed). Thus, IVC systems are seen as a preferred option to improve standards of environmental health for both staff (allergen containment) and animals (cross-contamination, environmental control) without investing heavily in facility refurbishment or in new facilities.

Ventilation is provided by plugging individual cages into an air-handling system that is either integral to the cage rack or is plumbed into the room air supply. Protection is afforded by maintaining either a positive or negative pressure within each cage. This works well while the cages are attached within the rack but the challenge to biocontainment status comes when the cages have to be removed in order to change bedding, food and water, or to handle the animals. Containment integrity after removal from the rack can be maintained, to some extent, by an airtight seal between the lid and the box. This airtight seal presents a potential threat to the welfare of the occupants should the air system fail or should the box not be replaced accurately on the rack. Manufacturers have overcome this problem by placing an additional filter on the lid of the box that will allow passive exchange of gases and by adding pressure alarms and emergency battery power that will allow continued operation for a finite time until power is restored and by engineering in accurate locating systems. The effect of various ventilation rates from 30 to 100 air changes per hour (ACH) has been evaluated (Reeb et al. 1998) and while all rates kept ammonia levels below 3 parts per million (ppm), carbon dioxide levels, relative humidity and temperature were found to vary according to air change rate. The authors concluded that ventilation rates of 30ACH were adequate if bedding was changed weekly, but this needed to be increased to 60ACH in case of a fortnightly change frequency.

Removal of the lid for any husbandry or procedural functions is generally performed within a safety cabinet (usually, Class II) but strict working protocols must be put in place to prevent cross-contamination between groups of animals. Any assessment of working practice should include the likelihood of contamination when handling the animals for operations such as cage changing or procedures; this is usually addressed either by changing gloves between each cage (very time-consuming) or using disposable forceps to pick up the mice. However, it should be considered that frequent handling by such methods is not considered as best practice as it will affect the welfare of the animals and more humane methods such as using a tunnel dedicated to each cage are preferable.

Other containment systems used for mice include:

- isolators;
- filter-top cages;
- ventilated cabinets;
- ventilated booths;
- Fully suited staff protection (Figure 11.3).

Welfare considerations with the use of containment systems for mice

Mice should be kept in groups wherever possible (Kappel et al. 2017). Bedding and nesting materials should be provided; this includes the consideration of the importance of location of nestboxes as described by Kostomitsopoulos et al. (2007). Plastic, autoclavable nestboxes are available specifically for containment systems and treats, disposable tunnels and mouse refuges are readily available (Figure 11.14).

Containment strategies should be selected that allow maximum observation of animals but minimise laborious clothing change procedures. Where ventilated containment systems are used due consideration must be given to avoid exposing mice to excessive air change rates or air velocities (see also Chapter 21: The laboratory mouse). All aspects of ergonomics should be considered so that staff are not reluctant to observe and care for animals. The preventative maintenance implications to keep containment systems running efficiently and safely for animal welfare should be considered.

Rats

IVCs are now manufactured at an appropriate size to maintain rats. Other suitable containment systems for rats include:

- isolators;
- IVCs;
- ventilated cabinets;
- ventilated booths;
- fully suited staff protection.

Welfare issues with the use of containment systems for rats

As with mice, rats should be housed in social groups of three to five (Patterson-Kane et al. 2001) wherever possible. Cage height is important to allow rats to stand erect. It has been noted that rats prefer a lower air change rate, below 80ACH (Krohn et al. 2003). Rats are also more adversely affected by ammonia build-up (Gamble & Clough 1976) compared to mice, who are thought to be more ammonia tolerant (Smith et al. 2004), so an optimal ventilation rate and cleaning regime needs to be established. While Teixeira et al. (2006) found that IVCs can prevent deleterious effects in the ciliated epithelium of airways, a study by Marchesi et al. (2017) showed that rats maintained in IVCs from birth to adulthood showed lower ciliary beat frequency and lower numbers of immune cells recovered from lung lavage, compared to those housed conventionally. Provision of refuge and shredded nesting materials are thought to provide the best environmental enrichment for rats, but they do not show any preference for tunnels or pipes (Bradshaw & Poling 1991). Recent developments in IVCs designed specifically for rats provide enhanced welfare through a two-level, three-dimensional environment that allow animals to climb, jump and stand in a bi-pedal posture (Figure 11.15).

Hamsters

Suitable containment systems for hamsters include:

- filter-top boxes;
- isolators;
- IVCs;
- ventilated cabinets;

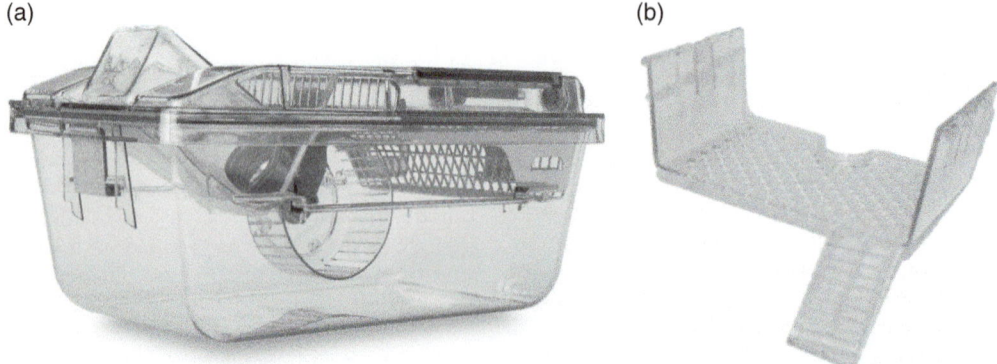

Figure 11.14 IVCs can now be fitted with additional enrichment such as (a) exercise wheels or (b) platforms (Source: Courtesy of Tecniplast UK).

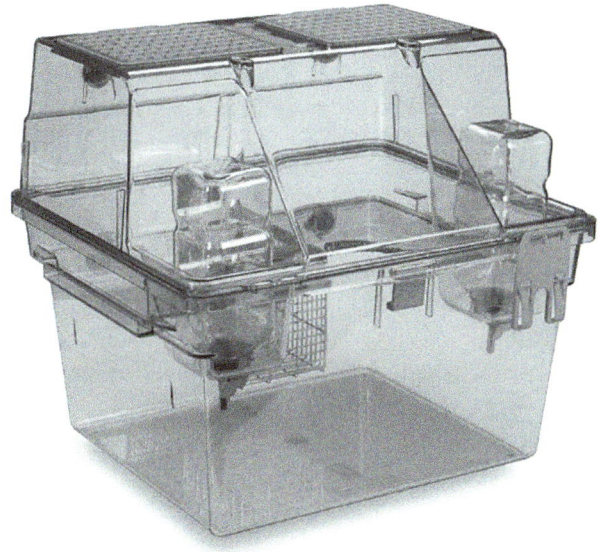

Figure 11.15 IVC system with improved height and enrichment for rats. Source: Courtesy of Tecniplast UK.

- ventilated booths;
- fully suited staff protection.

Welfare considerations with the use of containment systems for hamsters

Hamsters are more solitary than rats and mice and care is needed when housing them in social groups unless they are put together at an early age. See also Chapter 24: The Syrian hamster. They have a need to burrow or hide in shelters, so deep litter and appropriate nesting materials are of great benefit. It should be borne in mind that hamsters are very adept at chewing through cages.

Guinea pigs

Suitable containment systems for guinea pigs include:

- isolators;
- ventilated cabinets;
- ventilated booths;
- fully suited staff protection.

Welfare considerations with the use of containment systems for guinea pigs

Animals should be housed in groups or pairs with deep litter if possible. Sudden noises or movements should be avoided during husbandry or experimental procedures. Guinea pigs do well with a set routine and adapt poorly to changes, especially more mature animals. They may be upset by changes in the type of food hopper, water bottle or the type of food (Wolfensohn & Lloyd 2013), and they may be upset by a sudden move from conventional to contained housing.

Rabbits

Suitable containment systems for rabbits include:

- isolators;
- ventilated cabinets;
- ventilated booths;
- directional flow systems;
- fully suited staff protection.

Welfare considerations with the use of containment systems for rabbits

The use of senses such as smell or hearing may be impeded by the enclosure, by directional airflow or the use of protective clothing. A risk assessment taking into account the infectious agent may allow group housing in floor pens or large cages with deep litter if this results in no increased biological risk to handlers. This type of housing may be accommodated in a bespoke directional-flow system and will have the potential benefit of reducing stereotypic behaviours. Boxes or tubes should be provided as refuges from aggression. Cages should be of a size to allow the animals to stand on their hind legs, or climb on ledges to get a better view. See also Chapter 28: The laboratory rabbit. The housing should allow animals to get an early warning rather than be startled by the sudden appearance of an operator. Day time audible stimuli such as background music may help to remove this effect.

Ferrets

Ferrets are considered to be good models for several human respiratory infections, including influenza, to which they are naturally susceptible; they have been shown to respond to infection in the same way as humans. More recently, they have become a research model for Ebola and SARS COV-2 virus studies due to their susceptibility to the clinical isolates of these viruses (Cross *et al.* 2016; Muñoz-Fontela *et al.* 2020). See also Chapter 31: The ferret.

Suitable containment systems for ferrets include:

- ventilated cages (Figure 11.16);
- ventilated booths;
- directional flow systems;
- Plastic film isolators;
- Fully suited staff protection.

Welfare considerations with the use of containment systems for ferrets

Ferrets should be housed in social groups or pairs where possible. Risk assessments should be undertaken to give consideration to allowing pens with deep litter, tunnels, hammocks and disposable boxes if there is no increased risk to handlers. Consideration should be given to a bespoke system that will allow this while satisfying the experimental requirements for safe access to the animals for husbandry and procedures. Sullivan and Reardon (2008) report that ferrets used as a model for H5N1 influenza, requiring high-level containment, can be given the same level of enrichment as that provided prior to infection. Infection models of BCL4 agents, such as Ebola, require the highest level of containment (Figure 11.16) and safe handling strategies; nevertheless, housing in pairs or social groups is still possible and enrichment can be provided as described above (Figure 11.17).

Nonhuman primates

Suitable containment systems for nonhuman primates include:

- rigid isolators (New World only);
- directional flow systems: see Figure 11.13;
- negative pressure rooms plus RPE;
- fully suited staff protection

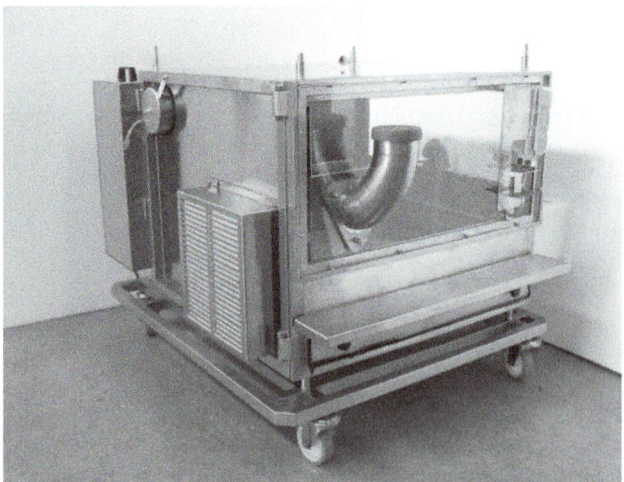

Figure 11.16 A ventilated unit for use with ferrets infected with a high-level pathogen (Source: Courtesy of Tecniplast UK).

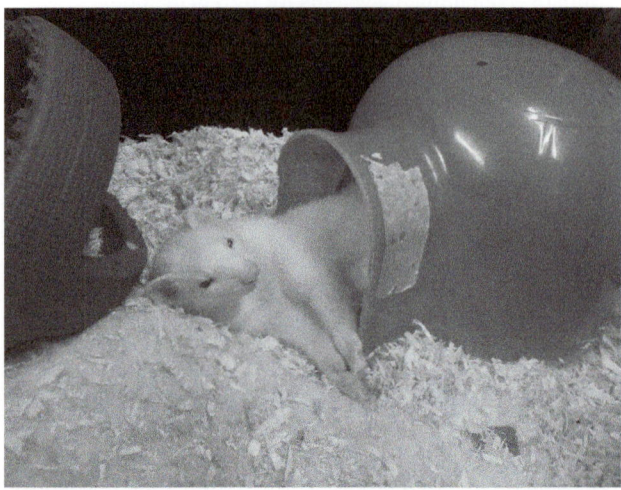

Figure 11.17 Ferret in high containment provided with shelter, toys and deep bedding. Source: Courtesy of UK Health Security Agency.

Welfare considerations with the use of containment systems for nonhuman primates

Primates should be housed in social groups wherever possible, and every opportunity should be taken to do this at lower containment housing levels so that after social groups have been established, sufficient time can be allowed before the start of a study to ensure that the groupings are compatible and stable.

Marmosets and tamarins are usually pair-housed for experimental work as a vasectomised male and female or with the female on birth control whereas Old World primates such as macaques can be successfully housed in single-sex social groups.

Provide foraging in deep litter or foraging tray/box; if not possible, vary the diet, add toys, puzzle feeders, mirrors, etc., and alternate these to maintain interest. The author has found that providing a TV can be useful enrichment. The TV should be visible for all individuals, with a range of DVDs. Duration and content should be varied to avoid losing the novelty value.

CCTV with a view of all animals and a zoom facility can be used to study abnormal behaviour or overt clinical signs without disturbing the animals. Far more subtle information about well-being can be acquired if the animals are not reacting to human presence. CCTV can also be used to record, so that any missed time-periods can be reviewed (Figure 11.18).

For primates, it is particularly important that staff familiar with individual animals should be those that assess clinical or behavioural signs such that humane endpoints are recognised at the earliest stage possible.

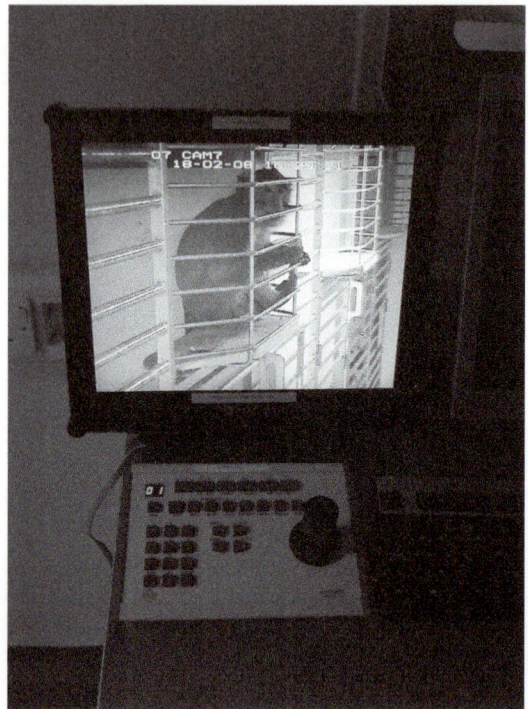

Figure 11.18 Animals being observed by CCTV. Source: Courtesy of UK Health Security Agency.

Where possible, train the animals to come to the front of cage or to the area where sedation will be given. Train them to take oral dose, use target training for groups, and use positive reinforcement. Train animals to allow them to be weighed by, for example, entering a detachable weighing box.

In addition to the above:

- Provide a nestbox or bucket for marmosets or tamarins to sleep in and hammocks for macaques.
- Maintain the same social groups throughout and plan experimental groups to allow same partners. Plan for eventuality of when humane endpoints are met. Plan necropsy schedules so that animals are not left alone if at all possible. It is good practice to establish an order on the bleed schedule throughout a study – NHPs generally establish an order so that quite often a confident one is last (never leave the least confident animal until last). Remote telemetry allows continuous data capture (temperature, blood pressure, ECG, respiration rate, activity), without repeated sedation. It provides improved experimental data and may assist in establishing early humane endpoints; but choose a system that allows group housing where possible and balance the harms to the animals in terms of surgical implantation, against the benefits (Figure 11.19).
- Design cages so that animals can be separated if aggressive, or isolated for sedation or veterinary treatment if injured. It is of little value having vast cages if animals cannot be captured/sedated without prolonged stress to the animals and staff. Brown and Hearson (2008) describe a humane way of restraining marmosets without stress or injury, using a netting cassette while Powell *et al.* (2014) report the successful use of a small capture box for marmosets infected with ABSL-3 agents.
- Make cages as complex as possible, using partitions and shelves, or perches for smaller species. This makes the environment more interesting and allows refuge from peers or more dominant animals (Figure 11.20).
- Feed in an appropriate manner, so that all members of the group can access adequate food: this avoids disrupting groups by minimising aggressive incidents at feeding.

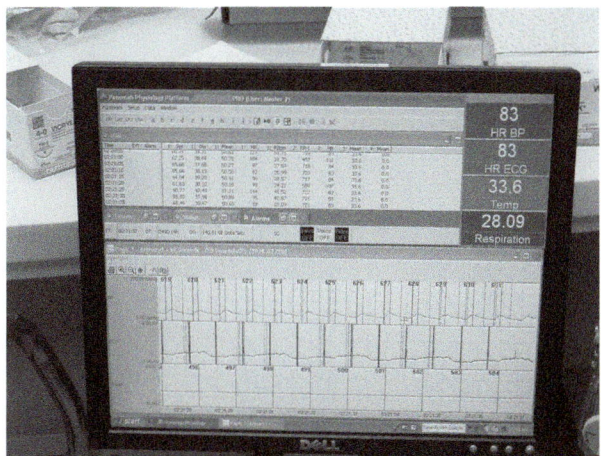

Figure 11.19 Real-time display of cardiac and respiratory data from a telemetry implant. Source: Courtesy of UK Health Security Agency.

Pigs

Young piglets can be housed in flexible film isolators, but will outgrow such limited accommodation within a few weeks to months (Figure 11.21). Powell *et al.* (2018) report the successful use of bio-bubble containment systems for the breeding and maintenance of specific pathogen-free immuno-deficient pigs.

Other suitable containment systems for pigs include:

- directional flow systems;
- negative pressure rooms plus RPE, or laboratories using fully suited staff protection.

Welfare considerations with the use of containment systems for pigs

Pigs are highly social animals and should be housed in groups. A deep substrate should be provided to permit natural behaviours such as rooting for food. Enrichment for pigs should be odorous, deformable, chewable and designed to sustain interest. It also needs to be destructible and ingestible (Van de Weerd *et al.* 2003) but can also include boxes, mirrors and play chains.

Interactions with handlers are important, so consider how high-quality interaction can be achieved. See also Chapter 32: Pigs and minipigs. It is important that there is a system to enable restraint for examination or sampling without causing stress. Powell *et al.* (2018) use clicker training with high value treats for routine procedures such as weighing and accepting a snare for restraint. They also report that the use of thick plastic mats adds comfort and variety to footing within the bio-bubble containment system (Sara Charley and Amanda Ahrens, Department of Animal Science Iowa State University personal communication).

Ruminants

Young calves and lambs have been reared in modified flexible film isolators either as germ-free animals or to contain an experimental infection. However, like piglets, they will outgrow this type of accommodation within a few weeks to months. Adult animals require negative pressure rooms plus RPE, or laboratories requiring fully suited staff protection.

Welfare considerations with the use of containment systems for ruminants

Unless permitted by regulatory approval through, e.g., a project licence, animals must be housed in isolators in pairs rather than as individuals as this type of containment gives a high degree of isolation from outside stimuli. The plastic canopy insulates from noise and the height of the base container limits vision of the external environment.

For containment of larger juveniles and adult ruminants, the most practicable alternative is the use of negative pressure rooms with staff wearing PPE (and RPE if necessary). In such accommodation, it is essential that consideration is given to providing more than just a concrete floor. Rubber matting, or straw or other bedding, if at all possible, should

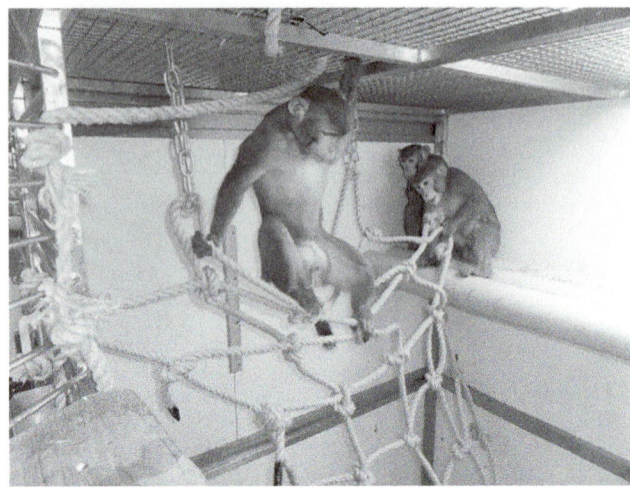
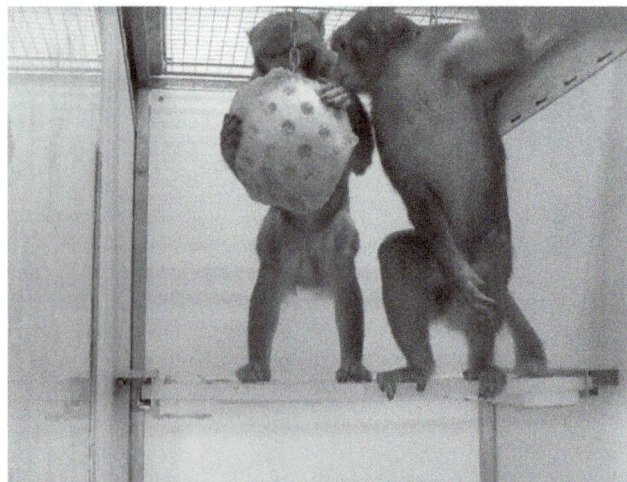

Figure 11.20 Enrichment provided at CL3. Source: Courtesy of UK Health Security Agency.

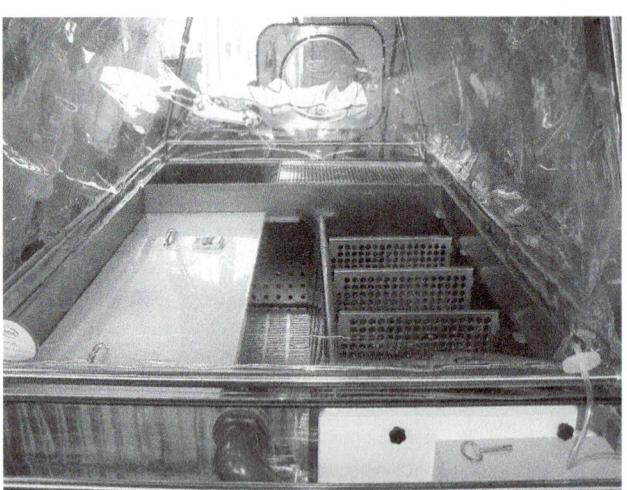

Figure 11.21 The interior of a containment isolator for piglets (Source: Courtesy of Bell Isolation Systems Ltd).

Birds

Suitable containment systems for birds include:

- rigid isolators (Figure 11.22);
- negative pressure rooms plus PPE/RPE or laboratories, using fully suited staff protection (Figure 11.23).

Welfare considerations with the use of containment systems for birds

Birds have very complex needs in terms of enrichment and environment. Two important behaviours of chickens are foraging and dustbathing so environmental enrichment, such as

be provided. It is important to ensure that systems are in place that allow the animals to be restrained for examination or sampling without stress. It is important also to ensure that a diet containing suitable fibre to prevent digestive problems can be provided without compromising any drainage/effluent treatment systems. In most cases, these problems can be addressed by the use of high-fibre, pelleted rations supplemented with mineral blocks and cubed hay. In addition, other strategies may be possible such as providing a bund around drains and removing bedding manually for incineration. Welfare monitoring systems been developed by the agricultural industry[2] and some have further developed this in biocontainment situations to capture video images and interpret the behaviour of individuals such that progression to disease can be monitored, allowing early humane interventions and linking to welfare assessment (Ryan *et al.* 2021).

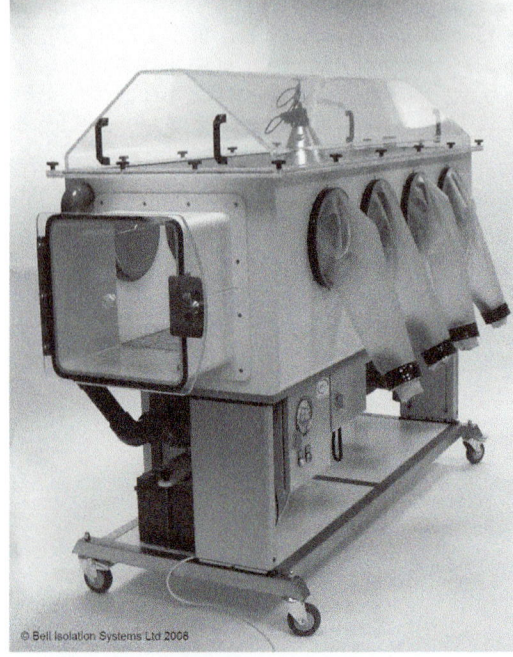

---

[2] https://www.postscapes.com/cattle-tracking-systems/ (Accessed June 28, 2022)

Figure 11.22 An isolator designed for use with poultry (Source: Courtesy of Bell Isolation Systems Ltd).

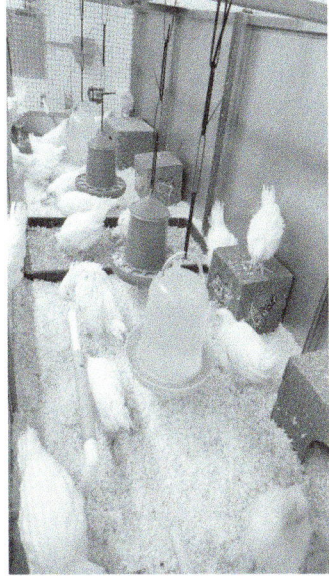
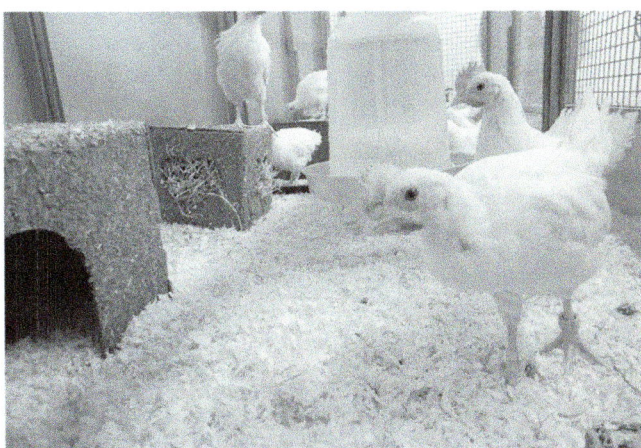

Figure 11.23 Enrichment for chickens in high containment (Source: Courtesy of Pirbright Institute, UK).

sand baths, artificial turf, provision of perches, has been shown to improve the condition of domestic hens (Abrahamsson et al. 1996) and it is possible to provide these substrates within a shallow wooden box or metal rings distributed evenly throughout the room.

Enrichment objects reduce aggression between birds (Gvaryahu et al. 1994). Increasing the complexity of the environment can reduce fear in poultry, thus improving animal welfare. This can be achieved by the provision of novel objects, such as coloured plastic balls, plastic bottles, mirrors, hanging bundles of string or other colourful items. The purpose of a novel object is to stimulate exploratory behaviour and activity, and possibly inducing play behaviour. Birds will be less fearful towards humans when they have had access to a variety of novel objects. Other strategies may include the use of radios or televisions.

Another important aspect to be considered in bird welfare is the provision of suitable lighting levels of appropriate wavelength (Lewis & Morris 2000; Campbell et al. 2015) and light and dark cycles that are suited to not only the species but the stage of development (EU Council Directives 2007/74/EC and 2007/43/EC.

Waterfowl are sometimes required for high containment studies (Wibawa et al. 2014) and, under these circumstances, consideration must be made of the requirement for access to water for swimming and the challenge of disposing of large volumes of potentially contaminated water.

Highly efficient ventilation systems will be required in enclosed systems to prevent ammonia build-up. The filters required for biocontainment can be affected by rapid clogging with dust.

Checklist for containment

The checklist below is designed to help avoid overlooking any important aspects when planning to use containment facilities.

- Is a containment system really necessary? Is its use going to decrease the risks associated with your experiment (Are the animals shedding infectious or allergenic particles? Are they infectious by aerosol or by direct contact?), or could you actually be increasing risks (e.g., needle-stick or bites due to decreased dexterity)?
- Does it do what it is supposed to do (contain or protect)?
- Does it still contain/protect during associated practices (e.g., feeding, watering, cage changing, experimental procedures) and does any ancillary equipment offer the same level of protection?
- Can you demonstrate/quantify the effectiveness of operator protection?
- Is it practical to use (ergonomics, dexterity)?
- Can you actually perform all the experimental requirements?
- Can the animals be housed in social groups?
- Can the animals engage in normal behaviours?
- Can they be accessed easily for food, water, health checks or handling?
- Can the animals be restrained or sedated without undue stress?
- Can they be readily observed for abnormal clinical signs, behaviour?
- Is rapid intervention practicable (e.g., humane killing at endpoint, separation if aggression observed, remedial veterinary care)?
- Can they escape, and, if so, can they be retrieved?
- Is air supply optimised for air changes, temperature and humidity?
- Can these conditions be sustained over an extended period?
- Are noise, odours, light, vibration levels acceptable at all times?
- What measures are necessary against power failures?

Legislative requirements

Each country will have its own legislative requirements (see Chapter 8: Legislation and oversight of the conduct of research using animals: a global overview) but there is general consistency especially in assigning containment levels to specific pathogens. In general, biological agents are assigned to a hierarchical grouping according to the perceived threat to human or animal health. These are normally called biocontainment or biosafety levels, or the hierarchy may be named after the national body that assigns these 'risk' or 'hazard' groups. Thus, for a particular infectious agent, you will encounter a number of risk assessment phrases such as biocontainment level (e.g., BCL3), biosafety level (e.g., BSL-3) in the US (Centers for Disease Control and Prevention and National Institutes for Health 2007) or, in the UK, Advisory Committee on Dangerous Pathogens level (e.g., ACDP3; Advisory Committee on Dangerous Pathogens (1995)). Criteria that affect this categorisation include: the ability of the pathogen to infect humans; the seriousness of disease; the ability to spread from person to person; and whether prophylaxis (e.g., a vaccine) or therapy is readily available. A good general outline of guidance on biohazard categories and the equipment and facilities required to operate safely is given in World Health Organization (2004).

To further complicate matters, many countries have assigned a similar hierarchical system to pathogens that may threaten the environment or agricultural species of economic importance. In this case, the hierarchy is based more upon the potential to infect such animals, the likelihood of escape into the environment and the consequences of infection, rather than the risk to human health. Here you will encounter categorisation of microbes under regulations such as Specified Animal Pathogen Order (e.g., SAPO3[3]) or BSL-3 Ag in the US (USDA Agricultural Research Service, Heckert & Kozlovac 2007). In some cases, e.g., anthrax, the pathogen may come under both human and animal pathogen legislation and the containment strategy will need to take both into account.

Yet more legislation applies to genetically modified organisms[4] and yet another hierarchy is applied based on the nature of the genetic alteration, whether this has enhanced or diminished the ability to infect or cause disease, whether the altered organism can survive outside the laboratory and whether the altered genes can be passed on to organisms in the outside environment. Be aware that this legislation will apply to genetically altered animals as well as microbes, so containment protocols and risk assessments will need to address the issue of escaped animals and how these might interact genetically with the wild population.

The future

As long as there are requirements for animal models of infectious diseases and for germ-free or SPF animals, there will be a need to use containment strategies to protect the operators or the animals. The principles underpinning current containment systems have changed little over the years, relying on some sort of physical barrier supplemented by a differential pressure regime: the main changes that have been seen relate mainly to improving the engineering associated with filtration, pressure and temperature control, alarm systems and emergency back-up capabilities. Thus, the use of isolators, IVCs and cabinets will continue to expand as the expectations of health and safety regulators increase. Furthermore, there is currently an explosion of investment worldwide in high-containment laboratories, driven in part by the perceived threats of bioterrorism, emerging diseases (e.g., H5N1 influenza, severe acute respiratory syndrome (SARS), large-scale outbreaks of Ebola and changing patterns in disease prevalence due to climate change and population mobility (e.g., vector-borne diseases). The main driver for improving these systems is always going to be minimising risk to the operators and will thus be focused on ergonomics and infection hazards. Many of these agents cause serious disease or death and there are some that have an infectious dose for humans of one organism. Thus, potentially lethal needle-stick injuries, bites or scratches must be prevented at all costs. Inevitably, any disease-containment strategy will add to the time taken to perform a given task. The challenge will be to optimise animals' welfare within these parameters.

The value of giving animals the ability to manipulate their environment and express preferences, even in a small way, should not be underestimated as it allows them to cope better with the housing conditions necessitated by the procedures. There are now several publications reviewing the impact of environmental enrichment on experimental outcomes (e.g. Bayne & Würbel 2014; Grimm 2018), and many conclude that less stressed animals are physiologically and immunologically more relevant to the clinical models they represent.

Given the range of materials available for the construction of cages and enrichment equipment there is little excuse for not addressing the welfare needs of all species of laboratory animals even under the most stringent biocontainment regimes. If animal-friendly materials cannot be sterilised for reuse, then they should be considered as disposable and destroyed or made safe in the most appropriate manner. Several laboratories that specialise in high containment have demonstrated that cage sizes can be maximised, that materials such as plastics and wood can replace stainless steel and that group housing is possible. Biotelemetry can be especially useful in the context of biocontainment, where human presence is kept to a minimum, as it allows continuous monitoring of physiological parameters that can be used to inform on humane endpoints or to indicate a point in the disease progression when extra monitoring or care will be required. Telemetric systems have now been developed that allow concurrent monitoring from multiple animals within group housing and a comprehensive bibliography of publications in this area for a wide range of species is provided on the NC3Rs website[5]. In addition, the creative use of CCTV can enable continuous monitoring of animals and can even be advantageous in observing natural behaviour that cannot be

---

[3] https://www.hse.gov.uk/biosafety/sapo.htm (Accessed February 21 2022)

[4] https://www.hse.gov.uk/biosafety/gmo/index.htm (Accessed February 21 2022)

[5] https://www.nc3rs.org.uk/refinement-rodent-and-non-rodent-housing-during-telemetry-recordings (Accessed 21 February 2022)

seen during human presence. Richardson (2015) reviewed the possibilities of refining studies involving laboratory mice by the use of automated behavioural technologies while high-quality video capture combined with software analysis of deviation from normal behaviour can be used to refine humane endpoints in disease studies involving cattle (Ryan *et al*. 2021).

References

Advisory Committee on Dangerous Pathogens (1995) Categorisation of Biological Agents According to Hazard and Categories of Containment, 4th edn. HSE books, Sudbury, UK.

Advisory Committee on Dangerous Pathogens (2015) Management of Hazard Group 4 viral haemorrhagic fevers and similar human infectious diseases of high consequence https://assets.publishing.service.gov.uk/government/uploads/system/uploads/attachment_data/file/534002/Management_of_VHF_A.pdf.

Abrahamsson, P., Tauson, R. and Appleby, M.C. (1996) Behaviour, health and integument of four hybrids of laying hens in modified and conventional cages. British Poultry Science, 37, 521–540.

Alexander, T.J.L., Lysons, R.J., Elliott, L.M. *et al*. (1973) Techniques for rearing gnotobiotic lambs. Laboratory Animals, 7, 239–254.

Basic, M. and Bleich, A. (2019) Gnotobiotics: past, present and future. Laboratory Animals, 53(3), 232–243.

Bayne, K. and Würbel, H. (2014, Apr) The impact of environmental enrichment on the outcome variability and scientific validity of laboratory animal studies. Revue scientifique et technique, 33(1), 273–280. doi: 10.20506/rst.33.1.2282. PMID: 25000800.

Bradshaw, A.L. and Poling, A. (1991) Choice by rats for enriched versus standard home cages: plastic pipes, wooden platforms, wood chips and paper towels as enrichment items. Journal of the Experimental Analysis of Behaviour, 55, 245–250.

Bridger, J.C., Hall, G.A. and Brown, J.F. (1984) Characterization of a calici-like virus (Newbury agent) found in association with astrovirus in bovine diarrhea. Infection & Immunity, 43, 133–138.

Brown, M. and Hearson, S. (2008) Refining handling for marmosets in high levels of biocontainment. Animal Technology and Welfare, 7, 39–41.

Butler, J.E., Francis, D.H., Freeling, J. *et al*. (2005) Antibody repertoire development in fetal and neonatal piglets. IX. Three pathogen-associated molecular patterns act synergistically to allow germ-free piglets to respond to type 2 thymus-independent and thymus-dependent antigens. Journal of Immunology, 175, 6772–6785

Burman, O., Buccarello, L., Redaelli, V. and Cervo, L. (2014) The effect of two different Individually Ventilated Cage systems on anxiety-related behaviour and welfare in two strains of laboratory mouse Physiology & Behavior, 124, 92–99.

Campbell, CL., Colton, S., Haas R. *et al*. (2015) Effects of different wavelengths of light on the biology, behaviour, and production of grow-out Pekin ducks. Poultry Science, 94, 1751–1757.

Centers for Disease Control and Prevention and National Institutes of Health (2007) Biosafety in Microbiological and Biomedical Laboratories (BMBL), 5th edn. US Government Printing Office, Washington, DC.

Chowdhury, S.R., King, D.E., Willing, B.P. *et al*. (2007) Transcriptome profiling of the small intestinal epithelium in germ-free versus conventional piglets. BMC Genomics, 8, 215–230.

Corning, B.F. and Lipman, N.S. (1991) A comparison of rodent caging systems based on microenvironmental parameters. Laboratory Animal Science, 41, 498–503.

Clough, G., Wallace, J., Gamble, M.R. *et al*. (1995) A positive, individually ventilated cage system: a local barrier system to protect both animals and personnel. Laboratory Animals, 29, 139–151.

Copps, J. (2005) Issues related to the use of animals in biocontainment research facilities. ILAR Journal, 46, 34–43.

Cross, R.W., Mire, C.E., Borisevich, V. *et al*. (2016) The Domestic Ferret (*Mustela putorius furo*) as a Lethal Infection Model for 3 Species of Ebolavirus. Journal of Infectious Diseases, 214(4), 565–569. doi: 10.1093/infdis/jiw209. Epub 2016 May 24.

David, J.M., Knowles, S., Lamkin, D.M. and Stout, D. (2013) individually ventilated cages impose cold stress on laboratory mice: a source of systemic experimental variability. Journal of the American Association for Laboratory Animal Science, 52(6), 738–744.

Dennis, M.J., Davies, D.C. and Hoare, M. (1976) A simplified apparatus for the microbiological isolation of calves. British Veterinary Journal, 132, 642–646.

Dennis, M., Parks, S., Taylor, I. *et al*. (2015) A flexible approach to imaging in ABSL-3 laboratories Applied Biosafety, 20(2), 89–99.

Feistenauer, S., Sander, I., Schmidt, J. *et al*. (2014) Influence of 5 different caging types and the use of cage-changing stations on mouse allergen exposure. Journal of the American Association for Laboratory Animal Science, 53(4), 356–363.

Gamble, M.R. and Clough, G. (1976) Ammonia build-up in animal boxes and its effect on rat tracheal epithelium. Laboratory Animals, 10, 93–104.

Grimm, D. (2018) Are happy lab animals better for science? Science. Available at https://www.sciencemag.org/news/2018/02/are-happy-lab-animals-better-science (Accessed 21 February 2022).

Gvaryahu, G., Ararat, E., Asaf, E. *et al*. (1994) An enrichment object that reduces aggressiveness and mortality in caged laying hens. Physiology & Behaviour, 55, 313–316.

Heckert, R.A. and Kozlovac, J.P. (2007) Biosafety levels for animal agricultural pathogens. Applied Biosafety, 12, 168–174.

Höglund, A.U. and Renström, A. (2001) Evaluation of individually ventilated cage systems for laboratory rodents: cage environment and animal health aspects. Laboratory Animals, 35, 51–57.

Hope, J.C., Thom, M.L., Villarreal-Ramos, B. *et al*. (2005) Vaccination of neonatal calves with *Mycobacterium bovis* BCG induces protection against intranasal challenge with virulent *M. bovis*. Clinical Experimental Immunology, 139, 48–56.

Ka, Y., Ogura, T., Tomiyama, K. *et al*. (2021) Creation of an experimental rearing environment for microbiome animal research using an individually ventilated cage system and bioBUBBLE enclosure. Experimental Animals, 70(2), 177–184. doi: 10.1538/expanim.20-0129. Epub 2020 Nov 25.

Kallnik, M., Elvert, R., Erhardt, N. *et al*. (2007) Impact of IVC housing on emotionality and fear learning in male C3HeB/FeJ and C57BL/6J mice. Mammalian Genome, 18, 173–186.

Kappel, S., Hawkins, P. and Mendl, M. (2017) To group or not to group? Good practice for housing male laboratory mice. Animals, 7(12), p. 88. https://www.mdpi.com/2076-2615/7/12/88

Keller, L.S., White, W.J., Snider, M.T. *et al*. (1989) An evaluation of intra-cage ventilation in three animal caging systems. Laboratory Animal Science, 39, 237–242.

Kim, A.H.J., Hogarty, M.P., Harris, V.C. and Baldridge, M.T. (2020) The complex interactions between rotavirus and the gut microbiota. Frontiers in Cellular and Infection Microbiology, 10, 08 January 2021 | https://doi.org/10.3389/fcimb.2020.586751

Kostomitsopoulos, N.G., Paronis, E., Alexakos, P. *et al*. (2007) The influence of the location of a nest box in an individually ventilated cage on the preference of mice to use it. Journal of Applied Animal Welfare Science, 10, 111–121.

Krohn, T.C. and Hansen, A.K. (2002) Carbon dioxide concentrations in unventilated IVC cages. Laboratory Animals, 36, 209–212.

Krohn, T.C., Hansen, A.K. and Dragsted, N. (2003) The impact of cage ventilation on rats housed in IVC systems. Laboratory Animals, 37, 85–93.

Lanni, F., Burton, N., Harris, D. *et al*. (2021) The potential of microdialysis to estimate rifampicin concentrations in the lung of guinea pigs. PloS one, 16(1), e0245922. https://doi.org/10.1371/journal.pone.024592

Leonhardt, P. and Domone, A. (2015) Improving animal welfare, reducing energy and increasing flexibility Animal Technology and Welfare, 14(1), 41–43.

Lewis, P.D. and Morris, T.R. (2000) Poultry and colored light. World's Poultry Science Journal, 56(3), 189–207.

Lipman, N.S., Corning, B.F. and Saifuddin, M.D. (1993) Evaluation of isolator caging systems for protection of mice against challenge with mouse hepatitis virus. Laboratory Animals, 27, 134–140.

Logge, W., Kingham, J. and Karl, T. (2013) Behavioural consequences of IVC cages on male and female C57Bl/6J mice. Neuroscience, 237, 285–293. http://dx.doi.org/10.1016/j.neuroscience.2013.02.012

Logge, W., Kingham, J. and Karl, T. (2014) Do individually ventilated cage systems generate problem for genetic mouse model research? Genes, Brain and Behavior, 13, 713–720.

Llonch, P., Troy, SM., Duthie, C-A. et al. (2016) Changes in feed intake during isolation stress in respiration chambers may impact methane emissions assessment. Animal Production Science, 58(6), 1011–1016. https://doi.org/10.1071/AN15563

Luczynski, P., McVey Neufeld, K.A., Oriach, C.S. et al. (2016) Growing up in a bubble: using germ-free animals to assess the influence of the gut microbiota on brain and behavior. International Journal of Neuropsychopharmacology, 19(8), 1–17.

Marchesi, G.D., Fatima de Soto, S., de Castro, I. et al. (2017) The effects of individually ventilated cages on the respiratory systems of male and female Wistar rats from birth until adulthood. Clinics, 72(3), 171–177.

Mellor, D.J. (2016) Updating animal welfare thinking: moving beyond the "Five Freedoms" towards "a Life Worth Living". Animals, 6(3), p. 21.

Memarzadeh, F., Harrison, P.C., Riskowski, G.L. et al. (2004) Comparison of environment and mice in static and ventilated isolator cages with different air velocities and ventilation designs. Contemporary Topics in Laboratory Animal Science, 43, 14–20.

Morrell, J.M. (1997) Efficacy of mini-containment units in isolating mice from micro-organisms. Scandinavian Journal of Laboratory Animal Science, 24, 191–199.

Muñoz-Fontela, C., Dowling, W.E. and Funnell, S.G.P. (2020, Oct) Animal models for COVID-19. Nature, 586(7830), 509–515. doi: 10.1038/s41586-020-2787-6. Epub 2020 Sep 23. PMID: 32967005; PMCID: PMC8136862.

Patterson-Kane, E.G., Harper, D.N. and Hunt, M. (2001) The cage preferences of laboratory rats. Laboratory Animals, 35, 74–79.

Powell, D.S., Walker, R.C., Heflin, D.T. et al. (2014) Development of novel mechanisms for housing, handling and remote monitoring of common marmosets at animal biosafety level 3 Pathogens and Disease, 71, 219–226.

Powell, E., Charley, S., Boettcher, A.N. et al. (2018) Creating effective biocontainment facilities and maintenance protocols for raising specific pathogen-free, severe combined immunodeficient (SCID) pigs. Laboratory Animals, 52(4), 402–412.

Reeb, C., Jones, R., Bedigan, H. et al. (1998) Microenvironment in ventilated animal cages with differing ventilation rates, mice populations and frequency of bedding changes. Contemporary Topics in Laboratory Animal Science, 37, 43–49.

Reeb-Whitaker, C.K., Paigen, B., Beamer, W.G. et al. (2001) The impact of reduced frequency of cage changes on the health of mice housed in ventilated cages. Laboratory Animals, 35, 58–73.

Renström, A., Björing, G. and Höglund, A.U. (2001) Evaluation of individually ventilated cage systems for laboratory rodents: occupational health aspects. Laboratory Animals, 35, 42–50.

Richardson, C.A. (2015) The power of automated behavioural homecage technologies in characterizing disease progression in laboratory mice: a review. Applied Animal Behaviour Science, 163, 19–27.

Roberts, A., McGlashan, J., Al-Abdulla, I. et al. (2012). Development and evaluation of an ovine antibody-based platform for treatment of Clostridium difficile infection. Infection and Immunity, 80(2), 875–882. https://doi.org/10.1128/IAI.05684-11

Ryan, M., Waters, R. and Wolfensohn, S. (2021) Assessment of the welfare of experimental cattle and pigs using the Animal Welfare Assessment Grid. Animals (Basel), 11(4), 999. doi: 10.3390/ani11040999. PMID: 33918263; PMCID: PMC8065713.

Smith, A.L., Mabus, S.L., Stockwell, J.D. et al. (2004) Effects of housing density and cage floor space on C57BL/6J mice. Comparative Medicine, 54, 656–663.

Spangenberg, E., Wallenbeck, A., Eklöf, A.C. et al. (2014) Housing breeding mice in three different IVC systems: maternal performance and pup development. Laboratory Animals, 48(3), 193–206.

Sullivan, A. and Reardon, H. (2008) The use of multiple species and models at MRC NIMR: care and welfare implications. Animal Technology & Welfare, 7, 35–38.

Teixeira, M.A., Chaguri, L.C.A.G. and Carissimi, A.S. (2006) Effects of an individually ventilated cage system on the airway integrity of rats (Rattus norvegicus) in a laboratory in Brazil. Laboratory Animals, 40, 419–431.

Timms, J.R., Cooper, D.M., Millard, B.J. et al. (1979) An isolator for avian disease research. Laboratory Animals, 13, 101–105.

Trexler, P.C. and Reynolds, L.I. (1957) Flexible film apparatus for the rearing and use of germfree animals. Applied Microbiology, 5, 406–412.

Tavernor, W.D., Trexler, P.C., Vaughan, L.C. et al. (1971) The production of gnotobiotic piglets and calves by hysterotomy under general anaesthesia. Veterinary Record, 88, 10–14.

Van de Weerd, H.A., Docking, C.M., Day, J.E.L. et al. (2003) A systematic approach towards developing environmental enrichment for pigs. Applied Animal Behaviour Science, 84, 101–118. http://dx.doi.org/10.1016/s0168-1591(03)00150-3.

Webster, J. (2005) Animal Welfare: Limping Towards Eden. Wiley-Blackwell; Chichester, UK.

Wolfensohn, S. and Lloyd, M. (2013) Handbook of Laboratory Animal Management and Welfare, 4th Edition, Wiley-Blackwell.

World Health Organization (2004) Laboratory Biosafety Manual, 3rd edn. WHO, Geneva.

Wyatt, R.G., Mebus, C.A., Yolken, R.H. et al. (1979) Rotaviral immunity in gnotobiotic calves: heterologous resistance to human virus induced by bovine virus. Science, 203, 548–550.

12 Transportation of laboratory animals

Sonja T. Chou, Donna Clemons, Nicolas Dudoignon, Guy Mulder and Aleksandar Popovic

Introduction

Laboratory animals represent a fraction of animals moved in commerce and they differ from many in usually having a more defined health status. A wide range of purpose-bred or wild-caught animals could be used in research, but, in practice, only a small number of species are used in significant numbers. Animals used, and transported for research purposes, include rats, mice, guinea pigs, gerbils, hamsters, rabbits, cats, dogs, swine, nonhuman primates (only a few species), fish (zebrafish, medaka, etc.), and rarely frogs, sheep, goats, cattle and poultry (mostly chickens). The greatest numbers of shipped containers holding laboratory animals, as well as the greatest number of shipments, are of rats and mice. This chapter is based on the original text in the 8th edition of the UFAW Handbook (White *et al.* 2010) and focuses on the transport of common laboratory animals although the principles can be applied across many species destined for research use. Species-specific information for less commonly used species can be found in other more comprehensive sources (International Air Transport Association [IATA] 2019a). While the general principles and considerations associated with laboratory animal transportation have not changed much in recent decades, animal rights campaigns and attacks on laboratory animal transportation have created significant transport logistic challenges, putting animal welfare and research quality at risk for the global research community. Therefore, the importance of journey planning cannot be overstated to ensure safe and efficient transport of laboratory animals.

General principles and requirements

When transporting laboratory animals, the objective is to move them in a manner that does not jeopardise their well-being or health status, minimises controllable sources of stress and ensures their safe arrival at their destination. Part of the stewardship of animal care and use is to understand, and provide for, needs and eventualities arising during transport.

There are various reasons for transporting laboratory animals. Animals are commonly produced in commercial facilities, using specialised housing and handling systems that can reliably exclude disease-causing and unwanted micro-organisms. These animals must be transported to the institutions that use them in research, testing or other activities. In the past, this traffic between commercial breeders and users comprised most of the transportation of laboratory animals. However, advances in techniques for genetic manipulation have led to increasing numbers of animals, with unique genotypes and phenotypes, being bred in small research colonies. These colonies have increasingly become a source of supply for other institutions, either as a small commercial enterprise, or for use on a collaborative basis. Collaborative studies between two or more institutions may require that animals are transported more than once in larger multi-institutional studies. The number of institutionally produced animals that must be transported may be relatively small for any given institution, when compared to commercial producers, but across institutions the aggregate may represent a substantial number of journeys.

Research institutions often have a limited number of options regarding methods for transporting animals between institutions. In the UK and continental Europe, ground transportation by contracted carriers is more common than air transport because of the relatively short distances within and between countries and a very limited number of air carriers willing to transport research animals. The majority of ground shipments involve journey times of less than 24 hours. Short water-borne voyages may be used in some circumstances, when species-specific needs have been appropriately considered. Carriage by air still remains the most rapid means of transport over long distances and represents the only practical option for transporting animals between continents.

The type of journey, its duration, the physical environment during carriage, the design of the container and other factors can influence the animals' safety and well-being during the journey. Transportation involves removal of animals from a controlled home environment and their placement in a varying and less controlled environment in which they may be transported with other animals from other locations and with non-animal freight. Even if proper arrangements and

---

The UFAW Handbook on the Care and Management of Laboratory and Other Research Animals, Ninth Edition.
Edited by Huw Golledge and Claire Richardson.
© 2024 John Wiley & Sons Ltd. Published 2024 by John Wiley & Sons Ltd.

procedures are followed, it is, unfortunately likely that some animals will experience some discomfort or stress and adverse events may occur, albeit very rarely. In order to minimise adverse events and stress, it is essential to understand the biological and behavioural requirements of the species, properly plan for the journey and provide adequate contingency provisions prior to commencing the journey. In practice, this means that the consignor should clearly understand all aspects of the procedures involved in transporting their animals as well as the variables that may be encountered during the journey. Since transporting animals between research institutions is not a daily or even a weekly event for most institutions, a detailed written set of procedures and a checklist can be very useful in assuring that all steps in the journey have been carefully considered and that appropriate actions have been taken.

Animal transportation includes the entire period from packing, through dispatch, carriage and receipt by the consignee to the unpacking of the animals at their final destination. It is important during the transportation process:

- That intended journey be planned well in advance of the intended shipping date. A professional shipper should generally be utilised to develop a route plan and address contingencies to protect animal welfare, should problems arise in transit;
- That a professional shipper specialising on animal transportation be contracted, one with good working knowledge and experience with the species being shipped;
- That species-appropriate containers be used, constructed of strong, durable materials which meet or exceed all national and international guidelines, and able to withstand the length of transport;
- That the animals and their shipping containers be protected from adverse weather conditions such as precipitation, direct sunlight and high winds which can affect the ambient conditions within the container or the security of the container;
- That the animals be provided with an adequate supply of fresh or conditioned ambient air that provides for their thermoregulatory, respiratory and metabolic needs;
- That the animals be protected from exposure to extremes in environmental conditions;
- That the animals be prevented from escaping, or from falling out of the container, or extending appendages outside the container, or from experiencing other conditions that result in physical harm, including illness, injury or death;
- That factors that may cause animal discomfort or stress during the journey are recognised and, as far as practically possible, be minimised;
- That appropriate documentation based on journey route, species, strain, number, sex, age/weight, identification numbers, microbiological status and any special requirements resulting from phenotype accompanies each shipment.

The health and welfare of animals

Animals to be shipped should be in good clinical health. Prior to packing, each animal should be examined by an appropriately trained animal care provider, experienced in recognising signs associated with illness in that species. For international transport, animals must be examined by an authorised veterinarian of the originating country to ensure they are fit for travel, as per Article 10 of the European Convention for the Protection of Animals during International Transport (Council of Europe 2003). Animals should be excluded from shipment if there is behavioural or other clinical evidence of abnormalities that would make them unsuitable for transportation. In some cases, transport may involve animals with inherited abnormalities due either to spontaneous mutations or genetic manipulation. If animals have adapted to these abnormalities so that there are no apparent functional deficits or if the phenotypic expression of these abnormalities, in the judgement of the health care provider, does not present a risk to their well-being in transit, then these animals may be considered for transport. This is subject, however, to appropriate documentation of their abnormalities and the granting of any necessary regulatory permission for their transport. Similarly, diseased or injured animals may be considered for transport only when the purpose of such transport is for the diagnosis or treatment of the condition.

Health and infectious status

Health is an important concern in the transport of laboratory animals. In general, we can place infections into three groups as they relate to transportation: (1) infections that pose a risk to domestic animals or humans; (2) infections that pose a risk to the transported animals themselves and (3) infections that may produce no clinical disease but make the animals unsuitable for some types of research. The health certifications for transport of animals, required to allow them to move in commerce and between countries, usually focus on infections that have human or agricultural/domestic animal significance. A health certificate issued by a competent veterinary authority prior to a journey or by virtue of customs inspection directed at assessing health during the journey, is the principal safeguard for assuring that the clinical health of the animal(s) is appropriate for them to make or continue a journey.

Infections that may not be harmful to the carrier animals, and which may not be regulated in transport may, nevertheless, make the animal unsuitable for its intended research purposes. The risk that animals can carry such infections, either as a result of infection at the source colony or during transportation, is a potential reason to hold newly received animals in quarantine housing until their health status can be verified.

Institutions transporting animals often provide health screening information for the source colony. While commercial suppliers of laboratory animals often perform extensive and frequent health screening of closed colonies, the health screening of animals may vary considerably between research institutions in accordance with professional guidelines and institutional needs (Berard et al. 2014; Collymore et al. 2016; Balansard et al. 2019; OIE 2019a). A thorough description of the health monitoring programme for the colony should be sought in order to determine what, if any, additional testing should be done upon the receipt of the animals by the consignee. Verifying health status on arrival is recommended as a reasonable precaution when receiving animals from unfamiliar sources. Such testing is generally performed while animals are segregated in quarantine and away from general research colonies.

IATA sets standards for air shipment of laboratory animals and has defined two health status categories for laboratory animals. They are (1) Conventional, and (2) Specific Pathogen Free (SPF), which is further subdivided into subcategories of (a) *Conditioned SPF* and (b) *Barrier-raised SPF* (IATA 2019a). Designation of health status classifications dictates the selection of appropriate shipping containers to maintain health status during transport, see Table 12.1.

During transport, animals of differing health status and of different species may be shipped together in the same cargo area of the aircraft (Figures 12.1 and 12.2). The IATA Live Animals Regulations (LAR) further recommends separation of animals that are natural enemies whenever possible in separate cargo areas (IATA 2019a). Similarly, depending upon whether dedicated ground transportation or a common carrier is used, animals from more than one source, and hence potentially of different health statuses, could be shipped in the same vehicle or aircraft cargo compartment. Commercial suppliers of SPF animals generally produce and ship only barrier-raised SPF animals (although the pathogens from which they are free can vary considerably between suppliers). Since the cargo compartment, whether it is in a ground transport vehicle or an aircraft, is one microbiological space, it is up to the shipping institution ('consignor/shipper') to select an appropriate container to maintain the microbiological status of the animals that are being shipped. No assumption should be made regarding the microbiological status of the outside of the shipping container when received at the consignee's institution: containers may have been exposed to unwanted micro-organisms during transit. In the case of SPF animals, surface disinfection of the container before unpacking is an important precaution to take in preventing unwanted introduction of contaminants. Aqueous halogen-based disinfectants are inexpensive and very useful for this purpose.

Laboratory animals, which have been infected with agents that pose a threat to humans, animals of agricultural importance, or other domestic animals or wildlife, always provide

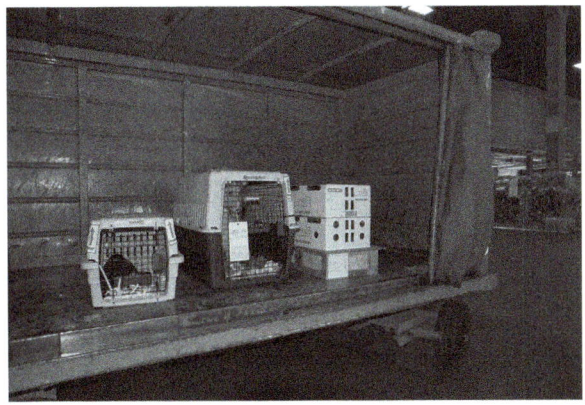

Figure 12.1 Example of multiple species being held together in a ramp cart in the same airport staging area prior to loading on an aircraft.

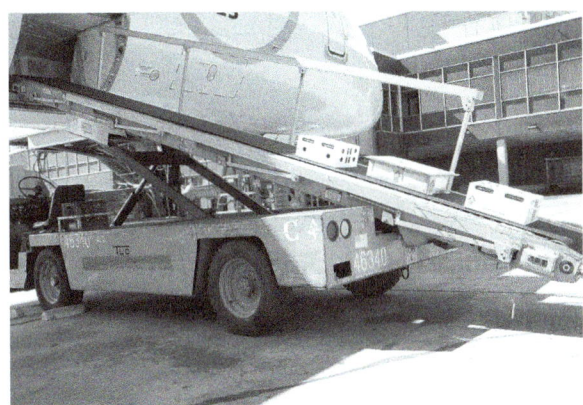

Figure 12.2 Containers of mice and rats being loaded into the climate-controlled hold of an aeroplane that contains other perishable goods.

a challenge for the shipper. An infectious substance is defined as any substance which is known or can be reasonably expected to contain pathogens which can cause disease in humans or animals.

Table 12.1 IATA Health Status Classifications for Laboratory Animals and Associated Shipping Container Requirements.

Health Status Classification	Examples	Shipping Container Requirement
1. **Conventional**: presence or absence of specific micro-organisms and parasites is unknown due to the absence of testing, treatment or vaccination.	Wild-caught and domestic animals maintained under uncontrolled microbiological conditions with a conventional health status.	Non-filtered shipping container.
2. **Specific Pathogen Free (SPF)**: Animals free of one or more specific infectious agents (parasites or infectious micro-organisms).		
a. **Conditioned SPF**: Animals that have undergone testing, vaccination or treatment to ensure absence of one or more specific infectious agents.	Nonhuman primates, dogs, cats, swine.	Non-filtered shipping container.
b. **Barrier-reared SPF**: Animals raised in specialised facilities (e.g. barriers, isolators) in the absence of one or more infectious agents, including agents of agricultural and human significance.	Rodents, rabbits.	Filtered SPF shipping container.

Source: Adapted from IATA (2019a).

Infectious substances can be divided into two categories: Category A – an infectious substance transported in a form that, if exposure to it occurs, is capable of causing permanent disability, life-threatening or fatal disease in otherwise healthy humans or animals; and Category B – an infectious substance that does not meet the criteria of Category A. The International Civil Aviation Organization (ICAO) Technical Instructions for the Transport of Dangerous Goods by Air (ICAO 2017–2018) and the IATA's Dangerous Goods Regulations (IATA 2019b) provide additional detail on the transportation of these substances.

Live animals that have been intentionally infected or are suspected to contain an infectious substance must not be transported unless the substance cannot be consigned by any other means. Under such circumstances, infected animals may only be transported under terms and conditions approved by the appropriate national authorities and the carrier.

Genetically modified animals such as laboratory mice, rats and zebrafish are frequently submitted for transportation. Their transport is regulated under IATA's Dangerous Goods Regulations (IATA 2019b) for genetically modified organisms. IATA defines genetically modified organisms (GMOs) as organisms in which genetic material has been purposely altered through genetic engineering in a way that does not occur naturally. GMOs, including laboratory animals that are capable of genetically altering natural populations of animals as a result of natural reproduction and which do not harbour or express pathogens or toxins are not considered to be 'dangerous goods' by the IATA, and may be shipped provided this is done in compliance with other live animal shipping requirements. Thus, such animals do not have to be packaged and labelled as dangerous goods or meet transport standards that differ from other animals of the same species. However, shipments of such animals could be required by the countries of origin, transit or destination to have authorisation (and perhaps additional labelling) to leave, transit through or enter these countries. It is the responsibility of the consignor (shipper) to ensure that the animals to be transported comply with regulations regarding genetic modification, including local regulations in the countries of origin and destination. In most countries, transport of genetically engineered laboratory animals is allowed. In some parts of the world, misunderstanding of the terms transgenic, genetically modified (GM), engineered or manipulated can cause delays in transportation. Shippers should ensure they have secured in advance the appropriate documentation and authorisation for the movement of their shipments. However, unforeseen welfare problems associated with their phenotypic expression may arise and this risk can be avoided by transporting GM animals as cryopreserved embryos or cryopreserved gametes. Such options should be considered when planning shipment of GM stock.

Considerations for Animal Models with Special Needs

Shipment of pregnant animals should be avoided when possible. Shipment during the last 20% of gestation is risky, as it may be associated with stress-induced abortion. It should be noted that there is some variation in guidance on shipment of pregnant animals. Article 9 of The European Convention for the Protection of Animals during International Transport (Council of Europe 2003) states that pregnant female mammals shall not be transported either during the last tenth of the gestation period or for at least 1 week after they have given birth. However, the Laboratory Animal Science Association (LASA) recommends that pregnant animals should not normally be transported during the last fifth (20%) of gestation to minimise the risk of abortion or parturition in transit (LASA 2005). The risk of adverse events occurring during transport increases with the increasing body size of the mother and the size of the foetal mass being carried also varies with the species. While time-mated rodents can be successfully shipped during the first two-thirds of the gestation period, shipping during the pre-implantation period, which is generally around gestation day (GD) 4 or 5, should be avoided. Upon arrival, exposure of time-mated rodents to chemical cues (e.g. the Bruce effect) should be avoided to minimise the risk of embryo losses. Larger species, such as dogs and nonhuman primates, can be transported nearer the time of parturition provided that the journey is direct, of relatively short duration and can be undertaken under appropriate veterinary direction and supervision. Guidance on this varies with different codes of practice, regulatory bodies and by species. In summary, and as a general rule, shipment during the last 20% of gestation is considered more risky, particularly for larger species (see Table 12.2).

Transport of unweaned (nursing) animals presents a considerable risk to their safety and well-being. Nursing animals with their young may be transported when the young are a minimum of 7 days of age and with additional bedding and nesting material (LASA 2005). Unweaned animals may, depending upon their age, have difficulty in regulating body temperature, be incapable of eating solid food and may be unfamiliar with, or unable to access, water sources within the container. Some species such as guinea pigs can be weaned at a very early age since they are precocious at birth and capable of regulating body temperature and consuming solid food within a few days of birth. While there is no universal minimum age for shipment, animals must be capable of functioning independently from their mothers, consuming solid food and water as well as maintaining normal physiological and metabolic functions. Shipping a lactating female with her young, especially over long distances, may result in her failing to care for her young and hence in their death.

Table 12.2 Recommended pregnancy shipping limits for common laboratory animal species (adapted from LASA 2005).

Species	Gestational Length (days)	Shipping Limit (days)
Mouse	21	17
Rat	21	17
Guinea pig	56–75	45
Rabbit	30–32	22
Dog	61–65	40
Cat	64–67	42
Pig	114	91
Common marmoset	144	96
Long-tailed macaque	153–167	102

The risk of this varies somewhat between species and with the age of the young but, as a general rule, shipping lactating females and young constitutes an unacceptable risk to their health and well-being and is not recommended.

Immunologically deficient, or immunocompromised animals, are commonly transported for research purposes. Some GM animals can possess unrecognised immune defects that may alter their susceptibility to disease. These animals may, as a result of acquiring human or environmental commensal organisms, develop illness that would not be experienced by animals that did not have immune dysfunction. Whenever immunologically deficient or immunologically compromised animals are transported, great care must be taken with all packing and handling and disinfection processes, to ensure that the animals will not be exposed to infectious agents. Other than these considerations, the requirements for successful transport of these animals are the same as for immunocompetent animals of the same species.

A number of physical conditions, such as obesity, cardiac disease, and elevated age may impact upon the metabolism and physiology of laboratory animals during transportation. The greater insulation provided by body fat in obese animals compromises their ability to dissipate heat and to adapt to elevated environmental temperatures. Similarly, models of cardiac disease and old age are more susceptible to elevated heat during transport. Reducing the number of such animals placed in a shipping container will help lessen the risk of excess heat by decreasing the total amount of heat generated within the container. Consideration should also be given to postponing shipments of such animals during abnormally warm weather if there is a possibility that the ambient environmental conditions could exceed acceptable ranges even for brief periods of time. If animals must be shipped internationally during periods of seasonally high heat, flights that depart and arrive in the evening and early morning when temperatures are generally more moderate should be considered whenever possible.

Certain strains of laboratory rodents lack a protective hair coat, and this compromises their ability to thermoregulate at lower environmental temperatures and also makes them more susceptible to cuts and abrasions from rough surfaces within their shipping containers. When hairless animals are transported, extra care must be taken to select a container that does not have exposed or rough edges that could injure unprotected skin. In addition, when hairless animals are shipped during periods of cold weather, the provision of extra bedding and nesting materials will help to provide insulation within the shipping container during transport. For animals that lack eyelashes, dust-free bedding should be considered to reduce the potential of animal eye irritation. In some instances, when hairless animals are produced as a result of breeding homozygous and heterozygous animals for the desired genotype, haired cage mates of the same microbiological status are also produced. Inclusion of some of these haired colony animals can also be used to provide additional thermal protection, as they huddle with the hairless animals.

Some laboratory animals can have metabolic or physiological conditions that may predispose them to challenges during transport. Diabetic animals, for example, require greater water intake than non-diabetic animals in order to maintain homeostasis. They also produce, as a result, large volumes of urine, which can result in unacceptably wet bedding in the transport container. In order to provide an appropriate environment, more bedding material or the addition of absorbent pads may be required. Consideration should also be given to decreasing the number of animals per container to help address this problem.

Zebrafish can be shipped during various stages of their life cycle. Shipping of live fish has the added challenges of maintaining water temperature and water quality parameters, such as oxygen, CO_2, and nitrogen, within a suitable range. Shipping of embryos is cost effective and generally offers better biosecurity, but embryos are also more sensitive to temperature fluctuations and shipment delays. Laboratories that distributing multiple lines of fish globally will often prefer to ship cryopreserved sperm instead.

Animal provisions during shipment

Direct or indirect contact bedding is provided for terrestrial laboratory animals in shipping containers. It serves several functions, the most important of which is the absorption of moisture from urine and faeces, water released from hydration sources such as water bottles or gelled water, as well as from animal sources such as condensation from insensible water loss on internal container surfaces. In the case of small mammals, bedding also provides a source of insulation. Using familiar bedding and nesting products in the shipping container may help reduce animal stress levels during transport. Due to positional changes of the container during various stages of the transportation process, as well as due to the disturbances caused by the transportation environment, nest building may not always occur.

Sufficient bedding materials must be provided to maintain a dry and sanitary environment during shipping. Care must be taken, however, not to place so much bedding within a shipping container that it occludes ventilation openings. In the case of SPF animals, it may be necessary to provide suitably disinfected bedding that matches their microbiological status.

Recently, concerns have been raised over wood products used for bedding, as well as in shipping container construction and in pallets used to support and secure shipping containers during transit, with respect to their potential to carry plant diseases and agricultural pests across borders. Additional requirements for the treatment of such materials to eliminate these risks, as well as other measures imposed by countries and carriers, may eventually affect the use of untreated wood products in transportation.

Animals in transit should be provided with access to food and water during the journey. Ideally, the food provided to the animals during shipment should be of the same type and microbiological status as that they were fed at the institution of origin. Barrier-raised SPF small mammals that are shipped in filtered containers must be provided with food and water of a compatible microbiological status. In such instances, since there will be no opportunity during the course of the journey to replenish the food and water without opening the container (and thus potentially altering their microbiological status), sufficient quantities must be placed within the container at the time of packing. Larger animals, such as nonhuman primates and dogs, are almost always shipped in non-filtered containers, which allow for food and water to be replenished at scheduled stops during shipment. The design of these shipping containers for larger animals usually includes devices built into the container for addition of feed and water during the course of the journey. When large domestic animals undergo ground transportation, regulatory bodies require provision of feed and water, observation of the animals and specified rest periods at prescribed intervals. In the case of air transport of larger laboratory animals, there is usually no access to the cargo hold by personnel for the purposes of feeding and watering during flight and this has to be done following landing.

In their home environments, common laboratory animals are usually fed a dry pelleted or extruded diet. For nonhuman primates this is often supplemented by fruits and vegetables. Such foods, with high water content, can serve as an additional source of water during shipment. Unfortunately, these can spoil easily and may require some level of preparation prior to being introduced into the container. Opening the shipping container during the journey for purposes of introducing or removing materials carries with it the risk of escape. Food and water containers that are built into the shipping container but accessible from the outside may provide a route for escape or entrapment and great care must be taken when re-feeding or replenishing water supplies during the journey. It is recommended to provide sufficient food and water for a journey of twice the anticipated journey time in case of any unforeseen delays.

Presentation of food and water should be done using a method that is appropriate to the past experience of the animals and to the behaviour patterns of the species. Purpose-bred dogs, for example, are accustomed to eating and drinking out of bowls in a lighted environment. Many common laboratory rodents, by contrast, feed principally at night; and despite the use of feeders in a laboratory environment, some rodents such as hamsters and gerbils will remove all feed from the feeder and hoard them in piles. Feeders or feed bowls are unnecessary for rodent transport since these animals forage for feed in the wild and do so quite readily when it is placed in with the bedding material.

Food consumption while in transit will often be less than when the animals are in their home environment. Commonly, this is reflected in weight loss, which will be rapidly regained during the first few days in their new home environment. The use of novel food items during transit may also contribute to reduced intake and weight loss.

Access to drinking water during transit is important to help animals maintain hydration and thermoregulate. Water in liquid form can be provided in refillable water bowls in the case of certain large animals (e.g. nonhuman primates) or through the use of water kits in the case of small animals (e.g. rodents). A water kit consists of a sealed flexible pouch of water of the appropriate microbiological quality that is placed in a holder affixed to the wall of the container. Animals access water through a disposable drinking valve that is inserted into the pouch by puncturing the wall of the pouch. When water bowls are used, substantial amounts of water can be spilled out of the bowl either through the course of drinking or by movements of the container or movements of the animal. Similarly, with a water kit much of the water can be spilled if there is leakage around the insertion point of the drinking valve or by animals brushing against the valve thereby releasing water. This can result in the bedding within the container becoming wet. If a water kit is to be used, the animals should be conditioned to the use of a drinking valve as compared to the use of water bottles or other means of providing water in their home environment.

Alternatively, a gelled water source can be provided. Gelled water is a hydrocolloid-stabilised material containing between 70 and 98% water by weight. Gelled water pouches and cups are available commercially (Figure 12.3). Various sources of calories in the form of carbohydrates can also be added to the gelled water as well as flavouring and stabilising ingredients to prevent spoilage. Animals have taste preferences and hence the presence or absence of certain nutrients may affect the consumption of gelled water during transit. A number of commercially available sources of this material have been shown to be accepted by various species. When using a gelled water product, it is important to cut the outer plastic, or remove the cap, at time of packing and expose the gel to the animals, as some animals won't naturally open the containers. When a large amount of gelled water is placed in a container in order to provide for extended journeys, it is important to assure that it is suitably affixed within the container as movement of this material within the container during transit could result in injury to small animals.

For shipment of laboratory fish, ensuring even temperature and water quality during transit can be the most challenging aspect of transport. Changes in temperature can alter fish metabolism and affect the consumption of oxygen and the production of CO_2 and nitrogenous waste. The level of dissolved oxygen can be maintained by ensuring the primary containment has a water to air (fresh air or pure oxygen) ratio of 1:3. Feeding should be withheld from adult and juvenile fish for 24 hours prior to shipment, or longer for larger fish, to avoid fouling of the water. If transit time is

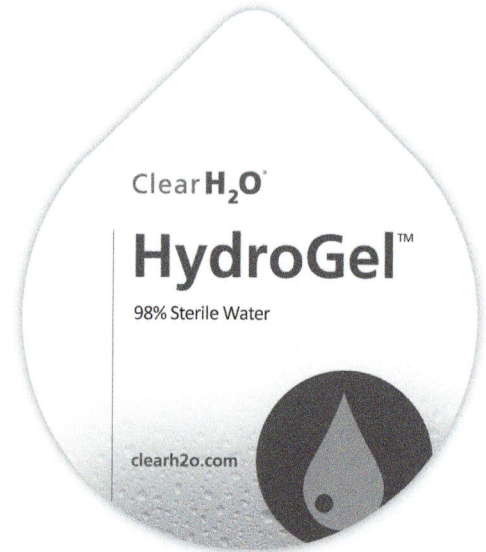

Figure 12.3 A gelled water pouch and gelled water cup, both sealed prior to use for use as a hydration source for research rodents and rabbits. Photo courtesy of ClearH2O, Portland, ME, USA.

expected to last more than 24 hours, ammonia binder such as ClorAm-X® or similar products may be added to condition the shipping water and reduce the impact on water quality.

Fish embryos are shipped in sterile embryo medium with methylene blue added to inhibit microbial growth. Prior to packing, the embryo surface should be disinfected using sodium hypochlorite (bleaching) or iodine solution to remove potential contaminants on the chorion. Protocols for fish embryo surface sanitation are readily shared among fish users (ZIRC 2019).

Having proper insulation/cushioning material will help maintain fish species in their preferred temperature zones. The insulation used, such as Styrofoam or inflatable air-filled liners, should reflect the best practices based on the ambient temperatures and other climactic conditions of the origin and destination locations. Cooling agents (e.g. ice or gel packs) or heating agents (e.g. hand warming heat packs) may be placed inside the insulated container, as appropriate, to maintain a steady temperature appropriate for the animals being shipped. Live fish must never be packed in direct contact with ice to avoid tissue damage.

Transport container design and construction

The most common design of research animal transport container is in the form of a rectangular box, the dimensions and shape of which are largely dictated by the species for which it is intended. Various types of containers have been developed commercially for transporting laboratory animals, some of which are illustrated in this text.

Adequate ventilation is essential for terrestrial animals, and the shipping container should be designed so that it can incorporate filtered or non-filtered ventilation apertures according to the microbiological status of the animals. The container and air vents should be designed so that vents cannot be occluded, even when stacked (Figure 12.4). Many containers have additional built-in features such as spacers or stand-offs to aid in ventilation (Figures 12.5, 12.6 and 12.7). Air vents should be sited on at least two opposite sides of the container. The combined area of the ventilation apertures should be determined according to the species, dimensions of the container, intended stocking density, whether filter material covers the ventilation apertures and the range of ambient conditions expected to prevail during transport. Ventilation apertures should be covered with wire mesh of such a gauge that no part of the animal can protrude, and be designed such that the animal cannot damage the mesh with its teeth or feet.

While non-filtered transport containers are available for rodents and rabbits (Figure 12.8), animals with restricted microbial status destined for research use should be transported under SPF conditions using microbiologically secure containers (Figures 12.6 and 12.7) to protect them from infectious agents. SPF transport containers have ventilation apertures that are covered with some form of filter material of a pore size and filtration efficiency selected according to the degree of filtration and airflow required. Since most infectious agents are carried on particulates of larger diameter than the mean pore diameter of standard filters and since air velocity across the filters is low, small pore-size filters such as High Efficiency Particular Air or High Efficiency Particulate Arresting (HEPA) filters are not usually required. It is important to remember that filter material can decrease the ventilation rate within a container by 70% or more depending on thickness and pore size. Other factors such as stocking density within the container should be adjusted accordingly to compensate for decreased ventilation imposed by the addition of filters.

Filtered containers require a viewing port (viewing window) to allow assessment of animals while in transit (Figure 12.9). This is particularly important for journeys that cross national borders where some form of official inspection may be required.

A variety of materials is available for container construction. For rodents and rabbits, the most commonly used materials are plastic or varying strengths of corrugated cardboard or corrugated polypropylene. Each container may be partitioned into separate compartments, or two or more separate, primary containers may be placed into an overshipper for transport (Figure 12.7). Corrugated cardboard and corrugated polypropylene are relatively cheap and easy to dispose of, or recycle, and therefore are commonly used in non-reusable containers. For transporting larger species, materials used to construct containers include wood, plastic, metal or fibreglass. Such containers when made of plastic can be injection or vacuum moulded or, in the case of wood or metal, constructed with a strong framework and joints sheathed with solid panels with reinforced ventilation openings (Figure 12.10). Care must be taken to avoid using materials which adversely affect the health or welfare of the animal(s) to be transported, such as wood that has been treated with preservatives.

The container should be durable, non-toxic and able to withstand stacking without causing damage or crushing. Wooden containers should be constructed so that the animal cannot bore, claw or bite them open at the seams or joints. Nails, bolts, staples, sharp edges or other protrusions, on which animals could injure themselves, should be avoided; all slats and uprights should have rounded edges and be installed so that the animals cannot entrap their extremities.

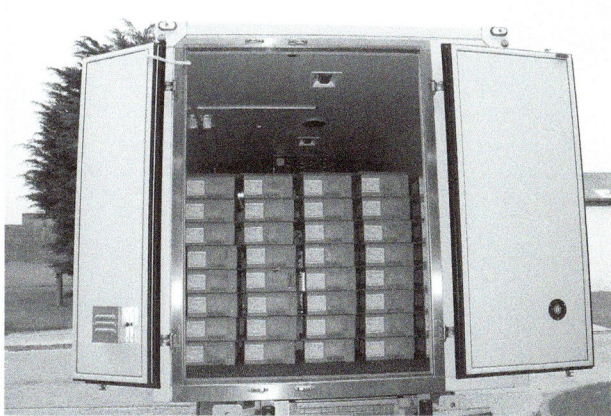

Figure 12.4 The back of a partially loaded, climate-controlled truck containing rodent shipping containers with integral ventilation stand-offs. The air channels between the containers allow circulation of air across the filtered openings.

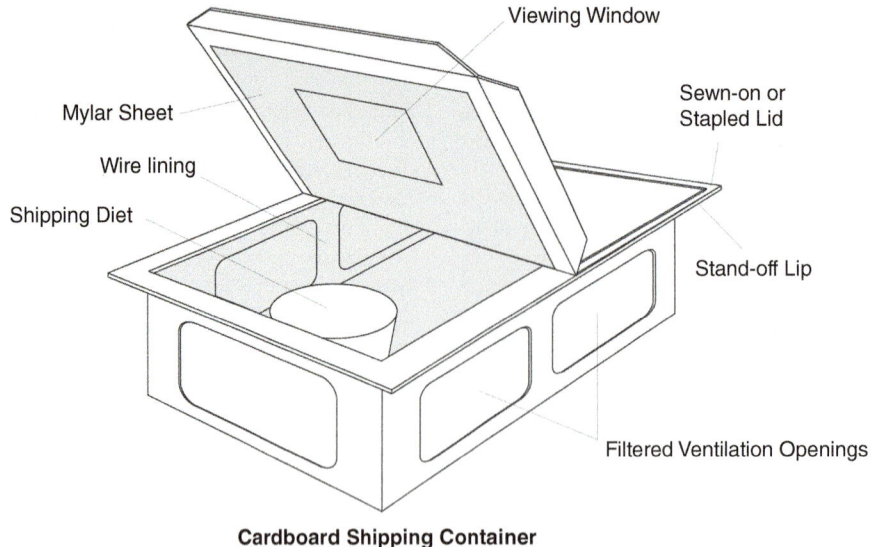

Figure 12.5 Diagram of a cardboard shipping container used for transport of mice and rats. The principal features of this design of container are noted on the illustration.

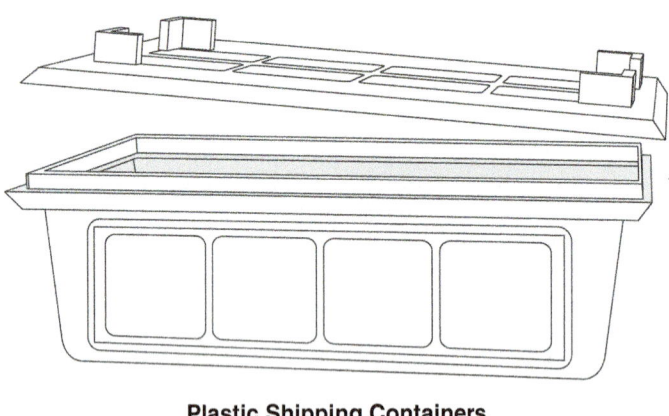

Figure 12.6 A drawing of a plastic shipping container used for transporting rodents. Ventilation openings (four) are visible along the side with similar ventilation openings located on the lid of the container. Plastic stand-offs are located on the top and a continuous stand-off runs around the top of the base of the container providing a channel for ventilation along the sides of the container.

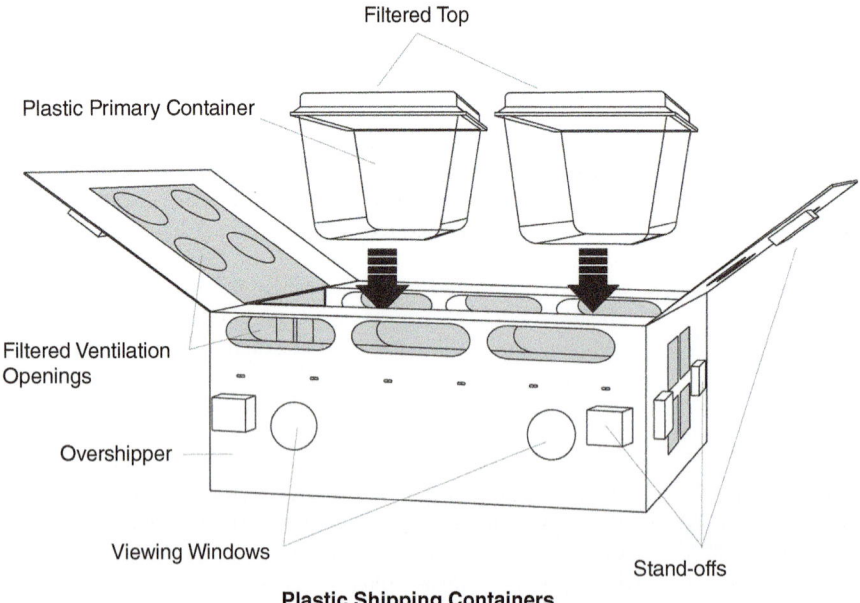

Figure 12.7 Two plastic filtered shipping containers are placed within a cardboard overshipper with filtered openings. The overshipper contains two viewing windows as well as rigid foam stand-offs to allow for unobstructed ventilation.

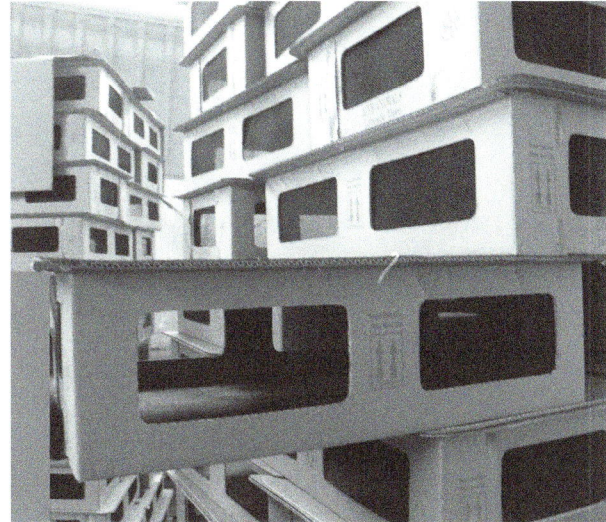

Figure 12.8 Unfiltered rodent shipping containers.

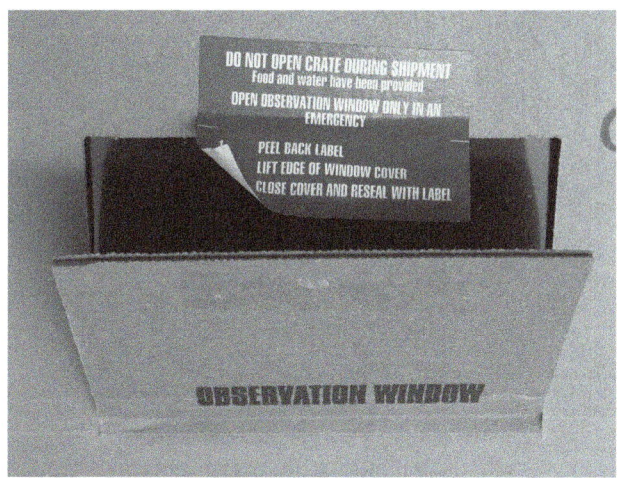

Figure 12.9 A disposable cardboard shipping container with a viewing window that can be accessed by peeling back an instruction label and lifting up a cut-out in the cardboard. The viewing window is constructed of Mylar™.

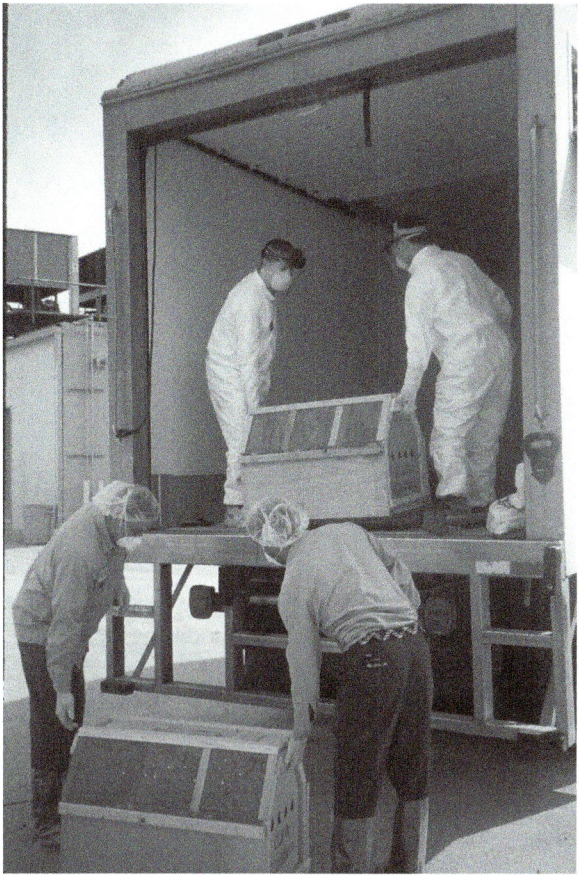

Figure 12.10 Wooden nonhuman primate shipping containers being loaded into a climate-controlled truck. The containers are designed to hold up to three nonhuman primates each with separate ventilation openings.

The interior surface of the container must be of solid construction and can be protected to some extent from the effects of moisture seepage due to urine by coating the inner surface with plastic or wax. For rodents that chew and gnaw, a wire mesh lining may be applied over all internal surfaces, including the floor and filtered ventilation openings, of disposable cardboard shipping containers to prevent escape. The wire should be applied so that the animals do not have access to loose or sharp edges. Some animals such as hamsters that aggressively dig and chew at surfaces must be shipped in containers with a double layer of wire lining covering all internal surfaces to prevent escape. Moulded plastic containers that provide a rugged smooth surface constructed such that corners and ventilation openings are not within the animals bite radius, do not require a wire lining when used with certain species. These are designed for specific species and may not work for others. Similarly, the lids of some shipping containers can be lined with a thick sheet of Mylar that, by its smooth surface design, does not fall within the animal's bite radius.

The lid or door of the container must fit the container securely to prevent accidental opening. Containers should have adequate hand holds or other lifting devices to enable them to be lifted without undue tilting or bringing the handlers in close contact with the animals. If containers are to be used on more than one journey, it must be possible to adequately clean and sterilise them. Although some shipping containers for laboratory rodents may be sanitisable, the integrity of cardboard and plastic containers may change after autoclaving, irradiation or chemical disinfection. The protective plastic or wax, for example, which lines corrugated cardboard is destroyed by heat sterilisation within an autoclave. After transport, the pores of the air filters covering the vents may be obstructed by debris such as food dust, bedding, animal fur and dander, or be compromised due to autoclaving, thereby reducing airflow into the container (Figure 12.11). Therefore, whenever possible, use new shipping crates which are commonly available through commercial sources to ensure safe animal transport and biosecurity.

Aquatic species must be packed with waterproof materials. Primary containment for adult fish typically uses strong polyethylene bags of at least 0.03 mm thick, with square or single seam bottom. One should fill the bag with appropriate amount of air and water then twist the top close while applying constant pressure to keep the bag inflated. Tie off the bag with a knot and secure with an additional fastener such as

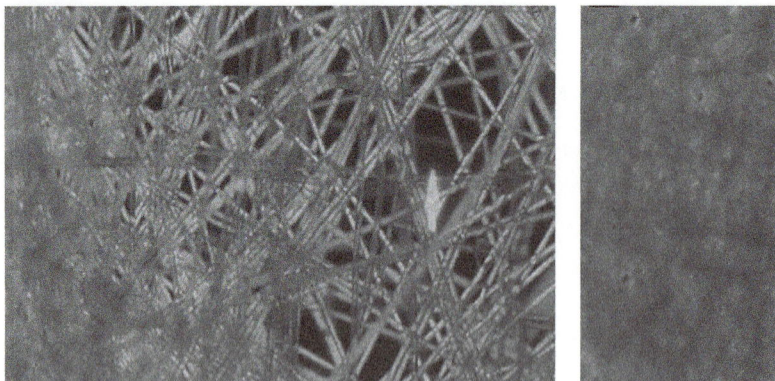

Figure 12.11 Top is a 10× magnification of a spun-bound polyester filter typically used to cover ventilation openings in shipping containers used for certain SPF laboratory animals. Note the varying pore-size openings. Bottom is the same filter material after being used to ship animals and subsequently autoclaved. Note that the remaining pores are very small in diameter. The use of moist heat has caramelised food particles and adhering dust has occluded most of the pores in the material. Effective ventilation is substantially reduced.

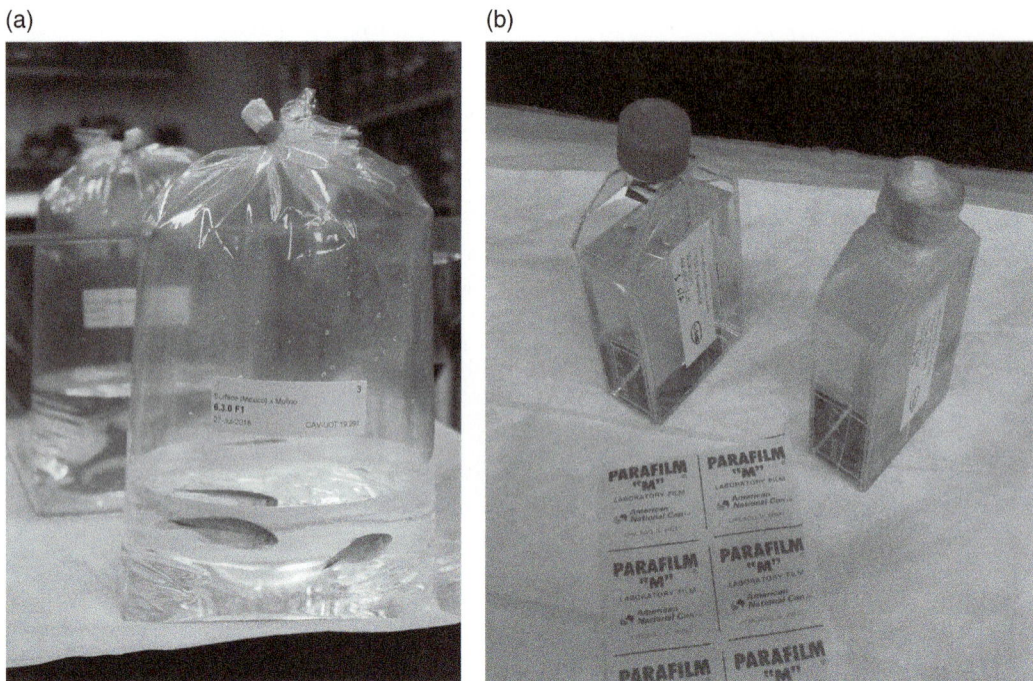

Figure 12.12 Illustrations of primary fish containment for transport. (a) Adult fish in polyethylene bags. (b) Fish embryos in 250 mL tissue culture flasks, cap reinforced with paraffin wax. Source: Courtesy of Stowers Institute for Medical Research, Kansas City, MO, USA.

heavy-duty rubber band or a plastic stable (Figure 12.12a). Check to make sure there are no leaks before reinforcing with an outer bag. Remove as much air as possible from the bag before sealing the outer bag to avoid water loss in case of leakage from the inner bag during transit. Alternatively, collapsible polyethylene cubitainers with a screw cap lid may be used instead of polyethylene bags (Figure 12.13a).

The primary containment for shipping fish embryos can use small rigid containers such as tissue culture flasks with solid sealed screw cap (Figure 12.12b). As with packaging for adults, flasks can be placed within another bag to serve as secondary containment. Absorbent material should be added in case the flasks break or leak. A label should be affixed to each of the bags or flasks with relevant content information.

The bags containing adult fish or flasks with fish embryos are placed into a rigid container with insulation and cushioning for protection. An expanded polystyrene (Styrofoam) container, or Styrofoam-liner of 3.8–5 cm (1.5–2 inches), that fits into a cardboard shipping container is typically used. Additional water-resistant packing material, such as bubble wrap, packing peanuts, air packs, should be used to fill unused space within the insulated container (Figure 12.13). As appropriate for the species of aquatic animals, it is common practice to add a small air-activated heat pack to the top of the packing material or affixed to the underside of the insulated container lid during colder months. A small hole must be drilled in the lid of the container, above the heat pack, to ensure oxygen supply necessary for continued heat pack activation.

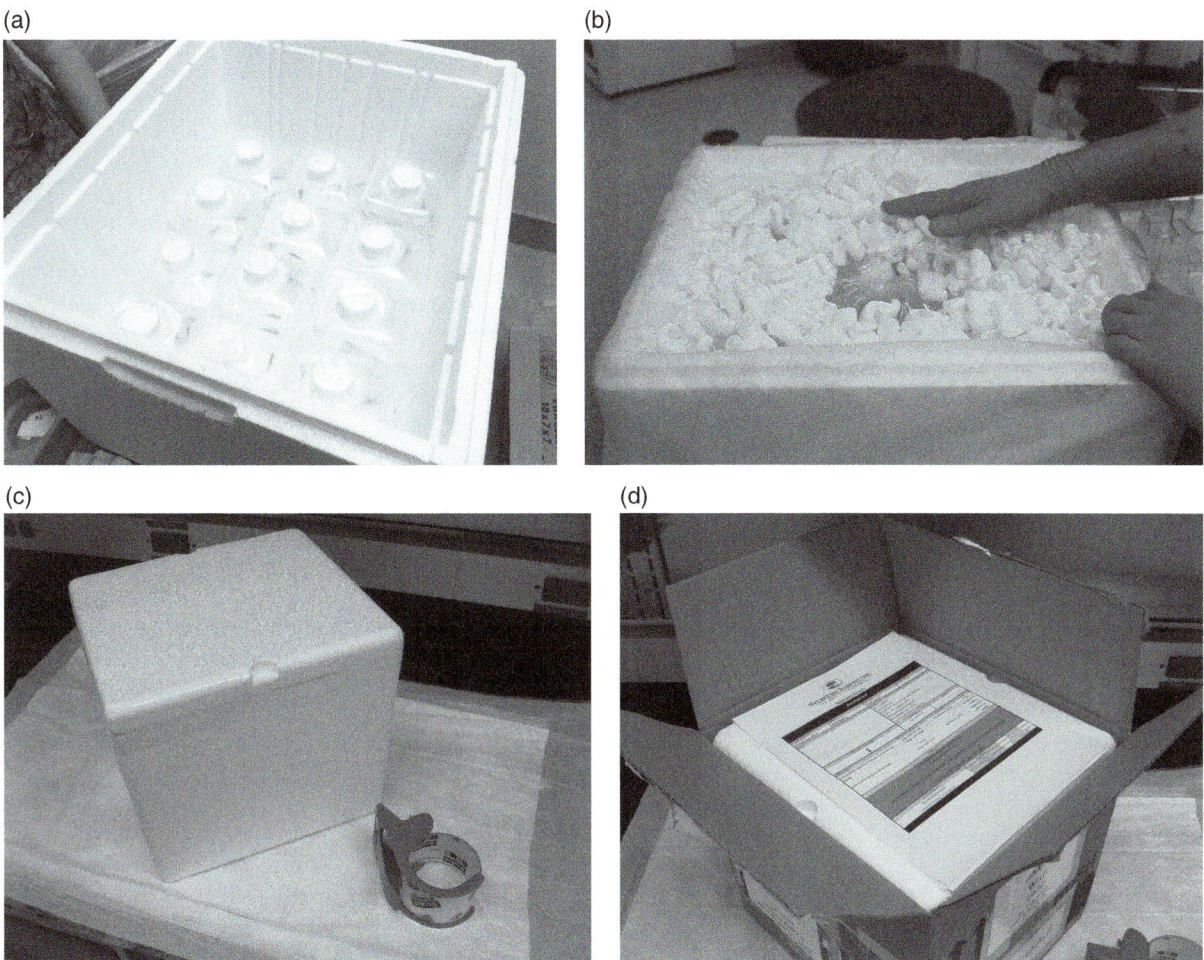

Figure 12.13 Illustrations of packing of containers of fish for shipment. (a) Placement of multiple cubitainers within a Styrofoam box. (b) Addition of packing material to insulate and protect the primary containers. (c) Securing and sealing the lid of the Styrofoam insulated shipper. (d) Placement of the insulated shipper within a cardboard shipping container and enclose a copy of the shipping documentation. Source: Courtesy of Stowers Institute for Medical Research, Kansas City, MO, USA.

Transport container stocking density

Terrestrial animals should have adequate space to provide for normal postures and postural adjustments within a transport container, including the ability to stand quadrupedally, stretch, turn around and lie down. Recommendations for transport container height and stocking density are based on species and body weight, as well as ambient temperature control and overall heat output of animals within a given area with ventilation apertures. The calculation of animal heat output is based in part on the work by Kleiber (1975) and Besch and Woods (1977), which is outlined by Swallow (1999). The results of these and other engineering studies, modified by experience using various stocking densities, have formed the basis for the current recommendations. Stocking density guidelines for shipping laboratory animals in filtered containers to maintain their SPF status as well as shipment using non-filtered containers are found in the LAR (IATA 2019a).

Compatible animals are best transported in a socially harmonious group within the same shipping container or container compartment. Species should never be mixed within the same transport container. Rodents shipped within a container should come from the same colony, be of similar age, of the same sex as appropriate and when possible be from the same weaning or social group. Similarly, when it is necessary to transport breeding adults and their offspring, they should travel in the same container, if possible. The maximum number of animals per compartment should be reduced when the ambient temperature at ground level exceeds 24 °C. Rabbits are usually transported singly or in divided boxes with or without filtered air vents.

Temperature within a filtered transport container for rodents, rabbits and guinea pigs is likely to be higher than ambient temperature due to heat load produced by animals and passive air exchange through filter. In one study, using data loggers during a ground transport of rats and guinea pigs in air acclimatised vehicles, measured temperatures differences between the interior of transport container and van's cargo space were 4.5°C and 2.4°C, respectively (M. Galasso, personal communication).

In some countries within continental Europe, dogs may travel in a loose housing system in small single-sex groups using the cargo area of a suitably equipped ground vehicle. However, this arrangement is forbidden in certain other countries when transporting dogs by air and by ground. In these cases, each dog must have its own shipping container, except when specifically permitted by the competent authority. Following IATA LAR guidance for calculating the appropriate size of the travelling container, it can be used to transport two compatible animals of comparable size (up to 14 kg each) or up to three animals not exceeding 6 months of age, from the same litter. To ensure compliance with current regulations, it is important to verify exceptions with the local competent authority (European Council 2004).

Same-sex adult macaques that have been maintained in an established compatible cohort should travel as pairs. Juveniles should be transported in pre-established single-sex pairs. Animals under 3 kg can be shipped using three-compartment containers, while those over 3 kg should be shipped in two-compartment containers (Figures 12.10 and 12.15). If cohousing is not feasible, then the animals should be shipped either in the company of compatible conspecifics in partitioned containers, or in separate containers loaded adjacent to each other. Pregnant females and females with suckling young are generally not accepted for air transport.

Adult fish shipments require a low density of fish. Institutional guidelines on shipping density should be developed, taking into consideration the duration of the transit and size of the fish. The typical recommendations can vary between fish users, but labs will typically use approximately 50 to 100 mL of water per adult fish and 1.5 to 2 ml of embryo medium per embryo (ILAR Roundtable 2014; Varga 2016; Aleström et al. 2019; Barton et al. 2020).

Stressors during animal transport

Current scientific knowledge supports the concept that stress is a real or perceived perturbation to an organism's physiological homeostasis or psychological well-being (NRC 2008). Stress can be harmful when prolonged and if animals fail to adjust (distress) (see also Chapter 6: Brief introduction to welfare assessment: A 'toolbox' of techniques). Stress can be characterised as acute or chronic, and acute or transient periods of stress are likely to occur during different phases of transport, such as preparation and packing, transportation and finally receipt at destination. While changes in heart rate, respiratory rate, behaviour, food and water consumption, and in the cellular and chemical composition of blood may occur, changes in one of these parameters are not necessarily diagnostic of stress nor is it practical to routinely assess these parameters during the transportation process. Moreover, there are species differences in what constitutes an environmental stress and the magnitude of its effects as well as the manifestation of those effects.

As examples, the effects of transportation as a stressor in mice and rats was studied by measuring a variety of parameters such as body weight, plasma corticosterone levels, faecal corticosterone metabolites (FCMs), mean arterial blood pressure (MAP) and heart rate (HR), locomotor activity, and by observation of social interaction and grooming behaviours post transport (Arts et al. 2012; Rumpel et al. 2019). Using prepuberal female mice from five genetic backgrounds, including C57BL/6J, C57BL/6NCrl, FVB/NCrl, Crl:CD1(ICR), and BALB/cAnCrl, Rumpel et al. (2019) found varied response based on genetic background. A significantly higher FCM levels was found one day post transport in C57BL/6NCrl, while all strains tested had increased FCM levels that returned to baseline within 4 days of transport except for FVB/NCrl (Rumpel et al. 2019). Using male Wistar Unilever rats (HsdCpb:Wu) with pre-implanted radio-telemetry devices, Arts et al. (2012) demonstrated that transportation affects rat physiology and behaviour. While some parameters such as MAP and HR stabilised after approximately 4 days post transport, the increase in plasma corticosterone levels did not return to baseline within the 16-day observation period, and social behaviours such as grooming and play-related behaviours were notably reduced, suggesting compromised welfare for at least 2 weeks (Arts et al. 2012).

Physiological response to environmental temperature may be a source of stress. The Thermoneutral Zone (TNZ) for rats and mice will vary in the scientific literature as it depends on the environments in which the animals are housed and assessed, but it is considered to be between 26 and 34°C. The TNZ can vary by strain, age and reproductive health status (NRC 2006). The highest temperature at which animal can maintain its core temperature is close to the upper limit of TNZ, this is because many research animals are non-sweating species and have a limited capacity for dissipating heat. When the ambient temperature rises above the upper limit of the TNZ, heat is dissipated by increasing radiant heat loss through increased peripheral vascular flow and evaporative heat loss via saliva spreading in rodents. Thermal stress, due to high environmental temperature and humidity within the transport box, is therefore likely to have high impact and may result in morbidity and mortality.

The length of the journey is an important variable affecting stress in shipment. Avoidance of delays in shipment and transfers by good journey planning is important to minimise the overall level of stress associated with the journey. From an animal welfare point of view, transport distance and time should be kept to a minimum, and an uninterrupted journey is preferable. In the periods where extreme weather conditions are forecasted (e.g. winter storms, summer heatwaves), it is prudent to have contingency procedures in place to prevent dispatch from the facility of origin.

Research on domestic farm animals suggests that the process of loading and unloading animals from shipping containers is more stressful than are other components of the journey (Knowles et al. 1995; Warriss et al. 1995). For this reason, acclimatisation of larger laboratory animals, such as domestic farm animals, to the container as well as to the loading and the unloading process may mitigate some of the stress encountered during the journey. For larger species, their efforts in counteracting the movements of the transport vehicle while in motion (Warriss et al. 1995) may cause additional stress. This may be less of a concern for smaller species that do not have to balance a large body mass at a substantial height above the floor. It is possible that species with more advanced cognitive abilities, such as nonhuman primates, may be more aware of their change in circumstances and be more predisposed to fear during transport, resulting in additional stress. Changes in presumptive measures of stress should be interpreted in context. For example, simply moving mice from one room or floor of a building to another can alter plasma cortisol levels (Tuli et al. 1995). Sheep undergoing a 24-hour journey showed increases in HR, plasma cortisol and glucose during loading and the initial stages of the journey but after 9 hours of travel, these had returned to normal levels (Knowles et al. 1995).

Experience has shown that there is considerable risk in sedating laboratory animals prior to transport in effort to counteract stress and destructive behaviours. Tranquillisers and other psychoactive drugs can reduce the ability of animals to respond to stresses during transport, affect their ability to thermoregulate and have unpredictable cardiovascular effects. In addition, the reaction of various species to these drugs cannot always be foreseen. For these reasons, the routine use of psychoactive medication is not recommended.

In order to enable animals to recover adequately from stress experienced during transport, it is very important that they are given a recovery period at their final destination prior to use in a research programme. An appropriate period of acclimatisation allows for recovery from the effects of stress during shipment and also allows the animals to adapt to changes in housing and husbandry. In the case of group-housed animals whose groups have changed prior to shipment, or which have a disrupted social structure, this period of acclimatisation permits the re-establishment of social order and resumption of natural behaviours. During this period, some presumptive measures of stress such as changes in electrolyte concentrations, haematological parameters, blood corticosteroid levels and a variety of physiological parameters can return to normal levels. Transportation-induced changes in the immune system may take longer to recover than fluid balance, electrolytes, plasma cortisol or glucose (Wallace 1976). The longer and more stressful the journey, the longer it may take for this stabilisation to occur.

During transport, animals can lose varying amounts of body weight, often of the order of 10% or sometimes even a little more. Most of this loss occurs early in the transport process, much of which is attributable to the voiding of faeces and urine as well as decreased food and water intake. Most, if not all, of this weight is normally recovered within a few days upon return to a more stable environment in the acclimatisation period post shipping. Grooming and exploratory behaviour in rats and mice are restored early in the acclimatisation period as are plasma cortisol concentrations, which may have been elevated upon receipt (Landi 1982; Arts et al. 2012). Various components of immune function may take longer to recover to pre-transport capability, as may certain other metabolic functions (Damon et al. 1986; Bean-Knudsen and Wagner 1987; Olubadeno 1994). Long-distance transport across different time zones may require extended periods of acclimatisation due to disturbance of the diurnal rhythm of the animals (Council of Europe 2006). Readers may refer to the ILAR special topics journal issue titled 'Preparation of Animals for Use in the Laboratory' for species-specific applicable recommendations aimed at minimising stress in transport (ILAR 2006). Ultimately, institutions should prepare carefully to avoid extreme situations wherein environmental control is lost.

Journey planning

The IATA LAR is the worldwide standard covering animal transport of all species. The information covered may be applied towards ground transport, with the exception that additional provisions, such as increase of space available per animal, decrease animal density, behavioural enrichment, and lighting, temperature, ventilation modifications, may be necessary to accommodate the longer length of travel. The IATA Live Animals Board developed the 'IATA Live Animals Acceptance Check List' for assisting shippers, agents and airlines to prepare shipments for air carriage (IATA 2019a). Airlines will only accept animals which appear to be in good health and condition and after verifying that the provisions specified within the LAR have been complied with by the shipper. They are not responsible, however, for making judgements on whether documentation has been completed correctly. For aquatic species being shipped in sealed solid-walled shipping containers, carriers are only responsible for ensuring that the outer surfaces of the shipping container meet the relevant provisions of the appropriate Container Requirements.

Ground transport

Purpose-bred laboratory animals such as rodents and rabbits must be transported in an environmentally controlled vehicle that can be easily sanitised and which provides ventilation rates and temperature parameters as set forth in European Union (EU) regulations. Council Regulation (EC) No 1/2005, requires that temperature within the cargo area be monitored and recorded throughout the journey (European Council 2004). This regulation also provides measures to ensure better enforcement of EU rules for transport. Article 3 and Article 27 of this regulation detail general conditions for the transport of animals, as well as requirements for inspections and for annual reports by the competent national authority. Authorisation is generally required for journeys but transporters undertaking journeys of less than 65 km from place of departure to place of destination do not require authorisation nor are they required to use drivers/attendants who have been trained and who hold a certificate of competency (Article 6.7). A journey log or appropriate satellite navigation record must be kept for each journey, and be in line with the Trade Control and Expert System (TRACES) (DEFRA 2010).

Council Regulation EC 1/2005 requires that all transported animals must be fit for travel. This applies to the transport of all laboratory animals including those undergoing regulated procedures under the authority of the Animals (Scientific Procedures) Act (ASPA 1986). Exceptions may be authorised under ASPA where there might be a compelling scientific need to move ill or injured animals. However, in such cases an appropriately certified veterinarian is required to confirm that such animals are fit for the intended journey. There are additional specific requirements regarding feeding and watering intervals and certain general loading requirements for cats, dogs, poultry, domestic birds and rabbits.

The journey log required by European regulation is the official record of the ground transportation journey. It includes sections on planning, place of departure, place of destination, a declaration by the transporter and an anomaly report. As envisioned, it would serve as a mechanism for approval by the competent authority prior to the journey beginning and would contain specifics of the actual journey as it occurred. This record would remain within the EU and be available for inspection for a period of 3 years.

For ground transport in other parts of the world, there are likely country-specific regulations, guidelines and oversight for the movement of laboratory animals within and between countries. A competent professional shipper with good working knowledge and regional experience should always be used to provide species-specific care during transit and to ensure safe and humane transport of laboratory animal species.

Air transport

The air transport process also has a ground transportation component which must meet applicable ground transport regulations. Air transport begins when the animal shipment arrives at the air cargo facility and is accepted by the carrier. Where international shipments are made outside the EU, and more generally for all cargo freight, a customs broker or freight forwarder must be engaged to assist in the export process. The air waybill is the official acceptance document used by the carrier for air transport wherein liability is accepted by the carrier. This liability is limited by international convention and should be supplemented by additional coverage if the animals are very valuable. The waybill is also the document used by the shipper to describe the contents of the shipment. Since the carrier and its personnel are not experts in animal biology and care or in taxonomy, they depend upon the shipper who is responsible to provide the necessary information on the waybill to indicate the required conditions for carriage. It is the duty of the shipper to use appropriate transport crates according to the current IATA LAR and to provide adequate amounts of food, bedding and water to sustain the animals during travel (IATA 2019a). The shipper must also supply the appropriate documents for export, carriage and import to satisfy existing laws and regulations in the countries of export, transit and import.

Animals are classified as sensitive cargo and are provided a climate-controlled environment in the aircraft. The consignor should provide the carrier with any specific environmental requirements for the animals being shipped. If there are no specific requirements given, general guidance for the species as found in the IATA LAR will be used. If very tight temperature or other environmental restrictions are required, the shipment may not be able to be accommodated. Air cargo personnel are provided training in handling animal containers as well as basic information on animals in transport. Typically, carrier personnel use a checklist to ensure that all the appropriate steps and paperwork have been completed. They are not responsible, however, for making judgements on whether documentation has been completed correctly.

Once the appropriate paperwork is completed, the shipment will be accepted by the carrier and moved to a section of the cargo facility where it can be held in a well-ventilated and quiet area. Not all airports, however, have dedicated areas for this purpose. Hence, animals may share space with other perishable cargo, live animals or personnel.

After holding in the cargo facility, typically 4 to 6 hours in advance of flight departure, the shipment will be transported to the flight line for loading on to the aircraft. Typically, animals are loaded on to the aircraft last, for a first-off unloading at the final destination. During summer months, extra care is required to minimise animal health impact resulting from direct exposure of shipping crates to excess heat during loading and unloading from aircraft. Use of temperature and humidity-controlled transfer vehicles is encouraged. Once on the aircraft, the animals are kept in a darkened environment. Even though space is reserved for animal shipments, circumstances can arise resulting in their being kept off a particular flight for a variety of reasons including incompatibility with other priority cargo (e.g. mail, human remains) and temperature embargos.

Upon arrival, the unloading process is a mirror image of the loading process. Animals will be transferred to a dedicated animal holding station, available in some airports, or designated holding area in smaller airports. Arrangements should be made by the consignee, the person receiving the shipment at the final destination, either directly or preferably through the use of a broker or customs agent, for pickup once the animals have cleared customs and veterinary services check. The vehicle used for this should be capable of providing a conditioned environment.

Due to the complexity of air transportation and the potential for intermediate stops and delays in flight schedules, it is important that contingency plans be made during the journey planning process. The carrier must be made aware of special requirements of the animals and must be given contact information for both the shipper and the consignee, in case of unforeseen delays or adverse events. Beyond these general considerations, airlines are entitled to establish their own additional rules and requirements related to the welfare of animals they are carrying.

Documentation

When animals are being transported, the shipping containers must affix relevant shipping labels (Figures 12.14 and 12.15) and be accompanied by the appropriate travel documentation. Depending on the animals to be transported, their health status, the mode of transportation and the final destination of the animals, a number of documents need to be prepared and authorised and should accompany the shipment. Some certifications are time sensitive and must be submitted as originals, not copies. It is highly recommended to keep copies of all documents required for shipment in case of loss during shipment – an event that could strand animals at border crossings or airports. The EUR-Lex website[1] offers readers searchable access to EU law for documents related to transport of animals within Europe.

One of the documents necessary for the shipment of laboratory animals is the Export Health Certificate (EHC). This is needed for the shipment of animals between countries. Guidance in relation to this requirement is generally given by the competent authority. As an example, in the UK, this is Animal and Plant Health Agency (APHA). An EHC is an

---

[1] https://eur-lex.europa.eu/homepage.html?locale=en (accessed 16 May 2020)

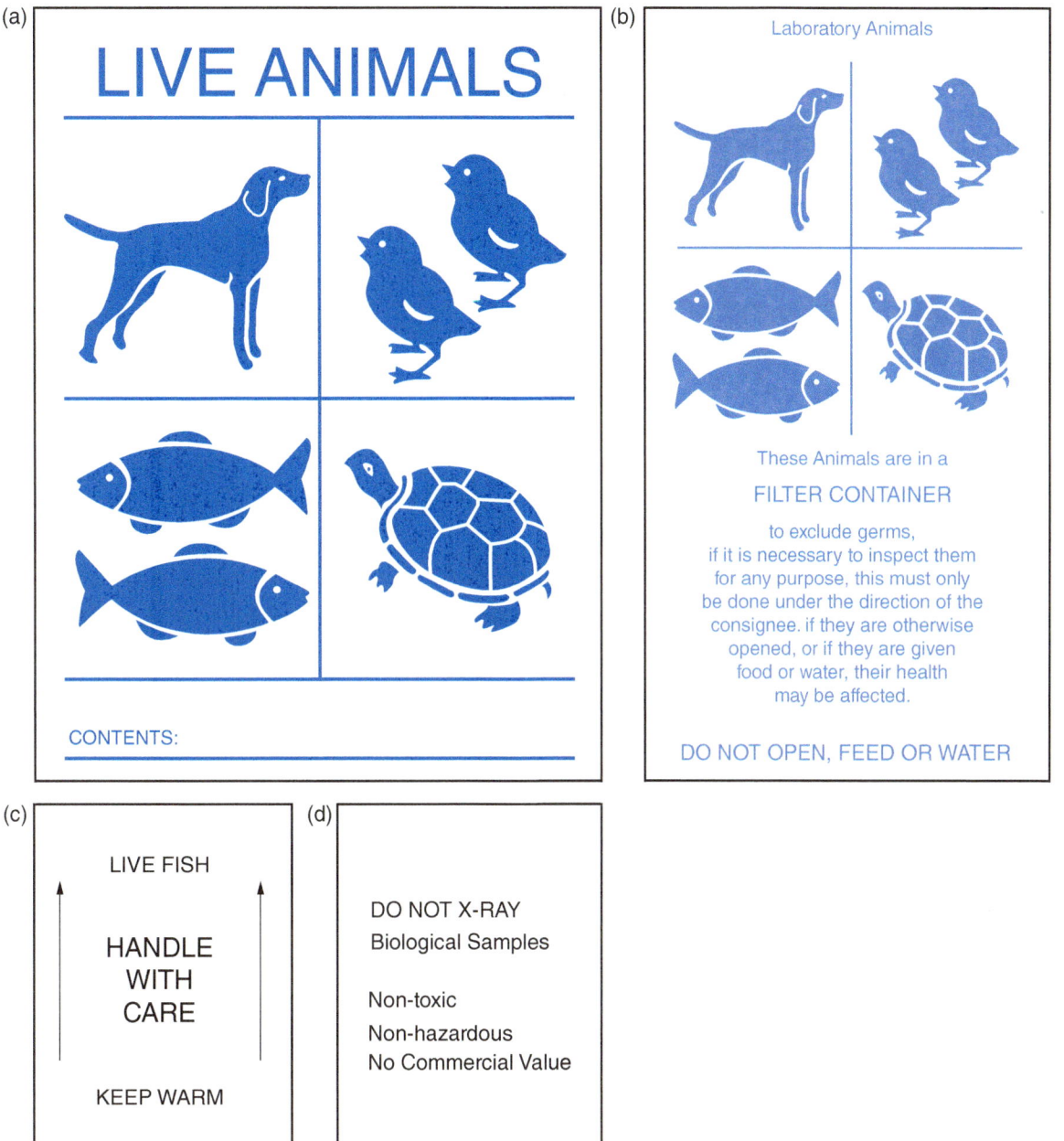

Figure 12.14 Illustrations of IATA-approved shipping labels. (a) The 'LIVE ANIMALS' label is used when shipping any live animal. (b) The 'LABORATORY ANIMALS' label must be used when shipping SPF laboratory animals. (c and d) Containers carrying live fish may affix additional labels or statements to emphasise package content.

official veterinary document used to confirm that a consignment of animals or animal products meets certain health criteria. Shippers wanting to export live animals, animal products or germ plasm to an EU member state will need the health certificate signed by a government-approved 'official veterinarian'. Further information on EHCs can be obtained by contacting APHA in the UK or similar competent authorities in exporting or receiving countries. In addition, on any journey of any length, an Animal Transport Certificate (ATC) is also required, for the purpose of helping transporters and inspectors ensure journeys are within the maximum journey times for the animals, and to inform the appropriate vehicle standards of vehicle being used (DEFRA 2010).

Other documents that may be required include: import licences issued by the state veterinary service; CITES permits where necessary; invoices for custom purposes; fitness to travel documents, including records of certain laboratory tests, vaccinations or treatments; quarantine labels, if applicable; transfer authorisations from specific bodies that regulate the use of laboratory animals; an ATC or group plan; and, in the case of ground transportation, vehicle registration details and insurance.

Information specific to the animals being transported, including species, strain, scientific name, number, sex, age, weight, individual identification and any special care requirements related to phenotype, should accompany each

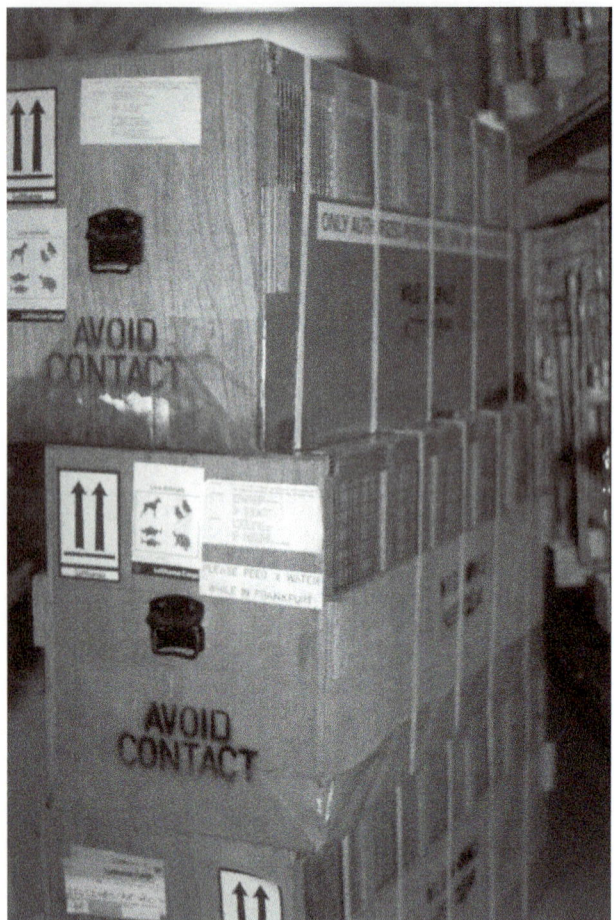

Figure 12.15 Wooden nonhuman primate shipping containers with directional arrow labelling, live animals labelling and transportation documents attached to the outside of the container. Other labelling imprinted on the container is used to advise personnel that only authorised individuals should handle these containers.

shipment. Some of this information is required on other documents and placing it in one location can prove helpful. In addition, the name, address, and 24-hour telephone contact numbers for the consignor (person with ultimate responsibility for the shipment), intermediaries, consignee and the shipper's attending veterinarian can also be helpful in case of difficulties during shipment.

All the required documents should be collated and attached to the first container of each consignment. It is advisable to make sure that the necessary documents have been aligned with the United Nations (UN) layout key for trade documents. These are internationally agreed standards that are easily translated because common information appears in standard positions on all forms.

Correct and complete documentation is essential to avoid delays in transit. Animal shipments are often delayed in customs due to failure to provide correct documents containing the appropriate wording, signatures and authorisations. Accompanying documents can be lost in transit, highlighting the need to keep copies of all necessary documents. There is currently an air freight industry initiative to make many documents electronic so that they can be sent in advance of shipment to the competent authorities at the point of entry (POE). Basic documentation requirements for international shipment for various countries can be found in The Air Cargo Tariff and Rules (TACT) (IATA 2019c) and the LAR (IATA 2019a). If a customs broker is employed to facilitate the shipment, they can also provide guidance on the required documents. Individual country embassies are also a source of information. It is also helpful to have the consignee at the destination assist in determining what documentation is required and for an electronic copy of all shipment documents to be sent in advance of the shipment to the consignee.

Points of entry

Most countries have a limited number of designated locations, or border inspection posts (BIPs), where animals can enter the country. For example, the EU and the USA, operate a system of BIPs or POE which are approved for the importation of different species such as farm livestock, equidae, rabies-susceptible animals, birds, fish or any combination of the above, including laboratory animals. Animal consignments may be inspected by officials upon arrival. Authorities often require advance notification of the import or export of live animals, especially in the case of larger animals, so that the appropriate inspection personnel can be available. Recipients of animals should note that such inspections take time and journey plans should allow for delays at BIPs.

Both consignor and consignee should agree in advance of any shipment the conditions of transportation, including the departure and arrival times so that, at their destination, the animals can be placed in previously prepared cages, fed, watered and rested as quickly as possible. On arrival, animals should be removed from their transport container and examined by a responsible person with the least possible delay.

Journey time

Most terrestrial laboratory animals travel within containers with food, water and bedding sufficient in quantity for the journey. Under these conditions, there is not usually a maximum permitted journey time. However, for some animals, particularly larger species, there can be specific restrictions regarding journey time and rest stops according to Council Regulation (EC) No 1/2005 of 22 December 2004 on the protection of animals during transport (European Council 2004). Given the broad definition of animals in this regulation, guidance might be included in future revisions to cover more traditional laboratory species.

Current laws, regulations and standards

Most regulations and standards apply to livestock animals which are, by far, the principal category of animals transported worldwide. However, general considerations are applicable to all species, especially vertebrates and additional guidance for laboratory animal species are also available. In Europe, Council Regulation (EC) No 1/2005 (European Council 2004) on the protection of animals during transport and related operations setting out minimum standards for the welfare of animals during transport came into force on 25 January 2005. This Regulation applies to the transport of all live vertebrate animals for the purposes of economic activity (i.e. business or trade). While EU Regulation is directly applicable, some national legislation is needed to provide for enforcement and penalty provisions, derogations from the rules and to levy the charges for authorisations. Hence, it is implemented in England by The Welfare of Animals (Transport) (England) Order 2006 by parallel legislation in Scotland, Wales and Northern Ireland (DEFRA 2010).

EU Regulation 1/2005 aims to improve animal welfare through raising transportation standards. In particular, it provides significant improvements in enforcement capability for all species transported. While its scope covers all live vertebrate animals, the regulation does not apply to the transport of non-vertebrate species such as insects, worms, crustaceans, cephalopods and molluscs. However, general welfare in transport provisions protecting non-vertebrates from injury or unnecessary suffering are contained in regulations for devolved administrations in the UK. In addition, cephalopods, being covered by the Directive 2010/63/EU on the protection of animals used for scientific purposes since 2010, are subject to new guidelines for their care and welfare, including transportation (Fiorito et al. 2015).

Considering transportation is typically a stressful experience for animals, the World Organization for Animal Health (OIE) have set up standards for use of animals in research and education, including their transportation, as well as more general guidance for transport of animals by sea, by land and by air (OIE 2019a, OIE 2019b). In addition, OIE and the Convention on International Trade in Endangered Species of wild flora and fauna (CITES) have agreed that the current version of LAR be employed as guidelines for the air transportation of animals. The LAR set standards concerning the transport of animals by air which include advice on general care and loading, the design and construction of containers together with appropriate packing, feeding and watering arrangements (IATA 2019a). Since 2004, the LAR have been adopted by the EU as minimum standards for transporting animals, and, globally, most airlines and countries will only accept animals packed and transported according to the LAR standards. In its latest edition, the LAR mandates recurrent training for all staff involved in the transport of live animals and reinforces the feeding and watering requirements (IATA 2019a). Other useful guidance is available; see for example the publications by Elmore (2008), Institute for Laboratory Animal Research (NRC 2006) or contact Animal Transportation Association[2].

On 31 January 2020, 'Brexit' took place, confirming the withdrawal of the UK from the EU. This begins a transition period that is set to end on 31 December 2020, during which time the UK and EU will negotiate their future relationship. In this transition period, the UK remains subject to EU law and remains part of the EU customs union and single market, but is no longer part of the EU's political bodies or institutions. In the preparation for Brexit, the UK and EU have worked together to limit potential disruption to the movement of research animals and biological samples. No significant changes will take place during the transition period. There are likely to be regulatory changes agreed by the end of 2020, but it is uncertain which regulations will change and how far the changes go. Current common legislation and implementation tools are based on EU Regulations; however, changes in the processes and the systems being used to transport animals will likely occur. The scientific community can thankfully rely on stakeholder organisations, such as the European Animal Research Association[3], which is carefully monitoring the Brexit discussions and will seek to limit the negative impacts from both animal welfare and research continuity perspectives.

Impact of animal rights movement on animal transport

Background and history

There is a long tradition of opposition to animal research based on a variety of philosophical positions. Historically, these efforts have been one component of a more general concern for the welfare of animals including animals kept as pets, wildlife, animals used for food, fibre and transportation, as well as research animals. Over time, the anti-vivisection movement has become a specific focus for some and led to more extreme activities and positions.

By 2016, most major airlines had created a policy against transporting nonhuman primates, dogs and cats for research purposes. Research rodent shipping was also impacted by a growing number of airlines publishing policies that stated they will not carry animals of any species intended for biomedical research. In a recent count, over 75 airlines refused to transport nonhuman primates for research. Air France, the most prominent major national airline that continues to carry nonhuman primates for biomedical research, supports the biomedical research community despite ongoing protests.

As success with airline policies grew, the emboldened antivivisection community broadened their efforts to include additional modes of transportation. At least three major ferry companies operating in Europe, citing animal rights pressure, refuse to accept shipments of animals bound for biomedical research, as does the Eurotunnel authority. One ferry company spokesman noted the need to preserve their reputation and assure the safety of their employees; the threat of violence was taken seriously[4]. Ground transportation remains a viable option in many situations but is not immune to targeting. Reports of arson and firebomb destruction of animal transport trucks are noted and while the majority impact the agriculture industry, there are instances where the target was research animal transporters.

---

[2]https://www.animaltransportationassociation.org/ (accessed 26 May 2020)

[3]www.eara.eu (accessed 26 May 2020)
[4]https://www.sciencemag.org/news/2012/03/no-ticket-ride-uk-animal-rights-campaigners-end-ferry-service-lab-animals (accessed July 6 2021)

The Animal Liberation Front (ALF) has claimed responsibility for destruction of vehicles and facilities belonging to research animal producers, citing their intent to cause monetary harm to research animal producers and to eliminate the means to transport animals to research facilities[5].

Current activity and general status

The airlines still willing to transport research animals face intermittent protests and disruption of airport activity, street theatre (with individuals dressed as animals in cages, fake blood), offensive posters, chanting, bombardment with email and phone calls, and customer harassment. This activity is not limited to airports, and is also conducted at airline offices, travel agencies and other public venues. Airline executives have been accosted in public and at their homes by protesters as a pressure tactic. Some airline executives claimed to have been concerned for the safety of their employees and passengers as a factor in their decisions to stop transporting research animals, citing the fear that the aircraft could be damaged by an escaped animal. This concern has not resulted in airlines refusal of pet, zoo, or sanctuary animals, however. While there is little evidence that targeting by animal rights groups has impacted airline revenues or reputation, most airlines continue to avoid perceived controversy connected to transporting some or all species of research animals.

Impact on animal welfare and research quality

Despite opposition, most research institutions can and do obtain the animals necessary for their scientific investigations. This does not mean that the institutions or the animals are unaffected by anti-transport activity. Faced with loss of traditional transportation routes and methods, researchers and animal providers are forced into necessary but regrettable transportation choices using convoluted air routes, connecting flights with layovers, extended lorry travel to/from alternate airports or excessively long ground transportation – all which create additional risk and stress to animals, including longer confinement in shipping crates. Research model providers report numerous examples and concerns regarding prolonged travel such as:

- An animal shipment that was a direct flight requiring 6 hours now requires three flights and nearly 24 hours to arrive at the same destination
- A shipment that had been a reasonable domestic trip by round vehicle now requires two flights and international/customs clearance
- Animal shipments routed to alternate airports, requiring much longer truck movement before and after a flight, adding hours or even days to trip duration
- For flights originating in non-US/EU countries, travel to distant alternate airports can be harrowing trips over poor quality roads

- Longer ground transportation carries increased risk to animals due to opportunities for mechanical problems, weather disruptions, customs issues and (statistically) vehicle accidents

A less recognised transportation impact on research is cost. Having fewer providers transporting research animals allows remaining providers to charge higher fees; the cost of transportation has reportedly increased by 30–40% in the past 5 years for all research animal species. Charter flights are expensive and often unfeasible options to replace commercial airlines. In cases where lack of airline options has forced increased ground transportation, the industry experts report significantly higher costs. A recent review of rodent transportation in the USA demonstrated that ground transportation by dedicated vehicle costs >$3/mile, charged round trip, as opposed to the relatively modest cargo fees for shipping containers in commercial air transport (W. White, personal communication, 2020). Breeding animals internally to avoid transportation costs and difficulties is not a viable alternative for most institutions. In addition to producing a limited variety of models, resources/labour/space requirements would displace a significant percentage of ongoing research and eliminate many institutions' access to GM rodent models. At the same time, creating duplicative breeding colonies undermines efforts to reduce total animal numbers. Another option for rodent models, reconstitution of frozen embryos, requires expertise and resources outside the reach of smaller institutions.

Longer transport, reduced ability to fully control conditions and increased handling heighten stress on animals which potentially impacts research. Fortunately, research facilities provide high quality environments, stable conditions and added time for animals to acclimate to their new environment and recover from shipping stress. Research professionals note fewer choices in selection of animal models and intermittent delays in their work due to longer waits for shipments and longer animal acclimation periods.

Attacks on transportation are intended to limit resources at research institutions, raise costs and influence public opinion. Transportation targeting is not limited to legal and peaceful protests, but includes property destruction, vandalism, harassment, slander, intimidation and character assassination. Without societal and legal support for transportation freedom, we can expect increasingly negative impacts on research, research animal welfare and the goal of fully employing the Three Rs principles. The research community faces perceived insecurity in research animal supply, inability to share and collaborate, increased budget constraints, and continued shift of research to non-EU countries.

Acknowledgements

We thank Dr William J. White, Mr Carl B. Kole, and Mr Roy Sutcliffe for use of the original text and figures from the 8th edition of the UFAW Handbook; Ms Diana Baumann and Stowers Institute for Medical Research for sharing illustrations related to fish shipment; Dr Marica Galasso of Charles River Laboratories Italia for sharing study data from a 2014 internal study on rodent ground transportation; and

---

[5] https://www.mississauga.com/news-story/5666768-updated-animal-rights-group-claims-responsibility-for-blaze-that-destroyed-two-trucks-in-west-mississauga/ (accessed July 6 2021)

Mr Carl B. Kole of Kole Consulting and Mr Tristan Bradfield of Heathrow Animal Reception Centre for their constructive review of this manuscript.

References

Aleström P., D'Angelo L., Midtlyng P.J. et al. (2019). Zebrafish: Housing and husbandry recommendations. *Laboratory Animals*, **0**, 1–12.

Animals (Scientific Procedures) Act (1986) *UK Public General Acts* (available at http://www.legislation.gov.uk/ukpga/1986/14/contents, accessed 10 March 2020).

Arts, J.W., Kramer, K., Arndt, S.S. et al. (2012). The impact of transportation on physiological and behavioral parameters in Wistar rats: Implications for acclimatization periods. *ILAR Journal*, **53**, E82–E98 (available at https://doi.org/10.1093/ilar.53.1.82, accessed 29 February 2020).

Balansard, I., Cleverley, L., Cutler, K.L. et al. (2019) Revised recommendations for health monitoring of non-human primate colonies (2018): FELASA Working Group Report. *Laboratory Animals*, **53**, 429–446.

Barton, C.L., Baumann, D.P. and Cox, J.D. (2020) Export and transportation of Zebrafish. In: *The Zebrafish in Biomedical Research*. Eds Cartner S.C., Eisen J.S., Farmer S.C. et al., pp. 443–450.

Bean-Knudsen, D.E. and Wagner, J.E. (1987) Effect of shipping stress on clinicopathologic indications in F344/N Rats. *American Journal of Veterinary Research*, **48**, 306–308.

Berard, M., Feinstein, R., Gallagher, A. et al. (2014) FELASA recommendations for the health monitoring of mouse, rat, hamster, guinea pig and rabbit colonies in breeding and experimental units. *Laboratory Animals*, **48**, 178–192.

Besch, B.E.L. and Woods, J.E. (1977) Heat dissipation biorhythms of laboratory animals. *Laboratory Animal Science*, **27**, 54–59.

Collymore, C., Crim, M.J., and Lieggi, C. (2016) Recommendations for health monitoring and reporting for zebrafish research facilities. *Zebrafish*, **13**, S-138–S-148.

Council of Europe (2003) *European Convention for the Protection of Animals during International Transport (Revised)*. European Treaty Series No. 193. (available at https://www.coe.int/en/web/conventions/full-list/-/conventions/treaty/193, accessed 24 February 2020)

Council of Europe (2006) *Appendix A of the European Convention for the Protection of vertebrate Animals Used for Experimental and other Scientific Purposes (ETS no. 123), Guidelines for Accommodation and Care of Animals (article 5 of the Convention)* Cons 123 (2006) (available at https://www.coe.int/en/web/conventions/full-list/-/conventions/treaty/123, accessed 24 February 2020).

Damon, E.G., Eidson, A.F., Hobbs, C.H. et al. (1986) Effect of acclimation on nephrotoxic response of rats to uranium. *Laboratory Animal Science*, **36**, 24–27.

Department for Environment, Food and Rural Affairs (DEFRA) (2010) *Welfare of Animals During Transport* (available at https://www.gov.uk/government/publications/welfare-of-animals-during-transport, accessed 01 March 2020).

Elmore, D.B. (2008) Quality management for the international transportation of nonhuman primates. *Veterinaria Italiana*, **44**(1), 141–147.

European Council (2004) *Council Regulation (EC) No 1/2005 of 22 December 2004 on the Protection of Animals during Transport and Related Operations and Amending Directives 64/432/EEC and 93/119/EC and Regulation (EC) No 1255/97* (available at https://eur-lex.europa.eu/legal-content/en/ALL/?uri=CELEX%3A32005R0001, accessed 01 February 2020).

Fiorito, G., Affuso, A., Basil, J. et al. (2015) Guidelines for the Care and Welfare of Cephalopods in Research – A consensus based on an initiative by CephRes, FELASA and the Boyd Group. *Laboratory Animals* **49**(2), 1–90.

International Air Transportation Association (2019a) *Live Animals Regulations*, 46th edn. IATA, Montreal.

International Air Transportation Association (2019b) *Dangerous Goods Regulations*, 61st edn. IATA, Montreal.

International Air Transportation Association (2019c) *The Air Cargo Tariff (TACT) and Rules* available via online subscription at https://www.iata.org/en/publications/tact/tact-online

International Civil Aviation Organization (2017–2018) *Technical Instructions for the Safe Transport of Dangerous Goods by Air* (Doc 9284). (available at https://www.icao.int/publications/pages/publication.aspx?docnum=9284, accessed 01 February 2020).

Institute for Laboratory Animal Research (2006) *Preparation of Animals for Use in the Laboratory*. *ILAR Journal*, **47**(4) (available at https://academic.oup.com/ilarjournal/issue/47/4, accessed 02 March 2020).

[Ilar Roundtable] (2014, September 26) *Transportation for Specific Species Presentations* [Video File]. Retrieved from https://www.youtube.com/watch?v=m6_guAW1ft0&list=PLhfetJ6qmFsUgZD9zbaNvN_E3Jj0sRFR-&index=13&t=0s

Kleiber, M. (1975) *The Fire of Life: an Introduction to Animal Energetics*. Robert E. Kreiger, Huntingdon.

Knowles, T.G., Brown, S.N., Warriss, P.D. et al. (1995) Effects on sheep of transport by road for up to 24 hours. *Veterinary Record*, **136**, 431–488.

Laboratory Animal Science Association (2005) Guidance on the transport of laboratory animals. Report of the Transport Working Group established by LASA. *Laboratory Animals*, **39**, 1–39.

Landi, M.S. (1982) Effects on shipping on the immune function in mice. *American Journal of Veterinary Research*, **43**, 1654–1657.

National Research Council (NRC) Committee on Guidelines for the humane Transportation of Laboratory Animals, Institute for Laboratory Animal Research (2006) *Guidelines for the Humane Transportation of Research Animals*. National Academies Press, Washington, DC.

National Research Council (NRC) Committee on Recognition and Alleviation of Distress in Laboratory Animals, Institute for Laboratory Animal Research (2008) *Recognition and Alleviation of Distress in Laboratory Animals*. National Academies Press, Washington, DC.

Olubadeno, J.O. (1994) The effects of stress on lipoproteins and catecholamines in rats. *Cellular Immunology and Molecular Biology*, **40**, 1201–1206.

Rumpel, S., Scholl, C., Göbel, A. et al. (2019) Effect of ground transportation on adrenocortical activity in prepuberal female mice from five different genetic backgrounds. *Animals*, **9**, 239 (available at https://doi.org/10.3390/ani9050239, accessed 24 February 2020).

Swallow, J.J. (1999) Transporting animals. In: *The UFAW Handbook on The Care and Management of Laboratory Animals, Vol 1 Terrestrial Vertebrates*, 7th edn. Ed. Poole, T., pp. 171–187. Blackwell Publishing, London.

The Welfare of Animals (Transport) (England) Order 2006 (2006) *UK Statutory Instruments 2006 No. 3260* (available at http://www.legislation.gov.uk/uksi/2006/3260/contents, accessed 10 March 2020).

Tuli, J.S., Smith, J.A. and Morton, D.B. (1995) Stress measurements after transportation. *Laboratory Animals*, **29**, 132–138.

Varga, Z.M. (2016) Aquaculture, husbandry, and shipping at the Zebrafish International Resource Center. In: *Methods in Cell Biology: The Zebrafish: Genetics, Genomics, and Transcriptomics*, Volume 135 4th edn. Eds Detrich, H.W., Westerfield, M., and Zon L.I., pp. 509–534. Academic Press, Cambridge, MA.

Wallace, M.E. (1976) Effects of stress due to deprivation and transport in different genotypes of house mouse. *Laboratory Animals*, **10**, 335–347.

Warriss, P.D., Brown, S.N., Knowles, T.G. *et al.* (1995) Effects on cattle of transport by road for up to 15 hours. *Veterinary Record*, **136**, 319.

White, W.J., Chou, S.T., Kole, C.B. *et al.* (2010) Transportation of laboratory animals. In: *The UFAW Handbook on The Care and Management of Laboratory and Other Research Animals*, 8th edn. Eds Hubrecht, R. and Kirkwood, J., pp. 169–182. The Universities Federation for Animal Welfare, Wiley-Blackwell, Oxford.

World Organisation for Animal Health (OIE) (2019a) Aquatic Animal Health Code. (available at https://www.oie.int/standard-setting/aquatic-code/, accessed 20 February 2020).

World Organisation for Animal Health (OIE) (2019b) Terrestrial Animal Health Code. (available at https://www.oie.int/standard-setting/terrestrial-code/, accessed 29 February 2020).

Zebrafish International Resource Center (ZIRC) (2019) ZIRC Protocols [ZIRC Public Wiki] (available at https://zebrafish.org/wiki/protocols/start, accessed 14 February 2020).

13 Nutrition, feeding and animal welfare

Graham Tobin and Annette Schuhmacher

Introduction

This chapter is not intended to be a general discussion on animal nutrition. For that, there are many excellent textbooks, particularly those by Wu (2018) and McDonald et al. (2011), which reflect US and European approaches to nutrition, respectively. Here we have selected nutrition topics in laboratory animal science that we consider closely related to animal welfare. We have discussed other, more general, practical aspects of laboratory animal nutrition elsewhere (Tobin & Schuhmacher 2021). We have largely excluded farm animals from our chapter, even though sometimes they may be used as experimental animals. The issue of nutrition and the welfare of farm animals has been reviewed by the FAO (2012) and Phillips (2016).

The contribution of diet and nutrition to good animal welfare begins with ensuring freedom from chronic thirst and hunger (Tolkamp & D'Eath 2016) though mild thirst and hunger are physiologically normal and are necessary to initiate drinking and feeding (Kyriazakis & Tolkamp 2011). As we describe later, hunger and thirst may form part of an experimental protocol but one that must be tightly regulated and approved independently of the investigators. Severe hunger and associated stereotypical behaviours have been a major concern in farm animals such as breeding sows and broiler breeders, where considerable feed restriction is often used to minimise body weight gain in 'normal' husbandry (D'Eath et al. 2009). Extreme restriction (<50% of ad libitum intake) has also been used with minipigs in experimental and regulatory studies to counter their tendency to become obese (Bollen et al. 2006; Ellegaard et al. 2010). This level of restriction is much greater than that used in rodent diet-restriction studies, which we discuss later and should never be considered 'normal' husbandry. Although some of the hunger associated with such severe diet restriction may be offset, at least in pigs, by access to hay or straw, some investigators consider that compensation is far from complete, and animals remain 'metabolically hungry' (D'Eath et al. 2009) and possibly stressed.

Laboratory animals should also not be subjected to unintended nutritional deficiencies and excesses. While many textbooks emphasise nutritional deficiencies and their severe effects on animal welfare, these are extremely rare in animals fed on diets formulated by specialist laboratory animal diet manufacturers, at least in developed countries. However, they may occasionally occur when diet is used inappropriately, and we discuss the most likely scenarios below. If the deficiencies or excesses are imposed as part of a pre-planned experimental protocol, like hunger and thirst, the protocol must be subject to independent approval and control (see Chapter 18: Ethical review), and there may be specific regulation or guidance in some jurisdictions. For example, in the UK, project licence authority is required for food restriction resulting in weight loss or reduced gain of >15% or where animals are maintained at a body weight below 85% of that of controls fed ad libitum[1]. The reader is also recommended to consult Chapter 8: Legislation and oversight of the conduct of research using animals: a global overview. Many of the experimental studies with farm animals are primarily nutrition-related and conducted by experienced nutritionists, so unintended deficiencies are extremely unlikely.

In our view, the greatest welfare issue related to diet lies in the inappropriate way it is often used in many animal-based investigations (see also Tobin 2004). In recent years, the scientific community has become increasingly concerned about the lack of reproducibility in animal-based investigations (Bomzon & Tobin 2021). This inability to reproduce published scientific results has considerable significance for animal welfare: at the very least, it may substantially increase the number of animal studies required to resolve a scientific question. We have focused on three broad dietary causes of diet-related irreproducibility in animal-based studies: poor scientific method, the use of diverse diets with different effects, and a failure to appreciate the variability that is possible within a single diet over time.

We frequently see major failings in the application of the scientific principle when investigators design or select

---

[1] Home Office Guidance Note Water and Food Restriction for Scientific Purposes https://www.med.hku.hk/images/document/04research/culatr/HomeOfficeGuide_WaterFoodRestriction.pdf (accessed 8 November 2019)

The UFAW Handbook on the Care and Management of Laboratory and Other Research Animals, Ninth Edition.
Edited by Huw Golledge and Claire Richardson.
© 2024 John Wiley & Sons Ltd. Published 2024 by John Wiley & Sons Ltd.

ill-matched diets for use in control and experimental treatments. These diets often differ by many more variables than the one singled out by the investigators for attention as the primary cause of any experimental outcomes. The effects of diets are also rarely just limited to their nutrient content. Different diets may vary in many factors that can affect study outcomes, including their physical nature (hardness), sensory properties including palatability, and the presence and levels of contaminants and bioactive substances. These may even vary in a single diet, with considerable batch-to-batch differences over time. Such variation may produce inconsistent responses in animals, possibly leading not only to between-laboratory irreproducibility but also to within-laboratory irreproducibility over time. These effects on reproducibility and the production of possibly erroneous data are not only financially profligate but are ethically unjustifiable in the waste of animals entailed. See also Chapter 2: The Three Rs.

We consider that some of the irreproducibility problems in animal-based research arise from a lack of knowledge of diet and nutrition by investigators, those providing study oversight in IACUCs and the like, and even editors and referees. A better understanding of diet and nutrition by those working in laboratory animal science should improve the quality of experimental design and research outcomes in animal-based studies, benefiting reproducibility, the more effective use of animals, and consequently better animal welfare. With these points in mind, we have discussed some of the more important basic elements of laboratory animal nutrition and diets.

Diet types: ingredient, formula, and physical form

Laboratory animal diets can be characterised by their ingredients, formula type, and manufacturing method, and we describe each type in detail below. Each of these characteristics has significant consequences for investigators. We also describe various supplementary items that are valuable in improving animal welfare in both laboratory animal husbandry and experimental studies.

Ingredient-based diet types

Diets can be divided into those manufactured from natural ingredients and those from purified ingredients. Natural-ingredient diets are the basis for most of the 'off-the-shelf' commercial diets fed to laboratory animals, while purified diets are largely used as the basis of custom research diets, i.e. diets which are made specifically to an individual customer request. Custom research diets are also sometimes manufactured from natural ingredients, but these are a small proportion of the total produced.

Natural-ingredient diets

The dominant type of diet used for laboratory animals is manufactured from typical agricultural products, including cereals (barley, maize, oats and wheat), cereal by-products (wheatfeed, middlings, bran), high-protein animal (primarily fish meal) and vegetable (soybean meal, corn gluten meal) sources, and fats. These primary ingredients are supplemented with vitamin and mineral premixes and often the amino acids methionine and lysine. The preferred term for such products is 'natural-ingredient diets', though less descriptive terms such as 'grain-based', 'chow' (particularly in the United States), 'stock', 'standard', or 'regular diets' have been used. There are several characteristics of natural-ingredient diets that may affect experimental studies: their nutrient analysis varies from batch-to-batch; nutrients in the diet are not completely available; it is almost impossible to vary individual nutrient levels without changing others; and they often contain non-nutrients that have biological effects and may confound an experimental study.

Purified Diets

The problems with natural-ingredient diets are largely overcome by using purified diets (sometimes referred to as synthetic or semi-synthetic diets, particularly in older publications). They are manufactured from ingredients that individually usually contribute a single nutrient type, so it is possible to create purified diets that are both accurate and precise in achieving desired nutrient levels, with negligible differences between batches. The most common protein source is casein, usually supplemented with either methionine or cystine, though others such as egg and soy protein may be occasionally used. Carbohydrates are usually supplied by corn starch and mono- or disaccharides such as glucose, sucrose, or fructose; dextrins may also be added to aid pelleting, particularly in high-fat diets. The main fibre source is cellulose. Soybean oil is the main fat source to supply essential fatty acids, but other vegetable oil types such as corn oil, coconut oil (unusually, a 'solid' oil), and animal fats such as lard and anhydrous milk fat may also be used for specific purposes. Vitamin and mineral premixes are also added to the diet, and these may be modified to introduce individual deficiencies and excesses. Klurfeld et al. (2021) have recently raised the possibility that more complex mixtures of dietary fibre, available carbohydrates, and fat might be necessary to improve the metabolic health of animals fed on purified diets. These changes remain to be determined in detail.

The manufacture of purified diets is quite different from that of natural-ingredient diets (Tobin et al. 2007; Coman & Vlase 2017). The manufacturing equipment is of a much smaller scale and considerably easier to decontaminate between batches. Process temperatures are much lower, which minimises losses of heat-labile components such as vitamins. Although most purified diets can be pelleted, those containing high levels of fat are fragile, and it is often more practicable to supply these in powdered form. Very high-fat ketogenic diets are supplied in dough form. Generally, purified diets are well accepted by rodents, though less so by other species such as rabbits and cats; for the latter, it is sometimes necessary to include small amounts of non-purified ingredients to enhance palatability.

Manufacturers have formulated thousands of purified diets to meet specific customer needs, and each year continue to add to that number. However, the American Institutes of Nutrition have proposed purified diets that, with simple modifications, can meet most requirements. The first of these was AIN76 (AIN 1977), but this was subsequently found to be vitamin K deficient (Bieri 1979; Roebuck et al. 1979). This was corrected in a modified version, AIN76A (Bieri 1979). Ten years later, two new diets were proposed to correct the weaknesses experienced with AIN76A, primarily by increasing essential fatty acid levels, substituting starch for sucrose to decrease the risk of hyperlipidaemia and nephrocalcinosis, and improving mineral levels (Reeves 1989). The change also gave the opportunity to increase the range to provide a version suitable for breeding and growth (AIN93G) and a lower protein and fat version (AIN93M) for maintenance (Reeves et al. 1993; Reeves 1997). Further development of these diets has been recommended (Klurfeld et al. 2021).

Chemically defined diets are a subset of purified diets in which the protein source is replaced by individual amino acids and/or the fat source is replaced by individual fatty acids. These diets are rarely used, but historically they were developed to determine fatty and amino acid requirements and effects (Baker 1992) and as the basis for minimum antigenic diets (Wostmann & Pleasants 1991). More recently, amino acid defined diets have been used to induce non-alcohol fatty liver disease in rodents (Teramoto et al. 1993; Ramadori et al. 2015; Hansen et al. 2017).

Formula types

There are two distinct approaches to classifying diet based on its formula. The first is whether the formula remains constant throughout its life (fixed formulation) or whether it can be changed to reflect changes in ingredient price (least-cost formulation) or ingredient nutrient composition, either year-to-year or batch-to-batch (variable-formula diets). The latter type may be described by manufacturers as optimised or constant-nutrition diets. It is impossible to maintain the nutrient composition of natural-ingredient diets constant even with variable-formula diets, which in practice seek largely to maintain a uniform level of dietary protein, though the evidence shows they provide little or no advantage over fixed-formula diets. The relative benefits of different diet types have been discussed by Tobin et al. (2007) and Barnard et al. (2009).

The second approach is the division of diets into open- and closed-formula types. Open-formula diets have their formula in the public domain, while those of closed-formula types remain confidential to the manufacturer. Closed-formula diets allow the manufacturer to create and sell products that may result from much background research and knowledge without the risk of them being copied. Purified diets are typically open formulas since it is often necessary to disclose full diet details in research publications. The other major open-formula diets are the natural-ingredient diets designed by the National Institutes of Health in the United States and manufactured by several producers. Their details can be found on the website of the NIH Office of Research Services[2].

Physical form

Laboratory animal diets are available in pellet, extruded, ground or powdered, or liquid form. Each has unique characteristics that help define its primary purpose. There are several reviews on diet manufacture (Tobin et al. 2007; Rokey et al. 2010).

Pellet

The pellet is the default form of product and results from the compression of ingredients, usually with steam treatment to gelatinise starches that bind the ingredients together. The pellets are made in a variety of diameters to suit different species, for example, about 3–4 mm for rabbits and guinea pigs and 9–12 mm for rodents. Pelleted purified diets are usually made by cold pressing after ingredients are mixed with a small amount of water.

Extruded

Extruded diets were first introduced into the pet food industry, primarily for cats and dogs. They are typically the standard type of diet used for such species in laboratory animal science, but in addition are usually used for non-human primates and, to a limited extent, for rodents. Much of the manufacturing process is like that for pelleted diets, but the ingredients are processed at a higher temperature and pressure, with higher moisture contents, and are cooked rather than just compressed. The resulting product is more brittle than a pelleted diet with much better digestibility of starches and is likely to have a lower microbiological load. It can hold a much higher level of fat than a pelleted diet without compromising physical quality. Grinding extruded diet produces a more uniform particle size than obtained by grinding pellets, and this is useful if compounds need to be homogeneously mixed with diet. While physically stronger, an extruded product is easier for animals to bite into than a pelleted diet (see 'Pellet hardness effects').

Ground and powdered diet

Prior to the development of pelleting, animals were fed blended ingredients with no further processing: this was described as mash. This process is still used for purified diets as described in the preceding text but referred to as powdered diet. Although a non-pelleted natural-ingredient diet is often useful in laboratory animals, for example, as an excipient for test, veterinary, and other compounds, it is now more commonly formed from ground pelleted or extruded diet. The exposure to heat and moisture during processing increases the digestibility of starches, decreases the microbiological load, and reduces or eliminates many non-nutrients, and these benefits are transferred to the ground product.

Liquid diets

Liquid diets either use purified water-soluble ingredients when this is practicable or are made by suspending ingredients in water (sometimes described as a slurry) with the aid of a substance such as xanthan gum (Ramirez 1987). They are

---

[2] https://www.ors.od.nih.gov/sr/dvr/drs/nutrition/Pages/Diets.aspx (accessed 3 September 2019)

primarily used to administer alcohol and water-soluble compounds. The most well-known liquid diet formulas are those based on the work of Lieber-DeCarli (Lieber & DeCarli 1982; Guo et al. 2018). Liquid diets have been used to create alcoholic and non-alcoholic liver disease in rodents and liver damage in non-human primates (Lieber & DeCarli 1974; Lieber et al. 2004).

Supplementary products

There are several other nutritionally related products that, while not complete diets, can prove useful in contributing to good animal welfare and which we include here for completeness.

Gels and pastes

Gels and pastes may be beneficial for overcoming palatability issues associated with the physical state of the diet, for example, with some powdered purified diets (Keane et al. 1962). Agar gel diets can be used to prevent atmospheric dispersion of fine powders and volatile compounds that need to be administered orally (Lang et al. 1984; Landrigan et al. 1989). Gels are now also commonly used as a water source during transportation, particularly of rodents.

While these materials are unlikely alone to overcome aversion to taste entirely (Hovard et al. 2015), many unpalatable drugs and compounds have been incorporated into highly palatable pastes such as Nutella, peanut butter, or sugar paste to improve acceptability to dosed animals (Abelson et al. 2012; Guarnieri et al. 2012; Diogo et al. 2015). Other attractive forms such as gelatine treats, cookie dough and honey have also been recommended as a palatable means of dosing compounds (Corbett et al. 2012; Küster et al. 2012; Zhang et al. 2012).

Hay

Although in principle the high-fibre requirements of rabbits and guinea pigs can be met in processed natural-ingredient diets, there is evidence that long fibre such as hay is beneficial, decreasing stress and fur chewing (Beynen et al. 1992). Hay must be carefully selected since it is a potential source of pathogens, may be contaminated with pesticides and heavy metals, and contain toxic weeds. Ideally, it should be gamma irradiated or autoclaved to destroy pathogens.

Energy, nutrient and water requirements

Energy and nutrient requirements

The most common source of information on nutrient requirements are publications produced by the National Research Council of the United States (NRC) and available on their website[3]. One covers small laboratory animals, including rats, mice, guinea pigs, hamsters, gerbils, and voles, while others cover rabbits, non-human primates, dogs and cats. The NRC website also provides access to nutrient requirements of agricultural animals such as pigs, cattle, and poultry that may occasionally be used in experimental studies. Except for that for rabbits, most of these publications are reasonably up to date. The sparse and outdated information for rabbits (last published in 1977) may be supplemented by reference to data published for pet and meat-producing rabbits (de Blas & Wiseman 2010; Lebas 2010; FEDIAF 2013). We have not included tables of requirements in this chapter because it is important that users read the NRC's supporting literature to put the reliability of these values into context, and the data are readily available. Clarke et al. (1977) published a practical assessment of nutrient requirements of laboratory animals, which is useful despite its age.

Nutrient requirement values in tables are commonly expressed on a gravimetric basis, for example, per 100 g or kg diet. If diets are likely to have very different energy densities (for example, control and high-fat diets), nutrient requirements may also be expressed relative to the metabolisable energy (ME) density of the diet, e.g., per 100 kJ ME. This ensures a consistent adequate nutrient intake if, as expected, animals adjust food intake to achieve a consistent energy intake when fed on diets with different energy densities.

There are often large gaps in our knowledge on requirements in many laboratory animal species for different physiological states such as gestation, lactation, and maintenance. It is assumed that most of the requirements expressed on a gravimetric basis for growth are also adequate for reproduction. The higher absolute nutrient requirements for reproduction are met by the associated increase in food intake (and perhaps a contribution from tissue catabolism). Nutrient requirements in ageing, even on a gravimetric basis, are almost certainly lower than for growth and reproduction, though there are few accurate nutritional requirement data for many ageing species. Nevertheless, most diet manufacturers produce maintenance diets for ageing animals based on assumed requirements. In contrast to most laboratory animal species, there are extensive, reliable data for cats and dogs for all phases, largely a consequence of substantial research into designing and producing better pet foods.

There are several ways of expressing nutrient requirements. The primary one is the minimum requirement, which is the lowest nutrient concentration required to achieve the optimum desired response (such as growth, reproductive indices, the blood or tissue concentration of a substance, or absence of a deficiency-related pathology). Usually, minimal nutrient requirements are determined by measuring the response to increasing doses of the nutrient in a purified diet (see below). However, in some cases, the estimate of minimal requirement may be flawed by the failure to use doses below the true minimum requirement. The broken stick method (Figure 13.1) was originally used as the best fit for the points since this required little or no computing power. Both the rising and horizontal lines could be easily fitted by eye. However, with increased access to computers, more complex saturation kinetics, dose-response, or growth fits are now preferred. The main alternatives are linear-quadratic, Gompertz, Weibull, or four-parameter logistic models. For these responses, the estimate of requirement has usually

---

[3] https://www.nap.edu/topic/278/biology-and-life-sciences (accessed 3 September 2019)

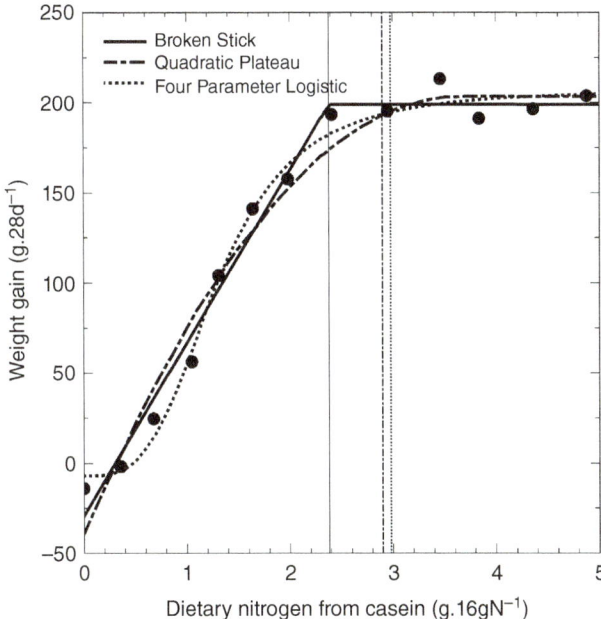

Figure 13.1 The effect of fitting different curves to predict the nitrogen (protein [Nx6.25]) requirements of rats fed on diets containing several levels of casein. The possible estimated requirements for maximum growth are where the three vertical lines intercept the x-axis. Source: The original data are from Phillips, R. D. (1981) Linear and nonlinear models for measuring protein nutritional quality. *Journal of Nutrition*, **111**(6), 1058–1066.

been set at 95% of the maximum response (this occurs at a steeper part of the curve and narrows the confidence limits of the estimate on the x-axis. This is illustrated in Figure 13.1). The relative merits of several curve fits have been reviewed by Pesti *et al.* (2009). The move to using sigmoidal or linear-quadratic responses has typically resulted in increased estimates of nutrient requirements compared to the broken stick method, and this effect can be seen in Figure 13.1. The change in the curve fit method resulted in an increase between the 1978 and 1995 editions of the NRC Requirements of Laboratory Animals of estimates of the requirement in rats for most amino acids from the same data. Baker (1986) has described many of the problems in determining nutrient requirements in a detail that is outside the scope of this chapter.

The second expression of nutrient requirements is 'recommended allowance'. This derives from the fact that the availability of nutrients in purified diets is typically higher than in natural-ingredient diets, and so underestimates the minimum amount of a nutrient required in a natural-ingredient diet. 'Recommended allowance' is determined by adjusting the minimal requirement for the lower availability of the nutrient in natural-ingredient diets. For example, if the minimum requirement of a nutrient is 10 units and its availability is 80%, the recommended allowance is 12.5 units.

The third expression of nutrient requirements is termed 'adequate intake'. It may be estimated from studies not specifically designed to measure minimal requirements and is the lowest nutrient value in a study not associated with any evidence of deficiency. As with 'minimal requirement', it may reflect the lowest dose used rather than the true minimal value. It may be determined from studies either with purified diets or natural-ingredient diets: those predicted from purified-diet studies may be subsequently adjusted to provide an estimate of the 'recommended allowance'.

Excessive nutrients

While most interest in nutrient levels is concerned with deficiencies of essential nutrients, many can have deleterious effects when fed at high levels. The most familiar problems have occurred with excesses of individual essential dietary amino acids (Harper *et al.* 1970), minerals and vitamins (NRC 1987; NRC 2005). Excessive levels of nonessential nutrients may also cause toxicity. Figure 13.2 summarises the response of an animal to deficiencies and excesses of essential and nonessential nutrients: the main difference is the absence of deficiency with nonessential nutrients. There are two critical points of inflexion in the response: the lowest critical concentration (LCC), which represents the optimum nutrient requirement (for an essential nutrient only); and the upper critical concentration (UCC), beyond which there is the possibility of declining benefit or adverse effects from additional concentrations of the nutrient. Generally, for an essential nutrient, the range between the lower and UCC is wide, providing a high degree of tolerance. However, in a few instances, the margin between requirement and toxicity may be very narrow. For example, the requirement for selenium for rats and mice is 0.15 mg kg^{-1} for growth and 0.4 mg kg^{-1} for breeding, yet the maximum allowable in diet is 0.5 mg kg^{-1}, though EFSA (2016) state that the tolerated levels in complete feed are 'markedly above the currently authorised maximum content'. We consider that 0.75 mg kg^{-1} would be a more realistic justifiable upper limit. Despite some

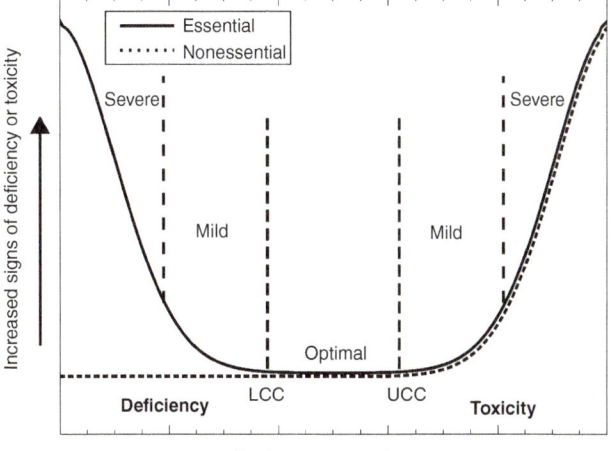

Figure 13.2 The response of animals to changing essential and nonessential nutrient concentrations and the potential for deficiencies and toxicity. The optimum nutrient concentration for essential nutrients is bounded by the lower critical concentration (LCC) and upper critical concentration (UCC). If the response to an essential nutrient is similar to an inverted normal distribution rather than the flat-valley shape shown here, the LCC and UCC can be taken as ±5% around the maximum value.

challenges like this, commercial laboratory animal diets formulated by professional nutritionists are unlikely to contain deleterious nutrient excesses or be nutritionally imbalanced.

Water

Thirst and the need for water

Thirst is probably one of the most stressful and powerful physiological drives to affect welfare and is exceeded only by severe pain and gasping for air (Fitzsimons 1979; von Keyserlingk et al. 2016). Water intake is generally closely associated with food intake in both amount and pattern of intake (Fitzsimons & Le Magnen 1969) and appears to be linked to the ingestion of dietary organic osmolytes and minerals, particularly sodium. However, drinking may also proceed eating as a learned response to a dry mouth that would make ingestion of food difficult or unpleasant (Fitzsimons & Le Magnen 1969; Rolls & Rolls 1982; Zimmerman et al. 2017).

Drinking follows the diurnal pattern of feeding in most animals (Siegel & Stuckey 1947; Tsuji et al. 1982), occurring mainly in the night in rats, mice, guinea pigs, and rabbits. Cats and dogs tend to drink in parallel to bouts of random eating rather than showing a fixed diurnal pattern (Robinson & Adolph 1943; Johnson et al. 1983; Ozon et al. 1987). The ratio of water intake to food intake is quite uniform within a species at any specific room temperature, though there may be considerable individual variation. Bachmanov et al. (2002) reported a mean value of about 1.34 g water per gram food (SD 0.19) for 28 strains of mice. Kutscher (1969) reported a similar overall mean value (1.43, SD 0.23) for rats, hamsters, and gerbils but a higher and slightly more variable estimate for guinea pigs (2.11, SD 0.44). Data on other laboratory animal species are sparse, and it is not possible to draw firm conclusions on ratios. Cats seem particularly sensitive to the availability of water since they do not adjust total water intake when transitioning from a highly digestible canned food to a dry diet (e.g. prior to experiments) and may develop feline urinary syndrome (Markwell et al. 1998; Buckley et al. 2011). Estimates for water requirements of several livestock species and poultry that might be used as experimental animals are summarised by Parker and Brown (2003).

Although animals commonly decrease water intake during food restriction, this is not a universal observation, and some stocks and strains of rodents, rabbits, pigs and perhaps non-human primates exhibit excessive drinking beyond their physiological needs (Cizek 1954; Cizek 1961; Kutscher 1974; Yang et al. 1981; Kemnitz 2011; Patience 2012), and to such an extent that it may be fatal (Cizek 1954). This diet-restriction or hunger-induced polydipsia is briefly described by Kyriazakis and Tolkamp (2011) and is one of several secondary drinking types primarily behavioural in causation (Rolls & Rolls 1982).

Water quality

Water quality is an important aspect of animal welfare, and the ILAR Guidelines for the Care and Use of Laboratory Animals state that 'Animals should have access to potable, uncontaminated drinking water according to their particular requirements' (ILAR 2011). Dysko et al. (2009) and Allen et al. (2018) provide comprehensive overviews of the sources, treatment, and distribution of water for use in an animal facility. Traditionally, the contaminants of most concern for drinking water are pathogenic microorganisms and chemicals such as nitrates, pesticides, polychlorinated biphenyls (PCB), dioxins, and heavy and other metals. These concerns are reflected in two primary pieces of legislation in the US and EU, namely the US EPA Safe Drinking Water Act[4] (and the associated National Primary Drinking Water Regulations[5]), and the EU Drinking Water Directive (Council Directive 98/83/EC of 3 November 1998 on the quality of water intended for human consumption)[6]. These list compounds of importance and recommendations on their safe upper limits. Similar guidance, intended for global use, has been given by WHO (2011).

The main sources of drinking water are groundwater (obtained through boreholes and wells) and surface water. In the EU, the ratio of drinking water origin is about 50:50, and almost all is disinfected (mainly with chlorination), though 20% of the groundwater is not (van der Hoek et al. 2013). In the United States, although groundwater systems form 80% of the sources of drinking water, they are of generally small scale and supply only about 34% of the population. All public water must be disinfected, which is achieved mainly by chlorination (Levin et al. 2002), but many private sources are exempt.

Decontamination of drinking water is carried out in drinking water treatment plants (DWTP) or wastewater treatment plants (WWTP) that produce recycled drinking water. Although the exact process varies from plant to plant, it will generally involve several stages that might include: screening to remove large particulate material, clarification, filtration, aeration, adsorption on activated carbon, ozone treatment, disinfection, and ammoniation[7,8]. These processes clarify the water, improve its taste, and remove much of the undesirable microbiological activity and inorganic and organic material to achieve levels stipulated in the legislation described in the preceding text.

The levels of many historically significant chemical contaminants in source water have declined in the US and Europe with their decreased industrial output and agricultural use. However, a new large group of contaminants is emerging for which regulation is lacking. These include pharmaceutical compounds, personal care products, surfactants and their residues, plasticisers and other additives (Petrović et al. 2003). Since about 2005, the American Chemical Society has published biennial reviews on emerging water contaminants and their method of measurement: at the time

---

[4] https://www.epa.gov/sdwa (accessed 12 November 2019)
[5] https://www.epa.gov/ground-water-and-drinking-water/national-primary-drinking-water-regulations (accessed 12 November 2019)
[6] https://eur-lex.europa.eu/legal-content/EN/TXT/?uri=CELEX:01998L0083-20151027 (accessed 12 November 2019)
[7] https://www.thameswater.co.uk/help-and-advice/water-quality/how-we-look-after-your-water/drinking-water-treatment (accessed 19 November 2019)
[8] http://dwi.defra.gov.uk/private-water-supply/installations/Treatment-processes.pdf (accessed 19 November 2019)

of writing, the latest was published in 2020 (Richardson & Kimura 2020). Traditional water treatment plants are only modestly effective at removing these emerging contaminants. Fortunately, modern water treatment plants are highly effective at removing most of these compounds, with an efficiency >85% for most (Ahmed et al. 2017). Some of the least well-eliminated are bisphenol A (70%) and antibiotics (50%), and some such as analgesics, anti-inflammatories, and beta-blockers appear to be particularly resistant to treatment, with a 30–40% removal rate (Deblonde et al. 2011). Chemical oxidation processes such as ozonisation are considered to be among the best of the 'newer' treatment processes (Ahmed et al. 2017).

Many animal facilities also have in-house water treatment, including mechanical filtration, acidification and chlorination, ozonisation, reverse osmosis, and UV germicidal irradiation to provide an additional level of biosafety (Dysko et al. 2009; Allen et al. 2018). Although non-barrier-reared laboratory animals are mainly supplied directly with potable water from municipal supplies, the possibility of the growth of pathogenic organisms in the distribution lines to the facility remains (Ramírez-Castillo et al. 2015; Prest et al. 2016), and some treatment such as acidification and/or chlorination is frequently carried out on site. Some facilities, even in the United States, obtain water from local boreholes or wells, and the regulation of water quality standards from such sources is highly variable (Dysko et al. 2009) with a risk of microbiological contamination (Allevi et al. 2013; Bradford & Harvey 2017). For these animal facilities, acidification or chlorination is almost always essential. Because of the variability in the quality of incoming water, Allen et al. (2018) recommend an assessment be carried out by laboratory facility management of likely microbiological risk from any source water and an appropriate level of decontamination applied. The water supply to animals reared in barriers should always be treated to a high standard using an appropriate combination of the methods listed above. The water may also be steam-sterilised or irradiated in systems that rely on non-automated watering systems such as bottles.

There is considerable variation in the chemical composition of water in different locations, and while many drinking water providers issue analytical certificates for water, routine verification checks of analytes in samples at the point of access by animals should be carried out periodically (Davidowitz et al. 1998). The absence of testing by municipal authorities for the emerging contaminants and the variable success in removing them implies a need to identify those likely to be a confounding factor in the experimental studies within an animal facility and to set up general or study-specific monitoring. Although details of water supply are not a high priority in the ARRIVE guidelines, Hooijmans et al. (2010) consider water to be a significant experimental variable and include it in a checklist of significant items to describe in reports of animal-based studies. Unfortunately, many published animal-based studies provide very little information on water delivery, quality, and decontamination. While there is little evidence to date that water treatment processes such as acidification or chlorination at typical levels have had consistent significant effects on research outcomes (Hall et al. 1980; Hermann et al. 1982; Jayaraman & Jayaraman 2018), it does affect the microbiome (Bidot et al. 2018; Barnett & Gibson 2019). Thus, with increasing interest in the microbiome and the risk that emerging contaminants might impact on research endpoints in animal-based studies, it is inevitable that including information on drinking water is essential in reports of animal-based studies.

Water delivery systems

The final stage of the delivery of drinking water to the animal has important welfare implications that include physical, behavioural, chemical, and microbiological aspects. Water bottles and nipple valve drinkers are most commonly used for rodents, guinea pigs, and rabbits and are highly practicable. Dysko et al. (2009) have discussed the relative merits of both. Nipple drinkers are commonly incorporated into automated watering systems. They provide a relatively hygienic method of water delivery and may be attractive to animals because they use the same chewing actions for drinking as those used for eating. Pigs appear to prefer nipple drinkers (Bøe & Kjelvik 2011), perhaps for this reason. Troughs, drinking bowls and push-paddle drinkers may be used for larger animals such as cats, dogs, and farm animals. Irrespective of type, drinkers should be positioned at an appropriate height, should not restrict natural behaviour (von Keyserlingk et al. 2016), and be present in sufficient numbers to satisfy the needs of all animals in a group.

Many animal facilities have replaced the use of water bottles by automated watering systems. Despite their convenience, these systems pose two major welfare concerns, foremost of which is the risk of leaks and cage flooding (Barley et al. 2004). Although this problem can occur with bottles, there is a perception that the problem may be greater with automated systems. The issue is of such concern that many caging systems now include leak detection. The problem of leakage is mainly caused by the nipple valve remaining open because of blockage by material such as bedding or damage to the valve or its seating (Gonzalez et al. 2011). Death may occur by drowning or hypothermia. Although the failure rate should not exceed 0.1% per annum, this may increase with inadequate monitoring or maintenance. Gonzalez et al. (2011) have provided a comprehensive description of the problem and a preventive maintenance programme that achieves a low failure rate. Additionally, the valves may become blocked by particles in the water line and fail to release water, causing dehydration, though inline filters reduce the risk of such blocking.

The selection of drinker type also needs to accommodate the natural behaviour of the animal to avoid unnecessary potential stress. For example, nipple drinkers do not allow the lapping or scooping method of drinking natural to some animals, such as chinchillas (Hagen et al. 2014), rabbits (Tschudin et al. 2011), and poultry (Houldcroft et al. 2008), which consequently prefer open drinking bowls. Some animals, such as the guinea pig, do not show any clear preference for drinker type (Hagen et al. 2014; Balsiger et al. 2017). A water supply may also fulfil functions other than satiating thirst. For example, The Council of Europe recommends that ducks can cover their heads with water and spread it over their feathers: they consistently select water sources that permit such behaviours (Rodenburg et al. 2005).

The last welfare concerns applicable to final water delivery are: chemical contamination from the materials in which the water is contained; growth of microorganisms in the water lines; and contamination from other animals' faeces and/or urine. These affect welfare directly through the health of the animal and as confounding factors in obtaining accurate, reliable experimental outcomes. These are discussed further below.

Allen *et al.* (2018) have drawn attention to the risk of chemical leaching from the materials used to deliver water. Most concern has been directed to the leaching of endocrine disruptors from polycarbonate water bottles, including bisphenol A (Le *et al.* 2008; Honeycutt *et al.* 2017) and, more recently, possibly bisphenol S (a replacement for bisphenol A in polycarbonate plastics) (Gorence *et al.* 2019). It now appears that a wide range of plastic materials can leach detectable amounts of oestrogenic compounds and also several elements (particularly antimony) and phthalates (Wagner & Oehlmann 2011; Yang *et al.* 2011), though the practical significance for laboratory animals has not been clearly established.

The risk of microbiological contamination of drinking water is not only a concern for external inputs to the facility from well or municipal water distribution systems. It may occur within the animal facility in automated watering systems (Meier *et al.* 2008) and even in components of water treatment such as reverse osmosis systems (Molk *et al.* 2013). The threat in all distribution systems is primarily from biofilms in which bacteria bind to wet surfaces, including stainless steel, and secrete a 'protective' glycocalyx. Although primarily bacterial in nature, biofilms may contain viruses, protozoa, fungi, and algae. Contamination is spread by particles of the biofilm becoming dislodged and spreading downstream. *P. aeruginosa* in biofilms may be a serious problem for immunocompromised rodents. The problem of biofilms has been discussed by Dysko *et al.* (2009) and Simões and Simões (2013). Development of biofilms in automated watering systems is almost inevitable, but careful design of the system and regular flushing with water can minimise the level of contamination (Dysko *et al.* 2009). The final microbiological risk comes from faecal and urinary contamination of drinking water, which is more common with larger animals (including experimental farm animals). Their water delivery is often from communal drinking bowls and troughs that can be contaminated from other animals that share access and from wild animals that gain access (von Keyserlingk *et al.* 2016). It is one of the disadvantages of providing standing water suitable for normal behaviour in ducks (Schenk *et al.* 2016). Contaminated unpalatable water is not only a health risk *per se* but may lead to decreased water intake and dehydration (Kyriazakis & Tolkamp 2011).

Voluntary food intake in laboratory animals

Investigators must consider two issues when reporting food intake: how to allow for body size; and whether the values include spillage. If values do not include spillage, the term 'food removed' should be used rather than 'food intake' and the extent to which ignoring spillage might affect the interpretation of experimental results should be considered carefully.

Body size effects

Intuitively, the size of the animal (even within a stock or strain) must influence energy and nutrient requirements. These, and particularly energy requirements, are often standardised to metabolic body size, usually expressed as $W^{0.75}$. This exponent is the slope of the regression of log metabolic rate on log body weight (kg) originally determined by Kleiber (1932), though he preferred using three-fourths power (see Hulbert (2014) for a historical view). There are several problems using metabolic body size: (a) $W^{0.75}$ was determined in mature animals while most laboratory animal studies, particularly those in rodents, are done in growing animals; (b) there is considerable doubt that the exponent of 0.75 applies universally within and between species and (c) it has no physiological basis. Within a species, an adjustment on body weight alone (i.e. per 100 g or kg body weight) is simpler and just as meaningful. However, Packard has argued that using any adjustment of measurements on some size-specific basis may grossly distort the interpretation of data and that body size differences between different experimental groups are best compensated for by the use of the analysis of covariance (ANCOVA) (Packard & Boardman 1999). Measurements in lean and obese animals should never be 'corrected' or 'adjusted' based on body weight since this may distort experimental observations and lead to incorrect conclusions (Butler & Kozak 2010).

Spillage

Many reports of voluntary food intake appear to include no allowance for food spillage (Cameron & Speakman 2010). Failure to determine spillage accurately may lead to substantial errors in estimates of food and energy intake and distort experimental findings. Spillage has been most studied in rats and mice and originates mainly from damaged pellets, breakage in the food hopper, dropped food, and the grinding activity of the animals during feeding. Larger components are often added back to the food hopper when measurements of intake are made; however, the remaining smaller material is often difficult to quantify accurately. In gridded cages, almost all spillage becomes inaccessible to the animals, while in solid bottom cages, at least some of the spilt food will be eaten during foraging. The main causes of variation in spillage levels are pellet quality and palatability. Although excessive spillage is undesirable, modest, accessible spillage is beneficial in breeding rodents, contributing to the early ingestion of solid food by young animals and supporting the weaning process.

Spillage of well-formed low-fat purified diets is less than 10% (Goodrick 1973) and considerably lower if carefully sorted and small pieces returned to the hopper (Cameron & Speakman 2010). But with softer high-fat and other diets, wastage can increase to 50–60% (Cameron & Speakman 2010). C57BL/6 mice tend to be particularly wasteful, which is of concern since it is one of the main mouse models used in studies of energy intake and balance. High wastage may also occur on unpalatable (Peck 1978) or nutrient-deficient diets (Tagliaferro & Levitsky 1982). The use of specialised food hoppers for powdered diets can substantially decrease spillage (Miller 1990; Matsuzawa *et al.* 1998).

Koteja et al. (2003) have shown that individual mice wasted 2–40% of their food pellets when fed natural-ingredient diets and that individual wastage was consistent across time and different treatments. Median wastage was 9.4% (mean 9.6%, SD 3.1), suggesting that the very high values were outliers, and visual inspection of their data suggests most values were less than 15%. Cameron and Speakman (2010) reported that wastage between and within mouse stock/strain ranged from 4% (SD 5) to 17% (SD 18), and Keenan et al. (1994) reported spillage of 8.4% by rats fed a standard pelleted diet over two years. These values are similar to those of 8.7% and 11.0% reported by Roe et al. (1995) for two standard commercial diets. Our unpublished data show spillage with well-formed pellets was about 12% (SD 2.4) in animals raised on mesh-bottomed cages. Overall, a spillage of about 10% seems a reasonable estimate for a well-formed diet.

Changing diet hardness significantly affects spillage: increasing hardness by autoclaving decreased spillage to about 7% (SD 1.3), while softening the diet by adding a few per cent of soybean oil increased wastage to 16.4% (SD 1.1). Increasing dietary fibre content, which makes the diet more fragile, progressively increases spillage: in the study by Roe et al. (1995), it rose from about 8% in a standard diet with 2.5% crude fibre to 20% with 7% crude fibre and 40% with 10% crude fibre. We observed that rats would discard fibrous material and access the more palatable parts of the pellet: a similar observation has been noted in other rodents (Peterson & Wunder 1997). This may result in an intake of nutrients very different from that expected from the composition of the diet.

Natural food intake patterns in non-reproducing animals

Food intake typically increases near-linearly from weaning, peaking between about 40 to 100 days of age in laboratory species, even though growth continues (Figure 13.3). Thereafter it remains moderately constant, though it may decline in old age (ageing anorexia). The cessation in the increase in food intake is unlikely to be due to the limited capacity of the gastrointestinal tract since, as we describe below, food intake can be further increased by other physiological and environmental conditions. Estimates of variation (expressed as the coefficient of variation (CV)) in food intake between 28 strains of mice was about 15% (Bachmanov et al. 2002) and 7% between 16 stocks and strains of rats (Walsh 1980). In our data, the CV for three stocks/strains of male mice was about 16%, and for four stocks/strains of rats, about 22%.

In most species, males are bigger and eat more food than females. We have calculated from the literature that compared to males, the intake of non-reproducing females is about 70–75% for rats and 90–95% for mice and guinea pigs. In contrast, female common marmosets and, usually, rabbits are larger than males at any age (Ralls 1976) and have a food intake about 20% greater.

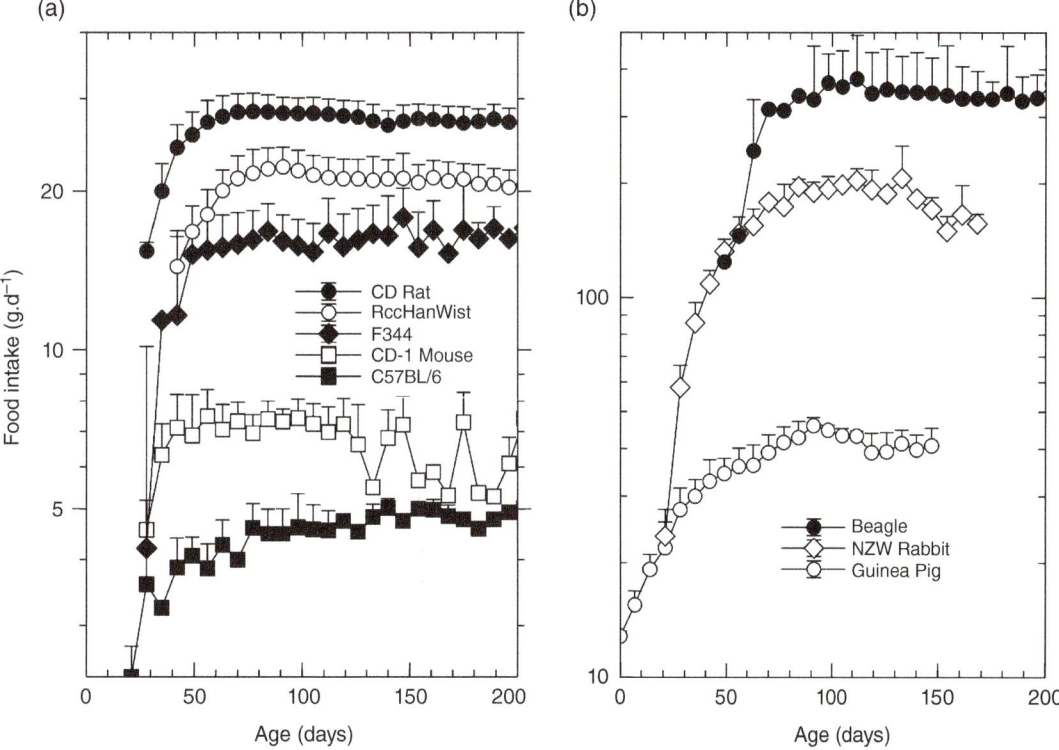

Figure 13.3 The change in food intake with age of (a) several stocks and strains of rats and mice, and (b) guinea pigs, rabbits, and beagles. Where sufficient data are available, standard deviations have been calculated and shown. The data were obtained from a substantial number of publications not referenced here.

Natural food intake patterns in reproducing animals

The rapid and often contrary changes in food intake and body weight in reproduction make any simple formulaic approach to expressing intake relative to body weight of little value. We prefer to express the magnitude of changes as a percentage of pre-mating levels. Figure 13.4 shows food intake data for reproduction in several species in this way. Estimates of food intake changes during reproduction for guinea pigs, rabbits and dogs are based on only a few studies, and their absolute accuracy should be treated with caution.

In the mouse, rat, and dog, there is little change during early gestation but a modest increase of about 20–40% in the third trimester. Intake in the rabbit (and perhaps other species) may decline in late gestation, possibly because the increasing size of the *in-utero* contents compresses the gastrointestinal tract. At parturition, there is a marked drop in food intake (Morrison 1956), but during lactation, food intake rises steeply. The increase beyond the initial pre-mating level is dependent on litter size and is species dependent. The relative increase is greatest in inbred mice such as the C57BL/6 (c. 400%), followed by outbred Swiss-type mice (c. 300%), outbred rats typified by the CD rat (c. 200%), beagles (c. 180%), and rabbit (c. 130%). The precocial nature of the guinea pig produces a different response to that seen in other laboratory animals, with a steady increase in food intake from the second trimester of gestation. The increase during lactation is the lowest (c. 120%) since the pups eat solid food soon after birth and have limited reliance on maternal milk (Jenness 1986; Künkele 2000).

Foraging for food

Foraging for food has been most studied in rodents. In the wild, mice may travel up to 100 metres in search of food (Wolton 2009). However, rodents will preferentially select a food source with easy access (Paronis et al. 2008) and preferably in a small search area or range (Akbar & Gorman 1993; Perrin & Monadjem 1998), avoiding unnecessary risk of predation. Foraging has been advocated as a method of environmental enrichment for laboratory animals (see also Chapter 10: Environmental enrichment: animal welfare and scientific validity), though its benefits for caged rodents are limited because the range (i.e. cage) is very small and the availability of feed is large. It has more potential for non-human primates, particularly when they have access to outdoor areas (Buchanan-Smith 1994). In smaller enclosed areas, foraging can be mimicked by various devices (Lutz and Novak 2005), though simple devices may not provide continuing interest from the animals (Bennett et al. 2016). It is unlikely that foraging significantly increases energy expenditure, so it remains important to ensure that provision of food items does not lead to overfeeding.

Diurnal feeding rhythms

Most laboratory species, except for non-human primates (Natelson & Bonbright 1978; Hansen et al. 1981) and pigs (de Haer and Merks 1992), are primarily nocturnal feeders. Rodents eat about 70–90% of their food at night with bursts of eating around lights off in the early evening and prior to lights on (Siegel & Stuckey 1947; Siegel 1961; Kersten et al. 1980). Rabbits and guinea pigs ingest about 50–60% of their intake at night, and display a tri-phasic feeding pattern with one feeding period prior to lights out, one mid-dark period, and a third after lights on, though the pattern is less pronounced in young rabbits (Hirsch 1973; Horton et al. 1974; Horton et al. 1975; Büttner 1992; Gidenne et al. 2010). Cats also eat about 60% of their intake in the dark, but the proportion varies significantly from about 28 to 80%, with some individuals showing strong diurnal patterns (Johnson et al. 1983). Dogs are usually fed a restricted diet once or twice per day but given *ad libitum* access, they show primarily nocturnal feeding in natural light: in controlled 12D:12N lighting, food intake is similar in the dark and light periods.

Many biological processes such as hormonal activity follow feeding patterns and disturbing the pattern, for example by acute or chronic diet restriction (Nelson 1988), may lead to abnormal metabolic and behavioural processes (Challet 2013; Patton & Mistlberger 2013). For example, feeding early in the morning rather than early in the dark period substantially decreased survival of severely food-restricted mice (Nelson

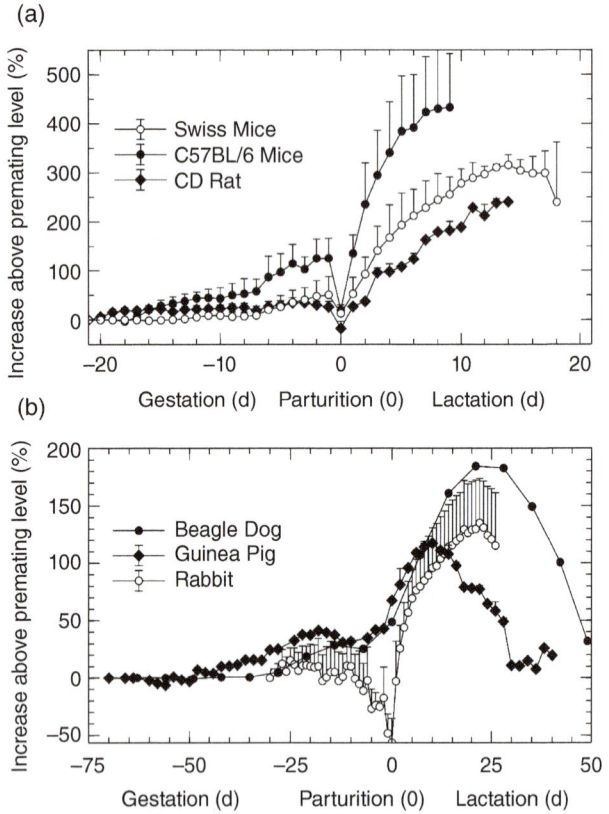

Figure 13.4 The change in food intake during gestation and lactation of (a) several stocks and strains of rats and mice, and (b) guinea pigs, rabbits, and beagles. The values are a percentage of the pre-mating food intake. Where sufficient data are available, standard deviations have been calculated and shown. There were few data for guinea pigs and dogs.

et al. 1973). And Krohn *et al.* (1999) noted that feeding rabbits at 2 pm decreased abnormal behaviour in the dark period compared to feeding at 8 am. Most animal manipulations such as measuring food intake and body weight occur in the early morning for the convenience of staff. In practice, more reliable data and improved welfare may be obtained by carrying out these processes just before switching off lighting or early in the dark cycle (Toth & Gardiner 2000). It is possible to compromise between the animal's usual diurnal pattern and staff requirements by shifting the onset of the dark period to mid or late afternoon. The evidence is that the animals' circadian rhythms will adjust to such change (Strubbe & Woods 2004).

Environmental effects

The two major environmental factors that affect food intake are environmental temperature (ET) and activity. Most animal rooms control ET within 3 °C of the desired setting, which would be in the range 20–24 °C for rats, mice, gerbils and hamsters, 15–21 °C for guinea pigs, rabbits, and cats, and 15–24 °C for dogs. These temperatures are below thermoneutrality, so an animal's energy requirement in normal housing includes a component for thermoregulation. Using data from Herrington (1940), Durrer and Hannon (1962) and Tobin *et al.* (2007), we calculated that across all the main laboratory species (except for rabbits and non-human primates for which we have insufficient data), metabolism increases about 2–5% per day for each one-degree decrease in ET.

The energy cost of activity in laboratory animals has been most studied in rats and mice. Spontaneous activity in laboratory animals is low, and generally, the additional energy expended in activity is much less than resting metabolism (Speakman & Selman 2003). In mice, activity contributes 10–20% of daily expenditure (Van Klinken *et al.* 2012; Virtue *et al.* 2012), which is similar to that in sedentary humans (Ravussin *et al.* 1986). Spontaneous activity is also low in pet dogs, with only about 13% of the time associated with non-sedentary activity (Michel & Brown 2014), and even high activity only increases energy expenditure about 14% above resting levels (Bermingham *et al.* 2014).

Palatability and variety effects

Palatability is difficult to define with certainty, but it is regarded as a hedonistic response to a combination of odour, taste and texture (Ramirez 1990). Palatability is rarely a problem *per se* with standard laboratory animal diets (though both rabbits and non-human primates may be selective in the laboratory diets they eat) but may be of importance when chemical compounds or ingredients are added to experimental diets. In our view, it is always important to measure food intake to determine to what extent it rather than some direct cellular effect of the compound or ingredient may be responsible for the endpoint. For example, the decrease in food intake in rats fed a high-protein diet may be ascribed to regulatory control of protein intake when the effect is almost certainly the low palatability of the protein (McArthur *et al.* 1993). The effect of palatability is often overlooked in the interpretation of experimental findings.

Increased palatability

Food variety has been well established as a means of increasing food intake (Johnson & Wardle 2014). It is used experimentally with rats and mice to induce obesity by presenting them a range of different food ingredients (supermarket or cafeteria feeding), usually together with the standard diet (Sclafani & Springer 1976; Rolls *et al.* 1980). It is effective in creating obesity (Armitage *et al.* 1983; Barr & McCracken 1984) and metabolic syndrome (Brandt *et al.* 2010; Carillon *et al.* 2013) in rodents and more so than purified high-fat diets (Sampey *et al.* 2011; Higa *et al.* 2014).

Decreased palatability

The most common cause of poor palatability is the addition of test or medicinal compounds to the diet. Unpalatable test compounds typically decrease food intake and body weight (Moran *et al.* 1955). Poor palatability may have surprising effects: Haseman (1998) showed that the decreased intake and body weight resulting from feeding a high concentration of carcinogenic o-nitroanisole paradoxically increased survival and equalised tumour rate to the control group.

Tamoxifen included in the diet has been used to activate ligand-dependent Cre recombinases in transgenic mouse models. However, it depresses food intake and body weight for about 3–5 days, after which animals usually start to eat again (Kiermayer *et al.* 2007). These effects are seen even if tamoxifen is administered in a normally highly palatable high-fat diet (Owen *et al.* 2013). The consequences of tamoxifen appear to be a CNS effect rather than taste *per se* since it occurs in a similar transient manner in rats even if the tamoxifen is injected (Wade & Heller 1993; Lopez *et al.* 2006).

Some compounds may be added to drinking water, but care must be taken that this does not decrease water intake, which in turn decreases food intake. For example, the inclusion of 2 mg mL^{-1} of the Tet-inducer doxycycline in drinking water decreased the body weight of mice by as much as 20% through dehydration (Cawthorne *et al.* 2007).

Fat rancidity is also a potential cause of decreased palatability. It lowered food intake and body weight in rats for about 2–3 weeks, after which, as with tamoxifen, food intake increased, and growth rate was restored (Greenberg & Frazer 1953). It is primarily associated with inappropriate diet storage and is discussed further in that section.

Pellet hardness effects

Researchers rarely ascribe differences in experimental observations to diet hardness, yet excessive hardness may significantly decrease food intake, especially in rodents. Rats are particularly sensitive to diet hardness, followed by inbred mice and then outbred mice (Tobin *et al.* 2007). Even in the absence of decreased food intake, growth rate in mice may be decreased, reflecting the additional work required to ingest the diet (Ford 1977). Hardness is affected by the composition of ingredients (Briggs et al. 1999) and by processing conditions such as the fineness of the ingredients, moisture content, and conditioning settings in the pellet press (Behnke 2001; Muramatsu et al. 2015). Adding increasing amounts of fat to pelleted diet decreases its hardness. This may be important in comparing the effects in rodents of a low-fat control diet with those on a much softer high-fat diet. Fat content has little or no effect on the hardness of extruded diet.

Planned deviations from ad libitum feeding

Calorie or diet restriction and longevity

The benefits of feeding amounts of food less than *ad libitum* levels (calorie or diet restriction) were recognised in the early twentieth century, but its current importance is largely traced back to the work of McCay in the 1930s and 1940s (Tobin et al. 2007; McDonald & Ramsey 2010). While most of the early studies were concerned with the question of ageing *per se*, in the mid-1970s, it was suggested that it could be a technique to correct the excessive weight gain, increasing tumour incidence, and declining longevity seen in many stocks and strains of rodents in 2-year chronic bioassay studies (Roe & Tucker 1974; Roe 1981; Rao et al. 1990; Turturro et al. 2016). See also Chapter 16: 3Rs considerations when using ageing animals in science. The increased incidence of these problems was ascribed to deliberate or inadvertent breeder selection for rapidly growing animals (Rao 1995; Allaben et al. 1996; Keenan et al. 1999) and/or improvements in the health status of rodents with the development of specific-pathogen-free models and improvements in diet hygiene. Declining survival was important because the FDA (and similar regulatory bodies) required a minimum of 25 surviving animals in the control group at the end of the study or 50% of those allocated to the group.

The terms diet and calorie restriction are used interchangeably though calorie restriction is often preferred because it emphasises that the beneficial effects are derived from decreased energy intake rather than decreased intake of specific nutrients such as protein, carbohydrate, or fat (Shanley & Kirkwood 2000; Keenan et al. 2013).

Calorie restriction may cause welfare issues because of the inability of the animal to satisfy hunger. However, its health benefits have become well established. They include decreased body weight, increased survival rates (particularly beyond 12 months of age), reduction of the incidence of some tumours and chronic progressive nephropathy, and improvements in plasma lipid levels and glucose tolerance (Reaven & Reaven 1981a; Reaven & Reaven 1981b; Kalant et al. 1988; Keenan et al. 1995a; Keenan et al. 1995b; Roe et al. 1995; Barzilai et al. 1998). There is a near-linear relationship in rats and mice between the magnitude of calorie restriction and a decrease in body weight (mainly body fat reduction), tumour incidence and improved longevity, at least down to 60% restriction (Klurfeld et al. 1989; Keenan et al. 1999; Duffy et al. 2001; Speakman & Hambly 2007). Calorie restriction for even a moderate part of the animal's life appears beneficial, though less than lifetime restriction (Weindruch & Walford 1982; Yu et al. 1985; Beauchene et al. 1986; Berrigan et al. 2002).

Calorie restriction is effective in a wide range of rodent models (Turturro et al. 1999), with about 70–80% of *ad libitum* intake being commonly used. However, the effect is highly variable: Swindell (2012) estimated that in rats, the average improvement in median life span was 30.2% (range 14–45%), with the maximum life span increased by 31.6% (range 18–36%). Improvement was less in mice with a median life span increase of 14.6% (range 4–27%) and an average of 17.8% in maximum life span (range 1–25%). The greatest benefits were for male animals and outbred stocks. Large strain differences in the effectiveness of calorie restriction have been reported by others (Lipman 2002; Forster et al. 2003; Hempenstall et al. 2010), with even decreased longevity in some strains (Liao et al. 2010). Sohal and Forster (2014) have made the important and logical point that the effectiveness of calorie restriction is greatest in stocks and strains that are predisposed to gain the greatest weight when fed *ad libitum*, and this may explain much of the variation seen.

Calorie restriction has also been beneficial in dogs (Kealy et al. 2002; Lawler et al. 2008) and non-human primates (Gresl et al. 2001; Colman et al. 2014; Mattison et al. 2017). Although longevity is increased, not all of the benefits seen in rodents have been confirmed, particularly decreased tumour incidence (Mattison et al. 2007). And in dogs, the major causes of death or euthanasia with ageing are not tumours but musculoskeletal disorders or problems with the gastrointestinal tract (Lawler et al. 2005).

A perceived problem of calorie restriction in carcinogenicity studies is the possibility that it reduces the development of treatment-induced tumours, conceivably obscuring the carcinogenic effects of compounds (Abdo & Kari 1996; Haseman 1998; Keenan et al. 1999). Though calorie restriction does compromise sensitivity to test compounds, Keenan (1996) argues that a balance can be achieved by using moderate restriction to about 70–80% of ad lib intake. If necessary, the doses of compounds can be increased since calorie-restricted animals tolerate doses several times higher than *ad libitum*-fed animals (Keenan 1998). Furthermore, increasing survival time by reducing spontaneous ageing-related diseases and tumours means that more animals are exposed to test compounds for longer periods of time, increasing the probability of compound-related pathology becoming apparent.

Although calorie restriction can be used with group-housed animals, unequal food intake is likely within the group, with dominant animals achieving the highest intake (Kasanen et al. 2009). While calorie restriction can be practised easily with singly housed rodents in the United States (Pugh et al. 1999), in the EU, there are perceived welfare issues with such housing, and alternative methods of restricting body weight have been sought.

One of the more useful forms of calorie restriction for group-housed rodents is intermittent, alternate-day, or every other day (EOD) feeding in which animals have *ad libitum* access on alternate days interspersed with total food deprivation (Anson et al. 2005). It is effective in many mouse (Goodrick et al. 1990) and rat stocks and strains (Carlson & Hoelzel 1946; Beauchene et al. 1986). Many of the studies have been reviewed by Varady and Hellerstein (2007). Intermittent feeding has beneficial effects in rats similar to those with calorie restriction even if introduced at 10 months of age (Goodrick et al. 1982; Goodrick et al. 1983), and the between-animal variation in food intake and body weight in a cage is little different from that seen with ad libitum-fed groups (Donati et al. 2009).

Acute food restriction/deprivation (fasting)

Relatively short-term removal of food for periods ranging from a few hours up to 48 hours, though more usually 4–24 hours, is used largely to decrease variability in measured clinical chemistry parameters and the metabolic state. It stabilises circadian rhythms in clinical chemistry blood values, particularly lipids, and eliminates irregular fluxes of absorbed analytes that follow periodic ingestion of food (Bertolucci et al. 2008). It is a standard procedure in blood glucose and insulin studies in diabetes. It may also be used before surgery to minimise vomiting or aspiration of gastric contents during anaesthesia, although that is a negligible risk with laboratory rodents and rabbits that lack a vomiting reflex (Horn et al. 2013), though they can gag or retch (Horn 2008).

It has become a standard procedure in both basic research and chronic bioassays in laboratory animals to apply food deprivation overnight prior to measuring clinical chemistry values. This is based on typical clinical practice in humans, where it corresponds to a period of minimal activity and fasting. But that is the opposite of the situation in most laboratory animals, particularly rats and mice, which are largely nocturnal (see 'Diurnal feeding rhythms' in the preceding text) (Andrikopoulos et al. 2008). This difference brings into question the validity of overnight food deprivation in animals. Although Rowland (2007) has shown no evidence of demonstrable physiological or apparent psychological distress in rodents that have been food-deprived for up to 24 hours, it would seem logical to use the shortest duration necessary to achieve stable levels of the clinical chemistry values (Matsuzawa & Sakazume 1994). This period may be different for different analytes and may also differ within and between species (Palou et al. 1981; Matsuzawa & Sakazume 1994). For example, recent studies have suggested that in mice, food deprivation of about 5–6 hours might be as effective as overnight deprivation without serious welfare issues (Andrikopoulos et al. 2008; Jensen et al. 2013; Jensen et al. 2019). However, in rats, a deprivation period of about 12 hours may be necessary for optimal results (Kale et al. 2009) and is achievable with minimal stress (Nowland et al. 2011). A slightly longer period, of 16 hours, might be required to achieve stability of plasma analytes in the beagle (Matsuzawa & Sakazume 1994). In contrast, the study of plasma lipid levels in rabbits seems to need no food deprivation, though minimum glucose levels were only achieved after 8 hours of deprivation (Wang et al. 2019). This variability between species casts doubt on whether a single restriction protocol is appropriate.

The ability of animals to withstand short-term severe food restriction or deprivation is a function of their metabolic rate and body energy reserves (mainly fat). And although after about 12–24 hours of restriction, animals may start to decrease their energy expenditure by physiological and behavioural mechanisms (Rowland 2007), this adaptation may be insufficient to protect small lean animals such as the common shrew (Sorex sinuosus) that have a high metabolic rate. As a result, they have been reported to die within 5–23 hours of food deprivation (Newman & Rudd 1978). Other species of shrew have a similarly low survival time after the onset of food restriction, and Hanski (1994) has estimated that may be a little as 5–10 hours in five species of European Sorex.

Torpor

Torpor is associated with acute and chronic energy restriction. It is characterised by a decrease in body temperature (to less than about 31-33°C) and metabolic rate (Hudson 1978; Webb et al. 1982; Ruf & Heldmaier 1992; Wilz & Heldmaier 2000). The torpor that follows acute restriction is termed daily torpor. Unintended daily torpor should be regarded as a significant welfare issue. Hibernation can be viewed as an extreme form of daily torpor but one that is an adaptative response of benefit to the animal. It occurs in response to a prolonged energy restriction that is sufficiently great to cause a loss of body fat content (Bieber et al. 2014). It may also be associated with low environmental temperatures and drought. The main difference between daily torpor and hibernation, apart from their cause, is the duration of the event and the extent of the drop in core body temperature. Daily torpor lasts about 3–21 hours (i.e. less than a day), while hibernation involves torpor for periods of about 40–770 hours and with a greater difference in core body and ambient temperature (Wilz & Heldmaier 2000). The third form of torpor is estivation, which is unique to a hot, dry environment, usually when conditions are extremely arid and is found in a wide range of species (Storey 2002).

In some animals in cold environments such as the Djungarian Hamster (Phodopus sungorus), torpor may allow a reprioritisation of energy utilisation from body temperature maintenance to locomotion so that the time for foraging can be extended (Ruf & Heldmaier 1992). A discussion of the mechanism of torpor is outside the scope of this chapter and has been well described in a series of reviews (Heldmaier & Elvert 2004; Staples & Brown 2008; Storey et al. 2010; Klug & Brigham 2015).

Food restriction as part of husbandry and other procedures

Rabbits, dogs, and non-human primates are often diet restricted as part of their normal husbandry. Laboratory rabbits frequently become overweight, and because they are very efficient at using fibre, low-density diets rarely prevent excessive weight gain. Feed restriction also decreases digestive disturbances in rabbits (Gidenne et al. 2012). Dogs are usually fed a fixed restricted amount of food each day, ranging in beagles from about 300 to 450 g per day, depending on size.

Food and water restriction have also been used in behavioural studies with both rodents and non-human primates to enhance the effect of food/drink rewards to encourage completion of tasks and other behavioural activities (Toth & Gardiner 2000). However, restriction of food or water can result in mild, moderate, or severe welfare impacts depending on the duration and degree of restriction. Protocols that rely on rewards alone rather in combination with restriction should be used where possible (Prescott et al. 2010), and where restriction is used, refinements to reduce the welfare impact should be considered.

Regulation of diet-restriction studies

Food and water restriction may be subject to regulatory approval in some jurisdictions and should always be subject to ethical approval. In the EU, general guidance is given in Directive 2010/63/EU for animals used for scientific purposes: in Article 33, 1(b) it requires Member States to ensure that *'any restrictions on the extent to which an animal can satisfy its physiological and ethological needs are kept to a minimum'*. The Directive provides examples in which withdrawal of food for <24 hours in adult rats is defined as a mild procedure, while withdrawal of food beyond 24 hours and up to 48 hours is classified as moderate. In the UK, these limited EU-level guidelines have been supplemented by the UK Home Office[9]. The Home Office stipulates that project licence authority is required for food deprivation of 16 hours or more for mice, young hamsters and rats under 100 g; 24 hours or more for rabbits, rats, dogs, cats and non-human primates weighing over 100 g and that food restriction should be avoided in guinea pigs, ferrets, and shrews. These are quite consistent with the scientific evidence presented above. These times may be shortened if additional factors that might cause suffering are superimposed. And if animals are subjected to repeated periods of deprivation, even shorter periods of restriction may require project licence approval.

In the United States, regulation of severity of diet restriction is generally determined by IACUCs. To the best of our knowledge, there is no mandated limit on the duration of restriction *per se*, and an IACUC will usually define an acceptable duration based on science and animal welfare. Although a duration in rodents of about 12 hours (up to 18 hours if specifically justified) is typically acceptable, a maximum 20% decline in body weight may be a more easily definable endpoint. Irrespective of what fixed endpoints are introduced, IACUCs usually emphasise the importance of careful and detailed monitoring of the condition, health, and behaviour of animals in deciding acceptable limits to food deprivation. The footnotes provide links to example IACUC guidelines from the Universities of Boston[10] and Michigan[11].

In addition to regulatory or institutional guidelines, several investigators and institutions have provided more detailed guidance, supported by scientific evidence, on food restriction for rats (Dietze et al. 2016) and non-human primates (Prescott et al. 2010).

Gavage

Gavage is the introduction of drugs or liquid diet through a feeding tube inserted via the oesophagus into the stomach and is mainly used in rodents. It can be used to introduce unpalatable compounds and fixed amounts of energy and nutrients with very high accuracy, though it does require good training and experience. Several studies have shown the procedure is not necessarily unduly stressful in rodents (Arantes-Rodrigues et al. 2012; Turner et al. 2012), and coating the gavage tube with sucrose may decrease measurable stress to negligible levels (Hoggatt et al. 2010). Though increases in plasma corticosterone (a marker of stress) were noted when various oils were administered to rats by gavage (Brown et al. 2000), an increase also occurred when rats were fed a high-fat diet (Cano et al. 2008; Namvar et al. 2016) suggesting Brown's observation may not be stress-related. Palatable compounds can be accurately administered by syringe into the animal's mouth rather than by gavage (Atcha et al. 2010; Tillmann & Wegener 2018).

Dogs are also often routinely gavaged in toxicology studies but may become averse to the procedure (Laule 2010). This adverse reaction is undoubtedly an indication that dogs find the procedure stressful. Although preparatory sham dosing has been commonly used to habituate dogs to dosing in experimental studies, it appears to increase stress rather than reduce it (Hall et al. 2015). However, positive reinforcement therapy (PRT), in which dogs are rewarded for accepting handling and dosing, was most effective. As with rodents, coating the gavage tube with a palatable substance improved acceptance of the procedure (Hall et al. 2015).

Pair feeding

Pair feeding can be used if food intake differences between the control group and any other groups are likely because of palatability or diet hardness effects. It requires a staggered start to the experiment: feeding of the group likely to show the lowest food intake commences on day 0. Food intake is measured over the first 24 hours, and then on day 1, the other group(s) are given the same amount of food. The staggered procedure continues for the duration of the study so that by the end, all the groups have received the same amount of food, and any experimental effects are independent of

---

[9]Home Office Guidance Note Water and Food Restriction for Scientific Purposes; https://www.med.hku.hk/images/document/04research/culatr/HomeOfficeGuide_WaterFoodRestriction.pdf (accessed 20 October 2019)

[10]http://www.bu.edu/researchsupport/compliance/animal-care/working-with-animals/food-regulation-and-restriction-in-rodents/ (accessed 7 November 2019)

[11]https://az.research.umich.edu/animalcare/guidelines/guidelines-experimental-food-or-water-restriction-or-manipulation-laboratory (accessed 7 November 2019)

differences in food intake. Despite its attractiveness, it does lead to gorging in the group(s) not eating to appetite, with the possibility of metabolic differences (Baker 1984; Harper 1986). To minimise gorging and its consequences, the typical diurnal feeding pattern may be mimicked in pair-fed restricted groups by giving a third of the food in the morning and two-thirds in the evening.

Unintended nutrient deficiency and excess

It is very rare to find unintended nutrient deficiencies when animals are fed *ad libitum* on standard laboratory animal diets that have been stored correctly and used according to the manufacturers' directions. We are aware of only a few incidences over many years: these included vitamin K deficiency in animals fed an irradiated diet that was well past its expiration date and vitamin C deficiency in guinea pigs as a result of either errors in formulation or poor storage of diet. The primary risk of nutrient deficiency comes from the misuse of diet, as described below.

Using diet as enrichment

Baumans *et al.* (2007) have described some of the ways in which the diets of laboratory animals have been enlivened by the addition of a range of highly palatable additional food items to the standard diet. The technique is most widely practised with non-human primates though application to a wider range of species is sometimes recommended. We need to add a note of caution on this practice based on our experience of cafeteria feeding in rodents (see 'Increased Palatability') and practical experience with marmosets where it can result in excessive weight gain and nutrient imbalances. We are not against the principle of food enrichment, but it must be tightly managed.

Non-human primates

Non-human primates encompasses a wide range of species with very different natural diets and differences in nutrient requirements, particularly with respect to vitamin D (Chun *et al.* 2008). Their gastrointestinal systems vary considerably across species and have become adapted to the nature of the diet (NRC 2003). In Europe, the primary non-human primates used in research are the rhesus macaque (*Macaca mulatta*) and Cynomolgus (*Macaca fascicularis*) monkeys and common marmosets (*Callithrix jacchus*). Our focus here is on these species.

The problems associated with feeding a mix of highly palatable foods, particularly fruits, are clearly demonstrated with cotton-top tamarins by Kirkwood (1983). Intake of the nutritionally complete diet decreased as fruit intake increased, with adverse effects on breeding. At the highest level of fruit inclusion, the protein intake of the animals was marginal and perhaps even deficient. Several facility managers have also reported nutritional deficiencies, including rickets, when insufficient control is maintained over supplementary feeding. We have found that supplementary foods may contribute as much as 75% of the dry matter food intake of laboratory-housed non-human primates. Even in the wild, non-human primates will gorge almost exclusively on fruit when it is readily available, substantially increasing their energy intake (Knott 1998). Plesker and Schuhmacher (2006) have calculated that dietary regimes for non-human primates that include high levels of fruit are likely to be low in protein and deficient in Ca, P, Zn, Cu, Se, and vitamins A, E, and folic acid. High levels of obesity are prevalent in many laboratory and zoo non-human primate colonies (Brent 1995; Schwitzer & Kaumanns 2001; Bauer *et al.* 2010), and excessive access to palatable foods is a significant factor.

The problem is not insurmountable: replacing fruits by vegetables and ensuring that only modest quantities are fed may be all that is required. Generally, vegetables contain lower levels of total sugars, fructose and sucrose, and higher levels of dietary fibre, calcium and iron than fruits. Schwitzer *et al.* (2009) has pointed out that fruits in the wild are much closer in nutrient composition to North American and European vegetables, with lower sugar and higher fibre content than fruits intended for humans. However, both vegetables and fruits contain low levels of vitamins, so a commercial non-human primate diet fed in appropriate amounts is essential.

In an unpublished study, substantial improvement in bone quality in a marmoset colony was observed when fruit in the diet was replaced by vegetables, probably as a result of increased calcium (from the commercial diet and vegetables) and vitamin D intake. It was notable that, as with Kirkwood's study, intake of the commercial non-human primate diet increased, boosting the intake of all the essential nutrients. Animals initially showed disappointment at the loss of the more palatable items but that was corrected by the introduction of a very small amount of melon (c. 3 cm cube) daily under strict control. In contrast to popular belief, vitamin C levels are low in most fruits except for oranges: the highest levels are in carrots. It has also been suggested that feeding whole or near-whole foods increases environmental enrichment and that inclusion of hard feed materials keeps animals occupied (Ceja & White 2010).

Rabbits

The use of coarse mixes is very common in feeding pet rabbits, though they are now referred to as 'muesli' feeds. They typically include cereals, oilseeds, and dried vegetables. The ingredients may be supplied whole or in crushed, flaked, or micronised form. Standard pellets are also included to provide a source of essential nutrients not delivered by the other individual ingredients. While visually more appealing than a complete pelleted diet, 'muesli' feeds have been associated with severe nutritional deficiencies, particularly calcium deficiency and skeletal problems (Tobin 1996). The problem was first noted by Harcourt-Brown (Harcourt-Brown 1996; Harcourt-Brown 2017) and presented as skeletal and dental problems associated with a low calcium intake brought about by the selection of the individual food items and rejection of the complete pellets. 'Muesli' feeds for rabbits are also associated with excessive weight gain (Prebble *et al.* 2015). While it may be tempting to feed such diets to laboratory rabbits, there are substantial risks.

Storage effects

Diet manufacturers define the shelf life of their products based on their own and published data, and generally the expiration date is 6–12 months after manufacture. The major nutrients most likely to be affected by storage conditions are amino acids, fats and oils, and vitamins. The rate of nutrient breakdown is mainly determined by storage temperature, and the effect can be expressed simplistically in the Q_{10} effect. This is the rate of change in nutrient loss per 10 °C: this is about 2 for laboratory diet nutrients, which means nutrient destruction doubles for every 10 °C increase, halving shelf life. Provided the product is stored under recommended environmental conditions, any nutrient losses with time should be insufficient to cause nutritional problems. In practice, the main problems with storage are more likely to be microbiological (fungi and bacteria) and biological (insects and mites) than nutritional and influenced by humidity as well as temperature. We have described the effects of environmental temperature and humidity in detail elsewhere (Tobin & Schuhmacher 2021).

Purified diets

Protein, fats, and vitamins in purified diets are vulnerable to damage. The main effects on protein amino acids result from Maillard reactions (browning), particularly between lysine and reducing sugars, which decrease the availability of amino acids and protein quality (Hurrell 1990). The risk of Maillard reactions is greater in purified diets containing casein and various sugars than in natural-ingredient diets. While Maillard reactions are primarily associated with heat treatment of ingredients, they may occur slowly at typical ambient conditions.

The damage to fats in purified diets arises from oxidative rancidity and the production of peroxides and other undesirable products (Choe & Min 2006). The main causes of rancidity are storage at ambient temperature rather than under refrigeration (Fullerton *et al*. 1982; Sun *et al*. 2012) and irradiation (Wills 1980b; Lee *et al*. 1999). The peroxides formed in irradiation create a chain reaction in which further peroxides are formed for many weeks thereafter while the diet is in storage (Takigawa *et al*. 1976). Because of the risk of rancidity in purified diets, it is quite common to include synthetic antioxidants such as tert-butylhydroquinone (TBHQ) and butylated hydroxyanisole (BHA). This is particularly important for diets with high-fat inclusions (Wills 1980a; Warner *et al*. 1982), which form a large proportion of purified diets produced. Although the most obvious effect of feeding a rancid diet is a reduction in food intake (Greenberg & Frazer 1953; Carpenter & L'Estrange 1966), peroxides generated early in the rancidification of unsaturated fatty acids may be toxic *per se* (Fekete *et al*. 2009).

Several vitamins in purified diets appear to be more susceptible to storage losses than those in natural-ingredient diets (Fullerton *et al*. 1982). A similar difference is seen with irradiation (Coates *et al*. 1969), probably because of the presence of natural antioxidants in natural-ingredient diets, as discussed below. Vitamin losses in purified diets can be reduced by the addition of antioxidants and by refrigeration (Q_{10} effect), preferably (if practicable) in sealed packages under vacuum or nitrogen.

Natural-ingredient diets

The storage conditions for natural-ingredient diets are largely dictated by the need to prevent microbiological growth. A reasonable target for diet storage is about 20–25 °C and a relative humidity of 65% or less (though short, infrequent periods up to 70–75% RH are unlikely to be a major problem).

In natural-ingredient diets, the main nutrient storage losses are of vitamins (Fullerton *et al*. 1982; Eva & Rickett 1983; Spencer 1985). However, in recent years there have been progressive improvements in vitamin stability, and average vitamin losses are now typically less than about 10% per month (Coelho 2002). Most diets have sufficient amounts of vitamins to allow for such losses up to the expiration date and usually beyond, and nutrient deficiencies are rare if storage is managed correctly.

Maillard reactions are of little importance in natural-ingredient diets. Nor is rancidity since natural-ingredient diets have intrinsic antioxidant capacity primarily from carotenoids, natural tocopherols and several other naturally occurring compounds in some of their ingredients (Brewer 2011; Shahidi & Ambigaipalan 2015), and from added vitamins such as A or C. Added vitamin E in the form of tocopherol acetate provides no antioxidant activity in the diet (Schuler 1990). Laboratory diet manufacturers seldom add synthetic antioxidants directly to natural-ingredient laboratory animal diets, but they may be present in high-fat dog and cat diets through their inclusion in bulk supplies of oils and fats used as ingredients (Joseph 2016).

Diet decontamination

Although irradiation results in some vitamin loss, it is usually 20% or less: the main risk in diet decontamination occurs with autoclaving, with particularly high losses in vitamin K, thiamine, pantothenate, vitamin B_{12}, and ascorbic acid (losses of ascorbyl-2-monophosphate are much lower). However, the problem is well-recognised by manufacturers who increase the amounts of vitamins and some amino acids in autoclavable diets to compensate for potential autoclaving losses. We are not aware of any nutrient deficiencies associated with autoclaving diets intended for that purpose if the procedure is correctly carried out. A fuller discussion of diet decontamination is provided by Tobin *et al*. (2007).

Diet and feeding as a basis for irreproducibility

Poor reproducibility in biomedical sciences has become an increasingly important issue in recent years (Collins & Tabak 2014). This is financially wasteful and leads to unnecessary use of animals. We describe here some of the potential pitfalls in the use of diets in the hope that increasing awareness will contribute to better animal welfare.

The use of control diets

One of the cardinal principles of experimental design is that the control group and experimental group(s) should differ only in the variable(s) that the investigator is testing. Any other differences, many of which will be unknown, make it difficult to ascribe experimental effects purely to the variable(s) under study.

Using a natural-ingredient diet as the control diet and one or more purified experimental diets fails this basic scientific requirement. This error is alarmingly common, particularly when comparing low-fat and high-fat diets (Warden & Fisler 2008). Substantial differences in phenotype are observed between animals fed equivalent natural-ingredient and purified control diets (Woods et al. 2003; Benoit et al. 2013; Del Bas et al. 2015) and between natural-ingredient and purified high-fat diets (Cheng et al. 2019). Rodents fed on purified diets commonly gain weight more quickly than those fed on nutritionally similar natural-ingredient diets (Anastasia et al. 1990; Lewis et al. 2003; Moraal et al. 2012; Cheng et al. 2019). The importance of using a purified diet as a control for purified experimental diets has been emphasised by Pellizzon and Ricci (2018). A single study that reported few differences between the two types of control diet (Almeida-Suhett et al. 2019) should not be taken as justification for the practice. First, it fails to address the issue of the scientific principle, and second, there is no certainty that differences will never occur in future studies. As we report in this chapter, there are differences between batches of the same product in nutrient, contaminant and other non-nutrients levels, and the formulas of some natural-ingredient diets may even be changed between batches. If natural-ingredient diets must be used, it is possible to produce balanced control and experimental natural-ingredient diets though it may be difficult. Some minor nutrient differences may remain, and their possible contribution to the endpoint of the study must be evaluated. Table 13.1 provides an example of balanced diets with and without soybean meal (the two formulas will change depending on the nutrient levels in the ingredients and are used here as an illustration).

Even if the control and experimental diets are identical in diet type and most nutrient levels, any large differences in food intake will cause differences in nutrient intake that may affect the experimental outcome *per se*. This occurs commonly in studies using high-fat diets when the higher energy density causes a decreased food intake compared with the control group because of the tendency of animals to 'eat for energy'. To maintain the level of intake of protein, minerals, and vitamins equal to that of the control, their concentrations are increased in the diet to a similar proportion of the dietary energy as in the control. These diets are referred to as 'calorie-adjusted'.

Nutrient levels in diet

Investigators sometimes choose to use nutrient values from manufacturers' data sheets or from tables of food composition in their studies rather than to measure them. These values are insufficiently accurate on which to base any important conclusions. They should be treated as indicative of typical

Table 13.1 An example of how natural-ingredients diets can be modified by experienced nutritionists to create nutritionally balanced soy-free control and soy-containing experimental diets to test the effect of bioactive substances in soybean meal. The ingredients are expressed as a percentage of the diet, and those changed to balance nutrient levels are highlighted. The amounts of ingredients would need to be adjusted to reflect any differences in the nutrient levels in the actual ingredients used. The minerals include major elements such as calcium, phosphorus and sodium and a trace element premix.

Ingredient (%)	Maize gluten-based control	Soy-containing experimental diet
Barley	23.00	23.00
Maize	**19.20**	**17.95**
Wheat	30.25	30.25
Maize Gluten Meal	**23.00**	**0.00**
Soy Meal	**0.00**	**24.00**
Corn Oil	**0.20**	**1.00**
Lysine	**0.60**	**0.10**
Methionine	0.10	0.15
Tryptophan	**0.10**	**0.00**
Minerals	3.00	3.00
Vitamin Premix	0.50	0.50
Choline Chloride	0.05	0.05
Calculated Nutrient Levels		
Crude Protein (%)	18.86	18.66
Crude Oil (%)	3.44	3.38
Crude Fibre (%)	3.21	3.22
Ash (%)	4.79	5.60
Calcium (%)	0.79	0.83
Phosphorus (%)	0.57	0.60
Zinc (mg/kg)	66	65
Copper (mg/kg)	14	16
Iron (mg/kg)	284	214
Vitamin A (iu/g)	15	15
Vitamin E (mg/kg)	91	89
Thiamine (mg/kg)	13	14
Pantothenate (mg/kg)	31	33
Lysine (%)	1.03	1.03
Methionine (%)	0.38	0.37
Tryptophan (%)	0.22	0.22

levels in the diet or food. If it is important to know such values accurately, they should always be measured in the batch of diet or food being used.

Since every manufacturer of laboratory diet will act independently, we cannot provide evidence of the extent to which individual nutrient values in datasheets are representative of actual measurements. When a diet is first developed, the datasheet values are calculated from the nutrient composition of the ingredients. Subsequently, these may be updated to reflect analytical data on multiple batches of the product. Most of the analytical data gathered by manufacturers cover the analytes typically required to support the use of batches of diet in good laboratory practice studies.

We have provided elsewhere calculations of variation in nutrient levels in almost 1000 batches of different laboratory animal diets (Tobin & Schuhmacher 2021). A summary of the data is shown in Table 13.2: overall, the average coefficient of variation (CV) between batches of a diet was about 7% for

Table 13.2 Variation in the levels of nutrients measured in almost 1000 batches of several laboratory animal diets from different manufacturers. The SD represents the variation in the coefficient of variation (CV) within the rodent, guinea pig, rabbit and dog diets tested.

Analyte	Mean CV ± SD	Analyte	Mean CV ± SD
Crude Protein	3.4 ± 0.6	Calcium	10.3 ± 1.5
Crude Fat	8.7 ± 1.4	Phosphorus	7.1 ± 0.4
Crude Fibre	9.6 ± 2.8	Magnesium	10.4 ± 2.0
Ash	5.5 ± 0.5	Sodium	9.6 ± 1.7
Vit A	18.1 ± 0.9	Potassium	8.1 ± 1.10
Vit E	17.7 ± 4.8	Chloride	7.4 ± 2.3
Vit C	18.1 ± 3.2	Iron	19.6 ± 8.5
		Zinc	11.5 ± 2.7
		Manganese	12.8 ± 2.4
		Copper	12.5 ± 2.8

proximate constituents, 9% for the major minerals, 14% for trace minerals, and about 18% for vitamins. The overall variation reflects the combination of true diet variation and analytical variation (accuracy and precision). The latter is inversely related to the magnitude of the value and its closeness to the detection or quantitation limit: thus, small values are usually associated with a large analytical variation (Horwitz & Albert 1995). This effect is often called the Horwitz Trumpet or Horn (Thompson 2004).

Non-nutrients in diet

Natural-ingredient diets commonly contain contaminants originally derived from soil and air. The main ones are: heavy metals such as arsenic, cadmium, lead and mercury; organic compounds, mainly pesticides and PCBs; and microbiological agents and their products such as mycotoxins (Tobin et al. 2007). Their potential to affect research studies was formally recognised in the 1970s, and organisations such as the FDA drew attention to their importance in toxicology studies in the statement of Good Laboratory Practice (GLP). There are well-defined limits on contaminant levels permissible in laboratory diet that should minimise any significant impact on studies. Diet manufacturers analyse individual batches of diet to confirm compliance with any relevant standards, but this usually only applies to those diets used in GLP studies. However, the data may be available to other users. Problems with dietary contaminants in North America, UK and EU are rare.

There are potentially deleterious non-nutrients in the diet that are not the result of environmental pollution (Cheeke 1998). In practice, they are more likely to be the cause of irreproducibility than the contaminants mentioned in the preceding text. The most important of these have been phytoestrogens associated with soybean meal (Csaky & Fekete 2004) and alfalfa and other forage legumes (Cornara et al. 2016).

Phytoestrogens potentially influence research results through their ability to bind to oestrogen receptors, particularly the β-oestrogen receptor. They are natural selective oestrogen receptor modulators (SERMS), having both agonist and antagonist effects (Setchell 2001), and they often show biphasic effects in which a greater response is invoked with the lower of two concentrations (Anderson et al. 1998; Almstrup et al. 2002).

In laboratory animal diets, the main phytoestrogens are isoflavones (mainly genistein and daidzein) found in soybean meal and coumestrol in alfalfa. Batch-to-batch variation of isoflavones, particularly those in soy, is considerable (Thigpen et al. 2007). There are other groups, such as lignans (found mainly in flaxseed), but these have received less attention (Setchell 1998). Mycoestrogens, such as resorcylic acid lactones (primarily zearalenone), are sometimes found in diet, originating from fungi growing on inappropriately harvested and stored cereals, mainly maize (Jimenez et al. 1996; Yazar & Omurtag 2008). Manufacturers can use test kits to check suspect raw materials for many mycotoxins: those ingredient batches that show measurable contamination should be rejected. Saponins in soybean meal and alfalfa also have biological effects on animals that may be incorrectly attributed to isoflavones (Price et al. 1987; Francis et al. 2002; Kang et al. 2010).

Although the existence of isoflavones in laboratory animal diets is well established, researchers are often unaware of their presence and the possibility that they can confound their experimental results (Setchell & Clerici 2010). The large variations in isoflavone concentration and their biphasic effects make it difficult for researchers to predict how their results may be affected by a diet containing soybean meal (Setchell & Clerici 2010). Measurement of isoflavones is possible but expensive. In practice, the only means of avoiding their confounding effects is to use diets devoid of soybean meal and alfalfa (Thigpen et al. 2004).

There have been several reviews describing the effects of phytoestrogens, mainly in rodents, and cautioning the use of soybean meal in laboratory animal diets for experimental work (Brown & Setchell 2001; Jensen & Ritskes-Hoitinga 2007; Tobin et al. 2007). Their effects can be seen at even low levels and well within the range found in laboratory diets (Menon et al. 1998; Delclos et al. 2001; Ju et al. 2001; Mentor-Marcel et al. 2001). Although they affect a wide range of physiological systems, most attention has been on their effects on cancer and metabolic syndrome. They may also interact with test compounds masking or exaggerating their effects (Ju et al. 2002; Constantinou et al. 2005; Ju et al. 2008; Du et al. 2012).

Their effects on tumour development are of particular importance, and nude mice, one of the main oncology models, may be potentially very sensitive (Setchell et al. 2011). Barnes (1995) has reported that the incidence of many tumours is typically decreased, and latency increased, by dietary genistein in animal studies. The experimental findings in animals are consistent with molecular (mainly in vitro) studies. Generally, isoflavones act by: (a) suppressing oxidative stress; (b) regulating cell signalling pathways involved in tumour growth and suppression, and cell apoptosis; (c) inhibiting the angiogenesis needed to support tumour growth, and (d) inhibiting the spread of tumour cells (metastasis); (Sarkar & Li 2004; Banerjee et al. 2008).

The ability of soy isoflavones to activate peroxisome proliferator-activated receptors such as PPARα and PPARγ has been well established (Dang et al. 2003; Ricketts et al. 2005; Patel & Barnes 2010). These receptors have widespread importance (Medjakovic *et al.* 2010), and by activating them, soy can inhibit processes such as metabolic syndrome (Mezei *et al.* 2003; Ronis *et al.* 2009), cardiovascular disease, and metastasis. Activation also increases fatty acid catabolism (Kim *et al.* 2004) and lowers blood lipids (Mezei *et al.* 2006) and proinflammatory genes (Sakamoto *et al.* 2016).

Several studies have been carried out on isoflavone effects on diabetes, atherosclerosis, behaviour and reproduction in non-human primates (Anthony *et al.* 1996; Simon *et al.* 2004; Wood *et al.* 2004a; Wood *et al.* 2004b; Adams *et al.* 2005; Walker *et al.* 2008) but the effects are not always consistent with those in rodents (Wood *et al.* 2006).

Continued use of laboratory animal diets containing phytoestrogens is sometimes justified on the basis that this may better reflect human diets. However, human intake, even in those with a high soybean intake, is a fraction of that in rodents fed on typical soya-containing diets. This is confirmed by comparing plasma isoflavone levels in rodents and humans (Brown & Setchell 2001; Grace *et al.* 2004). Additionally, the metabolism of daidzein to equol in the gastrointestinal tract is common in rodents but only occurs in about 25% of humans (Gu *et al.* 2006). Circulating levels of equol in soy-fed rodents are much higher than genistein or daidzein (Brown & Setchell 2001). This is important because equol may be a more potent oestrogen than genistein or daidzein (Setchell *et al.* 2002).

Research into the effects of phytoestrogens often suffers from the problem of inappropriate controls. Three approaches have been taken to diet studies: addition of pure isoflavone in controlled amounts to a purified diet; the use of intact soy protein in an experimental purified diet and a control diet containing soy protein from which isoflavones have been stripped; but mainly the use of two, usually natural-ingredient, diets one with soybean meal and the other without. In the latter case, the diets are often very different, and the possibility that other differences in the two diets might be responsible for the effects is ignored. We have described earlier how manufacturers can create soy-containing and soy-free natural-ingredient diets with similar nutrient levels, and while not perfect, that would be a better alternative to using two very different diets.

Concluding remarks

We have identified four major nutritional and dietary contributors to animal welfare. The first is ensuring an adequate intake of nutrients by feeding an appropriate diet, storing it at the required temperature and humidity, and not providing uncontrolled access to other nutritionally unbalanced foods that distract animals from the primary diet. Secondly, it is essential to use the correct control diet. This might seem a minor issue, but it is a widespread problem, and a strictly scientific view would be that failure to do so probably invalidates the study with an unacceptable waste of animals. Thirdly, care must be taken to consider the possible effects of physiologically active non-nutrients and, to a lesser extent, dietary contaminants that may confound experimental outcomes. Our final point is that of balancing the welfare benefits of providing animals with a 'happy environment' (we appreciate this is an anthropomorphic phrase) with one that gives health and longevity. For example, while diet restriction undoubtedly brings benefits to many stocks and strains of animals, it is associated with signs of hunger during periods of food deprivation (D'Eath *et al.* 2009). And providing highly palatable supplementary foods that are attractive to the animal without rigid control may be considered harmful. There is an argument that when it comes to feeding, animal welfare may sometimes be better served by 'beneficial austerity'.

References

Abdo, K.M. and Kari, F.W. (1996) The sensitivity of the NTP bioassay for carcinogen hazard evaluation can be modulated by dietary restriction. *Experimental and Toxicologic Pathology*, **48**, 129–137. doi: 10.1016/s0940-2993(96)80033-9.

Abelson, K.S.P., Jacobsen, K.R., Sundbom, R. *et al.* (2012) Voluntary ingestion of nut paste for administration of buprenorphine in rats and mice. *Laboratory Animals*, **46**, 349–351. doi: 10.1258/la.2012.012028.

Adams, M.R., Golden, D.L., Williams, J.K. *et al.* (2005) Soy protein containing isoflavones reduces the size of atherosclerotic plaques without affecting coronary artery reactivity in adult male monkeys. *The Journal of Nutrition*, **135**, 2852–2856. doi: 10.1093/jn/135.12.2852.

Ahmed, M.B., Zhou, J.L., Ngo, H.H. *et al.* (2017) Progress in the biological and chemical treatment technologies for emerging contaminant removal from wastewater: A critical review. *Journal of Hazardous Materials*, **323**, 274–298. doi: 10.1016/j.jhazmat.2016.04.045.

AIN (1977) Report of the American Institute of Nutrition ad hoc Committee on Standards for Nutritional Studies. *The Journal of Nutrition*, **107**, 1340–1348. doi: 10.1093/jn/107.7.1340.

Akbar, Z. and Gorman, M.L. (1993) The effect of supplementary feeding upon the sizes of the home ranges of woodmice *Apodemus sylvaticus* living on a system of maritime sand-dunes. *Journal of Zoology*, **231**, 233–237. doi: 10.1111/j.1469-7998.1993.tb01914.x.

Allaben, W.T., Turturro, A., Leakey, J.E. *et al.* (1996) FDA points-to-consider documents: the need for dietary control for the reduction of experimental variability within animal assays and the use of dietary restriction to achieve dietary control. *Toxicologic Pathology*, **24**, 776–781. doi: 10.1177/019262339602400622.

Allen, E.D., Czarra, E.F. and DeTolla, L. (2018) Water quality and water delivery systems. In: *Management of Animal Care and Use Programs in Research, Education, and Testing*. 2nd ed., Eds Weichbrod, R.H., Thompson, G.A.H. and Norton, J.N., pp. 655–672, CRC Press, Boca Raton, FL. doi: 10.1201/9781315152189-28.

Allevi, R.P., Krometis, L.A., Hagedorn, C. *et al.* (2013) Quantitative analysis of microbial contamination in private drinking water supply systems. *Journal of Water and Health*, **11**, 244–255. doi: 10.2166/wh.2013.152.

Almeida-Suhett, C.P., Scott, J.M., Graham, A. *et al.* (2019) Control diet in a high-fat diet study in mice: Regular chow and purified low-fat diet have similar effects on phenotypic, metabolic, and behavioral outcomes. *Nutritional Neuroscience*, **22**, 19–28. doi: 10.1080/1028415x.2017.1349359.

Almstrup, K., Fernández, M.F., Petersen, J.H. *et al.* (2002) Dual effects of phytoestrogens result in u-shaped dose-response curves. *Environmental Health Perspectives*, **110**, 743–748. doi: 10.1289/ehp.02110743.

Anastasia, J.V., Braun, B.L. and Smith, K.T. (1990) General and histopathological results of a two-year study of rats fed semi-purified diets containing casein and soya protein. *Food and Chemical Toxicology*, **28**, 147–156. doi: 10.1016/0278-6915(90)90003-6.

Anderson, J.J., Ambrose, W.W. and Garner, S.C. (1998) Biphasic effects of genistein on bone tissue in the ovariectomized, lactating rat model. *Proceedings of the Society for Experimental Biology and Medicine*, **217**, 345–350. doi: 10.3181/00379727-217-44243.

Andrikopoulos, S., Blair, A.R., Deluca, N. et al. (2008) Evaluating the glucose tolerance test in mice. *American Journal of Physiology: Endocrinology and Metabolism*, **295**, E1323–1332. doi: 10.1152/ajpendo.90617.2008.

Anson, R.M., Jones, B. and de Cabod, R. (2005) The diet restriction paradigm: a brief review of the effects of every-other-day feeding. *Age (Dordr)*, **27**, 17–25. doi: 10.1007/s11357-005-3286-2.

Anthony, M.S., Clarkson, T.B., Hughes, C.L., Jr. et al. (1996) Soybean isoflavones improve cardiovascular risk factors without affecting the reproductive system of peripubertal rhesus monkeys. *The Journal of Nutrition*, **126**, 43–50. doi: 10.1093/jn/126.1.43.

Arantes-Rodrigues, R., Henriques, A., Pinto-Leite, R. et al. (2012) The effects of repeated oral gavage on the health of male CD-1 mice. *Laboratory Animals*, **41**, 129–134. doi: 10.1038/laban0512-129.

Armitage, G., Hervey, G.R., Rolls, B.J. et al. (1983) The effects of supplementation of the diet with highly palatable foods upon energy balance in the rat. *Journal of Physiology*, **342**, 229–251. doi: 10.1113/jphysiol.1983.sp014848.

Atcha, Z., Rourke, C., Neo, A.H. et al. (2010) Alternative method of oral dosing for rats. *Journal of the American Association for Laboratory Animal Science*, **49**, 335–343.

Bachmanov, A.A., Reed, D.R., Beauchamp, G.K. et al. (2002) Food intake, water intake, and drinking spout side preference of 28 mouse strains. *Behavior Genetics*, **32**, 435–443. doi: 10.1023/a:1020884312053.

Baker, D.H. (1984) Equalized versus ad libitum feeding. *Nutrition Reviews*, **42**, 269–273. doi: 10.1111/j.1753-4887.1984.tb02354.x.

Baker, D.H. (1986) Problems and pitfalls in animal experiments designed to establish dietary requirements for essential nutrients. *The Journal of Nutrition*, **116**, 2339–2349. doi: 10.1093/jn/116.12.2339.

Baker, D.H. (1992) Applications of chemically defined diets to the solution of nutrition problems. *Amino Acids*, **2**, 1–12. doi: 10.1007/bf00806073.

Balsiger, A., Clauss, M., Liesegang, A. et al. (2017) Guinea pig (Cavia porcellus) drinking preferences: do nipple drinkers compensate for behaviourally deficient diets? *Journal of Animal Physiology and Animal Nutrition*, **101**, 1046–1056. doi: 10.1111/jpn.12549.

Banerjee, S., Li, Y., Wang, Z. et al. (2008) Multi-targeted therapy of cancer by genistein. *Cancer Letters*, **269**, 226–242. doi: 10.1016/j.canlet.2008.03.052.

Barley, J.B., Cherry, K.A., Garner, J.P. et al. (2004) Water leakage in rodent cages: a discussion by the Laboratory Animal Refinement and Enrichment Forum (LAREF). *Animal Technology and Welfare*, **3**, 111–114.

Barnard, D.E., Lewis, S.M., Teter, B.B. et al. (2009) Open-and closed-formula laboratory animal diets and their importance to research. *Journal of the American Association for Laboratory Animal Science*, **48**, 709–713.

Barnes, S. (1995) Effect of genistein on in vitro and in vivo models of cancer. *The Journal of Nutrition*, **125**, 777S–783S. doi: 10.1093/jn/125.3_Suppl.777S.

Barnett, J.A. and Gibson, D.L. (2019) H2Oh No! The importance of reporting your water source in your in vivo microbiome studies. *Gut Microbes*, **10**, 261–269. doi: 10.1080/19490976.2018.1539599.

Barr, H.G. and McCracken, K.J. (1984) High efficiency of energy utilization in 'cafeteria'- and force-fed rats kept at 29°. *British Journal of Nutrition*, **51**, 379. doi: 10.1079/bjn19840044.

Barzilai, N., Banerjee, S., Hawkins, M. et al. (1998) Caloric restriction reverses hepatic insulin resistance in aging rats by decreasing visceral fat. *Journal of Clinical Investigation*, **101**, 1353–1361. doi: 10.1172/jci485.

Bauer, S.A., Leslie, K.E., Pearl, D.L. et al. (2010) Survey of prevalence of overweight body condition in laboratory-housed cynomolgus macaques (*Macaca fascicularis*). *Journal of the American Association for Laboratory Animal Science*, **49**, 407–414.

Baumans, V., Coke, C., Green, J. et al. (eds.) (2007) *Making lives easier for animals in research labs*, Animal Welfare Institute, Washington, DC.

Beauchene, R.E., Bales, C.W., Bragg, C.S. et al. (1986) Effect of age of initiation of feed restriction on growth, body composition, and longevity of rats. *Journal of Gerontology*, **41**, 13–19. doi: 10.1093/geronj/41.1.13.

Behnke, K.C. (2001) Processing factors influencing pellet quality. *Feed Technology*, **5**, 1–7.

Bennett, A.J., Perkins, C.M., Tenpas, P.D. et al. (2016) Moving evidence into practice: cost analysis and assessment of macaques' sustained behavioral engagement with videogames and foraging devices. *American Journal of Primatology*, **78**, 1250–1264. doi: 10.1002/ajp.22579.

Benoit, B., Plaisancie, P., Awada, M. et al. (2013) High-fat diet action on adiposity, inflammation, and insulin sensitivity depends on the control low-fat diet. *Nutrition Research*, **33**, 952–960. doi: 10.1016/j.nutres.2013.07.017.

Bermingham, E.N., Thomas, D.G., Cave, N.J. et al. (2014) Energy requirements of adult dogs: a meta-analysis. *PloS One*, **9**, e109681. doi: 10.1371/journal.pone.0109681.

Berrigan, D., Perkins, S.N., Haines, D.C. et al. (2002) Adult-onset calorie restriction and fasting delay spontaneous tumorigenesis in p53-deficient mice. *Carcinogenesis*, **23**, 817–822. doi: 10.1093/carcin/23.5.817.

Bertolucci, C., Fazio, F. and Piccione, G. (2008) Daily rhythms of serum lipids in dogs: Influences of lighting and fasting cycles. *Comparative Medicine*, **58**, 485–489.

Beynen, A.C., Mulder, A., Nieuwenkamp, A.E. et al. (1992) Loose grass hay as a supplement to a pelleted diet reduces fur chewing in rabbits. *Journal of Animal Physiology and Animal Nutrition*, **68**, 226–234. doi: 10.1111/j.1439-0396.1992.tb00664.x.

Bidot, W.A., Ericsson, A.C. and Franklin, C.L. (2018) Effects of water decontamination methods and bedding material on the gut microbiota. *PloS One*, **13**, e0198305. doi: 10.1371/journal.pone.0198305.

Bieber, C., Lebl, K., Stalder, G. et al. (2014) Body mass dependent use of hibernation: why not prolong the active season, if they can? *Functional Ecology*, **28**, 167–177. doi: 10.1111/1365-2435.12173.

Bieri, J.G. (1979) AIN-76 diet. *The Journal of Nutrition*, **109**, 925–926. doi: 10.1093/jn/109.5.925.

Bøe, K.E. and Kjelvik, O. (2011) Water nipples or water bowls for weaned piglets: Effect on water intake, performance, and plasma osmolality. *Acta Agriculturae Scandinavica, Section A – Animal Science*, **61**, 86–91. doi: 10.1080/09064702.2011.599859.

Bollen, P.J.A., Lemmens, A.G., Beynen, A.C. et al. (2006) Bone composition in male and female Göttingen minipigs fed variously restrictedly and near ad libitum. *Scandinavian Journal of Laboratory Animal Sciences*, **33**, 149–158. doi: 10.23675/sjlas.v33i3.105.

Bomzon, A. and Tobin, G. (2021) Scholarly publishing and scientific reproducibility. In: *Experimental Design and Reproducibility in Preclinical Animal Studies*. Eds Sanchez, J. and Brønstad, A., pp. 185–211, Springer, Cham, Switzerland.

Bradford, S.A. and Harvey, R.W. (2017) Future research needs involving pathogens in groundwater. *Hydrogeology Journal*, **25**, 931–938. doi: 10.1007/s10040-016-1501-0.

Brandt, N., De Bock, K., Richter, E.A. et al. (2010) Cafeteria diet-induced insulin resistance is not associated with decreased insulin signaling or AMPK activity and is alleviated by physical training in rats. *American Journal of Physiology: Endocrinology and Metabolism*, **299**, E215–224. doi: 10.1152/ajpendo.00098.2010.

Brent, L. (1995) Feeding enrichment and body weight in captive chimpanzees. *Journal of Medical Primatology*, **24**, 12–16. doi: 10.1111/j.1600-0684.1995.tb00139.x.

Brewer, M.S. (2011) Natural antioxidants: Sources, compounds, mechanisms of action, and potential applications. *Comprehensive*

Reviews in Food Science and Food Safety, **10**, 221–247. doi: 10.1111/j.1541-4337.2011.00156.x.

Briggs, J.L., Maier, D.E., Watkins, B.A. *et al.* (1999) Effect of ingredients and processing parameters on pellet quality. *Poultry Science*, **78**, 1464–1471. doi: 10.1093/ps/78.10.1464.

Brown, A.P., Dinger, N. and Levine, B.S. (2000) Stress produced by gavage administration in the rat. *Contemporary Topics in Laboratory Animal Science*, **39**, 17–21.

Brown, N.M. and Setchell, K.D. (2001) Animal models impacted by phytoestrogens in commercial chow: implications for pathways influenced by hormones. *Laboratory Investigation*, **81**, 735–747. doi: 10.1038/labinvest.3780282.

Buchanan-Smith, H.M. (1994) Environmental enrichment in captive marmosets and tamarins. *Humane innovations and alternatives in animal experimentation*, **8**, 559–564.

Buckley, C.M., Hawthorne, A., Colyer, A. *et al.* (2011) Effect of dietary water intake on urinary output, specific gravity and relative supersaturation for calcium oxalate and struvite in the cat. *British Journal of Nutrition*, **106**, Suppl. 1, S128–130. doi: 10.1017/s0007114511001875.

Butler, A.A. and Kozak, L.P. (2010) A recurring problem with the analysis of energy expenditure in genetic models expressing lean and obese phenotypes. *Diabetes*, **59**, 323–329. doi: 10.2337/db09-1471.

Büttner, D. (1992) Social influences on the orcadian rhythm of locomotor activity and food intake of guinea pigs. *Journal of Interdisciplinary Cycle Research*, **23**, 100–112. doi: 10.1080/09291019209360134.

Cameron, K.M. and Speakman, J.R. (2010) The extent and function of 'food grinding' in the laboratory mouse (Mus musculus). *Laboratory Animals*, **44**, 298–304. doi: 10.1258/la.2010.010002.

Cano, P., Jimenez-Ortega, V., Larrad, A. *et al.* (2008) Effect of a high-fat diet on 24-h pattern of circulating levels of prolactin, luteinizing hormone, testosterone, corticosterone, thyroid-stimulating hormone and glucose, and pineal melatonin content, in rats. *Endocrine*, **33**, 118–125. doi: 10.1007/s12020-008-9066-x.

Carillon, J., Romain, C., Bardy, G. *et al.* (2013) Cafeteria diet induces obesity and insulin resistance associated with oxidative stress but not with inflammation: improvement by dietary supplementation with a melon superoxide dismutase. *Free Radical Biology and Medicine*, **65**, 254–261. doi: 10.1016/j.freeradbiomed.2013.06.022.

Carlson, A.J. and Hoelzel, F. (1946) Apparent prolongation of the life span of rats by intermittent fasting. *The Journal of Nutrition*, **31**, 363–375. doi: 10.1093/jn/31.3.363.

Carpenter, K.J. and L'Estrange, J.L. (1966) Effects of moderate levels of oxidized fat in animal diets under controlled conditions. *Proceedings of the Nutrition Society*, **25**, 25–31. doi: 10.1079/pns19660007.

Cawthorne, C., Swindell, R., Stratford, I.J. *et al.* (2007) Comparison of doxycycline delivery methods for Tet-inducible gene expression in a subcutaneous xenograft model. *Journal of Biomolecular Techniques*, **18**, 120–123.

Ceja, C. and White, J. (2010) Feeding behavior of *Saguinus oedipus* in relation to food hardness in a zoo setting: Possibilities for enrichment? *Laboratory Primate Newsletter*, **49**, 10.

Challet, E. (2013) Circadian clocks, food intake, and metabolism. *Progress in Molecular Biology and Translational Science*, **119**, 105–135. doi: 10.1016/b978-0-12-396971-2.00005-1.

Cheeke, P.R. (1998) *Natural Toxicants in Feeds, Forages, and Poisonous Plants*. Interstate Publishers, Inc, Danville, Il.

Cheng, H.S., Phang, S.C.W., Ton, S.H. *et al.* (2019) Purified ingredient-based high-fat diet is superior to chow-based equivalent in the induction of metabolic syndrome. *Journal of Food Biochemistry*, **43**, e12717. doi: 10.1111/jfbc.12717.

Choe, E. and Min, D.B. (2006) Mechanisms and factors for edible oil oxidation. *Comprehensive Reviews in Food Science and Food Safety*, **5**, 169–186. doi: 10.1111/j.1541-4337.2006.00009.x.

Chun, R.F., Adams, J.S. and Hewison, M. (2008) Back to the future: a new look at 'old' vitamin D. *Journal of Endocrinology*, **198**, 261–269. doi: 10.1677/joe-08-0170.

Cizek, L.J. (1954) Total water content of laboratory animals with special reference to volume of fluid within the lumen of the gastrointestinal tract. *American Journal of Physiology*, **179**, 104–110. doi: 10.1152/ajplegacy.1954.179.1.104.

Cizek, L.J. (1961) Relationship between food and water ingestion in the rabbit. *American Journal of Physiology*, **201**, 557–566. doi: 10.1152/ajplegacy.1961.201.3.557.

Clarke, H.E., Coates, M.E., Eva, J.K. *et al.* (1977) Dietary standards for laboratory animals: report of the Laboratory Animals Centre Diets Advisory Committee. *Laboratory Animals*, **11**, 1–28. doi: 10.1258/002367777780959175.

Coates, M.E., Ford, J.E., Gregory, M.E. *et al.* (1969) Effects of gamma-irradiation on the vitamin content of diets for laboratory animals. *Laboratory Animals*, **3**, 39–49. doi: 10.1258/002367769781071952

Coelho, M. (2002) Vitamin stability in premixes and feeds. A practical approach in ruminant diets. 13th Annual Florida Ruminant Nutrition Symposium. Gainesville, FL, University of Florida, from http://dairy.ifas.ufl.edu/rns/2002/coelho.pdf.

Collins, F.S. and Tabak, L.A. (2014) Policy: NIH plans to enhance reproducibility. *Nature*, **505**, 612–613. doi: 10.1038/505612a.

Colman, R.J., Beasley, T.M., Kemnitz, J.W. *et al.* (2014) Caloric restriction reduces age-related and all-cause mortality in rhesus monkeys. *Nature Communications*, **5**, 3557. doi: 10.1038/ncomms4557.

Coman, C. and Vlase, E. (2017) Formulation, preparation and chemical analysis of purified diets for laboratory mice and rats. *Scientific Works. Series C. Veterinary Medicine*, **63**, 149–154.

Constantinou, A.I., White, B.E., Tonetti, D. *et al.* (2005) The soy isoflavone daidzein improves the capacity of tamoxifen to prevent mammary tumours. *European Journal of Cancer*, **41**, 647–654. doi: 10.1016/j.ejca.2004.12.005.

Corbett, A., McGowin, A., Sieber, S. *et al.* (2012) A method for reliable voluntary oral administration of a fixed dosage (mg/kg) of chronic daily medication to rats. *Laboratory Animals*, **46**, 318–324. doi: 10.1258/la.2012.012018.

Cornara, L., Xiao, J. and Burlando, B. (2016) Therapeutic potential of temperate forage legumes: A review. *Critical Reviews in Food Science and Nutrition*, **56**, Suppl. 1, S149–161. doi: 10.1080/10408398.2015.1038378.

Csaky, I. and Fekete, S. (2004) Soybean: feed quality and safety. Part 1: Biologically active components. A review. *Acta Veterinaria Hungarica*, **52**, 299–313. doi: 10.1556/avet.52.2004.3.6.

D'Eath, R.B., Tolkamp, B.J., Kyriazakis, I. *et al.* (2009) 'Freedom from hunger' and preventing obesity: the animal welfare implications of reducing food quantity or quality. *Animal Behaviour*, **77**, 275–288. doi: 10.1016/j.anbehav.2008.10.028.

Dang, Z.C., Audinot, V., Papapoulos, S.E. *et al.* (2003) Peroxisome proliferator-activated receptor gamma (PPARgamma) as a molecular target for the soy phytoestrogen genistein. *Journal of Biological Chemistry*, **278**, 962–967. doi: 10.1074/jbc.m209483200.

Davidowitz, B.I., Boehm, K.M., Banovetz, S.E. *et al.* (1998) Increase in lead concentration in the drinking water of an animal care facility. *Contemporary Topics in Laboratory Animal Science*, **37**, 51–53.

de Blas, C. and Wiseman, J. (2010) *Nutrition of the Rabbit*. CAB International, Wallingford, United Kingdom.

de Haer, L.C.M. and Merks, J.W.M. (1992) Patterns of daily food intake in growing pigs. *Animal Production*, **54**, 95–104. doi: 10.1017/s0003356100020614.

Deblonde, T., Cossu-Leguille, C. and Hartemann, P. (2011) Emerging pollutants in wastewater: A review of the literature. *International Journal of Hygiene and Environmental Health*, **214**, 442–448. doi: 10.1016/j.ijheh.2011.08.002.

Del Bas, J.M., Caimari, A., Ceresi, E. *et al.* (2015) Differential effects of habitual chow-based and semi-purified diets on lipid metabolism in lactating rats and their offspring. *British Journal of Nutrition*, **113**, 758–769. doi: 10.1017/S0007114514004358.

Delclos, K.B., Bucci, T.J., Lomax, L.G. *et al.* (2001) Effects of dietary genistein exposure during development on male and female CD (Sprague-Dawley) rats. *Reproductive Toxicology*, **15**, 647–663. doi: 10.1016/s0890-6238(01)00177-0.

Dietze, S., Lees, K.R., Fink, H. *et al.* (2016) Food deprivation, body weight loss and anxiety-related behavior in rats. *Animals*, **6**, 4. doi: 10.3390/ani6010004.

Diogo, L.N., Faustino, I.V., Afonso, R.A. *et al.* (2015) Losartan voluntary oral administration in rats. *Journal of the American Association for Laboratory Animal Science*, **54**, 549–556.

Donati, A., Cavallini, G. and Bergamini, E. (2009) Methods for inducing and monitoring liver autophagy relative to aging and antiaging caloric restriction in rats. *Methods in Enzymology*, **452**, 441–455. doi: 10.1016/s0076-6879(08)03626-4.

Du, M., Yang, X., Hartman, J.A. *et al.* (2012) Low-dose dietary genistein negates the therapeutic effect of tamoxifen in athymic nude mice. *Carcinogenesis*, **33**, 895–901. doi: 10.1093/carcin/bgs017.

Duffy, P.H., Seng, J.E., Lewis, S.M. *et al.* (2001) The effects of different levels of dietary restriction on aging and survival in the Sprague-Dawley rat: implications for chronic studies. *Aging*, **13**, 263–272. doi: 10.1007/bf03353422.

Durrer, J.L. and Hannon, J.P. (1962) Seasonal variations in caloric intake of dogs living in an arctic environment. *American Journal of Physiology*, **202**, 375–378. doi: 10.1152/ajplegacy.1962.202.2.375.

Dysko, R.C., Huerkamp, M.J., Yrjanainen, K.E. *et al.* (2009) Plumbing: Special considerations. In: *Planning and Designing Research Animal Facilities*. Eds Hessler, J.R. and Lehner, N.D.M., pp. 425–453, Academic Press, Amsterdam, The Netherlands. doi: 10.1016/B978-0-12-369517-8.00032-3.

EFSA (2016) Safety and efficacy of selenium compounds (E8) as feed additives for all animal species: sodium selenite, based on a dossier submitted by Retorte GmbH Selenium Chemicals and Metals. *EFSA Journal*, **14**. doi: 10.2903/j.efsa.2016.4398.

Ellegaard, L., Cunningham, A., Edwards, S. *et al.* (2010) Welfare of the minipig with special reference to use in regulatory toxicology studies. *Journal of Pharmacological and Toxicological Methods*, **62**, 167–183. doi: 10.1016/j.vascn.2010.05.006.

Eva, J.K. and Rickett, M.J. (1983) Improvements in diet stability through processing. *Laboratory Animals*, **17**, 1–6. doi: 10.1258/002367783781070885.

FAO (2012) *Impact of Animal Nutrition on Animal Welfare – Expert Consultation 26-30 September 2011*. FAO, Rome, Italy.

FEDIAF (2013) *Nutritional Guidelines for Feeding Pet Rabbits*. European Pet Food Industry Federation, Brussels, Belgium.

Fekete, S.G., Andrasofszky, E. and Glavits, R. (2009) Pathological changes induced by rancid feed in rats and effects on growth and protein utilisation. *Acta Veterinaria Hungarica*, **57**, 247–261. doi: 10.1556/avet.57.2009.2.6.

Fitzsimons, J.T. (1979) The physiology of thirst and sodium appetite. *Monographs of the Physiological Society*, 1–572.

Fitzsimons, T.J. and Le Magnen, J. (1969) Eating as a regulatory control of drinking in the rat. *Journal of Comparative and Physiological Psychology*, **67**, 273.

Ford, D.J. (1977) Influence of diet pellet hardness and particle size on food utilization by mice, rats and hamsters. *Laboratory Animals*, **11**, 241–246. doi: 10.1258/002367777780936486.

Forster, M.J., Morris, P. and Sohal, R.S. (2003) Genotype and age influence the effect of caloric intake on mortality in mice. *FASEB Journal*, **17**, 690–692. doi: 10.1096/fj.02-0533fje.

Francis, G., Kerem, Z., Makkar, H.P. *et al.* (2002) The biological action of saponins in animal systems: a review. *British Journal of Nutrition*, **88**, 587–605. doi: 10.1079/bjn2002725.

Fullerton, F.R., Greenman, D.L. and Kendall, D.C. (1982) Effects of storage conditions on nutritional qualities of semipurified (AIN-76) and natural ingredient (NIH-07) diets. *The Journal of Nutrition*, **112**, 567–573. doi: 10.1093/jn/112.3.567.

Gidenne, T., Combes, S. and Fortun-Lamothe, L. (2012) Feed intake limitation strategies for the growing rabbit: effect on feeding behaviour, welfare, performance, digestive physiology and health: a review. *Animal*, **6**, 1407–1419. doi: 10.1017/S1751731112000389.

Gidenne, T., Lebas, F. and Fortun-Lamothe, L. (2010) Feeding behaviour of rabbits. In: *Nutrition of the Rabbit*. 2nd edn. Eds de Blas, C. and Wiseman, J., pp. 233–252, CABI, Wallingford, United Kingdom. doi: 10.1079/9781845936693.0233.

Gonzalez, D.M., Graciano, S.J., Karlstad, J., *et al.* (2011) Failure and life cycle evaluation of watering valves. *Journal of the American Association for Laboratory Animal Science*, **50**, 713–718.

Goodrick, C.L. (1973) The effects of dietary protein upon growth of inbred and hybrid mice. *Growth*, **37**, 355–367.

Goodrick, C.L., Ingram, D.K., Reynolds, M.A., *et al.* (1990) Effects of intermittent feeding upon body weight and lifespan in inbred mice: interaction of genotype and age. *Mechanisms of Ageing and Development*, **55**, 69–87. doi: 10.1016/0047-6374(90)90107-q.

Goodrick, C.L., Ingram, D.K., Reynolds, M.A., *et al.* (1982) Effects of intermittent feeding upon growth and life span in rats. *Gerontology*, **28**, 233–241. doi: 10.1159/000212538.

Goodrick, C.L., Ingram, D.K., Reynolds, M.A., *et al.* (1983) Differential effects of intermittent feeding and voluntary exercise on body weight and lifespan in adult rats. *Journal of Gerontology*, **38**, 36–45. doi: 10.1093/geronj/38.1.36.

Gorence, G.J., Pulcastro, H.C., Lawson, C.A., *et al.* (2019) Chemical contaminants from plastics in the animal environment. *Journal of the American Association for Laboratory Animal Science*, **58**, 190–196. doi: 10.30802/aalas-jaalas-18-000074.

Grace, P.B., Taylor, J.I., Low, Y.-L.L., *et al.* (2004) Phytoestrogen concentrations in serum and spot urine as biomarkers for dietary phytoestrogen intake and their relation to breast cancer risk in European Prospective Investigation of Cancer and Nutrition-Norfolk. *Cancer Epidemiology, Biomarkers & Prevention*, **13**, 698–708.

Greenberg, S.M. and Frazer, A.C. (1953) Some factors affecting the growth and development of rats fed rancid fat. *The Journal of Nutrition*, **50**, 421–440. doi: 10.1093/jn/50.4.421.

Gresl, T.A., Colman, R.J., Roecker, E.B., *et al.* (2001) Dietary restriction and glucose regulation in aging rhesus monkeys: a follow-up report at 8.5 yr. *American Journal of Physiology: Endocrinology and Metabolism*, **281**, E757–765. doi: 10.1152/ajpendo.2001.281.4.e757.

Gu, L., House, S.E., Prior, R.L., *et al.* (2006) Metabolic phenotype of isoflavones differ among female rats, pigs, monkeys, and women. *The Journal of Nutrition*, **136**, 1215–1221. doi: 10.1093/jn/136.5.1215.

Guarnieri, M., Brayton, C., DeTolla, L. *et al.* (2012) Safety and efficacy of buprenorphine for analgesia in laboratory mice and rats. *Laboratory Animals*, **41**, 337–343. doi: 10.1038/laban.152.

Guo, F., Zheng, K., Benede-Ubieto, R. *et al.* (2018) The Lieber-DeCarli Diet-a flagship model for experimental alcoholic liver disease. *Alcoholism, Clinical and Experimental Research*, **42**, 1828–1840. doi: 10.1111/acer.13840.

Hagen, K., Clauss, M. and Hatt, J.M. (2014) Drinking preferences in chinchillas (*Chinchilla laniger*), degus (*Octodon degu*) and guinea pigs (*Cavia porcellus*). *Journal of Animal Physiology and Animal Nutrition*, **98**, 942–947. doi: 10.1111/jpn.12164.

Hall, J.E., White, W.J. and Lang, C.M. (1980) Acidification of drinking water: its effects on selected biologic phenomena in male mice. *Laboratory Animal Science*, **30**, 643–651.

Hall, L.E., Robinson, S. and Buchanan-Smith, H.M. (2015) Refining dosing by oral gavage in the dog: a protocol to harmonise welfare. *Journal of Pharmacological and Toxicological Methods*, **72**, 35–46. doi: 10.1016/j.vascn.2014.12.007.

Hansen, B.C., Jen, K.L. and Kalnasy, L.W. (1981) Control of food intake and meal patterns in monkeys. *Physiology & Behavior*, **27**, 803–810. doi: 10.1016/0031-9384(81)90046-9.

Hansen, H.H., Feigh, M., Veidal, S.S. *et al.* (2017) Mouse models of nonalcoholic steatohepatitis in preclinical drug development. *Drug Discovery Today*, **22**, 1707–1718. doi: 10.1016/j.drudis.2017.06.007.

Hanski, I. (1994) Population biological consequences of body size in *Sorex*. In: *Advances in the Biology of Shrews*. Eds Merritt, J.F., Kirkland, G.L. and Rose, R.K., pp. 15–26, Carnegie Museum of Natural History, Special Publication No. 18, Pittsburgh, PA.

Harcourt-Brown, F. (2017) Reflections on rabbit diets. *Journal of Small Animal Practice*, **58**, 123–124. doi: 10.1111/jsap.12660.

Harcourt-Brown, F.M. (1996) Calcium deficiency, diet and dental disease in pet rabbits. *Veterinary Record*, **139**, 567–571. doi: 10.1136/vr.139.23.567.

Harper, A.E. (1986) Nutritional control in animal experiments. *Nutrition Reviews*, **44**, Suppl 175–184. doi: 10.1111/j.1753-4887.1986.tb07695.x.

Harper, A.E., Benevenga, N.J. and Wohlhueter, R.M. (1970) Effects of ingestion of disproportionate amounts of amino acids. *Physiological Reviews*, **50**, 428–558. doi: 10.1152/physrev.1970.50.3.428.

Haseman, J.K. (1998) National Toxicology Program experience with dietary restriction: Does the manner in which reduced body weight is achieved affect tumor incidence? *International Journal of Toxicology*, **17**, Suppl. 2, 119–134. doi: 10.1080/109158198226387.

Heldmaier, G. and Elvert, R. (2004) How to enter torpor: Thermodynamic and physiological mechanisms of metabolic depression. In: *Life in the Cold: Evolution, Mechanisms, Adaptation, and Application*. Eds Barnes, B.M. and Carey, H.V., pp. 185–198, Institute of Arctic Biology, University of Alaska, Fairbanks, AK.

Hempenstall, S., Picchio, L., Mitchell, S.E. et al. (2010) The impact of acute caloric restriction on the metabolic phenotype in male C57BL/6 and DBA/2 mice. *Mechanisms of Ageing and Development*, **131**, 111–118. doi: 10.1016/j.mad.2009.12.008.

Hermann, L.M., White, W.J. and Lang, C.M. (1982) Prolonged exposure to acid, chlorine, or tetracycline in the drinking water: effects on delayed-type hypersensitivity, hemagglutination titers, and reticuloendothelial clearance rates in mice. *Laboratory Animal Science*, **32**, 603–608.

Herrington, L.P. (1940) The heat regulation of small laboratory animals at various environmental temperatures. *American Journal of Physiology*, **129**, 123–129. doi: 10.1152/ajplegacy.1940.129.1.123.

Higa, T.S., Spinola, A.V., Fonseca-Alaniz, M.H. et al. (2014) Comparison between cafeteria and high-fat diets in the induction of metabolic dysfunction in mice. *International Journal of Physiology, Pathophysiology and Pharmacology*, **6**, 47–54.

Hirsch, E. (1973) Some determinants of intake and patterns of feeding in the guinea pig. *Physiology & Behavior*, **11**, 687–704. doi: 10.1016/0031-9384(73)90255-2.

Hoggatt, A.F., Hoggatt, J., Honerlaw, M. et al. (2010) A spoonful of sugar helps the medicine go down: a novel technique to improve oral gavage in mice. *Journal of the American Association for Laboratory Animal Science*, **49**, 329–334.

Honeycutt, J.A., Nguyen, J.Q.T., Kentner, A.C. et al. (2017) Effects of water bottle materials and filtration on bisphenol A content in laboratory animal drinking water. *Journal of the American Association for Laboratory Animal Science*, **56**, 269–272.

Hooijmans, C.R., Leenaars, M. and Ritskes-Hoitinga, M. (2010) A gold standard publication checklist to improve the quality of animal studies, to fully integrate the Three Rs, and to make systematic reviews more feasible. *Alternatives to Laboratory Animals*, **38**, 167–182. doi: 10.1177/026119291003800208.

Horn, C.C. (2008) Why is the neurobiology of nausea and vomiting so important? *Appetite*, **50**, 430–434. doi: 10.1016/j.appet.2007.09.015.

Horn, C.C., Kimball, B.A., Wang, H. et al. (2013) Why can't rodents vomit? A comparative behavioral, anatomical, and physiological study. *PloS One*, **8**, e60537. doi: 10.1371/journal.pone.0060537.

Horton, B.J., Turley, S.D. and West, C.E. (1974) Diurnal variation in the feeding pattern of rabbits. *Life Sciences*, **15**, 1895–1907. doi: 10.1016/0024-3205(74)90040-x.

Horton, B.J., West, C.E. and Turley, S.D. (1975) Diurnal variation in the feeding pattern of guinea pigs. *Nutrition and Metabolism*, **18**, 294–301. doi: 10.1159/000175607.

Horwitz, W. and Albert, R. (1995) Precision in analytical measurements: Expected values and consequences in geochemical analyses. *Fresenius' Journal of Analytical Chemistry*, **351**, 507–513. doi: 10.1007/bf00322724.

Houldcroft, E., Smith, C., Mrowicki, R. et al. (2008) Welfare implications of nipple drinkers for broiler chickens. *Animal Welfare*, **17**, 1–10.

Hovard, A., Teilmann, A., Hau, J. et al. (2015) The applicability of a gel delivery system for self-administration of buprenorphine to laboratory mice. *Laboratory Animals*, **49**, 40–45. doi: 10.1177/0023677214551108.

Hudson, J.W. (1978) Shallow, daily torpor: A thermoregulatory adaptation. In: *Strategies in Cold. Natural Torpidity and Thermogenesis*. Eds Wang, L.C.H. and Hudson, J.W., pp. 67–108, Academic Press, New York. doi: 10.1016/B978-0-12-734550-5.50008-9.

Hulbert, A. (2014) A sceptics view: "Kleiber's Law" or the "3/4 rule" is neither a law nor a rule but rather an empirical approximation. *Systems*, **2**, 186–202. doi: 10.3390/systems2020186.

Hurrell, R.F. (1990) Influence of the Maillard reaction on the nutritional value of foods. In: *The Maillard Reaction in Food Processing, Human Nutrition and Physiology*. Eds Finot, P.A., Aeschbacher, H.-U., Hurrell, R.F. et al., pp. 245–258, Birkhauser, Basel, Switzerland.

ILAR (2011) *Guide for the Care and Use of Laboratory Animals*. National Academies Press, Washington, DC. doi: 10.17226/12910

Jayaraman, S. and Jayaraman, A. (2018) Long-term provision of acidified drinking water fails to influence autoimmune diabetes and encephalomyelitis. *Journal of Diabetes Research*, **2018**. doi: 10.1155/2018/3424691.

Jenness, R. (1986) Lactational performance of various mammalian species. *Journal of Dairy Science*, **69**, 869–885. doi: 10.3168/jds.S0022-0302(86)80478-7.

Jensen, M.N. and Ritskes-Hoitinga, M. (2007) How isoflavone levels in common rodent diets can interfere with the value of animal models and with experimental results. *Laboratory Animals*, **41**, 1–18. doi: 10.1258/002367707779399428.

Jensen, T.L., Kiersgaard, M.K., Mikkelsen, L.F. et al. (2019) Fasting of male mice – Effects of time point of initiation and duration on clinical chemistry parameters and animal welfare. *Laboratory Animals*. doi: 10.1177/0023677218824373.

Jensen, T.L., Kiersgaard, M.K., Sorensen, D.B. et al. (2013) Fasting of mice: a review. *Laboratory Animals*, **47**, 225–240. doi: 10.1177/0023677213501659.

Jimenez, M., Manez, M. and Hernandez, E. (1996) Influence of water activity and temperature on the production of zearalenone in corn by three *Fusarium* species. *International Journal of Food Microbiology*, **29**, 417–421. doi: 10.1016/0168-1605(95)00073-9.

Johnson, F. and Wardle, J. (2014) Variety, palatability, and obesity. *Advances in Nutrition*, **5**, 851–859. doi: 10.3945/an.114.007120.

Johnson, R.F., Randall, S. and Randall, W. (1983) Free-running and entrained circadian rhythms in activity, eating and drinking in the cat. *Biological Rhythm Research*, **14**, 315–327. doi: 10.1080/09291018309359825

Joseph, P. (2016) Oxidative stability and shelf life of bulk animal fats and poultry fats. In: *Oxidative Stability and Shelf Life of Foods Containing Oils and Fats*. Eds Hu, M. and Jacobsen, C., pp. 233–249, AOCS Press, Amsterdam, The Netherlands. doi: 10.1016/b978-1-63067-056-6.00006-9.

Ju, Y.H., Allred, C.D., Allred, K.F. et al. (2001) Physiological concentrations of dietary genistein dose-dependently stimulate growth of estrogen-dependent human breast cancer (MCF-7) tumors implanted in athymic nude mice. *The Journal of Nutrition*, **131**, 2957–2962. doi: 10.1093/jn/131.11.2957.

Ju, Y.H., Doerge, D.R., Allred, K.F. et al. (2002) Dietary genistein negates the inhibitory effect of tamoxifen on growth of estrogen-dependent human breast cancer (MCF-7) cells implanted in athymic mice. *Cancer Research*, **62**, 2474–2477. doi: 10.1158/1078-0432.ccr-04-1130.

Ju, Y.H., Doerge, D.R., Woodling, K.A. et al. (2008) Dietary genistein negates the inhibitory effect of letrozole on the growth of aromatase-expressing estrogen-dependent human breast cancer cells (MCF-7Ca) in vivo. Carcinogenesis, 29, 2162–2168. doi: 10.1093/carcin/bgn161.

Kalant, N., Stewart, J. and Kaplan, R. (1988) Effect of diet restriction on glucose metabolism and insulin responsiveness in aging rats. Mechanisms of Ageing and Development, 46, 89–104. doi: 10.1016/0047-6374(88)90117-0.

Kale, V.P., Joshi, G.S., Gohil, P.B. et al. (2009) Effect of fasting duration on clinical pathology results in Wistar rats. Veterinary Clinical Pathology, 38, 361–366. doi: 10.1111/j.1939-165X.2009.00143.x.

Kang, J., Badger, T.M., Ronis, M.J. et al. (2010) Non-isoflavone phytochemicals in soy and their health effects. Journal of Agricultural and Food Chemistry, 58, 8119–8133. doi: 10.1021/jf100901b.

Kasanen, I.H., Inhila, K.J., Nevalainen, J.I. et al. (2009) A novel dietary restriction method for group-housed rats: weight gain and clinical chemistry characterization. Laboratory Animals, 43, 138–148. doi: 10.1258/la.2008.008023.

Kealy, R.D., Lawler, D.F., Ballam, J.M. et al. (2002) Effects of diet restriction on life span and age-related changes in dogs. Journal of the American Veterinary Medical Association, 220, 1315–1320. doi: 10.2460/javma.2002.220.1315.

Keane, K.W., Smutko, C.J., Krieger, C.H. et al. (1962) The addition of water to purified diets and its effect upon growth and protein efficiency ratio in the rat. The Journal of Nutrition, 77, 18–22. doi: 10.1093/jn/77.1.18.

Keenan, K.P. (1996) Commentary. The uncontrolled variable in risk assessment: ad libitum overfed rodents – fat, facts and fiction. Toxicologic Pathology, 24, 376–383. doi: 10.1177/019262339602400315.

Keenan, K.P. (1998) Effects of diet and overfeeding on body weight and survival in the rodent bioassay: The impact on pharmaceutical safety assessment. International Journal of Toxicology, 17, 101–117. doi: 10.1177/109158189801700206.

Keenan, K.P., Ballam, G.C., Soper, K.A. et al. (1999) Diet, caloric restriction, and the rodent bioassay. Toxicological Sciences, 52, 24–34. doi: 10.1093/toxsci/52.2.24.

Keenan, K.P., Smith, P.F., Hertzog, P. et al. (1994) The effects of overfeeding and dietary restriction on Sprague-Dawley rat survival and early pathology biomarkers of aging. Toxicologic Pathology, 22, 300–315. doi: 10.1177/019262339402200308.

Keenan, K.P., Soper, K.A., Hertzog, P.R. et al. (1995a) Diet, overfeeding, and moderate dietary restriction in control Sprague-Dawley rats: II. Effects on age-related proliferative and degenerative lesions. Toxicologic Pathology, 23, 287–302. doi: 10.1177/019262339502300306.

Keenan, K.P., Soper, K.A., Smith, P.F. et al. (1995b) Diet, overfeeding, and moderate dietary restriction in control Sprague-Dawley rats: I. Effects on spontaneous neoplasms. Toxicologic Pathology, 23, 269–286. doi: 10.1177/019262339502300305.

Keenan, K.P., Wallig, M.A. and Haschek, W.M. (2013) Nature via nurture: effect of diet on health, obesity, and safety assessment. Toxicologic Pathology, 41, 190–209. doi: 10.1177/0192623312469857.

Kemnitz, J.W. (2011) Calorie restriction and aging in nonhuman primates. ILAR Journal, 52, 66–77. doi: 10.1093/ilar.52.1.66.

Kersten, A., Strubbe, J.H. and Spiteri, N.J. (1980) Meal patterning of rats with changes in day length and food availability. Physiology & Behavior, 25, 953–958. doi: 10.1016/0031-9384(80)90316-9.

Kiermayer, C., Conrad, M., Schneider, M. et al. (2007) Optimization of spatiotemporal gene inactivation in mouse heart by oral application of tamoxifen citrate. Genesis, 45, 11–16. doi: 10.1002/dvg.20244.

Kim, S., Shin, H.J., Kim, S.Y. et al. (2004) Genistein enhances expression of genes involved in fatty acid catabolism through activation of PPARalpha. Molecular and Cellular Endocrinology, 220, 51–58. doi: 10.1016/j.mce.2004.03.011.

Kirkwood, J.K. (1983) Effects of diet on health, weight and litter-size in captive cotton-top tamarins Saguinus oedipus. Primates, 24, 515–520. doi: 10.1007/bf02381684.

Kleiber, M. (1932) Body size and metabolism. Hilgardia, 6, 315–353. doi: 10.3733/hilg.v06n11p315

Klug, B.J. and Brigham, R.M. (2015) Changes to metabolism and cell physiology that enable mammalian hibernation. Springer Science Reviews, 3, 39–56. doi: 10.1007/s40362-015-0030-x.

Klurfeld, D.M., Gregory, J.F. and Fiorotto, M.L. (2021) Should the AIN-93 rodent diet formulas be revised? The Journal of Nutrition, 151, 1380–1382. doi:10.1093/jn/nxab041.

Klurfeld, D.M., Welch, C.B., Davis, M.J. et al. (1989) Determination of degree of energy restriction necessary to reduce DMBA-induced mammary tumorigenesis in rats during the promotion phase. The Journal of Nutrition, 119, 286–291. doi: 10.1093/jn/119.2.286.

Knott, C.D. (1998) Changes in orangutan caloric intake, energy balance, and ketones in response to fluctuating fruit availability. International Journal of Primatology, 19, 1061–1079. doi: 10.1023/a1020330404983.

Koteja, P., Carter, P.A., Swallow, J.G. et al. (2003) Food wasting by house mice: variation among individuals, families, and genetic lines. Physiology & Behavior, 80, 375–383. doi: 10.1016/j.physbeh.2003.09.001.

Krohn, T.C., Ritskes-Hoitinga, J. and Svendsen, P. (1999) The effects of feeding and housing on the behaviour of the laboratory rabbit. Laboratory Animals, 33, 101–107. doi: 10.1258/002367799780578327.

Künkele, J. (2000) Energetics of gestation relative to lactation in a precocial rodent, the guinea pig (Cavia porcellus). Journal of Zoology, 250, 533–539. doi: 10.1017/s095283690000409x.

Küster, T., Zumkehr, B., Hermann, C. et al. (2012) Voluntary ingestion of antiparasitic drugs emulsified in honey represents an alternative to gavage in mice. Journal of the American Association for Laboratory Animal Science, 51, 219–223.

Kutscher, C.L. (1969) Species differences in the interaction of feeding and drinking. Annals of the New York Academy of Sciences, 157, 539–552. doi: 10.1111/j.1749-6632.1969.tb12906.x.

Kutscher, C.L. (1974) Strain differences in drinking in inbred mice during ad libitum feeding and food deprivation. Physiology & Behavior, 13, 63–70. doi: 10.1016/0031-9384(74)90307-2.

Kyriazakis, I. and Tolkamp, B.J. (2011) Hunger and Thirst. In: Animal Welfare. Eds Appleby, M.C., Mench, J.A., Olsson, A.S. et al., pp. 44–63, CABI, Wallingford, United Kingdom. doi: 10.1079/9781845936594.0044.

Landrigan, J., Patterson, F. and Batey, R. (1989) A histological study of the use of agar as a delivery vehicle for alcohol or iron to rats. Alcohol, 6, 173–178. doi: 10.1016/0741-8329(89)90044-x.

Lang, J.A., Lang, C.M. and White, W.J. (1984) Use of agar-based diet to fulfil the food and water requirements of mice. Laboratory Animals, 18, 40–41. doi: 10.1258/002367784780865045.

Laule, G. (2010) Positive reinforcement training for laboratory animals. In: The UFAW Handbook on the Care and Management of Laboratory and Other Research Animals. 8th ed., Eds Hubrecht, R. and Kirkwood, J., pp. 206–218, Wiley-Blackwell, Oxford, United Kingdom. doi: 10.1002/9781444318777.ch16.

Lawler, D.F., Evans, R.H., Larson, B.T. et al. (2005) Influence of lifetime food restriction on causes, time, and predictors of death in dogs. Journal of the American Veterinary Medical Association, 226, 225–231. doi: 10.2460/javma.2005.226.225.

Lawler, D.F., Larson, B.T., Ballam, J.M. et al. (2008) Diet restriction and ageing in the dog: major observations over two decades. British Journal of Nutrition, 99, 793–805. doi: 10.1017/S0007114507871686.

Le, H.H., Carlson, E.M., Chua, J.P. et al. (2008) Bisphenol A is released from polycarbonate drinking bottles and mimics the neurotoxic actions of estrogen in developing cerebellar neurons. Toxicology Letters, 176, 149–156. doi: 10.1016/j.toxlet.2007.11.001.

Lebas, F. (2010) Vitamins in rabbit nutrition: literature review and recommendations. World Rabbit Science, 8, 185–192. doi: 10.4995/wrs.2000.438.

Lee, K.H., Yook, H.S., Lee, J.W. et al. (1999) Quenching mechanism and kinetics of ascorbyl palmitate for the reduction of the gamma irradiation-induced oxidation of oils. *Journal of the American Oil Chemists' Society*, **76**, 921–925. doi: 10.1007/s11746-999-0107-2.

Levin, R.B., Epstein, P.R., Ford, T.E. *et al.* (2002) US drinking water challenges in the twenty-first century. *Environmental Health Perspectives*, **110**, 43–52. doi: 10.1289/ehp.02110s143.

Lewis, S.M., Johnson, Z.J., Mayhugh, M.A., *et al*. (2003). Nutrient intake and growth characteristics of male Sprague-Dawley rats fed AIN-93M purified diet or NIH-31 natural-ingredient diet in a chronic two-year study. *Aging Clinical and Experimental Research*, **15**, 460–468. doi: 10.1007/BF03327368.

Liao, C.Y., Rikke, B.A., Johnson, T.E. *et al.* (2010) Genetic variation in the murine lifespan response to dietary restriction: from life extension to life shortening. *Aging Cell*, **9**, 92–95. doi: 10.1111/j.1474-9726.2009.00533.x.

Lieber, C.S. and DeCarli, L.M. (1974) An experimental model of alcohol feeding and liver injury in the baboon. *Journal of Medical Primatology*, **3**, 153–163. doi: 10.1159/000459999.

Lieber, C.S. and DeCarli, L.M. (1982) The feeding of alcohol in liquid diets: two decades of applications and 1982 update. *Alcoholism, Clinical and Experimental Research*, **6**, 523–531. doi: 10.1111/j.1530-0277.1982.tb05017.x.

Lieber, C.S., Leo, M.A., Mak, K.M. *et al.* (2004) Model of nonalcoholic steatohepatitis. *The American Journal of Clinical Nutrition*, **79**, 502–509. doi: 10.1093/ajcn/79.3.502.

Lipman, R.D. (2002) Effect of calorie restriction on mortality kinetics in inbred strains of mice following 7,12-dimethylbenz[a]anthracene treatment. *Journals of Gerontology. Series A: Biological Sciences and Medical Sciences*, **57**, B153–157. doi: 10.1093/gerona/57.4.b153.

Lopez, M., Lelliott, C.J., Tovar, S. *et al.* (2006) Tamoxifen-induced anorexia is associated with fatty acid synthase inhibition in the ventromedial nucleus of the hypothalamus and accumulation of malonyl-coA. *Diabetes*, **55**, 1327–1336. doi: 10.2337/db05-1356.

Lutz, C.K. and Novak, M.A. (2005) Environmental enrichment for nonhuman primates: theory and application. *ILAR Journal*, **46**, 178–191. doi: 10.1093/ilar.46.2.178.

Markwell, P.J., Buffington, C.T. and Smith, B.H. (1998) The effect of diet on lower urinary tract diseases in cats. *The Journal of Nutrition*, **128**, 2753S–2757S. doi: 10.1093/jn/128.12.2753S.

Matsuzawa, T., Kitamura, K. and Iwasaki, M. (1998) Improvement of a mouse feeder for chemical toxicology testing. *Experimental Animals*, **47**, 123–126. doi: 10.1538/expanim.47.123.

Matsuzawa, T. and Sakazume, M. (1994) Effects of fasting on haematology and clinical chemistry values in the rat and dog. *Comparative Haematology International*, **4**, 152–156. doi: 10.1007/bf00798356.

Mattison, J.A., Colman, R.J., Beasley, T.M. *et al.* (2017) Caloric restriction improves health and survival of rhesus monkeys. *Nature Communications*, **8**, 14063. doi: 10.1038/ncomms14063.

Mattison, J.A., Roth, G.S., Lane, M.A. *et al.* (2007) Dietary restriction in aging nonhuman primates. In: *Mechanisms of Dietary Restriction in Aging and Disease*. Eds Mobbs, C.V., Yen, K. and Hof, P.R., pp. 137–158, Karger Publishers, Basel, Switzerland. doi: 10.1159/000096560.

McArthur, L.H., Kelly, W.F., Gietzen, D.W. *et al.* (1993) The role of palatability in the food intake response of rats fed high-protein diets. *Appetite*, **20**, 181–196. doi: 10.1006/appe.1993.1019.

McDonald, P., Edwards, R.A., Greenhalgh, J.F.D. *et al.* (2011) *Animal Nutrition*. Pearson Education, Harlow, United Kingdom.

McDonald, R.B. and Ramsey, J.J. (2010) Honoring Clive McCay and 75 years of calorie restriction research. *The Journal of Nutrition*, **140**, 1205–1210. doi: 10.3945/jn.110.122804.

Medjakovic, S., Mueller, M. and Jungbauer, A. (2010) Potential health-modulating effects of isoflavones and metabolites via activation of PPAR and AhR. *Nutrients*, **2**, 241–279. doi: 10.3390/nu2030241.

Meier, T.R., Maute, C.J., Cadillac, J.M. *et al.* (2008) Quantification, distribution, and possible source of bacterial biofilm in mouse automated watering systems. *Journal of the American Association for Laboratory Animal Science*, **47**, 63–70.

Menon, L.G., Kuttan, R., Nair, M.G. *et al.* (1998) Effect of isoflavones genistein and daidzein in the inhibition of lung metastasis in mice induced by B16F-10 melanoma cells. *Nutrition and Cancer*, **30**, 74–77. doi: 10.1080/01635589809514644.

Mentor-Marcel, R., Lamartiniere, C.A., Eltoum, I.E. *et al.* (2001) Genistein in the diet reduces the incidence of poorly differentiated prostatic adenocarcinoma in transgenic mice (TRAMP). *Cancer Research*, **61**, 6777–6782.

Mezei, O., Banz, W.J., Steger, R.W. *et al.* (2003) Soy isoflavones exert antidiabetic and hypolipidemic effects through the PPAR pathways in obese Zucker rats and murine RAW 264.7 cells. *The Journal of Nutrition*, **133**, 1238–1243. doi: 10.1093/jn/133.5.1238.

Mezei, O., Li, Y., Mullen, E. *et al.* (2006) Dietary isoflavone supplementation modulates lipid metabolism via PPARα-dependent and -independent mechanisms. *Physiological Genomics*, **26**, 8–14. doi: 10.1152/physiolgenomics.00155.2005.

Michel, K.E. and Brown, D.C. (2014) Association of signalment parameters with activity of pet dogs. *Journal of Nutritional Science*, **3**, e28. doi: 10.1017/jns.2014.49.

Miller, D.L. (1990) A new feeder for powdered diets. *Proceedings of the Society for Experimental Biology and Medicine*, **193**, 81–84. doi: 10.3181/00379727-193-1-rc1.

Molk, D.M., Karr-May, C.L., Trang, E.D. *et al.* (2013) Sanitization of an automatic reverse-osmosis watering system: removal of a clinically significant biofilm. *Journal of the American Association for Laboratory Animal Science*, **52**, 197–205.

Moraal, M., Leenaars, P.P., Arnts, H. *et al.* (2012) The influence of food restriction versus ad libitum feeding of chow and purified diets on variation in body weight, growth and physiology of female Wistar rats. *Laboratory Animals*, **46**, 101–107. doi: 10.1258/la.2011.011011.

Moran, T., Pace, J. and Hutchinson, J.B. (1955) Toxicity trials: Palatability of the diet as a factor in experiments on the rate of growth of rats. *Journal of the Science of Food and Agriculture*, **6**, 324–329. doi: 10.1002/jsfa.2740060606.

Morrison, S.D. (1956) The total energy and water metabolism during pregnancy in the rat. *Journal of Physiology*, **134**, 650–664. doi: 10.1113/jphysiol.1956.sp005672.

Muramatsu, K., Massuquetto, A., Dahlke, F. *et al.* (2015) Factors that affect pellet quality: a review. *Journal of Agriculture, Science and Technology* **9**, 717–722. doi: 10.17265/2161-6256/2015.09.002.

Namvar, S., Gyte, A., Denn, M. *et al.* (2016) Dietary fat and corticosterone levels are contributing factors to meal anticipation. *American Journal of Physiology: Regulatory, Integrative and Comparative Physiology*, **310**, R711–723. doi: 10.1152/ajpregu.00308.2015.

Natelson, B.H. and Bonbright, J.C. (1978) Patterns of eating and drinking in monkeys when food and water are free and when they are earned. *Physiology & Behavior*, **21**, 201–213. doi: 10.1016/0031-9384(78)90042-2.

Nelson, W. (1988) Food restriction, circadian disorder and longevity of rats and mice. *The Journal of Nutrition*, **118**, 286–289. doi: 10.1093/jn/118.3.284.

Nelson, W., Cadotte, L. and Halberg, F. (1973) Circadian timing of single daily "meal" affects survival of mice. *Proceedings of the Society for Experimental Biology and Medicine*, **144**, 766–769. doi: 10.3181/00379727-144-37678.

Newman, J.R. and Rudd, R. (1978) Minimum and maximum metabolic rates of *Sorex sinuosus*. *Acta Theriologica*, **23**, 371–380. doi: 10.4098/at.arch.78-28.

Nowland, M.H., Hugunin, K.M. and Rogers, K.L. (2011) Effects of short-term fasting in male Sprague-Dawley rats. *Comparative Medicine*, **61**, 138–144.

NRC (1987) *Vitamin Tolerance of Animals*. National Academies Press, Washington, DC. doi: 10.17226/949

NRC (2003) *Nutrient Requirements of Nonhuman Primates*. National Academies Press, Washington, DC. doi: 10.17226/9826

NRC (2005) *Mineral Tolerance of Animals*. National Academies Press, Washington, DC. doi: 10.17226/11309.

Owen, C., Lees, E.K., Grant, L. et al. (2013) Inducible liver-specific knockdown of protein tyrosine phosphatase 1B improves glucose and lipid homeostasis in adult mice. *Diabetologia*, **56**, 2286–2296. doi: 10.1007/s00125-013-2992-z.

Ozon, C., Dolisi, C., Ardisson, J.L. et al. (1987) Synchronization of dog drinking behaviour by light/dark rhythm and food availability. *Biological Rhythm Research*, **18**, 205–217. doi: 10.1080/09291018709359946.

Packard, G.C. and Boardman, T.J. (1999) The use of percentages and size-specific indices to normalize physiological data for variation in body size: wasted time, wasted effort? *Comparative Biochemistry and Physiology Part A: Molecular & Integrative Physiology*, **122**, 37–44. doi: 10.1016/s1095-6433(98)10170-8.

Palou, A., Remesar, X., Arola, L. et al. (1981) Metabolic effects of short term food deprivation in the rat. *Hormone and Metabolic Research*, **13**, 326–330. doi: 10.1055/s-2007-1019258.

Parker, D.B. and Brown, M.S. (2003) Water consumption for livestock and poultry production. In: *Encyclopedia of Water Science*. Eds Stewart, R.A., Howell, T. and Trimble, S.W., pp. 588–591, Marcel Dekker Inc, New York.

Paronis, E., Alexakos, P., Dimitriou, C. et al. (2008) Evaluation of the preference of mice on food intake-Preliminary study. *Journal of the Hellenic Veterinary Medical Society*, **59**, 168–174. doi: 10.12681/jhvms.14957.

Patel, R.P. and Barnes, S. (2010) Isoflavones and PPAR signaling: a critical target in cardiovascular, metastatic, and metabolic disease. *PPAR Research*, **2010**, 153252. doi: 10.1155/2010/153252.

Patience, J.F. (2012) Water in swine nutrition. In: *Sustainable Swine Nutrition*. Ed. Chiba, L.I., pp. 1–22, Wiley-Blackwell, Ames, IA. doi: 10.1002/9781118491454.ch1.

Patton, D.F. and Mistlberger, R.E. (2013) Circadian adaptations to meal timing: neuroendocrine mechanisms. *Frontiers in Neuroscience*, **7**, 185. doi: 10.3389/fnins.2013.00185.

Peck, J.W. (1978) Rats defend different body weights depending on palatability and accessibility of their food. *Journal of Comparative and Physiological Psychology*, **92**, 555–570. doi: 10.1037/h0077474.

Pellizzon, M.A. and Ricci, M.R. (2018) The common use of improper control diets in diet-induced metabolic disease research confounds data interpretation: the fiber factor. *Nutrition & Metabolism*, **15**, 3. doi: 10.1186/s12986-018-0243-5.

Perrin, M.R. and Monadjem, A. (1998) The effect of supplementary food on the home range of the multimammate mouse *Mastomys natalensis*. *South African Journal of Wildlife Research*, **28**, 1–3.

Pesti, G.M., Vedenov, D., Cason, J.A. et al. (2009) A comparison of methods to estimate nutritional requirements from experimental data. *British Poultry Science*, **50**, 16–32. doi: 10.1080/00071660802530639.

Peterson, J. and Wunder, B.A. (1997) Food sorting by collared lemmings (*Dicrostonyx groenlandicus*) and prairie voles (*Microtus ochrogaster*): a cautionary note for digestibility studies. *Comparative Biochemistry and Physiology – Part A: Molecular & Integrative Physiology*, **116**, 119–124. doi: 10.1016/s0300-9629(96)00161-2.

Petrović, M., Gonzalez, S. and Barceló, D. (2003) Analysis and removal of emerging contaminants in wastewater and drinking water. *TrAC Trends in Analytical Chemistry*, **22**, 685–696. doi: 10.1016/s0165-9936(03)01105-1.

Phillips, C.J.C. (Ed.) (2016) *Nutrition and the Welfare of Farm Animals*, Springer, Cham, Switzerland. doi: 10.1007/978-3-319-27356-3.

Plesker, R. and Schuhmacher, A. (2006) Feeding fruits and vegetables to nonhuman primates can lead to nutritional deficiencies. *Laboratory Primate Newsletter*, **45**, 1–5.

Prebble, J.L., Shaw, D.J. and Meredith, A.L. (2015) Bodyweight and body condition score in rabbits on four different feeding regimes. *Journal of Small Animal Practice*, **56**, 207–212. doi: 10.1111/jsap.12301.

Prescott, M.J., Brown, V.J., Flecknell, P.A. et al. (2010) Refinement of the use of food and fluid control as motivational tools for macaques used in behavioural neuroscience research: Report of a Working Group of the NC3Rs. *Journal of Neuroscience Methods*, **193**, 167–188. doi: 10.1016/j.jneumeth.2010.09.003.

Prest, E.I., Hammes, F., van Loosdrecht, M.C.M. et al. (2016) Biological stability of drinking water: controlling factors, methods, and challenges. *Frontiers in Microbiology*, **7**. doi: 10.3389/fmicb.2016.00045.

Price, K.R., Johnson, I.T. and Fenwick, G.R. (1987) The chemistry and biological significance of saponins in foods and feeding stuffs. *Critical Reviews in Food Science and Nutrition*, **26**, 27–135. doi: 10.1080/10408398709527461.

Pugh, T.D., Klopp, R.G. and Weindruch, R. (1999) Controlling caloric consumption: protocols for rodents and rhesus monkeys. *Neurobiology of Aging*, **20**, 157–165. doi: 10.1016/s0197-4580(99)00043-3.

Ralls, K. (1976) Mammals in which females are larger than males. *Quarterly Review of Biology*, **51**, 245–276. doi: 10.1086/409310.

Ramadori, P., Weiskirchen, R., Trebicka, J. et al. (2015) Mouse models of metabolic liver injury. *Laboratory Animals*, **49**, 47–58. doi: 10.1177/0023677215570078.

Ramírez-Castillo, F.Y., Loera-Muro, A., Jacques, M. et al. (2015) Waterborne pathogens: Detection methods and challenges. *Pathogens*, **4**, 307–334. doi: 10.3390/pathogens4020307.

Ramirez, I. (1987) Practical liquid diets for rats: effects on growth. *Physiology & Behavior*, **39**, 527–530. doi: 10.1016/0031-9384(87)90384-2.

Ramirez, I. (1990) What do we mean when we say "palatable food"? *Appetite*, **14**, 159–161. doi: 10.1016/0195-6663(90)90081-i.

Rao, G.N. (1995) Husbandry procedures other than dietary restriction for lowering body weight and tumor/disease rates in Fischer 344 rats. In: *Dietary Restriction: Implications for the Design and Interpretation of Toxicity and Carcinogenicity Studies*. Eds Hart, R., Neumann, D. and Robertson, R., pp. 51–62, ILSI Press, Washington, DC.

Rao, G.N., Haseman, J.K., Grumbein, S. et al. (1990) Growth, body weight, survival, and tumor trends in F344/N rats during an eleven-year period. *Toxicologic Pathology*, **18**, 61–70. doi: 10.1177/019262339001800109.

Ravussin, E., Lillioja, S., Anderson, T.E. et al. (1986) Determinants of 24-hour energy expenditure in man. Methods and results using a respiratory chamber. *Journal of Clinical Investigation*, **78**, 1568–1578. doi: 10.1172/jci112749.

Reaven, E.P. and Reaven, G.M. (1981a) Structure and function changes in the endocrine pancreas of aging rats with reference to the modulating effects of exercise and caloric restriction. *Journal of Clinical Investigation*, **68**, 75–84. doi: 10.1172/jci110256.

Reaven, G.M. and Reaven, E.P. (1981b) Prevention of age-related hypertriglyceridemia by caloric restriction and exercise training in the rat. *Metabolism*, **30**, 982–986. doi: 10.1016/0026-0495(81)90096-2.

Reeves, P.G. (1989) AIN-76 diet: should we change the formulation? *The Journal of Nutrition*, **119**, 1081–1082. doi: 10.1093/jn/119.8.1081.

Reeves, P.G. (1997) Components of the AIN-93 diets as improvements in the AIN-76A diet. *The Journal of Nutrition*, **127**, 838S–841S. doi: 10.1093/jn/127.5.838S.

Reeves, P.G., Nielsen, F.H. and Fahey, G.C., Jr. (1993) AIN-93 purified diets for laboratory rodents: final report of the American Institute of Nutrition ad hoc writing committee on the reformulation of the AIN-76A rodent diet. *The Journal of Nutrition*, **123**, 1939–1951. doi: 10.1093/jn/123.11.1939.

Richardson, S.D. and Kimura, S.Y. (2020) Water analysis: emerging contaminants and current issues. *Analytical Chemistry*, **92**, 473–505. doi: 10.1021/acs.analchem.9b05269.

Ricketts, M.L., Moore, D.D., Banz, W.J. et al. (2005) Molecular mechanisms of action of the soy isoflavones includes activation of promiscuous nuclear receptors. A review. *Journal of Nutritional Biochemistry*, **16**, 321–330. doi: 10.1016/j.jnutbio.2004.11.008.

Robinson, E.A. and Adolph, E.F. (1943) Pattern of normal water drinking in dogs. *American Journal of Physiology*, **139**, 39–44. doi: 10.1152/ajplegacy.1943.139.1.39.

Rodenburg, T.B., Bracke, M.B.M., Berk, J. et al. (2005) Welfare of ducks in European duck husbandry systems. *World's Poultry Science Journal*, **61**, 633–646. doi: 10.1079/wps200575.

Roe, F.J. (1981) Are nutritionists worried about the epidemic of tumours in laboratory animals? *Proceedings of the Nutrition Society*, **40**, 57–65. doi: 10.1079/pns19810010.

Roe, F.J., Lee, P.N., Conybeare, G. et al. (1995) The Biosure Study: influence of composition of diet and food consumption on longevity, degenerative diseases and neoplasia in Wistar rats studied for up to 30 months post weaning. *Food and Chemical Toxicology*, **33**, Suppl. 1, 1S–100S. doi: 10.1016/0278-6915(95)80200-2.

Roe, F.J.C. and Tucker, M.J. (1974) Recent developments in the design of carcinogenicity tests on laboratory animals. *Proceedings of the European Society for the Study of Drug Toxicity*, **15**, 171–177.

Roebuck, B.D., Wilpone, S.A., Fifield, D.S. et al. (1979) Hemorrhagic deaths with AIN-76 diet. *The Journal of Nutrition*, **109**, 924–925. doi: 10.1093/jn/109.5.924b.

Rokey, G.J., Plattner, B. and de Souza, E.M. (2010) Feed extrusion process description. *Revista Brasileira de Zootecnia*, **39**, 510–518. doi: 10.1590/s1516-35982010001300055.

Rolls, B.J. and Rolls, E.T. (1982) *Thirst*. Cambridge University Press, Cambridge, United Kingdom. doi: 10.1017/s0033291700050418.

Rolls, B.J., Rowe, E.A. and Turner, R.C. (1980) Persistent obesity in rats following a period of consumption of a mixed, high energy diet. *Journal of Physiology*, **298**, 415–427. doi: 10.1113/jphysiol.1980.sp013091.

Ronis, M.J., Chen, Y., Badeaux, J. et al. (2009) Dietary soy protein isolate attenuates metabolic syndrome in rats via effects on PPAR, LXR, and SREBP signaling. *The Journal of Nutrition*, **139**, 1431–1438. doi: 10.3945/jn.109.107029.

Rowland, N.E. (2007) Food or fluid restriction in common laboratory animals: balancing welfare considerations with scientific inquiry. *Comparative Medicine*, **57**, 149–160.

Ruf, T. and Heldmaier, G. (1992) The impact of daily torpor on energy requirements in the Djungarian Hamster, *Phodopus sungorus*. *Physiological Zoology*, **65**, 994–1010. doi: 10.1086/physzool.65.5.30158554.

Sakamoto, Y., Kanatsu, J., Toh, M. et al. (2016) The dietary isoflavone daidzein reduces expression of pro-inflammatory genes through PPARalpha/gamma and JNK pathways in adipocyte and macrophage co-cultures. *PloS One*, **11**, e0149676. doi: 10.1371/journal.pone.0149676.

Sampey, B.P., Vanhoose, A.M., Winfield, H.M. et al. (2011) Cafeteria diet is a robust model of human metabolic syndrome with liver and adipose inflammation: comparison to high-fat diet. *Obesity (Silver Spring)*, **19**, 1109–1117. doi: 10.1038/oby.2011.18.

Sarkar, F.H. and Li, Y. (2004) The role of isoflavones in cancer chemoprevention. *Frontiers in Bioscience*, **9**, 2714–2724. doi: 10.2741/1430.

Schenk, A., Porter, A.L., Alenciks, E. et al. (2016) Increased water contamination and grow-out Pekin duck mortality when raised with water troughs compared to pin-metered water lines using a United States management system. *Poultry Science*, **95**, 736–748. doi: 10.3382/ps/pev381.

Schuler, P. (1990) Natural antioxidants exploited commercially. In: *Food Antioxidants*. Ed. Hudson, B.J.F., pp. 99–170. Springer, Dordrecht, The Netherlands. doi: 10.1007/978-94-009-0753-9_4.

Schwitzer, C. and Kaumanns, W. (2001) Body weights of ruffed lemurs (*Varecia variegata*) in European zoos with reference to the problem of obesity. *Zoo Biology*, **20**, 261–269. doi: 10.1002/zoo.1026.

Schwitzer, C., Polowinsky, S.Y. and Solman, C. (2009) Fruits as foods–common misconceptions about frugivory. In: *Zoo Animal Nutrition IV*. Eds Clauss, M., Fidgett, A.L., Hatt, J.M., et al., pp. 131–168. Filander Verlag, Fürth, Germany.

Sclafani, A. and Springer, D. (1976) Dietary obesity in adult rats: similarities to hypothalamic and human obesity syndromes. *Physiology & Behavior*, **17**, 461–471. doi: 10.1016/0031-9384(76)90109-8.

Setchell, K.D.R. (1998) Phytoestrogens: the biochemistry, physiology, and implications for human health of soy isoflavones. *The American Journal of Clinical Nutrition*, **68**, 1333S–1346S. doi: 10.1093/ajcn/68.6.1333S.

Setchell, K.D.R. (2001) Soy isoflavones – benefits and risks from nature's selective estrogen receptor modulators (SERMs). *Journal of the American College of Nutrition*, **20**, 354S–362S. doi: 10.1080/07315724.2001.10719168.

Setchell, K.D.R., Brown, N.M. and Lydeking-Olsen, E. (2002) The clinical importance of the metabolite equol – a clue to the effectiveness of soy and its isoflavones. *The Journal of Nutrition*, **132**, 3577–3584. doi: 10.1093/jn/132.12.3577.

Setchell, K.D.R., Brown, N.M., Zhao, X. et al. (2011) Soy isoflavone phase II metabolism differs between rodents and humans: implications for the effect on breast cancer risk. *The American Journal of Clinical Nutrition*, **94**, 1284–1294. doi: 10.3945/ajcn.111.019638.

Setchell, K.D.R. and Clerici, C. (2010) Equol: history, chemistry, and formation. *The Journal of Nutrition*, **140**, 1355S–1362S. doi: 10.3945/jn.109.119776.

Shahidi, F. and Ambigaipalan, P. (2015) Phenolics and polyphenolics in foods, beverages and spices: antioxidant activity and health effects – a review. *Journal of Functional Foods*, **18**, 820–897. doi: 10.1016/j.jff.2015.06.018.

Shanley, D.P. and Kirkwood, T.B. (2000) Calorie restriction and aging: a life-history analysis. *Evolution*, **54**, 740–750. doi: 10.1111/j.0014-3820.2000.tb00076.x.

Siegel, P.S. (1961) Food intake in the rat in relation to the dark-light cycle. *Journal of Comparative and Physiological Psychology*, **54**, 294–301. doi: 10.1037/h0044787.

Siegel, P.S. and Stuckey, H.L. (1947) The diurnal course of water and food intake in the normal mature rat. *Journal of Comparative and Physiological Psychology*, **40**, 365–370. doi: 10.1037/h0062185.

Simões, L.C. and Simões, M. (2013) Biofilms in drinking water: problems and solutions. *RSC Advances*, **3**, 2520–2533. doi: 10.1039/c2ra22243d.

Simon, N.G., Kaplan, J.R., Hu, S. et al. (2004) Increased aggressive behavior and decreased affiliative behavior in adult male monkeys after long-term consumption of diets rich in soy protein and isoflavones. *Hormones and Behavior*, **45**, 278–284. doi: 10.1016/j.yhbeh.2003.12.005.

Sohal, R.S. and Forster, M.J. (2014) Caloric restriction and the aging process: a critique. *Free Radical Biology and Medicine*, **73**, 366–382. doi: 10.1016/j.freeradbiomed.2014.05.015.

Speakman, J.R. and Hambly, C. (2007) Starving for life: what animal studies can and cannot tell us about the use of caloric restriction to prolong human lifespan. *The Journal of Nutrition*, **137**, 1078–1086. doi: 10.1093/jn/137.4.1078.

Speakman, J.R. and Selman, C. (2003) Physical activity and resting metabolic rate. *Proceedings of the Nutrition Society*, **62**, 621–634. doi: 10.1079/PNS2003282.

Spencer, K.E.V. (1985) Long term storage of irradiated rodent diet. *8th ICLAS/CALAS Symposium*, pp 447–450.

Staples, J.F. and Brown, J.C. (2008) Mitochondrial metabolism in hibernation and daily torpor: a review. *Journal of Comparative Physiology. B: Biochemical, Systemic, and Environmental Physiology*, **178**, 811–827. doi: 10.1007/s00360-008-0282-8.

Storey, K.B. (2002) Life in the slow lane: molecular mechanisms of estivation. *Comparative Biochemistry and Physiology Part A: Molecular & Integrative Physiology*, **133**, 733–754. doi: 10.1016/s1095-6433(02)00206-4.

Storey, K.B., Heldmaier, G. and Rider, M.H. (2010) Mammalian hibernation: physiology, cell signaling, and gene controls on metabolic rate depression. In: *Dormancy and Resistance in Harsh Environments*. Eds Lubzens, E., Cerda, J. and Clark, M.S., pp. 227–252, Springer, Heidelberg, Germany. doi: 10.1007/978-3-642-12422-8_13.

Strubbe, J.H. and Woods, S.C. (2004) The timing of meals. *Psychological Review*, **111**, 128–141. doi: 10.1037/0033-295x.111.1.128.

Sun, G.S., Tou, J.C., Reiss-Bubenheim, D.A. et al. (2012) Oxidative and nutrient stability of a standard rodent spaceflight diet during long-term storage. *Laboratory Animals*, **41**, 252–259. doi: 10.1038/laban0912-252.

Swindell, W.R. (2012) Dietary restriction in rats and mice: a meta-analysis and review of the evidence for genotype-dependent effects on lifespan. *Ageing Research Reviews*, **11**, 254–270. doi: 10.1016/j.arr.2011.12.006.

Tagliaferro, A.R. and Levitsky, D.A. (1982) Spillage behavior and thiamin deficiency in the rat. *Physiology & Behavior*, **28**, 933–937. doi: 10.1016/0031-9384(82)90217-7.

Takigawa, A., Danbarra, H. and Ohyama, Y. (1976) Gamma ray irradiation to semi-purified diet – peroxide formation and its effects on chicks. *Japanese Journal of Zootechnical Science*, **47**, 292–302. doi: 10.2508/chikusan.47.292.

Teramoto, K., Bowers, J.L., Khettry, U. et al. (1993) A rat fatty liver transplant model. *Transplantation*, **55**, 737–741. doi: 10.1097/00007890-199304000-00010.

Thigpen, J.E., Setchell, K.D., Padilla-Banks, E. et al. (2007) Variations in phytoestrogen content between different mill dates of the same diet produces significant differences in the time of vaginal opening in CD-1 mice and F344 rats but not in CD Sprague-Dawley rats. *Environmental Health Perspectives*, **115**, 1717–1726. doi: 10.1289/ehp.10165.

Thigpen, J.E., Setchell, K.D., Saunders, H.E. et al. (2004) Selecting the appropriate rodent diet for endocrine disruptor research and testing studies. *ILAR Journal*, **45**, 401–416. doi: 10.1093/ilar.45.4.401.

Thompson, M. (2004) The amazing Horwitz function. *Royal Society of Chemistry AMC Technical Brief*, **17**.

Tillmann, S. and Wegener, G. (2018) Syringe-feeding as a novel delivery method for accurate individual dosing of probiotics in rats. *Beneficial Microbes*, **9**, 311–315. doi: 10.3920/bm2017.0127.

Tobin, G. (1996) Small pets – food types, nutrient requirements and nutritional disorders. In: *Manual of Companion Animal Nutrition and Feeding*. Eds Kelly, N. and Wills, J., pp. 208–225, British Small Animal Veterinary Association, Cheltenham, United Kingdom.

Tobin, G. (2004) The role of diet in the 3Rs. In: *Lifting the Veil: Finding Common Ground*. Eds Cragg, P., Stafford, K., Love, D. et al., pp. 145–162, Royal Society of New Zealand/ANZCCART, Christchurch, New Zealand.

Tobin, G. and Schuhmacher, A. (2021) Laboratory animal nutrition in routine husbandry, and experimental and regulatory studies. In: *Handbook of Laboratory Animal Science, 4th Edition*. Eds Hau, J. and Schapiro, S., pp. 269–311. CRC Press, Boca Raton, FL.

Tobin, G., Stevens, K.A. and Russell, R.J. (2007) Nutrition. In: *The Mouse in Biomedical Research*. Eds Fox, J.G., Barthold, S., Davisson, M., et al., pp. 321–383, Academic Press, New York. doi: 10.1016/b978-012369454-6/50064-9.

Tolkamp, B.J. and D'Eath, R.B. (2016) Hunger associated with restricted feeding systems. In: *Nutrition and the Welfare of Farm Animals*. Ed. Phillips, C.J.C., pp. 11–27, Springer, Cham, Switzerland. doi: 10.1007/978-3-319-27356-3_2.

Toth, L.A. and Gardiner, T.W. (2000) Food and water restriction protocols: physiological and behavioral considerations. *Contemporary Topics in Laboratory Animal Science*, **39**, 9–17.

Tschudin, A., Clauss, M., Codron, D. et al. (2011) Preference of rabbits for drinking from open dishes versus nipple drinkers. *Veterinary Record*, **168**, 190a. doi: 10.1136/vr.c6150.

Tsuji, K., Ebihara, S. and Ohkouchi, O. (1982) Strain differences in drinking and eating activities of the inbred mice. *Tohoku Psychologica Folia*, **41**, 147–157.

Turner, P.V., Vaughn, E., Sunohara-Neilson, J. et al. (2012) Oral gavage in rats: animal welfare evaluation. *Journal of the American Association for Laboratory Animal Science*, **51**, 25–30.

Turturro, A., Hass, B., Hart, R. et al. (2016) Body weight impact on spontaneous diseases in chronic bioassays. *International Journal of Toxicology*, **17**, 79–99. doi: 10.1177/109158189801700205.

Turturro, A., Witt, W.W., Lewis, S. et al. (1999) Growth curves and survival characteristics of the animals used in the Biomarkers of Aging Program. *Journals of Gerontology. Series A: Biological Sciences and Medical Sciences*, **54**, B492–B501. doi: 10.1093/gerona/54.11.b492.

van der Hoek, J.P., Bertelkamp, C., Verliefde, A. et al. (2013) Drinking water treatment technologies in Europe: state of the art–challenges–research needs. *Journal of Water Supply: Research and Technology – AQUA*, **63**, 124–130. doi: 10.2166/aqua.2013.007.

Van Klinken, J.B., van den Berg, S.A., Havekes, L.M. et al. (2012) Estimation of activity related energy expenditure and resting metabolic rate in freely moving mice from indirect calorimetry data. *PloS One*, **7**, e36162. doi: 10.1371/journal.pone.0036162.

Varady, K.A. and Hellerstein, M.K. (2007) Alternate-day fasting and chronic disease prevention: a review of human and animal trials. *The American Journal of Clinical Nutrition*, **86**, 7–13. doi: 10.1093/ajcn/86.1.7.

Virtue, S., Even, P. and Vidal-Puig, A. (2012) Below thermoneutrality, changes in activity do not drive changes in total daily energy expenditure between groups of mice. *Cell Metabolism*, **16**, 665–671. doi: 10.1016/j.cmet.2012.10.008.

von Keyserlingk, M.A.G., Phillips, C.J.C. and Nielsen, B.L. (2016) Water and the welfare of farm animals. In: *Nutrition and the Welfare of Farm Animals*. Ed. Phillips, C.J.C., pp. 183–197, Springer, Cham, Switzerland. doi: 10.1007/978-3-319-27356-3_9.

Wade, G.N. and Heller, H.W. (1993) Tamoxifen mimics the effects of estradiol on food intake, body weight, and body composition in rats. *American Journal of Physiology*, **264**, R1219–1223. doi: 10.1152/ajpregu.1993.264.6.r1219.

Wagner, M. and Oehlmann, J. (2011) Endocrine disruptors in bottled mineral water: estrogenic activity in the E-Screen. *Journal of Steroid Biochemistry and Molecular Biology*, **127**, 128–135. doi: 10.1016/j.jsbmb.2010.10.007.

Walker, S.E., Adams, M.R., Franke, A.A. et al. (2008) Effects of dietary soy protein on iliac and carotid artery atherosclerosis and gene expression in male monkeys. *Atherosclerosis*, **196**, 106–113. doi: 10.1016/j.atherosclerosis.2007.02.007.

Walsh, L.L. (1980) Differences in food, water, and food-deprivation water intake in 16 strains of rats. *Journal of Comparative and Physiological Psychology*, **94**, 775–781. doi: 10.1037/h0077698.

Wang, R., Liu, R., Li, L. et al. (2019) Fasting is not required for measuring plasma lipid levels in rabbits. *Laboratory Animals*, 0023677219855102. doi: 10.1177/0023677219855102

Warden, C.H. and Fisler, J.S. (2008) Comparisons of diets used in animal models of high-fat feeding. *Cell Metabolism*, **7**, 277–279. doi: 10.1016/j.cmet.2008.03.014.

Warner, K., Bookwalter, G.N., Rackis, J.J. et al. (1982) Prevention of rancidity in experimental rat diets for long-term feeding. *Cereal Chemistry*, **59**, 175–178. doi: 10.1016/0003-2697(78)90795-9.

Webb, G.P., Jagot, S.A. and Jakobson, M.E. (1982) Fasting-induced torpor in Mus musculus and its implications in the use of murine models for human obesity studies. *Comparative Biochemistry and Physiology. A: Comparative Physiology*, **72**, 211–219. doi: 10.1016/0300-9629(82)90035-4.

Weindruch, R. and Walford, R.L. (1982) Dietary restriction in mice beginning at 1 year of age: effect on life-span and spontaneous cancer incidence. *Science*, **215**, 1415–1418. doi: 10.1126/science.7063854.

WHO (2011) *Guidelines for Drinking-Water Quality*. WHO, Geneva, Switzerland.

Wills, E.D. (1980a) Effects of antioxidants on lipid peroxide formation in irradiated synthetic diets. *International Journal of Radiation Biology and Related Studies in Physics, Chemistry and Medicine*, **37**, 403–414. doi: 10.1080/09553008014550481.

Wills, E.D. (1980b) Studies of lipid peroxide formation in irradiated synthetic diets and the effects of storage after irradiation. *International Journal of Radiation Biology and Related Studies in Physics, Chemistry and Medicine*, **37**, 383–401. doi: 10.1080/09553008014550471.

Wilz, M. and Heldmaier, G. (2000) Comparison of hibernation, estivation and daily torpor in the edible dormouse, *Glis glis*. *Journal of Comparative Physiology B: Biochemical, Systemic, and Environmental Physiology*, **170**, 511–521. doi: 10.1007/s003600000129.

Wolton, R.J. (2009) The ranging and nesting behaviour of Wood mice, *Apodemus sylvaticus* (Rodentia: Muridae), as revealed by radio-tracking. *Journal of Zoology*, **206**, 203–222. doi: 10.1111/j.1469-7998.1985.tb05645.x.

Wood, C.E., Appt, S.E., Clarkson, T.B. *et al.* (2006) Effects of high-dose soy isoflavones and equol on reproductive tissues in female cynomolgus monkeys. *Biology of Reproduction*, **75**, 477–486. doi: 10.1095/biolreprod.106.052142.

Wood, C.E., Cline, J.M., Anthony, M.S. *et al.* (2004a) Adrenocortical effects of oral estrogens and soy isoflavones in female monkeys. *Journal of Clinical Endocrinology and Metabolism*, **89**, 2319–2325. doi: 10.1210/jc.2003-031728.

Wood, C.E., Register, T.C., Anthony, M.S. *et al.* (2004b) Breast and uterine effects of soy isoflavones and conjugated equine estrogens in postmenopausal female monkeys. *Journal of Clinical Endocrinology and Metabolism*, **89**, 3462–3468. doi: 10.1210/jc.2003-032067.

Woods, S.C., Seeley, R.J., Rushing, P.A. *et al.* (2003) A controlled high-fat diet induces an obese syndrome in rats. *The Journal of Nutrition*, **133**, 1081–1087. doi: 10.1093/jn/133.4.1081.

Wostmann, B.S. and Pleasants, J.R. (1991) The germ-free animal fed chemically defined diet: a unique tool. *Proceedings of the Society for Experimental Biology and Medicine*, **198**, 539–546. doi: 10.3181/00379727-198-43286d.

Wu, G. (2018) *Principles of Animal Nutrition*. CRC Press, Boca Raton, FL. doi: 10.1201/9781315120065.

Yang, C.Z., Yaniger, S.I., Jordan, V.C. *et al.* (2011) Most plastic products release estrogenic chemicals: a potential health problem that can be solved. *Environmental Health Perspectives*, **119**, 989–996. doi: 10.1289/ehp.1003220.

Yang, T.S., Howard, B. and Macfarlane, W.V. (1981) Effects of food on drinking behaviour of growing pigs. *Applied Animal Ethology*, **7**, 259–270. doi: 10.1016/0304-3762(81)90082-1.

Yazar, S. and Omurtag, G.Z. (2008) Fumonisins, trichothecenes and zearalenone in cereals. *International Journal of Molecular Sciences*, **9**, 2062–2090. doi: 10.3390/ijms9112062.

Yu, B.P., Masoro, E.J. and McMahan, C.A. (1985) Nutritional influences on aging of Fischer 344 rats: I. Physical, metabolic, and longevity characteristics. *Journal of Gerontology*, **40**, 657–670. doi: 10.1093/geronj/40.6.657.

Zhang, S., Ye, B., Zeng, L. *et al.* (2012) Drug-containing gelatin treats as an alternative to gavage for long-term oral administration in rhesus monkeys (Macaca mulatta). *Journal of the American Association for Laboratory Animal Science*, **51**, 842–846.

Zimmerman, C.A., Leib, D.E. and Knight, Z.A. (2017) Neural circuits underlying thirst and fluid homeostasis. *Nature Reviews Neuroscience*, **18**, 459–469. doi: 10.1038/nrn.2017.71.

14 Attaining competence in the care of animals used in research

Bryan Howard and Marcel Gyger

Introduction

In recent years, there has been very considerable improvement in our understanding of the needs of laboratory animals, although there is much still to learn, and many of the measures implemented to improve husbandry have been empirically formulated. Their introduction and application need to be addressed sensitively by dedicated, knowledgeable and skilled staff. The people who have most influence on the well-being of laboratory animals are those who care for them on a daily basis. Although the conduct of scientific procedures almost invariably impacts on animals' well-being, that impact is often transient or of relatively short duration. On the other hand, animals must be bred, transported and cared for before a study starts and during its progress; and at the end of the investigation, they must usually be humanely killed. Animal care staff and their supervisors are in the frontline of these processes, although their central contribution is sometimes overlooked (Greenhough & Roe 2017). There is an urgent need for more investigative work into the most appropriate husbandry conditions of many of these species and those who are routinely engaged in animal care are particularly well placed to carry out or assist in such research.

In addition to animal welfare-focused changes to the way animals are housed and cared for, other developments have brought science into the animal facility and technology into the day-to-day routines of staff working there. New ways of keeping animals include: the group housing of rabbits, primates and dogs; ventilated racks and other biocontainment facilities; high-intensity aquatic environments; computerised systems for monitoring the environment and maintaining animal records; and high-performance room ventilation systems, which minimise carbon costs while maintaining rigorously defined air quality within rooms and minimising the burden of aeroallergens. Changes such as these have coincided with the emergence of new experimental methods and models, including targeted genetic modification of animals, high health status and chronic studies on animals with instrumentation. Additionally, care staff may be required to become involved with research techniques such as tissue sampling for genetic monitoring, automated home cage monitoring (for example, using activity sensors or remote physiological data capture from bio-implants), the management of dosing and autosampling equipment and sophisticated data collection and processing techniques.

Training programmes should be designed, delivered and assessed with a view to developing and monitoring the knowledge and skills appropriate to the duties of individuals, while promoting the diversity and flexibility necessary for career development. This chapter reviews the considerations necessary for this, promoting the development of competent animal care staff dedicated to achieving the highest standards of animal welfare. The material should also be of interest to those designing and conducting programmes of work with experimental animals who must work closely with them. In addition, it is of relevance to specialists in laboratory animal science, those charged with overseeing standards and others who have an interest in this topic. For readers wishing to explore further the range of issues relating to staff development, there is an excellent text written by Knowles *et al.* (2015) and specific information about the development of learning in those caring for or using laboratory animals can be found in Howard *et al.* (2010).

Those delivering training to animal care staff have often not received formal teacher training, although they may be highly competent in a wide range of animal husbandry tasks. This aspect of staff development is often overlooked and deserves much more attention by those with overall responsibility for the management of biomedical facilities. The present text is not intended to be an exhaustive account of teaching methodologies but rather an introduction to the principal considerations to be addressed. Published literature in this discipline is sparse, although the education and training of those designing and conducting experiments has received more attention. Some parallels can be drawn between the skills, attitudes and knowledge of those engaged

---

The UFAW Handbook on the Care and Management of Laboratory and Other Research Animals, Ninth Edition.
Edited by Huw Golledge and Claire Richardson.
© 2024 John Wiley & Sons Ltd. Published 2024 by John Wiley & Sons Ltd.

in the nursing and paramedical professions, and the authors also draw on their own experience in this context. As in all occupational training, it is important to keep in mind that in a changing workplace, the objective is to prepare entrants for their role in the future rather than just the present time. This means the development of a culture of continual learning and the ability to identify and replace outdated methodologies. It involves discarding the concept of learning as acquiring, memorising and retrieval of knowledge and skills. Instead, the student must develop the ability to embrace the adaptive nature of thinking and processing, recalling information and experiences acquired at different times and incorporating these into a consistent and relevant course of action. In this text, the term 'teacher' is used to refer to a person who assists students in acquiring these abilities rather than simply providing information; the teacher may also be described as a facilitator or an educator, but the role goes beyond the act of instructing or training. Both teachers and learners need to work towards the parallel development of skills and knowledge and their application to tasks and situations relevant to their work-role (Mennin 2015).

Persons participating in an activity which to some extent is likely to compromise animal welfare and hence requires legislation to make it legal, must make ethical decisions and accept the consequences of those on an ongoing basis. For these reasons, as well as to ensure compliance with current legislative requirements most countries require those who care for and use animals to be knowledgeable about their responsibilities and also to demonstrate a high level of competence. Training programmes should be designed and delivered with a view to developing the knowledge and skills appropriate to the duties of personnel, while promoting the diversity and flexibility necessary for career development. Training helps staff to develop basic competencies and, in the case of ongoing training, to use new equipment and procedures. Training is important for maintaining and updating knowledge about legislative and regulatory developments, and for the renewal of competencies, particularly in techniques not frequently used (Pritt & Duffee 2007). The amount and nature of training required by individuals is likely to differ, which, with variation in preferred learning styles, resource allocation and conflicting work demands places a considerable load on those responsible for delivering training in the workplace.

For these reasons, all staff must commit at the outset to their own development, explicitly understand and accept the outcomes required and be clear about what constitutes satisfactory performance, the way and time at which this will be assessed and the ways in which both staff and the organisation will benefit (Kennedy et al. 2017). Training without follow-up is ineffective and a clear, transparent and objective means of measuring progress must be set in place that allows both staff and their supervisors to monitor progress and recognise success as learning objectives are achieved.

Legal and ethical considerations

All those working with laboratory animals need to be made aware of their obligations under national and regional legislation, and this is an essential part of the training process (see also Chapter 8: Legislation and oversight of the conduct of research using animals: a global overview). In most instances, legislation is based on the ethical framework of the Three Rs of Russell and Burch (Russell & Burch 1959). In general terms, this states that animals should only be used when no non-sentient alternatives exist, that then as few as possible should be used and that the experiments should be conducted in such a way as to minimise the adverse impact on each animal concerned (see Chapter 2: The Three Rs).

Animal care staff must clearly understand these ethical principles and also the concerns of wider society. While it may not always be appropriate to focus on the theoretical background of ethical decision making, all persons involved in animal experimentation should be able to apply ethical principles to rationalise and feel confident about their role, the activities of the institution and the regulatory systems within which they work. Moreover, within any establishment, those caring for and conducting experiments on animals should participate in a shared ethical framework thereby developing collective values, which underpin a pervasive 'culture of care'. Such an institutional culture is intolerant of acts which unnecessarily impair animal welfare, thereby supporting legal compliance, establishing ethical sustainability and ultimately enhancing the robustness of scientific studies. The implication is that staff involved in animal experimentation must be equipped with the necessary information, tools and materials to perform effectively alongside others (Romick et al. 2006) and be confident and able to take appropriate actions should problems arise. This responsibility can be communicated by a variety of means, including: team briefings, focused seminars addressing technical and scientific progress of projects, circulation of newsletters and information from social media, staff meetings and performance reviews. Whichever method is used, the regular flow of information is important to ensure that all staff are acquainted with the activities of the organisation.

For all these reasons animal care staff and others must be made aware of the ethical framework and the law as soon as they commence work. These are important topics in formal training courses, but should also be promoted by initiatives within establishments and by supervisors and colleagues. These are topics for which formal teaching based on lectures, seminars or study of online materials, is less effective than interactive learning, in which participants are prompted to ask questions and to solve problems. Good communication is central to developing shared ethical values and both care staff and scientists should be able to talk freely with each other using a common understanding focused on high-quality care routines, welfare issues and science and based on acceptance of individual responsibility and accountability.

Purposes of education and training

Training is a necessary prerequisite to achieving high-quality science and good animal welfare (Prescott & Lidster 2017). Consideration of the needs for education and training should not be restricted to ethical or regulatory requirements, which tend to be broadly drafted and include general statements such as the need for 'appropriate education'. Guidelines have not usually addressed details of curriculum content, the length and content of initial training or maintenance of up-to-date knowledge; approaches to skills development were usually overlooked (see for example European Parliament and the Council 2010; US National Institutes of Health, 2015[1]). However, in recent years, efforts have been made to provide more specific guidance on curriculum content.

University undergraduate and sometimes even graduate science curricula do not usually specifically address issues relating to animal welfare, good scientific practice or associated ethical subjects although a strong case can be made for including these topics, at least in outline. Many undergraduates pursuing biology-based courses will not progress to carry out research involving animals, and therefore do not need to gain manual skills or competences in these areas, but it is important that all who acquire or use such information in a scientific or technical way should appreciate how that information has been obtained not only for the ethical context underlying this, but also for the reliance that can be placed on the findings. The value to be gained by including such information in university courses has been explored by assessing student opinions (Franco & Olsson 2014; von Roten 2018) but more needs to be done to determine the most appropriate level and time of presentation.

The terminology surrounding education and training

There is much confusion about terminology in the fields of education and training, so it is appropriate to identify here the ways in which these terms are used in this chapter. In particular, the terms 'education' and 'training' are often used interchangeably, but here the term education describes a process of developing theoretical and conceptual knowledge to assist in the enhancement of judgement and reasoning whereas the term training is applied to the process of helping a person to develop specific practical skills or behaviours, usually involving hands-on experiences.

Knowing is the possession of knowledge and comprises the expertise and skill acquired by an individual through experience and education. It involves the commitment to memory of facts and information about relevant topics and the basic ability to recall that information. It may also imply an awareness of how to use a certain concept or object for an appropriate purpose. Knowing involves perception, learning, communication, association and reasoning.

Learning is the process by which an individual acquires or modifies existing knowledge, attitudes and/or behaviours. People learn in different ways – for example, they may most readily absorb, process, comprehend and retain information presented verbally, visually or by physical participation in a relevant activity. The ease of learning is influenced also by the environment within which it takes place and the learner's emotion and motivation at the time. For example, positive emotions encourage longer-term recall, whereas negative emotions can disrupt the process of learning. Acquisition of knowledge is not directly observable, and it becomes apparent only when expressed through some observable behaviour. A regular flow of information is required to ensure that staff are acquainted with the activities of the organisation and their immediate work environment so as to provide context for learning.

Memory is the ability to draw on past experiences in order to use information in the present. Learners assess and interpret information they acquire and make connections with pre-existing knowledge to make sense of it. Memory is commonly classified into short-term memory and long-term memory according to the duration of retention. Repetition of an experience or its utilisation, for example, by practice, tends to reinforce long-term memory. The formation of memory involves linking an experience to other mental representations and recall is facilitated if associated environmental cues can be recalled. Memory is facilitated if learners are encouraged to summarise, explain or use material in a variety of contexts.

Understanding is a more complex mental process than knowing and involves the ability to recall knowledge, assess its relevance and appropriateness and use it to address a particular purpose (Foshay & Tinkey 2007). It involves the ability to identify connections between pieces of information. When something is meaningfully understood, it is remembered much longer, and provides the basis for developing further understanding and its adaption for dealing with novel and perhaps more complex situations. For factual knowledge to become meaningful, it needs to be incorporated into a broader, previously learned and closely related context, a process known as assimilation. The stronger the association with that context, the more coherent is the resultant understanding.

Competency is the deployment of a set of related knowledge, skills and abilities to successfully perform functions or tasks in a defined work setting – the focus is on the personal attributes or inputs of the individual. The education, training and development of persons working with laboratory animals require the learning of skills, the presentation and assimilation of knowledge and the incorporation of all these into a framework of understanding and responsiveness that is competency. Many of the higher qualities associated with competency are acquired in the workplace rather than delivered by formal training although the quality of the latter is paramount in establishing a reliable platform for this development.

Competence has a broader context that encompasses demonstrable outputs of both performance and behaviour and may relate to a system or set of minimum standards required for effective performance (Albanese *et al.* 2008). As such, it encompasses not only technical skill and deep understanding of the rationale for courses of action, but an awareness of, and sensitivity to, societal interest in what is being done. In addition, there is a need to be able to respond to the unexpected in a scientifically and ethically appropriate way, to work professionally and effectively with colleagues from a wide range of disciplines and to maintain high personal and workplace standards.

As an example of the distinction between competency and competence, a technician possessing the former may be aware of the importance of feeding sterile diet to gnotobiotic

---

[1] National Institutes of Health, Office of Laboratory Animal Welfare (OLAW) PHS Policy on Humane Care and Use of Laboratory Animals. https://olaw.nih.gov/policies-laws/phs-policy.htm (accessed 1 February 2022)

mice in ventilated racks, be aware of the impact of sterilisation methods on the palatability and nutritional value of that diet and appropriately monitor and record its use. However, competence implies that the technician responds to deviations from the expected performance of such animals resulting from an anticipated or unanticipated change in diet in a way that is appropriate both to animal welfare and the scientific programme being pursued.

The term competence has been introduced into EU Directive 2010/63/EU (European Parliament and the Council 2010) and is frequently used in place of the word competency. In consequence, no distinction will be drawn here between two words in this text.

Many other terms have been introduced to identify levels of attainment, including skill, effectiveness, expertise, aptitude, capability and proficiency; their use has been inconsistent and definition of these is beyond the purpose of this chapter. However, it is appropriate to draw a distinction between the attainment of competence, the ability to train others to become competent and the ability to effectively and objectively assess the levels of competence in others. These attainments are not a reflection simply of greater depth and breadth of knowledge within the technical discipline, but demand additional skills. Teachers must be able to identify key issues, to assemble them in a meaningful way and present them using an array of appropriate media that makes logical sense and retains their inherent importance. They must be able to establish an empathy with learners, taking account of their individual backgrounds, motivations, and capabilities and ensure that they make themselves available for students who encounter difficulties in their learning. Those assessing learners must not only be highly competent but also able to gather evidence and make judgements on their ability using tools and metrics that are meaningful and objective, avoiding ambiguity. In addition, they must achieve this within an environment which allows the student to demonstrate his or her abilities within what will inevitably be a fairly stressful situation. The competencies required by trainers and assessors extend beyond the immediate subject discipline and require additional targeted learning.

Additionally, it may be necessary to develop specific competencies, for example, relating to the ability to administer compounds, withdraw biological samples, carry out specific observations or make measurements using validated equipment, under the direction of a scientist or other authorised person and subject to compliance with local and legal requirements. Those with aptitude may develop additional competencies such as managing staff, overseeing facilities or provision of specialist technical services.

The training programme

Fundamental considerations in designing a training programme are the learning objectives, the starting point of the learners, the resources available, the level of competence required and the ways in which this will be applied. Educational principles relevant to enhancing performance of the adult workforce differ substantially from those appropriate for children at school or indeed for undergraduates at the university level; they constitute a topic known as *andragogy*.

This topic was explored by Knowles (1973) who identified four major areas of difference between mature learners and school children. He argued that adult learners have a considerably wider background experience and diversity of prior life experiences than youngsters and so expect to take control of their own learning in this context. They learn most readily topics and skills for which they see a valid application and they construct their understanding around the nature of those tasks rather than theoretical scenarios. Consequently, formal classroom instruction is less effective or motivating than interactive and performance/problem-centred learning activities.

The effectiveness of learning is determined by cognitive, emotional and environmental factors (Tyng *et al*. 2017), as well as prior experience and may even vary from time to time in the same individual. To learn intentionally, people must *want* to learn, and positive motivation substantially increases the facility with which students can engage in complex learning. Basic technical procedures can be learned by following a series of steps without understanding why they are taken or the consequences of performing them; this is knowledge without understanding – for example, close adherence to a standard operating procedure (SOP).

In the case of animal care staff, a trained technician will have learned a wide range of topics, understand their relevance and should be competent in some or all of the following:

- Ethical issues associated with the scientific use of animals and application of the Three Rs;
- National and local legislation and regulations; insofar as these relate to the sourcing, care and use of the species concerned, including any requirements of local ethical, welfare or care and use oversight bodies;
- Basic biology of relevant animal species;
- Knowledge and skill in housing, handling and husbandry, nutrition, sexing and breeding of relevant species, including animals undergoing experiments;
- Appropriate provision for social interaction and optimising the environment of animals;
- Identifying and meeting special needs of animal models, including those genetically altered;
- Signs of well-being or poor health and actions to be taken if these are compromised;
- Selecting and conducting a suitable method of euthanasia if necessary and disposal of carcases;
- Effective communication with colleagues, supervisors and scientists conducting procedures;
- Measures for maintaining good hygiene and biosecurity;
- Compliance with appropriate health and safety procedures including personal hygiene, safe working practices and the occupational health programme;
- Store keeping and replenishment of stock items.

More senior staff will also be acquainted with a number of management topics, for example procedures and policies for the efficient and safe operation of the animal facility, including the sourcing of animals, involvement in staff development and establishing policies for effective management. In addition, he or she may directly assist the veterinarian in maintaining the health of the animals or treating those that are sick and also participate in the conduct of animal studies if they have completed the education and training necessary to acquire authorisation under relevant national rules.

The most effective method of delivering training is influenced by the topic to be addressed, the learner's background and preferred way of learning, the trainer's skills and preferences and the facilities available. Wherever possible, a mix of teachers and teaching styles is preferable to a continuous sequence of lectures, practical classes or seminars. Normally, formal lectures should last no more than 45 minutes to an hour and can then be followed by a contrasting activity such as a practical session, audiovisual presentation[2] or online lesson addressing a different topic, which assists assimilation of issues and material which has been presented formally. If the amount of material to be covered requires longer than this, it is advisable to break up the session by introducing brief supporting activities such as impromptu quizzes, brainstorming, a question-and-answer session or a 'think, pair and share' exercise. These need last no more than 5 minutes and also introduce learners to the value of collaboration and networking as well as enabling the teacher to assess the progress of learning.

Whatever method of training is adopted, students should be prompted to actively use information acquired, so encouraging participative learning which is a powerful way of reinforcing short-term memory and converting it to long-term memory appropriate to real-life issues (Weir *et al.* 2019).

Although all staff are ultimately responsible for developing their own knowledge and competence, legislation usually places additional responsibilities on those overseeing animal facilities. Primary responsibility may be placed on a named individual (e.g. the EU Directive 2010/63 or the Australian Code for the Care and Use of Animals for Scientific Purposes (NHMRC 2013)); shared between several persons (e.g. the Resource Manager and Study Director in Switzerland (Swiss Animal Welfare Ordinance 2008); or vested in a committee, such as an ethical review committee (ERC) or an Institutional Animal Care and Use Committee (IACUC) in the USA (NRC 2011).

Whatever the details of the arrangement, management of the facility should provide opportunities for all personnel to develop satisfactory standards of performance. This includes providing a framework to identify training needs and promoting both initial and lifelong learning opportunities (continuing professional development or CPD). There are three key components of such a framework:

1. planning and developing strategies to assure high standards of animal welfare and the quality of research;
2. maximising the effectiveness and efficiency of staff in the workplace;
3. reviewing the impact of the programme against predefined metrics.

One approach to establishing a training programme is to benchmark the provision of education and training against that of similar establishments undertaking similar work. Alternatively, or additionally, views may be sought of key individuals within the establishment such as line managers, veterinarians, senior scientists or their representatives, members of the IACUC or Animal Welfare Body (AWB) and perhaps other key individuals such as client representatives or officials concerned with regulatory compliance. Often such a body already exists, performing other functions and, in such cases, this is likely to be the most effective yardstick. The training plan must identify clear targets based on the Three Rs, quality of science and the business or academic objectives of the organisation.

Critical to this process is the identification of priorities for education and training. The programme should take account of the size and type of establishment, the current knowledge and skills of staff, the complexity of the work, the rate of staff turnover and the level of support and advice available within the workplace. Particular consideration should be given to perceived future skills requirements resulting from the introduction of new equipment, new technologies or changing workplace needs within a realistic timescale. While the training programme is being developed, there must be wide consultation with staff, particularly in large organisations or where staff work in distinct teams in relative isolation and in different parts of a single organisation, for example where strict biosecurity regimes are in place. Budgetary issues are always contentious but if inadequate provision is made, training will inevitably be compromised; in such cases, the training plan needs to be revisited to establish a realistic compromise that provides good value and satisfies the institution's needs. Poor quality training is completely unacceptable ethically, legally and from a business viewpoint.

A logically structured training programme offers many practical benefits including:

- The opportunity to review current policies and practices and to identify areas where improvement is possible.
- Increased productivity in terms of scientific output and the quality of publications generated by skilled and motivated people who work more effectively and consistently, delivering higher-quality scientific outputs.
- Enhanced motivation and greater understanding by staff of their role within the workplace. Motivation encourages teamwork in the conduct of scientific investigations, promoting closer liaison between animal care staff, scientists and those overseeing projects.
- Improved personal development and recognition of achievements which enhances morale, reduces staff turnover and absenteeism and creates a climate in which change is more readily embraced.
- Greater clarity in the planning of future strategies and developments.
- Recognition that the facility is staffed by effective and competent individuals aids recruitment and staff retention, makes it easier to attract grants or commissions and to identify promising research leads. Many academic establishments are focusing increasingly on the consistency and quality of scientific investigations that they undertake.

Developing knowledge and understanding

Teaching is nothing more than the facilitation of learning, but having said this it should be recognised that teachers bear a great deal of responsibility. Not only must they ensure that learners have a clear appreciation of what material needs to

---

[2] For example, see https://nc3rs.org.uk or https://norecopa.no (accessed 1 February 2022)

be learned and at what depth, but they need to take account of personal differences between learners to ensure that they are appropriately motivated and that the learning environment is conducive to the effective development of knowledge and skill. Teachers must not only be well versed in the relevant subject matter, but they should be inspirational, motivational and effective communicators. It is the responsibility of the teacher to negotiate positive yet realistic expectations with each student and to monitor progress. Learning is only relevant to the workplace if it has an application; focus on the responsibilities and duties of the learner provides a foundation for motivation, thereby maximising the scope and depth of learning. Finally, teachers serve as role models by adhering to the highest ethical and professional standards at all times.

Effective instruction depends on understanding the complex interplay in learners of their prior knowledge and experiences, motivation, manual and cognitive skills and preferred learning styles (Mennin 2015). Educators should carefully manage students' engagement, persistence and performance, e.g. by creating learning experiences they value, supporting their sense of control and autonomy and incorporating the values of teamwork. Students should be encouraged to develop their sense of competence, helping them to recognise, monitor and regulate their learning progress by providing critical but non-confrontational feedback on progress.

Various training opportunities are available to those wishing to find employment or to enhance their competence in laboratory care, including courses organised by specialist training providers, major laboratory animal breeders and equipment manufacturers; these deal with general laboratory animal care, as well as specific research techniques. In addition, national/regional laboratory animal science associations frequently hold symposia or conferences at which aspects of animal care and use are presented, discussed and placed within context. Attendance at such events should be framed as a learning opportunity and recognised formally so that credit can be given to individuals who take the time and effort to participate. The importance of recognition as a way of maintaining staff motivation and commitment is discussed by Symonowiez (2006).

While it is theoretically possible for students to develop the necessary knowledge by studying textbooks or online sources (or to follow online training courses), it often proves difficult to maintain steady progress in the absence of guidance and supervision by an experienced practitioner. This route may be attractive where specialised knowledge is required and the availability of information locally is sparse or lacking; for example, information on the management of particular strains of genetically altered animals may be obtained using websites such as that of the International Society for Transgenic Technologies[3]. Care should be taken to focus on reputable and verifiable sources. It is strongly recommended that those wishing to undertake self-study should initially secure the support of an experienced colleague who commits to devoting sufficient time and resources to the task of mentoring and occasionally tutoring. It should also be recognised that it can prove difficult for supervisors and institutions to assess the quality and effectiveness of such learning.

In-house training is often preferred where several people need to learn similar material. It has the advantage that hands-on training is usually easier to arrange, participants are already acquainted with each other, students may find domestic arrangements easier, and training can be targeted more precisely at the institution's needs. When necessary, an experienced trainer can be brought in from outside. 'External' courses allow networking by students who can share experiences from different environments.

Orienting the new employee

Recruitment of new employees is often regarded as a means of addressing a particular need within the establishment or department, but it should also be seen in the context of developing future talent and contributing to the overall culture of care (Klein & Bayne 2007). The first few days are important in setting ground rules, but also in shaping the attitude of a new colleague and integrating him or her into the workforce. Orientation is best done by the immediate line manager, who understands the role of the new employee but is not so senior as to appear remote from the work to be done; however, it is helpful to briefly introduce the recruit to senior management at an early stage (Silverman 2016). Sufficient time must be made available for the person to fully understand key aspects of their role. If it is not the immediate supervisor who is providing the orientation, new employees should be introduced to that person as soon as possible.

Right at the beginning of employment, the line manager should ensure that immediate work details such as the employment contract, pay roll, medical tests are dealt with; it may also be necessary for recruits to attend courses or be briefed about responses to emergencies, such as fire procedures and what to do in case of accidents. Where the organisation has a clear mission statement, this should be presented and placed in context. On a new employee's first day, it makes good managerial sense also to sit down and explain the organisation and the facility within which the employee will be working, the organisational culture, including responsibilities and what is expected of them, humane treatment of animals, sources of advice, whistle-blowing policies, etc. A clear, alternative channel of communication should be established wherever possible, although not for regular use. This personal touch demonstrates the manager's awareness of the activities of the department and informs recruits about the context of the role so that it is easier for them to come back with questions subsequently should that be necessary. The training expectations and opportunities and the routes for promotion should also be explained. Where it is anticipated that close supervision will be needed for some time, the arrangements for this should be explained clearly and agreed. It is a good idea to accompany new employees to the first rest break of the day to introduce him or her or to other staff. This is a relatively stress-free way of introducing the employee to colleagues and vice versa.

A check list should be developed for orientating new employees. This should identify what information needs to

---

[3] http://www.transtechsociety.org/.(accessed 1 February 2022)

be given upfront, and what new arrivals should work out for themselves. Examples of the former may include matters bearing on health and safety, current working routines (such as working hours, lunch and rest breaks), holiday entitlements, and key contacts both for gaining advice and seeking assistance when necessary. It is also helpful to have available written briefing materials appropriate to the role of the employee – ideally, this information would be a handbook so that misunderstandings can be avoided. The nature of material which new employees should work out for themselves depends upon the level of employment, and may be relatively basic or may relate to much more complex issues, for example staffing roles, workloads, and procedures and practices. Such materials may include information about staffing numbers, grades and competences, animal health records, SOPs, minutes of committee meetings; again, a checklist is helpful.

Developing practical skills

Competence in the care of animals depends crucially on practical skills, the development of which is an essential part of training in laboratory animal science. Hands-on exercises provide a means of relating theoretical understanding (taught alongside or previously) to hands-on skills. Despite this, the development of practical skills often receives less attention than that given to knowledge and understanding, probably because it involves a more complex learning environment, and it is more difficult to assess and record levels of performance. These obstacles are usually easier to overcome than is often assumed. No course can teach all of the practical skills required by someone working in laboratory animal science, so the objective is to equip students with sufficient theoretical understanding and skill to enable them to address practical issues in a safe, ethical and systematic way and to know when to seek help and from whom.

Practical skills may be developed by formal or informal training sessions followed by working under the supervision of enthusiastic, competent and experienced staff[4]. This helps to develop a commitment to achieving and sustaining practical competence in preparation for working independently or as a member of a team. In order to ensure the quality of the process, it is important that learning takes place within a structured framework, is overtly linked to underlying theoretical principles, is formally documented and is properly assessed. However, it must also be made clear that this basic training is only the first stage of a lifelong process of learning and improvement, during which time practices and procedures are likely to change.

Animal care staff can generally devote considerable time to developing expertise and competence, but throughout this process they should be supported and mentored by experienced colleagues. It is particularly important that new employees are made to feel part of a team and that the contribution of their work to the team and the animals for which they care is acknowledged. It is during this early period of training that a good working relationship with more experienced care staff is developed.

If it is proposed to use live animals to teach practical skills, the instructor should judge whether this is essential for development of the relevant skills and it is usually necessary to seek authorisation from the ethical review process, IACUC or AWB before commencing. Students must be made aware of their ethical and legal responsibilities and clearly understand what the session is expected to achieve and how they will be assessed. Animals used for teaching skills should be in good health and should never be subjected to unnecessary pain, suffering or harm. The use of animals to teach techniques such as handling, restraint, sexing and basic technical procedures can cause them distress and one way of dealing with this difficulty is to maintain a small stock of animals that have been habituated to being handled and are used principally for initial training. Such animals become compliant, their behaviour is more predictable and they are less likely to be perceived as threatening. Once the learner develops confidence in working with these, naïve animals should be introduced.

If possible, lessons should be organised to be species- or technique-specific, and learner groups kept as small as possible; one-to-one training is often best and allows attention to be given to the student's specific needs. In addition, only the smallest number of animals necessary to develop appropriate skills should be used and there must be adequate technical oversight so that each student is closely supervised during the learning period and given prompt assistance if necessary. Learners should be allowed to progress at their own pace, to ask questions, receive accurate, timely and supportive feedback, and helped to rectify faults. If a formal lesson is involved, it must allow sufficient time for a concluding question-and-answer session. This allows learners and teacher to critically assess progress and performance. In addition, tutors should reflect subsequently on how well the session went.

Before initiating lessons involving the handling of animals, it is a good idea first to explain the techniques (e.g. with the help of video presentations) then practise with surrogate or non-sentient models which are as realistic as possible. Sometimes, it may be appropriate to carry out a technique on a recently killed animal or possibly one that has been anaesthetised or sedated (in which case it is usually killed without recovering). These techniques allow tasks to be paused during their performance thereby allowing discussion of key aspects, which would not be possible using conscious animals. When this stage has been completed, or where sentient animals are not involved, the teacher usually proceeds with a demonstration of the practical task, accompanying this with a commentary explaining its purpose and importance, indicating possible health and safety issues and emphasising relevant refinement and reduction methods, safe working practices, etc. Skilled performance of a task is characterised by speed and dexterity, and it may be difficult to conduct some tasks at slow speed; examples include: capturing an animal in a large cage, opening the mouth of a rabbit or rat to examine its teeth or performing euthanasia. In such cases, pre-recorded video material, which can be replayed at slow speed, may be a useful alternative.

---

[4] https://www.lasa.co.uk/wp-content/uploads/2016/09/LASA_supervision_and_competence_2016.pdf (accessed 1 February 2022)

Table 14.1 Levels of competence recognised by three major care-staff associations.

Organisation	Qualification		
	Basic	Intermediate	Advanced
AALAS	Assistant laboratory animal technician	Laboratory animal technician	Laboratory animal technologist
IAT	First Certificate in Animal Husbandry	First Diploma in Animal Technology	National Certificate in Animal Technology
CALAS	Associate registered laboratory animal technician	Registered laboratory animal technician	Registered master laboratory animal technician

After demonstrating the task, each student should be asked to repeat it several times under close supervision and while doing so, to provide a commentary. Putting the process into words helps learners to remember the different stages involved. In addition, requiring students to demonstrate a technique immediately after it has been shown to them is a useful way of identifying deficiencies or problems that may have arisen in performance of the task so that these can be corrected before poor practices become assimilated; it also reinforces memory of the technique.

As with teaching theoretical knowledge, a list of practical skills to be learned should be presented to students at the beginning of their training. Also, each class should be logically structured, and one way of achieving this is to prepare a worksheet listing the stages and competencies expected. An assessment schedule should be prepared, based on those key points and the assessment process itself should be clearly separated from the process of learning. It is good practice to ask whether the trainee is ready for the assessment to begin or whether he or she would prefer to defer it until further experience has been gained; where possible the assessor should not be the person who delivered the training. The proficiency with which the task is performed should be judged using a formal check sheet which lists the key elements of its conduct (see the section on evaluating competence). A means should also be found of allowing the trainee to comment on the learning process and difficulties which he or she may have experienced so that future learning sessions can take account of these perceptions.

When training personnel who are already working with laboratory animals, for example at a different establishment, learning may be enhanced by inviting them to explain how the procedure is done at their home institution followed by an analytical and non-confrontational discussion about the strengths and weaknesses of various aspects of the method.

National training schemes

Several national training schemes for animal care staff have been established and some of these are recognised worldwide. Three will be considered in outline here: those organised by the American Association for Laboratory Animal Science (AALAS), the Institute of Animal Technology (IAT) and the Canadian Association for Laboratory Animal Science (CALAS). In general, the syllabus does not differ greatly from that recommended by the Federation of European Laboratory Animal Science Associations (FELASA 2010) which is discussed later.

Each scheme recognises three levels of competence, summarised in Table 14.1. The entry level in each case is appropriate for trainee technicians who have relatively recently entered the field and the experience required is generally basic. AALAS requires those seeking this qualification to have at least 6 months' experience of laboratory animal science, depending upon their academic qualifications at the outset. IAT does not lay down specific requirements; CALAS expects applicants to have a high school diploma or have worked in an animal facility full-time for at least 3 years and to have already successfully completed three basic study modules. At each level, assessment is based on written examinations. The IAT and CALAS also stipulate an oral examination and, in the case of the latter, a formal practical examination.

For all three organisations, the intermediate-level qualification is the basic qualification for experienced laboratory animal technicians. Entry requirements are rather more diverse. The stipulation by AALAS is for at least 6 months' work-experience, possibly extending up to 3 years, depending on previous formal educational experience. In the case of the IAT, a candidate would normally hold the First Certificate in Animal Husbandry, although this is not mandatory, and some exemptions are available for previous educational experience. CALAS is more prescriptive and requires 5 years of experience after successful completion of the basic qualification.

The most advanced level of qualification is intended for individuals entering senior management positions within animal care facilities. Entry requirements are generally more rigorous, and in the case of CALAS include completion of the intermediate qualification and 5 years of additional continued employment in the field of laboratory animal science.

All organisations encourage involvement with continuing educational programmes, and contribute to the provision of these, but CALAS is the only one requiring all persons holding registered qualifications to meet annual requirements in order to maintain their status. The IAT requires all those it has accepted as Registered Animal Technologists to undertake CPD.

In Australia, a national scheme for training animal care staff has been established by the National Training Information Service, and is delivered by a number of local providers at Certificate and Diploma levels over a period of 2 years. The process is competency-based and recognises three levels, corresponding to those who perform care tasks, those who manage them and persons who evaluate and revise practices[5].

---

[5] https://www.myskills.gov.au/Courses/Search?keywords=animal+technician&distance=25 (accessed 1 February 2022)

An alternative model for the development of expertise in laboratory animal care is common in Germany and based on the apprentice scheme. Persons interested in the care and welfare of animals are able to follow a two-year training course addressing topics including animal health and welfare, nutrition, housing and husbandry. A third year is then spent specialising in particular work areas, which may include laboratory animal care. In effect, standards reached by following this programme comply with those of the FELASA Category A. However, the broad background knowledge acquired makes the basic qualification appropriate also for those working in diverse areas, including farm animal work and caring for pet animals.

The FELASA training scheme

Efforts have been made in some areas to harmonise training, but this has proved easier for general topics than for specific research techniques because of the greater number of organised training opportunities, the much greater size of the target group and the development of national and international guidelines.

Harmonisation of general courses within countries has been achieved in some cases, but to achieve the same within a continent or globally is much more of a challenge. None the less, efforts in that direction have been initiated by the International Council for Laboratory Animal Science (ICLAS)[6]. In contrast, the quality and volume of specific training on offer is highly variable and it is difficult to conceive a mechanism for ensuring sufficient targeted training for the wide variety of specific procedures conducted.

The first focused attempt to introduce a transnational approach to the education and training of persons caring for laboratory animals was outlined by FELASA in 1995 (FELASA 1995) which also set out recommendations for the education and training of persons directing or designing experiments. Subsequent papers proposed recommendations for training persons carrying out animal experiments (FELASA 2000) and for specialists in laboratory animal science (FELASA 1999). Prior to this, as early as 1957, moves had been made to establish an internationally recognised programme for the education and training of laboratory animal veterinarians by the American College of Laboratory Animal Medicine (ACLAM) but there were no such moves for non-veterinarians engaged in the care and use of laboratory animals. None of these recommendations was made mandatory. The International Association of Colleges of Laboratory Animal Medicine (IACLAM), founded in 2005, has proposed a scheme for lifelong learning – but again only for veterinarians.

The FELASA proposals identified four different categories of persons working with experimental animals:

- Category A: persons taking care of animals;
- Category B: persons carrying out experimental procedures;
- Category C: persons responsible for directing or designing experiments;
- Category D: laboratory animal science specialists.

FELASA subsequently published further clarification of these requirements basing its recommendations on functions common to the different categories, rather than on nomenclature, which may vary from country to country (FELASA 1999; FELASA 2000). Recommendations for practical, theoretical and ethical topics were applicable for all categories of personnel. The Category A recommendations were subsequently revised (FELASA 2010) to take account of opportunities that had arisen for Category A persons to assume more managerial roles and the additional competences associated with this development. It proposed two different levels of education beyond basic training (level A0) which provided competency to undertake limited specific duties under supervision. Most A0 assistants were expected to continue their education and training for at least a year while in full-time employment. During this time, they would be supervised and regularly assessed and could take a final examination to become qualified at level A1. Laboratory animal technicians achieving Level A1 competency would be able to carry out routine animal care duties with minimal supervision and some would continue specific education for at least another year of full-time employment to obtain level A2. During this time, they would develop additional knowledge and expertise as well as supervisory and basic managerial skills.

Competence as an element of Directive 2010/63/EU

One key principle underlying introduction of Directive 2010/63/EU (European Parliament and the Council 2010) was to ensure that public concerns about animal experimentation were recognised and that appropriate measures were taken to ensure that high welfare standards were set in place. Central to this is the competence of staff. This emphasis on competence was intended both to satisfy ethical and societal concerns about animal well-being and to facilitate movement of personnel between Member States. In addition, scientific investigations designed and carried out by competent personnel are less likely to be flawed or to lack rigour (Romick et al. 2006). In particular, this Directive has the effect of harmonising the practices of all EU Member States – not only those who were members at the time of drafting but also any who joined subsequently. In 1993, the parties of the European Convention ETS 123 issued a resolution to further promote the development and uptake of training and educational programmes to meet the competency requirements of these personnel[7]. European Directive 2010/63/EU provides no detailed guidance as to what might be expected of a competent person, although it outlines the basic knowledge considered necessary (ANNEX V) and offers much more detailed information on the educational requirements than did the

---

[6] https://iclas.org/harmonization-committee/ (accessed 1 February 2022)

[7] Council of Europe (1986) *Convention for the Protection of Vertebrate Animals used for Experimental and other Scientific Purposes* (ETS 123). Strasbourg. https://www.coe.int/en/web/conventions/full-list/-/conventions/treaty/123 (accessed 1 February 2022)

Directive it replaced – 86/609/EEC[8]. The current Directive has modified the list of job roles adopted earlier and refers instead to 'Functions':

- Function A: carrying out procedures on animals;
- Function B: designing procedures and projects;
- Function C: taking care of animals;

and introduces a further function:

- Function D: killing animals.

The Directive also makes reference to additional functions that were previously referred to in FELASA Category D:

- Designated Veterinarians (Art. 25),
- Person(s) 'responsible for overseeing the welfare and care of animals in the establishment' (Art. 24.1.a),
- Person(s) ensuring that 'staff dealing with animals have access to information specific to the species housed in the establishment' (Art. 24.1.b), and
- Person(s) responsible for ensuring 'that staff are adequately educated, competent and continuously trained and that they are supervised until they have demonstrated the requisite competence' (Art. 24.1.c).

Article 23(2) of the Directive stipulates that function B persons shall have received instruction in a relevant scientific discipline and shall have species-specific knowledge but there are no stipulations about the prior experience of those carrying out functions A, C or D; all must be supervised after training until they have demonstrated the requisite competence. A list of core elements is provided in ANNEX V. although responsibility for education, training and competencies of these functions remain the remit of Member States.

In 2010, the European Commission established an Education and Training Platform for Laboratory Animal Science, ETPLAS[9] to assist Member States in promoting development of competence in the four primary functions and to facilitate mutual recognition of courses across European countries and therefore mobility of competent personnel.

To provide further guidance and to establish a more uniform approach to developing competence, the European Commission established a working group which published a guidance document in 2014 (European Commission 2014). This document proposed a common education and training framework to fulfil the Directive's requirements; it is based on a modular educational scheme that addresses the requirements of the four functions and indicates the expected learning outcomes. It comprises six basic core modules applicable to all four functions, and additional function-specific modules are outlined for each function. In addition, task-specific modules are identified that define training needs for those intending to conduct certain special procedures. Advice is also offered on the competences expected of specialists active in laboratory animal science such as veterinarians, inspectors or animal welfare officers. Some training modules are species (or group of species) specific and intended to lead to competence only in relation to the species studied; those proposing to work with other species must demonstrate attainment of learning outcomes for the new species within the relevant module(s).

Reflective and self-directed learning

Critical reflection is fundamental to establishing and maintaining full competence, including the development of higher cognitive skills and professional attitudes. It requires the learner to step back from events and to explore what has happened by examining his or her own performance, reflecting on how different approaches might have turned out if they had been taken[10]. This process brings the learner to realise that the interpretation of events following a particular action is simply one of many other possible outcomes. Learners may find it easier to reflect by documenting their experience of an event then identifying and exploring possible alternative approaches, attempting to reach a greater understanding of their actions. Subsequent review of this 'portfolio' may offer an assessor insight into the reflective performance of the learner. It is this continuing exploration of the bigger picture alongside personal experience that underpins real, sustainable knowledge and learning.

Reflection maximises the learning potential arising from relatively routine encounters in the workplace and is particularly valuable as a means of learning from errors or problems that may have arisen. The approach underlines why it is important to do more than just have an experience in order to truly learn. Reflection unlocks events and enables the learner to formulate concepts and generalisations that will provide guidance in future situations. However, this process must be ongoing and regularly applied so that newly acquired skills are repeatedly tested in the face of best practice (Pryce-Miller 2010).

Evaluating competence

It is important that supervisors can assess the competence of those for whom they are responsible. There is an outdated view that competency can be determined by measurable actions and that the effectiveness with which these are performed can be reliably assessed. In fact, the setting of written – or formally structured practical – examinations fail to take account of the attitudes of individuals, their use of appropriate skills in the workplace (rather than under examination conditions), the way they evaluate and respond to the needs of animals, their aptitude in identifying signs and causes of distress or disturbance and how to respond when a problem arises. No single test can assess all these elements, but careful and objective observation of performance will go far in achieving this.

---

[8] European Council (1986) Council Directive 86/609/EEC of 24 November 1966 on the approximation of laws, regulations and administrative provisions of the Member States regarding the protection of animals used for experimental and other scientific purposes. https://eur-lex.europa.eu/legal-content/EN/TXT/?uri=celex%3A31986L0609 (accessed 1 February 2022)

[9] https://www.etplas.eu/ (accessed 1 February 2022)

[10] http://infed.org/mobi/self-directed-learning/ (accessed 1 February 2022)

It is generally accepted that multiple choice questions (MCQs) including single best answer questions (SBAs) and extended matching questions (EMQs) are sufficiently effective for the evaluation of knowledge and levels of understanding providing they are carefully constructed (Coughlin & Featherstone 2017). This type of assessment allows a wide range of topics to be covered, ensures consistency of marking by different examiners (indeed they can be marked by anyone with a 'key' or by using IT) and permit psychometric analysis to determine ambiguities in questioning or group deficiencies in learning. Alternative ways of testing knowledge include short-answer questions, longer essays, group-projects, face-to-face discourse, oral presentations, case reports or viva-voce examinations. Several of these methods provide evidence about the ability of the learner to both understand and contextualise knowledge; each has strengths and weaknesses and often one or more is combined with an MCQ paper. Ideally, the assessment should take place at least a week after the training has been completed to ensure that long-term memory is being assessed rather than more transient memory.

Practical skills cannot usually be taught in a short course so methods are needed to assess progress over a longer time period and assessment is potentially much more difficult and susceptible to influence by context – for example, performance of a task under examination conditions may be much more stressful than if there is no assessor watching, or the learner may adhere more closely to good practice than he or she might otherwise. Educators in the medical sciences have been struggling for some time to improve practices for the evaluation of day-to-day competence in the educational, practitioner and clinical environment. Several assessment tools have been developed, principally Mini-Clinical Evaluation Exercises (Mini-CEXs) and Direct Observation of Procedural Skills (DOPS). DOPS were introduced in 2005 as assessment tools for evaluating the competence of specialist medical practitioners following an evaluation by Wragg et al. (2003). They have gained wide acceptance. In the field of laboratory animal science, some accreditation schemes (e.g. those managed by FELASA and the IAT) have for many years recommended the use of objective measures of technical skill by using score sheets and standardised examination procedures (Clifford et al. 2013). Identified features might include having minimal impact on the animal's well-being, successfully achieving the task being assessed, speed, precision, safe working practices, understanding the underlying rationale, etc. Introduction of the DOPS scheme formalises the use of score sheets by providing an explicit statement of expectations which can be shared between training providers and so ensure an element of consistency. For example, the UK Laboratory Animal Science Association (LASA) has established a library of DOPS as 'living documents' suitable for assessing laboratory animal science techniques, procedures and practical skills and these are freely available for use by those responsible for training[11].

DOPS are designed to objectively measure performance and are carefully drafted in order that trainees and trainers understand the minimum standard of performance required.

Not only do DOPS evaluate specific procedural skills but may also provide evidence about the attitudes of those caring for animals. They have been claimed to have an educational impact by ensuring that the learner understands what needs to be improved to reach competence. In the training of medical clinicians, this aspect has not always been realised (Bindal et al. 2013) and it is important that the relevance of DOPS is made clear to students at the outset and that feedback concerning areas of good and bad practice is provided immediately after the assessment is finished. A further drawback of DOPS is that the consistency of assessors must be carefully validated, because there is inevitably a degree of subjectivity in their application; videotaping can be a useful way of assessing the uniformity of different assessments (Khanghahr & Azar 2018).

In 2014, the National Competent Authorities for the implementation of the EU Directive 2010/63/EU produced a working document that envisaged uniform standards for the education and training of those caring for or using laboratory animals. This document emphasised the need to work towards common, acceptable standards based on detailed learning outcomes and an agreed understanding of assessment criteria[12]. Since then, a pilot project has been funded by the European Commission entitled *Promoting alternatives to animal testing through accessible and harmonised education and training*. It is led by ETPLAS and includes a number of initiatives, one of which is the establishment of a database of DOPS applicable to the assessment of persons conducting procedures on laboratory animals[13]. Over the coming years, this promotion of the use of DOPS is likely to result in increased integration of the approach into training courses at all levels.

However, competence is not simply the sum or some other derivative of understanding and skill. It involves a holistic combination of knowledge, skills, understanding, attitude and reflection (Schuwirth 2015). Simply adding up a student's responses to MCQ questions, his or her skill in picking up and handling a rodent, describing the importance of providing bedding and nesting materials and assessing its general health does not by some arithmetic magic provide an evaluation of the competence of that individual within a work environment. In order to draw such a conclusion, a number of factors have to be considered. First, the observations have to be quantified – for example, 4/5 or 80%, or 'good'. Then, an inference has to be made about the generality of these scores and finally a conclusion reached about the relevant competence of the individual that can be defended if challenged. Despite these difficulties, the competence of personnel must be assessed, not only because of the legal and ethical imperatives surrounding the care of animals, but also because supervisors need to monitor competence so as to direct the development of staff needing further training.

Most guidelines and recommendations in laboratory animal science advocate an examination at the end, and sometimes also during the training period. A good examination tests the understanding of students by requiring them to

---

[11] http://www.lasa.co.uk/dops/ (accessed 1 February 2022)

[12] https://ec.europa.eu/environment/chemicals/lab_animals/pdf/Endorsed_E-T.pdf (accessed 1 February 2022)

[13] https://ec.europa.eu/environment/chemicals/lab_animals/pdf/WG-Members_Description_Process-20190109.pdf (accessed 1 February 2022)

retrieve, evaluate, weigh and apply their knowledge and to demonstrate learned skills, e.g. by combining various taught elements in each question. The objective should be to assess how the student would deal with real-life situations. To this end EU Directive 2010/63/EU requires Member States to 'ensure that each breeder, supplier and user has one or several persons on site who are responsible for ensuring that the staff are adequately educated, competent and continuously trained and that they are supervised until they have demonstrated the requisite competence', and why the *Guide for the Care and Use of Laboratory Animals* (NRC 2011) requires that 'animal care staff should be sufficiently trained to facilitate effective implementation of the programme and the humane care and use of animals'. In the UK, for example, the function required under Directive 2010/63/EU rests with the Named Training and Competence Officer, whose responsibilities are outlined in a LASA document.[14]

No doubt efforts will continue to be made over the coming years to establish criteria for the determination of competence. One such method currently used in medical practice is mini-peer assessment, a simplified form of 360° appraisal, in which each trainee nominates a number of assessors from among those who are his/her supervisors or peers to complete a questionnaire addressing the trainee's knowledge, technical ability and interpersonal skills. The same questionnaire is completed by the trainee. Forms are submitted independently to an assessor to ensure confidentiality (Norcini & McKinkley 2007).

Records

In order for an establishment to provide evidence that measures have been taken to ensure the competence of staff working with laboratory animals it is important that appropriate records are maintained (Pritt *et al.* 2004). Records should cover all staff, including researchers, animal care staff, long-term visitors and students, maintenance, quality assurance and other technical staff whose work may directly or indirectly impact on the well-being of laboratory animals. At regular intervals, line managers should review progress with each employee to ensure that appropriate competences are either proven, or being addressed; this can take place at periodic staff appraisals or performance reviews.

Records of training and competence have a number of functions:

- They provide evidence that the facility regards competence as important thereby motivating staff and assuring others of staff proficiency;
- They enable each staff member to demonstrate measures taken to develop appropriate competencies and to chart progress;
- They provide staff members with a structured training programme which they will expect to complete over time;
- They enable supervisors and managers to gain an overview of the training and development currently undertaken, the resources required to meet these and future demands;
- They demonstrate compliance with the requirements of the Directive and national legislation;
- They save time by ensuring that staff and their supervisors can find relevant information easily;
- They provide a means of detecting and analysing areas where a particular focus on training is required in order to ensure that all staff are brought up to a satisfactory level of competence;
- They may be useful in allocating scientific and technical staff to particular projects for which they have demonstrated competence, thereby facilitating mobility.

A distinction should be made between records of competence and records of training, which are less immediate measures of performance. The training record should establish when employees started to learn about each task which they are expected to perform, when and by whom competence was deemed to have been achieved (and, where appropriate, the level of that competence) and record periodic update training. Moreover, an employee may be deemed competent to perform a task under supervision, unsupervised or to train others to do it. As competences progress, the trainer or line manager should sign off each task for each student. Personnel who attend external training sessions should ensure that certificates of attendance are maintained with the remainder of their file, in a scanned electronic format if appropriate.

Records may be kept as hard copy files – for example in loose-leaf folders – may be particularly convenient in the case of small facilities employing few personnel. This is a relatively simple process and can incorporate all relevant documents but suffers from the disadvantage that it is available only to the person who holds it and could be misplaced or destroyed.

There are several advantages to maintaining records of competence on relational databases. They can be set up to actively notify staff, supervisors and managers of the current status of training and the need for staff members to undertake additional requirements; they may also act as a reminder of upcoming education or training events and facilitate evaluation of courses attended by summarising assessment outcomes, incorporating course or course provider evaluations and assessments and comments. Electronic records are easily updated and retrieved and may be distributed by e-mail or printed out when necessary. However, it is important to ensure that electronic records are backed up, that they are accurate and kept up to date and can be accessed only by authorised personnel.

Lifelong learning or CPD

The necessity of lifelong learning, also called *continuing professional development* (CPD), cannot be over-emphasised. A lifelong desire to learn, stimulation to acquire new skills and promotion of critical and deep thinking should be part of the culture of care of any institution. Training and education in laboratory animal science must be seen as a continuum starting immediately after taking up employment and proceeding throughout an individual's career; this is illustrated in Figure 14.1. During this process, various quality assurance

---

[14] Guiding Principles for Named Training and Competency Officers (NTCO), Named Information Officers (NIO) and Home Office Liaison Contacts (HOLC) working under the Animals (Scientific Procedures) Act 1986 - via https://www.lasa.co.uk/wp-content/uploads/2018/05/Guiding-Principles-for-Named-Persons-2016.pdf (accessed1 February 2022)

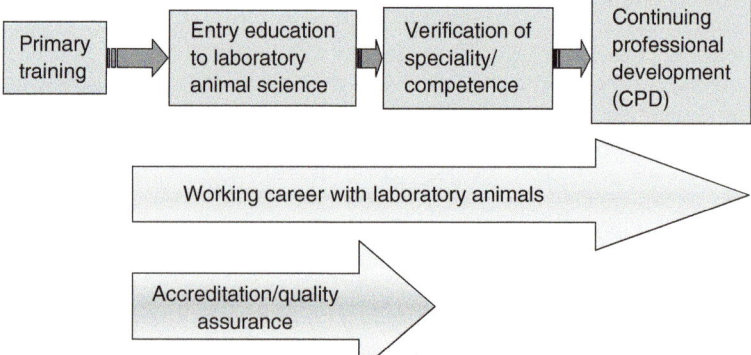

Figure 14.1 Schematic representation of lifelong education in laboratory animal science.

elements can be implemented (e.g. accreditation of entry education programmes, certification of individuals, specialty examinations and assessment of competence).

Lifelong learning relies critically on reflection but may also involve supplementary courses, such as those described for experimental design (Howard *et al.* 2009); seminars which are organised by several commercial companies; scientific meetings; workshops; home study of journals, books and technical articles; and electronic course offerings among other opportunities. The importance of supervision and CPD training in achieving and maintaining competence and in contributing to good science and welfare needs to be more widely recognised within the research community, both locally within research establishments and by those sponsoring or funding research.

In all training and education, there are some items which one is required to master, some with which one should be familiar and finally those which may be nice to know. Allocation of learning should be weighted accordingly with fundamental items filling a majority (typically up to 80%) of the allocated time.

Quality schemes

The delivery of training is a long-term process usually involving inputs from a number of different individuals. In view of this, it is most important that there is a mechanism in place to ensure high-quality delivery at an appropriate level and time, and that it is effective and within budget. Wherever possible, the assurance of quality should involve a mechanism quite independent of the training process, so as to avoid any conflict of interest. At its simplest, this may involve independent assessment or scrutiny of the assessment results by an uninvolved third party. People need to be competent in all aspects of animal care and use with which they will be involved. It has been seen that there are various ways of assessing competence and various problems to be overcome in doing this.

Regardless of the training method, feedback from trainees is a crucial part of the process. This should be gathered anonymously wherever possible and common approaches are by use of a paper form, online (using a dedicated PC) or by verbal communication; the latter precludes anonymity but allows deeper questioning about specific issues and may be used to supplement other methods. Responses may be solicited during the course (e.g. after each lesson) immediately after completion (either before or after the assessment) or several months later – or any combination of these. Focus groups can be a valuable way of reviewing training programmes or dealing with specific issues. Internet-based questionnaires are increasingly being used and an institution may adopt a standard format, which allows comparisons with other courses. It is important that issues raised during feedback are dealt with objectively and communicated to the course participants as well as being discussed by teachers. In addition, participants can be asked to carry out self-evaluation (i.e. do they feel that they truly learned and did the final outcome genuinely match their expectations). These reflections can be collated by the course organiser – if anonymity can be assured.

A more thorough approach is to also review the quality of students' work before and after training and their productivity which may be assessed by regular evaluation by supervisors or work colleagues – more frequently in the case of newly trained personnel. For those working at more senior levels, techniques such as 360° appraisal might be more appropriate.

An additional approach to assurance of training course quality is to secure accreditation from a recognised agency. Accreditation is a process that determines whether appropriate learning experiences are deployed; the process involves verification by an independent accrediting body which assesses course quality against predefined criteria. Such accreditation applies to courses and does not offer assurance about the competence of students. Accrediting bodies usually require courses to be regularly revalidated as a means of ensuring that quality is maintained.

As indicated above, some countries have established schemes to certify the education and training of animal technicians, researchers and also veterinary specialists in laboratory animal science or medicine. For example, in UK, the Home Office requires that Named Veterinary Surgeons have received appropriate post-graduate specialist training. Persons designing procedures and those carrying them out are required to have completed training on an appropriate course accredited by one of three UK accrediting bodies. In the US, veterinarians working in the field of Laboratory Animal Medicine are licensed only when they have completed certification training.

At present, there are few schemes with similar aims for those caring for animals, and attendance at a course of verified quality is often considered to be sufficient. Unfortunately, there are limited opportunities for research technicians to achieve specialist competence certification although there is an example of such a system in a related professional area: the Federation of European Toxicologists & European Societies of Toxicology (EUROTOX) administers a programme based on theoretical and practical training in toxicology, completion of which allows use of the title 'European registered toxicologist'[15].

The IAT[16] is an Awarding Body based in UK and recognised by the Office of Qualifications and Examinations Regulation (Ofqual) that encourages animal technologists to develop their knowledge, skills and attitudes. They are responsible for ensuring that regulated qualifications reliably indicate the knowledge, skills and understanding that students have attained. Courses accredited by the IAT include all levels of laboratory animal carers (EU Function C). Ofqual gathers information relating to the training offered, which it publishes for public use; they hold further data from awarding organisations which they do not publish. Ofqual monitors the IAT's internal processes and qualifications offered to ensure that the latter are fit for regulation.

At a European level, the first accreditation scheme to offer assurance about course quality was established by FELASA in 2002 and was intended to promote wider harmonisation of education and training provision in laboratory animal science (FELASA 2002; Gyger et al. 2018). The scheme was updated and is overseen by an Accreditation Board. It is open to courses which develop full competence in any of the four Functions identified in Directive 2010/63/EU and also provides for recognition of other well-established, non-European courses in laboratory animal science, provided they lead to the development of comparable competences. Course organisers wishing to apply for accreditation submit details of the course frequency, size, curriculum and teaching staff and describe the methodology and materials used in teaching. The Board also requests sight of assessment results, evaluations of the course by students and information about the background of teaching staff. Clarification or further information may be requested if necessary. Members of the Board visit each course and prepare a report which is considered by the full Board and also sent to the course organiser. Course organisers submit an annual (or for courses lasting more than 1 year, biennial) report. The accreditation process is conducted and maintained in strict confidence.

Future trends

Although there is an increasing awareness of the importance of animal care staff in safeguarding the welfare of animals used in biomedical studies, there is a need for greater appreciation of the impact that care routines can have on the quality of scientific output. Related to this is the need for those with overall responsibility for scientific programmes to provide appropriate teaching and assessment methodologies for care staff. In the face of declining budgets and the increasing complexity of investigations, those working at the 'coalface' must be suitably equipped for the changing environment. The importance of 'future-proofing' the competence of care staff argues for approaches to teaching that are not primarily didactic and subject-based but are participative, self-monitored and holistic. There must be regular reviews of the curriculum to ensure that it addresses the current and envisaged needs of the profession and the scientific community. The focus must be on desired learning outcomes and performance rather than programme structure, focusing on the essential competencies the learner will acquire during the programme. And after a period of formal training and the demonstration of competence, staff must be motivated to keep abreast of technical developments by committing to a programme of CPD. Although this may sometimes involve an element of formal instruction, it also requires personal commitment and self-motivation, the ability to network with others and regular horizon scanning to monitor changing practices and technologies. The increasing professionalism arising from such developments will require staff to be appropriately rewarded.

One driver of the changing scene is the increased complexity and expense of many scientific investigations, resulting from advances in research and technology. In addition, *ex-vivo* and *in-vitro* techniques are likely over time to displace many routine animal-based studies, for example in the assessment of toxicity. This will be partly offset by additional experimental approaches requiring the use of whole animals to answer questions that could not be approached in other ways. In order to satisfy budgets, it is likely that in the future collaborative projects between different organisations will become more common. Staff will need to work in conjunction with different facilities (possibly with several different ones at the same time) and will need to learn to adopt new techniques and routines to create a seamless research platform. This has implications for staff flexibility, communication skills and professionalism.

These pressures are likely to require those caring for animals to have an increasingly deep and wider knowledge base as well as deploying consistent, highly proficient practical skills and in part these will be reflected by changes to the methodology used for teaching. Already, remote learning programmes are being developed and it has been predicted that informatics and communication technologies would be a disruptor in education and that massive open online courses (MOOCs) will be among cutting-edge technologies in the current decade. This prediction appears to have become true already as a number of such courses have become available in laboratory animal science, although these are principally directed at those conducting scientific investigations rather those caring for animals. In the future, it is likely that such initiatives will become more widespread, involving strategies based not only on Moodle and Blackboard, but also embracing social media including blogging platforms such as WordPress, wikis and the use of chat rooms (Sandars 2015). Such developments would encourage more careful attention to integrating the learner's needs within the technological format. They demand a 'learning centric' focus within which responsibility for learning is transferred from the teacher (which is frequently the situation at the present time) to the learner, each with his or her own unique needs and preferred approach to

---

[15] http://www.eurotox.com/ert/what-is-ert/ (accessed 1 February 2022)
[16] https://www.iat.org.uk/ (accessed 1 February 2022)

learning. There are trends towards blended learning – flipping the classroom for more dialogue with experts and peers outside of the classroom. The challenge will be to maintain motivation to learn, ensuring the appropriateness of what is being learned and providing resources to enable the learner to chart progress. In contrast, the development of practical skills is likely to continue to involve close supervision and either one-to-one or small group training. Greater use will probably be made of models and visual aids including virtual reality or enhanced reality, before introduction to techniques involving living animals and particularly those of small body mass, which may be susceptible to inadvertent injury. In the words of Alkhatib *et al.* (2015), '*The future holds even more for the integration of work and education via augmented reality. For example, as someone is working, she will receive customized information that allows for progressive training. This scenario will revolutionize several sectors, including customer care training and learning new services and products*'; to which we may add 'animal care and use'.

With the increasing mobility of labour, it is likely that considerable efforts will be made to ensure that the process of assessing competence is increasingly benchmarked and objective although current approaches to assessing knowledge and understanding may well be retained. In contrast, assessment of practical skills needs to become more uniformly objective, and at the time of writing the EU ETPLAS has established a working group to develop an approach using DOPS to progress this[17]. The issue of assessing uniformity between assessors may require the preparation of guidelines and perhaps even the setting of standards. However, the greatest difficulty remains the development of reliable indices of competence. Attempts will undoubtedly be made to develop effective scoring schemes, but their acceptance and adoption appear to be some way off.

References

Albanese, M.A., Mejicano, G., Mullan, P. *et al.* (2008) Defining characteristics of educational competencies. *Medical Education*, **42**, 248–255.

Alkhatib, H., Faraboschi, P., Frachtenberg, E. *et al.* (2015) What will 2022 look like? The IEEE CS 2022 Report. *IEEE Computer*, **48**, 68–76.

Bindal, N., Goodyear, H., Bindal, T. *et al.* (2013) DOPS assessment: a study to evaluate the experience and opinions of trainees and assessors. *Medical Teacher*. **35**, 1230–1234.

Clifford, P., Melfi, N., Bogdanske, J. *et al.* (2013) Assessment of proficiency and competency in laboratory animal biomethodologies. *Journal of the American Association for Laboratory Animal Science*, **52**, 711–716.

Coughlin, P.A. and Featherstone, C.R. (2017) How to write a high quality multiple choice question (MCQ): a guide for clinicians. *European Journal of Vascular and Endovascular Surgery*, **54**, 654–658.

European Commission (2014) National Competent Authorities for the implementation of Directive 2010/63/EU on the protection of animals used for scientific purposes. A working document on the development of a common education and training framework to fulfil the requirements under the Directive. Brussels, http://ec.europa.eu/environment/chemicals/lab_animals/pdf/guidance/animal_welfare_bodies/en.pdf (accessed 25 January 2019).

European Parliament and the Council (2010) Directive 2010/63/EU on the protection of animals used for scientific purposes. *Official Journal of the European Union*, **L 276/33**. https://eur-lex.europa.eu/legal-content/EN/TXT/HTML/?uri=CELEX:32010L0063&from=EN (accessed 28 January 2019).

FELASA (1995) Federation of European Laboratory Animal Science Associations recommendations on the education and training of persons working with laboratory animals: categories A and C. *Laboratory Animals*, **29**, 121–131.

FELASA (1999) Federation of European Laboratory Animal Science Associations guidelines for education of specialists in laboratory animal science (Category D). *Laboratory Animals*, **29**, 1–15.

FELASA (2000) Federation of European Laboratory Animal Science Associations recommendations for the education and training of persons carrying out animal experiments (Category B). *Laboratory Animals*, **34**, 229–235.

FELASA (2002) FELASA recommendations for the accreditation of laboratory animal science education and training. *Laboratory Animals*, **36**, 373–377.

FELASA (2010). Federation of European Laboratory Animal Science Associations: recommendations for the education and training of laboratory animal technicians: Category A. *Laboratory Animals*, **44**, 163–169.

Foshay, W.R. and Tinkey, P.R. (2007) Evaluating the effectiveness of training strategies: performance goals and testing. *ILAR Journal*, **48**, 156–162.

Franco, N.H. and Olsson, I.A.S. (2014). Scientists and the 3Rs: attitudes to animal use in biomedical research and the effect of mandatory training in laboratory animal science. *Laboratory Animals*, **48**, 50–60.

Greenhough, B. and Roe, E. (2017) Exploring the role of animal technologists in implementing the 3Rs: an ethnographic investigation of the UK university sector. *Science, Technology, & Human Values*, **43**, 694–722.

Gyger, M., Berdoy, M., Dontas, I. *et al.* (2018) FELASA accreditation of education and training courses in laboratory animal science according to the Directive 2010/63/EU. *Laboratory Animals*, **52**, 137–147. https://doi.org/10.1177/0023677218788105 (accessed 8 September 2019).

Howard, B., Hudson, M. and Preziosi, R. (2009) More is less: reducing animal use by raising awareness of the principles of efficient study design and analysis. *ATLA*, **37**, 33–42.

Howard, B., Howard, K. and Sandøe, P. (2010) Education, training and competence. In: *The COST Manual of Laboratory Animal Care and Use: Refinement, Reduction, and Research*. Eds Howard, B., Nevalainen, T. and Perretta, G., pp. 369–391. CRC Press, Boca Raton, ISBN 9781439824924.

Kennedy, B.W. and Froeschl, K. (2017) Education and training. In: *Management of Animal Care and Use Programs in Research, Education, and Testing*. Eds Weichbrod, R.H., Thompson, G.A.H. and Norton, J.N. pp 221–266. CRC Press/Taylor & Francis.

Khanghahr, M.E. and Azar, F.E.F. (2018) Direct observation of procedural skills (DOPS) evaluation method: systematic review of evidence. *Medical Journal of the Islamic Republic of Iran*, **32**, 254–261.

Klein, H.J. and Bayne, K.A. (2007) Establishing a culture of care, conscience, and responsibility: addressing the improvement of scientific discovery and animal welfare through science-based performance standards. *ILAR Journal*, **48**, 3–11.

Knowles, M. (1973) *The Adult Learner: A Neglected Species*. Gulf Publishing Company, Houston, USA. Available at https://files.eric.ed.gov/fulltext/ED084368.pdf (accessed 28 August 2019).

Knowles, M.S., Holton, III E.F. and Swanson, R.A. (2015). *The Adult Learner: The Definitive Classic in Adult Education and Human Resource Development*, 8th edn. Routledge, New York, ISBN 0415739020.

---

[17] https://ec.europa.eu/environment/chemicals/lab_animals/pdf/WG-Members_Description_Process-20190109.pdf (accessed 1 February 2022).

Mennin, S. (2015) How can Learning be made more Effective in Medical Education? In: *Routledge Handbook of Medical Education: Global Perspectives and Best Practices*. Eds Abdulrahman, K.A.B., Mennin, S., Harden, R. *et al.*, pp. 207–220. Taylor and Francis (Abingdon, UK). ISBN 9780415815734.

NHMRC (2013) *Australian Code for the Care and Use of Animals for Scientific Purposes*, 8th edn. Canberra: National Health and Medical Research Council.

Norcini, J.J. and McKinkley, D.W. (2007) Assessment methods in medical education. *Teacher and Teaching Education*, **23**, 239–250.

NRC (2011) *National Research Council Guide for the Care and Use of Laboratory Animals*, 8th edn. Washington, DC, The National Academies Press.

Prescott, M.J. and Lidster, K. (2017) Improving quality of science through better animal welfare: the NC3Rs strategy. *Laboratory Animals*, **46**, 152–156.

Pritt, S., Samalonis, P., Bindley, L. *et al.* (2004) Creating a comprehensive training documentation program. *Laboratory Animals*, **33**, 38–41.

Pritt, S. and Duffee, N. (2007) Training strategies for animal care technicians and veterinary technical staff. *ILAR Journal*, **48**, 109–119.

Pryce-Miller, M. (2010) Are first year undergraduate student nurses prepared for self directed learning? *Nursing Times*, **106(46)**, 21–24.

Romick, M.L., Chavez, J. and Bishop, B. (2006) An interdisciplinary performance-based approach to training laboratory animal technicians. *Laboratory Animals*, **35**, 35–39.

von Roten, F.C. (2018). Laboratory animal science course in Switzerland: participants' points of view and implications for organizers. *Laboratory Animals*, **52**, 68–79.

Russell, W. and Burch, R. (1959) *The Principles of Humane Experimental Technique*. Methuen, London. (2nd edn. 1992 UFAW) http://altweb.jhsph.edu/publications/humane_exp/het-toc.htm (accessed 27 April 2008).

Sandars, J. (2015) New technologies can contribute to a successful educational programme. In: *Routledge Handbook of Medical Education: Global Perspectives and Best Practices*. Eds Abdulrahman, K.A.B., Mennin, S., Harden, R. *et al.*, pp. 221–234. Taylor and Francis (Abingdon, UK). ISBN 9780415815734.

Silverman, J. (2016) *Managing the Laboratory Animal Facility*, 3rd Edition. CRC Press, Boca Raton, London, New York, Washington DC.

Schuwirth, L. (2015) How to implement a meaningful assessment programme. In: *Routledge Handbook of Medical Education: Global Perspectives and Best Practices*. Eds Abdulrahman, K.B., Harden, R.M., Mennin, R.M.S., pp. 237–246. Taylor and Francis (Abingdon, UK).

Symonowiez, C. (2006) Motivation of animal care technicians through recognition. *Laboratory Animals*, **35**, 39–42.

Swiss Animal Welfare Ordinance (2008) https://www.admin.ch/opc/fr/classified-compilation/20080796/index.html (accessed 1 February 2022).

Tyng, C.M., Amin, H.U., Saad, M.N.M. *et al.* (2017) The influences of emotion on learning and memory. *Frontiers in Psychology*, **8**, 1454. Published online https://www.ncbi.nlm.nih.gov/pmc/articles/PMC5573739/ (accessed 14 August 2019).

Weir, L.K., Barker, M.K., McDonnell, L.M. *et al.* (2019) Small changes, big gains: a curriculum-wide study of teaching practices and student learning in undergraduate biology. *PLoS ONE*, **14**(8), e0220900. https://doi.org/10.1371/journal.pone.0220900 (accessed 14 August 2019).

Wragg, A., Wade, W., Fuller, G. *et al*. (2003). Assessing the performance of specialist registrars. *Clinical Medicine*, **3**, 131–134.

15 The use of positive reinforcement training techniques to enhance the care and welfare of laboratory and research animals

Gail Laule

Introduction

Concern for the welfare of animals in captivity by professionals, NGOs and the general public has increased significantly in the last 20 years, with a particular focus on both the zoological and biomedical research communities. This concern is based on the widespread recognition that every animal in captivity deserves the best care possible. Animals housed and managed in a laboratory setting have both individual needs (Capitanio 2011) and those specific to the species, and must cope with an array of potentially negative experiences. Despite efforts by the research community to provide more species-appropriate housing options and socialisation opportunities, many laboratory animals still live in small relatively barren cages, sometimes without social companions, are handled and restrained frequently, and are subjected to a wide range of invasive husbandry and medical procedures. These conditions create significant challenges to collective efforts to enhance animal welfare.

The fundamental premise of this chapter is that the application of positive reinforcement training techniques in the daily care and management of animals used in research, as well as in their participation in research studies, can lead to significant reductions in overall negative experiences while increasing positive ones. This directly contributes to refining the use of animals in research (see Chapter 2 – The three Rs) and improving the quality of data collected from them as less stressed animals make better research models.

The use of positive reinforcement training (PRT) has grown in acceptance over the last two decades to the point of being referred to as a best practice, 'gold standard', and key welfare refinement in the management of laboratory animals in the substantial body of literature describing the benefits of PRT for scientific, veterinary and husbandry purposes (Laule *et al.* 2003; Prescott & Buchanan-Smith 2003, 2007; Coleman *et al.* 2008; Bowell 2010; Perlman *et al.* 2010, 2012; Kemp *et al.* 2017; Martin *et al.* 2018; Fischer & Wegener 2018).

There has also emerged an increasing interest in measuring the effects of training through scientific studies. PRT techniques are now recommended as good practice by many legislative and professional research guidelines as well (e.g. Home Office 1989; Institute of Laboratory Animal Resources 1986); International Primatological Society 1989; Laboratory Animal Science Association/Medical Research Council 2004; National Research Council 1998).

This chapter provides a review of basic training methods and their application. It also includes practical suggestions for integrating a PRT approach into the management of animals in the laboratory setting.

When does training occur?

In day-to-day management activities, animals are being trained all the time, whether the humans realise it or not. Every time anyone interacts with an animal, there is some training/communication occurring. The more frequent the interaction, the more established resultant behaviours become. Caregivers, veterinarians, researchers, technicians and other staff can affect changes in behaviour (aka training). When a caregiver places a desirable food item in a cage, opens the door and the animal moves into that cage, training has occurred. While no 'intentional' training has been conducted, the animal's behaviour changes through a process of operant conditioning. However, much better results, whether for routine care or research, can be attained by consciously and deliberately implementing the training process.

Which species to train?

Most of the applications of training for management, husbandry, and medical purposes in the biomedical field have focused on nonhuman primates and dogs. As a domestic

---

The UFAW Handbook on the Care and Management of Laboratory and Other Research Animals, Ninth Edition.
Edited by Huw Golledge and Claire Richardson.
© 2024 John Wiley & Sons Ltd. Published 2024 by John Wiley & Sons Ltd.

species and common household pet, laboratory dogs are managed differently than other animals, with direct contact in the form of petting, playing, walking on a leash and manual restraint for simple procedures. Training is used to augment an inherently positive human–animal relationship where simple verbal praise has significant value to many individuals. There are many good resources on the training of dogs within the laboratory setting (Clark 1999; Prescott *et al.* 2004; Lindsay 2005; Meunier 2006), and many others on general dog training that present positive training techniques that can be applied to the laboratory setting (Donaldson 1996; Pryor 1999; McConnell 2002; Colflesh 2004; Overall & Dyer 2005; see also Chapter 30 – The laboratory dog), so this specific subject will not be covered in depth in this chapter.

Farm animals are also prime candidates for training. As domesticated animals, the emphasis is again on developing a positive human/animal relationship and using positive handling techniques to minimise stress during restraint and to gain voluntary cooperation to the extent of each species' cognitive abilities; swine being amenable to more complex training objectives (Sørensen *et al.* 2005; Sørensen 2010; Coleman & Hemsworth 2014).

Nonhuman primates, however, are not domesticated and do not have an inherent affiliation to humans; in fact, it is often quite the opposite. Therefore, training primates focuses on developing a positive human/animal relationship, gaining safe access to individuals whether singly housed (Reinhardt 1992) or in a group setting (Kemp *et al.* 2017), and gaining an animal's voluntary cooperation in husbandry and medical procedures (Brando 2012; Westlund 2015), so that more negative forms of restraint and coercion can be reduced or eliminated (Graham *et al.* 2012; McMillan *et al.* 2014).

Finally, rodents, rabbits and birds make up the vast majority of animals used in research. Although rodents are capable of learning a wide range of tasks as evidenced by numerous experiments by Skinner (1938) and others (Ferster 2002; Hernstein 1997), they are small enough to be easily handled and restrained. Therefore, training is primarily based on habituation or acclimation (see the section titled 'Using PRT techniques to address fear') through the practice of patience, empathy and a calm, gentle handling style rather than formal PRT (Annas *et al.* 2013).

The techniques discussed in this chapter are universal and apply to all species and individuals to varying degrees. PRT techniques can enhance the welfare of laboratory animals by contributing to the implementation of research procedures with as little stress for the animals as possible (Lambeth *et al.* 2006). Less stressed animals make better research models and produce the most reliable research results (Bloomsmith 1992; Reinhardt 1997, 1997a; Bassett *et al.* 2003). Therefore, these techniques should be applied whenever reasonable and feasible to do so.

Operant conditioning

Operant conditioning is defined as a type of learning in which the probability of a behaviour recurring is increased or decreased by the consequences that follow (Pryor 1999). These consequences include reinforcement, whether positive or negative, which increases the probability that the behaviour will occur again; and punishment, whose purpose is to reduce the likelihood that a behaviour will occur again. (Figure 15.1).

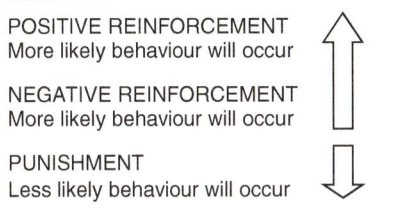

Figure 15.1 The behavioural consequences of positive and negative reinforcement and punishment.

There is sometimes confusion between the terms 'negative reinforcement' and 'punishment', primarily because of the term 'negative'. But the operative word is 'reinforcement' which defines the purpose and anticipated outcome of the action. The use of negative reinforcement in the management of laboratory animals is of particular significance because of its aversive qualities and will be addressed in detail later in this chapter.

Positive reinforcement training (PRT)

The training discussed and recommended in this chapter is based on the use of positive reinforcement in which animals are rewarded with something they like for responding appropriately to the caregiver's cues or commands (Pryor 1999). In practical terms, it means that when the animal performs the correct behaviour, for example laying down, presenting a leg, or moving into an adjacent cage, the behaviour is followed with something the animal wants: food, praise, tactile contact, favourite toy, release to a favoured place, etc. That sequence increases the chance of the response occurring again.

Voluntary cooperation by the animal is a key characteristic of a positive reinforced-based system (Laule & Desmond 1994), allowing animals greater choice and control in how and when they participate in procedures (Badihi 2006; Laule & Whittaker 2007). Even within the constraints of study designs and protocols, some measure of choice can and should be offered (Kurtycz 2015) (see the section titled 'Practical approach to training laboratory animals'). It should be emphasised that PRT does not require food or water deprivation – animals should be provided their daily allotment of food and water. Training rewards can be preferred diet items, or special treats reserved for training alone.

Negative reinforcement training (NRT)

Negative reinforcement (NRT) involves following an action or response by removing an unpleasant aversive stimulus, no matter how mild, that the subject wants to avoid (Pryor 1999). The aversive stimulus may be the threat of a net or glove, the side of a restraint chute moving inward or the presentation of a novel object that elicits even a mild fear response from the animal (Prescott & Buchanan-Smith 2007; Wergård *et al.* 2015). Fear of the aversive stimulus triggers an escape/avoidance response, which leads to performance of the desired behaviour. The proper use of NRT requires that the aversive stimulus is removed immediately after the correct behaviour is performed. For example, a net is used to threaten or coerce a monkey to move from one cage into another and then removed as soon as the monkey complies.

Animal management practices in the laboratory have traditionally included a high frequency of negative reinforcement. Devices like squeeze backs are used as a routine means of encouraging and/or forcing animals to the front of the cage for access and manipulation. Unfortunately, negative reinforcers are sometimes accompanied by other unpleasant stimuli like authoritative or loud voices and physical threats including chasing of animals (i.e. primates in large corral situations; livestock in pens) by animal care staff (Coleman & Hemsworth 2014).

NRT is quite effective in achieving behavioural results and can often do so faster than PRT (Laule *et al.* 2003; Perlman *et al.* 2012; Wergård *et al.* 2015). However, there is an inherent cost to the animal's welfare through the threat of a negative event or experience that elicits fear or anxiety (Reinhardt 1992; Laule & Desmond 1997; Pryor 1999; Bacon 2018) and, if used, such methods require ethical justification. For example, studies with farm animals have shown a high degree of fear response associated with negative handling methods. In one study on managing heifers using negative methods that included hits and slaps, fearful animals showed both acute and chronic stress responses (Breuer *et al.* 1998). Negative handling methods with chickens often leads to escape reactions with associated injury, decreased breeding behaviour and greater inter-flock aggression (Jones 1997).

In contrast, dogs trained exclusively using reward-based methods were reported to be significantly more obedient and to exhibit less problem behaviours like food stealing and over-excitement than dogs trained using negative methods (including punishment), or even a combination of positive and negative methods (Hiby *et al.* 2004).

Combined use of NRT and PRT

Operationally, it may not be feasible to utilise PRT exclusively in the laboratory setting, especially with the pressures of time and human resource constraints. However, despite the challenges, positive alternatives should be exhausted before any kind of NRT is employed. If an escape-avoidance technique is necessary, its use should be kept to a minimum and balanced by positive reinforcement (Laule *et al.* 2003; McKinley 2004; Warren-Smith & McGreevy 2007). For example, restraining an animal in a squeeze cage can be immediately followed by offering the animal a preferred food treat. Effort should also be made to use the least aversive stimuli in NRT. Wergård *et al.* (2015) achieved greater success in training naïve pair-housed rhesus macaques with a combination of NRT and PRT than with PRT alone to respond to a cue, enter a specific section of the cage and accept a gate board being closed. The mildly aversive stimuli were novel objects mounted on a stick and presented slowly from a distance of approximately 120 cm from the animals.

In another study, rhesus macaques were trained to cooperate for pole-and-collar transfer to a primate restraint chair using primarily PRT with supplemental use of the squeeze back as a negative reinforcer to accelerate training progress (McMillan *et al.* 2014). In both these cases, the use of NRT was limited and the goal was to eliminate its use over time.

Benefits of PRT

PRT can be used to enhance the care, management and welfare of laboratory animals in a number of ways (Kirkwood *et al.* 1989; Reinhardt 1997; Laule *et al.* 2003). From an animal welfare perspective, PRT is based on voluntary cooperation, which directly contributes to offering animals greater choice and control (Hanson *et al.* 1976; Buchanan-Smith & Badihi 2012; Whitehouse *et al.* 2013). It also provides animals the opportunity to work for their food (Neuringer 1969; Anderson & Chamove 1984; Laule & Desmond 1997). Both factors have been associated with enhanced welfare (Hanson *et al.* 1976; Markowitz 1982; Mineka *et al.* 1986; Perlman *et al.* 2012; Kurtycz 2015).

As an example, consider the animal who must receive an injection for a research protocol. Without training, the animal has no choice in how that event occurs. If NRT is used, the threat of a negative stimulus is necessary to achieve the desired behaviour of presenting a leg for the injection, thus exposing the animal to stress from both stimuli. Using a positive reinforcement approach, the animal is trained through shaping and rewards to voluntarily present a leg for an injection, and concurrently desensitised to the procedure to reduce the associated fear or anxiety (the processes of shaping and desensitisation are described in detail later in this chapter). It would seem logical to argue that having a clearer choice in how that event happens, and being less fearful of it, contributes to that animal's well-being. (Reinhardt *et al.* 1990; Turkkan *et al.* 1990; Perlman *et al.* 2004; Videan *et al.* 2005; Lambeth *et al.* 2006).

PRT allows many husbandry and veterinary procedures to be implemented with less disruption to the animals. It reduces the need to separate individuals from their social groups (Schapiro *et al.* 2003; Laule & Whittaker 2007) and the need for restraint and anaesthesia (Bloomsmith 1992; Reinhardt *et al.* 1995; McKinley *et al.* 2003). PRT provides the tools to improve husbandry and veterinary care (Laule & Desmond 1994; Bassett *et al.* 2003; Prescott *et al.* 2005; Schapiro *et al.* 2005; Coleman *et al.* 2008; Gillis *et al.* 2012; Graham *et al.* 2012; Westlund 2015); enhance cooperation in collection of urine, semen and blood samples (Phillipi-Falkenstein & Clarke 1992; VandeVoort *et al.* 1993; Stone *et al.* 1994; Laule *et al.* 1996; McKinley *et al.* 2003; Smith *et al.* 2004; Bloomsmith *et al.* 2015); reduce abnormal and/or stereotypic behaviour (Laule 1993; Laule 2005; Whittaker 2005; Bloomsmith *et al.* 2007; Baker *et al.* 2003; Coleman & Maier 2010); reduce aggression (Bloomsmith *et al.* 1994; Minier *et al.* 2011); improve socialisation (Desmond *et al.* 1987; Desmond & Laule 1994; Bloomsmith 1994; Baker 2004; Perlman *et al.* 2010); enhance enrichment programmes (Bloomsmith *et al.* 1997, 1999; Laule & Desmond 1997) and increase the safety of the attending personnel (Bloomsmith 1994; Martin *et al.* 2011).

Experience has shown that trained animals maintain a high degree of reliability in participating in procedures and are less stressed while doing so (Reinhardt *et al.* 1990; Turkkan *et al.* 1990; Lambeth *et al.* 2006). Evidence for this includes reports of reductions in cortisol levels, stress-related abortions, physical resistance to handling and fear responses such as fear-grinning, screaming and acute diarrhoea in a variety of primate species (Moseley & Davis 1989; Vertein & Reinhardt 1989; Reinhardt *et al.* 1990).

One area of great concern in primate husbandry is reduction of self-injurious behaviours (SIB). Bloomsmith *et al.* (2007, pp. 211) reviewed a number of studies that, '…although preliminarily in nature, indicate that stereotyped behaviour and SIB in nonhuman primates can be modified through the use of operant conditioning'. No studies achieved complete elimination of the problematic behaviour, but significant reductions were documented.

PRT objectives

The following are examples of training objectives relevant to the laboratory setting:

- achieve voluntary cooperation by animals in daily husbandry activities, and medical and research procedures (i.e. blood draw, injections, urine collection, enter restraint cage, move to different cage, blood pressure measurement, topical treatment, oral dosing, etc.)
- reduce fear and discomfort to a wide array of stimuli (medical procedures, human presence, handling and restraint, novel equipment, new places, conspecifics, etc.)
- decrease abnormal or stereotypic behaviour (locomotor, appetitive, SIB, etc.)
- reduce or eliminate aggressive behaviour towards conspecifics and/or caregivers
- facilitate introductions and socialisation with conspecifics (pair housing, group formation)
- create opportunities for greater choice and control (voluntary cooperation in wider array of activities, preference testing, etc.)

PRT methods – tools and techniques

To achieve all the potential benefits of PRT requires skillful and effective implementation. It is beyond the scope of this chapter to provide a step-by-step guide to the training of laboratory animals, however, some sample training protocols for specific behaviours have been provided. The following is a brief discussion of the basic tools and techniques of PRT, and suggested steps to be taken in the training process. Although these are used most often with primates, they apply to the management of all species and individual animals.

Basic tools of PRT

1. *Positive reinforcers* – A positive reinforcer is anything the animal likes. Food, tactile contact, verbal praise, a favoured enrichment item, access to conspecifics and play are all potential reinforcers. Food, which is the most often used reinforcer, can be part of the normal diet, enrichment allotment or an extra treat. It is always beneficial to have a variety of reinforcers to choose from and to know how the animal perceives their value (recognising that animals' preferences and perceptions can change over time).

2. *Conditioned reinforcer (Bridge)* – A conditioned reinforcer is an initially meaningless signal that, when repeatedly associated with a primary reinforcer (make the sound then offer the reward), takes on reinforcing properties of its own. The animal learns that every time it hears that signal, a reward will follow. The most commonly used bridge in animal training is a verbal 'good', hand-held clicker or dog whistle, but other bridges are also possible, and for each species and/or task the most appropriate can be chosen.

The bridge performs the following functions, it:

- provides precise information about which behaviour will be rewarded
- signals that the primary reinforcer is coming
- bridges the gap between the behaviour occurring and the food reward being delivered

The use of a conditioned reinforcer, particularly a mechanical bridge like the clicker, is highly recommended for training laboratory animals as it is much easier to closely associate a conditioned reinforcer with the desired behaviour. A clicker is preferred to a verbal 'good' because the sound is always the same no matter who uses it, voices are not. Furthermore, the sound occurs only in the context of training. It is also more precise, pinpointing an instant in time more effectively than the verbal 'good'. Finally, many trainers and care staff find it natural and useful to talk to the animal and encourage positive behaviour during training. The clicker remains a discreet sound delivering precise information, even if the trainer is simultaneously providing verbal encouragement to the animal.

During the training process, the bridge often coincides with the end of the behaviour but should not be the signal that the behaviour is complete. Other actions will indicate that the behaviour is finished, e.g. trainer reaches for food, trainer changes position or tone of voice, a verbal release like 'alright' is given or the trainer presents another cue.

Using the bridge *during* a behaviour (an 'intermediate bridge') is important for:

- building duration by incrementally reinforcing the continuation of the desired behaviour (e.g. stationing, positioning, body part presentation)
- delivering precise information throughout a sequence or chain of behaviours; (e.g. remaining still and calm during series of steps of blood draw)
- allowing delivery of intermediate food reinforcement throughout the behaviour in direct relation to animal's response
- allowing the use of a variable schedule for food reward, so the bridge reinforces the behaviour either alone or with the primary reinforcement

3. *Target* – A target is an object that the animal is trained to move towards, to follow, to remain nearby and to touch. Commonly used targets include a ball or flat object on the end of a stick, a plastic bottle, a wooden dowel or PVC

pipe, or any object that can be easily held by the trainer or attached to the enclosure, for example with a carabiner. Depending on the type of animal being trained, it may be useful to have various types of targets including stationary and movable, and targets of varying lengths.

Primates are normally trained to touch their hand to the target. Other species may be taught to touch the target with a limb or the nose. Contact usually first occurs spontaneously as most animals are curious to touch or sniff something new. However, if the animal is fearful or apprehensive of the target, the behaviour can be taught in small steps as follows:

- move the object towards the animal's hand or nose a little bit at a time and reinforce each time it gets closer
- hold the target stationary and reinforce any forward movement the animal makes towards the target
- or a combination of both

A target is used to achieve the following, to:

- control/elicit gross movement (move to cage front, shift between enclosures, present body part by moving foot, paw, arm, leg, chest, back, side, etc. to the target)
- control/elicit small or fine movement (open mouth, small adjustment of body positioning, etc.)
- stay at the target to achieve or extend stationing

Once stationing is established, socially housed animals can be trained to remain at their own individual target, allowing the trainer to access individual animals within the group.

PRT techniques – options for teaching behaviour

Shaping or successive approximation

Shaping is the process of breaking a behaviour into small, individual steps that build upon each other, eventually leading to the completed behaviour. Teaching an animal to touch a target by moving it incrementally closer and closer and reinforcing any movement the animal makes towards it, no matter how small or tentative, is a simple example of shaping. In some cases, shaping starts with reinforcing a naturally occurring behaviour. For example, to train a dog to open its mouth, the first step may be to hold a food treat up for it to see. When the mouth opens in anticipation, a quick 'Good' or a click followed by the delivery of the treat is the first step in the shaping process.

The following training protocol illustrates the potential approximations in training a pig to enter a squeeze cage:

- Choose a verbal and/or hand cue for the behaviour, such as 'inside'; use a hand-held clicker as a bridge.
- Place the squeeze cage in enclosure, or attach to door of home cage, and bridge and reinforce when pig looks at squeeze.
- Bridge and reinforce any movement towards the squeeze.
- A target can be used to direct the animal to the squeeze.
- Bridge and reinforce any exploratory behaviour such as sniffing the squeeze, looking inside, touching with nose or foot.
- Bridge and reinforce any forward movement into the squeeze; a target can be attached to inside back of squeeze and animal reinforced for moving towards it.
- Use verbal cue 'inside' whenever the animal initiates movement towards the squeeze or trainer encourages movement towards or into the squeeze.
- Once animal is entering the squeeze, send the animal in and out of the squeeze (reinforcing movement in both directions) to firmly establish cue and strengthen the desired behaviour.
- Reinforce animal for remaining in the squeeze for progressively longer periods of time.
- Begin to move door, small amount at a time for short periods of time, bridging and reinforcing each approximation, until pig will remain inside while door closes.
- Slowly increase the amount of time the door is closed.
- When pig is comfortable in the squeeze with the door closed, begin to repeat the last two steps with the squeeze back until pig will stand calmly when completely restrained.

The key to successful shaping is the ability to identify appropriate-sized steps. Steps that are too big can create confusion and frustration in the animal. Too small steps can lead to loss of motivation and boredom. Generally speaking, the most common mistake made by new trainers is to expect too much from the animal and attempt steps that are too big. The aim should always be to end each training session on a positive note, no matter how small the step achieved.

Capturing behaviour

Capturing is another option for training behaviour and involves reinforcing a behaviour when it naturally occurs. Some behaviours can only be trained by capturing (e.g. urination, defecation, vocalisation). The trainer must wait until the behaviour occurs, then immediately bridge and reinforce. Over several repetitions, the reward becomes associated with the behaviour which then slowly shifts from a naturally occurring even random act to a deliberate action by the animal. It is best to decide ahead of time a cue for the behaviour, and pair that verbal or visual cue with the bridge and reward.

For example, to capture urination on cue, whenever the monkey urinates, the trainer bridges, says the verbal cue or shows the visual cue (e.g. the collection cup) and gives the reward. Repetition is key, so it's useful to know an individual's pattern of urination, for example first thing in the morning, or some other relatively predictable time so that the trainer can be ready with reinforcers. To increase the likelihood of urination occurring, the trainer can give the monkey some water or juice and then return half an hour later to capture urination when it occurs. Capturing a behaviour such as urination takes initial time to train. However, once trained the benefits are significant, including saving staff hours to collect samples, allowing the collection of clean mid-stream samples from animals in their home cages and sampling without the need to separate animals from their social group. Additionally, there is very high reliability of the behaviour over time (Laule et al. 1996; Bloomsmith et al. 2015).

There are methods to shorten the training period to capture a behaviour. In one study with chimpanzees by Perlman *et al.* (2010), the pace of learning was accelerated by providing an opportunity for social learning through a video that showed female chimpanzees urinating into a collection cup and receiving a food reward. The experimental group that watched the video reached reliable performance (success four out of five times) significantly faster than those from the control group.

Regression – Training and learning are complex processes and progress is not linear. In fact, it occurs in steps forward *and* backward. The progress the animal makes one day seems to be forgotten the next. Then suddenly learning accelerates, and the animal moves two steps forward. Each of the backward steps is called regression, and it is a normal part of training.

Delivery of reinforcement

Schedules of reinforcement

Schedules of reinforcement govern when the reinforcement is delivered. There are many schedules of reinforcement that can be found in the operant conditioning literature (Pryor 1999), but two are most useful in practice.

- *Continuous schedule* – Reinforcement is given after every correct response. This schedule should be used when training new behaviour. In PRT, learning through successive approximations involves trial and error by the animal, so it's necessary to reinforce every correct response. Each time reinforcement is delivered, important information is provided that will help the animal learn. A continuous schedule is also recommended to maintain invasive or unpleasant behaviours, like an injection or blood draw. Behaviours that are important for daily management, for example shifting between areas, should also be reinforced every time.

    Experience has shown that a continuous schedule is most effective when the amount and type of reward given is varied based on the quality of the response being reinforced. (See also magnitude of reinforcement in the following text).
- *Variable or intermittent schedule* – Reinforcing correct behavioural responses by offering the *primary* reinforcement (food) on a random or unpredictable basis to the animal. This schedule is only appropriate for complete behaviours. It is useful when an animal is responding to a series of cues, for example with a body exam where the animal presents a series of body parts for examination. It is also an opportunity to reinforce with food (perhaps a more preferred food item) those behaviours that are more difficult, of higher quality, newer or have been problematic in previous sessions.

Selective or differential reinforcement

Effective training relies on good decision making on how and when to reinforce. Once an animal is responding correctly to the cue, reinforcing selected responses of higher quality will improve performance.

Magnitude of reinforcement

The magnitude of reinforcement refers to the type, size, amount of reinforcement used and its perceived value to the animal. PRT is based on voluntary cooperation, so an animal's motivation to cooperate can be positively impacted by choosing the best reinforcement for the task. In one study by Martin *et al.* (2018), rhesus macaques were more engaged in training sessions when their more preferred reinforcers were used. Subjects worked longer and more quickly when provided with a highly preferred food item as compared to a less preferred food item.

It is recommended to have a variety of reinforcers available for training that are used flexibly, based on the animal's preference for the different rewards, and the difficulty or complexity of the behaviour being reinforced.

Fisher and Wegener (2018) recognised the specific challenges of training primates in the behavioural tasks used in cognitive neuroscientific studies, that include: working outside familiar environments while restrained; attending to rather abstract cues; and the requirement to perform hundreds of consecutive trials. The researchers used a nonbinary, graded reward schedule, based on offering higher value reinforcers for all correct, desired behaviours and lesser value reinforcers for lesser quality behavioural responses. This increased the motivation of the animals by keeping unreinforced errors to a moderate level.

Preference testing is useful in assessing the perceived value of reinforcement items for each individual (Badihi 2006; Martin *et al.* 2018), although preferences can change over time (Clay *et al.* 2009). Incorporating preference testing into PRT sessions may also have welfare benefits, for example, decreasing the need for fluid and food restriction (Tulipa *et al.* 2017; Westlund 2015). Finally, allowing the animal to choose a reinforcer may, in itself, enhance the welfare of laboratory animals (Perdue *et al.* 2014).

Jackpot or bonus

A jackpot or bonus is a reward that is much bigger, in quantity and in value, than the normal reinforcer, and comes as a surprise to the subject. A well-placed jackpot can be a very powerful way of reinforcing desired behaviour. It should be special, so not overused.

Addressing undesirable behaviour

There are two appropriate and acceptable techniques that are well-suited for a laboratory environment and can be used in a PRT system to reduce or eliminate undesirable behaviour.

Time out

Punishment, by definition, is designed to decrease or eliminate behaviour by adding something the animal does not like or removing something the animal does like. In PRT, physical punishment is not appropriate except in a life-threatening situation for person or animal. The only acceptable punisher is a 'time out', which briefly takes away the animal's opportunity to participate in training and earn a reward.

Time out – Punishment, by definition, is designed to eliminate behaviour and occurs after the behavioural response. (Note: The term 'punishment' is often confused with 'negative reinforcement' which has the opposite effect and significantly different timing. Negative reinforcement is designed to increase the likelihood of a behaviour occurring and is used at the same time the behaviour occurs.) In PRT, the only acceptable punisher is a 'time out'. Physical punishment is not appropriate except in a life-threatening situation for person or animal. A time out is a very mild form of punishment in which reinforcement is withheld for a brief period of time immediately following an inappropriate response. A time out can vary in quality and length, from the trainer breaking eye contact for several seconds to walking away for a couple of moments. A time out is a very simple, powerful response to undesirable behaviour, with two basic rules:

- Do not use a time out too often or it will lose its effectiveness.
- Always follow a time out by giving the animal another chance to start fresh either by retrying the original behaviour or moving on to a different one.

Extinction

Extinction (no longer reinforcing a behaviour) is a very useful method of reducing or eliminating a problem behaviour. The trainer must determine what exactly the reinforcement is (food, attention, etc.) and then ensure that it is consistently withheld whenever the behaviour occurs. Extinction is most effective when paired with the reinforcement of a more desirable alternative behaviour. For example, a macaque has been inadvertently reinforced with attention for reaching out to grab people with her hand. All staff stop giving her attention whenever she reaches out, and simultaneously, the animal is given attention every time she keeps her hand inside the cage.

Improving the human/animal relationship

Because humans have almost complete control over the important features of a captive animal's life, the decisions and behaviour of humans have perhaps the greatest potential to both compromise and enhance animal welfare (Waiblinger *et al.* 2006; Mellor 2012; Brando & Buchanan-Smith 2018). A patient, empathetic handler with a gentle hand, quiet voice and measured approach will contribute much towards the well-being of an animal, no matter what the circumstance or the species. Wolfle (1985, pp. 450) argues, 'It is not an overstatement to say that the right animal technician instils qualities in the animals that make them better and more reliable research subjects'.

One of the most effective ways to establish a positive relationship with captive animals is to have some positive interaction with them on a daily basis. Bayne *et al.* (1993) found that 3–5 minutes of positive interactions and treat provisioning daily with singly housed rhesus macaques (*Macaca mulatta*) resulted in decreased abnormal behaviour and overall fear. Baker (2004) reported that 10 minutes a day of positive interactions and treat provisioning reduced aggressive responses to humans and the occurrence of abnormal behaviour in group-housed chimpanzees. PRT used as an enrichment strategy for primates resulted in similar reductions of abnormal behaviour and anxiety-related behaviour (Baker *et al.* 2003).

Studies have shown that petting a dog can have a calming effect and decrease heart and respiratory rates (Gantt *et al.* 1966) and may be effective in reducing cortisol responses to aversive situations such as physical examinations, injections and blood sampling (Hennessy *et al.* 1998). With gentle handling and positive reinforcement techniques, pigs can be readily trained to tolerate a simple physical examination, to walk out of their cages to another location, and to accept restraint, including manual, mechanical (i.e. a sling) and chemical (Smith & Swindle 2006).

PRT is a powerful vehicle for creating a positive bond between human and animal. The very nature of the process – gaining the voluntary cooperation of the animal and rewarding behavioural performance with something the animal likes – enhances both the behaviour and the motivation to perform it, and all within the context of a positive interaction. Furthermore, specific training techniques that are directed at reducing fear can serve the dual purpose of achieving a positive human–animal relationship while reducing stress for the animal.

Using PRT techniques to address fear

Animals in laboratory environments are faced with a wide array of fearful stimuli and experiences, with humans often the source of anxiety, pain and discomfort. When feeling threatened and/or fearful, flight is normally the first strategy employed by animals. However, in the confined spaces of the laboratory, escape is not possible. This tends to lead to either the fight response, which we label as aggression (Hediger 1950) or an avoidance behaviour (Boissey 1995), often seen as the rodent who retreats from the human hand, the dog that cowers in the corner of the kennel, the swine who emits a 'squeal' when approached or the primate who is pressed against the back of the cage and refuses to approach for a food treat.

Laboratory animals demonstrate fearful responses when subjected to invasive medical procedures like blood draws, dosing of medications and injections. Restraint procedures such as the use of a squeeze cage, tether, gloves, pole and collar, restraint chair, sling and restraint board will trigger varying degrees of fear, physical discomfort, and stress in most animals. Studies have shown repeatedly that even routine procedures by familiar personnel, traditionally viewed as neutral events, may result in persistent stress responses (Malinow *et al.* 1974; Line *et al.* 1989).

When ongoing fear is unresolved, the animal can remain in a chronic stress response or state of distress (Moberg 1985; Toates 1995). It can also lead to an array of abnormal behaviours (Erwin & Den 1979; Anderson & Chamove 1980; Laule 2005).

From a practical perspective, it will be difficult to gain the voluntary cooperation of an animal in any husbandry or research procedure if that animal is overwhelmed by fear.

The animal must be able to tolerate the stimulus to the degree that a reward is accepted and learning is possible.

Therefore, it is important for all staff responsible for the care of research animals to:

1. recognise fear
2. acknowledge its effects
3. adjust behavioural criteria and expectations accordingly
4. develop and implement strategies to reduce fear.

One of the most significant applications of PRT is the reduction of fear in the laboratory animal (Laule 2005; Laule & Whittaker 2007). Diminishing fear directly enhances welfare and increases the likelihood of achieving a greater degree of cooperation by the animal in behavioural objectives. PRT is most beneficial and effective in reducing fear by:

- providing a context for interactions that build a positive human/animal relationship
- applying the techniques of habituation and desensitisation to directly address the fear response.

Habituation or acclimation

Habituation is a widely accepted approach to managing laboratory animals and their fearful, painful or stressful experiences (Ruys *et al.* 2004). It refers to the process of gradually accustoming an animal to a situation that it normally avoids, by prolonged exposure. It differs from desensitisation in that there is no direct pairing of a positive reinforcer with the fear-inducing stimulus. Once the animal no longer displays the behavioural signs of fear or stress, it is assumed to have habituated or acclimated to the previous stressor. Habituation is often used rather than desensitisation, because of time and resource constraints.

For example, habituation is used to help primates like macaques or baboons to get used to chair restraint. It is readily acknowledged that forced restraint is stressful for an animal. Behavioural signs include physical resistance and struggling, heightened agitation, alarm vocalisations and facial expressions of fear and defensive threats (Reinhardt *et al.* 1995). Physiological changes include increased respiration and heart rate, and activation of the hypothalamic–pituitary–adrenal (HPA) axis, and the secretion of glucocorticoids in proportion to the intensity of the perceived threat (Bassett *et al.* 2003; Grissom *et al.* 2008).

With repeated exposure to the restraint, behavioural and physiological responses diminish, which is cited as evidence that the animal has become habituated to the experience. However, one study by Ruys *et al.* (2004) showed that after repeated chairing of rhesus macaques (*Macaca mulatta*) expected behavioural changes occurred, yet there was still an HPA response, albeit diminished, suggesting the animals may not be truly habituated.

Compliance on the part of the animal, therefore, may not be indicative of the level of stress the individual is experiencing (McMillan *et al.* 2014). Using habituation followed by desensitisation can help reduce this stress. This was demonstrated in a study by Lambeth *et al* (2006). Results showed that total white blood cell (WBC) counts, blood glucose (GLU) levels and absolute segmented neutrophils (SEG) levels were significantly lower in chimpanzees that voluntarily presented their arms for injection than in animals that received an injection through coercion or the use of a dart-gun. Moreover, a within-subject analysis showed that individuals had significantly lower WBC and GLU levels when they voluntarily presented for the injection than when they did not.

Habituation can be useful as a preliminary step before desensitisation and may shorten the time required for training and desensitisation. For example, in the sample training protocol for training a pig to enter a squeeze cage, the first step might be to attach the squeeze cage to the pig's enclosure and allow free access to it for a couple of days. Adding some food inside may make exploration of the cage more likely and hasten the habituation process. If habituation is the only method employed, caregivers should at the very least provide some positive reinforcements, i.e. food rewards, in conjunction with the experience as frequently and as generously as possible.

Desensitisation

Desensitisation is a process designed to 'train out', or overcome, fear. By pairing positive rewards with any action, object or event that causes fear, that fearful entity slowly becomes less negative, less frightening and less stressful. The effectiveness of desensitisation can be assessed in two ways. Is there a positive change in the animal's willingness to voluntarily cooperate in the event? And are there changes in the animal's behaviour in relation to the fearful entity that indicate reduced stress or fear? Through desensitisation, animals learn to tolerate and eventually accept a wide array of frightening or uncomfortable stimuli. Effective desensitisation relies on two elements: precise reinforcement, and good judgement in determining where the process should start and how fast to move through the steps to the desired outcome.

Precise reinforcement means bridging at the exact moment the animal experiences the stimulus. For example, when training an animal to accept an injection, training may include pairing positive rewards with the experience of being touched with a progression of items, starting with the trainer's finger or a wooden dowel, then a capped syringe, and then a needle with the end cut off so it is blunted, and finally the real needle. In each case, the bridge must occur at the exact moment the animal feels the object touch the skin. The bridge is then immediately followed by a reward. If desensitisation is done well, the animal will voluntarily accept the injection, or allow the blood draw, and recognisable signs of stress and fear will be diminished or absent.

The second key to effective desensitisation is determining the starting point, and how fast to progress. If fear of the syringe is so great that the animal cannot accept a food reward in its presence, then learning cannot occur. In that case, the first step may be to offer the animal a brief glimpse of the syringe or increase the distance between the syringe and the animal, and pair these experiences with the bridge and food reward. The next step would entail moving the syringe towards the animal in small increments, each one paired with the bridge and reward. How quickly progress occurs and how big each step should be depends on how the animal reacts to each approximation.

Desensitisation can and should be used whenever fear or discomfort is present or suspected. Animals can be desensitised to husbandry and research procedures, new enclosures, unfamiliar people, specific people like the veterinarian, novel objects, strange noises and other possible aversive stimuli. Experience with many different species has shown that the more specific stimuli animals are desensitised to, the less fearful they become overall (Laule & Desmond 1994). So, training efforts for one protocol can have a cumulative beneficial effect for other protocols.

The following sample shaping plan illustrates the progression of steps and accompanying desensitisation for training a primate for voluntary blood collection using a PVC-type blood sleeve attached to the cage front.

- Desensitise the subject to the presence of the blood sleeve.
- Reinforce progressive movement of animal towards the sleeve and then positioning in front of it.
- Reinforce exploratory behaviour – touching the sleeve, reaching into the sleeve, touching pin at the end of the sleeve. Drop treats through hole in top of sleeve to reinforce ventral forearm facing up.
- Target the hand to the end of the sleeve so that the hand is in position to clasp tightly around the pin.
- Once the subject is firmly holding onto the pin, begin to touch the forearm gently with a finger or hand. Slowly extend duration of both the arm position and tolerating the touch (up to 2 minutes).
- Desensitise to the increasing pressure of your hand on ventral forearm to expose the vein.
- Introduce materials needed during the blood collection procedure (e.g., alcohol swabs, gauze pads, vacutainers, butterfly needles, tubes, needles).
- Introduce a second person to the process and desensitise to the additional human presence.
- Desensitise to alcohol swab on the ventral forearm.
- Desensitise to a capped syringe touching the blood sampling location; increase duration.
- Desensitise to touching with blunted needle with the end cut off (18 g).
- Desensitise to two experiences with a blunted needle – extended steady pressure (duration of 1–2 minutes) and quick 'jab'.
- Desensitise to a sharp needle resting on top of the skin. Do not pierce the skin.
- Desensitise to small gauge real needle (25G) piercing skin next to vein. The first time you prick the skin, give a big bonus and end the session. Expect some possible regression in following sessions. If so, go back in the process, determine new starting point and rebuild.
- Do not use the real needle too often (no more than 1–2 times per week). Every needle prick reminds the animal that it hurts. Be aware that some animals are more sensitive to this step than others, therefore, adjust the schedule accordingly.
- Practise the entire process through the blunt needle with the vet technician or veterinarian who will be performing the blood draw.
- Attempt the actual blood draw. Use the smallest gauge needle possible to draw sufficient blood – the larger the needle the more it hurts. Bonus any level of cooperation.

Socialisation training

Social animals should be housed socially where possible to promote positive social opportunities and interactions. One PRT method, cooperative feeding, has been used successfully with a wide range of species to facilitate introductions, reduce aggression and increase the likelihood of maintaining stable groupings (Desmond & Laule 1994; Laule & Whittaker 2007).

Cooperative feeding

Cooperative feeding can be used to enhance positive social behaviour and reduce agonistic behaviour (Cox 1987; Desmond *et al.* 1987; Bloomsmith *et al.* 1994; Laule & Whittaker 2007). It is of particular value in managing socially housed primates in laboratories. Many caregivers of captive animals have used subterfuge and distraction to provide subordinate animals with food, enrichment or other desirable resources. However, these techniques actually exacerbate aggression, causing dominant animals to become more vigilant in order to maintain control of the desirable resources. In captivity, aggressive interactions can have serious consequences if group members or cage mates are unable to escape the aggressors.

In cooperative feeding, the dominant animal receives reinforcement, in the form of desirable foods, whenever the subordinate animal receives similar resources. This technique reinforces the dominant animal for behaviour that is cooperative rather than aggressive, thus strengthening cooperative behaviours. When consistently and skilfully applied, cooperative feeding has two positive outcomes:

- the dominant animal becomes less aggressive and more tolerant
- the subordinate animal becomes less fearful and more willing to accept rewards in the presence of the dominant animal.

Cooperative feeding can be used to enhance introductions of animals, prior to and after they are given physical access to each other. Initial training can be done with animals separated in adjacent cages. However, they must have visual access to each other so the dominant animal can see what is happening with the other animal and thus what s/he is being reinforced for. A housing situation with multiple animals may require more than one trainer in the initial stages so that one trainer can focus on the dominant animal and the other trainer feed the rest of the animals. In most cases, the training should progress to doing the feed with one person.

The following is a sample protocol for applying cooperative feeding to two pair-housed primates. Tools include a clicker and food, including some special food items for the dominant (target) animal.

- Cue target animal to 'sit', then reinforce.
- Give second animal a piece of food and as he takes it, bridge and reinforce the target animal with 2–3 pieces of food (if necessary, cut food smaller to keep volume down) for sitting and staying without interfering.
- Provide verbal and visual information to the target animal – look at him and say 'Good!' as you feed the other

animal, say 'No' if the target animal breaks position, immediately followed by the cue to 'sit' again.
- Ignore minor interferences (head bob, reaching for food, etc.) as long as second animal is successful in taking food.
- If the target animal aggresses or intimidates second animal so he won't take food, bring target animal back to sit/stay, then resume feed.
- Use a high rate of continuous reinforcement at first (1 piece for second animal, 2–3 pieces for target animal) then as progress is made, the amount and frequency of reinforcement for the target animal can be slowly reduced.
- Give target animal special treat at the end of every successful session.

Training programme development

Despite widespread recognition of the benefits of PRT and increased uptake, it is still not universally adopted (Perlman et al. 2012). Reasons for this include:

- Caregiver staff that are responsible for large numbers of animals, (Baker 2016) limiting the amount of time they can spend with individuals. Often staff are given only short periods of time to prepare animals for research procedures.
- Unsuitable housing, which can vary from small caging that severely restricts the animal's range of physical movement to big corrals with large numbers of animals that are difficult to access on an individual basis.
- Research protocols, which often dictate or restrict the amount and type of food animals can receive, the type of physical activity they can engage in and acceptable enrichment options.
- Lack of staff sufficiently trained in PRT.

The success of a PRT programme is dependent on the ability of personnel to understand the principles of operant conditioning and effectively apply PRT techniques. PRT is a skill that takes time and practice to develop. Poorly planned and implemented training will yield minimal benefits at best. Applications for research funding should include the need for time and money specifically dedicated to the animal training programme, to promote animal welfare and to achieve research goals.

Although it may not be feasible to develop equal training skills in all animal care personnel, one approach that is effective is to develop multiple levels of skills in staff (Perlman et al. 2012). For example, everyone who works with the animals should have a basic understanding of operant conditioning techniques and be capable of using and maintaining trained behaviour once it is complete. They should also be capable of implementing simple training protocols, for example, incorporating reinforcement into interactions with animals when they comply with daily cleaning and shifting activities as well as husbandry and medical procedures. A smaller subset of staff should have training skills that allow them to design training protocols and train new behaviour. These individuals can then plan and implement PRT to improve these daily handling and husbandry procedures and better prepare animals for research protocols. Finally, at least one individual on site should have sufficient training skills to coordinate and oversee PRT activities and problem-solve difficult situations as they arise.

Despite the complexity of this process, apparent costs of implementing a PRT programme can be turned into real benefits for the staff, animals and the institution (Prescott & Buchanan-Smith 2007). Training skills translate directly into problem solving skills (Whittaker 2005). A positive human–animal relationship can enhance learning and thus cooperation in the trained laboratory procedures (Bliss-Moreau & Moadab 2016; Wolflie 1985). Finally, animals voluntarily cooperating, can reduce the use of restraint and anaesthesia and save time, labour and money over the long term (Bloomsmith 1992; Luttrell et al. 1994; McKinley et al. 2003; Prescott & Buchanan-Smith 2007; Perlman et al. 2012).

Practical approach to training laboratory animals

Despite the challenges of implementing a PRT programme in the laboratory environment, there is a broad array of objectives that can be achieved and practical solutions that can be applied to maximise success. PRT in its purist form may not be practical in some settings but, with even basic skills, it is feasible to integrate positive reinforcement techniques into existing management procedures for all species to achieve a reasonable degree of success. In order to develop such a system, the following actions are recommended and ideally should be integrated into existing operational protocols.

1. Use the basic principles of PRT to reduce the animals' fear of humans and increase the likelihood of greater voluntary cooperation in future procedures. When moving through a room with multiple cages, stop for even a few seconds each day to say some kind words and deliver a food treat to each animal, remembering that learning is occurring all the time. This simple conditioning is well-suited for care routines at breeding centres and import/quarantine facilities as well.
2. Begin the process by incorporating the tools of PRT into daily activities. Teach a bridge, either mechanical (clicker) or verbal ('good') by pairing the sound with the delivery of a food treat. Once that is understood, introduce the target. Each day, ask the animal to come to the target for his treat. A stationary target attached to the cage side and slowly moved to the front can encourage timid or fearful animals to approach the trainer at the front of the cage. With a bridge and target, training can begin with simple cues and responses such as moving to the target, stationing, sitting, climbing on the cage front, presenting a hand, arm, leg, side, or chest and so on. The sooner this process is begun, the greater the benefits in the long term. During these early stages, the animal is learning that his actions are associated with rewards. Experience with many different species has shown that the more familiar animals are with the process of PRT, the faster they learn new behaviours (Laule & Desmond 1994).
3. Provide animals the opportunity and motivation to voluntarily cooperate in activities and procedures by following the basic steps of PRT. First, provide a cue or a

signal (e.g. the stimulus) that clearly tells the animal what he is being asked to do. If the animal can perceive and understand the signal, he can then respond with the correct behaviour and earn a reward.

stimulus → response → positive reinforcement

If the caregiver must resort to negative reinforcement to gain compliance, i.e., showing a net to elicit movement into an adjacent cage, as soon as the behaviour occurs, the negative reinforcement is immediately removed and the treat is given.

stimulus → response → negative reinforcement +positive reinforcement

Over time, the use of negative reinforcement is steadily decreased until it is no longer necessary. With a clear signal and regular reinforcement, the animal now has the information necessary to cooperate, and the motivation to do so.

4. Exercise patience – always give the animal a reasonable opportunity to voluntarily cooperate in the desired behaviour. Time constraints may be an issue, and numbers of animals that require training may be high, but training will not be successful without patience. For example, if a primate must be restrained in a squeeze cage, rather than immediately moving the cage wall all the way forward, the wall should be moved in increments, offering the animal the chance to cooperate by moving to the front of the cage after each increment. When it complies, a reward is given. Total cooperation will not be immediate, but over time the animal will learn what is expected. Similarly, when handling or restraint of a rodent or rabbit is required, a patient, gentle hand and a treat following the procedure is the most humane and positive way to carry out the task and gain greater cooperation.

5. Learning occurs through repetition, so find ways to train regularly and frequently. Fernstrom et al. (2009) found that training rhesus macaques every day rather than thrice a week enhanced learning. In this particular study, however, training twice a day did not have measurable benefits over just once a day. But before deciding to limit numbers of sessions, consider the content of the session itself. With significant pressure to complete behaviours as quickly as possible, the key is to make every session count. In practical terms, that means each training session may vary in length, objectives, expectations, content, sequence of responses, variety of reinforcement and so on. Maximising success in PRT involves practising good technique (the science of PRT) as well as instilling a healthy dose of creativity (the art of PRT).

6. Plan ahead. Prepare for research protocols by identifying which animals will be involved, what behaviours are needed, what equipment will be used, how long the procedure will take, how often it will occur and other relevant factors. Then focus some effort on a daily basis towards preparing the animals for the protocol. A couple of behavioural responses each day can have a beneficial impact and easily fit into the staff member's routine.

There are two fundamental objectives of this approach. First is to gain the voluntary cooperation of the animal in as much of the research protocol as possible, even if the entire procedure is not complete. Second is to habituate and/or desensitise the animal to individual components of the process that may be new, frightening or uncomfortable, thus increasing the likelihood of voluntary cooperation.

For example, during daily care, caregivers could show an instrument or apparatus that will be used in the procedure, to each animal prior to giving enrichment. Remember, animals are always learning.

Desensitisation can be incorporated into the process by directly pairing a bridge and treat with the experience of the event as has been described for injections. In the same fashion, one could hold the dog or cat's paw for a couple of seconds, pick up the rat or rabbit, and rub the pig's belly with the sling, pairing the bridge and reward with each action.

By working on these relatively small units on a daily basis, the animal is slowly conditioned to accept and cooperate with the process. Even if the final behaviour is not formally trained in its entirety, animals are likely to be more cooperative and less fearful when the actual procedure is implemented.

7. Consistency in methods applied and between staff is critical for the effectiveness of the training and how quickly new behaviours are completed. For best results, it is advisable to limit the number of staff training new behaviours. Consistency can be achieved by assigning individual caregivers to individual animals, training all new behaviours related to the protocol with their assigned animals. A secondary trainer can work on the behaviours on the primary trainer's days off, as long as good communication and record keeping are maintained. Another option is to divide responsibility for training new behaviour by individual behaviours. Several individuals may then work with each animal, but each person only works on his or her assigned behaviour.

8. Always look for and employ the least invasive methods to achieve objectives. Research protocols put great demands on animals and caregivers. Desired results are dependent upon consistent means of collecting samples and administering medications. However, it is often possible to meet the specific study requirements in a less invasive or stressful way. For example, collecting urine samples from group-housed callitrichids through training animals to urinate quickly and reliably into a vial (McKinley et al. 2003) or on a clean platform inside the cage (Smith et al. 2004) is less invasive than separating animals until they urinate. Similar results were attained with chimpanzees (Bloomsmith et al. 2015). In two studies, one with rats (Huang-Brown & Guhad 2002) and another with rabbits (Marr et al. 1993), animals were trained to take oral doses of medication in chocolate and a sucrose solution respectively, so avoiding the very stressful experience of gastric gavage. In both cases, drug absorption and serum levels were appropriate.

9. Explore other applications of PRT whenever possible. The application of automated PRT has shown significant

benefits when used in neuroscience studies (Wilson *et al.* 2005; Fagot & Paleressompoulle 2009; Gazes *et al.* 2012; Calapai *et al.* 2016). Tulip *et al.* (2017, pp.15) investigated the potential benefits of using an automated PRT system with rhesus macaques at a breeding facility and its effect on subsequent training performance at a research housing facility and in the laboratory. They found that 'automated training enabled animals to learn a high level of performance on simple tasks with minimal requirements for staff time and no food or fluid control'. Furthermore, subsequent performance at the research facility and in the laboratory suggested that 'automated training records could be used to identify animals suitable for behavioural experiments and assist in optimising the training process for each individual' (Tulip *et al.* 2017, pp. 17). Finally, in addition to the training benefits of the automated PRT, animals displayed sustained voluntary use of the systems suggesting they may prove effective as an environmental enrichment device as well.

Conclusions

The use of PRT as an animal care and management tool offers many opportunities to promote positive animal welfare, with great benefits to biomedical facilities, staff and researchers. Primary among these is the ability to gain the voluntary cooperation of animals in husbandry and research procedures. Through techniques like desensitisation, the fear and stress associated with these procedures can be significantly reduced. PRT can be applied in a wide array of situations with a wide variety of species. When appropriately and skilfully applied, positive reinforcement techniques can offer a viable alternative to more stressful traditional approaches to the management of laboratory animals in breeding, quarantine and research housing. By moving to a more positive reinforcement-based system, the welfare of the animals is significantly enhanced while providing better research models and data.

References

Anderson, J.R. and Chamove, A.S. (1980) Self-aggression and social aggression in laboratory-reared macaques. *Journal of Abnormal Psychology*, **89**, 539–550.

Anderson, J.R. and Chamove, A.S. (1984) Allowing captive primates to forage. In: *Standards in Laboratory Animal Science*, Vol. 2, pp.253–256. Universities Federation for Animal Welfare, Potters Bar, England.

Annas, A., Bengtsson, C. and Tornqvist, E. (2013) Group housing of male CD1 mice: reflections from toxicity studies. *Laboratory Animals*, **47**, 127–129.

Bacon, H. (2018) Behaviour-based husbandry – a holistic approach to the management of abnormal repetitive behaviors. *Animals*, **8**, 1–14.

Badihi, I. (2006) The effects of complexity, choice and control on the behaviour and the welfare of captive common marmosets (*Callithrix jacchus*). PhD Thesis, University of Stirling.

Baker, K.C. (2004) Benefits of positive human interaction for socially housed chimpanzees. *Animal Welfare*, **13**, 239–245.

Baker, K.C. (2016) Survey of 2014 behavioral management programs for laboratory primates in the United States. *American Journal of Primatology*, **78**, 780–796.

Baker, K., Bloomsmith, M., Griffis, C. and Gierhart, M. (2003) Self-injurious behaviour and response to human interaction as enrichment in rhesus macaques. *American Journal of Primatology*, **60**, 94–95.

Bassett, L., Buchanan-Smith, H., McKinley, J. and Smith, T.E. (2003) Effects of training on stress-related behaviour of the common marmoset (*Callithrix jacchus*) in relation to coping with routine husbandry procedures. *Journal of Applied Animal Welfare Science*, **6**, 221–233.

Bayne, K., Dexter, S. and Strange, D. (1993) The effects of food provisioning and human interaction on the behavioural well-being of rhesus monkeys (*Macaca mulatta*). *Contemporary Topics (AALAS)*, **32**, 6–9.

Bliss-Moreau, E. and Moadab, G. (2016) Variation in behavioral reactivity is associated with cooperative restraint training efficiency. *Journal of the American Association for Laboratory Animal Science*, **55**, 41–49.

Bloomsmith, M.A. (1992) Chimpanzee training and behavioural research: a symbiotic relationship. In: *Proceedings of the American Association of Zoological Parks and Aquariums Annual Conference*, 403–410, AAZPA. MD.

Bloomsmith, M.A. (1994) Evolving a behavioural management program in a breeding/research setting. In: *Proceedings of American Association of Zoological Parks and Aquariums Annual Conference*, 8–13, AAZPA. MD.

Bloomsmith, M.A., Marr, J.M. and Maple, T.L. (2007) Addressing nonhuman primate behavioural problems through the application of operant conditioning: Is the human treatment approach a useful model? *Applied Animal Behaviour Science*, **102**, 205–222.

Bloomsmith, M., Laule, G., Thurston, R. and Alford, P. (1994) Using training to modify chimpanzee aggression during feeding. *Zoo Biology*, **13**, 557–566.

Bloomsmith, M., Lambeth, S., Stone, A. and Laule, G. (1997) Comparing two types of human interaction as enrichment for chimpanzees. (Abstract) *American Journal of Primatology*, **42**, 96.

Bloomsmith, M.A., Baker, K.C., Ross, S.K. and Lambeth, S.P. (1999) Comparing animal training to non-training human interaction as environmental enrichment for chimpanzees. (Abstract) *American Journal of Primatology*, **49**, 23–116.

Bloomsmith, M., Neu, K., Franklin, A. *et al.* (2015) Positive reinforcement methods to train chimpanzees to cooperate with urine collection. *Journal of the American Association for Laboratory Animal Science*, **54**, 66–69.

Boissy, A. (1995) Fear and fearfulness in animals. *Quarterly Review of Biology*, **70**, 165–191.

Bowell, V.A. (2010) Improving the welfare of laboratory-housed primates through the use of positive reinforcement training: practicalities of implementation. PhD Thesis, University of Stirling.

Brando, S.I. (2012) Animal learning and training: implications for animal welfare. *Veterinary Clinics: Exotic Animal Practice*, **15**, 387–398.

Brando, S. and Buchanan-Smith, H.M. (2018) The 24/7 approach to promoting optimal welfare for captive wild animals. *Behavioural Processes*, **156**, 83–95.

Breuer, K., Coleman, G. and Hemsworth, P. (1998) The effect of handling on the stress physiology and behaviour of nonlactating heifers. In: *Proceedings of Australian Society for the Study of Animal Behaviour, 29th Annual Conference*, pp. 8–9, Institute of Natural Resources, Massey University, Palmerston North, New Zealand.

Buchanan-Smith, H.M. and Badihi, I. (2012) The psychology of control: effects of control over supplementary light on welfare of marmosets. *Applied Animal Behaviour Science*, **137**, 166–174.

Calapai, A., Berger, M., Niessing, M. *et al.* (2016) A cage-based training, cognitive testing and enrichment system optimized for rhesus macaques in neuroscience research. *Behavioral Research Methods.* http://dx.doi.org/10.3758/s13428-016-0707-3.

Capitanio, J.P. (2011) Nonhuman primate personality and immunity: mechanisms of health and disease. In: *Personality and Temperament in Nonhuman Primates. Developments in Primatology: Progress and Prospects,* Eds Weiss, A., King, J. and Murray, L. Springer, New York, NY.

Clark, J.M. (1999) The dog. In: *The UFAW Handbook on the Care and Management of Laboratory Animals,* Ed. Poole, T., pp. 423–444. Oxford, Blackwell Science.

Clay, A.W., Bloomsmith, M.A., Marr, J. and Maple, T.L. (2009) Systematic investigation of the stability of food preferences in captive orangutans: implications for positive reinforcement training. *Journal of Applied Animal Welfare Science,* **12,** 306–313.

Coleman, K. and Maier, A. (2010) The use of positive reinforcement training to reduce stereotypic behavior in rhesus macaques. *Applied Animal Behavior Science,* **1,** 142–148.

Coleman, G.J. and Hemsworth, P.H. (2014) Training to improve stockperson beliefs and behavior towards livestock enhances welfare and productivity. *Review of Science and Technology,* **33,** 131–137.

Coleman, K., Pranger, L., Maier, A. *et al.* (2008) Training rhesus macaques for venipuncture using positive reinforcement techniques: a comparison with chimpanzees. *Journal of the American Association for Laboratory Animal Science,* **47,** 37–41.

Colflesh, L. (2004) *Making Friends: Training Your Dog Positively.* Howell Book House, Hoboken, NJ.

Cox, C. (1987) Increase in the frequency of social interactions and the likelihood of reproduction among drills. In: *Proceedings of the American Association of Zoological Parks and Aquariums Western Regional Conference,* 321–328. AAZPA, MD.

Desmond, T. and Laule, G. (1994) Use of positive reinforcement training in the management of species for reproduction. *Zoo Biology,* **13,** 471–477.

Desmond, T., Laule, G. and McNary, J. (1987) Training for socialization and reproduction with drills. In: *Proceedings of the American Association of Zoological Parks and Aquariums Annual Conference,* 435–441. AAZPA, MD.

Donaldson, J. (1996) *The Culture Clash.* James and Kenneth, Berkley, CA.

Erwin, J. and Deni, R. (1979) Strangers in a strange land: abnormal behaviours or abnormal environments? In: *Captivity and Behaviour: Primates in Breeding Colonies, Laboratories, and Zoos,* Eds Erwin, J., Maple, T.L. and Mitchell, G., pp. 1–28. Nostrand Reinhold Co., New York.

Fagot, J. and Paleressompoulle, D. (2009) Automatic testing of cognitive performance in baboons maintained in social groups. *Behavior Research Methods,* **41,** 396–404.

Fernstrom, A.L., Fredlund, H., Spangberg, M. and Westlund, K. (2009) Positive reinforcement training in rhesus macaques – training progress as a result of training frequency. *American Journal of Primatology,* **71,** 373–379.

Ferster, C.B. (2002) Schedules of reinforcement with Skinner. 1970. *Journal of the Experimental Analysis of Behavior,* **77,** 303–311.

Fischer, B. and Wegener, D. (2018) Emphasizing the 'positive' in positive reinforcement: using nonbinary rewarding for training monkeys on cognitive tasks. *Journal of Neurophysiology,* **120,** 115–128.

Gantt, W.H., Newton, J.E., Royer, F.L. and Stephen, J.H. (1966) Effect of person. *Conditioned Reflex,* **1,** 18–35.

Gazes, R.P., Brown, E.K., Basile, B.M. and Hampton, R.R. (2012) Automated cognitive testing of monkeys in social groups yields results comparable to individual laboratory-based testing. *Animal Cognition,* **16,** 445–458.

Gillis, T.E., Janes, A.C. and Kaufman, M.J. (2012) Positive reinforcement training in squirrel monkeys using clicker training. *American Journal of Primatology,* **74,** 712–720.

Graham, M.L., Rieke, E.F., Mutch, L.A. *et al.* (2012) Successful implementation of cooperative handling eliminates the need for restraint in a complex non-human primate disease model. *Journal of Medical Primatology,* **41,** 89–106.

Grissom, N., Kerr, W. and Bhatnagar, S. (2008) Struggling behavior during restraint is regulated by stress experience. *Behavioural Brain Research,* **191,** 219–226.

Hanson, J., Larson, M. and Snowdon, C. (1976) The effects of control over high intensity noise on plasma cortisol levels in rhesus monkeys. *Behavioural Biology,* **16,** 333–340.

Hediger, H. (1950) *Wild Animals in Captivity.* Butterworth, London.

Hennessy, M.B., Williams, M.T., Miller, D.D. *et al.* (1998) Influence of male and female petters on plasma cortisol and behaviour: Can human interaction reduce the stress of dogs in a public animal shelter? *Applied Animal Behaviour Science,* **61,** 63–77.

Hernstein, R.J. (1997) *The Matching Law: Papers in Psychology and Economics,* Eds Rachlin, H. and Laibson, D.I. Harvard University Press, MA.

Hiby, E.F., Rooney, N.J. and Bradshaw, J.W. (2004) Dog training methods: their use, effectiveness and interaction with behaviour and welfare. *Animal Welfare,* **13,** 63–59.

Home Office (1989) Code of practice for the housing and care of animals used in scientific procedures. HMSO: London. http://scienceandresearch.homeoffice.gov.uk/animalresearch/publications/publications/code-of-practice/

Huang-Brown, K.M. and Guhad, F.A. (2002) Chocolate, an effective means of oral drug delivery in rats. *Laboratory Animals,* **31,** 34–36.

International Primatological Society (1989) IPS International guidelines for the acquisition, care and breeding of nonhuman primates. *Primate Report,* **25,** 3–27.

Institute of Laboratory Animal Resources (US), Committee on Care, & Use of Laboratory Animals (1986) *Guide for the care and use of laboratory animals* (No. 86). US Department of Health and Human Services, Public Health Service, National Institutes of Health.

Jones, R.B. (1997) Fear and distress. In: *Animal Welfare,* Eds Appleby, M.C. and Hughes, B.O., pp. 75–87. CAB International, UK.

Kemp, C., Thatcher, H., Farningham, D. *et al.* (2017) A protocol for training group-housed rhesus macaques (*Macaca mulatta*) to cooperate with husbandry and research procedures using positive reinforcement. *Applied Animal Behaviour Science,* **197,** 90–100.

Kirkwood, J., Kichenside, C. and James, W. (1989) Training zoo animals. In: *Proceedings of Animal Training Symposium: A Review and Commentary on Current Practices.* pp. 93–99. Universities Federation for Animal Welfare: Cambridge.

Kurtycz, L.M. (2015) Choice and control for animals in captivity. *The Psychologist On Line,* **28,** 11, 892–894.

Laboratory Animal Science Association/Medical Research Council. (2004) Principles of best practice in the breeding of macaques and marmosets for scientific purposes: a statement by the Laboratory Animal Science Association and the Medical Research Council. http://www.lasa.co.uk/position_papers.

Lambeth, S.P., Hau, J., Perlman, J.E. *et al.* (2006) Positive reinforcement training affects hematologic and serum chemistry values in captive chimpanzees (*Pan troglodytes*). *American Journal of Primatology,* **68,** 245–256.

Laule, G.E. (1993) The use of behavioural management techniques to reduce or eliminate abnormal behaviour. *Animal Welfare Information Center Newsletter,* **4,** 1–11.

Laule, G.E. (2005) The role of fear in abnormal behavior and animal welfare. In: *Proceedings of the Seventh International Conference on Environmental Enrichment,* pp. 120–125. ICEE, NY.

Laule, G.E. and Desmond, T.J. (1994) Use of positive reinforcement techniques to enhance animal care, research, and well-being. In: *Proceedings of Wildlife Mammals as Research Models: in the Laboratory and Field.* A seminar sponsored by the Scientists Center for Animal Welfare at the American Veterinary Medical Association Annual Meeting, pp. 53–59. SCAW: MD.

Laule, G.E. and Desmond, T.J. (1997) Positive reinforcement training as an enrichment strategy. In: *Second Nature: Environmental Enrichment for Captive Animals*, Eds Sheperdson, D., Mellen, J. and Hutchins, M., pp. 302–312. Smithsonian Institution Press, Virginia.

Laule, G.E. and Whittaker, M.A. (2007) Enhancing nonhuman primate care and welfare through the use of positive reinforcement training. *Journal of Applied Animal Welfare Science.* **10**, 31–38.

Laule, G.E., Bloomsmith, M.A. and Schapiro, S.J. (2003) The use of positive reinforcement training techniques to enhance the care, management, and welfare of primates in the laboratory. *Journal of Applied Animal Welfare Science*, **10**, 31–38.

Laule, G.E., Thurston, R.H., Alford, P.A. and Bloomsmith, M.A. (1996) Training to reliably obtain blood and urine samples from a diabetic chimpanzee (*Pan Troglodytes*). *Zoo Biology*, **15**, 587–591.

Lindsay, S.R. (2005) *Handbook of Applied Dog Behaviour and Training. Vol III. Procedures and Protocols*. Ames, Blackwell Publishing, UK.

Line, S., Morgan, K.N., Markowitz, H. and Strong, S. (1989) Heart rate and activity of rhesus monkeys in response to routine events. *Laboratory Primate Newsletter*, **28**, 9–12.

Luttrell, L., Acker, L., Urben, M. and Reinhardt, V. (1994) Training a large troop of rhesus macaques to co-operate during catching: analysis of the time investment. *Animal Welfare*, **3**, 135–140.

Malinow, M.R., Hill, J.D. and Ochsner, A.J. (1974) Heart rate in caged rhesus monkeys (*Macaca mulatta*). *Laboratory Animal Science*, **24**, 537–540.

Markowitz, H. (1982) *Behavioural Enrichment in the Zoo*. Van Nostrand Reinhold Co., New York.

Marr, J.M., Gnam, E.C., Calhoun, J. and Mader, J.T. (1993) A nonstressful alternative to gastric gavage for oral administration of antibiotics in rabbits. *Laboratory Animals*, **22**, 47–49.

Martin, A.L., Bloomsmith, M.A., Kelley, M.E. et al. (2011) Functional analysis and treatment of human-directed undesirable behavior exhibited by a captive chimpanzee. *Journal of Applied Behavior Analysis*, **44**, 139–143.

Martin, A.L., Franklin, A.N., Perlman, J.E. and Bloomsmith, M.A. (2018) Systematic assessment of food item preference and reinforcer effectiveness: enhancements in training laboratory-housed rhesus macaques. *Behavioural Processes*, **157**, 445–452.

McConnell, P. (2002) *The Other End of the Leash. Why We Do What We Do Around Dogs*. Valentine Books, New York, NY.

McKinley, J. (2004) Training in a laboratory environment: methods, effectiveness and welfare implications of two species of primate. PhD Thesis, University of Stirling.

McKinley, J., Buchanan-Smith, H.M., Bassett, L. and Morris, K. (2003) Training common marmosets (*Callithrix jacchus*) to cooperate during routine laboratory procedures: ease of training and time investment. *Journal of Applied Animal Welfare Science*, **6**, 209–220.

McMillan, J.L., Perlman, J.E., Galvan, A. et al. (2014) Refining the pole-and-collar method of restraint: emphasizing the use of positive training techniques with rhesus macaques (*Macaca mulatta*). *Journal of the American Association for Laboratory Animal Science.* **53**, 61–68.

Mellor, D.J. (2012) Animal emotions, behaviour and the promotion of positive welfare states. *New Zealand Veterinary Journal*, **60**, 1–8.

Meunier, L.D. (2006) Selection, acclimation, training, and preparation of dogs for the research setting. *ILAR Journal*, **47**, 326–347.

Mineka, S., Gunnar, M. and Champoux, M. (1986) The effects of control in the early social and emotional development of rhesus monkeys. *Child Development*, **57**, 1241–1256.

Minier, D.E., Tatum, L., Gottlieb, D.H. et al. (2011) Human-directed contra-aggression training using positive reinforcement with single and multiple trainers for indoor-housed rhesus macaques. *Applied Animal Behaviour Science*, **132**, 178–186.

Moberg, G.P. (1985) Influence of stress on reproduction: a measure of well-being. In: *Animal Stress*, Ed. Moberg, G.P., pp. 245–267. American Physiological Society, Bethesda, MD.

Moseley, J. and Davis, J. (1989) Psychological enrichment techniques and New World monkey restraint device reduce colony management time. *Laboratory Animal Science*, **39**, 31–33.

National Research Council (1998) *The Psychological Wellbeing of Nonhuman Primates*. National Academy Press: Washington DC, USA.

Neuringer, A. (1969) Animals respond for food in the presence of free food. *Science*, **166**, 339–341.

Overall, K.L. and Dyer, D. (2005) Enrichment strategies for laboratory animals from the viewpoint of clinical veterinary behavioral medicine: emphasis on cats and dogs. *ILAR Journal*, **46**, 202–216.

Perdue, B.M., Evans, T.A., Washburn, D.A. et al. (2014). Do monkeys choose to choose? *Learning & Behavior*, **42**, 164–175.

Perlman, J.E., Thiele, E., Whittaker, M.A. et al. (2004) Training chimpanzees to accept subcutaneous injections using positive reinforcement training techniques. *American Journal of Primatology*, **62(1)**. Wiley-Liss, NJ, USA.

Perlman, J., Horner, V., Bloomsmith, M. et al. (2010) Positive reinforcement training: social learning, and chimpanzee welfare. In: *The Mind of the Chimpanzee*, Eds Londsorf, E.V., Ross, S.R. and Matsuzawa, T., pp. 320–331. The University of Chicago Press, Chicago, IL.

Perlman, J.E., Bloomsmith, M.A., Whittaker, M.A. et al. (2012) Implementing positive reinforcement animal training programs at primate laboratories. *Applied Animal Behaviour Science*, **137**, 114–126.

Phillipi-Falkenstein, K. and Clarke, M. (1992) Procedure for training corral-living rhesus monkeys for fecal and blood sample collection. *Laboratory Animal Science*, **42**, 83–85.

Prescott, M.J. and Buchanan-Smith, H.M. (2003) Training non-human primates using positive reinforcement techniques. *Journal of Applied Animal Welfare Science*, **6**, 157–161.

Prescott, M., Morton, D., Anderson, D. et al. (2004) Refining dog husbandry and care: eighth report of the Joint Working Group on Refinement (British Veterinary Association's Animal Welfare Foundation/ Fund for Replacement of Animals in Medical Experimentation/ Royal Society for Protection of Cruelty to Animals/ University Federation for Animal Welfare). *Laboratory Animals*, **38**, 63–66.

Prescott, M.J., Bowell, V.A. and Buchanan-Smith, H.M. (2005) Training laboratory-housed non-human primates, Part 2: Resources for developing and implementing training programmes. *Animal Technology and Welfare*, **4**, 133–148.

Prescott, M.J. and Buchanan-Smith, H.M. (2007) Training laboratory-housed non-human primates, part I: a UK survey. *Animal Welfare*, **16**, 21–36.

Pryor, K. (1999) *Don't Shoot the Dog. The New Art of Teaching and Training*. Bantam Books, New York.

Reinhardt, V. (1992) Improved handling of experimental rhesus monkeys. In: *The Inevitable Bond: Examining Scientist–Animal Interactions*, Eds Davis, H. and Balfour, A., pp. 171–177. Cambridge University Press, Cambridge.

Reinhardt, V. (1997) Training nonhuman primates to cooperate during blood collection: a review. *Laboratory Primate Newsletter*, **36**, 1–4.

Reinhardt, V. (1997a) Training nonhuman primates to cooperate during handling procedures: a review. *Animal Technology*, **48**, 55–73.

Reinhardt, V., Liss, C. and Stevens, C. (1995) Restraint methods of laboratory nonhuman primates: a critical review. *Animal Welfare*, **4**, 221–238.

Reinhardt, V., Cowley, D. and Scheffler, J. et al. (1990) Cortisol response of female rhesus monkeys to venipuncture in home-cage versus venipuncture in restraint apparatus. *Journal of Medical Primatology*, **19**, 601–606.

Ruys, J.D., Mendoza, S.P., Capitanio, J.P. and Mason, W.A. (2004) Behavioural and physiological adaptation to repeated chair restraint in rhesus macaques. *Physiology and Behaviour*, **82**, 205–213.

Schapiro, S.J., Bloomsmith, M.A. and Laule, G.E. (2003) Positive reinforcement training as a technique to alter nonhuman primate behaviour: quantitative assessments of effectiveness. *Journal of Applied Animal Welfare*, **6**, 175–187.

Schapiro, S.J., Perlman, J.E., Thiele, E. and Lambeth, S. (2005) Training non-human primates to perform behaviours useful in biomedical research. *Laboratory Animals*, **34**, 37–42.

Skinner, B.F. (1938) *The Behaviour of Organisms*. Appleton-Century-Crofts, NY.

Smith, A.C. and Swindle, M.M. (2006) Preparation of swine for the laboratory. *ILAR Journal*, **47**, 358–363.

Smith, T.E., McCallister, J.M., Gordon, S.J. and Whittikar, M. (2004) Quantitative data on training New World primates to urinate. *American Journal of Primatology*, **64**, 83–93.

Sørensen, D.B. (2010). Never wrestle with a pig. *Laboratory Animals*, **44**, 159–161.

Sørensen, D.B., Dragsted, N. and Glerup, P. (2005) Positive reinforcement training in large experimental animals. *Altex Proceedings*, 1/12, Proceedings of WC8 477–479.

Stone, A.M., Bloomsmith, M.A., Laule, G.E. and Alford, P.L. (1994) Documenting positive reinforcement training for chimpanzee urine collection. (Abstract) *American Journal of Primatology*, **33**, 242.

Toates, F. (1995) *Stress. Conceptual and Biological Aspects*. John Wiley & Sons, Chichester, UK.

Tulip, J., Zimmermann, J.B., Farningham, D. and Jackson, A. (2017) An automated system for positive reinforcement training of group-housed macaque monkeys at breeding and research facilities. *Journal of Neuroscience Methods*, **285**, 6–18.

Turkkan, J., Ator, N., Brady, J. and Craven, K. (1990) Beyond chronic catheterization in laboratory primates. In: *Housing, Care and Psychological Well-being of Captive and Laboratory Primates*, Ed. Segal, E., pp. 305–322. Noyes Publishing, New York, NY.

VandeVoort, C., Neville, L., Tollner, T. and Field, L. (1993) Noninvasive semen collection from an adult orangutan. *Zoo Biology*, **12**, 257–265.

Vertein, R. and Reinhardt, V. (1989) Training female rhesus monkeys to cooperate during in-home cage venipuncture. *Laboratory Primate Newsletter*, **28**, 1–3.

Videan, E.N., Fritz, J., Murphy, J. *et al.* (2005) Training captive chimpanzees to cooperate for an anesthetic injection. *Laboratory Animals*, **34**, 43–48.

Waiblinger, S., Boivin, X., Pedersen, V. *et al.* (2006) Assessing the human–animal relationship in farmed species: a critical review. *Applied Animal Behaviour Science*, **101**, 185–242.

Warren-Smith, A.K. and McGreevy, P.D. (2007) The use of blended positive and negative reinforcement in shaping the halter response of horses (*Equus caballus*). *Animal Welfare*, **16**, 481–488.

Wergård, E.M., Temrin, H., Forkman, B. *et al.* (2015) Training pair-housed rhesus macaques (*Macaca mulatta*) using a combination of negative and positive reinforcement. *Behavioral Processes*, **113**, 51–59.

Westlund, K. (2015) Training laboratory primates – benefits and techniques. *Primate Biology*, **2**, 119–132.

Wilson, F.A., Kim, B.H., Ryou, J.W. and Ma, Y.Y. (2005) An automated food delivery system for behavioural and neurophysiological studies of learning and memory in freely moving monkeys. *Behavioural Research Methods*, **37**, 368–372.

Whittaker, M. (2005) Applied problem solving to diminish abnormal behavior. In: *Proceedings of the Seventh International Conference on Environmental Enrichment*, pp. 126–131. ICEE. NY.

Whitehouse, J., Micheletta, J., Powell, L.E. *et al.* (2013) The impact of cognitive testing on the welfare of group housed primates. *PLoS ONE*, **8(11)**, e78308.

Wolfle, T. (1985) Laboratory animal technicians: their role in stress reduction and human-companion animal bonding. *Veterinary Clinics of North America: Small Animal Practice*, **15**, 449–454.

16 3Rs considerations when using ageing animals in science

J. Norman Flynn, Linda Horan, Carl S. Tucker, David Robb and Michael J.A. Wilkinson

Introduction

Ageing is a natural and multi-factorial process, acting at many levels of the organism's physiological and functional organisation, driven by genetic, epigenetic and environmental factors (Jayanthi et al. 2010). Due to its multi-faceted nature, there is great heterogeneity in the ageing phenotype even among members of the same species and, consequently, producing a comprehensive list of 'common' signs of ageing is fraught with difficulties. Moreover, it is hard to differentiate between exclusively age-related changes and age-independent disease, as both processes result in impairment. The main difference between them is that the former is a normal, universal process affecting all individuals whereas the latter is an abnormal process affecting a subset. A further distinction is made in human medicine between ageing and age-related frailty, and the distinction has also been explored in laboratory mice (Parks et al. 2012; Whitehead et al. 2014).

In this chapter, we describe the reasons for the increased use of ageing animals in research, some of the purposes for which they are used and opportunities to apply the Three Rs (Russell and Burch 1959). We review the common clinical signs encountered when using ageing animals for scientific research purposes and suggest husbandry and veterinary refinements and interventions aimed at mitigation of age-related adverse effects. The main focus is on mice because this is the most commonly used species in ageing research worldwide.

The chapter also includes sections on zebra finches, zebrafish, dogs and non-human primates (NHPs). Dogs and NHPs are not generally used for ageing research *per se*, but are used in studies that often last several years. Animal care staff and scientists, therefore, need to be aware of the changing husbandry, dietary and veterinary needs of these ageing animals as these studies progress to completion.

In the last section of this chapter, we review and discuss when 'purposeful ageing' of animals should be considered as requiring authorisation under relevant legislation. We argue that the criteria for this cannot be based solely on the age of animals but should instead be based on the potential for the animals to experience adverse effects of pain, suffering, distress or lasting harm.

Research areas that require the study of ageing animals include:

1. Fundamental research on the molecular, genetic and cellular processes and pathways that are involved in the natural ageing process, exploring the potential to manipulate and exploit these processes to promote healthy ageing and prolong lifespan.
2. Research aimed at improving our understanding of how the natural process of ageing may impact on intercurrent diseases such as arthritis, cardiovascular disease and certain types of cancer.
3. Study types that result in the retention of animals for a significant period, which can be several years. The most common examples are the retention of dogs (typically, beagles in the UK) and macaques (typically, cynomolgus in the UK) for repeated use in pharmacokinetic studies and telemetry studies, following surgical preparation. Colonies of animals may also be retained as blood donors, to enable *in vitro* work such as protein binding studies. On rare occasions, such animals may also be retained until they are several years old for single use (up to 10 years in some instances), where the study in question requires use of older animals.
4. Lastly, ageing animals may be required not directly because there is a scientific question around the ageing itself, but simply because the animals involved will age naturally during the period of study.

Age-related research and animal models

Drivers for the increased use of ageing animals in research

Human life expectancy is increasing globally, and this is particularly marked in the developed world[1]. Between 2015 and 2030, the number of people in the world aged 60 years or over is projected to grow by 56 per cent, from 901 million to 1.4 billion, and by 2050, the global population of older persons is projected to more than double its size reaching nearly 2.1 billion (United Nations 2015). In the European Community alone, 21% of population was over 60 in 1996, and the percentage is projected to rise to over 33% by 2050 (Cracknell 2017). These demographics present significant medical, social and economic challenges for the future. The economic and social impact of our ageing society is evident because health-span, defined here as the period of life free from age-related disease, is not increasing at the same rate as lifespan. Consequently, more and more individuals within our society will spend a greater proportion of their life with poor health because age is the primary risk for many highly debilitating chronic diseases, such as cardiovascular disease, neurodegenerative diseases including Alzheimer's disease, osteoporosis, type 2 diabetes, obesity and many forms of cancer (Figueira et al. 2016). Typically, these age-associated diseases do not present clinically in isolation, with an estimated 60% of people over the age of 65 years suffering from multimorbidity (Vogeli et al. 2007).

As ageing is the primary risk factor for these diseases, research is being carried out to better understand the ageing process, to improve or maintain good quality health as the population ages. The hope is that by identifying potential points of intervention, the ageing process may be ameliorated, thereby extending health-span through the reduction in the incidence of, and/or the delaying of the onset of age-related disease. Ageing animals, particularly mice, are being used as research models in an attempt to recapitulate more accurately the disease processes and better understand the interplay between natural ageing processes and any age-related intercurrent disease. Many studies focus, in particular, on the reduced drug metabolism and reduced cardiovascular function potentially seen in ageing animals (and humans) that may, in turn, impact on pharmacokinetics and drug distribution.

The mouse as a model of ageing

Previously, the use of ageing rodents was mainly limited to the study of ageing itself, long-term carcinogenesis studies and neurodegenerative research. However, driven by the need to know more about 'healthy ageing', rodents are being increasingly used to examine age-related conditions. Although, the molecular and cellular mechanisms that underlie ageing are complex, multi-factorial and remain incompletely understood, the processes that underlie ageing appear conserved across species. It appears that these underlying processes and the genes involved in ageing are not random mutations; rather, these genes form tight-knit families that are conserved across animal species, hence the relevance of using the laboratory mouse, *Mus musculus* in these studies. However, it has also been possible to use relatively short-lived and easily maintained non-vertebrate replacement model organisms such as *Caenorhabditis elegans* and *Drosophila melanogaster* for some studies (Gems & Partridge 2013; Fontana & Partridge 2015).

It is now well established that a range of environmental, pharmacological and genetic interventions extend lifespan in these organisms, and importantly these interventions tend also to increase late-life health and vitality (Selman & Withers 2011; Gems & Partridge 2013; Fontana & Partridge 2015). The beneficial effects induced by these various interventions seem to be conserved across wide evolutionary distances and can elicit a wide number of health benefits in humans (Most et al. 2017).

In mice, for example, it is well established that interventions, such as dietary restriction, can extend health-span significantly. This appears to occur through several mechanisms including the attenuation of late-life glucose intolerance, insulin resistance, adiposity and systemic inflammation, the preservation of stem cell and mitochondrial function and the preservation of cognitive function in old age (Selman & Withers 2011). In addition, many of these interventions can rescue lifespan and health-span in rapidly ageing (progeroid) mouse models and in various mouse models of disease (Selman et al. 2016).

Finally, it has become clear that profound strain-specific, and indeed sex-specific, differences exist in lifespan, health-span and causes of death across different mouse strains and this must be borne in mind when choosing a particular chronological age to study (Yuan et al. 2009). While significant insights into the ageing process have been identified using progeroid mouse models (Liao & Kennedy 2014), these models do not appear to recapitulate all aspects of ageing typically seen in conventional mice over their lifespan. Therefore, to understand the fundamental mechanisms underlying natural ageing, and to define exactly how (and when) a particular intervention acts to modulate particular age-related traits or processes, there is presently still a requirement to study aged animals.

It is important that animal models are relevant and, with respect to mice, it is clear that particular age classes to be studied need to most appropriately reflect the ageing profile of that mouse strain wherever possible. A valuable and freely available resource that provides such information for a large number of mouse strains is the International Mouse Phenotyping Consortium (IMPC)[2]. In addition, many of the large commercial suppliers of genetically altered mice offer this type of information in their websites (see also Chapter 4: An introduction to laboratory animal genetics).

The Zebra finch as a model of ageing

Birds constitute an important class of animals used in scientific research across the globe. In Europe, almost 6% of the

---

[1] https://www.who.int/gho/mortality_burden_disease/life_tables/situation_trends_text/en/ (accessed 27 March 2019)

[2] https://www.mousephenotype.org/ (accessed 29 November 2019)

11.5 million animals used for scientific research in 2011 were birds[3]. They possess a number of features that make them particularly suitable in biogerontology, such as their greater longevity compared to mammals of equal size, moderately slow ageing and innate anti-ageing mechanisms (Holmes & Austad 1995; Holmes & Ottinger 2003). For these reasons, they have been widely used in studies of ageing processes and their prevention, and some authors believe they can be more suitable as models of longevity than short-lived laboratory rodents (Holmes & Ottinger 2003).

It is not surprising, therefore, that the zebra finch (*Taeniopygia guttata*), which has long been a very important species in biomedical and zoological research (Bateson & Feenders 2010), has also been involved in biogerontology. It has featured in multiple studies exploring – for example – the interplay between longevity and oxidative stress (Kim *et al.* 2010), telomere length (Heidinger *et al.* 2012), basal metabolic rate (Moe *et al.* 2009), neurogenesis and vocal control (Pytte *et al.* 2007; Wang *et al.* 2002), offspring lifespan (Noguera *et al.* 2018) and immunity (Haussmann *et al.* 2005).

Zebra finches are a hardy species, well adapted to captive environments, where they can typically live well beyond the 5 years of age that is more typical of their wild counterparts (see also Chapter 42: Zebra finches). However, their innate anti-ageing mechanisms notwithstanding, prolonged life comes at a price for them too.

The Zebrafish as a model of ageing

Aquatic species have also been employed for ageing studies, including fish, frogs (*Xenopus laevis* and *Xenopus tropicalis*) and axolotl (*Ambystoma mexicanum*). However, the most frequently used aquatic species is the zebrafish (*Danio rerio*), which represents 12% of the total number of scientific procedures conducted in 2018 in the UK alone. A 5% increase in the numbers of fish used over the last 10 years reflects the increasing popularity of this model species. The experimental use of zebrafish has shown that this species is recognised as an important and significant tool for biomedical research and for translatable medicine (Phillips & Westerfield 2014; Patton & Tobin 2019; see also Chapter 49: Zebrafish). Approximately 70% of human genes have at least one obvious zebrafish orthologue (Howe *et al.* 2013), and numerous reports have highlighted the benefits of using fish as an important research *in-vivo* model (Shin & Fishman 2002; Meeker & Trede 2008; Bradford *et al.* 2017; Collin & Martin 2017). Zebrafish are also important animal models of certain diseases of humans because, in contrast to adult mammalian species, they retain their natural physiological regenerative capability for all organs and tissues (Gemberling *et al.* 2016).

In its native environment, the zebrafish is considered an annual species (Spence *et al.* 2006, 2007; Engeszer *et al.* 2007), which inhabits shallow streams and rice paddies; their potentially curtailed life may be due to the harsh conditions encountered over 12 months, i.e. monsoon, drought, predation, disease and human intervention (Spence *et al.* 2008). In direct contrast, when maintained in a laboratory environment, with optimised husbandry environmental conditions, the zebrafish can live up to a maximum age of 66 months (Gerhard *et al.* 2002). It is important to consider and understand the consequences of ageing (Gerhard 2003; Carneiro *et al.* 2016) whether as a result of studies on senescence (Gilbert *et al.* 2014; Carneiro *et al.* 2016), or due to fish stocks being kept beyond a biologically prudent age.

Age-related conditions: signs and care for some commonly used species

There are many challenges associated with maintaining ageing cohorts of experimental animals. Some research groups have developed and are using 'in house' scoring systems to determine intervention points for potential refinements and to identify clear endpoints for ageing animals. Although many good systems are in use, variations between them could contribute to poor reproducibility of the scientific results and efforts should be made to adopt good practice worldwide.

In this chapter, we propose setting time points, where relevant, for enhanced monitoring and inclusion of husbandry and/or veterinary intervention for the care of ageing animals. In the case of mice, the trigger-point for enhanced monitoring is based on the phenotype and clinical signs shown by the animals when reaching a particular age. Given the number and variety of ageing mouse models and genotypes and phenotypes currently in use, it is clear that trigger-points will differ. Nevertheless, this approach will underpin the development of consistent scoring systems that can be widely adopted, with agreed refinement steps and intervention points designed to minimise the potential impact of age-related adverse effects on animal welfare. Furthermore, definition of clear, humane endpoints will help to ensure that animals are not maintained for longer than is scientifically necessary.

Frailty in humans is conceptually defined as *a clinically recognizable state of increased vulnerability to adverse health outcomes for people of the same chronological age as a result of ageing-associated decline across multiple physiological systems such that the ability to cope with every day or acute stressors is severely compromised* (Chen *et al.* 2014). As age is normally accompanied by frailty, it is important to remember that these additional monitoring and intervention steps should not, themselves, cause additional harms to the animals. Furthermore, wherever possible any sampling should be conducted as early in the life of the animals as possible – particularly when measuring a parameter that is not going to change, such as the genetic makeup – as sampling younger animals that are likely to be more robust is inherently more refined.

In all cases, careful analysis of the animals' quality of life and welfare should help keep the right harm/benefit balance and facilitate timely interventions, including application of humane end points. There are some excellent resources that can help scientists, animal care takers and veterinarians evaluate cumulative suffering and quality of life in their

---

[3] https://eur-lex.europa.eu/legal-content/EN/TXT/PDF/?uri=CELEX:52013DC0859&from=EN (accessed 26 July 2019)

experimental animals (Honess & Wolfensohn 2010; Hawkins et al. 2011; see also Chapter 6: Brief introduction to welfare assessment).

Mice

It is well known that different mouse strains have different predispositions to develop one or more health conditions as they grow older, and it behoves those who care for them to be familiar with these. There are several excellent data sources which can provide this information and act as repositories for further data (the aforementioned IMPC; the International Mouse Strain Resource[4]; Yuan et al. 2009; Pettan-Brewer & Treuting 2011; Brayton et al. 2012; McIness 2012). It is vitally important that researchers contribute to these repositories by recording, collating and reporting new information relating to the ageing phenotype – including histopathology – because they can significantly contribute to improvements in the care and welfare of ageing animals and greater scientific rigour.

Environmental factors also need to be taken into account since they can be predictive of certain age-related conditions. For example, the generalised practice of *ad-libitum* feeding of laboratory mice, together with very limited opportunity for exercise, is well known to predispose to obesity and obesity-related pathologies (Martin et al. 2010). Therefore, a clear understanding of the animals' past and present environment is a pre-requisite when assessing age-related health conditions. Using a commercial breeder that can supply pre-aged animals on demand, can reduce animal wastage through unnecessary over-breeding and save expense and time for scientists.

Signs of ageing and management of aged mice

Despite the heterogeneity in the ageing phenotype, there are some clinical/pathological manifestations that can be considered more or less typical in a given species. The impact of these various clinical/pathological manifestations on the animals' welfare will depend, to a large extent, on what organ/s and/or system/s are primarily affected but also on how well the animal can cope or compensate for them. Many age-related health conditions develop slowly over extended periods of time and the body – and the animal – adapts to them. However, clinical signs appear, when there is a decline in function (e.g. progressive heart or kidney failure) that can no longer be compensated for. Common age-related clinical signs, such as impaired vision, hearing loss or generalised hair loss, do not usually cause the same level of functional impairment in laboratory mice as they probably do in their wild counterparts or indeed in humans. By contrast, other clinical/pathological manifestations such as neoplasia or degenerative joint disease can profoundly affect their welfare. At a cellular and tissue level, age-related changes lead to reductions in function, such as muscle strength, epithelial renewal, alignment of the teeth and cardiovascular output. Similarly, alterations to collagen cross-links may predispose to some of the aforementioned pathology.

Initial signs of ageing in laboratory mice can typically include: thinning, texture change and/or colour change of the coat; reduced self-grooming; body mass change (middle-age obesity may be followed by loss of condition); hearing loss; deteriorating eyesight; reduced spontaneous activity and exercise intolerance. Taken separately, these changes may be of minor importance, but collectively they can have a significant impact on the animal's general wellbeing. The animal's decline can be measured by, for example, reductions in grip strength, endurance, voluntary movement, speed of walking, rate of wound healing and cardiovascular function. There may also be an increased anaesthetic risk, and these changes need to be taken into consideration in the study design, incorporating mitigating steps in order to minimise impact both on the animals' welfare and the study itself (Mimeault & Batra 2010; Liu et al. 2014). Some institutions, for example, routinely trim the animals' nails at a certain age, as this greatly reduces the risks of ulcerative dermatitis (Marshall & Melville 2015). Other factors that can be considered at the initial, planning stages include: increasing room temperature as the animals age, housing aged animals in a quieter/dedicated area of the facility, establishing baseline 'normal' values for welfare parameters such as activity levels or body condition, methods for evaluating health and welfare during the study, training for those conducting health and welfare assessments, cumulative severity and impact of other experimental interventions, ameliorating steps and humane end-points, etc.

We recommend that a monitoring regime is adopted either: (a) from the expected onset of one or more age-related adverse clinical signs where the mouse (wild type or genetically altered (GA)) is well characterised; or (b) an age-related time point of 15 months where no information is yet available to suggest that there will be adverse age-related clinical signs prior to this time or (c) a combination of these parameters. A simplified version of a matrix of clinical signs for ageing mice with suggested staged monitoring frequencies, potential interventions aimed at ameliorating or mitigating the expected adverse effects and humane endpoints is provided in Table 16.1 and some of the most common clinical signs are illustrated in Figure 16.1. A matrix of this sort can act as a basis for local numerical scoring systems tailored to the strain of mouse under investigation and the scientific question/s posed (Bugnon et al. 2016). Other authors have proposed the use of a clinical frailty index, with a particular focus on body weight and temperature as two objective measures that can predict impending death (Toth 2018), that could be adopted as a surrogate marker for ageing and used as an endpoint for an ageing study.

Semi-quantitative approaches offer certain advantages over other methods, including providing a basis for training and improved consistency between observers carrying out objective assessments (Hawkins 2002; see also Chapter 6: Brief introduction to welfare assessment: A toolbox of techniques). Adoption of this approach should improve animal welfare by providing more refined husbandry and management of ageing mice. It can also positively contribute to the science by providing research scientists with more information about the animals they use in their studies. For example, enhanced monitoring of ageing mice could contribute to the identification of subtle modulatory effects of, for instance,

---

[4] http://www.findmice.org/ (accessed 29 November 2019)

Table 16.1 Signs of ageing in mice and recommended action.

OBSERVATION	GENERAL ACTION TO BE TAKEN (in white) – in consideration with the project authorisation adverse effects and humane endpoints, the expected phenotype of the animal and the needs of the intended research. Note: Always use in partnership with the Establishment's Veterinarian (EV) and bear in mind that allowing animals to display many of the signs in this table will likely require specific legal authorisation.			
	ADVISE TO MONITOR EVERY TWO WEEKS FROM 15 MONTHS	WEEKLY MONITORING ADVISED FROM 20 MONTHS		DAILY MONITORING ADVISED FROM 30 MONTHS
	Initiate regular monitoring	Increase monitoring		Critical monitoring
Weight loss (compared to the animal's adult, stable weight)	**Column A:** Under 5% Check teeth; consider using softer or smaller food pellets if appropriate; look out for presence of other clinical signs and act accordingly	**Column B:** 5–10% As for column A; consider adding soft pellets and/or wet mash or other treats every few days; weigh weekly	**Column C:** 10–20% Correct underlying causes if known and if possible; offer pellets/wet mash/ treats and weigh daily ensure the water nozzle is within easy reach; start to prepare to use the animal at an earlier time point	**Column D:** 20%+ If body condition score is also low (e.g. 1 or 2), special justification normally required to keep the animal; otherwise cull
Weight gain (compared to the animal's adult, stable weight)	**Column A:** Above 5% Check for possible internal tumours, ascites or impactions and act accordingly; if appropriate, offer opportunity for exercise (e.g., running wheel, larger/play cages)	**Column B:** 5–10% As for column A; plus consider dietary or caloric restriction if appropriate and not already in place	10–20% Advice as for columns A and B	20%+ Watch out for other signs associated with gross obesity (e.g. difficulty moving, impaired respiration) and act accordingly
Hair loss	**Column A:** Generalised or localised hair thinning Look out for possible Barber and separate if skin becomes damaged	Alopecic (bald) patches As for column A; provide extra nesting material to help thermoregulation	Extensive alopecia Ensure plenty of nesting material and facilitate nest-building; ensure cage/nest is away from draughts	**Generalised and extensive alopecia affecting most of body surface** Follow advice in other columns; check skin remains in good condition
Ulcerative Dermatitis	**Column A:** Small area of skin affected (<5 mm); mostly excoriation and erythema Consider possible treatment/s with EV (e.g., green clay + clip or file nails; fatty acid supplement; diluted chlorhexidine; silver sulfadiazine cream; dust free bedding and so on)	Lesions of <3 mm affecting face or extremities; more extensive lesions over the body (0.5–1 cm) As for column A; try a different therapy from the list of possibilities. Monitor the condition daily	Lesions of >3 mm in face or extremities, extensive body lesions and/or clear discomfort Unlikely to respond to treatment at this stage, best to cull the animal.	

(Continued)

Table 16.1 (Continued)

OBSERVATION	GENERAL ACTION TO BE TAKEN (in white) – in consideration with the project authorisation adverse effects and humane endpoints, the expected phenotype of the animal and the needs of the intended research. Note: Always use in partnership with the Establishment's Veterinarian (EV) and bear in mind that allowing animals to display many of the signs in this table will likely require specific legal authorisation.						
	ADVISE TO MONITOR EVERY TWO WEEKS FROM 15 MONTHS		WEEKLY MONITORING ADVISED FROM 20 MONTHS		DAILY MONITORING ADVISED FROM 30 MONTHS		
	Initiate regular monitoring		Increase monitoring		Critical monitoring		
General appearance / coat condition	Grey hairs observed	No action required	Grey hairs; slightly dirty or unkempt or dry pelt; possible mild piloerection	Ensure adequate companionship to stimulate allogrooming; improve general condition (e.g. lower caloric intake, more exercise); if piloerection, investigate further (e.g., hypothermic?) and respond accordingly	Grey hairs; unkempt coat; piloerection; staining around penis/vagina	Advice as per other columns; if present, try to determine cause of piloerection and try to rectify. If other clinical signs are increasing in frequency, monitor daily prepare to cull	Very unkempt coat and marked piloerection; signs of incontinence	Cull
General appearance/ colour	Column A: Slight paleness noted in feet or tail or eyes	Investigate possible causes and act accordingly; look out for other clinical signs; provide extra heat/nesting	Moderate paleness	As for column A; if possible and appropriate, use other diagnostic tests (e.g. imaging, blood sampling) to help determine cause/s; monitor daily and prepare to cull	Marked paleness	Cull		
Spontaneous mobility – response to stimuli	Column A: Minor decrease noted in activity levels; slower to respond to stimuli	Perform more thorough examination and act accordingly (e.g. if arthritis involved, provide softer or deeper bedding; consider use of analgesics)	More obvious reluctance to move when cage lid removed or if prompted; less alert than normal	As for column A; if necessary and possible, carry out further diagnostic tests (e.g. imaging) to help determine cause/s. Accelerate to weekly monitoring	Moves when prompted but little voluntary activity noted; often isolated from others	Monitor daily, provide additional heat and thoroughly evaluate any other possible clinical signs (e.g. pain? swellings?) If no clear cause or treatment solution available, prepare to cull	Generally dull and inactive/ unresponsive or clear signs of pain	Cull

Abnormal movement	Slow/stiff	Perform more thorough examination and act accordingly (e.g. if arthritis involved, provide softer or deeper bedding; consider use of analgesics)	Stereotypy; limp; slight head tilt	Investigate further and act accordingly (e.g. environmental changes to treat stereotypic behaviours)	Paresis; ataxia; paralysis; unable to keep balance; worsening of some of the previous signs	If no clear cause-treatment solution available, cull
Hunching	Slight hunched posture, possibly intermittent	Investigate possible causes and act accordingly	Moderate hunched posture, possibly continuous	Monitor daily, thoroughly assess possible causes and other clinical signs and act accordingly; prepare to cull	Markedly hunched posture	If no clear cause-treatment solution available or no response to previous treatment, cull
General behaviour (e.g. interaction with cage mates/use of bedding/nest making)	**Column A:** Minor departure from normal (e.g., less interaction with peers; some neglect of nest-building; some signs of aggression)	Investigate possible causes (e.g. pain?, male-to-male aggression?) and act accordingly	Noticeable departure from normal (e.g., becoming isolated; more subdued or more aggressive)	As for column A; and monitor daily	Significant departure from normal	If no clear cause-treatment solution available, cull
Prolapse	**Column A:** Slightly protruding penis, vagina or rectum	Consider possible treatment/s with EV; consider change of bedding/nesting to avoid abrasion	More pronounced protrusion	As for column A if appropriate; otherwise consider termination	No resolution despite treatment/s; damaged organs	Cull
External lumps/masses	Small lumps/masses not affecting normal body functions	Consider possible treatment/s with EV if appropriate	Medium-size (0.5–0.8 cm) lumps/masses	As for column A; check for possible presence of other internal lumps and/or other clinical signs. Monitor body condition score weekly	Large lumps (0.8–1 cm); ulcerated or infected	If no clear cause-treatment solution available, monitor daily and prepare to cull	**Lumps/masses >1.1 cm or affecting body functions/mobility**	Cull
Internal lumps/masses	**Column A** Small palpable lumps/masses not affecting normal body functions	Consider possible treatment/s with EV if appropriate; check for other possible clinical signs	Medium-size (<0.5 cm) lumps/masses	As for column A, consider the possible use of other diagnostic tests (e.g. ultra sound imaging) Monitor body condition score weekly	Large lumps (>0.5 cm); concurrent presence of other clinical signs (e.g. pallour)	If no clear cause-treatment solution available, monitor daily and prepare to cull	**Large lumps/masses affecting body functions or causing other significant clinical signs**	Cull

(Continued)

Table 16.1 (Continued)

OBSERVATION	GENERAL ACTION TO BE TAKEN (in white) – in consideration with the project authorisation adverse effects and humane endpoints, the expected phenotype of the animal and the needs of the intended research. Note: Always use in partnership with the Establishment's Veterinarian (EV) and bear in mind that allowing animals to display many of the signs in this table will likely require specific legal authorisation.			
	ADVISE TO MONITOR EVERY TWO WEEKS FROM 15 MONTHS		WEEKLY MONITORING ADVISED FROM 20 MONTHS	DAILY MONITORING ADVISED FROM 30 MONTHS
	Initiate regular monitoring		Increase monitoring	Critical monitoring
Eye defects	Defects unlikely to affect normal body functions and behaviour (e.g. cataracts, one missing eye, conjunctivitis, small eye)	Consider possible treatment/s with EV if appropriate; check for possible behavioural changes or other clinical signs	Defects likely to result in pain or affect normal body functions (e.g., swollen, closed eye; protruding eye)	As per column A; monitor daily	Defects clearly affecting normal body functions or behaviour (e.g. ulceration)	If no clear cause-treatment solution available or no response to previous treatment, cull
Abnormal respiration	Slight departure from normal (e.g. slight increased or decreased respiratory rate; intermittent change; cough/sneeze)	Thoroughly evaluate possible causes with EV and act accordingly	Moderate departure from normal or more persistent changes	As per column A; monitor daily and check for presence of other possible clinical signs	Significant departure from normal (e.g. laboured breathing; nose bleeding; rapid shallow breathing)	If no clear cause-treatment solution available, or no response to previous treatment, cull
Abnormal stools	**Column A** Slightly softer than normal faeces; slight staining around anus	Thoroughly evaluate possible causes and act accordingly; provide clean bedding	Soft stools; stained perineal area	As for column A and check for presence of other possible clinical signs	Persistent diarrhoea; stained perineum; blood-stained stools	If no clear cause-treatment solution available, or no response to previous treatment, cull

Source: Adapted from Wilkinson et al. (2019).

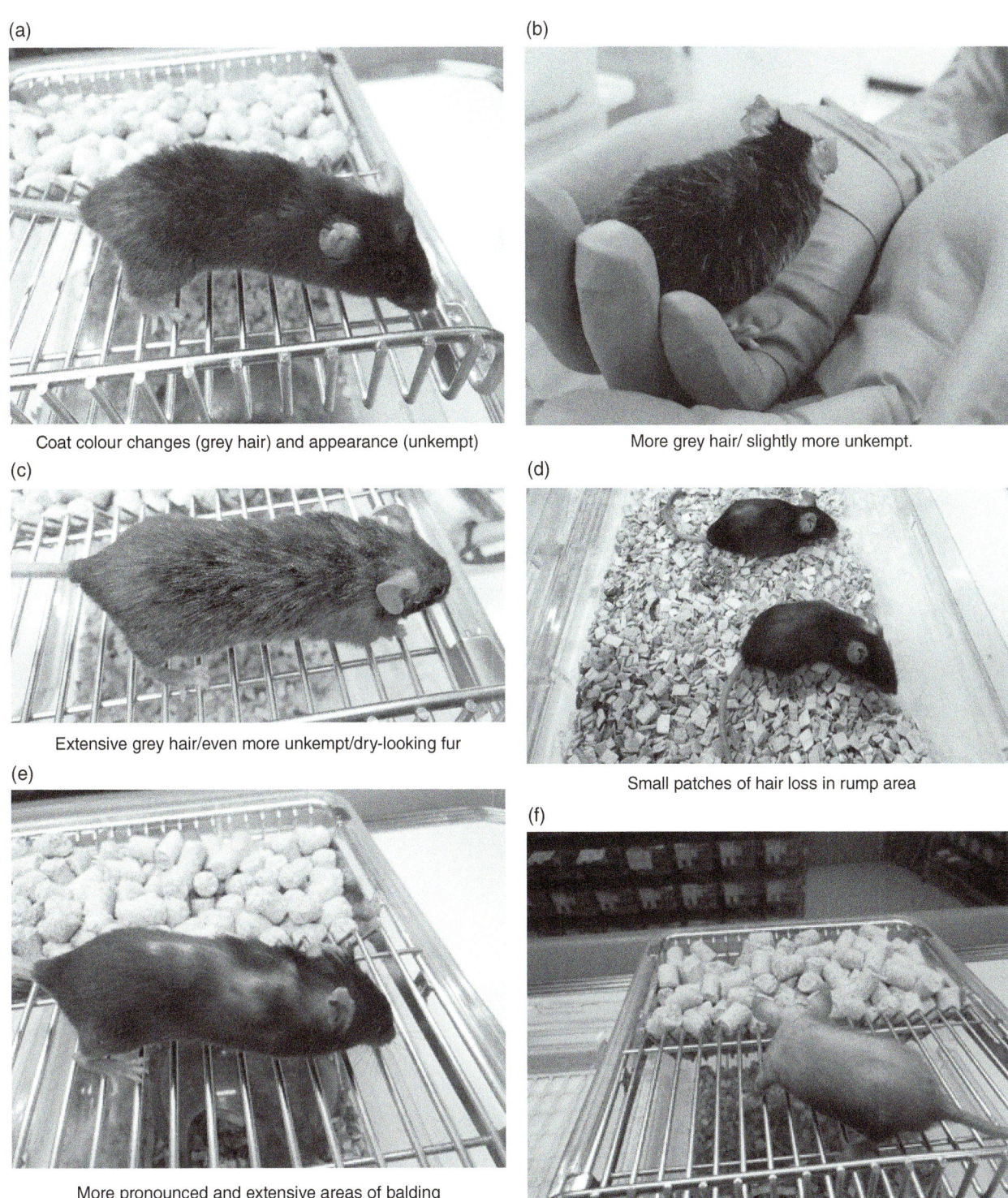

Figure 16.1 Common phenotypic ageing–related adverse effects in mice.

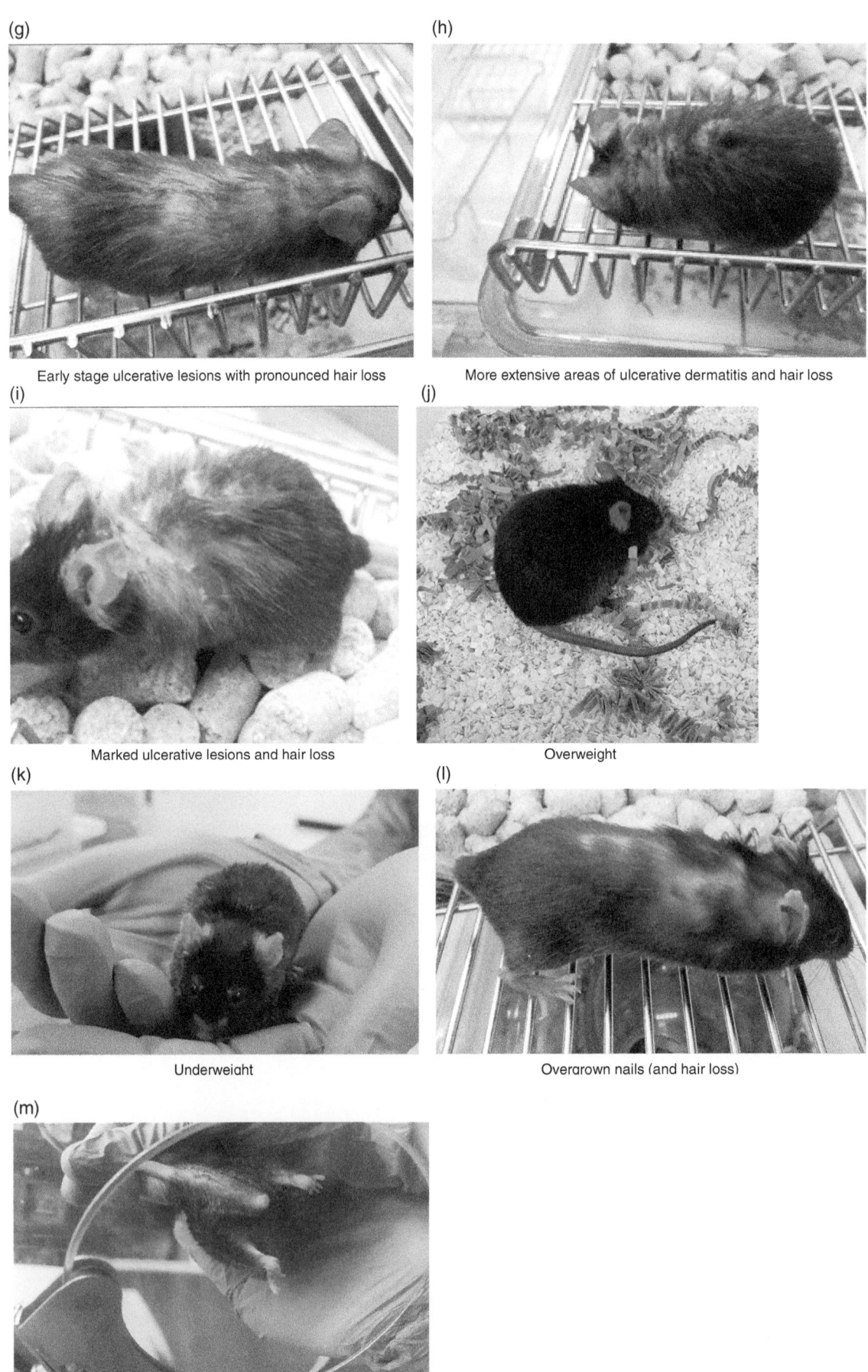

Figure 16.1 (Continued)

the putative therapeutic intervention under investigation and this, in turn, could ultimately translate into significant human patient benefits.

Depending on the knowledge of the particular mouse strain – be it wild type or GA – these enhanced monitoring regimes can be adapted to suit both the expected adverse effects and the scientific needs of each study (see also Chapter 5: Phenotyping of genetically modified mice). The chosen monitoring regime should be as non-invasive as possible given the age of the animals, designed to minimise stress, and should include the use of refined handling methods such as cupping and the use of tubes (Hurst & West 2010).

Zebra finches

In common with other avian species, aged zebra finches can develop a raft of conditions that are more or less typical of the geriatric bird. Arthritis, for example, is not an uncommon finding in zebra finches that have passed their fifth or sixth year of life and can manifest itself – among other signs – as reduced activity (including less flight or abnormal flight), lameness, difficulty perching or swollen joints (Figure 16.2). A condition that is often related to arthritis is pododermatitis, which can be inflammatory or degenerative in nature and is relatively common in aged birds. Older birds also have an increased risk of developing cataracts, poor plumage, chronic liver disease (especially, hepatic lipidosis), renal insufficiency, atherosclerosis and cardiac and pulmonary disease (Hoppes 2018). Since many of these conditions can be closely related to inadequate nutrition and/or husbandry, it is very important to periodically revise these when keeping birds on long-term studies. One example is the introduction of simple environmental enrichment measures that can keep birds more active, enhance exercise, reduce the risk of obesity and keep birds motivated (see also Chapter 42: Zebra finches).

An increased risk of developing neoplastic conditions is another hallmark of ageing. Neoplasia in passerine birds is

(a)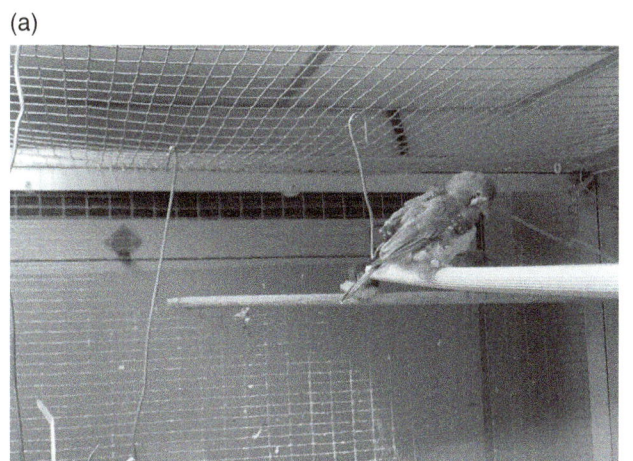
Body plumage and primary wing feather loss; dull eyes; fluffed

(b)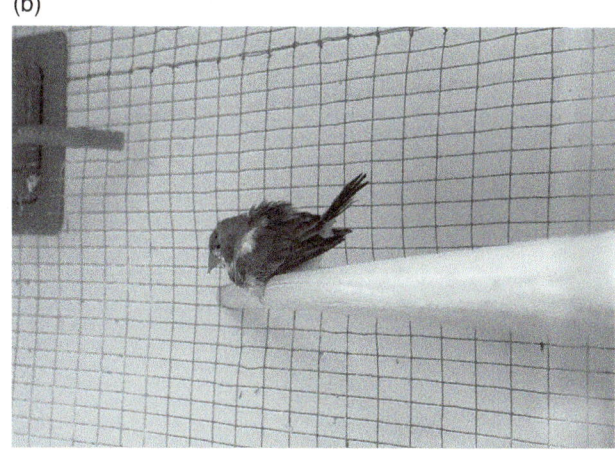
Overgrown bill and altered perching ability; fluffed up

(c)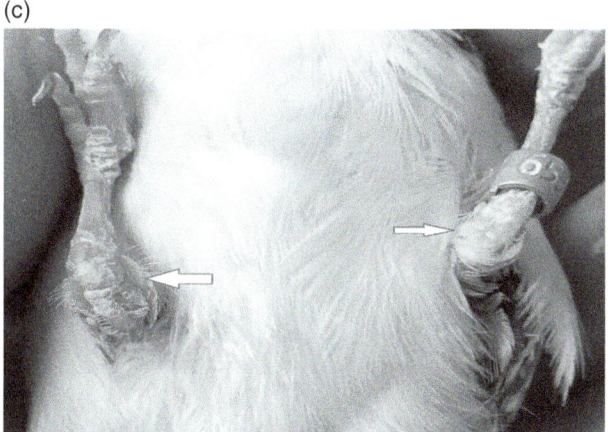
5-year-old zebra finch showing arthritic-like, swollen joints (white arrows)

(d)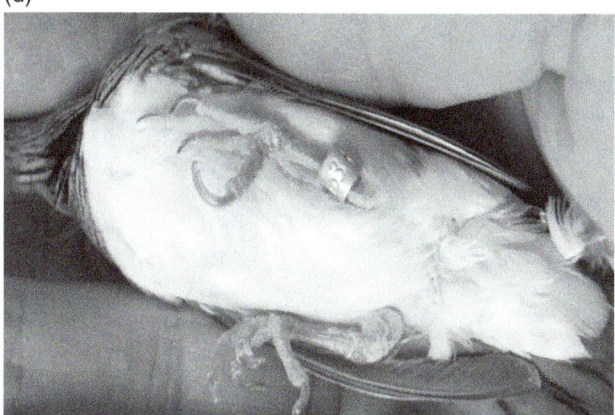
Overgrown nails due to bird not perching properly. Affected birds avoid perching and spend more time on the cage floor

Figure 16.2 Common phenotypic ageing–related adverse effects in zebra finches.

not as common as in psittacines and yet aged finches can and do develop a variety of neoplasms such as lymphosarcomas (commonly of liver and spleen), adenocarcinomas (commonly of gonads or kidneys), fibromas and haemangiosarcomas, among others (Best 2018). Moreover, captive colonies harbouring endemic infectious agents, be they primary or opportunistic, are likely to see reduced lifespans as a result of the insidious effects of these agents on the animals as they age. A classic example is Avian Gastric Yeast (AGY), a common organism in captive colonies of zebra finches, that can slowly erode the health of some individuals and often results in premature culling for welfare reasons.

Signs of ageing and management of aged zebra finches

The decision for when to humanely kill an aged bird that is being used as part of a longevity study will depend on numerous factors, including the severity limits imposed by regulatory authorities and institutional bodies (e.g., Animal Welfare Committees, Institutional Animal Care and Use Committees (IACUC)), the potential – or not – to alleviate some of the adverse manifestations of ageing and the purpose of the study. An example of a welfare assessment system used in a particular ageing study of zebra finches is given in Table 16.2. Clearly, any such system has to be interpreted in light of the limits imposed by project authorisation or experimental protocols and adapted to the nature of the particular study. But it is important to emphasise that its value will depend, in great measure, on good communication between scientists, animal care staff and institutional veterinarians, such that health and welfare issues can be spotted promptly and acted upon effectively. The veterinary care of geriatric birds is an incipient field that has been gradually growing and there are a variety of valuable information sources that can be consulted (Lightfoot 2011; Hoppes 2018). As mentioned before, many age-related conditions, such as obesity or arthritis, can be closely linked to erroneous nutrition and/or husbandry so it is imperative to carefully plan these factors before embarking on a longevity study. Other conditions, such as many malignant neoplasias or renal insufficiency, are probably not amenable to treatment in small birds, such as finches, especially after a harm/benefit analysis is performed. But, for many of them, simple measures can improve the quality of life of the geriatric bird. The provision of perches of the right (and varying) diameter and texture, positioned at multiple heights, allowing easy access to food and water can help non-flying birds or birds with swollen joints, plus help prevent pododermatitis. Similarly,

Table 16.2 Example of a welfare assessment system for zebra finches used in a longevity study.

	YELLOW	ORANGE	RED
General appearance and response	• Fluffed up some of the time* • Eyes slightly dull, not bright* • Normal escape/flight reactions when approached	• Fluffed up most of the time • Eyes semi-closed and dull most of the time • Possibly slower than normal reactions when approached	• Fluffed up all the time, eyes semi-closed or dull all the time, quite unresponsive (very slow or no escape reaction)
Weight loss (from when * signs above first noticed)	5–10%	10–15%	>15%
Respiration	Normal	Intermittent abnormal breathing	Persistent abnormal breathing
Vent	Slight staining around vent that can be easily cleansed/removed	Extensive and persistent staining around vent	Non-resolving prolapse
Flying and movement	Normal flying but some feathers may be damaged or missing	Moderate limb or wing abnormalities (e.g. swollen joints, bruising) Unable to fly (>1 week) Many feathers damaged or missing	Major limb/wing or other injuries (e.g. fractures, dislocations) Unable to keep normal balance
Feet and joints	Dry-looking or slightly damaged skin of feet Normal perching	Abnormal feet or joints (e.g. swollen) Difficulty perching	Unable to perch even after treatment (if appropriate)
Other	Small (e.g. 2–3 mm) palpable lump/mass/cyst	Medium-size (4–5 mm) lump/mass/cyst palpable or visible	Larger (>5 mm) lump/mass/cyst that is not amenable to treatment or any mass which interferes with normal functions or becomes ulcerated
ACTION	Start weighing the animal weekly when * signs noticed Alert vet and discuss possible treatments Closely monitor bird Mark colour card accordingly Enter information in individual health record	As for bird with yellow signs if not already being monitored If three or more orange signs are persistently present, discuss culling with stakeholders	Cull any bird showing a red sign

consideration of cage furniture arrangements (e.g. fixed position of perches and food and water sources), adequate companionship and provision of secluded/quiet areas can greatly help birds that have developed blindness as a result of cataracts or other eye abnormalities.

Zebrafish

Zebrafish undergo a gradual natural ageing process (Kishi et al. 2003), and many of the important age-related considerations given to mammalian model species are equally applicable to fish species; in particular, in ageing fish stocks the appearance of age-related phenotypes become more obvious, for example, scoliosis and muscle degeneration (see Figure 16.3; Gerhard et al. 2002; Gerhard 2003). There are age-related issues affecting zebrafish, as ageing, i.e. >18 months old, will markedly reduce fertility and fecundity and increase health problems (Ramsay et al. 2009a, b; Wilson 2012), which in turn will have a significant impact maintaining zebrafish lines (Lawrence 2007). Nasiadka and Clark (2012) report that once sexual maturity is reached, prime reproductive performance is maintained for several months, but then decreases with age. Aged stocks of ovigerous females are also more likely to become egg-bound. Age also increases susceptibility to disease (Kent et al. 2009; Borges et al. 2016; Collymore et al. 2016). Furthermore, inbreeding may have the consequence of premature ageing, which will also include loss of fecundity and difficulty with survival of offspring (Aleström et al. 2019) and should therefore also be taken into consideration.

In some cases, it may be better for both science and welfare to avoid using older fish in research. Because adult zebrafish retain their ability to regenerate organs and tissues, experimental conclusions following surgery, when examining, for example, infarcted adult myocardial wall, can be confused by the normal process of cellular remodelling during ageing (Yu et al. 2018). Although post-surgical recovery can be refined by the use of anaesthetics and analgesics (Schroeder & Sneddon 2016), their impact on studies, where the role of inflammation is recognised, has not fully been addressed. Further, outcomes of cancer models may be masked by age (Franceschi et al. 2018) or confounded by spontaneous neoplasia (Spitsbergen et al. 2012; Paquette et al. 2013) or age-related neoplasia (Carneiro et al. 2016; Cayuela et al. 2019).

Therefore, choosing, when relevant, a younger sample of fish may provide more robust science. As with all research models, good quality data will only be obtained when animals are maintained in a condition where chronic stressors, including age, are kept to a minimum to reduce any physiological change (see Vargesson 2007 and Reed and Jennings 2011 for a review of housing and care of zebrafish).

Signs of ageing and management of aged zebrafish

The identification of humane endpoints for zebrafish is as important as for other species, and ageing studies require clear welfare assessments and enhanced clinical monitoring similar to those described earlier in the section on ageing mice.

It is important to note that some GA zebrafish lines, like some GA mouse lines, are progeroid and have a predisposition to ageing, e.g. rag$^{-/-}$ (Novoa et al. 2019) and consequently enhanced clinical monitoring is required; here, the clinical scoring will be linked to actual severity. Such GA lines reinforce that there is not a 'one size fits all' approach (Wilkinson et al. 2019) when applying clinical phenotypic scoring as it will need to be applied individually to each different zebrafish line (Gerhard et al. 2002); fundamentally the biology of each line needs to be understood.

Dogs and macaques

In this section, we consider dogs and macaques together because both species are commonly used in long-term safety evaluation studies. In the UK, both species have special protection under the regulations controlling the use of animals for research purposes. Further, the ageing-related clinical issues that they develop are often similar. Indeed, one of the more common issues affecting both dogs and macaques held for years in the laboratory setting is effective weight management. Long-term holding in even the best examples of laboratory housing typically results in sub-optimal opportunities for exercise. Over time, this can result in a tendency to obesity. Enrichment strategies should be considered, to maximise potential for regular exercise of the animals. In the case of dogs, out of pen exercise should be a standard part of the husbandry practice. See also Chapter 30: The laboratory dog and Chapter 13: Nutrition, feeding and animal welfare.

(a) 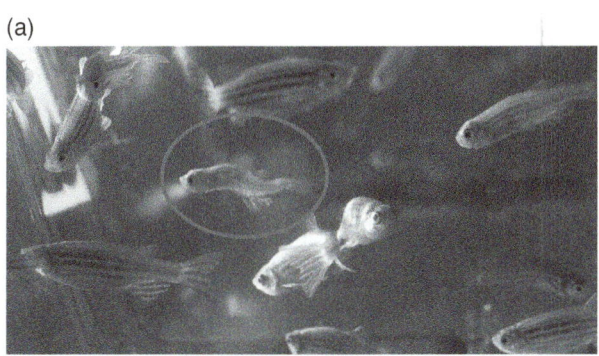 (b)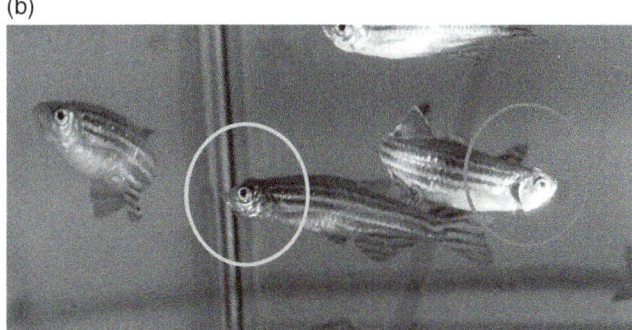

Figure 16.3 Common phenotypic ageing–related adverse effects in zebrafish.

Signs of ageing and management of aged dogs and macaques

Regular assessment of weight and body condition should be an established part of the veterinary oversight of the animals. This process will enable identification of animals which may require dietary management. Laboratory diets provide a standard energy ration to laboratory animals. The daily amount of food offered to the animals will be a standard. However, individual requirements vary, and for dogs, calorie restriction, in addition to exercise, can be an important part of managing body condition. Routine monitoring of weight and/or body condition enables early identification of animals losing condition, so that these individuals can be provided with increased diet or calories.

Management of caloric intake is much easier for group-housed dogs than group-housed macaques due first, to the differing feeding regimes of the two species (single daily meals for dogs as opposed to forage feeding of macaques). Second, high-value treats and edible enrichments may be used as part of positive reinforcement strategies for macaques. Judicious reduction in use of high calorie items such as some fruits and nuts should be established early in the management programme of animals identified for long-term holding. Colony monitoring should involve regular clinical chemistry assessment, which would identify any animals which may become diabetic.

Dental disease is a risk factor for both species, but more commonly seen in dogs. A build-up of plaque and dental calculus is common as dogs age, and this can result in gingivitis and periodontal disease. Husbandry strategies should include the provision of chews to reduce likely development of calculus. Many items are marketed specifically for this purpose in dogs, and are also considered to be enrichment items. These items can also be provided to macaques, although it is advisable to conduct small-scale trials to assess their safety and robustness. The husbandry programme should include a regular assessment of dental health, and preventative dental care such as brushing with enzymatic toothpaste to reduce periodontal disease that would otherwise require veterinary intervention. Tooth de-scaling and polishing under anaesthesia can be conducted under veterinary guidance as part of the health management programme.

A number of health concerns typically considered to be diseases of ageing may occasionally be seen in dogs. Cases of prostatic disease and osteoarthritis have been seen in the author's colony over the years. Theoretically, uterine pyometra of female dogs, and various neoplastic events may also occur. However, as long-term use animals should be regularly observed by animal care staff, routine assessment and recording of clinical findings, weight, food consumption, body condition, clinical pathology, together with regular veterinary assessments should enable early identification and resolution of adverse health-related issues in ageing animals.

Legal considerations when using ageing animals for scientific purposes

A final consideration when working with ageing animals is the question of when exactly should the 'purposeful ageing' of animals be considered to require authorisation under relevant legislation. This section aims to describe the criteria that need to be considered for a consistent approach with regard to setting the time point for commencing enhanced monitoring and determining when legal authorisation may be required to comply with local legislation. We describe this using European legislation as an example, but the underlying principles as to when authorisation should be required can be applied more generally, e.g., at a local authorisation level by an IACUC or similar oversight body.

In Europe, the relevant legislation is Directive 2010/63/EU (see also Chapter 8: Legislation and oversight of the conduct of research using animals: A global overview). The Directive defines a 'procedure' as any use, invasive or non-invasive, of an animal for experimental or other scientific purposes, with known or unknown outcome, or educational purposes, which may cause the animal a level of pain, suffering, distress or lasting harm equivalent to, or higher than, that caused by the introduction of a needle in accordance with good veterinary practice. Keeping animals alive, for a qualifying scientific purpose, beyond this point requires project authorisation. This is important because procedures can only be applied to a protected animal as part of a programme of work described in a project authorisation.

Where the scientific investigation relates to the physiological process of ageing, or investigates a disease mechanism or the metabolism of a drug in an ageing animal, then keeping animals beyond the age when they would normally be kept in standard efficient breeding programmes will be necessary in order to achieve the scientific goals. Mice need to be given additional consideration firstly because mice are currently the most commonly used species in ageing studies. Secondly because they, along with zebrafish, encompass a range of genetic types from non-GA, wild type, in-bred, to GA (where the genetic alteration may have been either created experimentally or occurs naturally and is potentially expected to be associated with a harmful phenotype). Some of these are very well characterised both genetically and phenotypically, others less so, particularly the phenotypes of ageing strains. Both in the EU and the UK, all mice kept for use in scientific procedures are protected animals whether they carry a genetic alteration or not. In the UK, the breeding and maintenance of virtually all GA mice, whether or not they have a harmful clinical phenotype associated with the genetic alteration or not, requires project authorisation. This is because it is assumed that all experimentally created mouse strains <u>may</u> cross the threshold requiring project authorisation and few welfare assessments have (as defined and required under the Directive) been completed on established strains to determine that do not have a harmful clinical phenotype. The Directive has been interpreted differently across EU member states, and in some, while all laboratory-created strains are produced under project authorisation, only GA mice with a manifest adverse phenotype require project authorisation. The assumption being that there is no overt harm unless it has been previously demonstrated. This situation has recently been reviewed by the EU Commission and no substantive changes are anticipated. Because of this difference between EU member states, some GA mice will already be under project authorisation and others not. Parallel situations exist with other national legislations, such as that in the USA, where mice are afforded protection under some federal laws but not others[5].

What about mice that are 'purposefully aged'? Does the 'purposeful ageing' of the animals, in itself, require project authorisation, as defined above? Should consideration be given to the effect – enhancement or diminishment – of the genetic alteration on the ageing process? Will they have different or additional adverse clinical effects as a consequence of the ageing process that may need to be defined in a project authorisation?

We consider that the requirement for project authorisation of ageing animals cannot be determined solely on age. Instead, it should be viewed as a performance standard, that is, when any age-associated clinical signs indicating pain, suffering, distress or lasting harm actually occur and the animal is not immediately culled. This is consistent with the definition of a procedure for qualifying scientific purpose (see the preceding text). Given that there is already published evidence of age-related 'watersheds' in some mouse colonies (Kitching 2008), we consider it reasonable to propose that, when no information is available from establishment health records or from the published literature on a particular mouse strain or new genotype, a point should be established for enhanced monitoring of any ageing mice. Having worked with the scientific and regulatory communities in the UK, comprised of a wide range of scientists and experienced animal care technologists, currently we propose that this age-related trigger-point for enhanced monitoring should be 15 months. As more information is generated from enhanced monitoring systems, it seems reasonable to predict that this time point may change. But presently, the recommendation is that from this age onwards, mice should undergo an enhanced regime of monitoring with additional husbandry or veterinary intervention steps aimed at identifying, recording and mitigating any ageing-associated adverse clinical signs. This general recommendation does not preclude the establishment of earlier points for enhanced monitoring when this is seen as a prudent decision, such as when expected progeroid mouse models are generated or when new GA models start showing signs of frailty or ageing earlier than expected.

Where there is information available on the phenotype of the mouse and the strain is already well characterised, with details available through – for example – the 'Mouse Passport Scheme[6]', establishment health records or published literature, then the trigger-point for enhanced monitoring and consideration given to project authorisation should coincide with the onset of any known adverse ageing-associated clinical or phenotypic sign(s). Obviously, the timing can vary widely depending on the onset of expected age-related clinical or phenotypic sign(s) in mice of that particular strain and need not coincide with the 15-month trigger-point mentioned in the preceding text. In all cases, information on the background strain must be taken into account as this is known to have an influence on the onset of age-related clinical signs. For instance, it may be asked: is it necessary to implement enhanced monitoring of mice from 15 months of age where no adverse phenotype is expected? We are of the opinion that if there is evidence (for example, from health records) to show that no adverse clinical or phenotypic signs are expected, then an informed decision can be taken that there is no need for enhanced monitoring because no signs of pain, suffering, distress or lasting harm are anticipated.

Summary

We have outlined the background to the marked increase in the number of ageing animals that are being used in scientific studies. Currently, there is an unmet need to ensure consistency in the husbandry and management of these ageing animals, thereby optimising their welfare and, at the same time, underpinning the achievement of good quality, reproducible scientific results (Toth 2018). It is often easy, when designing a scientific study that may last for several months or years, to overlook that the animals will age naturally during their time on study. When considering appropriate refinement, the changing physiological, behavioural and ethological needs of the animal, as well as refinements more directly related to the disease processes under primary investigation, need to be taken into account.

We have described some refinements mostly in the care of ageing mice but also in zebra finches, zebrafish and raised awareness of ageing-related issues in dogs, and NHPs used principally in the safety evaluation of novel pharmaceutical compounds. We believe that a significant way forward towards the achievement of improved animal welfare and better science is the adoption of enhanced clinical monitoring (as exemplified for ageing mouse colonies intended for scientific use in Table 16.1). However, there is a widespread applicability of these refinement principles and approaches to other species. For example, the use of a standardised tank-side scoring system for zebrafish has been described aimed at monitoring the health and welfare of laboratory zebrafish and highlighting clear endpoint determinations (Wilson et al. 2013; Wilson & Dunford 2018).

Given the diversity of research studies using ageing animals, it is clear that monitoring and intervention need to be tailored to the species, genetic background and strain, study design and scientific objectives without causing additional harms to the animals and without being too labour intensive. It is also important that monitoring, handling and use of ageing animals should cause as little stress as possible as any stressor may impact on the physiology of the animal. As for all animals used in research, thought needs to be given to reducing stress during handling, and the impact of procedures for example by the use of anaesthesia/analgesia (e.g., for fish, Schroeder & Sneddon 2016), and using the most refined way to take samples (e.g., mucus swabbing, Breacker et al. 2017) and by avoiding sampling later in the life of aged animals.

---

[5] National Research Council (US) Committee to Update Science, Medicine, and Animals (2004) *Regulation of Animal Research*: In: Science, Medicine, and Animals. National Academies Press (US), Washington (DC) ISBN-10: 0-309-08894-1. Available at: https://www.ncbi.nlm.nih.gov/books/NBK24650/ (accessed 29 November 2019)

[6] https://www.rspca.org.uk/webContent/staticImages/Downloads/3RsInitiativesForGAMice.pdf (accessed 29 November 2019)

Finally, this chapter is not intended to be an authoritative source of advice and guidance on international legislation regarding the regulation of ageing animals used in science. Instead, it is a reminder that such legislation exists and needs to be complied with wherever the studies are conducted. Legislative requirements vary between different countries or continents but the principles we describe are – we believe – widely relevant and applicable.

References

Aleström, P., D'Angelo, L., Midtlyng, P.J. et al. (2019). Zebrafish: Housing and husbandry recommendations. *Laboratory Animals*. https://doi.org/10.1177/0023677219869037

Bateson, M. and Feenders, G. (2010) The use of passerine bird species in laboratory research: implications of basic biology for husbandry and welfare. *Institute for Laboratory Animal Research*, **51**, 394–408.

Best, J.R. (2018) Passerine birds: approach to the sick individual. In: *BSAVA Manual of Avian Practice*. Eds Chitty, J. and Monks, D. pp. 80–97; BSAVA Publications, Gloucester, UK.

Borges, A.C., Pereira, N., Franco, M. et al. (2016) M. Implementation of a Zebrafish Health Program in a Research Facility: a 4-year retrospective study. *Zebrafish*, **13**, 115–126.

Bradford, Y.M., Toro, S., Ramachandran, S. et al. (2017) Zebrafish Models of Human Disease: Gaining Insight into Human Disease at ZFIN. *ILAR Journal*, **58**, 4–16.

Brayton, C.F., Treuting, P.M. and Ward, J.M. (2012) Pathobiology of ageing mice and GEM: background strains and experimental design. *Veterinary Pathology*, **49**, 85–105.

Breacker, C., Barber, I., Norton, W.H.J. et al. (2017) A low-cost method of skin swabbing for the collection of DNA samples from small laboratory fish. *Zebrafish*, **14**, 35–41.

Bugnon, P., Heimann, M. and Thallmair, M. (2016). What the literature tells us about score sheet design. *Laboratory Animals*, **50**(6), 414–417.

Carneiro, M.C., de Castro, I.P. and Ferreira, M.G. (2016) Telomeres in aging and disease: lessons from zebrafish. *Disease Models and Mechanisms*, **9**, 737–748.

Cayuela, M.L., Claes, K.B.M., Ferreira, M.G. et al. (2019) The Zebrafish as an emerging model to study DNA damage in aging, cancer and other diseases. *Frontiers in Cell and Developmental Biology*, **10**(6), 178.

Chen, X., Mao, G. and Leng, S.X. (2014) Frailty syndrome: an overview. *Clinical Interventions in Aging*, **9**, 433–441.

Collin, J. and Martin, P. (2017) Zebrafish as a research organism. *Basic Science Methods for Clinical Researchers*, 235–261.

Collymore, C., Crim, M.J. and Lieggi, C. (2016) Recommendations for health monitoring and reporting for zebrafish research facilities. *Zebrafish*, **13**(S1), S-138–S-148.

Cracknell, R. (2017) The ageing population. Key issues for the new parliament 2010. *Statistics UK Parliament*, 44–45. Available at https://www.parliament.uk/business/publications/research/key-issues-for-the-new-parliament/value-for-money-in-public-services/the-ageing-population/ (accessed 6 June 2019).

Engeszer, R.E., Patterson, L.B., Rao, A.A. et al. (2007) Zebrafish in the wild: a review of the natural history and new notes from the field. *Zebrafish*, **4**, 21–38.

EUD, *European Directive 2010/63/EU of the European Parliament and of the Council on the protection of animals used for scientific purposes*. Available at: https://eur-lex.europa.eu/legal-content/EN/TXT/?uri=celex%3A32010L0063 (accessed 27 March 2019).

Figueira, I., Fernandes, A., Mladenovic Djordjevic, A. et al. (2016) Interventions for age-related diseases: Shifting the paradigm. *Mechanisms of Ageing and Development*, **160**, 69–92.

Fontana, L. and Partridge, L. (2015) Promoting health and longevity through diet: from model organisms to humans. *Cell*, **161**, 106–118.

Franceschi, C., Garagnani, P., Parini, P. et al. (2018) Inflammaging: a new immune–metabolic viewpoint for age-related diseases. *Nature Reviews Endocrinology*, **14**, 576–590.

Gemberling, M., Bailey, T.J., Hyde, D.R. et al. (2013) The zebrafish as a model for complex tissue regeneration. *Trends Genetics*, **29**, 611–620.

Gems, D. and Partridge, L. (2013) Genetics of longevity in model organisms: debates and paradigm shifts. *Annual Review of Physiology*, **75**, 621–644.

Gerhard, G.S. (2003) Comparative aspects of zebrafish (*Danio rerio*) as a model for aging research. *Experimental Gerontology*, **38**, 1333–1341.

Gerhard, G.S., Kauffman, E.J., Wang, X. et al. (2002) Life spans and senescent phenotypes of zebrafish (*Danio rerio*). *Experimental Gerontology*, **37**, 1055–1068.

Gilbert, M.J., Zerulla, T.C. and Tierney, K.B. (2014) Zebrafish (*Danio rerio*) as a model for the study of aging and exercise: physical ability and trainability decrease with age. *Experimental Gerontology*, **50**, 106–113.

Haussmann, M.F., Winkler, D.W., Huntington, C.E. et al. (2005) Cell-mediated immunosenescence in birds. *Oecologia*, **145**, 269–274.

Hawkins, P. (2002). Recognizing and assessing pain, suffering and distress in laboratory animals: a survey of current practice in the UK with recommendations. *Laboratory Animals*, **36**(4), 378–395.

Hawkins, P., Morton, D.B., Burman, O. et al. (2011) A guide to defining and implementing protocols for the welfare assessment of laboratory animals: eleventh report of the BVAAWF/FRAME/RSPCA/UFAW Joint Working Group on Refinement. *Laboratory Animals*, **45**, 1–13.

Heidinger, B.J., Blount, J.D., Boner, W. et al. (2012) Telomere length in early life predicts lifespan. *Proceedings of the National Academy of Sciences*, **109**, 1743–1748.

Holmes, D.J. and Austad, S.N. (1995) Birds as animal models for the comparative biology of aging: a prospectus. *Journal of Gerontology*, **50A**, B59–B66.

Holmes, D.J. and Ottinger, M.A. (2003) Birds as long-lived animal models for the study of aging. *Experimental Gerontology*, **38**, 1365–1375.

Honess, P. and Wolfensohn, S. (2010) The extended welfare assessment grid: a matrix for the assessment of welfare and cumulative suffering in experimental animals. *ATLA*, **38**, 205–212.

Hoppes, S.M. (2018) Geriatric Diseases of Pet Birds. MSD Veterinary Manual. Available at: https://www.msdvetmanual.com/exotic-and-laboratory-animals/pet-birds/geriatric-diseases-of-pet-birds (accessed 26th July 2019).

Howe, K., Clark, M.D., Torroja, C.F. et al. (2013) The zebrafish reference genome sequence and its relationship to the human genome. *Nature*, **496**, 498–503.

Hurst, J.L. and West, R.S. (2010) Taming anxiety in laboratory mice. *Nature Methods*, **7**, 825–826.

Jayanthi, P., Joshua, E. and Ranganathan, K. (2010) Ageing and its implications. *Journal of Oral Maxillofacial Pathology*, **14**, 48–51.

Kent, M.L., Feist, S.W., Harper, C. et al. (2009) Recommendations for control of pathogens and infectious diseases in fish research facilities. *Comp. Biochem. Physiol Part C (Toxicol. Pharmacol.)*, **149**, 240–248.

Kim, S-Y., Velando, A., Sorci, G. et al. (2010) Genetic correlation between resistance to oxidative stress and reproductive life span in a bird species. *Evolution*, **64**, 852–857.

Kishi, S., Uchiyama, J., Baughman, A.M. et al. (2003) The zebrafish as a vertebrate model of functional aging and very gradual senescence. *Experimental Gerontology*, **38**, 777–786.

Kitching, A. (2018) A retrospective review of the causes of deaths in an aged mouse colony. IAT Congress, Harrogate, England. Poster presentation.

Lawrence, C. (2007) The husbandry of zebrafish (*Danio rerio*): a review. *Aquaculture*, **269**, 1–20.

Liao, C.Y. and Kennedy, B.K. (2014) Mouse models and aging: longevity and progeria. *Current Topics in Developmental Biology*, **109**, 249–285.

Lightfoot, T. (2011) Geriatric Avian Medicine (Proceedings). CVC Kansas City Proceedings. Available at: http://veterinarycalendar.dvm360.com/geriatric-avian-medicine-proceedings (accessed 28th July 2019).

Liu, H., Graber, T.G., Ferguson-Stegall, L. *et al.* (2014) Clinically relevant frailty index for mice. *The Journals of Gerontology Series A Biological Science and Medical Science*, **69**, 1485–1491.

Marshall, C. and Melville, G. (2015) Refinement and reduction in pruritic aged C57/Bl6 mice. IAT Congress, Glasgow, Scotland. Poster presentation.

Martin, B., Ji, S., Maudsley, S. *et al.* (2010) 'Control' laboratory rodents are metabolically morbid: why it matters. *Proceedings of the National Academy of Sciences USA*, **107**, 6127–6133.

McIness, E.F. (2012) *Background Lesions in Laboratory Animals A Color Atlas 1st edition*. Saunders, Elsevier, Edinburgh.

Meeker, N.D. and Trede, N.S. (2008) Immunology and zebrafish: spawning new models of human disease. *Dev Comp Immunol*. **32**(7), 745–757.

Mimeault, M. and Batra, S.K. (2010) Recent advances on skin-resident stem/progenitor cell functions in skin regeneration, aging and cancers and novel anti-aging and cancer therapies. *Journal of Cellular and Molecular Medicine*, **14**, 116–134.

Moe, B., Ronning, B., Verhulst, S. *et al.* (2009) Metabolic ageing in individual zebra finches. *Biol. Lett.*, **5**, 86–89.

Most, J., Tosti, V., Redman, L.M. *et al.* (2017) Calorie restriction in humans: An update. TORC1 inhibition enhances immune function and reduces infections in the elderly. *Ageing Research Review*, **39**, 36–45.

Nasiadka, A. and Clark, M.D. (2012) Zebrafish Breeding in the Laboratory Environment. *ILAR Journal*, **53**, 161–168.

Noguera, J.C., Metcalfe, N.B. and Monaghan, P. (2018) Experimental demonstration that offspring fathered by old males have shorter telomeres and reduced lifespans. *Proceedings of the Royal Society of London Series B: Biological Sciences*, **285**(1874), 20180268.

Novoa, B., Pereiro, P., López-Muñoz, A. *et al.* (2019) Rag1 immunodeficiency-induced early aging and senescence in zebrafish are dependent on chronic inflammation and oxidative stress. *Aging Cell*, doi: 10.1111/acel.13020.

Paquette, C.E., Kent, M.L., Buchner, C. *et al.* (2013) A retrospective study of the prevalence and classification of intestinal Neoplasia in Zebrafish (*Danio Rerio*). *Zebrafish*, **10**(2), 228–236.

Parks, R.J., Fares, E., MacDonald, J.K. *et al.* (2012) A procedure for creating a frailty index based on deficit accumulation in ageing mice. *The Journals of Gerontology Series A Biological Science and Medical Science*, **67**, 217–227.

Patton, E.E. and Tobin, D.M. (2019) Spotlight on zebrafish: the next wave of translational research. *Disease Models & Mechanisms*, **12**, 1–4.

Pettan-Brewer, C. and Treuting, P.M. (2011) Practical pathology of aging mice. *Pathobiology of Aging and Age-related Diseases*, **1**, 7202.

Phillips, J.B. and Westerfield, M. (2014) Zebrafish models in translational research: tipping the scales toward advancements in human health. *Disease Models & Mechanisms*, **7**, 739–743.

Pytte, C.L., Gerson, M., Miller, J. *et al.* (2007) Increasing stereotypy in adult zebra finch song correlates with a declining rate of adult neurogenesis. *Developmental Neurobiology*, **67**, 1699–1720.

Ramsay, J.M., Watral, V., Schreck, C.B. *et al.* (2009a) Husbandry stress exacerbates mycobacterial infections in adult zebrafish, *Danio rerio* (Hamilton). *Journal of Fish Diseases*, **32**, 931–941.

Ramsay, J.M., Watral, V., Schreck, C.B. *et al.* (2009b) *Pseudoloma neurophilia* infections in zebrafish Danio rerio: Effects of stress on survival, growth, and reproduction. *Diseases of Aquatic Organisms*, **88**, 69–84.

Reed, B. and Jennings, M. (2011) RSPCA Guidance on the housing and care of zebrafish. Available at: https://science.rspca.org.uk/documents/1494935/9042554/Guidance+on+the+housing+and+care+of+zebrafish.pdf/a4982df2-1499-52bd-d866-9c5706ddda09?t=1552901798437 (accessed 4th September 2019).

Russell, W.M.S. and Burch, R.L. (1959) *The Principles of Humane Experimental Technique*. Special Edition, Universities Federation for Animal Welfare, Potters Bar.

Selman, C. and Withers, D.J. (2011) Mammalian models of extended healthy lifespan. *Philosophical Transactions of the Royal Society of London Series B: Biological Sciences*, **366**, 99–107.

Selman, C., Sinclair, A., Pedroni, S.M. *et al.* (2016) Evidence that hematopoietic stem cell function is preserved during aging in long-lived S6K1 mutant mice. *Oncotarget*, **7**, 29937–29943.

Schroeder, P.G. and Sneddon, L.U. (2016) Exploring the efficacy of immersion analgesics in zebrafish using an integrative approach. *Applied Animal Behaviour Science*, **187**, 93–102.

Shin, J.T. and Fishman, M.C. (2002) From zebrafish to human: modular medical models. *Annual Review of Genomics and Human Genetics*, **3**(1), 311–340.

Spence, R., Fatema, M.K., Reichard, M. *et al.* (2006) The distribution and habitat preferences of the zebrafish in Bangladesh. *Journal of Fish Biology*, **69**, 1435–1448.

Spence, R., Fatema, M.K., Ellis, S. *et al.* (2007) The diet, growth and recruitment of wild zebrafish (*Danio rerio*) in Bangladesh. *Journal of Fish Biology*, **71**, 304–309.

Spence, R., Gerlach, G., Lawrence, C. *et al.* (2008) The behaviour and ecology of the zebrafish, *Danio rerio*. *Biological Reviews* **83**, 13–34.

Spitsbergen, J.M., Buhler, D.R., Peterson, T.S. *et al.* (2012) Neoplasia and Neoplasm Associated Lesions in Laboratory Colonies of Zebrafish Emphasizing Key Influences of Diet and Aquaculture System Design. *ILAR Journal*, **53**(2), 114–125.

Toth, L.A. (2018) Identifying and implementing endpoints for geriatric mice. *Comparative Medicine*, **68**, 439–451.

United Nations, Department of Economic and Social Affairs, Population Division (2015) *World Population Ageing 2015* (ST/ESA/SER.390).

Vargesson, N.A. (2007) 'Zebrafish'. In: *Manual of Animal Technology*, Ed. Barnett, S. Blackwell Publishing Ltd, Oxford, UK.

Vogeli, C. Shields, A.E., Lee, T.B. *et al.* (2007) Multiple chronic conditions: prevalence, health consequences, and implications for quality care management and costs. *Journal of General Internal Medicine*, **22**, 391–395.

Wang, N., Hurley, P., Pytte, C. *et al.* (2002) Vocal control neuron incorporation decreases with age in the adult zebra finch. *Journal of Neuroscience*, **22**, 10864–10870.

Whitehead, J.C., Hildebrand, B.A., Sun, M. *et al.* (2014) A clinical frailty index in ageing mice: Comparisons with frailty index data in humans. *The Journals of Gerontology Series A Biological Science and Medical Science*, **69**, 621–632.

Wilkinson, M., Horan, L., Selman, C. *et al.* (2019) Progressing the care, husbandry and management of ageing mice used in scientific studies. *Laboratory Animals*, e-pub ahead of print, 1–14.

Wilson, C. (2012) Aspects of larval rearing. *ILAR Journal*, **53**, 169–178.

Wilson, C. and Dunford, K. (2018) Refining severity limits for laboratory zebrafish. LASA Meeting, Birmingham, England. Poster presentation.

Wilson, C., Dunford, K., Nichols, C. *et al.* (2013) Body condition scoring for laboratory zebrafish. *Animal Technology and Welfare*, **12**, 1–7.

Yu, J.K., Sarathchandra, P., Chester, A. *et al.* (2018) Cardiac regeneration following cryoinjury in the adult zebrafish targets a maturation-specific biomechanical remodeling program. *Scientific Reports*, **8**, 15661.

Yuan, R., Tsaih, S.W., Petkova, S.B. *et al.* (2009) Aging in inbred strains of mice: study design and interim report on median lifespans and circulating IGF1 levels. *Aging Cell*, **8**, 277–287.

17 Euthanasia and other fates for laboratory animals

Huw Golledge

Introduction

For animals that undergo scientific procedures, it is now extremely unusual for death to be the endpoint of the study. The widespread use of humane endpoints (see below) and refinement of research procedures means that in most cases, animals will survive until the end of their research use.

> **Euthanasia or killing? A note on terminology**
>
> The killing of an animal after being used in research is often referred to as euthanasia, and the title of this chapter 'Euthanasia and other fates for laboratory animals' reflects that common usage. The title has been retained for consistency with previous editions of this book. However, the term 'euthanasia' is perhaps best reserved for the process of ending an animal's suffering, and this is the definition frequently used by the veterinary profession. The Royal College of Veterinary Surgeons in the UK defines euthanasia as 'painless killing to relieve suffering'. Most commonly when animal's lives are ended as a consequence of their use in scientific research and testing, it is more accurate to say that they are *killed*, although in some cases, animals used in research do undergo euthanasia to end their suffering. This can happen, when they have reached a predetermined humane endpoint, but many others are killed when they are not suffering. Euthanasia also means 'a good death', and this is usually taken to mean one that does not involve suffering. As will be seen later in this chapter, some of the methods used to kill laboratory animals also involve suffering and, therefore, fail to meet the definition of euthanasia on this basis.
>
> Neither UK nor EU legislation uses the term 'euthanasia' for ending the life of laboratory animals, whereas US and Canadian guidelines do use the term.

In addition, a significant number of animals are bred for use in research but never actually used in scientific procedures. For both these groups of animals, amounting to many millions a year worldwide, an active decision about their fate must be taken, making it one of the major issues in research animal welfare.

There are three possible fates for animals that have been used or bred for research purposes:

- Reuse or continued use – the animal is used for further scientific purposes.
- Release or rehoming – the animal continues its life but is not used for any further research purposes.
- Killing – the animal is actively killed.

All of the fates carry potentially negative consequences for the animals' welfare. Therefore, the choice of what happens to an animal after being used for research should involve the same careful weighing of the harm involved against the benefits as any other procedure carried out during research. The difference being that in the case of release, re-homing or killing the benefits are to the individual animal rather than for the advancement of science.

The decision process should be a considered one, taking into account the welfare consequences of all the possible fates for the animal. Wherever possible, the eventual fate of an animal used for a scientific purpose should be predetermined, although in some cases the decision to euthanise an animal may be an emergency one. Even in this case, a plan should be in place for such emergencies.

In this chapter, I will consider all three fates with particular emphasis on the animal welfare implications of each. Recommended humane killing techniques are included in the species- or taxon-specific chapters of this book (Chapters 19–51); in this chapter, I consider the general principles, which should guide selection of the most humane possible fate for animals at the end of their use for research or testing purposes.

The UFAW Handbook on the Care and Management of Laboratory and Other Research Animals, Ninth Edition.
Edited by Huw Golledge and Claire Richardson.
© 2024 John Wiley & Sons Ltd. Published 2024 by John Wiley & Sons Ltd.

Humane and scientific endpoints

As well as deciding *what* the fate of an animal should be at the end of its use in research, it is also crucial to first have clear criteria for deciding *when* that fate will occur. In most cases, this can be formalised into the concept of an endpoint – a point in time where for one reason or another, the animal must move from the research study onto its fate (be that killing or some other fate). There are two types of endpoint – scientific and humane. The scientific endpoint is reached when all the data for which the animal was used have been collected. A humane endpoint is a defined level of suffering, which should not be exceeded (Hendriksen *et al*. 2010).

If an animal reaches a humane endpoint before the scientific endpoint is reached, its welfare must take precedence and the suffering be reduced even if this jeopardises the experiment. If the suffering cannot be rapidly ameliorated, the animal must be killed to prevent further suffering.

Both scientific and humane endpoints should be clearly defined at the outset of a study, and they should be agreed between researchers and animal care staff to ensure that both scientific and animal welfare concerns are considered. Animals should be regularly monitored throughout a study to ensure that the humane endpoint is not being approached. Ideally, this should be a formal process of recording welfare indicators on a score sheet (Golledge & Jirkof 2016).

There should be a clearly defined set of actions, which are taken without undue delay when a humane endpoint is approached (for instance attempts to treat any suffering to avoid the endpoint being reached). If, despite remedial actions the endpoint is reached, decisive action should be taken to humanely kill the animal. The method of killing in such circumstances should be predefined and may differ from the method chosen to kill the animal when the scientific endpoint is reached.

Deciding whether to keep an animal alive after research

If an animal does not reach a humane endpoint and either reaches the scientific endpoint or is a surplus animal that is not required or not suitable for research use, a considered decision about the most appropriate fate must be taken. While humane killing is still by far the most common fate, other options are possible in many cases, and these should be carefully considered before a decision to kill the animal is taken.

Animals may be kept alive after their use in research either to allow them to be used for further scientific purposes or to be rehomed or released into the wild. In all cases, it must be ensured that, firstly, the animal is fit to be reused, released or rehomed and, if so, that it does not pose a risk to the environment or human safety before rehoming or release can be considered.

Further use in scientific research

Animals may be used for further scientific purposes under two scenarios: *continued use* where they are used for further research where the data gained are linked to their first use or *reuse* where they are used for a new purpose that has no linkage to the previous use of the animal. In either case, it must be established that the animal is fit to be kept alive and that the further use in research will not lead to excessive suffering. If this is not the case, the animal should be humanely killed.

Continued use

Continued use occurs where the animal continues to undergo scientific procedures as part of the same purpose as the initial study. For instance, in a crossover study, an individual animal could move from the control group to the experimental group or vice versa, whereas in a longitudinal study, further observations or measurements of the effect of a drug could be made. In such cases, the continued use of the animal could not be substituted by the use of a naïve animal, and the ethical consideration is simply whether any additional suffering likely to be experienced by the animal is outweighed by the benefits of the additional data collected.

Reuse

Reuse of an animal involves using the animal for a further scientific procedure, where the data are not linked to the first use of the animal. In this scenario, the animal could be substituted by a naïve animal, and hence, the ethical consideration is more complex.

Keeping animals alive for reuse is an interesting case where two of the 3Rs can be in conflict. Gaining the maximal amount of information from an animal clearly contributes to *reduction*, but this may come at the cost of *refinement* because the individual animal may suffer more.

The concepts of lifetime experience and cumulative severity are particularly important when considering reuse. The lifetime experience of the animal should be considered such that it does not experience an unacceptable level of suffering over its lifetime. Animals that have already undergone procedures may suffer more when undergoing further procedures; this can mean that a reused animal will suffer more than a naïve one when undergoing an identical procedure (this is often termed 'cumulative severity' or 'cumulative suffering'). For a detailed consideration of this issue, see Nunamaker *et al*. (2021). There is no simple way to balance the two concerns, but in general the presumption should be that the reuse is not justified if the level of suffering of the individual will be greater than that of a naïve animal. In other words, reduction should not come at the cost of increased suffering.

Scientific consideration should also be given to whether the effects of an animal's first use in research could compromise the quality of data obtained during the animals' reuse. If naïve animals are likely to produce better quality data, it is unlikely that reuse can be justified.

Deciding whether reuse or continued use is justified

Careful consideration of whether reuse or continued use is justified must be undertaken, and in most jurisdictions, this will be governed by laws and/or regulations, which should be consulted before any reuse is considered.

In the UK, a detailed flow chart is used for deciding whether an animal can be reused[1]. First and foremost, any animal that is suffering or likely to suffer if reused must not be reused and should be humanely killed. Animals cannot be reused for procedures classified as severe (in general, animals cannot be reused if they have already undergone a procedure that was retrospectively classified as severe either); these preclusions attempt to ensure that animals do not undergo an unacceptable level of cumulative suffering. Animals can only be used on protocols where the use of animals that have undergone prior scientific procedures is authorised. Once reuse is approved, a veterinary surgeon with knowledge of the lifetime experience of the animal must certify that the animal's 'general state of health and well-being has been restored' such that it is fit to be used in the new procedure.

A useful set of example scenarios is provided in the UK Home Office guidance on the reuse of animals[1].

Release or rehoming

Release or rehoming allows animals used in research to continue their lives for a non-scientific purpose. Rehoming involves passing the animal into human care/captivity as a companion animal or into a sanctuary or zoological collection. Livestock animals may also be rehomed into a production setting. Release, on the other hand, involves releasing an animal into the wild where its life will continue outside human care.

While allowing an animal to continue its life outside of research is an appealing one which most people would instinctively prefer to humanely killing the animal, it is crucial to consider whether keeping the animal alive is actually best for its welfare. In many cases, keeping the animal alive may entail welfare challenges, which cannot be justified.

For an animal to be released or rehomed, it must be in an adequate state of health; pose no danger to humans, other animals, or the environment; and be socialised to enable it to adapt to its new home. In many cases, these criteria are unlikely to be met. Many animals kept in a research setting will be difficult or impossible to socialise for life as a companion animal even if they are from a species that is commonly kept as a companion. Similarly, animals potentially releasable to the wild may be unfit for release if they have been bred or kept in captivity because they may lack the ability to adapt to free living and would thus be unlikely to survive. A veterinary assessment of the suitability of each individual animal to be rehomed or released considering all the above factors should be made before any animal is permitted to be released. In the case of rehoming, the assessment should also consider the adequacy of the proposed new home and the keeper before permitting the animal to be rehomed. At the institutional level the ethical review body should oversee the policy on release and rehoming of animals and monitor the programme.

If animals cannot be kept alive, either because they do not meet the criteria for further scientific use, release, or rehoming or because they are not practicable, then they must be humanely killed (see below).

For those animals that can be rehomed or released, they should be adequately prepared for their destination. In the case of animals that are rehomed, the establishment from which the animal is rehomed should check on the success of the rehoming after a reasonable interval. Contingency plans should be in place in case the animal does not settle into its new home, which may include plans for euthanasia if the situation cannot be remedied.

Extensive guidance from the UK Home Office, which includes an informative flow chart on the steps to be taken to decide if an animal can be released, is available. While this guidance is specific to the legal requirements in the UK, the general principles and advice are more widely applicable (Home Office 2015).

Killing

Animals may be killed for scientific purposes for a range of reasons; some are killed to end their suffering (euthanasia), some are killed because there is simply no further scientific use for them (and they cannot be rehomed or released) and still others are killed because it is necessary to take samples or undertake some other procedure that necessitates their death to achieve the scientific purpose for which they were used. Whatever the reason for killing an animal used in research, there is a moral and, in most jurisdictions, a legal imperative to ensure that the animal's death is as humane as possible. A humane death is widely defined as one that involves the minimal possible pain, suffering or distress (see Table 17.1).

Constraints on the selection of killing methods

The choice of killing method is constrained by a number of factors when animals are used for research purposes.

Legal constraints

Many jurisdictions produce legislation or guidelines, which regulate the use of killing methods for animals used for research purposes (see Table 17.1 for examples). In other cases, a general animal welfare law may also enforce the use of humane methods to kill animals. In all cases, local guidance or legislation must be consulted and followed when deciding how and when an animal used for research should be killed; it is beyond the scope of this chapter to detail all the requirements of legislation in various jurisdictions. However, there are some common themes in most legislation and guidance as well as some notable differences. Typically, guidance or legislation lists permissible methods that are considered

---

[1] Advice Note 02/2015: Animals (Scientific Procedures) Act 1986 Use, Keeping Alive and Reuse. https://assets.publishing.service.gov.uk/government/uploads/system/uploads/attachment_data/file/660236/Use__Keeping_Alive_and_Re-use_Advice_Note.pdf (Accessed November 13, 2023)

Table 17.1 Examples of legislation and guidance documents from various jurisdictions, which regulate the way in which animals used for scientific purposes may be killed.

Jurisdiction/Authority	Type of regulation	Title	Specification of methods	Requirement for humane killing
Canada – Canadian Council on Animal Care (2010, 2020)	Guidance	CCAC Guidelines on euthanasia of animals used in science	Acceptable, Acceptable with conditions, unacceptable for species/taxa, developmental stage, etc.	'...the method likely to cause the least distress and pain to the animal should be selected, consistent with the nature of the experimental protocol'.
European Union (EU) (European Parliament and Council 2010)	Legislation	European Directive 2010/63/EU (Annex IV)	Permissible methods listed for species/taxa, developmental stage and weight	'Member States shall ensure that animals are killed with minimum pain, suffering and distress'.
UK – Home Office (2014)	Legislation	Animals (Scientific Procedures) Act, 1986 (Schedule 1)	Permissible methods listed for species/taxa, developmental stage and weight	'The methods of humane killing listed... are appropriate for the animals listed'.
USA – American Veterinary Medical Association (Leary et al. 2020)	Guidance	AVMA Guidelines for the Euthanasia of Animals: 2020 Edition	Acceptable, Acceptable with conditions, unacceptable for species/taxa, developmental stage, etc.	'The Guidelines set criteria for euthanasia, specify appropriate euthanasia methods and agents, and are intended to assist veterinarians in their exercise of professional judgment'. The POE's objective in creating the Guidelines is to provide guidance for veterinarians about how to prevent and/or relieve the pain and suffering of animals that are to be euthanised.'
USA – National Institutes of Health (Institute of Laboratory Animal Resources 2011)	Guidance	Guide for the Care and Use of Laboratory Animals	Refer to latest edition of AVMA Guidelines on Euthanasia	'Euthanasia is the act of humanely killing animals by methods that induce rapid unconsciousness and death without pain or distress. Unless a deviation is justified for scientific or medical reasons, methods should be consistent with the AVMA Guidelines on Euthanasia (AVMA 2007 or later editions). In evaluating the appropriateness of methods, some of the criteria that should be considered are ability to induce loss of consciousness and death with no or only momentary pain, distress, or anxiety; reliability; irreversibility; time required to induce unconsciousness; appropriateness for the species and age of the animal; compatibility with research objectives; and the safety of and emotional effect on personnel.'

broadly acceptable for a given species, developmental stage and, in the case of some physical methods, weight. Sometimes a little extra nuance is included, for instance by classifying methods as acceptable with conditions (see Table 17.1). Usefully, some documents also specify which methods are unacceptable or should be avoided if possible.

When selecting a method of killing, an essential first step is to check which methods are permissible in the jurisdiction where the animal is kept. However, if there is good justification for using a non-approved method, such as a specific scientific need (see below) or the adoption of a new method that can be shown to be at least as humane as listed methods, then permission can often be sought to use a non-approved method. In the EU and UK, the use of a method not specified in the legislation may be allowed as a licensed procedure as part of the project licence under which experimental procedures are permitted.

It is often also permissible to use other methods on animals that are unconscious provided that consciousness is not regained prior to death. This allows for the use of more appropriate methods for animals undergoing terminal (non-recovery) procedures under general anaesthesia, where, for instance an overdose of potassium chloride can be used to induce cardiac arrest, a procedure that would not be humane in a conscious animal. Another common reason for killing an animal under anaesthesia is to allow trans-cardiac perfusion of fixatives to allow for histological studies to be performed on fixed tissue such as the brain.

The European Directive and Animals (Scientific Procedures) Act (European Parliament and Council 2010) also allow for the use of methods allowed for the slaughter of livestock species under the legislation covering slaughter of animal if the animals are kept under farm conditions and killed by a person licensed to carry out slaughter.

Animal welfare constraints

As outlined in Table 17.1, legislation and guidelines often lack detailed information about which accepted methods are most humane. When selecting from a range of permitted methods, the most appropriate method to choose is the most humane method. It is not sufficient to simply select the most convenient method from the permitted list or to use the same method in all circumstances.

Some information on the animal welfare impacts of various methods is provided in the following sections of this chapter.

Scientific constraints

In some cases, the achievement of some or all of the scientific aims of the use of an animal for research may not be possible if certain killing methods are used.

For example, if researchers wish to examine the anatomical structure of the brain, it will not be possible to use a mechanical method that causes damage to the brain. On the other hand, the use of chemical methods, such as anaesthetic overdoses, may be precluded in scenarios where these drugs may interfere with biochemical analyses. In some cases, death may need to be very rapid to avoid physiological changes that occur during death, for instance when living brain tissues needs to be recovered, preventing the use of an overdose of anaesthetic.

These constraints are easy to justify on ethical grounds since ignoring them would invalidate the use of the animal for research. Nonetheless, where methods that are known to not be the most humane are used, the use of such methods should be factored into the assessment about whether the use of animals for the entire procedure is justified. An example is the use of decapitation of conscious rodents to allow the recovery of fresh brain tissue uncontaminated by drugs. The EU legislation specifically notes that decapitation of rodents may only be used if other methods are not possible (European Parliament and Council 2010). By contrast, in the UK, the method is entirely omitted from the list of permissible methods for adult animals, meaning that specific permission to use the method would need to be sought as part of the project licence (Home Office 2014).

Financial and technical constraints

Some killing methods are expensive, requiring sophisticated equipment and technical skill to use them. For instance, the use of volatile anaesthetics typically requires an anaesthetic vaporiser, and safety equipment to extract waste anaesthetic gas will also be required. Other methods are considerably cheaper; some physical methods require little or no equipment, but nonetheless require good training of staff to ensure they can restrain the animal and apply the method confidently.

Compromising animal welfare for lack of resources is hard to justify on ethical grounds, and ethical committees or other authorities should carefully consider such compromises, using their influence to ensure that the means to employ best practice are made available wherever possible.

Safety and environmental constraints

Many of the agents used to kill animals pose risks to humans and the environment.

Halogenated volatile anaesthetics are often used as part of the killing process. These agents are potent greenhouse gases (Varughese & Ahmed 2021). Some volatile anaesthetic agents exert more potent greenhouse effects than others and if they are to be used without scavenging the least damaging agent should be used and the minimal volume used for each animal killed. Desflurane is significantly more potent as a greenhouse gas than isoflurane and sevoflurane and, therefore, should be avoided if possible. Volatile anaesthetic agents also pose significant human health risks (Varughese & Ahmed 2021), and for this reason, excess agents should either be scavenged using an activated charcoal absorber (which can also reduce environmental impact) or vented through a fume cupboard.

Inert gases pose a risk of asphyxia in humans, so steps should be taken to ensure that the area where they are used is well ventilated; this also applies to the use of carbon dioxide.

Physical methods pose dangers to those handling the animal both from the equipment used (e.g. guillotines or captive bolt guns) and from the animals themselves that can bite or scratch the handler.

Injectable agents can be accidentally injected into the handler if the animal struggles, and as with physical methods there is a risk from the animal scratching or biting.

The way the animal is handled prior to killing can affect it's response to handling at the time of death. Habituation of animals to handling and good handling technique can greatly reduce the animal's stress at the time of killing. It should also be borne in mind that animals which have reached a humane end point may be in pain and/or distress which may mean they react in a fearful or aggressive manner to handling.

In all cases, good technique and training are essential to minimise the risk of injury and environmental harm.

Selection of killing methods

The method of killing should be carefully considered at the outset of the study and the most humane method that will allow the scientific aims of the study selected, taking into account the constraints listed in the preceding section.

The method should be chosen carefully for the specific animal that must be killed. Different species will have different responses to the various methods based upon their physiology, anatomy, developmental stage, life history, etc. For instance, burrowing mammals may respond to killing methods, which induce hypoxia in a vastly different way to ground-dwelling species. As an example, pigs tolerate hypoxia induced by argon-filled environments (Raj & Gregory 1995), whereas rats are profoundly averse to similar conditions (Makowska et al. 2008). Even within species, sex or strain differences in the response of animals to killing methods have been demonstrated (Creamer-Hente et al. 2018; Munro et al. 2023) as have significant variations in the responses of individuals to killing agents (Améndola & Weary 2019).

In certain emergency situations, the need to kill the animal may take precedence over the use of the most humane method, for instance where there is a major risk to animal welfare, public or animal health or a serious threat to the environment. Every effort should be used to prevent the occurrence of such situations, and contingency plans including equipment should be available. In the EU and the UK, the restrictions on which methods are permissible do not apply to the killing of animals in an emergency.

In the following section, the most commonly used techniques for common laboratory species are considered in terms of their welfare impacts.

Common methods for killing laboratory animals and their welfare impacts

Gases and controlled atmospheres

Controlled atmosphere methods expose animals to a modified atmosphere, which renders them unconscious either through the deprivation of oxygen by displacement of air with another gas (for instance in the case of the inert gases Argon and Nitrogen) or because of the direct physiological effects of the inhaled gas (carbon dioxide or carbon monoxide, for instance). Low atmospheric pressure stunning (LAPS) can also be used to induce unconsciousness due to the low partial pressure of oxygen followed by death by exposing animals to a reduced atmospheric pressure. This novel method has been approved for slaughter of poultry in Europe and is currently being investigated as a method for killing rodents used in research (Clarkson et al. 2023).

The use of carbon dioxide to kill rodents is by far the most commonly used method to kill rats and mice but is also the most controversial. For decades, researchers have debated the animal welfare impacts of CO_2, and debate about whether it is less humane than other controlled atmosphere methods is ongoing (Conlee et al. 2005; Hawkins et al. 2006, 2016; Shomer et al. 2020; Turner et al. 2020).

Advantages

Controlled atmosphere methods share many practical advantages. Typically, since they are applied by pumping gas into a chamber (or in the case of LAPS by reducing the pressure in an airtight chamber), they do not involve restraint of the animals. Handling and restraint stress can be significant, especially for animals that are not well habituated to human handling. Controlled atmosphere methods allow the animal either to be placed into the chamber where they are to be killed or, in some cases, to be killed in their home cages either by placing the home cage into a larger chamber or by introducing the gas into the home cage, further reducing the amount of disturbance required. Killing animals in groups is also possible with these methods. This is clearly an advantage in terms of efficiency. Group killing may also offer welfare advantages by avoiding separating social animals such as rats from their cage mates, although studies have not shown significant welfare advantages of this approach (Hickman 2018, 2021)

Controlled atmosphere methods require less operator skill than some other methods such as physical or injectable methods. Some modern systems for controlled atmosphere killing are fully automated (Mcintyre et al. 2007). Once animals are introduced to the chamber, an automated cycle that introduces the gas is initiated, and the concentration is monitored until a period of time sufficient to ensure that all animals are killed elapses, reducing the chance of operator error.

Controlled atmosphere methods also kill the animal without causing any physical damage to the body of the animal meaning that they are well suited to studies where postmortem anatomical examination is required. In contrast, physical methods typically cause trauma to the brain and spinal cord, which may be unacceptable for some studies. The carcase also remains uncontaminated meaning that the carcase of an animal killed with CO_2, inert gas or LAPS can be used for food for reptiles or other carnivores.

Disadvantages

Many of the agents used for controlled atmosphere killing appear to cause significant welfare challenges. In particular, carbon dioxide causes a range of issues. At high concentrations, CO_2 directly activates nociceptive neurons (Peppel & Anton 1993), suggesting that it is likely to cause pain in non-human animals, as it has been shown to do in humans. Humans who breathe in high concentrations of CO_2 describe a stinging sensation, which becomes increasingly painful as the concentration increases (Danneman et al. 1997). The mechanism for CO_2-induced pain is well understood. CO_2 dissolves into water forming carbonic acid. This reaction occurs within moist tissues such as the lining of the respiratory tract, corneal surface or nasal epithelium. Nociceptive neurons in these tissues are activated by protons liberated as carbonic acid dissociates.

Both animal and human studies suggest that CO_2 only causes pain when used in high concentrations (>~50%), and therefore, pain can be avoided by using a gradually rising concentration of CO_2 to kill animals such as rodents. When applied in a rising concentration, consciousness is lost before noxious levels of CO_2 are reached. Most legislation and guidance, therefore, mandate that CO_2 is used in a gradually rising concentration rather than allowing animals to be placed into chambers pre-filled with CO_2. The optimal flow rate that minimises the duration of aversion (see below) while avoiding causing pain remains the subject of ongoing study and debate (Niel et al. 2008; Moody et al. 2014; Boivin et al. 2016a; Hickman et al. 2016). The latest AVMA guidelines recommend 30–70% of the chamber volume per minute as an appropriate flow rate (Leary et al., 2020), whereas the previous edition recommended 10–30% (Leary et al. 2013).

At concentrations well below those likely to induce pain, CO_2 is strongly aversive in many mammals. Experimental evidence has shown that rats, mice and pigs all show pronounced aversion to CO_2, avoiding CO_2 wherever possible, even foregoing rewards (Raj & Gregory 1995; Niel & Weary 2007; Makowska et al. 2009) or exposing themselves to stressful environments (Wong et al. 2013) to avoid exposure. This aversion occurs at concentrations lower than those thought to cause pain. Strikingly, humans also show aversion and anxiety-like responses when exposed to low concentrations of CO_2 (7.5%) and when asked to describe how CO_2 exposure makes them feel frequently describe a strong desire to avoid the environment where they are exposed to CO_2 (Bailey et al. 2005), suggesting that aversion to CO_2 is a widely conserved vertebrate response.

A recent systematic review concluded that the evidence for welfare impacts of CO_2 such as those cited above was inadequate to conclude that it is an unacceptable method for killing animals (Turner et al. 2020). However, it should be noted that this study only considered studies specifically aimed at assessing the welfare impacts of CO_2 for killing laboratory rodents. There is an extensive body of literature, which indirectly informs the debate as a result of the use of CO_2 as an experimental anxiogen in pre-clinical pharmacology, where it is used to induce anxiety or panic in rodents to test the efficacy of potential anxiolytic drugs for anxiety and panic disorders (Leibold et al. 2016; Améndola & Weary 2020). These studies typically employ relatively low concentrations of CO_2 to induce anxiety-like behaviours in mice or rats. Extensive evidence from studies in rodents suggests that CO_2 in concentrations as low as 5% or even less is an anxiogen, producing behavioural responses such as escape behaviours that are strongly indicative of negative affective states. This research has also elucidated a range of physiological mechanisms by which the brain detects CO_2 and translates this into behavioural responses based upon the detection of the lowered pH in the cerebrospinal fluid by acid-sensitive ion channels (Quagliato et al. 2018)

The use of CO_2 remains hotly debated, but, given the significant body of evidence that it has serious consequences for animal welfare, a strong case can be made for giving animals the benefit of the doubt by using an alternative method where practical. The Canadian Council on Animal Guidelines on euthanasia (2020) stipulate that CO_2 should 'not be used where other methods are practical for the experiment and the species'; however, the method is still listed as permissible or acceptable with conditions in EU, UK and US guidelines (Home Office 2014; European Parliament and Council 2010; Institute of Laboratory Animal Resources 2011).

Inert gases, such as argon or nitrogen, can also be used to kill animals and are a potential alternative to CO_2. Unlike CO_2, which induces a state of anaesthesia before death, these agents simply displace air and kill the animals by hypoxia. Nitrogen is less dense than air and, therefore, requires an airtight chamber to maintain a hypoxic environment; an advantage of argon is that it is heavier than air and thus, like CO_2, can be used in a less than airtight chamber. Some species such as pigs appear largely unable to detect hypoxic environments. Pigs that self-exposed themselves to an argon-filled chamber in return for a food reward lost consciousness without apparent signs of aversion (Raj & Gregory 1995). On the other hand, rats show pronounced aversion to chambers filled with argon (Makowska et al. 2008), perhaps as a result of being a burrowing species evolved to avoid hypoxic environments in contrast to surface-dwelling species such as pigs and humans.

LAPS has been shown to be relatively humane for stunning chickens (McKeegan et al. 2013) and is now permitted by the European Food Safety Agency for stunning broiler chickens in commercial chicken slaughter. However, the method was shown to cause significant welfare problems when used with pigs (Baxter et al. 2022a, 2022b). Ongoing research is seeking to establish whether LAPS might be a humane method for killing laboratory rodents (Clarkson et al. 2023).

Inhaled volatile anaesthetics

Volatile anaesthetic agents, such as isoflurane and sevoflurane, can be used as part of a humane killing procedure, inducing unconsciousness before the animal is killed by another method. Inhaled agents can also be used in overdose to kill the animal, but generally this requires a lengthy exposure to the agent to induce cardiac arrest (Golledge 2012). It is more practical to deeply anaesthetise animals and then kill them using a secondary method such as a physical technique. The advantage of this approach is that any welfare impacts of the secondary methods are irrelevant as long as the animal remains anaesthetised.

Typically, anaesthesia is induced in the same way as recovery anaesthesia for surgery with the agent delivered to the animal vaporised in oxygen or a nitrous oxide/oxygen mixture. Induction can either be in a chamber for rodents and other smaller species or by mask. Alternatively, since safe recovery of the animal is not a concern, induction can be via the so-called 'drop method', whereby high concentrations of the inhaled agent are achieved by pouring the liquid agent onto a cotton swab and allowing it to vaporise into a chamber (Risling et al. 2012). This can lead to a much more rapid induction of unconsciousness and requires less equipment.

Volatile anaesthetic agents have been shown to be less aversive to rodents than CO_2 (Wong et al. 2013; Moody & Weary 2014). In some cases, rodents showed little to no aversion, remaining in the presence of volatile anaesthetics until they lost consciousness. However, animals that had been previously exposed to a volatile anaesthetic showed stronger aversion upon re-exposure (Wong et al. 2013; Moody & Weary 2014). This evidence suggests that caution should be used when using a volatile anaesthetic to kill an animal that has previously been exposed to the same agent (e.g. for surgery).

An additional disadvantage of volatile anaesthetics is that they contaminate tissues precluding their use in some studies and preventing carcases being used for food.

Physical methods

Animals can be killed using mechanical or physical methods, which render them unconscious or kill them, typically by causing damage to the nervous system. These methods can be used to induce a rapid and potentially very humane death, but they often require handling of individual animals, necessitating a degree of technical skill not required by inhalation methods. Methods for rodents and other small vertebrates include decapitation, cervical dislocation and concussion.

Physical methods also include those for dispatch of livestock such as captive bolt devices or firearms. Firearms are tightly regulated in most jurisdictions and regulations may also apply to captive bolt devices that are typically powered by an explosive cartridge (although pneumatic or spring-powered devices are also available).

Advantages

Physical methods do not contaminate the animal's body with drugs or other substances, and the rapidity of death may also mean that peri-mortem physiological changes are minimised, both of which may be important for some uses of animals. When carried out correctly, some physical methods, such as concussion, captive bolt and firearms, should cause instantaneous unconsciousness or death, ensuring a humane death. Some physical methods are also relatively cheap, requiring little or no specialist equipment but are reliant on excellent operator technical skills and good training.

Disadvantages

Not all physical methods cause instantaneous death or loss of consciousness. Following decapitation or cervical dislocation, activity in the brain of rodents persists for several seconds following application of the method (Cartner *et al.* 2007; Kongara *et al.* 2014) as revealed by ongoing EEG activity. If the animal is not killed immediately, there is a possibility that they may consciously experience severe pain as a result of the injury inflicted, although it remains unclear whether the persistent EEG activity is consistent with consciousness. However, given the possibility that they do remain conscious, a precautionary approach would suggest that the use of such methods should be avoided unless they are applied to animals already rendered unconscious by anaesthesia.

Cervical dislocation requires skill to accomplish correctly, and there is considerable scope for the technique to fail. One study using anaesthetised mice suggested a high failure rate as evidenced by the finding that over 20% of mice continued to breathe following attempted cervical dislocation (Carbone *et al.* 2012). As part of the training to use this method, operators should be taught to confirm by palpation that the cervical vertebrae have been fully separated.

Concussion in rodents is typically performed by striking the animal's head against a rigid surface such as a table causing lethal damage to the brain. The method is also commonly used for fish. Concussion has been little studied in rodents but performed well it would be expected to cause instantaneous loss of consciousness as do mechanically assisted concussion methods such as captive bolt devices when used in livestock species such as cattle. As with the other physical methods, technical proficiency and accuracy of the blow is likely to be crucial and practice with cadavers of animals killed by non-physical methods may be helpful.

Parenteral anaesthetic overdose

An injected overdose of anaesthetic can be used via parenteral routes to kill animals. This method is also commonly used for euthanasia of animals in routine clinical veterinary practice. For many larger species such as primates, it may be the only practical method available in a laboratory setting, and it is also widely used for smaller species. The most commonly used agent is the barbiturate anaesthetic pentobarbital; this agent is available in preparations specifically formulated for euthanasia (e.g. Euthatal (Dopharma Research B.V.) or Dolethal (Veotquinol, UK)). These solutions contain a high concentration of pentobarbital, typically 200 mg in 1 ml, suitable for rapid induction of unconsciousness if administered intravenously at a dose of 0.7 ml per kg bodyweight. Other anaesthetic drugs can also be used in overdose for killing, and they may be combined with sedative agents to ensure a more smooth and/or rapid induction of unconsciousness. Sedatives may also be administered prior to killing to reduce anxiety and make the animal easier to handle, which may be particularly helpful when intravenous access is required.

Advantages

Anaesthetic overdose can be used to induce very rapid unconsciousness followed by death. The method does not cause any physical damage to the animal allowing for post-mortem examination/necropsy.

Disadvantages

To administer the drug, the animals must be handled (unless the animal has been fitted with an indwelling cannula for other research purposes). Handling may be stressful and, for larger species, may also pose risks to the personnel administering the agent. Training of animals to tolerate handling injections can reduce both these risks.

Injection causes minor pain due to the physical insertion of the needle. Some agents also cause pain around the injection site, and this may be particularly problematic if the agent is administered by the intraperitoneal (i.p.) route. Intraperitoneal injection is a popular route of administration, especially in smaller species where intravenous administration may be difficult or impossible. Use of the i.p. route means that loss of consciousness will be considerably slower than for an intravenous injection, taking several minutes as opposed to seconds. In addition, i.p. injection of barbiturates has been shown to cause behavioural signs such as abdominal writhing indicative of pain (Reimer *et al.* 2020). Svendsen *et al.* (2007) showed that pentobarbitone injection activated nociceptive pathways; the alkalinity of pentobarbitone solutions is likely responsible for this effect. Some studies suggest that pain caused by i.p. injection of pentobarbital can be ameliorated by the addition of the local anaesthetic lidocaine to the injected solution (Svendsen *et al.* 2007; Khoo *et al.* 2018) or by buffering the solution to reduce the alkalinity; however, in both cases, it has been suggested that there is a danger of the pentobarbitone being precipitated by these modifications

(Reimer et al. 2020). A recent study has shown that a higher dose of pentobarbitone (800 mg/kg) delivered in a larger volume than conventional euthanasia solutions can more rapidly induce unconsciousness in rats (Zatroch et al. 2017) reducing the duration of any period of pain or distress. Intraperitoneal administration also comes with a risk of accidental injection into organs rather than the peritoneal space, which may lead to a significant delay in the induction of unconsciousness.

In addition to potential animal welfare impacts, a further disadvantage of anaesthetic overdose is that it contaminates tissue with the agent used for overdose, which may preclude its use for some scientific purposes and prevents the use of the animal's carcase for food. Many drugs used for anaesthetic overdose will be strictly controlled in many jurisdictions, limiting the availability of the agents and/or restricting their use to licensed professionals.

Special cases

Much of the above information is specific to adult mammals; in the following section I consider some other scenarios.

Aquatic species

Fish and other aquatic species including amphibians provide a unique challenge when they must be humanely killed.

One approach that can be employed with aquatic species is to add an agent to the tank water. This method can be used to carry out an overdose of anaesthetic. The advantage of this approach is that the animals do not need to be handled other than moving them to a tank where they are to be killed. However, as is the case with rodents, fish display aversion to many commonly used anaesthetic agents (for instance, zebrafish are averse to MS-222, which is routinely used to kill or anaesthetise them (Readman et al. 2013, 2017; Wong et al. 2014)). However, unlike rodents, some studies have shown that there are anaesthetic agents that will be tolerated by some fish species, for instance zebrafish do not appear to be averse to etomidate or 2,2,2 tribromoethanol.

Unsurprisingly, given the huge diversity in fish species, agents that are non-aversive to some fish species can be strongly aversive in others (Readman et al. 2017), demonstrating the necessity of carefully researching the appropriate agent for the species under study.

Other acceptable methods for killing fish include concussion/percussive blow to the head and electrical stunning. See also Chapter 48: Fishes and Chapter 49: Zebrafish.

Birds

The physiology and anatomy of birds means that they may respond very differently to agents commonly used to kill mammals. Appropriate methods for birds can include an overdose of anaesthetic, concussion, cervical dislocation and exposure to inert gases. See Chapters 40–45 for detail on specific bird species.

Carbon dioxide is widely used to kill poultry species slaughtered for food and can be used for killing birds used in research. However, as with mammals, CO_2 appears to be aversive to birds (McKeegan et al. 2006). Inert gases or mixtures of CO_2 and inert gases (Sandilands et al. 2011) and the newly developed LAPS system (Mackie & McKeegan 2016) are also used in poultry slaughter and appear to cause less aversion than CO_2.

Methods such as thoracic compression that are sometimes used to kill birds are unacceptable.

Neonatal chicks and fertilised eggs are often killed by maceration in commercial settings, and while this method is aesthetically unappealing, it is likely to cause instantaneous death if the equipment is used correctly.

Non-human primates

Under EU legislation, only an overdose of anaesthetic is permitted for killing non-human primates. Sedation, where appropriate, may also be administered to ensure a smooth induction of unconsciousness. See Chapters 36–39 for detail on specific non-human primate species.

Euthanasia of neonates

The physiology of neonatal animals means that the method used to kill them may need to differ from that needed to kill adults of the same species. For instance, neonatal rodents are highly resistant to hypoxia and will, therefore, take many times longer than adults to die in hypoxic conditions induced by CO_2 (Pritchett et al. 2005), as do newborn chicks (Burton & Carlise 1969).

It has been argued that altricial species, such as mice, are less capable of suffering during euthanasia due to the lack of development of their nervous system. As evidence for this assertion, the lack of an adult-like EEG response of neonatal rodents to painful stimulation is often cited (e.g. Diesch et al. 2009). This has been used to argue that some neonatal animals lack the capacity to suffer in the first few days after birth, with pain sensitivity developing gradually over the following days (Mellor 2019).

Nonetheless, regulations and guidelines typically mandate that neonatal animals should be killed using methods expected to be humane, giving the benefit of the doubt to the animal that it may have developed some form of sentience by the time it is born.

Foetal forms

It is sometimes necessary to kill pregnant animals. Neurobiological evidence suggests that in the earlier stages of pregnancy, foetuses are unlikely to be sentient. Indeed, it has been argued that in some altricial species, sentience may develop some days after birth (see above). Birth itself may be the trigger for the onset of sentience (Mellor & Diesch 2006). It is thus thought that foetal forms will not suffer if they remain in utero following the killing of a pregnant adult. Nonetheless, there is a presumption in legislation that foetal vertebrates are protected in the later stages of development.

If removed from the uterus, foetuses must be humanely killed.

Handling of animals for humane killing

Regardless of the method used to kill animals, a number of other factors can affect the welfare of animals at the time of killing.

The way in which animals are handled can profoundly change their stress levels. Picking up mice in tunnels or cupped hands rather than by the tail greatly reduces their stress (Hurst & West 2010). Mice being moved into a euthanasia chamber should be moved in tubes or cupped hands rather than by the tail to prevent unnecessary stress before the procedure begins. In general, every effort should be made to minimise handling or restraint stress by using best practice handling techniques appropriate for the species during killing procedures, just as for any other procedure. See also Chapter 6: Brief introduction to welfare assessment and Chapter 21: The laboratory mouse. In some cases sedation can be used to reduce handling stress prior to killing.

Other factors can also cause stress at the time of killing, of particular importance is smell. Equipment used for killing, including chambers or cages where animals are killed should be thoroughly cleaned and dried after each use to remove stress pheromones. Animals should also be handled with gloved hands and gloves changed or cleaned after each animal is handled.

It is often assumed that animals may be negatively affected by witnessing the death of other animals, especially conspecifics. The evidence that this is the case is not strong, for instance Boivin et al. (2016b) examined the effect on C57BL/6N mice of witnessing conspecifics being killed with CO_2 and found no signs of agitation or stress. Being in the presence of animals killed by decapitation did elevate heart rate and activity, but this was shown to be a result of the noise generated by the guillotine as the effect was similar when the device was operated without being used to kill an animal. Similarly, studies of pigs and sheep in an abattoir setting did not detect stress responses in animals witnessing conspecifics (Anil et al. 1996, 1997).

Nonetheless, wherever possible animals should not be killed in the presence of other animals as there is evidence for emotional contagion in a number of species (Reimert et al. 2013; Hernandez-Lallement et al. 2022), including rodents.

Many species are social, and if they are normally housed in groups will suffer stress if separated from their cage mates (Ferland & Schrader 2011). Although it may not always be possible, it can be good practice to kill animals in their home-cage groups, especially if using a controlled atmosphere method where animals can be killed simultaneously in the same chamber.

Use of dead animals

Once any necessary research procedures have been carried out on the animal's body, consideration should be given to whether any further use can be made of it before it is disposed of.

A number of schemes have been launched to enable the sharing of tissue or organs from animals with other researchers. The use of such tissue can prevent other animals being killed to provide samples and, therefore, can make a significant contribution to reduction. Many institutions will have mechanisms for sharing tissue, and there are also larger scale systems that can facilitate the exchange of material between institutions such as AniMath[2]. Researchers should consider the fate of the carcases of the animals they use at the outset of the research so that plans to collect, preserve, and distribute the tissue are in place before the animal is killed.

The bodies of animals may also be useful for training purposes, e.g. to practise surgery or other experimental techniques.

Assuming that the body of the animal is not required for further scientific or training purposes after death, it may still be possible to find a use for the cadaver. For instance, birds and small mammals that have been killed by a physical method or by CO_2 may be used as food for carnivores such as reptiles and raptors. Care must be taken to ensure that animals that have been administered drugs, exposed to infectious agents, or toxic substances are never fed to other animals.

Once all other uses have been exhausted, carcases should be disposed of as clinical waste following local regulations.

Human factors

Training

Many methods used to kill animals require considerable technical skill. If methods are applied incorrectly, there is a considerable danger that animals can be injured but not killed, causing significant avoidable suffering. Many techniques also pose health and safety risks, including physical injury from the animals being killed or the devices used alongside chemical hazards from agents used for killing. Therefore, for all techniques, training is essential and personnel should not carry out the techniques until they have been trained and assessed as competent (see also Chapter 14: Attaining competence in the care of animals used in research). Competence should be reassessed periodically. Alongside proficiency in the killing procedure, staff killing animals should also be well trained and proficient in the gentle handling and restraint of the species which they intend to kill.

Training should include not only how to apply the killing method effectively and safely but also what to do in the event that an animal is not killed by the method. This can include reapplication of the method or use of an emergency method (e.g. cervical dislocation in the case of a failure of equipment for controlled atmosphere stunning). Those carrying out euthanasia should also be trained to confirm that animals are dead. In most cases, especially the non-physical methods, it is essential to apply a secondary method to ensure that there is no possibility of the animal recovering consciousness prior to any post-mortem procedures or disposal of the carcase. The European Directive (2010/63/EU) stipulates that killing

---

[2] www.animatch.eu. Accessed November 14, 2023

of animals should be completed by one of the following methods: confirmation of permanent cessation of the circulation; destruction of the brain; dislocation of the neck; exsanguination; or confirmation of the onset of rigor mortis (European Parliament and Council 2010).

Following theoretical training, it may be possible to practice physical techniques on dead animals before moving on to killing live animals under supervision.

Effects of killing animals on those who kill them

Killing animals should not be taken lightly, and indeed, the process of killing animals used in research can weigh heavily on those involved (Scotney et al. 2015). Compassion fatigue can occur in those involved in working with laboratory animals and specifically among those who are tasked with killing them (Newsome et al. 2019). Steps should be taken to minimise compassion fatigue due to carrying out killing procedures both to prevent the effect on human health and to ensure that those charged with the undeniably unpleasant task of killing animals are not desensitised to the potential welfare consequences (Newsome et al. 2019). It is important that staff carrying out killing are well-trained, well-supported and clearly understand the reason why the animals are being killed. One study has shown that compassion fatigue is lower among staff who are involved in the choice of how or when the animals are killed (LaFollette et al. 2020). Personnel should also clearly understand the reason for use of a particular killing method, especially when that method may be one they find distasteful. Wherever possible, the task of killing animals should be shared among as many staff as possible to avoid a single person or small number of people spending significant amounts of their working time on killing animals. Appropriate support for staff in terms of peer-support or professional psychological help may be necessary.

It is important, however, that the feelings of those carrying out killing methods do not override the welfare of animals. The methods considered to be least aesthetically unpleasant by operators may not necessarily be those with the least welfare impact on animals. This is evidenced by the preference of staff to avoid physical methods. Those carrying out physical methods of euthanasia report higher levels of compassion fatigue (LaFollette et al. 2020) and when surveyed on which methods are least aesthetically acceptable prefer non-physical methods (Hickman & Johnson 2011). In some cases, physical methods are likely to be considerably more humane than alternatives such as the use of CO_2 in rodents. In such scenarios where there is a discrepancy between the methods preferred by staff and the most humane method, it is important to justify the choice of the more humane method rather than allowing a less-humane method to be used.

Considerations for ethical committees

Although the method by which animals are killed is not considered a scientific procedure in many regulations and guidelines, an argument can be made that the killing process should undergo the same scrutiny as any other procedure such as a surgical intervention or the administration of a drug. The fate of the animal, be it killing, rehoming, release or reuse, forms a part of the potential harms which an animal undergoes to achieve the benefits of the research and is, therefore, deserving of harm–benefit analysis.

Animal ethics committees should consider the method of killing for each project which they scrutinise. In particular, they should consider whether the most humane method is being used and if not whether the use of a less-humane method is justified for a scientific reason. If the reason for the choice of a less-humane method is due to financial constraints, lack of equipment or simply because the researchers have always used a particular method, a committee should use its influence to encourage or require that a more humane method is used. Ethical committees should also pay close attention to the killing of those animals not used directly for scientific/experimental procedures such as surplus animals and animals used for breeding, scrutinising the methods by which these animals are killed and ensuring that the number of animals needing to be killed is minimised.

Ethical committees should stay ahead of developments in the field; new information on the existing methods of killing and new methods are constantly emerging, so it important that guidelines and approved methods are regularly reviewed. See also Chapter 18: Ethics review of animal research.

Conclusion

The fate of animals used in research is an important but often under-considered part of the harms inflicted upon animals used in research. Careful consideration should be given to select the least harmful fate for the animal at the end of its experimental use. The harm of killing or any other fate should be a factor in the initial decision as to whether or not the use of the animal is justified and should be decided at the outset of the animal's use in research wherever possible. Where there is any uncertainty about the animal welfare impacts upon an animal, the benefit of the doubt should be given to the animal, and wherever possible a method known to be humane should be used.

Killing methods vary greatly in the degree of suffering that they cause, meaning that careful thought should be given to selecting the least harmful method. Given that for some species there are few if any accepted methods that do not cause significant welfare concerns, there is a pressing need for further research to both assess which current methods are least harmful and to develop new methods which minimise harm while allowing scientific objectives to be achieved.

References

Améndola, L. and Weary, D.M. (2019). Evidence for consistent individual differences in rat sensitivity to carbon dioxide. PLOS ONE, **14**(4), e0215808.

Améndola, L. and Weary, D.M. (2020). Understanding rat emotional responses to CO_2. Translational Psychiatry, **10**, 253.

Anil, M.H., McKinstry, J.L., Field, M. and Rodway, R.G. (1997). Lack of evidence for stress being caused to pigs by witnessing the slaughter of conspecifics. Animal Welfare, **6**(1), 3–8.

Anil, M.H., Preston, J., McKinstry, J.L., Rodway, R.G. and Brown, S.N. (1996). An assessment of stress caused in sheep by watching slaughter of other sheep. *Animal Welfare*, **5**(4), 435–441.

Bailey, J.E., Argyropoulos, S.V., Kendrick, A.H. and Nutt, D.J. (2005). Behavioral and cardiovascular effects of 7.5% CO_2 in human volunteers. *Depression and Anxiety*, **21**(1), 18–25.

Baxter, E.M., McKeegan, D.E.F., Farish, M., *et al*. (2022a). Characterizing candidate decompression rates for hypobaric hypoxic stunning of pigs. Part 2: pathological consequences. *Frontiers in Veterinary Science*, **9**, 1027883. doi:10.3389/fvets.2022.1027883

Baxter, E.M., McKeegan, D.E.F., Farish, M., *et al.* (2022b). Characterizing candidate decompression rates for hypobaric hypoxic stunning of pigs. Part 2: pathological consequences. *Frontiers in Veterinary Science*, **9**.

Boivin, G.P., Bottomley, M.A., Dudley, E.S., Schiml, P.A., Wyatt, C.N. and Grobe, N. (2016a). Physiological, behavioral, and histological responses of male C57BL/6N mice to different CO_2 chamber replacement rates. *Journal of the American Association for Laboratory Animal Science: JAALAS*, **55**(4), 451–461.

Boivin, G.P., Bottomley, M.A. and Grobe, N. (2016b). Responses of male C57BL/6N mice to observing the euthanasia of other mice. *Journal of the American Association for Laboratory Animal Science: JAALAS*, **55**(4), 406–411.

Burton, R.R. and Carlisle, J.C. (1969). Acute hypoxia tolerance of the chick. *Poultry Science*, **48**(4), 1265–1269.

Canadian Council on Animal Care (2010). CCAC guidelines on euthanasia of animals used in science. Available at: https://ccac.ca/Documents/Standards/Guidelines/Euthanasia.pdf (Accessed November 13, 2023)

Canadian Council on Animal Care (2020). CCAC revised guidance on euthanasia using carbon dioxide. Available at: https://ccac.ca/Documents/Standards/Guidelines/CCAC_Revised_Guidance_on_Euthanasia_Using_Carbon_Dioxide.pdf/ (Accessed November 13, 2023)

Carbone, L., Carbone, E.T., Yi, E.M., *et al.* (2012). Assessing cervical dislocation as a humane euthanasia method in mice. *Journal of the American Association for Laboratory Animal Science: JAALAS*, **51**(3), 352–356.

Cartner, S.C., Barlow, S.C. and Ness, T.J. (2007). Loss of cortical function in mice after decapitation, cervical dislocation, potassium chloride injection, and CO_2 inhalation. *Comparative Medicine*, **57**(6), 570–573.

Clarkson, J.M., Martin, J.E., Sparrey, J., Leach, M.C. and McKeegan, D.E.F. (2023). Striving for humane deaths for laboratory mice: hypobaric hypoxia provides a potential alternative to carbon dioxide exposure. *Proceedings of the Royal Society B: Biological Sciences*, **290**(1997), 20222446.

Conlee, K.M., Stephens, M.L., Rowan, A.N. and King, L.A. (2005). Carbon dioxide for euthanasia: concerns regarding pain and distress, with special reference to mice and rats. *Laboratory Animals*, **39**(2), 137–161.

Creamer-Hente, M.A., Lao, F.K., Dragos, Z.P. and Waterman, L.L. (2018). Sex- and Strain-related Differences in the Stress Response of Mice to CO_2 Euthanasia. *Journal of the American Association for Laboratory Animal Science: JAALAS*, **57**(5), 513–519.

Danneman, P.J., Stein, S. and Walshaw, S.O. (1997). Humane and practical implications of using carbon dioxide mixed with oxygen for anesthesia or euthanasia of rats. *Laboratory Animal Science*, **47**(4), 376–385.

Diesch, T.J., Mellor, D.J., Johnson, C.B. and Lentle, R.G. (2009). Electroencephalographic responses to tail clamping in anaesthetized rat pups. *Laboratory Animals*, **43**(3), 224–231.

European Parliament and Council (2010) Directive 2010/63/EU of the European Parliament and of the Council of 22 September 2010 on the Protection of Animals Used for Scientific Purposes. *Official Journal of the European Union*, L 276/33–79. https://eur-lex.europa.eu/LexUriServ/LexUriServ.do?uri=OJ:L:2010:276:0033:0079:EN:PDF (Accessed 13 November 2023)

Ferland, C.L. and Schrader, L.A. (2011). Cage mate separation in pair-housed male rats evokes an acute stress corticosterone response. *Neuroscience Letters*, **489**(3), 154–158.

Golledge, H.D.R. (2012). Response to Roustan *et al.* 'Evaluating methods of mouse euthanasia on the oocyte quality: cervical dislocation versus isoflurane inhalation': animal welfare concerns regarding the aversiveness of isoflurane and its inability to cause rapid death. *Laboratory Animals*, **46**(4), 358–359.

Golledge, H. and Jirkof, P. (2016). Score sheets and analgesia. *Laboratory Animals*, **50**(6), 411–413.

Hawkins, P., Playle, L., Golledge, H., *et al.* (2006). Newcastle consensus meeting on carbon dioxide euthanasia of laboratory animals. In *Newcastle Consensus Meeting on Carbon Dioxide Euthanasia of Laboratory Animals*, pp. 1–17. Newcastle upon Tyne, UK. Available online: http://www.nc3rs.org.uk/sites/default/files/documents/Events/First%20Newcastle%20consensus%20meeting%20report.pdf [Google Scholar]

Hawkins, P., Prescott, M.J., Carbone, L., *et al.* (2016). A good death? Report of the second newcastle meeting on laboratory animal euthanasia. *Animals*, **6**(9), 50. doi:10.3390/ani6090050

Hendriksen, C., Morton, D. and Cussler, K. (2016). Use of humane endpoints to minimise suffering. In *The COST Manual of Laboratory Animal Care and Use*. Eds. Howard, B., Nevalainen, T. and Perretta, G., pp. 333–353. CRC Press, Boca Raton.

Hernandez-Lallement, J., Gómez-Sotres, P. and Carrillo, M. (2022). Towards a unified theory of emotional contagion in rodents— A meta-analysis. *Neuroscience & Biobehavioral Reviews*, **132**, 1229–1248.

Hickman, D.L. (2018, November). Home cage compared with induction chamber for euthanasia of laboratory rats [Text]. doi:info:doi/10.30802/AALAS-JAALAS-17-000160

Hickman, D.L. (2021). Wellbeing of mice euthanized with carbon dioxide in their home cage as compared with an induction chamber. *Journal of the American Association for Laboratory Animal Science*, **60**(1), 72–76.

Hickman, D.L., Fitz, S.D., Bernabe, C.S., *et al.* (2016). Evaluation of low versus high volume per minute displacement CO_2 methods of euthanasia in the induction and duration of panic-associated behavior and physiology. *Animals: An Open Access Journal from MDPI*, **6**(8), 45.

Hickman, D.L. and Johnson, S.W. (2011). Evaluation of the aesthetics of physical methods of euthanasia of anesthetized rats. *Journal of the American Association for Laboratory Animal Science : JAALAS*, **50**(5), 695–701.

Home Office (2014) Guidance on the Operation of the Animals (Scientific Procedures) Act 1986. Her Majesty's Stationary Office: London. Available at https://assets.publishing.service.gov.uk/media/5a8211e1ed915d74e62359f4/Guidance_on_the_Operation_of_ASPA.pdf (Accessed November 13, 2023)

Home Office (2015) Advice Note: 03/2015 Animals (Scientific Procedures) Act 1986 Re-homing and setting free of animals Animals in Science Regulation Unit. Her Majesty's Stationary Office: London. Available at: https://assets.publishing.service.gov.uk/media/5a82e2ab40f0b6230269d373/Advice_Note_Rehoming_setting_free.pdf (Accessed November 13, 2023

Hurst, J.L. and West, R.S. (2010). Taming anxiety in laboratory mice. *Nature Methods*, **7**(10), 825–826.

Institute of Laboratory Animal Resources (2011) *Guide for the Care and Use of Laboratory Animals*. The National Academies Press, Washington, D.C.

Khoo, S.Y.-S., Lay, B.P.P., Joya, J. and McNally, G.P. (2018). Local anaesthetic refinement of pentobarbital euthanasia reduces abdominal writhing without affecting immunohistochemical endpoints in rats. *Laboratory Animals*, **52**(2), 152–162.

Kongara, K., McIlhone, A.E., Kells, N.J. and Johnson, C.B. (2014). Electroencephalographic evaluation of decapitation of the anaesthetized rat. *Laboratory Animals*, **48**(1), 15–19.

LaFollette, M.R., Riley, M.C., Cloutier, S., Brady, C.M., O'Haire, M.E. and Gaskill, B.N. (2020). Laboratory animal welfare meets human welfare: a cross-sectional study of professional quality of life, including compassion fatigue in laboratory animal personnel. *Frontiers in Veterinary Science*, **7**. Retrieved from https://www.frontiersin.org/articles/10.3389/fvets.2020.00114

Leary, S.L., Underwood, W., Anthony, R., et al. (2013) *AVMA Guidelines for the Euthanasia of Animals: 2013 edition*. AVMA, Schaumburg. Available at: https://www.in.gov/boah/files/AVMA_Euthanasia_Guidelines.pdf (Accessed November 13, 2023)

Leary, S.L., Underwood, W., Anthony, R., et al. (2020) *AVMA Guidelines for the Euthanasia of Animals: 2020 edition*. AVMA, Schaumburg. Available at: https://avmajournals.avma.org/view/journals/javma/261/5/javma.22.08.0373.xml#ref3 (Accessed November 13, 2023)

Leibold, N.K., van den Hove, D.L.A., Viechtbauer, W., et al. (2016). CO_2 exposure as translational cross-species experimental model for panic. *Translational Psychiatry*, **6**(9), e885–e885.

Mackie, N. and McKeegan, D. (2016) Behavioural responses of broiler chickens during low atmospheric pressure stunning. *Applied Animal Behaviour Science*, **174**, 90–98.

Makowska, I.J., Niel, L., Kirkden, R.D. and Weary, D.M. (2008). Rats show aversion to argon-induced hypoxia. *Applied Animal Behaviour Science*, **114**(3–4), 572–581.

Makowska, I.J., Vickers, L., Mancell, J. and Weary, D.M. (2009). Evaluating methods of gas euthanasia for laboratory mice. *Applied Animal Behaviour Science*, **121**(3–4), 230–235.

Mcintyre, A.R., Drummond, R.A., Riedel, E.R. and Lipman, N.S. (2007). Automated mouse euthanasia in an individually ventilated caging system: system development and assessment. *Journal of the American Association for Laboratory Animal Science*, **46**(2), 65–73.

McKeegan, D.E.F., McIntyre, J., Demmers, T.G.M., Wathes, C.M. and Jones, R.B. (2006). Behavioural responses of broiler chickens during acute exposure to gaseous stimulation. *Applied Animal Behaviour Science*, **99**(3), 271–286.

McKeegan, D.E.F., Sandercock, D.A. and Gerritzen, M.A. (2013). Physiological responses to low atmospheric pressure stunning and the implications for welfare. *Poultry Science*, **92**(4), 858–868.

Mellor, D.J. and Diesch, T.J. (2006). Onset of sentience: the potential for suffering in fetal and newborn farm animals. *Applied Animal Behaviour Science*, **100**(1–2), 48–57.

Mellor, D.J. (2019). Welfare-aligned sentience: enhanced capacities to experience, interact, anticipate, choose and survive. *Animals*, **9**(7), 440.

Moody, C., Chua, B. and Weary, D. (2014). The effect of carbon dioxide flow rate on the euthanasia of laboratory mice. *Laboratory Animals*, **48**(4), 298–304.

Moody, C.M. and Weary, D.M. (2014). Mouse aversion to isoflurane versus carbon dioxide gas. *Applied Animal Behaviour Science*, **158**, 95–101.

Munro, B.A., Merenick, D.R., Gee, J.M. and Pang, D.S. (2023). Use of loss of righting reflex to assess susceptibility to carbon dioxide gas in three mouse strains. *Journal of the American Association for Laboratory Animal Science: JAALAS*. doi:10.30802/AALAS-JAALAS-23-000035

Newsome, J.T., Clemmons, E.A., Fitzhugh, D.C., et al. (2019). Compassion fatigue, euthanasia stress, and their Management in laboratory animal research. *Journal of the American Association for Laboratory Animal Science*, **58**(3), 289–292.

Niel, L., Stewart, S.A. and Weary, D.M. (2008). Effect of flow rate on aversion to gradual-fill carbon dioxide exposure in rats. *Applied Animal Behaviour Science*, **109**(1), 77–84.

Niel, L. and Weary, D.M. (2007). Rats avoid exposure to carbon dioxide and argon. *Applied Animal Behaviour Science*, **107**(1–2), 100–109.

Nunamaker, E.A., Davis, S., O'Malley, C.I. and Turner, P.V. (2021). Developing recommendations for cumulative endpoints and lifetime use for research animals. *Animals*, **11**(7), 2031.

Peppel, P. and Anton, F. (1993). Responses of rat medullary dorsal horn neurons following intranasal noxious chemical stimulation: effects of stimulus intensity, duration, and interstimulus interval. *Journal of Neurophysiology*, **70**(6), 2260–2275.

Pritchett, K., Corrow, D., Stockwell, J. and Smith, A. (2005). Euthanasia of neonatal mice with carbon dioxide. *Comparative Medicine*, **55**(3), 275–281.

Quagliato, L.A., Freire, R.C. and Nardi, A.E. (2018). The role of acid-sensitive ion channels in panic disorder: a systematic review of animal studies and meta-analysis of human studies. *Translational Psychiatry*, **8**(1), 185. doi:10.1038/s41398-018-0238-z

Raj, A.B.M. and Gregory, N.G. (1995). Welfare implications of the gas stunning of Pigs 1. determination of aversion to the initial inhalation of carbon dioxide or argon. *Animal Welfare*, **4**(4), 273–280.

Readman, G.D., Owen, S.F., Knowles, T.G. and Murrell, J.C. (2017). Species specific anaesthetics for fish anaesthesia and euthanasia. *Scientific Reports*, **7**(1), 7102.

Readman, G.D., Owen, S.F., Murrell, J.C. and Knowles, T.G. (2013). Do fish perceive anaesthetics as aversive? *PLOS ONE*, **8**(9), e73773.

Reimer, J.N., Schuster, C.J., Knight, C.G., Pang, D.S.J. and Leung, V.S.Y. (2020). Intraperitoneal injection of sodium pentobarbital has the potential to elicit pain in adult rats (Rattus norvegicus). *PLOS ONE*, **15**(9), e0238123.

Reimert, I., Bolhuis, J.E., Kemp, B. and Rodenburg, T.B. (2013). Indicators of positive and negative emotions and emotional contagion in pigs. *Physiology & Behavior*, **109**, 42–50.

Risling, T.E., Caulkett, N.A. and Florence, D. (2012). Open-drop anesthesia for small laboratory animals. *The Canadian Veterinary Journal*, **53**(3), 299–302.

Sandilands, V., Raj, A.B.M., Baker, L. and Sparks, N.H.C. (2011). Aversion of chickens to various lethal gas mixtures. *Animal Welfare*, **20**(2), 253–262.

Scotney, R.L., McLaughlin, D. and Keates, H.L. (2015). A systematic review of the effects of euthanasia and occupational stress in personnel working with animals in animal shelters, veterinary clinics, and biomedical research facilities. *Journal of the American Veterinary Medical Association*, **247**(10), 1121–1130.

Shomer, N.H., Allen-Worthington, K.H., Hickman, D.L., et al. (2020). Review of Rodent Euthanasia Methods. *Journal of the American Association for Laboratory Animal Science*, **59**(3), 242–253.

Svendsen, O., Kok, L. and Lauritzenä, B. (2007). Nociception after intraperitoneal injection of a sodium pentobarbitone formulation with and without lidocaine in rats quantified by expression of neuronal c-fos in the spinal cord – a preliminary study. *Laboratory Animals*, **41**(2), 197–203.

Turner, P.V., Hickman, D.L., van Luijk, J., et al. (2020). Welfare impact of carbon dioxide euthanasia on laboratory mice and rats: a systematic review. *Frontiers in Veterinary Science*, **7**. Retrieved from https://www.frontiersin.org/articles/10.3389/fvets.2020.00411

Varughese, S. and Ahmed, R. (2021). Environmental and occupational considerations of anesthesia: a narrative review and update. *Anesthesia and Analgesia*, **133**(4), 826–835.

Wong, D., Makowska, I.J. and Weary, D.M. (2013). Rat aversion to isoflurane versus carbon dioxide. *Biology Letters*, **9**(1), 20121000. doi:10.1098/rsbl.2012.1000

Wong, D., von Keyserlingk, M.A.G., Richards, J.G. and Weary, D.M. (2014). Conditioned place avoidance of Zebrafish (Danio rerio) to three chemicals used for euthanasia and anaesthesia. *PLoS ONE*, **9**(2), e88030.

Zatroch, K.K., Knight, C.G., Reimer, J.N. and Pang, D.S.J. (2017). Refinement of intraperitoneal injection of sodium pentobarbital for euthanasia in laboratory rats (Rattus norvegicus). *BMC Veterinary Research*, **13**(1), 60.

18 Ethics review of animal research

I. Anna S. Olsson and Peter Sandøe
Penny Hawkins and Maggy Jennings (Appendix)

Introduction

This chapter is about ethics review of animal use for experiments. In most jurisdictions, such review is legally required, and experiments with animals can generally only go ahead after they have undergone an ethics review with a favourable outcome.

The chapter aims to provide an overview of ethics review within animal experimentation. We begin by looking briefly at the history of ethics review and its philosophical underpinning, including a reflection on the different public perspectives that form the backdrop, in order to understand why ethics review has become part of animal experimentation regulation. We then go on to examine how ethics review is done. On the one hand, we address where in the regulatory system that review takes place, and who is involved in doing it. On the other hand, we ask what, exactly, is being reviewed. This part is to a great extent about ethics committees and how they work, and draws on published research of ethics committee functioning.

The chapter has been written with an international audience in mind, and uses examples from many different countries and systems in Europe, America and Australia. There is not a single right way to do ethics review, and the variety of approaches referred to here are examples of different ways of meeting the challenges faced by ethics committees.

This chapter is not meant primarily as a practical guide on how to do ethics review. Rather, it aims to provide insight and critical reflection for people who are involved in ethics review, in particular those who perform review and those who are in control of its organisation.

The chapter is accompanied by an appendix written by Penny Hawkins and Maggy Jennings, which through its self-assessment checklist aims to provide more practical guidance for ethics committees (Appendix 18.1). Also, whereas we provide a wider background and context to the practice of ethics review in our text, we acknowledge that ethics review does not capture all ethical issues related to animal use in experiments, and consequently this chapter is not a comprehensive overview of animal research ethics.

Why is ethics review required for animal research?

Across the world, the use of live animals for research or testing is regulated by law. Legal regulations typically require those who conduct experiments with animals to submit a proposal describing their research to a committee for 'ethical review'. The review process is ethical because the committee is required to weigh up the potentially conflicting interests of those doing the experiments, those for whose sake the experiments are done, and the animals being used. Actually, there is a little more to it than this, but before we unpack the ethical issues further, we want to look at where the idea of ethics review came from.

The idea that research should undergo ethical or ethics review is likely to have originated in research involving humans. A brief look at the history of its development will explain its origins and why it was introduced.

The origin of ethics review in research

The first half of the twentieth century saw a series of experiments on humans in which the people involved were not provided with information or asked for their consent. In the worst cases – such as the experiments on concentration camp inmates during Second World War – human subjects were seriously harmed or killed. The prosecution of the Nazi experimenters at the Nuremberg Trials after the war was the first step in the development of a series of international codes and treaties, including the so-called Declaration of Helsinki, first published in 1964. In its second iteration of 1975, the Declaration included the requirement for review by an independent committee to take place before medical researchers were allowed to undertake experiments on human subjects.

In parallel with the international process, in the USA a series of medical research scandals triggered similar developments, so that since the mid-1970s any medical research involving human subjects has been required to undergo review, mostly by what are known in the USA as Institutional

The UFAW Handbook on the Care and Management of Laboratory and Other Research Animals, Ninth Edition.
Edited by Huw Golledge and Claire Richardson.
© 2024 John Wiley & Sons Ltd. Published 2024 by John Wiley & Sons Ltd.

Review Boards. One of the more important purposes of the review is to check that the research subjects are not facing unreasonable risks, and that the risks they are facing are proportionate to the expected benefits to society.

The development of a system for ethics review of human research was part of a global shift in legal frameworks in the post-war period that recognised universal human rights (UN Declaration on Human Rights 1948), implying that no human being can be sacrificed for the sake of the general good. In the Declaration of Helsinki, this is evident in Article 5: 'In medical research on human subjects, considerations related to the well-being of the human subject should take precedence over the interests of science and society'.

The idea of using ethics review in connection with animal experimentation was clearly influenced by the developments just described. And just as the emergence of ethical review for human experiments reflected acceptance that moral standing should be accorded to all human beings, so the ethical review of animal experiments was driven by a growing consensus that non-human animals have moral status.

In Western countries until around the start of the nineteenth century when the first laws for the protection of animals were put in place, the dominant view was that animals are there for us to use. It was felt that the only protection animals merited was that given to a person's property. With the introduction of so-called anti-cruelty legislation in the nineteenth century (see Kelch, 2013 for an overview), meaningless cruelty (as it was called) was banned, but the use of animals for food and fur production was not regulated.

Interestingly, discussions of animal experimentation in the nineteenth century often framed the experiments as cruel and meaningless. The framing was not entirely unjustified: since anaesthesia was unavailable, there was no way at that time to prevent the animals experiencing pain, and this was not restricted to scientific experiments – live animals were also used in demonstrations of anatomy and physiology.

In fact, this use of animals was controversial among nineteenth-century scientists. Famously, while Charles Darwin defended some animal experimentation as necessary, he also denounced much of it as meaningless cruelty. On the other hand, his French contemporary Claude Bernard dismissed critics, arguing that 'a man of science should attend only to the opinion of men of science who understand him, and should derive rules of conduct only from his own conscience' (Bernard 1927, p. 103). And still today there continues to be genuine discussion of how we should balance the wish to protect the interests of animals against the right of the scientists to pursue their research. Academic freedom is an important value alongside animal welfare and an important part of the debate is concerned with which is most important. Today a statement like that quoted from Bernard would not pass public scrutiny, and it is widely believed that academic freedom must be subordinate to considerations of animal welfare.

In the UK, unregulated animal experimentation came to an end with the Cruelty to Animals Act 1876, which required animal experiments to be licensed. There is wide international variation, but around the mid-1980s legislation regulating animal experimentation had been passed in most Western countries. In many countries, a requirement for ethics review was part of this legislation already then.

Underlying philosophy

The legislation regulating the use of animals in experiments from the outset permitted this use with two provisos: (1) that the experiment served a decent and useful purpose; and (2) that the animals were not exposed to more suffering than was necessary to achieve this purpose. In the jurisdictions where ethics committees were responsible for evaluating if proposed experiments or projects met these requirements, their role was initially, therefore, mainly of a technical nature.

It was felt that they should assess, first, whether the animals were being used in the best possible way to achieve the stated goals (i.e. whether the experiments were novel and properly designed, whether the research questions were scientifically relevant, etc.), and second, whether animal suffering had been minimised as much as possible, relative to the goal of the experiments. The second assessment has gradually been linked to the 3Rs principle of Replacement, Reduction and Refinement. This principle was first introduced in 1959 (Russell and Burch) but only started to gain attention in the scientific community in the 1980s (Stephens and Mak 2013). Consequently, ethics reviews of research with animals were initially dominated by technical expertise, and the role of the few lay, non-expert committee members involved in them was mainly to oversee that the reviews were undertaken in a fair manner.

The notion that animals may be used for experimentation if this is necessary to deliver important human benefits, principally benefits to human health, will generally ensure that serious human interests prevail over animal interests. The political scientist Robert Garner has dubbed this ethical hierarchy, in which human and animal interests belong to different orders of moral worth, 'animal welfarism' (Garner et al. 2017). There can be different varieties of this notion, which differ regarding the level of animal discomfort, pain or other forms of suffering tolerated to pursue vital human interests.

In considering human and animal interests as morally distinct, this view differs strikingly from the philosophical theory known as 'utilitarianism'. The idea of balancing harm and benefit and striving for the best possible aggregate outcome is central to utilitarian thinking. However, utilitarians believe that human and animal interests are on par. For them, animal harm matters as much as human harm. Whether or not this implies that animal experiments are morally acceptable will depend on the value one attaches to harm and benefit. Some well-known utilitarian philosophers, notably Peter Singer, oppose much animal experimentation on the grounds that the benefit in general is much too small to outweigh the harm caused to the animals (Singer 1975).

Other critics of animal experimentation argue that it is morally unacceptable because it is in principle wrong to inflict harm on living animals. This view finds support in the philosophical theory of animal rights. According to this view, the question of human interests is irrelevant for the discussion of how to treat animals, because animals have rights which should not be violated no matter what gains are expected. The American philosopher Tom Regan, who is an adherent of the view that animals have rights, argues like this: 'The rights view is categorically abolitionist. Lab animals are not our tasters; we are not their kings. Because these animals are treated routinely, systematically as if their value were reducible to their usefulness to others, they are routinely, systematically treated with lack of respect, and thus are their rights routinely, systematically violated. This is just as true when they are used in trivial, duplicative, unnecessary or unwise research as it is when they are used in studies that hold out real promise for human benefits' (Regan 2007, p. 210).

There are other ethical positions which are potentially relevant here – the virtue ethics that underpins many codes of professional ethics and care ethics that has come to inform the adoption of ideas around a culture of care. These may be very important preconditions for ensuring the best possible level of animal welfare. However, for the issue of ethical review here under scrutiny the main issue when deliberating on whether to accept a specific experiment will be whether everything practically possible has been done to limit animal discomfort, pain and other forms of suffering and whether there is a decent balance between the expected human benefit and the anticipated animal harm. A stance here will reflect an ethical stance.

Public perspectives

The animal rights perspective that attributes animals' absolute rights which are not to be overruled by human interests is present in the public debate. It is also represented among some Non-Governmental Organizations (NGOs) which take a more radical stance on human use of animals. But the fact that animal experimentation is not socially condemned suggests that animal rights-based thinking is not widespread in society. Indeed, this has been confirmed in empirical research.

Studies by Thomas Lund and colleagues (Lund et al. 2012, 2014) identify three kinds of stance on animal experimentation among members of the Danish public: Disapprovers (16%) uphold the view that animal research cannot be accepted despite potential benefits to humans; reserved people (49%) occupy an ambivalent position and typically shift between approval and disapproval of specific experiments, depending on harm–benefit evaluations; approvers (35%) tend to attach more weight to potential human benefits than they do to protecting animals against suffering. Another relevant result of the studies is that most people seem to accept the harm–benefit framework as a basis for making decisions about the use of animals in research and testing. There seems to be substantial national variation both in general attitudes to animal use and in attitudes to the use of particular species (von Roten 2013). Still, the general picture is that in most countries a clear majority favours using animals for important biomedical research, but also that the support reduces if animals are used for purposes perceived by the respondents to be less important and if the animals have to endure significant suffering.

In short, then, changing societal views of animal use have implications for animal research regulation in that there is: (1) Growing concern over whether the suffering or discomfort imposed on animals in experiments is proportional to the human benefits which the research aims to achieve; (2) A growing awareness that in some cases the suffering imposed on animals may not be acceptable despite the expected human benefits and (3) A concern about the use of some species of animal, notably primates, which are seen as more worthy of protection than others (see Olsson and Sandøe 2021 for a more extensive discussion of this).

With these changes, the kinds of skill and expertise required in ethical review also develop – for example, to focus balancing human benefits against animal suffering; and technical expertise – important as it is, for example, to ensure that harm is minimised relative to the goal set – will not suffice. What are called for are also general competencies which can be well-represented by persons without a role and background in science. Not surprisingly, during the period since committees were first introduced some countries have seen evolution in the composition of animal ethics committees, with more lay and other members joining who are not technical experts on animal experimentation.

So, there is a clear link between the requirements that ethics review should fulfil and the way a review is organised. In the following three sections, we will first give an overview of the role of the review and the ways in which the process can be organised. We will then turn to the different requirements of the review. Finally, in the concluding section, we will discuss the interaction between the two.

How is the ethics review of animal research undertaken?

Ethics reviews play a significant role in the process leading to the authorisation of animal experiments. How large that role is differs between jurisdictions (Olsson *et al.* 2017). The decisions of the animal research ethics committees in some countries are legally binding, hence the legal authorisation can be said to be based entirely on the outcome of the ethics review. In other countries, ethics committees provide advice but there is a different competent authority which issues the legal authorisation. Even in the USA, where most laboratory animals are not covered by federal legislation and the legal status of the committees is unclear (Tannenbaum 2017), in practice the committee decision is decisive within an institution. It seems fair to say that across jurisdictions, experiments with animals can generally only go ahead after they have undergone an ethics review with a favourable outcome and approval.

Prospective reviews – of planned studies with animals – represent the largest proportion of ethics reviews. Normally, these reviews focus on the scientific work in which animals are used. The research team and the physical infrastructure are considered in this context, in the sense that skilful and experienced personnel and adequate facilities are important for maximising the quality of the research and minimising the harm caused to the animals. But there are usually separate licensing procedures for animal facilities, on the one hand, and research personnel, on the other. These licensing procedures are not addressed in this chapter.

Applications for approval are submitted by the responsible researcher. Usually, what is being reviewed is not an individual experiment, but a larger body of proposed work – what in the USA is called an 'animal study protocol' and in the European Union simply a 'project'. We discuss the type of information that an application needs to provide in the next section. Applications usually enter the system through an administrative entry point – they are submitted to a secretariat and then sent out for ethics review. In addition to receiving the information that applicants provide in written format in the original application, ethics review committees are usually permitted to ask for further information which clarifies matters or adds details that are necessary to complete the review. Some committees also have a mechanism enabling direct dialogue with researchers, including meetings or teleconferences in which the committee members can raise questions and the applicant provides further detail and explanations.

Animal research ethics committees

The term introduced in the preceding paragraph – 'ethics committee' – describes a central concept in the currently predominant organisation of the review. As we will see in the following paragraphs, many different aspects of animal ethics review revolve around the committee.

In most countries, applications are analysed and discussed by a group of people. The group is often referred to as an 'Animal Ethics Committee' (variants of this label are used throughout Europe and Australia), or an 'Animal Care and Use Committee (a label predominantly used in North and Latin America). We will focus here on more general considerations pertaining to committee composition and functioning, with examples from different countries and regions. For a more comprehensive international overview, the reader is referred to Röcklinsberg et al. (2017, Chapter 5).

The first animal research ethics committees were introduced in Sweden in 1979. At that time, there was a political wish to move from a system where decisions over animal use in experiments were left entirely to the scientific community to one where society has insight into the activity and influence. The outcome was a system of advisory ethics committees composed by scientists, animal care personnel and lay people in equal proportions (Alexius Borgström 2009). The US committee system, introduced in 1985, also included representation of wider society through its so-called unaffiliated members (Dresser 1999).

The establishment of committee systems introduced two important features: the first was that the authorisation of animal experiments would now require assessment by a group of people, and the second was that this group would involve lay persons or persons without a stake in animal experimentation. As will become clear in the following text, there are some significant differences in the composition of ethics committees between countries.

There is no international standard on the composition of animal ethics committees. In fact, this aspect is not even covered in the only supranational legislation for animal experimentation, the EU Directive 2010/63/EU (European Union 2010). Article 38, which regulates the authorisation of projects, establishes the kinds of expertise that need to be considered in the review process (the scientific area in which animals will be used, the application of the 3Rs in this area, veterinary practice, and animal husbandry and care, for the species in question). But how these requirements are met in the practical operation of ethics committees is left to the individual EU member states to decide.

When we reviewed the European situation in 2015, we did indeed find great variation between countries, but also some patterns (Olsson et al. 2017). In terms of expertise, all EU member states included scientific and veterinary and/or animal welfare experts on the committees reviewing projects. The same is true in North America and Australia. Even in the absence of a comprehensive up-to-date overview of animal ethics committees across the world, it seems reasonable to assume that these two areas of expertise are universally included. They are the minimum expertise one would want to have in order to be able to work for the best possible balance between scientific objectives and the minimisation of animal suffering.

But we also found that in European ethics committees, other areas of expertise are being required by some countries. The most common were expertise in ethics, law, alternatives to animal experiments, and the design and statistical methodology of animal experiments. It is easy to see how the last two of these will contribute to the objective of optimising science and minimising animal suffering. The inclusion of an ethicist seems very reasonable for a process that is called ethics review which is performed by an ethics committee. And where legal experts participate, that is often in countries where the animal ethics review is part of the legal system itself.

However, if we return to the introduction of the ethics committee system in Sweden and the USA more than 30 years ago, we see that more than expertise was at stake. Already, at the introduction of the system, both countries considered the desirability of having broader representation on the committee. Lay or independent members also sit on committees in Canada and Australia, and in some – but far from all – other European countries. In some cases, they are asked to represent the interests of society. In others, they are representatives of special interest groups, typically animal protection organisations.

A third aspect of committee composition is the balance between different groups and interests. We saw that the original approach in Sweden asked for equal proportions of scientists, animal care personnel and lay persons. This has since changed to a distribution of 50% scientists and animal care personnel and 50% lay representation. There are other approaches to composition. It is mainly experts that sit on the national committee reviewing animal experiments in Denmark, but the entities mandated to nominate members reflect an ambition to balance representation between research stakeholders and animal protection stakeholders. Outside Scandinavia, we are not aware of committees which are fully balanced between members who are internal and those who are external to the research community. In general, members from outside the research community are in the minority, and in a considerable number of countries animal research ethics committees only include people nominated for their expertise rather than stakeholder representation (Olsson et al. 2017).

When and where does ethics review take place?

There is also variation regarding at what administrative level animal ethics committees operate, although it seems safe to say that institutional committees, i.e. committees run by the universities or other academic institutions themselves, predominate internationally. The USA, Canada, Latin American countries and Australia all operate systems where the mandate to review and authorise experiments with animals lies with institutional committees. In Europe, there is again greater variation, and also some overlapping mandates. Directive 2010/63/EU introduced the animal welfare body as a requirement for all institutions. This body, which was tasked with ensuring implementation of the 3Rs in the institution, was not intended to be involved in reviewing for authorisation, and not meant to have the role of an ethics committee. However, it is difficult to avoid a reviewing role for an entity which is responsible for making sure that the 3Rs are respected in work with animals. As we will see in the Portuguese example below, in some countries animal welfare bodies also play a formal role in project authorisation.

Some countries have a system with national, or federal, review; in other words, a single committee for the entire country. This is the case in, for example, Denmark and Hungary. Sweden and Germany are examples of countries with regional, or state, review systems, with a committee for each part of the country. There are also systems which combine different levels, and especially institutional and national evaluations. For example, Portuguese legislation requires institutional animal welfare bodies to issue non-binding recommendations for project authorisation. In Ireland, a local review is not a legal requirement, but it is nevertheless encouraged as a step preceding project authorisation at national level.

How committees deliberate when they carry out the ethics review is another important aspect of ethics committee operation. Again, we possess no comprehensive overview of how committees operate, which criteria and methods they use in review, etc. This kind of information is often difficult to find and not necessarily made public in terms other than the vernacular language of a country. In general, committees have procedures of some sort which distribute work among their members. One approach is to have a smaller group, or even a single member, performing an in-depth review of a project first. On the basis of that review, the project is presented for discussion and a final decision by the full committee. In the USA, an individual member may decide whether the decision is straightforward enough for approval through the so-called designated member review. Of course, the member may decide that a full committee review is required. We will explore the question of different methods for deliberation and decision-making in more detail in the last section of this chapter.

The focus so far has been on prospective review for the authorisation of projects with animals. However, many of the review committees have a wider range of tasks. Institutional ethics review bodies often also perform inspections of the facilities where animals are housed and experiments carried out, and they may also be responsible for promoting good practice and 3Rs knowledge in the institution. In Denmark, the national committee makes site visits and may also ask researchers to demonstrate the relevant competencies before they are authorised to use certain procedures.

In the EU, the current legal framework also includes a requirement for retrospective assessment to be carried out by the same entities that perform prospective reviews. The retrospective assessment is linked to the prospective review and provides an opportunity to compare what actually happened with what was expected in a number of relevant aspects. These include the comparison of project outcome with research objectives, actual versus predicted harm to the animals and the number of animals used. In this way, retrospective review provides an opportunity to identify new avenues of refinement and other measures to improve the harm–benefit balance in future projects of a similar nature.

Retrospective assessments are mandatory in the EU both for experiments involving non-human primates and for severe experiments. It is possible for committees to require them in other cases too. Given that a retrospective assessment provides a structure in which it is made clear how recent experiences can be used to improve future projects, it is particularly relevant for projects where models or methods are being used for the first time.

What is included in the ethics review of animal research?

As a consequence of its regulatory role, one of the most important functions of animal ethics review is to make sure that the proposed research will comply with the conditions laid down in legislation. This process entails assessing the information provided by the applicants, asking for additional information, providing feedback on issues that need addressing and giving a final ethics approval.

An important first step of this assessment is provision, to the assessment committee, of the appropriate information. This is largely determined by the application form. Unsurprisingly, there is no standard format for application forms. They vary not only between jurisdictions but even between committees. Some guidance can, however, be found in legislation. Here we will use the requirements set out in EU Directive 2010/63/EU as an example illustrating the kinds of information that need to be provided for ethics review (Table 18.1).

What, then, is this information used to assess? Although there is room for some variation in criteria and assessment methods, a set of general conditions must be met for research with animals to be ethically acceptable within the EU legislative framework. The research must be of a kind that is expected to generate benefit by producing information that is relevant and reliable. Therefore, the expected benefits must be assessed, and ideally maximised. The harm the animals are expected to endure as a consequence of the research also needs to be assessed, as must the measures that are will be taken to minimise this harm. Finally, there should be proportionality between harm and benefit. This must be assessed by weighing the total expected harm against the total expected benefit. In the following, we will look at benefit assessment, focusing on validity and experimental design. When we examine harm assessment, we will focus on the 3Rs and harm–benefit weighing. Detailed analysis of each of these topics individually is beyond the scope of this chapter, but it can be found in, for example, Hubrecht (2014) and Röcklinsberg et al. (2017).

Table 18.1 EU Directive 2010/63/EU (Article 37c + Annex VI) requires applications for project authorisation to include information on the following elements of the proposed project with animals.

1	Relevance and justification of the following:
	a. use of animals including their origin, estimated numbers, species and life stages;
	b. procedures.
2	Application of methods to replace, reduce and refine the use of animals in procedures.
3	The planned use of anaesthesia, analgesia and other pain-relieving methods.
4	Reduction, avoidance and alleviation of any form of animal suffering, from birth to death where appropriate.
5	Use of humane endpoints.
6	Experimental or observational strategy and statistical design to minimise animal numbers, pain, suffering, distress and environmental impact where appropriate.
7	Reuse of animals and the accumulative effect thereof on the animals.
8	The proposed severity classification of procedures.
9	Avoidance of unjustified duplication of procedures where appropriate.
10	Housing, husbandry and care conditions for the animals.
11	Methods of killing.
12	Competence of persons involved in the project.

Benefit – what it is and how to ensure it is maximised

Traditionally, the focus when it comes to research benefit has been on conventional standard measures of scientific potential and quality, of the same kind that are used in evaluating applications for funding. Thus in order to assess the potential benefit of the proposed project, members of the Federation of European Laboratory Animal Science Associations (FELASA) working group on ethics review Smith *et al.* (2007) have recommended that committees should ask how original, timely and realistic the objectives are; whether there is replication of previous work and how the work being proposed relates to other work in the field. To assess the likelihood of achieving the potential benefits, committees are advised to consider the choice of animal model and scientific approach, the competence of researchers, the appropriateness and quality of facilities, and the way the results will be communicated.

In academic research, questions about how original, timely and realistic the objectives are, and how those objectives relate to other work in the field, are typically addressed in the scientific evaluation of funding applications. And in animal testing for safety purposes, this question does not really apply – beyond the need to confirm whether there is a legal requirement for testing, there is no room to discuss whether this is a relevant objective. Therefore, it may be reasonable that in many cases the review committees for animal experiments will focus on addressing the likelihood that the benefits will be achieved in practice. In animal research, the suitability of animal models is often critical in determining whether or not the expected scientific and medical benefits are secured (Olsson and Sandøe 2021).

Choosing the right research model

Often researchers study animals of one species with the aim of gaining understanding with wider application, or with application to another species (typically, humans). This is especially true for fundamental biology and biomedical research, where animals are used to model a phenomenon of interest. Choosing the right research model is not only a question of choosing the species but often also of making sure that the phenomenon occurs, by inducing for example a disease or a genetic mutation. In this section, we refer to an animal model in the conceptual sense, as a model of study. Of course, not all animal research is of this sort. In fields such as animal and veterinary sciences, or ecology and conservation biology, animals are usually studied in their own right rather than being used as models.

Determining what the right model is for a given research question requires expertise within the research field itself that is usually more specialised than the expertise present in an animal ethics committee. In practice, therefore, ethics committees will sometimes have little alternative other than to take the applicant's information at face value. A possible approach for a committee at this point is to ask the applicant to provide information about how valid their chosen model is for addressing the research questions they aim to answer. The concept of model validity has been best developed in the field of neurobehaviour, following Paul Willner's (Willner 1984) critical analysis of depression models.

The ultimate measure of validity is how well the results obtained in the model predict outcomes in the species of interest – in biomedical research, usually humans. However, predictive validity can only be assessed once comparable studies in humans exist, and it will often be a long time before such information is available. Therefore, researchers tend to look for earlier theoretical indications of model validity. The notion of 'construct validity', recording how similar the underlying mechanisms of the model and the other species of interest are, is useful here. There is no quantitative method of ascertaining the construct validity of an animal model. Instead, researchers are obliged to identify critical features of what is being studied – e.g. a disease mechanism in humans – and ask whether these are present in the animal model (see also Chapter 2: The Three Rs).

Unavoidably, scientists also operate under practical constraints. Most research is to some extent dependent on existing technologies. It is shaped by factors such as what models have been used before, what models the researcher has expertise in, whether an animal colony has already been set up at high cost and so on. In practice, therefore, scientists are rarely choosing from the full range of existing animal models. Given this, an understanding of the feasibility constraints on a project is vital in discussions of its validity. It has even been suggested that the most appropriate framework for critically assessing model choice, model limitations and their consequences for research is to focus on not what is modelled but what is being ignored in the model (Garner *et al.* 2017).

Experimental design

In contrast to the choice of model, where there are many practical constraints, experimental planning and design are fully under the control of researchers. Shortcomings in these aspects have a considerable impact on research benefits, as has become painfully evident from work performed during the first decade of the twenty-first century, much of which involved animal research underpinning the development of treatments for stroke in humans (Van der Worp et al. 2010). Problems became apparent after a number of compounds had shown neuroprotective effects in animal models but then turned out to be ineffective in clinical trials on humans (van der Worp et al. 2005).

When researchers reviewed the animal research data, they found that in many of the experiments, for example, the efficacy of the prospective treatment had probably been overestimated as a result of design bias. Animals had not been randomly allocated to treatments, or the researchers had not blinded themselves when they administered treatments (drug or control) or assessed outcomes. As a consequence, the odds of positive treatment effects were higher than they would have been had such measures been in place. Significant clinical differences were also an unwelcome factor, in that the animals used were generally young and healthy before the experimentally induced condition. This has been found to be the case in studies of stroke. While the animals used were young, human stroke patients are often elderly and hypertensive (Van der Worp et al. 2010).

In the vocabulary of validity, the kind of problem we have just considered raises issues of internal and external validity (see Garner et al. 2017 and Würbel 2017 for more detail). Briefly, internal validity has to do with whether the observed differences between treatment groups are indeed due to the treatment and not some other factor of which the researchers are unaware, such as unconscious bias among researchers involved in the experiment. External validity refers to whether the results will also apply in contexts other than that of the study – e.g. whether the results in the young and healthy experimental animals would also apply to elderly, hypertensive patients.

Issues of validity, in choice of animal model and experimental design, certainly lie within the remit of ethics review. They arise at a level of detail that will not have been assessed in the peer review for funding, and they are of critical importance in ensuring that animals are used to produce valuable information. However, despite the relevance of experimental design and planned measures against bias, it is unclear to what extent ethics committees actually assess them. In an analysis of 1277 applications submitted for authorisation in Switzerland, Vogt et al. (2016) found that very few provided any information on measures against bias. The authors suggest that 'authorization of animal experiments is based on confidence rather than evidence of scientific rigour'.

In this section, we have focused on scientific aspects of planning as important measure to ensure research benefit. Well-designed experiments using scientifically valid approaches can be expected to deliver reliable knowledge. In the section on harm–benefit weighing, we will discuss how issues related to purpose are also considered by some to be relevant when benefit is assessed. Of course, whether the knowledge produced in research will actually translate into new treatments or otherwise changed health practice is also relevant (Davies et al. 2017).

Minimising animal harm

The next set of questions to be asked are about how the experimental animals are affected by the research, and what can be done to minimise any harm done to them. These are mainly – although not exclusively – questions about the 3Rs. At the beginning of this section, we pointed out benefits and harms as key determinants of ethically acceptable research. Ethical concerns about the use of animals in research centre mainly on the harm that such research may inflict on animals, and measures to minimise this harm are crucial in improving ethical acceptability – this generalisation applies within all of the views considered here.

The 3Rs principle of Replacement, Reduction and Refinement was introduced by Russell and Burch (1959) as a way to perform biological and biomedical research with minimum harm to animals. Although animal-based research has undergone enormous change over the 60 years which have passed since the 3Rs principle was first presented, the principle continues to offer a highly relevant framework for assessing research methods (see also Chapter 2: the Three Rs). We will now look at the roles of each of the 3Rs in the ethics review.

Replacement, reduction, refinement

Replacement enjoys particularly high standing among the 3Rs. It was the first of the Rs to be introduced by Russell and Burch (1959), reflecting the intended order in which the Rs were to be considered. Questions about reduction and refinement only become relevant when replacement has been considered and found impossible in the given case. The goal of replacement is also the only goal to gain support from opponents of the use of animals in research, including the more radical NGOs which advocate that all animal use for human purposes is unacceptable. Interestingly, however, this is probably also the R that is most challenging in the animal ethics review.

In the case of animal use in toxicology and safety testing, determining whether there is a replacement alternative is fairly straightforward. Regulatory requirements define what is to be considered a validated test method, and there are searchable databases where these methods can be found.

However, the concept of a validated non-animal alternative does not apply in typical biomedical research. It is true that it is usually possible to pursue a research question using different methods, but these are different approaches, not methods that directly substitute one another. Also, the composition of animal ethics committees, where veterinary and animal care expertise is always included but expertise on replacement alternatives is provided only very occasionally, indicates that they are prepared primarily to review research in which it is not expected that animals will be replaced.

It is, therefore, common for the information on Replacement in an application for approval of an experiment to be limited to a brief statement that entire living organisms are necessary for the proposed experiment. Often this is provided together with an outline of the complementary non-animal methods that are being used in the same research project.

Let us turn to the Reduction principle. Although it is seemingly straightforward, reduction is probably the most controversial of the 3Rs. There is often political value in bringing down the numbers of animals used in experimental procedures as a whole, as the number of animals reported in annual statistics is a very visible and easily understood aspect of research animal ethics. (This is also true of replacement. The fact that fewer experiments are being conducted is similar in that it is immediately recognisable in the statistics.) However, the problem with reduction is that, as detailed analyses have repeatedly shown, in actual research the number of animals used in an individual experiment is often too small for results to be reliable.

From the perspective of the animal ethics review – which, we must remember, is also tasked with ensuring that the research produces relevant results – it is, therefore, often appropriate to ask if the number of animals is appropriate in the context of each proposed experiment. This is usually approached by asking applicants to prepare a power analysis. A power analysis is a way of statistically determining the number of animals to be used on the basis of information about the variability between animals, the effect size the researcher wishes to be able to detect and how large a risk of missing a real difference can be tolerated (see also Chapter 3: The design of animal experiments).

The ethics review, however, can also help to ensure that animal numbers are kept down through the avoidance of unnecessary animal experiments. This can be done by requiring applicants to perform, and present the findings of, a systematic review of previously published experiments addressing the research question in which they interested (de Vries *et al.* 2014).

The third of the 3Rs, and arguably the one that animal ethics review seems best designed to focus on, is Refinement – specifically, the refinement of interventions on animals in order to minimise suffering. The order of the 3Rs is indicative mainly of the chronology of 3Rs consideration: once it has been shown that a research aim cannot be pursued without animal use, and once the animal numbers have been optimised, it is time to look at how to minimise the suffering of any animals that actually will be used.

Refinement is a central issue in most of the chapters in this book, so for the purpose of this chapter we will only provide a very general overview. The most obvious refinement option will generally be to adjust or adapt experimental procedures to cause as little pain or distress as possible. This may include proper use of analgesia and anaesthesia for invasive procedures. But it also implies taking animal welfare into account when deciding on blood sampling methods and routes of administration, including volumes and frequencies for sampling and administration. In the case of conditions that are expected to be progressive, refinement implies planning for euthanasia interventions before animals reach unacceptable levels of suffering, so-called humane endpoints. That will generally include the preparation of score sheets for systematic monitoring of the state of these animals.

Refinement of housing conditions is relevant for all animals, including those which are not subject to experimental interventions such as breeding animals. Animals which are expected to be debilitated or have other issues of mobility as a consequence of procedures they have undergone or conditions they are developing will require special housing adaptations. Standard animal husbandry such as feeding and breeding management needs to be considered from the perspective of animal welfare. The way animals are transported affects their welfare as does the way they are handled, and here refinement measures are certainly possible (see also Chapter 12: Transportation of laboratory animals). In short, many chapters of this book present areas of intervention with the potential to be refined, and specific guidance on applying such refinement measures.

The primary argument for refinement is to improve animal welfare. But interestingly, refinement measures are often also scientifically motivated. Environmental enrichment can be employed to create systematic variation for improved external validity (Bayne and Würbel 2014; see also Chapter 10: Enrichment: Animal welfare and scientific validity). Tail-handled mice show less explorative behaviour than mice handled using non-aversive methods, which in turn affects their performance in many behaviour tests (Gouveia and Hurst 2017).

Severely affected animals that are not offered the refinements of housing adaptation and humane endpoints are likely to die from secondary causes (e.g. dehydration or malnutrition in rodents unable to feed and drink from the cage top) rather than the disease being studied (Franco *et al.* 2012). Survival/mortality when the cause of death is unknown, or only indirectly related to the disease, is not a high-quality variable to measure. As demonstrated by Scott and colleagues (2008), failure to consider non-disease-related mortality in a neurodegenerative disease model may even account for false treatment effects.

The differing R principles do not operate in isolation, and sometimes they may conflict. Perhaps the most likely conflict is that between reduction and refinement, because lowering the total number of animals used will sometimes place a greater burden on each animal that continues to be used. Examples include the reuse of animals in different experiments versus naïve animals for each experiment, taking more blood from fewer animals versus smaller amounts from a greater number, or, in toxicology, testing the use of a higher dose (which produces a greater effect and thus requires fewer animals, but can cause more serious harm to each animal used) versus using lower doses on more animals (De Boo *et al.* 2005).

People have different opinions as to whether Reduction or Refinement should take precedence when they conflict. However, as we have argued elsewhere, if animal research ethics is to be consistent with ethical standards for other animals in society, Refinement should be the priority. By extending the way of thinking applied to farm animals, where we accept that animals are killed as long as they are given a good life, one could argue that killing more animals is acceptable if it allows each used animal to live a better life – perhaps especially if focusing on keeping numbers down results in living conditions in which the animal is considered unfortunate to be alive (Sandøe et al. 2015). This way of looking at the relative significance of animal numbers and the burdens placed on each individual animal can also be supported by the moral view that 'fairness to the individual animal' (Tannenbaum 1999), and thus spreading the load of suffering, is important.

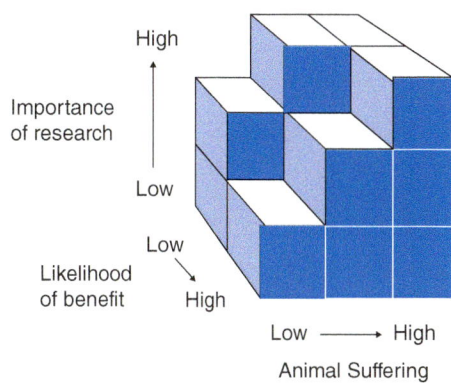

Balancing harm and benefit

In the section on how to maximise benefit, we looked at the benefits derived from animal experimentation from a technical perspective. It is obvious that a poorly designed experiment that cannot give a reliable answer to the questions it poses will not be beneficial; it may indeed be harmful if it produces misleading results. But technical quality is only one of the many aspects of benefit. The question what it means for an experiment to be beneficial leads to a complex discussion involving various notions of benefit. That discussion becomes even more complex when we move from estimating a given benefit to weighing this estimated benefit against the predicted animal harm.

There has traditionally been some reluctance in ethics committees to enter into this discussion, sometimes even in the committees' handling of the benefit evaluation and weighing (Olsson et al. 2015). But increasingly it is becoming necessary not just to minimise harms and maximise benefits, but to weigh the two against each other – and to see the ethical acceptability as something determined by the balance. With this approach, research should only be allowed if its expected benefits, in terms of the knowledge and improved treatment options (etc.) that can reasonably be expected, are proportionate to the predicted harm to the animals. The concept of harm–benefit analysis (HBA) is now used more or less globally. HBA is embedded as an explicit requirement in a series of regulatory documents across the world, including EU legislation, AAALAC International requirements and the Guide for the Care and Use of Laboratory Animals, which regulates publicly funded research in the USA (Grimm et al. 2019).

Traditionally, this weighing has taken place through (a generally loosely structured) reflection and discussion on the merit of the project, taking into account the harm caused to animals. However, a number of authors have proposed more specific methodologies, and there seems to be a perceived need for a more structured system. The idea of a more systematic approach to analysis was originally developed in a seminal paper in which Patrick Bateson argued that harms imposed on animals must be proportionate to the scientific value of the experiment. Bateson (1986) introduced the decision cube as a way to work out the acceptable level of animal suffering in an experiment relative to the value it has to humans, where the latter is defined in the two dimensions of 'importance of research' and 'likelihood of benefit'.

The Bateson Cube (Bateson 1986) The cube has three axes indicating importance of research, likelihood of benefit and animal suffering. Research, where combinations of these fall in the solid part of the cube, should not be carried out.

In 2016, an expert working group made up of North American and European laboratory animal scientists proposed that benefits should be defined according to a set of overarching domains: social benefits (human health, animal health, environmental health), socioeconomic benefits, scientific benefits, educational benefits, and safety and efficacy. In the assessment, benefit is further modulated by a set of factors: importance of outcome, clarity of objectives, translational potential, likelihood of success, continuity of recognised scientific efforts, quality of experimental design, innovation level and dissemination results (Laber et al. 2016).

In their effort to develop a systematic approach, the working group brought together components from a number of previously presented approaches. The resulting framework for benefit assessment was very broad. A broad definition of this sort has not found support everywhere. Several recent papers, based primarily on the extensive critical analysis of research methodology that we refer to in the section on how to maximise benefit, propose instead exclusively scientific methods of benefit assessment. Briefly, they favour a parallel to the 3Rs as an approach to benefit assessment – the 3Vs. V here stands for *validity*: validity of construct, internal validity and external validity (Würbel 2017; Sena and Currie 2019).

Definitions and the assessment of harm are less controversial and rely on a large body of research in animal welfare science. The transatlantic working group on harm–benefit analysis define harm through the Five Freedoms – a close to 50-year-old framework originally proposed in the context of farm animal welfare regulation (Farm Animal Welfare Council 2009). Thus, the assessment process should consider to what extent experimentation would impact on the animals' freedom from pain/injury, fear/distress, hunger/thirst and discomfort as well as the animals' ability to express normal behaviour. To this assessment is then added a layer of modulating factors related to the animals, their environment and the experiment. Animal-related modulating factors are animal species, number of animals, whether the animals are suited to the environment and animal health status. Experimental modulating factors include the intensity and duration of the harm inflicted through the experiment, the cumulative experience of the animals, the application of endpoints to curtail suffering, the possibility of complications and phenotypic manipulations. Environmental modulating factors are housing, husbandry and personnel competence (Laber et al. 2016).

Although severity assessment is closely related to harm assessment, they are not synonymous. Severity refers to the experience of the individual animal, whereas harm is aggregative and thus also takes the number of animals into account. Especially within the EU, several tools and initiatives have been developed to aid severity assessments of animal studies in the context of ethics review. One is a workshop run regularly by FELASA in different countries and venues and based on work developed by an international expert group (Smith et al. 2018).

The real challenge in the harm–benefit analysis lies in the weighing of total expected harm against total expected benefit. This is where the analysis moves from being mainly a technical exercise to one really involving ethical deliberation. This is also where we see substantial disagreement among both practitioners and scholars. One contentious issue is about what to include in the definition of benefit. We have seen in the preceding text that some approaches favour a broad definition whereas others focus more narrowly on scientific aspects. On the surface, a broader definition which considers the purpose for which animals are used seems better aligned with the public perception of what matters in decisions over the ethical acceptability of animal use in research. As we saw in the introduction, research purpose matters, and it would appear that the more highly valued research purposes justify a greater degree of animal harm in the view of the public. Others argue against this approach, alleging that this will favour applied research in a way that is poorly aligned with the role of knowledge production in scientific research (Eggel and Grimm 2018).

Indeed, it is unclear whether the differentiation of basic and applied research is really what was intended by legislators or actually what is applied in practice. For example, the European Commission Expert Working group on ethics review and harm–benefit analysis saw the need to express its own 'acknowledgement that without basic/fundamental research, many of the subsequent applied benefits would not have occurred' (Anonymous 2013). A recent review of HBA in the UK regulatory system reports the proportion of animals in severe studies in 2016 to be 2.1% for basic research, 2.9% for translational/applied research and 15.8% for regulatory testing (Davies et al. 2017). In other words, there is a negligible difference between basic and applied research as regards the acceptance of severe experiments, but severe experiments are much more common in regulatory testing, where they are not necessarily more beneficial but are often legally required.

Beyond the 3Rs

Whereas most of the ethics review will focus on benefit, 3Rs and harm–benefit analysis, it is not limited to these issues alone (see also Appendix 18.1). We will now touch upon two further issues that sometimes come up for consideration: the issue of animal species and the absolute banning of experiments above a certain level of suffering.

The relevance of animal species in the context of ethics review is often highlighted with reference to sentience. This is sometimes made explicit in regulation, as is the case when EU Directive 2010/63/EU requires the researcher to choose procedures which 'involve animals with the lowest capacity to experience pain, suffering, distress or lasting harm' (Article 13, b). However, the significance of sentience as a criterion of species selection can be seriously doubted. It is relatively poorly understood, and it is attributed to animals largely on the basis of imperfect analogies. Worse, a systematic checklist of scientifically respectable indicators shows that sentience is possessed by all vertebrates and possibly some invertebrates. That is not of much help if one is trying to determine which species to use in a potentially painful in vivo procedure.

Another issue is that some species may be ethically more challenging to use than others. For example, it is not uncommon for cats, dogs and non-human primates to be classified as a distinct category in legislation and formal requirements for the approval of experiments. Taking into consideration their biology, with the possible exception of some of the primate species, this separation can hardly be based on the idea that these animals are more sentient than, or have more important needs from, animals of other species. It is rather a result of a difference in how we, as humans, relate to them.

Throughout human culture, there is clearly a perception of hierarchy among animals – quasi-moral ordering that gives some species higher status than others. This hierarchy has been labelled 'the socio-zoological scale' (Arluke and Sanders 1996). The central idea of the scale is that people rate animal species as morally more or less important, and, therefore, more or less worth protecting, on the basis of a number of factors. These include how useful an animal is, how closely people typically associate with it, and how 'cute' it is. They also include how dangerous the animal is capable of being and how 'demonic' it is perceived to be.

Clearly, the socio-zoological scale varies from place to place and time to time but, today, at least in Western societies, some companion animal species, notably dogs, cats and horses, together with some charismatic wild animals such as apes and elephants, seem to be at the top of it. The socio-zoological scale is, in many ways, based on traditions and unexamined prejudice, and its use as a basis of animal protection can be criticised both scientifically and ethically. However, it undoubtedly affects public attitudes. There is in many countries some support, in the regulatory guidance, for a differentiation between animal species in line with the socio-zoological scale. For example, the Recitals of EU Directive 2010/63/EU refer to the higher public sensitivity regarding research with dogs, cats and primates.

Whereas it is a universal requirement in ethics review to minimise animal suffering, in some places in the world there is a move towards a new standard for animal research ethics that involves putting an absolute cap on the suffering that animals may endure as part of an experiment (Olsson et al. 2019). According to this requirement, experiments should never be allowed if they involve severe suffering. Such a requirement has been in place in Danish legislation for more than two decades. It is also included in the recent EU directive which defines the minimum standards of the regulation of animal experimentation to be put in place in each of the

28 EU countries. Thus in the directive (Article 15(2)), it is stated that 'Member States shall ensure that a procedure is not performed if it involves severe pain, suffering or distress that is likely to be long-lasting and cannot be ameliorated' (European Union 2010). This wording in the legal text gives clear guidance to the ethics review: experiments which are expected to result in long-lasting severe suffering must not be approved.

How to make ethics reviews function well in practice?

In the previous sections, we have examined how ethics review is done and asked what, exactly, is being reviewed. We will finish the chapter with a reflection on how these two aspects may interact. This will require us to consider the different roles that ethics review play.

There are two fundamentally different ways to understand the role of ethics reviews and the committees undertaking them. They revolve around the question how we are to understand the word 'ethics' in 'ethics review'. On one understanding, the role of the review is to apply the standards and principles enshrined in the laws regulating the use of animals for research and testing – and the only way ethics comes into this process is through the deliberation of the politicians who originally defined the standards and principles. We will call this the 'restricted' view of the role of ethics committees. On the other understanding, there is a significant grey area, undecided by the standards and principles enshrined in law, which has to be filled out by the ethics reviews typically undertaken by ethics committees. And in filling out this grey area, the committees undertaking the ethics reviews engage in ethical deliberation. We will call this the 'expansive' view of the role of ethics review.

It is fair to say that traditionally the restricted view prevailed. This was reflected in the sorts of requirement that ethics committees were supposed to enforce, all of which were of a rather technical nature. However, recently – at least in the EU – the committees have been given the task of applying requirements that are less technical and seem to leave more room for ethical deliberation. This is especially true of harm–benefit assessments, but to some extent it also applies to limitations on the use of some animal species. In some countries, notably but not exclusively in Scandinavia, there has also been a shift in the composition of the committees undertaking ethics reviews, and there is now a larger role for people without first-hand experience of animal experimentation. Typically, these people do not only have less of a direct stake in animal experimentation, their involvement may also be a way of representing the views of society, providing public insight into the review process and in some cases also providing competencies of a non-technical, 'ethical' nature.

Challenges

There seem to be room for genuine discussion of the merits of different approaches to ethics review. In the following, which is a brief recapitulation of a previous paper (Grimm et al. 2019), we will approach this discussion from a philosophical as well as an empirical angle. We will consider the restricted (limiting the ethics review to ensuring that standards and principles are applied as established in legislation) and the expansive (encompassing ethical deliberation) view of ethics review, and we will further discuss two different models for organising the review.

The empirical angle is provided by studies of the actual functioning of ethics reviews. It is common to find, in these studies, reports of the dominance of scientists in the committee's deliberation and decisions. This is partly the upshot of scientists being present in greater numbers than any other type of member on many committees, but there is more to it than this. Studies of deliberation within US committees showed that scientists on average contributed 50% more comments than community members, and discussion in Canadian committees was found to be dominated by the committee president, scientists and veterinarians. Even in Swedish committees, with their balanced composition, scientists have been described as controlling the agenda. Both Swedish and Canadian committee members commented that the discussion is more technical than ethical, and that the committees rarely engage in real harm–benefit assessment.

The findings in these studies of how ethics committees operate (Grimm et al. 2019) also show the need for a more philosophical angle: the extent to which the above findings can be seen to document problems and the answer to the question of what to do about them very much depends on what is seen as the ideal ethics review. If the role of the committee is to ensure that harms are minimised through implementation of the 3Rs, and that benefits are maximised through an appropriate choice of animal model and experimental methodology, then it is hardly a problem if scientists and other technical experts dominate the discussion. Similarly, if the role of members with no professional interest in animal experiments 'is that of public witness to the activities of the research facility (. . .) as reminders that animal research and education activities must be defensible to the broader society' (Dresser 1999), it is enough that these members are present and pose questions, and there is no need for them to really influence the discussion. But if the aim really is to have decisions influenced by a broader discussion in which there is room for a genuinely pluralistic ethical dialogue reflecting the multifaceted views that exist in society, ethics committees seem not to be living up to the expectations.

Another important question about the functioning of ethics committees is consistency in decision-making. Within a system where ethics approval is required for research to be lawful, ethics review has legal implications. As such, applicants should know what is expected for an application to be approved and for that approval to be granted under similar conditions within the same jurisdiction irrespective of which ethics committee is making the assessment. Relatively little is known about consistency in practical decisions, but an experimental study of IACUCs (Institutional Animal Care and Use Committees) in the USA showed wide variation when two independent committees evaluated the same application (Plous and Herzog 2001). The only aspect over which there was good evidence of agreement was pain assessment, which was also the only aspect for which detailed criteria and a scale were available.

We have elsewhere discussed two different models for ethics review and more particularly harm–benefit assessment, which we call the discourse model and the metric model (Grimm et al. 2019). The discourse model depicts the classic functioning of an ethics committee, with a relatively loosely structured dialogue over applications. The underlying idea is that if one brings together people with different backgrounds and perspectives to discuss proposals for animal experiments, they will be able to engage in a discussion where the different perspectives feed into the final decision in a way that is fair and generally acceptable. The ideal here is 'a sensible middle ground where disagreements about animal use can be argued out between fair-minded people' (Grimm et al. 2019). The empirical data suggest that this ideal is far from being achieved in practice. It can also be questioned from a theoretical perspective: not all views on animal research can be reconciled, and the model is bound to result in minority views being overruled by the majority.

The metric model is more of a theoretical construct than an actual practice. The idea is to set up a system with scores strictly linked to predefined criteria and computational algorithms to generate an aggregate output that takes all relevant aspects into account. The ideal is a transparent, consistent and standardised decision-making system. Several variations on this model have been proposed in research papers, but the only real attempt to realise the metric ideal in practice was made in Austria as the EU Directive 2010/63/EU was being implemented. Here, the ambition was to engage all stakeholders in the development, so that the system would be based on a consensus across different groups of society. Not surprisingly, this attempt failed at the developmental stage: it was simply not possible to get stakeholder agreement on the criteria to base the metrics on. This is not the only problem with the metrics model: there is also the challenge of setting up an algorithm to compute concepts for which there is no common 'currency' and the likely impossibility of fitting the complex and variable nature of projects into a single predefined mathematical framework.

In Grimm et al. (2019), we proposed a combination of the discourse and the metric model as a way forward that overcomes a number of the limitations which are apparent when each model is applied in isolation. This can be achieved if deliberation is done in a committee setting, as happens in the discourse model, but also draws on the metric model approach to structure the discussion and to ensure that all relevant aspects are systematically assessed, and that this assessment is documented. Ideally, this approach should prevent the agenda from being set by one group of committee members. It should also help to structure the discussion and provide a transparent record of what was discussed and how that fed into the final decision.

The combined model may be one way to secure better ethics deliberation in committees, but it is unlikely to address all of the problems. One significant challenge which is rarely addressed is the workload associated with ethics review. Under EU legislation, where review is conducted on projects with a maximum duration of 5 years, it is not uncommon for applications to run to 50–100 pages and include tens of experiments using several thousand animals. Properly evaluating such an application is no small piece of work.

For many members, ethics committee membership is a service commitment that comes on top of one's normal work, and one that is not necessarily remunerated or compensated for by a reduction in other tasks. As animal model research becomes increasingly sophisticated and complex, and as the number of issues included in review increase, there is danger that the system is moving towards a situation where what committees are expected to do is not realistically possible with the resources they are given. The situation is worsened by many committee members being left to work out for themselves how to do the job, and are expected to deal with highly complex and specialised information often going well beyond their own area of expertise.

These challenges affect all committee members, but perhaps they are a bigger problem for non-expert members than they are for others. Stuart G. Mondschein, a long-term unaffiliated member (UM) of an IACUC in the USA, captures several of the challenges vividly:

> "UMs are supposed to be non-laboratory-animal users (and quite often are not scientists), but nonetheless are expected to understand that a 'power analysis' suggests the minimum number of animals required in a project to achieve a reliable scientific result. UMs are expected to be independent, unbiased, free of conflicts of interest, and uncompensated, but also able to read and understand complex scientific experiments. UMs are expected to bring the general interests of the community to a research approval process that itself is a balance of scientific, legal, and ethical standards and interests. Some members of the public would allow no research involving animals. Others focus on the benefits they see such research brings to human medicine, agriculture, or the environment. Still others reject any connection between research on animals and advances in human affairs. Determining the sense of the community is not simple."
>
> (Mondschein 2007)

In summary, a well-functioning ethics review seems to call for a stronger support infrastructure than is in place in many systems today. This infrastructure should include guidance criteria for evaluation, the training of ethics committee members and appropriate time allocation, and recognition for the work invested in ethics review. A system of communication and dialogue between committees also seems to be a good idea, given the need to achieve consistency across hundreds of committees in the same jurisdiction (as may be the case in big countries operating a review system based on institutional committees). Initiatives to promote interactions between committees and training for committee members exist or are under development in, for example, the Netherlands, Portugal and the UK.

In describing the challenges in representing a diverse community, Mondschein also points to a fundamental dilemma for the form of ethics review we earlier referred to as 'expansive'. In contemporary Western society, the range of views on how humans should treat animals is so wide that consensus is simply not possible. Setting up a review system which accommodates this plurality of views in its decision-making is a huge challenge – arguably one that it is simply impossible to meet if, at the same time, we are striving to ensure fair treatment of applications and some predictability of outcome for researchers needing approval for their work. There is an obvious conflict between the view of some opponents of animal experimentation (that no, or almost no, experiments are acceptable) and the present expectation from the research community that most proposed research can be made acceptable by maximising scientific quality and minimising negative impacts on the animals. The present system may be able to go a long way towards delivering improved practice and increasing the acceptability of animal research, but realistically it will not be possible to guarantee the fair treatment of applications while at the same time allowing sufficient room for manoeuvre in which committees can make decisions on the basis of a real ethical deliberation with several perspectives.

Further guidance

In this chapter, we have provided a general overview of the history and underlying philosophy of animal research ethics review. We have considered its different aspects and asked how it can best be done. We concluded by discussing some of the tensions that are inherent in ethical decision-making over animal experiments in a pluralistic society – one containing widely differing views on animal experimentation. However serious or surmountable these tensions are, animal ethics committees and other decision-making entities are required to come to concrete decisions over proposed animal experiments, and the people involved need guidance on how to carry out this activity. Appendix 18.1 provides a Self-Assessment checklist for ethics committees.

Given the different national settings, ideally this guidance will be provided specifically within the jurisdiction where the ethics review takes place. In practice, we know that access to country-specific guidance varies widely, and that in many countries the committees are left to work out for themselves how to review and decide over projects. These committees may still be helped by resources that have been developed for other places. We suggest the following:

https://science.rspca.org.uk/sciencegroup/researchanimals
The animal protection NGO RSPCA plays an active role in supporting animal ethics review bodies in the UK, and provides study materials as well as training.

https://ec.europa.eu/environment/chemicals/lab_animals/index_en.htm
This website presents all of the official information on animal research and testing regulation in the European Union, including guidance documents for different aspects of animal ethics review.

https://olaw.nih.gov/home.htm
The Office for Laboratory Animal Welfare provides general guidance on animal research ethics review and committee operation in the USA.

http://www.felasa.eu/working-groups/working-groups-past/
FELASA has coordinated two working groups on different aspects of ethics review, and their outputs can be consulted.

https://www.nature.com/laban/
Until the end of 2020, the journal Lab Animal had a regular section entitled Protocol Review where case studies were presented and discussed by members of IACUCs in the USA.

For further in-depth reading with a theoretical as well as practical perspective, we recommend two books: Hubrecht (2014) and Röcklinsberg et al. (2017).

Acknowledgements

Parts of this chapter are based on material from the following papers or chapters of ours. We are grateful to our co-authors for their contribution to the original work and permission to re-use it in this chapter. Thanks are also due to the late Jesper Lassen, who collaborated on the work on EU animal ethics review.

Grimm, H., Olsson, I.A.S. and Sandøe, P. (2019). Harm–benefit analysis – what is the added value? A review of alternative strategies for weighing harms and benefits as part of the assessment of animal research. Laboratory Animals, 53(1), 17–27.

Olsson, I.A.S., da Silva, S.P., Townend, D. and Sandøe, P. (2017). Protecting animals and enabling research in the European Union: an overview of development and implementation of directive 2010/63/EU. ILAR Journal, 57(3), 347–357.

Olsson, I.A.S., Varga, O. and Sandøe, P. (2015). A matter of importance: considering benefit in animal ethics review. ALTEX Proc, 4, 33–36.

Sandøe, P., Franco, N.H., Lund, T.B. et al. (2015). Harms to animals – can we agree on how best to limit them. Altex, 4(1), 28–32.

Olsson, I.A.S. and Sandøe, P. (2021). Animal research ethics. In: Handbook of Laboratory Animal Science: Essential Principles and Practices, Vol. I., 4th edn. Eds J. Hau and S.J. Schapiro, pp. 3–22. CRC Press LLC.

References

Anonymous (2013). Working document Project Evaluation and Retrospective Assessment. edited by European Commission.

Arluke, A. and Sanders, C.R. (1996). Regarding Animals. Philadelphia: Temple University Press.

Bateson, P. (1986). When to experiment on animals. New Scientist, 109(1496), 30–32.

Bayne, K. and Würbel, H. (2014). The impact of environmental enrichment on the outcome variability and scientific validity of laboratory animal studies. Revue scientifique et technique-Office international des epizooties, 33(1), 273–280.

Bernard, C. (1927). An Introduction to the Study of Experimental Medicine. New York: Macmillan.

Borgström, K.A. (2009). Animal experiment regulations as a part of Public Law. European Public Law, 15(2), 197–205.

Davies, G.F., Golledge, H., Hawkins, P. et al. (2017). Review of Harm–Benefit Analysis in the Use of Animals in Research. London: Home Office.

De Boo, M.J., Rennie, A.E., Buchanan-Smith, H.M. and Hendriksen, C.F.M. (2005). The interplay between replacement, reduction and refinement: considerations where the Three Rs interact. Animal Welfare, 14(4), 327.

de Vries, R.B., Wever, K.E., Avey, M.T. et al. (2014). The usefulness of systematic reviews of animal experiments for the design of preclinical and clinical studies. ILAR journal, 55(3), 427–437. doi: 10.1093/ilar/ilu043

Dresser, R. (1999). Community representatives and nonscientists on the IACUC: what difference should it make?. ILAR journal, 40(1), 29–33.

Eggel, M. and Grimm, H. (2018). Necessary, but not sufficient. The benefit concept in the project evaluation of animal research in the context of Directive 2010/63/EU. Animals, 8(3), 34.

European Union. (2010). Directive 2010/63/EU of the European Parliament and of the Council of 22 September 2010 on the protection of animals used for scientific purposes. Official Journal of the European Union L276 53, 33–79.

Farm Animal Welfare Council. (2009). Farm animal welfare in Great Britain: past, present and future: Farm Animal Welfare Council.

Franco, N.H., Correia-Neves, M. and Olsson, I.A.S. (2012). How "humane" is your endpoint? – Refining the science-driven approach for termination of animal studies of chronic infection. PLoS Pathogens, 8(1), p.e1002399.

Garner, J.P., Gaskill, B.N., Weber, E.M. et al. (2017). Introducing Therioepistemology: the study of how knowledge is gained from animal research. Lab Animal, 46(4), 103–113.

Gouveia, K. and Hurst, J.L. (2017). Optimising reliability of mouse performance in behavioural testing: the major role of non-aversive handling. Scientific Reports, 7(1), 1–12.

Grimm, H., Olsson, I.A.S. and Sandøe, P. (2019). Harm–benefit analysis – what is the added value? A review of alternative strategies for weighing harms and benefits as part of the assessment of animal research. Laboratory Animals, 53(1), 17–27.

Hubrecht, R.C. (2014). The Welfare of Animals Used in Research: Practice and Ethics. The UFAW Animal Welfare Series: Wiley-Blackwell.

Kelch, T.G. (2013). A short history of (mostly) western animal law: Part II. Animal Law Review, 19, 347–390.

Laber, K., Newcomer, C.E., Decelle, T. et al. (2016). Recommendations for addressing harm–benefit analysis and implementation in ethical evaluation – report from the AALAS–FELASA working group on harm–benefit analysis – part 2. Laboratory Animals, 50(1_suppl), 21–42.

Lund, T.B., Lassen, J., and Sandøe, P. (2012). Public attitude formation regarding animal research. Anthrozoös, 25, 475–490.

Lund, T.B., Mørkbak, M.R., Lassen, J., et al. (2014). Painful dilemmas: A study of the way the public's assessment of animal research balances costs to animals against human benefits. Public Underst Sci, 23, 428–444.

Mondschein, S.G. (2007). A current perspective on the role and needs of IACUC unaffiliated members. Lab Animal, 36(6), 21–26.

Olsson, I.A.S., Nicol, C.J., Niemi, S.M. and Sandøe, P. (2019). From unpleasant to unbearable – Why and how to implement an upper limit to pain and other forms of suffering in research with animals. ILAR Journal, 60(3), 404–414.

Olsson, I.A.S., Silva, S.P.D., Townend, D. and Sandøe, P. (2017). Protecting animals and enabling research in the European Union: An overview of development and implementation of directive 2010/63/EU. ILAR Journal, 57(3), 347–357.

Olsson, I.A.S., Varga, O. and Sandøe, P. (2015). A matter of importance: considering benefit in animal ethics review. ALTEX Proc, 4(1), 33–36.

Olsson, I.A.S. and Sandøe, P. (2021). Animal research ethics. In: Handbook of Laboratory Animal Science. Eds J. Hau and S.J. Schapiro, pp. 3–22. Boca Raton: CRC Press.

Plous, S. and Herzog, H. (2001). Reliability of protocol reviews for animal research. Science, 293(5530), 608–609.

Regan, T. (2007). The case for animal rights. In: Ethics in Practice, 3rd ed. Ed H. Lafollette, pp. 205–211. Oxford: Blackwell Publishing.

Röcklinsberg, H., Gjerris, M. and Olsson, I.A.S. (2017). Animal Ethics in Animal Research. New York: Cambridge University Press.

Russell, W.M.S. and Burch, R.L. (1959). The Principles of Humane Experimental Technique. London: Methuen.

Sandøe, P., Franco, N.H., Lund, T.B. et al. (2015). Harms to animals – can we agree on how best to limit them. ALTEX Proc, 4, 28–32.

Scott, S., Kranz, J.E., Cole, J., et al. (2008). Design, power, and interpretation of studies in the standard murine model of ALS. Amyotroph Lateral Sc, 9, 4–15.

Sena, E.S. and Currie, G.L. (2019). How our approaches to assessing benefits and harms can be improved. Animal Welfare, 28(1), 107–115.

Singer, P. 1975. Animal Liberation. London: Harper Collins.

Smith, D., Anderson, D., Degryse, A.D. et al. (2018). Classification and reporting of severity experienced by animals used in scientific procedures: FELASA/ECLAM/ESLAV Working Group report. Laboratory Animals, 52(1_suppl), 5–57.

Smith, J.A., Van Den Broek, F.A.R., Martorell, J.C. et al. (2007). Principles and practice in ethical review of animal experiments across Europe: summary of the report of a FELASA working group on ethical evaluation of animal experiments. Laboratory Animals, 41(2), 143–160.

Stephens, M.L. and Mak, N.S. (2013). History of the 3Rs in toxicity testing: from Russell and Burch to 21st century toxicology. In: Reducing, Refining and Replacing the Use of Animals in Toxicity Testing. Eds D. Allen and M.D. Waters. Cambridge: Royal Society of Chemistry Publishing.

Tannenbaum, J. (1999). Ethics and pain research in animals. ILAR Journal, 40(3), 97–110.

Tannenbaum, J. (2017). Ethics in biomedical animal research: the key role of the investigator. In Animal Models for the Study of Human Disease, 2nd edn, Ed. P.M. Conn, pp. 1–44. Cambridge: Academic Press.

van der Worp, H.B., de Haan, P., Morrema, E. and Kalkman, C.J. (2005). Methodological quality of animal studies on neuroprotection in focal cerebral ischaemia. Journal of Neurology, 252(9), 1108–1114.

Van der Worp, H.B., Howells, D.W., Sena, E.S. et al. (2010). Can animal models of disease reliably inform human studies? PLoS Medicine, 7(3), e1000245.

Vogt, L., Reichlin, T.S., Nathues, C., et al. (2016). Authorization of animal experiments is based on confidence rather than evidence of scientific rigor. PLoS Biol, 14, e2000598.

von Roten, F.C. (2013). Public perceptions of animal experimentation across Europe. Public Understanding of Science, 22(6), 691–703. doi: 10.1177/0963662511428045.

Willner, P. (1984). The validity of animal models of depression. Psychopharmacology, 83(1), 1–16.

Würbel, H. (2017). More than 3Rs: the importance of scientific validity for harm–benefit analysis of animal research. Lab Animal, 46(4), 164–166.

Appendix 18.1

Self-assessment checklist for ethics committees

There are different kinds of ethics committee worldwide that oversee and review animal use in research and testing, including Institutional Animal Care and Use Committees (IACUCs), Animal Welfare Bodies (AWBs), Animal Ethics Committees (AECs) and Animal Welfare and Ethical Review Bodies (AWERBs). The membership, role and status of these can vary, but each one has a responsibility to undertake its list of tasks and is entitled to receive the support it needs to achieve this. This Appendix uses the term 'ethics committee' to cover all the different bodies listed above.

The generic checklist below, based on the preceding chapter and the references listed at the end, is intended to help ethics committees assess how effectively they are operating and whether they are fulfilling their overall roles and specific tasks. The 22 example topics set out under the 4 subheadings are suitable for consideration by individuals or small groups drawn from the committee, or they could be used as meeting agenda items. Clearly, the committee should receive timely and adequate resources if any remedial actions are necessary.

1. The role, tasks and composition of the committee

a. Is the committee effectively implementing all its tasks? If the regulator or competent authority has set out a list of functions, whether or not it is fulfilling these will obviously be a good starting point for self-assessment. There may also be tasks that the committee has set itself. It is good practice to review whether any tasks are not addressed in sufficient depth, or neglected, e.g. because standards have drifted or resources are limited, and to set out a plan to remedy this.

b. Does the committee include the requisite competencies to ensure that it is functioning effectively? The regulator may have listed a minimum membership, but it is helpful to regard this as the absolute minimum and ensure that there is a range of seniority, roles, expertise and viewpoints. Lay, or independent, members are especially useful with respect to asking insightful questions and challenging accepted norms.

c. Does the committee have a good collective understanding of each of the 3Rs, and does it advise on all of these? 'The 3Rs' is often viewed as a single concept, but each 'R' is achieved using different approaches, and may encounter different obstacles limiting its implementation. It is essential to assess whether the committee is genuinely advising on all three Rs, with positive outcomes and impacts for each, or whether in practice it is mainly (or only) addressing Refinement. This applies to both project review (if the committee does this) and general advice to the establishment.

d. Are committee members aware that there is more to 'doing ethics' than applying the 3Rs? Harms should be identified and minimised (as in the R of refinement) but benefits should also be critically assessed. Committees sometimes believe they have performed a full 'ethical review', when in fact all they have done is identified a couple of refinements. It is important to recognise and address this.

e. If the committee conducts a harm–benefit analysis of proposed animal studies, is this done in a way that is understandable and that everyone can relate to?

f. Do members know about the Culture of Care, and the role of the committee in helping to define, develop and maintain this locally?

g. If the committee is expected to (or wishes to) look at wider ethical issues (e.g. as is the case in the UK AWERB), does it actually do this? This involves going beyond addressing the 3Rs and the harm–benefit analysis within specific projects. For example, in the case of pre-clinical research, the committee could explore whether research groups liaise effectively with clinicians and patient groups, to discuss whether project outcomes would be wanted and needed, and to see how their research objectives would complement other approaches to solving the human health problem. For further information, see [2] in the following text.

h. Does the committee also review animal use that is out of scope in the legislation? Examples include non-invasive behavioural or observational studies; use of out-of-scope invertebrates or developmental stages; or the use of 'protected' animals in third countries. Some committees do this to demonstrate the establishment's commitment to responsible practice and recognition of the intrinsic worth of all animals.

2. Processes

a. If there is also a regulator or competent authority that licenses and/or reviews animal use, does everyone understand how its role, and the role of the committee, relate to one another? Understanding the legal framework is important for effective committee functioning and should help ensure that activities are complementary, avoiding unnecessary duplication of roles.

b. Does the committee have defined Terms of Reference and an annual work plan, including objectives relating to all its tasks? These can be used to assess and monitor the committee's performance.

c. Is enough time devoted to planning and holding meetings? For example, papers should be circulated sufficiently in advance; and committee meetings should be frequent enough, and long enough, for all business to be dealt with. If it is not always possible to discuss agenda items in full, or meetings end up rushed, remedial action will be needed, e.g. devolving some tasks to sub-groups. This may require additional resource, which should be provided (see [3] in the following text).

d. Are there effective channels of information into the committee, and do people who are responsible for accessing and providing information, either to staff dealing with animals or to the committee, have the resources they need? This includes information on animal behaviour, welfare, the 3Rs, training resources and opportunities, regulations and codes of practice, and the Culture of Care.

3. Experiences of committee members

a. Are members well informed about the establishment's own animal use? This includes basic knowledge about species, numbers used, severity of procedures, and broad research fields and objectives. All committee members should visit the animal unit regularly to see animals and interact with staff, to help familiarise them with 'local' values, perspectives and resources.

b. Are discussions balanced, with all members feeling that they are able to speak and will be listened to? People should know other committee members and understand one another's roles. 'Awaydays' are a good way of facilitating this (run over half a day or a couple of hours if time is limited). Are members' expectations of the committee being met?

c. Is adequate induction and training provided for all members, including the chair? For further information, see [4] in the following text.

d. How do committee members feel about their individual workloads? For example, if the committee reviews project applications, it is a useful exercise to examine their workload. This could include checking how many applications they are asked to assess and asking them how long they spend on each one, and whether they feel that they have enough time to perform a proper evaluation.

4. Communications, engagement and support

a. Is the committee well supported by senior management? For example, is it granted sufficient financial budget and staff time? Senior members of staff should attend meetings and show their support for the committee's conclusions and recommendations.
b. Are communications, and engagement, good between the ethics committee and the rest of the establishment? The committee should not exist in isolation, but should liaise with other internal bodies that may have overlapping roles such as research governance, 3Rs and animal welfare committees, to ensure that it adds value. One way of helping to achieve this is to invite representatives of these bodies to attend committee meetings. Internal communications should clearly explain what the committee is for, why it is important, who is involved and how it benefits the establishment.
c. Do researchers view the committee positively and are they prepared to act on its advice? It is important to understand the needs, and feelings, of researchers, and to foster good relations and two-way communications. Asking for feedback about the committee and its advice will help to identify any issues of concern. If the committee reviews projects, it is good practice for researchers to be able to present and discuss their work. Providing clear forms, templates and timelines to researchers is also helpful when asking for information.
d. Are staff rewarded for participating in the committee and its activities? For example, is it included in their objectives, or is there any other kind of internal recognition?
e. Does the committee have dialogue with other committees at other establishments, either ad hoc or as part of a regional or national network? A number of countries have set up networks to enable committees to meet and discuss good practice for running committees and fulfilling different tasks. It may be worth considering whether, and to what extent, the committee participates in available networks. If none exist, it may be possible to initiate a liaison with one or more other committees.
f. What role does the committee play with respect to internal and external openness? This includes reviewing the potential to hold meetings that are partly, or entirely, open to all staff, and ensuring that the committee is properly represented on the establishment's intranet.

The committee should play a role in any activities aiming to promote openness with the public, ensuring that messaging from the establishment includes the harms and limitations of animal research, as well as a realistic assessment of the benefits. The public should be able to access information about the committee.

Further reading on ethics committees

1. RSPCA/LASA Guiding principles on good practice for Animal Welfare and Ethical Review Bodies (3rd edn, 2015). Although this was written for the UK AWERB, much of the content applies to other ethics committees. tinyurl.com/AWERB-RSPCA-LASA
2. Delivering effective ethical review: the AWERB as a 'forum for discussion' by Penny Hawkins and Pru Hobson-West (2017). view.pagetiger.com/AWERB/AWERB
3. European Commission Working Document on Animal Welfare Bodies and National Committees (2014). Helpful for all types of ethics committee, especially the section on achieving a successful AWB on pp 18–19. ec.europa.eu/environment/chemicals/lab_animals/pdf/endorsed_awb-nc.pdf
4. Developing induction materials for AWERB members (1st edn, 2017) by RSPCA/LASA. As above, the content is widely applicable. tinyurl.com/RSPCA-LASA-induct
5. RSPCA web pages on ethical review: science.rspca.org.uk/sciencegroup/researchanimals/ethicalreview – for an international audience
6. A resource book for lay members of ethical review and similar bodies worldwide (3rd edn, 2015) by Maggy Jennings and Jane A Smith. tinyurl.com/RSPCALMRB
7. International Culture of Care Network website, hosted by Norecopa: norecopa.no/coc

Further reading on the ethics of animal use in research and testing

- The Ethics of Research Involving Animals by the Nuffield Council on Bioethics (2005). Download at nuffieldbioethics.org/publications/animal-research
- The Welfare of Animals Used in Research: Practice and Ethics by Robert C Hubrecht (2014). UFAW/Wiley-Blackwell, Bognor Regis, UK. ISBN: 978-1-119-96707-1
- Animal Ethics in Animal Research edited by Helena Röcklinsberg, Mickey Gjerris and I Anna S Olsson (2017. Cambridge University Press, UK. doi.org/10.1017/9781108354882
- Principles of Animal Research Ethics by Tom L Beauchamp and David DeGrazia (2020). Oxford University Press, UK. ISBN 978-0-19-093912-0

All downloads are free and URLs last viewed 20 May 2020.
Penny Hawkins and Maggy Jennings, RSPCA Animals in Science Department

PART 2
SPECIES KEPT IN THE LABORATORY

Mammals

19 The laboratory opossum

John L. VandeBerg and Sarah Williams-Blangero

Biological overview

General biology of marsupials

The term marsupial derives from the Latin word *marsupium*, meaning little pouch. However, the word is somewhat deceptive because males of most species and even females of some species, including *Monodelphis* species, have no pouch.

Metatherian (marsupial) mammals diverged from eutherian mammals an estimated 160 million years ago (Graves & Renfree 2013). Of the 388 extant marsupial species listed in the ASM Mammal Diversity Database (MDD)[1] 251 are native to Australasia and 137 are native to the Americas. Only one species, the Virginia opossum (*Didelphis virginiana*), is native to North America. With the exception of monito del monte (*Dromiciops gliroides*) and two congeneric species, all of which reside in small region of Chile and Argentina, all of the American marsupial species are opossums (Family Didelphidae) or shrew opossums (also known as rat opossums) (Family Caenolestidae). The genus *Monodelphis* (Family Didelphidae) comprises 24 species, including the grey short-tailed opossum (*Monodelphis domestica*), the laboratory stocks and strains of which are collectively known as laboratory opossums.

The first known reference to any marsupial was in 1607–1609, when Captain John Smith used the word from the Pohatan (Virginia Indian language), which he wrote as 'opassom', in reference to the species now known as the Virginia opossum (Mithun 2001). Recognising that females have an internal uterus like those of other mammals and that embryos and foetuses were found in the pouch, Linneas in 1758 designated the genus name as *Didelphis*, derived from Greek, meaning two wombs (internal and external) (Tyndale-Biscoe 1973). The short-tailed opossums were named *Monodelphis* (meaning single womb) in 1830 by Burnett (Pine & Handley 2008) who recognised them as being closely related to *Didelphis* but without a pouch (external womb). The species name, *domestica*, is said to have been given because the animals were frequently observed in and around the small, open-air, rural houses, where they played a welcome role in controlling insect and rodent populations (Nowak 1999). However, currently, these animals are infrequently found in human dwellings (Ilmar Santos, personal communication).

The most important feature of marsupials from the standpoint of unique experimental research opportunities is the early developmental stage at which they are born. The gross anatomy of a newborn *Monodelphis domestica* resembles that of a mouse at 11.5 days of gestation and that of a human at five to six weeks of gestation (Cardosa-Moreira et al. 2019). Each neonate quickly attaches to a teat, which swells in its mouth. The neonate is unable to release the teat until it has developed a functional jaw at 14 days of age. The lungs, as well as other organs of the newborns, are at an early developmental stage; much or most of gas exchange is accomplished in newborns via the skin (see Ferner 2018; Modepalli et al. 2018). An early developmental stage at birth is common to all marsupials and renders the newborn marsupial, essentially an extrauterine embryo that can be manipulated and observed throughout much of embryonic and all of foetal development in ways that are not possible with eutherian mammals.

In addition, marsupials have a variety of unique anatomical characteristics of the jaw, skull, teeth and reproductive system (Tyndale-Biscoe 1973). The early developmental stage of marsupials at birth and their distinctive anatomy are interpreted not as reflecting a more primitive stage in evolutionary development than eutherians, but rather as alternative strategies for achieving an equally adaptive endpoint. Thus, marsupials are useful for comparative research designed to improve the understanding of the evolution of genetic and physiological mechanisms in mammals generally. *Monodelphis domestica* is a marsupial species that is well suited for research in the laboratory environment, and it has become the most widely utilised laboratory marsupial.

Only three other American marsupial species, all opossums, have been used extensively as laboratory animals, although the adaptability of many other species to laboratory conditions has never been thoroughly explored. Two of the three species are large pouched opossums (genus

---
[1] https://mammaldiversity.org/ (Accessed 20 July, 2022)

Didelphis), and the other one is a small pouchless opossum (*Marmosa robinsoni*).

Marsupials in the laboratory

Australian marsupial species

Two species of Australian marsupials have been propagated in the laboratory over many generations. They are the fat-tailed dunnart (*Sminthopsis crassicaudata*) and the tammar wallaby (*Macropus eugenii*) (see, e.g., Suarez *et al.* 2017, and Modepalli *et al.* 2014, for publications that utilised animals produced in breeding colonies of the two species, respectively). Although neither species is widely available, both are used in a variety of research applications in Australia.

The initial captive breeding colony of fat-tailed dunnarts was established in the 1960s, but this species has never been propagated in the laboratory in large numbers nor has it been heavily used in research. Fat-tailed dunnarts tend to be anxious and easily agitated in captivity, and they are not nearly fecund as *Monodelphis*. Another impediment to their use in many types of research is their small size: 10–20 g at adulthood (Garrett *et al.* 2019).

Tammar wallabies have been produced in outdoor pens for research purposes, also since the 1960s. Adult females weigh 4–6 kg, while adult males weigh up to 9 kg (Hickford *et al.* 2009). While their relatively large size is an asset for some types of research, for example, when large blood sample quantities are required, it is an impediment to the economical maintenance of large numbers of animals. Another major impediment to the propagation of this species and its use in research is that females can produce and rear only one progeny per year. In spite of these impediments, tammar wallabies have been and continue to be produced in captivity and used in research.

Didelphis species

Didelphis virginiana has been used extensively as a laboratory animal in North America, and a close relative, *Didelphis marsupialis*, has been used in South America. The care, experimental manipulation, and use of these species in laboratory research were reviewed in detail by Jurgelski (1987). However, *Didelphis* have limited utility because they are relatively large (1.0–5.5 kg), are aggressive towards one another, and are seasonal breeders. Moreover, reproductive success is low among captive-born animals, particularly males (VandeBerg 1990). No one has developed a long-term, self-propagating breeding colony of *Didelphis*. Therefore, experimental animals or breeders needed to produce first-generation captive progeny are usually captured from the wild. Wild-caught animals have additional disadvantages in that they are of unknown age and health status and generally carry a heavy parasite load. Furthermore, they are a potential source of pathogens that are causal agents of a variety of serious human diseases (Jurgelski 1987; Civen & Ngo 2008). Despite the shortcomings of *Didelphis* species, they are likely to continue to be used as experimental animals for research that requires a relatively large marsupial or depends on the unique characteristics of these species.

Marmosa robinsoni

Robinson's mouse opossum, *Marmosa robinsoni* (40–70 g for adult females and 60–130 g for adult males), was bred in captivity for several generations during the 1960s and 1970s and appeared to have promise as a potential laboratory marsupial (Barnes & Barthold 1969; Barnes 1977). However, fecundity decreased with each successive generation, and satisfactory conditions, including a nutritionally adequate diet, for long-term propagation of this species were never identified.

Monodelphis domestica

Monodelphis domestica are broadly distributed below the southern rim of the Amazon basin in much of central and eastern Brazil, the eastern half of Bolivia, the northern half of Paraguay and the northern tip of Argentina (Macrini 2004). The natural habitat of *Monodelphis domestica* encompasses the relatively dry Chaco, Cerrado and Caatinga biomes, where they are most frequently found among rock outcrops (Streilein 1982). Even though population densities are low, zero to four adults per hectare in the Caatinga region of Brazil (Streilein 1982), the species is not endangered or threatened. The grey short-tailed opossum is the only American marsupial species that has proven to be successful as a long-term self-perpetuating population in captivity. It has many characteristics that render it ideally suited as a laboratory animal, and it is widely used in North America and Europe. Some stocks of this species have been produced in captivity for more than 50 generations (maximum of 62 generations to date) with no apparent detrimental effects on health status, fertility or fecundity in random bred stocks, although fecundity is negatively associated with the level of inbreeding. Because of the selection and genetic drift that have undoubtedly taken place over these generations, *Monodelphis domestica* presently in captive colonies may be genetically, physiologically and behaviourally quite different from their wild counterparts. It is for these reasons that laboratory stocks of this species are collectively designated as the laboratory opossum. Figure 19.1 shows an adult female laboratory opossum.

Monodelphis domestica has been inappropriately designated in the scientific literature as the Brazilian opossum, grey opossum or short-tailed opossum. The term Brazilian opossum is incorrect because dozens of opossum species are native to Brazil; *Monodelphis domestica* also are found in much of Bolivia and Paraguay, and the northernmost tip of Argentina (Macrini 2004). The grey opossum is not an appropriate designation for *Monodelphis domestica* because many other opossum species also have grey pelage. The short-tailed opossum also is not appropriate because six of the other *Monodelphis* species have names that include the phrase 'short-tailed opossum'. The only appropriate names for this species are grey short-tailed opossum, laboratory opossum (when used in reference to laboratory stocks rather than wild animals) and *Monodelphis domestica*. The genus name,

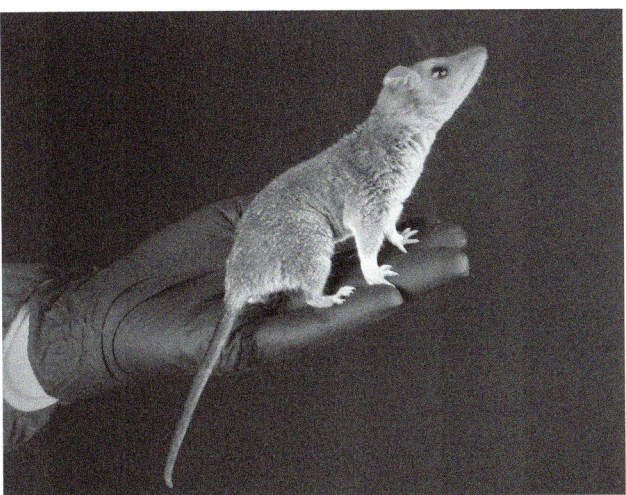

Figure 19.1 An adult female laboratory opossum.

Monodelphis, may be used as an abbreviation without the species name when it is clear that *Monodelphis domestica* is implied, much as *Drosophila* is often used in reference to *Drosophila melanogaster*.

Biological data

The body size of *Monodelphis domestica* is among the largest of the *Monodelphis* species. Adult laboratory-reared females typically weigh 60–100 g and males 90–150 g, although some individuals of some stocks may exceed these ranges (VandeBerg 1990). Growth curves for males and females have been developed (Cothran *et al*. 1985; Rousmaniere *et al*. 2010). Laboratory opossums begin to show physical signs of senescence at approximately three years of age and, in the laboratory setting, generally die of natural causes during the fourth year of life. The oldest individual maintained in the authors' colony reached the age of 55.5 months. Normal serum chemistry and hematologic values, and the effects of diet and age on them, have been described (VandeBerg *et al*. 1986; Cothran *et al*. 1990; Evans *et al*. 2010). Biological data are summarised in Table 19.1.

Social organisation

Grey short-tailed opossums are nocturnal, and individuals are most active during the first few hours of the evening (Streilein 1982). Individuals are difficult to capture because they are solitary and nomadic, and the estimated population density in the wild is less than four per hectare (2.47 acres) in areas where the animals are most common (Streilein 1982). Furthermore, they are terrestrial and do not congregate at isolated trees where species of semi-arboreal marsupials are more easily found.

Both in the wild and in captivity, grey short-tailed opossums are non-seasonal breeders. Females are induced ovulators, and they do not normally undergo oestrus in the absence of a male. When mature reproductive animals of both sexes come into close proximity to one another, mating typically occurs five to nine days later (most often, at seven days),

Table 19.1 Laboratory opossum biological data.

Parameter	Normal value
Weight at birth (mg)	~100
Weight at 2 weeks (mg)	~840
Weight at 8 weeks (g)	~20
Weight of adult female (g)	60–100
Weight of adult male (g)	90–150
Dental formula (van Nievelt & Smith 2005)	$I^5_4 C^1_1 Pm^3_3 M^4_4$
Typical range of litter size at weaning	4–12
Normal age at weaning (weeks) in the laboratory	8–9
First oestrus (in presence of a male) (days)	~140
Full sexual maturity (months)	6
Time of ovulation after exposure to male (days)	5–10
Time from copulation to fertilisation (days)	1
Gestation (days)	13.5
Minimum inter-birth interval (with successful weaning) (weeks)	11
Typical age of reproductive failure, females (months)	18–24
Typical age of reproductive failure, males (months)	24–30
Typical lifespan (months)	36–42
Body temperature (°C) (Dawson & Olson 1988)	~32.6 °C
Respiratory rate at rest (breaths/minute) (Kraus & Fadem 1987)	~54
Systolic blood pressure (mmHg) (Kraus & Fadem 1987)	~188
Heart rate (beats/minute) (Krauss & Fadem 1987)	~345
Maximal hearing sensitivity (kHz) (Frost & Masterson 1994)	8–64
Number of chromosomes (2N)/G-bands (Pathak *et al*. 1993)	18/233

followed by ovulation approximately 20 hours later, and fertilisation by 24 hours after mating (Mate *et al*. 1994). The gestation period from fertilisation to birth is 13.5 days (Mate *et al*. 1994).

Reproduction

Female laboratory opossums of some genetic stocks can reach sexual maturity as early as five months of age (Stonebrook & Harder 1992), and males achieve sexual maturity two to three weeks later. The youngest female reported to have given birth was 141 days old, but few females conceive prior to 140 days of age. In our breeding program, we do not pair animals for breeding until they are at least six months of age, when the females are considerably larger than at their earliest possible age of conceiving. For most females, the prime reproductive period is prior to 18 months. Not all successful breeders continue to reproduce that long, and most females cease to reproduce by 24 months of age. Older females tend to produce smaller litters and to have a lower rate of success in rearing them to weaning. Some of them also become highly aggressive towards males that are introduced to them. Males are frequently successful breeders until 24–30 months of age, and sometimes slightly longer.

Litters that contain fewer than four pups are usually lost within a week after birth, and rarely survive to weaning. If a litter is lost and the female is immediately paired with a male, mating typically takes place in five to nine days. This loss of small litters may be an evolutionary adaptation that affords a female the opportunity to produce and rear a large litter with little loss of time, rather than investing eight weeks in rearing a small litter.

Dead pups up to the age of three weeks are almost never found in the cages. They are eaten by the mother; even furred pups may be cannibalised. This characteristic may also be an evolutionary adaptation by which a mother is able to acquire nutrition with no expenditure of energy. The requirement for protein and other nutrients is especially high for lactating mothers that still have many remaining pups, whose combined weights by the age of weaning can be double or even triple the weight of the mother.

Normal behaviour

Wild *Monodelphis domestica* are solitary animals, except when females and males come together for short periods of time during which mating occurs. In the laboratory environment, they are housed singly after four months of age except when females are paired with males after six months of age for two-week intervals for the purpose of breeding.

Wild animals of both sexes build fully enclosed nests of bark, leaves and other materials, with an opening just large enough to allow entry, in hollow logs or fallen tree trunks, or among rocks (Nowak 1999). Animals in the laboratory are provided with nesting material, such as shredded paper towelling or crinkle paper. Both males and females use their semi-prehensile tails to carry nesting material to the nest. Females tend to build more elaborate and tightly woven nests than males.

The animals are nocturnal; they are most active during the first few hours of the darkness. Copulation normally occurs during the dark cycle.

Genetics and genomics

Early surveys of genetic variants among laboratory opossums revealed that the laboratory populations derived from the four founding sites in Brazil had significantly different allele frequencies at many loci, and that some alleles are specific to one population or another (van Oorschot *et al.* 1992a).

A peculiarity that was discovered during the early genetic analyses of *Monodelphis* (van Oorschot *et al.* 1992b, 1993) and confirmed during the creation of a physically anchored genetic linkage map with 150 highly polymorphic loci (Samollow *et al.* 2007) is that females exhibit greatly reduced rates of recombination by comparison with males and that the sex-averaged recombination rate is among the lowest documented for all mammals. This reduced rate of recombination might be responsible, at least in part, for the difficulty in producing inbred strains, that is, since the generational recombination rate is lower for *Monodelphis* than for eutherian mammals, new gene combinations that are favourable for fecundity under inbreeding cannot be generated as quickly as in eutherian laboratory species.

A cytogenetic bacterial artificial chromosome (BAC) map was developed (Duke *et al.* 2007), as was a high-quality draft of the genome sequence (Mikkelsen *et al.* 2007). Two *Monodelphis* genome assemblies were released in 2007; MonDom5 is a RefSeq Assembly (GCF_000002295.2), and ASM229v1 is a GenBank Assembly (GCA_000002295.1). More than 21,000 coding and 12,000 non-coding genes are annotated in MonDom5 by NCBI (release 103) and ASM229v1 by Ensembl (release 99). The genome sequence was instrumental in revealing the complexities of the marsupial immune system, and a prominent role for the evolution non-protein-coding sequences in mammalian diversification (Gentles *et al.* 2007; Gu *et al.* 2007; Lemos 2007; Mikkelsen *et al.* 2007). It also has proven vital to many other research disciplines.

Genetic stocks and strains

The laboratory opossum, like the Syrian hamster, differs from other laboratory animals in that the details of its origins are precisely known and well documented (see Table 19.2) (VandeBerg & Robinson 1997; see also Chapter 24: The Syrian hamster). The first captive animals ancestral to the present laboratory population were four males and five females captured in 1978 near the town of Exu in the state of Pernambuco, Brazil. They were transported to the National Zoological Park in Washington, DC, where all of them reproduced. Twenty pedigreed first- and second-generation descendants were provided to one of the authors (JLV) in 1979. Genetic material from all nine of the original wild-caught founders from Exu is present in the laboratory stock known as Purebred Population 1.

Table 19.2 summarises the populations present in the laboratory opossum colony maintained by the authors. The authors believe that these populations are the original source of all of the other extant laboratory colonies of *M. domestica* in the world.

A single shipment of 40 fully pedigreed laboratory opossums, all derived from the nine original founders from

Table 19.2 Laboratory populations of *Monodelphis domestica*.

Laboratory code for wild populations	Year of importation to the USA	Town of origin	Number of founders	Purebred laboratory population currently maintained (number of founders)
1	1978	Exu	9	Yes (9)
2	1984–1988	Piraua	14	Yes (7)
3	1990	Joaima	2	No
4	1992	Conselheiro Mota	1	No
5	1993	Brecha (Bolivia)	2	No

Exu (Purebred Population 1) and from the LL1 stock (see Table 19.3), was sent from the authors' colony to the Zoological Society of London, Regent's Park, London, in 1983. A successful breeding colony was established there and became a source of animals for European investigators. Several shipments totalling 56 descendants of the founders of Populations 1 and 2 were also made to German institutions during the 1980s. It is believed that all populations of *Monodelphis domestica* in Europe are derived from those shipments to London and Germany.

In 1992, laboratory opossums were exported from the UK to Australia. The Australian animals were descended from the 40 individuals sent to London in 1983, and thus, all trace their ancestry to the original nine founders of Purebred Population 1. This colony was disbanded in 2020,

Another colony outside North America was initiated in 2007 with 16 descendants of the founders of Population 1, also from the LL1 stock, shipped to the Federal University of Mato Grosso do Sul in Campo Grande, Brazil. Previously, there had been no self-sustaining captive colonies of this species in Brazil. This colony continues to be accessible to researchers in Brazil.

The most recent colony to be established outside North America was populated with a breeding nucleus of 24 females and 12 males from the LL1 and LL2 stocks, sent in 2013 from the authors' laboratory to Japan. This breeding colony continues to be maintained at the Riken Center for Biosystems Dynamics Research in Japan, and currently has more than 500 animals (H. Kiyonari, personal communication, September 5, 2021).

Table 19.2 summarises some pertinent information about the five cohorts of animals captured at different locations and imported to the USA. The animals collected at each site are designated numerically as a population. Populations 1–4 were collected at locations in Brazil, and Population 5 was collected in Bolivia. Purebred stocks derived from Populations 1 and 2 have been maintained, but it was necessary to integrate some animals from Population 1 into the breeding groups of Populations 3–5.

At the present time, there are eight random bred genetic stocks derived from these five populations of animals (see Table 19.3).

Because the number of founders is limited, all laboratory opossums within a random bred genetic stock are partially inbred. However, it is possible to produce animals with inbreeding coefficients of zero by mating animals of the PBP stock (Purebred Population 2) with animals of the LL1 stock (Purebred Population 1), or with the FD6, FD7, or FD8X stocks (Admixed Populations 1 and 3, 1 and 4 and 1 and 5, respectively).

In addition, there are three fully inbred strains (inbreeding coefficient >0.99), two of which, LSD and LSD1 are sibling strains, and eight partially inbred strains (inbreeding coefficients ranging from 0.78 to 0.95) (see Table 19.4). Despite many attempts to establish inbred strains by sequential full-sib matings, success was never achieved. The strains typically experienced diminishing litter sizes and diminishing litter survival rates, until they were lost after 6–10 generations of full-sib matings. One line that was promulgated by full-sib matings achieved an average inbreeding coefficient (F) of 0.911 (equivalent to just over 11 generations of full-sib matings) before it was lost (VandeBerg & Robinson 1997).

The difficulty in developing fully inbred strains of this species, by comparison with mice or rats, may be a consequence of its low rate of recombination. It is possible that the low number of linkage groups (i.e., chromosomes), combined with the low recombination rate, precludes sufficiently rapid selection of combinations of chromosomally linked alleles required to maintain a sufficient level of fecundity to overcome inbreeding depression. However, a breeding strategy that involves interspersing several generations of full-sib matings with several generations of less severe inbreeding has enabled the development of fully inbred strains. Efforts are continuing to transform the partially inbred strains into fully inbred strains.

The genetic and genomic architecture of seven of the extant stocks and strains, and one (FD2M4) that no longer exists, has been defined in detail via DNA sequencing, which identified 66,640 high-quality single-nucleotide polymorphisms (SNPs) (Xiong et al. 2021). SNP density, average heterozygosity, nucleotide diversity and the population differentiation parameter F_{st} were analysed in relation to pedigree history and ancestral founder populations, and in relation to the reference genome monDom5 (derived from the sequence of an ATHL animal determined by Mikkelsen et al. 2007).

Table 19.3 Random bred genetic stocks of laboratory opossums as of February 2020. Populations are defined in Table 19.2.

Stock Designation	Proportion of Ancestry by Population					Mean Inbreeding Coefficient
	1	2	3	4	5	
FD2M	0.24	0.76	-	-	-	0.63
FD345	0.32	0.68	-	-	-	0.40
FD6	0.68	-	0.32	-	-	0.48
FD7	0.75	-	-	0.25	-	0.08[1]
FD8X	0.62	-	-	-	0.38	0.46
LL1	1.00	-	-	-	-	0.44
LL2	0.28	0.78	-	-	-	0.23
PBP	-	1.00	-	-	-	0.59

[1] Until recently the FD7 stock had been derived primarily from Population 4 and was substantially inbred, but animals from the LL1 stock were added to ameliorate low fecundity. Hence, the mean inbreeding coefficient is currently low.

Table 19.4 Partially and fully inbred strains of laboratory opossums as of February 2020. Populations are defined in Table 19.2.

Strain Designation	Proportion of Ancestry by Population		Mean Inbreeding Coefficient
	1	2	
A1HH	1.00	-	0.80
AH11L	1.00	-	0.81
ATHHC	1.00	-	0.83
ATHHN	1.00	-	0.86
ATHL	1.00	-	0.95
DNAH	1.00	-	0.81
DNAL	1.00	-	0.84
FD2M1	0.25	0.75	>0.99
LSD	1.00	-	>0.99
LSD1	1.00	-	>0.99
PBPi	-	1.00	0.78

Cell, tissue and embryo culture

Cells, tissues and organs from *Monodelphis* have been cultured for a variety of research purposes under culture conditions suitable for eutherians, but *Monodelphis* cultures are typically conducted at 32–33 °C (the approximate body temperature of an adult *Monodelphis* at rest is 32.6 °C; Dawson & Olson 1988). Cell types that have been cultured include lymphocytes (Robinson et al. 1996), fibroblasts (Merry et al. 1983; Robinson et al. 1994), melanocytes (Dooley et al. 1995) and melanoma cells (Robinson et al. 1994). Recently, long-term primary cortical neuronal cultures have been established from neonates (Petrovic et al. 2021; Ban & Mladinic 2022).

Procedures for long-term (10-day) culture of the intact central nervous system of two-day-old pups have been developed and used to investigate the actions of amines and transmitters, and the activation and inactivation of gamma-aminobutyric acid (GABA) receptors (Stewart et al. 1991; Mollgard et al. 1994).

Embryos have been cultured by several groups (Moore & Taggart 1993; Johnston et al. 1994; Selwood et al. 1997; Keyte & Smith 2008a, b; Rousmaniere et al. 2010). Embryos cultured at 32.6 °C progress further than those cultured at 37 °C (Selwood & VandeBerg 1992). Parthenogenic development to the two-cell stage occurred in 8% of oocytes cultured at 32.6 °C. However, the rate embryo development from 1 cell to 16 cells was slower at 32.6°C (Selwood et al. 1997) than at 37°C (Moore & Taggart 1993), suggesting that more research is required to determine the optimal temperature for culturing embryos of this species.

Even whole limbs of neonates have been cultured for the purpose of investigating the mechanisms that drive differential growth rates of the forelimbs and hindlimbs (Dowling et al. 2016).

Impediments to creating induced pluripotent stem cells (iPSCs) of laboratory opossums also have been overcome recently, leading to the establishment of iPSC lines derived from fibroblasts of two inbred strains (Kumar et al. 2022).

Developmental biology

The embryonic development of *Monodelphis* has been described in detail (Baggott & Moore 1990; Mate et al. 1994; Selwood et al. 1997). According to Mate et al. (1994), ovulation and fertilisation occur about 24 hours after mating. Between two and three days later (days 3 and 4 after mating), most embryos are at the four-cell stage, and on day 5, most are at the 16–32-cell stage. Complete unilaminar blastocysts are present on day 7 and bilaminar blastocysts on day 8. The first somites are formed in the primitive streak by day 10, the heart and blood vessels by day 11 and paddle-shaped forelimbs by day 12. By day 14, the forearm is well developed with claws on the digits, and birth occurs on post-mating day 15 (~13.5 days post conception). Thus, development from the bilaminar blastocyst stage to birth takes place in mere seven days. The most obvious distinctive feature of marsupials, the birth at such an early stage of development, was a major driving force for establishing a laboratory marsupial.

Uses in research

The continuous availability and non-seasonal reproduction of laboratory opossums have made possible the large-scale experimental use of a marsupial species. Consequently, the laboratory opossum has become by far the most extensively used marsupial in research. A total of 1477 publications citing *Monodelphis domestica* were indexed in Web of Science/BIOSIS Citation Index under the search terms 'monodelphis domestica' (Topic) OR 'laboratory opossum' (Topic) OR 'grey short-tailed opossum (Topic)' between 1978, the year in which the first *Monodelphis domestica* arrived in the USA as founders of existing laboratory stocks and strains, and 2022. Most of those reports are based on research with laboratory opossums.

Comparative developmental stages of laboratory opossums, mice and humans

For the appropriate use of animals in comparative biological research among species, or as models for aspects of human biology, it is critical to know the ages at which key life history events occur in each species. Table 19.5 presents the ages of laboratory opossums that approximately correspond to the ages of humans and mice at some critical time points in development. Beyond the very early stages of development, the developmental equivalencies between laboratory opossums and humans are approximately one laboratory opossum year per 25 human years. For example, a six-month-old opossum is similar to a 12.5-year-old human adolescent in being able to reproduce but not having reached the size of an adult; a one-year-old opossum resembles a 25-year-old human in being in

Table 19.5 Developmental timetable comparisons of laboratory opossums, laboratory mice, and humans (adapted in part from Dutta & Sengupta 2016, and Cardoso-Moreira et al. 2019). E = Embryonic age in days (d), weeks (w), or years (y).

Opossums	Mice	Humans	Life History Event (for all three species, except where specified)
E13.5d	E10.5d	E4-5w	
0d	E11.5d	E5-6w	Birth of opossum
2d	E13d	E7w	
4d	E15d	E8-11w	
6d	E16.5d	E12w	
14d	0d	E16w	Detachment of opossums from nipples; birth of mouse (after 20 days of gestation)
21d	3d	E20w	Opossum fur growth well-initiated
30d	6d	0d	Birth of human (after 40 weeks of gestation)
8w	3.5w	3y	Natural weaning
12w	4w	6y	
18w	5w	9y	
22w	6w	12y	Onset of puberty
26w	8w	15y	Adolescence
52w	17w	25y	Physically and reproductively prime
2y	52w	50y	Loss of female fertility
3y	2y	75y	Elderly
4y	3y	100y	Near maximum lifespan

the prime of young adulthood; a two-year-old opossum is comparable to a 50-year-old human in having reached the stage of female reproductive senescence; and a four-year-old opossum corresponds to a 100-year-old human in that only a small proportion of individuals reach that age even under ideal living conditions.

Research in developmental biology

The altricial features of the newborn laboratory opossum (see Figure 19.2) have been exploited in many areas of research in developmental biology, including function of the embryonic nervous system in long-term cell culture (Stewart et al. 1991), healing of the neonatal spinal cord after complete transection or crushing (Fry & Saunders 2000; Mladinic et al. 2005; Lane et al. 2007; Noor et al. 2011; Wheaton et al. 2011, 2021; Saunders et al. 2014; Tomljanovic et al. 2022), effects of oestrogen on testicular development (Fadem & Tesoriero 1986), ontogeny of skin healing and development of capacity for scarring (Armstrong & Ferguson 1995), development of neuropeptides, steroid receptors and the visual system (reviewed by Kuehl-Kovarik et al. 1995), regulation of differential rates of limb growth (Sears et al. 2012; Beiriger & Sears 2014; Dowling et al. 2016) and biological mechanisms that contribute to birth defects (Molineaux et al. 2015; Sorensen et al. 2017).

Other research uses

Laboratory opossums are used for research in a wide variety of disciplines, in addition to those mentioned above. Some historical research applications were summarised by VandeBerg and Williams-Blangero (2010), and Samollow (2008) provided a comprehensive review of the earlier literature on *Monodelphis* genomics, and its applications in many fields of research.

Some of the other areas of research with laboratory opossums that have been highly active during the past decade, and selected recent references for each, are as follows: Immunobiology (Schraven et al. 2020; Morrissey et al. 2021),

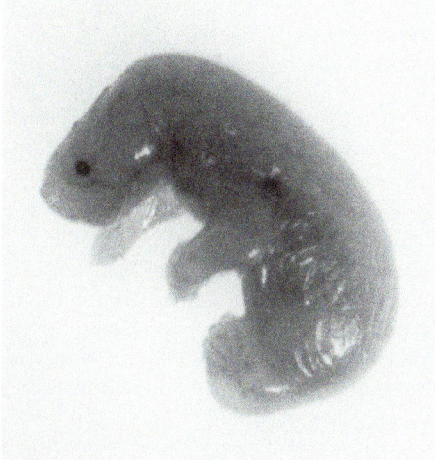

Figure 19.2 A newborn laboratory opossum.

sex chromosome dosage compensation (Wang et al. 2014; Mahadevaiah et al. 2019), UVB-induced melanoma and efficacy of sunscreen in protecting from it (Nair & VandeBerg 2012; Nair et al. 2014), diet and genetic interactions leading to hypercholesterolemia, non-alcoholic fatty liver disease and steatohepatitis (NASH) (Chan et al. 2008, 2010, 2012), mechanisms of resistance to snake venoms (Drabeck et al. 2020), biological factors that impede the development of AIDS vaccines (Yang et al. 2013; Finney et al. 2019) and neurobiological determinants of behaviour (Gil et al. 2019; Tepper et al. 2019). The recent publication of a detailed three-dimensional stereotaxic atlas of the brain of *Monodephis domestica* (Majka et al. 2018) will facilitate investigations that relate behavioural abnormalities to brain lesions and is likely to stimulate increased use of this species for research in other areas of neurobiology.

Laboratory opossums also have been demonstrated to be useful models for infectious diseases, including Rickettsial diseases (Dias Cordeiro et al. 2019; Blanton et al. 2022), Chagas disease (American trypanosomiasis) (Roellig et al. 2010) and Zika virus disease (Thomas et al. 2019).

Recently, several impediments to creating gene knockout laboratory opossums have been overcome, and the first knockout opossums were produced by CRISPR/Cas9 genome editing (Kyonari et al. 2021). The gene for tyrosinase was disrupted, so homozygotes for the altered gene were albino. This is the first heritable coat colour variant of this species. The capability to create targeted gene knockouts will add enormous utility and scientific value to the laboratory opossum in research on genes that may not exist in other laboratory animals (such as a recently discovered T-cell receptor gene; Morrissey et al. 2021) or that may function in different ways in other laboratory animals.

General husbandry

Enclosures

Polypropylene and polycarbonate cages (mouse shoebox cages) of two standard sizes are generally used: 'large cages' of approximately 870–950 sq. cm × 13–22 cm in height; and 'small cages' of approximately 460–485 sq. cm × 12–16 cm in height (see Figure 19.3a). Taller cages are not recommended unless long sipper tubes are used, because the distance from the bottom of the cage to the end of the sipper tube on the water bottle may make it difficult for some animals, particularly pups around the time of weaning, to easily reach the sipper tube.

Individual animals are kept in the small cages, whereas paired animals, mothers with litters and group-housed littermates up to four months of age are kept in large cages. Beyond four months of age, or slightly less than that age for some genetic stocks and strains, the animals begin to become more aggressive towards one another, and they are separated into single cages (mimicking natural dispersal of wild juveniles) in order to avoid injury and possible death.

When conventional cages fitted with a standard stainless steel grid used for rodents are used, the tops used in breeding colonies must fit within 0.75 cm of the cage edges, and

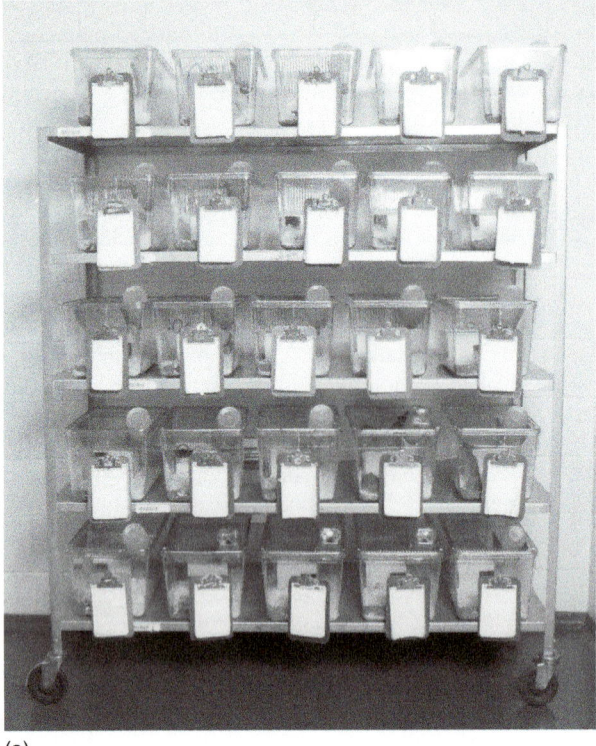
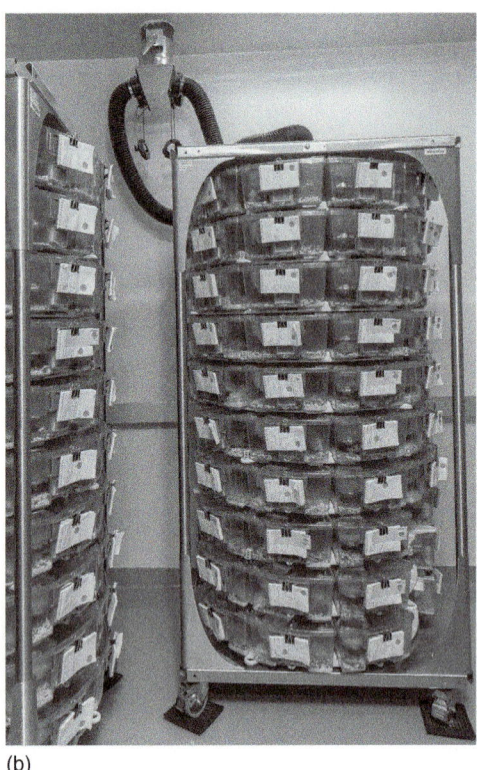

(a) (b)

Figure 19.3 (a) A rack of conventional cages, each containing a pair of animals and a nest box. (b) (UTRGV Photo by David Pike) A rack of Optimice® ventilated cages, each containing a single animal. For both types of racks, the I.D. number of the animal and a record of every life history event and every experimental procedure conducted with that animal is kept in a spiral notebook affixed to the front of each cage. The details are uploaded daily to a computerised database so they can be accessed remotely. Coloured tags and stickers are affixed temporarily to the fronts of the notebooks to distinguish among animals in different treatment groups or animals scheduled for upcoming manipulations.

the space between the bars on the top must not exceed 0.75 cm. Pre-weanlings can escape through openings as small as 1.0 cm, which is a standard distance between bars on some tops sold for use with rodents.

Although the animals managed by the authors fared well and were free of infectious diseases for more than three decades in conventional caging, usually without filter covers, they have been maintained since 2015 in individually ventilated cages (Optirat® and Optimice® cages, Animal Care Products, Inc.) (see Figure 19.3b). Because ammonia and other airborne waste products are removed from the cages continuously, the cages need to be changed only every two weeks rather than every week for conventional cages (Allison et al. 2011). In addition to maintaining high air quality for the animals, ventilated cages maintain high air quality for the caretakers minimising their risk of developing allergies. Additionally, the risk of any cross-contamination of cages with infectious organisms is also minimised.

Environmental provisions and enrichment

The cage bottom should be covered with bedding to a depth of approximately 2.5 cm. The authors have used pine or aspen shavings without adverse consequences, but shredded aspen causes foot irritation of some animals. The authors now use ground corn cob bedding, which has less fine particulate matter than wood shavings, thus affording higher air quality for the animals and the caretakers. The animals generally choose a single corner of their cage as a toilet area. In addition to bedding, each cage in our facility is provided with paper towelling, cut into 5 mm × 18 cm strips by a paper shredder, for nesting material. The amount of nesting material provided is about 3 g for a single animal, 5–6 g for a pair or a female with a litter and 10–12 g for a group of weanlings caged together. Some colony managers provide crinkle paper, which is commonly used for rodents, instead of shredded paper towelling. Nests made with crinkle paper tend to be more highly structured and robust than those made with shredded paper towelling. The early stage of development at birth, incapability of thermoregulation at birth and lack of a maternal pouch make nesting material especially important for neonatal survival.

A nest box is essential for paired animals to provide a haven in which one member of the pair may be able to protect itself from an aggressive mate, and for providing seclusion for mothers with litters. Animals should be paired in the morning and monitored frequently for aggressive behaviour throughout the day. If a high level of aggression occurs, the animals should be separated. Either sex can be the more aggressive in any given pairing, and in cases of extreme aggression, it is as likely for the smaller female to kill the male as vice versa. For this reason, a nest box or other shelter should be provided in cages that contain a breeding pair, a female with a litter or a group of weanlings. If cage size is large enough, two nest boxes for a pair of breeders are preferred in order to minimise

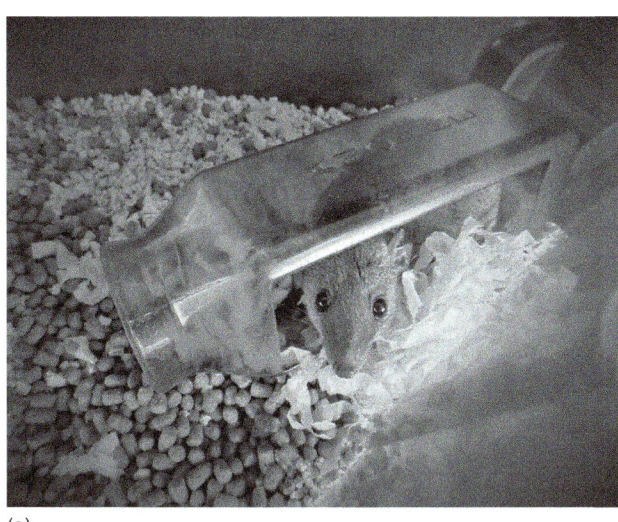
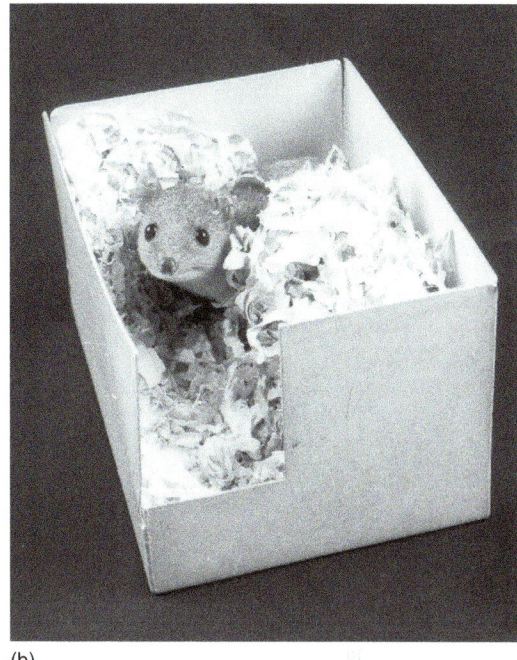

(a) (b)

Figure 19.4 (a) A female with a nest constructed in an Ancare Enrichment Unit. (b) A female with a four-week-old litter in an aluminium nest box from which the lid has been removed. The nest is well-formed except across the top where the lid contacted the sides of the nest itself.

the risk of aggression. Nest boxes can be constructed of any material that can be easily cleaned and, for females that have been recently paired with a male, that permit the female to be checked for the presence of a litter with minimal disruption. Each pair of breeders in the authors' colony is provided with an Ancare Enrichment Unit (Model MH16RDRC) (7 inches long and 2.4 inches on each side) to serve as a nest box (see Figure 19.4). These enrichment devices are transparent and red, so animals inside them can be observed, but the animals cannot see through the walls. Some colony managers use polypropylene plastic food containers with a doorway (approximately 4.5 cm square) cut into them, open ended translucent cylinders, or quart-size wide mouth glass Mason jars as nest boxes. It has not been documented whether these nest boxes with a single opening or the Ancare Enrichment Units with two openings are more effective in reducing deaths of paired animals from aggression. These devices, with intact nests, are transferred with the female to a clean cage when she is separated from the male, and they continue to be transferred with the mother and litter at the time of cage changes until the litter is three weeks of age.

In the authors' colony, groups of littermates are provided aluminium nest boxes (18 cm × 13 cm × 10 cm) at weaning. Unlike the Ancare Enrichment Units, these boxes are large enough for a large group of littermates to occupy together. Each box has a removable 'shoe box' type lid and an entrance measuring 5 cm × 4.5 cm (w × h). Polypropylene or plastic food storage boxes with removable lids and an entrance hole cut from one side will also suffice for weaned siblings.

A convenient and inexpensive alternative is a round glass Mason jar 16.5 cm long, 8.9 cm in diameter, with an opening 8.3 cm in diameter (wide-mouth, US quart size). The animals seem to adapt well to a jar, but it is easier to check females for the presence of litters if an Ancare Enrichment Unit or a nest box with a removable lid is used (see Figure 19.4). On the other hand, the use of Mason jars as nest boxes for weaned litters is thought to promote faster growth, perhaps because, when the littermates are huddled together in a jar, they lose less body heat and can commit more energy to growth (P.B. Samollow, personal communication).

From the perspectives of psychological well-being and environmental enrichment, ample nesting material is essential for all animals whether they are single- or pair-housed. Both males and females may spend many hours per day assembling bundles of nesting material, curling their semi-prehensile tails around a bundle and carrying it around the cage. In some instances, bundles of nesting material are woven into elaborate nests, even by animals that are not in breeding situations.

Food treats may be provided as enrichment. Some treats that are commonly used are hard-boiled eggs (whites and yolks), boiled chicken (light and dark meat) and seedless grapes, cut in half (P.B. Samollow, personal communication); as well as apple, pear, banana, grapefruit and oranges (Rousmaniere et al. 2010). Lean ground beef supplemented with calcium carbonate and potassium iodide also may be used for enrichment (Rousmaniere et al. 2010). It is speculated that the meat supplement might reduce the incidence of cannibalism of young pups by their mothers (Rousmaniere et al. 2010).

Feeding/watering

Monodelphis domestica are omnivorous and in the wild have been documented to consume rodents, lizards, snakes, frogs, insects and a wide variety of other invertebrates, and fruits (Streilein 1982).

In captivity, *Monodelphis* will consume virtually any small animal, such as cockroaches, crickets, earthworms, infant mice and *Tenebrio* larvae. They will also eat many fruits, but exhibit marked individual preferences in this regard.

Dietary experiments have been conducted with commercially prepared foods for cats, dogs, marmosets, mink and foxes, as well as more natural diets containing meat, insects, eggs, milk, infant mice and fruit (Cothran *et al.* 1985; J.L. VandeBerg, unpublished data). However, the currently recommended diet is Purina LabDiet® Short Tailed Opossum #2, 5ATD, 3/16-inch pellet[2]) for which no supplements are required. This diet contains not less than 30.0% protein, 9.5% fat, and 5.0% fibre, and not more than 9.55% water. It was developed by Purina in collaboration with one of the authors (JLV). In controlled experiments where several variations of this diet were fed for two generations, animals fed the **5ATD** formulation outperformed animals on the other formulations in growth and reproductive success (J.L. VandeBerg, unpublished data).

Prior to the adoption of the 5ATD diet, the animals in the authors' colony performed well for many years while fed a reproductive grade of commercial fox chow (see Cothran *et al.* 1985), which contained not less than 35% protein, 13.0% fat and 4.5% fibre, dry weight.

Some colonies have fared well when the animals were fed dried cat chow (e.g., Saunders *et al.* 1989). However, in an early experiment on effects of diet, a cat chow used by one of the authors proved not to be nutritionally adequate; the consequences were small body size and a high level of aggression of the animals towards humans and towards one another when they are paired for mating. Therefore, if cat chow is going to be fed to a newly established colony, it is advised to test several different brands and to select those that approximate the protein, fat and fibre contents specified above.

Feeders designed for rodents are unsatisfactory for laboratory opossums. Food pellets may be placed in a shallow bowl, but the animals are prone to scatter the pellets in the bedding. Hence, for the authors' colony, pellets are placed directly on the bedding in a clean area of the cage. A sufficient quantity of pellets to last a week is added to each cage weekly, and replenished if necessary, during the daily inspections of each cage.

When it is necessary to wean animals prior to the developmental stage normally reached at eight weeks of age, for example, because of spontaneous death of the mother, the pups are able to eat by the age of six to seven weeks if the pelleted food if it is mixed with water to form a pasty mush. Soft food supplements such as the whites of hard-boiled eggs and seedless grapes, cut in half, may be beneficial until the pups are able to eat un-moistened pellets.

For experimental research that requires a diet enriched in saturated fat and cholesterol to investigate the genetics of lipid metabolism and non-alcoholic fatty liver disease (e.g., see Chan *et al.* 2010, 2012), Purina TestDiet® diet[3] designated as Modified 5ATD w/0.7% cholesterol and 19% Fat (Lard), 5AM9, is fed. Other diets can be custom made by the same manufacturer. All of the Purina diets can be purchased from the distributor, LabSupply[4].

Although tap water was provided to animals in the authors' colony for many years, the current practice is to provide water that is purified by reverse osmosis.

Social housing

Because *Monodelphis domestica* are naturally solitary animals and may behave aggressively towards one another, they are generally housed individually. While some colony managers have established protocols for gradually acclimating the two members of a pair intended to be bred (e.g., see Keyte & Smith 2008c), for the authors' colony, a male and a female are placed in a clean cage with a nest box in the morning and are observed frequently during the day for signs of excessive aggression. Occasionally, the two animals must be separated to avoid serious injuries. Excessively aggressive animals are euthanised. This practice is believed to have been responsible for strong selection for lack of aggression over the many generations in captivity. The pairmates are separated after 14 days.

Litters are weaned typically at eight weeks of age, and under optimal conditions, the animals are caged individually (a small cage is sufficient). Littermates, preferably of the same sex, may be caged communally in a large cage containing a nest box, but there is risk of aggression. If caged communally beyond four months of age, many animals, especially males, become aggressive towards one another, and severe injuries or death are likely outcomes. Therefore, individual caging is mandatory after four months of age, or as early as three months for some stocks that exhibit a high level of aggression.

Identification and sexing

After littermates are separated into individual cages, the only contact between animals occurs during the pairing of females and males. Therefore, after the separation of littermates, each individual can be tracked by an ID number that is recorded in a cage record booklet or on a cage card that is maintained with each animal as it is moved from cage to cage.

Ear punching and shearing off fur to create identification patterns on the back are practical short-term methods of identifying individuals if there is a need to do so with group-housed littermates, provided that the identification patterns are monitored and renewed as needed. Over a longer term, subcutaneous microchip transponders may also provide an efficient means for the identification of individual juvenile and adult *Monodelphis* throughout life.

Monodelphis can be easily sexed long before weaning because the testicles are enclosed in a pendulous scrotum attached to the body by a thin stalk. An experienced observer can determine sex visually as early as 10 days post-partum.

---

[2] https://www.labdiet.com/ (Accessed 13 September 2022)
[3] https://www.testdiet.com/ (Accessed 13 September 2022)

[4] https://www.labsupplytx.com (Accessed 13 September 2022)

Physical environment

The ideal room temperature is generally considered to be 24–27 °C, slightly higher than that recommended for rodents. Some colony managers maintain their colonies at the high end of that range (e.g., 26–27 °C; see Rousmaniere et al. 2010; Busse et al. 2014), and a temperature range as high as 25–30 °C has been recommended (Benato et al. 2010). Although no controlled experiments have been reported, the neonatal survival rate is believed to be higher at the more elevated temperatures, and pups are believed to grow faster.

Fluorescent lighting is used in a cycle of 14 h light and 10 h dark, and humidity is maintained at 45–70%. Humidity levels below 35% may lead to desiccation and necrosis of the distal region of ear pinnae and tails of some individuals (see Benato et al. 2010 for a detailed case report of a pet *Monodelphis* that was maintained at 25% humidity).

The animal rooms should be kept as quiet as practicable. Loud noises and vibrations such as those that occur during construction cause stress that may lead to increased levels of aggression and cannibalism. Additionally, *Monodelphis domestica* can hear at ultrasound frequencies inaudible to humans, so sources of high-frequency noise should be monitored and minimised (see Sales et al. 1988).

Hygiene

Every two weeks (for ventilated cages; every week for conventional cages), all animals should be moved to clean cages with fresh bedding. Nest boxes and well-constructed nests may be moved to the new cage if they are not heavily soiled. Care should be taken to disturb mothers and their nests as little as possible, at least while the litters are less than three weeks old, and preferably until after they are five weeks old, to discourage cannibalism. Some colony managers do not change nests at all until the pups are weaned. Nest boxes are generally washed in a cage washer every two weeks, and at a time when young litters are not present.

Health monitoring and quarantine

Laboratory opossums are exceptionally healthy laboratory animals and usually require no other health monitoring procedures than routine daily observation. Nevertheless, a quarantine of 30 days is recommended for animals coming into a facility from other research colonies.

Animals captured from wild populations typically carry endoparasites and should be kept in quarantine, while the bedding is changed three times per week to break the life cycle of the parasites. Endoparasites are generally eliminated within a few weeks by this procedure.

Ectoparasites have not been documented on newly captured animals but, recently, mites of the species *Archemyobia (Nearchemyobia) latipilis* were discovered throughout a breeding colony (Smith 2016) and subsequently in the authors' colony (unpublished data), which was the source of the founders of the colony in which the mites were discovered. Since mites are generally species specific to their hosts, and since the *Monodelphis* in both colonies have never been housed in the same room with another species, it is inferred that these mites were present on at least some of the initial wild-caught founders. The mites appear to have no impact on the health or well-being of the animals, but they can be eradicated by topical application of 2.0 mg/kg in mineral oil or propylene glycol, which does not cause any apparent toxicity to the animals (Smith 2016).

Care of aged animals

Aged animals do not have special needs, except that they may develop difficulty in eating the hard food pellets. The remedy is to develop a pasty mush by softening the pellets with water. Of course, soft food treats, examples of which are provided in a previous section, are appropriately provided as supplements, but do not by themselves constitute a nutritionally adequate diet.

Breeding

Female laboratory opossums reach sexual maturity by five months of age (Stonebrook & Harder 1992), two to three weeks earlier than males. Oestrus is induced at any time of the year by the introduction of a male, generally 5–10 days after the animals are caged together. The induction of oestrus occurs even immediately after a litter dies or is removed prior to weaning, if a female is provided with a male. This characteristic is highly advantageous in comparison to many marsupial species that are seasonal breeders. This characteristic also facilitates timed pregnancies and the collection of staged embryos.

Females are biologically capable of rearing up to four litters per year, although this level of success is rare. Since the reproductive performance of most females declines or ceases by 18 months of age (12 months after full sexual maturity), four weaned litters in the lifetime of a female is judged to be excellent reproductive performance. In the authors' colony, the largest number of progeny weaned by a female during her life was 49, just short of the theoretical maximum of 52 (13 progeny/litter × 4 litters = 52 progeny) that could be weaned in one year. More than four litters can be produced by a single female in a year if the pups are removed for experimental purposes prior to weaning and the female is immediately paired with a mate. One female subjected to this protocol produced 67 progeny in one year. Since females are induced to ovulate approximately seven days after pairing, and birth occurs 14 days later; a female could conceivably produce a litter every month if the pups were removed within the first week of life for experimental (or other) purposes. The most fecund strains produce an average of 10 pups per litter so, in theory, an average female of such a strain could produce 120 pups in a year if all of them were removed within the first week of life.

A single male can be paired with a different female every two weeks and could in theory sire up to 26 litters per year. The largest number of weaned progeny sired by a single male in the authors' colony was 105.

The only practical strategy for determining if an animal is fertile is to pair it with a member of the opposite sex that has a recent history of fertility. In the author's colony, if an animal does not reproduce after four such opportunities, it is judged to be unlikely to succeed in subsequent opportunities and is removed from the breeding program.

Pairing

Monogamous pairings are made to minimise aggressive behaviour and to prevent interference with mating. In the authors' colony, under normal conditions, a mature male and female are placed together in a large clean cage (with bedding, nesting material, a nest box and fresh feed and water (see Figure 19.5). Pairing should be done early in the day so that animal care staff can be alert for undue aggression for at least a few hours after pairing. A low level of aggression is common and does not pose a serious risk, but occasionally the animals must be separated due to highly aggressive fighting. Some colony managers attempt to minimise aggression by introducing females and males to one another by placing them for a few days in a large cage with a partition that allows air flow between the two compartments, and then removing the partition. Others prefer to place the male into the female's cage after she has occupied it for several days and may feel more secure in interactions with the male. Finally, a method wherein the individually housed female and male are swapped between one another's cages for a day or two prior to placing them together a clean cage (female first, then male) has been successful in reducing aggressive behaviour in some colonies.

Conceptions are not likely to occur more than 10–12 days after pairing, so males are typically removed after two weeks, at which time they may be paired with another female. After the removal of the male from the cage, and depending on requirements of the breeding program or experimental protocol, the female is kept solitary for at least two weeks (the gestation period), preferably in a large cage with a nest box. If a litter has not been born (or has died or been removed), the female may be paired immediately with the same or a different male.

The day of mating cannot be precisely ascertained by techniques that are used for rodents. There is no vaginal plug, and sperm are rarely detected in vaginal smears. Furthermore, the time of ovulation is difficult to predict from vaginal smears because cornified cells from the lateral vaginae may infiltrate the posterior vaginal sinus, masking changes in the cytology of the cells that line the posterior vaginal sinus (Fadem & Rayve 1985). Therefore, video systems have been used to determine the precise timing of mating (Baggott & Moore 1990; Mate *et al.* 1994; Kuehl-Kovarik *et al.* 1995; Selwood *et al.* 1997; Rousmaniere *et al.* 2010; Yoshida *et al.* 2019). Generally, a group of cages is filmed under red light or infrared light during the dark phase when most matings occur. The film can be fast forwarded for examination each day to identify the exact time of copulations. Another strategy has been to keep the paired animals separated by a perforated plexiglass partition except for 1–2 hour at the end of the light period and at 12-hour intervals after that until mating occurs (Kuehl-Kovarik *et al.* 1995). Mating usually takes place within 20 minutes of removal of the partition.

Pregnancy can be detected beginning on the ninth day of gestation by ultrasound (Miles *et al.* 1997).

Generally, no harm arises from leaving a male paired with a female longer than two weeks, provided he is removed within the first two weeks after a litter is born to prevent him from eating the pups when they are left alone by the mother. However, there is little chance of conception from a prolonged pairing, and there is always risk of aggression.

Fertility decline and aggression

Risk of aggression is especially high among older animals, particularly females. For most females, the prime reproductive age is up to 18 months, and most cease to reproduce by 24 months of age. Cessation of reproductive success is often

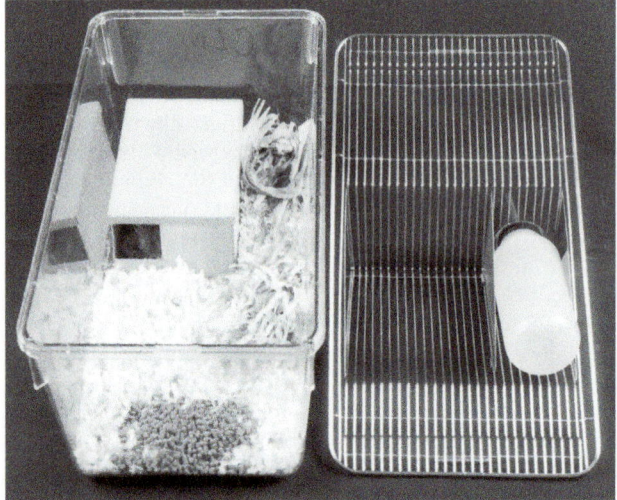
(a)

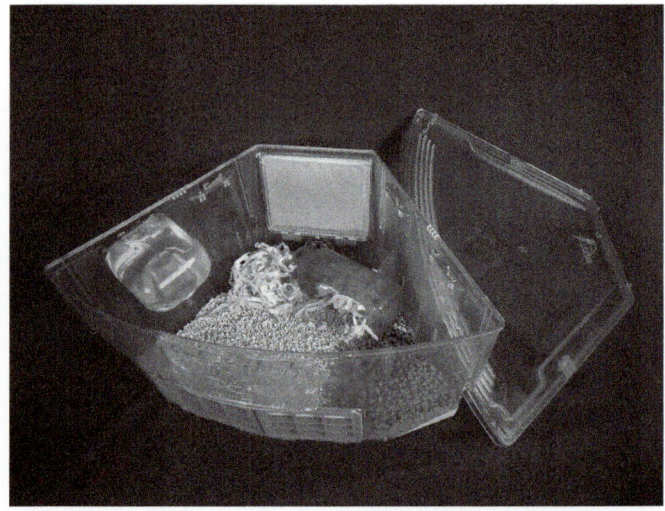
(b)

Figure 19.5 (a) A large conventional cage ready for a pair of animals. (b) An Optirat® cage ready for a pair of animals. Feed pellets are placed on the bedding near the front of the cage. Nesting material is divided into two portions to limit competition for it. Frequently, one animal builds a nest inside the nesting box and the other builds a nest outside.

accompanied by aggressive behaviour towards prospective mates. Females in the authors' colony are routinely removed from the breeding programme at between 18 and 24 months of age depending on their reproductive history, history of aggression towards potential mates and importance of a particular animal to its breeding programme. However, the oldest female that produced a litter in the authors' colony was 34 months old at the time of conception, and she succeeded in rearing the litter to weaning.

Some elderly males become aggressive to their potential mates, so a judgement is made as to which males are allowed to continue as breeders beyond two years of age. The oldest male that sired a litter in the authors' colony was 40 months old at the time the litter was conceived.

Birth and newborn pups

Birth occurs approximately 14.5 days after copulation and 13.5 days after ovulation and fertilisation (Mate *et al.* 1994). Under normal circumstances, birth probably occurs in the seclusion of the nest, and nesting material should be provided to allow for this behaviour. Pregnant females may be observed giving birth if deprived of nests, for example when it is necessary to harvest pups for experimental purposes immediately after birth and before attachment to a nipple.

Females may become more active for a few minutes before birth. At the moment of birth, the female places one side of the dorsal surface of her rump on the floor, with hindfeet in the air; props the anterior part of her body by placing a forepaw on the floor; and curves her spine so her head is near the urogenital opening, which is raised to extrude the neonates on to the mammary area.

As many as 18 neonates have been observed in a newborn litter. However, the maximum number of newborns that are capable of surviving is equal to the number of teats of the mother; that number is 13 in most individuals but may be only 11 or 12 (Robinson *et al.* 1991). Typical litter size (determined after attachment to the nipples) varies among stocks, but 7–8 is common for many stocks, and 9–12 is not unusual. Occasionally, a litter of 13 is reared to weaning.

The neonates are light grey at birth and are licked vigorously by the mother while they flail from side to side in worm-like movements. Attachment to the nipples generally occurs within seconds, or a few minutes at most, and the colour of the skin turns to a bright pink shortly thereafter. Neonates that do not find a teat continue crawling, generally in an upward direction and remain light grey. After the unattached neonates reach the dorsal side of the mother, they are cannibalised. This behaviour is probably an evolutionary adaptation that enables the mother to acquire an immediate source of protein from those pups that have no chance of survival.

Litter survival is highly variable, depending on the breeding stock, the age and reproductive experience and age of the dam and the size of the litter. In general, it well exceeds 50%, but survival is reduced in highly inbred litters and in litters born to older females (approaching two years of age and beyond). Small litters tend to be lost more frequently than large litters; litters with fewer than four pups rarely survive to weaning. If it is desired to return a female with a small litter immediately to breeding, rather than to hope for the survival of a litter of one to three pups, the litter can be euthanised. It is important that nest disturbance and extraneous noise be kept to a minimum in breeding colonies to reduce the risk of cannibalism of litters by their mothers.

The newborn marsupial has an embryonic two-layered forebrain, no cerebellum, embryonic eyes, no ears and hindlimbs at the paddle stage of development. Anatomically, it resembles a mouse at 10.5 days of gestation. Newborn *Monodelphis* weigh approximately 100 mg and are approximately 1 cm in length. Each newborn remains attached to the same nipple for the first two weeks after birth. At two weeks of age, each pup weighs about 840 mg (VandeBerg 1990) and may be left alone in the nest, although pups are frequently present on the nipples during the third week of life both when the mother is resting and when she is active. The pups begin to grow fur at the beginning of the third week of life and their eyes open about 33–35 days postnatally.

Laboratory opossums are routinely weaned at eight weeks of age, when they weigh about 20 g. Some colony managers feed pellets softened with water to lactating mothers, enabling the pups to begin eating solid food at an earlier age and stimulating faster growth (P. B. Samollow, personal communication). In addition, they continue to feed the pups water-softened pellets for a month after weaning. As per Dr. Samollow, 'the water-softened feed also helps maintain a good hydration level in the lactating female (perhaps reducing the likelihood of [cloacal] prolapse) and reduces the probability of pups dying of dehydration in the event there is a water bottle problem, or during the early stages of weaning when they might not obtain an adequate supply of water through nursing alone'.

Lactation can continue for as long as 15 weeks after birth (Rousmaniere *et al.* 2010), and pups may be left with their mothers up to 16 weeks of age without adverse consequences (P.B. Samollow, personal communication). Reasons for leaving pups with their mothers longer than eight weeks are: 1) the size (and developmental state) of the pups is smaller than normal for their age, in which case they should be left with their mother until they are able to function independently, and 2) cage space is too limited to enable the separation of the pups from their mother. Indeed, it may be that 'pups left with their mothers grow faster than those that are weaned/separated at younger ages (eight to nine weeks), probably a result of the added body heat from the mother enabling the pups to channel more calories into growth' (P.B. Samollow, personal communication).

Weaning is accomplished simply by placing littermates, preferably of the same sex, in a large cage by themselves or by placing each one in a small cage. If mixed sex groups are housed together, there is more risk of aggression, and as they approach puberty, there is risk of a physiological response to pheromones of the opposite sex. Animals must be singly-housed by the age of four months to prevent serious aggressive behaviour. The weanlings continue to grow rapidly for 200–250 days, after which growth plateaus (see growth curves in Cothran *et al.* 1985; Rousmaniere *et al.* 2010). Growth of females and onset of puberty may be stimulated if they are paired with males prior to six months of age (Stonebrook & Harder 1992). Conversely, females exhibit pronounced growth retardation if they are deprived of mates after six months of age (Cothran *et al.* 1985; VandeBerg 1990).

Breeding systems

Most aspects of breeding systems are similar to those for rodents, with the exception of inbreeding.

For stocks where the number of animals and reproductive success are especially limited, a useful practice is to pair proven breeders with animals that are virgin or have failed to reproduce. This practice helps to ensure that animals capable of reproduction are provided the best opportunity for success before they are culled on the basis of reproductive performance.

More than 140,000 laboratory opossums have been produced and weaned in the authors' colony over the 42 years since its inception in 1979. Pedigree data are maintained for each individual in a computerised database, and the inbreeding coefficient of each individual is calculated using software specifically developed for that purpose (Dyke 1989). Because the number of founders was small, all individuals of the non-inbred strains are partially inbred except those that can be produced by intercrosses between several stocks (as discussed in the section headed 'Genetic stocks and strains').

For all breeding stocks, an effort is made to select for the highest possible fecundity by replacing breeders with animals from litters that had the highest number of surviving pups at weaning. For example, for the LL2 stock that is the most genetically heterogeneous and most fecund stock in the authors' colony, only animals from litters with 10 or more surviving progeny at weaning are retained for breeding. For stocks with the lowest fecundity, only animals with five or more surviving progeny at weaning are retained for breeding. To maximise the retention of genetic variation and to minimise inbreeding, for a given breeding stock, a small and equal number of animals are retained for breeding from each litter that meets the required minimum size at the time of weaning. Of course, breeding schemes for other colonies need to be tailored to the individual space and size constraints, and to the experimental objectives of the investigators utilising those colonies.

Transport

For general advice on transport, see Chapter 12: Transportation of laboratory animals. Local transportation in a climate-controlled vehicle approved for animal transport can be safely conducted with the *Monodelphis* in their standard cages. Temperature should be maintained as constant as is practical and within the normal laboratory range for this species.

Monodelphis are typically shipped by road or by air in boxes that are used for air transportation of mice. A standard mouse shipping box purchased from a commercial mouse supplier can be subdivided with plywood partitions to enable the transport of up to six *Monodelphis* (see Figure 19.6). Each animal must be placed singly into a partitioned enclosure to prevent fighting en route. Even littermates that have been caged together since weaning are likely to be aggressive during transport, so they should be housed individually during transport. Care must be taken in constructing partitions to ensure that a portion of each compartment has open access to at least one ventilation opening. The authors typically partition each box into six compartments, the dimensions of

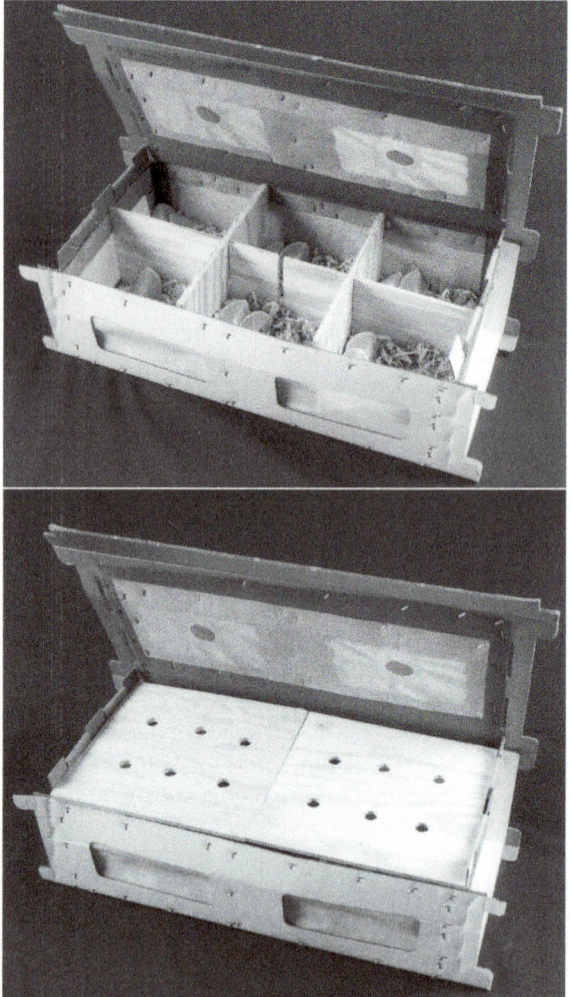

Figure 19.6 Top: a shipping box ready for six animals to be placed inside. Note the nesting material on top of the wood shavings and the two orange quarters in each. Bottom: two plywood covers with holes for air exchange are placed side-by-side inside the box before closing the cardboard top in order to ensure that animals cannot gain access to an adjacent compartment and to facilitate putting individual animals into, and retrieving them from, the compartments.

which are 18 cm × 13 cm × 18 cm (l × w × h). The box is divided into four compartments if fewer than five animals are to be transported.

The floor of each compartment should be covered with about 2.5 cm of bedding, and about 15 g of nesting material provided for each animal. Provision of feed in the form of orange quarters, apple quarters or pieces of watermelon have been used successfully. In addition, water gel packs can be used, especially for trips of extended duration. If water gel packs are used, it is recommended that they be used to augment rather than replace fruit, because fruit provides a source of nutrition, in addition to moisture.

Attempts to ship females with suckling pups have had limited success because of cannibalism. However, the authors have encountered no problems in shipping pregnant females, even in the late stages of pregnancy.

Animals should be acclimated to a new environment in solitary cages. Pairings of breeders that arrive from a single breeding colony should not occur less than one week after arrival to minimise the risk of aggressive behaviour. However, animals should be quarantined for the standard 30-day period if they are going to be paired with animals other than those that were shipped together with them.

Monodelphis were routinely transported nationally and internationally by air in the partitioned mouse shipping boxes for many years. Some years ago, the International Air Transport Association (IATA) classified *Monodelphis* together with large opossums, such as *Didelphis* species, which require large and complex shipping box designs. However, IATA now groups *Monodelphis* together with rats and mice, and allows them to be shipped in standard rodent shipping containers (International Air transport Association 2020), enabling the economical distribution of animals from existing breeding colonies.

Laboratory procedures

Handling

Monodelphis domestica are gentle and docile in response to human handling. Even individuals captured from wild populations can be picked up by experienced handlers with little risk of being bitten. The only hand coverings typically used for routine handling are disposable latex or nitrile gloves. Under most circumstances the animal is picked up by the tail, as has typically been done with laboratory mice in the past (see Figure 19.7). Animals may also be picked up by placing the fingers under the midsection and the index finger and thumb on the two sides of the neck to secure the head so the animal cannot bite the handler, as shown Figure 19.8.

Despite its generally docile nature, a laboratory opossum that is not handled properly may bite. Unlike rodents, laboratory opossums have small incisors and do not inflict severe lacerations. Nevertheless, they do have sharp, needle-like teeth and most adults, particularly the larger males, are capable of puncturing human skin. Inexperienced or careless handlers are generally bitten under either of two circumstances. One is when they move their hand too quickly in attempting to capture an animal. The animals have an extremely fast reflex to bite anything that moves rapidly, whether it be prey (presumably a hunting adaptation) or a human hand. The biting reflex is often quicker than the initial movement of the human hand attempting to grab the tail (or animal). In contrast, moving the hand slowly to the animal and picking the animal up slowly will almost never elicit a bite, even though some animals back into the corner of the cage hissing with an open mouth and displaying their teeth. The second circumstance in which an inexperienced or careless handler is likely to be bitten is when an attempt is made to restrain any part of the body of the animal. If the body of an unanaesthetised animal must be restrained, light leather gloves, such as golf gloves, should be used.

Monitoring and sampling methods

Body temperature can be assessed by thermocouples as a deep colonic measure at an insertion depth of 3–4 cm (Dawson & Olson 1988). However, since marsupials have a cloaca,

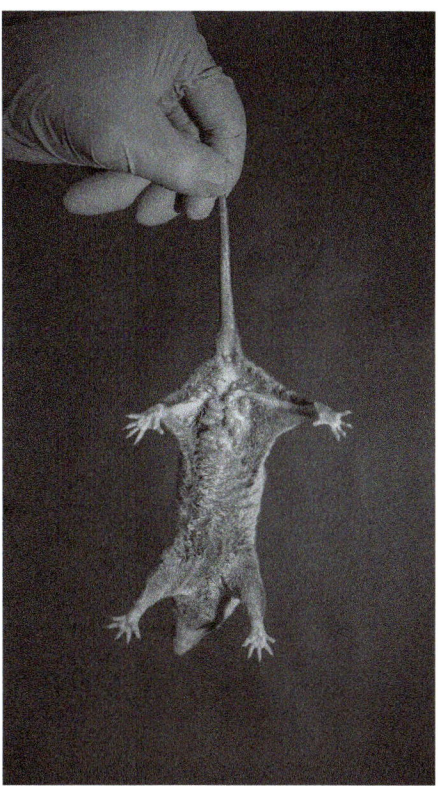

Figure 19.7 (UTRGV Photo by David Pike) Picking up an animal by the tail. This female has a newborn litter. The proper placement of the thumb and forefinger would be less distal on the tails of rodents, which are susceptible to de-gloving injuries, but those injuries do not occur with *Monodelphis*. Animals of this species may be held by the tail with the fingers in either position, but holding the tail more distally reduces the capacity of animal to curl its body sufficiently to bite the handler.

extreme care must be taken to ensure that the thermocouple is inserted into the colon and not into a genital or urinary tract opening. A temperature-sensitive microchip transponder also can be used.

The least invasive method of collecting small volumes of blood is to hold the tail tightly near the base so as to constrict venous blood flow to the body and to puncture the tail with a hypodermic needle pointed towards the rump of the animal (and with the bevel towards the skin). After the removal of the needle, blood (typically up to 0.5 ml) can be aspirated into capillary tubes or collected with a micropipette. Anaesthesia is not required if a rodent restrainer designed for the collection of blood from the tail and of an appropriate size is used.

Although the anatomy of the skull and soft tissue around the eyeballs of laboratory opossums is quite different from those of rodents, similar quantities of blood can be collected from anaesthetised animals by inserting a 27-g needle on a 1-ml tuberculin syringe into front corner of the eye socket, manipulating it into the highly vascularised area under the front portion of the eyeball and slowly withdrawing blood into the syringe.

Substantial volumes of blood can be collected easily and routinely by cardiac puncture of anaesthetised animals. This method also has the advantage in that a consistent quantity

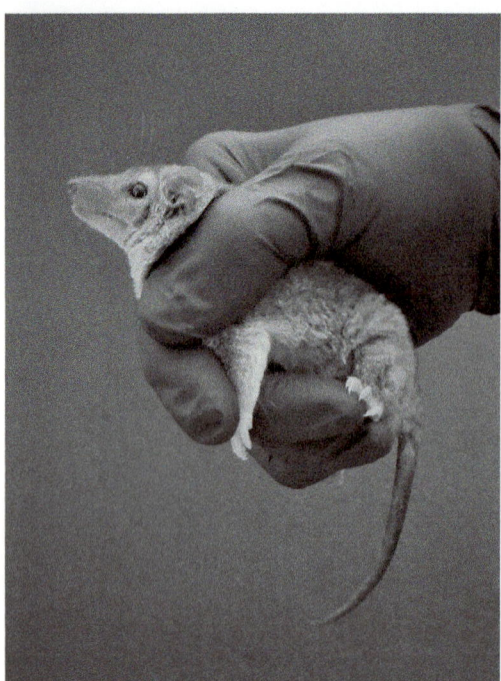

Figure 19.8 Picking up an animal by placing the fingers under the midsection with thumb and index finger on the two sides of the neck.

of blood can be collected from each animal. A 1.27 cm, 27G (0.406 mm nominal outside diameter) needle on a 1-ml tuberculin syringe is typically used, although a larger syringe may be used for collecting larger volumes of blood. Experienced technical staff collecting blood routinely are able to obtain 0.8–1.0 ml of blood in 95% of attempts, with no obvious adverse impact on health (Robinson & VandeBerg 1994).

Cardiac puncture, under anaesthetic, has been conducted repeatedly over time on an animal without apparent ill effects. In an investigation of the effects of chronic blood loss, 2 ml of blood was removed weekly for 13 weeks from each of 20 adult animals that weighed 89.0 ± 5.7 g (Manis et al. 1992). No apparent changes in health status occurred, although haematopoietic characteristics were altered. Although this species is remarkable tolerant of chronic blood loss, the volume collected for routine purposes is generally limited to 2 ml per 100 g of body weight for single blood collections, and 10 ml per 100 g of body weight over 13 weeks of multiple blood collections. Removal of more than the routine amount defined above should require scientific justification as well as ethics approval, since haematopoietic characteristics can be altered when larger quantities of blood are removed.

When survival of the animal is not an objective, large volumes of blood can be collected by lethal exsanguination using the cardiac puncture method under general anaesthesia. Experienced personnel can routinely collect at least 5 ml and often as much as 6–7 ml from an animal that weighs 100 g or more (Robinson & VandeBerg 1994). After exsanguination, a secondary method of euthanasia must be performed, for example, thoracotomy or cervical dislocation, while the animal remains anesthetised, in order to ensure death.

Urine may be collected by putting individual animals in cages with wire mesh bottoms placed over collection pans as described by Christian (1983). The collection pans should contain a layer of mineral oil to prevent evaporation of urine and faeces.

The only way to collect milk within two weeks postpartum is to remove the sucklings from the teats. Because they cannot be reattached, the sucklings must be euthanised. For older litters, the mothers can be separated from their litters temporarily. Two hours after the separation of mothers from their litters, dams are anaesthetised with isoflurane and injected intramuscularly with 0.75-ml oxytocin (Samples et al. 1986). Milk droplets are exuded by manually squeezing the mammary glands, and they are collected in capillary tubes. Between 5 and 10 µl of milk can be collected during the first few days of lactation, and up to 80 µl during the later stages (Crisp et al. 1989).

Ovulation of Monodelphis can be induced by the injection of exogenous hormones (Hinds et al. 1996; Witt & Rodger 2018). An effective regimen of injections is 1 I.U. of equine serum gonadotropin (eSG) on Day 0 to elicit the development of follicles, followed by 3 × 10 ug of gonadotropin-releasing hormone (GnRH) at 1.5-hour intervals on Day 2 or Day 3 to promote oocyte maturation and ovulation.

Administration of substances

Substances can be administered to laboratory opossums by the same procedures that are used for rodents. For administration of fluid by gavage, animals can be held as shown in Figure 19.8, and the fluid can be administered slowly to the back of the throat from a fine-bore soft plastic tube that is fitted to a syringe. Less stressful alternatives, including administration of tablets and voluntary ingestion from syringes, are being developed for use with rodents (Walker et al. 2012; Kuster et al. 2012) and may be effective with Monodelphis.

Anaesthesia and analgesia

Light anaesthesia by inhalation is recommended for all injections because it is difficult to restrain an active Monodelphis for this purpose. The procedures for injections of Monodelphis are the same as those for rodents. Subcutaneous injections are generally given in the shoulder area, intramuscular injections in the hindlimb area and intraperitoneal injections in the caudal abdomen.

The most satisfactory inhaled anaesthetic in the authors' experience is isoflurane. Barnett et al. (2017) compared isoflurane with six injectable anaesthetics for anaesthetising laboratory opossums and also concluded that isoflurane provided the most consistent and reliable results. Although considerable care must be taken to maintain depth of anaesthesia for a few minutes or more without killing the animal, isoflurane is relatively safe in the hands of experienced personnel using anaesthesia equipment for short-term anaesthesia (up to 1 hour). Animals may be anaesthetised without having been fasted without adverse consequences, although they are more prone to defecate if they have not been fasted. For that reason, in the authors' laboratory, the animals are typically provided with water but no food during the 4–6 hours prior to anaesthesia. While we formerly fasted animals overnight, we switched to a shorter fasting period because the animals are most active during the dark cycle, and absence of food during an overnight fast, which might last for 14–19 hours prior to anaesthesia, might be expected to be unnecessarily stressful to the animals. Moreover, it has been established in mice that gastric content is reduced equally after 4–6 hours of fasting as after 12–18 hours, and that cardiovascular, hormonal and metabolic parameters are significantly altered after as little as 7 hours of fasting (Jensen et al. 2013). Although *Monodelphis* are three or four times as large as mice, the data from mice are probably indicative of the responses of other small mammals to fasting. An additional advantage to a shorter duration of fasting is that *Monodelphis* generally recover more quickly from the effects of anaesthesia after a shorter fast. For all of those reasons combined, a fast of 4–6 hours is preferred over a longer duration.

In the authors' laboratory, up to six animals to be anaesthetised are placed in separate compartments of an acrylic six-compartment chamber, with each compartment lined with paper towels to absorb urine and faeces. The chamber (six side-by-side compartments, each with inside dimensions of 25.5 cm L × 10.0 cm W × 10.0 cm H), which is placed in a biosafety hood, is flooded with a mixture of isoflurane/oxygen delivered from an anaesthesia machine (see Figure 19.9). The oxygen flow rate is set at 0.8 l/min and the isoflurane level is set at 4% V/V. The animals can be monitored through the clear acrylic sides of the chamber. The length of time required to sedate the animals is variable, but most animals are thoroughly sedated within 5 minutes. Animals are removed from the chamber based on their apparent depth of anaesthesia.

For quick procedures, such as collecting a small sample of ear pinna for DNA extraction, the animal may be lightly anesthetised with isoflurane prior to the procedure and returned immediately to its home cage (provided that it is singly housed). Most animals are up and ambulatory within a minute, and fully recovered within 2-5 minutes.

Depth of anaesthesia can best be judged, after the body is limp, by toe pinching and respiratory rate. Deep anaesthesia sufficient for cardiac puncture or surgical procedures is indicated by failure to withdraw a foot in response to a pinch. Respiratory rate should be watched continuously during the procedure and during the recovery period; a sudden reduction in rate of breathing or sporadic breathing indicates that an animal is at high risk of death. If respiration ceases, an animal can often be resuscitated by placing one or two drops of doxapram hydrochloride (20 mg/ml) on the tongue of the animal. If respiration does not commence within a few seconds, one end of a 20 cm length of plastic tubing is placed over the animal's nostrils and snout, firmly against the skin, and the person conducting the procedure blows gently into the other end at intervals of 1–2 seconds so that that the animal's lungs inflate on each occasion. The tubing has an external diameter of 15 mm and an inside diameter of 11 mm.

For recovery from anaesthesia, an animal is placed in an acrylic observation chamber or small plastic animal cage (e.g., mouse cage) so that its ventral surface is resting on a heating pad covered with absorbent paper and maintained at 30 °C. If there is any sign of respiratory distress, the procedures for resuscitation are immediately performed. Most animals are fully recovered and able to walk without losing balance within 10–30 minutes, when they are returned to their cages.

For inducing deep anaesthesia for a prolonged period of time, a combination of inhalation and injection anaesthesia has been developed (Dooley et al. 2013). In this protocol, the animal is anaesthetised in a chamber flooded with isoflurane, and then removed from the chamber and fitted with a mask placed over its snout. Isoflurane is delivered through the mask at 1–2%. Just prior to surgery, the animal is injected intramuscularly with dexamethasone (0.4–2.0 mg/kg) and atropine (0.04 mg/kg).

Light anaesthesia of dams and litters with isoflurane is used for procedures that can be completed quickly. However, litter loss is unacceptably high when dams with attached litters are subjected to deep anaesthesia in a chamber flooded with isoflurane.

Another approach to anaesthesia of a mother with attached pups is to anaesthetise it lightly using a 50-ml conical tube delivering the regulated anaesthetic mixture over the head of the mother (Wang & VandeBerg 2003). This procedure enables anaesthesia of the dam without affecting the pups, greatly reducing the risk of losing the litter. Alternatively, the mother's head and front half of the body can be lowered into a semi-covered 2-liter beaker that contains anaesthetic vapour, while the attached pups remain outside of the beaker.

Hypothermia has been recommended for surgical procedures on altricial neonates that have not developed effective thermoregulation capabilities (National Research Council 1992; reviewed by Martin 1995). Because neurones in mammals cease to function when body temperature is reduced to 20 °C, as compared with 0–4 °C in poikilotherms, cooling is an effective form of anaesthesia for altricial mammalian neonates which are incapable of effective thermoregulation. Anaesthesia of *Monodelphis* pups within the first three weeks of life has been accomplished by cooling them with ice (Morykwas et al. 1991; Stewart et al. 1991; J.L. VandeBerg, unpublished data) or by using a series of puffs of dry ice dust (Taylor & Guillery 1995), prior to rapid inoculations or surgeries. The methods are appropriate not only

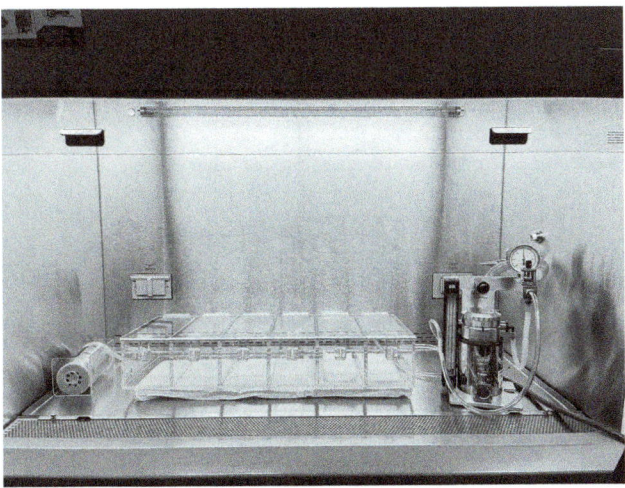

Figure 19.9 Anaesthetic chamber for anaesthesia of multiple animals.

because the neonates have poor thermoregulation capacity, but also because they are developmentally equivalent to a human foetus at 20 weeks of gestation, at which time the nervous system is poorly developed and the cerebellum is not yet developed.

Another method of anaesthetising pups that are still attached to their mothers' nipples has been developed for rapid surgical procedures by Dr. Ben Wheaton (Wheaton et al. 2011, 2021; details provided here, with permission, via personal communication). The mother is placed in an anaesthesia box until she is subdued but still awake and moving. She is then transferred to a warm pad in a supine position with an anaesthetic mask placed over her nose to induce a deep plane of anaesthesia. Then, surgery can be conducted sequentially on each pup after it is anesthetised individually, until it stops moving and reacting to touch, by placing a 1.5-ml tube containing cotton soaked in isoflurane over the nose. For surgical procedures that last up to 10 minutes per pup, the pup is positioned around the circumference of a short, round bar in order to stabilise it, while maintaining the anaesthesia tube in place. Anaesthesia is judged to be becoming too shallow if the pup begins to move and too deep if the skin colour begins to change from pink to grey (indicating anoxia). The anaesthesia tube is adjusted appropriately when these observations are made. This procedure has been applied to seven-day-old pups and probably would serve for pups within a few days of that age, perhaps nearly to the age of 14 days, when the pups are able to detach from the nipples (and could be surgically manipulated independently of anaesthesia of their mother). The wounds are closed with tissue glue (3M Vetbond tissue adhesive).

It has been reported that feeding a mother mealworms immediately after recovery from anaesthesia may reduce the incidence of cannibalism (Saunders et al. 1995).

Surgery and blood sampling

Procedures for ovariectomy, castration, partial hepatectomy, unilateral hysterectomy, vasectomy and embryo transfer have been described in detail (Kraus & Fadem 1987; Robinson & VandeBerg 1994). In addition, procedures have been developed for tail amputations and eye removals, which are sometimes necessary following trauma (usually fighting) or infection (Robinson et al. 1994). A procedure for anaesthesia by inhalation and injection is generally used for major surgery, but simple procedures can be conducted under isoflurane anaesthesia alone. Techniques are similar to those used for rodent surgery. However, incisions must be closed with sutures rather than surgical clips, because the animals are adept at removing the clips.

Buprenorphine may be administered as a post-surgical analgesic, intraperitoneally at a dose of 0.6 mg/kg, or intramuscularly at a dose of 0.3 mg/kg (Wheaton et al. 2011; Dooley et al. 2013).

Ear pinna sampling for DNA extraction is less invasive and less time-consuming than blood sampling. Care must be taken to excise the sample form the outer minimally vascularised edge of the ear pinna. If any bleeding occurs, it can be stopped by the application of silver nitrate.

Euthanasia

Animals beyond three weeks of age

Euthanasia of animals beyond three weeks of age is most easily accomplished by inhalation because the animals are difficult to restrain for physical methods of euthanasia. Carbon dioxide (administered by the gradual fill method, which is approved by the AVMA Guidelines for the Euthanasia of Animals 2020) and isoflurane are suitable inhalants for the purpose of euthanasia (see also Chapter 17: Euthanasia and other fates for laboratory animals). Alternatively, after induction of anaesthesia using injectable agents (e.g., tiletamine/zolazepam mixture), animals can be euthanised with an overdose of intravenous or intra-cardiac barbiturates (Pye 2006). Regardless of the primary method of euthanasia, after the animal has ceased to breathe, cervical dislocation or another physical procedure is performed to ensure that the animal is dead.

Animals up to three weeks of age

Up to three weeks of age, when they are equivalent to a 20-week human foetus, laboratory opossums are resistant to carbon dioxide and isoflurane. Although they can easily be euthanised by decapitation, that process is time-consuming when dealing with large numbers of animals. Therefore, just as hypothermia is recommended for anaesthesia of pups up to three weeks of age, so also it is appropriate to euthanise pups up to that age by placing them in a freezer or on dry ice (but not in direct contact with dry ice or any cold surface). As with older animals that die from inhalation of a gas after first becoming unconscious, these embryos and early foetuses first become unconscious from hypothermia, and then die from hypothermia seconds or, at most, a minute or two later. An alternative is to submerge the pups in liquid nitrogen, which causes instant death. Pups may also be put in an ice water bath in which they become immobilised and anaesthetised almost instantly and expire soon after from anoxia. However, for pups placed in an ice water bath, a secondary method of euthanasia, such as decapitation or freezing the carcasses, should be performed to ensure death.

When whole carcasses are needed from pups for the purpose of fixation and whole-body sectioning for histology, they may be subjected to prolonged carbon dioxide or isoflurane inhalation (i.e., for at least 10 minutes) prior to immersing them in fixative. When whole carcasses are needed from pups for the purpose of freezing for histology, they may be euthanised by placing them on a weigh boat on dry ice.

Common welfare problems

Health

Infectious diseases

Infectious diseases are virtually non-existent in laboratory opossums that are properly managed and fed a nutritionally adequate diet. If, however, the diet is suboptimal, some animals may be prone to respiratory infections (J.L. VandeBerg, unpublished data).

As is the standard procedure with other small laboratory animals, a colony can be protected from transmissible diseases by euthanising animals suspected of being infected and conducting a complete pathological and microbiological evaluation. Appropriate prevention measures can be implemented on the basis of the results. Comprehensive texts on wild animal medicine are available (e.g., Holz 2015).

Common clinical signs of infectious disease include rapid breathing, poor coat condition and loss of body weight. If an animal suspected of having an infectious disease is discovered in a colony, it should be necropsied by a veterinary pathologist, and all husbandry procedures and conditions, including nutritional adequacy of the diet, should be carefully assessed.

Wild-caught *Monodelphis* may harbour a variety of endoparasites, including *Capillaria*, *Trichuris*, *Cruzia*, *Strongylus* and fluke-like and *Hymenolepis*-like species, although no disease states induced by these parasites have been observed (Hubbard et al. 1997). There have been no published reports of ectoparasites in wild or captive populations of *Monodelphis domestica*, although a mite species, *Archemyobia (Nearchemyobia) latipilis*, has been detected in colonies of laboratory opossums (Smith 2016). Inasmuch as this mite species has been isolated from other wild South American marsupials of the family Didelphidae (Fain et al. 1981, 1996), these mites were probably present on the wild *Monodelphis domestica* that were imported to the USA. The mites are not known to have any impact on the health and well-being of the opossums, but they can be eliminated by treating the animals topically with ivermectin in mineral oil or polypropylene at a dose of 2.0 mg/kg (Smith 2016).

Non-infectious diseases

Based on 150 necropsies of *Monodelphis* that became ill or died spontaneously, the most prevalent pathological changes were in the digestive (38%), urogenital (19%), cardiovascular (12%) and respiratory (19%) systems (Hubbard et al. 1997). The primary disease problems were rectal prolapse, congestive heart failure and dermatitis.

Cloacal prolapse was a common problem in laboratory opossum females in earlier years, particularly in lactating females (Cothran et al. 1985), but this condition has become much less common in the authors' colony. It is possible that animals resistant to this condition under laboratory conditions have been highly favoured by selection. It also is possible that the incidence of cloacal prolapse was reduced when the standard diet fed to the animals in this colony was switched from commercial fox chow to the Purina diet that is fed today (see section on 'Feeding/watering'). Other husbandry practices that might have impacted the incidence of cloacal prolapse were the change from wood shavings to ground corn cobs as bedding, and the change from providing tap water to providing water purified by reverse osmosis. The incidence of cloacal prolapse at another colony (P.B. Samollow, personal communication) was eliminated by providing grapes and laxatone ('a quarter-sized dollop') on a petri dish to nursing mothers a few times per week and feeding them water-softened chow. It was noted that the presence of water-softened chow had the added benefit of stimulating more rapid growth of the suckling pups.

Recently, two novel species of *Helicobacter* were isolated from laboratory opossums, some of which had developed cloacal prolapses; however, it is not known if these *Helicobactor* species are associated in any way with cloacal prolapses (Shen et al. 2020).

The most common neoplasia is pituitary adenoma, followed by uterine lesions and cutaneous lipomas (Kuehl-Kovarik et al. 1994; Hubbard et al. 1997).

No zoonoses have been identified.

As stated previously, desiccation and necrosis of the extremely thin and poorly vascularised ear pinnae frequently occurs when humidity levels are at 35% or lower. Tails, which also are poorly vascularised, are also prone to necrosis at low humidity levels. This problem can be prevented or arrested by maintaining the humidity at the recommended level of 45–70%.

Loss of hair (alopecia), most frequently near the tail on the rump, occurs commonly in females, especially when they are lactating, and rarely in males. There is no apparent detriment to health from hair loss.

Reproductive problems

In addition to those animals that fail to reproduce (see the section entitled 'Breeding'), some females that readily produce litters routinely cannibalise them during the first two weeks after parturition. In the authors' colony, females that fail to wean three consecutive litters are generally culled.

When the mother of a valuable litter dies, cross-fostering to another mother can be employed to rear the litter to weaning if the pups are old enough to release the teat. However, milk production may not be sufficient for survival of members of an existing litter in addition to foster pups. Therefore, fostering is generally practised only when the mother of an especially valuable litter dies. In that case, a foster mother is required whose pups are at the same age as the orphaned litter and whose litter size is at least as large as the litter to be fostered. The foster mother's pups are euthanised and replaced in the nest by the foster pups.

Cross-fostering has been successful for litters between two and four weeks of age. Beyond four weeks of age, orphaned litters can be reared by feeding Purina pellets liquefied with water; the liquefied feed is fed via an eye dropper three to four times per day. In addition, half-and-half cow's milk may be provided in a shallow dish, such as a Petri dish, along with small pieces of hard-boiled eggs. As the animals mature, the amount of water added to the pellets is gradually reduced until the feed has a pasty consistency by the time the animals are six weeks old. By six to seven weeks of age, the animals can eat moistened pellets in a shallow dish. By eight weeks, the age at which they are normally weaned, most pups are able to consume unsoftened pelleted feed.

Behavioural/abnormal behaviour

While aggressive behaviour often occurs when adults are paired for mating, it was noted in the early years of seeking a nutritionally adequate diet that animals fed diets that were sub-optimal behaved even more aggressively towards their mates and towards human handlers. In addition, mothers fed sub-optimal diets exhibited a higher rate of cannibalism of their pups.

Some laboratory opossums may exhibit various stereotypic behaviours when housed in standard rodent cages. These behaviours include bar chewing, tail chasing, rolling onto the back and head spinning (Wilkinson et al. 2010). In addition, the authors have observed repetitive summersaulting. When some opossums that exhibited these behaviours were moved into a larger enclosure (145 × 83 cm versus 56 × 38 cm) that was highly enriched, the animals did not exhibit stereotypic behaviours (Wilkinson et al. 2010). It is not known which of the environmental conditions – cage size, enrichment materials and devices and change to a novel environment – contributed to the change in behaviour.

Signs of poor welfare or poor health

Stereotypic behaviour, which can be caused by deficiencies in diet or housing, is a sign of poor welfare. Behaviour should be monitored, and changes in diet, housing, enrichment practices and caretaking practices should be considered and implemented in an effort to reduce stereotypic behaviour.

As stated previously, rapid breathing, poor coat condition and loss of body weight are signs of poor welfare due to infectious diseases, and poor coat condition and loss of body weight may also be indicative on non-infectious diseases.

Haematological and serum chemical values have been determined for healthy laboratory opossums maintained under standard conditions (VandeBerg et al. 1986; Cothran et al. 1990; Evans et al. 2010). These values may be useful as reference values in instances where health problems are suspected.

References

Allison, S.O., Criley, J.M., Kim, J.Y. et al. (2011) Cage change intervals for opossums (Monodelphis domestica) in individually ventilated cages. Journal of the American Association for Laboratory Animal Science, 50, 647–652.

Armstrong, J.R. and Ferguson, M.W.J. (1995) Ontogeny of the skin and the transition from scar-free to scarring phenotype during wound healing in the pouch young of a marsupial, Monodelphis domestica. Developmental Biology, 169, 242–260.

AVMA Guidelines for the Euthanasia of Animals: 2020 Edition.

Baggott, L.M. and Moore, H.D.M. (1990) Early embryonic development of the grey short-tailed opossum, Monodelphis domestica, in vivo and in vitro. Journal of Zoology, 222, 623–639.

Ban, J. and Mladinic, M. (2022) Monodelphis domestica: A new source of mammalian primary neurons in vitro. Neural Regeneration Research, 17, 1726–1727.

Barnes, R.D. (1977) The special anatomy of Marmosa robinsoni. In: The Biology of Marsupials. Ed. Hunsaker, D., II, pp. 387–413. Academic Press, New York.

Barnes, R.D. and Barthold, S.W. (1969) Reproduction and breeding behaviour in an experimental colony of Marmosa mitis Bangs (Didelphidea). Journal of Reproduction and Fertility, 6 S, 477–482.

Barnett, G.J., Barnett, I.J., Wilson, S.R. (2017) Comparison of 6 injectable anesthetic regimens and isoflurane in gray short-tailed opossums (Monodelphis domestica). Journal of the American Association for Laboratory Animal Science, 56, 544–549.

Beiriger, A. and Sears K.E. (2014) Cellular basis of differential limb growth in postnatal gray short-tailed opossums (Monodelphis domestica). Journal of Experimental Zoology. Part B, Molecular and Developmental Evolution, 322, 221–229.

Benato, L., Eatwell, K. and Stidworthy, M.F. (2010) Necrosis of the pinnae in a grey short-tailed opossum (Monodelphis domestica). Veterinary Record, 166, 121–122

Blanton, L.S., Quade, B.R., Ramirez-Hernandez, A. et al. (2022) Experimental Rickettsia typhi infection in Monodelphis domestica: Implications for opossums as an amplifying host in the suburban cycle of murine typhus. American Journal of Tropical Medicine and Hygiene, 107, 102–109.

Busse, S., Lutter, D., Heldmaier, G. et al. (2014) Torpor at high ambient temperature in a neotropical didelphid, the grey short-tailed opossum (Monodelphis domestica). Naturwissenschaften, 101, 1003–1006.

Cardoso-Moreira, M., Halbert, J., Valloton, D. et al. (2019) Gene expression across mammalian organ development. Nature, 571, 505–509.

Chan, J., Donalson, L.M., Kushwaha, R.S. et al. (2008) Differential expression of hepatic genes involved in cholesterol homeostasis in high- and low-responding strains of laboratory opossums. Metabolism, 57, 718–724.

Chan, J., Mahaney, M.C., Kushwaha, R.S. et al. (2010) ABCB4 mediates diet-induced hypercholesterolemia in laboratory opossums. Journal of Lipid Research, 51, 2922–2928.

Chan, J., Sharkey, F.E., Kushwaha, R.S. et al. (2012) Steatohepatitis in laboratory opossums exhibiting a high lipemic response to dietary cholesterol and fat. American Journal of Physiology. Gastrointestinal and Liver Physiology, 303, G12–19.

Christian, D.P. (1983) Water balance in Monodelphis domestica (Didelphidae) from the semiarid caatinga of Brazil. Comparative Biochemistry and Physiology, 74(A), 665–669.

Civen, R. and Ngo, V. (2008) Murine typhus: an unrecognized suburban vectorborne disease. Clinical Infectious Diseases, 46, 913–918.

Cothran, E.G., Aivaliotis, M.J. and VandeBerg, J.L. (1985) The effects of diet on growth and reproduction in the gray short-tailed opossum (Monodelphis domestica). Journal of Experimental Zoology, 236, 103–114.

Cothran, E.G., Haines, C.K. and VandeBerg, J.L. (1990) Age effects on hematologic and serum chemical values in gray short-tailed opossums (Monodelphis domestica). Laboratory Animal Science, 40, 192–197.

Crisp, E.A., Messer, M. and VandeBerg, J.L. (1989) Changes in milk carbohydrates during lactation in a didelphid marsupial, Monodelphis domestica. Physiological Zoology, 62, 1117–1125.

Dawson, T.J. and Olson J.M. (1988) Thermogenic capabilities of the opossum Monodelphis domestica when warm and cold acclimated: similarities between American and Australian marsupials. Comparative Biochemistry and Physiology, 89(A), 85–91.

Drabeck, D.H., Rucavado, A., Hingst-Zaher, E. et al. (2020) Resistance of South American opossums to vWF-binding venom C-type lectins. Toxicon. 2020 Mar 2. pii: S0041-0101(20)30069-6. doi: 10.1016/j.toxicon.2020.02.024. [Epub ahead of print].

Dias Cordeiro, M., de Azevedo Baêta, B., Barizon Cepeda, M. et al. (2019) Experimental infection of Monodelphis domestica with Rickettsia parkeri. Ticks and Tick Borne Diseases, 2019 Dec 24: 101366. doi: 10.1016/j.ttbdis.2019.101366. [Epub ahead of print].

Dooley, T.P., Mattern, V.L., Moore, C.M. et al. (1995) UV-induced melanoma: a karyotype with a single translocation is stable after allografting and metastasis. Cancer Genetics and Cytogenetics, 83, 155–159.

Dooley, J.C., Franca, J.G., Seelke, A.M.H. et al. (2013) A connection to the past: Monodelphis domestica provides insight into the organization and connectivity of the brains of early mammals. Journal of Comparative Neurology, 521, 3877–3897.

Dowling, A., Doroba, C., Maier, J.A. et al. (2016) Cellular and molecular drivers of differential organ growth: insights from the limbs of

Monodelphis domestica. *Development Genes and Evolution*, **226**, 235–243.

Duke, S.E., Samollow, P.B., Mauceli, E. *et al.* (2007) Integrated cytogenetic BAC map of the genome of the gray, short-tailed opossum, Monodelphis domestica. *Chromosome Research*, **15**, 361–370.

Dyke, B. (1989) *PEDSYS. A Pedigree Data Management System. Users Manual*. PGL Technical Report No. 2. Southwest Foundation for Biomedical Research, San Antonio, Texas.

Dutta, S. and Sengupta, P. (2016) Men and mice: Relating their ages. *Life Sciences*, **52**, 244–248.

Evans, K.D., Hewett, T.A., Clayton, C.J. *et al.* (2010) Normal organ weights, serum chemistry, hematology, and cecal and nasopharyngeal bacterial cultures in the gray short-tailed opossum (Monodelphis domestica). *Journal of the American Association of Laboratory Animal Science*, **49**, 401–406.

Fadem, B.H. and Rayve, R.S. (1985) Characteristics of the oestrous cycle and influence of social factors in gray short-tailed opossums (*Monodelphis domestica*). *Journal of Reproduction and Fertility*, **73**, 337–342.

Fadem, B.H. and Tesoriero, J.V. (1986) Inhibition of testicular development and feminization of the male genitalia by neonatal estrogen treatment in a marsupial. *Biology of Reproduction*, **34**, 771–776.

Fain, A., Méndez, E. and Lukoschus, F.S. (1981) Archemyobia (Nearchemyobia) latipilis sp.n. (Acari: Prostigmata: Myobiidae) parasitic on marsupials in Panama and Brazil. *Revista de Biologia Tropical*, **29**, 77–81.

Fain, A., Zanatta-Coutinho, M.T. and Fonseca, M.T. (1996) Observations on a small collection of mites (Acari) parasitic on mammals from Brazil. *Entomologie*, **66**, 57–63.

Ferner, K. (2018) Skin structure in newborn marsupials with focus on cutaneous gas exchange. *Journal of Anatomy*, **233**, 311–327.

Finney, J., Yang, G., Kuraoka, M. *et al.* (2019) Cross-reactivity to kynureninase tolerizes B cells that express the HIV-1 broadly neutralizing antibody 2F5. *Journal of Immunology*, **203**, 3268–3281.

Frost, S.B. and Masterton, R.B. (1994) Hearing in primitive mammals: *Monodelphis domestica* and *Marmosa elegans*. *Hearing Research*, **76**, 67–72.

Fry, E.J. and Saunders, N.R. (2000) Spinal repair in mammals, a novel approach using the South American opossum *Monodelphis domestica*. *Clinical and Experimental Pharmacology and Physiology*, **27**, 542–547.

Garrett, A., Lannigan, V., Yates, N.J. *et al.* (2019) Physiological and anatomical investigation of the auditory brainstem in the fat-tailed dunnart (*Sminthopsis crassicaudata*). *PeerJ*, 2019 Sep 30; **7**, e7773. doi: 10.7717/peerj.7773. eCollection 2019.

Gentles, A.J., Wakefield, M.J., Kohany, O. *et al.* (2007) Evolutionary dynamics of transposable elements in the short-tailed opossum Monodelphis domestica. *Genome Research*, **17**, 992–1004.

Gil, M., Torres-Reverón, A., Ramirez, A.C. *et al.* (2019) Influence of biological sex on social behavior, individual recogntion, and non-associative learning in the adult gray short-tailed opossum (Monodelphis domestica). *Physiology & Behaviour*, **211**, 112659. doi: 10.1016/j.physbeh.2019.112659. Epub 2019 Aug 26.

Graves, J.A. and Renfree M.B. (2013) Marsupials in the age of genomics. *Annual Review of Genomics and Human Genetics*, **14**, 393–420.

Gu, W., Ray, D.A., Walker, J.A. *et al.* (2007) SINEs, evolution and genome structure in the opossum. *Gene*, **396**, 46–58.

Hickford, D., Frankenberg, S. and Renfree, M. (2009) The tammar wallaby, *Macropus eugenii*: A model kangaroo for the study of developmental and reproductive biology. *Cold Spring Harbor Protocols*, 2009, doi. 10.1101/pdb.emo137.

Hinds, L.A., Fletcher, T.P. and Rodger, J.C. (1996) Hormones of oestrus and ovulation and their manipulation in marsupials. *Reproduction, Fertility, and Development*, **8**, 661–672.

Holz, P. (2015) Marsupials. In: *Zoo and Wild Animal Medicine*, vol. 8. Eds Miller, R.E. and Fowler, M.E., pp. 255–274. Elsevier Saunders, St. Louis.

Hubbard, G.B., Mahaney, M.C., Gleiser, C.A. *et al.* (1997) Spontaneous pathology of the laboratory opossum (*Monodelphis domestica*). *Laboratory Animal Science*, **47**, 19–26.

International Air Transport Association (2020) *Live Animals Regulations*, 47th edn. International Air Transport Association, Montreal-Geneva.

Jensen T, Kiersgaard M, Sørensen D. and Mikkelsen L. (2013) Fasting of mice: A review. *Laboratory Animals*, **47**, 225–240.

Johnston, P.G., Dean, A., VandeBerg, J.L. *et al.* (1994) HPRT activity in embryos of a South American opossum *Monodelphis domestica*. *Reproduction, Fertility and Development*, **6**, 529–532.

Jurgelski, W. (1987) American marsupials. In: *The UFAW Handbook on the Care and Management of Laboratory Animals*, 6th edn. Ed. Poole, T.B., pp. 189–206. Longman Scientific and Technical, Harlow.

Keyte, A.L. and Smith, K.K. (2008a) Harvesting Monodelphis embryos. *CSH Protocols*, Oct 1; 2008: pdb.prot5074. doi: 10.1101/pdb.prot5074.

Keyte, A.L. and Smith, K.K. (2008b) Monodelphis whole-embryo culture. *CSH Protocols*, Oct 1; 2008: pdb.prot5075. doi: 10.1101/pdb.prot5075.

Keyte, A.L. and Smith, K.K. (2008c) Basic maintenance and breeding of the opossum Monodelphis domestica. *CSH Protocols*, Oct 1; 2008: pdb.prot5073. doi: 10.1101/pdb.prot5073.

Kraus, D.B. and Fadem, B.H. (1987) Reproduction, development and physiology of the gray short-tailed opossum (*Monodelphis domestica*). *Laboratory Animal Science*, **37**, 478–482.

Kuehl-Kovarik, C., Sakaguchi, D.S., Iqbal, J. *et al.* (1995) The gray short-tailed opossum: a novel model for mammalian development. *Lab Animal*, **24**, 24–29.

Kuehl-Kovarik, M.C., Ackermann, M.R., Hanson, D.L. *et al.* (1994) Spontaneous pituitary adenomas in the Brazilian gray short-tailed opossum (*Monodelphis domestica*). *Veterinary Pathology*, **31**, 377–379

Kumar, S., De Leon, E.M., Granados, J. *et al.* (2022) *Monodelphis domestica* induced pluripotent stem cells reveal metatherian pluripotency architecture. *International Journal of Molecular Science*, **23**, 12623. doi: 10.3390/ijms232012623

Küster, T., Zumkehr, B., Hermann, C. (2012). Voluntary ingestion of antiparasitic drugs emulsified in honey represents an alternative to gavage in mice. *Journal of the American Association for Laboratory Animal Science*, **51**, 219–223.

Kyonari, H., Kaneko, M., Shiraishi, A. *et al.* (2021) Targeted gene disruption in a marsupial, Monodelphis domestica, by CRISPR?Cas9 genome editing. *Current Biology*, 2021 Jul 13;S0960-9822(21)00885-X. doi: 10.1016/j.cub.2021.06.056. Online ahead of print 10.1016/j.cub.2021.06.056. Online ahead of print.

Lane, M.A., Truettner, J.S., Brunschwig, J.P. *et al.* (2007) Age-related differences in the local and molecular responses to injury in developing spinal cord of the opossum, *Monodelphis domestica*. *European Journal of Neuroscience*, **25**, 1725–1742.

Lemos, B. (2007) The opossum genome reveals further evidence for regulatory evolution in mammalian diversification. *Genome Biology*, **8**, 223.

Macrini, T.E. (2004) *Monodelphis domestica*. *Mammalian Species*, **760**, 1–8.

Mahadevaiah, S.K., Royo, H., VandeBerg, J.L. *et al.* (2009) Key features of the X inactivation process are conserved between marsupials and eutherians. *Current Biology*, **19**, 1478–1484.

Majka, P., Chlodzinska, N., Turlejski, K. *et al.* (2018) A three-dimensional stereotaxic atlas of the gray short-tailed opossum (Monodelphis domestica) brain, *Brain Structure & Function*, **223**, 1779–1795.

Manis, G.S., Hubbard, G.B., Hainsey, B.M. *et al.* (1992) Effects of chronic blood loss in a marsupial (*Monodelphis domestica*). *Laboratory Animal Science*, **42**, 567–571.

Martin, B.J. (1995) Evaluation of hypothermia for anesthesia in reptiles and amphibians. *ILAR Journal*, **37**, 186–190.

Mate, K.E., Robinson, E.S., VandeBerg, J.L. et al. (1994) Timetable of *in vivo* embryonic development in the grey short-tailed opossum (*Monodelphis domestica*). *Molecular Reproduction and Development*, **39**, 365–374.

Merry, D.E., Pathak, S. and VandeBerg, J.L. (1983) Differential NOR activities in somatic and germ cells of *Monodelphis domestica* (Marsupialia, Mammalia). *Cytogenetics and Cell Genetics*, **35**, 244–251.

Mikkelsen, T.S., Wakefiled, M.J., Aken, B. et al. (2007) Genome of the marsupial *Monodelphis domestica* reveals innovation in non-coding sequences. *Nature*, **447**, 167–177.

Miles, K.G., Sonea, I.M., Jackson, L.L. et al. (1997) Ultrasonographic pregnancy detection and inhalation anesthesia in the gray short-tailed opossum (Monodelphis domestica). *Laboratory Animal Science*, **47**, 280–282.

Mithun, M. (2001). *The Languages of Native North America*. Cambridge University Press. p. 332. ISBN 978-0-521-29875-9.

Mladinic, M., Wintzer, M., Del Bel, E. et al. (2005) Differential expression of genes at stages when regeneration can and cannot occur after injury to immature mammalian spinal cord. *Cellular and Molecular Neurobiology*, **25**, 407–426.

Modepalli, V., Kumar, A. Hinds, L. et al. (2014) BMC Genomics 2014 Nov 23;15(1):1012. doi: 10.1186/1471-2164-15-1012.

Modepalli, V., Kumar, A., Sharp, J.A. et al. (2018) Gene expression profiling of postnatal lung development in the marsupial gray short-tailed opossum (Monodelphis domestica) highlights conserved developmental pathways and specific characteristics during lung organogenesis. *BMC Genomics*, **19**, 732.

Molineaux, A.C., Maier, J.A., Schecker, T. et al. (2015) Exogenous retinoic acid induces digit reduction in opossums (Monodelphis domestica) by disrupting cell death and proliferation, and apical ectodermal ridge and zone of polarizing activity function. *Birth Defects Research. A, Clinical and Molecular Teratology*, **103**, 225–234.

Mollgard, K., Blaslev, Y., Stagaard, J. et al. (1994) Development of spinal cord in the isolated CNS of a neonatal mammal (the opossum *Monodelphis domestica*) maintained in longterm culture. *Journal of Neurocytology*, **23**, 151–165.

Moore, H.D.M. and Taggart, D.A. (1993) *in vitro* fertilization and embryo culture in the grey short-tailed opossum *Monodelphis domestica*. *Journal of Reproduction and Fertility*, **98**, 267–274.

Morrissey, K.A., Wegrecki, M, Praveena, T. et al. (2021) The molecular assembly of the marsupial γμ T cell receptor defines a third T cell lineage. *Science*, 2021 Mar 26; **371**(6536), 1383–1388. doi: 10.1126/science.abe7070.

Morykwas, M.J., Ditesheim, J.A., Ledbetter, M.S. et al. (1991) *Monodelphis domesticus*: a model for early developmental wound healing. *Annals of Plastic Surgery*, **27**, 327–331.

Nair, H.B., and VandeBerg, J.L. (2012) Laboratory opossum (*Monodelphis domestica*) model for melanoma chemoprevention. *Journal of Cancer Science and Therapy*, **4**, xiv–xv.

Nair, H.B., Ford, A., Dick, E.J. Jr. et al. (2014) Modeling sunscreen-mediated melanoma prevention in the laboratory opossum (Monodelphis domestica). *Pigment Cell and Melanoma Research*, **27**, 843–845.

National Research Council (1992) *Recognition and Alleviation of Pain and Distress in Laboratory Animals*, p. 83. National Academy Press, Washington, DC.

Noor, N.M., Steer, D.L., Wheaton, B.J. et al. (2011) Age-dependent changes in the proteome following complete spinal cord transection in a postnatal South American opossum (*Monodelphis domestica*). *PLoS One* 2011; **6**(11), e27465. doi: 10.1371/journal.pone.0027465. Epub 2011 Nov 16.

Nowak, R.M. (1999) *Walker's Mammals of the World*, 6th edn. The Johns Hopkins University Press, Baltimore.

Pathak, S., Ronne, M., Brown, C.L. et al. (1993) A high-resolution banding ideogram of *Monodelphis domestica* chromosomes (Marsupialia, Mammalia). *Cytogenetics and Cell Genetics*, **63**, 181–184.

Petrovic, A., Ban, J., Tomljanovic, I. et al. (2021) Establishment of long-term primary cortical neuronal cultures from neonatal opossum *Monodelphis domestica*. *Frontiers in Cellular Neuroscience* 2021 Mar 18;15:661492. doi: 10.3389/fncel.2021.661492. eCollection 2021.

Pine, R.H. and Handley, C.O. Jr. (2008) Genus *Monodelphis* Burnett, 1830. In: *Mammals of South America, Volume 1: Marsupials, Xenarthrans, Shrews, and Bats*. Ed. Gardner, A.L., pp. 82–85. University of Chicago Press, Chicago.

Pye, G.W. (2006) *Marsupials*. In: *Guidelines for Euthanasia of Nondomestic Animals*. Ed. Kirk-Baer, C., pp. 52–56. American Association of Zoo Veterinarians (AAZV) http://www.aazv.org

Robinson, E.S., Renfree, M.B., Short, R.V. et al. (1991) Mammary glands in male marsupials. 2. Development of teat primordia in *Didelphis virginiana* and *Monodelphis domestica*. *Reproduction, Fertility, and Development*, **3**, 295–301.

Robinson, E.S. and VandeBerg, J.L. (1994) Blood collection and surgical procedures for the laboratory opossum (*Monodelphis domestica*). *Laboratory Animal Science*, **44**, 63–68.

Robinson, E.S., VandeBerg, J.L., Hubbard, G.B. et al. (1994) Malignant melanoma in ultraviolet-irradiated laboratory opossums: initiation in suckling young, metastasis in adults, and xenograft behavior in nude mice. *Cancer Research*, **54**, 5986–5991.

Robinson, E.S., VandeBerg, J.L., Watson, C.M. et al. (1996) Intersexual phenotypes and sex chromosome complements of five gray short-tailed opossums. *Laboratory Animal Science*, **46**, 555–560.

Roellig, D.M., McMillan, K., Ellis, A.E. et al. (2010) Experimental infection of two South American reservoirs with four distinct strains of Trypanosoma cruzi. *Parasitology* 2010 May; **137**(6), 959–66. doi: 10.1017/S0031182009991995. Epub 2010 Feb 4.

Rousmaniere, H., Silverman, R., White, R.A. et al. (2010) Husbandry of Monodelphis domestica in the study of mammalian embryogenesis. *Laboratory Animals*, **39**, 219–226.

Sales, G.D., Wilson, K.J., Spencer, K.E. and Milligan, S.R. (1988) Environmental ultrasound in laboratories and animal houses: a possible cause for concern in the welfare and use of laboratory animals. *Laboratory Animals*, 1988 Oct; **22**(4), 369–375. doi: 10.1258/002367788780746188.

Samollow, P.B. (2006) Status and applications of genomic resources for the gray, short-tailed opossum, *Monodelphis domestica*, an American marsupial model for comparative biology. *Australian Journal of Zoology*, **54**, 173–196.

Samollow, P.B. (2008) The opossum genome: insights and opportunities from an alternative mammal. *Genome Research*, **18**, 1199–1215.

Samollow, P.B., Gouin, N., Miethke, P. et al. (2007) A microsatellite-based, physically anchored linkage map for the gray, short-tailed opossum (*Monodelphis domestica*). *Chromosome Research*, **15**, 269–281.

Samples, N.K., VandeBerg, J.L. and Stone, W.H. (1986) Passively acquired immunity in the newborn of a marsupial (*Monodelphis domestica*). *American Journal of Reproductive Immunology and Microbiology*, **11**, 94–97.

Saunders, N.R., Adam, E., Reader, M. et al. (1989) Monodelphis domestica (grey short-tailed opossum): an accessible model for studies of early neocortical development. *Anatomy and Embryology (Berl)*, **180**, 227–236.

Saunders, N.R., Deal, A., Knott, G.W. et al. (1995) Repair and recovery following spinal cord injury in a neonatal marsupial (*Monodelphis domestica*). *Clinical and Experimental Pharmacology and Physiology*, **22**, 518–526.

Saunders, N.R., Noor, N.M., Dziegielewska, K.M. et al. (2014) Age-dependent transcriptome and proteome following transection of neonatal spinal cord of Monodelphis domestica (South American grey short-tailed opossum). *PLoS One*, **9**(6), e99080. doi: 10.1371/journal.pone.0099080. eCollection 2014.

Schraven, A.L, Stannard, H.J., Ong, O.T.W. et al. (2020) Immunogenetics of marsupial B-cells. *Molecular Immunology*, **117**, 1–11.

Sears, K.E., Patel, A., Hübler, M. *et al.* (2012) Disparate Igf1 expression and growth in the fore- and hind limbs of a marsupial mammal (Monodelphis domestica). *Journal of Experimental Zoology. Part B, Molecular and Developmental Evolution*, **318**, 279–293.

Selwood, L., Robinson, E.S., Pedersen, R.A. *et al.* (1997) Development *in vitro* in marsupials: a comparative review of species and a timetable of cleavage and early blastocyst stages of development in *Monodelphis domestica*. *International Journal of Developmental Biology*, **41**, 397–410.

Selwood, L. and VandeBerg, J.L. (1992) The influence of incubation temperature on oocyte maturation, parthenogenetic and embryonic development *in vitro* of the marsupial *Monodelphis domestica*. *Animal Reproduction Science*, **29**, 99–116.

Shen, Z., Mannion, A, Lin, M. *et al.* (2020) *H. monodelphidis* sp. nov. and *Helicobacter Didelphidarum* sp. nov., isolated from grey short-tailed opossums (*Monodelphis domestica*) with endemic cloacal prolapses. *International Journal of Systematic and Evolutionary Microbiology*, **70**, 6032–6043.

Smith, B.D. (2016) Diagnosis and treatment of the mite *Archemyobia* (*Nearchemyobia*) *latipilis* found in the Brazilian opossum (*Monodelphis domestica*). *Journal of the American Association for Laboratory Animal Science*, **55**, 618 (abstract).

Sorensen, D., Sackett, A., Urban, D.J. *et al.* (2017) A new mammalian model system for thalidomide teratogenesis: Monodelphis domestica. *Reproductive Toxicology*, **70**, 126–132.

Stewart, R.R., Zou, D.-J., Treherne, J.M. *et al.* (1991) The intact central nervous system of the newborn opossum in long-term culture: fine structure and GABA-mediated inhibition of electrical activity. *Journal of Experimental Biology*, **161**, 25–41.

Stonebrook, M.J. and Harder, J.D. (1992) Sexual maturation in female gray short-tailed opossums, *Monodelphis domestica*, is dependent upon male stimuli. *Biology of Reproduction*, **46**, 290–294.

Streilein, K.E. (1982) Behavior, ecology, and distribution of South American marsupials. In: *Mammalian Biology in South America*. Eds Mares, M.A. and Genoways, H.H., pp. 231–250. Pymatuning Symposia in Ecology. Special Publications Series. Linesville, PA: Pymatuning Laboratory of Ecology, University of Pittsburgh.

Suárez, R., Paolino, A., Kozulin, P. *et al.* (2017) Development of body, head and brain features in the Australian fat-tailed dunnart (Sminthopsis crassicaudata; Marsupialia: Dasyuridae); A postnatal model of forebrain formation. *PLoS One*. 2017 Sep 7; **12(9)**, e0184450. doi: 10.1371/journal.pone.0184450. eCollection 2017.

Tepper, B., Aniszewska, A., Bartkowska, K. *et al.* (2019) Aged opossums show alterations in spatial learning behavior and reduced neurogenesis in the dentate gyrus. *Frontiers in Neuroscience*. 2019 Nov 12; **13**, 1210. doi: 10.3389/fnins.2019.01210. eCollection 2019.

Thomas, J.M. III, Garcia, J., Terry, M. *et al.* (2019) *Monodelphis domestica* as a fetal intra-cerebral inoculation model for Zika virus pathogenesis. bioRxiv preprint doi: https://doi.org/10.1101/785220 .

Taylor, J.S.H. and Guillery, R.W. (1995) Does early monocular enucleation in a marsupial effect the surviving uncrossed retinofugal pathway? *Journal of Anatomy*, **186**, 335–342

Tomljanovic, I., Petrovic, A., Ban, J. and Mladinic, M. (2022) Proteomic analysis of opossum *Monodelphis domestica* spinal cord reveals the changes of proteins related to neurodegenerative diseases during developmental period when neuroregeneration stops being possible. *Biochemical and Biophysical Research Communications*, **587**, 85–91.

Tyndale-Biscoe, C.H. (1973) *Life of Marsupials*. Edward Arnold, London.

van Nievelt, A.F.H. and Smith, K.K. (2005) Tooth eruption in *Monodelphis domestica* and its significance for phylogeny and natural history. *Journal of Mammalogy*, **86**, 333–341.

van Oorschot, R.A.H., Birmingham, V., Porter, P.A. *et al.* (1993) Linkage between complement components 6 and 7 and glutamic pyruvate transaminase in the marsupial *Monodelphis domestica*. *Biochemical Genetics*, **31**, 215–222.

van Oorschot, R.A.H., Porter, P.A., Kammerer, C.M. *et al.* (1992b) Severely reduced recombination in females of the South American marsupial *Monodelphis domestica*. *Cytogenetics and Cell Genetics*, **60**, 64–67.

van Oorschot, R.A.H., Williams-Blangero, S. and VandeBerg, J.L. (1992a) Genetic diversity of laboratory gray short-tailed opossums (*Monodelphis domestica*): effect of newly introduced wild-caught animals. *Laboratory Animal Science*, **42**, 255–260.

VandeBerg, J.L. (1990) The gray short-tailed opossum (*Monodelphis domestica*) as a model didelphid species for genetic research. *Australian Journal of Zoology*, **37**, 235–247.

VandeBerg, J.L., Cothran, E.G. and Kelly, C.A. (1986) Dietary effects on hematologic and serum chemical values in gray short-tailed opossums (*Monodelphis domestica*). *Laboratory Animal Science*, **36**, 32–36.

VandeBerg, J.L. and Robinson, E.S. (1997) The laboratory opossum (*Monodelphis domestica*) in biomedical research. In: *Recent Advances in Marsupial Biology*. Eds Saunders, N. and Hinds, L., pp. 238–263. University of New South Wales Press, Sydney.

VandeBerg, J.L., and Williams-Blangero, S. (2010) The Laboratory Opossum, in The UFAW Handbook on the Care and Management of Laboratory and Other Research Animals, Eighth Edition (eds R. Hubrecht and J. Kirkwood), Wiley-Blackwell, Oxford, UK. doi: 10.1002/9781444318777.ch19.

Walker, M.K., Boberg, J.R., Walsh, M.T. *et al.* (2012) A less stressful alternative to oral gavage for pharmacological and toxicological studies in mice. *Toxicology and Applied Pharmacology*, **260**, 65–69.

Wang, Z. and VandeBerg, J.L. (2003) Survival anesthetic and injection procedures for neonatal opossums. *Contemporary Topics in Laboratory Animal Science*, **42**, 41–43.

Wang, X., Douglas, K.C., VandeBerg, J.L. *et al.* (2014) Chromosome-wide profiling of X-chromosome inactivation and epigenetic states in fetal brain and placenta of the opossum, Monodelphis domestica. *Genome Research*, **24**, 70–83.

Wheaton, B.J., Callaway, J.K., Ek, C.J. *et al.* (2011) Spontaneous development of full weight-supported stepping after complete spinal cord transection in the neonatal opossum, Monodelphis domestica. *PLoS One*, 2011; **6(11)**, e26826. doi: 10.1371/journal.pone.0026826. Epub 2011 Nov 2.

Wheaton, B.J., Sena, J., Sundararajan, A. et al. (2021) Identification of regenerative processes in neonatal spinal cord injury in the opossum (Monodelphis domestica): A transcriptomic study. *Journal of Comparative Neurology*, 2021 Apr 1; **529(5)**, 969–986. doi: 10.1002/cne.24994. Epub 2020 Aug 4.

Wilkinson, M., Stirton, C. and McConnachie, A. (2010). Behavioural observations of singly-housed grey short-tailed opossums (Monodelphis domestica) in standard and enriched environments. *Laboratory Animals*, **44**, 364–369.

Witt, R.R. and Rodger, J.C. (2018) Recent advances in tools and technologies for monitoring and controlling ovarian activity in marsupials. *Theriogenology*, **109**, 58–69.

Xiong, X., Samollow, P.B., Cao, W. *et al.* (2021). Genetic and genomic architecture in eight strains of the laboratory opossum, Monodelphis domestica. BioRxiv preprint doi: https://doi.org/10.1101/2021.09.02.458745 .

Yang, G., Holl, T.M., Liu, Y. *et al.* (2013) Identification of autoantigens recognized by the 2F5 and 4E10 broadly neutralizing HIV-1 antibodies. *Journal of Experimental Medicine*, **210**, 241–256.

Yoshida, K., Line, J., Griffith, K. *et al.* (2019) Progesterone signaling during pregnancy in the lab opossum, Monodelphis domestica. *Theriogenology*, **136**, 101–110.

20 Tree Shrews

Eberhard Fuchs

Biological overview

General biology

The first report of tree shrews dates back to 1780. The description and an accompanying sketch were from William Ellis, who maintained a naturalist's journal during Captain Cook's third Pacific voyage on the ship *Discovery*. Uncertainties concerning the taxonomic affinities of tree shrews originated with this description, in which tree shrews were designated 'squirrels', a confusion that still occasionally persists today. About 80 years ago, a variety of reports described similarities between tree shrews and primates, and the conclusion that there was a direct phylogenetic relationship between modern tree shrews and primates was predominantly made by Le Gros Clark (1924), largely on the basis of brain anatomy. His view was endorsed in G.G. Simpson's classification of the mammals (Simpson 1945). In the following years, several authorities (Luckett 1980) had doubts about this phylogenetic link and, as a result, excluded tree shrews from primates. An intensive discussion of tree shrews and their phylogenetic relationships is provided in Luckett (1980), Martin (1990) and Emmons (2000). Despite their name, tree shrews have nothing to do with real shrews and most species of tree shrews are much more active on the ground than in trees. Today, tree shrews are placed in their own order, Scandentia, and according to recent molecular phylogenetic studies they are placed together with primates and dermoptera within the clade Euarchonta (Kriegs *et al.* 2007). In 2008, the Board Institute provided the first assembly of the genome of *Tupaia belangeri*[1]. On the basis of more advanced genome information of the Chinese tree shrew (*Tupaia belangeri chinensis*), Fan *et al.* (2014a) postulated that tree shrews have a relatively close relationship to non-human primates. Nevertheless, the long-running debate regarding the phylogenetic position of the tree shrew within eutherian mammals is still not fully settled.

Tree shrews (family Tupaiidae) are subdivided in two subfamilies: the diurnal subfamily Tupaiinae containing five genera (*Tupaia, Anathana, Dendrogale, Lyonogale, Urogale*) and the nocturnal subfamily Ptilocercinae, with a single genus the pen-tailed tree shrew *Ptilocercus*. The geographic distribution of the Tupaiidae extends from India to the Philippines, and from Southern China to Java, Borneo, Sumatra and Bali. Natural habitats are tropical forests and plantation areas (Table 20.1).

In general, tree shrews are similar to squirrels in their external appearance and habits and the Malay word 'tupai' (from which the name *Tupaia* is derived) is used for both tree shrews and squirrels, whereas the Malay word 'tana' (found in the species *Lyonogale tana*) is used only for tree shrews. Although there are clear differences between tree shrew species, they share a basic common pattern that can be described with reference to the relatively well-known Belanger's tree shrew *Tupaia belangeri* (Figure 20.1). All are relatively small and agile, and are in general omnivorous with a preference for small fruits and invertebrates, especially arthropods. Tree shrews range from the predominantly arboreal (*Dendrogale, Tupaia minor, Ptilocercus*) to the predominantly terrestrial (*Lyonogale, Urogale*). But most tree shrew species are semi-arboreal and usually forage on the ground. The terrestrial tree shrews have a long snout and sharp claws both of which are used to obtain food by rooting through the leaf litter on the forest floor. Species which are more arboreal are smaller than the terrestrial species. They have shorter snouts, smaller or poorly developed claws, long tails and more forward-facing eyes. When eating, all species will hold food between the front paws. In general, tree shrews have a well-developed visual system and colour vision has been documented in some species. The vocal repertoire of *Tupaia belangeri* consists of eight distinct sounds. Within this repertoire, four basic acoustic structures can be distinguished which can be associated with functional categories such as alarm, attention contact and defence (Binz & Zimmermann 1989). Tree shrews evaluate social calls linked to sound-associated context, unusualness and acoustic cues (Konerding *et al.* 2011). No ultrasonic vocalisations have been found in *Tupaia belangeri* (Kirchhof *et al.* 2001). The same authors report that during

---

[1] http://ensembl.org/Tupaia_belangeri/Info/Index (accessed 14 July 14 2021)

The UFAW Handbook on the Care and Management of Laboratory and Other Research Animals, Ninth Edition.
Edited by Huw Golledge and Claire Richardson.
© 2024 John Wiley & Sons Ltd. Published 2024 by John Wiley & Sons Ltd.

Table 20.1 Tree shrews, Scandentia, their biological data and distribution.

	Body	Reproduction	Life history	Distribution
Subfamily Tupaiinae *Tupaia* (tree shrews) *T. belangeri*, *T. glis*, *T. gracilis*, *T. javanica*, *T. longipes*, *T. minor*, *T. montana*, *T. nicobaria*, *T. palawanensis*, *T. picta*, *T. splendidula*	BW: 50–270 g HBL: 12–21 cm TL: 14–20 cm NN: 1–3 pairs	GP: 41–55 days L: 1–5 BIW: 6–10 g	W: around 30 days P: around 2 months L: 9–12 years	Tropical forests, semi-terrestrial
Lyonogale (Malaysian tree shrews) *L. tana*, *L. dorsalis*	BW: approx. 300 g HBL: approx. 22 cm TL: approx. 17 cm NN: 2 pairs	GT: 45–55 days L: 1–4 BIW: approx. 10 g	W: around 30 days P: around 2 months L: Unknown	Mainly terrestrial, primary and secondary forests
Urogale (Philippine tree shrew) *U. everetti*	BW: 220–350 g HBL: approx. 20 cm TL: approx. 15 cm NN: 2 pairs	GP: approx. 55 days L: 1–4 BIW: approx. 10 g	W: around 30 days P: probably 2 months L: 6 years	Terrestrial
Anathana (Indian tree shrew) *A. ellioti*, *A. ellioti pallida*, *A. ellioti wroughtoni*	BW: approx. 180 g HBL: approx. 19 cm TL: approx. 18 cm NN: 3 pairs	Unknown	Unknown	Tropical forests, semi-terrestrial
Dendrogale (smooth-tailed tree shrew) *D. melanura*, *D. murina*	BW: approx. 60 g HBL: approx. 13 cm TL: approx. 13 cm NN: 1 pair	Probably like *Tupaia*	Probably like *Tupaia*	Mainly arboreal
Subfamily Ptilocercinae *Ptilocercus lowii* (pen-tailed tree shrew)	BW: approx. 15 g HBL: approx. 14 cm TL: approx. 17 cm NN: 2 pairs	GP: unknown L: probably 1–4 BIW: unknown	Unknown	Nocturnal, arboreal, tropical forests

Source: With modifications from von Holst (1988).
BW, body weight; HBL, head-body length; TL, tail length; NN, number of nipples; GP, gestation period; L, litter size; BIW, birth weight; W, weaning; P, puberty; L: longevity in captivity.

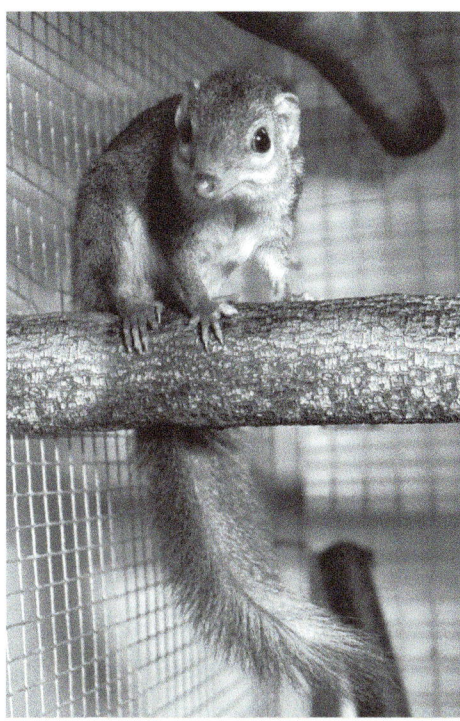

Figure 20.1 Adult male *Tupaia belangeri* from the German Primate Center.

agonistic encounters, adult males produce five distinct call types, partially with graded variants. The calls show harmonic or noisy spectra ranging from 0.4 to 20 kHz. The call structure depends on the dominant status and the motivation of the individuals. Increasing pitch indicates increasing fear, while decreasing pitch and larger frequency range indicate increasing aggression (Kirchhof *et al.* 2001). Recent bioacoustic studies have revealed that valence and emotional arousal is conveyed and recognised in tree shrews (Schehka *et al.* 2007; Schehka & Zimmermann 2012). In addition, tree shrews convey individual identity and emotions acoustically (Schehka *et al.* 2007; Schehka & Zimmermann 2009) and are able to recognise affect intensity via social calls (Schehka & Zimmermann 2012).

All tree shrews seem to use nests both for sleeping and rearing of offspring. Nests may be located in trees or on the ground level. Even tree shrews which spend most of their time in trees avoid climbing on fine branches and do not leap within or between trees. Typically, they use broad branches as support and use trees as a vertical extension of the terrestrial substrate (Martin 1990).

Size range and lifespan

Depending on the species, the body weight of tree shrews ranges between 45 and 350 grams (see Table 20.1) with adult males being usually heavier than adult females (own observation). Their lifespan in the wild is still unknown but in captivity, *Tupaia glis* (Bever & Sprankel 1986) and *Tupaia belangeri* (own observations) can live 10 years or more.

Social organisation

Despite extensive morphological description and behavioural studies in the laboratory, remarkably little is known about the behaviour and the ecological roles of tree shrews in the wild (Emmons 1991; Emmons & Biun 1991; Emmons 2000). Based on observations of Kawamichi and Kawamichi (1979), males of the common tree shrew *Tupaia glis*, which are close relatives to the Belanger's tree shrew, have relatively stable home ranges of about 0.8 ha. The territory of an adult male overlaps to a certain extent with the home range of one adult female and also includes the ranges of a small number of juveniles. This suggests that common tree shrews are basically monogamous in the wild, which is in agreement with observations made in the laboratory where tree shrews can be effectively maintained in pairs. The same authors also reported territorial marking behaviour using the chest gland, and territorial fights between adults of the same sex. Chemical signals play an important role in territorial behaviour of male tree shrews. Scent substances are found in glandular secretions, urine, faeces and saliva, and contain information concerning the identity and physiological state of the individual. Laboratory experiments have shown that in males, both the production of the scent substances and the marking behaviour are controlled by androgens (von Holst & Buergel-Goodwin 1975; von Holst & Eichmann 1998; Eichmann & Holst 1999).

Biological data

The dental formula of the Tupaiidae is: I^2_3 C^1_1 Pm^3_3 M^3_3 (Butler 1980). Core body temperature and its circadian rhythm have been studied by telemetry in *Tupaia belangeri*. Minimal body temperature during the night was about 36°C while during daytime the core temperature increased to a maximum of about 40°C (Refinetti & Menaker 1992; Coolen et al. 2012; Schmelting et al. 2014) (Figure 20.2c). This day/night difference of about 4°C is much larger than of most endotherms.

Systolic blood pressure recorded using the tail-cuff method similar to that often used in rats yielded a mean systolic blood pressure of 125 mmHg (Fuchs et al. 1993). When using this technique, it is not necessary, as is the case with rats, to warm the tree shrew's tail before measurement. In *Tupaia belangeri chinensis*, telemetric recordings revealed a systolic blood pressure of 156 mmHg and a diastolic pressure in the range of 88 mmHg (Wang et al. 2013a).

Heart rates in tree shrews show a surprising pattern of variance. Telemetric analysis has revealed that heart rate is

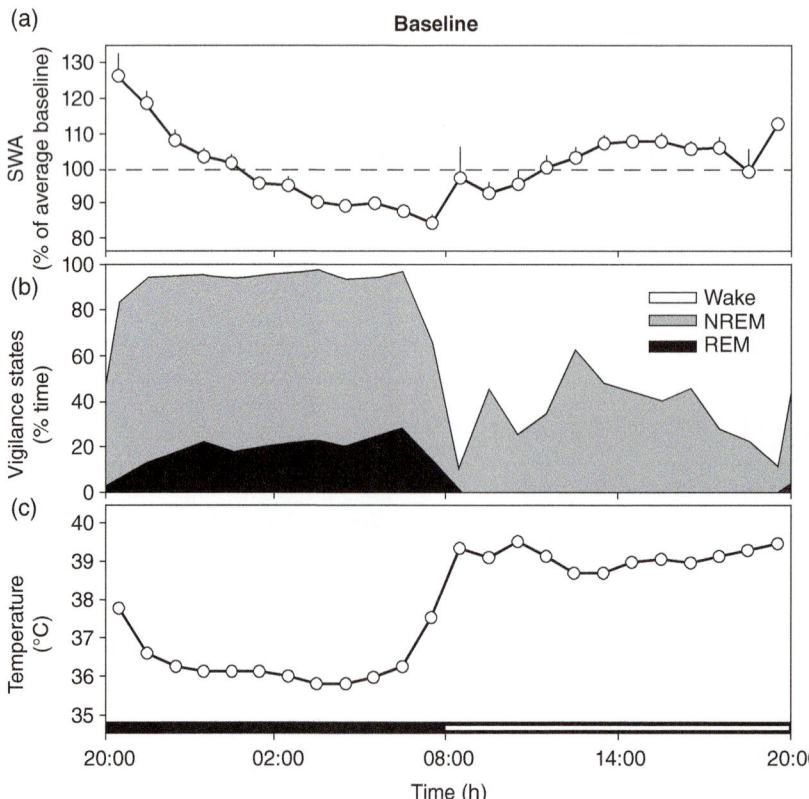

Figure 20.2 Daily rhythms of sleep and body temperature in the tree shrew (*Tupaia belangeri*) under baseline conditions. (a) NREM sleep EEG slow-wave activity; (b) distribution of vigilance states; (c) core body temperature. Data shown are the average of eight animals ±SEM. The black-and-white bar at the bottom of the graph indicates the 12-hr dark/12-hr light cycle (light from 08:00 to 20:00) (from Coolen et al. 2012).

strictly correlated with the behaviour and the emotional status of the animals. A heart rate between 240 and 300 beats/min (own observations) is characteristic of resting periods, while during physical activity, heart rate is in the range between 250 and 350 beats/min and can increase up to 650 beats/min in emotionally exciting situations (Stohr 1986; Muller & Hub 1992; Wang *et al.* 2013a). *Tupaia belangeri* shows a high locomotor activity revealing a clear bimodal pattern with a clear trough in the early afternoon (Kurre & Fuchs 1988) (Figure 20.3).

Sleep architecture and sleep homeostasis in male *Tupaia belangeri* was investigated in detail by telemetry (Coolen *et al.* 2012). The animals share most of the characteristics of sleep structure and sleep homeostasis that have been reported for other mammalian species (Figures 20.2 and 20.4) indicating that the day-active tree shrews may be a valuable model species for studies of sleep regulation and sleep function.

Reliable data on serum constituents are available for *Tupaia belangeri*. Table 20.2 summarises serum values reported by Schwaier (1975). Further, an overview of serum and endocrine data is given by von Holst (1977). Erythrocyte numbers are in the range of $8 \times 10^6/mm^3$, leukocytes in the range of $3 \times 10^3/mm^3$ and mean thrombocyte numbers in the range of $170 \times 10^3/mm^3$ (Zou *et al.* 1983). Basal concentrations for plasma norepinephrine (noradrenaline) range from 2.8 to 36.3 ng/ml and for epinephrine (adrenaline) from 1.3 to 19.1 ng/ml (Fuchs 1984). Corticosterone is the principal corticosteroid (mean 9 ng/ml) in the peripheral plasma and in unstressed animals the ratio corticosterone:cortisol is 4.5:1 (Collins *et al.* 1984). Values of urinary hormones for *Tupaia belangeri* are summarised in Table 20.2.

For the closely related species, *Tupaia belangeri chinensis* basal physiological parameters were reported by Wang *et al.* (2013a).

Breeds, strains and genetics

When selecting a breeding stock for tree shrews, it is important to know the exact origin of the animals. Sometimes, it can be extremely difficult to distinguish between closely related species since traditional classifications do not provide substantial help. Based on their external morphology alone, *Tupaia glis* and *Tupaia belangeri* are difficult to distinguish from one another. The exact taxonomic classification could be ascertained by means of geographical origin, morphological criteria, cytogenetic analysis and analysis of acoustic signals (Toder *et al.* 1992; Esser *et al.* 2008).

Sources of supply

To easily manage the tree shrew genome and physiological data researchers of the Kunming Institute of Zoology, Chinese Academy of Sciences have launched a freely accessible tree shrew data base[2] (Fan *et al.* 2014b).

The Three Rs are a fundamental ethical requirement in laboratory animal science (see Chapter 2, The Three Rs). To refine animal experiments and to reduce the number of animal subjects to a minimum, full control over the genetic background and lifespan of the subjects is required. Therefore, it is strongly recommended that animals should only be obtained from laboratory breeding colonies.

Use in research

Evidence derived from studies on the brain of *Tupaia* by Sir Wilfred Le Gros Clark played a major role in the acceptance of the classification of Tupaiids as primates. Their popularity as experimental subjects in neurobiology, in particular neuroanatomy, has been a direct consequence of their former phylogenetic status in which they were classified as primitive primates (Campbell 1980). The vast majority of experimental work with *Tupaia* has been on the visual system since they were considered ideal subjects to gain insight into the organisation of the early primate visual system. However, it became clear from comparative studies that *Tupaia* possesses none of the features that are characteristic of primate visual systems (Campbell 1980).

Tree shrews have proved to be useful animal models in many instances where a small omnivorous non-rodent species is required for studying fundamental biological functions and disease mechanisms (Cao *et al.* 2003; Yao 2017). Of course, they should only be used where it is appropriate and necessary for the study. They can be used in many fields of preclinical research such as infectious diseases (Li *et al.* 2018) and published a first study of a successful genetic manipulation of tree shrews. This approach could provide the possibility for the generation of various disease models and facilitate the wider application of tree shrews in biomedical research. Further, various aspects of behaviour, infant development, communication and social structures can be investigated in tree shrews (for details: Martin 1968a; Martin 1968b; Hertenstein *et al.* 1987; Benson *et al.* 1992). Based on a study by von Holst (1972), psychosocially stressed male tree shrews were thought to be a suitable model to study the mechanisms

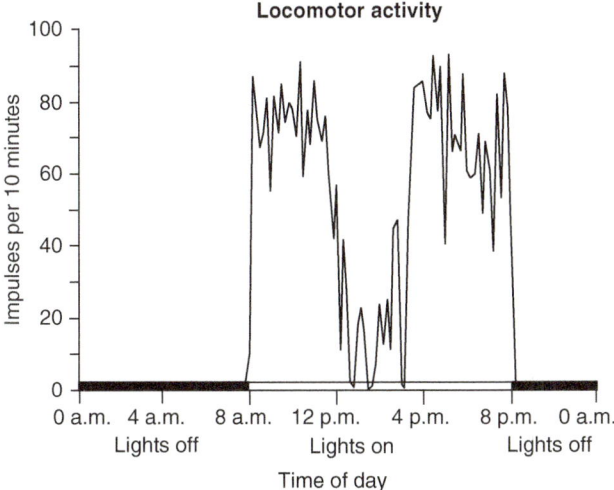

Figure 20.3 Circadian pattern of locomotor activity (with modifications from Kurre & Fuchs 1988).

[2] http://www.treeshrewdb.org (accessed 23 April 2019)

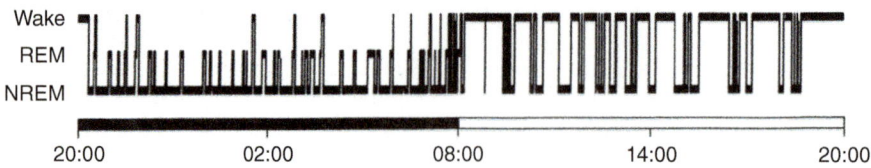

Figure 20.4 Representative 24-hr hypnogram showing the distribution of wakefulness, nonrapid eye movement (NREM) sleep and rapid eye movement (REM) sleep of an individual tree shrew (*Tupaia belangeri*) under baseline conditions. The bar below the hypnogram indicates the light-dark cycle and the time of day (from Coolen et al. 2012).

Table 20.2 Physiological data of adult *Tupaia belangeri*. Blood serum values from Schwaier (1975) and morning urine values from Fuchs (1988).

Parameter	Serum/plasma			Urine			
	Unit	mean	SD	Gender	Unit	mean	SD
Na+	mmol/l	141	2.7	M	mol/ml	95	34
				F	mol/ml	120	48
K+	mmol/l	5.2	0.75	M	mol/ml	85	65
				F	mol/ml	152	43
Na+/K+				M		1.05	0.5
				F		0.82	0.3
Mg^{2+}	mmol/l	2.12	0.24	M	mol/ml	3.5	2
				F	mol/ml	4.3	2.2
Ca^{2+}	mmol/l	5.58	0.88	M	mol/ml	1.25	0.6
				F	mol/ml	1.35	0.5
Fe^{2+}	μmol/l	95					
Cl-	mmol/l	105	3.3				
Osmolarity	mOsmol/l	318	7.8	M	mOsmol/kg H_2O	2000	750
				F	mOsmol/kg H_2O	1950	350
pH				M		6.75	0.6
				F		6.75	0.4
Creatinine	μmol/l	62		M	mol/ml	10.5	4.4
				F	mol/ml	11.2	3.8
Urea		25.8	7.8	M	mol/mol Crea	0.9	0.8
				F	mol/mol Crea	0.9	0.2
Uric acid	mol/l	48		M	g/mol Crea	16	14
				F	g/mol Crea	15	8
Cholesterol	mmol/l	2					
Triglycerides	mol/l	1					
Glucose	mg/100 ml	115.9	16.3	M	mg/mol Crea	0.1	0
				F	mg/mol Crea	0.08	0
Protein	g/100 ml	6.5		M	mg/ml	2.65	1.1
				F	mg/ml	0.3	0.2
Protein/Crea				M	mg/mol Crea	0.25	0.1
				F	mg/mol Crea	0.27	0.1
Prolactin	ng/ml	12					
Cortisol	g/ml	8.8					
Corticosterone				M	pg/mol Crea	335	130
Gastrin	pg/ml	55					
GPT	U/l	10.9	6.2				
GOT	U/l	58	16.8				
LDH	U/l	1872	802				
AP (14-27 month age)	U/l	90.8	48.2				
GH	ng Eq/ml	>50					
Epinephrine (adrenaline)	ng/l	7.5-11		M	pg/mol Crea	47	39
Norepinephrine (noradrenaline)	ng/l	5-6.9		M	pg/mol Crea	103	75
ACTH	pg/ml	65					
TSH	pg/ml	3.5					
FSH	pg/mg	89					
LH	ng/ml	24					

of acute renal failure. However, we and others (Steinhausen *et al.* 1978; Fuchs 2015) were unable to replicate these results.

The pronounced territoriality of, especially in, male tree shrews can be used to establish natural challenging situations under experimental control in the laboratory. When living in visual and olfactory contact with a male conspecific by which it has been defeated, the subordinate Belanger's tree shrew shows dramatic behavioural, physiological and neuroendocrine changes. As we know today, these stress-induced alterations result entirely from the continuous visual presence of the dominant conspecific. In contrast, dominant tree shrews show no noticeable biobehavioural alterations. It is an interesting aspect of preclinical research that many of the alterations in subordinate tree shrews are similar to the symptoms observed in depressed patients and be counteracted by several classes of antidepressant drugs (Fuchs 2005; Wang *et al.* 2013b).

There is a high degree of genetic homology between tree shrews and primates for several receptor proteins of neuromodulators (Fuchs & Flugge 2002) and the amyloid-beta precursor protein (Pawlik *et al.* 1999); this and the three to four times longer lifespan of tree shrews than that of rodents (Keuker *et al.* 2005) suggest that this species may possibly come to be used in future studies focusing on ageing-related brain changes in socially homogenous and stable cohorts.

General Husbandry

Housing

Tree shrews have been housed in enclosures of various sizes. Cages and cage equipment should be adapted to the natural behaviour patterns of the animals, providing enough space for their locomotor activities. The cage equipment thus should include substrates for climbing such as suitable branches and wire mesh. A broad branch (diameter ca 7 cm), board or tube should be fixed near the top of the cage where the animals can rest during their siestas. Objects for scent marking such as branches, pasteboard tubes for hiding and marking should also be offered. It is important that the caging, enrichment items and resting areas are of different sizes and textures to help avoid ulcer formations on the foot pads or potential injury. Outside the cages, wooden sleeping boxes and, for breeding pairs, a separate nest box and nesting material should be provided. The sleeping boxes are made from marine plywood and thus can be thoroughly sanitised. Schwaier (1973) recommended the installation of tunnels made out of flexible plastic tubing, of suitable diameter, which can be fixed outside the cages allowing opportunities for greater travel. Cages should not be side by side and touching unless new animals are being introduced to each other so as to avoid harm. When cages are side by side, they must be separated by opaque screens which prevent interactions other than the exchange of calls and dispersed odours. Cages face to face separated by a corridor are quite satisfactory because they allow visual interactions without the threat of an immediate attack. Below the cages are waste trays lined with paper to catch excrements and food. In general, the caging conditions should allow control and observation of the animals during the active period by the animal care staff. Construction of the animal facilities should allow each room to be emptied of animals from time to time to allow for cleaning, disinfection and repairs. In the rooms, all possible routes of escape must be screened with small diameter wire mesh. To avoid startling the animals, it is recommended that staff should give a sign to the animals before entering an animal room, for example, by knocking on the door. In general, any new items or individuals should be gradually introduced to the animal holding room because tree shrews are very aware of different people and objects.

Tree shrews are best housed at a temperature between 23 and 25°C. Temperatures less than 20°C can be dangerous for the offspring. Humidity is also critical. Experience suggests that minimal levels required are in the range 30–50%.

Little systematic research has been carried out on housing of tree shrews; a description of a successful facility is provided here.

In the German Primate Center, Göttingen, *Tupaia belangeri* are housed in steel cages size 50 cm × 80 cm × 130 cm (w × d × h), (Figure 20.5), or 65 cm × 85 cm × 85 cm (w × d × h). Outside the cages are wooden nest boxes with removable covers (18 cm × 15 cm × 15 cm (w × d × h); entrance 6 cm diameter). These boxes are made from waterproof plywood, which is highly resistant to water and heat and can be effectively cleaned. As the animals stay in the box the whole night, moisture arises and the animals become damp unless open-pored material is used for the nest box. Therefore, boxes made of plastic or metal are inappropriate. The animals can be locked in the box by a shutter and the box can be removed from the cage. Breeding pairs are housed in modular units (two units with nest boxes) which can be separated by a wire mesh frame.

The animal quarters in the German Primate Center are air-conditioned with a relative humidity of 60±7%, a temperature of 27±1°C, and a tenfold air-exchange per hour. The animal rooms are illuminated (L:D=12:12) from 8:00 am to 8:00 pm with six neon lamps (58 W each, light intensity about 900 lux). After lights are on and before lights are shut down, a 30-minute 'sunrise' and a 30-minute 'sunset' with reduced light intensity are programmed. In addition to the neon lamps, each room is equipped with two ultraviolet lamps which are regulated by a separate timer. The total UV exposure time per day is 2 h (four intervals of 30 minutes each). During the night, there is no natural or artificial illumination of the rooms. Each animal room is equipped with one loudspeaker which is active from 8:30 am to 7:30 pm broadcasting news, reports and some music at low volume for background sounds including human voices. Cages are cleaned once a week with water, and the paper under the cages is changed daily. From time to time and depending on the degree of contamination, cages are cleaned in an automatic cage washer. No detergents are used in the animal rooms.

The above description should be considered as an example. Other facilities have somewhat different housing regimes for tree shrews (Schehka & Zimmermann 2012; Nair *et al.* 2014; Shen *et al.* 2014) such as different cage sizes, light cycles or the lack of a loudspeaker in the animal rooms.

Feeding

Tree shrews of the genus *Tupaia* are predominantly insectivorous, but they also eat fruit to add extra calories or nutrients such as calcium to a high protein diet.

At the author's colony, as basic food *Tupaia belangeri* are provided with a specially developed pelleted *Tupaia* diet. In

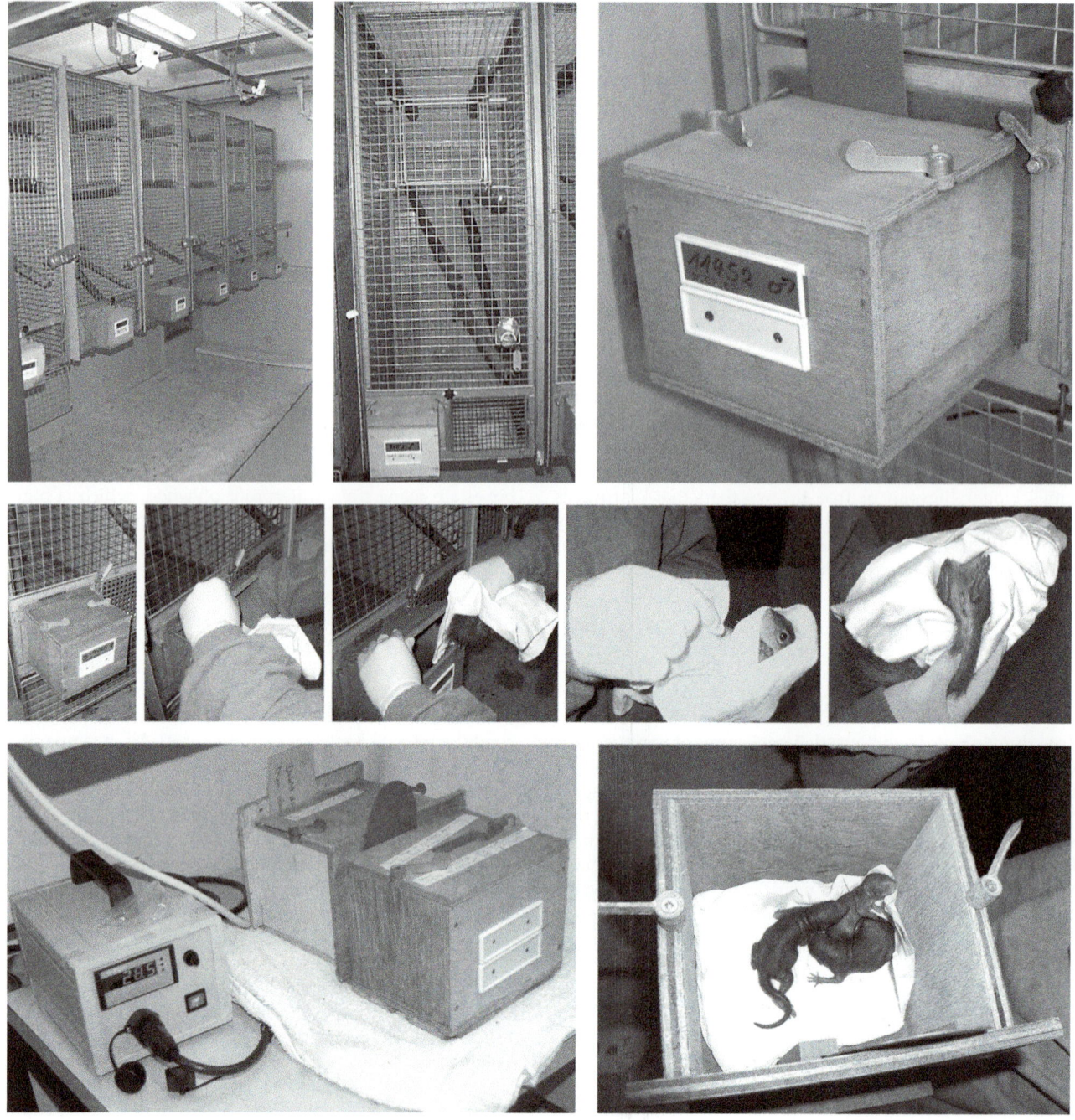

Figure 20.5 Housing and rearing *Tupaia belangeri* in the German Primate Center. Upper row: Animal room, a single cage and a nest box closed with a slider. Middle row: Catching a tree shrew from its nest box with a cloth. Lower row: Housing for newborn tree shrews.

addition, the animals get small pieces of fruit (such as apples, bananas, grapes, kiwi) and vegetables twice a week. Once a week, they get fruit juice and vitamins, cooked eggs or baby food and on weekends, small pieces of crisp bread. As rewards, they get mealworms, raisins, pieces of banana, dates and figs. Breeding pairs or recovering animals get, in addition to the standard food, cat chow or mashed bananas.

In the laboratory, tree shrews are reported to eat almost anything. Therefore, when pellets are not available, they can be fed with steamed rice and chopped beef heart; especially they prefer soft, fat and sweet food, and all kinds of fruits and vegetables. There are, however, indications for allergic mechanisms against soybean products and oat flakes (Brack *et al.* 1990).

Food is supplied in glazed stoneware or stainless-steel dishes (diameter about 8 cm, height about 3 cm) which are changed and cleaned daily.

Water

As judged from the water content of their faeces, tree shrews absorb little water from their ingesta, and they cannot stay without water for more than one day without serious problems. Consequently, water bottles must be controlled daily, and water must always be present *ad libitum*; the mean water intake is 350 ml/kg. Bottles and nipples should be washed with hot water or sterilised between changes. No detergents should be used.

Identification and sexing

Animals should be individually marked which can be achieved by subcutaneous implantation of microchips or by cutting patterns into the tail hair. Tattooing is hard to perform, and the marks often do not last long. Other methods such as notching the inside of the ear or even amputation of claws are prohibited by law in most countries.

The external genitalia of adult male tree shrews consist of a slender and elongate penis which is posterior to scrotal testes. Retraction of the testes in the abdominal cavity can occur under experimental conditions of stress. In female *Tupaia*, *Lyonogale*, *Urogale*, and *Dendrogale*, the clitoris is greatly elongated and grooved on its ventral surface. In neonatal *Tupaia*, the urethra enters the clitoris and extends throughout its length as the clitoral urethra whereas in the adult, the urethra opens together with the vagina as a urogenital sinus at the base of the clitoris. Therefore, infant and juvenile females and males might sometimes be mixed up because the vaginal orifice at the base of the clitoris is sealed. In contrast to the penis, the clitoris does not have a tubular sheath (Figure 20.6).

Health monitoring, quarantine and barrier systems

From the information available to date, the maintenance of tree shrews involves very little risk to human health but, nevertheless, they should be handled with caution. Routine colony health-screening procedures should be carried out and veterinary assistance must be available. Newly acquired animals must be kept in quarantine and require veterinary treatment for external and internal parasites. As pointed out earlier, environmental and social stressors may be a cause of health problems in tree shrews. They may induce sudden and dramatic weight loss or even wounds. Therefore, animal care staff should routinely monitor the animals for signs of illness, such as reduced or no food and water intake, diarrhoea, weight loss, aberrant body posture or movements, rough fur and lethargy or apathy. When the animals are handled for the routine weighing procedure (at least once a month), they should also be checked for signs of cataracts or tumours.

Transport

The shipping of animals should be done in the warmer months to avoid extreme temperature variations and to remain within the guidelines set by the carriers. For shipment, each individual should be confined to a small dark wooden compartment or its nest box. The size of the compartment is determined by the body weight of the animal

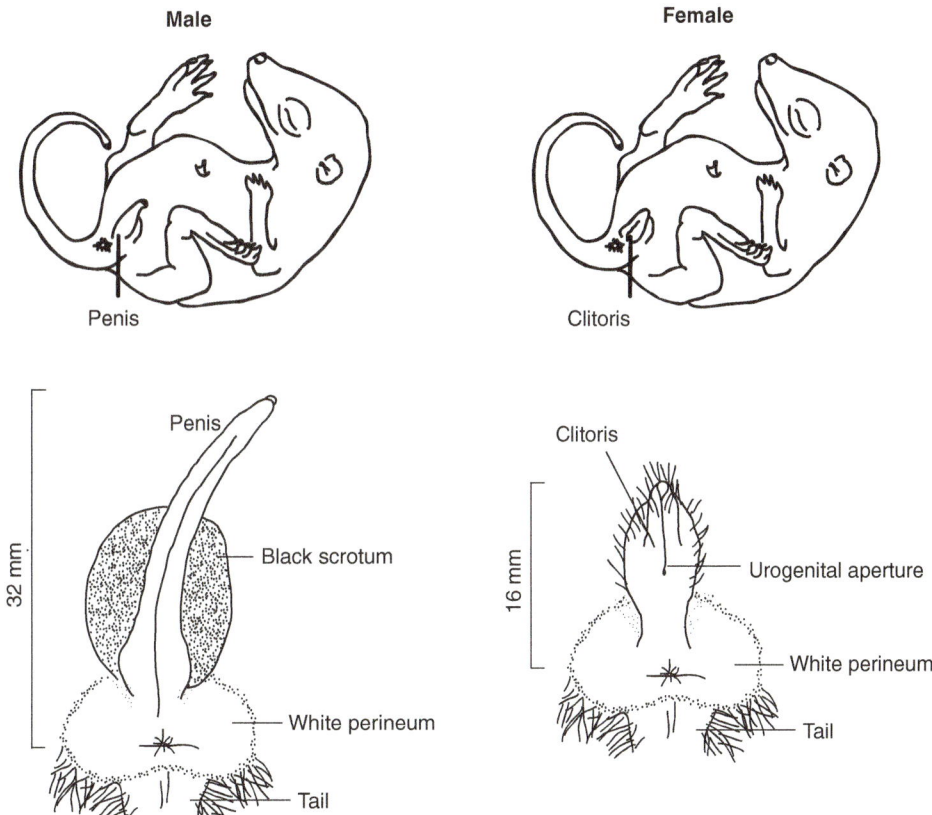

Figure 20.6 Ventral view of the external genitalia of infant and adult tree shrews (*Tupaia belangeri*). Note the penis of the infant tree shrew is twice as long as the clitoris and the anterior position of the scrotum in the adult male tree shrew (Bearder and Pitts 1987 adapted from Martin 1968a).

and both national and international regulations (see also Chapter 12: Transportation of laboratory animals). It must have openings for sufficient ventilation and should be lined with nesting material such as shredded paper. Moist fruits, cooked moist rice and water in gel form (available commercially) should be provided. Before shipping, animals should be habituated to water provided in gel form.

Upon arrival, the animal should be examined for any health issues. Due to the high metabolic rate and the sensitivity of tree shrews to disturbances, newly arrived animals may be exhausted. For recovery, they should be supplied with sugar water or apple juice and high-calorie diet. Sleeping boxes should be warmed with an electric cushion (30°C), lights in the room should be dimmed and disturbances should be avoided to promote a positive transition and reduced stress level for the animal.

Breeding

Adults

Females can give birth to their first litter at an age of about 4 months. Males become fertile between 4 and 5 months. The best age for first pregnancy seems to be between 6 and 9 months. Many females are able to produce offspring until ~3–4 years of age with no issues. If the animal is older, problems such as infertility, stillbirth, cannibalism or abortion occur more often. In males, stress can result in testicular inactivity (Fischer et al. 1985; Brack & Fuchs 2000).

Identifying fertile state

Based on the length of the intervals between copulation periods observed in laboratory conditions, several authors have suggested an 8–12-day (anovulatory) oestrous cycle in various species of Tupaia and ovulation is supposed to be induced by copulation (Martin 1990). However, it is still a matter of discussion whether ovulation is triggered by copulation (induced ovulation) and/or whether an oestrus cycle exists. No cyclic changes in vaginal smears have been detected by the author's group or others. In addition, the author could not find any cyclic alterations in urinary excretion of sex hormones. According to Cao et al. (2001), ovulation can be induced by combined injections of pregnant mare serum gonadotrophin and human chorionic gonadotrophin.

Mating systems

In tree shrews, mating is one of the critical and in many cases most difficult part of breeding. If a female accepts a male, copulation may be observed within a few hours. In many cases, however, placing an adult male and an adult female together in one cage will result in aggressive interactions. There are two main reasons for these fights. One is that the individuals just do not like each other; 'love at first sight' and its cardiovascular consequences have been described by von Holst (1987). Another reason is territoriality. If the mating cage is the territory of one partner this animal – male or female – defends its area against the intruder. In many cases, the animals become gradually familiar with another, and amicable physical attractions can be observed at the 'border' between the cages so that the partition can be removed after some days. However, if aggressive interactions or fights do not cease, other partners have to be tested. When a well-matched couple is found and stable pair-bonding is established, constant reproductive success is guaranteed. Under natural and laboratory conditions, breeding may occur at any time of the year and no seasonal breeding peaks have been described.

When the female leaves the nest after giving birth and having suckled the young, copulation with the male usually occurs within a few hours. Therefore, leaving a couple together is convenient and ensures regular births. Repeated pregnancy cycles are typical of a highly successful breeding colony of Tupaia belangeri, and female receptivity and copulation are often confined to the post-partum oestrus (Martin 1968a; Martin 1968b).

Conception and pregnancy

In Tupaia belangeri, pregnancy can be detected by palpation from the second week of gestation onwards. A significant weight gain (30 – 50 g) and a marked swelling of the abdomen are observed within 2 weeks before term. Duration of pregnancy in regular breeding pairs is within the range of 41–45 days. Breeding success is a good indicator of the general condition of the colony. But even with harmonious, healthy and well-nourished breeders, successful breeding is disrupted by all sorts of disturbances. Tree shrews are highly susceptible to stress and many of the problems in housing them are related to this. Loud noises, strange persons and unfamiliar care staff, overcleaning, inadequate furnishing of the cages and crowding have all been shown to be the reasons for abortion, shortened pregnancies, cannibalism or reduced amounts of milk resulting in starvation of the offspring.

Nesting

About 1 week before term, the female starts to carry nesting material into one of the two nesting boxes. For nesting material, we offer shredded paper, wood-wool or dry leaves. If no nesting material is available, the females will use pellets or any enrichment items that are available in the cage. However, not all females carry out nesting behaviour, yet the offspring appear to be well cared for and healthy.

Parturition

After a relatively short gestation period of 41–45 days, litters consist of 1–5 infants per pregnancy, tree shrews give birth to mostly naked and altricial pups. In most cases, births occur in the morning hours, but sometimes they also occur in the afternoon.

Early development

The infants are born without fur with some sparse hairs on their body; their ears open around 10 days and their eyes after 20 days. The development strongly depends on the milk supply and health condition. The nipple count for all species of Tupaiids falls within the range of one to three pairs. Field and laboratory studies indicate that the number of pups per litter is one to four (in some cases in the author's colony, there were five young per litter which were successfully raised). The birth weight is about 10 g.

Immediately after birth, the young are nursed and the weight of optimally fed babies is in the range of 14–20 g. Females tend to be a little heavier than males. Schwaier (1973) reports a litter size of 2.23 and sex ratio of 0.82 (males: females). For another colony of *Tupaia belangeri*, a sex ratio of 1.8 and a litter size of 2.4 was reported (Hertenstein *et al.* 1987). A survey of the *Tupaia belangeri* colony at the German Primate Center, Göttingen, (1984-2007, total 2962 animals) revealed a sex ratio of 0.95 (m:f) and the following litter sizes: singletons: 158; twins: 462; triplets: 461; quadruplets: 113; quintuplets: 9.

A detailed description of growth and reproductive development in *Tupaia belangeri* from birth to sexual maturity is given by Collins and Tsang (1987) and Hertenstein *et al.* (1987).

The maternal behaviour in *Tupaia* is unusual among mammals and has been described in detail by Martin (1968a, 1968b). The tree shrew species that have been investigated (*Tupaia belangeri*, *Tupaia minor*, *Lyonogale tana*) all show an unusual nursing schedule with the infants kept in separate nests and visited by the mother for suckling only once every 24 to 48 hours.

The pups receive about 5–10 ml milk. Due to the thin skin, the dilated stomach appears as a light patch in the abdomen (Figure 20.7). The fat content in tree shrew milk is very high (about 25 %) while the sugar concentration is low. The energy content of the tree shrew milk lies within the range of other mammals which is in general related to body size (Martin 1990). Since any suckling visit takes only 5–10 minutes, a tree shrew infant will be in contact with its mother less than 2 h during the 30-day nest phase, following which the infant is independent of its mother for milk supply. Thus, tree shrews have the lowest mother-infant contact and parental investment yet described for viviparous mammals (Martin 1990). The pattern of minimal mother-infant contact is strikingly different from the characteristic primate pattern of elaborated maternal care, juvenile dependence and enhanced social organisation (Martin 1990). In a field study, Emmons and Biun (1991) investigated the maternal behaviour of the Malaysian tree shrew *Tupaia (Lyonogale) tana*. Their observations confirmed the peculiar 'absentee' system previously demonstrated only in the laboratory. For the first month of life, the pups stay in a nest apart from the mother, who visits them every other day to nurse them for about 2 minutes. After leaving the nest, the mother spends much time with them daily for at least 3 weeks. The male that shared the mother's territory frequently interacted with the mother during the nestling phase of the pups, but had no contact with them.

Death of young can be due to premature birth (noninflated lungs, interstitial pneumonia), cannibalism or starvation. Cannibalism of the newborn young by the mother or other adults occurs under stressful laboratory conditions which contribute to high mortality and leads also to modifications of maternal suckling behaviour. It has been observed by von Holst (1969) that increasing stress in the group modifies the suckling intervals and leads to increased cannibalism of young *Tupaia belangeri* under laboratory conditions.

According to reports in the literature, newborn *Tupaia belangeri* are marked by a maternal scent substance which protects against cannibalism (von Stralendorff 1982). In contrast to these observations, the author's group was successful with cross-fostering strategies in cases where the mothers were unable to suckle and raise their offspring.

In order to avoid cannibalism and to control suckling success, neonates are separated from the parents immediately after birth. For the next 3 weeks, they are kept in a nest box elsewhere in the animal facility (Figure 20.5). Since temperature regulation is immature in newborn tree shrews, the floor of the nest box is warmed by a temperature-controlled heating cushion (temperature about 27°C) during the first 10 days (Figure 20.5). Alternatively, the newborn animals can be transferred in a nest box in an incubator at 23–25°C and ~30–50% humidity. Mothers are transferred to their litter every

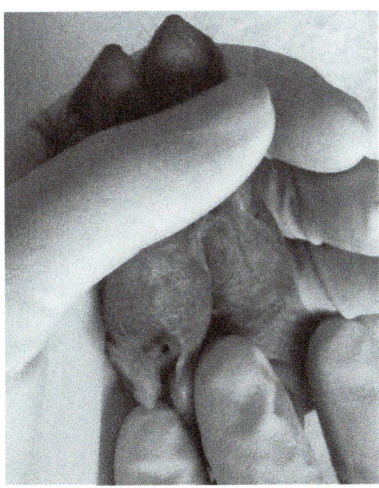
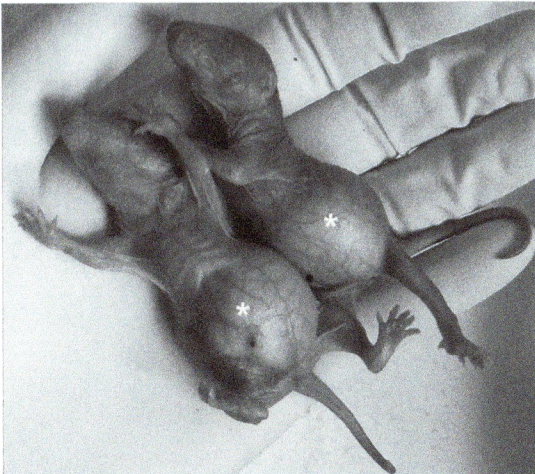

Figure 20.7 Newborn *Tupaia belangeri* before (left) and after suckling (right). Due to the thin skin the dilated stomachs appear as light patches (*) in the abdomen.

day for a maximum of 30 minutes. It is important to note that some females suckle their young only every second day; others have very clear daily time windows within which suckling will take place. The best suckling rhythm for each breeder can only be found by careful observation of individual animals.

Hand rearing

The extremely high fat content of the tree shrew milk is probably one reason why hand rearing is regarded as being very difficult. For successful hand rearing, Tsang and Collins (1985) developed a liquid formula and a protocol which conforms to the natural weaning pattern of *Tupaia belangeri*.

Weaning and rearing

Tupaia belangeri can be weaned around day 35. In the author's colony, the young are separated from the parents at 50–60 days of age.

Depending on cage size, weaned tree shrews of the same sex and close proximity in age should be housed in groups of up to three animals. At 8–10 weeks of age, females and males gradually become fertile with a greater potential for fighting as they are establishing hierarchy. If this fighting becomes an ongoing issue, including substantial wounds, the animals should be separated to avoid any further stress/trauma for themselves as well as surrounding animals. In several cases, smaller all-female groups (three animals) are stable. Males are housed singly or together with a female.

Laboratory Procedures

Handling and training

For quick and easy catching, tree shrews can be locked in their nesting boxes as the animals usually slip into the boxes as soon as somebody enters the room. When removing the animals and to protect the experimenter's hands, the animal is gently wrapped in a cloth (e.g., 40 cm x 40 cm) (Figure 20.5). Since their teeth are small, bites are not dangerous but can be painful. Using this technique, no difficulties occur with the usual procedures such as regular external body inspection, weighing, urine and blood collection, temperature and blood pressure recording, and application of substances by different routes. Tree shrews can be easily trained for memory tests, for example, by positive reinforcement techniques (Ohl *et al.* 1998; Bartolomucci *et al.* 2001). Results from behavioural studies suggest multiple stages of spatial memory formation in tree shrews that are associated with various forms of behavioural responses to novelty (Nair *et al.* 2014).

Monitoring methods

Body temperature (rectal or ear) can easily be measured by thermometers of the type used in humans. For long-term studies, various transmitters can be implanted to register various physiological parameters such as EEG, heart rate, blood pressure or body temperature (Coolen *et al.* 2012; Wang *et al.* 2013a; Schmelting *et al.* 2014). Single photon emission computed tomography (SPECT) and magnetic resonance imaging (MRI) can be used to study central nervous process *in vivo* (see e.g. Michaelis *et al.* 2001; Geisler *et al.* 2015). Stereotaxic ^{18}F-FDG PET and MRI templates (Huang *et al.* 2018) as well as a diffusion tensor imaging atlas of white matter (Dai *et al.* 2017) may facilitate the use of tree shrews in the neuroimaging field.

Collection of specimens – blood, urine

Blood withdrawal (about 500 μl) by puncturing the venous plexus of the tail with a small scalpel is recommended by some authors. Prior to puncture, the fur of the tail can be shaved and is impregnated with a silicon paste which improves blood collection. Blood flow can be enhanced by holding the tail under a heating lamp. This technique, however, requires experience and is therefore often unsatisfactory. Another approach is described by Schwaier (1974) taking blood from the saphenous vein. A cephalic or jugular vein can also be utilised, but this is more challenging. Following the recommendations of GV-SOLAS for small laboratory animals (Dülsner *et al.* 2017), not more than 0.7 ml blood per 100 g body weight at a time should be collected. In cases of repeated blood sampling (e.g. over 2 weeks) not more than 0.07 ml/100 g body weight should be collected within 24 h (Dülsner *et al.* 2017). Despite being completely relaxed during blood sampling, the procedure *per se* seems to be stressful for the animals as documented by increased basal heart rate over several days after one blood sampling procedure (Stohr 1986). There are several general principles which apply to any procedure carried out on an animal. Concerning removal of blood, the Joint Working Group on Refinement (1993) provides a summary of good practice rules.

Morning urine can easily be collected from animals which have been confined to their nest box shortly before the lights turns on in the animal rooms. A slight massage of the hypogastrium gives between 1 and 7 ml of urine. Another approach is to place plastic mats with wells under the cages and to collect the urine later with a pipette out of the wells.

Urine analysis has proved to be a stress-free and reliable procedure for long-term monitoring of the physiological status of *Tupaia belangeri*. Among these are parameters for metabolic activity (Johren *et al.* 1991), various bioactive compounds (Collins *et al.* 1989; Fuchs & Schumacher; 1990, Fuchs *et al.* 1992) and urinary proteins which play a crucial role in olfactory communication (Weber & Fuchs 1988). Age and time of the day may have an impact on the values (Fuchs 1988; Van Kampen & Fuchs 1998). For urinary data, see Table 20.2.

Administration of substances

Most routes of applications such as subcutaneous, intramuscular, intraperitoneal or oral via a bulb-headed cannula are easy to perform. For intravenous injections, it is recommended to use the saphenous vein (Schwaier 1974).

Anaesthesia and analgesia

Adequate anaesthesia is a prerequisite for using an animal species in the laboratory for a wide range of experiments. Early studies used pentobarbital in a comparatively high dose of 75 mg/kg.

A quick and safe injection anaesthetic is the so-called Goettinger Mixture II (GM II) consisting of ketamine (50 mg/ml), xylazine (10 mg/ml) and atropine (0.1 mg/ml) to reduce secretions. The dosage is 0.1 ml/100 g body weight. Anaesthesia usually occurs within 5 minutes of the intramuscular injection and a general anaesthesia lasts about 20–45 minutes. In an alternative protocol described by Huang et al. (2014), tree shrews are initially anaesthetised with midazolam (100 mg/kg, i.m.), ketamine (100 mg/kg, i.m.) and atropine (0.5 mg/kg, s.c.). For a longer general anaesthesia, inhalation anaesthesia is recommended. For inhalation anaesthesia, animals had to be artificially ventilated through an endotracheal tube (home-made from high-med-PE-microtube, inner diameter 1.75 mm, outer diameter 2.08 mm). Our experiences with a respirator for small animals show that 0.5–2% isoflurane in a mixture of 30% oxygen and 70% N_2O, with a respiration rate of 35 per minute with an inspiratory phase of 35% and plateau phase of 5% work fine for *Tupaia belangeri*.

Inhalation anaesthesia is introduced following induction by injection anaesthesia (e.g. GMII). The jawbone is deposited on the fingers and the head is fixated by placing the thumbs behind the skull. The mouth is opened by introducing the laryngoscope. Sometimes the epiglottis can be held down with the tip. After inserting the tube, correct placement must be checked by auscultation; once correct placement is confirmed, the tube can be held in place with a strip of adhesive tape (Figure 20.8). Under inhalation anaesthesia, animals should be kept on temperature-regulated heating blankets to avoid cooling and eyes should be protected against dehydration by an ophthalmic ointment. For immediate vein access, should emergency drugs be needed an iv catheter can also be placed for administration of lactate Ringer's/5% dextrose solution during procedures.

Managing pain during and after surgery, the use of non-steroidal anti-inflammatory drugs (NSAID) such as Meloxicam (0.5 mg/kg) or Flunixin (2.5 mg/kg) is recommended. Alternatively, slow-release buprenorphine

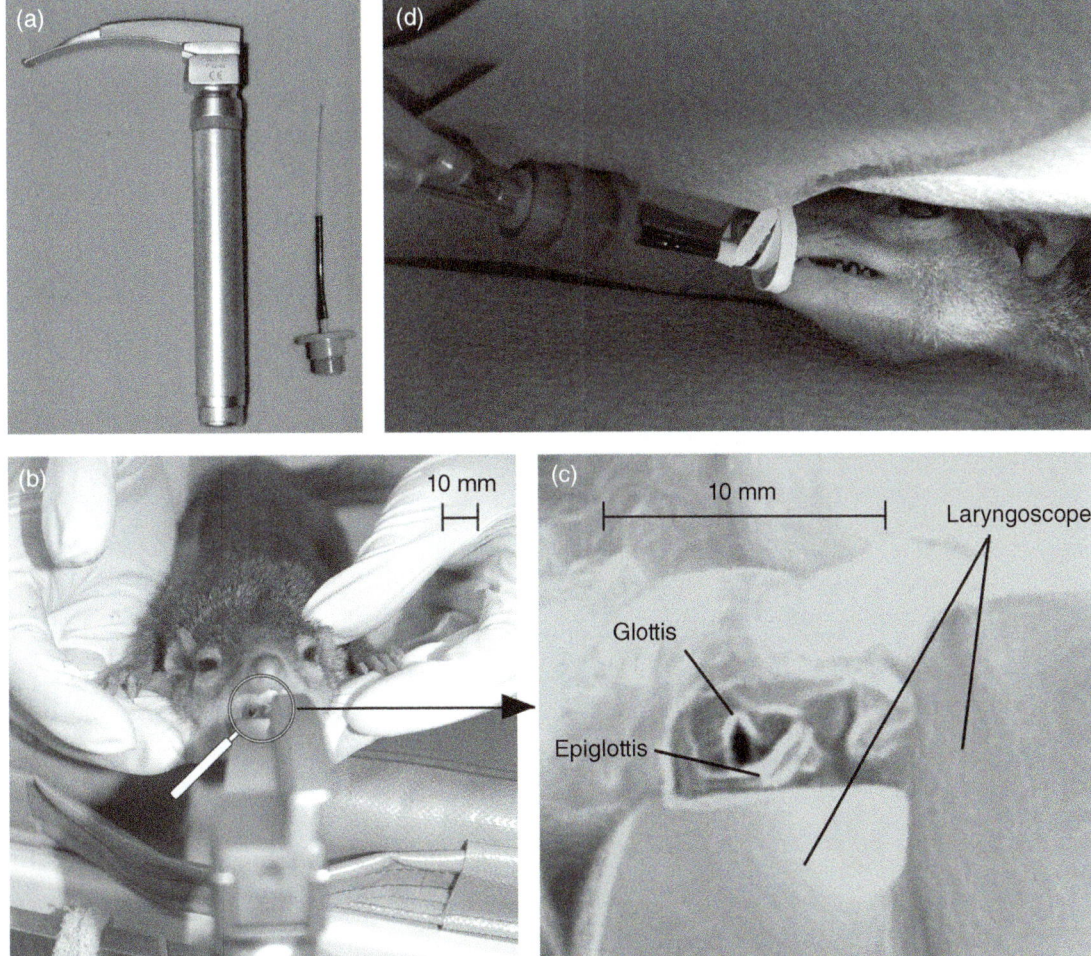

Figure 20.8 Intubation of a tree shrew (*Tupaia belangeri*) for inhalation anaesthesia (a) Laryngoscope and home-made micro-tube (for details, see text). (b) Fixation of the head and position of the laryngoscope. (c) Enlarged view of (b) showing glottis and epiglottis. (d) After successful intubation, the tube is held in place with a strip of adhesive tape.

(0.2–1.2 mg/kg) can also be used for analgesia. The treatment (subcutaneous injection) should start with the onset of anaesthesia and continued for about three days after surgical intervention. An overview of the effective use of analgesics is given by Flecknell (2018).

Euthanasia

The use of animals in research, including euthanasia, is a sensitive issue. While there may be differences in national regulations, permissions may need to be received from local or national ethical committees for research leading to euthanasia (see also Chapter 17: Euthanasia and other fates for laboratory animals). In our opinion, cervical dislocation is not an appropriate method of euthanasia for tree shrews. there are increasing concerns regarding carbon dioxide as a means of euthanasia. Carbon dioxide is known to be anxiogenic and at certain concentrations can be aversive to various species. An appropriate means of euthanasia for infants to adult tree shrews is induction by isoflurane until surgical plane of anaesthesia is obtained, followed by overdose of sodium pentobarbital. A combination of injectable medications such as midazolam (100 mg/kg, i.m.) followed by ketamine or dexdomitor can also be used as an induction prior to overdose with sodium pentobarbital or Euthasol®. In any case, after exposing animals to an overdose of anaesthetics it is always mandatory to confirm death by, for example, cervical dislocation as an appropriate secondary means of euthanasia.

Common welfare problems

Health problems

Tree shrews experience relatively few health problems. However, our experience shows that gastritis can be a frequent problem. In this case, animals stop eating and a lack of faeces can also be observed. Gastritis can be effectively treated with cimetidine (10 mg/kg body weight, twice daily orally).

Diarrhoea is another symptom often seen in a colony. Mostly, *Escherichia coli variatio haemolytica*, Klebsiella *pneumonia* or protozoa (*Giardia, Trichomonas, Entamoeba*) is the reason for this symptom. Before antibiotic treatment of diarrhoea, appropriate diagnostic and a resistance test are strongly recommended.

Infection with the cestode *Tupaia taenia quentini* was successfully treated with praziquantel (Brack *et al.* 1987). Intestinal trichomoniasis with *Tiritrichomonas mobilensis* (mostly in the caecum) has been described as well (Brack *et al.* 1995). Enteropathy of the upper digestive tract was due to a foodstuff allergy against oat flakes and soybean products (Brack *et al.* 1990).

Penis prolapse is another possible health problem. We found this in several males of different age with unknown cause. The prolapse is not lethal by itself, but since there is no effective treatment and the penis becomes irritated and swollen, in most cases, the animal has to be euthanised.

Automutilation can often be found if the cages are too small, overcrowded or the animals are disturbed too much. Moving the animal to a quieter area in the facility is the first step in treatment. In some cases, standard antibiotic treatment and amputation of the affected body part (e.g. a toe or the distal part of the tail) is necessary.

Tupaia seems to be prone to the spontaneous development of gallstones with fatty and cholesterol-rich diets (Schwaier 1979). In two reports, mite infestations were described (Bever 1985; Brack *et al.* 1989).

Most tumours of the genital system of male animals have a Leydig cell origin and occur unilaterally. Tumours of the female genital system are predominantly mammary tumours or sometimes ovarian tumours. Tumours of the haematopoietic system are malignant lymphomas; tumours of the integument occur mostly in the jugulo-sternal gland. Similar to humans, the incidence of tumours increases with the age (Brack 1998). The most common spontaneous tumours are summarised in Figure 20.9.

Two tree-shrew-specific viruses are known and reported by the literature so far: The Tupaia herpes virus (THV) (five different types), which might be a cause for tumours (Darai *et al.* 1982), and the potentially non-pathogenic Tupaia paramyxovirus (TPMV) (Tidona *et al.* 1999).

Signs of poor welfare

Signs of poor welfare are automutilation and stereotyped behaviour; they can often be found if the cages are too small, overcrowded or the animals are disturbed too much. Treatment of automutilation is described in the preceding text. Animals showing stereotyped behaviour such as circling should be moved to a quieter area in the facility. Other important indications are significant weight loss or rough fur. Signs of pain are aberrant body postures or movements, lethargy or apathy. In all cases, a veterinarian should be consulted for optimal treatment.

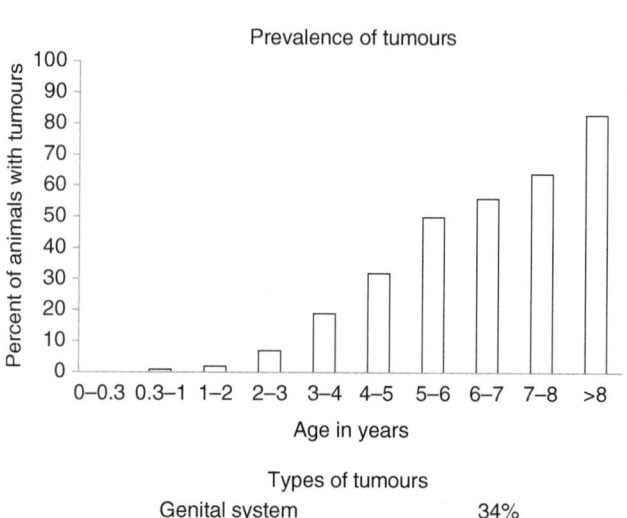

Figure 20.9 Common spontaneous tumours and incidence of tumours, which rises with the age (Brack 1998).

Conclusions

Despite their obvious attractiveness, there are limitations to the use of tree shrews in research. Major limitations are housing and breeding, both of which are time consuming and expensive. However, the implementation of transgenic technology is making tree shrews an interesting species for biological and medical research programmes and their use may increase. Laboratories considering keeping tree shrews should seek advice from institutions that have expertise.

Acknowledgement

Revised from Fuchs E. and Corbach-Söhle S.: Tree shrews. In: Hubrecht R., Kirkwood J. (eds.) *The UFAW Handbook on the Care and Management of Laboratory Animals and Other Research Animals*. 8th Ed. Chichester, Wiley-Blackwell, 262-275, 2010.

References

Bartolomucci, A., de Biurrun, G. and Fuchs, E. (2001) How tree shrews perform in a searching task: Evidences for strategy use? *Journal of Comparative Psychology*, **115**, 344–350.

Bearder, S. and Pitts, R.S. (1987) Prosimians and tree shrews. In: *The UFAW Handbook on the Care and Management of Laboratory Animals*, Ed. Poole, T.B., pp. 551–567. Longman Scientific & Technical, Harlow.

Benson, B., Binz, H. and Zimmermann, E. (1992) Vocalization of infant and developing tree shrews (*Tupaia belangeri*). *Journal of Mammalogy*, **73**, 106–119.

Bever, K. (1985) Mite infestation of *Tupaia glis* DIARD, 1820. *Primate Report*, **13**, 69–70.

Bever, K. and Sprankel, H. (1986) A contribution to the longevity of *Tupaia glis* DIARD, 1820 in captivity. *Zeitschrift für Versuchstierkunde*, **28**, 3–5.

Binz, H. and Zimmermann, E. (1989) The vocal repertoire of adult tree shrews (*Tupaia belangeri*). *Behavior*, **109**, 142–162.

Brack, M. (1998) Spontaneous tumours in tree shrews (*Tupaia belangeri*): population studies. *Journal of Comparative Pathology*, **118**, 301–316.

Brack, M., Naberhaus F. and Heyman E. (1987) *Tupaia taenia quentini* (Schmidt and File, 1977) in *Tupaia belangeri* (Wagner, 1841): transmission experiments and praziquantel treatment. *Laboratory Animals*, **21**, 18–19.

Brack, M., Gatesman, T.J. and Fuchs E. (1989) Otacariasis in tree shrews (*Tupaia belangeri*) caused by *Criokeron quintus*. *Laboratory Animal Science*, **39**, 79–80.

Brack, M., Fooke, M., Wirth, H. and Fuchs E. (1990) Futtermittelallergie bei Spitzhörnchen (*Tupaia belangeri*). In: *Verhandlungsbericht des 32. Internationalen Symposiums über die Erkrankungen der Zoo- und Wildtiere Eskilstuna*, pp. 99–105. Akademie-Verlag, Berlin.

Brack, M., Kaup, F.J. and Fuchs E. (1995) Intestinal trichomoniasis due to tritrichomonas mobilensis in tree shrews (*Tupaia belangeri*). *Laboratory Animal Science*, **45**, 533–537.

Brack, M. and Fuchs, E. (2000) Incidence of testicular lesions in a population of tree shrews (*Tupaia belangeri*). *Comparative Medicine*, **50**, 212–217.

Butler, P.M. (1980) The Tupaiid dentation. In: *Comparative Biology and Evolutionary Relationships of Tree Shrews*. Ed. Luckett, W.P., pp. 171–204. Plenum Press, New York.

Campbell, C.B.G. (1980) The nervous system of the Tupaiidae: Its bearing on phyletic relationships. In: *Comparative Biology and Evolutionary Relationships of Tree Shrews*. Ed. Luckett W.P., pp. 219–242. Plenum Press, New York.

Cao, X., Ben, K. and Wang, X. (2001) Ovulation in the tree shrew (*Tupaia belangeri*) induced by gonadotrophins. *Reproduction, Fertility and Development*, **13**, 377–382.

Cao, J., Yang, E.B., Su, J.J. et al. (2003) The tree shrews: adjuncts and alternatives to primates as models for biomedical research. *Journal of Medical Primatology*, **32**, 123–130.

Collins, P.M., Tsang, W.N. and Metzger J.M. (1984) Influence of stress on adrenocortical function in male tree shrew (*Tupaia belangeri*). *General and Comparative Endocrinology*, **55**, 450–457.

Collins, P.M. and Tsang, W.N. (1987) Growth and reproductive development in the male tree shrew (*Tupaia belangeri*) from birth to sexual maturity. *Biology of Reproduction*, **37**, 261–267.

Collins, P.M., Dobyns, R.J. and Tsang W.N. (1989) Urinary immunoreactive androgen levels during sexual development in the male tree-shrew (*Tupaia belangeri*). *Comparative Biochemistry and Physiology*, **92A**, 489–494.

Coolen, A., Hoffmann, K., Barf, R.P. et al. (2012) Telemetric study of sleep architecture and sleep homeostasis in the day-active tree shrew *Tupaia belangeri*. *Sleep*, **35**, 879–888.

Dai, J.K., Wang, S.X., Shan, D. et al. (2017) A diffusion tensor imaging atlas of white matter in tree shrew. *Brain Structure and Function*, **222**, 1733–1751.

Darai, G, Koch, H.G., Flugel, R.M. and Gelderblom, H. (1982) Tree shrew (*Tupaia*) herpesviruses. *Developments in Biological Standardization*, **52**, 39–51.

Dülsner, A., Hack, R., Krüger, C. et al. (2017) Empfehlung zur Blutentnahme bei Versuchstieren, insbesondere kleinen Versuchstieren. *Fachinformation der GV-SOLAS*.

Eichmann, F. and Holst, D.V. (1999) Organization of territorial marking behavior by testosterone during puberty in male tree shrews. *Physiology and Behavior*, **65**, 785–791.

Emmons, L.H. (1991) Frugivory in treeshrews (*Tupaia*). *The American Naturalist*, **138**, 642–649.

Emmons, L.H. (2000) *Tupai: A Field Study of Bornean Treeshrews*. University of California Press, Berkeley.

Emmons, L.H. and Biun, A. (1991) Malaysian treeshrews. Maternal Behavior of a wild treeshrew, *Tupaia tana*, in Sabah. *National Geographic Research & Exploration*, **7**, 70–81.

Esser, D., Scheka, S. and Zimmermann, E. (2008) Species-specificity in communication calls of tree shrews (*Tupaia*: Scandentia). *Journal of Mammalogy*, **89**, 1456–1463.

Fan, Y., Huang, Z.Y., Cao, C.C. et al. (2014a). Genome of the Chinese tree shrew. *Nature Communication*, **4**, 1426. doi: 10.1038/ncomms2416.

Fan, Y., Yu, D. and Yao, Y.G. (2014b) Tree shrew database (TreeshrewDB): a genomic knowledge base for the Chinese tree shrew. *Science Reports*, **4**, 7145. doi: 10.1038/srep07145.

Fischer, H.D., Heinzeller, T. and Raab, A. (1985) Gonadal response to psychosocial stress in male tree shrews (*Tupaia belangeri*) morphometry of testis, epididymis and prostate. *Andrologia*, **17**, 262–275.

Flecknell, P. (2018) Analgesics in small mammals. *Veterinary Clinics of North America. Exotic Animal Practice*, **21**, 83–103.

Fuchs, E. (1984) Activity of the sympatho-adrenomedullary system in male *Tupaia belangeri* under control and stress situations. In: *Stress – The Role of Catecholamines and Other Neurotransmitters*. Eds Usdin, E., Kvetnansky, R. and Axelrod, J., pp. 595–602. Gordon and Breach, Langhorne.

Fuchs, E. (1988) *Physiologische Charakterisierung von Spitzhörnchen (Tupaia belangeri) unter besonderer Berücksichtigung nichtinvasiver Untersuchungsmethoden*. Habilitationsschrift, Universität Karlsruhe.

Fuchs, E. (2005) Social stress in tree shrews as an animal model of depression: an example of a behavioral model of a CNS disorder. *CNS Spectrum*, **10**, 182–189.

Fuchs, E. (2015) Tree shrews at the German Primate Center. *Primate Biology*, **2**, 1–8.

Fuchs, E. and Schumacher, M. (1990) Psychosocial stress affects pineal function in the tree shrew (*Tupaia belangeri*). *Physiology and Behavior*, **47**, 713–717.

Fuchs, E., Johren, O. and Goldberg, M. (1992) Psychosocial stress affects urinary pteridines in tree shrews. *Naturwissenschaften*, **79**, 379–381.

Fuchs, E., Johren, O. and Flugge G. (1993) Psychosocial conflict in the tree shrew: effects on sympathoadrenal activity and blood pressure. *Psychoneuroendocrinology*, **18**, 557–565.

Fuchs, E. and Flugge, G. (2002) Social stress in tree shrews: effects on physiology, brain function, and behavior of subordinate individuals. *Pharmacology Biochemistry Behavior*, **73**, 247–258.

Geisler, S., Beindorff, N., Cremer, M. et al. (2015) Characterization of [^{123}I]FP-CIT binding to the dopamine transporter in the striatum of tree shrews by quantitative *in vitro* autoradiography. *Synapse*, **69**, 497–504.

Hertenstein, B., Zimmermann, E. and Rahmann H. (1987) Zur Reproduktion und onogenetischen Entwicklung von Spitzhörnchen. *Zeitschrift des Kölner Zoo*, **30**, 119–133.

Huang, X., Elyada, Y.M., Bosking, W.H. et al. (2014) Optogenetic assessment of horizontal interactions in primary visual cortex. *Journal of Neuroscience*, **34**, 4976–4990.

Huang, Q., Nie, B., Ma, C. et al. (2018) Stereotaxic ^{18}F-FDG PET and MRI templates with three-dimensional digital atlas for statistical parametric mapping analysis of tree shrew brain. *Journal of Neuroscience Methods*, **293**, 105–116.

Hunt, R.D. (1993) Herpesviruses of primates: an introduction. In: *Nonhuman Primates*. Eds Jones, T.C., Mohr, T.U. and Hunt, R.D., pp. 74–78. Springer-Verlag, Berlin.

Johren, O., Topp, H., Sander, G. and Schoch, G. (1991) Social stress in tree shrews increases the whole-body RNA degradation rates. *Naturwissenschaften*, **78**, 36–38.

Joint Working Group on Refinement (1993) Removal of blood from laboratory mammals and birds. First Report of the BVA/FRAME/RSPCA/UFAW Joint Working Group on Refinement. *Laboratory Animals*, **27**, 1–22.

Kawamichi, T. and Kawamichi, M. (1979) Spatial organization and territory of tree shrews (*Tupaia glis*). *Animal Behavior*, **27**, 381–393.

Keuker, J.I.H., Keijser, J.N., Nyakas, C. et al. (2005) Aging is accompanied by a subfield-specific reduction of serotonergic fibers in the tree shrew hippocampal formation. *Journal of Chemical Neuroanatomy*, **30**, 221–229.

Kirchhof, J., Hammerschmidt, K. and Fuchs E. (2001) Aggression and dominance in tree shrews (*Tupaia belangeri*). Agonistic pattern is reflected in vocal patterns. In: *Prevention and Control of Aggression and the Impact on its Victims*. Ed. Martinez, M., pp. 409–414, Kluwer Academic/Plenum Publishers, New York.

Konerding, W.S., Brunke, J., Schehka, S. and Zimmermann, E. (2011) Is acoustic evaluation in a non-primate mammal, the tree shrew, affected by context? *Animal Cognition*, **14**, 787–795.

Kriegs, J.O., Churakov, G., Jurka, J. et al. (2007) Evolutionary history of 7SL RNA-derived SINEs in Supraprimates. *Trends in Genetics*, **23**, 158–161.

Kurre, J. and Fuchs, E. (1988) Messung der Spontanaktivität von Spitzhörnchen (*Tupaia belangeri*) mit Passiv-Infrarot-Detektoren. *Zeitschrift für Versuchstierkunde*, **31**, 105–110.

Le Gros Clark, W.E. (1924) On the brain of the tree shrew (*Tupaia minor*). In: *Proceedings of the Zoological Society of London*, pp. 1053–1074.

Li, C.H., Yan, L.Z., Ban, W.Z. et al. (2017) Long-term propagation of tree shrew spermatogonial stem cells in culture and successful generation of transgenic offspring. *Cell Research*, **27**, 241–252.

Li, R., Zanin, M., Xia, X. and Yang, Z. (2018) The tree shrew as a model for infectious diseases research. *Journal of Thoracic Disease*, Suppl. 19, S2272–S2279.

Luckett, W.P. (1980) *Comparative Biology and Evolutionary Relationships of Tree Shrews*. Plenum Press, New York and London.

Martin, R.D. (1968a) Reproduction and ontogeny of tree-shrews (*Tupaia belangeri*), with reference to their general behaviour and taxonomic relationships. *Zeitschrift für Tierpsychologie*, **25**, 409–495.

Martin, R.D. (1968b) Reproduction and ontogeny in tree-shrews (*Tupaia belangeri*), with reference to their general behaviour and taxonomic relationships. *Zeitschrift für Tierpsychologie*, **25**, 505–532.

Martin, R.D. (1990) *Primate Origins and Evolution*. Chapman & Hall, London.

Michaelis, T., de Biurrun, G., Watanabe, T. et al. (2001) Gender-specific alterations of cerebral metabolites with aging and cortisol treatment. *Journal of Psychiatric Research*, **35**, 231–237.

Muller, E.F. and Hub, T. (1992) O_2-uptake and heart rate in tree shrews. In: *IPS Congress Strasbourg*, abstract 370.

Nair, J., Topka, M., Khani, A. et al. (2014) Tree shrews (*Tupaia belangeri*) exhibit novelty preference in the novel location memory task with 24-h retention periods. *Frontiers in Psychology*, **5**, 303. doi: 10.3389/fpsyg.2014.00303. eCollection 2014.

Ohl, F., Oitzl, M.S. and Fuchs, E. (1998) Assessing cognitive functions in tree shrews: visuo-spatial and spatial learning in the home cage. *Journal of Neuroscience Methods*, **81**, 35–40.

Pawlik, M., Fuchs, E., Walker, L.C. and Levy, E. (1999) Primate sequence of amyloid-b protein in tree shrew that do not develop cerebral amyloid deposition. *Neurobiology of Aging*, **20**, 47–51.

Refinetti, R. and Menaker, M. (1992) Body temperature rhythm of the tree shrew, *Tupaia belangeri*. *The Journal of Experimental Zoology*, **263**, 453–457.

Schehka, S. and Zimmermann, E. (2009) Acoustic features to arousal and identity in disturbance calls of tree shrews (*Tupaia belangeri*). *Behavioural Brain Research*, **203**, 223–231.

Schehka, S. and Zimmermann, E. (2012) Affect intensity in voice recognized by tree shrews (*Tupaia belangeri*). *Emotion*, **12**, 632–639.

Schehka, S., Esser, K.H. and Zimmermann, E. (2007) Acoustical expression of arousal in conflict situations in tree shrews (*Tupaia belangeri*). *Journal of Comparative Physiology A*, **193**, 845–852.

Schmelting, B., Corbach-Söhle, S., Kohlhause, S. et al. (2014) Agomelatine in the tree shrew model of depression: effects on stress-induced nocturnal hyperthermia and hormonal status. *European Journal of Neuropsychopharmacology*, **24**, 437–447.

Schwaier, A. (1973) Breeding Tupaias (*Tupaia belangeri*) in captivity. *Zeitschrift für Versuchstierkunde*, **15**, 255–271.

Schwaier, A. (1974) Method of blood sampling and intravenous injection in Tupaias (tree shrews). *Zeitschrift für Versuchstierkunde*, **16**, 35–36.

Schwaier, A. (1975) *Die Verwendung von Tupaias (Praeprimaten) als neues biologisches Testobjekt in der Präventivmedizin und angewandten medizinischen Forschung*. Bericht für das Bundesministerium für Forschung und Technologie, Bonn.

Schwaier, A. (1979) Tupaias (tree shrews) a new animal model for gall stone research. 1st observation of gall stones. *Research in Experimental Medicine*, **176**, 15–24.

Shen, F., Duan, Y., Jin, S. and Sui, N. (2014) Varied behavioral responses induced by morphine in the tree shrew: a possible model for human opiate addiction. *Frontiers in Behavioral Neuroscience*, **8**, 333. doi: 10.3389/fnbeh.2014.00333. eCollection 2014.

Simpson, G.C. (1945) The principles of classification and a classification of mammals. *Bulletin of the American Museum of Natural History*, **85**, 1–350.

Steinhausen, M., Thederan, H., Nolinski, D. et al. (1978) Further evidence of tubular blockage after acute ischemic renal failure in *Tupaia belangeri* and rats. *Virchows Archiv Part A. Pathological Anatomy and Histology*, **381**, 13–34.

Stohr, W. (1986) Basic values, diurnal pattern and variance of heart rate in tree shrews. *Journal of the Autonomic Nervous System*, 177–181.

Tidona, C.A., Kurz, H.W., Gelderblom, H.R. and Darai, G. (1999) Isolation and molecular characterization of a novel cytopathogenic paramyxovirus from tree shrews. *Virology*, **258**, 425–434.

Toder, R., von Holst, D. and Schempp, W. (1992) Comparative cytogenetic studies in tree shrews (*Tupaia*). *Cytogenetic and Cell Genetics*, **60**, 55–59.

Tsang, W.N. and Collins, P.M. (1985) Techniques for hand-rearing tree-shrews (*Tupaia belangeri*) from birth. *Zoo Biology*, **4**, 23–31.

van Kampen, M. and Fuchs, E. (1998) Age-related levels of urinary free cortisol in the tree shrew. *Neurobiology of Aging*, **19**, 363–366.

von Holst, D. (1969) Sozialer Stress bei Tupajas (*Tupaia belangeri*). Die Aktivierung des sympathischen Nervensystems und ihre Beziehung zu hormonal ausgelösten ethologischen und physiologischen Veränderungen. *Zeitschrift für vergleichende Physiologie*, **63**, 1–58.

von Holst, D. (1972) Renal failure as the cause of death in *Tupaia belangeri* exposed to persistent social stress. *Journal of Comparative Physiology*, **78**, 236–273.

von Holst, D. (1977) Social stress in tree shrews: Problems, results, and goals. *Journal of Comparative Physiology*, **120**, 71–86.

von Holst, D. (1987) Physiologie sozialer Interaktionen – Sozialkontakte und ihre Auswirkungen auf Verhalten sowie Fertilität und Vitalität von Tupaias. *Physiologie aktuell*, **3**, 189–208.

von Holst, D. and Buergel-Goodwin, U. (1975) Chinning by male *Tupaia belangeri*: The effects of scent marks of conspecifics and other species. *Journal of Comparative Physiology*, **103**, 153–171.

von Holst, D.V. and Eichmann, F. (1998) Sex-specific regulation of marking behavior by sex hormones and conspecifics scent in tree shrews (*Tupaia belangeri*). *Physiology and Behavior*, **63**, 157–164.

von Stralendorff, F. (1982) Maternal odor substances protect newborn tree shrews from cannibalism. *Naturwissenschaften*, **69**, 553.

Wang, J., Xu, X.L., Ding, Z.Y. et al. (2013a). Basal physiological parameters in domesticated tree shrews (*Tupaia belangeri chinensis*). *Dongwuxue Yanjiu*, **34**, E69–74.

Wang, J., Chai, A., Zhou, Q. et al. (2013b) Chronic clomipramine treatment reverses core symptom of depression in subordinate tree shrews. *PLoS One*, **8**, e80980.

Weber, M.H. and Fuchs, E. (1988) 1D-micro-slab-PAGE of urinary proteins of tree shrews (*Tupaia belangeri*). A tool for non-invasive physiological studies. *Zeitschrift für Versuchstierkunde*, **31**, 55–63.

Yao, Y.G. (2017) Creating animal models, why not use the Chinese tree shrew (*Tupaia belangeri chinensis*)? *Zoological Research*, **38**, 118–126.

Zou, R., Dai, W., Ben, K. and Song, B. (1983) Blood picture of the tree shrew *Tupaia belangeri*. *Zoological Research*, **4**, 291–294.

Rodentia and Lagomorpha

21 The laboratory mouse
Biology, behaviour, enrichment and welfare: first principles and real solutions for laboratory mice

Kathleen R. Pritchett-Corning and Joseph P. Garner

Preamble – Why we should care?

There is an ongoing crisis in biomedical research – on the one hand, there is growing evidence that a significant proportion, if not the majority, of basic science results in preclinical models cannot be replicated (i.e. the reproducibility crisis) (Prinz et al. 2011; Begley 2013; Rosenblatt 2016; Scannell et al. 2022), and, on the other hand, that the majority of preclinical discoveries in animals fail to translate into effective human therapies regardless of disease area (i.e. attrition or the translation crisis) (Kola & Landis 2004; Paul et al. 2010; Sena et al. 2010; van der Worp et al. 2010; Zahs & Ashe 2010; Garner 2014; Hay et al. 2014; Kannt & Wieland 2016; Wong et al. 2019). For instance, in cancer, roughly 10% of preclinical results are replicable between laboratories (Begley 2013), and estimates of successful translation to humans are 5% or less (Kola & Landis 2004; Kane & Kimmelman, 2021). When we dig into these data sets, it is clear that the greatest cause of these failures is a lack of sufficient efficacy (Kola & Landis 2004; Paul et al. 2010) – in other words, every drug that fails in human trials 'worked' in an animal model, and thus, false positive results from animal models are driving attrition and the translation crisis (Garner et al. 2017).

This failure rate should not be dismissed as the cost of doing business. Not only does it fundamentally undermine the harm–benefit ratio justifying animal research (Garner et al. 2017; Würbel 2017; Garner 2020), but the incredible financial cost of these failures (Kola & Landis 2004) drives human public health decision-making, and many healthcare disparities.

Furthermore, we should ask ourselves whether the fundamental biology of cancer (for instance) is so radically different in rodents and humans that a 95% failure rate is believable. If it is, then there seems little value to preclinical work in rodents given the unresolved pain and distress typical in such models. Conversely, perhaps the underlying biology is in fact very similar, but the stress psychology and physiology of traditional animal models and human patients is sufficiently different to explain the failure of animal models to translate to humans (Shemesh & Chen 2023).

Indeed, this is the fundamental argument of this chapter – that mice (and animals in general) fail to be good models of humans when we think of them as tools, reagents or little furry test tubes, and that conversely when we think of animals as patients and design their housing, care and experiments as if they were human patients, reproducibility and translation are radically improved (Würbel 2000; Würbel & Garner 2007; Richter et al. 2009; Richter et al. 2010; Garner et al. 2017; Gaskill & Garner 2017; Würbel 2017; Garner 2020). Doing so involves a paradigm shift that covers almost all areas of animal work (Garner et al. 2017), but of particular relevance to this chapter, providing animals with control over their environment, through enrichment and other forms of behavioural management, is absolutely critical to normalising their physiology and psychology and ensuring the best chance of translation (Gaskill & Garner 2017).

What does it mean to be an animal? Stress, control and well-being

The understanding of stress and distress in the context of animal physiology, animal welfare and animal husbandry has advanced considerably in recent years (National Research Council (US) Committee on Recognition and Alleviation of Distress in Laboratory Animals 2008; Gaskill & Garner 2017), particularly due to the earlier work of Moberg (Carstens & Moberg 2000; Moberg 2000). Simply put, animals exist in

The UFAW Handbook on the Care and Management of Laboratory and Other Research Animals, Ninth Edition.
Edited by Huw Golledge and Claire Richardson.
© 2024 John Wiley & Sons Ltd. Published 2024 by John Wiley & Sons Ltd.

four states: comfort, where no additional resources are required to maintain homeostasis; stress, where resources must be spent to maintain homeostasis; distress, where animals run out of internal resources and must compromise one biological function to maintain homeostasis in others; and ultimately death. Animals meet these challenges to homeostasis with behavioural, autonomic, neuroendocrine and immune responses (Moberg 2000). Thermoregulation serves as a clear example, especially since a failure to thermoregulate is fatal. Mice prefer temperatures of 30–38 °C depending on sex, age, strain, time of day and behavioural activity, and their thermoneutral zone (where they show minimal energy expenditure) typically ranges from 30 to 32 °C, again depending on a variety of factors (Gordon 1993; Gaskill et al. 2009; Gaskill et al. 2013a; Gaskill et al. 2013b; Gaskill et al. 2013c; Gaskill et al. 2013d; Johnson et al. 2017). In humans, physiological thermoneutrality is the temperature at which we feel subjectively comfortable (Gordon 1993). Yet, we house mice at 20–26 °C, and more typically at the colder end of this range. Even at 23 °C, mice increase their metabolic rate by 60%, and we begin to see the first signs of distress (in terms of compromise of other biological systems) at around 20 °C (Gaskill et al. 2009; Gordon 1993; Gaskill et al. 2013a; Gaskill et al. 2013b; Gaskill et al. 2013c; Gaskill et al. 2013d; Johnson et al. 2017). However, these physiological limits miss the point – lethal lower temperatures for mice depend on the method of exposure and acclimation and, most particularly, behaviour. Thus, mice are significant pests (i.e. they survive and reproduce) in meat freezers held at −30 °C (Randall 1999; Latham & Mason 2004), because they build nests. Without nests, similar temperatures are lethal. Thus, even for something as fundamental as thermal homeostasis, the temperature at which a mouse becomes distressed depends entirely on its ability to control it behaviourally.

The classic yoked-control paradigm illustrates the centrality of this phenomenon. In yoked-control experiments, two animals experience identical stressors (usually foot shocks), but one can predict or control the shock. Animals that can predict or control stressors are essentially unaffected, whereas the animals experiencing identical but unpredictable stressors show chronic elevated stress responses that can be fatal (Weiss 1970; Weiss 1971). This phenomenon makes intuitive sense. Behaviour is the thing that makes animals animals (their telos, philosophically speaking), and the telos of behaviour is to overcome the narrow physiological limitations of the organism. Thus, a thirsty animal walks to water, a freezing animal builds a nest and an animal threatened by predators will burrow, climb or flee. A thirsty plant dies, a freezing plant dies and a plant exposed to herbivores gets eaten. Unsurprisingly then, if animals exist to behave, and behaviour exists to predict and control stressors, an animal that cannot predict and control stressors in the wild will surely die. Consequently, animals are designed to do everything in their power, via behavioural, autonomic, neuroendocrine and immunological responses, to control a stressor, and they persist in these efforts until all these systems change and ultimately fail (Moberg 2000). Other than evolution, it is hard to think of a more consistent general theoretical point in biology – for instance, across species, yoked experiments show fundamental changes in everything from immune function (Laudenslager et al. 1983) to reproductive biology (Holmer et al. 2003), and in the case of routine husbandry, something as simple as changing the visually available social companions affects disease progression in simian immunodeficiency virus (SIV) (Capitanio & Lerche 1998; Capitanio et al. 1998; Capitanio et al. 1999).

The universality of this phenomenon – that animals that cannot control stressors become abnormal in every aspect of their behaviour and physiology (Moberg 2000) – is not an esoteric point. Animals that cannot control stressors are abnormal and simply cannot function as meaningful models of humans. Furthermore, given the centrality of this phenomenon in humans too (Kroenke et al. 2006), any animal that does not benefit from control is *a priori*, a fundamentally unsuitable model of humans. For instance, when some zebrafish researchers claim that enrichment is 'mammocentric' and irrelevant for fish, they are claiming that fish models are of little-to-no translational relevance. In short, researchers cannot have their cake and eat it – if a model is worth using, behavioural management and enrichment are not luxuries – they are necessary for reproducible, translatable and responsible science.

Good behavioural management – including enrichment – is therefore focused on providing animals with control over stressors that are important to them, which may be radically different from things that are easy or convenient for humans to measure or manage. Accordingly, developing a comprehensive, evidence based, behavioural management plan for any animal involves a consistent process, namely:

1. Understanding the ecological niche, basic biology, sensory world and behaviour of the animal in order to understand what it finds stressful, how it detects stressors and how the animal attempts to control them.
2. Understanding the unique signs that the animal may be mismatched to its environment, particularly problem and abnormal behaviours specific to the species.
3. Understanding how the animal indicates further distress in terms of failing health or disease.
4. Understanding how the animal is used in research, both in terms of its husbandry and the common procedures it may undergo in the name of science.
5. Understanding the housing system from the animal's point of view so that stressors, failures of control and opportunities to provide control can be identified.
6. And finally, using this holistic insight, designing behavioural management and enrichment strategies that address these issues.

The rest of this chapter works this process through for the laboratory mouse.

What does it mean to be a mouse? Our secretive super-flexible companion

The mouseness of mouse: natural history, domestication and use in research

House mice (*Mus*, Linnaeus 1758) evolved in arid grasslands, originating in the Indian subcontinent, and spreading from there around the world with humans. The most recent taxonomic classification of *Mus* gives *Mus musculus* as the species name, with several subspecies differentiated from that species. For example, *M. m. domesticus* is the Western European house mouse, while *M. m. musculus* is the Eastern and Southern European house mouse. The two species share a hybrid zone in a swathe reaching from Scandinavia to the Black Sea. The native mouse-like animal for North and South America is a species differentiated from mice and rats several million years earlier, *Peromyscus* (Bedford & Hoekstra 2015), and will not be discussed further in this chapter. For further information on *Peromyscus*, the reader is directed to several resources (Wiedmeyer *et al.* 2014; Bedford & Hoekstra 2015; Machtinger & Williams 2020; Pritchett-Corning & Winnicker, 2021).

The domestication of *Mus* into the laboratory mouse began much earlier than is widely realised. While many pre-modern cultures, both agrarian and hunter-gatherer, were familiar with mice and incorporated them into their stories, we do not have surviving records of mice being kept in captivity by these cultures, although we do have acknowledgement of their status as common pests and documentation of their being used as medicine by ancient Egyptians (Bryan & Joachim 1930). However, slightly later cultures with still-extant written sources documenting mouse captivity, such as ancient Greeks, ancient Romans and Chinese, have documented their management of mice in captivity (Keeler 1931). In ancient Greece, (some) mice were sacred to the god Apollo, and there are stories from the mid-seventh-century BCE of a colony of albino mice kept in the temple of Apollo Smintheus, located in modern-day Turkey. In China, in the third century BCE, an encyclopaedia/glossary/dictionary known as the *Erya* has a section that translates as 'explaining beasts' (221 BCE). In that section are clear descriptions of dancing (waltzing) mice, mice with spots and yellow mice. To be able to describe these mice so clearly, the Chinese must have domesticated house mice and were breeding them to obtain certain traits. The Romans incorporated the Greek god Apollo into their pantheon, and in the first century CE, the Roman historian Strabo described the temple of Apollo Smintheus and the statue there of Apollo with his foot on a mouse (Strabo *et al.* 1903).

The organised mouse fancy that led to laboratory mice as we know them – the colours, varieties and their use as experimental subjects – should be acknowledged as originating in Asia, and more specifically China and Japan. Chobei Zeniya, a moneychanger in Kyoto, wrote a small book called Chingan-sodategusa (how to breed fancy mice) in 1787, which is before the opening of Japan to the West. This book was brought back to Western notice by a publication in 1935 in the *Journal of Heredity* (Tokuda 1935; Keeler & Fuji 1937). Tokuda's translation of this small treatise in his manuscript describes many types of fancy mice, and this book states that fancy mice were introduced to Japan in 1654 by a Buddhist priest from China. Fancy mice likely made their way to Europe and the US under the auspices of sailors returning from Japan and China.

As the idea of fancy mice as pets spread, they rapidly increased in number and popularity, particularly in the UK. In 1877, Walter Maxey, the father of the mouse fancy, acquired his first mice. In 1895, he was the founder of the National Mouse Club in England, still extant today and still using a show cage of his design. The National Mouse Club set standards for the different varieties and held judged shows. Their first show was in 1895 in Lincoln and was won by Miss Ursula Dickenson with a Dutch Even. Maxey published books on mouse-keeping and breeding and the books later expanded to cover rats as well (Maxey *et al.* 1920). Maxey's books, although ignorant of genetics *sensu strictu*, did contain practical tips on obtaining desired coat colours and traits, as well as information on line-breeding. Mouse fanciers did keep records on their colonies, and this might have led to the discovery of Mendelian genetics earlier than Mendel, according to some sources.

Roughly contemporaneously to the importation of fancy mice to the UK and the beginning of the mouse fancy, in the 1860s in Austria, Brother Gregor Mendel was codifying the concept of how heritable traits were inherited. At least one author suggests that some of the earliest work on genetics might have been performed in mice if Br. Mendel's superiors had not decided that his religious calling meant that the monk should study something that did not actively copulate (Henig 2000). Mendel's work, published in a botany journal in 1866 (Mendel 1866), lay undiscovered for many years, but was first verified in mammals (after its rediscovery in 1900 by De Vries, Correns and von Tschermark, all independent of each other) by Cuénot, using mice (Cuénot 1902). As noted earlier, mouse fanciers bred mice and kept documents about their colonies, and there is a legitimate claim that a Swiss pharmacist, J.A. Colladon, bred white and grey mice and recorded results in line with classical Mendelian ratios about 40 years before Mendel (Rostand 1960). Our current laboratory mice originate from the intersection of the mouse fancy and the burgeoning field of genetics.

This intersection happened in the early 1900s in the mouse breeding barn of a retired Massachusetts schoolteacher, Miss Abigail Lathrop, who supplied mice to both researchers and the mouse fancy (McNeill 2018). William Castle, a professor at Harvard's now defunct Bussey Institute, and his student, Clarence Cook Little, began to study genetics in mice. In 1909, C. C. Little and William Castle created the first inbred line for use in cancer research, the DBA (Castle & Little 1909). Little, who would go on to found the Jackson Laboratory in 1929, first published a link between genetic inheritance and resistance to the growth of certain tumours using these mice (Little 1915a; Little 1915b). In 1913, J. Halsey Bagg purchased albino mice from an Ohio dealer for behavioural studies and in 1920–1921, shared them with Leonell Strong. Leonell Strong crossed the DBA line with Bagg's albino mice to form hybrids, and those hybrids are the source of the CBA and C3H strains, as well as others (Beck *et al.* 2000). In the same year, at Harvard, Little crossed female 57 with male 52 from the farm of Miss. Lathrop. The mice obtained were segregated into two populations, one black and one brown, thereby creating the respective C57BR and C57BL lines. MacDowell also raised Bagg's albinos and sent some of them to George D. Snell in 1932. Snell used the lowercase 'c' to indicate that the animals were albino. The name 'BALB/c' for this strain stuck, and this relic of prior naming conventions is retained today. Any historic stock or strain of Swiss origin was derived from mice that were originally acquired in 1926 by Clara J. Lynch at the Rockefeller Institute from A. Coulon of Lausanne in Switzerland (Chia *et al.* 2005). Descendants of these mice were spread across different laboratories, and during the 1950s, other lines of mice were created including the inbred SWR/J and SJL/J and the outbred ICR and CD1. Also, in the 1950s, to assess the risk of the use of nuclear energy on reproductive outcomes, millions of mice were irradiated at the Oak Ridge National Laboratory in Tennessee and the Medical Research Council laboratory at Harwell in Oxfordshire, UK (Gondo 2008). Irradiation of mice and breeding them allowed for the discovery of hundreds of new mutations, which, when coupled with Rosalind Franklin's discovery of the structure of DNA, ushered in a new era of mammalian genetics.

Most of the inbred mice in use today were initially developed for use in cancer research to study the heritability of the disease and tumour transplantation (Paigen 2003b). By using brother x sister mating, mouse lines were obtained that had a higher frequency of tumour occurrence, whereas others were resistant. Unknowingly, researchers were actually studying the action of a retrovirus (Bittner 1941), but the work continued, as mice bred for these studies were found to have other illnesses. In some of these inbred lines, there were increased incidences of other diseases, such as skeletal malformations, metabolic diseases, eye and ear defects, or neuromuscular disorders. Mouse geneticists also acquired animals with metabolic or other oddities that had been preserved by the mouse fancy. It was through the power of sheer numbers of mice that many disorders were first linked to genetic factors. Additionally, these studies led to a Nobel Prize for George Snell as he worked to elucidate the mechanisms of tissue acceptance or rejection in transplantation (Snell 1948).

As the mouse became established as the premier mammalian genetics model in the early twentieth century, its contributions to science began to mount. Mice have been used to study transplantation biology, sex determination, mammalian physiology, embryo cryopreservation, the mechanisms of mutagenesis, transgenesis, targeted homologous recombination, and other methods of genetic modification (Paigen 2003a; Paigen 2003b). Mice are used in toxicology work, in basic discovery, in safety studies and as models for a wide number of human conditions and diseases. After researchers realised that infectious agents were likely interfering with their research beyond parasitic infections or the diseases that outright killed mice, the gnotobiotic revolution was underway (Stehr et al. 2009; Yi & Li 2012; Brand et al. 2015; Kennedy et al. 2018) leading to mice free of infectious agents, and the elucidation of how those infectious agents may affect research. The microbiome of the mouse has come under intense scrutiny of late, and manipulation of the microbiome through antibiotics, rewilding or colonisation with defined flora has yielded insights into how gut flora affect all parts of an organism and how excessively clean mice may be less relevant models (Rosshart et al. 2019; Graham 2021).

As with other rodents, such as the Norway rat, mice live synanthropically with humans. To occupy this niche and follow us around the world, mice have had to be as adaptable to differing environments as humans. Their short generation times, phenotypic and genotypic plasticity and behavioural flexibility all allow them to rapidly exploit new human environments. Their biology, sensory physiology and behaviour are all tuned to living in stealth mode, existing alongside us while only rarely detected. Mice have evolved their phenotypic plasticity for the same reasons that humans have, which is part of what makes them such versatile models. As a result, there is very little one can say about 'mice' as a class that is generally consistent. Almost everything about them can change in response to their environment, which is why investigators sometimes see wildly inconsistent results from continent to continent, from institution to institution and even from hallway to hallway within the same institution (Crabbe et al. 1999; Wahlsten et al. 2003; Wahlsten et al. 2006; Richter et al. 2009; Richter et al. 2010). When this human-like plasticity is seen as a feature, not a bug, and experiments and assays are designed to take this into account, essentially treating them as human patients, results are more consistent and translatable.

Basic biology

To move back to basic biology from history, *Mus musculus* (Linnaeus 1758) is a small fossorial rodent, native to the Palearctic. They are typically short-lived (2 years in the laboratory; 6–12 months in the wild) and occupy an important place in the food webs of many animals. They are quadrupedal with a tail they use for balance, thermoregulation and communication. Wild mice have a short, plush haircoat and are typically brown, black or grey and usually have white or buff undersides. Domesticated mice have a wider variety of colours and coat textures. There are several subspecies of *Mus musculus*, including *M. m. musculus*, *M. m. domesticus*, *M. m. castaneus* and *M. m. molossinius* (Wade et al. 2002; Wade & Daly, 2005). Domesticated laboratory *Mus* used in research are derived from all four of those subspecies, plus elements from a closely related species, *Mus spretus* (Zhao et al. 1996; Greene-Till et al. 2000; Hardies et al. 2000). They are properly called 'laboratory mice', rather than giving them classical binomial nomenclature (Didion & de Villena 2013).

Laboratory mice can be divided into inbred lines, called strains, and outbred lines, called stocks (Figure 21.1). Inbred strains are maintained by brother x sister mating, while

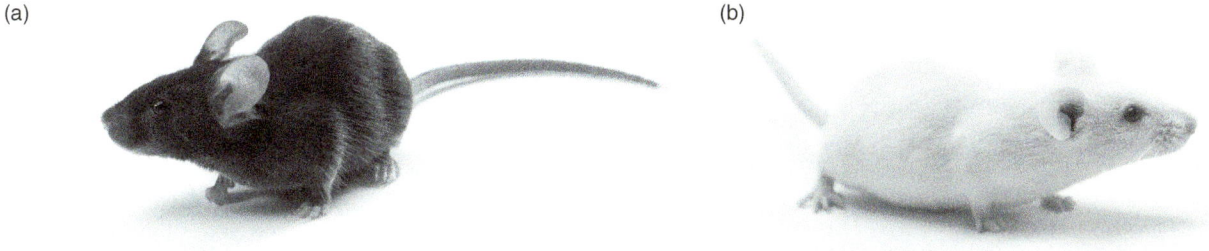

Figure 21.1 (a) C57BL/6NCrl mouse, an inbred strain. (b) Crl:CD1(ICR), an outbred stock.

outbred stocks are maintained through matings that maximise genetic diversity, albeit within a closed colony with a strong founder effect (for example, many outbred stocks are definitely homozygous at the tyrosinase locus). Wild *Mus* vary in size based on species. *M. m. musculus* and *M. m. domesticus* are larger than *M. m. castaneus*, *M. spretus* or *M. m. molossinius*. Similarly, domesticated laboratory mice vary in size depending on strain/stock, and this characteristic is both strongly associated with genetic background and readily manipulated by breeders, sometimes inadvertently. Adult laboratory mice have a body length of 7.5–10 cm, and their tail adds another 5–6 cm. Outbred stocks tend to be more robust, with adult body weights up to 90 g (pregnant adult outbred female at term), while inbred strains are smaller in weight and length. Average inbred mouse adult weights are 20–30 g but range from 10 to 48 g (Reed *et al.* 2007). Inbred mice with genetic modifications affecting appetite or energy regulation can weigh more – some genetic models of obesity can weigh 55–65 g at adulthood. Table 21.1 outlines basic biologic parameters for laboratory mice.

In the wild, mice can obtain water from various sources, including natural ones such as streams, puddles or lakes. They may also drink dew or other sources of condensation, and in homes, pet water dishes and water left in sinks are also sources. In some environments, mice obtain all moisture they need from the foods they consume, including metabolic water derived from fat metabolism. Laboratory mice drink about 8 ml per 30 g of body weight per day (Bachmanov *et al.* 2002; Tordoff *et al.* 2007) and will show signs of acute dehydration after 24 h with no access to water but may live as long as 48 h with no water intake (Bekkevold *et al.* 2013). Mice seemingly adapt well to water restriction as part of behavioural training paradigms (Bekkevold *et al.* 2013). Although water restriction is commonly used to motivate behaviour in mice, this practice is misguided – the behaviour motivated is unlikely to be task-focused, especially for complex paradigms. Accordingly, there are effects on research associated with water deprivation; water deprivation should be avoided, and refinements should be sought (Goltstein *et al.* 2018; Reinagel 2018; Urai *et al.* 2021).

The mouse kidney follows a standard mammalian plan, but functioning of the kidney may differ between strains (Hackbarth & Hackbarth 1982). Urine production varies in mice by age, weight and sex, but mice typically produce a total of 2–3 ml of urine per day (Drickamer 1995). Consideration should be given to the fact that urine collection may take place in metabolic cages, which are stressful to mice and to which they do not acclimate, perhaps affecting these values (Kalliokoski *et al.* 2013). Urine collection for biological sampling can be trained or non-aversive methods may be used allowing mice on such studies to live in normal caging (Kurien *et al.* 2004).

Although classified as granivores, mice consume almost anything present in their environment. Wild mouse diets vary by season and may include grains, seeds, fungi, insects, fruit and (opportunistically) other mice (Rowe *et al.* 1974; Morris *et al.* 2012). Cannibalism is a normal behaviour in mice and usually occurs after cage-mates or newborns have died (Brajon *et al.* 2021). Mice do not hunt and kill other mice for food. Cannibalism is a way to dispose of dead pups, or mice may be driven to cannibalise cage-mates if food or water to the cage is interrupted. Different strains of inbred mice have different preferences for fat and protein levels in food (Smith *et al.* 2000; Bachmanov *et al.* 2002), sucrose (Lewis *et al.* 2005) and bitter compounds (Tordoff 2007). Mouse diets, overall, are lacking in levels of several important amino acids (Greenfield & Briggs 1971) and may contain contaminants and non-nutrients that will affect research (Pellizzon & Ricci 2020). Where reproducibility or dietary manipulation is desired, purified diets should be sought out and 'chow' diets eschewed (Reeves *et al.* 1993; Nielsen 2018; Weiskirchen *et al.* 2020). Regardless of source, mouse diets are low in sulphur-containing amino acids and would benefit from supplementation with DL-methionine, an essential amino acid (Klurfeld *et al.* 2021). Diet may be further manipulated as an enrichment source or as an attempt to manage maladaptive behaviours (Pritchett-Corning *et al.* 2013).

The mouse stomach has two distinct areas – a non-glandular portion, where the oesophagus enters, and a glandular portion, where the duodenum exits. Mice cannot vomit, likely due to a change in the brainstem conserved in rodents (Horn *et al.* 2013), and the phenomenon of pica may be a sign of nausea in non-vomiting animals (Yamamoto *et al.* 2002). Mice are hindgut fermenters, with a relatively large cecum, where much of their digestion occurs. The mouse pancreas is diffuse, and the mouse has a gallbladder. Mice produce between 0.5 and 1 g of faeces per day, and the amount is dependent on the type of diet (Kalliokoski *et al.* 2012).

Table 21.1 Basic biological parameters of laboratory mice.

Diploid chromosome number	40
Lifespan (years)	2–3
Body temperature	35.8–37.6 °C (96.4–99.7 °F)
Thermoneutral zone	30–32 °C
Heart rate (beats per minute, resting)	500–700
Heart rate (beats per minute, anaesthetised)	350–450
Respiration rate (per minute, resting)	90–220
Respiration rate (per minute, anaesthetised)	55–65
Weights, possible: adult (g)	12–90
Weight range (g): typical adult male	25–40
Weight range (g): typical adult female	20–40
Weight: neonate (g)	1–2
Body length (cm)	7.5–10
Tail length (cm)	5–10
Water consumption (daily; ml)	4–7
Food consumption (daily; g)	3–6
Life span (years)	1–3
Type of dentition	Monophydont hypsodont
Dental formula	1 0 0 2
Vertebral formula	7 cervical, 13 thoracic, 6 lumbar, 4 sacral, ≥ 10 caudal
Urine production (daily; ml)	1–4
Urine specific gravity	1.030
Faecal production (daily; g)	0.5–1

As a typical mammal, the mouse has a four-chambered heart with nothing unusual about the circulation of blood within the heart or between the heart and lungs. The heart rate of the mouse varies between 350 and 700 beats/min. Coronary arteries in mice are located within the myocardium and surface vessels tend to be veins, and that, along with their size, makes surgical induction of myocardial infarction in mice more difficult than in some other species. However, these technical difficulties have been overcome, and mice are widely used as a model of infarction (De Villiers & Riley 2020) although they are apparently of limited utility as models of atrial fibrillation (Fu et al. 2022). Mice have a circulating blood volume of approximately 8% of their body weight (Diehl et al. 2001), and there are guidelines in place in countries and institutions as to how much blood may be sampled and how frequently.

The mouse respiratory system also follows a generally conserved mammalian pattern. The right lung of the mouse has four lobes, while their left lung is only one lobe. They do not have cartilaginous airways within the lung itself; only their trachea and primary bronchi contain cartilage. Mice are obligate nasal breathers and cannot pant. The respiratory rate of mice is 80–230 breaths/min, but a basal respiratory rate should be distinguished from sniffing (Grimaud & Murthy, 2018).

Ambient temperature requirements for mice vary widely. Although they do not have physiologic thermoregulatory methods similar to other animals, mice can still live and thrive at a variety of temperatures. As noted earlier, they are a persistent pest in meat lockers and also reside comfortably in conditions of high heat and humidity, despite their inability to pant or sweat. The thermoneutral zone for mice is approximately 30–32 °C (Gordon 2012; Škop et al. 2020), but this can vary based on age, sex, time of day, and adaptation to ambient temperature. While keeping mice warm may make them better models for many human diseases (Ganeshan & Chawla 2017; Hankenson et al. 2018), this is often best accomplished by the mice themselves through the provision of copious amounts of biologically useful nesting material (Gaskill et al. 2009; Gaskill et al. 2013a) rather than warming the environment.

The above paragraphs reference serve as an overview of some basic aspects of mouse anatomy as they relate to mouse biology. For further information on mouse anatomy, we recommend the following works. For line drawing introductions to mouse anatomy, Margaret Cook's book, *The Anatomy of the Laboratory Mouse* (Cook 1965), is available on the Jackson Laboratory's website[1]: For more detailed anatomical illustrations and photomicrographs of normal mouse tissues, including comparisons with human and rat anatomy and tissues, the reader is further directed to *Comparative Anatomy and Histology: A Mouse, Rat, and Human Atlas* by Treuting et al. (2018). Finally, for examination of the anatomy of other rodents (and a lagomorph) for comparative purposes, the two-volume Popesko, Raťjova, and Horak set, *A Colour Atlas of Anatomy of Small Laboratory Animals*, also addresses rats, rabbits, guinea pigs and hamsters (Popesko et al. 1990a; Popesko et al. 1990b). General exposure to mice does not mean an investigator is a laboratory animal veterinarian, veterinary pathologist or ethologist, and the input of knowledgeable parties ideally before experimental design or at the least before publication can prevent inadvertent errors (Ward et al. 2017; Cooper et al. 2021; Hoenerhoff et al. 2021; Meyerholz et al. 2021).

The sensory world of the mouse

Mice perceive the world differently than humans, and knowledge and understanding of this is crucial in adapting environments to suit mice as well as troubleshooting mouse behavioural or reproductive issues. It is natural, of course, for humans to explain the world through what human senses can perceive, hence the terms 'ultraviolet' or 'infrared' or 'ultrasonic'. All of these relate radiation or sound waves to human sensory input but are not necessarily valid descriptors when the range of perception of mice is considered. The terms are used below regardless.

Mouse senses: vision

Mice are commonly used to study various highly conserved aspects of mammalian vision such as development or the function of various homologous genes as they relate to the eye. The vision of mice in and of itself, however, is related to their niche as a nocturnal/crepuscular prey species, although they lack a tapetum lucidum unlike other nocturnal animals (Rodriguez-Ramos Fernandez & Dubielzig 2013). Mice are dichromats having two colour vision cones and have fewer cones compared to rods, typical for a nocturnal animal. Their cones are sensitive at different frequencies than human cones, with one cone having peak sensitivity in the UV at 360 nm and the other in 'green' at 508 nm (Wang et al. 2011). Mouse colour vision is also concentrated in the ventral retina, meaning that they perceive colours best when presented in the upper part of their field of vision (Nadal-Nicolás et al. 2020). When compared to typical human vision, mice are ferociously nearsighted (Histed et al. 2012), and their vision is low-resolution. As a result, what humans can see at a 50-m distance, mice would not see clearly until they were a metre from the object. Mice have a visual field that lets them see above their heads, below their muzzles, and laterally behind their heads to the opposite side of the body. They, therefore, have a large binocular field both in front of their snout and above their heads and a monocular visual field of about 200° (Holmgren et al. 2021). They have a fixed focal point with a very deep field of focus, but they are also 3–5× more sensitive to movement in their field of vision than humans (Douglas et al. 2006). Various strains of inbred mice also carry alleles that affect retinal function, including ones that render them blind by weaning or that affect retinal development differently on different genetic backgrounds (Pritchett-Corning et al. 2012). Since docile mice that did not startle from human hands would have been selected for breeding early on, it is not surprising blindness became fixed in many strains. Many common strains and stocks of mice are also albino, meaning that their vision is negatively affected by the bright lights present in animal facilities (De Vera Mudry et al. 2013).

---

[1] http://www.informatics.jax.org/cookbook/ (Accessed 29 March, 2023)

Understanding the limits of mouse vision helps us to understand how mice will perceive visual cues in mazes or behavioural tasks. A sighted mouse will check itself at a visual cliff but will supplement its eyesight with its whiskers and likely proceed. A blind mouse will not hesitate in a visual cliff task, as its whiskers will inform it of the solid surface underfoot. In a Morris water task, most mice cannot see cues placed on the walls of a room but can probably distinguish simple geometric shapes placed on the walls of the water maze itself (Wong & Brown 2006). Mouse visual limitations also mean that cues that would be different to humans, such as purple versus blue, are not distinguished by mice. Because the frequencies of red, green, and blue light used in LCD and other displays are tuned to human color vision the faithful illusion of color only works for humans. Colors distinguishable by humans, especially those relying on red, may be indistinguishable or invisible to mice. Many behavioural tasks would likely yield different results if performed under UV light. However, while mice cannot 'see' red light, it is still detected by a variety of means and can disrupt circadian rhythm, potentially affecting research results. Light, including colour, intensity and duration, is a crucial facility variable that may affect the health and suitability of animals used for research and should be considered as such (Peirson *et al.* 2018; Barabas *et al.* 2022b).

Mouse senses: hearing

The decibel (dB) is a unit of proportion used to measure sound pressure (loudness) on a logarithmic scale. dB measurements range from 0, considered inaudible, to about 140, which is the pain threshold as reported by humans. Generally, a hearing range is defined as the frequencies, defined in hertz or kilohertz (Hz or kHz) audible to an animal at a level of 60 dB. Within those audible frequencies are frequencies to which animals are more sensitive, meaning those sounds audible to an animal at 10 dB. For ease of consideration, 60 dB is a shout, while 10 dB is a whisper. Animal communication tends to fall into the frequencies at which their hearing is most sensitive. Human hearing range is 31 Hz to 17.6 kHz with the most sensitive parts of our hearing reserved for sounds from 2 to 4 kHz. Mouse hearing starts at 2.3 kHz and goes to 85.5 kHz, with the most sensitive part of their hearing spectrum at 12–20 kHz (Heffner & Heffner 2007) (Figure 21.2). Mice both hear and communicate well into the ultrasound (Portfors & Perkel 2014).

Communication in the ultrasound is of vital importance to mice throughout life (Peleh *et al.* 2019). Mouse pups call to their dam for retrieval if they are out of the nest (Hahn & Lavooy 2005), while male mice produce ultrasonic calls when exposed to female mouse urine (Holy & Guo 2005). Mice vocalise during both affiliative and agonistic encounters (Panksepp *et al.* 2007; Chabout *et al.* 2017). Fewer inbred mouse strains have alleles for total deafness fixed than for blindness; however, an allele fixed in various strains renders mice deaf with age (Johnson *et al.* 2000; Johnson *et al.* 2006), although age is relative, with B6J mice having high-frequency hearing loss as early as 3–6 months of age (Kane *et al.* 2012). This may affect their social or maternal behaviour since cues emitted by other animals

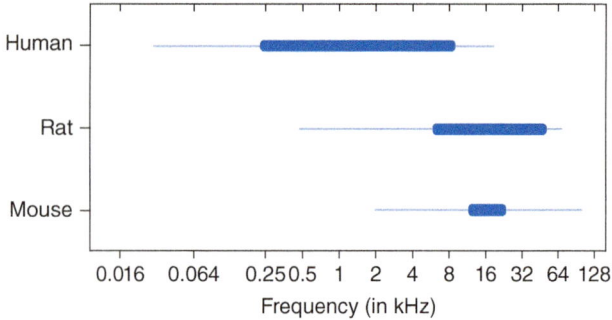

Figure 21.2 Mouse, rat and human hearing ranges. The thin blue lines indicate sensitivity to sound at a 60-dB sound pressure level, while the thick red lines indicate sensitivity to sounds at a 10-dB sound pressure level. The decibel (dB) scale is a logarithmic scale. Source: Adapted from (Heffner & Heffner 2007).

are no longer audible. Mice that are profoundly deaf earlier also often have problems with balance since their deafness may be due to abnormalities of the inner ear (Leibovici *et al.* 2008).

Can we hear mouse squeaks? Yes, some of them. To study mouse vocalisations well, however, means ultrasonic microphones and software that can shift those vocalisations to human hearing or provide digital output for analysis. Can mice hear human voices? Yes. Can mice also hear a great deal of noise from objects that are silent to human hearing? Also, yes. Disruption of mouse behaviour by noise produced by normal husbandry, construction or malfunctioning equipment has been widely recognised and reported in the literature (Turner *et al.* 2005; Rasmussen *et al.* 2009).

Considering sound and vibration separately, vibration is a mechanical phenomenon where oscillations occur around an equilibrium, and sound is the movement of air through vibration. Vibration of animals is generally considered an unwanted occurrence and may be used as a source of chronic stress, although there are some indications that vibration may also serve as a therapeutic modality (Reynolds *et al.* 2018). Consistent vibration (e.g. from an individually ventilated rack) is generally considered to be less distressing than sudden, intermittent vibration, as can be seen with construction, and slower vibrations less distressing than faster (Carman *et al.* 2007; Atanasov *et al.* 2015). Noise and vibration are likely to affect research outcomes in mice and should be considered as part of a facility plan (Turner 2020). Although not all sources of noise and vibration can be mitigated, they can be reported to investigative groups and as part of publications.

Mouse senses: touch

Touch is an essential sense, mediated through specialised neurons called mechanoreceptors present in both haired and glabrous skin. These mechanoreceptors each detect different types or qualities of touch and may be broadly divided into low-threshold mechanoreceptors and nociceptors (Jenkins & Lumpkin 2017). Low-threshold mechanoreceptors may have subtypes as diverse as the detection of hair follicle movement, pressure or skin stretching (Jenkins & Lumpkin 2017). Mice have a keen sense of touch, not only mediated by their vibrissae, specialised touch-sensitive hairs, but by guard hairs present on the body. These hairs detect the presence of surfaces against the body, including cover. Since mice rely on thigmotaxis for protection, having specialised body hair types to detect surface contact is important (Walsh et al. 2015). Mice also have small C-fibres in the skin that react to gentle pressure, so mice probably enjoy petting, as other mammals do (Liu et al. 2007). Indeed, mice can be trained using gentle stroking ('affective touch' in the literature) as a reward (Cho et al. 2021).

Mice have more vibrissae than just their micro and macro mystacial vibrissae (their 'whiskers') (Prescott et al. 2011). There are vibrissae located on various parts of the head, including above the eye and between the rami of the mandible, and near the palmar and plantar surfaces of the paws. Vibrissae are extremely sensitive and acute touch sensors, not passive receptors. Using active 'whisking' movements of the mystacial vibrissae, mice can detect and discriminate textures (e.g. grades of sandpaper), edges (e.g. sizes and shapes of openings) and obstacles (Garner et al. 2006). Each of the large whiskers in the mouse maps to a particular part of the sensory cortex called the barrel cortex. The barrel cortex has been used to study neuronal plasticity, as, since vibrissae are hairs, they are regularly shed by the mouse, and the underlying neurons must adapt to a lack of or change in input as the vibrissa grows back (Erzurumlu & Gaspar 2020). Sensory maps in the cortex reflect neuronal number, and hence acuity and processing power, meaning that mouse whiskers use about as much relative brain processing power for sensory input as human fingers (Campagner et al. 2018) (Figure 21.3).

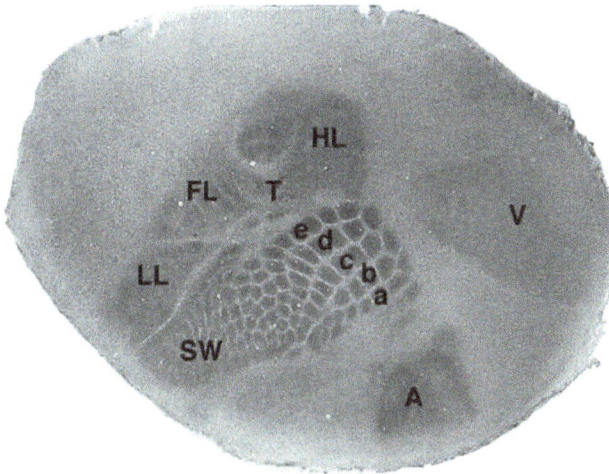

Figure 21.3 This figure shows the flattened left hemisphere of a wild-type genetically modified mouse. It has been immunostained with a serotonin transporter. The layer IV thalamocortical afferents show a complete body map: V: visual, A: auditory, a-e, large mystacial vibrissae ("whiskers"), SW: small whiskers of the snout, LL: lower lip, FL: forelimb, HL hindlimb, T: trunk. Source: Photo used courtesy of Dr. S.L. Donovan and Dr. J.S. McCasland.

Mouse senses: smell and taste

Olfaction is the most important mouse sense (Shepherd 2004). Mice have two ways to receive olfactory input: olfactory receptor neurons in the olfactory epithelium and the vomeronasal organ (Zeppilli et al. 2021). Both inputs connect to the brain, with the receptor neurons connecting to the main olfactory bulb and from thence to other brain regions, while the neurons from the vomeronasal organ connect to the accessory olfactory bulb and then to the amygdala. Pheromones, used for communication within a species, generally act through the vomeronasal organ (Rodriguez & Boehm 2009), while other odorants are perceived through the olfactory epithelium. Mice rely on their sense of smell to locate food and mates, identify relatives, avoid predators (Ferrero et al. 2011) and other sources of danger and determine territory holders. They use their sense of smell to navigate their environment, to assess the health of other mice and to parent appropriately. Besides general odours that identify individual mice, mice also have a robust system of pheromonal production involving urine, faeces and sebaceous and eccrine glands present around the genitals and on the surfaces of the paws. These pheromones and other odorants allow communication of fear (Brechbühl et al. 2013), illness (Arakawa et al. 2011), sexual receptivity (Lenschow & Lima 2020) and sexual attraction (Ramm et al. 2008). The same pheromones may act differently on each mouse dependent on sex, experience and internal state (Tan & Stowers 2020).

One of the most important ways laboratory mice use odorant cues in their environment is the maintenance of the hierarchical relationship of animals within the cage, and even highly inbred mice can differentiate between closely related animals (Arakawa et al. 2007). Dominant mice deposit urine at multiple sites around the cage, while subordinate mice tend to urinate in larger amounts in corners (Desjardins et al. 1973; Drickamer 2001). Disruption of these scent marks at cage change is related to the scuffling and injury sometimes seen at cage change. Different compound profiles appear when odours from toileting sites are compared to nesting sites and between inbred strains (Barabas et al. 2021b). Affiliative behaviours are associated with nesting sites, and transfer of nesting material at cage change may promote affiliative behaviour or at least decrease fighting in cages of males (Lidster et al. 2019; Van Loo et al. 2000).

Mouse senses: magnetoreception

Mice are apparently sensitive to the Earth's magnetic field (Prato et al. 2013), but studying this is challenging as low-level radiofrequency fields may interfere with magnetoreception (Phillips et al. 2022). When mice were trained through the use of a light gradient to build nests in one of four orientations and the local magnetic field was then rotated by 90°, 180°, or 270°, mice built their nests in the same magnetic orientation, not the physical location (Muheim et al. 2006). A similar manipulation of nearby magnetic fields was used to show that mice could orient to goal platforms in a water maze in the same fashion (Phillips et al. 2013). At least one strain of laboratory mice is also reported to spend more time exploring an active magnet when placed in the enclosure (Malewski *et al.* 2018).

Mouse behaviour

An excellent review of behaviour in mice, including social behaviour, can be found in several publications. Although many of them are older or focus on wild mice, their utility cannot be denied (Berry 1970; Berry 1981; Mackintosh 1981; Berry & Bronson 1992; Latham & Mason 2004; Würbel *et al.* 2009). The study of mice as an organism in their own right, rather than as just a general mammalian model, arguably began with the publication of *Mice all Over* by Peter Crowcroft (Crowcroft 1966). This book builds on material produced by Crowcroft in the 1950s combatting the infiltration of grain stores during post-war rationing, outlined in a more scientific fashion in a paper from 1963 (Crowcroft & Rowe 1963). A more recent reference is (MacLellan *et al.* 2021), which provides an overview of the behavioural biology of mice. A comprehensive resource for analysing mouse behaviour is the 'Mouse Ethogram'[2], which provides a detailed ethogram for mice. We cannot emphasise strongly enough that general exposure to mice or a PhD in a field that uses mice does not render an investigator an ethologist, so when a need to evaluate mouse behaviour arises, consultation with an ethologist is not just wise, but essential (Garner *et al.* 2017). Ethologists can be particularly helpful in mediating conversations with clinical psychologists and psychiatrists with regard to the validity of a mouse behaviour as a potential model, and again, doing so would have avoided many unwise suggestions made in the literature with real impacts on human patients (such as suggesting bone marrow transplants as a cure for trichotillomania) (Greer & Capecchi 2002; Chen *et al.* 2010).

Mouse maintenance behaviour

Mouse general maintenance behaviour includes ingestive behaviour (eating or drinking), sleeping or resting (usually coded as 'inactive' in time budgets) and grooming. C57BL/6J in standard laboratory housing are described as spending approximately 66% of their time inactive, about 10% of their time eating or drinking and 23% of their time in other behaviours, which may include grooming, social interactions, stereotypies or other locomotory activities (Goulding *et al.* 2008). This time budget may vary by genetic background, but it is a good place to start. As noted above, mice are functionally omnivores, but are not often allowed to express this behaviour in the lab. Most mouse ingestive behaviour takes place immediately after the lights turn off in the animal room with a second bout occurring right before the lights turn on. These patterns of circadian food intake also lead to circadian patterns in body weight (Ahloy-Dallaire *et al.* 2019). Knowing that most mice eat and drink sparingly with the lights on, that there is both a behavioural and metabolic demand for food at the end of the light-period, and that mice naturally forage and eat at these times means that behavioural assays can be timed accordingly, negating the need for additional artificial and aggressive water or food restriction (Pioli *et al.* 2014).

Mice are episodic sleepers, rousing to move about relatively frequently. During the day, 30–70% of their time in a 2-h period may be spent asleep (Robinson-Junker *et al.* 2018). This work was performed with singly housed mice, and group-housed mice may have different sleeping patterns (Febinger *et al.* 2014). As nocturnal animals, disruption of their sleep by husbandry activities during the light cycle is inevitable. Cage changing disrupts sleep for approximately 3 h (Febinger *et al.* 2014), and welfare is not improved by limiting such disturbance to predictable times of day (Robinson-Junker *et al.* 2019).

Grooming, both auto- and allo-, is an important part of mouse behaviour. Grooming of cage-mates can be an affiliative behaviour (Du *et al.* 2020) or an aggressive one (Kudryavtseva *et al.* 2000). Dams groom pups extensively and female mice often groom each other. Autogrooming by mice is a fixed action pattern, proceeding in a rostro-caudal direction and is very well described (Berridge *et al.* 1987; Fentress 1988; Sachs 1988). This self-grooming may also serve a social function in mice, as the act releases chemosensory cues that other mice find attractive (Zhang *et al.* 2022).

Mouse social behaviour

Sociality among animals may be defined in different ways. From completely solitary to colony living, mice may be placed in almost every social niche, depending on sex, resource availability and stage of life (Greenberg 1972). In environments where resources are sparse, spread-out and indefensible, mice occupy large overlapping 'home ranges' (of up to 80,000 m^2) and tolerate intruders (Latham & Mason 2004). Here, we consider wild mice living in resource-dense environments as most relevant to laboratory conditions. In these environments, mice live in loose kin groups called 'demes', where one male owns the territory above ground, and this male has established this territory through scramble competition – the first male into an unoccupied territory generally establishes it as his (Crowcroft & Rowe 1963). The territory is marked through urine deposition by both males and females (Hurst 1990a; Hurst 1990b). Mice have a strong exploratory desire and can travel great distances to both find and defend territory and mates. Territory is centred on nest sites and burrows, and all resident adults defend the territory. Females, especially, are vicious defenders of pups in the nest. Although there is usually only one male maintaining a territory with several females, the females have their own clear dominance hierarchy as well (Williamson *et al.* 2019). Within the territory, mice use structures present to mount a defence of the space. They use holes, chokepoints, and elevated areas to ambush intruders and drive other mice away. These natural defence points around desired territories leave most mice, males especially, living in a no-man's land, overcrowded and under-resourced (Crowcroft 1955; Crowcroft 1966; Calhoun 1973).

---

[2] https://mousebehavior.org/ (Accessed March 30, 2023)

Once pups are born and weaned, they begin to explore in anticipation of establishing their own territories. Males usually disperse singly, while females may disperse singly or in pairs or more. If related females enter a male's territory, he may mate with them both and the females will alloparent each other's offspring. Having more than one female in a territory, though, especially if unrelated, may result in reproductive suppression of one female. Two plus one does not always equal three (Garner *et al*. 2016; Chatkupt *et al*. 2018).

Generally, mice become more territorial, more aggressive and more infanticidal as population density increases. While mice are territorial when they have the space to be, they can establish stable dominance hierarchies if conditions dictate (Williamson *et al*. 2016). Population density in mice is driven by dense, clumped food resources (c.f. Australian mouse plagues) such as those present in human homes or agricultural buildings. Regardless, a dense population in a house with each mouse having a 2-m^2 territory is still approximately 85 standard laboratory cages, putting into relief how densely mice are housed in laboratories and further illustrating the behavioural plasticity of mice in their general tolerance of these conditions.

Territoriality, and hence aggression, may also vary with season, especially in colder environments. In colder environments, resources fluctuate with the season, meaning that mice become practically seasonally reproductive. This means that as the days lengthen, mice disperse from the nest and attempt to establish their own territories. Although laboratory mice are isolated from seasonal changes, an uptick in aggressive behaviour is noted by some animal caretakers in the late spring and early summer, when animals would disperse in the wild.

Breeding behaviour and biology

Mice are litter-bearing and incredibly fecund, capable of bearing a litter of 4–12 pups every 19–21 days after they reach sexual maturity at 42–48 days of age (Figure 21.4). A table of basic reproductive values in mice may be found in Table 21.2. Mice have a 4–5-day estrous cycle with a typical mammalian cycle of changes in vaginal cytology (Figure 21.5). Vaginal cytology may be examined either by use of a paediatric urethral swab to directly collect cells from the vaginal vault or by instilling sterile saline into the vault and collecting shed material (Cora *et al*. 2015). These changes are also reflected externally, and excellent photos to aid in staging the estrous cycle in order to maximise production can be found in Byers *et al*. (2012).

Male mice are alerted to receptive females through urinary odours and direct examination. Male mice vocalise when presented with the urine of receptive females (Musolf *et al*. 2010), and these vocalisations may affect the listening females in a way that enhances fertility (Asaba *et al*. 2017). As noted earlier, noise in the ultrasonic in the vivarium may have negative effects on animals that can be difficult to quantify.

The mating event in mice is necessary, but not sufficient, for natural conception and a successful pregnancy. Male mice approach female mice, and if the female is not

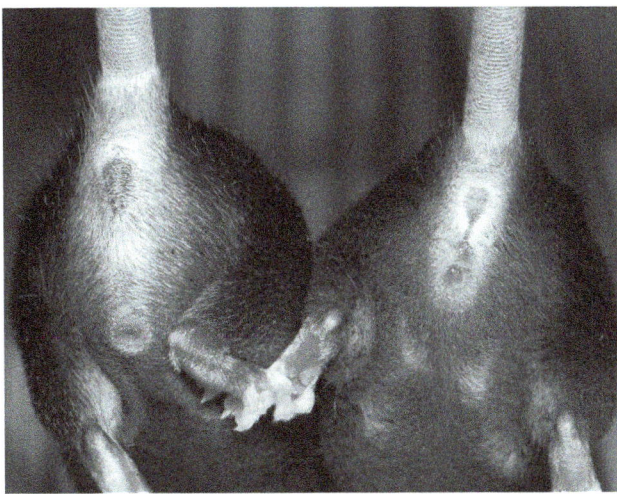

Figure 21.4 External female and male genitalia of adult C57BL/6 mice. The male is on the left, while the female is on the right. Female mice have nipples, while male mice do not. The anogenital distance in females is shorter than that in males.

Table 21.2 Basic reproductive and developmental values for mice.

Age at sexual maturity (days)	40–60
Uterus type	Bicornuate
Estrous cycle frequency (days)	4–5
Duration of oestrus (h)	10–12
Gestation period (days)	19–21
Placentation type	Discoid, haemochorial
Average litter size	4–10
Nursing frequency (per day)	>10 bouts
Hair erupts (days)	5–7
Milk production/day (ml)	5–16
Peak milk yield by dam (days)	10–16
Peak milk consumption by pups (d)	10
Teeth erupt (days)	10–11
Ears open (days)	12
Eyes open (days)	11–12
Vaginal closure membrane opens (days)	~30–35
Preputial separation (days)	~30
Young begin eating solid food (days)	10–12
Age at weaning (days)	21–28
Breeding life in captivity	8 months

receptive, the male is quickly driven away. If the female is receptive, she allows the male to sniff her extensively and perform a behaviour called 'rooting' where the male investigates the underside of the female, sometimes even moving entirely underneath her (McGill 1962). Eventually, she will stand in a lordotic posture for mating, allowing the male to mount. The male thrusts repeatedly and on ejaculation will clasp the female with all four feet, sometimes falling over to the side, taking the female with him (McGill 1962). During ejaculation, the male mouse's penis expands to resemble an inside-out umbrella, allowing for stimulation of mechanoreceptors in the female's vagina (McGill & Coughlin 1970). Concurrent with ejaculation, the male mouse deposits a copulation plug comprised of secretions from the prostate,

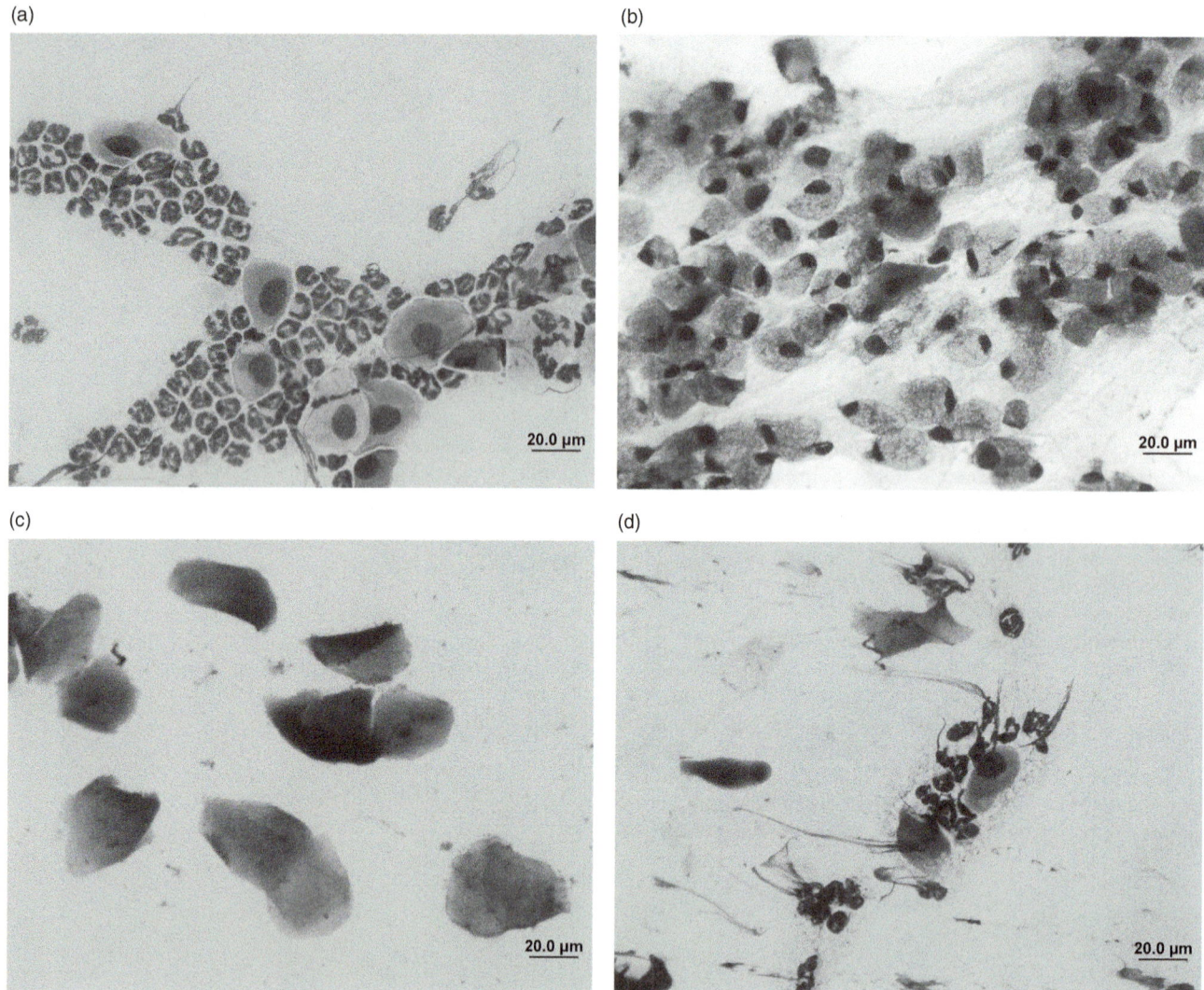

Figure 21.5 Progression of mouse vaginal epithelium through the stages of the estrous cycle. These are direct swabs of the vaginal mucosa, stained with Diff-Quik, a modified Wright-Giemsa stain and taken at 400×. There may be slight differences in cytology appearance when saline instillation of the vagina is used to assess cytology when compared to swabs. After mating, sperm may be visible on vaginal cytology. (a) diestrus, characterised by nucleated epithelial cells and large numbers of neutrophils. If cycling has ceased, cytology will usually reflect diestrus. (b) proestrus, characterised by large numbers of nucleated epithelial cells. Mice are usually in behavioural oestrus in late cellular proestrus. (c) oestrus, characterised by cornified epithelial cells. (d) metestrus, in which all three cell types appear, although the neutrophils are degenerate and tend to appear as smears of eosinophilic material.

seminal vesicles and the coagulating gland (Figure 21.6). Although female mice can remove the plug by grooming, and heteropaternity is common in wild mice (Dean et al. 2006), a copulation plug is a male mouse evolutionary tactic to decrease the chance of subsequent matings (Sutter et al. 2015). The pattern of intromission before ejaculation and the deposition of the copulation plug is necessary for the formation of the corpus luteum and maintenance of early pregnancy in mice. Ovulation in mice is spontaneous and not dependent on copulation. The male mouse has a copulation clock that changes his behaviour from aggressive to paternal towards pups when he encounters pups approximately 19 days after his last copulation event (Vom Saal & Howard 1982; McCarthy & Vom Saal 1986; Perrigo et al. 1992)

Nest building activity increases before parturition and female mice become defensive of the nest (Weber & Olsson 2008; Weber et al. 2016). Parturition is initiated by foetal signals (Reinl & England 2015) and mice usually give birth overnight. Mouse parturition takes place over several hours with each pup delivered and the membranes consumed before the next pup is born. Mice have a fertile post-partum oestrus 4–12 h after birth, dependent on the light cycle and their time of parturition (Runner & Ladman 1950), and will often immediately become pregnant again if a male is in the cage. In fact, most mouse production relies heavily on this fact (Lerch et al. 2015). Stillbirths are common in laboratory mice, and cannibalism as a means of disposing of dead pups can be misinterpreted by investigators as infanticide (Weber et al. 2013; Brajon et al. 2021). Infanticide may occur,

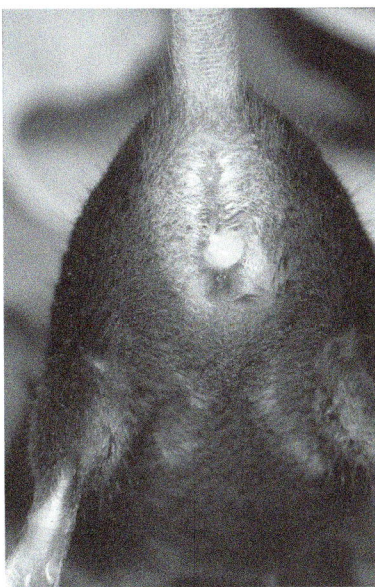

Figure 21.6 A typical copulation plug, deposited after mating. This is composed of secretions from the male's prostate, seminal vesicles and coagulating glands. The copulation plug is supposed to prevent a second mating event, but females may groom it away.

but it is uncommon in laboratory circumstances, as stable mating pairs decrease the incidence in male mice (Soroker & Terkel 1988).

The litter size of inbred mice is smaller than that of outbred mice and is a strain trait likely genetically determined, as is gestation period (Murray *et al.* 2010). Several inbred strains have issues with conception, placentation, fertility retention with age, or other aspects of successfully delivering a litter of pups (as an example: Hino *et al.* 2009). In outbred mice, litter sizes are typically 10–12 pups and the gestation period is shortened based on litter total weight, which usually correlates with litter size (Biggers *et al.* 1963; McLaren & Michie 1963) (Figure 21.7). Pups weigh 1–2 g at birth.

After giving birth, mice exhibit several highly conserved maternal behaviours (Weber & Olsson 2008). They maintain elaborate nests, are more aggressive towards strange conspecifics, groom and maintain pups and retrieve pups to the nest. Female mice have five pairs of mammary glands and feed their pups exclusively via lactation for at least the first 10 days of life. Mouse lactation peaks between days 10–16 and mice produce between 8 and 16 ml of milk per day (Knight *et al.* 1986). Mouse milk is relatively concentrated with a low water content, a fat level of around 20% and a protein level of about 14% (Meier *et al.* 1965; Gors *et al.* 2009). These percentages vary with the age of the litter (Knight *et al.* 1986).

Mice give birth to altricial pups that develop to weaning in 21–28 days. Major milestones of pup development are readily apparent on examination, and these cues can be used to accurately age a litter missed on daily checks. However, outbred mice develop 12–24 h more rapidly, that is, a 2-day-old outbred mouse pup will better resemble a 3-day-old inbred mouse pup until about post-natal day (PND) 7. The Jackson Laboratory has created a poster that illustrates these developments in pigmented and albino mice. On the day of birth (PND 0 and PND 1), mice are bright red and a milk spot – the full stomach – should be readily visible through the skin of the abdomen. The ear flaps are attached to the head at birth but shift to be perpendicular to the head around PND 3 and PND 4 and assume their usual backward appearance around PND 5. Fur begins erupting through the skin at about PND 6, starting behind the ears, and often giving the mice a linty or fuzzy appearance. By PND 10, all fur has fully erupted, and animals are more active, leaving the nest and attempting to eat food other than milk. The teeth erupt around PND 11, and by PND 12, the eyes are open, the ears are open and the animals are eating solid food. Mice can be successfully weaned at PND 14, but this gives rise to changes in behaviour when compared to animals weaned at PND 21 or PND 28, with the 7-day intervals above being a convenience of husbandry (Richter *et al.* 2016; Gaskill *et al.* 2017). In the wild, weaning

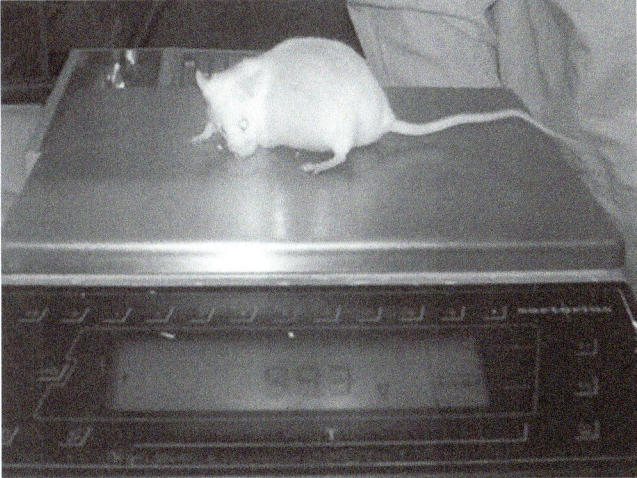
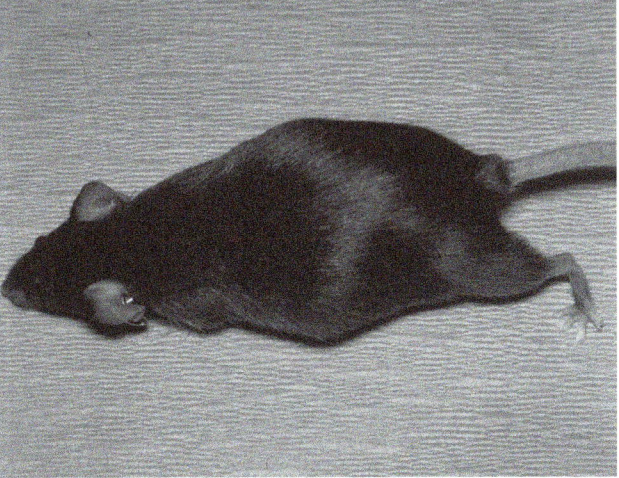

Figure 21.7 A pregnant CD1, weighing in at 99 g. The evening of this photo, she delivered 14 pups. The pregnant C57BL/6 pictured here delivered 6 pups later that day.

is a more gradual process, occurring between PND 28 and up to PND 86, where adolescent animals stop nursing and are allowed to hang around the territory, mostly ignored by adults, until their sexual maturity tips them towards dispersal (Gerlach 1996; Bechard & Mason 2010).

The rise of the genetically modified mouse as the most common mammal used in research today was at least partially down to the ease of manipulation of mouse reproduction. As well as artificially inducing oestrus through the administration of pregnant mare serum gonadotropin (PMSG) followed by human chorionic gonadotropin (hCG), manipulation of the mouse estrous cycle may be accomplished through natural means. The three most commonly described methods for manipulating mouse reproduction are known as the Bruce effect, the Whitten effect and the Lee-Boot effect. The Bruce effect is the termination of early pregnancy in a female when exposed to a strange male (Bruce 1960). The Whitten effect is the induction of oestrus in females exposed to male mouse urine (Whitten 1956; Whitten 1958). Finally, the Lee-Boot effect is the cessation of estrous cycling in female mice kept in groups with no male input (van der Lee & Boot 1955; van der Lee & Boot, 1956). The Whitten and Lee-Boot effects are often combined by housing female mice together for several days to allow them to cease cycling and then separating them and exposing them to male mouse urine to bring them into oestrus. As for PMSG/hCG administration, the responsiveness of mice to this regimen varies with genetic background, and refinements in time of administration may result in more successful outcomes (Byers *et al.* 2006; Luo *et al.* 2011).

Problem and abnormal behaviour

As discussed above, as animals fail to cope with chronic stress, every aspect of their biology changes and they cease to be a meaningful model (Garner *et al.* 2017; Gaskill & Garner 2017). Such animals can be hard to detect, especially if the population in general is under uncontrollable stress, and thus, what we think is normal is actually abnormal. In this scenario, even control animals are abnormal, and the 'internal validity' of the model is compromised (Garner *et al.* 2017; Gaskill & Garner 2017; Würbel 2017). For instance, non-obese diabetic (NOD) mice housed on the top of the rack are sufficiently stressed and immune compromised, that their development of type I (autoimmune) diabetes is significantly delayed (Ader *et al.* 1991). When abnormal physiology and immunology goes unnoticed because it is the statistical norm, abnormal or problem behaviours can often serve as the tell-tale signal that something is wrong. For instance, barbering used to be considered normal in C57BL/6 mice (The Jackson Laboratory 1987; Garner *et al.* 2004b) before its status as an abnormal behaviour was recognised (Garner *et al.* 2004a; Garner *et al.* 2004b; Dufour & Garner 2010; Garner *et al.* 2011).

Problem behaviours and abnormal behaviours are important to distinguish (Mills 2003; Mason & Latham 2004). Problem behaviours are perfectly normal behaviours that happen to annoy humans or otherwise cause inconvenience for humans, such as normal chewing in teething puppies. In mice, a good example is cannibalism of pups – this is a perfectly normal behaviour in mice when pups die (Weber & Olsson 2008; Weber *et al.* 2013). Conversely, abnormal behaviours do deviate from the normal expression of behaviour or normal behaviour repertoire in the wild. There is no one feature of a behaviour that makes it abnormal. Instead, in direct parallel to human psychiatry, we apply five criteria that are neither necessary nor sufficient and take a 'weight of evidence' approach (Garner 2005), namely:

1. Is the behaviour seen only in captivity (e.g. stereotypy in mice)?
2. If seen in the wild as well as captivity, is the behaviour performed in inappropriate circumstances, or performed excessively (e.g. food grinding)?
3. Is the behaviour peculiar to a subset of individuals (e.g. barbering in mice)?
4. Does the behaviour impair function? For example, does it involve self-injury (e.g. ulcerative dermatitis in mice), affect social interactions, or have deleterious consequences on health, growth, or reproduction?
5. Does the behaviour induce signs of distress in the animal or its companions (e.g. injurious aggression in mice)?

For instance, barbering meets criteria 1, 3, 4 and 5; stereotypies meet 1, 3 and 4; food grinding meets 1, 2 and 3. Abnormal behaviours can be further subdivided into 'maladaptive' and 'malfunctional behaviour' (Mills 2003). In maladaptive behaviour, the animal is perfectly normal, and the abnormality of their behaviour merely reflects the abnormality of the environment, in particular the persistence of a cue, or the blocking of the final culmination of the behaviour. Food grinding in mice (described below) is a great example; see (Pritchett-Corning *et al.* 2013). Conversely, in malfunctional behaviours, the behaviour reflects a fundamental underlying change in physiology, and the abnormality of the behaviour reflects the abnormality of the animal, as in the case of stereotypies and barbering (Garner *et al.* 2011). Note that the veterinary behaviour literature is inconsistent in the use of these terms and may refer to all three categories of behaviour as 'problem behaviours' or 'abnormal behaviours', but nevertheless typically separates them into the same three concepts (e.g. Mills 2003).

These distinctions matter because they have direct implications for behavioural management. Problem behaviours may require no management at all but rather education in species-typical behaviours such as disposing of dead pups by consumption or providing substrates for the behaviour so that the behaviour is not bothersome to humans. In either case, the real issue with problem behaviours is a human one not an animal one, and the onus is on the human to manage their expectations for the animal and their response to the behaviour – the animal itself is perfectly normal and should not be penalised for inadequate husbandry or our lack of understanding. In the case of maladaptive behaviours, given that the animal is normal, changing the environment to remove persistent cues, or allow the culmination of behaviour, can resolve the behaviour. For instance, with food grinding in mice, addressing the underlying deficiencies in mouse diets, which lead to this behaviour, resolves it (Pritchett-Corning et al. 2013). In the case of malfunctional behaviours, it is essential to recognise that because these behaviours reflect a fundamental, and potentially permanent, harm to the animal, animals showing these behaviours can be worthless as research subjects (Garner 2005). Thus, not only has the animal's life been wasted, but so have research funds and time, even to the point of potentially producing spurious results (Garner 2005; Garner et al. 2017). Therefore, malfunctional behaviours represent a turnabout of the old saying 'good welfare is good science'. In the case of malfunctional behaviours, 'bad welfare is bad science', and behavioural management and enrichment is not a luxury but a necessity.

Mouse illnesses

Mouse illnesses: infectious agents and health monitoring

Mice are prey to a number of different infectious agents including fungal, protozoan, metazoan, viral and bacterial (Fahey & Olekszak, 2015; Mahler et al. 2015; Marx et al. 2017; Cooper et al. 2021). Most of these have been eliminated from modern vivaria (Albers et al. 2023; Pritchett-Corning et al. 2009), often with clear unintended negative consequences for research (Abolins et al. 2017; Graham 2021). Table 21.3 lists information on a limited number of viral, bacterial and parasitic agents still prevalent in vivaria. These agents remain prevalent due to their biology, relatively recent discovery or perceived lack of effects on research. In modern vivaria, 'prevalent' can be defined very differently for each agent. For example, approximately 20% of samples submitted to a large diagnostic laboratory over 10 years tested positive for mouse norovirus, while 0.25% of samples tested positive for mouse parvoviruses (Albers et al. 2023). Despite differences in these absolute values, both are considered 'prevalent' for health-monitoring purposes. The reader is pointed to *The Mouse in Biomedical Research* (vol 2) (Fox et al. 2008) and *The Laboratory Mouse* (Hedrich & Bullock 2004) for more detailed information on mouse infectious agents, including those which are mainly of historical interest, and their potential consequences for research. Parasitic infections and infestations of mice are further covered in *Flynn's Parasites of Laboratory Animals* (Baker 2007). Texts should be supplemented with information from more recent sources as well. Charles River's infectious agent technical information sheets[3] and University of Missouri's DORA[4] are two examples. As new infectious agents are discovered, facilities must decide whether they will tolerate the presence of these agents in their colonies. An example of this is the newly described mouse kidney parvovirus/murine chapparvovirus (Ge et al. 2020), which is actually associated with lesions in immunocompetent animals unlike many other parvoviruses (Edmondson et al. 2020).

Health monitoring is an important part of maintaining the welfare of mice used in research. Although most infectious agents that cause acute illness or death in mice have been eliminated from modern vivaria (e.g. *Salmonella* or ectromelia), other infectious agents are not tolerated due to their putatively negative effects on research. For modern vivaria, a widely used list of infectious agents to monitor in facilities is propagated by the Federation of European Laboratory Animal Science Associations (FELASA) (Mähler et al. 2014). The FELASA guidelines are updated regularly and are likely due to be updated soon. In some cases, excluding these agents may be affecting research in an unexpected fashion, as the full development of the mouse's immune system is dependent on exposure to infectious agents (Hamilton et al. 2020).

The most basic type of health monitoring is sending sick mice for euthanasia and necropsy and attempting to diagnose illness. This may be supplemented by examination of apparently healthy colony mice. Classical health monitoring involves exposing clean mice, called sentinels and usually sourced from vendors, to either colony mice (direct) or their dirty bedding (indirect) (Thigpen et al. 1989). After the sentinels have been exposed to the colony, they are euthanised and sampled for the presence of infectious organisms via culture, exam, polymerase chain reaction (PCR) or serology, depending on the agent and the availability of the technology. Live sentinel mice have been supplanted in many vivaria with environmental sampling of exhaust dust of individually ventilated cages (IVCs) racks or other animal-sparing technologies (Miller et al. 2016; Niimi et al. 2018; Miller & Brielmeier, 2018; Luchins et al. 2020; Mailhiot et al. 2020; Buchheister & Bleich 2021; Winn et al. 2022).

Any concerns related to infectious illness or parasitism should also be addressed through a robust pest control programme. Wild and feral mice entering the vivarium may serve as a source of contamination of research colonies (Parker et al. 2009; Williams et al. 2018), as may items not treated to eliminate contamination (Reuter et al. 2011) or inadvertently contaminated (Lindstrom et al. 2018).

Mouse illnesses: non-infectious diseases

Non-infectious diseases of mice are relatively common. These are typically disorders of development (hydrocephalus and microphthalmia) or disorders associated with behaviour (wounding secondary to fighting). Some of these disorders may have a basis in genetics, as they appear more commonly in some strains when compared to others, but this may also be a confirmation bias, as some strains are much more commonly used in research than others. Several of these disorders and potential treatments, if available, will be addressed below. They are illustrated in Figure 21.8.

Anophthalmia/microphthalmia/congenital cataract

The failure of development of one or both eyes is a common finding in C57BL background mice with reported incidences of up to 12% (Smith et al. 1994). Mice are valuable models in the

---

[3] https://www.criver.com/products-services/research-models-services/animal-health-surveillance/infectious-agent-information (Accessed April 3, 2023)

[4] http://dora.missouri.edu/mouse/ (Accessed April 3, 2023)

Table 21.3 Some mouse infectious agents prevalent in modern vivaria.

Agent	Class	Clinical signs in immunocompetent animals	Treatment	Possible effects on research[5]
Pinworms	Metazoan parasite, various species	None	Avermectins, benzimidazoles	Potentiate Th2 immune system activation, changes in haematopoietic system (Bugarski et al. 2006)
Fur mites	Metazoan parasite, various species	None, mild pruritus alopecia	Avermectins, +/– insect growth regulators	Dermatitis, alopecia, IgE production (Pochanke et al. 2006; Moats et al. 2016)
Protozoa	Protozoan parasites	None, non-specific weight loss	Fostering, embryo transfer rederivation, some chemical treatments available, depending on agent	Dependent on type, for example, Th1 response (Escalante et al. 2016) or change in intestinal morphology (Brett & Cox 1982)
Parvoviruses	DNA viruses, non-enveloped	None	Embryo transfer rederivation	May suppress tumour formation (Cornelis et al. 2006), other immunomodulatory effects (Janus & Bleich 2012)
Coronaviruses	RNA viruses, enveloped	None to mortality	Embryo transfer rederivation	Dependent on type, prior presence in colony; neurotropic viruses are rarely seen but may cause fatality, while enterotropic viruses may result in death of young animals; may also have an immunomodulatory effect (Korner et al. 2020)
Murine norovirus	DNA virus, non-enveloped	None	Embryo transfer rederivation	Interactions with host enteric microbiome, (Karst & Wobus 2015), mild intestinal inflammation (Mumphrey et al. 2007)
Rodentibacter spp.	G- coccobacillus	None, respiratory infections, retrobulbar and other abscesses as an opportunist	Rederivation is possible and often pursued; enrofloxacin in drinking water also possible (Benga et al. 2018)	Generalised inflammatory effects would seem to be possible (Patten et al. 2010), but severe outcomes in immunodeficient mice are sometimes seen (Towne et al. 2014)
Helicobacter spp.	G- spiral-shaped bacteria	None, rectal prolapse, potentiation of hepatic tumours	Fostering, embryo transfer rederivation, oral 'triple therapy'(amoxicillin, metronidazole, bismuth) (Foltz et al. 1996)	May affect fertility (Bracken et al. 2017), induce hepatitis (Fox et al. 2004), induce liver tumours (Canella et al. 1996), cause gastritis and typhlocolitis (Whary & Fox 2006)
Staphylococcus aureus	G+ cocci	None, secondary skin infections if open wounds, preputial adenitis	Usually not recommended, but susceptibility and antibiotics might be considered. Most *S. aureus* found in mice are mouse-adapted, not from humans (Mrochen et al. 2018)	Secondary infection of wound sites, damage to prepuce secondary to preputial gland adenitis (Hong & Ediger 1978; Holtfreter et al. 2013), unsuitable for use in *S. aureus* modelling research (Schulz et al. 2017)

Source: Albers et al. 2023; Pritchett-Corning et al. 2009; Marx et al. 2017.

study of human ocular dysgenesis, and both spontaneously occurring, and genetically engineered animals are used to this end (Graw 2019). Mice can apparently have these problems to little ill effect, but their appearance can be disconcerting.

Barbering

Mice occasionally pull their own or their cage-mates' hair and whiskers, resulting in bald patches (e.g. Kahnau et al. 2022). C57BL/6 mice of any type are notorious for this behaviour, and female mice barber more than males (Garner et al. 2004b). Barbering is not dominance-related (Garner et al. 2004a) but is likely a disease of oxidative stress in mice (Vieira et al. 2017). Animals may barber other animals, adults or pups, as well as themselves, and these patterns may vary from cage to cage but are often consistent within a cage (Garner et al. 2004a). Barbering in and of itself is not harmful.

[5] By no means exhaustive and for many agents, references are sparse or not current.

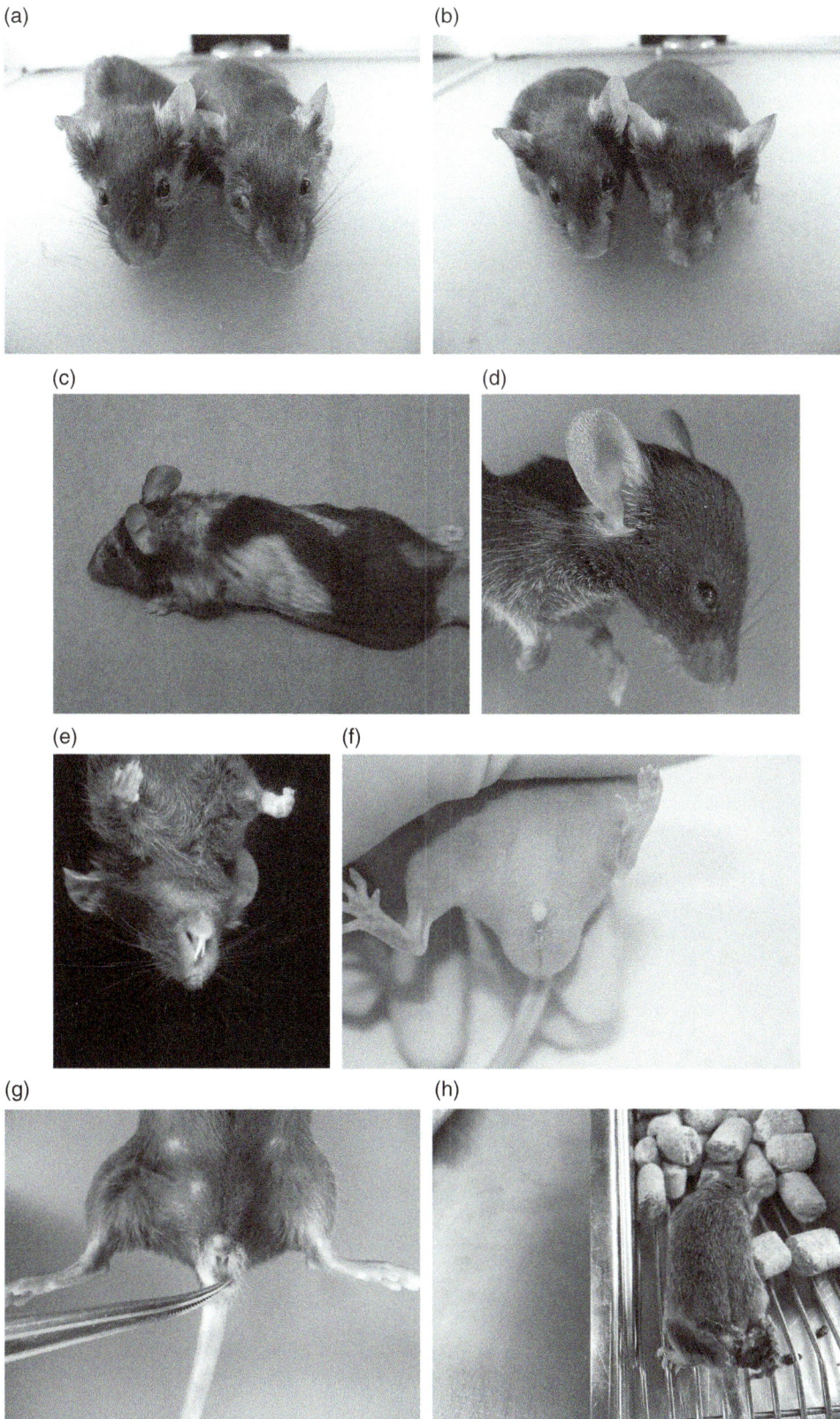

Figure 21.8 Photos of several conditions described below. (a) and (b) Micro- and anophthalmia in young C57BL/6 mice. In both photos, the normal mouse is on the left. (c) Barbering (flanks; hair is missing) and ulcerative dermatitis (scruff; open wounds) in a retired C57BL/6 breeder. (d) The domed head characteristic of hydrocephalus, as presented in a weanling-age C57BL/6 mouse. This is a common age for presentation and the domed head is produced when the intracranial pressure puts strain on the open cranial sutures. (e) A photo of a mouse with malocclusion. The mouse's open-rooted incisors should meet and the hard enamel should wear on the occlusal surfaces. When the jaw or teeth are damaged, the teeth continue to grow, resulting in pain, issues with eating, and weight loss. (f) The failure of the vaginal membrane to dissolve at puberty results in a build-up of fluids in the vagina. A vaginal septum may interfere with the animal's suitability for breeding use as shown in a nude mouse. (g) Imperforate vagina in a C57BL/6 mouse. (h) A very common presentation of wounds secondary to fighting in male mice. The tail, hind feet and genitals may also be targeted by the aggressor.

However, the behavioural deficits that may be caused by the loss of whiskers or the potential thermoregulatory issues associated with hair loss are of concern. Barbering can serve as a model of trichotillomania in humans (Garner et al. 2004b; Kurien et al. 2005).

Hydrocephalus

Hydrocephalus is characterised by the accumulation of cerebrospinal fluid in the ventricles of the brain, resulting in enlargement of the ventricles and damage to cerebral tissue (Vogel et al. 2012). In mice, hydrocephalus is a not unexpected finding, with a reported incidence of 0.03% in C57BL/6J mice (Pritchett 2003a). Although cases can be secondary to viral or other insults, most cases are found by noting the characteristic domed head at weaning. These animals should be euthanised when found as the condition is likely to be painful, and it is incompatible with maturation and normal life in mice.

Malocclusion

Malocclusion in mice is usually seen in the incisors, although molar malocclusion and tongue entrapment is theoretically possible. The open-rooted teeth of mice grow rapidly, with documented rates of 2 mm/week for upper incisors and 2.8 mm/week for lower incisors (Zegarelli 1944). The enamel of rodents is very hard, containing iron, which can give the teeth a yellow cast. Typically, the incisors wear on each other, and the mouse maintains normal dentition; although gnawing is an exploratory behaviour in mice, as well as an ingestive one, it is not necessary for normal tooth wear. If the occlusion of the incisors is damaged in any way, this wear does not occur, and the teeth overgrow. The incidence of spontaneous incisor malocclusion found at weaning in C57BL/6J mice is reported to be approximately 0.05% (Pritchett 2003b). Rates in older mice are unknown and dependent on a myriad of factors. If the animal is valuable, its teeth may be trimmed regularly, and it will likely do well if provided with a soft diet. Breeding is not advised, however, as the condition may be heritable.

Ulcerative dermatitis

Ulcerative dermatitis is a descriptive, catchall term for all moist skin lesions of uncertain aetiology in mice. Although some may be bacterial in origin, associated with Staphylococcal infections, most are behavioural. Typical ulcerative dermatitis lesions are seen on the ears and scruff and are associated with hindlimb scratching related to aberrant grooming behaviour. Trimming the hind nails seems to break the scratch/itch cycle for long enough for these lesions to heal on their own (Adams et al. 2016; Alvarado et al. 2016; Davison et al. 2022). Ulcerative dermatitis lesions seen on the flank or lower forelimbs, seem to be due to chewing and are difficult to resolve (Adams et al. 2016). Anecdotally, we have seen some resolution of flank lesions with nail trims on all four feet, as the normal grooming pattern of mice on the flanks does involve the forefeet. Ulcerative dermatitis is a significant cause of morbidity and mortality (through euthanasia) in mouse colonies (Marx et al. 2013), and subsequently, a welfare issue that should be vigorously addressed. If treatments turn out to be ameliorative rather than curative or if the disease recurs, animals should be scored as to severity (Hampton et al. 2012), and the quality of life evaluated with respect to pre-determined humane endpoints.

Unexpected genetic effects

'Unexpected genetic effects' covers a myriad of situations from off-target CRISPR effects (Anderson et al. 2018) to infertility or subfertility (Fei & Zhou 2022) to embryonic lethality (Ward et al. 2012) to leaky Cre-lox systems (Prabhakar et al. 2019) to inactivation of transgenes by methylation (Sapienza et al. 1987). The citations provided are hardly comprehensive. When genetically modified animals do not breed, have unexpected Mendelian ratios in offspring, or do not perform as expected in assays, evaluate the environment, of course, but also look into what might be going wrong genetically. Many genes have variable expression dependent on background (Rivera & Tessarollo 2008), genetic contamination is common (Nitzki et al. 2007; Yang et al. 2011), investigators are not always aware of how commercially available substrains of mice differ (Zurita et al. 2011) and substrain formation within labs is rampant (Benavides et al. 2020). All of these factors may affect behaviour and research outcomes (see also Chapter 4: An introduction to laboratory animal genetics).

Vaginal septa and imperforate vagina

The mouse has a bicornuate uterus with one uterine body, cervix, and vagina, formed from the paramesonephric ducts (Müllerian ducts) in the embryo (Kurita 2010). Any issues with fusion of this tissue may result in vaginal septa, typically longitudinal in the mouse (Cunliffe-Beamer & Feldman 1976). Vaginal septa occur at different frequencies in different inbred strains (Gearhart et al. 2004; Shire 1984). Breeding mice with vaginal septa is not recommended due to decreased reproductive success and likely heritability (Chang et al. 2013). Imperforate vagina is a separate issue, related to the failure of the vaginal closure plate to dissolve at the onset of puberty (Eisen et al. 1989; Sundberg & Brown 1994) leading to abdominal and perineal distention, secondary to mucometra (Ginty & Hoogstraten-Miller 2008). Although this condition may be repaired with surgery, its likely heritability (Didion et al. 1991) makes surgery only useful to keep a valuable animal on study (Masangkay & Kondo 1983).

Wounding secondary to aggression

As noted later, fighting in mice is a problem behaviour, but not an unnatural one. Mice are territorial and hierarchical, so aggressive behaviour comes as part of the installed firmware. Males are more likely to show home-cage aggression (Garner 2005; Gaskill et al. 2017; Lidster et al. 2019; Weber et al. 2017; Jirkof et al. 2020), but it is not limited entirely to males as females will defend pups and do establish hierarchies within a cage. Animals can kill each other over the course of a night, so any signs of aggression should be dealt with swiftly (Blankenberger et al. 2018). Housing animals at lower densities such as three to a standard cage rather than five may also help (Van Loo et al. 2003a; Jirkof et al. 2020).

Laboratory procedures

As the most commonly used mammal in research, there is a plethora of resources available describing common laboratory or research procedures. Before any studies using mice are undertaken, the authors recommend the use of the PREPARE guidelines (Smith *et al.* 2018) and subsequently, for reporting work completed, the ARRIVE 2.0 guidelines (Percie du Sert *et al.* 2020). See also Chapter 2: The design of animal experiments.

Identification

Individual mice within a cage may be identified in a myriad of ways. The most common tend to involve the ears, either ear punches or ear tags. Punch patterns are available widely online and one of the more commonly used may be found at the Jackson Laboratory's website[6]. Ear punching is likely to cause brief pain (Taitt & Kendall 2019; Burn *et al.* 2021) and in some strains, the hole will heal over, rendering this method useless (Rajnoch *et al.* 2003). If the laboratory uses ear punches, be sure to send the key with any mice exported to other institutions and be sure to ask for a key should mice be imported. Tags are also widely available and may be made of metal or plastic. They may be numbered, printed with bar codes or QR codes, or contain RFID chips, allowing them to be read by smartphones or other devices in use in the animal room. Ear tags are not suitable for all mice, as they may potentiate tumour formation in some strains or serve as a nidus of infection (Waalkes *et al.* 1987; Cover *et al.* 1989).

For more permanent identification, and uniquely for use on nude animals, tattoos may be applied to the body. For identification of very young animals, footpad tattoos may be of use, and some labs also identify older animals in this fashion. Automatic tattoo machines may also be used to apply consistent tattoos to the tails of animals. Microchips (actually RFID transponders) inserted subcutaneously on the dorsum or tail are also in use for some applications. These require outlay in implanting devices, chips and readers in order to output information, but are unique to animals and have the advantage of being removable at the end of study, where they can be stored with tissues to continue unique identification of any samples collected.

Depending on the coat colour, mice may be dyed or shaved if short-term markings are desired. Although human hair dye may be used, a better option is animal fur markers, which are available in a variety of colours. For very brief identification, tails or ears may be marked with permanent laboratory marker, although animals groom this away quickly. Although there is some evidence that rats may find this marking distressful, mice seem to mind it less when compared to ear punching (Burn *et al.* 2008; Burn *et al.* 2021).

In some localities, the removal of the distal portion of the toes from young mice is allowed as a means of identification as well as DNA sample collection, albeit with caveats. The main caveat is often that the tissue collected at toe removal must be used for another purpose; toe clipping is rarely allowed solely as an identification method. Furthermore, typical guidelines include an upper and lower age bound on animals for this procedure, the removal of only the third phalanx from only one digit of each paw and scientific justification for why other methods of identification are not suitable. When performed appropriately and with care, it does not seem to have long-term impacts on mouse health or welfare (Castelhano-Carlos *et al.* 2010; Schaefer *et al.* 2010; Paluch *et al.* 2014; Frezel *et al.* 2019). The same concerns related to ensuring clear communication about the assigned number for ear punched animals using varying systems also apply to toe clipping.

Handling

Mice must be regularly removed from their primary enclosures for husbandry and experimental reasons, and they come equipped with a convenient handle in the tail. Predators, including humans, find the tail an irresistible target, but mice find handling by the tail aversive (Hurst & West 2010). Adapting handing to minimise mouse anxiety can effect changes in behaviour that affect research results (Gouveia & Hurst 2013; Gouveia & Hurst 2017; Clarkson *et al.* 2018; Nakamura & Suzuki 2018) (Figure 21.9). Eschewing tail handling does not necessarily result in increased husbandry time or tasks (Doerning *et al.* 2019), but there is a potential biosecurity consideration. Refinement of mouse handling has been shown to increase breeding performance in C57BL/6 mice (Hull *et al.* 2022). Wider adoption of these methods must be driven by scientists and animal facilities together (O'Malley *et al.* 2022).

After the mouse is lifted to the top of the cage non-aversively, such as by tunnel or cupped hand, there are other means to grasp the mouse safely to allow for research manipulations with minimal risk to human handlers (Machholz *et al.* 2012; Attanasio *et al.* 2022). The most typical means is through 'scruffing', or restraining the mouse in one hand by pinching the scruff between the thumb and forefingers and threading the tail between the last two fingers. A

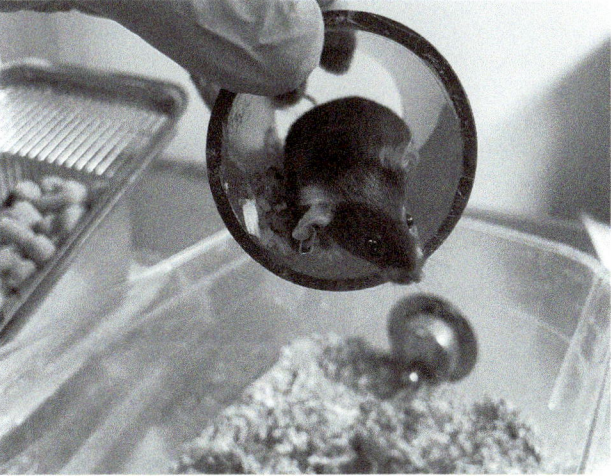

Figure 21.9 Handling mice using a polycarbonate tube. Mice readily adapt to such handling and the tube can be left in the cage and serve as a retreat, visual barrier and self-rescue apparatus in case of floods.

---

[6]https://www.jax.org/jax-mice-and-services/customer-support/technical-support/breeding-and-husbandry-support/mouse-identification (Accessed April 4, 2023)

commercially available method to aid scruffing is also possible, which allows for restraint as well as protecting the hand[7]. The slit in the item also allows for subcutaneous injection. If dangerous substances are to be injected peritoneally, thin plastic restrainers, typically used to allow for decapitation, can firmly restrain the mouse. For other injections, such as tail vein, intramuscular or procedures such as toenail clipping, a wide variety of plastic restrainers are available. One of the more common, and least expensive, involves melting holes in a standard 50-ml conical tube using a soldering iron.

Training

Mice can be trained, a trait they share with more charismatic megafauna. Training of mice to perform behavioural tasks is routine in many neuroscience laboratories, for example. Mice may be trained to press levers, poke their noses into holes or perform other behaviours in response to stimuli as varied as odour, foot shock or the presence of conspecifics. The rewards are just as varied: food, water, addictive substances or access to desired resources. In many cases, mice are acclimated to handling for research reasons (Gaskill et al. 2013b), trained to better perform certain tasks (Dickmann et al. 2022) or trained as part of an enrichment programme (Leidinger et al. 2017). If a scientist wishes to learn more about shaping mouse behaviour using positive reinforcement to meet a husbandry or research aim, an excellent reference may be found at Karen Pryor's website[8]. A further explanation of how this training may work can be found in (Feng et al. 2016); see also Chapter 15: The use of positive reinforcement training techniques to enhance the care and welfare of laboratory and research animals. A subtly different paradigm, negative reinforcement, can be used to train mice to void urine or faecal pellets for collection – in this case, the natural anti-predator response of voiding urine and faeces is shaped, during handling, and reinforced by return to the cage or cessation of handling.

Substance administration

Experimental requirements may mean that substances must be administered to mice. Standard routes are reviewed in Table 21.4, but the routes possible are limited only by research or anaesthesia requirements (Diehl et al. 2001; Turner et al. 2011a; Turner et al. 2011b; Attanasio et al. 2022). Volumes of substances administered should be appropriate to the route and any vehicles or diluents used adjusted to an appropriate temperature and pH (Gad et al. 2016) to avoid tissue damage.

Blood collection

A mouse's estimated total blood volume is 6–8% of their body weight or approximately 77–80 ml/kg. Without fluid replacement, approximately 0.007–0.008 ml of blood/g of body weight can be safely withdrawn (about 0.18–0.2 ml of blood from a 25-g mouse); with fluid replacement, approximately 0.014–0.016 ml blood/g of body weight can be withdrawn (about 0.35–0.4 ml blood from a 25-g mouse). All non-terminal blood collection without replacement of fluids is limited up to 10% of total circulating blood volume in healthy, normal, adult animals on a single occasion and collection may be repeated after 3–4 weeks. When repeated blood samples are required at short intervals, a maximum of 0.6 ml/kg/day or 1.0% of an animal's total blood volume can typically be removed every 24 h subject to local legal requirements (Diehl et al. 2001; Parasuraman et al. 2010). Common sampling routes, volumes obtainable and other details can be found in Table 21.5. Route of sampling may affect welfare and should be considered for non-terminal bleeds (Tsai et al. 2015; Meyer et al. 2020; Ahrens Kress et al. 2022).

Excellent web-based resources on mouse blood sampling can be found at NC3Rs[9] and JoVE.[10,11]

Anaesthesia and analgesia

Entire texts have been written on analgesia and anaesthesia of mice. The reader is referred specifically to Flecknell 2023. Anaesthetic and analgesic agent availability may vary from country to country; investigators should follow relevant laws or guidelines as necessary. As new anaesthetics and analgesics are regularly introduced to the market, and old drugs are combined in new ways, a review of current literature to ensure best practice is always warranted (Flecknell 2018; Foley et al. 2019; Navarro et al. 2021; Oates & Tarbert 2023). Tables 21.6

Table 21.4 Compound administration guidelines for mice.

Route	Abbreviation	Volume	Gauge/length of needle
Intranasal	IN	5–50 µl	N/A
Intramuscular	IM	0.00005 ml/g	<23 ga, 5–12.7 mm (3/16–1/2 in.)
Intraperitoneal	IP	0.02 ml/g	<21 ga, 19–25 mm (3/4 to 1 in)
Intradermal	ID	0.05–0.1 ml	<26 ga, 12.7 mm (1/2 in)
Subcutaneous	SC or SQ	0.01 ml/g	<22 ga, 12.7–25 mm (1/2 to 1 in)
Intravenous	IV	0.005–0.025 ml/g*	<25 ga, 12.7–19mm (1/2 to 3/4 in)
Oral gavage or per os	PO	0.01 ml/g	20–22 ga feeding needle, length determined by measurement of animal

Source: Machholz et al. 2012; Turner et al. 2011a; Turner et al. 2011b.

---

[7]https://researchdevices.com/scruffguard/ (Accessed April 4, 2023)
[8]www.clickertraining.com (Accessed April 4, 2023)
[9]https://www.nc3rs.org.uk/3rs-resources/blood-sampling/blood-sampling-mouse (Accessed April 4, 2023).
[10]https://www.jove.com/v/10246/blood-withdrawal-i (Accessed April 4. 2023)
[11]https://www.jove.com/v/10247/blood-withdrawal-ii (Accessed April 4, 2023)

Table 21.5 Blood withdrawal routes for mice.

Route	Anaesthesia required	Terminal only	Appropriate for repeated sampling	Other caveats
Tail vein	No	No	Yes	Nick the lateral tail vein with a needle or scalpel (Moore et al. 2017)
Tail snip	No	No	Yes	Care must be taken to remove only minimal amounts of skin, avoiding bone. For repeated sampling, disrupt the scab (Moore et al. 2017)
Facial vein/submandibular	No	No	Yes	Concerns have been raised about the humane aspects of this route (Frohlich et al. 2018)
Chin/submental vein	No	No	Yes	Relatively large volume obtainable compared to some other routes (Regan et al. 2016)
Saphenous vein	No	No	Yes	Difficult to collect large volumes and may cause concerns with repeated sampling (Aasland et al. 2010)
Retro-orbital sinus	Yes	Perhaps	Limited	Necessary for haemophilia models (Holmberg et al. 2011)
Jugular vein	No	No	Limited	Relatively limited data on welfare effects (Shirasaki et al. 2012; Tsai et al. 2015)
Cardiac puncture	Yes	Perhaps	No	Has been described as a non-terminal method in wild *Peromyscus* (Williams et al. 2020) and was used as a repeat sampling method for lab mice in the past (Hicks & Little 1931)

Source: Ahrens Kress et al. 2022; Hoggatt et al. 2016; Joslin 2009; Parasuraman et al. 2010; Whittaker and Barker 2020.

Table 21.6 Anaesthetics for mice: doses and routes.

Agent(s)	Dose	Route	Caveats
Single agents			
Halogenated anaesthetics (isoflurane, sevoflurane, desflurane)	Given in per cent mixed with oxygen – usually 1–5%	Inhaled	Quick onset, quick recovery, no residual pain management
Pentobarbital	40–50 mg/kg	IP	
Tribromoethanol	250 mg/kg	IP	Not available commercially, must be prepared, cannot be used twice in the same animal or top-up doses given (not advised, but still in use occasionally)
Cocktails			
Ketamine/xylazine	80–100 mg/kg ketamine, 10 mg/kg xylazine	IP	Dissociative (ketamine) + alpha-2 agonist (xylazine), slow recovery; anaesthetic dose cannot be easily or safely adjusted intra-operatively. Xylazine provides some analgesia. Potential for profound hypoxia with longer anaesthetic lengths. Xylazine reversible with atipamezole (1–2.5 mg/kg)
Ketamine/medetomidine	50–75 mg/kg ketamine, 0.5–1 mg/kg medetomidine	IP	Dissociative (ketamine) + alpha-2 agonist (medetomidine). Male mice more sensitive to this combination. Potential for profound hypoxia with longer anaesthetic lengths. Medetomidine reversible with atipamezole (1–2.5 mg/kg)
Ketamine/xylazine/acepromazine	80–100 mg/kg ketamine, 10 mg/kg xylazine, 3 mg/kg acepromazine	IP	Dissociative (ketamine) + alpha-2 agonist (xylazine) + sedative (acepromazine). Longer duration of surgical anaesthesia when compared to k + x alone. Xylazine reversible with atipamezole (1–2.5 mg/kg).

Source: Bennett & Lewis 2022; Flecknell 2023; Gargiulo et al. 2012a; Gargiulo et al. 2012b; Navarro et al. 2021.

and 21.7 provide a very truncated overview of some anaesthetic and analgesic agents commonly used in mice.

Surgery

Rodents are some of the few animals subject to surgery by people who are not medical professionals. Any proposed surgery should be reviewed and approved by the relevant authority (ethical board, Institutional Animal Care and Use Committee (IACUC), etc.). Before investigators undertake surgery, institutions should ensure that there is good training in surgical techniques, suture choice and asepsis as well as an understanding of perioperative and postoperative care of rodents (Hoyt et al. 2001a; Hoyt et al. 2001b; Hoogstraten-Miller & Brown 2008; Bernal et al. 2009;

Table 21.7 Analgesics for mice: doses and routes.

Agent(s)	Dose	Route	Caveats
Local			
Lidocaine	2–4 mg/kg, typically once	SC, ID, periosteally, splash block	Dilute human or animal product to 0.5%. Do not exceed 7 mg/kg total dose, administer subcutaneously before making incision. Typical onset of effects in 2–5 min, but duration of 2–3 h
Bupivacaine	1–2 mg/kg, typically once	SC, ID, periosteally, splash block	Dilute human or animal product to 0.25%. Do not exceed 8 mg/kg total dose. Administer subcutaneously along incision line before making incision. Typical onset of effects in 5–10 min, but duration of 4–8 h
Non-steroidal anti-inflammatory			
Ketoprofen	10 or 20 mg/kg	SC	Administer once every 12 h at 10 mg/kg OR every 24 h at 20 mg/kg
Carprofen	5 or 20 mg/kg	SC	Administer once every 12 h at 5 mg/kg OR every 24 h at 20 mg/kg
Meloxicam	5 or 10 mg/kg	SC	Administer once every 12 h at 5 mg/kg OR every 24 h at 10 mg/kg
Opioid			
Buprenorphine HCl	0.1–0.5 mg/kg	SC	Administer every 4–6 h
Ethiqa XR	3.25 mg/kg	SC	Administer, then repeat at 72 h if needed. Do not use on mice with pre-existing respiratory deficiencies. Do not dilute
Buprenorphine-ER-LAB	0.6 mg/kg	SC	Administer once every 24–48 h. Do not dilute.

Source: Flecknell 2023; Foley *et al.* 2019; Gargiulo *et al.* 2012a; Gargiulo *et al.* 2012b; Navarro *et al.* 2021; Oates & Tarbert 2023.

Lyons & Waterman 2012; Pritchett-Corning *et al.* 2011; Beckett 2015; Clevenger *et al.* 2017). Ideally, this training will improve animal welfare by minimising perioperative complications and improving outcomes and reproducibility. A broad overview of common rodent surgical techniques may be found in (Hayward *et al.* 2007), but, in general, laboratories would be best served by close examination of recent publications on the surgery they would like to undertake, and then consultation with veterinary staff in order to apply principles of aseptic technique and animal care referenced above (Gantenbein *et al.* 2022).

Euthanasia

Most scientific work relies on the humane killing of animals at the end of the study, either as a final data collection point or because the study is over, and space or time constraints preclude the natural lifespan of the mouse. Euthanasia is also used for intractable health issues in mice and may be necessary if depopulation is required. The premier reference for the euthanasia of animals is the AVMA Panel on Euthanasia document, *AVMA Guidelines for the Euthanasia of Animals: 2020 edition* (Leary *et al.* 2020). This document recommends several acceptable methods for mice, including physical methods such as cervical dislocation, overdose of injected anaesthetics and overdose of inhaled anaesthetics, including carbon dioxide. However, there is controversy as to whether or not death via inhaled carbon dioxide is truly euthanasia (Shomer *et al.* 2020; Turner *et al.* 2020). The balance of work continues to recommend its use, especially given that there are few alternatives that are as safe for human operators or as feasible for high-throughput applications. There are groups investigating alternatives, however, and solutions such as hyperbaric chambers may soon be in wide use (Clarkson *et al.* 2022). European workers must abide by EU Directive 2010/63/EU (European Parliament and Council, 2010) and its euthanasia recommendations (Close *et al.* 1996; Close *et al.* 1997), researchers in the UK by Home Office recommendations and relevant statutes (1986)[12] and the Canadian Council on Animal Care also promulgates its own euthanasia document (Canadian Council On Animal Care 2010).

Necropsy

In many cases, the ultimate disposition of the mouse at the end of a study is the provision of tissues for further analysis. A structured necropsy to either harvest relevant tissues or for examination of experimental changes is a valuable tool every investigator should have in their toolbox. Several publications provide templates for systematic evaluation of a mouse carcass (Silva & Sundberg 2012; Scudamore *et al.* 2014; Hampshire & Rippy 2015; Treuting & Snyder 2015; Knoblaugh & Randolph-Habecker 2018), and video assistance may also be found on the web (Parkinson *et al.* 2011). Special consideration may be given to newborn mice due to their small size and friable tissue (Capas-Peneda *et al.* 2021). In some cases, a terminal surgery in which mice are perfused with fixative is necessary and video protocols are available (Gage *et al.* 2012). Regardless, we cannot stress enough the importance of consulting and collaborating with veterinary staff on both the science and logistics of mission-critical necropsy. Adult mice autolyse rapidly, and even small delays between death and necropsy can severely affect the data attainable from necropsy.

General husbandry

Enclosures, enrichment, feeding and watering

In laboratories, mice are generally kept in solid-bottomed cages made of some type of plastic. Historically, wood and metal have both been used, and in other situations, ceramic vessels

---

[12]https://www.gov.uk/guidance/research-and-testing-using-animals (Accessed August 3, 2023)

have also come into play. Naturalistic and semi-naturalistic habitats are also used in research and may lead to the ascertainment of more subtle effects than can be seen in the cage environment (Lewejohann et al. 2009; Ruff et al. 2013; Mieske et al. 2021). These cages are usually fitted with a wire bar lid from which food and water are provided. Animals with head implants for research purposes should not be housed in cages with wire bars. Other types of feeders are available, should the course of research require it. These include J-feeders and feeders for powdered diet. If the cages are fitted to an individually ventilated rack, water and air may be delivered via various means peculiar to each caging system manufacturer. Cages that are not attached to an IVC rack are usually called static and these may be open, with no lid, or may have a filtered plastic microisolation lid placed on the cage. The filtered lid may be fitted with a perforated metal insert to protect the filter if mice are placed in a cage with no wire bar lid.

Mice are usually kept on a contact bedding, although wire-bottomed cages or cage inserts are still occasionally used. The ideal mouse substrate would be easy to handle, absorbent, allow for species-specific behaviours and be easy to dispose. Wood-based bedding is preferred by mice, and a shaving bedding is often vigorously used by the mice. Corncob-based bedding is frequently used as it is both inexpensive and absorbent but, as is shown later, is far from ideal. Paper beddings have their place, such as a chipped white paper product that allows for easy visualisation of urine abnormalities, or pressed paper cut to fit an entire cage, which can be used for animals with paresis or paralysis.

Nesting material should be provided for all mice, as it is a highly conserved species behaviour. Mice will preferentially use a long-fibre nesting material, whether provided loose or in a puck, and if allowed, will then line this nest with a short-fibre material, such as a compressed cotton square. If provided with more natural substrates, such as hay or straw, they will also incorporate those into their nests, and if given sand or another digging substrate, avidly excavate.

Enrichment is necessary for mice, and nesting material should not be considered enrichment, but rather another necessary component of the cage (see also Chapter 10: Animal welfare and scientific validity). See Figure 21.10 for a "normally" enriched mouse cage. Shelters can be enriching but may also be associated with fighting in groups of male mice. Care should be taken in their deployment, but the use of plastic tubes is well-accepted by most groups of mice and can also allow for non-aversive handling. Mice benefit from food enrichments, with sunflower seeds and mealworms being popular items. They may also investigate seedpods present in irradiated timothy hay. These not only add variety and micronutrients to the standard mouse diet, but also allow for foraging behaviour. Mice also relish the chance to gnaw on items and wood blocks, sticks or nylon objects are all used if provided.

Mice are typically fed a pelleted or extruded standard diet *ad libitum*. These diets are usually divided into two categories: standard and breeder. Standard mouse diets have similar macronutrient breakdowns of something like 22% protein, 5% fat and 5% fibre, while breeder diets are often higher in fat (see also Chapter 13: Nutrition, feeding and animal

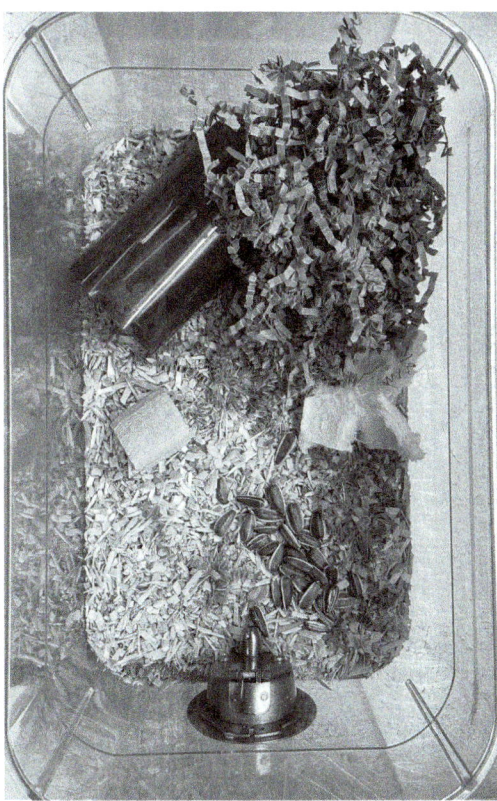

Figure 21.10 An example of an enriched cage (75 cm^2) for mice. As part of basic husbandry, this cage contains two types of nesting material and a wood-based contact bedding. This cage also contains a polycarbonate tube for handling and retreat, a gnawing item, and a foraging enrichment (sunflower seeds). Further enrichment for larger cages may include climbing items (manzanita wood is often used, as is certified aspen) or running wheels.

welfare). *Ad libitum* feeding of this unvarying diet to mice is likely not ideal, neither metabolically nor for their intended use as research subjects (Tuck et al. 2020; Weiskirchen et al. 2020). Mice eat 3–6 g of food (about a standard mouse pellet) per day. Occasionally, a non-ingestive food grinding behaviour is seen, which can be difficult to manage and may confound researchers' ability to accurately measure ingestion. While mice in the wild do not drink often, if at all, rather obtaining their water through food they ingest, laboratory mice need constant access to fresh water. This can be provided via automatic watering system or water bottle, and they will drink about 5 ml per day.

As noted in the behaviour section, mice are social animals and should be housed socially wherever possible. If their use precludes this (e.g. male mice for pseudopregnancy induction), they should be provided with extra enrichment at a minimum. Unfortunately, due to their territorial nature, if male mice are separated from a group housing situation after weaning, they are often unable to regroup without severe fighting. This may not be an insurmountable obstacle if the overall group size in the cage is reduced. However, other conditions, such as head implants, should not preclude social housing. Allowable group size per cage is often controlled by law or regulation; consult local authorities as to the allowable mouse density in the cages in use.

Mice do not have one fixed temperature at which they thrive. Given opportunity, mice become pests in almost any condition and can be found on every continent save Antarctica. If mice are provided with an adequate amount of nesting material, temperatures comfortable for humans in protective equipment are fine within the mouse room (20–22 °C), but without a substantial increase in food intake and nesting material, temperatures below 18 °C can be problematic. Mice cannot pant and do not sweat, as noted above in the biology section, so overly warm temperatures are also problematic.

Breeding and colony management

Mouse breeding and related behaviours are covered in an earlier section. This section will deal entirely with breeding paradigms, not mechanisms. If breeding genetically altered mice, the genotype used for breeding is related to: 1) viability and fertility of hemi-, hetero- or homozygotes, 2) the desired genetic composition of the offspring, and 3) the background on which the mice are maintained. A review of some of these considerations may be found in several publications (Murray & Parker, 2005; Ayadi et al. 2011; Pritchett-Corning & Landel 2015; see also Chapter 4: An introduction to laboratory animal genetics). Mice in laboratories are typically bred in one of three fashions: pair, trio or harem. Observed or controlled mating is also used, but usually only to generate timed pregnancies or pseudopregnant recipients for embryo transfer. Pair mating, in which a pair of mice are set up at an appropriate age (~8 weeks) and remain paired throughout their reproductive lifespan, is the most efficient way to generate mice but can limit the potential number of offspring of males. Pair mating is required for pedigreed matings or if no confusion as to the dam is desired. This mating paradigm allows for the male to assist the female in pup rearing, resulting in more normative social interactions that enhance the development of female offspring. It also allows for mating at the post-partum oestrus.

Trio mating, in which one male is mated with two females, is also commonly used in the laboratory setting. The perception that twice the females in the cage results in twice the number of weaned pups is incorrect (Kedl et al. 2014; Wasson 2017; Chatkupt et al. 2018). One female is usually reproductively suppressed (Garner et al. 2016). This breeding paradigm allows for communal nesting and nursing, should litters be born simultaneously, and alloparenting has been shown to enhance pup survival in wild mice. Unless coat colours allow, alloparenting behaviour may mean that the female parent cannot be definitively determined. In many localities, animal housing density regulations mean that if both females are pregnant, one must be removed in order to avoid overcrowding the cage. This deprives the offspring of one mouse from male parenting contributions and usually means the post-partum oestrus will be missed for that mouse as well.

Finally, harem breeding is sometimes used to maximise the reproductive potential of one male or to quickly build up a colony. In this case, one male is mated with up to four females, and females are removed to separate cages when pregnancy becomes obvious. The disadvantages to separating females as noted above apply here, as does the failure to use the post-partum oestrus.

Colony management as a topic deserves its own chapter, if not book, and several have been written to that end (The Jackson Laboratory 2007; Pritchett-Corning et al. 2015).

The lab from a mouse's point of view: glass tower blocks and tyrannosaurs

Abnormal behaviour and physiology can serve as *post hoc* indicators of issues in a husbandry system, but as argued above, this is often too late for the animal, or the research. Thus, good husbandry and good behavioural management should proactively consider the match (or mismatch) between the animal and its environment. As summarised above, house mice (from which lab mice are derived) are the epitome of a synanthropic animal, exquisitely adapted to both exploit human environments and avoid human detection and interaction. Viewing current mouse housing and husbandry from this point of view immediately reveals critical mismatches where demonstrably 'bad welfare is bad science'.

The undesirable penthouse shoebox

For ease of monitoring and 'footprint efficiency', we house mice in stacks of brightly lit cages. However, mice find brightly lit elevated spaces highly aversive – after all, this is the basis of measures of fear and anxiety used throughout behavioural neuroscience such as the open field test, the elevated plus maze, the light/dark box, and many other arguably more ethologically valid tests lost to the PDF event horizon (Archer 1973). Unsurprisingly, rack row (i.e. how high mice are housed from the floor) has major impacts on mice. Thus, mice housed higher on the rack are more fearful/anxious, and fear/anxiety and rack row are the major predictors of disease progression in Type I Diabetic mice (Ader et al. 1991) implicating a progressive immune suppression in mice housed higher on the rack. Similarly, aggression and barbering increase in rack rows further from the floor (Garner et al. 2004a; Theil et al. 2020). Rack and row effects have long been known as a confound in toxicologic pathology (Young 1987; Young 1989).

Aside from fear and anxiety, light exposure tends to increase with higher placement on a rack (Ader et al. 1991). Light exposure leads to induced retinal damage in most albino strains/stocks of mice (De Vera Mudry et al. 2013). This is a not a trivial matter, as the degree of visual acuity/impairment is actually the primary predictor of performance in the Morris water maze (Brown & Wong 2007) – far more so than genetics. In other words, confounds in visual acuity induced by lighting and cage position can easily masquerade as treatment effects, and differences in Morris water maze performance should be better interpreted as differences in visual acuity than differences in 'memory' (Brown & Wong 2007).

Too drafty for comfort?

IVCs have taken the mouse world by storm due to their ability to control infectious disease and decrease mouse handling requirements, but the available evidence indicates that they are detrimental for mouse welfare and, thus, represent an engineering solution in search of a performance standard problem. Indeed, this is a wonderful example for a generic problem that plagues the mouse housing and husbandry industry – engineers inventing solutions for problems that only exist in pedantic interpretation of regulatory guidelines, without ever considering the actual impact on mouse welfare.

In fact, when given the choice, mice vote with their feet and almost completely avoid IVC cages in favour of static cages (Baumans et al. 2002) although this effect is reduced if the IVC cage contains nesting material, once again emphasising the importance of control to animal welfare. Although behavioural preference can be an important indicator, it tells us relatively little about the impact on welfare compared with measures of demand (Mason et al. 1998). Nevertheless, the negative impact of IVC systems on welfare is clear: mice in IVC housing show increased anxiety in multiple studies (Kallnik et al. 2007; Burman et al. 2014; Ahlgren & Voikar 2019), hypothalamic–pituitary–adrenal axis sensitisation and associated immune suppression (Neigh et al. 2005), increased variability in breeding performance (Tsai et al. 2003; Spangenberg et al. 2014; Stover & Villano 2022), increased aggression (Theil et al. 2020) and changed implanted tumour biology (David et al. 2013). A switch to IVC caging has been shown to affect ongoing behavioural and neuroscience studies (Mineur & Crusio 2009; Logge et al. 2014). Furthermore, the effects of IVC on mice can vary between manufacturers, with the age of the equipment, and the location of the equipment within the room or facility (Barabas et al. 2022b). Accordingly, IVCs may represent an uncontrolled and unacknowledged source of variability between laboratories.

What is it about IVCs that might induce this level of distress in mice? Four potential stressors spring to mind. First, mice find puffs of air highly aversive (Krohn & Hansen 2010), a fact exploited in many behavioural phenotyping measures. *The Guide* (Institute of Laboratory Animal Resources 2011) recommends 10–15 air changes per hour (ACH) for the room, not the cage. Yet, IVC system manufacturers recommend air exchange rates of 40–75 ACH (Spangenberg et al. 2014), and internal industry comparisons similarly run cages at 60 ACH. An air exchange rate of 60 ACH represents a wind speed of 3.6 m/s through a 0.25-in inlet for a typical shoebox. To add further irony to injury, *The Guide* (Institute of Laboratory Animal Resources 2011) actively cautions against excessive air speeds within animal enclosures. Worse still, some systems inject air through smaller inlets around the drinker, effectively forcing mice to choose between water and a predation cue. Accordingly, in preference tests, mice actively avoid draughty IVCs (Krohn & Hansen 2010).

Second, IVCs do not actually control ammonia, resulting in serious ammonia burns and associated histopathology in the nose (DiVincenti et al. 2012). IVCs are designed to limit ammonia levels in the cage, not ammonia production or exposure itself. Thus, by removing ammonia from the cage, IVCs prevent the self-limiting effects of ammonia on ammonia-producing bacteria and allow ammonia production and bacterial growth to continue unchecked. The higher the manufacturer recommended ACH to achieve a steady state of ammonia in the cage, the higher the actual ammonia production, and cumulative ammonia exposure to the mice. Accordingly, cumulative ammonia exposure predicts the severity of nasal lesions (DiVincenti et al. 2012).

Third, some IVCs do not have wire top-lids, preventing climbing behaviour. Preventing highly motivated behaviours such as climbing can induce and modify the form of stereotypies (Würbel 2006). The direct effect of the lack of climbing in IVCs is not well investigated. However, available evidence suggests that climbing enrichments may provide a small benefit but are not able to overcome the negative impacts of IVCs (Kallnik et al. 2007).

Fourth, rack-mounted blowers, and air flow through the rack plenums, produce vibration in IVC cages (Reynolds et al. 2018). In mice, such vibration causes increases in heart rate and blood pressure, elevated corticosterone, breeding failure and post-natal pup mortality, disturbed sleep and acute behavioural responses consistent with fear and anxiety (Garner et al. 2018; Reynolds et al. 2018). In the case of behaviour and sleep disturbance at least, these responses often do not habituate over time (Garner et al. 2018). While the effects of vibration are consistent with the negative effects of IVCs in general, we are unaware of any study explicitly linking the two.

Why do we persist in using IVCs when the negative impacts on mouse health and welfare are so clear? The simple answer is that once a facility is designed around (or retrofitted for) IVCs, it is nigh impossible to return to static caging, whether investigators would like to or not. This is due to a widely held set of beliefs driven by the claims of manufacturers, an unwillingness to challenge those claims, and few if any studies which attempt to link ACH, ammonia or other stressors to measures of mouse health and welfare.

Ventilated cages supposedly aid in infectious agent containment, reduce labour costs via extended cage-change intervals, reduce bedding costs and increase mice housed per square foot of floor space. These claims are inherently problematic. First, similar, if not superior, levels of pathogen containment can be obtained in static cages in isolator cabinets. Furthermore, overly clean mice do not recapitulate human immune system development and function (Beura et al. 2016). Similarly, the overly restricted microbiota typical of lab mice actively creates false results, whereas 'wildling' mice with reconstituted microbiota correctly predict human outcomes (Rosshart et al. 2019). Second, the remaining claims are central to the use-case justification for switching to IVCs – namely that the much higher cost of installing IVCs pays for itself within the life of the equipment. This payoff is based on assumptions that may work on the back of an envelope for an engineer (assume a spherical cow in a vacuum) but are unrealistic in the real world – namely that cages are stocked at a maximum density of only five adult mice of uniform size, and that cages of five mice can go 14 days between changes. In the real world, the majority of mouse cages do not contain four or five mice (Theil et al. 2020), which is enough to ruin the math. Furthermore, the claim that cages can go 14 days between changes is not just incorrect, but also a serious welfare issue.

In the wild, and in complex housing systems, mice will form a latrine distant from the nest site (Makowska et al. 2019). Conventional mouse cages do not provide enough space for this behaviour, but still typically mice latrine and nest at the opposite end of the cage (Makowska et al. 2019). IVCs only make this problem worse. In reality, mice on average eat around 3–6 g of food per day, or 350 g for a cage of five mice over 14 days. 70 (14 × 5) mouse-days of faecal production far exceed any level of minimal hygiene. Mice produce faeces at the same rate whether they are ventilated or not, and living in a cage littered with faeces is inherently problematic. Similarly, this level of urine output inevitably results in permanently wet bedding. As a result, cages of four to five mice (or breeding cages with pups) typically end up being spot changed at some point in the second week. Spot changing is very inefficient in terms of technician time *versus* all-in-all-out changing. Thus, IVCs result in the same average cage-change rate (i.e. two changes per 14 days), but at the expense of increased technician costs, the expense of increased variability between cages, and the expense of exposing mice to increased levels of soiling.

Too cold for comfort?

As discussed earlier, typical cage temperatures of 20–22 °C represent a significant cold stress for mice (Gaskill et al. 2013a). Accordingly, mice prefer warmer cages and avoid 20 °C (Gaskill et al. 2009). Cold temperatures affect all aspects of mouse biology if there is no behavioural means for mice to modify temperatures, and this is reflected in research results (Hylander & Repasky 2016; Hylander et al. 2022). Unfortunately, mice are much more likely to fight as ambient temperature increases (Greenberg 1972), and the energetic burden of lactation means that lactating females are heat stressed at warmer temperatures (Krol et al. 2007). Thus, simply raising ambient temperature is not an option. Instead, nests provide an elegant and ecologically relevant solution to this problem. Mice alter nest building to attain thermoneutrality at different temperatures (Gaskill et al. 2009; Gaskill et al. 2013a). Nests eliminate preference for warmer cages (Gaskill et al. 2012) and eliminate the physiological burden of cold stress (Gaskill et al. 2013c). Accordingly, reproductive output increases and pup mortality decreases (particularly in C57BL/6 mice), through the reallocation of energy resources to lactation (Gaskill et al. 2013c). And nests create a thermoneutral microenvironment that benefits pups (and adults), but also allows mothers to cool off (Kolbe et al. 2022). Accordingly, we consider nests not to be an enrichment, but as necessary as food and water to mouse health and welfare.

Too toxic for comfort?

Housing and husbandry provide a wealth of opportunities to expose mice to a wide variety of chemicals that can impact health and welfare. Something as simple as alcohol-based hand sanitiser or quaternary ammonium compounds used for cleaning can have complex strain and sex dependent impacts on behaviour and reproduction (Melin et al. 2016; López-Salesansky et al. 2021). Perhaps, the most common and impactful issue (at least in North America) is corncob bedding. Corncob bedding contains biologically active oestrogen disruptors (THF- and LTX-diols) (Markaverich et al. 2002; Markaverich et al. 2005). Housing on corncob bedding reduces uterine weight, inhibits the estrous cycle and inhibits male and female sexual behaviour in rats, with major impacts on reproductive performance as well as elevating fasting blood glucose readings (Markaverich et al. 2002; Mani et al. 2005; Kondo et al. 2022). Extracts of these diols from corncob promote cancer cell growth *in vitro*, and housing mice on corncob similarly promotes tumour growth (Markaverich et al. 2002). Corncob also has profound behavioural effects. Rats housed on corncob show less slow-wave sleep (Leys et al. 2012), while deer mice (*Peromyscus*) housed on corncob show suppressed oestrogen receptor expression and increased territorial aggression (Villalon Landeros et al. 2012). Corncob also appears to be uncomfortable to mice that avoid corncob cages particularly when sleeping (Krohn & Hansen 2008). Although the majority of work showing problems with corncob bedding has not been performed in mice, the combination of corncob bedding with IVC housing is the strongest predictor of aggression in mice in a large-scale epidemiological study (Theil et al. 2020).

Enrichment and behavioural management

The telos of animals (i.e. the animalness of animals) is behaviour, and the telos of behaviour is to provide control so that animals can survive outside of their narrow physiological limits. Animals denied these opportunities are fundamentally abnormal and poor models of human patients. Therefore, we (Würbel & Garner, 2007; Garner et al. 2017; Gaskill & Garner, 2017) have argued that experimental lab animal welfare science and real-world enrichment should focus on 'biologically relevant enrichments' – that is, enrichments that allow animals to gain control over stressors in their environment. This argument extends to behavioural management in general – we should understand problem behaviours such as cannibalism and abnormal behaviours such as stereotypies, from the animal's point of view, and design behavioural management accordingly. The telos of the house mouse is arguably described as the only synanthropic animal that has followed humans around the world, surviving in every environment we have ever created, and doing so without the benefits of tools, clothing and language, solely relying on phenotypic plasticity. We have discussed how their biology is finely tuned to this niche, how mouse housing and husbandry is often mismatched to mouse behaviour and biology and how this results in a variety of health and behavioural issues. We have repeatedly hinted that behavioural management, starting with enrichment, can help with many of these problems.

Nesting material is not an enrichment – it is a basic need

As discussed above, we have argued that nesting material is as basic a need as food and water to mice, due to its clear ability to provide a thermal microenvironment, provide control over cold stress and accordingly eliminate the first-litter loss that was for a long time viewed as an unavoidable issue with C57BL/6 mice. However, it is critical to provide enough material (nominally 8–10 g), and it is common for programmes to provide less than this amount over concerns for daily visual checks. However, multiple studies have now shown that a wide range of morbidities present as mice failing to build nests (Gallo et al. 2020; Giménez-Llort & Torres-Lista 2021). Thus, nests aid in the detection of health and welfare issues – that is, a well-maintained nest indicates healthy mice that do not need to be disturbed. Poorly built nests can be further examined using the time to integrate into nest (TINT) assay to screen for potential health or welfare issues (Gallo et al. 2020).

Indeed, nests benefit mice in ways other than thermoregulation. They provide comfort when mice are housed on uncomfortable bedding such as corncob (Krohn & Hansen 2008). They provide shelter from predators, yet another reason not to disturb nests. They provide shelter from the elements beyond just cold, and accordingly, nesting material can reduce the aversion mice have to IVCs (Baumans et al. 2002). Unsurprisingly, mice housed with nesting material show lower cortisol than barren-housed mice (Brochu et al. 2018). Furthermore, these welfare benefits can be obtained without nesting material negatively affecting a variety of toxicological measures (Brochu et al. 2018).

Behavioural management

Aside from enrichment, a growing number of behavioural management options are becoming available for mice. Of particular note, non-aversive handling with a tube or a cupped hand has been shown to reduce anxiety and avoidance of humans (Hurst & West 2010), increase tolerance of restraint and injection (Gouveia & Hurst 2019), increase the number of pups born and weaned, and reduce litter loss, with major operational and financial benefits (Hull et al. 2022). In a similar vein, positive reinforcement training (PRT) is perfectly viable in mice. Not only can mice be trained to take part in their own care and husbandry, but like tunnel handling, PRT reduces anxiety in general, and reduces anxiety-related confounds in experimental measures for which the mice are not specifically trained (Leidinger et al. 2017). Unfortunately, it seems mice do not always generalise positive experiences between handlers, so care must be taken to acclimate mice to all potential handlers (Gaskill & Pritchett-Corning 2016).

There is growing interest in automated environments that attach to the home cage, collecting data or performing experiments (Pioli et al. 2014; Ahloy-Dallaire et al. 2019). Such devices often exploit mouse foraging behaviour and are, thus, inherently enriching. They also reduce stress from handling or forcing mice to work in the light phase. Indeed, many high-throughput tasks produce very different results when performed in the dark phase (Hossain et al. 2004; Tsao et al. 2022). Automated environments are also a refinement, producing more accurate and fine-grained data faster, including detecting sick animals faster than conventional cage checks (Pioli et al. 2014; Ahloy-Dallaire et al. 2019).

Social housing is a simple but highly impactful form of behavioural management. In humans, we know that for many diseases, the quality of a patient's social network has incredible impacts on outcomes. For instance, in one of the largest epidemiological studies of breast cancer, the top three predictors of 1 year-survival are all measures of social network quality and combined confer an extraordinary degree of protection (Kroenke et al. 2006). In mice, we see the same effects – socially housed mice have lower tumour burdens, longer survival times and better responses to chemotherapy in a variety of cancer models (Grimm et al. 1996; Kerr et al. 1997; Jirkof 2015). Social housing clearly benefits both welfare and science but comes at the cost of aggression.

Home-cage aggression remains the gorilla in the room for behavioural management of mice – for an extensive review, see (Weber et al. 2017). Injurious aggression is rare in breeding pairs and groups of female mice, but many if not most other results have been hard to reproduce (Van Loo et al. 2003b; Gaskill & Garner 2017; Weber et al. 2017; Theil et al. 2020). The most comprehensive study to date (a 12-month epidemiological study) (Theil et al. 2020) identified the usual suspects in mouse welfare problems – IVC caging, corncob bedding, time of year, row (i.e. height from the floor) and exposure to human traffic – but failed to detect factors that have been replicated in experimental studies (e.g. group size) (Van Loo et al. 2001; Van Loo et al. 2003b; Blankenberger et al. 2018). Epidemiological studies are limited by the variation present in the population, and by confounding husbandry practices – indeed, the failure to replicate the group size result in this study probably reflects the fact that fighting mice are routinely split into smaller groups (Blankenberger et al. 2018). Three important factors were also missing from this work (because they did not vary or could not be measured): enrichment type, cage-change method and kinship. Experimental literature does provide some consensus that nesting enrichment reduces fighting, while structural enrichment often increases it (Van Loo et al. 2002; Howerton et al. 2008). One possible explanation is that structural enrichment often introduces a highly valued resource that can be defended and/or choke points and ambush positions that mice naturally use to establish territories (Crowcroft 1966; Howerton et al. 2008), whereas nesting material's benefits increase from being shared or a dominant mouse can establish a secondary nest site (Barabas et al. 2021a). Moving the nest site to a clean cage during cage change reduces fighting, presumably by transferring affiliative pheromones and excluding territorial pheromones left at the borders of the cage (Van Loo et al. 2000; Barabas et al. 2021b; Barabas et al. 2022a, Barabas et al. 2022c). Although the Van Loo study is not current, and was performed in very different caging systems, the practice of nest site transfer is widely adopted. Reassuringly, recent surveys of mouse facilities confirmed that moving the nest site at cage change is highly effective in reducing aggression (Litvin et al. 2007; Lidster et al. 2019). Similarly, this work confirms earlier reports that mixing or consolidating litters at weaning increases aggression (Litvin et al. 2007; Van Loo et al. 2000).

Breeding failure is poorly studied, despite being a major concern in mouse facilities. To our knowledge, experimental work is limited to nesting material and trio breeding. Nesting material eliminates the first-litter loss typical of C57BL/6 mice (Gaskill et al. 2013c). Trio and harem breeding, though widely used, typically leads to reproductive suppression of one female (Garner et al. 2016), and the loss of the opportunity to capitalise on post-partum-oestrus if the male is removed (Pritchett & Taft 2007). Accordingly, trios typically have similar per-cage production and half the per-female production of pair-housed breeders (Garner et al 2016; Braden et al. 2017), and the crowding of trio cages leads to a wide variety of health and welfare issues (Braden et al. 2017). Other studies report no difference between trios and pairs, are unclear on whether per-cage or per-female production is reported, show very low productivity and/or have a range of methodological issues (e.g. Kedl et al. 2014; Wasson 2017). In our opinion, the only justification for breeding in trios is to take advantage of 'aunting' when a mutant female is unable to mother her pups (Garner et al. 2016). However, this can often be avoided by breeding mutant males against wild-type females, which is possible even for complex genetics such as Cre-lox systems (see Chapter 4: An introduction to laboratory animal genetics). Otherwise, managing breeding failure involves minimising stressors (e.g. moving breeders to the bottom of the rack and away from human traffic, checking for ultrasound, checking for interruption of the dark phase, etc.) and general physiological support such as provision of breeder diets (Pritchett & Taft 2007), but we stress that the evidence for the effectiveness of these interventions is anecdotal. In our experience, breeding failure is often also associated with genetic issues unappreciated by the typical investigator, such as the flanking gene problem (Crusio 2004); overlapping genes (Sanna et al. 2008); and issues arising from brother–sister mating including inbreeding suppression, background drift, background selection and the inadvertent generation of recombinant-inbred lines (Sigmund 2000). Finally, it is important to emphasise that cannibalism is a normal response of mothers to dead pups, and that cannibalism indicates a failure to thrive, not infanticide (Weber & Olsson, 2008; Weber et al. 2013).

Conclusion: three consistent trends

We hope this chapter illustrates the detailed steps and understanding required to avoid preventable welfare impacts of housing and husbandry, monitor for physical and behavioural health problems and develop a behavioural management plan. In the case of mice in particular, their telos and the examples above, three consistent trends appear that we would argue require constant attention in the behavioural and welfare management of any mouse housing and husbandry system.

First, cage position – in terms of height from the floor (row), exposure to human traffic (e.g. rack orientation relative to the wall, or proximity to the door), exposure to light and exposure to odour and pheromones (e.g. adjacency to the cage-change station) – is consistently associated with a variety of physiological, immunological and behavioural impacts. In existing facilities, there is little that can be done about these confounds in terms of room design. Instead, planning for their impact on experimental design, breeding performance and welfare, and mitigating where possible is paramount. For experimental mice, this means making sure that mice of different treatments are allocated to cage position in a randomised and balanced manner and especially making sure that treatment and row are not confounded, and ideally adopting randomised block or split plot designs that control for these confounds statistically and correctly analyse the data (Festing 2002; Würbel & Garner 2007; Richter et al. 2009; Festing & Nevalainen 2014; Garner et al. 2017). In terms of managing breeding failure, moving sensitive or genetically precious mice to the least threatening positions in the room (e.g. low on the rack and away from human traffic) can often be helpful. Moving forward, we can avoid inherently problematic room layouts such as long narrow rooms with racks parallel to the wall, which maximise light and human exposure, but again this requires active pushback against convenient engineering and architectural 'solutions' at the point of facility design.

Second, housing design provides opportunities to both positively and negatively affect mouse physiology, behaviour and welfare. As discussed above, IVCs are inherently problematic for many reasons. Similarly, the inability to use vertical space in many modern systems is an unnecessary and avoidable insult to a highly agile and three-dimensional animal. While issues related to physical infrastructure may be harder to change, other clearly detrimental husbandry practices, such as the use of corncob bedding, can be easily corrected. Other aspects of housing design can present a more complex mix of costs and benefits. For instance, structural enrichment such as shelters can both provide opportunities for mice to escape aggressors but can also provide cues that increase aggression (Weber et al. 2017). On the other hand, nesting material, providing that mice can actually build functional nests with it, appears to be universally beneficial. Indeed, nest structure can be used as an indicator of mouse health without requiring visual inspection of the mice themselves (Gallo et al. 2020).

Third, current mouse diets represent several challenges. As discussed above, many current diet formulations may not be well balanced in macronutrients, and amino acid profile and protein and lipid sources can vary and introduce phytoestrogens or other physiologically active compounds. Food grinding in mice appears to be an extreme but natural and adaptive response to a mismatch between the diet and the macronutrient (particularly lipid) needs of individual mice. Furthermore, essential micronutrients are destroyed by autoclaving, requiring that those diets be supplemented to make up for this loss. Indeed, adding n-acetylcysteine to diet or water both prevents and cures barbering and ulcerative dermatitis (George et al. 2015; Vieira et al. 2017). Microflora can radically alter mouse phenotypes, and restoring 'wild' microflora improves the ability of mice to predict human outcomes (Rosshart et al. 2019). Macronutrient balance, especially fibre content, impacts microfloral balance, and current diets have been criticised for insufficient fibre and microbiotal support (Morrison et al. 2020) and for contamination with pesticides and heavy metals (Mesnage et al. 2015). Indeed, the monotonous overly standardised diets fed to mice represent a great example of 'one size fits nobody', as dietary preferences and needs differ between different strains, sexes, ages and breeding status (Smith et al. 2000; Starr & Saito 2012; Maric et al. 2022). Indeed, cafeteria diets, used to show these differences, represent both a simple solution and an enrichment (because they provide control).

The authors hope that this chapter has both given an overview of how mice are currently cared for and how they might be better cared for in the future. When you know better, you do better – research and mice will both benefit when we understand the animal's point of view and acknowledge centrality of control to the mouse's lived experience. Progress in welfare and refinement of care for mice has been too slow, hampered by financial considerations, institutional inertia, the adoption of 'sexy' engineering solutions to problems that do not exist and without consideration of mouse welfare and, at the same time, the contrarian spectre of 'historical controls'. As people who work with and care for mice, we know what to do to improve welfare and, therefore, improve reproducibility and translation. Progress in this arena cannot come too soon.

References

Aasland, K.E., Skjerve, E. and Smith, A.J. (2010) Quality of blood samples from the saphenous vein compared with the tail vein during multiple blood sampling of mice. *Laboratory Animals*, **44**, 25–29.

Abolins, S., King, E.C., Lazarou, L., et al. (2017) The comparative immunology of wild and laboratory mice, *Mus musculus domesticus*. *Nature Communications*, **8**, 14811.

Adams, S.C., Garner, J.P., Felt, S.A., et al. (2016) A "pedi" cures all: toenail trimming and the treatment of ulcerative dermatitis in mice. *PLoS One*, **11**, e0144871.

Ader, D.N., Johnson, S.B., Huang, S.W., et al. (1991) Group size, cage shelf level, and emotionality in non-obese diabetic mice: impact on onset and incidence of IDDM. *Psychosomatic Medicine*, **53**, 313–321.

Ahlgren, J. and Voikar, V. (2019) Housing mice in the individually ventilated or open cages-does it matter for behavioral phenotype? *Genes, Brain and Behavior*, **18**, e12564.

Ahloy-Dallaire, J., Klein, J.D., Davis, J.K., et al. (2019) Automated monitoring of mouse feeding and body weight for continuous health assessment. *Laboratory Animals*, **53**, 342–351.

Ahrens Kress, A.P., Zhang, Y., Kaiser-Vry, A.R., et al. (2022) A comparison of blood collection techniques in mice and their effects on welfare. *Journal of the American Association for Laboratory Animal Science*, **61**, 287–295.

Albers, T.M., Henderson, K.S., Mulder, G.B., et al. (2023) Pathogen prevalence and health monitoring trends in laboratory mice and rats from 2003 to 2020. *Journal of the American Association for Laboratory Animal Science*, in press.

Alvarado, C.G., Franklin, C.L. and Dixon, L.W. (2016) Retrospective evaluation of nail trimming as a conservative treatment for ulcerative dermatitis in laboratory mice. *Journal of the American Association for Laboratory Animal Science*, **55**, 462–466.

Anderson, K.R., Haeussler, M., Watanabe, C., et al. (2018) CRISPR off-target analysis in genetically engineered rats and mice. *Nature Methods*, **15**, 512–514.

Arakawa, H., Arakawa, K., Blanchard, D.C., et al. (2007) Scent marking behavior in male C57BL/6J mice: sexual and developmental determination. *Behavioural Brain Research*, **182**, 73–79.

Arakawa, H., Cruz, S. and Deak, T. (2011) From models to mechanisms: odorant communication as a key determinant of social behavior in rodents during illness-associated states. *Neuroscience & Biobehavioral Reviews*, **35**, 1916–1928.

Archer, J. (1973) Tests for emotionality in rats and mice: a review. *Animal Behaviour*, **21**, 205–235.

Asaba, A., Osakada, T., Touhara, K., et al. (2017) Male mice ultrasonic vocalizations enhance female sexual approach and hypothalamic kisspeptin neuron activity. *Hormones and Behavior*, **94**, 53–60.

Atanasov, N.A., Sargent, J.L., Parmigiani, J.P., et al. (2015) Characterization of train-induced vibration and its effect on fecal corticosterone metabolites in mice. *Journal of the American Association for Laboratory Animal Science*, **54**, 737–744.

Attanasio, C., D'angelo, L. and Corsi, L. (2022) Chapter 5 – methods of handling and procedures. In: *Practical Handbook on the 3Rs in the Context of the Directive 2010/63/EU*. Eds Dal Negro, G. and Sabbioni, S. Academic Press, London.

Ayadi, A., Ferrand, G., Cruz, I.G.D., et al. (2011) Mouse breeding and colony management. *Current Protocols in Mouse Biology*, **1**, 239–264.

Bachmanov, A.A., Reed, D.R., Beauchamp, G.K., et al. (2002) Food intake, water intake, and drinking spout side preference of 28 mouse strains. *Behavior Genetics*, **32**, 435–443.

Baker, D.G. (ed.) (2007) *Flynn's Parasites of Laboratory Animals*. Blackwell, Ames.

Barabas, A.J., Aryal, U.K. and Gaskill, B.N. (2022a) Protein profiles from used nesting material, saliva, and urine correspond with social behavior in group housed male mice, *Mus musculus*. *Journal of Proteomics*, **266**, 104685.

Barabas, A.J., Darbyshire, A.K., Schlegel, S.L., et al. (2022b) Evaluation of ambient sound, vibration, and light in rodent housing rooms. *Journal of the American Association for Laboratory Animal Science*, **61**, 660–671.

Barabas, A.J., Lucas, J.R., Erasmus, M.A., et al. (2021a) Who's the boss? Assessing convergent validity of aggression based dominance measures in male laboratory mice, *Mus musculus*. *Frontiers in Veterinary Science*, **8**, 695948.

Barabas, A.J., Soini, H.A., Novotny, M.V., et al. (2022c) Assessing the effect of compounds from plantar foot sweat, nesting material, and urine on social behavior in male mice, *Mus musculus*. *PLoS One*, **17**, e0276844.

Barabas, A.J., Soini, H.A., Novotny, M.V., et al. (2021b) Compounds from plantar foot sweat, nesting material, and urine show strain patterns associated with agonistic and affiliative behaviors in group housed male mice, *Mus musculus*. *PLoS One*, **16**, e0251416.

Baumans, V., Schlingmann, F., Vonck, M., et al. (2002) Individually ventilated cages: beneficial for mice and men? *Contemporary Topics in Laboratory Animal Science*, **41**, 13–19.

Beck, J.A., Lloyd, S., Hafezparast, M., et al. (2000) Genealogies of mouse inbred strains. *Nature Genetics*, **24**, 23–25.

Beckett, J. (2015) How to suture – types and patterns in veterinary surgery. *The Veterinary Nurse*, **6**, 620–628.

Bedford, N.L. and Hoekstra, H.E. (2015) *Peromyscus* mice as a model for studying natural variation. *eLife*, **4**, e06813.

Begley, C.G. (2013) Six red flags for suspect work. *Nature*, **497**, 433–434.

Bekkevold, C.M., Robertson, K.L., Reinhard, M.K., et al. (2013) Dehydration parameters and standards for laboratory mice. *Journal of the American Association for Laboratory Animal Science*, **52**, 233–239.

Benavides, F., Rülicke, T., Prins, J.-B., et al. (2020) Genetic quality assurance and genetic monitoring of laboratory mice and rats: FELASA working group report. *Laboratory Animals*, **54**, 135–148.

Benga, L., Sager, M. and Christensen, H. (2018) From the [*Pasteurella*] *pneumotropica* complex to *Rodentibacter* spp.: an update on [*Pasteurella*] *pneumotropica*. *Veterinary Microbiology*, **217**, 121–134.

Bennett, K. and Lewis, K. (2022) Sedation and anesthesia in rodents. *Veterinary Clinics: Exotic Animal Practice*, **25**, 211–255.

Bechard, A. and Mason, G. (2010). Leaving home: a study of laboratory mouse pup independence. *Applied Animal Behaviour Science*, **125**, 181–188.

Bernal, J., Baldwin, M., Gleason, T., et al. (2009) Guidelines for rodent survival surgery. *Journal of Investigative Surgery*, **22**, 445–451.

Berridge, K.C., Fentress, J.C. and Parr, H. (1987) Natural syntax rules control action sequence of rats. *Behavioural Brain Research*, **23**, 59–68.

Berry, R.J. (1970) The natural history of the house mouse. *Field Studies*, **3**, 219–262.

Berry, R.J. (1981) Town mouse, country mouse – adaptation and adaptability in *Mus domesticus* (*M. musculus domesticus*). *Mammal Review*, **11**, 91–136.

Berry, R.J. and Bronson, F.H. (1992) Life-history and bioeconomy of the house mouse. *Biological Reviews*, **67**, 519–550.

Beura, L.K., Hamilton, S.E., Bi, K., et al. (2016) Normalizing the environment recapitulates adult human immune traits in laboratory mice. *Nature*, **532**, 512–516.

Biggers, J.D., Curnow, R.N., Finn, C.A., et al. (1963) Regulation of the gestation period in mice. *Journal of Reproduction and Infertility*, **6**, 125–138.

Bittner, J.J. (1941) The preservation by freezing and drying in vacuo of the milk-influence for the development of breast cancer in mice. *Science*, **93**, 527–528.

Blankenberger, W.B., Weber, E.M., Chu, D.K., et al. (2018) Breaking up is hard to do: does splitting cages of mice reduce aggression? *Applied Animal Behaviour Science*, **206**, 94–101.

Bracken, T.C., Cooper, C.A., Ali, Z., et al. (2017) *Helicobacter* infection significantly alters pregnancy success in laboratory mice. *Journal of the American Association for Laboratory Animal Science*, **56**, 322–329.

Braden, G.C., Rasmussen, S., Monette, S., et al. (2017) Effects of breeding configuration on maternal and weanling behavior in laboratory mice. *Journal of the American Association for Laboratory Animal Science*, **56**, 369–376.

Brajon, S., Morello, G.M., Capas-Peneda, S., et al. (2021) All the pups we cannot see: cannibalism masks perinatal death in laboratory mouse breeding but infanticide is rare. *Animals*, **11**, 2327.

Brand, M.W., Wannemuehler, M.J., Phillips, G.J., et al. (2015) The altered Schaedler flora: continued applications of a defined murine microbial community. *ILAR Journal*, **56**, 169–178.

Brechbühl, J., Moine, F., Klaey, M., et al. (2013) Mouse alarm pheromone shares structural similarity with predator scents. *Proceedings of the National Academy of Sciences*, **110**, 4762–4767.

Brett, S.J. and Cox, F.E.G. (1982) Immunological aspects of *Giardia muris* and *Spironucleus muris* infections in inbred and outbred strains of laboratory mice: a comparative study. *Parasitology*, **85**, 85–99.

Brochu, C.P., Winnicker, C.L., Provencher, A.L., et al. (2018) Effects of nesting material on the toxicologic assessment of cyclophosphamide in Crl:CD1(ICR) mice. *Journal of the American Association for Laboratory Animal Science*, **57**, 340–349.

Brown, R.E. and Wong, A.A. (2007) The influence of visual ability on learning and memory performance in 13 strains of mice. *Learning and Memory*, **14**, 134–144.

Bruce, H.M. (1960) A block to pregnancy in the mouse caused by proximity of strange males. *Journal of Reproduction and Fertility*, **1**, 96–103.

Bryan, C.P. and Joachim, H. (1930) *The Papyrus Ebers*. G. Bles, London.

Buchheister, S. and Bleich, A. (2021) Health monitoring of laboratory rodent colonies-talking about (r)evolution. *Animals (Basel)*, **11(5)**, 1410. https://doi.org/10.3390/ani11051410.

Bugarski, D., Jovčić, G., Katić-Radivojević, S., et al. (2006) Hematopoietic changes and altered reactivity to IL-17 in *Syphacia obvelata*-infected mice. *Parasitology International*, **55**, 91–97.

Burman, O., Buccarello, L., Redaelli, V., et al. (2014) The effect of two different individually ventilated cage systems on anxiety-related behaviour and welfare in two strains of laboratory mouse. *Physiology & Behavior*, **124**, 92–99.

Burn, C.C., Deacon, R.M. and Mason, G.J. (2008) Marked for life? Effects of early cage-cleaning frequency, delivery batch, and identification tail-marking on rat anxiety profiles. *Developmental Psychobiology*, **50**, 266–277.

Burn, C.C., Mazlan, N.H.B., Chancellor, N., et al. (2021) The pen is milder than the blade: identification marking mice using ink on the tail appears more humane than ear-punching even with local anaesthetic. *Animals (Basel)*, **11(6)**, 1664; https://doi.org/10.3390/ani11061664.

Byers, S.L., Payson, S.J. and Taft, R.A. (2006) Performance of ten inbred mouse strains following assisted reproductive technologies (arts). *Theriogenology*, **65**, 1716–1726.

Byers, S.L., Wiles, M.V., Dunn, S.L., et al. (2012) Mouse estrous cycle identification tool and images. *PLoS One*, **7(4)**, e35538. https://doi.org/10.1371/journal.pone.0035538.

Calhoun, J.B. (1973) Death squared: the explosive growth and demise of a mouse population. *Proceedings of the Royal Society of Medicine*, **66**, 80–88.

Campagner, D., Evans, M.H., Loft, M.S.E., et al. (2018) What the whiskers tell the brain. *Neuroscience*, **368**, 95–108.

Canadian Council on Animal Care (2010) CCAC guidelines on: euthanasia of animals used in science. Ottawa.

Canella, K.A., Diwan, B.A., Gorelick, P.L., et al. (1996) Liver tumorigenesis by *Helicobacter hepaticus*: considerations of mechanism. *In Vivo*, **10**, 285–292.

Capas-Peneda, S., Munhoz Morello, G., Lamas, S., et al. (2021) Necropsy protocol for newborn mice. *Laboratory Animals*, **55**, 358–362.

Capitanio, J.P. and Lerche, N.W. (1998) Social separation, housing relocation, and survival in simian aids: a retrospective analysis. *Psychosomatic Medicine*, **60**, 235–244.

Capitanio, J.P., Mendoza, S.P. and Baroncelli, S. (1999) The relationship of personality dimensions in adult male rhesus macaques to progression of simian immunodeficiency virus disease. *Brain, Behavior, and Immunity*, **13**, 138–154.

Capitanio, J.P., Mendoza, S.P., Lerche, N.W., et al. (1998) Social stress results in altered glucocorticoid regulation and shorter survival in simian acquired immune deficiency syndrome. *Proceedings of the National Academy of Sciences U S A*, **95**, 4714–4719.

Carman, R., Quimby, F. and Glickman, G. (2007) The effect of vibration on pregnant laboratory mice. INTER-NOISE 2007, 2007 Istanbul, Türkiye.

Carstens, E. and Moberg, G.P. (2000) Recognizing pain and distress in laboratory animals. *ILAR Journal*, **41**, 62–71.

Castelhano-Carlos, M.J., Sousa, N., Ohl, F., et al. (2010) Identification methods in newborn C57BL/6C57BL/6 mice: a developmental and behavioural evaluation. *Laboratory Animals*, **44**, 88–103.

Castle, W.E. and Little, C.C. (1909) The peculiar inheritance of pink eyes among colored mice. *Science*, **30**, 313–314.

Chabout, J., Jones-Macopson, J. and Jarvis, E.D. (2017) Eliciting and analyzing male mouse ultrasonic vocalization (USV) songs. *Journal of Visualized Experiments* (**123**), 54137. doi: 10.3791/54137.

Chang, T.K., Ho, P., Liang, C.T., et al. (2013) Effects of vaginal septa on the reproductive performance of BALB/cByJNArl mice. *Journal of the American Association for Laboratory Animal Science*, **52**, 520–523.

Chatkupt, T.T., Libal, N.L., Mader, S.L., et al. (2018) Effect of continuous trio breeding compared with continuous pair breeding in "shoebox" caging on measures of reproductive performance in estrogen receptor knockout mice. *Journal of the American Association for Laboratory Animal Science*, **57(4)**, 328–334. doi: 10.30802/AALAS-JAALAS-17-000125.

Chen, S.K., Tvrdik, P., Peden, E., et al. (2010) Hematopoietic origin of pathological grooming in *hoxb8* mutant mice. *Cell*, **141**, 775–785.

Chia, R., Achilli, F., Festing, M.F., et al. (2005) The origins and uses of mouse outbred stocks. *Nature Genetics*, **37**, 1181–1186.

Cho, C., Chan, C. and Martin, L.J. (2021) Can male mice develop preference towards gentle stroking by an experimenter? *Neuroscience*, **464**, 26–32.

Clarkson, J.M., Dwyer, D.M., Flecknell, P.A., et al. (2018) Handling method alters the hedonic value of reward in laboratory mice. *Scientific Reports*, **8**, 2448.

Clarkson, J.M., Martin, J.E. and Mckeegan, D.E.F. (2022) A review of methods used to kill laboratory rodents: issues and opportunities. *Laboratory Animals*, **56**, 419–436.

Clevenger, R.R., Bernal, J., Talcott, M., *et al.* (2017) Surgery. In: *Management of Animal Care and Use Programs in Research, Education, and Testing*, 2nd edn. Eds Weichbrod, R.H., Thompson, G.a.H. and Norton, J.N. CRC Press, Boca Raton.

Close, B., Banister, K., Baumans, V., *et al.* (1996) Recommendations for euthanasia of experimental animals: Part 1. DGXI of the European Commission. *Laboratory Animals*, **30**, 293–316.

Close, B., Banister, K., Baumans, V., *et al.* (1997) Recommendations for euthanasia of experimental animals: Part 2. DGXI of the European Commission. *Laboratory Animals*, **31**, 1–32.

Cook, M.J. (1965) *The Anatomy of the Laboratory Mouse*. Academic Press, San Diego.

Cooper, T.K., Meyerholz, D.K., Beck, A.P., *et al.* (2021) Research-relevant conditions and pathology of laboratory mice, rats, gerbils, guinea pigs, hamsters, naked mole rats, and rabbits. *ILAR Journal*, **62**, 77–132.

Cora, M.C., Kooistra, L. and Travlos, G. (2015) Vaginal cytology of the laboratory rat and mouse: review and criteria for the staging of the estrous cycle using stained vaginal smears. *Toxicologic Pathology*, **43**, 776–793.

Cornelis, J.J., Deleu, L., Koch, U., *et al.* (2006) Parvovirus oncosuppression. *Parvoviruses*, 365–378.

Cover, C.E., Keenan, C.M. and Bettinger, G.E. (1989) Ear tag induced *Staphylococcus* infection in mice. *Laboratory Animals*, **23**, 229–233.

Crabbe, J.C., Wahlsten, D. and Dudek, B.C. (1999) Genetics of mouse behavior: interactions with laboratory environment. *Science*, **284**, 1670–1672.

Crowcroft, P. (1955) Territoriality in wild house mice, *mus musculus* l. *Journal of Mammalogy*, **36**, 299–301.

Crowcroft, P. (1966) *Mice All Over*. The Chicago Zoological Society, Brookfield.

Crowcroft, P. and Rowe, F.P. (1963) Social organization and territorial behavior in the wild house mouse (*mus musculus* l.). *Proceedings of the Zoological Society of London*, **140**, 517–531.

Crusio, W.E. (2004) Flanking gene and genetic background problems in genetically manipulated mice. *Biological Psychiatry*, **56**, 381–385.

Cuénot, L. (1902) La loi de Mendel et l'hérédité de la pigmentation chez les souris. *Archives de Zoologie Expérimentale et Générale, 3e ser*, **10**, xxvii–xxx.

Cunliffe-Beamer, T.L. and Feldman, D.B. (1976) Vaginal septa in mice: incidence, inheritance, and effect on reproductive, performance. *Laboratory Animal Science*, **26**, 895–898.

David, J.M., Knowles, S., Lamkin, D.M., *et al.* (2013) Individually ventilated cages impose cold stress on laboratory mice: a source of systemic experimental variability. *Journal of the American Association for Laboratory Animal Science*, **52**, 738–744.

Davison, S.E., Emmer, K.M., Ugiliweneza, B., *et al.* (2022) Evaluation of topical oclacitinib and nail trimming as a treatment for murine ulcerative dermatitis in laboratory mice. *PLoS One*, **17**, e0276333.

De Vera Mudry, M.C., Kronenberg, S., Komatsu, S., *et al.* (2013) Blinded by the light: retinal phototoxicity in the context of safety studies. *Toxicologic Pathology*, **41**, 813–825.

De Villiers, C. and Riley, P.R. (2020) Mouse models of myocardial infarction: comparing permanent ligation and ischaemia-reperfusion. *Disease Models & Mechanisms*, **13**(11), dmm046565. https://doi.org/10.1242/dmm.046565

Dean, M.D., Ardlie, K.G. and Nachman, M.W. (2006) The frequency of multiple paternity suggests that sperm competition is common in house mice (*Mus domesticus*). *Molecular Ecology*, **15**, 4141–4151.

Desjardins, C., Maruniak, J.A. and Bronson, F.H. (1973) Social rank in house mice – differentiation revealed by ultraviolet visualization of urinary marking patterns. *Science*, **182**, 939–941.

Dickmann, J., Gonzalez-Uarquin, F., Reichel, S., *et al.* (2022) Clicker training mice for improved compliance in the catwalk test. *Animals (Basel)*, **12**(24), 3545. doi: 10.3390/ani12243545.

Didion, B.A., Hauser, M.E. and Eisen, E.J. (1991) Use of in vitro fertilization and embryo transfer to circumvent infertility caused by an inherited imperforate vagina in mice. *Journal of in vitro Fertilization and Embryo Transfer*, **8**, 167–172.

Didion, J.P. and De Villena, F.P. (2013) Deconstructing *mus gemischus*: advances in understanding ancestry, structure, and variation in the genome of the laboratory mouse. *Mamm Genome*, **24**, 1–20.

Diehl, K.H., Hull, R., Morton, D., *et al.* (2001) A good practice guide to the administration of substances and removal of blood, including routes and volumes. *Journal of Applied Toxicology*, **21**, 15–23.

Divincenti, L., Moorman-White, D., Bavlov, N., *et al.* (2012) Effects of housing density on nasal pathology of breeding mice housed in individually ventilated cages. *Laboratory Animals*, **41**, 68–76.

Doerning, C.M., Thurston, S.E., Villano, J.S., *et al.* (2019) Assessment of mouse handling techniques during cage changing. *Journal of the American Association for Laboratory Animal Science*, **58**, 767–773.

Douglas, R.M., Neve, A., Quittenbaum, J.P., *et al.* (2006) Perception of visual motion coherence by rats and mice. *Vision Research*, **46**, 2842–2847.

Drickamer, L.C. (1995) Rates of urine excretion by house mouse (*Mus domesticus*) – differences by age, sex, social-status, and reproductive condition. *Journal of Chemical Ecology*, **21**, 1481–1493.

Drickamer, L.C. (2001) Urine marking and social dominance in male house mice (*mus musculus domesticus*). *Behavioural Processes*, **53**, 113–120.

Du, R., Luo, W.J., Geng, K.W., *et al.* (2020) Empathic contagious pain and consolation in laboratory rodents: species and sex comparisons. *Neuroscience Bulletin*, **36**, 649–653.

Dufour, B. and Garner, J.P. (2010) An ethological analysis of barbering behavior. In: *Neurobiology of Grooming Behavior*. Eds Kalueff, A.V., Laporte, J.L. and Bergner, C.L. Cambridge University Press, Cambridge.

Edmondson, E.F., Hsieh, W.T., Kramer, J.A., *et al.* (2020) Naturally acquired mouse kidney parvovirus infection produces a persistent interstitial nephritis in immunocompetent laboratory mice. *Veterinary Pathology*, **57**, 915–925.

Eisen, E., Hauser, M., Pomp, D., *et al.* (1989) A recessive mutation causing imperforate vagina in mice. *The Journal of Heredity*, **80**, 478–482.

Erzurumlu, R.S. and Gaspar, P. (2020) How the barrel cortex became a working model for developmental plasticity: a historical perspective. *The Journal of Neuroscience*, **40**, 6460–6473.

Escalante, N.K., Lemire, P., Cruz Tleugabulova, M., *et al.* (2016) The common mouse protozoa *Tritrichomonas muris* alters mucosal t cell homeostasis and colitis susceptibility. *Journal of Experimental Medicine*, **213**, 2841–2850.

European Parliament and Council (2010) Directive 2010/63/EU of the European Parliament and of the Council of 22 September 2010 on the Protection of Animals Used for Scientific Purposes. *Official Journal of the European Union*, 2010; L 276/33–79. https://eur-lex.europa.eu/LexUriServ/LexUriServ.do?uri=OJ:L:2010:276:0033:0079:EN:PDF (accessed 3 August 2023).

Fahey, J.R. and Olekszak, H. (2015) An overview of typical infections of research mice: health monitoring and prevention of infection. *Current Protocols in Mouse Biology*, **5**, 235–245.

Febinger, H.Y., George, A., Priestley, J., *et al.* (2014) Effects of housing condition and cage change on characteristics of sleep in mice. *Journal of the American Association for Laboratory Animal Science*, **53**, 29–37.

Fei, C.-F. and Zhou, L.-Q. (2022) Gene mutations impede oocyte maturation, fertilization, and early embryonic development. *BioEssays*, **44**, 2200007.

Feng, L.C., Howell, T.J. and Bennett, P.C. (2016) How clicker training works: comparing reinforcing, marking, and bridging hypotheses. *Applied Animal Behaviour Science*, **181**, 34–40.

Fentress, J.C. (1988) Expressive contexts, fine structure, and central mediation of rodent grooming. *Annals of the New York Academy of Sciences*, **525**, 18–26.

Ferrero, D.M., Lemon, J.K., Fluegge, D., *et al.* (2011) Detection and avoidance of a carnivore odor by prey. *Proceedings of the National Academy of Sciences U S A*, **108**, 11235–11240.

Festing, M.F. (2002) The design and statistical analysis of animal experiments. *ILAR Journal*, **43**, 191–193.

Festing, M.F.W. and Nevalainen, T. (2014) The design and statistical analysis of animal experiments: introduction to this issue. *ILAR Journal*, **55**, 379–382.

Flecknell, P. (2018) Rodent analgesia: assessment and therapeutics. *Veterinary Journal*, **232**, 70–77.

Flecknell, P. (2023) *Laboratory Animal Anaesthesia*, 5th edn. Academic Press, London.

Foley, P.L., Kendall, L.V. and Turner, P.V. (2019) Clinical management of pain in rodents. *Comparative Medicine*, **69**, 468–489.

Foltz, C.J., Fox, J.G., Yan, L., et al. (1996) Evaluation of various oral antimicrobial formulations for eradication of *Helicobacter hepaticus*. *Laboratory Animal Science*, **46**, 193–197.

Fox, J.G., Barthold, S.W., Davisson, M.T., et al. (eds) (2008) *The Mouse in Biomedical Research*. Academic Press, New York.

Fox, J.G., Rogers, A.B., Whary, M.T., et al. (2004) Helicobacter bilis-associated hepatitis in outbred mice. *Comparative Medicine*, **54**, 571–577.

Frezel, N., Kratzer, G., Verzar, P., et al. (2019) Does toe clipping for genotyping interfere with later-in-life nociception in mice? *Pain Reports*, **4**, e740.

Frohlich, J.R., Alarcón, C.N., Toarmino, C.R., et al. (2018) Comparison of serial blood collection by facial vein and retrobulbar methods in C57BL/6 mice. *Journal of the American Association for Laboratory Animal Science*, **57**, 382–391.

Fu, F., Pietropaolo, M., Cui, L., et al. (2022) Lack of authentic atrial fibrillation in commonly used murine atrial fibrillation models. *PLoS One*, **17**, e0256512.

Gad, S.C., Spainhour, C.B., Shoemake, C., et al. (2016) Tolerable levels of nonclinical vehicles and formulations used in studies by multiple routes in multiple species with notes on methods to improve utility. *International Journal of Toxicology*, **35**, 95–178.

Gage, G.J., Kipke, D.R. and Shain, W. (2012) Whole animal perfusion fixation for rodents. *Journal of Visualized Experiments*, **(65)**, 3564. doi: 10.3791/356410.3791/3564.

Gallo, M.S., Karas, A.Z., Pritchett-Corning, K., et al. (2020) Tell-tale TINT: does the time to incorporate into nest test evaluate postsurgical pain or welfare in mice? *Journal of the American Association for Laboratory Animal Science*, **59**, 37–45.

Ganeshan, K. and Chawla, A. (2017) Warming the mouse to model human diseases. *Nature Reviews Endocrinology*, **13**, 458–465.

Gantenbein, F., Buchholz, T., Wever, K.E., et al. (2022) Protocol for a systematic review of good surgical practice guidelines for experimental rodent surgery. *BMJ Open Science*, **6**, e100280.

Gargiulo, S., Greco, A., Gramanzini, M., et al. (2012a) Mice anesthesia, analgesia, and care, part I: anesthetic considerations in preclinical research. *ILAR Journal*, **53**, E55–69.

Gargiulo, S., Greco, A., Gramanzini, M., et al. (2012b) Mice anesthesia, analgesia, and care, part ii: anesthetic considerations in preclinical imaging studies. *ILAR Journal*, **53**, E70–81.

Garner, A.M., Norton, J.N., Kinard, W.L., et al. (2018) Vibration-induced behavioral responses and response threshold in female C57BL/6 mice. *Journal of the American Association for Laboratory Animal Science*, **57**, 447–455.

Garner, J.P. (2005) Stereotypies and other abnormal repetitive behaviors: potential impact on validity, reliability, and replicability of scientific outcomes. *ILAR Journal*, **46**, 106–117.

Garner, J.P. (2014) The significance of meaning: why do over 90% of behavioral neuroscience results fail to translate to humans, and what can we do to fix it? *ILAR Journal*, **55**, 438–456.

Garner, J.P. (2020) The mouse in the room: the critical distinction between regulations and ethics. In: *Principles of Animal Research Ethics*. Eds Beauchamp, T.L. and Degrazia, D. Oxford University Press, London.

Garner, J.P., Dufour, B., Gregg, L.E., et al. (2004a) Social and husbandry factors affecting the prevalence and severity of barbering ('whisker trimming') by laboratory mice. *Applied Animal Behaviour Science*, **89**, 263–282.

Garner, J.P., Gaskill, B.N. and Pritchett-Corning, K.R. (2016) Two of a kind or a full house? Reproductive suppression and alloparenting in laboratory mice. *PLoS One*, **11**, e0154966.

Garner, J.P., Gaskill, B.N., Weber, E.M., et al. (2017) Introducing therioepistemology: the study of how knowledge is gained from animal research. *Laboratory Animals (NY)*, **46**, 103–113.

Garner, J.P., Thogerson, C.M., Dufour, B.D., et al. (2011) Reverse-translational biomarker validation of abnormal repetitive behaviors in mice: an illustration of the 4P's modeling approach. *Behavioural Brain Research*, **219**, 189–196.

Garner, J.P., Thogerson, C.M., Würbel, H., et al. (2006) Animal neuropsychology: validation of the intra-dimensional extra-dimensional set shifting task for mice. *Behavioural Brain Research*, **173**, 53–61.

Garner, J.P., Weisker, S.M., Dufour, B., et al. (2004b) Barbering (fur and whisker trimming) by laboratory mice as a model of human trichotillomania and obsessive-compulsive spectrum disorders. *Comparative Medicine*, **54**, 216–224.

Gaskill, B.N. and Garner, J.P. (2017) Stressed out: providing laboratory animals with behavioral control to reduce the physiological effects of stress. *Laboratory Animals (NY)*, **46**, 142–145.

Gaskill, B.N., Gordon, C.J., Pajor, E.A., et al. (2012) Heat or insulation: behavioral titration of mouse preference for warmth or access to a nest. *PLoS One*, **7**, e32799.

Gaskill, B.N., Gordon, C.J., Pajor, E.A., et al. (2013a) Impact of nesting material on mouse body temperature and physiology. *Physiology & Behavior*, **110–111**, 87–95.

Gaskill, B.N., Karas, A.Z., Garner, J.P., et al. (2013b) Nest building as an indicator of health and welfare in laboratory mice. *Journal of Visualized Experiments*, **(82)**, 51012. doi: 10.3791/5101210.3791/51012, 51012.

Gaskill, B.N. and Pritchett-Corning, K.R. (2016) Nest building as an indicator of illness in laboratory mice. *Applied Animal Behaviour Science*, **180**, 140–146.

Gaskill, B.N., Pritchett-Corning, K.R., Gordon, C.J., et al. (2013c) Energy reallocation to breeding performance through improved nest building in laboratory mice. *PLoS One*, **8**, e74153.

Gaskill, B.N., Rohr, S.A., Pajor, E.A., et al. (2009) Some like it hot: mouse temperature preferences in laboratory housing. *Applied Animal Behaviour Science*, **116**, 279–285.

Gaskill, B.N., Stottler, A.M., Garner, J.P., et al. (2017) The effect of early life experience, environment, and genetic factors on spontaneous home-cage aggression-related wounding in male C57BL/6 mice. *Laboratory Animals*, **46**, 176–184.

Gaskill, B.N., Winnicker, C., Garner, J.P., et al. (2013d) The naked truth: breeding performance in nude mice with and without nesting material. *Applied Animal Behaviour Science*, **143**, 110–116.

Ge, Z., Carrasco, S.E., Feng, Y., et al. (2020) Identification of a new strain of mouse kidney parvovirus associated with inclusion body nephropathy in immunocompromised laboratory mice. *Emerging Microbes & Infections*, **9**, 1814–1823.

Gearhart, S., Kalishman, J., Melikyan, H., et al. (2004) Increased incidence of vaginal septum in C57BL/6j mice since 1976. *Comparative Medicine*, **54**, 418–421.

George, N.M., Whitaker, J., Vieira, G., et al. (2015) Antioxidant therapies for ulcerative dermatitis: a potential model for skin picking disorder. *PLoS One*, **10**, e0132092.

Gerlach, G. (1996) Emigration mechanisms in feral house mice: a laboratory investigation of the influence of social structure, population density, and aggression. *Behavioral Ecology and Sociobiology*, **39**, 159–170.

Giménez-Llort, L. and Torres-Lista, V. (2021) Social nesting, animal welfare, and disease monitoring. *Animals*, **11**, 1079.

Ginty, I. and Hoogstraten-Miller, S. (2008) Perineal swelling in a mouse. Diagnosis: imperforate vagina with secondary mucometra. *Laboratory Animals (NY)*, **37**, 196–199.

Goltstein, P.M., Reinert, S., Glas, A., et al. (2018) Food and water restriction lead to differential learning behaviors in a head-fixed two-choice visual discrimination task for mice. *PLoS One*, **13**, e0204066.

Gondo, Y. (2008) Trends in large-scale mouse mutagenesis: from genetics to functional genomics. *Nature Reviews Genetics*, **9**, 803–810.

Gordon, C.J. (1993) *Temperature Regulation in Laboratory Rodents*. Cambridge University Press, New York.

Gordon, C.J. (2012) Thermal physiology of laboratory mice: defining thermoneutrality. *Journal of Thermal Biology*, **37**, 654–685.

Gors, S., Kucia, M., Langhammer, M., et al. (2009) Technical note: milk composition in mice-methodological aspects and effects of mouse strain and lactation day. *Journal of Dairy Science*, **92**, 632–637.

Goulding, E.H., Schenk, A.K., Juneja, P., et al. (2008) A robust automated system elucidates mouse home cage behavioral structure. *Proceedings of the National Academy of Sciences U S A*, **105**, 20575–20582.

Gouveia, K. and Hurst, J.L. (2013) Reducing mouse anxiety during handling: effect of experience with handling tunnels. *PLoS One*, **8(6)**, e66401. doi: 10.1371/journal.pone.0066401.

Gouveia, K. and Hurst, J.L. (2017) Optimising reliability of mouse performance in behavioural testing: the major role of non-aversive handling. *Scientific Reports*, **7**, 44999. https://doi.org/10.1038/srep44999

Gouveia, K. and Hurst, J.L. (2019) Improving the practicality of using non-aversive handling methods to reduce background stress and anxiety in laboratory mice. *Scientific Reports*, **9**, 20305.

Graham, A.L. (2021) Naturalizing mouse models for immunology. *Nature Immunology*, **22**, 111–117.

Graw, J. (2019) Mouse models for microphthalmia, anophthalmia and cataracts. *Human Genetics*, **138**, 1007–1018.

Greenberg, G. (1972) The effects of ambient temperature and population density on aggression in two inbred strains of mice, *Mus musculus*. *Behaviour*, **42**, 119–130.

Greene-Till, R., Zhao, Y. and Hardies, S.C. (2000) Gene flow of unique sequences between *Mus musculus domesticus* and *mus spretus*. *Mammalian Genome*, **11**, 225–230.

Greenfield, H. and Briggs, G.M. (1971) Nutritional methodology in metabolic research with rats. *Annual Review of Biochemistry*, **40**, 549–572.

Greer, J.M. and Capecchi, M.R. (2002) *Hoxb8* is required for normal grooming behavior in mice. *Neuron*, **33**, 23–34.

Grimaud, J. and Murthy, V.N. (2018) How to monitor breathing in laboratory rodents: a review of the current methods. *Journal of Neurophysiology*, **120**, 624–632.

Grimm, M.S., Emerman, J.T. and Weinberg, J. (1996) Effects of social housing condition and behavior on growth of the Shionogi mouse mammary carcinoma. *Physiology & Behavior*, **59**, 633–642.

Hackbarth, H. and Hackbarth, D. (1982) Genetic analysis of renal function in mice. 2. Strain differences in clearances of sodium, potassium, osmolar and free water, and their correlations with body and kidney weight. *Laboratory Animals*, **16**, 27–32.

Hahn, M.E. and Lavooy, M.J. (2005) A review of the methods of studies on infant ultrasound production and maternal retrieval in small rodents. *Behavior Genetics*, **35**, 31–52.

Hamilton, S.E., Badovinac, V.P., Beura, L.K., et al. (2020) New insights into the immune system using dirty mice. *The Journal of Immunology*, **205**, 3–11.

Hampshire, V. and Rippy, M. (2015) Optimizing research animal necropsy and histology practices. *Laboratory Animals*, **44**, 170–172.

Hampton, A.L., Hish, G.A., Aslam, M.N., et al. (2012) Progression of ulcerative dermatitis lesions in C57BL/6Crl mice and the development of a scoring system for dermatitis lesions. *Journal of the American Association for Laboratory Animal Science*, **51**, 586–593.

Hankenson, F.C., Marx, J.O., Gordon, C.J., et al. (2018) Effects of rodent thermoregulation on animal models in the research environment. *Comparative Medicine*, **68**, 425–438.

Hardies, S.C., Wang, L., Zhou, L., et al. (2000) Line-1 (l1) lineages in the mouse. *Molecular Biology and Evolution*, **17**, 616–628.

Hay, M., Thomas, D.W., Craighead, J.L., et al. (2014) Clinical development success rates for investigational drugs. *Nature Biotechnology*, **32**, 40–51.

Hayward, A.M., Lemke, L.B., Bridgeford, E.C., et al. (2007) Chapter 13 – Biomethodology and surgical techniques. In: *The Mouse in Biomedical Research*, 2nd edn. Eds Fox, J.G., Davisson, M.T., Quimby, F.W., et al. Academic Press, Burlington.

Hedrich, H.J. and Bullock, G. (Eds) (2004) *The Laboratory Mouse*. Elsevier, Amsterdam.

Heffner, H.E. and Heffner, R.S. (2007) Hearing ranges of laboratory animals. *Journal of the American Association for Laboratory Animal Science*, **46**, 20–22.

Henig, R.M. (2000) *The Monk in the Garden : The Lost and Found Genius of Gregor Mendel, the Father of Genetics*. Houghton Mifflin, Boston.

Hicks, R.A. and Little, C.C. (1931) The blood relationships of four strains of mice. *Genetics*, **16**, 397–421.

Hino, T., Oda, K., Nakamura, K., et al. (2009) Low fertility in vivo resulting from female factors causes small litter size in 129 inbred mice. *Reproductive Medicine and Biology*, **8**, 157–161.

Histed, M.H., Carvalho, L.A. and Maunsell, J.H.R. (2012) Psychophysical measurement of contrast sensitivity in the behaving mouse. *Journal of Neurophysiology*, **107**, 758–765.

Hoenerhoff, M.J., Meyerholz, D.K., Brayton, C., et al. (2021) Challenges and opportunities for the veterinary pathologist in biomedical research. *Veterinary Pathology*, **58**, 258–265.

Hoggatt, J., Hoggatt, A.F., Tate, T.A., et al. (2016) Bleeding the laboratory mouse: not all methods are equal. *Experimental Hematology*, **44**, 132–137.

Holmberg, H., Kiersgaard, M.K., Mikkelsen, L.F., et al. (2011) Impact of blood sampling technique on blood quality and animal welfare in haemophilic mice. *Laboratory Animals*, **45**, 114–120.

Holmer, H.K., Rodman, J.E., Helmreich, D.L., et al. (2003) Differential effects of chronic escapable versus inescapable stress on male Syrian hamster (*Mesocricetus auratus*) reproductive behavior. *Hormones and Behavior*, **43**, 381–387.

Holmgren, C.D., Stahr, P., Wallace, D.J., et al. (2021) Visual pursuit behavior in mice maintains the pursued prey on the retinal region with least optic flow. *eLife*, **10**, e70838.

Holtfreter, S., Radcliff, F.J., Grumann, D., et al. (2013) Characterization of a mouse-adapted *Staphylococcus aureus* strain. *PLoS One*, **8**, e71142.

Holy, T.E. and Guo, Z. (2005) Ultrasonic songs of male mice. *PLoS Biology*, **3**, e386.

Hong, C.C. and Ediger, R.D. (1978) Preputial gland abscess in mice. *Laboratory Animal Science*, **28**, 153–156.

Hoogstraten-Miller, S.L. and Brown, P.A. (2008) Techniques in aseptic rodent surgery. *Current Protocols in Immunology*, **82**, 1.12.11–11.12.14.

Horn, C.C., Kimball, B.A., Wang, H., et al. (2013) Why can't rodents vomit? A comparative behavioral, anatomical, and physiological study. *PLoS One*, **8**, e60537.

Hossain, S.M., Wong, B.K.Y. and Simpson, E.M. (2004) The dark phase improves genetic discrimination for some high throughput mouse behavioral phenotyping. *Genes, Brain and Behavior*, **3**, 167–177.

Howerton, C.L., Garner, J.P. and Mench, J.A. (2008) Effects of a running wheel-igloo enrichment on aggression, hierarchy linearity, and stereotypy in group-housed male CD-1 (ICR) mice. *Applied Animal Behaviour Science*, **115**, 90–103.

Hoyt, R.F., Jr., Clevenger, R.R. and Mcgehee, J.A. (2001a) Introduction to microsurgery: an emerging discipline in biomedical research. *Laboratory Animal (NY)*, **30**, 26–35.

Hoyt, R.F., Jr., Clevenger, R.R. and Mcgehee, J.A. (2001b) Microsurgical instrumentation and suture material. *Laboratory Animal (NY)*, **30**, 38–45.

Hull, M.A., Reynolds, P.S. and Nunamaker, E.A. (2022) Effects of non-aversive versus tail-lift handling on breeding productivity in a C57BL/6J mouse colony. *PLoS One*, **17**, e0263192.

Hurst, J.L. (1990a) Urine marking in populations of wild house mice *Mus domesticus* Rutty. I. Communication between males. *Animal Behaviour*, **40**, 209–222.

Hurst, J.L. (1990b) Urine marking in populations of wild house mice *Mus domesticus* Rutty. II. Communication between females. *Animal Behaviour*, **40**, 223–232.

Hurst, J.L. and West, R.S. (2010) Taming anxiety in laboratory mice. *Nature Methods*, **7**, 825–826.

Hylander, B.L. and Repasky, E.A. (2016) Thermoneutrality, mice, and cancer: a heated opinion. *Trends in Cancer*, **2**, 166–175.

Hylander, B.L., Repasky, E.A. and Sexton, S. (2022) Using mice to model human disease: understanding the roles of baseline housing-induced and experimentally imposed stresses in animal welfare and experimental reproducibility. *Animals*, **12**, 371.

Institute of Laboratory Animal Resources (2011) *Guide for the Care and Use of Laboratory Animals*. The National Academies Press, Washington, D.C.

Janus, L.M. and Bleich, A. (2012) Coping with parvovirus infections in mice: health surveillance and control. *Laboratory Animals*, **46**, 14–23.

Jenkins, B.A. and Lumpkin, E.A. (2017) Developing a sense of touch. *Development*, **144**, 4078–4090.

Jirkof, P. (2015) Effects of experimental housing conditions on recovery of laboratory mice. *Laboratory Animals*, **44**, 65–70.

Jirkof, P., Bratcher, N., Medina, L., et al. (2020) The effect of group size, age and handling frequency on inter-male aggression in CD 1 mice. *Scientific Reports*, **10**, 2253.

Johnson, J.S., Taylor, D.J., Green, A.R., et al. (2017) Effects of nesting material on energy homeostasis in BALB/cAnnCrl, C57BL/6NCrl, and Crl:CD1(ICR) mice housed at 20 degrees c. *Journal of the American Association for Laboratory Animal Science*, **56**, 254–259.

Johnson, K.R., Zheng, Q.Y. and Erway, L.C. (2000) A major gene affecting age-related hearing loss is common to at least ten inbred strains of mice. *Genomics*, **70**, 171–180.

Johnson, K.R., Zheng, Q.Y. and Noben-Trauth, K. (2006) Strain background effects and genetic modifiers of hearing in mice. *Brain Research*, **1091**, 79–88.

Joslin, J.O. (2009) Blood collection techniques in exotic small mammals. *Journal of Exotic Pet Medicine*, **18**, 117–139.

Kalliokoski, O., Jacobsen, K.R., Darusman, H.S., et al. (2013) Mice do not habituate to metabolism cage housing-a three week study of male balbBALB/c mice. *PLoS One*, **8**, e58460.

Kalliokoski, O., Jacobsen, K.R., Teilmann, A.C., et al. (2012) Quantitative effects of diet on fecal corticosterone metabolites in two strains of laboratory mice. *In Vivo*, **26**, 213–221.

Kallnik, M., Elvert, R., Ehrhardt, N., et al. (2007) Impact of IVC housing on emotionality and fear learning in male C3HeB/FeeJ and C57BL/6J mice. *Mammalian Genome*, **18**, 173–186.

Kane, K.L., Longo-Guess, C.M., Gagnon, L.H., et al. (2012) Genetic background effects on age-related hearing loss associated with *Cdh23* variants in mice. *Hearing Research*, **283**, 80–88.

Kane, P.B. and Kimmelman, J. (2021) Is preclinical research in cancer biology reproducible enough? *eLife*, **10**, e67527.

Kannt, A. and Wieland, T. (2016) Managing risks in drug discovery: reproducibility of published findings. *Naunyn-Schmiedeberg's Archives of Pharmacology*, **389**, 353–360.

Kahnau, P., Jaap, A., Hobbiesiefken, U., et al. (2022) A preliminary survey on the occurrence of barbering in laboratory mice in Germany. *Animal Welfare*, **31(4)**, 433–436. https://doi.org/10.7120/09627286.31.4.009

Karst, S.M. and Wobus, C.E. (2015) Viruses in rodent colonies: lessons learned from murine noroviruses. *Annual Review of Virology*, **2**, 525–548.

Kedl, R.M., Wysocki, L.J., Janssen, W.J., et al. (2014) General parity between trio and pairwise breeding of laboratory mice in static caging. *Journal of Immunology*, **193**, 4757–4760.

Keeler, C.E. (1931) *The Laboratory Mouse: Its Origin, Heredity, and Culture*. Harvard University Press, Cambridge.

Keeler, C.E. and Fuji, S. (1937) The antiquity of mouse variations in the Orient. *Journal of Heredity*, **28**, 93–96.

Kennedy, E.A., King, K.Y. and Baldridge, M.T. (2018) Mouse microbiota models: comparing germ-free mice and antibiotics treatment as tools for modifying gut bacteria. *Frontiers in Physiology*, **9**, 1534.

Kerr, L.R., Grimm, M.S., Silva, W.A., et al. (1997) Effects of social housing condition on the response of the shionogi mouse mammary carcinoma (sc115) to chemotherapy. *Cancer Research*, **57**, 1124–1128.

Klurfeld, D.M., Gregory, J.F., Iii and Fiorotto, M.L. (2021) Should the AIN-93 rodent diet formulas be revised? *The Journal of Nutrition*, **151**, 1380–1382.

Knight, C.H., Maltz, E. and Docherty, A.H. (1986) Milk yield and composition in mice: effects of litter size and lactation number. *Comparative Biochemistry Physiology A Comparative Physiology*, **84**, 127–133.

Knoblaugh, S.E. and Randolph-Habecker, J. (2018) Necropsy and histology. In: *Comparative Anatomy and Histology: A Mouse, Rat, and Human Atlas*. 2nd edn. Eds Treuting, P., Dintzis, S. and Montine, K.S. London: Academic Press.

Kola, I. and Landis, J. (2004) Can the pharmaceutical industry reduce attrition rates? *Nature Reviews Drug Discovery*, **3**, 711–716.

Kolbe, T., Lassnig, C., Poelzl, A., et al. (2022) Effect of different ambient temperatures on reproductive outcome and stress level of lactating females in two mouse strains. *Animals (Basel)*, **12(16)**, 2141. https://doi.org/10.3390/ani12162141.

Kondo, S.Y., Kropik, J. and Wong, M.A. (2022) Effect of bedding substrates on blood glucose and body weight in mice. *Journal of the American Association for Laboratory Animal Science*, **61**, 611–614.

Korner, R.W., Majjouti, M., Alcazar, M.A.A., et al. (2020) Of mice and men: the coronavirus MHV and mouse models as a translational approach to understand SARS-CoV-2. *Viruses*, **12(8)**, 880. doi: 10.3390/v12080880.

Kroenke, C.H., Kubzansky, L.D., Schernhammer, E.S., et al. (2006) Social networks, social support, and survival after breast cancer diagnosis. *Journal of Clinical Oncology*, **24**, 1105–1111.

Krohn, T.C. and Hansen, A.K. (2008) Evaluation of corncob as bedding for rodents. *Scandinavian Journal of Laboratory Animal Science*, **35**, 231–236.

Krohn, T.C. and Hansen, A.K. (2010) Mice prefer draught-free housing. *Laboratory Animals*, **44**, 370–372.

Krol, E., Murphy, M. and Speakman, J.R. (2007) Limits to sustained energy intake. X. Effects of fur removal on reproductive performance in laboratory mice. *Journal of Experimental Biology*, **210**, 4233–4243.

Kudryavtseva, N.N., Bondar, N.P. and Alekseyenko, O.V. (2000) Behavioral correlates of learned aggression in male mice. *Aggressive Behavior*, **26**, 386–400.

Kurien, B.T., Everds, N.E. and Scofield, R.H. (2004) Experimental animal urine collection: a review. *Laboratory Animals*, **38**, 333–361.

Kurien, B.T., Gross, T. and Scofield, R.H. (2005) Barbering in mice: a model for trichotillomania. *British Medical Journal*, **331**, 1503–1505.

Kurita, T. (2010) Developmental origin of vaginal epithelium. *Differentiation*, **80**, 99–105.

Latham, N. and Mason, G. (2004) From house mouse to mouse house: the behavioural biology of free-living *Mus musculus* and its implications in the laboratory. *Applied Animal Behaviour Science*, **86**, 261–289.

Laudenslager, M.L., Ryan, S.M., Drugan, R.C., et al. 1983. Coping and immunosuppression: inescapable but not escapable shock suppresses lymphocyte proliferation. *Science*, 221, 568–570.

Leary, S.L., Underwood, W., Anthony, R., et al. (2020) *AVMA Guidelines for the Euthanasia of Animals: 2020 edition*. AVMA, Schaumburg.

Leibovici, M., Safieddine, S. and Petit, C. (2008) Chapter 8 Mouse models for human hereditary deafness. *Current Topics in*

Developmental Biology, Vol. 84, pp. 385–429. Academic Press. ISBN 9780123744548.

Leidinger, C., Herrmann, F., Thone-Reineke, C., *et al.* (2017) Introducing clicker training as a cognitive enrichment for laboratory mice. *Journal of Visualized Experiments*, **(121)**, 55415. doi: 10.3791/55415.

Lenschow, C. and Lima, S.Q. (2020) In the mood for sex: neural circuits for reproduction. *Current Opinion in Neurobiology*, 60, 155–168.

Lerch, S., Brandwein, C., Dormann, C., *et al.* (2015) Bred to breed?! Implications of continuous mating on the emotional status of mouse offspring. *Behavioural Brain Research*, 279, 155–165.

Lewejohann, L., Reefmann, N., Widmann, P., *et al.* (2009) Transgenic Alzheimer mice in a semi-naturalistic environment: more plaques, yet not compromised in daily life. *Behavioural Brain Research*, 201, 99–102.

Lewis, S.R., Ahmed, S., Dym, C., *et al.* (2005) Inbred mouse strain survey of sucrose intake. *Physiology & Behavior*, 85, 546–556.

Leys, L.J., Mcgaraughty, S. and Radek, R.J. (2012) Rats housed on corncob bedding show less slow-wave sleep. *Journal of the American Association for Laboratory Animal Science*, 51, 764–768.

Lidster, K., Owen, K., Browne, W.J., *et al.* (2019) Cage aggression in group-housed laboratory male mice: an international data crowd-sourcing project. *Scientific Reports*, 9, 15211.

Lindstrom, K.E., Henderson, K.S., Mayorga, M.S., *et al.* (2018) Contaminated shipping materials identified as the source of rotaviral infection of exported mice. *Journal of the American Association for Laboratory Animal Science*, 57, 529–533.

Little, C.C. (1915a) Cancer and heredity. *Science*, 42, 218–219.

Little, C.C. (1915b) The inheritance of cancer. *Science*, 42, 494–495.

Litvin, Y., Blanchard, D.C., Pentkowski, N.S., *et al.* (2007) A pinch or a lesion: a reconceptualization of biting consequences in mice. *Aggressive Behavior*, 33, 545–551.

Liu, Q., Vrontou, S., Rice, F.L., *et al.* (2007) Molecular genetic visualization of a rare subset of unmyelinated sensory neurons that may detect gentle touch. *Nature Neuroscience*, 10, 946–948.

Logge, W., Kingham, J. and Karl, T. (2014) Do individually ventilated cage systems generate a problem for genetic mouse model research? *Genes, Brain and Behavior*, 13, 713–720.

López-Salesansky, N., Chancellor, N., Wells, D., *et al.* (2021) Handling mice using gloves sprayed with alcohol-based hand sanitiser: acute effects on mouse behaviour. *Animal Technology and Welfare*, 20, 11–20.

Luchins, K.R., Bowers, C.J., Mailhiot, D., *et al.* (2020) Cost comparison of rodent soiled bedding sentinel and exhaust air dust health-monitoring programs. *Journal of the American Association for Laboratory Animal Science*, 59, 508–511.

Luo, C., Zuñiga, J., Edison, E., *et al.* (2011) Superovulation strategies for 6 commonly used mouse strains. *Journal of the American Association for Laboratory Animal Science*, 50, 471–478.

Lyons, B.L. and Waterman, L.L. (2012) General considerations formouse survival surgery. *Current Protocols in Mouse Biology*, 2, 263–271.

Machholz, E., Mulder, G., Ruiz, C., *et al.* (2012) Manual restraint and common compound administration routes in mice and rats. *Jove-Journal of Visualized Experiments*, **(67)**, 2771. doi 10.3791/2771.

Machtinger, E.T. and Williams, S.C. (2020) Practical guide to trapping *Peromyscus leucopus* (Rodentia: Cricetidae) and *Peromyscus maniculatus* for vector and vector-borne pathogen surveillance and ecology. *Journal of Insect Science*, **20(6)**. https://doi.org/10.1093/jisesa/ieaa028

Mackintosh, J.H. (1981) Behaviour of the house mouse. In: *Biology of the House Mouse*. Ed. Berry, R.J. Academic Press, London.

Maclellan, A., Adcock, A. and Mason, G. (2021) Behavioral biology of mice. In: *Behavioral Biology of Laboratory Animals*. 1st edn. Eds Coleman, K. and Shapiro, S.J. CRC Press, Boca Raton.

Mähler, M., Berard, M., Feinstein, R., *et al.* (2014) FELASA recommendations for the health monitoring of mouse, rat, hamster, guinea pig and rabbit colonies in breeding and experimental units. *Laboratory Animals*, **48(3)**, 178–192. doi: 10.1177/0023677213516312. Epub 2014 Feb 4. Erratum in: *Laboratory Animals*, 2015 Jan; **49(1)**, 88.

Mailhiot, D., Ostdiek, A.M., Luchins, K.R., *et al.* (2020) Comparing mouse health monitoring between soiled-bedding sentinel and exhaust air dust surveillance programs. *Journal of the American Association for Laboratory Animal Science*, 59, 58–66.

Makowska, I.J., Franks, B., El-Hinn, C., *et al.* (2019) Standard laboratory housing for mice restricts their ability to segregate space into clean and dirty areas. *Scientific Reports*, 9, 6179.

Malewski, S., Malkemper, E.P., Sedláček, F., *et al.* (2018) Attracted by a magnet: exploration behaviour of rodents in the presence of magnetic objects. *Behavioural Processes*, 151, 11–15.

Mani, S.K., Reyna, A.M., Alejandro, M.A., *et al.* (2005) Disruption of male sexual behavior in rats by tetrahydrofurandiols (THF-diols). *Steroids*, 70, 750–754.

Maric, I., Krieger, J.P., Van Der Velden, P., *et al.* (2022) Sex and species differences in the development of diet-induced obesity and metabolic disturbances in rodents. *Frontiers in Nutrition*, 9, 828522.

Markaverich, B.M., Alejandro, M.A., Markaverich, D., *et al.* (2002) Identification of an endocrine disrupting agent from corn with mitogenic activity. *Biochemical and Biophysical Research Communications*, 291, 692–700.

Markaverich, B.M., Crowley, J.R., Alejandro, M.A., *et al.* (2005) Leukotoxin diols from ground corncob bedding disrupt estrous cyclicity in rats and stimulate MCF-7 breast cancer cell proliferation. *Environ Health Perspect*, 113, 1698–1704.

Marx, J.O., Brice, A.K., Boston, R.C., *et al.* (2013) Incidence rates of spontaneous disease in laboratory mice used at a large biomedical research institution. *Journal of the American Association for Laboratory Animal Science*, 52, 782–791.

Marx, J.O., Gaertner, D.J. and Smith, A.L. (2017) Results of survey regarding prevalence of adventitial infections in mice and rats at biomedical research facilities. *Journal of the American Association for Laboratory Animal Science*, 56, 527–533.

Masangkay, J.S. and Kondo, K. (1983) Imperforate vagina in mice: per cent incidence and surgical repair. *Jikken Dobutsu*, 32, 139–144.

Mason, G., Mcfarland, D. and Garner, J. (1998) A demanding task: using economic techniques to assess animal priorities. *Animal Behaviour*, 55, 1071–1075.

Mason, G.J. and Latham, N.R. (2004) Can't stop, won't stop: is stereotypy a reliable animal welfare indicator? *Animal Welfare*, 13, S57–S69.

Maxey, W., Thomas, A.S. and Douglas, M. (1920) *Fancy Mice and Rats, How to Breed and Exhibit*. Fur and Feather, Bradford.

Mccarthy, M.M. and Vom Saal, F.S. (1986) Inhibition of infanticide after mating by wild male house mice. *Physiology & Behavior*, 36, 203–209.

Mcgill, T.E. (1962) Sexual behavior in three inbred strains of mice. *Behaviour*, 19, 341–350.

Mcgill, T.E. and Coughlin, R.C. (1970) Ejaculatory reflex and luteal activity induction in *mus musculus*. *Journal of Reproduction and Fertility*, 21, 215–220.

Mclaren, A. and Michie, D. (1963) Nature of the systemic effect of litter size on gestation period in mice. *Journal of Reproduction and Fertility*, 6, 139–141.

Mcneill, L. (2018) The history of breeding mice for science begins with a woman in a barn. *Smithsonian Magazine*. Smithsonian Institute, Washington D.C.

Meier, H., Hoag, W.G. and McBurney, J.J. (1965) Chemical characterization of inbred-strain mouse milk. I. Gross composition and amino acid analysis. *Journal of Nutrition*, 85, 305–308

Melin, V.E., Melin, T.E., Dessify, B.J., *et al.* (2016) Quaternary ammonium disinfectants cause subfertility in mice by targeting both male and female reproductive processes. *Reproductive Toxicology*, 59, 159–166.

Mendel, G. (1866) Versuche über pflanzen-hybriden. Verhandlungen des naturforschenden vereines. *Abhandlungen, Brünn*, 4, 3–47.

Mesnage, R., Defarge, N., Rocque, L.-M., et al. (2015) Laboratory rodent diets contain toxic levels of environmental contaminants: implications for regulatory tests. *PLoS One*, **10**, e0128429.

Meyer, N., Kröger, M., Thümmler, J., et al. (2020) Impact of three commonly used blood sampling techniques on the welfare of laboratory mice: taking the animal's perspective. *PLoS One*, **15**, e0238895.

Meyerholz, D.K., Adissu, H.A., Carvalho, T., et al. (2021) Exclusion of expert contributors from authorship limits the quality of scientific articles. *Veterinary Pathology*, **58**, 650–654.

Mieske, P., Diederich, K. and Lewejohann, L. (2021) Roaming in a land of milk and honey: life trajectories and metabolic rate of female inbred mice living in a semi naturalistic environment. *Animals*, **11**, 3002.

Miller, M. and Brielmeier, M. (2018) Environmental samples make soiled bedding sentinels dispensable for hygienic monitoring of IVC-reared mouse colonies. *Laboratory Animals*, **52**, 233–239.

Miller, M., Ritter, B., Zorn, J., et al. (2016) Exhaust air dust monitoring is superior to soiled bedding sentinels for the detection of *Pasteurella pneumotropica* in individually ventilated cage systems. *Journal of the American Association for Laboratory Animal Science*, **55**, 775–781.

Mills, D.S. (2003) Medical paradigms for the study of problem behaviour: a critical review. *Applied Animal Behaviour Science*, **81**, 265–277.

Mineur, Y.S. and Crusio, W.E. (2009) Behavioral effects of ventilated micro-environment housing in three inbred mouse strains. *Physiology & Behaviour*, **97**, 334–340.

Moats, C.R., Baxter, V.K., Pate, N.M., et al. (2016) Ectoparasite burden, clinical disease, and immune responses throughout fur mite (*Myocoptes musculinus*) infestation in C57BL/6 and RAG1(-/-) mice. *Comparative Medicine*, **66**, 197–207.

Moberg, G.P. (2000) Biological response to stress: implications for animal welfare. In: *The Biology of Animal Stress: Basic Principles and Implications for Animal Welfare*. Eds Moberg, G.P. and Mench, J.A. CABI Publishing, New York.

Moore, E.S., Cleland, T.A., Williams, W.O., et al. (2017) Comparing phlebotomy by tail tip amputation, facial vein puncture, and tail vein incision in C57BL/6 mice by using physiologic and behavioral metrics of pain and distress. *Journal of the American Association for Laboratory Animal Science*, **56**, 307–317.

Morris, C.F., Mclean, D., Engleson, J.A., et al. (2012) Some observations on the granivorous feeding behavior preferences of the house mouse (*Mus musculus* L.). *Mammalia*, **76**(2), 209–218. https://doi.org/10.1515/mammalia-2011-0121.

Morrison, K.E., Jašarević, E., Howard, C.D., et al. (2020) It's the fiber, not the fat: significant effects of dietary challenge on the gut microbiome. *Microbiome*, **8**, 15.

Mrochen, D.M., Grumann, D., Schulz, D., et al. (2018) Global spread of mouse-adapted *Staphylococcus aureus* lineages cc1, cc15, and cc88 among mouse breeding facilities. *International Journal of Medical Microbiology*, **308**, 598–606.

Muheim, R., Edgar, N.M., Sloan, K.A., et al. (2006) Magnetic compass orientation in C57BL/6J mice. *Learning & Behaviour*, **34**, 366–373.

Mumphrey, S.M., Changotra, H., Moore, T.N., et al. (2007) Murine norovirus 1 infection is associated with histopathological changes in immunocompetent hosts, but clinical disease is prevented by stat1-dependent interferon responses. *Journal of Virology*, **81**, 3251–3263.

Murray, K.A. and Parker, N.J. (2005) Breeding genetically modified rodents: tips for tracking and troubleshooting reproductive performance. *Laboratory Animal (NY)*, **34**, 36–41.

Murray, S.A., Morgan, J.L., Kane, C., et al. (2010) Mouse gestation length is genetically determined. *PLoS One*, **5**, e12418.

Musolf, K., Hoffmann, F. and Penn, D.J. (2010) Ultrasonic courtship vocalizations in wild house mice, *Mus musculus musculus*. *Animal Behaviour*, **79**, 757–764.

Nadal-Nicolás, F.M., Kunze, V.P., Ball, J.M., et al. (2020) True s-cones are concentrated in the ventral mouse retina and wired for color detection in the upper visual field. *eLife*, **9**, e56840.

Nakamura, Y. and Suzuki, K. (2018) Tunnel use facilitates handling of ICR mice and decreases experimental variation. *Journal of Veterinary Medical Science*, **80**, 886–892.

National Research Council (US) Committee on Recognition and Alleviation of Distress in Laboratory Animals 2008. *Recognition and Alleviation of Distress in Laboratory Animals*. National Academies Press, Washington, D.C.

Navarro, K.L., Huss, M., Smith, J.C., et al. (2021) Mouse anesthesia: the art and science. *ILAR Journal*, **62**, 238–273.

Neigh, G.N., Bowers, S.L., Korman, B., et al. (2005) Housing environment alters delayed-type hypersensitivity and corticosterone concentrations of individually housed male C57BL/6 mice. *Animal Welfare*, **14**, 249–257.

Nielsen, F.H. (2018) 90th anniversary commentary: the AIN-93 purified diets for laboratory rodents – the development of a landmark article in the *Journal of Nutrition* and its impact on health and disease research using rodent models. *The Journal of Nutrition*, **148**, 1667–1670.

Niimi, K., Maruyama, S., Sako, N., et al. (2018) The Sentinel (tm) EAD(r) program can detect more microorganisms than bedding sentinel animals. *Japanese Journal of Veterinary Research*, **66**, 125–129.

Nitzki, F., Kruger, A., Reifenberg, K., et al. (2007) Identification of a genetic contamination in a commercial mouse strain using two panels of polymorphic markers. *Laboratory Animals*, **41**, 218–228.

O'malley, C.I., Hubley, R., Moody, C., et al. (2022) Use of nonaversive handling and training procedures for laboratory mice and rats: attitudes of American and Canadian laboratory animal professionals. *Frontiers in Veterinary Science*, **9**, 1040572.

Oates, R. and Tarbert, D.K. (2023) Treatment of pain in rats, mice, and prairie dogs. *Veterinary Clinics: Exotic Animal Practice*, **26**, 151–174.

Paigen, K. (2003a) One hundred years of mouse genetics: an intellectual history. I. The classical period (1902–1980). *Genetics*, **163**, 1–7.

Paigen, K. (2003b) One hundred years of mouse genetics: an intellectual history. II. The molecular revolution (1981–2002) (Reprinted from *The New Yorker*, 2003). *Genetics*, **163**, 1227–1235.

Paluch, L.R., Lieggi, C.C., Dumont, M., et al. (2014) Developmental and behavioral effects of toe clipping on neonatal and preweanling mice with and without vapocoolant anesthesia. *Journal of the American Association for Laboratory Animal Science*, **53**, 132–140.

Panksepp, J.B., Jochman, K.A., Kim, J.U., et al. (2007) Affiliative behavior, ultrasonic communication and social reward are influenced by genetic variation in adolescent mice. *PLoS One*, **2**, e351.

Parasuraman, S., Raveendran, R. and Kesavan, R. (2010) Blood sample collection in small laboratory animals. *Journal of Pharmacology & Pharmacotherapeutics*, **1**, 87–93.

Parker, S.E., Malone, S., Bunte, R.M., et al. (2009) Infectious diseases in wild mice (*Mus musculus*) collected on and around the University of Pennsylvania (Philadelphia) campus. *Comparative Medicine*, **59**, 424–430.

Parkinson, C.M., O'Brien, A., Albers, T.M., et al. (2011) Diagnostic necropsy and selected tissue and sample collection in rats and mice. *Journal of Visualized Experiments*, **(54)**, 2966. doi: 10.3791/2966.

Patten, C.C., Myles, M.H., Franklin, C.L., et al. (2010) Perturbations in cytokine gene expression after inoculation of C57BL/6 mice with *Pasteurella pneumotropica*. *Comparative Medicine*, **60**, 18–24.

Paul, S.M., Mytelka, D.S., Dunwiddie, C.T., et al. (2010) How to improve R&D productivity: the pharmaceutical industry's grand challenge. *Nature Reviews Drug Discovery*, **9**, 203–214.

Peirson, S.N., Brown, L.A., Pothecary, C.A., et al. (2018) Light and the laboratory mouse. *Journal of Neuroscience Methods*, **300**, 26–36.

Peleh, T., Eltokhi, A. and Pitzer, C. (2019) Longitudinal analysis of ultrasonic vocalizations in mice from infancy to adolescence: insights into the vocal repertoire of three wild-type strains in two different social contexts. *PLoS One*, **14**, e0220238.

Pellizzon, M.A. and Ricci, M.R. (2020) Choice of laboratory rodent diet may confound data interpretation and reproducibility. *Current*

Developments in Nutrition, **4**(4), nzaa031–nzaa031. doi: 10.1093/cdn/nzaa031

Percie Du Sert, N., Hurst, V., Ahluwalia, A., et al. (2020) The ARRIVE guidelines 2.0: updated guidelines for reporting animal research. *PLoS Biology*, **18**, e3000410.

Perrigo, G., Belvin, L. and Vom Saal, F.S. (1992) Time and sex in the male mouse: temporal regulation of infanticide and parental behavior. *Chronobiology International*, **9**, 421–433.

Phillips, J., Muheim, R., Painter, M., et al. (2022) Why is it so difficult to study magnetic compass orientation in murine rodents? *Journal of Comparative Physiology A*, **208**, 197–212.

Phillips, J.B., Youmans, P.W., Muheim, R., et al. (2013) Rapid learning of magnetic compass direction by C57BL/6 mice in a 4-armed 'plus' water maze. *PLoS One*, **8**(8), e73112. doi: 10.1371/journal.pone.0073112

Pioli, E.Y., Gaskill, B.N., Gilmour, G., et al. (2014) An automated maze task for assessing hippocampus-sensitive memory in mice. *Behavioural Brain Research*, **261**, 249–257.

Pochanke, V., Hatak, S., Hengartner, H., et al. (2006) Induction of IgE and allergic-type responses in fur mite-infested mice. *European Journal of Immunology*, **36**, 2434–2445.

Popesko, P., Rajtova, V. and Horak, J. (1990a) *A Colour Atlas of Anatomy of Small Laboratory Animals: Volume 1: Rabbit, Guinea Pig*. W. B. Saunders, London.

Popesko, P., Rajtova, V. and Horak, J. (1990b) *A Colour Atlas of Anatomy of Small Laboratory Animals: Volume 2: Rat, Mouse, Golden Hamster*. W. B. Saunders, London.

Portfors, C.V. and Perkel, D.J. (2014) The role of ultrasonic vocalizations in mouse communication. *Current Opinion in Neurobiology*, **28**, 115–120.

Prabhakar, A., Vujovic, D., Cui, L., et al. (2019) Leaky expression of channelrhodopsin-2 (ChR2) in AI32 mouse lines. *PLoS One*, **14**(3), e0213326. doi: 10.1371/journal.pone.0213326

Prato, F.S., Desjardins-Holmes, D., Keenliside, L.D., et al. (2013) Magnetoreception in laboratory mice: sensitivity to extremely low-frequency fields exceeds 33 nT at 30 Hz. *Journal of the Royal Society Interface*, **10**, 20121046.

Prescott, T.J., Mitchinson, B. and Grant, R.A. (2011) Vibrissal behavior and function. *Scholarpedia*, **6**, 6642.

Prinz, F., Schlange, T. and Asadullah, K. (2011) Believe it or not: how much can we rely on published data on potential drug targets? *Nature Reviews Drug Discovery*, **10**, 712–712.

Pritchett-Corning, K.R., Chou, S.T., Conour, L.A., et al. (2015) *Guidebook on Mouse and Rat Colony Management*. Charles River Laboratories, Wilmington, MA.

Pritchett-Corning, K.R., Clifford, C.B., Elder, B.J., et al. (2012) Retinal lesions and other potential confounders of ocular research in inbred mice. *Investigative Ophthalmology & Visual Science*, **53**, 3764–3765.

Pritchett-Corning, K.R., Cosentino, J. and Clifford, C.B. (2009) Contemporary prevalence of infectious agents in laboratory mice and rats. *Laboratory Animals*, **43**, 165–173.

Pritchett-Corning, K.R., Keefe, R., Garner, J.P., et al. (2013) Can seeds help mice with the daily grind? *Laboratory Animals*, **47**, 312–315.

Pritchett-Corning, K.R. and Landel, C.P. (2015) Genetically modified animals. In: *Laboratory Animal Medicine*. 3rd edn. Eds Fox, J., Anderson, L., Otto, G., et al. Academic Press, New York.

Pritchett-Corning, K.R., Mulder, G.B., Luo, Y., et al. (2011) Principles of rodent surgery for the new surgeon. *Journal of Visualized Experiments*, **(47)**, e2586. doi: 10.3791/2586

Pritchett-Corning, K.R. and Winnicker, C. (2021) Behavioral biology of deer and white-footed mice, Mongolian gerbils, and prairie and meadow voles. Behavioral Biology of Laboratory Animals. CRC Press, Boca Raton.

Pritchett, K.R. (2003a) Hydrocephalus in laboratory mice. *JAX Notes*, July 12.

Pritchett, K.R. (2003b) Malocclusion in laboratory mice. *JAX Notes*, April 8.

Pritchett, K.R. and Taft, R.A. (2007) Reproductive biology of the laboratory mouse. In: *The Mouse in Biomedical Research: Normative Biology, Husbandry, and Models*. 2nd edn. Eds Fox, J., Barthold, S., Davisson, M., et al. Academic Press, New York.

Rajnoch, C., Ferguson, S., Metcalfe, A.D., et al. (2003) Regeneration of the ear after wounding in different mouse strains is dependent on the severity of wound trauma. *Developmental Dynamics*, **226**, 388–397.

Ramm, S.A., Cheetham, S.A. and Hurst, J.L. (2008) Encoding choosiness: female attraction requires prior physical contact with individual male scents in mice. *Proceedings of the Royal Society B: Biological Sciences*, **275**, 1727–1735.

Randall, C. (Ed.) (1999) Vertebrate pest management – a guide for commercial applicators (extension bulletin e-2050). Michigan State University, East Lansing.

Rasmussen, S., Glickman, G., Norinsky, R., et al. (2009) Construction noise decreases reproductive efficiency in mice. *Journal of the American Association for Laboratory Animal Science*, **48**, 363–370.

Reed, D.R., Bachmanov, A.A. and Tordoff, M.G. (2007) Forty mouse strain survey of body composition. *Physiology & Behavior*, **91**, 593–600.

Reeves, P.G., Nielsen, F.H. and Fahey, G.C., Jr. (1993) AIN-93 purified diets for laboratory rodents: final report of the American Institute of Nutrition ad hoc writing committee on the reformulation of the AIN-76a rodent diet. *Journal of Nutrition*, **123**, 1939–1951.

Regan, R.D., Fenyk-Melody, J.E., Tran, S.M., et al. (2016) Comparison of submental blood collection with the retroorbital and submandibular methods in mice (*Mus musculus*). *Journal of the American Association for Laboratory Animal Science*, **55**, 570–576.

Reinagel, P. (2018) Training rats using water rewards without water restriction. *Frontiers in Behavioral Neuroscience*, **12**, 84. doi: 10.3389/fnbeh.2018.00084

Reinl, E.L. and England, S.K. (2015) Fetal-to-maternal signaling to initiate parturition. *The Journal of Clinical Investigation*, **125**, 2569–2571.

Reuter, J.D., Livingston, R. and Leblanc, M. (2011) Management strategies for controlling endemic and seasonal mouse parvovirus infection in a barrier facility. *Laboratory Animals*, **40**, 145–152.

Reynolds, R.P., Li, Y., Garner, A., et al. (2018) Vibration in mice: a review of comparative effects and use in translational research. *Animal Models and Experimental Medicine*, **1**, 116–124.

Richter, S.H., Garner, J.P., Auer, C., et al. (2010) Systematic variation improves reproducibility of animal experiments. *Nature Methods*, **7**, 167–168.

Richter, S.H., Garner, J.P. and Würbel, H. (2009) Environmental standardization: cure or cause of poor reproducibility in animal experiments? *Nature Methods*, **6**, 257–261.

Richter, S.H., Kastner, N., Loddenkemper, D.H., et al. (2016) A time to wean? Impact of weaning age on anxiety-like behaviour and stability of behavioural traits in full adulthood. *PLoS One*, **11**(12), e0167652. doi: 10.1371/journal.pone.0167652

Rivera, J. and Tessarollo, L. (2008) Genetic background and the dilemma of translating mouse studies to humans. *Immunity*, **28**, 1–4.

Robinson-Junker, A., O'Hara, B., Durkes, A., et al. (2019) Sleeping through anything: the effects of unpredictable disruptions on mouse sleep, healing, and affect. *PLoS One*, **14**(1), e0210620.

Robinson-Junker, A.L., O'Hara, B.F. and Gaskill, B.N. (2018) Out like a light? The effects of a diurnal husbandry schedule on mouse sleep and behavior. *Journal of the American Association for Laboratory Animal Science*, **57**, 124–133.

Rodriguez-Ramos Fernandez, J. and Dubielzig, R.R. (2013) Ocular comparative anatomy of the family Rodentia. *Veterinary Ophthalmology*, **16**, 94–99.

Rodriguez, I. and Boehm, U. (2009) Pheromone sensing in mice. *Results and Problems in Cell Differentiation*, **47**, 77–96.

Rosenblatt, M. (2016) An incentive-based approach for improving data reproducibility. *Science Translational Medicine*, **8**, 336ed335. doi:10.1126/scitranslmed.aaf5003

Rosshart, S.P., Herz, J., Vassallo, B.G., et al. (2019) Laboratory mice born to wild mice have natural microbiota and model human immune responses. *Science*, 365, eaaw4361.

Rostand, J. (1960) Du nouveau sur Colladon: Précurseur de Mendel. *Revue d'histoire des sciences et de leurs applications*, 13, 259–262.

Rowe, F.P., Bradfield, A. and Redfern, R. (1974) Food preferences of wild house-mice (*Mus musculus* L.). *Journal of Hygiene*, 73, 473–478.

Ruff, J.S., Suchy, A.K., Hugentobler, S.A., et al. (2013) Human-relevant levels of added sugar consumption increase female mortality and lower male fitness in mice. *Nature Communications*, 4, 2245.

Runner, M.N. and Ladman, A.J. (1950) The time of ovulation and its diurnal regulation in the post-parturitional mouse. *Anatomical Record*, 108, 343–361.

Sachs, B.D. (1988) The development of grooming and its expression in adult animals. *Annals of the New York Academy of Sciences*, 525, 1–17.

Sanna, C.R., Li, W.-H. and Zhang, L. (2008) Overlapping genes in the human and mouse genomes. *BMC Genomics*, 9, 169.

Sapienza, C., Peterson, A.C., Rossant, J., et al. (1987) Degree of methylation of transgenes is dependent on gamete of origin. *Nature*, 328, 251–254.

Scannell, J.W., Bosley, J., Hickman, J.A., et al. (2022) Predictive validity in drug discovery: what it is, why it matters and how to improve it. *Nature Reviews Drug Discovery*, 21, 915–931.

Schaefer, D.C., Asner, I.N., Seifert, B., et al. (2010) Analysis of physiological and behavioural parameters in mice after toe clipping as newborns. *Laboratory Animals*, 44, 7–13.

Schulz, D., Grumann, D., Trube, P., et al. (2017) Laboratory mice are frequently colonized with *Staphylococcus aureus* and mount a systemic immune response-note of caution for in vivo infection experiments. *Frontiers in Cellular and Infection Microbiology*, 7, 152.

Scudamore, C.L., Busk, N. and Vowell, K. (2014) A simplified necropsy technique for mice: making the most of unscheduled deaths. *Laboratory Animals*, 48, 342–344.

Sena, E.S., Van der Worp, H.B., Bath, P.M., et al. (2010) Publication bias in reports of animal stroke studies leads to major overstatement of efficacy. *PLoS Biology*, 8, e1000344. https://doi.org/10.1371/journal.pbio.1000344

Shemesh, Y. and Chen, A. (2023) A paradigm shift in translational psychiatry through rodent neuroethology. *Molecular Psychiatry*, 28, 993–1003.

Shepherd, G.M. (2004) The human sense of smell: are we better than we think? *PLoS Biology*, 2(5), e146. https://doi.org/10.1371/journal.pbio.0020146

Shirasaki, Y., Ito, Y., Kikuchi, M., et al. (2012) Validation studies on blood collection from the jugular vein of conscious mice. *Journal of the American Association for Laboratory Animal Science*, 51, 345–351.

Shire, J.G. (1984) Studies on the inheritance of vaginal septa in mice, a trait with low penetrance. *Journal of Reproduction and Fertility*, 70, 333–339.

Shomer, N.H., Allen-Worthington, K.H., Hickman, D.L., et al. (2020) Review of rodent euthanasia methods. *Journal of the American Association for Laboratory Animal Science*, 59, 242–253.

Sigmund, C.D. (2000) Viewpoint: are studies in genetically altered mice out of control? *Arteriosclerosis, Thrombosis, and Vascular Biology*, 20, 1425–1429.

Silva, K.A. and Sundberg, J.P. (2012) Chapter 5.6 – Necropsy Methods a2. In: *The Laboratory Mouse*, 2nd edn. Ed. Hedrich, H.J. Academic Press, Boston.

Škop, V., Guo, J., Liu, N., et al. (2020) Mouse thermoregulation: introducing the concept of the thermoneutral point. *Cell Reports*, 31, 107501.

Smith, A.J., Clutton, R.E., Lilley, E., et al. (2018) PREPARE: guidelines for planning animal research and testing. *Laboratory Animals*, 52, 135–141.

Smith, B.K., Andrews, P.K. and West, D.B. (2000) Macronutrient diet selection in thirteen mouse strains. *American Journal of Physiology – Regulatory Integrative and Comparative Physiology*, 278, R797–R805.

Smith, R.S., Roderick, T.H. and Sundberg, J.P. (1994) Microphthalmia and associated abnormalities in inbred black mice. *Laboratory Animal Science*, 44, 551–560.

Snell, G.D. (1948) Methods for the study of histocompatibility genes. *Journal of Genetics*, 49, 87–108.

Soroker, V. and Terkel, J. (1988) Changes in incidence of infanticidal and parental responses during the reproductive cycle in male and female wild mice *Mus musculus*. *Animal Behaviour*, 36, 1275–1281.

Spangenberg, E., Wallenbeck, A., Eklöf, A., et al. (2014) Housing breeding mice in three different IVC systems: maternal performance and pup development. *Laboratory Animals*, 48, 193–206.

Starr, M.E. and Saito, H. (2012) Age-related increase in food spilling by laboratory mice may lead to significant overestimation of actual food consumption: implications for studies on dietary restriction, metabolism, and dose calculations. *Journals of Gerontology Series A Biological Sciences and Medical Sciences*, 67, 1043–1048.

Stehr, M., Greweling, M.C., Tischer, S., et al. (2009) Charles River altered Schaedler flora (CRASF (R)) remained stable for four years in a mouse colony housed in individually ventilated cages. *Laboratory Animals*, 43, 362–370.

Stover, M.G. and Villano, J.S. (2022) Evaluation of various IVC systems according to mouse reproductive performance and husbandry and environmental parameters. *Journal of the American Association for Laboratory Animal Science*, 61, 31–41.

Strabo, Hamilton, H.C. and Falconer, W. (1903) *The Geography of Strabo*. George Bell & Sons, London.

Sundberg, J.P. and Brown, K.S. (1994) Imperforate vagina and mucometra in inbred laboratory mice. *Laboratory Animal Science*, 44, 380–382.

Sutter, A., Simmons, L.W., Lindholm, A.K., et al. (2015) Function of copulatory plugs in house mice: mating behavior and paternity outcomes of rival males. *Behavioral Ecology*, 27, 185–195.

Taitt, K.T. and Kendall, L.V. (2019) Physiologic stress of ear punch identification compared with restraint only in mice. *Journal of the American Association for Laboratory Animal Science*, 58, 438–442.

Tan, S. and Stowers, L. (2020) Bespoke behavior: mechanisms that modulate pheromone-triggered behavior. *Current Opinion in Neurobiology*, 64, 143–150.

The Jackson Laboratory (1987) Alopecia (loss of hair) in C57BL/6J and related strains. *JAX|NOTES*. The Jackson Laboratory.

The Jackson Laboratory (2007) *Breeding Strategies for Maintaining Colonies of Laboratory Mice*. The Jackson Laboratory, Bar Harbor, ME.

Theil, J.H., Ahloy-Dallaire, J., Weber, E.M., et al. (2020) The epidemiology of fighting in group-housed laboratory mice. *Scientific Reports*, 10, 16649.

Thigpen, J.E., Lebetkin, E.H., Dawes, M.L., et al. (1989) The use of dirty bedding for detection of murine pathogens in sentinel mice. *Laboratory Animal Science*, 39, 324–327.

Tokuda, M. (1935) An eighteenth century Japanese guide-book on mouse-breeding. *Journal of Heredity*, 26, 481–484.

Tordoff, M.G. (2007) Taste solution preferences of C57BL/6J and 129X1/SvJ mice: influence of age, sex, and diet. *Chemical Senses*, 32, 655–671.

Tordoff, M.G., Bachmanov, A.A. and Reed, D.R. (2007) Forty mouse strain survey of water and sodium intake. *Physiology & Behavior*, 91, 620–631.

Towne, J.W., Wagner, A.M., Griffin, K.J., et al. (2014) Elimination of *Pasteurella pneumotropica* from a mouse barrier facility by using a modified enrofloxacin treatment regimen. *Journal of the American Association for Laboratory Animal Science*, 53, 517–522.

Treuting, P., Dintzis, S. and Montine, K.S. (Eds) (2018) *Comparative Anatomy and Histology: A Mouse, Rat, and Human Atlas*. Academic Press, London.

Treuting, P.M. and Snyder, J.M. (2015) Mouse necropsy. *Current Protocols in Mouse Biology*, 5, 223–233.

Tsai, P.P., Oppermann, D., Stelzer, H.D., *et al.* (2003) The effects of different rack systems on the breeding performance of DBA/2 mice. *Laboratory Animals*, **37**, 44–53.

Tsai, P.P., Schlichtig, A., Ziegler, E., *et al.* (2015) Effects of different blood collection methods on indicators of welfare in mice. *Laboratory Animals (NY)*, **44**, 301–310.

Tsao, C.-H., Flint, J. and Huang, G.-J. (2022) Influence of diurnal phase on behavioral tests of sensorimotor performance, anxiety, learning and memory in mice. *Scientific Reports*, **12**, 432.

Tuck, C.J., De Palma, G., Takami, K., *et al.* (2020) Nutritional profile of rodent diets impacts experimental reproducibility in microbiome preclinical research. *Scientific Reports*, **10**, 17784.

Turner, J.G. (2020) Noise and vibration in the vivarium: recommendations for developing a measurement plan. *Journal of the American Association for Laboratory Animal Science*, **59**, 665–672.

Turner, J.G., Parrish, J.L., Hughes, L.F., *et al.* (2005) Hearing in laboratory animals: strain differences and nonauditory effects of noise. *Comparative Medicine*, **55**, 12–23.

Turner, P.V., Brabb, T., Pekow, C., *et al.* (2011a) Administration of substances to laboratory animals: routes of administration and factors to consider. *Journal of the American Association for Laboratory Animal Science*, **50**, 600–613.

Turner, P.V., Hickman, D.L., Van Luijk, J., *et al.* (2020) Welfare impact of carbon dioxide euthanasia on laboratory mice and rats: a systematic review. *Frontiers in Veterinary Science*, **7**, 411. doi: 10.3389/fvets.2020.00411

Turner, P.V., Pekow, C., Vasbinder, M.A., *et al.* (2011b) Administration of substances to laboratory animals: equipment considerations, vehicle selection, and solute preparation. *Journal of the American Association for Laboratory Animal Science*, **50**, 614–627.

Urai, A.E., Aguillon-Rodriguez, V., Laranjeira, I.C., *et al.* (2021) Citric acid water as an alternative to water restriction for high-yield mouse behavior. *eNeuro*, **8(1)**, ENEURO.0230-20.2020. doi: 10.1523/ENEURO.0230-20.2020.

Van der Lee, S. and Boot, L.M. (1955) Spontaneous pseudopregnancy in mice. *Acta Physiologica et Pharmacologica*, **4**, 442–444.

Van der Lee, S. and Boot, L.M. (1956) Spontaneous pseudopregnancy in mice II. *Acta Physiologica et Pharmacologica*, **5**, 213–215.

Van der Worp, H.B., Howells, D.W., Sena, E.S., *et al.* (2010) Can animal models of disease reliably inform human studies? *PLoS Medicine*, **7**, e1000245.

Van Loo, P.L., Kruitwagen, C.L.J.J., Koolhaas, J.M., *et al.* (2002) Influence of cage enrichment on aggressive behaviour and physiological parameters in male mice. *Applied Animal Behaviour Science*, **76**, 65–81.

Van Loo, P.L., Kruitwagen, C.L.J.J., Van Zutphen, B.F., *et al.* (2000) Modulation of aggression in male mice: influence of cage cleaning regime and scent marks. *Animal Welfare*, **9**, 281–295.

Van Loo, P.L., Mol, J.A., Koolhaas, J.M., *et al.* (2001) Modulation of aggression in male mice: influence of group size and cage size. *Physiology & Behavior*, **72**, 675–683.

Van Loo, P.L., Van Zutphen, L.F. and Baumans, V. (2003a) Male management: coping with aggression problems in male laboratory mice. *Laboratory Animals*, **37**, 300–313.

Van Loo, P.L.P., Van Der Meer, E., Kruitwagen, C., *et al.* (2003b) Strain-specific aggressive behavior of male mice submitted to different husbandry procedures. *Aggressive Behavior*, **29**, 69–80.

Vieira, G.L.T., Lossie, A.C., Lay, D.C., Jr., *et al.* (2017) Preventing, treating, and predicting barbering: a fundamental role for biomarkers of oxidative stress in a mouse model of trichotillomania. *PLoS One*, **12(4)**, e0175222. https://doi.org/10.1371/journal.pone.0175222

Villalon Landeros, R., Morisseau, C., Yoo, H.J., *et al.* (2012) Corncob bedding alters the effects of estrogens on aggressive behavior and reduces estrogen receptor-alpha expression in the brain. *Endocrinology*, **153**, 949–953.

Vogel, P., Read, R., Hansen, G., *et al.* (2012) Congenital hydrocephalus in genetically engineered mice. *Veterinary Pathology*, **49**, 166–181.

Vom Saal, F.S. and Howard, L.S. (1982) The regulation of infanticide and parental behavior: implications for reproductive success in male mice. *Science*, **215**, 1270–1272.

Waalkes, M.P., Rehm, S., Kasprzak, K.S., *et al.* (1987) Inflammatory, proliferative, and neoplastic lesions at the site of metallic identification ear tags in Wistar [Crl:(WI)br] rats. *Cancer Research*, **47**, 2445–2450.

Wade, C.M. and Daly, M.J. (2005) Genetic variation in laboratory mice. *Nature Genetics*, **37**, 1175–1180.

Wade, C.M., Kulbokas, E.J., 3rd, Kirby, A.W., *et al.* (2002) The mosaic structure of variation in the laboratory mouse genome. *Nature*, **420**, 574–578.

Wahlsten, D., Bachmanov, A., Finn, D.A., *et al.* (2006) Stability of inbred mouse strain differences in behavior and brain size between laboratories and across decades. *Proceedings of the National Academy of Sciences USA*, **103**, 16364–16369.

Wahlsten, D., Metten, P., Phillips, T.J., *et al.* (2003) Different data from different labs: lessons from studies of gene-environment interaction. *Journal of Neurobiology*, **54**, 283–311.

Walsh, C.M., Bautista, D.M. and Lumpkin, E.A. (2015) Mammalian touch catches up. *Current Opinion in Neurobiology*, **34**, 133–139.

Wang, Y.V., Weick, M. and Demb, J.B. (2011) Spectral and temporal sensitivity of cone-mediated responses in mouse retinal ganglion cells. *The Journal of Neuroscience: The Official Journal of the Society for Neuroscience*, **31**, 7670–7681.

Ward, J., Elmore, S. and Foley, J. (2012) Pathology methods for the evaluation of embryonic and perinatal developmental defects and lethality in genetically engineered mice. *Veterinary Pathology*, **49**, 71–84.

Ward, J.M., Schofield, P.N. and Sundberg, J.P. (2017) Reproducibility of histopathological findings in experimental pathology of the mouse: a sorry tail. *Laboratory Animals*, **46**, 146–151.

Wasson, K. (2017) Retrospective analysis of reproductive performance of pair-bred compared with trio-bred mice. *Journal of the American Association for Laboratory Animal Science*, **56**, 190–193.

Weber, E.M., Algers, B., Hultgren, J., *et al.* (2013) Pup mortality in laboratory mice – infanticide or not? *Acta Veterinaria Scandinavica*, **55(1)**, 83. doi: 10.1186/1751-0147-55-83

Weber, E.M., Dallaire, J.A., Gaskill, B.N., *et al.* (2017) Aggression in group-housed laboratory mice: why can't we solve the problem? *Laboratory Animals (NY)*, **46**, 157–161.

Weber, E.M., Hultgren, J., Algers, B., *et al.* (2016) Do laboratory mouse females that lose their litters behave differently around parturition? *PLoS One*, **11(8)**, e0161238. doi: 10.1371/journal.pone.0161238. Erratum in: *PLoS One*. 2016 Oct; **11(10)**, e0165578.

Weber, E.M. and Olsson, I.a.S. (2008) Maternal behaviour in *Mus musculus* spp.: an ethological review. *Applied Animal Behaviour Science*, **114**, 1–22.

Weiskirchen, S., Weiper, K., Tolba, R.H., *et al.* (2020) All you can feed: some comments on production of mouse diets used in biomedical research with special emphasis on non-alcoholic fatty liver disease research. *Nutrients*, **12(1)**, 163. doi: 10.3390/nu12010163.

Weiss, J.M. (1970) Somatic effects of predictable and unpredictable shock. *Psychosomatic Medicine*, **32**, 397–408.

Weiss, J.M. (1971) Effects of coping behavior with and without a feedback signal on stress pathology in rats. *Journal of Comparative and Physiological Psychology*, **77**, 22–30.

Whary, M.T. and Fox, J.G. (2006) Detection, eradication, and research implications of *Helicobacter* infections in laboratory rodents. *Laboratory Animals (NY)*, **35**, 25–27, 30–26.

Whittaker, A.L. and Barker, T.H. (2020) The impact of common recovery blood sampling methods, in mice (*Mus musculus*), on well-being and sample quality: a systematic review. *Animals (Basel)*, **10(6)**, 989. doi: 10.3390/ani10060989.

Whitten, W.K. (1956) Modification of the oestrous cycle of the mouse by external stimuli associated with the male. *Journal of Endocrinology*, **13**, 399–404.

Whitten, W.K. (1958) Modification of the oestrous cycle of the mouse by external stimuli associated with the male – changes in the oestrous cycle determined by vaginal smears. *Journal of Endocrinology*, **17**, 307–313.

Wiedmeyer, C.E., Crossland, J.P., Veres, M., *et al.* (2014) Hematologic and serum biochemical values of 4 species of *Peromyscus* mice and their hybrids. *Journal of the American Association for Laboratory Animal Science*, **53**, 336–343.

Williams, S.C., Linske, M.A. and Stafford, K.C., 3rd (2020) Humane use of cardiac puncture for non-terminal phlebotomy of wild-caught and released *Peromyscus* spp. *Animals (Basel)*, **10**(5), 826. doi: 10.3390/ani10050826.

Williams, S.H., Che, X., Garcia, J.A., *et al.* (2018) Viral diversity of house mice in New York City. *mBio*, **9**(2), e01354–17. doi: 10.1128/mBio.01354-17.

Williamson, C.M., Lee, W. and Curley, J.P. (2016) Temporal dynamics of social hierarchy formation and maintenance in male mice. *Animal Behaviour*, **115**, 259–272.

Williamson, C.M., Lee, W., Decasien, A.R., *et al.* (2019) Social hierarchy position in female mice is associated with plasma corticosterone levels and hypothalamic gene expression. *Scientific Reports*, **9**, 7324.

Winn, C.B., Rogers, R.N., Keenan, R.A., *et al.* (2022) Using filter media and soiled bedding in disposable individually ventilated cages as a refinement to specific pathogen-free mouse health monitoring programs. *Journal of the American Association for Laboratory Animal Science*, **61**, 361–369.

Wong, A.A. and Brown, R.E. (2006) Visual detection, pattern discrimination and visual acuity in 14 strains of mice. *Genes Brain Behav*, **5**, 389–403.

Wong, C.H., Siah, K.W. and Lo, A.W. (2019) Estimation of clinical trial success rates and related parameters. *Biostatistics*, **20**, 273–286. Erratum in: *Biostatistics*. 2019 Apr; **20**(2), 366.

Würbel, H. (2000) Behaviour and the standardization fallacy. *Nature Genetics*, **26**, 263–263.

Würbel, H. (2006) The motivational basis of caged rodents' stereotypies. In: *Stereotypic Animal Behavior: Fundamentals and Applications to Welfare*. Eds Rushen, J. and Mason, G. CABI, Wallingford, UK.

Würbel, H. (2017) More than 3Rs: the importance of scientific validity for harm–benefit analysis of animal research. *Laboratory Animals*, **46**, 164–166.

Würbel, H., Burn, C. and Latham, N. (2009) The behavior of laboratory mice and rats. In: *The Ethology of Domestic Animals, 2nd edition: An Introductory Text*. Ed. Jensen, P. Oxford University Press, Oxford.

Würbel, H. and Garner, J.P. (2007) Refinement of rodent research through environmental enrichment and systematic randomization. *NC3Rs*, **9**, 1–9.

Yamamoto, K., Matsunaga, S., Matsui, M., *et al.* (2002) Pica in mice as a new model for the study of emesis. *Methods and Findings in Experimental and Clinical Pharmacology*, **24**, 135–138.

Yang, H., Wang, J.R., Didion, J.P., *et al.* (2011) Subspecific origin and haplotype diversity in the laboratory mouse. *Nature Genetics*, **43**, 648–655.

Yi, P. and Li, L. (2012) The germfree murine animal: an important animal model for research on the relationship between gut microbiota and the host. *Veterinary Microbiology*, **157**, 1–7.

Young, S.S. (1987) Are there local room effects on hepatic-tumors in male-mice – an examination of the NTP eugenol study. *Fundamental and Applied Toxicology*, **8**, 1–4.

Young, S.S. (1989) Are there location cage systematic nontreatment effects in long-term rodent studies – a question revisited. *Fundamental and Applied Toxicology*, **13**, 183–188.

Zahs, K.R. and Ashe, K.H. (2010) 'Too much good news' – are Alzheimer mouse models trying to tell us how to prevent, not cure, Alzheimer's disease? *Trends in Neurosciences*, **33**, 381–389.

Zegarelli, E.V. (1944) Adamantoblastomas in the Slye stock of mice. *American Journal of Pathology*, **20**, 23–87.

Zeppilli, S., Ackels, T., Attey, R., *et al.* (2021) Molecular characterization of projection neuron subtypes in the mouse olfactory bulb. *eLife*, **10**, e65445.

Zhang, Y.-F., Janke, E., Bhattarai, J.P., *et al.* (2022) Self-directed orofacial grooming promotes social attraction in mice via chemosensory communication. *iScience*, **25**, 104284.

Zhao, Y., Daggett, L.P. and Hardies, S.C. (1996) *Mus spretus* LINE-1s in the *Mus musculus domesticus* inbred strain C57BL/6J are from two different *Mus spretus* LINE-1 subfamilies. *Genetics*, **142**, 549–555.

Zurita, E., Chagoyen, M., Cantero, M., *et al.* (2011) Genetic polymorphisms among C57BL/6 mouse inbred strains. *Transgenic Research*, **20**, 481–489.

22 The laboratory rat

Sietse F. de Boer and Jaap M. Koolhaas

Biological overview

General biology and history

For well over a century, rats have been the most important model organisms for studying (patho)physiological processes of virtually every organ system in human health and disease. Rats gained popularity due to their docility, ability to breed well in the laboratory, and robust cognitive, emotional, social and reproductive behaviours. In addition, they are large enough for allowing physiological measurements and manipulations as well as (neuro)anatomical investigations. The genus *Rattus* contains 66 species and belongs to the family of the Muridea and the order of Rodentia, the largest within the class Mammalia. The laboratory rat is the domesticated form of the species *Rattus norvegicus* or brown Norway rat. The wild *Rattus norvegicus* has agouti-coloured fur, meaning that it has the agouti gene which produces hairs with colour bands varying between brown–black and red–yellow. *Rattus rattus* may have a more variable coat colour but is mainly dark brown or black. The most conspicuous difference between the two species concerns the relatively large, mouse-like ears of *R. rattus*. The two species share more or less the same habitat, but *R. norvegicus* lives mainly in burrow systems at ground level, whereas *R. rattus* tend to occupy higher areas in trees and roofs.

Whereas most species of *Rattus* are indigenous in subtropical and tropical areas, *R. norvegicus* is cosmopolitan and can be found on all continents where humans are present. Human settlements are now the ecological niche of the wild rat: the farm, the city, the garbage dump, the sewer, the subway. The brown Norway rat has a rather interesting recent evolutionary history. The species seems to have originated on the central Asian steppes, where they first learned they could eat well by living in proximity to humans and then has spread over almost all of the world during the last two or three centuries (Hedrich 2000). This spread was strongly facilitated by the increase in long-distance trading along the Silk Road, and rats were established in parts of Europe in the early eighteenth century. (The misnomer 'Norway rat' may have arisen when an infested ship that happened to be Norwegian docked in an English port.) Early *R. norvegicus* colonies were established by Russian ships and wrecks in the Baltic region. *R. norvegicus* reached North America by 1755, the north-eastern part of the United States in 1775 and the Pacific coast in 1851, arriving on ships with early settlers. In all of these areas, they rapidly displaced *R. rattus*, and often became a major pest. In eighteenth-century Europe, wild brown rats ran rampant and this infestation fuelled the industry of rat-catching. Rat-catchers would not only make money by trapping the rodents, but also by selling them for food, or more commonly, for rat-baiting. Rat-baiting was a popular sport which involved filling a pit with rats and timing how long it took for a terrier to kill them all. Over time, breeding the rats for these contests may have produced variations in coat colour, notably the albino and hooded varieties. The first time one of these albino mutants was brought into a laboratory for a study was in 1828, in an experiment on fasting. Over the next 30 years, rats were used for several more experiments and eventually the laboratory rat became the first animal domesticated for purely scientific reason.

The Brown Norway rat is a generalist which is able to survive in a wide variety of habitats and climatic conditions. The species greatly benefits from the presence of human beings and may live in buildings, harvest stores, sewer systems and on rubbish dumps (Feng & Himsworth 2014; Traweger et al. 2006). Wild rats live in colonies and it prefers to live in burrow systems usually located near water. The burrow system occupies 2–4 m^2 and consists of tunnels 5–7 cm in diameter and 0.25–1.5 m long (Pisano & Storer 1948; Calhoun 1962). The tunnels usually end in small chambers used for nesting and storage of food. The area around the burrow system can be considered as the territory and will be defended against unfamiliar conspecifics. However, the home range of the animals (i.e. the range in which they search for food) may be about 100 m^2. The rat is a nocturnal animal and generally has three activity periods, one at the beginning, one in the middle and one at the end of the night (Figure 22.1). It feeds during these activity periods taking three to five separate meals. The worldwide success of the

---

The UFAW Handbook on the Care and Management of Laboratory and Other Research Animals, Ninth Edition.
Edited by Huw Golledge and Claire Richardson.
© 2024 John Wiley & Sons Ltd. Published 2024 by John Wiley & Sons Ltd.

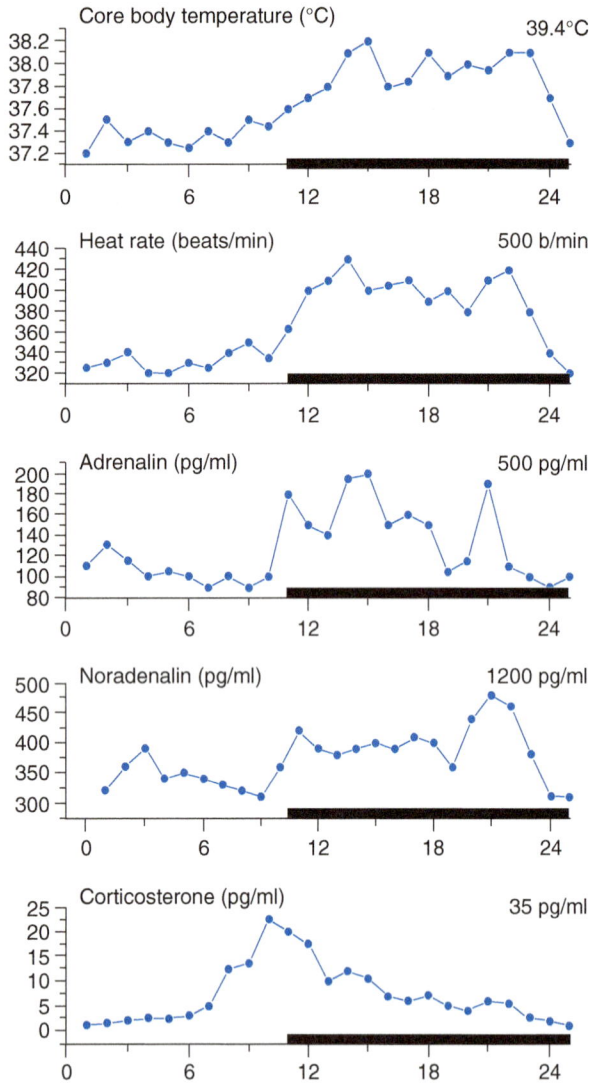

Figure 22.1 Circadian variation in plasma corticosterone, noradrenaline and adrenaline levels, heart rate and core body temperature in adult male Wistar rats. The black bar indicates the dark period of the light–dark cycle. The data on the right-hand side of each graph indicate the maximum response levels obtained during 15 minutes restraint stress.

Norway rat is partially due to the fact that the species is omnivorous, having a remarkable capacity to balance its nutrient intake in a broad range of dietary conditions (Klemann & Peltz 2006).

Sensory systems

The rats' senses of smell, taste, hearing and touch are highly developed (Burn 2008), and its behaviour is strongly determined by olfactory signals. In a social setting, male rats are able to recognise social status of other males, reproductive status of females and kinship solely on the basis of olfactory cues (Beynon & Hurst 2004). Moreover, rats are very sensitive to olfactory signals from predators such as cats and alarm pheromones from other rats (Dielenberg & McGregor 2001). The crucial role of odours should be considered in every ethological study of rat behaviour, but this is not always the case. The sense of taste in rats appears to be similar to that of humans. The rat's robust approach and avoidance responses to taste compounds, as well as its innate oromotor reflexes to chemical stimuli, parallel the hedonic reactions of humans (Spector & Kopka 2002).

Rats have a large vocal repertoire, and many of these are in the ultrasonic spectrum, as rats can hear frequencies up to at least 80 kHz. Different categories of ultrasonic vocalisations (USVs) have been associated with different functions and affective states (Brudzynski 2013; Wöhr & Schwarting 2013). Rat pups emit 40 kHz sounds when left alone by the nursing mother, eliciting pup retrieval by the dam (Portfors 2007). Aversive situations can give rise to USVs in the 22kHz range, whereas vocalisations in the 50 kHz range have been associated with a state of positive affect (a positive emotional state; Barker 2018), as these are emitted during social play, as appeasement, and in response to rewarding conditions (Panksepp 2007; Burgdorf et al. 2008; Kisko et al. 2017).

Tactile receptors are particularly well-developed on the head, around the whiskers, on the paws and on the tail. Studies indicate that the rat whisker system has a sensitivity of less than 90 μm, which is comparable to that of primate fingertips (Carvell & Simons 1990). Rats use their vibrissae to perform a variety of tactile discriminations and behaviours.

Acuity and contrast sensitivity of rats are lower than that of other small mammals such as cats and ferrets, and the rat does not have trichromatic colour vision, a fovea or the elaborate functional divisions of the lateral geniculate nucleus and visual cortex that many primates do, including human. The rat retina contains both rods and cones, with the proportion of cones being about 1 % (LaVail 1976). One type of cone in the retina has a photo pigment with a maximal sensitivity at a wavelength of 510 nm (green) (Neitz & Jacobs 1986), which declines rapidly at wavelengths above 560 nm (red–infrared). A second type of cone has its maximal sensitivity in the near ultraviolet range (360 nm) (Jacobs et al. 2001). Rats are frequently housed with a lighting schedule using red light to mimic the dark period. Sensitivity to red light is reduced in rats, but they can still detect it (Akula et al. 2003). Although lights in the red spectrum may not be equivalent to darkness for rodents, certain types of lighting are sufficient to mimic darkness, i.e. induce the behaviour and physiology usually seen during the nocturnal period. For rodents, this can be obtained by using low pressure sodium bulbs (McLennan & Taylor-Jeffs 2004), which have a very narrow bandwidth of 589 nm wavelength, emitting a soft yellowish light that is bright enough for humans to read in.

Visual acuity (the smallest spatial pattern that can be resolved) is generally low (approx. 1.0 cycle/degree compared to 30 c/d for humans), with albino strains being more variable and often lower in visual acuity than pigmented laboratory strains, and about half of those of wild rats (Prusky et al. 2002). All of the above may be complicated by the fact that many commonly used strains of laboratory rodent are albino, leading to a risk of phototoxic retinopathy if light levels in the holding facility are too high.

Size range and lifespan

The size of a rat is usually expressed in terms of body weight. Growth rate depends not only on strain, but also on quality and availability of food, as well as environmental factors such as temperature and social housing situation. Because of the *ad libitum* feeding regimens of nutritious food, standard in most rodent facilities, combined with little opportunity for exercise in standard laboratory cages, male laboratory rats are particularly prone to excessive fat deposition or develop obesity and can easily reach weights exceeding 800 g, occasionally over one kg. Many standard control laboratory rats used in biomedical research are sedentary, obese, glucose intolerant and on a trajectory to premature death which may confound data interpretation and outcomes of human studies (Martin *et al.* 2010).

Size can also be determined using morphological parameters such as body and tail length. Body length is measured from the tip of the nose to the middle of the anus and tail length from the middle of the anus to the tip of the tail. Although the body length to tail length ratio is rather constant in adult rats, the absolute values, particularly the length of the tail, may be influenced by the environmental temperature during rearing.

Rats do not live long in the wild, the average lifespan is probably less than a year. In one study, it was found that 95% of rats living at a farm were no longer alive a year later (Calhoun 1962). So, rats suffer very high mortality in the wild. However, their birth rate is high as well, ranging from 1% to 6% of the carrying capacity per month during population recovery after an artificial reduction. The maximum lifespan of wild rats kept in a semi-natural enclosure is about 600 days for males and 700 days for females, whereas the median lifespan (50% survival) is 300 days for males and 550 days for females[1] (Calhoun 1962). In laboratory strains, longevity may vary considerably depending on the strain and diet. The maximum lifespan of the Wistar strain, for example, is about 1200 days (3.2 years) for males and 1400 days (3.8 years) for females. Median lifespan for the Wistar rat is 850 days for males and 900 days for females (Ghirardi *et al.* 1995)

Social organisation

When environmental conditions such as weather, food supplies, nesting opportunities, infectious and predatory pressures are favourable, wild rats crowd together in colonies that rapidly increase and eventually may number many hundreds. The fact that the Norway rat is a social species by nature has often been under-emphasised, if not ignored, in the design and interpretation of laboratory experiments. In their classic works, Calhoun (1962), Barnett (1963) and Telle (1966) gave a detailed account of the social interactions and ecology of wild brown Norway rats. Generally, in groups of wild rats, the social system of males is territorial or despotic depending on the population density (number of rats per m^2). At low population densities, one adult dominant male rat can be distinguished which lives together with a small group of females and young rats. The dominant rat vigorously marks, patrols and defends the region (called the territory) around their feeding and underground nest sites (burrows) from other male intruders. Outside these territories, neutral areas exist where fighting is minimal and avoidance occurs. In general, a colony comprises a number of territories and neutral areas. In case of an encounter with an intruder, the male displays fierce territorial aggressive behaviour often causing the intruder to flee. Although it is mainly the resident male who drives away male intruders, lactating female rats defend their nest, both against males and females. Such dispersive territorial behaviour can only persist when invasions of a territory are infrequent. With increasing population densities (e.g. 1 rat per 5 m^2), rats become socially more tolerant and cohesive, and adapt to a despotic social structure, with one male being socially dominant (the *alpha* rat) and prevailing most often over rival or *beta* males and over subordinate or *omega* animals in aggressive confrontations. The attacks and threats exerted by dominant individuals are responded to by defensive, evasive and submissive postures in the beta and omega animals that decrease the probability of being attacked further. Although overt aggression may initially be necessary to obtain a dominance-subordinate relationship, once established a stable hierarchy suppresses further aggressive conflicts and unwanted fights among the group members. Yet, most male lab rats can generally be housed together without any major or problematic signs of aggression. This is largely due to the general loss of aggressiveness in the highly domesticated rat strains (de Boer *et al.* 2003).

Mating system and reproduction

The rat has an exceptionally high reproductive capacity. Both males and females are, on average, sexually mature at the age of 2–3 months. The oestrous cycle is 4–5 days. At the time of oestrus, receptivity occurs in the second half of the dark period (Barbacka-Surowiak *et al.* 2003). In the wild, a receptive female will be followed and mounted by the dominant male and often by a number of other male colony members as well (McClintock & Adler 1978). Since a promiscuous mating system is evident in both wild and domesticated rats, multiple paternity is common. At low densities, Norway rats are territorial and polygynous, one male mates with multiple females. At high densities, they are despotic and polygynandrous, multiple males mate with multiple females, through group mating and rushing. After several successful copulations, the female's willingness starts to decline; this is indicated by aggressive actions and escape behaviour by the female (for more details of male and female rats' sociosexual behaviours, see Chu & Agmo 2014, 2015). Gestation is 20–22 days, and during the few days prior to delivery of the pups, the pregnant female starts to build a nest and will defend her nest against both male and female colony members. This maternal aggression will continue throughout the

---

[1] Note that the maximum and median lifespan are different measures of longevity, which cannot be compared directly.

first week of nursing, after which it gradually declines and another reproductive cycle may start (Rosenblatt et al. 1994). In temperate regions, wild rats have a clear seasonal variation in reproduction governed by day length and food availability. Some studies of laboratory rats indicate the presence of an intrinsic annual cycle (Claassen 1994; De Boer et al. 2003). The average litter size is approximately 10 and in the wild, sex ratio depends on season, population density and food availability (Bacon & McClintock 1994; Parshad 1997).

Standard biological data

Some of the basic physiological and morphological data of the Wistar rat are presented in Table 22.1 (see also Suckow et al. 2019; Krinke et al. 2000 for more extensive information). These data should, however, be used with some caution, as many of the parameters are not static but highly dynamic in time, varying both diurnally and throughout life. Moreover, there are significant strain differences, and within strains there may be broad individual differences as well as large differences between suppliers, in particular where outbred or random-bred strains are concerned.

Most physiological parameters show a strong circadian variation and are highly responsive to environmental arousing and stressful situations (see Hawkins & Golledge 2018 for a discussion on how circadian rhythms might affect welfare and scientific research outcomes). Figure 22.1 shows the circadian variation in some neuroendocrine and physiological parameters of 4-month-old male Wistar rats, measured using undisturbed methods (permanent jugular vein cannulation for blood sampling and wireless radiotelemetric physiological recording). The number in the right-hand part of each graph shows the maximum value of these parameters obtained during a 15-minute period of physical restraint (de Boer et al. 1990; unpublished data collected by the authors).

Breeds, strains and genetics

The use of rats for research in the laboratory began at the end of the nineteenth century, by a number of French and English scientists. The first known breeding experiments with rats using albino rats were performed in Germany from 1877–1885 by Crampe (see Lindsey and Baker 2006 for excellent historical review of the history of the laboratory rat). The first experiments known to use rats in the USA were neuroanatomical studies performed during the early 1890s by Hatai and other faculty members in Henry Donaldson's department of Neurology at the University of Chicago. After moving to the Wistar Institute in Philadelphia, Donaldson together with genetic researcher Helen King began efforts to standardise the albino rat resulting in the Wistar rat colony (Lindsey & Baker 2006). This rat strain is one of the most popular laboratory albino rat breeds for use in biological and medical research, and is notably the first rat developed to serve as a model organism at a time when laboratories primarily used the common house mouse (*Mus musculus*). More than half of all laboratory rat strains are descended from this original Wistar rat colony. Recent genetic analysis of 117 albino rat strains collected from all parts of the world carried out by a team led by Takashi Kuramoto at Kyoto University in 2012 showed that the albino rats descended from hooded rats and all the albino rats descended from a single ancestor. In other words, several millions of albino rats used worldwide have descended from a single ancestor. An analysis, using DNA markers, of the genetic relationships or genetic distance between 60 inbred rat strains has been published by Otsen et al. (1995).

More recent studies confirm the general idea that laboratory strains of rats must be considered as a rather narrow selection from the original wild species *Rattus norvegicus* (De Boer et al. 2003). Figure 22.2 shows the frequency distribution of the individual level of aggressive behaviour in a population of Wistar rats and a population of a laboratory-bred wild-type rats (De Boer et al. 2003). Compared to this semi-wild population, even the use of the outbred Wistar strain shows a strong selection bias for docility. In virtually all commercially available laboratory rat strains today, the aggressive behavioural traits, including the putatively underlying molecular genetic components, are dramatically compromised in terms of absolute level and variation. Most likely, this is the result of artificial selection for tame and tractable behaviour during the century-long domestication process of this wild-caught animal, being kept, reared and bred in captivity (de Boer et al. 2003).

Currently, more than 200 inbred strains are available and about 50 outbred or random-bred stocks. A list of available

Table 22.1 Basic biological data of Wistar rats.

Parameter	Normal value
Chromosome number (2n)	42
Lifespan (years)	2–4
Body weight at birth (g)	4.5–6
Body weight at weaning (g)	40–50
Weaning age (days)	21
Puberty (weeks)	6–8
Breeding age (weeks)	12–16
Duration of pregnancy (days)	20–22
Adult body weight (g)	400–800
Total body fat (%)	25–40
Daily food intake (g/100 g BW)	10
Daily water intake (ml/100 g BW)	10–15
Defecation (g/24 h)	9–13
Urine production (ml/24 h)	10–15
Blood volume (ml/kg)	60
Haemoglobin (g/100 ml)	14–20
Haematocrit (vol%)	36–48
Weight of organs (in % BW)	
Adrenal (single)	0.02
Blood	5–7
Brain	1
Heart	0.5
Kidney (single)	0.5
Liver	3
Lung	1
Ovary (single)	0.05
Spleen	0.2
Testis (single)	0.5
Thymus	0.07
Thyroid	0.005

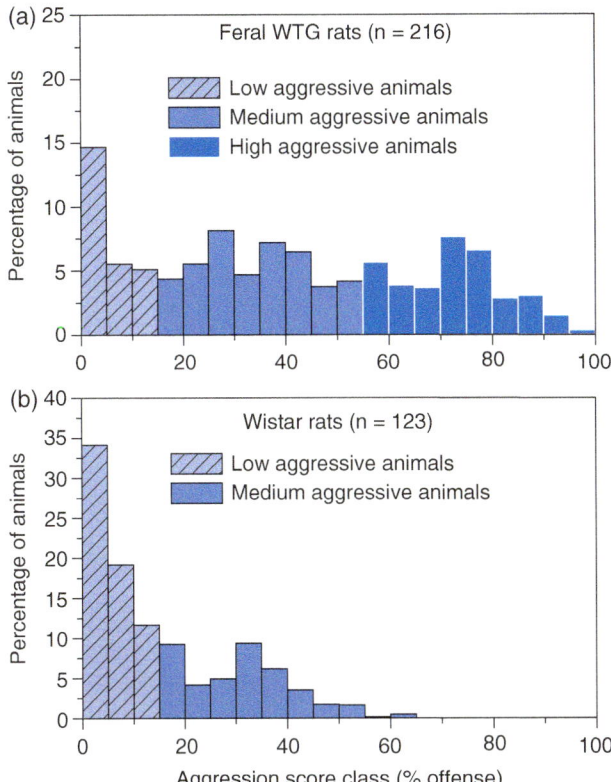

Figure 22.2 Frequency distribution of offensive aggression in a population of unselected feral Wild-Type Groningen rats (a) and in standard Wistar Han laboratory rats (b). Note that the highly aggressive phenotype is mostly absent in the domesticated rat strain.

Examples of frequently used strains:

- Wistar albino. This strain was developed at the Wistar Institute in 1906. The animals are easy to handle, and male aggressive behaviour develops relatively late. Wistar rats are available as inbred (e.g. Wistar Kyoto), outbred (Wistar Han) or random-bred strains and a large number of varieties exist worldwide, and are currently one of the most popular rat strains used for laboratory research.
- Sprague-Dawley albino. This strain originates from R.W. Dawley from Wisconsin in 1925. Originally, female Wistar rats were crossed with males from an unknown origin. The animals are gentle and may grow to a large size. This random- or outbred strain may vary considerably across breeders.
- Long-Evans hooded. This strain was originally developed by Drs Long and Evans at Berkeley, California in 1915 by crossing Wistar females with wild male rats. The head and extremities are black, and the rest of the body is white. It has pigmented eyes, and, although this outbred strain can be easily handled, the level of aggressive behaviour is generally higher than Wistar or SD rats.

Apart from the traditional inbred and outbred strains, a wide variety of genetic selection lines are available. These lines are artificially selected for the presence or absence of certain behavioural or (neuro)physiological characteristics. For example, the Roman High Avoidance (RHA) and the Roman Low Avoidance (RLA) lines are selected for their behavioural performance in an active shock avoidance paradigm, using the Roman Wistar as the parental population. The Kyoto Wistar was used to select the Spontaneous Hypertensive Rat (SHR) line, using high sympathetic reactivity and consequent high blood pressure as a selection criterion. Several of these genetic selection lines are not commercially available, and can only be obtained via the specific research institutes that breed and select these lines.

Genetics and genomics

Recent developments in rat genomics, the availability of genetically defined strains and the recent availability of molecular genetic manipulation tools allow the functions of genes to be established not only by linking clinical phenotypes, physiology and genetics but also by using comparative mapping techniques switching between rat, mouse and human, as well as by targeted suppression/enhancement of gene expression. The analysis of the full rat genome was an important development, a joint project of 13 research institutes coordinated by the American National Institute of Health to produce the Rat Genome Database (RGD)[3] The RGD provides access to a wide variety of curated rat data including disease associations, phenotypes, pathways, molecular functions, biological processes and cellular components for genes, quantitative trait loci and strains, as well as data for comparative genomics between rat, human and mouse. A genome-wide analysis of single nucleotide polymorphisms (SNPs) has also become available for 35 different rat strains including wild rats (Nijman et al. 2008). Finally, the

inbred strains is presented in the International Index of Laboratory Animals (Festing 1993), and a more recent overview can be found at the MGI website[2]. A more extensive description of the origin and stockholders of these strains is given by Hedrich (1990). Provided a constant monitoring of the genetic stability of an inbred strain is carried out, they have the advantage that they remain genetically stable over a long period of time. However, it is important to be aware that the use of inbred strains depends on the nature of the experiments. The main disadvantage of inbred strains is that each of them represents a very narrow selection of the wide and functional genetic variation observed in a wild population. Consequently, one may question the general external validity of the results (Richter et al. 2009). Therefore, if the results of the experiments are to be extrapolated to the human population, as for example in toxicity testing, the use of at least two inbred strains is often preferable.

The disadvantage of outbred stocks is that each breeding colony may be different due to genetic drift. Hence, a Wistar or Sprague-Dawley rat from one breeder may be genotypically and phenotypically different from those obtained from a different source. Considerable differences in neuroanatomy, behaviour and pharmacology have been reported, for example, in Sprague-Dawley rats obtained from different commercial breeders (Rex et al. 2007).

---

[2] http://www.informatics.jax.org/external/festing/rat/STRAINS.shtml (Accessed 5 April 2022).

[3] http://rgd.mcw.edu. (Accessed 5 April 2022).

increased availability of genetic manipulation tools for rats, including N-ethyl-N-nitrosourea (ENU) mutagenesis, zinc-finger nucleases, transcription activator-like effector nucleases (TALENs) homologous recombination and CRISPR/Cas-mediated genome editing are leading to a rapid increase in new genetic rat models. This important development obsoletes the necessity to alter the experimental protocols and designs to fit mice (Ellenbroek & Youn 2016).

Laboratory management and breeding

General husbandry

In the past, laboratory rats have been housed under a wide variety of conditions and in cages of all sorts of materials. Currently, most countries have formal rules and guidelines for accommodation and care of laboratory animals, for example: the European *Directive for the Protection of Animals used for Experimental and Scientific Purposes* (2010/63/EU) (European Directive 2010), The Directive is firmly based on the principle of the Three Rs, to replace, reduce and refine the use of animals used for scientific purposes (see Chapter 2: The Three Rs). For example, these guidelines specify floor area required per animal in relation to weight and number of cage mates, and the minimum cage height. These guidelines have led to a considerable degree of standardisation of housing conditions and putative improvement of welfare. However, it is difficult to scientifically specify the minimum sizes of pens and cages for maintaining laboratory rats as much depends on the strain, group size and age of the animals, their familiarity with each other and their reproductive status. Rats are unusual in that even the adults still play on occasion, so space to play may remain important for this species (Pellis & Pellis 1987). However, increasing the available floor area per animal does not necessarily improve housing conditions, because in some more socially active strains, well-defined dominance relationships with associated aggressiveness may develop. This in turn may lead to a larger variation between individuals and even the development of social stress-related pathologies (Tamashiro *et al.* 2005; de Boer *et al.* 2017).

In view of the importance of play in the development of adult social behaviour and adaptive capacity, it is recommended that animals are provided with sufficient space during the first 3–4 weeks after weaning with a maximum of seven or eight animals on a floor space of about 0.2 m^2 (Yildiz *et al.* 2007). For most strains, this density will be adequate until the animals reach a body weight of around 300 g. As the animals grow older and become larger, the number of animals may be reduced to three per 0.2 m^2 cage. There is general agreement on stocking densities in the various European, American and Australian regulations and codes of practice. When changing to a different housing system or different rat strains, it is generally recommended that all animals are carefully monitored in terms of their behaviour, breeding performance and general health condition.

Most modern cages have their walls and floor made from a variety of thermoplastic materials (e.g. polycarbonate) with a stainless-steel mesh lid. Many cage designs now no longer use a stainless-steel lid and may use plastic feeders and water bottle holders. These cages are available in different sizes and are relatively cheap and easy to clean. Although stainless-steel cages with a wire mesh floor may be easier to clean, the rats have no opportunity for behavioural thermoregulation; consequently, they should only be used when temperature, humidity and ventilation (draught) are well-controlled. Indeed, when given a choice, rats prefer solid floors for resting (Manser *et al.* 1995). Within the ambient temperature range of 20–28 °C no thermoregulatory differences have been observed between animals housed on acrylic floors or metal floors. Below this range, however, animals housed on metal floors show a significant increase in metabolism, whereas above 28 °C animals housed on acrylic floors have problems controlling their body temperature (Gordon & Fogelson 1994). In addition, wire mesh floors may cause serious foot damage (Zochodne *et al.* 1995) and hence are banned as permanent housing system.

Environmental provisions

In general, cages should be provided with adequate bedding material. The main function of bedding is to absorb urine and faeces. However, bedding material seems to be essential for certain biological needs as well. It provides insulation and with some materials the opportunity for nest-building. Therefore, using appropriate bedding material may be an easy way to improve the well-being of laboratory rats. A variety of bedding materials is commercially available, ranging from wood chips, wood shavings and sawdust to absorbent paper. Experiments using preference tests have shown that male rats generally prefer bedding which consists of large fibrous particles (Blom *et al.* 1996). This preference may be due to several factors. Experimental evidence suggests that rats prefer bedding material which they can manipulate. Certain types of bedding material should be avoided if they contain irritating dust, hormonal disrupters or produce high levels of ultrasound in a frequency range for which rats are extremely sensitive when the animal moves (Blom *et al.* 1996). For example, aspen woodchip bedding was shown to be associated with significantly worse respiratory pathology than was compressed paper bedding (Burn *et al.* 2006). Corn cob bedding contains potent oestrogen disrupters and causes health issues (Garner *et al.* 2017).

Certain experimental conditions preclude the use of bedding material, for example in experiments where diet is critical and where the ingestion of bedding could affect the experimental results. In these conditions, it may be necessary to use paper bedding or a wire mesh floor and carefully controlled environmental conditions.

Several studies show that environmental enrichment may be another important provision for the animals. Animals raised from weaning in an environment enriched with objects such as ladders, balls, tubes and boxes are better in several learning tasks, are less defensive, show more exploration, better welfare and have a thicker cerebral cortex and a higher synaptic density than rats raised under standard conditions (Smith & Corrow 2005; Abou-Ismail & Mahboub 2011; Brydges *et al.* 2011; Abou-Ismail & Mendl 2016). There are several enrichments that can be safely recommended, e.g.

shelters, social housing, gnawing items, nesting material and structural complexity (Patterson-Kane 2001).

Social housing

Rats are social animals by nature, and an extensive literature shows that they are very sensitive to social isolation (Hall 1998; Heidbreder *et al.* 2000; Toth *et al.* 2008). Although isolation at any age can have permanent effects on behaviour and physiology, some periods seem to exist throughout which rats are particularly vulnerable to social isolation. In particular, pre-weaning maternal separation and handling affects a wide variety of adult behavioural and neurobiological processes (see Sandi & Haller 2015 for review). Another sensitive period is the one when juveniles spend much time playing, particularly post-natal weeks 5 and 6. Even brief social isolation during these 2 weeks has a significant effect on subsequent adult social behaviour and stress reactivity (Gutman & Nemeroff 2002). In adulthood, long-term social isolation is well-known to induce a number of behavioural disturbances such as increased locomotor activity, learning deficits, anxiety and aggression (Arakawa 2005; Malkesman *et al.* 2006; Sandi & Haller 2015). Some experiments have indicated that isolation at adulthood may induce a state of anxiety or depression which is presumably due to changes in central serotonergic neurotransmission, and which are difficult to restore with resocialisation (Maisonnette *et al.* 1993; Silva *et al.* 2003). Although these data indicate that the social environment has a strong and often lasting impact on behaviour and physiology, the consequences for animal welfare are not always clear and have not been studied very well (Krohn *et al.* 2006). Great care should be taken in standardising the social environment and, wherever possible, rats should be housed in a social group of familiar subjects to ensure their welfare and consequently that they are normal both behaviourally and physiologically. In the author's experience, a reliable standardised method of avoiding the effects of social isolation, without encountering problems with dominance relationships, is to house individual male rats with a hormonally intact female sterilised by ligation of her fallopian ducts.

In the breeding colony, rats are usually housed in all male and all female groups. These groups should be of a standard size and composed of littermates. Mixing litters may affect the social relations between group members and may induce social stress. Mixing groups of adult male rats should be avoided, as it can result in serious dominance fights, and consequently in injury and social stress. Actually, regular mixing of social groups has been used as an experimental procedure to study the adverse health effects of social stress (Mormede 1997; Beery *et al.* 2020).

Feeding/watering

The Norway rat is omnivorous by nature and has a remarkable capacity to adjust its diet and food intake for specific dietary deficiencies (Markison 2001). The rat is widely used to study the mechanisms of food intake and body weight regulation (Schwartz *et al.* 2000). Feeding occurs in a specific daily pattern (Figure 22.3). Most of the food intake takes place during the dark period with a higher incidence of feeding in the

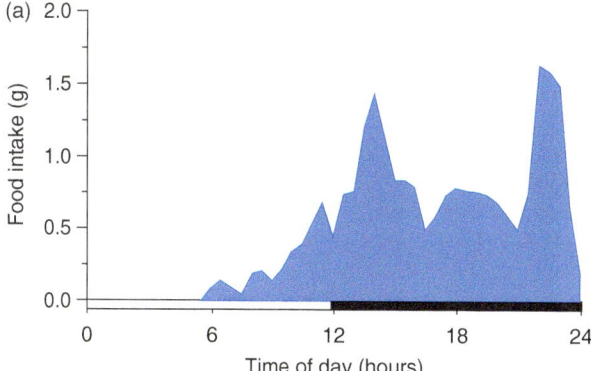

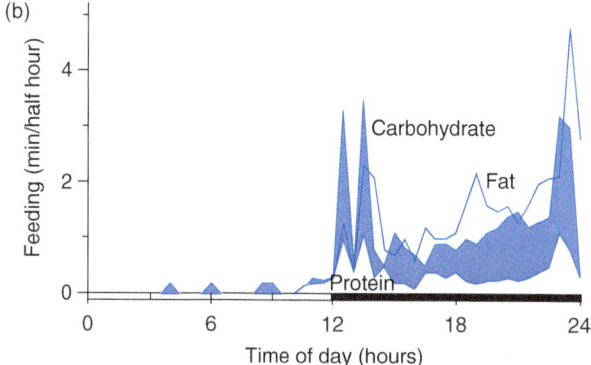

Figure 22.3 Circadian variation in food intake (a) and nutrient preference (b) in male Wistar rats. The black bar indicates the dark period of the light–dark cycle.

first and last 2 h of the dark period (Strubbe & Woods 2004). Rats exhibit a clear preference for certain diets and, in the laboratory, they show preferences for specific nutrients, which vary across the light–dark cycle (Tempel *et al.* 1989; Shor-Posner *et al.* 1994). Figure 22.3 also shows the daily variation in preference for carbohydrate, fat and protein-enriched lab chow. Nutrient balance and in particular amino acid intake are also maintained by coprophagia. Depending on the nutritional balance of their food, rats may eat 10–50% of their own faeces (Fajardo & Hornicke 1989). Moreover, studies show a strong influence of the social environment on food preference, i.e., individual rats rapidly adopt the food preference of their cage mates (Galef 2003). The latter aspect is likely the result of the fact that rats are highly neophobic. In addition, the rat is well-known for its conditioned taste aversion, namely its capacity to associate a certain type of food or taste with sickness (Mediavilla *et al.* 2005).

Within laboratory housing conditions, food is generally presented in food trays forming part of the lid of the cage in order to avoid contact with soiled bedding, and standard procedure is to provide a standard feed *ad libitum*. However, rats prefer varied diets (Galef & Whiskin 2005) and also show contra-freeloading where they are very willing to work for food even though food is freely available (Carder & Berkowitz 1970). Furthermore, a large number of experiments show that health and longevity is increased when food availability and/or caloric intake is restricted (for reviews see Roe *et al.* 1995; Goto *et al.* 2007; Martin *et al.* 2010). In a well-controlled study, Roe *et al.* (1995) found that a restriction of food intake to 80% of the *ad libitum* intake increased the 30 months survival from 42% to 68%. In one study, the average lifespan of rats was increased from 2.4 years for those housed under standard conditions to 4 years for those maintained on a reduced energy diet. Moreover, under such food restriction regimes, the incidence of neoplasms is significantly reduced, in particular in the ageing animal. This suggests that welfare and health may beimproved with a restricted diet if the animal is to be kept into its old age. Providing nesting material and cage mates to help the animal keep warm, and enrichment to give it something to do, are especially important for food restricted rats. Despite these studies, rats are still bred with *ad libitum* food availability. Commercially available diets are generally made from natural ingredients. Although most manufacturers specify the formula of their diets, the exact concentration of dietary components, nutrients and contaminants may vary considerably. This variation may either be due to different brands or to the use of different natural ingredients within the same brand. If such variations are likely to have an adverse or unpredictable effect on the experimental results, it may be necessary to use a chemically defined or purified diet. See also Chapter 13: Nutrition, feeding and animal welfare.

Various behavioural experiments for neurocognitive research, whereby animals must perform activities to obtain an insight into the activity of the functioning brain, are frequently employed. To motivate animals to perform these activities, their food or fluid intake is restricted to such an extent that they become hungry or thirsty. Generally, restriction protocols should be applied that prevent animals from decreasing their body weights below 85–80 % of normal *ad libitum* body weights, and contingencies should be in place to increase feed intake when body weight drops below the set lower acceptable threshold (Toth *et al.* 2011). Water should always be given *ad libitum*. However, in a review, Rowland (2007) argued that 12–24 h of water deprivation falls well within the regulatory range of physiological and behavioural adaptive mechanisms of the rat. Although physiological adaptation cannot be taken as evidence that the welfare of the animals have not been compromised, the behavioural and physiological adjustments to these periods of water deprivation seem to minimise the additional physiological and psychological stress of deprivation. Water is usually given in containers with a stainless-steel nipple. This allows the water intake in individual cages to be monitored and controlled. Several sizes of water bottles for rats are available commercially. In large animal facilities, automatic watering systems may be used. However, these systems must be checked regularly to ensure that the water valves are functioning properly to avoid the possibility of the animals becoming dehydrated or the cage flooding. Automatic watering systems must also be sanitised routinely to avoid biofilm accumulation.

Identification and sexing

Many experimental procedures require individual marking of animals for which several methods can be used. Consideration should be given to using the least invasive method that is compatible with the study. The easiest way is to write a number at the base of the tail with a permanent marker. However, as a result of tail skin growth and renewal, these marks have to be replaced every 2 weeks. Research is needed to identify inks that are permanent and not aversive to the animals, but even though some inks are avoided, rats do habituate to the process. This is also the case with coloured dyes applied to the fur. Tattooing numbers or codes on the tail ears or toes is an invasive and more permanent way of marking. Another method of individual marking is to use an ear notch or ear-punch code, or to use numbered metal ear tags. However, because of the important role of auditory information in the social communication of rats, and because ears can be damaged by fighting and the markings obliterated, these methods are often unsuitable. Rats can also be identified by means of injectable microchips or transponders. These chips are commercially available and sufficiently miniaturised for use in rats at weaning. Each chip is provided with a unique code, and in some systems an additional code for the experiment can be added. The chip can be read without handling the animal using a portable reader provided with a display. Data from the reader can also be downloaded on to a computer. These electronic identification systems are reliable, and further developments are to be expected. For example, some systems include the option to also monitor body temperature or heart rate in association with the individual code of the animal.

The sexes of rat pups can readily be distinguished on the basis of the anogenital distance (Figure 22.4). In males, the distance between the urethra and the anus is greater than in females. Moreover, males can be distinguished by the wrinkled, sparsely haired scrotum at the root of the tail. In a cool environment, the testes may be retracted. The presence of testes in pre-weanling pups cannot be reliably used to aid in sex determination because the testes normally descend into the scrotum at approximately 15 days of age. Observation of mammae can be used to positively identify females, as males do not possess nipples. The vagina of the female is an orifice at some distance caudal to the urethra.

Physical environment and hygiene

Rats are normally housed in well-ventilated rooms in which temperature, light and humidity are controlled. They can be bred and maintained in a wide range of environmental temperatures, provided that a sufficient degree of behavioural thermoregulation such as nest-building is possible (Gordon 1990). Most codes of practice specify a room temperature of 20–24 °C mainly for the purpose of standardising laboratory experiments. Temperature should be measured in the cage because this may deviate strongly from room temperature, depending on the ventilation, the density of animals per cage and the location of the cage with respect to the heating system of the room. When rats are kept in wire mesh cages (although strongly discouraged, see above), the environmental temperature should not drop below 22 °C, and there should be no draughts.

The animal room should be well-ventilated without creating draughts. It is difficult to give a standard recommendation on the number of air changes per hour, as it depends on: the number of animals kept in the room, their size, the

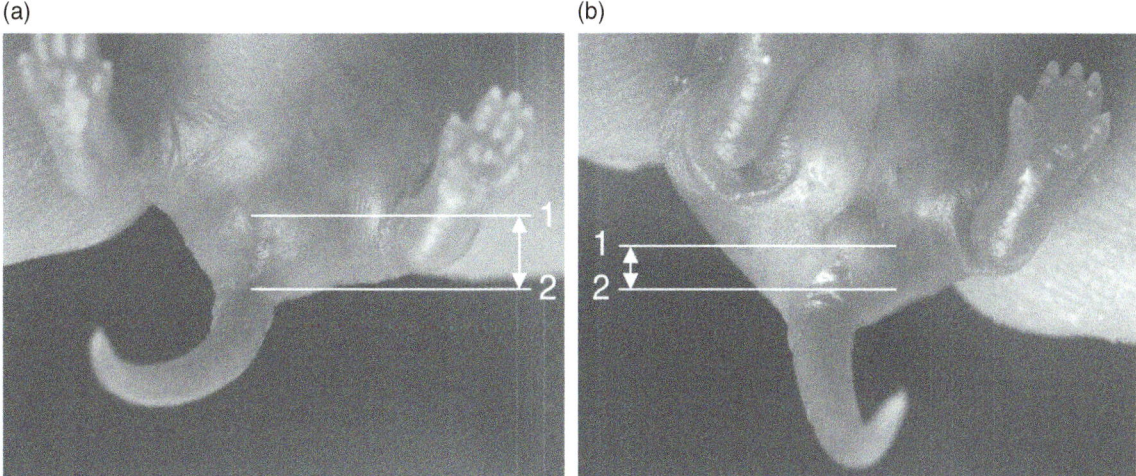

Figure 22.4 Sex differentiation of newborn rats. (a) male, (b) female. Note the longer anogenital distance between urethra (1) and anus (2) in the male.

humidity of the air and the cage cleaning routine. However, a few general guidelines can be provided. The main purpose of ventilation is to provide the animals with air of good quality, as well as personnel working in the room. Apart from the obvious requirements of sufficient oxygen and low levels of carbon dioxide, the concentration of ammonia should be kept as low as possible. Ammonia is a breakdown product of urea and is harmful to the animals because it may facilitate bacterial infections of *Mycoplasma pulmonis* in the mucous membranes of the eyes, nose and the respiratory tract (Schoeb *et al*. 1982). As long as the bedding remains dry, ammonia will not be formed. This, in turn, depends on the number of animals per cage, the humidity, the ventilation and the frequency of cleaning. A smell of ammonia in the animal room, however, is a good indication that the animals are overcrowded or the cages need cleaning. Humidity should be around 50% (range 45–65 %). When it drops below 30%, young animals tend to develop ring tail (Njaa *et al*. 1957). Cages should not be cleaned more often than once a week, because cleaning in itself is a considerable stressor and may disrupt the existing social structure in the cage. Around parturition, it is important not to clean cages (Burn & Mason 2008). However, any increase in ventilation should not result in draught. On average, 8–20 air changes per hour should suffice for a normally populated animal room (Clough 1984).

The use of individually ventilated cages (IVC) is increasingly common. A wide variety of systems is commercially available. Ventilated caging strongly improves the working conditions of animal care staff in terms of exposure to allergens. However, few studies have addressed the question of rat welfare in these housing systems. Depending on the system, ventilation rate may range between 40 and 50 air changes per hour, but 120 air changes per hour can also be found. In a study on the impact of cage ventilation on rats, Krohn *et al*. (2003) concluded that the number of air changes should be kept below 80 changes per hour according to preference tests and telemetric measurements of heart rate and blood pressure. It is not clear why the ventilation rate of IVC systems differ so strongly from the recommended ventilation rate of animal rooms. Most likely, this discrepancy arise from the ventilation rate of small cages being technically easier to increase than that of a whole animal room. Nevertheless, from a biological point of view, the currently used ventilation rates of individual ventilated cages might be considered as a rather artificial laboratory condition, since feral rats live in underground burrow systems with hardly any ventilation of the nesting chambers.

Rats are generally kept in light-controlled rooms with a photoperiod of 12 h light and 12 h dark. Different photoperiods such as 16 h light and 8 h dark are sometimes employed to improve for example breeding results. However, it is important to realise that the photoperiod may strongly affect experimental results (Prendergast *et al*. 2007; Prendergast & Kay 2008; Hawkins & Golledge 2018).

Rats are extremely sensitive to light, in particular albino strains. Retinal damage in albino rats due to light exposure is frequently reported (Perez & Perentes 1994). On the basis of the analysis of retinal damage, it is recommended that the light intensity as measured at the level of the bedding of the cage should not exceed 50 lux (Semple-Rowland & Dawson 1987; Perez & Perentes 1994) and provision of dark shelters is essential. However, when behavioural measures are also considered, such as activity and light avoidance, welfare of the animal seems to be optimised at levels below 25 lux. As a result of their sensitivity to light, rats may differ in the degree of retinal damage depending on the distance between the cage and the light source. A recent study also showed that the age of the rat at the onset of exposure to bright light also impacts degree of retinal damage (Polosa *et al*. 2016).

Health monitoring, quarantine and barrier systems

Infections of laboratory animals can severely influence the outcome of experiments. Therefore, a health monitoring policy is essential to ensure reliability and reproducibility of research data. The Federation of European Laboratory Animal Science Associations (FELASA) advises that breeding units of laboratory rats should be screened every 3–6 months with

Table 22.2 Recommended infectious agents to be monitored and frequencies of monitoring for rats (FELASA 2014).

Viruses	Test frequency
Kilham rat virus	3 months
Rat minute virus	3 months
Rat parvovirus	3 months
Toolan's H-1 virus	3 months
Pneumonia virus of mice	3 months
Rat coronavirus/Sialodacryoadenitis virus	3 months
Rat theilovirus	3 months
Sendai virus	Annually
Hantaviruses	Annually
Mouse adenovirus type 1 (FL)	Annually
Mouse adenovirus type 2 (K87)	Annually
Reovirus type 3	Annually
Bacteria and fungi	
Pneumocystis spp.	Annually
Clostridium piliforme	3 months
Cilia-associated respiratory bacillus	Annually
Mycoplasma pulmonis	3 months
Pasteurella pneumoniae	3 months
Salmonella spp.	Annually
Streptobacillus moniliformis	Annually
Streptococci β-haemolytic	3 months
Streptococcus pneumoniae	3 months
Helicobacter spp.	3 months
Parasites	
Endo- and ectoparasites	3 months

respect to serology, bacteriology, parasitology and pathology with a sample size that depends on population size in the room (FELASA 2014). Table 22.2 summarises the recommended viral, bacterial and parasitic infections to be monitored. It is recommended that positive serological results should be confirmed using another method or a repeated investigation. Bacterial and fungal infections should be investigated in samples from nasal turbinates/nasopharynx, trachea, prepuce/vagina and caecum. In addition, serum samples should be tested for *mycoplasmas* and *Leptospira* spp. Parasitology should be based on a microscopic examination of the skin, and of fresh wet samples of the caecalcontents, the inner lining of the ileum and of faecal flotation.

Depending on the requirements of the experiments, rats can be housed under different regimes with respect to microbiological control. In many experiments, it is sufficient to keep the animals under conventional clean conditions. This means that there are no special barrier systems, banning of specific pathogens, and that the microbiological status of the animals is not guaranteed. However, with regular health monitoring and some precautions with respect to cleaning regime, quarantine and traffic of animal care staff, healthy and highly standardised animals can usually be obtained.

Other experiments require a stricter microbial status. To guarantee the microbiological status of the animals, a strict barrier system is required. These systems usually consist of physical barriers, combined with strict rules regarding disinfection of cages, utensils and personnel. A microbiologically defined breeding colony is started with animals obtained by caesarean section and fostered with microbiologically defined or germ-free mothers kept in isolators, according to standard procedures.

In some highly controlled experiments, it is necessary to keep rats in germ-free conditions. Special isolators are required to prevent contamination. These animals are, however, highly abnormal because they lack the natural micro-organisms involved in essential processes such as digestion and heat production. Accumulating recent evidence suggests that symbiotic micro-organisms, specifically the microbiota that reside within the gastrointestinal system, may influence neurodevelopment and programming of behaviour and physiology across diverse animal species, including rats. This holobiont-level hypothesis is substantiated by evidence documenting how changes in gut microbiota composition can affect behaviour and physiology in laboratory animals and in some cases wild animals (see for review: Sherwin *et al*. 2019).

Transport

Long-distance transportation of rats should be avoided wherever possible because of the long-lasting effects of stress on behaviour and physiology (Koolhaas *et al*. 1997). When rats are obtained from a commercial breeder, they should be allowed a recovery period of at least 1 week, but preferably 2–3 weeks. Although the animals can be transported in cages used for standard laboratory housing, special disposable transport cages are available as well. When the rats are shipped by air, the transport cage should meet the criteria of the International Air Transport Association *Dangerous Goods Regulations Manual* (IATA 2010). Although it is unlikely that animals will drink or eat, owing to the stress involved in transportation, if the journey is expected to last longer than 24 h, they must be provided with food and water. For a general discussion of transport issues, see Chapter 12: Transportation of laboratory animals.

Breeding

Adults

Rats are sexually mature at around 2 months of age. The rat's oestrous cycle averages four to six days in length, occurs throughout the year without seasonal influence in laboratory colonies and occurs from the pubertal onset until senescence, including during the postpartum period (Kohn & Clifford 2002). The fertile state of the female is most easily recognised by her behaviour in the presence of a male rat. Females in oestrus perform a highly characteristic soliciting behaviour, consisting of hopping and ear-wiggling and presenting the anogenital region to the male (Erskine 1989). When the male attempts to mount her, a receptive female adopts the lordosis position. For a detailed description of male and female rat sexual behaviour, see (Heijkoop *et al*. 2018). Experienced animal care staff can induce lordosis in the female rat by gently palpating her flanks. A more elaborate way of determining the fertility state of the female is by monitoring the oestrous cycle by means of daily vaginal smears. These smears are taken by flushing the vagina with a drop of saline using a small drip

Table 22.3 Reproductive parameters.

Female	Normal value
Mammary glands	6 pairs
Vaginal opening (day)	28–60
First oestrus (day)	40–65
Oestrous cycle	Polyoestrus
Length of oestrous cycle (days)	4–6
Stage 1 dioestrus	6 h
Stage 2 pro-oestrus (early)	60 h
Stage 3 pro-oestrus (late)	12 h
Stage 4 oestrus	12 h
Stage 5 metoestrus	21 h
Age at first mating (day)	50–100
Gestation period	21–23
Size of litter	3–18

Male	Normal value
Descent of testes (day)	15–50
Age at sexual maturity (day)	40–50
Age at aggressive maturity (day)	90–120
Age at end of mating (months)	9–24
Minimum number of intromissions	3–10
Length of ejaculation (s)	10–20

pipette, or by taking a sample with a small flexible spatula. The sample is subsequently put on a glass slide, dried and stained with cresyl violet. The phase of the oestrous cycle can be determined under the microscope on the basis of the presence and quantity of cornified epithelial cells and leucocytes. Table 22.3 summarises some of the basic data on reproduction in the rat.

The male will frequently mount an oestrous female and, after several intromissions, an ejaculation occurs. This sequence of events may be repeated two or three times with a post-ejaculatory interval of 5–10 minutes. After a while, the female ceases courtship behaviour and defends herself from the male. Simultaneously, the vaginal fluid and the ejaculate coagulate and form a plug. The presence of such a plug is often used as evidence of mating. If the time of conception has to be determined accurately, the behaviour of the male and female can be observed directly or recorded for subsequent viewing. When this is not possible, a series of vaginal smears can be taken and monitored for the presence of sperm.

Sperm cells can be detected microscopically in the vaginal smear up to 12 h after conception. It is difficult to detect pregnancy before the 15th day post conception. After day 15, foetuses can be detected by palpation, body weight rapidly increases, the female starts to perform nest-building behaviour and maternal aggression towards males gradually develops.

On the day of delivery, the pregnant rat becomes restless, and nest-building behaviour reaches its maximum. Pups are delivered at intervals of 5–10 minutes, usually during the last hours of the dark period and the beginning of the light phase. After delivery of a pup, the mother bites the umbilical cord, eats the placenta and cleans the neonate. A weak or stillborn neonate will usually be eaten immediately, but the occurrence of this can be difficult to determine unless the birth is continuously monitored.

The young

A healthy rat neonate begins to suckle within the first few hours after birth. Disturbance of the delivery process should be avoided, because this may lead to infanticide by the mother. From the second day onwards, a beige spot shining through the abdominal wall of the pup indicates the amount of milk it has consumed. Normally, mothers nurse their pups for about 1 h, after which she leaves the nest for several hours to rest and eat. The mother keeps the pups together in the nest, and when one escapes from the nest, she rapidly retrieves it. Pup retrieval is facilitated by ultrasonic vocalisations emitted by pups which have become separated from their mother and littermates (see Stern and Lonstein (2001) for a review on maternal behaviour). A healthy neonate has a pink colour and a well-filled abdomen. Pups with a dark pink, violet or cyanotic, often wrinkled skin are indicative of a mother with insufficient milk supply. A somewhat disturbed nest and the absence of pup retrieval is indicative of a mother who is not nursing her pups properly.

Pups are extremely sensitive to rearing conditions. A large amount of literature shows that the adult behavioural, neurobiological, immunological and neuroendocrine reactivity (Tang et al. 2006) is affected by quality of nursing, neonatal handling, maternal separation, environmental enrichment and social isolation. Increasing evidence shows that these effects are mediated by epigenetic processes like DNA methylation resulting in permanent blockade of the expression of specific genes (Meaney & Szyf 2005; Szyf et al. 2008). Furthermore, several studies have demonstrated that acquired epigenetic modifications can be inherited and cause trans-generational behaviour and physiological changes, i.e., epigenetic inheritance (Skinner et al. 2010). In view of these lasting influences of early-life rearing conditions, it is recommended that neonates are raised with as little disturbance as possible, and that the cleaning regime, number of pups and sex ratio per nest are standardised. Cages should not be cleaned in the 3 days before and after birth, to avoid infanticide (Burn & Mason 2008). Any manipulation of the litter, such as reducing size or mixing with others, should be done on the first day after birth and ideally nesting material should be transferred with pups.

At birth, the pups are hairless, toothless and blind. The newborn is essentially poikilothermic and rely upon the maternally maintained microenvironment and huddling of the litter to achieve thermal homeostasis. Within 2 weeks, thermoregulation matures, the fur coat develops and the eyes open. By day 9, the incisor teeth are sufficiently developed to gnaw and by day 11 the first solid food is usually eaten.

The young are generally weaned at the age of 21 days, and subsequently housed in groups of the same sex. The period immediately after weaning till the age of about 60 days is characterised by intense play fighting, in both sexes but seen more in male rats (Kisko et al. 2021). This is essential for the development of normal adult social behaviour (Pellis & Pellis 1998).

Breeding systems

Several systems can be used for breeding rats depending on whether inbred or outbred strains are used. The main purpose of any breeding system is to maintain a standard genetic quality of animals over generations. Inbreeding requires the crossing of closely related animals, usually brother × sister mating. To maintain adequate control over the genetic quality of the foundation stock, monogamous mating is recommended. In random-bred colonies, inbreeding is inevitable, but the degree of inbreeding depends on the breeding system used. When a monogamous mating system is used, the inbreeding coefficient, which represents the loss of genetic variation in the colony (ΔF) will be $1/(2N)$, where N is the total number of breeding animals. This means that the smaller the breeding colony, the greater will be the degree of inbreeding. Polygamous mating can be used for the expansion or production stock. However, using one male with several females for foundation stock, increases not only the risk of inbreeding, but also the likelihood of uncontrolled selection, and selection based on breeding performance. It is, therefore, better to use a monogamous rotation mating scheme. Rotation schemes are designed to reduce the degree of inbreeding by 50%. If a random-bred colony is maintained as a closed colony for at least four generations, and the number of breeding animals is sufficiently large for a $\Delta F <1\%$, the colony may be designated as an outbred stock (Willis & Dalton 1998; Zimmermann *et al.* 2000).

Random-bred and outbred strains have a certain degree of genetic heterogeneity. In some experiments, this heterogeneity may be desirable, for example when results should have some degree of general validity in a population. It has the advantage that the results are based upon a broad spectrum of genotypes. In other experiments, genetically homogeneous inbred strains are required. This has the advantage that the individual variation is reduced and hence the number of animals required per experiment. However, it is important to realise that the results may only be valid for the particular genotype in question. To minimise this problem, F1 hybrids of two inbred strains can be used; they are still genetically homogeneous, but share the genetic characteristics of two different genotypes. See also Chapter 3: The design of animal experiments.

Laboratory procedures

Handling and training

Rats can usually be handled easily without the use of steel-reinforced gloves. Rats recognise humans as individuals, so it is always best if they are handled by a familiar person, usually the animal care staff or experimenter. Before handling a rat, it is important to ensure that the animal is awake and alert. Rats should be trained to be handled, first by touching them without picking them up. Stroking the back and neck region of the animals will comfort them, and after a few minutes, the animal is usually willing to be picked up with the hand around its body (Figure 22.5). The rat should immediately be put on the arm of the handler, while gently holding the tail (Figure 22.6), and comforted by stroking. After being accustomed to being handled, rats can be lifted short distances, e.g. between adjacent cages, without needing to rest on the arm of the handler.

Rats like being petted and most rats like being tickled, during which they emit ultrasonic 50 kHz vocalisations as a sign of positive affect (Panksepp 2007; LaFollette 2017). If rats are

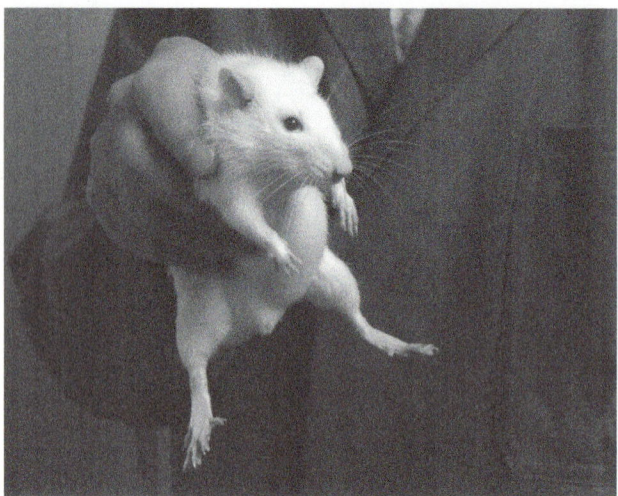

Figure 22.5 Holding a friendly rat or one accustomed to handling. Note that in case institutional regulations require the use of gloves to prevent allergic reactions, these can be employed accordingly.

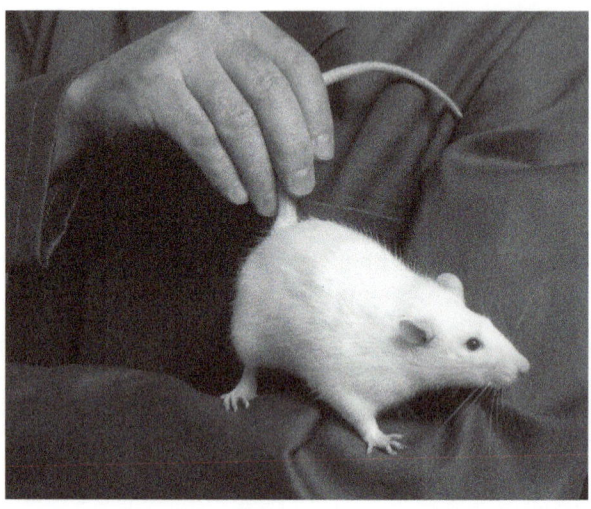

Figure 22.6 Method of holding a rat which has not been handled previously, placing a rat by its tail-base on handlers arm to provide support. Note that in case institutional regulations require the use of gloves to prevent allergic reactions, these can be employed accordingly.

routinely gently handled and petted, they are much less likely to be stressed by routine experimental procedures such as injections. A good relationship with a handler makes an important contribution to the welfare of these animals. Force should not be necessary and avoided as much as possible, because it will result in stress to the rat and likely elicit defensive responses like biting. However, some strains of rats may be more aggressive or nervous and relatively difficult to handle, and these rats require more training to enable handling them without inducing stress. If a rat has to be restrained, the best way of doing so is presented in Figure 22.7. The animal should be approached from the back, with one hand grasping the base of the tail and the other hand should be laid on the back of the animal. The thumb and forefinger should form a circle around the neck of the animal, with one

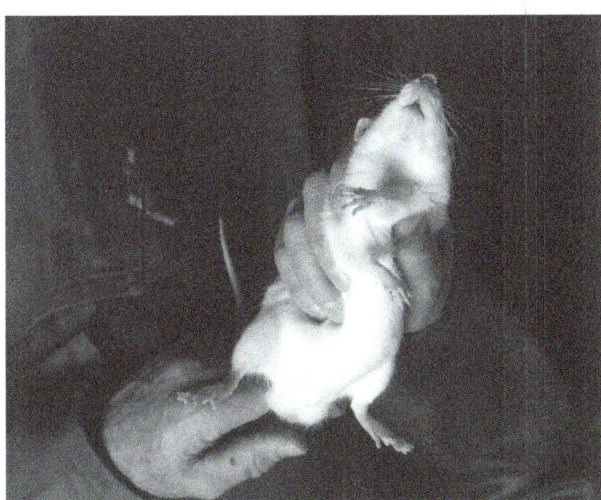

Figure 22.7 Restraining a rat. Note that in case institutional regulations require the use of gloves to prevent allergic reactions, these can be employed accordingly.

forepaw included in the ring. The other forepaw can be fixed between the forefinger and the middle finger. This type of handling should be the exception, as in general, rats are very easily trained to co-operate. It is recommended, therefore, to habituate the animals to the handling procedure several days before the animal will be used for experimentation. It is well-known that rats are very trainable and positive reinforcement should be much more widely used for training rats housed in labs (Eriksson 2019 and see also Chapter 15: The use of positive reinforcement training techniques to enhance the care and welfare of laboratory and research animals).

Physiological monitoring

A wide variety of techniques is available to monitor physiological processes in rats. A summary of the most common experimental and surgical techniques is presented by Waynforth and Flecknell (1992), whereas a more advanced manual of microsurgical techniques is presented by Dongen et al. (1990). However, many of these techniques are too complex to be suitable as a standard daily laboratory procedure. Because stress from handling significantly affects their physiology, data should be obtained from undisturbed animals. Body temperature, for example, is often recorded using a thermistor inserted into the rectum to a depth of 3–5 cm. However, handling is unavoidable for this procedure; so, in fact it measures stress-induced hyperthermia (Olivier et al. 2003). Recent developments in chip technology using implanted transponders combine the identification of the individual with a body temperature measurement in the freely moving animal. More detailed and permanent recordings of body temperature can be obtained using permanently implanted radio transmitters or data loggers. Transmitter systems are also suitable for monitoring heart rate, blood pressure, respiratory rate, electroencephalograms (EEG) and electrocardiograms (ECG) in freely moving animals.

Blood samples can be collected in several ways. A decision tree for the choice of the best method can be found on the website of the National Centre for the Replacement, Refinement and Reduction of Animals in Research[4]. Microsampling using a capillary tube without restraint has recently been promoted (Jonsson et al. 2019). However, for the assay of stress-sensitive and rapidly changing substances in the blood, a permanently implanted jugular vein canula is generally recommended (Waynforth & Flecknell 1992). This technique allows repeated sampling over a period of several weeks. Another method of sampling to obtain reliable baseline values of stress-sensitive substances is to collect trunk blood from rapidly decapitated animals. This method, of course, has the disadvantages that it is fatal for the animal and does not allow repeated measures from the same individual. Moreover, great care should be taken that the whole procedure from catching, handling and decapitation of one animal does not affect stress levels in the subsequently sampled animals (Zethof et al. 1995). There are also potential welfare consequences of decapitation unless done under anaesthesia – see Chapter 17: Euthanasia and other fates for laboratory animals. For the assay of less reactive substances, blood may be collected with a syringe from the tail vein. When a large volume of blood is required, a cardiac puncture can be used with the animal under deep anaesthesia, usually only permitted by ethical review committees as a terminal procedure.

Urine and faeces can be collected by housing the animals in commercially available metabolism cages. Alternatively, as wire-floor cages are strongly discouraged, hydrophobic sand may be employed (Hoffman et al. 2018). Faeces can be used to measure baseline concentrations of steroid hormones (Lepschy et al. 2007).

Administration of compounds

Most of the commonly used techniques to administer substances to rats are extensively described in Waynforth and Flecknell (1992) and by the Joint Working Group on Refinement (2001). As most of these procedures are stressful to the animal and, therefore, may interfere with the experiment, the least stressful methods will be indicated here. Although not yet frequently applied, there are several effective oral drug delivery methods that employ voluntary oral consumption of palatable vehicles like sucrose or chocolate (Huang-Brown & Guhad 2002; Atcha et al. 2010; Fitchett et al. 2012).

Intravenous (iv) injections can be given via the sublingual vein or the lateral vein at the root of the tail in an anesthetised rat (needle size: 0.5–0.6 mm (25–23 G)). When frequent iv injections are required or the injection is to be combined with subsequent blood sampling, the implantation of a permanent jugular vein catheter is recommended. This method allows a relatively stress-free iv injection to be given to freely moving animals.

Intraperitoneal (ip) injections are given in the lower left quadrant of the abdomen, to avoid damage to vital organs such as liver, stomach and spleen (needle size: maximum 0.9 mm (20 G)). It is not usually necessary to restrain the animal so that an animal which is used to handling can be given an ip injection as depicted in Figure 22.8. More nervous, defensive animals will need to be held more firmly, including their hindquarters, and a second person may be needed to give the injection.

Subcutaneous (sc) injections can be given by placing the animal on top of the cage or on a table and raising a fold of the skin of the neck (needle size: 0.5–0.6 mm (25–23 G)). The needle

---

[4] https://www.nc3rs.org.uk/rat-decision-tree-blood-sampling/. (Accessed 12 April 2022.)

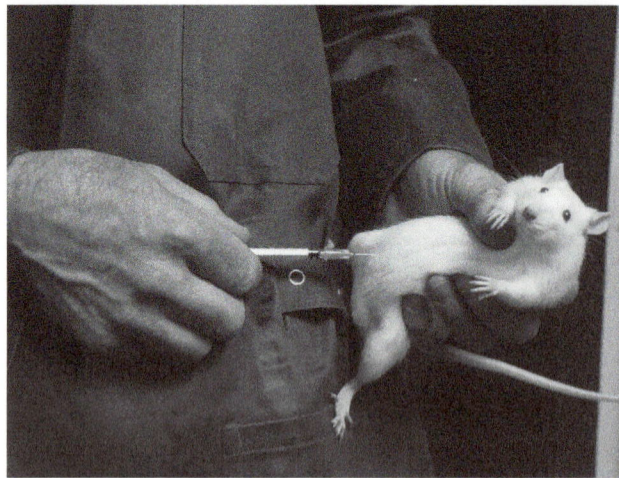

Figure 22.8 Giving an intraperitoneal injection to a well-handled rat. Note that in case institutional regulations require the use of gloves to prevent allergic reactions, these can be employed accordingly.

should be slid into the fold with its tip parallel to the body surface. When a more chronic administration of substances is required, it may be better to use osmotic mini pumps, the implantation of pellets or silicon capsules, in preference to a frequent injection schedule. Osmotic mini pumps are commercially available in a broad range of volumes and infusion rates.

Intragastric administration of fluids can be performed by gavage of the oesophagus using a curved needle with a small bulb at the tip. Different sized rats need different sizes of gavage needle (Waynforth & Flecknell 1992). For per oral administration, the rat is held firmly by the skin of the neck and the back so that the head is kept immobile and in line with the back. Great care should be taken that the injection fluid does not enter the trachea. When frequent intragastric administrations are required, a permanent intragastric catheter may be surgically implanted. However, voluntary ingestion of substances as described above should be promoted as a very useful refinement of oral administration of drugs.

Intranasal drug administration is one of the promising options to bypass blood-brain barrier, to reduce the systemic

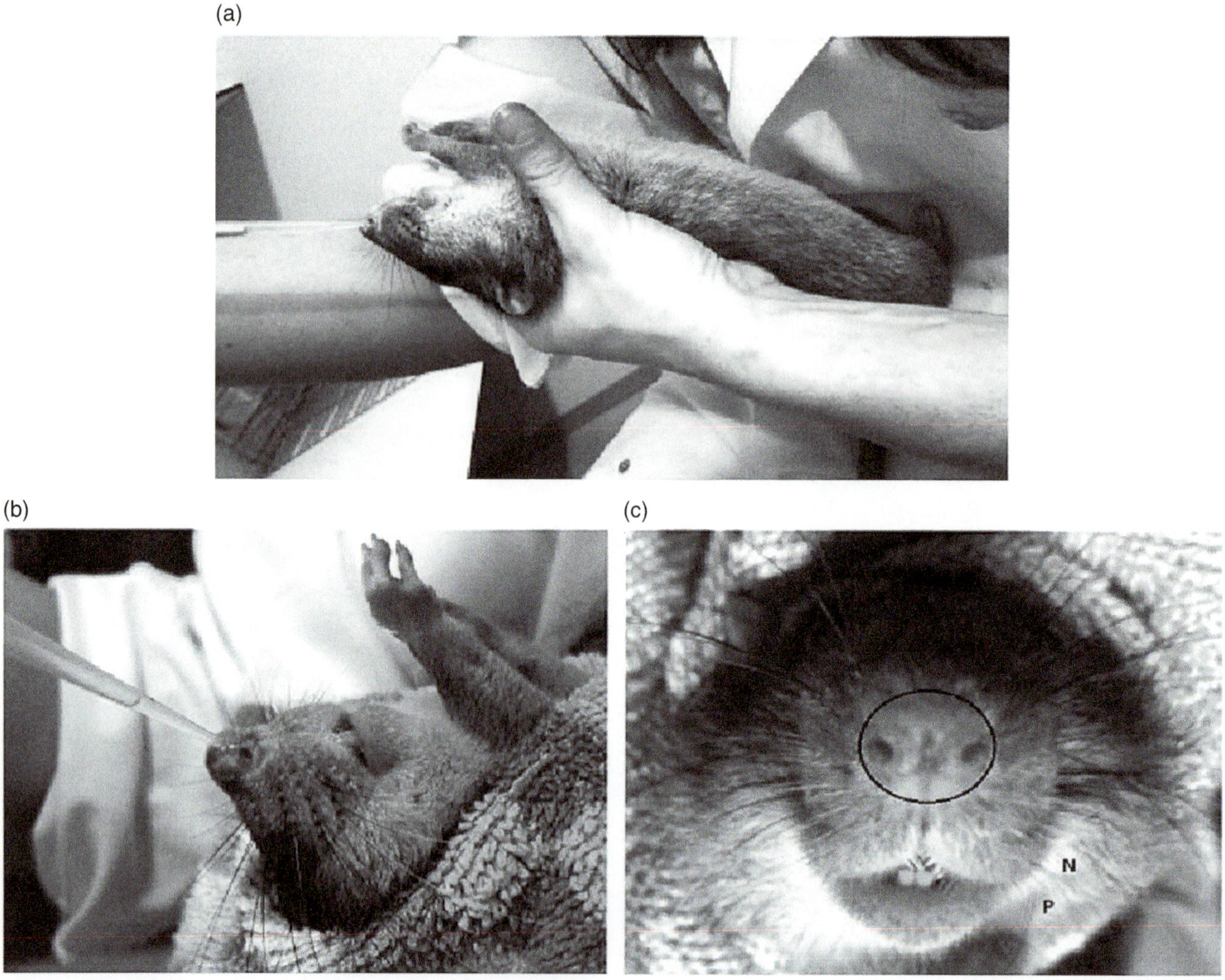

Figure 22.9 Holding of a conscious well-handled rat during nasal administration (a) while applying the solution intranasally (b) and magnification of the nose region (c). Note that in case institutional regulations require the use of gloves to prevent allergic reactions, these can be employed accordingly.

adverse effects of the drugs and to lower the doses to be administered. Figure 22.9 demonstrates this rather easy and convenient route of drug administration in rats (Calcagnoli et al. 2015). It is important to habituate the animals to the holding position, as well as training them to the intranasal procedure to minimise stress responses. A rat is held in a supine position with a horizontal head position. Drug solutions (maximal 10 µl per rhinarium) are applied using a pipette and equally distributed in the squamous epithelium of both the left and right rhinarium (see Figure 22.9). Direct contact of the pipette with the rhinarium, or direct application into one of the nostrils or in proximity of the philtrum, should be avoided to limit the drainage of the liquid into the oesophagus and trachea.

Anaesthesia and analgesia

General anaesthesia can be induced either by inhalation or by injection of anaesthetics by intraperitoneal, intramuscular or intravenous route. There are excellent standard works available with all the detailed information on anaesthesia and pain management (Flecknell & Waterman-Pearson 2000; Fish et al. 2011). Reference to these books is strongly recommended. Table 22.4 summarises the inhalation and injection anaesthetics recommended for use in rats.

Inhalational anaesthetics are generally preferable because they have the advantage of easy adjustment of the depth of anaesthesia and rapid recovery. Induction of anaesthesia with volatile anaesthetics can be achieved using an induction chamber connected to a vaporiser. After induction of anaesthesia, gas can be delivered through a face mask or via an endotracheal tube; a calibrated vaporiser should be used. The volatile anaesthetic is mixed with air, 100% oxygen or a mixture of N_2O and O_2 (1:1). If using nitrous oxide in the delivery gas mixture, a lesser amount of volatile anaesthetic should be needed.

Several types of injectable anaesthetics are suitable for rats. The selection of these anaesthetics depends on a variety of factors such as: the duration of the surgery; the preferred degree of muscle relaxation and the appropriate level of analgesia. In rats, the anaesthetic is generally given as a single intraperitoneal injection. Only very small volumes can be administered intramuscularly and ketamine in particular can cause pain upon injection and subsequent muscle damage. However, it is important to appreciate that the response to these injectable anaesthetics may vary strongly between individual animals and between sexes and strains. Therefore, when using a new anaesthesia regimen for the first time, the dosage required should be carefully assessed and tested in a few animals initially.

It is sometimes useful to reduce possible side effects of the anaesthetic compound by administering certain drugs as premedication. Sedatives or tranquillisers can be used to reduce the stress associated with the induction of anaesthesia, reduce the dose of primary anaesthetic needed and to promote a smooth recovery. However, most of these compounds have little or no analgesic properties and cannot be used to reduce post-operative pain. Anticholinergic agents may be used to reduce the production of saliva and to reduce undesirable autonomic responses.

During surgery, the depth of the anaesthesia should be monitored frequently. This can be assessed easily by checking some reflexes of the animal. A correctly anaesthetised rat shows a regular deep respiration and an absence of the righting reflex when being placed on its back. Pinching the tail with the fingernails does not induce a flick of the tail or vocalisations and a puff of air on the eyes does not induce an eye blink reflex. In view of the sensitivity of the rat's eyes for bright light, they should be protected from the surgical light. Eyes should be protected with a lubricating ophthalmic ointment during any anaesthetic episode lasting more than five minutes, to help prevent corneal drying and opacification., and a drop of saline in the eye will prevent the eye from dehydration during long surgical procedures.

Many anaesthetics interfere with the thermoregulation of the animal. Therefore, body temperature should be carefully monitored during anaesthesia. An electric blanket or other warming device controlled by a thermostat and integrated with a rectal temperature probe should be used.

Generally, rats recover rapidly from major surgery. However, a post-operative recovery period of at least 1 week is recommended. Moreover, pain should be relieved using analgesic treatment and should be administered pre-emptively and at appropriate dosing intervals throughout to avoid break-through pain. The most common analgesics for rats are summarised in Table 22.5 (Bertens et al. 1993; Flecknell &

Table 22.4 Inhalation and injection anaesthetics recommended for use in rats.

Drug and indication	Dose and route of administration
Premedication (anticholinergics)	
Atropine	0.05 mg/kg sc, ip
Premedication (sedatives)	
Diazepam	2.5 mg/kg ip
Acepromazine	2.5 mg/kg sc, ip
Hypnorm (fentanyl/fluanisone)	0.3–0.6 ml/kg ip
Xylazine	1–3 mg/kg sc, ip
Dexmedetomidine	0.02–0.05 mg/kg sc, ip
Medetomidine	0.05–0.1 mg/kg sc
Anaesthesia (short duration, 5–10 minutes)	
Alphaxalone (Alfaxan)[1]	10–12 mg/kg iv
Propofol	10 mg/kg iv
Methohexital	7–10 mg/kg iv
Anaesthesia (injection agents, medium duration, 20–60 minutes)	
Hypnorm/ midazolam	2 ml/kg ip (1 part Hypnorm, 1 part midazolam and 2 parts sterile water for injection)
Ketamine/ xylazine	75–90 mg/kg ip 10 mg/kg ip
Ketamine/ medetomidine	75 mg/kg ip 0.5 mg/kg ip
Ketamine/ dexmedetomidine	75 mg/kg ip 0.25 mg/kg ip
Pentobarbital	40–55 mg/kg ip
Anaesthesia (inhalation agents, short/medium/long duration)	
Isoflurane	Induction concentration 4–5% Maintenance concentration 1–2%
Sevoflurane	Induction concentration 4% Maintenance

[1] Not a recommended anaesthetic and should only be used when scientifically justified.

Table 22.5 Alphabetical list of analgesics and local anaesthetics for post-operative pain relief.

Drug	Dose
Aspirin[1]	100 mg/kg per os, 4 hourly
Bupivacaine	0.1–0.2 ml 0.25% infiltrated sc into incisional area
Buprenorphine	0.01–0.05 mg/kg sc 6–8 hourly
Butorphanol[2]	2 mg/kg sc, 4 hourly
Carprofen	5 mg/kg sc, 12–24 hourly
Codeine[2]	60 mg/kg sc, 4 hourly
Flunixin	2.5 mg/kg sc, im, 12 hourly
Ketoprofen	5 mg/kg sc, 24 hourly
Meloxicam	1–3 mg/kg sc, q 12–24 hourly
Morphine[2]	2.5 mg/kg sc, 2–4 hourly
Nalbuphine[2]	1–2 mg/kg im, 3 hourly
Paracetamol[2]	100–300 mg/kg per os, 4 hourly
Pentazocine[2]	10 mg/kg sc, 4 hourly
Phenacitin[2]	100 mg/kg per os, 4 hourly
Pethidine[2]	10–20 mg/kg sc or im, 2–3 hourly

[1] Weak analgesic; only effective for very minor procedures and requires frequent dosing.
[2] Not recommended due to frequency of administration needed.

Waterman-Pearson 2000). In some countries, sustained-release formulations of analgesics are commercially available and should be considered.

Analgesics administered systemically may have side effects which interfere with the experiment. In these situations, the use of long-acting local anaesthetics to infiltrate the surgical area such as 0.25% bupivacaine should be considered. Local analgesic ointment to treat surgical wounds topically may also be beneficial, and will sometimes prevent the animal from biting surgical wounds and stitches if applied repeatedly. Recovery is improved after a few days when group housing can be re-established.

Euthanasia

The Animal Welfare Act (AWA) and Animal Welfare Regulations (AWR)[5] define euthanasia as the humane destruction of an animal accomplished by a method that produces rapid unconsciousness and subsequent death without evidence of pain or distress, or a method that utilises anaesthesia produced by an agent that causes painless loss of consciousness. The most appropriate way of euthanising rats is, to some degree, determined by the type of experiment involved. The most common way of killing the animal is using a rising concentration of carbon dioxide and oxygen (6:4). After the animal has lost consciousness, the concentration of carbon dioxide is raised to 100% and kept at this level for at least 10 minutes. Although this method is widely used throughout the world, there is a significant debate on the stressful nature of this technique (Conlee et al. 2005; Hawkins et al. 2016; Boivin et al. 2017). CO_2 should be administered to chambers containing animals to be euthanised at a displacement rate of 10%–30% chamber volume per minute (AVMA Panel on Euthanasia 2013). It has been determined that this rate allows for rapid euthanasia of animals. Animals are usually left in the chamber until visible movement has ceased. Because CO_2 is heavier than atmospheric air, it is important to purge the chamber of remaining CO_2 between groups so that it does not build up to levels that would cause pain and distress to the animals. Because immature animals tolerate low oxygen levels better than adults, they require extended exposure time to CO_2 for death to result (Klaunberg et al. 2004). The immediate use of 100% carbon dioxide is not permitted by the EU directive 2010/63/EU and most other guidelines, like the American Veterinary Medical Association's (AVMA), because it induces severe dyspnoea and signs of stress. Alternative methods include pre-euthanasia anaesthesia and the use of argon rather than carbon dioxide (Valentim et al. 2016). Carbon dioxide should not be used as the sole method to kill neonatal rats because they are relatively resistant to hypoxemia. When specimens have to be obtained, administering a lethal dose of anaesthetic is usually an appropriate method. Although many anaesthetics could be used to induce death by overdose, some of the most common injection agents are sodium pentobarbital, phenytoin and potassium chloride (see Sivula & Suckow 2018 for more detailed info). In all cases, it is recommended that a method to confirm death is used such as: (a) confirmation of permanent cessation of the circulation; (b) destruction of the brain; (c) dislocation of the neck; (d) exsanguination or (e) confirmation of the onset of rigor mortis (stiffening of muscles). Physical methods of euthanasia may be necessary when use of anaesthetic agents could interfere with the experimental results. Methods include concussion of the brain, cervical dislocation and decapitation (using a special guillotine or sharp scissors); these are only permitted for rodents under 1 kg and rodents over 150 g shall be sedated. The choice of method will depend on the size of the animal and local regulations. See also Chapter 17: Euthanasia and other fates for laboratory animals.

Common welfare problems

The most common welfare problems in rats relate to disease, and behavioural and reproductive problems. These are detailed below. A guide to defining and implementing protocols for the welfare assessment of laboratory animals, including rats, was published by Hawkins et al. (2011).

Disease

Rats can be kept free of disease relatively easily under conventional husbandry conditions, provided that these conditions meet certain criteria. For example, it is essential to avoid overcrowding not only in the breeding cages, but also in the animal room. Moreover, proper ventilation, humidity control, a cleaning regime using dust-free bedding material and the use of filter caps are the best prophylactic precautions that can be taken. Strict attention to the macro-environment including pest control and stringent sanitation practices, and effective sanitation of cage components are essential components to maintaining a rodent pathogen-free facility. Reports in the literature suggest that a restricted feeding regime can reduce the incidence of neoplasm in

[5] https://www.aphis.usda.gov/animal_welfare/downloads/AC_BlueBook_AWA_508_comp_version.pdf. (Accessed 25 August 2022.)

ageing rats (Roe et al. 1995). Compared to those that are fed less, exercise more, and have a stimulating environment, animals maintained under the usual standard laboratory conditions are relatively overweight, insulin resistant, hypertensive and are likely to experience premature death (Martin et al. 2010). Reducing daily food intake 20–40% below the *ad libitum*, or providing food intermittently rather than continuously, has been shown to significantly reduce the risk of developing diseases such as cancer, type 2 diabetes, renal failure, and extend lifespan by up to 40 % in rats (Martin et al. 2010).

The most important indicators of disease and/or lack of well-being in rats are summarised below.

- Appearance. Piloerection and a rough greasy or matted pelage, sometimes with loss of hair, a loose skin, muscle wastage on the back, dehydration and reduced body weight may all be observed. Eyelids are half or fully closed and the eyes have the appearance of being sunken. Reddish-brown secretion from the lacrimal (Harderian) glands accumulates around the eyes and/or nose (chromodacryorrhoea).
- Faeces. Soft faeces, or diarrhoea, a dirty tail and an unpleasant smell are indicative of an intestinal infection.
- Body weight. Along with decreased food and water consumption, loss in body weight can signal a decline in the animal's health. Humane end points are determined prior to a study involving animals, and these often include that a rat should be euthanised when they lose 15% or 20% of their body weight (compared with age-matched controls) within a short period of time (24–48 h).
- Behaviour. Initially, animals may be more alert and aggressive, but will become progressively more passive and listless; they stop eating and drinking and reduce exploratory behaviour (Roughan & Flecknell 2003). Sometimes, rats excessively gnaw affected parts of the body.
- Posture. The animal frequently lies down, initially curled up with the head touching the abdomen, later stretched with the tail extended. A hard belly indicates abdominal pain. A tilted head is indicative of an infected middle ear or vestibular issue.
- Locomotion. A diseased rat, if it moves, does so slowly with a stiff-legged gait and arched back.
- Vocalisation. Squeaking when handled.
- Physiology. Regular sneezing may be the first sign of a respiratory infection. When the condition of the animal worsens, breathing is audible and laboured and the respiratory frequency increases. Hypothermia indicates a serious condition and a pale appearance is indicative of anaemia or loss of blood.
- In rats, like many rodents, Harderian glands next to the orbits secrete porphyrins, lipids and other compounds. High levels of secretion lead to chromodacryorrhoea (red or 'bloody' tears), often taken as a sign of stress or disease (Mason et al. 2004).

Sick animals must always be examined by a veterinarian for a complete clinical and *post-mortem* diagnosis. However, many diseases may take a subclinical course with no apparent signs of illness. It is important to be aware of such subclinical diseases, such as latent viral infections, because they may interfere with the standardisation or outcomes of the experiments.

Regular microbiological monitoring of the rat population is, therefore, essential (see guidelines by FELASA 2014).

The most common infectious diseases of rats involve infections of the respiratory tract by *Mycoplasma pulmonalis*, *Pasteurella* spp. and *Pneumococcus* spp. Under proper husbandry conditions, the disease will only be apparent in some animals. However, the disease may become a serious problem under less optimal husbandry conditions, or when experimental procedures compromise the physical condition of the animals. If the disease cannot be controlled by chemotherapy or by antibiotics, sick animals must be removed from the colony as soon as possible. Respiratory diseases are transmitted by air or by contact between the animals. Reducing the pH (or chlorination) of drinking water is sometimes used to reduce the spread of the infection in a colony through contaminated drinking spouts. See Krinke et al. (2000), Fox et al. (2002) or Suckow et al. (2019) for more extensive information on diseases and their treatment and control.

Abnormal behaviour

Rats rarely show obvious signs of abnormal behaviour. The incidence of stereotypies is very low under standard housing conditions. Abnormal behaviour is usually expressed as an increase in reactivity to environmental stimuli leading to panic reactions, or as increased passivity, listlessness or state of depression. Occasionally, abnormal aggressive behaviour may occur in group-housed males. One male may continuously attack one of his cage mates, leading to serious wounding or death, and sometimes to cannibalism. There are no known solutions to this problem, other than euthanising the particular group of animals.

Hair loss due to obsessive barbering refers to the abnormal grooming behaviour of an animal chewing and tearing the fur and whiskers of either itself or another animal. Barbering is known to occur in most companion rodent species, including guinea pigs, rats and mice. When one animal barbers another animal, it is used as a display of dominance, meaning that the more dominant member of the group chews on the fur and whiskers of the less dominant members. However, excessive barbering in mice is an expression of abnormal repetitive behaviour (Garner et al. 2004). Barbering results in alopecia (loss of hair) in the affected areas and sometimes skin irritation or even wounds. Some rodents will barber themselves due to stress, inappropriate caging, boredom and even heredity. This behaviour is more commonly seen in mice than rats.

Reproductive problems

Rats, in particular the outbred strains, generally reproduce without any problems. After giving birth, the mothers of some strains may be infanticidal. This usually results from disturbance to the nest, and the nursing mother caused by cage cleaning or other activities in the animal unit. Sensitive strains should be bred in separate, quiet breeding facilities, and pregnant females should be provided with nest boxes and nesting material. Excessive noise or vibrations such as those associated with nearby construction projects may also be stressful to the dams.

References

Abou-Ismail, U.A. and Mahboub, H.D. (2011). The effects of enriching laboratory cages using various physical structures on multiple measures of welfare in singly-housed rats. *Laboratory Animals*, **45(3)**, 145–153.

Abou-Ismail, U.A. and Mendl, M.T. (2016). The effects of enrichment novelty versus complexity in cages of group-housed rats (Rattus norvegicus). *Applied Animal Behaviour Science*, **180**(Supplement C), 130–139.

Akula, J.D., Lyubarsky, A.L. and Naarendorp, F. (2003). The sensitivity and spectral identity of the cones driving the b-wave of the rat electroretinogram. *Visual Neuroscience*, **20**, 109–117.

Arakawa, H. (2005). Interaction between isolation rearing and social development on exploratory behavior in male rats. *Behavioral Processes*, **70**, 223–234.

Atcha, Z., Rourke, C., Neo, A.H.P. et al. (2010). Alternative method of oral dosing for rats. *Journal of the American Association for Laboratory Animal Science*, **49(3)**, 335–343.

Bacon, S.J. and McClintock, M.K. (1994). Multiple factors determine the sex ratio of postpartum-conceived Norway rat litters. *Physiology & Behavior*, **56**, 359–366.

Barbacka-Surowiak, G., Surowiak, J. and Stoklosowa, S. (2003). The involvement of suprachiasmatic nuclei in the regulation of estrous cycles in rodents. *Reproductive Biology*, **3**, 99–129.

Barker, D.J. (2018). Ultrasonic vocalizations as an index of positive emotional state. In: *Handbook of Ultrasonic Vocalization: A Window into the Emotional Brain*, Ed. Brudzynski, S., pp. 253–260. Academic Press, London.

Barnett, S.A. (1963). *The Rat, a Study in Behavior*. Univ. of Chicago Press, Chicago.

Beery, A.K., Holmes, M.M., Lee, W. and Curley, J.P. (2020). Stress in groups: Lessons from non-traditional rodent species and housing models. *Neuroscience and Biobehavioral Reviews*, **113**, 354–372.

Bertens, A.P.M.G., Booij, L.H.D.J., Flecknell, P.A. et al. (1993). Anaesthesia, analgesia and euthanasia. In: *Principles of Laboratory Animal Sciences*. Eds Zutphen, L.F.M., Baumans, V. and Beynen, A.C., pp. 267–298. Elsevier, Amsterdam.

Beynon, R.J. and Hurst, J.L. (2004). Urinary proteins and the modulation of chemical scents in mice and rats. *Peptides*, **25**, 1553–1563.

Blom, H.J.M., Van Tintelen, G., Van Vorstenbosch, C.J.A.H.V. et al. (1996). Preferences of mice and rats for types of bedding material. *Laboratory Animals*, **30**, 234–244.

Boivin, G.P., Hickman, D.L., Creamer-Hente, M.A. et al. (2017). Review of CO_2 as a euthanasia agent for laboratory rats and mice. *Journal of the American Association for Laboratory Animal Science*, **56(5)**, 491–499.

Brudzynski, S.M. (2013). Ethotransmission: communication of emotional states through ultrasonic vocalization in rats. *Current Opinion in Neurobiology*, **23**, 310–317.

Brydges, N.M., Leach, M., Nicol, K. et al. (2011). Environmental enrichment induces optimistic cognitive bias in rats. *Animal Behaviour*, **81(1)**, 169–175.

Burn, C.C. (2008). What is it like to be a rat? Rat sensory perception and its implications for experimental design and rat welfare. *Applied Animal Behaviour Science*, **112**, 1–32.

Burgdorf, J., Kroes, R.A., Moskal, J.R. et al. (2008). Ultrasonic vocalizations of rats (Rattus norvegicus) during mating, play, and aggression: behavioral concomitants, relationship to reward, and self-administration of playback. *Journal of Comparative Psychology*, **122**, 357–367. doi: 10.1037/a0012889

Burn, C.C., Day, M.J., Peters, A. and Mason, G.J. (2006). Long-term effects of cage-cleaning frequency and bedding type on laboratory rat health, welfare, and handleability: a cross-laboratory study. *Laboratory Animals*, **40(3)**, 353–370.

Burn, C.C. and Mason, G.J. (2008). Effects of cage-cleaning frequencies on rat reproductive performance, infanticide, and welfare. *Applied Animal Behaviour Science*, **114**, 235–247.

Calcagnoli, F., De Boer S.F., Althaus, M. and Koolhaas, J.M. (2015). Acute and repeated intranasal oxytocin administration exerts anti-aggressive and pro-affiliative effects in male rats. *Psychoneuroendocrinology*, **51**, 112–121. doi: 10.1016/j.psyneuen.2014.09.019

Calhoun, J.B. (1962). *The Ecology and Sociology of the Norway Rat*. Government Printing Office, Washington DC.

Carder, B. and Berkowitz, K. (1970). Rats' preference for earned in comparison with free food. *Science*, **167(922)**, 1273–1274.

Carvell, G.E. and Simons, D.J. (1990). Biometric analyses of vibrissal tactile discrimination in the rat. *Journal of Neuroscience*, **10**, 2638–2648.

Chu, X. and Agmo, A. (2015). Sociosexual behaviors of male rats (Rattus norvegicus) in a seminatural environment. *Journal of Comparative Psychology*, **129(2)**, 132–144.

Chu, X. and Agmo, A. (2014). Sociosexual behaviours in cycling, intact female rats (Rattus norvegicus) housed in a seminatural environment. *Behaviour*, **151(8)**, 1143.

Claassen, V. (1994). *Neglected Factors in Pharmacology and Neuroscience Research*. Elsevier, Amsterdam.

Clough, G. (1984). Environmental factors in relation to the comfort and well-being of laboratory rats and mice. In: *Standards in Laboratory Animal Management*, Vol. 1, pp. 7–24. UFAW, Potters Bar.

Conlee, K.M., Stephens, M.L., Rowan, A.N. et al. (2005). Carbon dioxide for euthanasia: concerns regarding pain and distress, with special reference to mice and rats. *Laboratory Animals*, **39**, 137–161.

De Boer, S.F., Slangen, J.L. and Van der Gugten, J. (1990). Effects of chlordiazepoxide and buspirone on plasma catecholamine and corticosterone levels in rats under basal and stress conditions. *Endocrinologia Experimentalis*, **24**, 229–239.

De Boer, S.F., Van Der Vegt, B.J. and Koolhaas, J.M. (2003). Individual variation in aggression of feral rodent strains: a standard for the genetics of aggression and violence? *Behavior Genetics*, **33**, 485–501.

De Boer, S.F., Buwalda, B. and Jaap M. Koolhaas (2017). Untangling the Neurobiology of Coping Styles in rodents: towards neural mechanisms underlying individual differences in disease susceptibility. *Neuroscience Biobehavioral Reviews*, **74**, 401–422.

Dielenberg, R.A. and McGregor, I.S. (2001). Defensive behavior in rats towards predatory odors: a review. *Neuroscience and Biobehavioral Reviews*, **25**, 597–609.

Dongen, J.J.V., Remie, R., Rensema, J.W. et al. (1990). *Manual of Microsurgery on the Laboratory Rat*. Elsevier, Amsterdam.

Ellenbroek, B. and Youn, J. (2016). Rodent models in neuroscience research: is it a rat race? *Disease Models & Mechanism*, **9(10)**, 1079–1087.

Eriksson, M. (2019). *Handling and Training Techniques for Less Stressed Laboratory Rodents*. Paper presented at the NC3Rs/IAT Animal Technicians' Symposium, London, UK. https://www.nc3rs.org.uk/news/highlights-2019-nc3rsiat-animal-technicians-symposium

Erskine, M.S. (1989). Solicitation behavior in the estrous female rat: a review. *Hormones and Behavior*, **23**, 473–502.

European Parliament and Council (2010). Directive 2010/63/EU of the European Parliament and of the Council of 22 September 2010 on the Protection of Animals Used for Scientific Purposes. *Official Journal of the European Union*, 2010; L 276/33–79. https://eur-lex.europa.eu/LexUriServ/LexUriServ.do?uri=OJ:L:2010:276:0033:0079:EN:PDF. (Accessed 5 March 2020).

Fajardo, G. and Hornicke, H. (1989). Problems in estimating the extent of coprophagy in the rat. *British Journal of Nutrition*, **62**, 551–561.

Federation of European Laboratory Animal Science Associations (FELASA) (2014). FELASA recommendations for the health monitoring of rodent and rabbit colonies in breeding and experimental units. *Laboratory Animals*, **48**, 178–192.

Feng, A.Y.T. and Himsworth, C.G. (2014). The secret life of the city rat: a review of the ecology of urban Norway and black rats (Rattus norvegicus and Rattus rattus). *Urban Ecosystems*, **17(1)**, 149–162.

Festing, M.F.W. (1993). *International Index of Laboratory Animals*, 6th edn. Festing, Leicester.

Fish, R., Danneman, P.J., Brown, M. and Karas, A. (Eds) (2011). *Anesthesia and Analgesia in Laboratory Animals*. Academic Press, London.

Fitchett, A.E., Judge, S.J. and Morris, C.M. (2012). Using olive oil to orally dose laboratory rats. *Animal Technology and Welfare*, **10(1)**, 39–41.

Flecknell, P.A. (2009). *Laboratory Animal Anaesthesia*, 4th edn. Academic Press, London.

Flecknell, P.A. and Waterman-Pearson, A. (2000). *Pain Management in Animals*. W.B. Saunders, London.

Fox, J.G., Anderson, L.C., Loew, F.M. et al. (Eds) (2002). *Laboratory Animal Medicine*. American College of Laboratory Animal Medicine, Academic Press, New York.

Galef, B.G. Jr. (2003). Social learning of food preferences in rodents: rapid appetitive learning. *Current Protocols in Neuroscience*, **8**, 5.

Galef, B.G., Jr. and Whiskin, E.E. (2005). Differences between golden hamsters (*Mesocricetus auratus*) and Norway rats (*Rattus norvegicus*) in preference for the sole diet that they are eating. *Journal of Comparative Psychology*, **119(1)**, 8–13.

Garner, J.P., Gaskill, B.N., Weber, E.M. et al. (2017). Introducing Therioepistemology: the study of how knowledge is gained from animal research. *Laboratory Animals*, **46(4)**, 103.

Garner, J.P., Dufour, B., Gregg, L.E. et al. (2004). Social and husbandry factors affecting the prevalence and severity of barbering ('whisker trimming') by laboratory mice. *Applied Animal Behaviour Science*, **89(3–4)**, 263–282.

Ghirardi, O., Cozzolino, R., Guaraldi, D. et al. (1995). Within- and between-strain variability in longevity of inbred and outbred rats under the same environmental conditions. *Experimental Gerontology*, **30**, 485–494.

Gordon, C.J. (1990). Thermal biology of the laboratory rat. *Physiology & Behavior*, **47**, 963–991.

Gordon, C.J. and Fogelson, L. (1994). Metabolic and thermoregulatory responses of the rat maintained in acrylic or wire-screen cages: implications for pharmacological studies. *Physiology & Behavior*, **56**, 73–79.

Goto, S., Takahashi, R., Radak, Z. et al. (2007). Beneficial biochemical outcomes of late-onset dietary restriction in rodents. *Annals of the New York Academy of Sciences*, **1100**, 431–441.

Gutman, D.A. and Nemeroff, C.B. (2002). Neurobiology of early life stress: rodent studies. *Seminars in Clinical Neuropsychiatry*, **7**, 89–95.

Hall, F.S. (1998). Social deprivation of neonatal, adolescent, and adult rats has distinct neurochemical and behavioral consequences. *Critical Reviews in Neurobiology*, **12**, 129–162.

Hawkins, P. and Golledge, H.D.R. (2018). The 9 to 5 Rodent – Time for Change? Scientific and animal welfare implications of circadian and light effects on laboratory mice and rats. *Journal of Neuroscience Methods*, **300**, 20–25.

Hawkins, P., Prescott, M.J., Carbone, L. et al. (2016). A good death? Report of the Second Newcastle Meeting on Laboratory Animal Euthanasia. *Animals (Basel)*, **6(9)**, pii: E50.

Hawkins, P., Morton, D.B., Burman, O. et al. (2011). A guide to defining and implementing protocols for the welfare assessment of laboratory animals: eleventh report of the BVAAWF/FRAME/RSPCA/UFAW Joint Working Group on Refinement. *Laboratory Animals*, **45(1)**, 1–13.

Hedrich, H.J. (1990). Inbred strains in biomedical research. In: *Genetic Monitoring of Inbred Strains of Rats*. Ed. Hedrich, H.J., pp. 1–7. Gustav Fisher Verlag, Stuttgart

Hedrich, H.J. (2000). History, strains and models. In: *The Laboratory Rat*. Eds Krinke, G., Bullock, G. and Bunton, T., pp. 3–16. Academic Press, New York.

Heidbreder, C.A., Weiss, I.C., Domeney, A.M. et al. (2000). Behavioral, neurochemical and endocrinological characterization of the early social isolation syndrome. *Neuroscience*, **100(4)**, 749–768.

Heijkoop, R., Huijgens, P.T. and Snoeren, E.M.S. (2018). Assessment of sexual behavior in rats: the potentials and pitfalls. *Behavioural Brain Research*, **352**, 70–80.

Hoffman, J.F., Fan, A.X., Neuendorf, E.H. et al. (2018). Hydrophobic sand versus metabolic cages: a comparison of urine collection methods for rats (*Rattus norvegicus*). *Journal of the American Association for Laboratory Animal Science*, 2018 Jan; **57(1)**, 51–57.

Huang-Brown, K.M. and Guhad, F.A. (2002). Chocolate, an effective means of oral drug delivery in rats. *Laboratory Animals*, **31(10)**, 34–36.

International Air Transport Association (IATA) (2010). *Dangerous Goods Regulations*. http://www.iata.org/ps/publications/dangerous-goods-regulations-dgr

Jacobs, G.H., Fenwick, J.A. and Williams, G.A. (2001). Cone-based vision of rats for ultraviolet and visible lights. *Journal of Experimental Biology*, **204**, 2439–2446.

Joint Working Group on Refinement (2001). Refining procedures for the administration of substances. Report of the BVAAWF/FRAME/RSPCA/UFAW Joint Working Group on Refinement. *Laboratory Animals*, **35**, 1–41.

Jonsson, O., Villar, R.P., Nilsson, L.B. et al. (2012). Capillary microsampling of 25 μl blood for the determination of toxicokinetic parameters in regulatory studies in animals. *Bioanalysis*, **4(6)**, 661–674.

Kisko, T.M., Schwarting, R.K.W. and Wöhr, M. (2021). Sex differences in the acoustic features of social play-induced 50-kHz ultrasonic vocalizations: a detailed spectrographic analysis in wild-type Sprague–Dawley and Cacna1c haploinsufficient rats. *Developmental Psychobiology*, **63**, 262–276. DOI: 10.1002/dev.21998

Kisko, T.M., Wöhr, M., Pellis, V.C. and Pellis, S.M. (2017). From play to aggression: high-frequency 50-kHz ultrasonic vocalizations as play and appeasement signals in rats. *Current Topics in Behavioral Neurosciences*, **30**, 91–108.

Koolhaas, J.M., Meerlo, P., Boer, S.F.D. et al. (1997). The temporal dynamics of the stress response. *Neuroscience & Biobehavioral Reviews*, **21**, 775–782.

Krinke, G., Bunton, T. and Bullock, G. (Eds) (2000). *The Laboratory Rat*. Academic Press, New York.

Klaunberg, B.A., O'Malley, J., Clark, T. and Davis, J.A. (2004). Euthanasia of mouse fetuses and neonates. *Contemporary Topics in Laboratory Animal Science*, **43(5)**, 29–34.

Klemann, N. and Pelz, H.J. (2006). The feeding pattern of the Norway rat (*Rattus norvegicus*) in two differently structured habitats on a farm. *Applied Animal Behaviour Science*, **97(2–4)**, 293–302

Kohn, D.F. and Clifford, C.B. (2002). Biology and diseases of rats. In: *Laboratory Animal Medicine*. Eds Fox, L.C., Anderson, C., Leow, F.M. and Quimby, F.W., pp. 121–165, Academic Press, San Diego.

Krohn, T.C., Hansen, A.K. and Dragsted, N. (2003). The impact of cage ventilation on rats housed in IVC systems. *Laboratory Animals*, **37**, 85–93.

Krohn, T.C., Sorensen, D.B., Ottesen, J.L. et al. (2006). The effects of individual housing on mice and rats: a review. *Animal Welfare*, **15**, 343–352.

Kuramoto, T., Nakanishi, S., Ochiai, M. et al. (2012). Origins of albino and hooded rats: implications from molecular genetic analysis across modern laboratory rat strains. *PLoS One*, **7**, e43059.

LaFollette, M.R., Cloutier, S., Brady, C. et al. (2019). Laboratory animal welfare and human attitudes: a cross-sectional survey on heterospecific play or 'rat tickling'. *PLoS One*, **14(8)**, p.e0220580.

LaVail, M.M. (1976). Survival of some photoreceptors in albino rats following long-term exposure to continuous light. *Investigative Ophthalmology and visual Science*, **15**, 64–70.

Lepschy, M., Touma, C., Hruby, R. et al. (2007). Non-invasive measurement of adrenocortical activity in male and female rats. *Laboratory Animals*, **41**, 372–387.

Lindsey, J.R. and Baker, H.J. (2006). Historical foundations. In: *The Laboratory Rat*. Eds Suckow, M.A., Weisbroth, S.H. and Franklin C.L., pp. 1–53. Elsevier, Amsterdam.

Maisonnette, S., Morato, S. and Brandao, M.L. (1993). Role of resocialization and of 5-HT1A receptor activation on the anxiogenic effects induced by isolation in the elevated plus-maze test. *Physiology & Behavior*, **54**, 753–758.

Malkesman, O., Maayan, R., Weizman, A. *et al.* (2006). Aggressive behavior and HPA axis hormones after social isolation in adult rats of two different genetic animal models for depression. *Behavioral Brain Research*, **175**, 408–414.

Manser, C.E., Morris, T.H. and Broom, D.M. (1995). An investigation into the effects of solid or grid cage flooring on the welfare of laboratory rats. *Laboratory Animals*, **29**, 353–363.

Markison, S. (2001). The role of taste in the recovery from specific nutrient deficiencies in rats. *Nutritional Neuroscience*, **4**, 1–14.

Martin, B., Ji, S., Maudsley, S. and Mattson, M.P. (2010). 'Control' laboratory rodents are metabolically morbid: why it matters. *Proceedings of the National Academy of Sciences*, **107**, 6127–6133.

Mason, G., Wilson, D., Hampton, C. and Wurbel, H. (2004). Non-invasively assessing disturbance and stress in laboratory rats by scoring chromodacryorrhoea. *Alternatives to Laboratory Animals*, **32(Suppl. 1)**, 153–159.

McClintock, M.K. and Adler, N.T. (1978). The role of the female during copulation in wild and domesticated Norway rats (*Rattus norvegicus*). *Behaviour*, **67**, 67–96.

McLennan, I.S. and Taylor-Jeffs, J. (2004). The use of sodium lamps to brightly illuminate mouse houses during their dark phases. *Laboratory Animals*, **38**, 384–392. http://dx.doi.org/10.1258/0023677041958927

Meaney, M.J., Aitken, D.H., Bhatnagar, S. *et al.* (1991). Postnatal handling attenuates certain neuroendocrine, anatomical and cognitive dysfunctions associated with aging in female rats. *Neurobiology of Aging*, **12**, 31–38.

Meaney, M.J. and Szyf, M. (2005). Environmental programming of stress responses through DNA methylation: life at the interface between a dynamic environment and a fixed genome. *Dialogues in Clinical Neuroscience*, **7**, 103–123.

Mediavilla, C., Molina, F. and Puerto, A. (2005). Concurrent conditioned taste aversion: a learning mechanism based on rapid neural versus flexible humoral processing of visceral noxious substances. *Neuroscience & Biobehavioral Reviews*, **29**, 1107–1118.

Mormede, P. (1997). Genetic influences on the responses to psychosocial challenges in rats. *Acta Physiologica Scandinavica. Suppl*, **640**, 65–68.

Neitz, J. and Jacobs, G.H. (1986). Reexamination of spectral mechanisms in the rat (*Rattus norvegicus*). *Journal of Comparative Psychology*, **100**, 21–29.

Nijman, I.J., Kuipers, S., Verheul, M. *et al.* (2008). A genome-wide SNP panel for mapping and association studies in the rat. *BMC Genomics*, **9**, 95.

Njaa, L.R., Utne, F. and Braekkan, O.R. (1957). Effect of relative humidity on rat breeding and ringtail. *Nature*, **180**, 290–291.

Olivier, B., Zethof, T., Pattij, T., *et al.* (2003). Stress-induced hyperthermia and anxiety: pharmacological validation. *European Journal of Pharmacology*, **463(1–3)**, 117–132.

Otsen, M., Bieman, M.-D., Winer, E.-S. *et al.* (1995). Use of simple sequence length polymorphisms for genetic characterization of rat inbred strains. *Mammalian Genome*, **6**, 595–601.

Panksepp, J. (2007). Neuroevolutionary sources of laughter and social joy: modeling primal human laughter in laboratory rats. *Behavioural Brain Research*, **182**, 231–244.

Parshad, R.K. (1997). Effect of restricted feeding of prepubertal and adult male rats on fertility and sex ratio. *Indian Journal of Experimental Biology*, **31**, 991–992.

Patterson-Kane, E.G. (2001). Environmental enrichment for laboratory rats: a review. *Animal Technology*, **52(2)**, 77–84.

Pellis, S.M. and Pellis, V.C. (1998). Play fighting of rats in comparative perspective: a schema for neurobehavioral analyses. *Neuroscience & Biobehavioral Reviews*, **23**, 87–101.

Pellis, S.M. and Pellis, V.C. (1987). Play-fighting differs from serious fighting in both target of attack and tactics of fighting in the laboratory rat *Rattus-norvegicus*. *Aggressive Behavior*, **13(4)**, 227–242.

Perez, J. and Perentes, E. (1994). Light-induced retinopathy in the albino rat in long-term studies. An immunohistochemical and quantitative approach. *Experimental and Toxicologic Pathology*, **46**, 229–235.

Pisano, R.G. and Storer, T.I. (1948). Burrows and feeding of the Norway rat. *Journal of Mammalogy*, **29**, 374–383.

Polosa, A., Bessaklia, H. and Lachapelle, P. (2016). Strain differences in light-induced retinopathy. *PLoS One*, **11(6)**, e0158082.

Portfors, C.V. (2007). Types and functions of ultrasonic vocalizations in laboratory rats and mice. *Journal of the American Association of Laboratory Animal Sciences*, **46**, 28–34.

Prendergast, B.J., Kampf-Lassin, A., Yee, J.R. *et al.* (2007). Winter day lengths enhance T lymphocyte phenotypes, inhibit cytokine responses, and attenuate behavioral symptoms of infection in laboratory rats. *Brain Behavior and Immunity*, **21**, 1096–1108.

Prendergast, B.J. and Kay, L.M. (2008). Affective and adrenocorticotrophic responses to photoperiod in Wistar rats. *Journal of Neuroendocrinology*, **20**, 261–267.

Prusky, G.T., Harker, K.T., Douglas, R.M. *et al.* (2002). Variation in visual acuity within pigmented, and between pigmented and albino rat strains. *Behavioural Brain Research*, **136**, 339–348.

Rex, A., Kolbasenko, A., Bert, B. *et al.* (2007). Choosing the right wild type: behavioral and neurochemical differences between 2 populations of Sprague-Dawley rats from the same source but maintained at different sites. *Journal of the American Association of Laboratory Animal Sciences*, **46**, 13–20.

Richter, S.H., Garner, J.P. and Wurbel, H. (2009). Environmental standardization: cure or cause of poor reproducibility in animal experiments? *Nature Methods*, **6(4)**, 257–261

Roe, F.J.C., Lee, P.N., Conybeare, G. *et al.* (1995). The Biosure Study: Influence of composition of diet and food consumption on longevity, degenerative diseases and neoplasia in Wistar rats studied for up to 30 months post weaning. *Food and Chemical Toxicology*, **33**, 1S–100S.

Rosenblatt, J.S., Factor, E.M. and Mayer, A.D. (1994). Relationship between maternal aggression and maternal care in the rat. *Aggressive Behavior*, **20**, 243–255.

Roughan, J.V. and Flecknell, P.A. (2003). Evaluation of a short duration behaviour-based post-operative pain scoring system in rats. *European Journal of Pain*, **7**, 397–406.

Rowland, N.E. (2007). Food or fluid restriction in common laboratory animals: balancing welfare considerations with scientific inquiry. *Comparative Medicine*, 57, 149–160.

Sandi, C. and Haller, J. (2015). Stress and the social brain: behavioural effects and neurobiological mechanisms. *Nature Reviews Neuroscience*, **16(5)**, 290–304.

Schoeb, T.R., Davidson, M.K. and Lindsey, J.R. (1982). Intracage ammonia promotes growth of *Mycoplasma pulmonis* in the respiratory tract of rats. *Infection and Immunity*, **38**, 212–217.

Schwartz, M.W., Woods, S.C., Porte, D., Jr. *et al.* (2000). Central nervous system control of food intake. *Nature*, **404**, 661–671.

Semple-Rowland, S.L. and Dawson, W.W. (1987). Cyclic light intensity threshold for retinal damage in albino rats raised under 6 lux. *Experimental Eye Research*, **44**, 643–661.

Sherwin, E., Bordenstein, S.R., Quinn, J.L. *et al.* (2019). Microbiota and the social brain. *Science*, **366**, 587.

Shor-Posner, G., Brennan, G., Ian, C. *et al.* (1994). Meal patterns of macronutrient intake in rats with particular dietary preferences. *American Journal of Physiology*, **266**, R1395–402.

Silva, R.C., Santos, N.R. and Brandao, M.L. (2003). Influence of housing conditions on the effects of serotonergic drugs on feeding behavior in non-deprived rats. *Neuropsychobiology*, **47**, 98–101.

Sivula, C.P. and Suckow, M.A. (2018). Euthanasia (Chapter 35). In: *Management of Animal Care and Use Programs in Research, Education, and Testing*. 2nd edn. Eds Weichbrod, R.H., Thompson, G.A.H. and Norton, J.N. CRC Press/Taylor & Francis, Boca Raton (FL).

Skinner, M.K., Manikkam, M. and Guerrereo-Bosagne, C. (2010). Epigenetic transgenerational actions of environmental factors in disease etiology. *Trends in Endocrinology and Metabolism*, 21, 214–222.

Smith, A.L. and Corrow, D.J. (2005). Modifications to husbandry and housing conditions of laboratory rodents for improved well-being. ILAR Journal, 46, 140–147.

Spector, A.C. and Kopka, S.L. (2002). Rats fail to discriminate quinine from denatonium: implications for the neural coding of bitter-tasting compounds. *Journal of Neuroscience*, **22(5)**, 1937–1941.

Stern, J.M. and Lonstein, J.S. (2001). Neural mediation of nursing and related maternal behaviors. *Progress in Brain Research*, **133**, 263–278.

Strubbe, J.H. and Woods, S.C. (2004). The timing of meals. *Psychological Review*, **111**, 28–141.

Suckow, M.A., Hankenson, F.C., Wilson, R. and Foley, P. (2019). *The Laboratory Rat*, 3rd edn. Academic Press, London.

Szyf, M., McGowan, P. and Meaney, M.J. (2008). The social environment and the epigenome. *Environmental and Molecular Mutagenesis*, **49**, 46–60.

Tamashiro, K.L., Nguyen, M.M. and Sakai, R.R. (2005). Social stress: from rodents to primates. *Frontiers in Neuroendocrinology*, **26**, 27–40.

Tang, A.C., Akers, K.G., Reeb, B.C. et al. (2006). Programming social, cognitive, and neuroendocrine development by early exposure to novelty. *Proceedings of the National Academy of Sciences, USA*, **103**, 15716–15721.

Telle, H.J. (1966). Beitrag zur Kenntnis der Verhaltensweise von Ratten vergleichend dargestellt bei Ruattus norvegicus und Rattus rattus. *Zeitschrift angewende Zoologie*, **53**, 126–196.

Tempel, D.L., Shor-Posner, G., Dwyer, D. et al. (1989). Nocturnal patterns of macronutrient intake in freely feeding and food deprived rats. *American Journal of Physiology*, **256**, R541–R548.

Toth, M., Halasz, J., Mikics, E. et al. (2008). Early social deprivation induces disturbed social communication and violent aggression in adulthood. *Behavioral Neuroscience*, **122**, 849–854.

Toth, L.A. et al. (2011). Environmental enrichment of laboratory rodents: the answer depends on the question. *Comparative Medicine*, **61**, 314–321.

Traweger, D., Travnitzky, R., Moser, C. et al. (2006). Habitat preferences and distribution of the brown rat (*Rattus norvegicus* Berk.) in the city of Salzburg (Austria): implications for an urban rat management. *Journal of Pest Science*, **79(3)**, 113–125.

Valentim, A.M., Guedes, S.R., Pereira, A.M. and Antunes, L.M. (2016). Euthanasia using gaseous agents in laboratory rodents. *Laboratory Animals*, **50(4)**, 241–253.

Waynforth, H.B. and Flecknell, P.A. (1992). *Experimental and Surgical Technique in the Rat*, 2nd edn. Academic Press, London.

Willis, M.B. and Dalton, C. (1998). *Dalton's Introduction to Practical Breeding*. Blackwell Publishing, Oxford.

Wöhr, M. and Schwarting, R.K.W. (2013). Affective communication in rodents: ultrasonic vocalizations as a tool for research on emotion and motivation. *Cell and Tissue Research*, **354**, 81–97.

Yildiz, A., Hayirli, A., Okumus, Z. et al. (2007). Physiological profile of juvenile rats: effects of cage size and cage density. *Laboratory Animals*, **36**, 28–38.

Zethof, T.J.J., Van der Heyden, J.A.M., Tolboom, J.T.B.M. et al. (1995). Stress-induced hyperthermia as a putative anxiety model. *European Journal of Pharmacology*, **294**, 125–135.

Zimmermann, F., Weiss, J. and Reifenberg, K. (2000). Breeding and assisted reproduction techniques. In: *The Laboratory Rat*. Eds Krinke, G., Bullock, G. and Bunton, T., pp. 177–198. Academic Press, New York.

Zochodne, D.W., Murray, M.M., van der Sloot, P. and Riopelle, R.J. (1995). Distal tibial mononeuropathy in diabetic and nondiabetic rats reared on wire cages: an experimental entrapment neuropathy. *Brain Research*, **698**, 130–136.

23 The laboratory gerbil

Elke Scheibler

Biological overview

Taxonomy

The Mongolian gerbil (*Meriones unguiculatus*) is the most widely used species for laboratory purposes within the subfamily of Gerbillinae. Members of this subfamily are distributed in deserts and semi-deserts of Asia and Africa including the near East. Their ecological niche is that of a granivorous, non-hibernating, fossorial, commonly social small mammal. To a small degree, gerbils propose a threat as pest species, or disease vector species, or by destabilising dams and foundations as results of extensive underground digging. The genus *Meriones* (sandrat, 14 species) contains the subgenera *Meriones*, *Parameriones*, *Pallasiomys* and *Cheliones*. Various authors have recently discussed gerbil taxonomy and phylogeny (Michaux *et al*. 2001; Palinov 2001; Jansa & Weksler 2003; Steppan *et al*. 2004; Chevret & Dobigny 2005; Musser & Carleton 2005). This chapter will be limited to the Mongolian gerbil, or jird. The gerbil's scientific name *Meriones unguiculatus* means 'little clawed warrior' after Meriones, a marshal and relative of the Cretan king Idomeneus in the Trojan War, said to have been one of the warriors in the Trojan horse.

Standard biological data

Basic data on the gerbil have been described by McManus (1972a), Thiessen and Yahr (1977), Tumblebrook Farm (1979) and Field and Sibold (1999). Gerbils have 44 chromosomes, 4 pairs of mammary glands, and have a typical rodent dental formula (1 incisor, a diastema and 3 molars in each half mandible (I C P M: 1 0 0 3 in upper and lower jaw)). Dental anomalies are rare. An adult male weighs between 80 and 130 g, and a female between 60 and 100 g under laboratory conditions. At birth, pups weigh about 3–4 grams, at 20 days around 16 g, at 30 days 25 g, at 40 days 40 g, at 3 months: 65 g, at 6 months: 70–90 g. The life expectancy in the laboratory is usually 3–4 years but may reach up to 6 years. In the wild, the mortality rate for the first year of life is assumed to be 80% mainly due to predation (Liu *et al*. 2009, also personal communication). Gerbils' body temperature is 38.1–38.4 °C (measured by rectal probe), heart rate is 360 per min (range 260–600 per min) and respiration rate 90 per min with a range of 70 up to 160 per min. Gerbils drink 9.63 +/− 1.95% of body weight per day, which corresponds to 4–7 ml per day. The urine is highly concentrated with a volume of about 3–4 ml per day. Caloric uptake is 40.32 +/− 4.92 kcal per day per 100 g body weight, which corresponds to 5–8 g common standard food per day per 100 g body weight. All measures are valid under standard conditions but vary with ambient temperature and humidity. Increased water uptake can be observed in lower humidity, while lower ambient temperatures cause an increase in food uptake (Thiessen & Yahr 1977; Tumblebrook Farm 1979; Field & Sibold 1999). Gerbils have a body length of 11–13.5 cm, and a tail length of 9.5–12 cm. Gerbils often show an upright posture for exploration and vigilance (Figure 23.1). They also feed and autogroom in this posture. When upright, gerbils are about 15 cm tall.

External features

The fur colour is agouti with a crème-coloured belly, with some black markings close to the claws and tail tip. The tip of the tail may form a small tuft. During seasonal change of fur or shedding, a black line running across the body is often recognisable. However, this is unsuitable for individual identification as it is only temporary.

Hindfeet are longer than forefeet, which may support efficiency of digging, food manipulation and vigilance. In the digging process, the forefeet are usually used in an alternating manner, while the hindfeet are used simultaneously to remove loose material. Although the hindlegs appear longer, there is no bipedal jumping. Gerbils show a quadrupedal type of locomotion with a gallop-like foot order (left front, then right front, then both hind legs; or in case of escape the two front and then the hindfeet). Gerbils may overcome taller obstacles via jumping; 30 cm with ease, while up to 50 cm may be possible if the animal is frightened. In the laboratory, gerbils do not readily climb, at least not upside down at the cage top as mice do

---

The UFAW Handbook on the Care and Management of Laboratory and Other Research Animals, Ninth Edition.
Edited by Huw Golledge and Claire Richardson.
© 2024 John Wiley & Sons Ltd. Published 2024 by John Wiley & Sons Ltd.

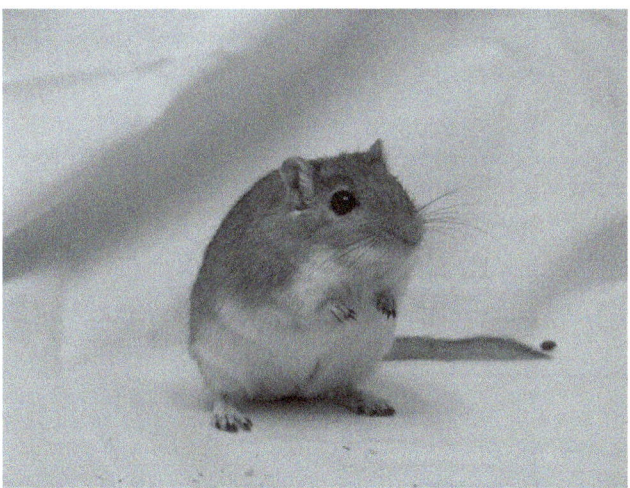

Figure 23.1 Mongolian gerbil (*Meriones unguiculatus*) in erected posture. The name-giving long, black claws are recognisable. The ventral gland is covered by hair and not visible from this angle.

(Lerwill 1974; Roper & Polioudakis 1977). However, gerbils are skilled climbers under more natural conditions.

Senses and communication

Acoustic communication

Although gerbils vocalise in a range of about 100 Hz up to 150 kHz, the majority (about 80%) of calls fall into the human audible frequency of 20 Hz to 20 kHz. It is assumed that calls in the ultrasonic range are mainly alarm calls, as gerbils are more sensitive in this range (Nakayama & Riquimaroux 2017). Sound pressure ranges from 2 to 106 dB (Lerwill 1978; Thiessen et al. 1978). Ultrasonic calling rate in gerbil pups increases from birth until day 4, then decreases. No vocalisations in the ultrasonic range and in context of parental behaviour were detected in adults when studied by De Ghett (1974) and Broom et al. (1977). Gerbils are altricial, and therefore their ears are not mature at birth. The sound-conducting apparatus and inner-ear structures develop between day 16 and 20 (Finck et al. 1969). The first cochlear microphonic potentials have been seen at day 12, with a very high 103 dB threshold (Woolf & Ryan 1984). Juvenile gerbils first approach an auditory stimulus (low-intensity tape-recorded gerbil social call compared to broadband white noise or silence) at 16 days of age (Kelly & Potash 1986). Hearing sensitivity then increases up to the age of 9 months.

Holman (1980) and Holman and Seale (1991) described sexual-specific differences with females vocalising in a lower range than males during mating. Additionally, they documented a variation of vocalisation between pre-, within- and postcopulatory conditions with upsweep (28–35 kHz), unmodulated (26 kHz) and modulated (28–38 KHz) calls.

Overall, adult gerbils respond to frequencies from 100 Hz to 60 kHz (Ryan 1976; Nakayama & Riquimaroux 2017), with maximum sensitivity (<10dB) between 4 and 44 kHz. In older gerbils (between 12 and 28 months), sensitivity is reduced at the range of 8–24 kHz. However, this is only the case in domesticated, rather than wild gerbils (Stuermer & Wetzel 2006; Eckrich et al. 2008). Minimum resolvable angles (MRAs) for sound localisation in azimuth for broadband noise is 23 degrees (if the animal is stimulated from the front) and 45 degrees (stimulated from the back; Maier & Klump 2006). Gerbils use both phase and intensity differences to localise sounds (Heffner & Heffner 1988).

Vision

Visual information is highly important for gerbils and they have been described as 'visually alert rodents' (Jacobs & Deegan 1994). They have good stereopsis, depth perception and cliff responses (Collins et al. 1969; Wilkinson 1984) and seem to be well adapted to diurnal life. Yang et al. (2015) found that the retinal structure of Mongolian gerbils is more analogous to the human eye than to mice. About 13% of the photoreceptors are of cone type (nocturnal mice: 1–3%). Two types of cones are reported: 95.0–97.5% are green sensitive (peak sensitivity at 493 nm, very close to the rod sensitivity, but at high illumination levels), 2.5–5.0% are blue-sensitive (sensitivity: 420 and 430 nm). Gerbils are therefore dichromatic with blue-green colour discrimination abilities (Govardovskii et al. 1992; Jacobs & Nietz 1989; Bytyqi & Layer 2005; Yang et al. 2015).

The majority (about 87%) of the photoreceptors are rods (peak sensitivity at 499–501 nm, Jacobs & Nietz 1989; Yang et al. 2015). General receptor density was found to be 314,000–332,000 per mm^2 for rods and 45,000–50,000 per mm^2 for cones (Govardovskii et al. 1992). Gerbils are also sensitive to ultraviolet light (Jacobs & Deegan 1994) and have retinal ganglion cells (Zhang et al. 2016).

Visual acuity is 1.8–2 cycles/degree at 70 cd/m^2 (Baker & Emerson 1983; Wilkinson 1984), with the acuity for horizontal gratings being better than for vertical gratings.

Olfaction and scent marking

Gerbils are classified as macrosmatic animals, as they have a highly developed sense of smell due to high densities of olfactory receptors and a well-developed olfactory bulb (Loskota et al. 1974; Thiessen & Yahr 1977; Radtke-Schuller et al. 2016). Gerbil pups show responses to odours as early as day 4, and strongly prefer home cage odour between days 8 and 14 (Cornwell-Jones & Azar 1982). Although all individuals have a ventral gland, it is only visible in adult and/or higher-ranking individuals. Scent marking, i.e. smearing sebum, of their ventral gland on objects in their territory and on group members is extensively described by Thiessen and Yahr (1977). The family odour is essential to distinguish between familiar and unfamiliar individuals (Wallace et al. 1973; Tang Halpin 1975; Roper & Polioudakis 1977; Yahr 1977; Yahr & Anderson-Mitchell 1983). Social stress, social defeat and ageing result in a decrease of scent-marking behaviour in male gerbils (Yamaguchi et al. 2005; Shimozuru et al. 2006b).

In the wild, gerbils predominantly mark along the border of their territory, with the dominant breeding male marking most, followed by the breeding female and adult male offspring (Agren et al. 1989a,b). A comparative study by Gromov (2015) found that females marked more often near burrow entrances, pathways and feeding sites. In contrast, males scent mark predominantly within the home range of reproductively active females rather than exclusively at the borders of their own territory. This supports the neighbour-mating hypotheses for Mongolian gerbils (see section on Social organisation). In same-sex groups of males, scent-mark frequency can be used as an indicator of rank (Shimozuru et al. 2006a), whereas body weight is usually taken as correlate of rank in mixed-sex groups (Weinandy 1995).

Activity patterns

Gerbils show polyphasic, diurnal and crepuscular activity patterns depending on environmental conditions. A bimodal pattern with a peak in the activity after dawn in the morning and around dusk is most frequent. Kept in LD 12:12 or long photoperiods with LD 16:8 will result in this bimodal pattern. Short photoperiods trigger a disruption of that pattern and several short activity periods can be measured including diurnal activity (Juarez-Tapia et al. 2015). This can be explained by climatic restrictions and the need to forage under natural conditions. In laboratory conditions, even the method of measurement may influence the activity observed pattern (Figure 23.2) as the use of running wheels results in a strengthening of a bimodal pattern (Refinetti 2006; Weinert et al. 2007). Under natural or semi-natural conditions, the activity pattern seems to be temperature dependent with a diurnal activity pattern only during winter, which may be a strategy against overheating during the hot summer months as found in other species (Leont'ev1954; Randall & Thiessen 1980). The thermoneutral zone of gerbils is between 26.5 and 38.9 °C and an atrophy of brown fat tissue can be observed in temperatures above 37 °C (Guo et al. 2019).

Social organisation

Extended family groups and sexual suppression

In the wild, gerbils live in extended families with one breeding pair and its offspring of overlapping generations. A family consists of a minimum of 2 and a maximum of 40 individuals in semi-natural conditions (Agren et al. 1989a,b; Scheibler et al. 2005a). Typically, group sizes tend to be smaller than 17 animals per group due to predation and dispersal, but group sizes of 26 animals in one burrow have been reported (Leont'ev 1954). Family members take part in foraging, territorial defence, vigilance, digging the communal burrow and alloparental care (Roper & Polioudakis 1977; Agren et al. 1989a,b; Ellard and Byers 2005). Although there is reproductive suppression of the offspring, neighbour-mating and mating of the founder female with male offspring have been reported (Agren et al. 1989a; Scheibler et al. 2006b). The offspring remain in the family and provide support for the younger offspring as helpers at the nest (Roper & Polioudakis 1977; Swanson & Lockley 1977; Agren et al. 1989a,b; Solomon & Getz 1996). Reproductive suppression is recognisable by lack of an oestrous cycle. Vaginal smears of non-reproductive daughters show characteristics of the met-oestrus stage (Figure 23.3, Nishino & Totsukawa 1996). Reproductive suppression is mediated by dominance display of the dominant female but is

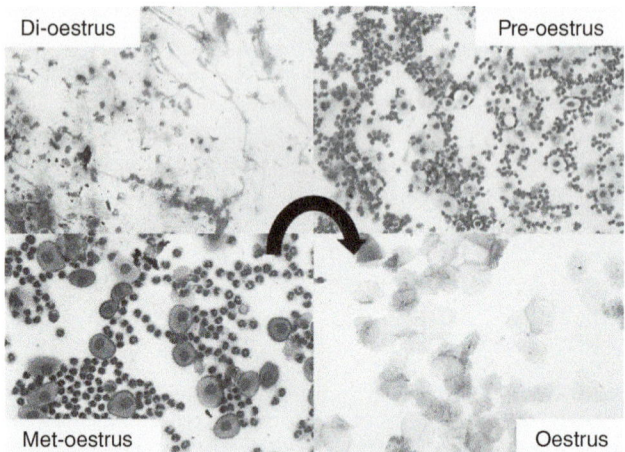

Figure 23.3 Vaginal smears of Mongolian gerbils during the oestrous cycle. Di-oestrus features prominent proteinaceous fluid 'slime' along with leucocytes and epithelial cells. During pre-oestrus, no slime can be found, only leucocytes and predominantly nucleated epithelial cells with rare cornified epithelial cells. In oestrus, only cornified epithelial cells are visible. In met-oestrus, again leucocytes and epithelial cells are visible, similar to pro-oestrus. Important: the number and composition of leucocytes vary.

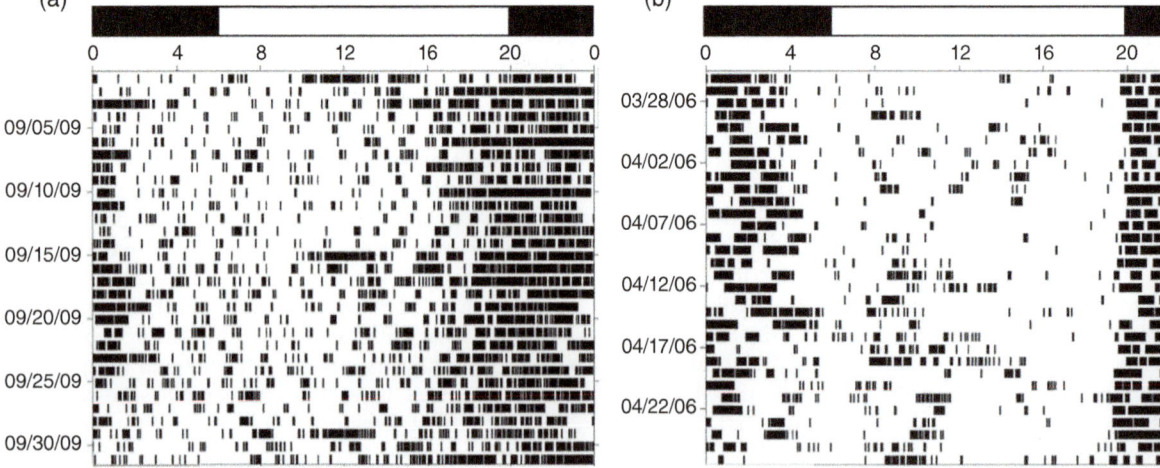

Figure 23.2 (a) Actograms of a pair of Mongolian gerbils measured with a passive infrared sensor (PIR) and (b) activity of a single Mongolian gerbil measured by running wheel. In both diagrams, activity is indicated in black in 3 min bouts. LD-bars corresponds to LD 14:10 with Lights-on at 6 am.

not necessarily completely effective (Clark & Galef 2002). Litters of other high-ranking daughters may be born under semi-natural, ad libitum conditions (French 1994; Scheibler *et al.* 2005b) and oestrous synchronisation and communal nesting may even occur (Scheibler unpubl.). Mating with close relatives such as siblings still results in vital offspring (Scheibler *et al.* 2006b); however, under natural conditions neighbour-mating would be more common. Wang *et al.* (2011) described seasonal variation in the territory size with larger overlap during breeding season.

Philopatry and intra-family aggression

Philopatry, i.e. remaining in the family, is a phenomenon that is widely explained by a direct and indirect fitness gain (Solomon 2003). The direct fitness gain occurs when the offspring starts to reproduce, as the increase in parental care experience is advantageous (Salo & French 1989). The indirect fitness gain is especially of importance as this species lives in habitats with limited and partially unpredictable resource availability, and predation pressure (Ostermeyer & Elwood 1984).

Although gerbils are highly social and cooperative breeders, severe outbreaks of aggression can lead to the death of family members. Aggressive behaviour is shown by the founder female and occasionally by the founder male. Attacked animals are mature males and females; however, maturity alone is not a trigger for those outbreaks (Scheibler *et al.* 2004, 2006b). The loss of one or both dominant, breeding animals (particularly the loss of the founder female) results in severe fights between remaining females until one (female) is left, irrespective of their reproductive status. If the founder male is lost, intragroup aggression may occur, but is not as severe as in case of the females (Scheibler *et al.* 2004).

A third context is aggression in same-sex litter groups, thought to be caused by a change in the ranking order and/or reproductive frustration. It is more frequent in female litter groups than in male ones. The presence of odours from the opposite sex is not essential or a valid trigger nor can the aggression be explained by overcrowding as frequency of aggressive outbreaks is not associated with the number of individuals (Clark & Galef 2001a; Scheibler *et al.* 2005a,b).

Under natural conditions, aggressive behaviour may occur in the same contexts, but instead leads to forced dispersal of fertile, reproductively active individuals.

Reproduction

Under laboratory conditions, gerbils reproduce all year round, whereas in the wild, the main reproductive season is from April to August, with only 2–3 litters per year (Naumov & Lobachev 1975; Liu *et al.* 2017). Females born in the first litter mature in the same summer, while later born ones overwinter with their families mature and disperse in the following year (Liu *et al.* 2017). Even under constant laboratory conditions, animals may show seasonal variation in their reproductive effort. The mediating factor is supposedly the prevailing humidity. In the light of discoveries of non-photic stimuli and their impact on circannual rhythms, systematic research is needed.

Vaginal opening of females is at 40–76 days of age, depending on their social surroundings (Norris & Adams 1979b). Sexual maturity occurs at 63–84 days of age if the female is separated from her mother. The mean number of litters per reproductive life span in females is 7.6 ± 3.8, but up to more than 15 litters have been observed. Lifetime reproductive success is 33–48 young born per female (maximum 54). Older females (2 years of age and more) tend to have smaller litters and longer interbirth intervals than younger females. However, the weaning rate is often higher in older females, reflecting a higher intensity of parental care (Thiessen & Yahr 1977). The sex ratio is affected by several factors such as population structure, food availability, stress level and/or health status.

Females are receptive directly after having given birth (post-partum oestrus). Beyond that, the oestrous cycle is suppressed until the end of lactation. Therefore, a common timeframe between litters under laboratory conditions is either 25–28 days or 50–60 days. The duration of the oestrous cycle ranges from 9 to 21 days. Abortion, infanticide and/or variation of the oestrous cycle can be triggered by the presence of unfamiliar males, social instability, change in housing conditions, even change of the position of the cage in the rack (Rohrbach 1982; Scheibler unpubl.). In male laboratory gerbils, testes descend at 30–45 days of age. A rapid increase of testosterone can be measured after day 42 indicating activity of Leydig cells. Spermatozoa are visible from day 60, the maximum sperm production is reached by day 70. Around this time, mating behaviour begins (70–84 days), and fertility can be assumed by day 90, when sperm is distributed in the epididymis (Pinto-Fochi *et al.* 2016).

Paternal care

Male gerbils take an active role in parental care from day 2 to 4 after birth, with nest-building, warming the young, attempts to retrieve them and allogrooming described (Waring & Perper 1980; Clark *et al.* 2001a; Clark & Galef 2001b; Weinandy *et al.* 2001; Martínez *et al.* 2015, 2019), which enhances the offspring's development (Piovanotti Arua & Vieira 2004). Moreover, the breeding male becomes the social centre for the older offspring when the female gives birth in a second nest. In a case study, the body temperature of a male has been reported to increase slightly during paternal care, similar to lactation hyperthermia of females (Weinandy and Gattermann (1996). Martínez *et al.* (2015) demonstrated an association of higher concentrations of testosterone, oestradiol and dihydrotestosterone with an inhibition of aggression towards pups. A follow-up study showed an association of testosterone increase during copulation with an increase of oestrogen and androgen receptors in the olfactory bulb and medial preoptic area possibly facilitating the parental response (Martínez *et al.* 2019).

Impact of uterine position on reproductive performance

Mertice Clark and Bennett Galef have demonstrated in a series of experiments that gerbil males strongly differ in their reproductive performance depending on their position in their mother's wombs (Clark *et al.* 1992, 1997, 1998; Clark & Galef 1994, 1999, 2000).

Males gestated between two sisters ('dud' males) will have much lower adult circulating testosterone levels, low territorial and sexual activity levels, but very high nest-bound activity levels (nest-building and caring for pups), whereas males gestated between two brothers ('stud' males) will develop into sexually and territorially very active adults, but with less interest in pup care. According to these authors, this phenomenon leads to a testosterone-mediated trade-off between parental and sexual efforts. In contrast, more recent studies by Martínez et al. (2015, 2019) show that higher testosterone levels have a positive influence on the level paternal care. This suggests that hormone concentration alone cannot be sufficient to determine behaviour, and that receptor sensitisation and modification of the endocrine response are also likely to be critical.

Uses in research

Gerbils have been mainly kept under laboratory conditions for research purposes in the fields of parasitology, medicine and to a lesser degree for behavioural studies. Research in neurobiology, bioacoustics, behavioural biology, eco-physiology and immunology/toxicology/parasitology involving gerbils is among the most common areas of study.

Breeds, strains and genetics

Breeding history

The French missionary Abbé Armand David produced the first systematic description of the species in 1866, while exploring Northern China. He sent three specimens of what he described as 'yellow rats with long, hair-covered tails' to Henry Milne-Edwards of the Natural History Museum in Paris. The first scientific description and scientific name *Meriones unguiculatus* was then published in 1867. Between World Wars 1 and 2, an increasing need for laboratory animals for medical research purposes lead to the introduction of new laboratory species. In case of the Mongolian gerbil, the original request came from the Kitasato Institute in Japan. Their breeding stock was based on 20 pairs from Manchuria delivered by C. Kasuga in 1935 (Rich 1968). In 1949, M. Nomura established a second breeding stock at the Central Laboratories for Experimental Animals, Tokyo. Only 5 years later, 11 pairs of gerbils were sent to the 'West Foundation'/Tumblebrook Farm in Brant Lake (USA) to Victor Schwentker. Their breeding is only based on 9 reproductive individuals (4 males, 5 females) from the original 11 pairs. Nevertheless, breeding was successful, and several universities and commercial laboratories were supplied. The European laboratory and later pet gerbils primarily originated from the US breeding stock, but it is likely that gerbils were also introduced via Russia and Eastern Europe even though documentation shows some gaps due to language barriers.

Another introduction of wild animals was the result of a German–Mongolian expedition led by Ingo W. Stuermer in 1995. Here, 60 animals were imported and a breeding stock (Strain Ugoe:MU95) was established to facilitate fresh genetic material and to allow comparisons to the established laboratory breeding stock (Stuermer 1998; Stuermer et al. 1998, 2003; Blottner et al. 2000; Blottner & Stuermer 2006; Neumann et al. 2001). Most animals used today are descendants of these two founder colonies. Studies conducted at the Zoological institute of Beijing are descendants of wild caught animals from the associated research stations in Manchuria (Wang & Zhong 2006; Zhang & Wang 2007; Liu et al. 2007 2017).

Domestication

Behavioural responses and physiological and anatomical features were compared between generation F0, F1 and F2 versus established laboratory strains (Stuermer 1998; Blottner et al. 2000; Neumann et al. 2001; Stuermer et al. 2003; Stuermer et al. 2006). Domesticated gerbils have higher body weight with higher variability, higher testes, liver and total fat weight, lower brain weight (17.7% less in laboratory gerbils), lower heart, lung, kidney and stomach weights, shorter intestinal tract length, higher testicular hormonal activity, bigger litters (mean 5.6 pups in lab gerbils versus 4 in first-generation wild gerbils bred in the lab), but also faster auditory discrimination learning in laboratory gerbils compared to wild gerbils. As expected, a reduced microsatellite variability and therefore genetic variability in general was also documented in domesticated gerbils. Epileptic seizures do not occur in wild gerbils but started to appear in their offspring/F1. Stuermer (Stuermer et al. 2003; Stuermer et al. 2006) observed rapid changes towards domestication characteristics with only a few generations of breeding wild gerbils in the laboratory. Behaviourally, slightly higher activity levels were observed in wild animals. Remarkably, wild gerbils (F0) tend to develop less stereotypic digging in the corner of the cage. This may be because stereotypical digging develops at a relatively young stage when F0 gerbils are not housed in a cage.

Colour mutations

Since the occurrence of the first coat colour mutations ('spotted', and 'white/Himalayan'), a wide variety of coat colours has emerged (15 in 2019, Waring et al. 1978; Swanson 1980; Waring & Poole 1980; Henley & Robinson 1981; Leiper & Robinson 1984, 1985, 1986; Matsuzaki et al. 1989). To date, there are at least seven known loci coding for gerbil coat colour, some with up to four alleles. Agouti, black, grey and spotted are the most frequent colours in laboratory gerbils. Apparently, differences exist in behaviour and physiology between the agouti and black gerbils (Dizinno & Clancy 1978) as well as in seizure propensity in gerbils (Gray-Allan & Wong 1990; Fujisawa et al. 2003). Waring et al. (1978) reported that homozygous 'spotted' is lethal, causing abortion in about 25% of cases. Females also seem to prefer males of their own fur colour (Wong et al. 1990).

Gerbil suppliers and available strains

Four main providers of laboratory gerbil strains exist: Charles River Laboratories UK (Crl:MON (Tum)), Elevage Janvier, B&K Universal Ltd. and Harlan Netherlands

(Hsd: MON). Hsd: MON are derived from a nucleus colony obtained from the University of Missouri, Columbia, in 1991. Crl:MON (Tum) were obtained at Tumblebrook Farms in 1995, and were rederived in 1996. Both strains are predominantly agouti with some black animals. Though listed as outbred by vendors, most of these gerbils can be considered inbred due to several bottlenecks and founder effects in the history of laboratory gerbil breeding. Several authors have described and bred seizure-prone gerbils (Gray-Allan & Wong 1990; Buckmaster & Wong 2002; Fujisawa et al. 2003). However, these animals are not currently available from the large laboratory animal breeding companies (see above) and the original authors would have to be contacted for these strains.

General husbandry

Enclosures

Gerbils should be kept in solid-bottomed cages with a thick layer of substrate (at least 5 cm) to allow for digging/moving material. Cages should be made out of gnaw-resistant material, for example polycarbonate. Height should be at least 15 cm, but preferably 18 cm, to allow an erect posture. The EU Council's Group of Experts on Rodents and Rabbits suggested a minimum cage floor area of 1200 cm^2 and a height of 18 cm for gerbils, with 150 cm^2 per animal weighing less than 40 g, and 250 cm^2 per animal weighing more than 40 g, either for same-sex groups or breeding pairs and their offspring (ETS No. 123 Appendix A). If an artificial burrow (nest box and 20 cm access tube) is fitted in a cage, minimum floor area for breeding pairs should be 1500–1800 cm^2 (Cage type 4).

Environmental provisions – Burrows and shelters

Captive and domesticated gerbils show pronounced burrow digging behaviour, and this appetence to dig and hide from light is a challenge in terms of animal welfare under laboratory conditions. In the wild, gerbils have extensive burrow systems with several entrances and foraging chambers and one nesting chamber. The number of entrances and depth of burrow varies by type of burrow, season and location (Scheibler et al. 2006a). Raising gerbils without a burrow or burrow-like structure in the laboratory has a profound effect on their behaviour. Wiedenmayer (1995,1996, 1997a and 1997b) found that the lack of an adequate burrow structure consisting of at least a nest chamber and access tunnel leads to stereotypic digging in the corner of the cage. This behaviour was exhibited for up to 21% of active time with bout lengths from 12 sec up to several minutes at a time. It did not develop in gerbils with access to a burrow structure. Moreover, upon presentation of a startling visual stimulus, shelter-reared gerbils respond by fleeing, foot-drumming and concealment, whereas open-reared gerbils approach the stimulus. After 24 h of access to a shelter, open-reared gerbils also start to flee into the shelter (Clark & Galef 1977; Cheal & Foley 1985; Cheal et al. 1986).

Minimum provision should be a dark nesting chamber of at least 13 cm × 13 cm × 13 cm accessible via a dark tunnel (length about 15–20 cm, diameter about 5 cm). The Council of Europe ETS No. 123 (European Convention for the Protection of Vertebrate Animals Used for Experimental and Other Scientific Purposes 2006) recommends either a thick layer of substrate for digging or a burrow substitute for gerbils. No such artificial burrow system is commercially available to date. One simple solution is to connect standardised type IV cages with tunnels. The height can be modified by cutting of the bottom of the cage and connecting 2 or 3 cages together. This facilitates the use of commercial racks and established cage materials.

Although provision of burrowing materials and systems for laboratory breeding stock requires additional costs and effort in the daily caretaking routines, it is important for the quality of any study that the animals be able to express their natural behaviours (see also Chapter 10: Environmental enrichment: animal welfare and scientific validity).

Environmental enrichment

Digging and chewing opportunities

Since gerbils are proficient diggers and gnawers, they should be provided with digging and gnawing opportunities: digging substrate such as wood chip bedding, and chewable materials such as hay, straw, tissues, paper, cardboard, branches and wood sticks; which can all be autoclaved. Wood chips and wood shavings, of for example aspen, are commonly used as bedding material. However, dust development due to the constant gnawing and digging may be challenging with respect to health and safety.

Sand bath

Offering a sand bath (bird or chinchilla sand) has proven very successful for fur cleanness and fur shine. Pendergrass and Thiessen (1983) have shown that sandbathing helps thermoregulation in gerbils. In the experience of the author, gerbils use the sand bath regularly – first to wallow and roll in, then to use as a latrine, and it should therefore be cleaned regularly. This initial additional effort pays off, as the exchange of the complete bedding can be reduced. It should be mentioned here that change of a cage means stress for an animal due to the loss of its familiar odours. Weinandy and Gattermann (1996) compared different stressors using implanted heart-rate transmitters and found that cage change is less stressful than group restructuring, but more so than handling, confrontation with an intruder or confrontation with a resident animal. Gerbils need about 30 min for their heart rate to return to baseline after cage cleaning when done in their active time, and 120 min if cages are cleaned during their resting time. Partial cleans should therefore be considered and lactating and gravid females should not be disturbed.

Nesting

The female builds the pup nest, but the male is also involved in nest-building. For that purpose, males and females shred material (tissues, straw, hay, textiles) into small pieces, collect these in their mouth and carry bundles of them to their nest. If a nest box or shelter is available, gerbils also pad it out with nesting material. Although females generally prefer a nest box for parturition, they may move the nest if disturbed by handling or caretakers. A nest is either globular or more frequently hemispherical, with a depression in the centre. Globular nests are constructed if the gerbils are kept at low ambient temperatures, as it serves thermoregulatory and reproductive function.

Running wheels

As outlined in the preceding text, running wheels seem to have an impact on the activity pattern of gerbils (Figure 23.2). Beyond that, they may provide some value as enrichment and an opportunity for physical exercise. However, running wheels placed in larger semi-enclosures were not heavily used (author's observation). If running wheels are used, they should have a 30 cm diameter, with a solid surface that provides grip and with no rails. Textile covers can be used, but they are usually transformed into nesting material and then gaps in the fabric can cause serious risk of injuries. In comparison with hamsters, gerbils don't seem to have the same tendency for the stereotypic wheel running (own observation).

Feeding/Watering

Water

Gerbils exhibit several adaptations to dry climate: they excrete relatively low amounts of highly concentrated urine (3–4 ml/day) in ad libitum water conditions and dry faecal pellets (McManus 1972a). They tolerate high salt concentrations (McManus 1972a). Mongolian gerbils are able to survive without drinking water or fresh, green food by the use of metabolic water, for example via the oxidation of lipids (Wang et al. 2003). If provided with ad libitum water, gerbils consume 4–10 ml/day (McManus 1972a; Field & Sibold 1999). Experiments by Thiessen and Yahr (1977) show that depending on the composition of the food, i.e. its fat content, water-deprived gerbils die after losing 30% of their body weight. Water deprivation also results in a halt of reproduction in breeding pairs. Pregnant and lactating females are especially susceptible to water undersupply. In general, it is easier to provide water ad libitum via bottles or an automated drinking system than by regular supply from greens and vegetables. In case of social instability, monopolised access should be avoided by providing two or more water sources at different, distant places. Sprinkling water on the bedding is sometimes practised as it enhances water uptake. Due to the latrines, the bedding is usually very clean; therefore, no health hazard is associated.

Feeding

Gerbils are granivorous-herbivorous animals (Wang et al. 2003); seeds and grains are complemented by green parts of plants like alfalfa, and various other, locally available plants with the occasional insect or larva (Figure 23.4, Bannikov 1954; Naumov & Lobachev 1975; Scheibler et al. 2006a). Gerbils also learn food preferences from familiar or related conspecifics (Galef et al. 1998; Valsecchi et al. 1996, 2002), and hunger influences the acquisition of food preferences (Forkman 1995).

Gerbils hoard food extensively, both in the wild and in the laboratory (Naumov & Lobachev 1975; Agren et al. 1989b; Tsurim & Abramsky 2004). Hoarding of up to 20 kg of food for the winter makes them a pest species on agricultural land (Naumov & Lobachev 1975). When providing food, it must be considered that the animals will hoard (and cover it) so this may act as a health hazard eventually due to fouling and moulding.

In the laboratory, gerbils can be fed standard mouse, rat or hamster breeding chow. The protein content should be 18–22%, and fat content only 4% to prevent the development of metabolic syndrome and obesity. If none of the brands provided fulfils the criteria, a mix can be fed. It is advisable to differentiate between food for non-breeding and breeding animals. The latter needs a higher energy and protein content. Gerbils eat about 18 times during the day at random times. Therefore, their stomachs always contain a small amount of food (Kanarek et al. 1977). As a rule, food should be presented ad libitum and not be time restricted. However, it needs to be considered that feed presentation method can affect weight gain in gerbils. Mulder et al. (2010) showed that weight gain after weaning was significantly higher when fed was provided on cage floor or in J-style feeder compared to the wire bar lid feed hopper. The authors recommended feeding from cage floor or using the J-style feeder.

Pellet diet can be supplemented with grains and seed mixtures, and/or greenery for the intake of vitamins, trace elements and to allow natural behaviour. If a treat is needed for training purposes, sunflower or pumpkin seeds are the most desired seeds. It must be clear that these seeds have a very high fat content. It is recommended to feed these only sparingly and evaluate non-caloric or low-caloric baits of different suppliers as alternatives.

Dietary enrichment, such as salad, dandelion leaves, cucumber, carrots, pumpkin (seeds and flesh), zucchini, fennel, and fruits, such as apples, pears, melon, fulfil a stimulation function. In the wild, gerbils consume a wide variety of aromatic herbal plants like mugworts (*Artemisia*, Scheibler et al. 2006a). In contrast to degus or hamsters, gerbils have not been found to be susceptible to type 2 diabetes mellitus (Besselmann & Hatt 2004); therefore, sweet fruit and vegetables can be offered occasionally. In order to avoid the risk of introducing food-borne pathogens, particularly bacterial agents, it is recommended to sanitise the exterior of fresh food items.

Social housing

Gerbils are social animals and should be housed in groups or pairs. Neonatal maternal separation triggers behavioural and neurochemical, depression-like alterations that differ in males and females with male offspring responding more sensitively (Jaworska et al. 2008). Loss of a partner or separation of a harmonious breeding pair can also lead to depression- and anxiety-like symptoms, and even body mass increase/obesity (Starkey & Hendrie 1997, 1998a,b; Hendrie & Starkey 1998; Hendrie & Pickles 2000; Starkey et al. 2007). Singly housed gerbils show increased activity and heart rate (Weinandy 1995), as well as pathological changes in the

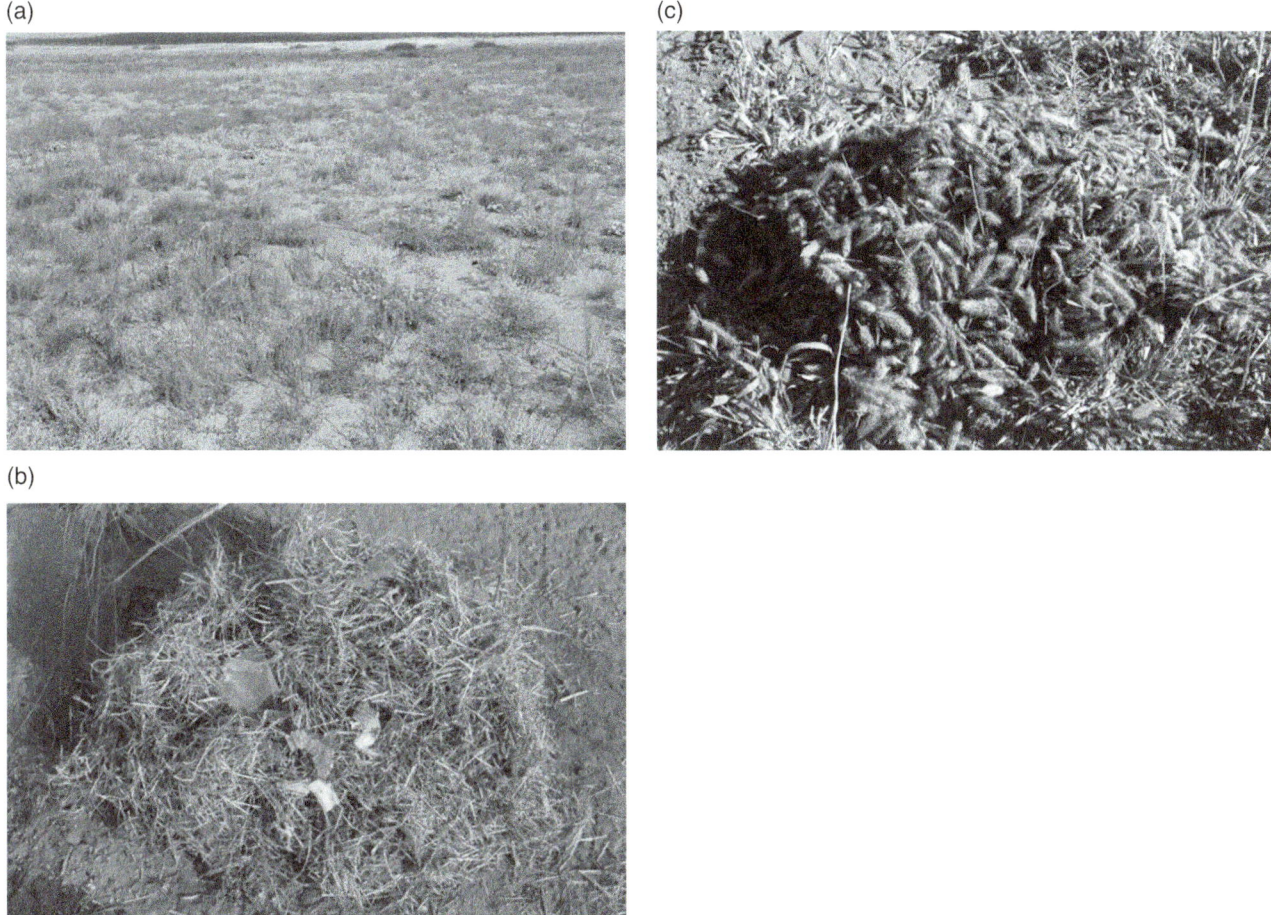

Figure 23.4 (a) Natural habitat of Mongolian gerbils, picture taken in Inner Mongolia, China near Xilinhot. The loose soil may indicate the close location of the nesting chamber. (b) Bedding material of an excavated burrow. (c) Food storage of an excavated burrow.

dopamine innervation of their prefrontal cortex that impair learning and working memory (Winterfeld *et al.* 1998). If gerbils of a group are separated for too long (roughly 1.5 hours), they may react with aggression upon regrouping with their groupmates. This is enhanced if the smell of the returning animal is modified, which can arise from some experimental protocols. Breeding pairs should not be disrupted at all (Norris 1985) and older offspring can be left in the cage beyond the birth of a new litter if the cage size and enrichment allows the opportunity for the animals to build a second nest. If cage size and enrichment are insufficient, an increase of infanticide can be observed, usually due to stress, inquisitive behaviour and/or accidental injuries.

It is common practice to keep same-sex litter groups under laboratory conditions, as well as in private households when keeping them as pets. As mentioned previously, same-sex male groups are usually more harmonious than same-sex female groups. Pair-housing of adult, non-familiar animals for non-reproductive purposes is extraordinarily difficult.

Identification and sexing

Gerbils can easily be marked by clipping their fur/hair tips in defined patterns or at pre-defined locations. This marking is visible for about two weeks. Colour dyes can also be used, but the intense grooming needs to be considered and it is not recommended as it can change the smell of individuals. Injection of subcutaneous microchips needs a short anaesthesia but marks the animals permanently. The newest generation of microchips are only 4 mm long and less than 1 mm in diameter. Nevertheless, animals should be adult when microchipped due to the potential risks of the anaesthetic and the presence of subcutaneous fat tissue in adult animals which embeds the transponder. Ear notching is not reliable due to the size of the ears and the fur. The animal itself or companions may remove ear tags, as gerbils usually respond very vigorously to anything attached to their body. Dahlborn *et al.* (2013) provide a comprehensive comparison of the available techniques.

Sexing of gerbils is easiest in juveniles and adults although handling of the juveniles can be challenging. Animals that are used to handling can be gently grasped and sat in an upright position, exposing the ventral side and the genitals. Another possibility is to lift the tail, but this requires great sensitivity as the tail and skin is extremely thin in juveniles and subadults. Alternatively, the animal can be placed in a transparent box or bag (with air holes!), allowing visual inspection without direct handling.

As in other rodents, the distance between genital papilla and anus is double in males, and the connecting line is thin and covered with fur. Scrotal sacs are darkly coloured in agouti males and already visible in older juveniles/ subadults.

Physical environment

Mongolian gerbils are distributed in the temperate steppes of East Asia. The climate is characterised by hot summers and cold winters. Precipitation is low in general, and gerbils require those dryer conditions under laboratory conditions (35–45%). Gerbils do not hibernate which means that they are able to tolerate these extreme temperature ranges. However, as a fossorial species, gerbils escape from unfavourable conditions into their burrows. The nesting chamber of winter burrows lies under the frozen layer and is well insulated with dry grass. Juvenile gerbils are unable to thermoregulate before the age of 12 days, and their endothermic capacity increases until the age of 21 days (McManus 1972b). Current guidelines require temperatures of 20–24 °C (ETS No. 123 Appendix A). During autogrooming, the secretion of the Harderian gland is distributed over the fur. At higher humidity, the fur cannot dry properly, and thermoregulation is negatively affected as the thin fur loses its insulation capacity. This is visually recognisable as matted, ruffled fur (Thiessen & Yahr 1977; Grant & Thiessen 1989).

Health monitoring and quarantine

Hormone analyses, immune parameters, body temperature, heart rate and parasite load are all valuable ways to assess gerbil health status. However, costs and the invasive nature of the methods need to be considered. Gerbils received from other colonies should be put in quarantine, or at least be observed for 7–14 days in a separate holding area. Non-invasive indicators of health status are the animals' appearance (fur shiny, smooth and not matted, ruffled fur), hair loss on the tail (sign of stress), body weight (i.e. weight loss as an indicator of poor health), and behaviour (esp. body posture). Gerbils should be inquisitive, active, and should eat and drink normally.

Transport

Only healthy animals should be transported. Special care must be taken if pregnant or lactating females are transported. Only animals compatible with each other should be transported together. Sufficient air circulation and protection from environmental influences have highest priority. It cannot be stressed enough that gerbils, like many other rodents, cannot sweat, and risk of overheating and dehydration is therefore substantial. Additionally, stress-triggered seizures often occur.

Gnaw-proof boxes of non-toxic material are necessary. Often, type II or III cages are used for gerbil transport. Time in transit must be minimised as much as possible. Food and water should be provided on both short and long journeys, since delays can always occur. Water can be offered in the form of gel packs ('solid drink'), moistened food and /or vegetables of high-water content such as cucumbers, apple or lettuce. See also Chapter 12: Transportation of laboratory animals.

Breeding

Gerbils are less prolific breeders than mice or rats, due to a combination of longer interbirth intervals, smaller litter sizes and higher pre- and postnatal pup mortality, reproductive skew and cooperative breeding. Future breeding animals should remain with their parents as long as possible. This is advantageous for their breeding performance, providing experience in pup care (Salo & French 1989; French 1994).

When pairing animals, the age, weight/size and social housing conditions need to be considered, as well as the genetic background. Norris and Adams (1972) found the shortest interval (40 days) from pairing to parturition if mature, sexually experienced males were paired with either inexperienced or experienced females. Clark et al. (2002) introduced females of various ages (35, 70, 90 and 100 days) to experienced males and found latency to parturition being 34, 36, 45 and 78 days, respectively. The probability of getting impregnated by the first male they were paired with was much higher among the younger females. Body weight and size seem to have an influence, as females usually avoid mating with a male that is younger or lighter (Scheibler unpubl.). If both partners or the male are less experienced, then parturition takes place later (about 60 days, but can be up to 90 days, Norris & Adams 1972). If a pair does not produce a litter within three months of being paired, it is very unlikely that they will successfully breed, and alternative breeding pairings should be considered. Ideally, the animals are paired at an age of 60–90 days, as they show a higher appetence for mating, less territorial behaviour and are usually fertile. It can be beneficial to monitor the oestrous cycle. The optimal time to mate is during pro-oestrus. Gerbils should not be paired too early, since familiarity resulting from growing up together can inhibit or delay reproduction in females (Clark & Galef 2001a; Clark et al. 2002; Clark & Galef 2002). Suggested breeding age for males is 75–85 days (Field & Sibold 1999). It is good practice to choose those males from same-sex litter groups that have larger and/or clearly visible testicles/scrotum. Females often reject group members that are subordinate or submissive. For the first encounter, a contact mesh can be used to prevent territorial aggression. As a minimum precaution, it is recommended to place both animals in an unfamiliar cage. If no new cage is used, then the female should be placed in the male's cage and not vice versa. Intensive anogenital sniffing and moderate chasing is normal. Aggression is demonstrated by grinding teeth which may be followed by biting attacks. In that case, animals should be separated immediately. Second attempts with the same animals should be avoided. Positive signs of a successful pairing are poking the head under the snout of another, greeting calls, allogrooming, rubbing the ventral gland and finally huddling together in a nesting box. It is debatable whether enrichment should be provided or not in this situation; the best compromise is to provide nesting material, but not a chamber for the first 24 hours. This allows visual inspection, as a nesting chamber could be used as an escape location. The quality of the nest can be a good indicator, with more harmonious pairs typically producing better nests. Following a successful initial pairing, breeding pairs typically remain harmonious.

Conception and pregnancy

Basic reproductive data presented in this section come from a range of sources (Marston & Chang 1965; Norris & Adams 1972, 1974, 1981a,b; Norris 1987; Tumblebrook Farm 1979; Burley 1979; Scheibler unpubl.). Mating occurs during oestrus, post-partem oestrus (13 hours after parturition, 80% fertility) and after weaning. The duration of the oestrous cycle varies between 4 and 9 days. While duration of pro-oestrus, oestrus and di-oestrus is comparably stable, the duration of met-oestrus varies. Any form of stress and disturbance can lead to a prolongation of the met-oestrous stage. Gerbils become active around sundown and females are then most active when in oestrus, and mate with males in their own family and presumably with neighbouring males.

The oestrous cycle is characterised by a short, 12–18 hrs oestrus, followed by 24–48 hrs met-oestrus (can be prolonged to 5 days), a very short 4–12 hrs di-oestrus, and a pro-oestrus of about 24–36 hrs. The oestrous stages can be differentiated based on the cell composition seen on vaginal cytology. During oestrus, only cornified epithelial cells are visible with a complete lack of leukocytes. Met- and pro-oestrus are challenging to differentiate if taken out of the sequence, as epithelial cells and leukocytes are visible during both stages and their number is individual – rather than stage-specific. However, there is tendency that the number and size of horny epithelial cells is larger in met-oestrus. Di-oestrus can be differentiated from met- and pro-oestrus by the presence of proteinaceous fluid 'slime' (Figure 23.3). The behaviour of females changes during pro-oestrus and oestrus. Females show a higher social appetence, and more allogrooming. After mating, sperm can be found in vaginal smears and a vaginal plug can persist for hours (Weinandy et al. 2002). Post-partum oestrus has been studied by Prates and Guerra (2005). They described a short-duration oestrus of 7–9 hours beginning about 13.5 hrs after parturition. Ovulation average is 6.6 ova (range 4–9). The phase is dominated by maternal behaviour including allogrooming, nest-building and warming the young. Copulatory behaviour patterns of females on the day of oestrus were described by Burley (1979). These include piloerection, presenting posture (lordosis), darting and foot-drumming, as well as an increase of female-initiated allogrooming and sniffing of the male's head and anogenital region. During oestrus, the male shows piloerection posture, presenting posture, intensive sniffing and chasing before mounting the female, who responds with lordosis. Mounting occurs many times during about 6 hrs. Mating is accompanied by the male regularly foot-drumming. Duration of a mount is about 2 sec. After mounting, both male and female lick their genitalia.

Implantation usually occurs 7–8 days after fertilisation. Pregnancy duration is between 24 and 28 days. However, if fertilisation occurred during post-partum oestrus, implantation of the blastocyst is delayed. According to Norris and Adams (1981a,b), pregnancy duration is increased by 1.9 days per neonate if three or more pups of the previous litter are suckled. Pregnancy duration can increase to a maximum of 48 days. Pregnancy itself has a strong impact on maternal resources, especially if females are pregnant and continuing to nurse their last litter; these animals are typically less fecund (smaller, more female-based litters) and show lower attachment to their mates (Clark et al. 2006). Pregnancy can be detected from day 15, and the teats are clearly visible from day 14. The female gains 10–30 g of weight during pregnancy. Mating with unfertile males can lead to a pseudo-pregnancy of 13–23 days. Embryo-transfer in gerbils has been described by Norris and Adams (1986).

Behaviour of males during parturition varies and largely depends on the female's behaviour. If older offspring is present, the female usually gives birth in a second nest that she defends against the older litter. The male is often tolerated but does not stay in the nest the whole time. Alternatively, the male is as close as is accepted by the female and undertakes attempts to mate whenever possible.

Parturition and infanticide

Parturition usually occurs during the night. The birth of one pup lasts about 10–15 min, and parturition for an entire litter somewhat longer than 1 hr. The female eats placentae and stillbirths. The number of pups depends on the age and condition of the female, with very young and older females delivering smaller litters. The role of males during parturition can be classified as a passive bystander, as they do not take an active part. Infanticide is rare in gerbils and independent of sex. It occurs spontaneously (Saltzman et al. 2006) or under poor husbandry conditions, for example if the female is undernourished during lactation. Social instability is another circumstance that may trigger the behaviour. Offspring may serve as a food source, as food-deprived males may become infanticidal (Elwood & Ostermeyer 1984).

Litter size and development

Neonatal mortality is around 20%, with most pups dying in the first 5 days. Larger litters (more than seven pups), litters of unexperienced females or litters with older offspring present tend to exhibit higher infant mortality with rates of up to 57% or 75% for single pup litters. Average pup sex ratio is 1.03 (M:F) at birth, decreasing to 1.0 at weaning due to higher mortality in male pups (Field & Sibold 1999). Causes for pup mortality are lack of care, hypothermia, milk undersupply, suffocation, older pups not reaching food or water due to cage layout/provision of pellets in elevated rack and infanticide. Ear opening in gerbil pups occurs between day 12 and 14, the first hair appears at 5–7 days, incisors erupt at 10–16 days, and the eyes open between days 16 and 20 (earliest eye opening at 14 days). Gerbil pups then begin to venture out of the nest box, start digging and eating solid food. Birth weight is inversely correlated with litter size. Singletons can weigh up to 3.3 g, pups in big litters (over 10 pups) only 2.6 g. Males are about 5% heavier than females, a sexual dimorphism that increases to 10% at older ages. Adult weight is reached at the age of about 3 months.

Weaning age

Gerbil pups are artificially weaned between 20 and 30 days. Weaning as early as 21 days requires specific justification and should only be considered if the breeding female is already heavily pregnant, and parturition is expected soon. A later weaning is advised, as the time between three and four weeks is critical both physiologically and mentally. Weaning weight should ideally be 25 g with 15–18 g being the minimum acceptable range, and the pups should be checked for irregularities in their growth rate. In the laboratory routine, it is good practice to wean pups before the next litter is born; however, in preparation of forming new breeding pairs it can be beneficial to leave planned future breeding animals with their mother for one breeding cycle to allow them to gain experience in alloparental care. It is always advisable to provide a small amount of food directly in the cage, as smaller or weaker animals can reach it without effort and older animals can display foraging behaviour. Pups start to ingest vegetables and salad from day 16 of age, and dry pelleted food from day 18 onwards.

Laboratory procedures

Handling

In many laboratories, gerbils are caught at the base of their tail, and then the body is immediately supported with the other hand. However, an easy way to catch gerbils is to use tubes since they will readily enter any tube provided. Also, if carefully habituated, gerbils can be caught with cupped hands. If gerbils are caught as part of a frequent procedure (weighing etc.), it can be beneficial to end the procedure with a treat (sunflower or pumpkin seed) to create a positive association. Over time, if routine handling is managed efficiently and without stress for the animals, gerbils habituate to the handling and are then more willing to participate. Gerbils should never be caught at the tip of their tail as they tend to struggle and kick vigorously, resulting in 'degloving' of the tail: i.e. the skin is shed and the gerbil escapes with the bloody remains of muscle and bones.

Gerbils can be restrained by neck-grip, i.e. holding by the fold of loose skin in the neck towards the shoulder region with thumb, index finger and middle finger, securing them also at the base of the tail ('scuffing') with the little finger and palm but as restraint induces stress, it should only be applied if necessary. Wild gerbils are usually transferred in a cotton bag from the trap. Gerbils can then be restrained through the fabric, the bag can be opened and used to wrap around the handler's hand/fist. This is advantageous as direct contact is avoided, and impact of the individuals' odour and ectoparasite transfer is minimised. In small animal veterinary practice, a soft towel is often used to restrain adult gerbils. They are tightly wrapped in a towel from behind and will often hold still as long as not too much pressure is applied around their body. A similar product is available as DecapiCones (Braintree Scientific, Inc., USA).

Monitoring methods

Recording body temperatures

As noted before, gerbils have a body temperature of 38.1–38.4 °C. Body temperature can be measured by using a rectal probe, but this requires handling and manipulation of the animal, which in itself might induce stress and temperature changes. For regular temperature readings, subcutaneous temperature-sensitive passive transponders, injected under isoflurane anaesthesia between the shoulder blades, can be used (Kort et al. 1998; Newsom et al. 2004). Infrared thermography can also be used to measure body surface temperature in lightly restrained animals. If gerbils are implanted with heart-rate transmitters in the peritoneum, core temperature is usually measured simultaneously (Weinandy 1995; Moons et al. 2007). However, the implantation is a major surgery, and a recovery period needs to be planned, as thermoregulation is affected due to the metabolic effects and the requirement to clip fur from the animal for aseptic surgery.

Blood sampling

For haematological and clinical chemistry values in gerbils, see Field and Sibold (1999). Blood volume is 6.7% of body weight or 66–78 ml/kg (van Zutphen et al. 2001). Conservatively, maximal blood volume collected should not exceed 10% of the calculated total blood volume. European guidelines (Directive 2010/63/EU) on the basis of Diehl et al. (2001) allow up to 15%, if the animal has at least a 4-week recovery period. If blood collection is planned on a weekly basis, then not more than 7.5% of the blood volume should be taken. Clearly, additional blood loss from the wound must be included and needs to be considered in the experimental design (Diehl et al. 2001).

Blood collection routes have been summarised by Field and Sibold (1999) and Diehl et al. (2001) on a more general basis. Blood can be collected from the lateral tail vein after warming the tail, either by placing it in warm water, by placing the animal under an infrared lamp or in a warmed chamber (30–35 °C for 10–15 min) to allow for vasodilation. Another accepted method is the puncture of the saphenous vein (Hem et al. 1998). Small amounts of blood (0.1–0.2 ml) can also be attained by cutting the tip of the tail, a procedure which should be avoided and never performed more than once per animal according to animal welfare guidelines. Retro-orbital sinus blood collection is also possible in gerbils, but it needs to be performed under anaesthesia, and should only be performed with recovery in rare circumstances with exceptional scientific justification because of its potential impact on the animal. Additionally, it must only be performed every 2 weeks at the same eye and is only an option if other peripheral veins are used for dosing but a large blood volume is needed[1]. Cardiac puncture should be reserved for terminal blood collection and must always be performed under anaesthesia.

---

[1] https://nc3rs.org.uk/hamster-retro-orbital-non-surgicalterminal (Accessed November 15, 2021)

Urine and faecal sampling

To collect urine, gerbils can be placed individually in metabolic cages. Gerbils can also be placed in wire mesh bottom cages with a sheet of metal below to collect urine for a maximum of 24 hrs (Fenske 1990, 1996; Waiblinger & König 2004). Handling stress can also induce urination, although this should not be used as a method of choice for urine collection.

Faecal samples can be easily collected, since gerbils eat frequently and therefore also defecate frequently. Therefore, fresh faeces (0.5–1 g) can be collected within an hour by placing an animal in a fresh cage or separated from the group (separation should not last longer than 1.5 hours to avoid social disturbance). Faecal pellets are dry and do not stick to the bedding.

Milk

Collection of milk in gerbils has been described by Rassin *et al.* (1978). For the exact method of collecting milk from small rodents, see Feller and Boretos (1967) and Raffel and König (1999).

Administration of substances

Routine handling procedures used in mice and rats can generally also be used in gerbils. Subcutaneous injections are usually given in the loose skin between the shoulder blades. To administer a substance by subcutaneous injection, the animal is placed on the wire top of a cage, where it will try to walk away. The base of the tail is picked up with one hand, and the hindquarters of the animal lifted slightly off the grid. With the same hand, thumb and forefinger, the loose skin at the neck and backline is picked up and the animal can be raised to an upright, vertical position (head up), at which time the injection can be made with the free hand or by an additional person. This provides secure restraint and is advantageous as movement of the animal is minimised, allowing injection to be performed efficiently and with low risk for the animal. Intravenous injection in the femoral vein and the external jugular vein, both under anaesthesia, have been described since the lateral tail vein is not as easily accessible for injections in gerbils as in mice or rats due to their furry tail (Pérez-García *et al.* 2003; Kakol Palm & Hollaender 2007). When choosing an appropriate needle for injection, the viscosity, duration of application and volume must be considered. Typically, 23–25-gauge needles are preferred. Details on dosing substances by common routes can be found in Field and Sibold (1999) and Diehl *et al.* (2001).

Anaesthesia and analgesia

In small animal veterinary practice, isoflurane and sevoflurane inhalation anaesthesia via precision vaporiser is generally used as the method of choice in small mammals such as gerbils. A common regimen for these inhaled anaesthetics is 2–5% in oxygen for induction, and 1.2–2.3% in oxygen for maintenance. Isoflurane is not metabolised to a great degree; therefore, recovery is very quick. Importantly, it needs to be considered that isoflurane accumulates more slowly in a bodyfat. This means anaesthesia of obese animals is challenging, as initially more isoflurane is needed, and it takes longer until the desired state of anaesthesia is accomplished. But with the delayed accumulation in the fat body, a deeper state of narcosis is finally reached, and this may lead to apnoea. It is to be noted that these gaseous anaesthesia agents do not have analgesic properties, and therefore pre- and post-surgery analgesia must be administered. Field and Sibold (1999) present a list of commonly used injectable anaesthetics and their combinations. Some common intraperitoneally injectable anaesthetics for gerbils are: 50 mg/kg Ketamine and 2 mg/kg Climazolam; 50 mg/kg Ketamine and 2 mg/kg Xylazine or Pentobarbital 60–80 mg/kg (duration 30–45 min).

Postoperative pain should in any case be relieved, using appropriate analgesia, which is required by most countries' animal welfare guidelines. Multimodal analgesia has become the standard of care, for example incorporating subcutaneous buprenorphine (Temgesic) 0.05–0.2 mg/kg subcutaneous before surgery and every 8–12 hours, with a non-steroidal anti-inflammatory (NSAID) such as carprofen or meloxicam (dosing varies). Field and Sibold (1999), Carpenter and Marion (2017), Quesenberry *et al.* (2020) list suitable analgesia agents for gerbils.

Euthanasia

Methods to kill gerbils must be painless, safe to apply and ensure a quick loss of consciousness. In the recommendations for euthanasia of experimental animals, the EU-commission working party suggests the following methods of euthanasia for rodents in general, not specifically for gerbils (Close *et al.* 1996, 1997; AVMA 2020).

Chemical methods, injectable agents

Generally, if venepuncture and intravenous injection can be used, this application route is recommended, since they act faster than intraperitoneal injections, which might lead to irritation of the peritoneum based on studies in mice and rats (Laferriere & Pang 2020). Gerbils can be killed by an overdose of sodium pentobarbitone, for example by intraperitoneally injecting Pentobarbital (> 270 mg/kg, max. 200 mg/ml injectable solution; Field & Sibold 1999). Three times the anaesthetic dose is recommended. T61 must be injected intravenously very slowly, and prior sedation is required, as otherwise, the criterion of a painless death is not fulfilled.

Chemical methods, inhalational agents

A frequent method is the usage of inhalation anaesthesia agents such as isoflurane. The animals must be left long enough in the chamber, and death must be confirmed, when or, alternatively, an adequate state of anaesthesia is reached, the animal can be killed by another method, for example decapitation or exsanguination. Animal welfare aspects of using carbon dioxide for euthanasia have been discussed widely (see Conlee et al. 2005 for a review, but also Leach et al. 2005; Hawkins et al. 2016; Turner et al. 2020).

Physical methods

Decapitation via guillotine is within the physical methods the most common one. However, it must be emphasised that this method is only an option if all other possibilities are exhausted. Moreover, the animal needs to be anaesthetised, in order to ensure that the process is safe and fast process as required. If microwaves are used for euthanasia, only specialised apparatuses adapted to the size of the animal can be used to focus the irradiation exactly to the brain. Unless the animal is anesthetised, cervical dislocation is not a method of choice, as the criterion of ensuring a painless death cannot be fulfilled because of the high probability of degloving the tail.

Euthanasia of neonates

Neonates cannot be reliably killed by CO_2 alone, since they have a high tolerance for hypoxia based on studies in rats and mice. Physical methods, such as decapitation, are therefore needed for euthanasia of neonates (Klaunberg et al. 2004).

Common welfare problems

Health

In general, gerbils adapt well to captivity and are typically healthy. The animals should be checked daily for their health status and weighed at least once a week. Stressed animals are more susceptible to disease than unstressed ones.

Signs of disease

Diseased gerbils show a reduction of activity, and will often have a ruffled fur, a hunched posture and may have diarrhoea and loss of body weight. Elderly animals tend to become emaciated (> 3 years old) and to sink in at their flanks. Increased drinking might be indicative of either diabetes or renal failure.

Common diseases

Gerbils can contract Tyzzer's disease (*Clostridium piliforme*). Affected animals become apathetic and huddle in a hunched position in the corner of the cage with ruffled fur (Field & Sibold 1999). Sometimes, diarrhoea can be seen. Since these animals do not feed, weight loss is quite severe, and the animals die within 1–3 days. Tyzzer's disease can be spread among animals by soiled bedding. If an outbreak occurs, affected animals, cages and rooms should be quarantined immediately. Tetracycline has been used to treat mice and might also be effective in gerbils. Oxytetracycline added to drinking water can be used, and dehydrated animals should be given rehydration therapy, if they are not euthanised. Since *C. piliforme* is spore-forming, animal bodies, bedding, food and nesting material must be incinerated and cages, equipment and rooms thoroughly sterilised to eliminate the pathogen.

A much less severe condition is the red or sore nose disease, where the animals develop reddish sores (erythema) around the nose. Red nose disease is caused by a staphylococcal infection of the nose (*S. aureus*, Peckham et al. 1974) rather than a reaction to substrate or from gnawing on the bars. Treatment can be conducted by application of odourless topical antiseptics creams or a systemic antibiotic treatment (Chloromycetin 0.083 g/1100 ml water, or tetracycline 0.3 g/100 ml water for 14 days, as suggested by Field & Sibold 1999). However, good hygiene should prevent outbreak of this disease. As a rule, most gerbils recover from red nose disease; however, a change of the animals' management and how they are housed in terms of enrichment but also animals per cage and group constellation should be considered, as stress level and immune status contribute to the outbreak of the disease. Animals should only be killed if the sores spread to larger areas of front paws and face.

As previously mentioned, some gerbils are prone to epileptic seizures and are used as a model to screen for antiepileptic drugs. Juveniles develop seizures at 2 months of age. If an animal has not shown sign of seizures by the age of about 10 months, then is it unlikely to develop them later in life. There is a strong hereditary component, and breeding lines can be established with up to 80% of the animals exhibiting seizures to various degrees (Kaplan & Miezejes 1972; Loskota et al. 1974; Kaplan 1975; Frey 1987; Cutler & Mackintosh 1989; Kupferberg 2001). For research not concerned with epilepsy, known seizure-eliciting stimuli such as handling stress, dangling by the tail, novelty, blasts of air or sudden noise should be avoided, and it is particularly important to avoid seizure-prone strains (Fujisawa et al. 2003). Habituation to handling procedures, experience and development of coping mechanisms to deal with new stimuli, social support may reduce the occurrence of epileptic seizures.

Aged animals

In aged animals, sebaceous gland carcinomas are occasionally observed (Raflo & Diamond 1980; Matsuoka & Suzuki 1995; da Costa et al. 2007). In early stages, the tumour does not appear to affect the animal. As the mass grows, gerbils may scratch and groom more frequently, leading to open wounds, blood loss and secondary infections. Definitive treatment of the tumour involves surgical removal.

Chronic interstitial nephritis is occasionally diagnosed in aged gerbils. Affected gerbils lose weight and exhibit polyuria and polydipsia (Johnson-Delaney 1998). Histopathological lesions of the ventral prostate have also been observed in aged gerbils (Campos et al. 2008).

Abnormal behaviour

The two most common abnormal behaviours which develop in laboratory gerbils in response to inappropriate environments are stereotypic digging and bar-gnawing. Stereotypic digging is caused by the lack of an appropriate burrow structure, either self-dug or artificial. Therefore, provision with a dark nest box and access tube can significantly reduce the incidence of this behaviour (Wiedenmayer 1996, 1997a,b,c). The development of bar-gnawing can be prevented if juvenile gerbils are not separated from their parents before the next litter is born, i.e. if the juveniles are left with the parents for at least 5 weeks (Wiedenmayer 1997c; Waiblinger & König 2001, 2004; Waiblinger 2002, 2003). As discussed in the previous breeding sections, this might present some problems with standard laboratory routine.

A further factor that needs to be considered is light. Gerbils are usually housed in LD 12:12, if breeding is desired, then 14:10. A study by Juarez-Tapia et al. (2015) suggested an induction of anxiety and depressive-like behaviours in gerbils with a short-day light cycle (LD 8:16), as measured by established rodent behavioural tests.

Humane endpoints

If an animal shows signs of morbidity (disease or illness) or is found moribund (dying), then its condition should immediately be evaluated. The decision to treat or euthanise should be made with due consideration for the welfare of the animal by the qualified personnel (Toth 2000).

Acknowledgements

I want to thank Eva Waiblinger for valuable and inspiring conversations about gerbils in the past and providing the former edition of this book chapter, which was an enormous help. I also want to thank Robert Hubrecht and Claire Richardson for their support, objective proof reading, editing and patience during the writing process, otherwise this chapter had never been finished (most likely). Moreover, Birte Nielsen, Huw Golledge and two referees unknown by name provided valuable feedback and helped massively to shape this book chapter.

References

Agren, G., Zhou, Q. and Zhong, W. (1989a) Ecology and social behaviour of Mongolian gerbils, *Meriones unguiculatus*, at Xilinhot, Inner Mongolia, China. *Animal Behaviour*, **37**, 11–27.

Agren, G., Zhou, Q. and Zhong, W. (1989b) Territoriality, cooperation and resource priority: hoarding in the Mongolian gerbil, *Meriones unguiculatus*. *Animal Behaviour*, **37**, 28–32.

AVMA (American Veterinary Medical Association) (2020). *AVMA Guidelines for the Euthanasia of Animals*, 2020 edition. AMVA, Schaumburg, Illinois.

Baker, A. and Emerson, V.F. (1983) Grating Acuity of the Mongolian Gerbil (*Meriones unguiculatus*). *Behavioural Brain Research*, **8**, 195–209.

Bannikov, A.G. (1954) The places inhabited and natural history of *Meriones unguiculatus*. Mammals of the Mongolian People's Republic, USSR Academy of Sciences – Committee of the Mongolian People's Republic. Trudy Mongol'skoi Komissii Nr.53: 410–415.

Besselmann, D. and Hatt, J.M. (2004) Diabetes mellitus in rabbits and rodents. *Tierärztliche Praxis Ausgabe Kleintiere / Heimtiere*, **32**(6), 370–376.

Blottner, S., Franz, C., Rohleder, M. et al. (2000) Higher testicular activity in laboratory gerbils compared to wild Mongolian gerbils (*Meriones unguiculatus*). *Journal of the Zoological Society of London*, **250**, 462–466.

Blottner, S. and Stuermer, I.W. (2006) Reproduction of wild gerbils bred in the laboratory in dependence on generation and season: II. Spermatogenic activity and testicular testosterone concentration. *Animal Science*, **82**, 388–395.

Broom, D., Elwood, R.W., Lakin, J. et al. (1977) Developmental changes in several parameters of ultrasonic calling by young Mongolian gerbils (*Meriones unguiculatus*). *Journal of Zoology*, **183**, 281–290.

Buckmaster, P.S. and Wong, E.H. (2002) Evoked responses of the dentate gyrus during seizures in developing gerbils with inherited epilepsy. *Journal of Neurophysiology*, **88**(2), 783–793.

Burley, R.A. (1979) Pre-copulatory and copulatory behaviour in relation to stages of the oestrus cycle in the female Mongolian gerbil. *Behaviour*, **72**(3–4), 211–241.

Bytyqi, A. and Layer, P.G. (2005) Lamina formation in the Mongolian gerbil retina (*Meriones unguiculatus*). *Anatomy and Embryology*, **209**, 217–225.

Campos, S.G.P., Zanetoni, C., Scarano, W.R. et al. (2008) Age-related histopathological lesions in the Mongolian gerbil ventral prostate as a good model for studies of spontaneous hormone-related disorders. *International Journal of Experimental Pathology*, **89**(1), 13–24.

Carpenter, J. and Marion, C.J. (Ed.) (2017) *Exotic Animal Formulary*, 5th edn. Elsevier.

Cheal, M. and Foley, K. (1985). Developmental and experiential influences on ontogeny: The gerbil (*Meriones unguiculatus*) as a model. *Journal of Comparative Psychology*, **99**(3), 289.

Cheal, M., Foley, K. and Kastenbaum, R. (1986). Brief periods of environmental enrichment facilitate adolescent development of gerbils. *Physiology & Behavior*, **36**(6), 1047–1051.

Chevret, P. and Dobigny, G. (2005) Systematics and evolution of the subfamily *Gerbillinae* (Mammalia, Rodentia, Muridae). *Molecular Phylogenetics and Evolution*, **35**, 674–688.

Clark, M.M., Desousa, D., Vonk, J. and Galef, B.G. (1997) Parenting and potency: alternative routes to reproductive success in male Mongolian gerbils. *Animal Behaviour*, **54**, 635–642.

Clark, M.M. and Galef, B.G. (1977) The role of the physical rearing environment in the domestication of the Mongolian gerbil (*Meriones unguiculatus*). *Animal Behaviour*, **25**, 298–316.

Clark, M.M. and Galef, B.G. (1994) A male gerbil's intrauterine position affects female response to his scent marks. *Physiology & Behavior*, **55**(6), 1137–1139.

Clark, M.M. and Galef, B.G. (1999) A testosterone-mediated trade-off between parental and sexual effort in male Mongolian gerbils (*Meriones unguiculatus*). *Journal of Comparative Psychology*, **113**(4), 388–395.

Clark, M.M. and Galef, B.G. (2000) Why some male Mongolian gerbils may help at the nest: testosterone, asexuality and alloparenting. *Animal Behaviour*, **59**, 801–806.

Clark, M.M. and Galef, B.G. (2001a) Socially-induced infertility: Familial effects on reproductive development of female Mongolian gerbils. *Animal Behaviour*, **62**, 897–903.

Clark, M.M. and Galef, B.G. (2001b) Age-related changes in paternal responses of gerbils parallel changes in their testosterone concentrations. *Developmental Psychobiology*, **39**, 179–187.

Clark, M.M. and Galef, B.G. (2002) Socially induced delayed reproduction in female Mongolian gerbils (*Meriones unguiculatus*): Is there anything special about dominant females? *Journal of Comparative Psychology*, **116**(4), 363–368.

Clark, M.M., Liu, C. and Galef, B. G. (2001) Effects of consanguinity, exposure to pregnant females, and stimulation from young on male gerbils' responses to pups. *Developmental Psychobiology*, 39, 257–264.

Clark, M.M., Moghaddas, M. and Galef, B.G. (2002) Age at first mating affects parental effort and fecundity of female Mongolian gerbils. *Animal Behaviour*, 63, 1129–1134.

Clark, M.M., Stiver, K., Teall, T. and Galef, B.G. (2006) Nursing one litter of Mongolian gerbils while pregnant with another: Effects on daughters' mate attachment and fecundity. *Animal Behaviour*, 71(1), 235–241.

Clark, M.M., Tucker, L. and Galef, B.G. (1992) Stud males and dud males: intrauterine position effects on the success of male gerbils. *Animal Behaviour*, 43, 215–221.

Clark, M.M., Vonk, J.M. and Galef, B.G. (1998) Intrauterine position, parenting, and nest-site attachment in male Mongolian gerbils. *Developmental Psychobiology*, 32(3), 177–181.

Close, B., Banister, K., Baumans, V. *et al.* (1996) Recommendations for euthanasia of experimental animals: Part 1. *Laboratory Animals*, 30(4): 293–316.

Close, B., Banister, K., Baumans, V. *et al.* (1997) Recommendations for euthanasia of experimental animals: Part 2. *Laboratory Animals*, 31(1), 1–32.

Collins, A., Lindzey, G. and Thiessen, D.D. (1969) The regulation of cliff responses in the Mongolian gerbil (*Meriones unguiculatus*) by visual and tactual cues. *Psychonomic Science*, 16, 227–229.

Conlee, C.M., Stephens, M.L., Rowan, A.N. and King, L.A. (2005) Carbon dioxide for euthanasia: concerns regarding pain and distress, with special reference to mice and rats. *Laboratory Animals*, 39, 137–161.

Cornwell-Jones, C.A. and Azar, L.M. (1982) Olfactory development in gerbil pups. *Developmental Psychobiology*, 15(2), 131–137.

Cutler, M.G. and Mackintosh, J.H. (1989) Epilepsy and behaviour of the Mongolian gerbil – an ethological study. *Physiology & Behavior*, 46(4), 561–566.

da Costa, R.M., Rema, A., Payo-Puente, P. and Gaertner, E. (2007) Immunohistochemical characterization of a sebaceous gland carcinoma in a gerbil (*Meriones unguiculatus*). *Journal of Comparative Pathology*, 137(2–3), 130–132.

Dahlborn, K., Bugnon, P., Nevalainen, T. *et al.* (2013) Report of the Federation of European Laboratory Animal Science Associations Working Group on animal identification. *Laboratory Animals*, 47(1), 2–11.

De Ghett, V. (1974) Developmental changes in the rate of ultrasonic vocalization in the Mongolian gerbil. *Developmental Psychobiology*, 7, 267–272.

Diehl, K.-H., Hull, R., Morton, D. *et al.* (2001). A good practice guide to the administration of substances and removal of blood, including routes and volumes. *Journal of Applied Toxicology*, 21, 15–23.

Dizinno, G. and Clancy, A.N. (1978) Ventral marking in black and agouti gerbils (*Meriones unguiculatus*). *Behavioural Biology*, 24, 545–548.

Eckrich, T., Foeller, E., Stuermer, I.W. *et al.* (2008) Strain-dependence of age-related cochlear hearing-loss in wild and domesticated Mongolian gerbils. *Hearing Research*, 235, 72–79.

Ellard, C.G. and Byers, R.D. (2005) The influence of the behaviour of conspecifics on responses to threat in the Mongolian gerbil, *Meriones unguiculatus*. *Animal Behaviour*, 70, 49–58.

Elwood, R.W. and Ostermeyer, M.C. (1984) The effects of food deprivation, aggression, and isolation on infanticide in the male Mongolian gerbil. *Aggressive Behavior*, 10(4), 293–301.

European Commission (2010) Directive 2010/63/EU of the European Parliament and of the council of 22 September 2010 and of the council of 22 September 2010 on the protection of animals used for scientific purposes. Available at: http://eurlex.europa.eu/LexUriServ/LexUriServ.do?uri=OJ:L:2010:276: 0033:0079:EN:PDF

European Convention for the Protection of Vertebrate Animals Used for Experimental and Other Scientific Purposes (2006). ETS No. 123, Strasbourg, 18.3.1986. Appendix A of the European Convention for the Protection of Vertebrate Animals Used for Experimental and Other Scientific Purposes (ETS No. 123), Guidelines for the Accommodation and Care of Animals, Strasbourg, 15.6.2006 (entry into force: 15.6.2007).

Feller, W.F. and Boretos, J. (1967) Semiautomatic apparatus for milking mice. *Journal of the National Cancer Institute*, 38(1), 11.

Fenske, M. (1990) Excretion of electrolytes, free cortisol and aldosterone-18-oxo-glucuronide in 24-hr urines of the Mongolian gerbil (*Meriones unguiculatus*): effect of lysine-vasopressin and adrenocorticotrophin administration, and of changes in sodium balance. *Comparative Biochemistry & Physiology A-Comparative Physiology*, 95(2), 259–265.

Fenske, M. (1996) Dissociation of plasma and urinary steroid values after application of stressors, insulin, vasopressin, ACTH, or dexamethasone in the Mongolian gerbil. *Experimental and Clinical Endocrinology and Diabetes*, 104(6), 441–446.

Field, K.J. and Sibold, A.L. (1999) *The Laboratory Hamster and Gerbil*. CRC Press Ltd., Washington DC.

Finck, A., Schneck, C.D. and Hartman, A.F. (1969) Development of auditory function in the Mongolian gerbil. *Journal of the Acoustical Society of America*, 64(1), 107.

Forkman, B.A. (1995) The effect of hunger on the learning of new food preferences in the Mongolian gerbil. *Behaviour*, 132(7–8), 627–639.

French, J.A. (1994) Alloparents in the Mongolian gerbil: Impact on long-term reproductive performance of breeders and opportunities for independent reproduction. *Behavioural Ecology*, 5(3), 273–279.

Frey, H-H. (1987) Induction of seizures by air blast in gerbils: stimulus duration/effect relationship. *Epilepsy Research*, 1, 262–264.

Fujisawa, N., Maeda, Y., Yamamoto, Y. *et al.* (2003) Newly established seizure susceptible and seizure-prone inbred strains of Mongolian gerbil. *Experimental Animals*, 52(2), 169–172.

Galef, B.G., Rudolf, B., Whiskin, E.E. *et al.* (1998) Familiarity and relatedness: Effects on social learning about foods by Norway rats and Mongolian gerbils. *Animal Learning and Behavior*, 26(4), 448–454.

Govardovskii, V., Röhlich, P., Szél, A. and Khokhlova, T.V. (1992) Cones in the retina of the Mongolian gerbil (*Meriones unguiculatus*): An immunocytochemical and electrophysiological study. *Vision Research*, 32, 19–27.

Grant, M. and Thiessen, D. (1989) The possible interaction of Harderian material and saliva for thermoregulation in the Mongolian gerbil, *Meriones unguiculatus*. *Perceptual and Motor Skills*, 68(1), 3–10.

Gray-Allan, P. and Wong, R. (1990) Influence of coat color genes on seizure behavior in Mongolian gerbils. *Behavioural Genetics*, 20(4), 481–485.

Gromov, V.S. (2015) Scent marking in gerbils and its possible functions. *Russian Journal of Theriology*, 14(1), 113–126.

Guo, Y-Y., Chia, Q.-S., Zhang, X.-Y. *et al.* (2019) Brown adipose tissue plays thermoregulatory role within the thermoneutral zone in Mongolian gerbils (*Meriones unguiculatus*). *Journal of Thermal Biology*, 81, 137–145.

Hawkins, P., Prescott, M.J., Carbone, L. *et al.* (2016) A Good Death? Report of the Second Newcastle Meeting on Laboratory Animal Euthanasia. *Animals*, 6(9), 50.

Heffner, R. and Heffner, H. (1988) Sound Localization and Use of Binaural Cues by the Gerbil (*Meriones unguiculatus*). *Behavioural Neuroscience*, 102, 422–428.

Hem, A., Smith, A.J. and Solberg, P. (1998) Saphenous vein puncture for blood sampling of the mouse, rat, hamster, gerbil, guinea pig, ferret and mink. *Laboratory Animals*, 32, 364–368.

Hendrie, C.A. and Pickles, A.R. (2000) Short-term individual housing in female gerbils as a putative model of depression. *Society for Neuroscience Abstracts*, 26(1–2): Abstract No.-103.12.

Hendrie, C.A. and Starkey, N.J. (1998) Pair-bond disruption in Mongolian gerbils: effects on subsequent social behaviour. *Physiology & Behavior*, 63(5), 895–901.

Henley, M. and Robinson, R. (1981) Non-agouti and pink-eyed dilution in the Mongolian gerbil. *The Journal of Heredity*, **72**, 60–61.

Holman, S.D. (1980) Sexually dimorphic ultrasonic vocalizations of Mongolian gerbils. *Behavioural and Neural Biology*, **28**, 183–192.

Holman, S.D. and Seale, W.T.C. (1991) Ontogeny of sexually dimorphic ultrasonic vocalisations in Mongolian gerbils. *Developmental Psychobiology*, **24**(2), 103–115.

Jacobs, G. and Deegan II, J.F. (1994) Sensitivity to ultraviolet light in the gerbil (*Meriones unguiculatus*): Characteristics and mechanisms. *Vision Research*, **34**, 1433–1441.

Jacobs, G. and Nietz, J. (1989) Cone monochromacy and a reversed Purkinje shift in the gerbil. *Experientia*, **45**, 317–319.

Jansa, S. and Weksler, M. (2003) Phylogeny of muroid rodents: relationships within and among major lineages as determined by IRBP gene sequences. *Molecular Phylogenetics and Evolution*, **31**, 256–276.

Jaworska, N., Dwyer, S.M. and Rusak, B. (2008) Repeated neonatal separation results in different neurochemical and behavioural changes in adult male and female Mongolian gerbils. *Pharmacology, Biochemistry and Behavior*, **88**, 533–541.

Johnson-Delaney, C.A. (1998) Disease of the urinary system of commonly kept rodents: Diagnosis and treatment. *Seminars in Avian and Exotic Pet Medicine*, **7**(2), 81–88.

Juarez-Tapia, C.R., Torres-Mendoza, D., Duran, P. and Miranda-Anaya, M. (2015) Short-day photoperiod disrupts daily activity and facilitates anxiety-depressive behaviours in gerbil *Meriones unguiculatus*. *Biological Rhythm Research*, **46**(6), 919–927.

Kakol Palm, D. and Hollaender, P. (2007) A procedure for intravenous injection using external jugular vein in Mongolian gerbil (*Meriones unguiculatus*). *Laboratory Animals*, **41**, 403–405.

Kanarek, R.B., Ogilby, J.D. and Mayer, J. (1977) Effects of dietary caloric density on feeding behavior in Mongolian gerbils (*Meriones unguiculatus*). *Physiology & Behavior*, **19**(4), 497–501.

Kaplan, H. (1975) What triggers seizures in the gerbil, *Meriones unguiculatus*? *Life Sciences*, **17**, 693–698.

Kaplan, H. and Miezejes, C. (1972) Development of seizures in Mongolian gerbils (*Meriones unguiculatus*). *Journal of Comparative and Physiological Psychology*, **81**(2), 267–269.

Kelly, J. and Potash, M. (1986) Directional Responses to sounds in young gerbils (*Meriones unguiculatus*). *Journal of Comparative Psychology*, **100**, 37–45.

Klaunberg, B.A., O'Malley, J., Clark, T. and Davis, J.A. (2004) Euthanasia of Mouse Fetuses and Neonates. *Contemporary Topics*, **43**(5), 29–34.

Kort, W.J., Hekking-Weijma, J.M., TenKate, M.T. et al. (1998) A microchip implant system as a method to determine body temperature of terminally ill rats and mice. *Laboratory Animals*, **32**(3), 260–269.

Kupferberg, H. (2001) Animal models used in the screening of antiepileptic drugs. *Epilepsia*, **42**(4), 7–12.

Laferriere, C.A. and Pang, D.S.J. (2020) Review of Intraperitoneal Injection of Sodium Pentobarbital as a Method of Euthanasia in Laboratory Rodents. *Journal of the American Association for Laboratory Animal Science*, **59**(3), 254–263.

Leach, M., Raj, M. and Morton, D. (2005) Aversiveness of carbon dioxide. *Laboratory Animals*, **39**(4), 452–453.

Leiper, B.D. and Robinson, R. (1984) A case of dominance modification in the Mongolian gerbil. *The Journal of Heredity*, **75**, 323.

Leiper, B.D. and Robinson, R. (1985) Gray mutant in the Mongolian gerbil. *The Journal of Heredity*, **76**, 473.

Leiper, B.D. and Robinson, R. (1986) Linkage of albino and pink-eyed dilution genes in the Mongolian gerbil and other rodents. *The Journal of Heredity*, **77**, 207.

Leont'ev, A.N. (1954) K. ekologii kogtistoi, peschanki v Buryat Mongol'skoi [Ecology of the clawed gerbil in Buryat Mongolia]. *Izvestiya Irkutskogo osudarstvennyi nauchno-issledovatel'skogo protivochumnogo instituta Sibiri ii Dal'nogo Vostoka*, **12**, 137–149.

Lerwill, C.J. (1974) Activity rhythms of Golden hamsters (*Mesocricetus auratus*) and Mongolian gerbils (*Meriones unguiculatus*) by direct observation. *Journal of Zoology*, **174**, 520–523.

Lerwill, C.J. (1978) Ultrasound in the Mongolian gerbil, *Meriones unguiculatus*. *Journal of Zoology*, **185**, 263–266.

Liu, W., Wan, X. and Zhong, W. (2007) Population dynamics of the Mongolian gerbils: Seasonal patterns and interactions among density, reproduction and climate. *Journal of Arid Environments*, **68**(3), 383–397.

Liu, W., Wan, G., Wang, Y. et al. (2009) Population ecology of wild Mongolian gerbils, *Meriones unguiculatus*. *Journal of Mammalogy*, **90**(4), 832–840.

Liu, W., Zhong, W. and Wan, X. (2017) Sex- and cohort-specific life-history strategies in Mongolian gerbils (*Meriones unguiculatus*). *Journal of Arid Environments*, 146, 18–26.

Loskota, W.J., Lomax, P. and Verity, M.A. (1974) A stereotaxic Atlas of the Mongolian gerbil Brain (*Meriones unguiculatus*). Ann Arbor Science, Ann Arbor, Michigan.

Maier, J.K. and Klump, G.M. (2006) Resolution in azimuth sound localization in the Mongolian gerbil (*Meriones unguiculatus*). *Journal of the Acoustical Society of America*, **119**(2), 1029–1036.

Marston, J.H. and Chang, M.C. (1965) The breeding, management and reproductive physiology of the Mongolian gerbil (*Meriones unguiculatus*). *Laboratory Animal Care*, **15**(1), 34–48.

Martínez, A., Ramos, G., Martínez Torres, M. et al. (2015) Paternal behavior in the Mongolian gerbil (*Meriones unguiculatus*): Estrogenic and androgenic regulation. *Hormones and Behavior*, **71**, 91–95.

Martínez, A., Arteaga-Silva, M., Bonilla-Jaime, H. et al. (2019) Paternal behavior in the Mongolian gerbil, and its regulation by social factors, T, ERα, and AR. *Physiology and Behaviour*, **199**, 351–358.

Matsuoka, K. and Suzuki, J. (1995) Spontaneous tumors in the Mongolian gerbil (*Meriones unguiculatus*). *Experimental Animals*, **43**(5), 755–760.

Matsuzaki, T., Yasuda, Y. and Nonaka, S. (1989) The genetics of coat colors in the Mongolian gerbil (*Meriones unguiculatus*). *Experimental Animals*, **38**, 337–341.

McManus, J.J. (1972a) Water relations and food consumption of the Mongolian gerbil, *Meriones unguiculatus*. *Comparative Biochemistry and Physiology*, **43A**, 959–967.

McManus, J.J. (1972b) Early postnatal growth and development of temperature regulation in Mongolian gerbils, *Meriones unguiculatus*. *Journal of Mammalogy*, **51**(4), 782.

Michaux, J., Reyes, A. and Catzeflis, F. (2001) Evolutionary history of the most species mammals: Molecular phylogeny of muroid rodents. *Molecular Biology and Evolution*, **18**, 2017–2031.

Milne-Edwards, A. (1867) Sur quelques mammifières du nord de la chine: *Gerbillus unguiculatus*. *Annales des Science Naturelles (Zoologie)*, **7**, 375–377.

Moons, C.P.H., Hermans, K., Remie, R. et al. (2007) Intraperitoneal versus subcutaneous telemetry devices in young Mongolian gerbils (*Meriones unguiculatus*). *Laboratory Animals*, **41**(2), 262–269.

Mulder, G.B., Pritchett-Corning, K.R., Gramlich, M.A. and Crocker, A.E. (2010) Method of feed presentation affects the growth of Mongolian gerbils (*Meriones unguiculatus*). *Journal of the American Association of Laboratory Animal Science*. 49(1): 36–39.

Musser, G.G. and Carleton, M.D. (2005) Mammal Species of the World, A Taxonomic and Geographic Reference. Eds Wilson, D.E. and Reeder, D.M., 3rd edn, Vol. 2, pp. 894–1531. Johns Hopkins University Press.

Nakayama, A. and Riquimaroux, H. (2017) Sensitivity to high frequency communication sounds in the inner ear enhanced by selective attention: Preliminary findings in Mongolian gerbils. *Journal of Computational Acoustics*, **25**(3), 1750016-1-11

Naumov, N.P. and Lobachev, S.V. (1975) Ecology of the desert rodents of the USSR (Jerboas and Gerbils). In: *Rodents in Desert Environments*. Eds Prakash, I. and Gosh, P.K., pp. 529–536. Dr. W. Junk b.v. Publishers, The Hague.

Neumann, K., Maak, S., Stuermer, I.W. et al. (2001) Low microsatellite variation in laboratory gerbils. *Journal of Heredity*, **92**(1), 71–74.

Newsom, D.M., Bolgos, G.L., Colby, L. and Nemzek, J.A. (2004) Comparison of body surface temperature measurement and conventional methods for measuring temperature in the mouse. *Contemporary Topics in Laboratory Animal Science*, **43**(5), 13–18.

Nishino, N. and Totsukawa, K. (1996) Study on the estrous cycle in the Mongolian gerbil (*Meriones unguiculatus*). *Experimental Animals*, **45**(3), 283–288.

Norris, M.L. (1981) Portable anaesthetic apparatus designed to induce and maintain surgical anaesthesia by Methoxyflurane inhalation in the Mongolian gerbil (*Meriones unguiculatus*). *Laboratory Animals*, **15**(2), 153–155.

Norris, M.L. (1985) Disruption of pair bonding induces pregnancy failure in newly mated Mongolian gerbils (*Meriones unguiculatus*). *Journal of Reproduction and Fertility*, **75**, 43–47.

Norris, M.L. (1987) Gerbils. In: *The UFAW Handbook on the Care and Management of Laboratory Animals*. Ed. Poole, T., pp. 360–376. Agricultural and Food Research Council, Cambridge.

Norris, M.L. and Adams, C.E. (1972) Aggressive behaviour and reproduction in the Mongolian gerbil, *Meriones unguiculatus*, relative to age and sexual experience at pairing. *Journal of Reproduction and Fertility*, 31, 447–450.

Norris, M.L. and Adams, C.E. (1974) Sexual development in the Mongolian gerbil (*Meriones unguiculatus*), with particular reference to the ovary. *Journal of Reproduction and Fertility*, 36, 245–248.

Norris, M.L. and Adams, C.E. (1979b) Vaginal opening in the Mongolian gerbil, *Meriones unguiculatus*: normal data and the influence of social factors. *Laboratory Animals*, **13**, 159–162.

Norris, M.L. and Adams, C.E. (1981a) Pregnancy concurrent with lactation in the Mongolian gerbils (*Meriones unguiculatus*). *Laboratory Animals*, **15**, 21–23.

Norris, M.L. and Adams, C.E. (1981b) Mating post partem and length of gestation in the Mongolian gerbil (*Meriones unguiculatus*). *Laboratory Animals*, **15**, 189–191.

Norris, M.L. and Adams, C.E. (1986) Embryo transfer to Mongolian gerbils during post-partum pregnancy and pseudopregnancy. *Animal Reproduction Science*, **11**, 63–67.

Ostermeyer, M.C. and Elwood, R.W. (1984) Helpers (?) at the nest in the Mongolian gerbil. *Meriones unguiculatus. Behaviour*, **91**, 61–77.

Palinov, I. (2001) Current concepts of Gerbillid phylogeny and classification. In: *African Small Mammals, Proceedings of the 8th International Symposium on African Small Mammals, Paris, 1999*. Eds Denys, C., Granjon, L. and Poulet, A., pp. 141–149. Institute de Recherche pour le Dévelopment, Paris.

Peckham, J.C., Cole, J.R., Chapman, W.L. et al. (1974) Staphylococcal dermatitis in Mongolian gerbils (*Meriones unguiculatus*). *Laboratory Animal Science*, **24**(1), 43–47.

Pendergrass, M. and Thiessen, D.D. (1983) Sandbathing is thermoregulatory in the Mongolian gerbil, *Meriones unguiculatus. Behavioural and Neural Biology*, **37**(1), 125–133.

Pérez-García, C.C., Peña-Penabad, M., Cano-Rábano, M.J. et al. (2003) A simple procedure to perform intravenous injections in the Mongolian gerbil (*Meriones unguiculatus*). *Laboratory Animals*, **37**, 68–71.

Pinto-Fochi, M.E., Negirn, A.C., Scarano, W.R. et al. (2016) Sexual maturation of the Mongolian gerbil (*Meriones unguiculatus*): a histological. Hormonal, and spermatic evaluation. *Reproduction, Fertility, and Development*, **28**, 815–823.

Piovanotti Arua, M.R. and Vieira, L.M. (2004) Presence of the father and parental experience have differentiated effects on pup development in Mongolian gerbils (*Meriones unguiculatus*). *Behavioural Processes*, **66**(2), 107–117.

Prates, E.J. and Guerra, R.F. (2005) Parental care and sexual interactions in Mongolian gerbils (*Meriones unguiculatus*) during the post-partum estrus. *Behavioural Processes*, **70**(2), 104–112.

Quesenberry, K., Mans, C. and Orcutt, C. (2020) In: *Ferrets, Rabbits, and Rodents: Clinical Medicine and Surgery*. Ed. Carpenter, J., 4th edn. Saunders Publishers.

Radtke-Schuller, S., Schuller, G., Angenstein, Grosser, O.S. et al. (2016). Brain atlas of the Mongolian gerbil (*Meriones unguiculatus*) in CT/MRI-aided stereotaxic coordinates. *Brain Structure and Function*, **221**(Suppl. 1), 1–272.

Raffel, M. and König, B. (1999) Influence of body weight on reproduction in female house mice (*Mus domesticus*). *Zoology*, **102**(Suppl. II), 33.

Raflo, C.P. and Diamond, S.S. (1980) Metastatic squamous-cell carcinoma in a gerbil (*Meriones unguiculatus*). *Laboratory Animals*, **14**(3), 237–239.

Randall, J.A. and Thiessen, D.D. (1980) Seasonal activity and thermoregulation in *Meriones unguiculatus* – a gerbil's choice. *Behavioural Ecology and Sociobiology*, **7**(4), 267–272.

Rassin, D.K., Sturman, J.A. and Gaull, G.E. (1978) Taurine and other free amino acids in milk of man and other mammals. *Early Human Development*, **2**(1), 1–13.

Refinetti, R. (2006) Variability in diurnality in laboratory rodents. *Journal of Comparative Physiology*, 192, 701–714.

Rich, S.T. (1968) The Mongolian gerbil (*Meriones unguiculatus*) in research. *Laboratory Animal Care*, **18**(2), 235–243.

Rohrbach, C. (1982) Investigation of the Bruce effect in the Mongolian gerbil (*Meriones unguiculatus*). *Journal of Reproduction and Fertility*, **65**, 411–417.

Roper, T.J. and Polioudakis, E. (1977) The behaviour of Mongolian gerbils in a semi-natural environment, with special reference to ventral marking, dominance and sociability. *Behaviour*, **61**(3–4), 205–237.

Ryan, A. (1976) Hearing sensitivity of the Mongolian gerbil, *Meriones unguiculatus. Journal of the Acoustical Society of America*, **59**, 1222–1226.

Salo, A.A. and French, J.A. (1989) Early experience, reproductive success, and development of parental behaviour in Mongolian gerbils. *Animal Behaviour*, **38**, 693–702.

Saltzman, W., Ahmeda, S. Fahimi, A. et al. (2006) Social suppression of female reproductive maturation and infanticidal behavior in cooperatively breeding Mongolian gerbils. *Hormones and Behavior*, **49**, 527–537.

Scheibler, E., Weinandy, R. and Gattermann, R. (2004) Social categories in families of Mongolian gerbils. *Physiology & Behavior*, **81**(3), 455–464.

Scheibler, E., Weinandy, R. and Gattermann, R. (2005a) Social factors affecting litters in families of Mongolian gerbils, *Meriones unguiculatus. Folia Zoologica*, **54**(1–2), 61–68.

Scheibler, E., Weinandy, R. and Gattermann, R. (2005b) Intra-family aggression and offspring expulsion in Mongolian gerbils (*Meriones unguiculatus*) under restricted environments. *Mammalian Biology – Zeitschrift fur Säugetierkunde*, **70**(3), 137–146.

Scheibler, E., Liu, W., Weinandy, R. and Gattermann, R. (2006a) Burrow systems of the Mongolian gerbil (*Meriones unguiculatus* Milne Edwards, 1867). *Mammalian Biology – Zeitschrift fur Säugetierkunde*, **71**(3), 178–182.

Scheibler, E., Weinandy, R. and Gattermann, R. (2006b) Male expulsion in cooperative Mongolian gerbils (*Meriones unguiculatus*). *Physiology & Behavior*, **87**(1), 24–30.

Shimozuru, M., Kikusui, T., Takeuchi, Y. and Mori, Y. (2006a) Scent-marking and sexual activity may reflect social hierarchy among group-living male Mongolian gerbils (*Meriones unguiculatus*). *Physiology & Behavior*, **89**(5), 644–649.

Shimozuru, M., Kikusui, T., Takeuchi, Y. and Mori, Y. (2006b) Social-defeat stress suppresses scent-marking and social-approach behaviors in male Mongolian gerbils (*Meriones unguiculatus*). *Physiology & Behavior*, **88**(4–5), 620–627.

Solomon, N.G. (2003) A re-examination of factors influencing philopatry in rodents. *Journal of Mammalogy*, **84**(4), 1182–1197.

Solomon, N.G. and Getz, L.L. (1996) Examination of alternative hypotheses for cooperative breeding in rodents. In: *Cooperative breeding in Mammals*. Eds Solomon, N.G. and French, J.A., pp. 199–230. Cambridge University Press.

Starkey, N.J. and Hendrie, C.A. (1997) Parallels between pairbond disruption in gerbils and human depression. *Behavioural Pharmacology*, **8**, 663–664.

Starkey, N.J. and Hendrie, D.C. (1998a) Importance of gender for the display of social impairment in pairbond disrupted gerbils. *Neuroscience & Biobehavioral Reviews*, **23**(2), 273–277.

Starkey, N.J. and Hendrie, C.A. (1998b) Disruption of pairs produces pair-bond disruption in male but not female Mongolian gerbils. *Physiology & Behavior*, **65**(3), 497–503.

Starkey, N.J., Normington, G. and Bridges, N.J. (2007) The effects of individual housing on 'anxious' behaviour in male and female gerbils. *Physiology & Behavior*, **90**(4), 545–552.

Steppan, S., Adkins, R.M. and Anderson, J. (2004) Phylogeny and divergence-date estimates of rapid radiations in muroid rodents based on multiple nuclear genes. *Systematic Biology*, **53**, 533–553.

Stuermer, I.W. (1998) Reproduction and developmental differences in offspring of domesticated and wild Mongolian gerbils (*Meriones unguiculatus*). *Mammalian Biology – Zeitschrift für Säugetierkunde*, **63**, 57–58.

Stuermer, I.W., Kluge, R., Nebendahl, K. *et al.* (1998) Genetic base and successful breeding of wild gerbils (*Meriones unguiculatus*) captured during an expedition to Outer Mongolia in 1995. *Mammalian Biology – Zeitschrift für Säugetierkunde*, **63**, 58–59.

Stuermer, W.I., Plotz, K., Leybold, A. *et al.* (2003) Intraspecific allometric comparison of laboratory gerbils with Mongolian gerbils trapped in the wild Indicates domestication in *Meriones unguiculatus* (Milne-Edwards, 1867) (Rodentia: Gerbillinae). *Zoologischer Anzeiger – A Journal of Comparative Zoology*, **242**(3), 249–266.

Stuermer, I.W., Tittmann, C., Schilling, C. and Blottner, S. (2006) Reproduction of wild gerbils bred in the laboratory in dependence on generation and season: I. Morphological changes and fertility. *Animal Science*, **82**, 377–387.

Stuermer, I.W. and Wetzel, W. (2006) Early experience and domestication affect auditory discrimination learning, open field behaviour and brain size in wild Mongolian gerbils and domesticated Laboratory gerbils (*Meriones unguiculatus forma domestica*). *Behavioural Brain Research*, **173**(1), 11–21.

Swanson, H.H. and Lockley, R.M. (1977) Population growth and social structure of confined colonies of Mongolian gerbils: Scent gland size and marking behaviour as indices of social status. *Aggressive Behaviour*, **4**, 57–89.

Swanson, H.H. (1980) The 'hairless' gerbil: A new mutant. *Laboratory Animals*, **14**, 143–147.

Tang Halpin, Z. (1975) The role of individual recognition by odours in the social interactions of the Mongolian gerbil (*Meriones unguiculatus*). *Behaviour*, **58**(1–2), 117–129.

Thiessen, D., Graham, M. and Davenport, R. (1978) Ultrasonic Signalling in the gerbil (*Meriones unguiculatus*): Social Interaction and Olfaction. *Journal of Comparative Physiology and Psychology*, **92**, 1041–1049.

Thiessen, D.D. and Yahr, P. (1977) *The Gerbil in Behavioural Investigations*. University of Texas Press, Austin, Texas.

Toth, L.A. (2000) Defining the Moribund Condition as an Experimental Endpoint for Animal Research. *ILAR Journal*, **41**(2).

Tsurim, I. and Abramsky, Z. (2004) The effect of travel costs on food hoarding in gerbils. *Journal of Mammalogy*, **85**(1), 67–71.

Tumblebrook Farm Inc. (1979) Physiological parameters and selected general data. *The Gerbil Digest*, **6**(2).

Tumblebrook Farm Inc. (1980) The gerbil as a stroke model. *The Gerbil Digest*, **7**(2).

Turner, P.V., Hickman, D.L., van Luijk, J. *et al.* (2020). Welfare impact of carbon dioxide euthanasia on laboratory mice and rats: A systematic review. *Frontiers in Veterinary Sciences*, **7**, article 411.

Valsecchi, P., Choleris, E., Moles, A. *et al.* (1996) Kinship and familiarity as factors affecting social transfer of food preferences in adult Mongolian gerbils (*Meriones unguiculatus*). *Journal of Comparative Psychology*, **110**(3), 243–251.

Valsecchi, P., Razzoli, M. and Choleris, E. (2002) Influence of kinship and familiarity on the social and reproductive behaviour of female Mongolian gerbils. *Ethology, Ecology and Evolution*, **14**, 239–253.

Van Zutphen, L.F.M., Baumans, V. and Beynen, A.C. (Eds) (2001) *Principles of Laboratory Animal Science, Revised Edition: A Contribution to the Humane Use and Care of Animals and to the Quality of Experimental Results*. Elsevier Health Sciences.

Waiblinger, E. and König, B. (2001) Housing and husbandry affect stereotypic behaviour in laboratory gerbils. 3R-Info-Bulletin 16 and Alternatives to Animal Experiments (Special Issue 07): 67–69. http://www.forschung3r.ch/de/publications/bu16.html

Waiblinger, E. (2002) Comfortable Quarters for Gerbils in Research Institutions. In: *Comfortable Quarters for Laboratory Animals*. Eds Reinhardt, V. and Reinhardt, A. Animal Welfare Institute, Washington D.C.

Waiblinger, E. (2003) Stereotypic behaviours in laboratory gerbils: Causes and solutions. PhD Thesis. Department of Animal Behaviour, Zoology Institute, University of Zurich.

Waiblinger, E. and König, B. (2004) Refinement of gerbil housing and husbandry in the laboratory. *Animal Welfare*, **13**, S229–235.

Wallace, P., Owen, K. and Thiessen, D.D. (1973) The control and function of maternal scent marking in the Mongolian gerbil. *Physiology & Behavior*, **10**, 463–466.

Wang, G. and Zhong, W. (2006) Mongolian gerbils and Daurian pikas responded differently to changes in precipitation in the Inner Mongolian grasslands. *Journal of Arid Environments*, **66**(4), 648–656.

Wang, D.H., Pei, Y.X., Yang, J.C. and Wang, Z.W. (2003) Digestive tract morphology and food habits in six species of rodents, *Folia Zoologica*, **52**(1), 51–55.

Wang, Y., Liu, W., Wan, X. and Zhong, W. (2011) Home-range sizes of social groups of Mongolian gerbils *Meriones unguiculatus*. *Journal of Arid Environments*, **75**(2), 132–137.

Waring, A.D. and Poole, T.W. (1980). Genetic analysis of the black pigment mutation in the Mongolian gerbil. *The Journal of Heredity*, **71**, 428–429.

Waring, A.D., Poole, T.W. and Perper, T. (1978). White spotting in the Mongolian gerbil. *The Journal of Heredity*, **69**, 347–349.

Waring, A.D. and Perper, T. (1980) Parental behaviour in Mongolian gerbils (*Meriones unguiculatus*). II. Parental interactions. *Animal Behaviour*, **28**, 331–340.

Weinandy, R. (1995) Untersuchungen zur Chronobiologie, Ethologie und zu Stressreaktionen der Mongolischen Wüstenrennmaus, *Meriones unguiculatus*. PhD Thesis (German). Zoologisches Institut, Martin Luther-Universität Halle-Wittenberg.

Weinandy, R., Hofmann, S. and Gattermann, R. (2001). Mating behaviour during the estrous cycle in Mongolian gerbils (*Meriones unguiculatus*). *Mammalian Biology*, **66**, 116–120.

Weinandy, R., Hofmann, S. and Gattermann, R. (2002) The oestrus of female gerbils, *Meriones unguiculatus*, is indicated by locomotor activity and influenced by male presence. *Folia Zoologica*, **51**(1), 145–155.

Weinandy, R. and Gattermann, R. (1996) Time of day and stress response to different stressors in experimental animals. 2. Mongolian gerbil (*Meriones unguiculatus* Milne Edwards, 1867). *Journal of Experimental Animal Science*, **38**(3), 109–122.

Weinert, D., Weinandy, R. and Gattermann, R. (2007) Photic and non-photic effects on the daily activity pattern of Mongolian gerbils. *Physiology & Behavior*, **90**(2–3), 325–333.

Wiedenmayer, C. (1995) The ontogeny of stereotypies in gerbils. PhD Thesis (partly in German). Zoologisches Institut, Universität Zürich.

Wiedenmayer, C. (1996) Effects of cage size on the ontogeny of stereotyped behaviour in gerbils. *Applied Animal Behaviour Science*, **47**, 225–233.

Wiedenmayer, C. (1997a) Causation of the ontogenetic development of stereotypic digging in gerbils. *Animal Behaviour*, **53**, 461–470.

Wiedenmayer, C. (1997b) Stereotypies resulting from a deviation in the ontogenetic development of gerbils. *Behavioural Processes*, **39**, 215–221.

Wiedenmayer, C. (1997c) The early ontogeny of bar-gnawing in laboratory gerbils. *Animal Welfare*, **6**, 273–277.

Wilkinson, F. (1984) The development of visual acuity in the Mongolian gerbil (*Meriones unguiculatus*). *Behavioural Brain Research*, **13**(1), 83–94.

Winterfeld, K.T., Teucert-Noodt, G. and Dawirs, R.R. (1998) Social environment alters both ontogeny of dopamine innervation of the medial prefrontal cortex and maturation of working memory in gerbils (*Meriones unguiculatus*). *Journal of Neuroscience Research*, **52**(2), 201–209.

Wong, R., Gray-Allan, P., Chiba, C. and Alfred, B. (1990) Social preference of female gerbils (*Meriones unguiculatus*) as influenced by coat color of males. *Behavioural and Neural Biology*, **54**(2), 184–190.

Woolf, N.K. and Ryan, A.F. (1984). The development of auditory function in the cochlea of the Mongolian gerbil. *Hearing Research*, **13**, 277–283.

Yahr, P. (1977) Social subordination and scent-marking in male Mongolian gerbils (*Meriones unguiculatus*) *Animal Behaviour*, **25**(2), 292–297.

Yahr, P. and Anderson-Mitchell, K. (1983). Attraction of gerbil pups to maternal nest odours: duration, specificity and ovarian control. *Physiology & Behavior*, **31**, 241–247.

Yamaguchi, H., Kikusui, T., Takeuchi, Y. *et al.* (2005) Social stress decreases marking behavior independently of testosterone in Mongolian gerbils. *Hormones & Behavior*, **47**(5), 549–555.

Yang, S., Luo, X., Xiong, G., So, K.F., Yang, H. and Xu, Y., (2015). The electroretinogram of Mongolian gerbil (Meriones unguiculatus): comparison to mouse. *Neuroscience Letters*, **589**, 7–12.

Zhang, Z. and Wang, D. (2007) Seasonal changes in thermogenesis and body mass in wild Mongolian gerbils (*Meriones unguiculatus*). *Comparative Biochemistry and Physiology – Part A: Molecular & Integrative Physiology*, **148**(2), 346–353.

Zhang, T., Huang, L., Zhang, L. *et al.* (2016) ON and OFF retinal ganglion cells differentially regulate serotonergic and GABAergic activity in the dorsal raphe nucleus. *Scientific Reports*, **6**, Article number: 26060.

24 The Syrian hamster

Christina Winnicker and Kathleen R. Pritchett-Corning

Biological overview

Taxonomy

Hamsters as a group can be described as stout-bodied, stubby-tailed, broad-headed, cheek-pouched, burrowing and nest-building rodents. Hamsters are of the mammalian order Rodentia, suborder Myomorpha, superfamily Muroidea of the family Cricetidae. The family Cricetidae includes 681 species distributed worldwide except Australia (Smith 2012). The most commonly used species in the laboratory is the Syrian hamster (*Mesocricetus auratus* [Waterhouse, 1839]), known also as the Golden Hamster. The Chinese (*Cricetulus griseus*), Djungarian, Siberian, or Siberian Dwarf (*Phodopus sungorus*) and European hamsters (*Cricetus cricetus*) are less often used in research. For this reason, the remainder of the chapter relates to the Syrian hamster, unless otherwise indicated. Those using hamsters in research should be aware that accurate identification of the species used is essential for correct reproducibility of work and interpretation of results.

Comparative anatomy and physiology

Species within the various hamster genera vary in body size. Hamsters in the genus *Cricetus* are the largest, *Mesocricetus* are medium sized whilst *Phodopus* are dwarf, mouse-like animals. Typically, adult Syrian hamsters reach weights of 114–140 g, Chinese hamsters 120–150 g and Siberian 100–130 g. Larger European hamsters may reach 400–500 g.

Hamsters generally have shorter lifespans than rats and mice routinely used for long-term studies; Bernfeld *et al.* (1986) provide data from over 600 control F1 hybrid Syrian hamsters. There are also marked sex and strain differences, with males tending to live longer than females. Most reports of longevity record deaths from 1 year onwards with only 50% or less survival at 2 years. Hamsters rarely survive beyond 3 years, this age being more typically reached by Chinese rather than Syrian hamsters.

Adult females (Syrian) are larger than males, and Syrian hamsters have abundant, loose skin. Both sexes possess paired, bilateral scent or flank glands (Figure 24.1), consisting of sebaceous glands, pigment cells and terminal hair. These glands are most prominent in the male, but are poorly developed in females. Females typically have six paired mammary glands. Hamsters have 7 cervical vertebrae, 13 thoracic, 6 lumbar, 4 sacral and 13–14 caudal, despite their tail's stubby appearance. They have four digits on their front paws and five on their hind (Murray 2012).

The hamster's dental formula is: 1/1 incisors, 0/0 canines, premolars 0/0 and molars 3/3. They have only one set of teeth (monophyodont), and the cheek teeth are roughly quadrate and low crowned (bunodont and brachyodont). The incisors are open-rooted, while the molars are rooted. Primary eruption is regular. Some but not all genera possess buccal pouches extending dorso-laterally from the oral cavity on either side of the shoulder region (Figure 24.1). These structures are used experimentally as immunologically privileged sites. A detailed account of anatomy, physiology, haematology and clinical chemistry is available in Suckow *et al.* (2012).

Ecology

Hamsters are native to dry, rocky plains and minimally vegetated slopes of western Asia where resources are scarce. A terrestrial species hamsters dig burrows for protection from both environment and predation, where they store foraged feed and other resources. These burrows are generally individually inhabited, limited to a female and her litter (Gatterman *et al.* 2001). Hamsters spend a significant amount of time foraging for food and nesting materials when out of the burrow.

Behaviour

Syrian hamsters live singly or with their mother and siblings in the wild. Both males and females will mark and defend territories against intruders. Females are larger and more aggressive than males.

The UFAW Handbook on the Care and Management of Laboratory and Other Research Animals, Ninth Edition.
Edited by Huw Golledge and Claire Richardson.
© 2024 John Wiley & Sons Ltd. Published 2024 by John Wiley & Sons Ltd.

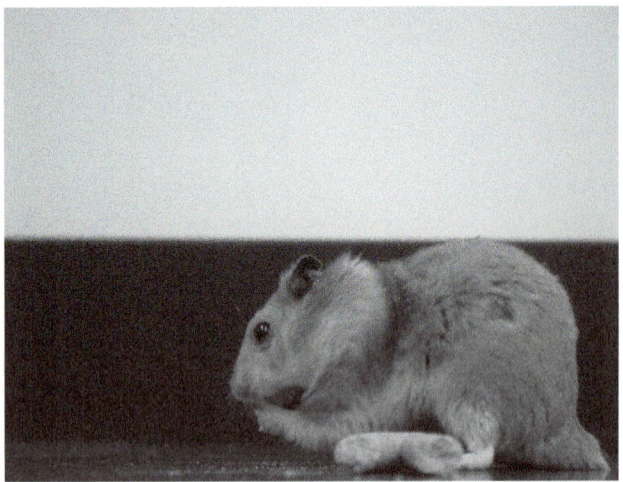

Figure 24.1 Syrian hamster showing flank gland and cheek pouch loaded with food pellet. (Figure used courtesy of KPC.)

Some species of hamsters hibernate under certain environmental conditions. Although this is of research interest, it is not an important feature with respect to their husbandry in most laboratory situations. Hibernation can be induced in hamsters by a number of environmental stimuli including low temperature, short days, solitude, nesting material and adequate food stores. Aspects of behaviour that are of importance for their husbandry include their solitary nature, propensity to burrow and nest build, hoarding behaviour and their nocturnal lifestyle, although in the wild, Syrian hamsters are reportedly diurnal (Gatterman et al. 2008). These are important factors in considering their housing and husbandry. More information on behaviour may be found in Winnicker and Pritchett-Corning (2021).

Uses in the laboratory

Syrian hamsters have a number of unusual and unique features, which historically made them particularly useful for certain experimental studies. The Syrian hamster has immuno-genetic characteristics that underlie marked tolerance to homologous, heterologous and human tumours, parasites, viruses and bacteria. As the Syrian hamsters' immune response to many infectious diseases is similar to humans, they also serve as a useful model for various infectious diseases, including multiple viral, bacterial and parasitic infections. An excellent summary can be found in Miao (2019). Perhaps once a niche or minor animal model, the COVID-19 pandemic fuelled search for relevant animal models of the disease once again focused on the hamster. Able to mimic much of the array of symptoms and varying disease courses seen in humans, they became a valuable tool in understanding the disease (Bryche et al. 2020; Chan et al. 2020; Gruber et al. 2021). Moreover, the presence of reversible cheek pouches, which in the Syrian hamster appear to be immunologically privileged, allowed tumour grafts from other species, including man, to grow freely and symmetrically without the need to induce immunosuppression. With the advent of immunodeficient mice, the usefulness of this model has declined.

The Syrian hamster has also been used for dental research as the form and occlusion of their molar teeth closely resemble those of humans and the induction of lesions is possible without fracturing of the teeth, as in rats. Other areas of use include teratology and reproductive biology. Chijioke et al. (1990) described the use of the Syrian hamster oocyte in assessing human spermatozoal fertilising potential. They concluded that it was a relatively precise method of quantifying the effects of various factors affecting human sperm function in vivo (Hirose & Ogura 2019). The Syrian hamster has been used in thermophysiology and circadian rhythm studies, since as hibernating animals they are subject to jet lag (Gibson et al. 2010).

Laboratory management and breeding

General husbandry

Housing and caging

For routine purposes, cages and equipment designed for rats can be used for housing hamsters, although the smaller species, such as Siberian, can use a shorter cage. European hamsters require more space and stronger cages due to their size and aggressiveness towards each other. Table 24.1 sets out the space requirements for Syrian hamsters as per Annex III to Directive 2010/63/EU. The US Guide for the Care and Use of Laboratory Animals published by the National Research Council (2011) outlines cage sizes in table 3.1 of the environment, housing and management section, summarised here in Table 24.2. The differences between these guidelines illustrate the more general point that it is difficult to specify scientifically the minimal sizes of cages for maintenance. However, the European guidelines took note of research indicating that hamsters were chronically stressed when housed in small enclosures, a condition likely to affect their welfare and the quality of science obtained from these animals (Kuhnen 1999a, 1999b).

While sufficient space is needed to allow appropriate enrichment and to give the animals some control over social interactions, other aspects of housing such as material of construction, floor type, provision of furniture and bedding, as well as appropriate social enrichment are equally important. Arnold and Estep (1994) explored the caging preferences of Syrian hamsters. Whilst their research showed that most Syrian hamsters preferred solid floors with bedding, they also demonstrated that previous housing conditions can affect cage type preference.

Hamster housing should provide bedding substrate deep enough to burrow in, such as wood shavings (pine or aspen), or shredded paper. If a less structural bedding is chosen, such as corn cob, shelter structures can be provided to serve as a burrow. Hamsters build nests, so nesting material, particularly for breeding hamsters, is recommended. Lanteigne and Reebs found that in a study of male hamsters, bedding preference depended on what material could be made into a nest; thus, hamsters of both sexes should be provided material suitable for nest building (Lanteigne & Reebs 2006). Further information on environmental enrichment for

The Syrian hamster

Table 24.1 Minimum enclosure dimensions and space allowances for Syrian hamsters according to Appendix A of the Council of Europe Convention, ETS/123 (Council of Europe 2006) and the European Directive 86/609 (European Commission 2007).

	Body weight (g)	Minimum enclosure size (cm²)	Floor area/animal (cm²)	Minimum enclosure height (cm)
In stock and during procedures	Up to 60	800	150	14
	From 60 to 100	800	200	14
	Over 100	800	250	14
Breeding		800 mother or monogamous pair with litter		14
Stock at breeders (*)	Less than 60	1500	100	14

(*) Post-weaned hamsters may be kept at these higher stocking densities, for the short period after weaning until issue provided that the animals are housed in larger enclosures with adequate enrichment, and these housing conditions do not cause any welfare deficit such as increased levels of aggression, morbidity or mortality, stereotypes and other behavioural deficits, weight loss or other physiological or behavioural stress responses.

Table 24.2 Minimum enclosure dimensions and space allowances for Syrian hamsters according to the US Guide for the Care and Use of Laboratory Animals (National Research Council 2011)*.

Weight (g)	Floor area/animal (cm²)	Cage height (cm)
< 60	65	15
Up to 80	84	15
Up to 100	103	15
> 100	≥123	15

*Dimensions in this table are to the nearest whole number as US measurements are in inches.

Syrian hamsters can be found: *Comfortable Quarters for Laboratory Animals* (Liss et al. 2015) and *Management, Husbandry and Colony Health* (Mulder 2012).

The Syrian hamster does not conform to the generalisation concerning other hamsters that males are more aggressive than females. Both sexes are highly aggressive, making group housing for welfare or experimental purposes challenging. Grelk et al. (1974) investigated the influence of caging conditions and hormone treatments on fighting in male and female Syrian hamsters. They found that sex, hormonal state and caging condition interact in a complex manner. Arnold and Estep (1994) explored the effects of housing on social preference and behaviour in male Syrian hamsters. Their results showed that they spent more time in social proximity than out of proximity, especially if they had prior group-housing experience. In addition, singly housed animals showed more aggressive behaviour with conspecifics and lower weight gains than group-housed animals, which showed more evidence of wounding. Thus, early housing experience can profoundly affect later social preference and behaviour, and most laboratory hamsters can be group housed (Krause & Schüler 2010) including breeder pairs without incident (Pritchett-Corning & Gaskill, 2015).

In summary, solid-bottomed cages with bedding material of sufficient depth and structure for burrowing or structures that can substitute as burrows should be provided. In general, group housing may be preferable to individual caging so long as the groups are formed early in life and are stable and harmonious. Where this is not possible, it is better to single house animals, either from the start of the study or immediately upon arrival, if purchased from a commercial breeder. When group housing, there should be room for hiding or escaping from cage-mates.

Environmental conditions

Conditions suitable for maintaining rats and mice are also suitable for Syrian hamsters. Generally, seasonal variability in the Syrian hamster can be reduced by the provision of a constant temperature of 21–22 °C. While hamsters in captivity can be kept in a 12:12 (12 h day and 12 h night) light cycle, a 14:10 light cycle is recommended for breeding colonies (Mulder 2012). Such conditions will eliminate hibernation. Extraneous noise should be kept to a minimum, consideration being given to sources of ultrasound. Excessive deviance from the normal environmental parameters should always be avoided if at all possible, especially in breeding colonies when it may contribute to lowered breeding efficiency and maternal cannibalism.

Identification and sexing

Individual animals can be identified by ear punch, ear tag, tattooing of the ear or toe or microchipping. Ear punching can be performed as in other rodents, with similar welfare considerations, and the ears of animals without dark pigmentation can be tattooed using a tattooing machine. Toe tattooing is used regularly in other species to identify newborn animals but may be complicated in hamsters by their tendency to kill litters if disturbed. Microchip implants have now become the preferred method for identifying many species of animals, including Syrian hamsters. Whilst they have the distinct advantage of being a reasonably permanent means of identification, microchip implants do have some disadvantages including cost, subcutaneous (SC) migration or chip failure.

The sex of mature Syrian, Chinese and Siberian hamsters can be easily distinguished by the prominent testes of the male, even in pubescent animals, and the greater anogenital distance in the male (Figures 24.2 and 24.3). Sexing the European hamster, however, presents some problems during the season when sexual activity ceases – usually October to February. It is difficult to tell the sexes apart at this time as the vulva of the female is closed and the testes of the male are drawn up into the abdominal cavity. At other times, the criteria used for sexing other hamster species can be used.

Breeding

An overall review of reproductive parameters for the Syrian, Chinese, and Siberian hamsters can be found in Table 24.3. Sexual maturity of the Syrian hamster is reached by 42 days

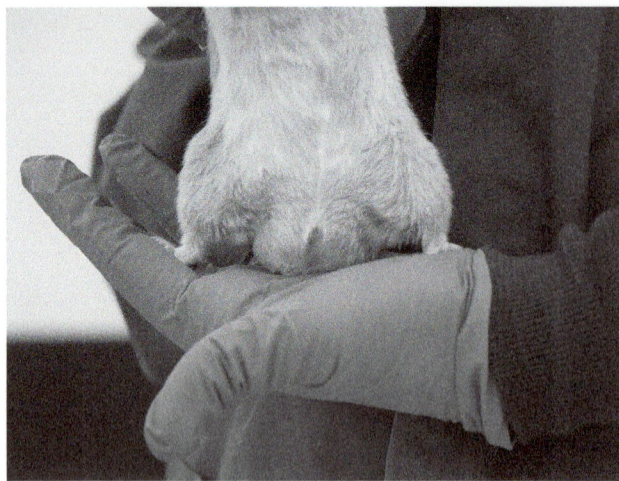

Figure 24.2 A male Syrian hamster. Note the prominent testicles and the greater anogenital distance. (Figure used courtesy of KPC.)

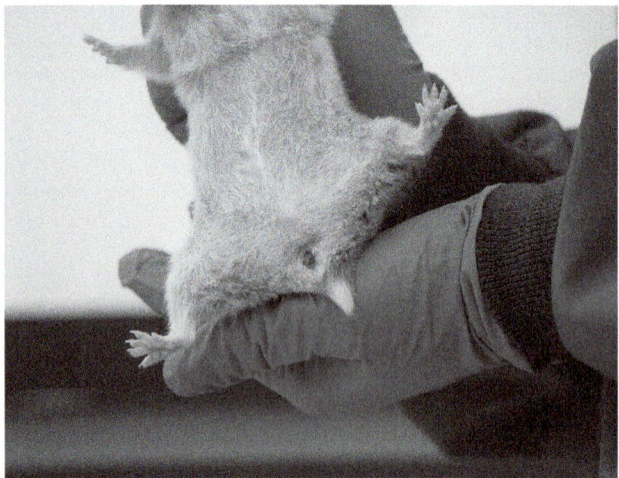

Figure 24.3 A female Syrian hamster. The anogenital distance is much shorter than in the male. (Figure used courtesy of KPC.)

of age or earlier (see later in this section) and can be confirmed using the penile smear technique to look for the presence of sperm on the glans penis. While sexual maturity is reached by 6–7 weeks of age in Syrian hamsters, optimal reproductive age is reached at 8–10 weeks of age for females and 10–12 weeks for males (Whitaker 2010).

The oestrous cycle is regular, lasting four days. Two lateral pouches lined with cornified epithelial cells in the vagina of hamsters can make the vaginal cytology method of evaluating the phase of the cycle difficult. External indications of the cycle include the presence of a white, stringy, opaque discharge with a distinct odour on the second day of the cycle followed by a waxy secretion on the third day (Figure 24.4). It is, therefore, possible to determine the day for mating by screening females for the stringy, opaque discharge. This indicates that the female reached peak oestrus the day before, and therefore, she can be reliably mated on the third day after disappearance of the discharge. Large groups of females for timed mating purposes can be selected in this way with up to 90% conception rates.

Adult hamsters are solitary and both sexes are aggressive, coming into contact for mating. Female Syrian hamsters are aggressive towards males during late oestrus and early dioestrus; during a receptive period that lasts about a week (Marques & Valenstein 1977), she attracts a mate by leaving a vaginal scent trail, tolerates the male's presence and shows lordosis, a posture of flattened back and elevated tail. Shortly afterwards copulation will take place, lasting around 30 minutes.

Harem mating, using a breeding system in which females are selected for mating by handlers via assessment of receptiveness, can be employed. One male can serve a harem of 12 females. This is a common method of breeding Syrian hamsters but is very labour intensive. The hamsters are mated soon after dark, when they are naturally most active. The female is placed in the same cage as the male and the pair observed to ensure mating occurs. Should fighting start, the pair must be immediately separated. Once confirmed pregnant, females are separated from the harem and housed singly through parturition and weaning. Fighting will occur, however, when reintroduced to the harem.

Table 24.3 Reproductive data for Syrian, Chinese and Siberian hamsters. (Reproduced with permission from the National Academies Press, Copyright (1996), National Academy of Sciences.)

Character	Syrian	Chinese	Siberian
Age at puberty	45–60 days	48–100 days	45–60 days
Min. breeding age	50 days	70–84 days	50 days
Breeding season	All year, may be a decrease in winter	All year in laboratory conditions	All year in laboratory conditions
Oestrous cycle	Polyoestrus: all year	Polyoestrus: all year	Polyoestrus: all year
Duration of oestrous cycle	4 days	4 days	4 days
Duration of oestrus	4–23 h	6–8 h	Unknown
Gestation	16 days	21 days	18 days
Average litter size	6	5	3.2
Ovulation time	Early oestrus	Shortly before oestrus	Unknown
Copulation	About 1 h after nightfall	About 1 h after nightfall	Unknown
Implantation	5 or more days	5–6 days	Unknown
Birth weight	2 g	1.5–2.5 g	1.5–2.0 g
Weaned	21 days	21 days	18 days
Chromosome no.	44	22	28
Return to oestrus post-partum	5–10 min	Post-partum mating does occur	Post-partum mating does occur
Number of mammae	12–16	8	8

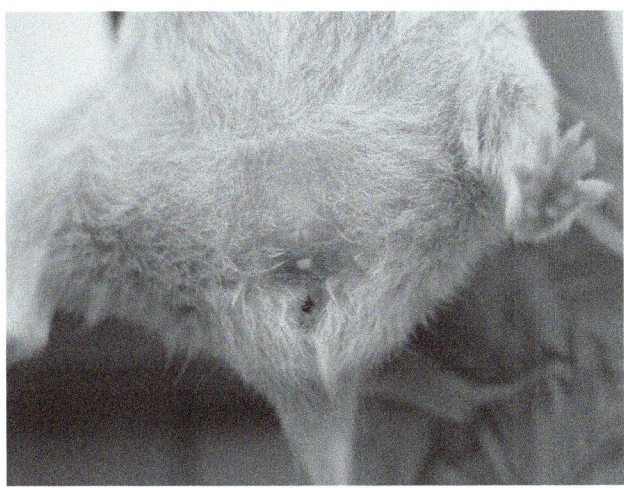

Figure 24.4 A female Syrian hamster showing the typical waxy secretion on the third day of the Syrian hamster oestrus cycle.

Monogamous pairing of hamsters at weaning is now considered the most satisfactory and labour-efficient method of breeding Syrian hamsters. Females can be placed in the cage with a male on the third day after the appearance of postovulatory discharge. Females that are receptive to mating will assume a lordosis posture and mating generally occurring within 5 minutes. Gestation is an average of 16 days (range 15–18) with litters ranging from 4 to 12 pups. Estrous cycles resume one to eight days post parturition (Battles 1985).

Implantation of the fertilised ovum takes place approximately six days post-coitus. It is important that at this time, the animal is handled as little as possible. The Syrian hamster has a short gestation period (~16 days) and the period is generally very regular, varying by only 2 or 3 h with hamsters primarily giving birth during the day (Viswanathan & Davis 1992). Pregnant females build nests beginning in late gestation (Swanson & Campbell 1979) and so should be placed in clean cages with additional nesting material approximately two days prior to parturition. Enough food should be made available in the cage to last the female 7–10 days so that there is minimal disturbance of the newborn litter. Any interference frequently results in the female killing her litter. Litter size normally increases with parity.

Newborn hamsters are altricial with closed eyes and ears and are hairless but have teeth. Fostering newborn Syrian hamsters onto other rodents is usually unsuccessful due to this characteristic. Ears begin to open at 4 days, solids begin to be taken at 7–10 days and eyes open at 14–16 days of age. Water must be available to animals from 10 days of age. Hamsters are normally weaned around 21 days and the female re-mated. Figure 24.5 shows typical growth curves for the Syrian hamster.

The optimal reproductive life of a Syrian hamster is considered to be around 10 months and a significant reduction in reproductive capacity occurs from 1 year of age onwards. During her reproductive lifetime, a female hamster will produce four to six litters. It is commonly thought that cross-fostering to other hamsters is not possible; however,

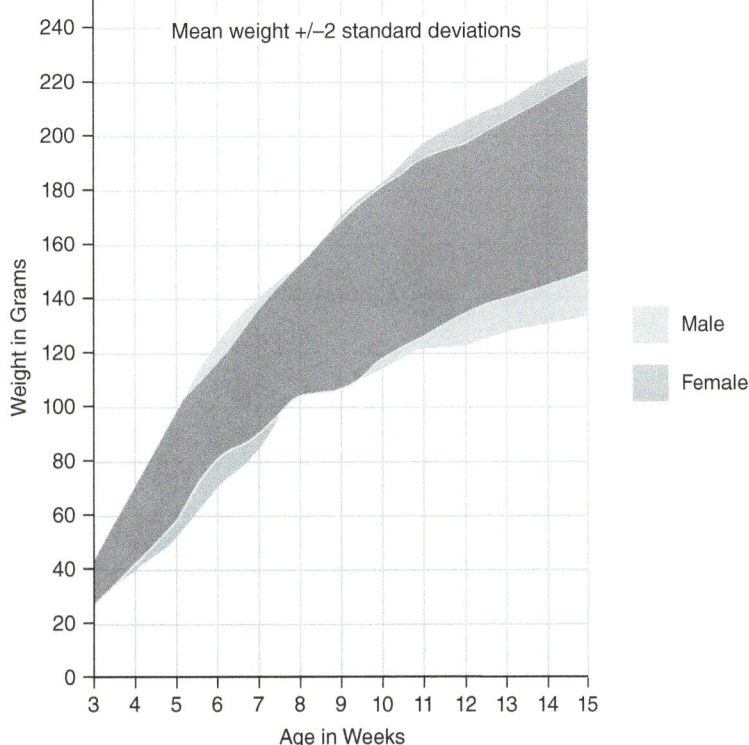

Figure 24.5 Typical growth curves for Syrian hamsters. (From: https://www.criver.com/products-services/find-model/lvg-golden-syrian-hamster?region=3611; accessed 24 April, 2023)

Grainger and Plotkin (1987) investigated cross-fostering and maternal care in Syrian hamsters and concluded that it can be successfully undertaken at three different ages – soon after birth, at about 1 week of age and around 2 weeks of age. They found nest quality, survival and pup weights to correlate well. Cross-fostering could prove useful in disease control or eradication, and the establishment of an SPF colony of caesarean-derived hamsters has been reported (Burke *et al.* 1970; Huaqiong *et al.* 2005).

Feeding

Natural and laboratory diets

Hamsters are omnivorous and coprophagous and hoard food as a survival strategy in the wild. Hamsters leave the safety of the burrow to forage for food, stuffing their cheek pouches and retrieving food back to the burrow to be deposited in their resource hoard. Natural diets consist of mainly grains, plant roots, shoots, insects and fruit (Whittaker 2010). In the laboratory and intensive breeding situations, complete diets of known formulation and quality are advised on both scientific and welfare grounds. Diets specifically formulated for rats and mice are adequate for the maintenance and breeding of hamsters. Providing that a good-quality, complete rodent diet is available, nutritional deficiencies are unlikely to occur. Vitamin E deficiency has been described by West and Mason (1958) and Keeler and Young (1979), but in both papers, the deficiency was experimentally induced. Mooij *et al.* (1992) have also described experimentally induced disturbed reproductive performance in extremely folic-acid-deficient Syrian hamsters. Due to their short, wide snouts and hoarding behaviour, feeding from the floor or other direct-access feeding method is preferred to the wire-bar feeders used for many other rodents.

Water

A fresh, clean, *ad libitum* supply of water must be provided to hamsters either by means of water bottles or through automatic watering devices. The average daily consumption of water by an adult Syrian hamster is 10–20 ml depending upon the housing conditions, the type of feed and the hamster's physiological condition (e.g. pregnancy and suckling).

Laboratory procedures

Handling

The Syrian hamster can have an unjustified reputation for being difficult to handle, but this is usually due to poor or intensive husbandry and startling sleeping animals. For routine handling, the Syrian hamster can be picked up by a firm but gentle grasp across the back of the animal. Picking up by placing the thumb across the abdomen enables sexing to be carried out. Turning the animal over so that it lies in the palm of the hand, ventral side up, tends to inactivate most animals and has a quietening effect. This handling technique is illustrated in Figures 24.6 and 24.7. All species of hamsters can be picked up in a similar way, but the use of cupped hands is preferred when minimal restraint is required.

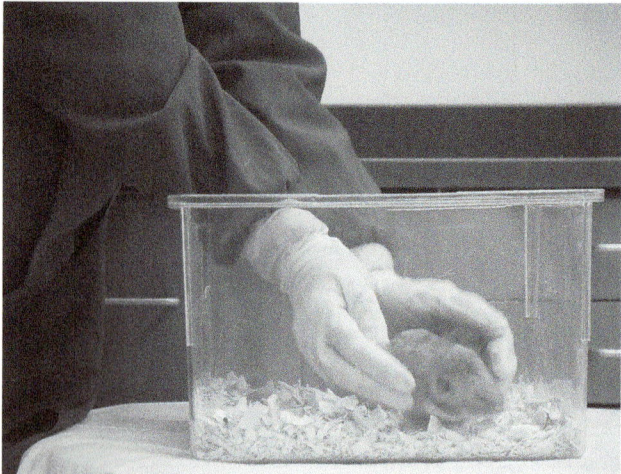

Figure 24.6 Approaching a Syrian hamster to pick it up in cupped hands. If hamsters are approached slowly and not abruptly grabbed from a sound sleep, they are usually easy to handle. (Figure used courtesy of KPC.)

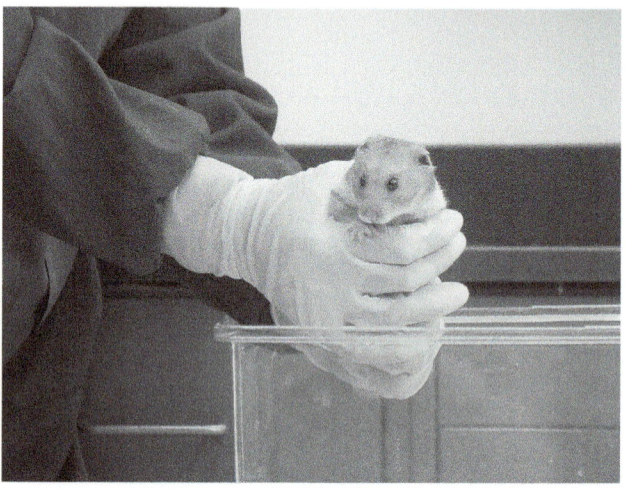

Figure 24.7 Successful lifting of a hamster from the cage using cupped hands. (Figure used courtesy of KPC.)

For oral dosing, intraperitoneal injections and other manipulations, most hamsters can be held by the dorsal skin ensuring that a firm grip is made at the scruff of the neck (Figure 24.8).

Hamsters can inflict serious bites, especially during the breeding season, so while protective gloves may be prudent, animals do become tamer with frequent handling. When handling hamsters, it should be remembered that, under normal conditions, they spend long periods sleeping during the day when little activity will be seen. After diurnal handling, they often appear aggressive towards their cage-mates and emit loud screeching noises and aggressive movements, disproportionate to the degree of interference.

Physiological monitoring

With care, a standard thermometer may be used to determine rectal temperature (37–38 °C) but it is far more convenient to use an electronic, semi-rigid probe thermometer. In

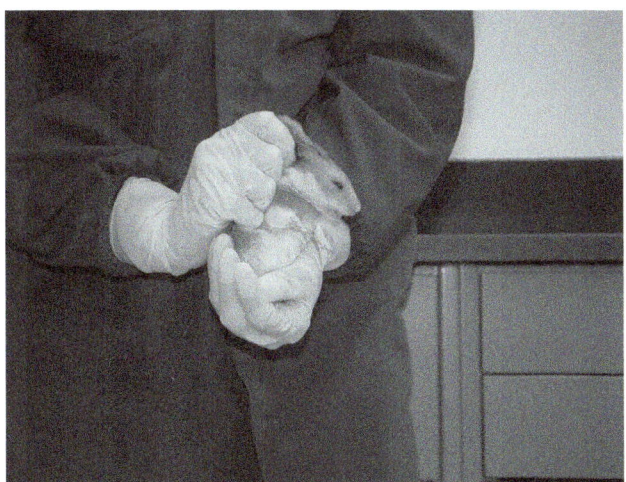

Figure 24.8 Scruffing a Syrian hamster from a cupped hold. Figure used courtesy of KPC.

addition, body temperature, motor activity and heart rate can all be monitored via telemetric devices.

Blood sampling

Small blood samples can be collected from the saphenous vein in hamsters. Orbital venous sinus puncture, gingival vein (Rodriguez et al. 2017) and cardiac puncture are also recognised routes for blood sampling in the hamster. An excellent summary of blood collection sites, with recommended technique and equipment described and volumes obtainable can be found on the NC3Rs blood sampling website[1]. The circulating blood volume of the Syrian hamster is around 78 ml/kg body weight. Generally, removal of no more than 10% of the circulating blood volume is advised at any one time.

Urine, faeces and expired gases

Standard glass, metal, or plastic metabolism cages can be used to separate urine from faeces, whereas only glass is recommended for the trapping of expired respiratory gases. The nesting of hamsters in feeders or other areas of metabolism cages should be avoided when possible. Cages that provide either access for liquid diets or closure of the access to the feeder may be used. An excellent summary of additional biological specimen collection can be found in Silverman (2012).

Administration of substances

Anaesthesia

As with all anaesthesia, the condition of the individual animal and requirements of the procedure should be taken into account when determining an appropriate anaesthetic regimen. Hamsters present similar anaesthetic challenges as other small rodents, including difficult IV access and the risk of hypothermia. Fasting prior to anaesthesia is unnecessary as vomiting does not occur.

The most common dose routes in hamsters are injected or inhaled. For injection, safe and effective anaesthesia can be achieved by fentanyl-fluanisone (hypnorm) (1 ml/kg) + midazolam or diazepam (5 mg/kg); see Flecknell 2023 Appendix 3 for mixing instructions. Additionally, ketamine in combinations (ketamine 150 mg/kg + acepromazine 5 mg/kg; ketamine 75–100 mg/kg + medetomidine 0.25–1 mg/kg or ketamine 80–200 mg/kg + zylazine 5–10 mg/kg) can provide between 30 and 120 min duration of anaesthesia (Flecknell 2023). Inhaled anaesthetic is usually isoflurane delivered via nosecone, after induction in a chamber.

Sources of in depth information on anaesthesia in the Syrian hamster include Flecknell (2023) and Flecknell et al. (2015).

Dosing routes

Dosing routes for hamsters include SC, intramuscular (IM), intravenous (IV) and intraosseous (IO) injections. Administration via the cheek pouch, oral administration (per os [PO]) and intratracheal (IT) dosing are also possible. The copious loose skin on the back and flanks of hamsters makes for easy SC injections. Care should be taken to properly restrain animals for injection, as hamsters are agile and may twist around to bite. A small gauge needle, such as a 30 g, is recommended. Hamsters have little muscle mass in their hind limbs making IM injection in the quadriceps difficult. IM injections are ideally restricted to a volume of 0.1–0.2 ml per site with a maximum number of two injection sites per day[2]. IV injection can be achieved via the cephalic, lateral saphenous, jugular and lingual veins. Injection directly into the bloodstream has been described via the retro-orbital venous sinus in the anaesthetised hamster, through caution must be exercised not to penetrate the thin skull or inject material that may clump or induce neoplasia if left behind, such as cell suspensions. Where IV injection is difficult, IO injection or catheterisation into the tibia or femur under anaesthesia is a possible alternative. Post-procedural analgesia is recommended.

Hamster cheek pouches, thin walled and well vascularised, are utilised mostly for feed and bedding storage and transport. It is, however, their characteristics of being 'immunologically privileged' (lacking lymphatic drainage) and well vascularised that has been used in research models for tumour growth. Cheek pouches are easily inverted, for sample implantation and subsequent inspection for examination, even in the awake hamster.

Gastric intubation in hamsters is similar to that in other small rodents. Ball-tipped intubation tubes should be measured to the bottom of the rib cage, slid along the roof of the restrained animals' mouth, and passed with gentle pressure into the oesophagus and stomach.

With the increased use of hamsters as a model for the respiratory virus that causes COVID-19, intratracheal installation has become a more prevalent route of experimental exposure. While this route of administration can be achieved via

---

[1] https://www.nc3rs.org.uk/3rs-resources/blood-sampling/blood-sampling-hamster (Accessed April 24, 2023)

[2] https://iqconsortium.org/images/LG-3Rs/IQ-CRO_Recommended_Dose_Volumes_for_Common_Laboratory_Animals_June_2016_%282%29.pdf (Accessed April 25, 2023)

multiple methods, exposure through the oropharynx under anaesthesia is the most straightforward. Multiple methods, equipment required and techniques are summarised in (Driscoll et al. 2000). Additional techniques and recommended volumes are well summarised by Silverman (2012).

Diseases

Commercially sourced hamsters are generally of good health, but may harbour commensal viral and bacterial pathogens. Similar to other rodent species, the Federation of European Laboratory Animal Science Associations has published recommendations on health monitoring in the species (FELASA 2014).

Non-infectious concerns

Infanticide or pup injury is common, especially when hamsters are stressed. Primiparous females are renowned for their tendency to eat their young. Injuries can vary from limb amputation to death (Griffin et al. 1989).

Amyloidosis, the polymerisation of normally soluble proteins, is found in the liver, kidney, stomach, adrenal, thyroid and spleen (Coe & Ross 1990) of older hamsters. Ascites, SC oedema and hydrothorax due to hypoalbuminemia and proteinuria are evidence of nephrotic syndrome.

Atrial thrombosis is common in older hamsters in some colonies. Females are usually affected earlier than males. The syndrome is often associated with amyloidosis (McMartin & Dodds 1982) and changes also occur in coagulation and fibrinolytic parameters consistent with consumptive coagulopathy (Wechsler & Jones 1984).

Polycystic disease is characterised by multiple hepatic cysts and is a common finding in older hamsters at necropsy (Gleiser et al. 1970; Somvanshi et al. 1987). Cysts can be found in other organs (cecum, kidneys, ovaries and spleen) and are generally asymptomatic, though occasional abdominal distension can be seen.

Hepatic cirrhosis is a spontaneous disorder occurring sporadically among hamsters, reaching an incidence of up to 20% in some colonies (Chesterman & Pomerance 1965). Brunnert and Altman (1991) describe the laboratory assessment of chronic hepatitis.

The incidence of neoplasms in hamsters is relatively rare but varies markedly between strains. The majority of tumours are benign and frequently arise from the endocrine system or alimentary tract. Malignant neoplasms reported in hamsters include adrenocortical carcinoma, renal cell carcinoma, SC sarcoma and most frequently lymphosarcoma (Homburger 1983). For extensive information on neoplasms in hamsters, see Pour et al. (1976a, 1976b, 1976c, 1976d, 1979), Van Hoosier and Trentin (1979), Turusov and Mohr (1982), Bernfeld et al. (1986) and Barthold (1992).

Viral infections

Whilst hamsters are susceptible to a number of viral infections, few are of practical importance. Serological recommendations include screening for lymphocytic choriomeningitis virus (LCMV), *Protoparvovirus* spp., murine pneumonia virus (MPnV), Mammalian orthoreovirus (Reo 3), Sendai virus (SV) and hamster polyomavirus (HAPyV).

LCMV, whilst an important zoonosis (Cassano et al. 2012), is not found in commercially sourced animals. LCMV can be transmitted vertically or horizontally; however, the transmission to laboratory hamsters has been through the implantation of unknowingly infected tumours. Hotchin et al. (1974) describe an outbreak in hospital personnel attributable to a research colony of Syrian hamsters, and Skinner and Knight (1979) review the potential role of Syrian hamsters and other small mammals as a reservoir of LCMV.

Hamster parvovirus (HaPV, closely related to mouse parvovirus 3), is typically an asymptomatic infection in adults (Christie et al. 2010). Young hamsters may be runted, with dental loss (Gibson 1983).

Sendai virus causes clinical respiratory disease in hamsters and may reduce productivity in a breeding colony. While hamsters can be infected, mice are considered the host species (Percy & Palmer 1997).

Hamster polyomavirus causes spontaneous skin epitheliomas as well as lymphoma. Clinical syndromes are associated with the particular organs infiltrated. Due to the stability of the virus in the environment, culling and environmental decontamination is recommended.

Syrian hamsters are also permissive hosts to SARS-CoV-2 (Imai et al. 2020), which makes them a valuable model for human infection as well as prone to spontaneous infection. Infected hamsters show clinical signs similar to those of humans including weight loss, fever, and signs of upper respiratory infections. Lung pathology is also similar. Hamsters have served as a source of human infection (Yen et al. 2022), and so care should be taken to both isolate hamsters from potentially infective humans as well as humans from potentially infective humans.

Bacterial infections

A wide variety of pathogenic or opportunistic bacterial infections may cause disease in hamsters if predisposing factors such as concurrent viral infection, stress, immunosuppression, etc. are present. Case reports are too numerous to mention but Amao et al. (1991) reports the isolation of *Corynebacterium kutscheri* from aging Syrian hamsters, and Shoji-Darkye et al. (1991) describe the pathogenesis of cilia-associated respiratory (CAR) bacillus (*Filobacterium rodentium*) in Syrian hamsters.

The most common bacterial infection in hamsters is proliferative ileitis (transmissible ileal hyperplasia) caused by *Lawsonia intracellularis* (Stills 1991). This is the most commonly recognised disease in Syrian hamsters and usually results in high morbidity and high mortality. The term 'wet-tail' should not be used because this descriptive term includes virtually all the conditions that may cause diarrhoea.

Other bacteria that may give rise to enteritis include *Salmonella* spp, *Clostridia piliformis* (Tyzzer's disease) and *Clostridium difficile* (non-antibiotic – associated). Barthold, Griffen and Percy (2016) provide an excellent overview of bacterial disease in hamsters together with further references.

Parasitic infestations

Commercially sourced hamsters should for the most part be free of pathogenic parasites. Discovery of ectoparasites, nematodes and cestodes in purchased animals should trigger an investigation for alternative sources whilst intestinal protozoa are usually non-pathogenic.

Hamsters are susceptible to infection by multiple species of internal parasites. Pinworms include *Syphacia mesocriceti*, *Syphacia criceti*, *Syphacia stroma*, *Syphacia peromysci*, *Syphacia obvelata*, *Syphacia muris*, *Aspiculuris tetrapetra* and *Dentostomella translucida* (Burr *et al*. 2012). Specific studies for the treatment for pinworm in hamsters are lacking. Treatment regimens successful in mice (Pritchett 2007; Pritchett & Johnston 2002) may be effective. Taylor (1992) describes the elimination of pinworms (*Syphacia obvelata*) using a combination of piperizine hydrate and thiabendazole. *Rodentoleptis nana*, *Hymenolepis diminuta* and *Rodentoleptis microstoma* infections have also been reported (Pinto *et al*. 2001).

Euthanasia

Methods of euthanasia suitable for other small rodents can also be used for hamsters and specific methods can be found in AVMA Guidelines for the Euthanasia of Animals: 2020 Edition[3] and Home Office (1997), and a thoughtful review of rodent euthanasia methods by Shomer *at al*. (2020). See also Chapter 17: *Euthanasia and other fates for laboratory animals*. It is important to ensure that staff are competent to perform the procedure, especially when using physical methods. When using carbon dioxide, it is essential that the animals are placed in a rising concentration of carbon dioxide and not a saturated atmosphere. Finally, whatever method is chosen, death must be confirmed via either severance of a major blood vessel, dislocation of the neck, or by observing rigor mortis before disposing of the carcase.

Acknowledgements: The authors would like to acknowledge Dr. David Whittaker, the author of the previous version of this chapter, for his work and for allowing them to edit and update.

References

Amao, H., Akimoto, T., Takahashi, W. *et al*. (1991) Isolation of *Corynebacterium kutscheri* from aged Syrian hamsters (*Mesocricetus auratus*). *Laboratory Animal Science*, **41**, 265–268.

Arnold, E.C. and Estep, Q.D. (1994) Laboratory caging preference in golden hamsters. *Laboratory Animals*, **28**, 232–238.

AVMA Guidelines for the euthanasia of animals, 2020 Edition: https://www.avma.org/sites/default/files/2020-02/Guidelines-on-Euthanasia-2020.pdf

Barthold, S.W. (1992) Haemolymphatic tumours. In: *The Pathology of Tumours of Laboratory Animals. III. Tumours of the Hamster*. Eds Mohr, U. and Turnsov, V., pp. 318–344. IARC Scientific Publication, Lyon, France.

Barthold, S.W., Griffen, S.M. and Percy, D.H. (2016) Hamsters. In: *The Pathology of Laboratory Rodents and Rabbits*, pp. 173–198. Wiley-Blackwell, Ames, Iowa.

Battles, A.H. (1985) The biology, care and diseases of the Syrian hamster. *Compendium on Continuing Education for the Practising Veterinarian*, **7**, 815–825.

Bernfeld, P., Homburger, F., Adams, R.A. *et al*. (1986) Base-line data in a carcinogen-susceptible first generation hybrid strain of golden hamsters: F1D Alexander. *Journal of the National Cancer Institute*, **77**, 165–171.

Brunnert, S.R. and Altman, N. (1991) Laboratory assessment of chronic hepatitis in Syrian hamsters. *Laboratory Animal Science*, **41**, 559–562.

Bryche, B., St Albin, A., Murri, S. *et al*. (2020) Massive transient damage of the olfactory epithelium associated with infection of sustentacular cells by SARS-CoV-2 in golden Syrian hamsters. *Brain, Behavior, and Immunity*, **89**, 579–586. doi: 10.1016/j.bbi.2020.06.032

Burke, J.G., Van Hoosier G.L. Jr. and Trentin J.J. (1970). Cesarean derivation and foster nursing of strain LSH inbred hamsters. *Laboratory Animal Care*, **20(2)**, 238–241.

Burr, H.N., Paluch, L.R., Roble, G.S. and Lipman, N.S. (2012) Parasitic diseases. In: *The Laboratory Rabbit, Guinea Pig, Hamster and Other Rodents*. Eds Suckow, M.A., Stevens, K.A. and Wilson, R.P., pp. 839–866. Academic Press, Waltham MA.

Cassano, A., Rasmussen, S. and Wolf, F.R. (2012). Viral diseases. In: *The Laboratory Rabbit, Guinea Pig, Hamster, and Other Rodents*. Eds Suckow, M.A., Stevens, K.A. and Wilson, R.P., pp. 821–837. Academic Press, Waltham, MA.

Chan, J., Zhang, A.J., Yuan, S. *et al*. (2020) Simulation of the clinical and pathological manifestations of coronavirus disease 2019 (COVID-19) in a golden Syrian hamster model: implications for disease pathogenesis and transmissibility. *Clinical Infectious Diseases*, **71(9)**, 2428–2446.

Chesterman, F.C. and Pomerance, A. (1965) Cirrhosis and liver tumours in a closed colony of golden hamsters. *British Journal of Cancer*, **1980**, 802–811.

Chijioke, C.P., Mansfield K.J. and Pearson, R.M. (1990) The reproducibility of the hamster egg penetration test for the assessment of human spermatozoal fertilising potential. *Animal Technology*, **41**, 49–58.

Christie, R.D., Marcus, E.C., Wagner, A.M. *et al*. (2010). Experimental infection of mice with hamster parvovirus: Evidence for interspecies transmission of mouse parvovirus 3. *Comparative Medicine*, **60**, 123–129.

Coe, J.E. and Ross, J.J. (1990) Amyloidosis and female protein in the Syrian hamster. Concurrent regulation by sex hormones. *Journal of Experimental Medicine*, **171**, 1257–1266.

Council of Europe (2006) Multilateral Consultation of Parties to the European Convention for the Protection of Vertebrate Animals used for Experimental and other Scientific Purposes (ETS 123) Appendix A. Cons 123 (2006) 3. http://www.coe.int/t/e/legal_affairs/legal_co-operation/biological_safety,_use_of_animals/laboratory_animals/2006/Cons123(2006)3AppendixA_en.pdf (accessed 31 July 2008).

Driscoll, K.E., Costa, D.L., Hatch, G. *et al*. (2000) Intratracheal Installation as an Exposure Technique for the Evaluation of Respiratory Tract Toxicity: uses and limitations. *Toxicological Sciences*, **55**, 24–35.

European Commission (2007) Commission recommendations of 18 June 2007 on guidelines for the accommodation and care of animals used for experimental and other scientific purposes. Annex II to European Council Directive 86/609. See 2007/526/EC. http://eurlex.europa.eu/LexUriServ/site/en/oj/2007/l_197/l_19720070730en00010089.pdf (accessed 13 May 2008).

Federation of European Laboratory Animal Science Associations (FELASA) (2014) Report of the FELASA Working Group on

---

[3]https://www.avma.org/resources-tools/avma-policies/avma-guidelines-euthanasia-animals (Accessed June 28, 2023)

Animal Health: recommendations of the health monitoring of mouse, rat, hamster, guinea pig and rabbit breeding colonies. *Laboratory Animals*, **48(3)**, 178–192.

Flecknell, P.A. and Mitchell, M. (1984) Midazolam and fentanyl-fluanisone. Assessment of anaesthetic effects in laboratory rodents and rabbits. *Laboratory Animals*, **18**, 143–146.

Flecknell, P.A. (2023) *Laboratory Animal Anaesthesia*, 5th edn. Academic Press, London.

Flecknell, P., Lofgren, J. L. S., Dyson, M. C. et al. (2015). Chapter 24 – Preanesthesia, anesthesia, analgesia, and euthanasia. In: *Laboratory Animal Medicine*, 3rd edn. Eds Fox, J.G., Anderson, L.C. and Otto, G.M. et al., pp. 1135–1200. Academic Press, Boston.

Gatterman, R., Fritzsche, P., Neumann, K., et al. (2001) Notes on the current distribution and the ecology of wild golden hamsters (*Mesocricetus auratus*). *Journal of Zoology London*, **254**, 359–365.

Gatterman, R., Johnston, R. E., Yigit, N. et al. (2008). Golden hamsters are nocturnal in captivity but diurnal in nature. *Biology Letters*, **4**, 253–255.

Gibson, S.V. (1983). Mortality in weanling hamsters associated with tooth loss. *Laboratory Animal Science*, **33**, 497.

Gibson, E.M., Wang, C., Tjho, S., et al. (2010) Experimental 'Jet Lag' inhibits adult neurogenesis and produces long-term cognitive deficits in female hamsters. *PLoS ONE*. https://doi.org/10.1371/journal.pone.0015267.

Gleiser, C.A., Van Hoosier, G.L. Jr. and Sheldon, W.G. (1970). A polycystic disease of hamsters in a closed colony. *Laboratory Animal Care*, **20**, 923–929.

Grainger, L.J. and Plotkin, H.C. (1987) Cross-fostering and maternal care in Syrian hamsters. *Animal Technology*, **38**, 25–30.

Grelk, D.F., Papson, B.A., Cole, J.E. et al. (1974) The influence of caging conditions and hormone treatments on fighting in male and female hamsters. *Hormones and Behaviour*, **5**, 355–366.

Griffin, H.E., Gbadamosi, S.G., Perry, R.L. et al. (1989) Hamster limb loss. *Laboratory Animal*, **18**, 19–20.

Gruber, A.D., Firsching, T.C., Trimpert, J. and Dietert, K. (2021) Hamster models of COVID-19 reviewed: how human can they be? *Veterinary Pathology*, **59(4)**, 528–545.

Hirose, M. and Ogura, A. (2019) The golden (Syrian) hamster as a model for the study of reproductive biology: past, present and future. *Reproductive Medicine and Biology*, **18**, 34–39.

Homburger, F. (1983) Background data on tumor incidence in control animals (Syrian hamsters). *Progress in Experimental Tumor Research*, **26**, 259–265.

Home Office (1997) *Code of Practice: The Humane Killing of Animals under Schedule 1 to the Animals (Scientific Procedures) Act 1986*. HMSO, ISBN 0102653976.

Hotchin, J., Sikora, E. and Kinch, W. (1974) Lymphocytic choriomeningitis in a hamster colony causes infection of hospital personnel. *Science*, **185**, 1173–1174.

Huaqiong, Z., Lin, H., Sulan, L., et al. (2005) Establishment of SPF golden hamster colony by cesarean section. (*Sichuan Dong wu= Sichuan Dongwu=) Sichuan Journal of Zoology*, **24(1)**, 85–87.

Imai, M., Iwatsuki-Horimoto, K., Hatta, M., et al. (2020). Syrian hamsters as a small animal model for SARS-CoV-2 infection and countermeasure development. *Proceedings of the National Academy of Sciences*, **117**, 16587–16595.

Krause, S. and Schüler, L. (2010) Behavioural and endocrinological changes in Syrian hamsters (*Mesocricetus auratus*) under domestication. *Journal of Animal Breeding and Genetics*, **127(6)**, 452–461.

Kuhnen, G. (1999a) The effect of cage size and enrichment on core temperature and febrile response of the golden hamster. *Laboratory Animals*, **33**, 221–227.

Kuhnen, G. (1999b) Housing-induced changes in the febrile response of juvenile and adult golden hamsters. *Journal of Experimental Animal Science*, **39**, 151–155.

Lanteigne, M. and Reebs, S.G. (2006) Preference for bedding material in Syrian hamsters *Laboratory Animals*, **40**, 410–418.

Liss, C., Litwak, K., Tilford, D. and Reinhardt, V. (eds) (2015) *Comfortable Quarters for Laboratory Animals*, 10th edn. Animal Welfare Institute, Washington, DC

Marques, D.M. and Valenstein, E.S. (1977) Individual differences in aggressiveness of female hamsters – response to intact and castrated males and to females. *Animal Behaviour*, **25(FEB)**, 131–139.

McMartin, D.N. and Dodds, W.J. (1982) Animal model of human disease: atrial thrombosis in ageing Syrian hamsters. *American Journal of Pathology*, **107**, 277–279.

Mooij, P.N.M., Wouters, M.G.A.J., Thomas, C.M.G. et al. (1992) Disturbed reproductive performance in extreme folic acid deficient golden hamsters. *European Journal of Obstetrics, Gynaecological Reproductive Biology*, **43**, 71–75.

Mulder, G.B. (2012) Hamsters: management, husbandry, and colony health. In: *The Laboratory Rabbit, Guinea Pig, Hamster and Other Rodents*. Eds Suckow M.A., Stevens K.A. and Wilson, R.P., pp. 765–777. Academic Press, Waltham, MA.

Murray, K.M. (2012) Hamsters: anatomy, physiology, and behavior. In: *The Laboratory Rabbit, Guinea Pig, Hamster and Other Rodents*. Eds Suckow M.A., Stevens K.A. and Wilson, R.P., pp. 753–763. Academic Press, Waltham, MA.

National Research Council (1996) *Guide for the Care and Use of Laboratory Animals*. National Academies Press, Washington, DC. Available from URL: http://www.nap.edu/readingroom/books/labrats/

Percy, D.H. and Palmer, D.J. (1997). Pathogenesis of Sendai virus infection in the Syrian hamster. *Laboratory Animal Science*, **47**, 132–137.

Pinto, R.M., Goncalves, I., Gomes, D.C. and Noronha, D. (2001). Helminth fauna of the golden hamster *Mesocricetus auratus* in Brazil. *Contemporary Topics in Laboratory Animal Science*, **40**, 21–26.

Pour, P., Mohr, U., Cardesa, A. et al. (1976a) Spontaneous tumours and common diseases in two colonies of Syrian hamsters. II. Respiratory tract and digestive system. *Journal of the National Cancer Institute*, **56**, 937–948.

Pour, P., Mohr, U., Althoff, J. et al. (1976b) Spontaneous tumours and common diseases in two colonies of Syrian hamsters. III. Urogenital system and endocrine glands. *Journal of the National Cancer Institute*, **56**, 949–960.

Pour, P., Mohr, U., Althoff, J. et al. (1976c) Spontaneous tumours and common diseases in two colonies of Syrian hamsters. IV. Vascular and lymphatic systems and lesions of other sites. *Journal of the National Cancer Institute*, **56**, 963–974.

Pour, P., Kmoch, N., Greiser, E. et al. (1976d) Spontaneous tumours and common diseases in two colonies of Syrian hamsters. I. Incidence and sites. *Journal of the National Cancer Institute*, **56**, 931–935.

Pour P., Mohr U., Althoff, J. et al. (1979) Spontaneous tumours and common diseases in three types of hamsters. *Journal of the National Cancer Institute*, **63**, 797–881.

Pritchett, K.R. (2007). Helminth parasites of laboratory mice. In: *The Mouse in Biomedical Research, vol. Diseases*, 2nd edn. Eds Fox, J.G., Barthold, S.W., Davisson, M.T. et al., pp. 551–564. Academic Press, New York.

Pritchett, K.R. and Johnston, N.A. (2002). A review of treatments for the eradication of pinworm infections from laboratory rodent colonies. *Contemporary Topics in Laboratory Animal Science*, **41**, 36–46.

Pritchett-Corning, K.R. and Gaskill, B.N. (2015) Lack of negative effects on Syrian hamsters and Mongolian gerbils housed in the same secondary enclosure. *Journal of the American Association for Laboratory Animal Science*, **54(3)**, 261–266.

Rodriguez, M.V., de Castro, S.O., de Albuquerque, C.Z., et al. (2017) The gingival vein as a minimally traumatic site for multiple blood sampling in guinea pigs and hamsters. *PLoS ONE*, **12(5)**, e0177967. https://doi.org/10/1371/journalpone.0177967.

Shoji-Darkye, Y., Itoh, T. and Kagiyama, N. (1991) Pathogenesis of CAR bacillus in rabbits, guinea pigs, Syrian hamsters and mice. *Laboratory Animal Science*, **41**, 567–571.

Shomer, N.H., Allen-Worthington, K.H., Hickman, D.L. *et al.* (2020) Review of rodent euthanasia methods *Journal of the American Association for Laboratory Animal Science*, **59(3)**, 242–253.

Silverman, J. (2012) Biomedical Research Techniques. In: *The Laboratory Rabbit, Guinea Pig, Hamster and Other Rodents*. Eds Suckow, M.A., Stevens, K.A. and Wilson, R.P., pp. 779–795. Academic Press, Waltham, MA.

Skinner, H.H. and Knight, E.H. (1979) The potential role of Syrian hamsters and other small animals as reservoir of lymphocytic choriomeningitis virus. *Journal of Small Animal Practice*, **20**, 145–161.

Smith, G.D. (2012) Taxonomy and history. In: *The Laboratory Rabbit, Guinea Pig, Hamster and Other Rodents*. Eds Suckow, M.A., Stevens, K.A. and Wilson, R.P., pp. 747–752. Academic Press, Waltham, MA.

Somvanshi, R., Iyer, P.K.R., Biswas, J.C. *et al.* (1987) Polycystic liver disease in golden hamsters. *Journal of Comparative Pathology*, **97**, 615–618.

Stills, H.F. Jr. (1991). Isolation of an intracellular bacterium from hamsters (*Mesocricetus auratus*) with proliferative ileitis and reproduction of the disease with a pure culture. *Infection and Immunity*, **59**, 3227–3236.

Suckow, M.A., Stevens, K.A. and Wilson, R.P. (eds) (2012) *The Laboratory Rabbit, Guinea Pig, Hamster and Other Rodents*. Academic Press, London.

Swanson, L.J. and Campbell, C.S. (1979) Maternal behavior in the primiparous and multiparous golden hamster. *Zeitschrift für Tierpsychologie*, **50(1)**, 96–104.

Taylor, D.M. (1992) Eradication of pinworms (*Syphacia obvelata*) from Syrian hamsters in quarantine. *Laboratory Animal Science*, **42**, 413–414.

Turusov, V.S. and Mohr, U. (1982) *Pathology of Tumours in Laboratory Animals III. Tumours of the Hamster*. IARC Scientific Publications, Lyon, France.

Van Hoosier, G.L., Jr. and Trentin, J.T. (1979) Naturally occurring tumours of the Syrian hamster. *Progress in Experimental Tumour Research*, **23**, 1–12.

Viswanathan, N. and Davis, F.C. (1992) Timing of birth in Syrian hamsters. *Biology of Reproduction*, **47(1)**, 6–10.

Wechsler, S.J. and Jones, J. (1984) Diagnostic exercise. *Laboratory Animal Science*, **34**, 137–138.

West, W.T. and Mason, K.E. (1958) Histopathology of muscular dystrophy in the vitamin E deficient hamster. *American Journal of Anatomy*, **102**, 323–363.

Whittaker, D. (2010) The Syrian hamster. In: *The UFAW Handbook on the Care and Management of Laboratory and Other Research Animals*. 8th edn. Eds Hubrecht, R. and Kirkwood, J., pp. 348–358. Wiley-Blackwell, New York.

Winnicker, C.W. and Pritchett-Corning, K.R. (2021) Behavioral biology of hamsters. In: *Behavioral Biology of Laboratory Animals*. Eds Coleman, K. and Schapiro, S.J., pp. 165–171. CRC Press, Boca Raton.

Yen, H.-L., Sit, T. H. C., Brackman, C.J., et al. (2022). Transmission of SARS-CoV-2 delta variant (AY.127) from pet hamsters to humans, leading to onward human-to-human transmission: a case study. *The Lancet*, **399**, 1070–1078.

25 Voles

Petra Kirsch

Biological overview

Origins

Voles belong to the sub-family Arvicolinae (comprising voles, lemmings and muskrats) within the family Cricetedae of the Rodentia. Cricetids originated in Eurasia during the mid-Miocene epoch, from ancestors that resemble modern squirrels. The voles themselves arose during the Pliocene epoch, and rapidly diversified during the Pleistocene. There are now about 70 species found in grassland, open forest and tundra. Voles are Paleartic and Neartic in distribution being found in Europe, Asia, Northern Africa and North America. The most numerous genus in terms of species is the *Microtidae*, which include the short-tailed or field vole (*Microtus agrestis*), one of the most common mammals of north-west Europe and the prairie vole (*Microtus ochro-gaster*) of North America (Musser & Carleton 2005). Other genera include *Avicola*, the water voles, and *Myodes* (formally, *Clethrionomys*) including the red-backed voles, such as the bank vole (*Myodes glareolus*).

General biology

Voles are often confused with mice. Voles have been classified as Muridae (rats, mice and their relatives) (MacDonald 2001) and some species are locally described as mice. For example, the meadow vole (*Microtus pensylvanicus*) of North America is often called the field or meadow mouse. Compared with mice, voles tend to have a stouter body, a shorter hairy tail, a rounder head with a blunt snout, and smaller ears and eyes. They tend to be grey–brown to reddish brown in colour often with paler grey or silvery fur on the underside. While some species such as *water voles* can be considerably larger, most vole species maintained under laboratory conditions are about the size of mice. For example, adult field or short-tailed voles have a body approximately 90–110 mm long and weigh between 20 and 40 g, while bank voles are between 80 and 120 mm long, weighing between 15 g and 40 g.

A distinguishing feature of voles is their molars, which, unlike those of many rodents, are rootless and continue to grow during their entire life. While superficially many vole species appear similar, their teeth can be used to identify modern and ancestral species. For this reason, they can be useful to archaeologists for dating strata, in a method referred to as the 'vole clock', based on extraction of vole teeth from substrates (Jernvall *et al*. 2000; Martin 2014). Most vole species can be identified by the structure and patterns of wear on their cheek or molar teeth, and distribution of ancestral species can be used to date sediments. Voles are largely herbivorous and their teeth structure allows them to chew large quantities of abrasive grasses. The diet of the field vole, a largely grassland species, consists for the most part of green leaves and stems of grass, herbs, sedges and bark, while the bank vole, which is associated with woodland habitats, has a more varied diet of grass, flowers, fruits, seeds, leaves, roots, fungi, moss, insects and worms (Flowerdew *et al*. 1985; Harris & Yalden 2008).

Reproduction

In the wild, many vole species have a high population turnover, with few individuals surviving from one year to the next (Chitty 1952, 1996). They have a large number of natural predators, including foxes, cats, weasels and stoats, birds of prey and owls. Average lifespan is in the order of 3–6 months and it is rare for wild voles to live for longer than 12 months, though laboratory colonies can include individuals over 18 months of age (Cooper *et al*. 1996). Voles tend to be more active at night than during the daytime, though daytime activity can still be noticeable in the wild and laboratory setting. Voles do not hibernate, and will continue to be active beneath lying snow. They are capable of rapid population growth in favourable conditions, and exhibit large cyclic fluctuations in population density similar to those of the closely related lemmings (Chitty 1996). Voles breed from early spring until early autumn, and their gonads are generally in a much less active state in the late autumn and winter, when they are not usually fertile. In the wild, voles do not normally have an oestrous cycle, though this can be induced under laboratory conditions by housing females in close visual contact with adult males. Ovulation in voles is normally caused by stimuli provided by mating and

The UFAW Handbook on the Care and Management of Laboratory and Other Research Animals, Ninth Edition.
Edited by Huw Golledge and Claire Richardson.
© 2024 John Wiley & Sons Ltd. Published 2024 by John Wiley & Sons Ltd.

occurs 6–12 h later. There are normally two components of the mating process, one causing ovulation and another causing corpora lutea to become functional (Clarke 1985). Gestation lasts 16–28 days depending on species.

Vole infants or pups are altricial being born blind, hairless and heavily dependent on maternal care. Nestling voles use ultrasonic vocalisations to communicate with their mother. These signals include distress calls, which change with the developmental stage, and with ambient and body temperature (Blake 1992; Mandelli & Sales 2004). Maturation is rapid with many species weaning pups within 3 weeks of age. Voles reach sexual maturity soon afterwards. For example, male field voles are sexually mature by the age of 6–7 weeks, while females are sexually mature by 4 weeks of age (Spears & Clarke 1987). Female field voles have, however, been known to have perforate vaginas, and to be capable of conceiving at the age of 18 days (Chitty 1952). On weaning, most vole species are solitary and do not form stable reproductive pairs. In many species, males are promiscuous or polygamous and court females for as long as is necessary to successfully mate. There is no paternal care of the young, whereas females are highly protective of their pups.

The prairie vole is a notable exception with regard to reproduction. These voles naturally live in multigenerational family groups with a single breeding pair. The offspring remain sexually suppressed so long as they remain within their natal group, and sexual maturity in the females (rather than developing with age as with other voles) depends on exposure to chemical cues in the urine of an unrelated male. Within 24 h of this cue, repeated mating can occur and thereafter they form a long-lasting relationship in which they tend to be monogamous, and the males share in the raising of pups (Insel 1997; Roberts et al. 1997).

Sources of supply

If it is not possible to obtain breeding stock from an established laboratory colony, a new colony can be started with voles caught from the wild, though it may take about 3 months for the wild-caught animals to begin producing litters (Cooper & Nicol 1996). Voles can be easily caught in their natural habitats, using 'Longworth' traps (Gurnell & Flowerdew 1982). Traps should be baited with cereals such as rolled oats or whole wheat grain, and fresh vegetable matter such as discs of carrot. A bedding material such as hay should be provided in the trap's nest box. It is advisable to cover the traps with foliage, or if that is sparse, with a small amount of hay, to give insulation against extremes of climate. Such traps will also catch insectivorous shrews, which can die in traps unless reasonable precautions are taken. These include provision of warm bedding such as hay and suitable food. Blowfly (*Calliphora*) puparia are normally adequate for overnight survival of shrews. Such precautions are not only in the interest of animal welfare, but are a legal requirement for mammal trapping in many countries (Little & Gurnell 1989). As with any other forms of live trapping, permission should be sought from landowners, and it is advisable to liaise with local ecology or naturalist groups in choosing trapping sites. However, it is also obligatory to note that for the removal of animals from the wild, it must be clarified before whether the capture of the animals requires an official permit on the basis of the nature conservation law and the animal welfare law. The authorisation may be accompanied by regulations that specify, among other things, the expertise of the trappers an how frequently the traps must be inspected to ensure that the trapped animals do not experience additional harm, apart from the stress of the trapping itself (European Parliament and Council 2010).

Uses in the laboratory

While not as common a laboratory animal as mice and rats, voles have been housed under laboratory conditions for a number of purposes, including studies of reproductive biology, disease and behavioural biology. Voles have been used in the laboratory to investigate their population ecology, for example their bioenergetics as well as various aspects of their reproductive biology (Leslie & Ranson 1940; Clarke 1985). There is also considerable interest in the ecto- and endoparasites of voles (e.g. Kaplan et al. 1980; Randolph 1995). Voles have been intensively studied since they appear to be the reservoir hosts of cowpox virus (Crouch et al. 1995; Burthe et al. 2008). The occurrence in field voles of very large sex chromosomes has encouraged their use in studies upon heterochromatin (Kalscheuer et al. 1996). Voles have also been proposed as a potential tool for detecting the accumulation of toxic minerals in herbage (Beardsley et al. 1978). Voles have been used to investigate rodent communication and as a model to investigate the control of behaviour (Fentress 1968). Bank voles, in particular, have been used as a model species to investigate of the causes and effects of abnormal behaviour patterns in captive animals such as stereotypic behaviour (Ödberg 1987; Cooper et al. 1996; Schoenecker & Keller 2000) and polydipsia (Sorensen & Randrup 1986; Schoenecker et al. 2000). However, bank voles have also been used to study tuberculosis (Jespersen 1954), hantaviruses (Olsson et al. 2003; Voutilainen et al. 2015) and Ljungan virus-associated type 1 diabetes (Niklasson et al. 2003) and have been emerged as a powerful infection model for prion diseases (Di Bari et al. 2013; Watts et al. 2014; Paul et al. 2018).

Prairie voles and meadow voles have been used to investigate genetic and hormonal factors involved in sexual fidelity. Male prairie voles show some variation in tendency to monogamy. Extra-pair copulations can occur and the likelihood of engaging in such behaviour has been related to genetic and physiological factors (Ophir et al. 2008). Those males most likely to be monogamous and engage in paternal care have longer strings of repetitions of microsatellite DNA (Hammock & Young 2005). Microsatellite DNA from prairie voles has been inserted into the genome of meadow voles and found to reduce promiscuity and increase pair-bonding behaviour in males (Lim et al. 2004). Similarly, the hormonal control of sexual fidelity involving vasopressin, oxytocin and dopamine has been investigated by manipulating their levels in male prairie voles (Cushing et al. 2001; Young et al. 2005). Finally, prairie voles have been promoted as a model for anxiety and depression (Kim & Kirkpatrick 1996; Stowe et al. 2005; Grippo 2009) as socially isolating adults leads to elevated corticosteroid concentrations, prolonged sensitivity to stress-inducing challenges, and affects their performance in tests of negative affective state (Grippo et al. 2008, 2014).

General husbandry

The bulk of this section will concentrate on laboratory management of the short-tailed or field vole (*Microtus agrestis*) and the bank vole (*Myodes glareolus*). The chapter will cover their basic biology, care and management in laboratory conditions, as well as application of laboratory procedures to these species. The chapter will illustrate issues that arise from the captive rearing of rodent species, which have not been intentionally selected for laboratory conditions.

Physical environment

In general, it should be remembered that appropriate animal welfare regulations apply to the keeping and breeding of voles for scientific purposes and, if required, a licence to keep them must be obtained from an authority. As with other laboratory rodents, it is important that voles be housed in controlled, secure, protected environments, with reliable access to food, water, shelter and/or nesting materials, where risks of infection are minimised and avoiding extremes of climatic variation (Figure 25.1). Vole rooms should be designed to provide suitable enclosures for the animals, ease of management and safety for the researchers. A well-designed room should minimise disturbing noises, and be able to maintain constant temperature and humidity. A temperature of 20 °C and relative humidity of about 60%, with 15–20 changes of warm air per hour is an adequate atmosphere for a vole colony. A photoperiod of 16 h light per day is appropriate for a breeding colony. To reduce noise, bins for food, bedding and rubbish should be made of heavy-duty plastic.

The colony room should be large enough to allow cages to be placed along one wall and sufficient space for basic husbandry procedures such as changing the cages or sexing pups. A room of about 4.5 m length, 3.0 m width and 2.5 m height should be adequate for colonies of 100 cages. This would provide sufficient space for a bench along one wall and the cages on shelving along the opposite wall, or fitted into racks mounted on castors. Cleaning of cages should be done in a separate area to avoid stressing the bank voles with the noise of cage washing. If the vole colony is housed in windowless rooms, then artificial lighting can be provided. For example, in a room laid out as above, a central 180 cm long 75 W fluorescent tube connected to a time switch, gives a light intensity of 105–735 lux at the front of cages in the absence of natural daylight. This light level seems adequate for basic husbandry procedures without flooding the cages with light, though it would be advisable to cover the top cages on a rack from direct lighting.

Housing

Voles can be housed in plastic, opaque polypropylene, or transparent polycarbonate cages designed for mice or rats. The largest possible cages should be used and not too many animals should be kept in one cage to avoid the development of stereotypic behaviour (Paul *et al.* 2018). Litter can be conventional bedding for use in rodent laboratory colonies or similar absorbent material. Nesting material should be provided to allow nesting behaviour. This is particularly important for pregnant or lactating females, which construct spherical nests 5–10 cm in diameter in which litters are born and reared. However, all voles will build nests and provision of nesting material or other opportunities for sheltering and enrichment materials considerably reduces the incidence of stereotypic behaviour in bank voles (Ödberg 1987; Cooper *et al.* 1996; Paul *et al.* 2018). Meadow hay makes a good nesting material, but is not suitable for systems requiring high hygiene and can evoke allergic responses in some people. In these situations, shredded paper or commercially produced rodent nesting material (e.g. nestlets) may be an

(a)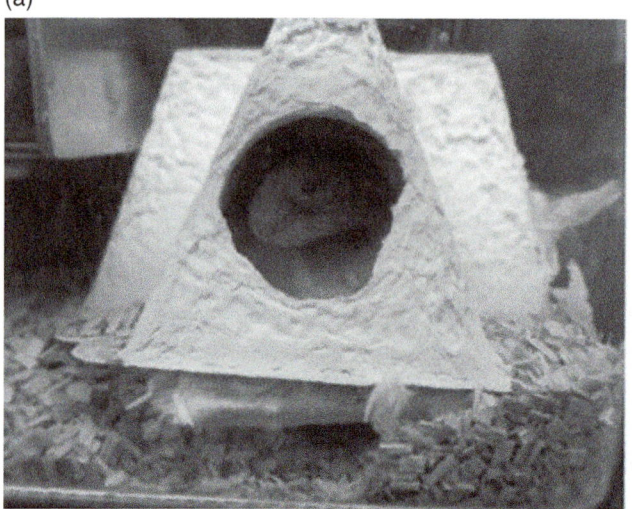

(b)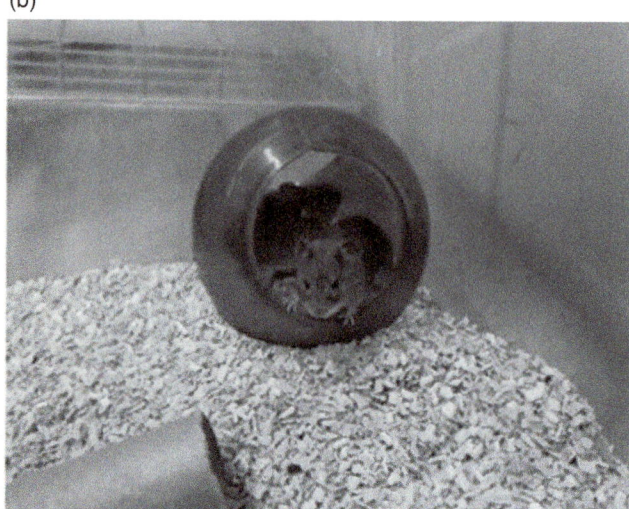

Figure 25.1 Environmental enrichment provision for bank voles. (a) Bank vole looking from inside a mini mouse maze. (b) Two bank voles inside a crawl ball. Source: Photo: Michael Beekes, reprinted with permission from Paul *et al.* (2018).

adequate substitute. A nest can last for a number of weeks, particularly if it is kept at the end of a cage away from the water bottle spout and can be transferred with the voles during cage cleaning.

Social grouping

It is possible to group house voles in single-sex groups following weaning, though groups should be monitored for signs of aggression (Clarke 1956; Sorensen & Randrup 1986; Lee et al. 2019). This is most prevalent in groups of unfamiliar males, though can arise in males housed together from weaning. Singly housed animals can be kept in standard cages such as those measuring 33 cm × 15 cm × 13 cm (l × w × h). Unless there has been significant spoilage of bedding (e.g. from flooding), these can be cleaned once per week. Cages run the risk of flooding as voles are prone to rapidly emptying water bottles (possibly in association with stereotypic licking and/or locomotion) (Schoenecker et al. 2000, 2011). For this reason, cages should be inspected at least once every 24 h. Lactating females or breeding pairs benefit from housing in larger cages (e.g. 48 cm × 15 cm × 13 cm), which again only need to be cleaned once per week unless significant spoilage has occurred. For bank voles, more frequent cleaning appears to be disturbing and may contribute to poor reproduction and infanticide. Wild-caught voles should be handled and their cages cleaned less frequently at least in the first months of introduction to the colony.

Food and water

Where problems of bulk and supply make the precise replication of wild diet impracticable for a laboratory colony, standard laboratory rodent diets can be used to meet the voles' nutritional requirements. Field voles should be given 8% or more protein in their diet, as a reduction to 4% has been shown to retard growth and sexual development (Spears & Clarke 1987). This can be provided by feeding whole oats, meadow hay, carrots and a few pellets of a rat and mouse laboratory diet. These supplies should be replenished every week or when cages are cleaned out. Field voles can be primarily fed a commercial pelleted standard rat and mouse breeding and grower diet *ad libitum*, though once per week a handful of commercial hamster food or toasted wheatgerm should be added to each cage. Although bank voles naturally eat a more varied diet than field voles, they can also be maintained on simple diets such as whole oats augmented by pellets of rat and mouse breeding diet. Bank voles will sample from a wide range of food items and this basic diet can be supplemented by hamster mix including nuts and seeds such as rolled corn, barley, peanuts and sunflower seeds. Fresh forage can be also given to voles including chopped apples, pears and carrots, as well as meadow hay. When feeding fresh, hygienically unprepared food, note that there is a risk of introducing undesirable microorganisms into the colony. When feeding nuts or seeds, there is a risk that the animals will quickly become fat.

Water can be supplied in standard laboratory drinking bottles and these should be checked daily. In addition to regular replacement with fresh water, the hygienic standards of laboratory animal husbandry should also be applied when keeping voles to protect them from pathogens. Voles are particularly susceptible to water shortage and total deprivation of water for 48 h will cause death. Daily water consumption is about 10 ml/24 h in both bank and field voles, so conventional water bottles should be adequate for many days. However, field and vole colonies often develop water bottle-related stereotypies (Sorensen & Randrup 1986; Schoenecker et al. 2000), and this behaviour is also known in other vole species (Kruckenburg et al. 1973). This involves the rapid emptying of water bottles, and repeated emptying of water can flood the cage and spoil litter. Voles showing this behaviour often develop the hunched posture associated with illness. This behaviour has also been termed 'polydipsia' though evidence of over-consumption of water is sparse (Schoenecker et al. 2000). However, infection with the Ljungan virus in bank voles is known to cause a condition similar to type 1 diabetes in humans and may explain the polydipsia (Niklasson et al. 2003). Changing the drinker spout to a design less likely to allow siphoning may solve this problem, though animals that engage in this behaviour are often culled once they show overt signs of illness.

Identification and sexing

Toe clipping as a method of identification of animals is no longer either acceptable or necessary in voles as microchips can be used where individual identification is desirable (Association for the Study of Animal Behaviour/Animal Behavior Society, 2020). However, unless individuals need to be identified from groups then a cage card system, supported by a computer database, would be adequate for keeping records for breeding colonies and for identifying individually caged animals. Each cage should carry, in a metal holder, a card bearing the cage number and giving details of animals' identification, birth date and parents. Breeding records should be monitored to ensure that breeding stock comprise females and males descended from mothers of high fertility. Care should be taken to ensure paper cards are kept out of reach of the cage's occupants as voles have a tendency to chew these records.

The sexes can be distinguished by the greater ano-genital distance of males (about 10 mm) compared to that of females (about 5 mm). Sexually mature males have testes bulging in the perineal region to form the typical rodent scrotum. The penis is immediately anterior to the scrotum. The vaginal opening of sexually mature females has the clitoris at its anterior border. The ano-genital distance is very much smaller in newborn and sucking young of either sex, but with practice can be used to distinguish males from females. Newborn and suckling females can also be recognised by rudimentary nipples, which are slightly better developed than in males. In prepubertal animals or those whose sexual development has been retarded by exposure to natural or artificial winter photoperiods, overlap in the frequency distribution of the ano-genital distance of the two sexes can cause difficulties in sexing. However, slight pressure on the lower abdomen may cause testes to descend more fully into the perineal region, where they can be seen through the skin or will cause slight bulging. Females that are not yet perforate often have a small scale of skin marking the future vaginal opening.

Reproduction and breeding

If wild-caught voles are to be used to found a colony, they should be caught during the breeding season, though even in these situations females may take several months to produce their first laboratory conceived litter. Animals brought from the wild to create a colony should be disturbed as little as possible and, provided cages are not damp through leakage of a water bottle or are otherwise unsavoury, the cage should be cleaned infrequently. Quiet conditions in the animal room probably shorten the acclimatisation time.

Voles do not have long life expectancies, and long-term studies of their biology can be more efficiently conducted by establishing a breeding colony. A common breeding system is to house pairs permanently together until there is evidence that a pairing is not regularly producing litters or reliably rearing young: in these circumstances partners of different pairs can be swapped around. At the first and any subsequent pairing, the male can be introduced to the cage already occupied by the female. Recruitment for breeding should be reviewed once a month and animals should be removed from the breeding colony once they reach 12 months old, since by about that age fertility of females has declined. Colony records can be used to predict the likely fertility of stock animals, as a guide for the recruitment of new females and males for the breeding colony. The male and female of a pair should not be closely related. Breeding schemes can be outbreeding schemes, as applied to laboratory mice, see Chapter 4: An introduction to laboratory animal genetics. In the field vole, it is advisable to select females and males with short upper (as well as lower) incisors. From time to time, animals of either sex may develop overgrown upper incisors. This causes difficulties in feeding, and these animals can become trapped when gnawing the wire mesh of cages.

A long photoperiod consistent with natural breeding season (e.g. 16L : 8D for field voles) is necessary for sexual development and maximum efficiency of breeding colonies of voles (Clarke 1985; Spears & Clarke 1987). Under these conditions, male field voles have spermatozoa in the testes, epididymides and vasa deferentia by the age of 42–49 days. Sexually mature males have well-developed patches of sebaceous tissue on their hindquarters. These are secondary sexual characters which in laboratory stock frequently became bare, pink areas 20 × 15 mm, with folding of the skin, producing abundant sebaceous secretion giving off a musty odour and making the adjacent fur greasy. Females will develop perforate vaginas and be fertile by 28 days of age under a 16L:8D light regime, though some can be fertile by as little as 18 days of age. In an established colony, females can be recruited to breeding stock from 2 months of age, and males from about 2.5 months of age.

Voles from laboratory colonies are generally heavier than animals from natural populations. For example, by the age of 24 weeks male and female field voles are considerably heavier than comparable wild animals, where mean maximum body weight during the breeding season has been recorded as 30 g for males and 26 g for females (Chitty 1952). The males most suitable for recruitment for breeding weigh 30–40 g and have somewhat spare bodies without much subcutaneous fat. In sexually mature males, the penis is well-developed, about 3 mm long within its prepuce; and the testes produce paired bulges in the perineal region, so forming a typical rodent scrotum. The scrotum may develop dark pigmentation in animals, which have been sexually mature for several months, but this is not a prerequisite condition for the fertile state. Suitable sexually mature females have a perforate vagina, which in the oestrous state is pink, gaping and slightly rugose. A vaginal smear made up of cornified epithelial cells is a good indication that the animal is fertile. Among virgin female field voles with these vaginal characteristics, those weighing from 25–35 g are usually more fertile than lighter or heavier animals. Females with abundant subcutaneous and abdominal fat (apparent from their 'feel' and conformation) tend to be less fertile than those with a more spare body.

When a sexually mature female, even one with an oestrous vaginal smear, is paired with a sexually mature male, the early interactions of the animals can appear aggressive. The male may pursue the female, attempting to mount her and, at the outset, the female will often turn on the male, squeaking vigorously and lunging defensively at him. This seeming antagonism may be part of courtship behaviour. After a period ranging from a few minutes to half an hour, the squabbling interactions usually end, and copulations commence. The male usually mounts the female a number of times within a few minutes. After each mounting, the female often runs ahead of the male and stops: the male follows and mounts again. Bouts of leading by the female and mounting by the male are usually separated from each other by intervals of 5–15 minutes, during which the animals appear not to respond to each other.

Following copulation, a white or cream-coloured vaginal plug, formed from the male's ejaculate, can be found in the vagina, though not invariably: whether this is because it has fallen out before the female is examined, or because it has not formed, is not known. Sperm are detectable in vaginal smears for a few hours after copulation. The likelihood that a female has become pregnant or pseudopregnant can be gauged from the vaginal smear. The oestrous smear is made up of cornified epithelial cells which will change 24–48 h after mating to one consisting almost exclusively of many leucocytes, and by day 5 or day 6 after copulation there are very few cells of any sort. Pregnancy can also be reliably gauged by a gain in body weight of 2–4 g in pregnant females, which occurs at about the 10th day of pregnancy, so weighing breeding females once per week (for example during cage cleaning) can avoid the need to conduct vaginal smears. Blastocysts implant 90–96 h post-coitus and pregnancy lasts 20–21 days. Pregnancy will be blocked if a female is exposed to an unfamiliar male 48–72 h after mating. Females have a post-partum oestrus, and implantation of the resulting blastocysts is only slightly delayed by concurrent suckling by the young. By full term, pregnant female field voles may weigh between 35 and 50 g. As females are fertile post-partum and throughout lactation, and where males are permanently present in breeding cages, females will produce litters at 20–23-day intervals for much of their breeding lives. To monitor births, females in the later stages of pregnancy should be checked daily for young with minimal disturbance using soft plastic tweezers.

Bank voles also have a breeding season to field voles lasting generally from early spring until early autumn, so a photoperiod of 16L : 8D is suitable to maintain a breeding colony. Under these conditions, spermatogenesis takes 31 days in males. The general pattern of sexual behaviour in bank voles is similar to that of field voles and has been described by Christiansen and Døving (1976) and Milligan (1979). Ovulation is induced by mating and occurs 6–14 h thereafter. There is no oestrous cycle of the sort occurring in the laboratory mouse but, as in the field vole, cycles of change in the vaginal smear lasting 4–10 days, accompanied by ovulations, can occur through the remote influence of males. Compared with field voles, a smaller proportion of bank voles are likely to be in oestrus at any one time, though oestrus can be rapidly induced by nearby males. Multiple sets of corpora lutea occur in wild females, as well as young laboratory bred females kept permanently with one male, and in females mated with a succession of males at 2-day intervals, as well as through the remote influence of males. Young, perforate, virgin females are less fertile than older, perforate, virgin animals, and bank voles take longer, generally, than field voles to become pregnant for the first time. This has been attributed either to the need to have the reproductive tract primed by ovarian hormones, or to the failure of corpora lutea at first mating to become functional. Implantation of blastocysts in non-lactating females occurs 105–107 h after coitus (Clarke 1985).

Pregnancy lasts 18–19 days in primigravida (first-time pregnant) bank voles and a high proportion of females will be in oestrus and fertile immediately post-partum; the proportion declining a day or two later and rising after the young are weaned. Permanently paired voles produce a steady stream of litters, but because implantation of blastocysts arising from post-partum mating of lactating females is delayed, pregnancies last from 19–22 days. Although bank voles can deliver litters of five to six pups, smaller litter sizes (mean of 3.5 pups) are more commonly reported (Clarke 1985).

Parturition, rearing and weaning

Young are born in the nest during the day or night. Occasionally, litters of permanently mated pairs are found dead and/or damaged. In these situations, it is not clear if the pups have been attacked while alive, or if they have died from neglect or poor cage conditions and subsequently been eaten by the adults. Changing the pairing or removing the male before parturition can reduce this problem, but can also cause some loss of breeding efficiency since their reintroduction or the introduction of another male to the lactating female's cage can in itself cause the death of her young. An unpaired lactating female vole usually vigorously attacks any male added to her cage, and, in the following mayhem, young can be neglected, damaged or killed by the adults. Increasing the cage size, providing a more natural diet and nest materials (use of meadow hay) and reducing the frequency of cage cleaning may also be effective in reducing pup mortality. Randrup et al. (1988) reported that in bank vole colonies with little cover or nesting material, high pup mortality was associated with mothers repeatedly moving pups around the cage. Again, providing ample, suitable nesting material may reduce this problem.

Newborn vole pups are bright pink in colour, have sealed eyelids and limited capacity for movement, though development is rapid in the subsequent days (Spears & Clarke 1987). At 2 days of age, the head and back change from bright pink to grey. By about 4 days, the young are able to crawl, and at 7 or 8 days, they show uncoordinated walking. At this stage, the coat is made up of smooth, very fine hair, brown above, light cream beneath, and the eyes have opened. When the young are 12–13 days old, walking becomes coordinated as in an adult. It is possible to cross foster suckling young by choosing a female with a small litter of about the same age as the young to be fostered. Suckling young are quite hardy and if they are found in a cold, wet, moribund state, may revive if placed with their mother, or a suitable foster mother, in a clean, dry cage with adequate nesting material.

Field voles can be weaned by about 14 days, although they can be kept in the parental cage until 16 days, after which there is an increasing risk of juvenile females becoming fertile. At this age, they have fine grey juvenile fur. From about 21 days, the coarser adult coat develops on the head and then spreads down the body. It is grey with yellow–brown or reddish brown tips and black guard hairs on the upper side, and on the underside cream to pale grey. Bank voles are born in essentially the same state as the young of field voles, and the pelage goes through the same stages as in field voles, though the hair colour is a richer brown. Because suckling bank voles develop a little more slowly than field voles, they can be removed from the parental cage at the age of 18 days rather than 16 days. Following weaning, males and females should be housed separately to avoid unwanted pregnancies. Adult females, which have been living separately, can be put together in a cage without the risk of stressful interactions, but if sexually mature males from different cages are put together they will fight vigorously, with consequent severe wounding. Even those which have been living together since weaning can start fighting when they become sexually mature (Sorensen & Randrup 1986).

Laboratory procedures

Transport and handling

Clear national guidelines covering transport of laboratory and other animals can be found elsewhere (e.g. for UK, see Laboratory Animal Science Association (LASA) 2005). See also Chapter 12: Transportation of laboratory animals. This section will provide some practical advice to support these guidelines. As with other species, voles should be transported in escape-proof containers that protect the animals from unfavourable environmental conditions, ensuring they arrive alive and well at their destination. In general, voles can be transported in a similar fashion to laboratory mice. Containers should be made of rigid plastic, or similar escape-proof materials such as metal. Adequate bedding (for warmth and the absorption or containment of urine and faeces), food and a source of water must be provided, and the container should have a means of inspection. Voles caught from the wild can be transported for short periods (up to 3 h) in the 'Longworth' traps in which they had been caught. Traps should always be well-stocked with oats, fresh carrot and meadow hay.

For transport over long distances and lasting some hours, by road in a supervised vehicle, or by air freight, a purpose-built carrier can be used. A good practical example could consist of 12 metal boxes, each 15 cm × 9 cm × 8 cm lightly welded together to give container of overall dimensions of about 45 cm × 36 cm, with a wire mesh lid (4 mm square mesh). A more convenient, though less portable solution would be to use conventional cages for short distances only. In all cases, each compartment should be provided with a little bedding and some non-absorbent cotton wool or paper wool and pellets of laboratory rodents diet. In order to eliminate aggressive encounters, only one animal should be housed in each compartment, except if the animals were intended for a breeding colony, where one female and one male can travel together satisfactorily. It is said that voles are less stressed if the familiar bedding from their cage is transferred to transport boxes, rather than if they are furnished with fresh material. If animals are to be sent abroad, a health certificate (from the relevant government department) for the animals will be needed, and the rules regulating importation into the destination country will need to be observed. See also Chapter 12: Transportation of laboratory animals.

Voles are easily picked up by the loose skin of the neck. They should be quite decisively and firmly grasped, and, retaining the grip, can be cradled upside down in the palm of the hand for examination (Figure 25.2). A struggling animal, in these circumstances, can be calmed momentarily by blowing on its nose. Under laboratory housing, bank voles are more 'lively' than field voles, even after many generations of laboratory breeding. This can make bank voles more challenging to handle. Paul *et al.* (2018) describe a handling procedure that reduced the stress of handling bank voles in laboratory animal husbandry over extended periods of time. The key element of this procedure was the handling of bank voles from birth by individual female personnel who permanently handled the animals in a calm manner. Attracting the animals with sunflower seeds in polycarbonate bottles reduced the stress of potentially stressful grabbing and picking up the bank voles (Paul *et al.* 2018).

For experienced personnel, bites are very rare, but painful and potentially hazardous if inflicted. Voles like other rodents can carry a number of serious infectious diseases (see the following text) and precautions should be taken to avoid bites in first instance and treat rapidly to minimise risk from infectious or parasitic diseases.

Physiological monitoring

Blood samples

Blood sampling for voles must be carried out under anaesthesia and analgesics must be administered (see next sections for recommendations) for all methods of blood sampling. It has been reported that (in a warm room and with practice) up to 200 μl of blood can be obtained by snipping no more than 1 mm from the tip of the tail of a vole. Alternatively, blood can be obtained by puncture of the retrobulbar venous plexus. Blood samples can also be taken from the external jugular vein 0.5 mm × 16 mm needle attached to a 1 ml plastic syringe. Clotting of blood in the syringe can be prevented by wetting the inside of the syringe with a solution of heparin (1000 U/ml, made up in 0.9% saline), then shaking out fluid remaining in the nozzle. To facilitate blood collection, an incision should first be made in the neck, then the fat overlying the external jugular parted, and the hypodermic needle inserted into the vein by passing it under the delicate pectoral muscle. This muscle, by its tension, serves to reduce bleeding which, with practice in delicate manipulations, becomes virtually non-existent. Nevertheless, the neck incision normally needs to be sutured, following sampling.

Terminal samples can be obtained from the heart under isoflurane anaesthesia, using 0.8 mm × 16 mm needle, and a 1 or 2 ml syringe. It is much easier to take such samples if the manipulations are carried out while observing the site with an operating or a dissecting microscope. The needle is inserted in the midline, directly behind the sternum, at an angle of about 30° to the horizontal. It is possible routinely to get 0.75–1.25 ml of blood from field voles in this way. Taking terminal blood samples requires that an overdose of anaesthetic is given at the end of the procedure or the use of cervical dislocation.

Valuable general information and principles about collection of blood samples is provided by the NC3Rs at their blood sampling microsite[1].

Vaginal smears

These can be easily taken using a small wire loop (c.1.0 mm diameter) fixed into a glass or metal rod. After flaming the loop to remove debris (and cooling in air), it can be used to

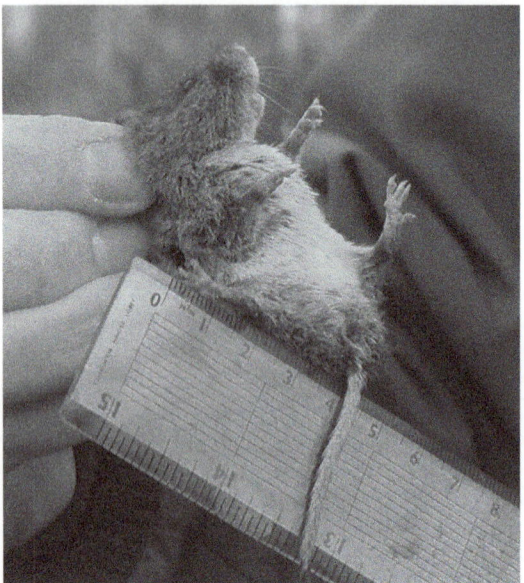

Figure 25.2 Adult female bank vole following capture in Longworth trap. Note small ano-genital distance, and restraint by firm grasp of fur at back of next, while supporting weight of body. Source: Photo: Charles Deeming.

---

[1] https://www.nc3rs.org.uk/3rs-resources/blood-sampling (Accessed 13 April 2022)

transfer a drop of physiological saline onto a clean microscope slide, again dipped in saline and then carefully inserted into the vagina. The loop is then dabbed in the drop of saline on the slide. Cells from the vagina are thus transferred to the slide, which can be immediately examined as a wet, unstained preparation with the simplest of monocular microscopes (total magnification × 60). Smears comprise: nucleated epithelial cells; or cornified epithelial cells; or leucocytes; or a mixture of two or all three cell types. Air-dried smears can be stained, for example, with 0.04% aqueous toluidine blue, and made into permanent preparations.

Administration of substances

Subcutaneous injections are easily given under the skin of the neck or back. It is helpful to shave the site, or part the fur by blowing, in order to guide the needle subcutaneously, to see the bleb at the injection site or to detect any leakage. Light anaesthesia with isoflurane makes the procedure less stressful for lively voles and the experimenter. The skin of the back or neck is held between index finger and thumb, the needle of the syringe inserted low down between finger and thumb through the fold of skin, and checked by touch and visually for correct positioning. Volumes of up to 0.2 ml can be injected in this fashion.

Intraperitoneal injections can be given by first grasping the vole by the loose skin of the back with the index finger and thumb which can then rotated so that the animal, with its belly uppermost, is supported by the palm. The needle should be inserted a couple of millimetres at an angle of about 45 °, then the angle changed so that the needle is nearly parallel to the surface of the belly, and finally the needle should be pushed a little forward before discharging the fluid.

Intravenous injections can be made into the external jugular vein, accessed as described above for taking a blood sample. The neck incision should be sutured following surgery. See the Procedures with Care website[2] for detailed information about administration of substances.

Anaesthesia

As there are no anaesthetics or analgesics with veterinary licences for use in voles, when selecting anaesthetics and analgesic agents, common substances that are also used for small rodents such as mice should be considered. See, for example, Chapter 21: The laboratory mouse.

Euthanasia

It is possible for trained personnel to cull sick individuals in emergencies using dislocation of the neck by instantaneous sharp pressure using the index finger and thumb, though researchers and technicians may prefer euthanasia by injection or inhalation for aesthetic reasons. If inhalation is to be used, the same guidelines and advice apply to voles as to similar sized mice (AVMA 2020). High concentration of carbon dioxide within a chamber connected to a carbon dioxide cylinder causes rapid loss of consciousness followed by death in voles, though it is not known how aversive they find the short exposures to this potentially noxious gas. In other rodents, euthanasia using a rising concentration of carbon dioxide has been recommended as this appears to render animals unconscious before they experience highly noxious concentrations of carbon dioxide. More recent work, however, has suggested that some rodents can detect carbon dioxide and find it aversive even at these low concentrations (Hawkins *et al.* 2006; Hawkins *et al.* 2016). As voles are an uncommon laboratory species no systematic research has been conducted into their perception of euthanising agents and if small numbers of animals are to be killed, then an overdose of an injectable or inhaled anaesthetic agent such as isoflurane as a humane means of killing should be considered. See also Chapter 17: Euthanasia and other fates for laboratory animals.

Finally, if surplus stock need to be disposed of, and if local regulations permit, then it may be worthwhile considering releasing them back into the wild. However, this introduces a number of welfare and ethical issues, in particular whether captive-reared voles will be equipped with the skills required to forage and avoid predation, and also the potential disturbance to resident voles. For these reasons, the matter would need to be carefully researched and it is likely also that there would be a need for careful screening for infectious diseases which might affect released animals or those with which they may come in contact. To date, no studies have tracked survival of laboratory-reared voles, following release into the wild, or their impact on resident populations. In may jurisdictions, several regulatory requirements must be met before animals used for research purposes can be released into the wild. See also Chapter 7: Welfare and 'best practice' in field studies of wildlife.

Common welfare problems

Health, disease and zoonosis

Voles in a healthy state have a shiny coat and are vigorous. Ill animals often adopt a hunched posture with fluffed-up, dull fur. It is essential that any animals showing signs of illness be examined and then either treated or euthanised promptly. The abdomen of adult voles may occasionally become greatly enlarged without any matching increase in body weight, so that the females in such cases are clearly not pregnant. Such animals should be culled, as this is a symptom of severe digestive problems. *Post-mortem* examination normally reveals that the small intestine is grossly distended with gas, or that the caecum is greatly engorged with digesta.

Wild voles can carry a number of ectoparasites, including fleas, ticks and mites, the human ringworm fungus, endoparasitic protozoa (including *Toxoplasma*), trematodes, cestodes and nematodes, as well as *Mycobacterium microti* and the spirochaete *Leptospira*. Tuberculosis can be endemic in wild populations of voles, and infected animals may have extensive caseous areas in subcutaneous tissue, lungs and elsewhere in the body. Antibody reacting with orthopoxvirus

---

[2] http://www.procedureswithcare.org.uk/administration-of-substances/ (Accessed 13 April 2022)

(cowpox virus) has been detected in both field and bank voles from the wild and both species are susceptible to a number of other viruses, including spontaneous mouse encephalomyelitis and encephalo-myocarditis and various hantaviruses (Kaplan *et al.* 1980; Flowerdew *et al.* 1985; Bennett *et al.* 1997; Barnard *et al.* 2002; Olsson *et al.* 2003; Harris & Yalden 2008; Kipar *et al.* 2014; Voutilainen *et al.* 2015; Jeske *et al.* 2019; Binder *et al.* 2020). The latter group is responsible for public health problems in some parts of Europe and Asia, including Korean haemorrhagic fever and nephropathia epidemica. The infective agent(s) can occur in both wild and laboratory populations. Voles can also be infected with the Ljungan virus, which is responsible for a condition similar to type 1 diabetes in humans (Nikklasson *et al.* 2003; Fevola *et al.* 2017) The mite *Laelaps hilaris* (Koch) is often found in small numbers in the perineal region of field voles, feeding on host body secretion, though apparently causing little harm to the host. Voles are hosts for the sheep tick (*Ixodes ricinus*) which transmits the spirochaete *Borrelia burgdorferi*, which is responsible for Lyme disease (Randolph & Craine 1995). Early symptoms are flu like and if untreated infection can have arthritic, cardiac and neurological consequences for people. Voles are also competent hosts for the protozoan *Babesia microti* (Baker *et al.* 1963), which can cause illness in people. This protozoan is transmitted by the ectoparasitic tick *Ixodes trianguliceps* (Randolph 1995; Brown *et al.* 2008) which can also carry the spirochaete responsible for Lyme disease.

When wild voles are brought into the laboratory for outcrossing of the breeding stock or for experimental purposes, a protocol for quarantine, screening and, where appropriate, treatment, for any parasitic or other infectious agents should be carefully devised and implemented. In order to guard against infection of laboratory workers, colonies of wild voles should be kept well-separated from breeding colonies of the same or other laboratory rodent species.

Behaviour and welfare

Aggressive interactions

Sexually mature male voles from laboratory stock are often very aggressive towards each other. This has been seen in groups of male voles housed in laboratory cages (Sorensen & Randrup 1986) as well as larger more naturalistic enclosures with high stocking densities (Clarke 1955, 1956). Sexually mature males may fight viciously if they are put together and fighting can also occur among sexually mature males which have cohabited since weaning (whether from the same or different litters). In cages with high levels of aggressive encounters, the problem can be moderated by identifying and removing the principal aggressor(s). It may be possible to identify such individuals from size, muscle tone and bite marks. They will tend to be larger animals with a muscular feel when handled due to little subcutaneous or abdominal fat. They may have small wounds on the nose inflicted by the defensive actions of subordinate voles. The latter, in contrast tend to have wounds anywhere on the body but especially on the hindquarters, incurred as they flee from the aggressor. Alternatively, given the risk of aggressive encounters in group-housed males and the potential for harm, avoid group housing males in stock cages. Females do not tend to have serious aggressive interactions, except perhaps when they are pregnant or lactating, so group housing is less problematic with female voles.

Social isolation and distress

The prairie vole has been used to investigate the effects of social isolation on stress physiology (Kim & Kirkpatrick 1996). Under laboratory conditions, pairs of prairie voles develop close relationships, spending much of their time sitting side by side (Insel & Shapiro 1992; Insel 1997). This contrasts markedly with the closely related, but polygamous, montane vole (*Microtus montanus*), as well as the meadow, field and bank voles described earlier, which generally avoid contact with conspecifics in both laboratory and natural conditions except when mating. Housing adult female prairie voles in isolation causes chronic distress, anxiety and depression, and consequently has been used as a model for these responses in man (Grippo 2009). Isolation leads to elevated serum corticosteroid and reduced body weight and a number of behavioural changes. These include anhedonia as measured by decreased sucrose intake; a decline in swimming in a forced swimming task, which are used as measures of depression and also reduced time in open arms of the elevated plus maze, which has been developed as a measure of anxiety (Stowe *et al.* 2005; Grippo *et al.* 2008, 2014). This extreme response to social isolation indicates the importance of maintaining prairie voles in stable pairs in breeding colonies both in terms of their welfare and in terms of successful breeding programmes.

Stereotypic behaviour

Stereotypic behaviour can be reliably induced in bank voles and consequently they have been used as a model species to investigate the causes and effects of repetitive, invariant apparently functionless activities. These behaviours, especially the sustained gnawing of the wire mesh of cages, as well as some weaving, jumping and somersaulting (Sorensen & Randrup 1986) are more commonly observed in bank voles (Ödberg 1987), where they can lead to injuries such as broken tails and facial lesions due to repeated collision with cage features.

Voles readily develop stereotypies in standard laboratory conditions without the use of drug treatments. In addition, vole stereotypy can be varied by manipulation of dopamine activity in a similar way to rat and mouse stereotypy, with dopamine antagonists blocking the performance of stereotypies, and agonists increasing their occurrence (Randrup *et al.* 1988). Stereotypic behaviour can be reduced in bank voles by simple changes to cage conditions, for example by increasing cage size or more effectively by providing cover in the form of hay or straw (Ödberg 1987; Cooper & Nicol 1991; Cooper *et al.* 1996). For example, rearing voles in 33cm × 15cm × 13cm cages with sawdust litter and no bedding leads to an incidence of locomotor stereotypic behaviour approaching 100%; whereas providing a handful of bedding (e.g. hay) results in only 50% of the population exhibiting the behaviour (Cooper & Nicol 1991). The use of larger cages (e.g. 45 cm × 28 cm × 13 cm or larger) with ample bedding, nesting and/or sheltering substrates, and other enrichment materials results in a very low incidence of stereotypic behaviour (Cooper et al. 1996; Paul et al. 2018). Additionally, stress-reducing, calm handling of the animals also leads to less stereotypic behaviour (Paul et al. 2018).

The motivation underlying the performance of stereotypies in voles appears to be persistence of locomotor behaviour, possibly related to motivation to escape from the cage (Cooper & Nicol 1991, 1993). Stereotypies can be initiated by an alarming stimulus (for example running a pen along the cage bars), and providing extensive shelter appears to be the most effective means of reducing the behaviour. Fine detailed observation of responses and the development of the behaviour suggests those voles which show the highest amount of locomotor behaviour following disturbance in the absence of cover are most likely to develop stereotypies, suggesting a development from this active response (Cooper & Nicol 1994, 1996). Finally, while environmental enrichment such as housing voles in larger cages with more shelter can prevent the performance of stereotypies, this is less effective for older voles (Cooper et al. 1996). It is, therefore, recommended that to minimise stereotypic activities, voles should be housed from weaning in large cages provided with both shelter and nesting material.

Acknowledgements

This chapter has been adapted from the chapter on voles published in the 8th edition of this handbook, written by Jonathan Cooper.

References

AVMA (American Veterinary Medical Association) (2020). *AVMA Guidelines for the Euthanasia of Animals*, 2020 edition. AMVA, Schaumburg, Illinois.

Association for the Study of Animal Behaviour/Animal Behavior Society (2020). Guidelines for the treatment of animals in behavioral research and teaching. *Animal Behaviour*, **159**, I–IX.

Baker, J., Chitty, D. and Phipps, E. (1963). Blood parasites of wild voles, Microtus agrestis, in England. *Parasitology*, **53(1–2)**, 297–301. doi:10.1017/S0031182000072772

Barnard, C.J., Behnke, J.M., Bajer, A. et al. (2002). Local variation in endoparasite intensities of bank voles (*Clethrionomys glareolus*) from ecologically similar sites: morphometric and endocrine correlates. *Journal of Helminthology*, **76**, 103–112.

Beardsley, A., Vagg, M.J., Beckett, P.H.T. et al. (1978). Use of the field vole (*M. agrestis*) for monitoring potentially harmful elements in the environment. *Environmental Pollution*, **16**, 65–71.

Bennett, M., Crouch, A.J., Begon, M. et al. (1997). Cowpox in British voles and mice. *Journal of Comparative Pathology*, **116**, 35–44.

Binder, F., Reiche, S., Roman-Sosa, G. et al. (2020). Isolation and characterization of new Puumala orthohantavirus strains from Germany. *Virus Genes*, **56(4)**, 448–460.

Blake, B.H. (1992). Ultrasonic vocalization and body temperature maintenance in infant voles of three species (Rodentia: Arvicolidae). *Developmental Psychobiology*, **25**, 581–596.

Brown, K.J., Lambin, X., Telford, G.R. et al. (2008). Relative Importance of *Ixodes ricinus* and *Ixodes trianguliceps* as Vectors for *Anaplasma phagocytophilum* and *Babesia microti* in Field Vole (*Microtus agrestis*) Populations. *Applied and Environmental Microbiology*, **74**, 7118–7125; DOI: 10.1128/AEM.00625-08

Burthe, S., Telfer, S., Begon, M. et al. (2008). Cowpox virus in natural field vole Microtus agrestis populations: significant negative impacts on survival. *Journal of Animal Ecology*, **77**, 110–119.

Chitty, D.H. (1952). Mortality among voles (*Microtus agrestis*) at Lake Vyrnwy, Montgomeryshire in 1936–39. *Philosophical Transactions of the Royal Society B*, **236**, 505–520.

Chitty, D.H. (1996). *Do Lemmings Commit Suicide? Beautiful Hypotheses and Ugly Facts*. Oxford University Press, New York.

Christiansen, E. and Døving, K.B. (1976). Observations of the mating behaviour of the bank vole, *Clethrionomys glareolus*. *Behavioural Biology*, **17**, 263–266.

Clarke, J.R. (1955). The influence of numbers on reproduction and survival in two experimental vole populations. *Proceedings of the Royal Society of London*, **144**, 68–85.

Clarke, J.R. (1956). The aggressive behaviour of the vole. *Behaviour*, **9**, 1–23.

Clarke, J.R. (1985). The reproductive biology of the bank vole (*Clethrionomys glareolus*) and the wood mouse (*Apodemus sylvaticus*). In: *The Ecology of Woodland Rodents Bank Voles and Wood Mice*. Eds Flowerdew, J.R., Gurnell, J. and Gipps, J.H.W., pp. 33–59. Symposia of the Zoological Society of London Number 55. Clarendon Press, Oxford.

Cooper, J.J. and Nicol, C.J. (1991). The effect of stereotypic behaviour on environmental preference in bank voles (*Clethrionomys glareolus*). *Animal Behaviour*, **41**, 977–987.

Cooper, J.J. and Nicol, C.J. (1993). The 'coping' hypothesis of stereotypies. *Animal Behaviour*, **45**, 616–618.

Cooper, J.J. and Nicol, C.J. (1994). Neighbour effects on the development of locomotor stereotypies in bank voles (*Clethrionomys glareolus*). *Animal Behaviour*, **47**, 222–224.

Cooper, J.J. and Nicol, C.J. (1996). Stereotypic behaviour in wild caught and laboratory bred bank voles (*Clethrionomys glareolus*). *Animal Welfare*, **5**, 245–257.

Cooper, J.J., Ödberg, F.O. and Nicol, C.J. (1996). Limitations on the effectiveness of environmental improvement in reducing stereotypic behaviour in bank voles (*Clethrionomys glareolus*). *Applied Animal Behaviour Science*, **48**, 237–248.

Crouch, A.C., Baxby, D., McCracken, C.M. et al. (1995). Serological evidence for the reservoir hosts of cowpox virus in British wildlife. *Epidemiology of Infection*, **115**, 185–191.

Cushing, B.S., Martin, J.O., Young, L.J. et al. (2001). The effects of peptides on partner preference formation are predicted by habitat in prairie voles. *Hormones and Behavior*, **39**, 48–58.

Di Bari, M.A., Nonno, R., Castilla, J. et al. (2013). Chronic wasting disease in bank voles: characterisation of the shortest incubation time model for prion diseases. *PLoS Pathogens*, **9**, e1003219.

European Parliament and Council (2010). Directive 2010/63/EU of the European Parliament and of the Council of 22 September 2010 on the Protection of Animals Used for Scientific Purposes: https://eur-lex.europa.eu/legal-content/EN/TXT/?uri=celex%3A32010L0063 (Accessed 10 April, 2022).

Fentress, J.C. (1968). Interrupted ongoing behaviour in two species of vole (*Microtus agrestis* and *Clethrionomys brittanicus*). I. Response as a function of preceding activity and the context of an apparently 'irrelevant' motor pattern. *Animal Behaviour*, **16**, 135–153.

Fevola, C., Rossi, C., Rosà, R. et al. (2017). Distribution and seasonal variation of Ljungan virus in bank voles (Myodes glareolus) in Fennoscandia. *Journal of Wildlife Diseases*, **53(3)**, 552–560.

Flowerdew, J.R., Gurnell, J. and Gipps, J.H.W. (Eds) (1985). *The Ecology of Woodland Rodents: Bank Voles and Wood Mice*. Symposia of the Zoological Society of London. Number 55. Clarendon Press, Oxford.

Grippo, A.J. (2009). Mechanisms underlying altered mood and cardiovascular dysfunction: the value of neurobiological and behavioral research with animal models. *Neuroscience and Biobehavioral Reviews*, **33**, 171–180.

Grippo, A.J., Wu, K.D., Hassan, I. and Carter, C.S. (2008). Social isolation in prairie voles induces behaviors relevant to negative affect: toward the development of a rodent model focused on co-occurring depression and anxiety. *Depress. Anxiety*, **25**, E17–E26. doi:10.1002/da.20375

Grippo, A.J., Ihm, E., Wardwell, J. et al. (2014). The effects of environmental enrichment on depressive and anxiety-relevant behaviors in socially isolated prairie voles. *Psychosomatic Medicine*, **76**, 277–284. doi:10.1097/PSY.0000000000000052

Gurnell, J. and Flowerdew, J.R. (1982). *Live Trapping Small Mammals: A Practical Guide*. Occasional Publications of the Mammal Society, Harvest House, Reading.

Hammock, E.A.D. and Young, L.J. (2005). Microsatellite instability generates diversity in brain and sociobehavioral traits. *Science*, **308**, 1630–1634.

Harris, S. and Yalden, D.W. (Eds) (2008). *Mammals of the British Isles*, 4th edn. The Mammal Society, Southampton.

Hawkins, P., Prescott, M.J., Carbone, L. et al. (2016). A Good Death? Report of the Second Newcastle Meeting on Laboratory Animal Euthanasia. *Animals Open Access Journal*, **6(9)**, 50.

Hawkins, P., Playle, L., Golledge, H. et al. (2006). Newcastle consensus meeting on carbon dioxide euthanasia of laboratory animals. *Animal Technology and Welfare*, **5**, 125–134.

Insel, T.R. (1997). A neurological basis of social attachment. *American Journal of Psychiatry*, **154**, 726–735.

Insel, T.R. and Shapiro, L.E. (1992). Oxytocin receptor distribution reflects social organisation in monogamous and polygamous voles. *Proceedings of the National Academy of Sciences of the United States of America*, **89**, 5981–5985.

Jeske, K., Weber, S., Pfaff, F. et al. (2019). Molecular detection and characterization of the first cowpox virus isolate derived from a bank vole. *Viruses*, **11(11)**, 1075.

Jespersen, A (1954). Immunity to tuberculosis in red mice (Clethrionomys G. glareolus Schreb.). *Acta Pathologica et Microbiologica Scandinavica*, **34**, 87–96.

Jernvall, J., Keranen, S.V.E. and Thesleff, I. (2000). Evolutionary modification of development in mammalian teeth: quantifying gene expression patterns and topography. *Proceedings of the National Academy of Sciences of the United States of America*, **97**, 14444–14448.

Kalscheuer, V., Singh, A.P., Nanda, I. et al. (1996). Evolution of the gonosomal heterochromatin of *Microtus agrestis*: rapid amplification of a large, multimeric, repeat unit containing a 3.0-kb $(GATA)_{11}$ – positive, middle repetitive element. *Cytogenetics and Cell Genetics*, **73**, 171–178.

Kaplan, C., Healing, T.D., Evans, N. et al. (1980). Evidence of infection by viruses in small British field rodents. *Journal of Hygiene*, **84**, 285–294.

Kim, J. and Kirkpatrick, B. (1996). Social isolation in animal models of relevance to neuropsychiatric disorders. *Biological Psychiatry*, **40**, 918–922.

Kipar, A., Burthe, S.J., Hetzel, U. et al. (2014). Mycobacterium microti Tuberculosis in Its Maintenance Host, the Field Vole (Microtus agrestis) Characterization of the Disease and Possible Routes of Transmission. *Veterinary Pathology*, **51(5)**, 903–914.

Kruckenburg, S.M., Gier, H.T. and Dennis, S.M. (1973). Post-natal development of the prairie vole. *Microtus ochrogaster. Laboratory Animal Science*, **23**, 53–55.

Laboratory Animal Science Association (2005). Guidance on the transport of laboratory animals. Report of the Transport Working Group established by LASA. *Laboratory Animals*, **39**, 1–39.

Lee, N.S., Goodwin, N.L., Freitas, K.E. and Beery, A.K. (2019). Affiliation, aggression, and selectivity of peer relationships in meadow and prairie voles. *Frontiers in Behavioral Neuroscience*, **13**, art. no. 52.

Leslie, P.H. and Ranson, R.M. (1940). The mortality, fertility and rate of natural increase of the vole (*Microtus agrestis*) as observed in the laboratory. *Journal of Animal Ecology*, **9**, 27–52.

Little, J.L. and Gurnell, J. (1989). Shrew captures and rodent field studies. *Journal of Zoology*, **218**, 329–331.

Lim, M.M., Wang, Z., Olazabel, D.E. et al. (2004). Enhanced partner preference in a promiscuous species by manipulating the expression of a single gene. *Nature*, **429**, 754–757.

Macdonald, D.W. (Ed.) (2001). *The New Encyclopaedia of Mammals*. Oxford University Press, Oxford.

Mandelli, M.-J. and Sales, G. (2004). Ultrasonic vocalizations of infant short-tailed field voles, *Microtus agrestis*. *Journal of Mammalogy*, **85**, 282–289. https://doi.org/10.1644/1545-1542 (2004)085<0282:UVOISF>2.0.CO;2

Martin, R.A. (2014). A critique of vole clocks. *Quaternary Science Reviews*, **94**, 1–6.

Milligan, S.R. (1979). The copulatory pattern of the bank vole (*Clethrionomys glareolus*) and speculation on the role of penile spines. *Journal of Zoology*, **188**, 279–300.

Musser, G.G. and Carleton, M.D. (2005). Superfamily muroidea. In: *Mammal Species of the World a Taxonomic and Geographic Reference*, Eds Wilson, D.E. and Reeder, D.M., pp. 894–1531. Johns Hopkins University Press, Baltimore.

Niklasson, B., Heller, K.E., Schonecker, B. et al. (2003). Development of type 1 diabetes in wild bank voles associated with islet autoantibodies and the novel Ljungan virus. *International Journal of Experimental Diabetes Research*, **4**, 35–44.

Ödberg, F.O. (1987). The influence of cage size and environmental enrichment on the development of stereotypies in bank voles (*Clethrionomys glareolus*). *Behavioural Processes*, **14**, 155–173.

Olsson, G.E., Ahlm, C., Elgh, F. et al. (2003). Hantavirus antibody occurrence in bank voles (Clethrionomys glareolus) during a vole population cycle. *Journal of Wildlife Diseases*, **39**, 299–305.

Ophir, A.G., Wolff, J.O. and Phelps, S.M. (2008). Variation in neural V1aR predicts sexual fidelity and space use among male prairie voles in semi-natural settings. *Proceedings of the National Academy of Sciences of the United States of America*, **105**, 1249–1254.

Paul, L., Kirsch, P., Thomzig, A. et al. (2018). Practical approaches for refinement and reduction of animal experiments with bank voles in prion research. *Berl Münch Tierärztl Wochenschrif*, **131(9–10)**, 359–367.

Randolph, S.E. (1995). Quantifying parameters in the transmission of *Babesia microti* by the tick *Ixodes trianguliceps* amongst voles (*Clethrionomys glareolus*). *Parasitology*, **110**, 287–295.

Randolph, S.E. and Craine, N.G. (1995). General framework for comparative quantitative studies on transmission of tick-borne diseases using Lyme borreliosis in Europe as an example. *Journal of Medical Entomology*, **32**, 765–777.

Randrup, A., Sorensen, G. and Kobayashi, M. (1988). Stereotyped behaviour in animals induced by stimulant drugs or by a restricted cage environment: relation to disintegrated behaviour, brain dopamine and psychiatric disease. *Japanese Journal of Psychopharmacology*, **8**, 313–327.

Roberts, R.L., Williams, J.R., Wang, A.K. et al. (1997). Cooperative breeding and monogamy in prairie voles; influence of the sire and geographical variation. *Animal Behaviour*, **55**, 1131–1140.

Schønecker, B., Freimanis, T. and Sørensen, I.V. (2011). Diabetes in Danish Bank Voles (M. glareolus): survivorship, influence on weight, and evaluation of polydipsia as a screening tool for hyperglycaemia. *PLoS ONE*, **6(8)**, e22893. https://doi.org/10.1371/journal.pone.0022893

Schoenecker, B. and Heller, K.E. (2000). Indication of a genetic basis of stereotypies in laboratory-bred bank voles (*Clethrionomys glareolus*), *Applied Animal Behaviour Science*, **68**, 339–347.

Schoenecker, B., Heller, K.E. and Freimanis, T. (2000). Development of stereotypies and polydipsia in wild caught bank voles (*Clethrionomys glareolus*) and their laboratory-bred offspring: is polydipsia a symptom of diabetes mellitus? *Applied Animal Behaviour Science*, **68**, 349–357.

Sorensen, G. and Randrup, A. (1986). Possible protective value of severe psychopathology against lethal effects of an unfavourable milieu. *Stress Medicine*, **2**, 103–105.

Spears, N. and Clarke, J.R. (1987). Effect of nutrition, temperature and photoperiod on the rate of sexual maturation of the field vole (*Microtus agrestis*). *Journal of Reproduction and Fertility*, **80**, 175–181.

Stowe, J.R., Liu, Y., Curtis, J.T. *et al.* (2005). Species differences in anxiety-related responses in male prairie and meadow voles: The effects of social isolation, *Physiology & Behavior*, **86**, 369–378.

Voutilainen, L., Sironen, T., Tonteri, E. *et al.* (2015). Life-long shedding of Puumala hantavirus in wild bank voles (Myodes glareolus). *Journal of General Virology*, **96**, 1238–1247.

Watts, J.C., Giles, K., Patel, S. *et al.* (2014). Evidence that bank vole PrP is a universal acceptor for prions. *PLoS Pathogens*, 10, e1003990.

Young, L.J., Young, A.Z.M. and Hammock, E.A.D. (2005). Anatomy and neurochemistry of the pair bond. *The Journal of Comparative Neurology*, **493**, 51–57.

26 The naked mole-rat (*Heterocephalus glaber*)

Chris G. Faulkes

Biological overview

General biology and natural history

The naked mole-rat (*Heterocephalus glaber*, NMR) is the only known species in its genus, among more than 30 African mole-rats (Faulkes *et al*. 1997a, 2004, 2010, 2011, 2017; Ingram *et al*. 2004; Van Daele *et al*. 2004, 2007, 2013). Traditionally, all these species were grouped as the family Bathyergidae, but more recently the nomenclature has changed and NMRs are now considered a separate taxonomic family (Heterocephalidae), but still within a monophyletic clade (Superfamily: Bathyergoidea) which includes the remaining African mole-rats as the Bathyergidae (Patterson & Upham 2014). African mole-rats are classified within the Hystricomorpha, a suborder of rodents distinct from mice and rats, and divided into South American caviomorphs (e.g. guinea pigs) and African phiomorphs (including mole-rats). Thus, NMRs are more closely related to guinea pigs than laboratory rats and mice. The six genera of African mole-rats – eusocial *Heterocephalus*, solitary-dwelling *Heliophobius*, *Bathyergus* and *Georychus*, social *Cryptomys* and social/eusocial *Fukomys* – constitute an extensive adaptive radiation of subterranean rodents across sub-Saharan Africa, with the genus *Fukomys* being particularly speciose. The occurrence of mole-rats is determined primarily by food availability, in the form of underground tubers, bulbs and corms, and to a lesser extent the soil type (Jarvis *et al*. 1994; Bennett & Faulkes 2000; Faulkes & Bennett 2013). Despite the speciose nature of the family, the biology of the NMR is in many aspects distinctive even when compared to other bathyergids, in particular its lack of a pelage and overall appearance. In the first formal description and naming of the species by Eduard Rüppell, *Heterocephalus glaber* translates as 'differently shaped head and smooth/naked skin'. Rüppell noted that it 'differs altogether from any other known rodent' and 'the whole form of the body makes a more unpleasant impression because of the hairlessness of the animal' (Rüppell 1842; Figure 26.1). Such are the differences and deep evolutionary divergence of *H. glaber*, that it has led to the aforementioned changes in taxonomic nomenclature with the NMR now considered as a separate taxonomic family (Patterson & Upham 2014).

Historically, the study of the NMR is of interest. After the initial species description by Rüppell, NMRs were largely ignored by biologists until Jennifer Jarvis began studying them as a graduate student in 1967 – first at the University of Nairobi in Kenya, and subsequently at the University of Cape Town in South Africa, including aspects of their social behaviour. Meanwhile, in the 1970s, University of Michigan professor Richard Alexander, in an attempt to explain why vertebrates had not evolved eusociality, hypothesised that such a mammal would probably be a subterranean rodent that fed on large tubers and lived in burrows protected from most predators. When he presented his thoughts in a lecture in 1976, a member of the audience (T.L. Vaughan) pointed out that Alexander's hypothetical eusocial mammal was a perfect description of the NMR, and put him in touch with Jarvis, now at the University of Cape Town. The seminal paper describing the social behaviour of NMRs and the occurrence of eusociality in a mammal was published by Jarvis in 1981. During the late 1970s and the 1980s, colonies of NMRs caught in the wild were established in captivity in universities in both Cape Town in South Africa and in the USA. These colonies are the ancestors of many of the captive stocks of NMRs across the world today (see the following text). In the intervening years, long-term study of captive colonies began to reveal the exceptional longevity and healthspan of the NMR, together with a host of other unique adaptations to the subterranean niche (Sherman & Jarvis 2002; Lewis & Buffenstein 2016). Notable among these are their low metabolic rate and inability to regulate body temperature (see Biological data section in the preceding text) and tolerance of prolonged exposure to low (3%) oxygen (Nathaniel *et al*. 2009), or even no oxygen at all (for up to 18 minutes; Park *et al*. 2017). They can also tolerate high levels of carbon dioxide (up to 50%), with adaptations in the lungs (Maina *et al*. 1992) preventing oedema induced by high levels of carbon dioxide (see Anaesthesia, analgesia and euthanasia section in the preceding text). Carbon dioxide produces an acidic solution when dissolved, likely to occur in the moisture laden air of humid burrows. Possibly as an

---

The UFAW Handbook on the Care and Management of Laboratory and Other Research Animals, Ninth Edition.
Edited by Huw Golledge and Claire Richardson.
© 2024 John Wiley & Sons Ltd. Published 2024 by John Wiley & Sons Ltd.

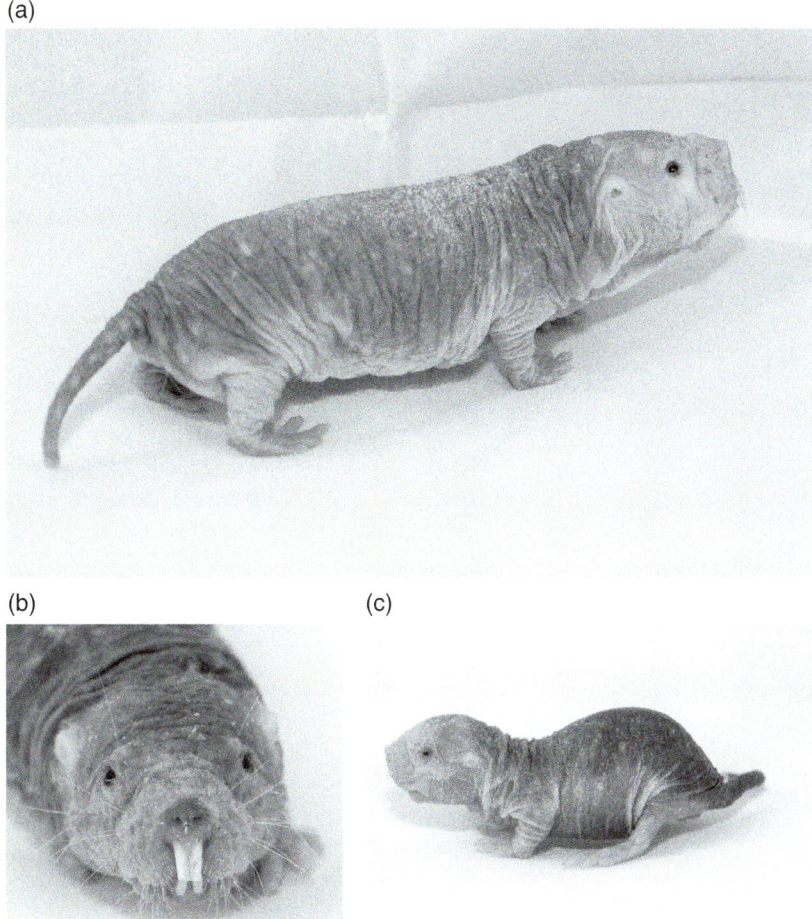

Figure 26.1 The naked mole-rat *Heterocephalus glaber*. (a) adult aged approximately 10 years, (b) close-up showing facial whiskers and (c) juvenile aged 3 months. Source: Photos: Lorna Faulkes.

adaptation to prevent constant irritation due to acid burn, NMRs are insensitive to certain types of pain due to a mutation in the gene for the Nav1.7 voltage-gated sodium channel (Park *et al*. 2008; Smith *et al*. 2011). Furthermore, they also lack substance P in their skin (Brand *et al*. 2010) and do not show thermal hyperalgesia due to changes in the protein structure of the TrkA signalling pathway, which normally sensitises TRPV1 ion channels in sensory neurons acting in pain reception (Omerbašić *et al*. 2016). Other African mole-rats, largely unstudied before 1981, have also received much subsequent attention, and the Damaraland mole-rat (*Fukomys damarensis*) was later shown to fulfil the classic definition of eusociality, together with the NMR (Jarvis & Bennett 1993). Much debate has also ensued about the social systems in these and other mole-rats, and how their sociality might best be defined and quantified (Faulkes *et al*. 1997a; Burda *et al*. 2000; O'Riain & Faulkes 2008).

Both the limited fossil record and DNA-based molecular clock estimates of divergence times suggest an ancient East Africa origin for mole-rats, with *Heterocephalus* forming an early diverging lineage within the clade. Huchon and Douzery (2001), using DNA sequence data and a molecular clock calibration based on the occurrence of the first caviomorph fossil in South America, estimated that the common ancestor of the mole-rat family dates to approximately 40–48 million years ago (myr). More recently, estimates have used fossils of a mole-rat (*Proheliophobius*; Lavocat 1973) as a calibration point for the molecular clock. These have put the common ancestor for the family at a younger date of 33–35 myr (Ingram *et al*. 2004) which seems a reasonable estimate given the occurrence of *Heterocephalus* fossils at Napak in Uganda dated at 17.8 million years ago (Bishop 1962; Bishop *et al*. 1969). Earlier fossil bearing rock strata from the Oligocene period are not present in the areas where mole-rats occur in East Africa, so pre-Miocene mole-rat fossils that might fill in the gap between these Napak *Heterocephalus* fossil dates and the aforementioned molecular estimates for the common ancestor of the family may never be found. Extant populations of NMRs do not extend into Uganda, but are widespread across the arid regions of Kenya, Ethiopia and Somalia (Figure 26.2).

Size range and lifespan

Body mass among adult NMRs is variable, dependent on food availability, age, colony size and composition, as well as social (dominance) and reproductive status (breeders versus

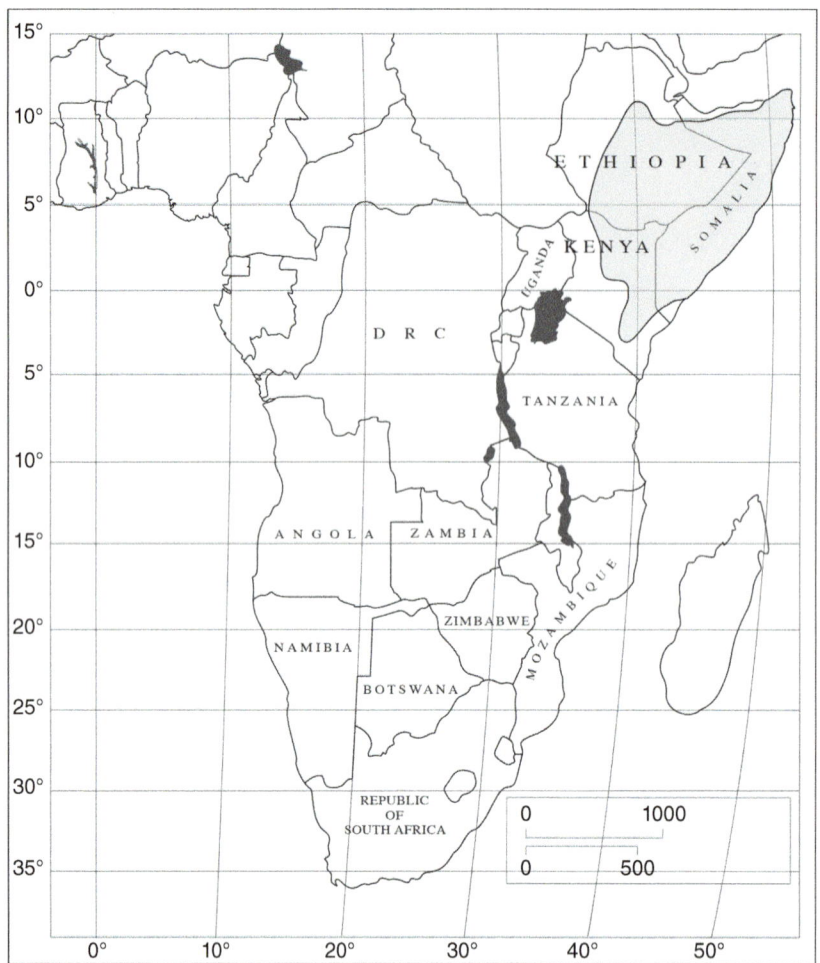

Figure 26.2 Approximate geographic distribution of the NMR in East Africa. Source: Modified from Bennett & Faulkes (2000).

non-breeders), though not sex – males and female non-breeders do not show differences in body size (Jarvis 1985; Jarvis et al. 1991; Lacey & Sherman 1991, 1997; O'Riain & Jarvis 1998; O'Riain et al. 2000; Jarvis & Sherman 2002). The mean ± SEM body mass of wild-caught adults is 33.9 ± 1.3 g (range, 9–69 g; n = 651; Brett 1991a). In captive colonies, body mass of most adults similarly ranges from 30 to 60 g but can occasionally be up to 80 g (Jarvis et al. 1991; Lacey & Sherman 1991). There are reports of zoo-housed animals attaining non-pregnant body weights of >100 g, and a single study records animals weighing up to 160 g (Johansen et al. 1976), but such cases may be unusual. Figure 26.3 illustrates body mass distributions with age among 13 captive colonies of NMRs at Queen Mary University of London (QMUL). Standard body size measurements (mm) of wild-caught adults (n = 42) are (mean ± SEM, range in parentheses): total length: 155.8 ± 1.4 (137–180); length of head and body, 116.2 ± 1.1 (103–136); length of tail, 39.3 ± 0.5 (32–47); length of hind foot, 20.5 ± 0.3 (15–31) (Jarvis & Sherman 2002). Naked mole-rats are unusual among African mole-rats in having a significant tail, which is 25% of the total body and tail length compared with approximately 12% in *Fukomys damarensis* (Bennett & Jarvis 2004). However, while the tail of the NMR is (proportionately) more than twice that of other mole-rats, it is relatively shorter than the laboratory mouse (where the tail may be longer than the body), and the rat (where the tail is almost the length of the body).

The long lifespan and lack of senescence is becoming one of the most studied aspects of NMR biology, and this has led to an increase in the number of captive populations kept in laboratories. The NMR is the longest-lived rodent (Buffenstein & Jarvis 2002; Buffenstein 2005, 2008), with maximum lifespan in captivity exceeding 30 years (Lewis & Buffenstein 2016; Ruby et al. 2018). This is approximately 10 times longer than an equivalently sized mouse, and five times longer than predicted by their body mass. At the time of writing, some NMRs are still alive in captivity aged 33 (R. Buffenstein, personal communication) with a single male animal aged 37 in the Buffenstein lab (Lee et al. 2020). Furthermore, NMRs are apparently unique among mammals in that they defy Gompertz's Law by not showing increased risk of mortality with age (Ruby et al. 2018). The extreme longevity and health span are likely due to a mosaic of adaptations, many of which have arisen from their subterranean lifestyle (see Lewis & Buffenstein 2016 for a review). Among others, these traits include the well-publicised resistance to cancer (Seluanov et al. 2009; Lewis et al. 2012; Tian et al. 2013), resistance to hypoxia and hypercapnia (Smith et al. 2011; Park et al. 2017; Faulkes et al. 2019), avoidance of sarcopenia (Stoll et al. 2016), and healthy heart function (Grimes et al. 2012).

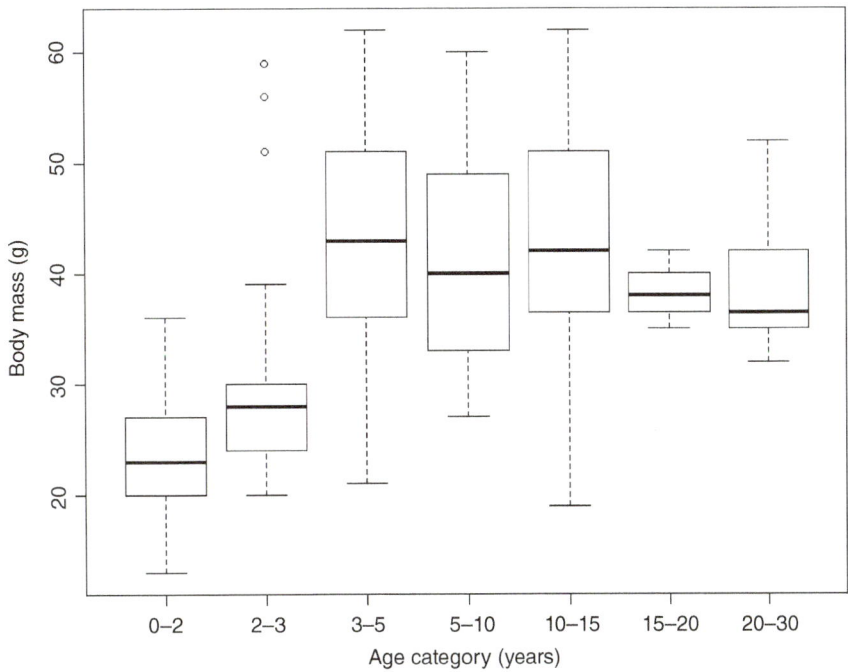

Figure 26.3 Body mass by age category in QMUL NMR colonies (n = 252 animals). The box-plot midline is the median, with the upper and lower limits of the box being the third and first quartile (75th and 25th percentile), respectively. Whiskers extend up to 1.5 times the interquartile range from the top or bottom of the box or to the furthest data point within that distance, whichever is closest (beyond that distance, they are represented individually as points/'outliers').

The publication of the first NMR genome (Kim et al. 2011) paved the way for an increase in studies looking at the molecular and genetic basis of the extraordinary biology of the NMR. Despite their lack of senescence and long healthspan, the NMR has recently been shown to exhibit the epigenetic signatures of ageing seen in other mammals (Horvath et al. 2022; Lowe et al. 2020).

Social organisation

Naked mole-rats are renowned for their social organisation, resembling that of eusocial insects such as bees, ants, wasps and termites. This led Jarvis (1981) to term them a eusocial mammal based on the presence of a reproductive division of labour, overlapping generations and cooperative care of offspring (Michener 1969). The breeding female and her breeding male consorts form a clearly defined caste within the colony. More than 99% of NMRs never reproduce – less than 0.1% of over 4000 animals captured as non-breeders were subsequently re-caught as breeding queens (Jarvis et al. 1994). Instead, these non-breeders help the closely related queen to rear litters, thereby passing on their genes indirectly (and increasing their inclusive fitness). The non-breeding animals within the colony (of both sexes) may show varying patterns of task specialisation, depending on colony age and size, producing a complex relationship between animal age, body mass and the role of an individual within a colony. Generally, differences in the frequencies of cooperative 'worker' (colony maintenance) behaviour correlate with body size, with small animals doing more. Although there can be considerable variation among colonies, behavioural role may change progressively as animals grow, with frequency of work often declining with increasing body size, while conversely, defence-related activities increase in larger animals (Jarvis 1981; Lacey & Sherman 1991; Faulkes et al. 1991a). Recent studies have emphasised the complex nature of the relationship between individual phenotype and worker behaviour (Gilbert et al. 2020). Behavioural plasticity within colonies is also evident, for example when task specialists were experimentally removed, the remaining animals switched tasks and adjusted their behaviour to fill the needs of the colony (Mooney et al. 2015). Vocal behaviours are also extensive with at least 18 context-specific vocalisations categorised (Pepper et al. 1991; Judd & Sherman 1996). Common vocalisations include bird-like 'soft chirps', often given during routine activities, and 'loud chirps' produced during mild conflicts. No purely ultrasonic sounds have been recorded for NMRs (Pepper et al. 1991). Other behaviours in NMRs are well-characterised and an established ethogram published for non-vocal behaviours (Lacey et al. 1991); these are summarised in Appendix A. The most commonly observed behaviours, apart from locomotory, sleeping and feeding related, are sweeping (the kicking of loose items like wood chips behind the animal while it moves backward down a tunnel) and digging (gnawing at tunnels and corners with the incisors, combined with foreleg digging).

Colonies in the wild can number up to almost 300 individuals although, commonly, colony size is around 90–100 (Brett 1991a). In captivity, colonies of up to around 70 can be housed in appropriately sized artificial burrow systems (see the following text) before pup survival becomes compromised or queens cease breeding. Some zoo-housed colonies are reported to have reached up to around 200 individuals.

Individuals may be housed singly, but they do not thrive in isolation. When non-breeders are removed from their parent colonies, reproductive activation occurs, and these isolated individuals will go through puberty to attain breeding status. Pairs of opposite sex individuals housed together will likewise (if they are initially non-breeders) become reproductively active and breed to form a new colony (Jarvis 1991a; Faulkes et al. 1990; Faulkes & Abbott 1991).

Biological data

As with many aspects of NMR biology, growth is atypical for a mammal. O'Riain and Jarvis (1998) and O'Riain et al. (2000) highlight the key points. Growth rates show considerable plasticity within and among colonies. While there is a correlation between body mass and age at all stages of a colony's history, growth varies significantly between litters, and there is an inverse trend between litter order and asymptotic body mass: individuals in successive litters grow more slowly. Unusually, 'adult' and aged (but reproductively pre-pubertal) non-breeders may put on a growth spurt following the death of breeders or older siblings, and the magnitude of this growth response is greater for older litter members (O'Riain & Jarvis 1998). Moreover, lumbar vertebrae lengthening can occur in adult females after the onset of transitioning into a queen role and the production of offspring, leading to the suggestion that queens constitute a morphological caste, as seen in social insects (O'Riain et al. 2000).

One of the characteristic features of NMRs are their procumbent, extra-buccal incisors, but there are also three upper and lower molar teeth on each side of the jaw within the mouth. The dental formula is thus i 1/1, c 0/0, p 0/0, m 3/3 (total = 16). As with other rodents, incisors grow continuously, but estimates of the growth rate do not differ from laboratory rodents. Daily impeded eruption rates (with teeth in occlusion) were 228.7 ± 17.5 µm, while mean daily unimpeded rates (with teeth trimmed to the gum) were higher at 624.7 ± 10.4 µm. These findings suggest that tooth wear sustained during their 'chisel-toothed digging' of burrows is not a limiting factor in the wild, as there does appear to have been selection for accelerated incisor growth (Berkovitz & Faulkes 2001). The procumbent incisors of the NMR are also important in processing tactile information, with nearly one-third of the primary somatosensory cortex of the brain allocated to representation of the incisors. Curiously, the lower incisors of the NMR are able to move independently of one another due to their mandibular symphysis remaining flexible and unfused (Catania & Remple 2002; Cain et al. 2019), although the functional significance of this trait is unclear.

To date, a comprehensive set of standard haematological data for the NMR has not been published. There is evidence for adaptations of the blood to the subterranean niche, with a high affinity of NMR haemoglobin for oxygen (compared to the mouse) being reported by Johansen et al. (1976). However, mean percentage (± SEM) red blood cell packed cell volume (PCV), the fraction of blood composed of red blood cells, from a total of 75 samples collected from 18 animals in captivity was 40.94 ± 0.64 (range 35.3–45.3). This is not far from the mean value of 42.6% calculated from a comparative study of 116 species of mammals (Hawkey 1975). Naked mole-rats have a relatively small heart compared to mice, and a resting heart rate that is less than half that predicted for its average body size at 229.28 ± 7.89 beats per minute (Grimes et al. 2012). It is likely that other well-known traits exhibited by the NMR may also contribute to the lower heart rate, including their low body temperature and basal metabolic rate (see the following text). Interestingly, the heart muscle of NMRs is extremely rich in glycogen, compared to the mouse and rat, even exceeding the concentration found in the mouse liver (the main storage organ for glycogen), an adaptation enabling NMRs to tolerate periods of hypoxia (Faulkes et al. 2019).

Naked mole-rats have a low body temperature (32 °C) and are essentially 'cold blooded' or poikilothermic – they are unable to regulate their body temperatures independently of ambient temperature across the range 12–37 °C (Buffenstein & Yahav 1991). Thermoregulation is achieved mainly through behavioural means, i.e. basking or moving to cooler areas and gaining/losing heat by thermal conduction. The latter is facilitated by their naked skin and lack of an extensive subcutaneous fat layer. Basal metabolic rate is also very low in relation to body size (30% lower than predicted by body mass), at approximately 1 ml/O_2/hour/g body weight, and unusually does not appear to decline with age (up to at least 20 years; O'Connor et al. 2002).

Neurobiological data has been published for the NMR, including a stereotaxic atlas of the brain (Xiao et al. 2006; Xiao 2007), and a multidimensional MRI-CT-based atlas of the brain (Seki et al. 2013).

Reproduction

Naked mole-rats are unusual in their extreme reproductive division of labour and skew in lifetime reproductive success. Normally a single female (the queen) breeds within colonies, although plural breeding (>1 queen) has very occasionally been observed in both captive and, more rarely, wild colonies. While Brett (1991a) and Jarvis (1985) only found single queen colonies, Braude (1991) records two instances of plural breeding (two queens) from a total of 2051 NMRs captured from 23 colonies in Meru National Park, Kenya, over a four-year period. Jarvis (1991a) has reported some incidences of plural breeding in captive colonies at the University of Cape Town (normally, two queens, once three), and they have been observed periodically over the 30-year history of captive colonies in London (at Queen Mary, University of London). Periods of plural breeding are generally short-lived and may result in fighting between the queens, and litters born have low survival rates (Jarvis 1991a).

The mating system of NMRs may be described as monogamous or polyandrous, as the queen can mate with more than one male (normally 1–2, but occasionally 3; Jarvis 1991a; Lacey & Sherman 1991; Faulkes et al. 1997b). Although the queen may mate with more than one male, it is important to note that the mating system is not promiscuous in the usual sense of the word, as the queen forms a long-term pair bond with the breeding male(s). While there are distinctive breeding male consorts to the queen, colonies may contain male dispersive morphs that are behaviourally, hormonally and morphologically distinctive. These so-called 'disperser males' do not reproduce in their home colony, but instead will attempt to emigrate and join a neighbouring colony and outbreed in a dispersal event (O'Riain *et al.* 1996). Disperser male phenotypes have also been observed in the wild, although similar numbers of female dispersers have also been recorded, suggesting that dispersal may not necessarily be male biased (Braude 2000).

Naked mole-rats are also unusual among African mole-rats in that they will facultatively inbreed, although out-breeding may be preferred in captivity if given a choice of unrelated/unfamiliar partners (Clarke & Faulkes 1999; Ciszek 2000) and in wild populations (Braude 2000). In captive colonies, if the queen is removed or dies, she will be replaced from within the colony by another high-ranking female (Clarke & Faulkes 1997). Occasionally, queens may be killed and replaced by previously non-breeding daughters or sisters. Examples of queen succession from within the colony, which may give rise to possible consanguineous matings, have also been described in 3 of 23 wild colonies studied by Braude (1991) and later by Hess (2004).

In females, first conception has been recorded in individuals as young as 7.5 months and mating in males may be from 9 months should opportunities arise in their cooperatively breeding social system (Sherman & Jarvis 2002). The ovarian cycle of a queen is approximately 34 days, with a follicular phase of 6 days and a luteal phase of 28 days (Figure 26.4; Faulkes *et al.* 1990). In a regularly breeding colony, the queen may exhibit oestrus approximately 10 days post-partum, while still lactating (which can continue for 5 weeks). There is no breeding season, and queens can have litters every 76–84 days (as a minimum; Jarvis 1991a), although interbirth intervals can be much less frequent than this, and highly variable among colonies.

As well as having a long ovarian cycle, gestation is also long for a small rodent, at 66–74 days and, during pregnancy, a breeding queen can increase in body mass by up to 84% (Jarvis 1991a). This is a reflection of the exceptionally large litter sizes that NMRs can produce. Average litter size in both captive and wild colonies is 11, with maximum litter sizes of 28 in the wild and 27 in captivity; a breeding queen can often produce more than 50 offspring per year (Jarvis & Sherman 2002). In an often-cited example, a single queen was known to have given birth to over 900 pups during her 11 years in captivity in the University of Cape Town (Sherman & Jarvis 2002). Despite these potentially large litters, the numbers of mammae (males and females) average (range 9–15) meaning that pups may need to share mammae during feeding. Such a disparity between maximum litter size and maximum number of mammae is unusual if not unique among non-domesticated mammals (Sherman *et al.* 1999). At birth, the sex ratio is equal, although it may become more male biased among adults to give a ratio of 1.4:1 in both wild (Brett 1991a) and captive colonies (Jarvis 1985), possibly as a result of higher mortality among female pups, or more likely higher mortality among adults arising from fighting among females for dominance and reproductive status. When born, pups have a body mass of 1–2 g and they become more active and coordinated after about two weeks, after which weaning gradually progresses and they beg faeces from other colony members (allocoprophagy). This ingestion of caecotrophes is important, as NMRs have an enlarged caecum with characteristic endosymbionts to facilitate hind-gut fermentation of their cellulose rich diet (Porter 1957; Jarvis & Bennett 1991; Debebe *et al.* 2017). Autocoprophagy occurs from the age of around 4–5 weeks, after which time the pups are fully weaned (Jarvis 1991a; Jarvis & Sherman 2002). Newly born pups are cared for communally by non-breeding members of the social group, who retrieve them when they begin to wander out of the communal nest chamber, pick them up and carry them during disturbances and groom them (Jarvis 1991a; Appendix).

Naked mole-rats do not appear to show any reproductive senescence and can continue breeding into very old age. Lewis and Buffenstein (2016) report that both males and females aged over 30 years can regularly produce large litters of live-born young, although pup survival is poor. Despite the ability to produce large numbers of offspring over a long lifespan, because of their characteristic reproductive division

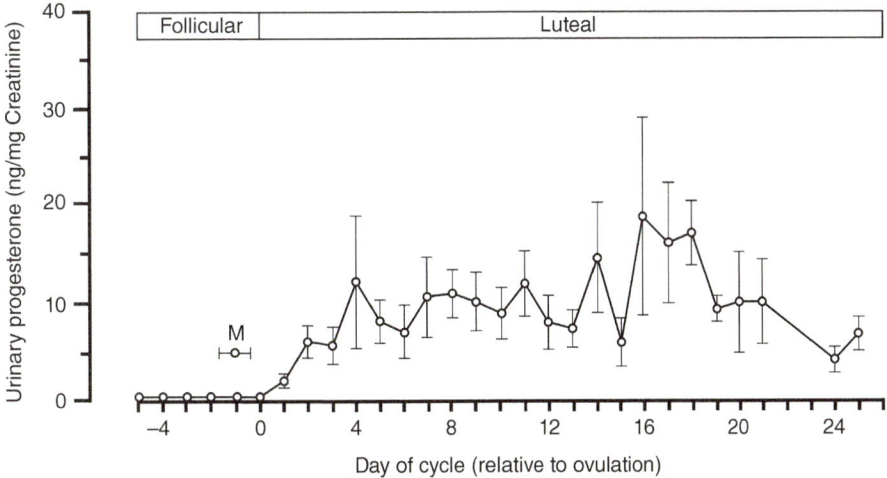

Figure 26.4 Composite ovarian cycle of the NMR based on mean ± SEM urinary progesterone concentrations (from 121 samples taken from 19 cycles from 9 breeding queens). M = mean ± SEM. time of 6 matings observed in 4 females. Ovulation is assumed to be around Day 0. Source: Adapted from Faulkes *et al.* (1990).

of labour and high reproductive skew, most NMRs will never breed. Instead, most are destined to a lifetime of suppressed reproduction and, although they are 'adults' in terms of age and body size, reproductively speaking most remain pre-pubertal, with underdeveloped gonads.

In males, most non-breeders have relatively small testes and reduced numbers of spermatozoa within the reproductive tract that lack normal levels of motility. In female non-breeders, ovarian cyclicity and ovulation are blocked. In both sexes, this diminished activity of the gonads is due to inadequate stimulation by pituitary gonadotrophins (Faulkes et al. 1990; Faulkes & Abbott 1991; Faulkes et al. 1991b). These extreme, and potentially life-long, reproductive blocks are brought about by the presence of the socially dominant queen, who may periodically initiate physical threats and aggression towards non-breeders. Non-breeders are not irreversibly suppressed but are 'totipotent' and can become reproductively active in the appropriate social environment. For example, if non-breeders are removed from their parent colony (and the suppressing influence of the queen) and, either housed singly or paired with an animal of the opposite sex in a new burrow system, they may reproductively activate and come into breeding condition. In females, urinary progesterone profiling shows that ovarian cyclicity commences for the first time (Faulkes et al. 1990). In males, urinary testosterone and plasma luteinising hormone levels may rise to concentrations comparable to those of breeding males (Faulkes & Abbott 1991). If social contact with the queen is removed by taking her out of the colony, or if the queen dies, one or more non-breeding females will become reproductively active and take over as the new queen. Queen successions can be accompanied by intense aggression and fatal fighting among these females, and sometimes among females and males (but male-male conflict is uncommon) although peaceful takeovers are possible (Jarvis 1991a; Lacey & Sherman 1991). The queen is usually succeeded by a high-ranking (dominant female) in the colony hierarchy (Clarke & Faulkes 1997). Reproductive suppression in NMRs is mediated by dominance and agonistic interactions between the queen and the non-breeders rather than primer pheromones released by the queen (Faulkes & Abbott 1993; Smith et al. 1997). However, smell is an important sensory modality in NMRs and it is likely that the individual 'signature' odour of the queen reinforces her physical presence. It is clear that dominance-based face-to-face passing in tunnels is always preceded by facial sniffing in dyadic encounters (Clarke & Faulkes 1997; Appendix). Agonistic behaviours initiated by the queen that potentially mediate reproductive suppression include open-mouth gaping, incisor fencing, biting and shoving, with the latter normally being highly queen-specific (Lacey et al. 1991; Clarke & Faulkes 1997; Appendix). Observations of shoving among non-breeders may be an indication of colony instability and/or changes in the hierarchy during queen succession.

Normal behaviour (wild and captive)

As highly social communally living mammals, NMRs have a rich behavioural repertoire, with 72 non-vocal behaviours characterised into an ethogram within 17 functional categories (Lacey et al. 1991). Comparative studies, although limited, suggest that NMRs behave broadly similarly in captivity to in the wild. However, direct comparisons of some behaviours are difficult to ascertain, for example, reactions to predators and colony defence (Lacey & Sherman 1991; Brett 1991a). A striking aspect of NMRs in captivity is their overall activity and industrious nature. When not dozing or resting in the nest chamber, common behaviours relate to colony maintenance and include sweeping and backward kicking in the tunnels, gnawing the substrate (especially, corners) and transporting food. Individuals will rapidly return to performing these activities following disturbances or translocation into a new environment or burrow system.

Non-experienced observers may be concerned by the preference of NMRs to cram into tight spaces (sometimes corners and tunnel sections) to sleep together, and in nest chambers where animals may recline to form multiple layers. However, this 'huddling' behaviour when animals are reclining together in close body contact (Lacey et al. 1991; Appendix) is an important feature of a normal social group and may constitute around 60% of a non-breeder's daily activity (Lacey et al. 1991; Lacey & Sherman 1991). Huddling has thermoregulatory and energetic benefits and reduces evaporative water loss (Withers & Jarvis 1980), as well as facilitating social interactions and social bonding especially between the queen and breeding male(s) (Jarvis 1991a).

If NMRs are kept in constant dim light, they do not exhibit regular sleep-wake cycles as do other laboratory rodents (e.g. nocturnal or free-running activity cycles), although they do show some synchrony of activity, preferring to sleep and arise simultaneously (Davis-Walton & Sherman 1994; C.G. Faulkes unpublished data). While many rodents show robust and predictable patterns of circadian activity, NMRs are typical subterranean rodents in showing high levels of variation in individual patterns of activity. Riccio and Goldman (2000) report that among NMRs that engaged in environmentally controlled wheel-running experiments to log activity patterns, over half (65%) showed clear circadian activity patterns in wheel-running. Moreover, these individuals could be entrained to varying light–dark (LD) cycles or showed free-running cycles when in constant darkness. The other 35% of animals exhibited free-running patterns of activity under controlled LD cycles, or were arrhythmic. Interestingly, circadian rhythms of locomotor activity were not seen in animals in a normal colony setting. Far from being more sedentary, breeding queens are highly active and spend considerable amounts of non-resting time patrolling the burrow system and interacting with other colony members (Reeve & Sherman 1991; Davis-Walton & Sherman 1994). In a long-term continuous activity monitoring study of one colony, over a 14-month period the queen was found to be approximately twice as active as the next most active colony member and travelled three times the distance patrolling the burrow, covering a total of almost 180 km (J. Freeman and C.G. Faulkes, unpublished data). In terms of any seasonality of breeding, NMRs breed continuously in the wild (Jarvis 1985; Brett 1991a) and in captivity (Jarvis 1991a), with no evidence of any effect of day length or light–dark cycle on reproduction.

Sources/supply/conservation status

Across the distribution of NMRs (Figure 26.2), in the past Kenya has been the main focus of field trips to capture wild animals (e.g. at Meru and Mtito Andei; Braude 1991, 2000; Brett 1991a,b). The majority of NMRs held in laboratories and zoos are derived from captive-bred animals captured during field trips organised and conducted by J.U.M. Jarvis, P.W. Sherman and R.D. Alexander in the 1980s. These took place at Mtito Andei (southern Kenya) and Lerata (northern Kenya). Various pure-bred and hybrid colonies (from northern and southern Kenyan animal pairings) were formed from these original animal stocks. Later in 1991, additional wild-caught NMRs became available from a collecting expedition in northern Kenya (Meru) organised by the Philadelphia Zoological Garden. Few, if any, new wild-caught animals appear to have contributed to the captive gene pool in recent years, due to the difficulty in capture, export and import of animals from East Africa (exacerbated by security concerns over parts of the NMR's range). Details regarding capture methods and transportation are outlined in Jarvis (1991b). Briefly, for transportation, containers must be IATA approved if air freighting, and insulated with a 2–3 cm thick layer of polystyrene with appropriate ventilation at the top. A box measuring (38 cm × 38 cm × 30 cm) can transport approximately 10–30 NMRs without them over heating or becoming too cold. Smaller boxes should be used for fewer animals allowing them to huddle. Hot water bottles (glass or plastic) at around 50 °C placed in a separate section in the box and inaccessible to the animals will keep the container temperature sufficiently warm for about 12 hours (but this should be carefully tested with the box in question beforehand). Large pieces of food should be provided as it will stay fresher, and no water should be given as the moisture in their food is sufficient. Laboratory mouse transportation boxes could be used for shorter, supervised journeys where ambient temperatures are 20–30 °C. See also Chapter 12: Transportation of laboratory animals.

In terms of their IUCN conservation status, NMRs are currently classed 'Least Concern' (2016 assessment) and are not CITES listed. This is probably due, in part, to their preference for semi-arid habitat where pressure from human encroachment is reduced.

Use in research

General husbandry

Enclosures/Artificial burrow systems

Naked mole-rat burrow systems in the wild can total 3–4 km of tunnel length for a large colony, interspersed with communal nest and toilet chambers (Brett 1991b). Much of the burrow system is composed of foraging tunnels built in search of the underground roots and tubers that form the staple diet of the NMR. Colonies can number from 10 to 290 individuals, with an average of 75–80 animals per colony (Braude 1991, 2000; Brett 1991a,b). In captivity, NMRs exhibit normal social and reproductive behaviour if given much less space, but will do best in an artificial burrow system that mimics (on a smaller scale) the wild burrow. This can be accomplished by using a system of interconnecting Perspex®/acrylic tubing with boxes for the nest, toilet and food chambers. Glass tubing of appropriate dimensions can also be used but is more expensive. Such a set-up allows the animals to express many of their natural behaviours (burrowing, digging, sweeping of debris along the tunnels, foraging and food carrying). For a typical set-up employed in a number of institutions, tunnels are normally constructed from various lengths of 5 cm external diameter tubes (with, e.g., a 3 mm wall thickness) connected by corners, X-pieces and T-pieces made from 6 cm external diameter tubing (with a 4 mm wall thickness), terminating or interspersed with round (15–20 cm) diameter or square 25 cm × 25 cm × 15 cm chambers. Connecting pieces can be made by careful cutting of lengths of tubing, using a mitre and band saw, and gluing components together. Alternatively, right-angled bends and T-pieces used for plumbing can be utilised (although these are opaque and can obscure observations). Round or square chambers can similarly be constructed from sheets of Perspex or large diameter tubing. Chambers should have a fixed bottom and removable top for accessing the animals, cleaning and feeding (Figure 26.5). The tops of the chambers must be drilled with a few 6–10 mm holes to provide ventilation. A colony of 40 individuals can be maintained in a burrow system with approximately six chambers. Nest chambers should have three entry/exit tunnels, food chambers two or three entry/exit tunnels and toilet chambers a single entry/exit located at a dead end in the burrow system. Total tunnel length for a burrow of this size should be approximately 8–10 metres. Tunnels with gentle gradients (5°) are desirable and offer the possibilities of more than one level. Naked mole-rats will eventually chew through parts of their burrow system over time (especially, at tunnel and box corners), so repairs or replacement sections will need to be made as necessary. When colony sizes begin to outgrow their space, high percentages of infant mortality may occur,

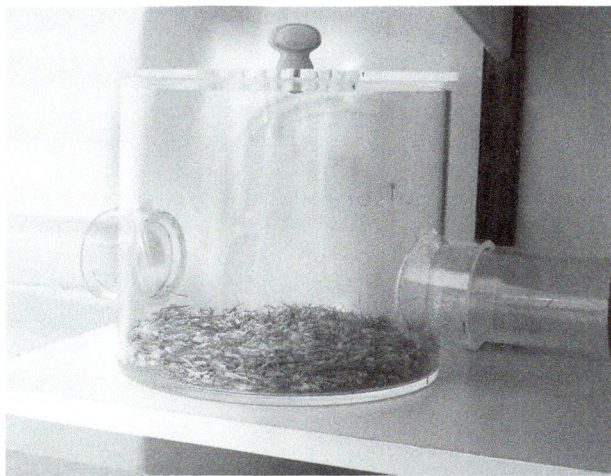

Figure 26.5 Food chamber constructed from 20 cm diameter acrylic tubing. Nest chambers can be similarly made with three entry/exit points, and toilet chambers with a single-entry tunnel.

and that the queen may at times shut down reproduction completely.

Suitable substrates for the burrow system chambers include soft wood shavings and other commercially available laboratory rodent options. Nest chambers should also include bedding material like hay or shredded paper. The fresh husks from sweetcorn provided as food form excellent bedding material when dry, and also act as an item for behavioural enrichment as NMRs shred and transport them around the burrow system. For the toilet chamber, examples of materials for litter include wood shavings and wood fibre derivatives like Lignocel Select®.

Environmental provisions

Room

A room approximately 3 × 4 m with appropriate benches and shelving can easily house 10–15 colonies totalling around 300 animals. Ideally, it should be situated in a quiet area away from vibrations, with a water supply and tiled or waterproof floor to enable proper cleaning. Windows are not essential, but maintenance of a stable temperature is crucial, so adequate insulation is important and air conditioning or some kind of environmental control highly desirable. Numerous hourly air changes of the kind required for mouse or rat rooms are not required for NMRs and may even be detrimental to their health and well-being as their natural habitat is claustrophobic and may often be low in oxygen and high in carbon dioxide.

Temperature

Naked mole-rats are unable to regulate their body temperature independently of the environment and are therefore essentially poikilothermic (Buffenstein & Yahav 1991). One of the most important factors for successfully keeping animals in captivity is maintaining the correct temperature. This is most easily achieved by controlling the temperature of the entire room. Other options could involve placing the artificial burrow systems (see the following text) in clear-sided temperature-controlled boxes. Enclosure temperature range must be maintained between 28 and 32 °C, using thermostatically controlled heaters or air conditioning. In a tropical climate, keeping the room cool may be more of an issue. A selection of warmer and cooler areas can be produced through the use of electrical heat pads under nest boxes or other sections of the burrow, but these are not essential. Sustained temperatures above the recommended range may cause overheating and lead to deaths by heat stroke. Although lower temperatures are less immediately harmful, anecdotal evidence suggests that at sustained temperatures below 25 °C, NMRs stop reproducing.

Humidity

Naked mole-rats should be maintained at a relatively high humidity level of over 50%; if the humidity level becomes too low for extended periods, NMRs will quickly develop dry, flakey skin (burrow humidity levels of 80% or more have been recorded in the wild; McNab 1966; Withers & Jarvis 1980). Experience has shown that the best way to attain this is to keep humidity high within the burrow systems, rather than trying to keep the entire room at high humidity. A well-fitted artificial burrow with few gaps and holes will do this; moisture released by the animals and the food keeps the local humidity up to the required levels.

Lighting

As a result of their complete subterranean lifestyle, NMRs have a limited visual sense, capable of light detection but only poorly equipped for imaging (Hetling et al. 2005). In the wild, they see daylight periodically via open molehills, so housing them in 24-hour light or 24-hour darkness is not desirable (the latter making routine husbandry difficult). Arguably, a natural approach is to turn lights on and off on entering/leaving the room, mimicking the dark burrows, but occasional burst of light from mole-hill production. Normal daylight cycles have also been implemented in zoos, apparently to no ill effect.

Environmental enrichment

A striking feature of NMRs in captivity is their industrious nature and abnormal, stereotypic behaviours resulting from their captive environment have not been reported. Interspersed among short periods of sleep, all colony members engage in periods of often intense activity. While the queen does not normally carry out any worker-related behaviour, she is nevertheless very active in patrolling the burrow system (see the preceding text). Other colony members carry out burrow maintenance behaviours as described in the preceding text (see Appendix), digging and chewing at the substrate and sweeping the tunnels. NMRs need little encouragement to undertake these activities, but they can be easily stimulated to dig, remove and transport material around the burrow if tunnels are blocked with wood shavings or similar materials. Rodent chew blocks can also be provided and running wheels have been successfully deployed by some labs. Modifications to the burrow system that circulate soil for digging trials have been described (Jarvis et al. 1991) but require time to maintain and soil/sand needs to be sterilised prior to addition to the burrow.

Feeding/Watering and daily upkeep

Naked mole-rats, like all of the African mole-rats, are strictly herbivorous. Their natural diet is made up of underground storage organs of geophytes, including swollen roots and tubers, corms, bulbs and rhizomes. Naked mole-rats (like other African mole-rats) are unusual for a mammal in that they do not drink and therefore do not need to be supplied with any separate supply of water, instead obtaining all their water requirements from the food they eat. This is presumably due to the lack of free-standing water in the subterranean burrow systems. This makes their diet especially important, as it is their only source of fluid. Interestingly, the kidney of the NMR does not appear to be morphologically adapted as in some terrestrial desert rodents (with long loops of Henle), suggesting that water is not a limiting factor within their particular niche and diet. Their kidney only has moderate kidney concentrating ability, and experiments have shown that they cannot maintain body mass or plasma osmolality with either salt loading or extreme water stress (Urison & Buffenstein 1994). Due to their high cellulose diet, the gut of NMRs contains a complex microbiome to aid with digestion (Porter 1957; Debebe et al. 2017) and both auto- and allocoprophagy is an essential component of their behaviour (Lacey et al. 1991; Appendix). In captivity, NMRs should be provided with a variety of food items such as butternut squash (and other squashes as available), yams, carrots, sweet corn, apple, and sweet potatoes (which NMRs will eat in the wild if near to cultivated areas). Banana is also favoured by the animals, but spoils quickly in the hot and humid conditions of the burrow system. Food should be given/replaced daily in the food chamber, which is normally a box with two or three entry/exit points and provided in excess so animals can feed *ad libitum* at any time to prevent dehydration. Large pieces of food stay fresher for longer and provide enrichment for the animals as they gnaw it into smaller pieces and transport it around the burrow. Laboratory rodent food (e.g. PMI Nutrition: Lab Diet (R) cat. no. 5LF2[1];) soaked in water is also readily consumed by NMRs but should not be given on a regular basis. Nutritional supplements such as the high-protein cereal-based Pronutro® have also been routinely fed to NMRs in the past in some laboratories and are still used by some, but should be used carefully as they may cause an excess of some vitamins and minerals, leading to health problems (see the following text). Sudden dietary changes should also be avoided to avoid upsetting the gut microbiome. Prior to presentation to the animals, food should be carefully washed with clean drinking quality water or soaked in a sterilising solution such as that used for baby bottles.

To service a room with 10–12 colonies and approximately 200 animals takes one person about an hour a day at most. Routine husbandry is straightforward; any remaining food should be removed from the food chamber and replaced with fresh. The food chamber should also be wiped clean if necessary and any soiled substrate replaced as appropriate. Likewise, 50–75% of soiled litter from the toilet chamber(s) should be replaced daily, while the nest should be inspected for any food remains and other soiling, and the substrate replaced as appropriate. More extensive cleaning should be avoided as it may upset the colony odour.

Social housing

It is important that NMRs are maintained in social groups of at least two animals but preferably as a full colony with a breeding pair and overlapping generations. Singly housed animals lose weight and become listless. Note that reintroducing animals that may have been isolated due to fighting and injury can be difficult and lead to further aggression. In such cases, it is best to find an opposite sexed partner to pair with the separated individual.

Identification and sexing

Naked mole-rats can easily be implanted with an RFID microchip in the loose skin between the shoulders and around the neck (e.g. AVID FriendChip-Mini®; AVID Plc, East Sussex, UK) enabling unambiguous identification. Microchips can be implanted from when individuals attain a body weight of 10 g. A permanent marker pen (e.g. Sharpie®) can be used to mark animals temporarily for up to a week to facilitate behavioural observations.

Sexing of NMRs can be difficult because males do not have external testes (they remain undescended due to the low body temperature of NMRs), and the fact that non-breeding males and females are socially suppressed and in a prepubertal state. External differentiation of the genitalia between the sexes is minimal in most animals, although sometimes more dominant females are easier to sex. Sexing is most easily accomplished by holding the animal upside down by the tail. In females, the horizontal line roughly equidistant between the anus and urethral openings tends to be thicker and redder than in males, where this horizontal line is less obvious (Figure 26.6). Breeding males are not obviously different from non-breeders in terms of their genitalia, although over time they can be recognised from their long but thin bodies and paler skin. Breeding queens have very prominent external genitalia with a perforate vagina. Phenotypically, they are large, long bodied and have well-developed teats. They are also more dominant and aggressive and may be seen to exhibit shoving behaviour (see Appendix), a trait uncommon or not normally seen at all in other colony members. It is noteworthy that, in some colonies, some or all non-breeding males and/or females may possess prominent teats that may be well-developed. The cause of this is unknown, and non-breeding animals do not lactate. It is also possible to use a simple multiplex PCR-based genetic assay to sex NMRs, using a Y-chromosome-linked *DBY* gene (Katsushima et al. 2010).

Hygiene and health monitoring

Normal hygiene procedures should be adhered to, for example, disposable shoe coverings and lab coats should be worn when in the animal room. Face masks and disposable gloves are not routinely required. Food must be clean (as described in the preceding text) and heavy soiling must not be allowed to accumulate within chambers and tunnels. Health monitoring is best achieved by daily observation and routine weighing to look for individuals injured from fighting, or listless/suffering from weight loss.

Care of aged animals

Geriatric mole-rats do not require any special treatment. Aged breeders will continue to reproduce into old age and

---
[1] http://www.labdiet.com/cs/groups/lolweb/@labdiet/documents/web_content/mdrf/mdi4/~edisp/ducm04_028052.pdf (Accessed 21 May, 2020)

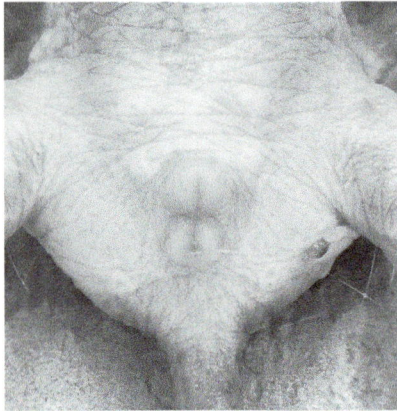 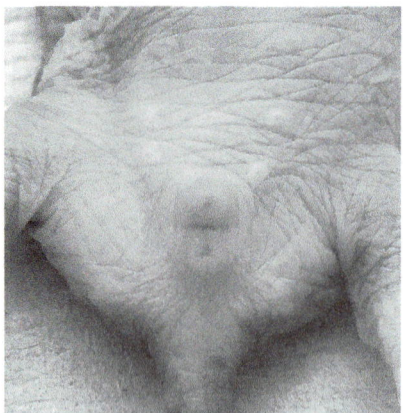 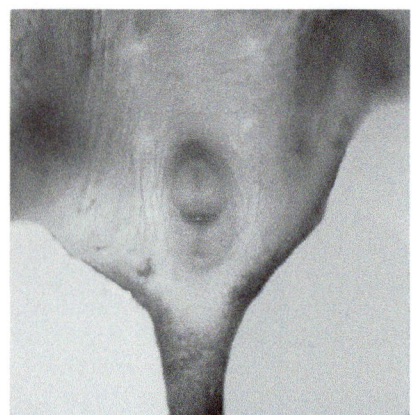

Figure 26.6 External genitalia of non-breeding male (left), non-breeding female (middle) and breeding queen (right)

are still capable of producing litters at over 30 years old (Lewis & Buffenstein 2016).

Breeding

In an established social group, the single breeding queen NMR forms a long-term pair bond with 1–3 males, with whom she breeds throughout the year (Jarvis 1985, 1991a; Brett 1991a; Lacey & Sherman 1991; Faulkes et al. 1997b). In a regularly breeding colony, litters are normally born at 80–90-day intervals, following a gestational period of around 72 days. It has been noted in most captive collections of NMRs that some queens may stop breeding for a year or more and then suddenly commence again, for reasons that remain unclear.

New breeding groups can be established by removing and pairing non-breeding males and females. Once removed from the suppressing influence of their parent colony, non-breeders can rapidly become reproductively active sometimes in as little as 8 days for females and 5 days for males (Faulkes et al. 1990, 1991b). Pairs can be formed from animals taken from different colonies by careful introduction, initially in a box, so that aggression can be monitored and rapid intervention is possible if fighting should occur. Generally, unfamiliar animals accept one another within 30 minutes.

Naked mole-rats prefer to outbreed (Clarke & Faulkes 1999; Braude 2000; Cisek 2000), but differ from other African mole-rats in that they will facultatively inbreed. Initial estimates of extremely high relatedness values (Reeve et al. 1990; Faulkes et al. 1997b) now seem to be more likely due to founder stock coming from a genetically bottlenecked population (Ingram et al. 2015). Detrimental effects of inbreeding have not been extensively investigated in NMRs, and it is thought that harmful recessive traits are at very low frequency having been purged from populations. However, Ross-Gillespie et al. (2007) opportunistically investigated factors affecting mortality in a captive population of NMRs, at the University of Cape Town, struck by a coronavirus outbreak. They found that among the colonies (of known pedigree), the calculated inbreeding coefficient strongly predicted mortality, with closely inbred NMRs over 300% more likely to die than those in the collection that were more outbred. These findings strongly argue for the presence of inbreeding depression in some NMRs.

Environmental disturbance must be minimised when newborn pups are present, as colonies become very sensitive at this time. Disruption leads to increased frequency of pup movement and carrying by other colony members, which can lead to injury, a reduction in nursing time and ultimately, decreased pup survival. Hand-rearing of pups has not been reported, and is not advisable due to the disturbance and the difficulty of reintroducing separated animals back into their parent colony. Attempts at cross-fostering of pups into a foreign colony with existing pups of different ages have been successful, with new pups accepted and fed by the recipient queen (Ke et al. 2014).

Laboratory procedures

Handling and habituation

Naked mole-rats readily become habituated to handling for routine procedures and husbandry. Regular catching of colonies for monitoring of body weight and general health will ensure that animals do not become stressed during the process; it is possible to catch and number animals with a marker pen on a weekly basis without any apparent ill effects. NMRs can be picked up and held by the scruff of very loose, stretchy skin around the neck and shoulders without causing them distress and should also be supported by a cupped hand (Figure 26.7). When catching, NMRs can also be safely lifted by their tail. When animals are unhappy (perhaps stressed) during handling, they will emit 'Hiss' and/or 'Grunt' vocalisations, with the latter often preceding attempts to bite (Pepper et al. 1991). These vocalisations are a useful indicator of aggression. There are no reports of NMRs being trained to take part in or to undergo procedures.

Monitoring methods

Urine sampling has been used successfully in the past for non-invasive monitoring of reproductive status (Figure 26.4; Faulkes et al. 1990, 1991a; Faulkes and Abbott 1991; Clarke & Faulkes 1997, 1998, 2001). Collection of samples can be accomplished by partitioning the toilet chamber litter to one end of

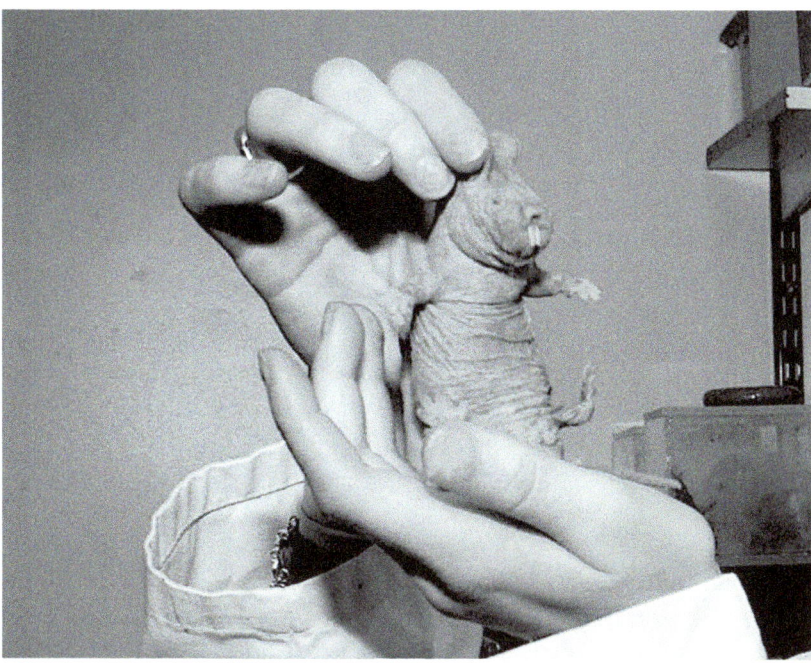

Figure 26.7 Lifting and holding an NMR by their loose skin.

the box with a plastic screen, wiping the floor clean with a wet tissue, and then retrieving samples following urination of known individuals with a pipette. Differing concentrations of urine can be corrected for by expressing hormone concentrations relative to urinary creatinine concentrations.

Blood sampling should not exceed 10% of the individual's total blood volume at any one collection. A sample of 200–300 μl whole blood (of which approximately half will be plasma) is within these limits and sufficient for most purposes. Blood can be taken from a gently held non-anaesthetised animal by pricking the blood vessels in the foot (saphenous or intermetatarsal veins) with a narrow-gauge hypodermic needle, or from a small incision in the skin at the tip of the tail (Figure 26.8). Blood can then be collected in heparinised or non-heparinised microhematocrit tubes (depending on whether clotted, or un-clotted blood for separation of plasma is needed).

Administration of substances

Oral dosing of NMRs is potentially more awkward than in a mouse due to the arrangement of their extra-buccal incisors, but it is possible to administer liquids using a 1 ml syringe. Other routes, including intraperitoneal and subcutaneous, are straightforward, particularly the latter given the loose skin around the neck and shoulders of NMRs. Administration of substances to NMRs through an intravenous route has not been reported.

Anaesthesia, analgesia and euthanasia

During any anaesthesia, NMRs need to be kept warm using a thermostatically controlled heat pad (set at approx. 30 °C) or equivalent, and their temperature carefully monitored.

NMRs can be anaesthetised using an inhalation anaesthetic such as halothane if available or isoflurane (e.g. Fluothane®) for short procedures such as X-raying (C.G. Faulkes, unpublished data). Goldman *et al.* (2006) also report using an inhalant anaesthetic (isoflurane) to implant and remove steroid releasing capsules, and for performing ovariectomies, with Tribromoethanol (avertin) anaesthesia (at a dose of 30 mg/100 g body weight given intraperitoneally) being used for castrations. In the same study, analgesia was administered by subcutaneous injection of Meloxicam at a dosage of 50 μg/100 g. Another study by Catania and Remple (2002) used an i.p. injection of 15% urethane diluted in PBS at a dosage of 1.5 g/kg for anaesthesia. It should be noted that there are relatively few published studies that report surgical procedures in NMRs. Similarly, there are a small number of reports of anaesthetic use during surgery in other African mole-rats (e.g. Nemec *et al.* 2004; Streicher *et al.* 2011). One systematic study investigated the use of anaesthesia more fully in African mole-rats of the *Fukomys* genus (Garcia Montero *et al.* 2015).

Recently, several detailed studies that focus on the use and effects of commonly used small mammal anaesthetics have been published for NMRs. Eshar *et al.* (2019) compared intramuscular (i.m.) administration of alfaxalone–ketamine–dexmedetomidine (AKD) with alfaxalone–butorphanol–midazolam (ABM) and concluded that AKD provided more consistent and deeper anaesthesia (dosage: 2 mg/kg A; 20 mg/kg K; 0.02 mg/kg D). A follow-on study by Huckins *et al.* (2020) assessed an i.m. dexmedetomidine-ketamine-midazolam (DKM) combination (0.06 mg/kg D; 20 mg/kg K; 1.0 mg/kg M). One of the 10 animals in the study died 40 min after apparent recovery from the anaesthetic and was suspected to be an anaesthetic-related death. Thus, while DKM is another suitable alternative to inhalant anaesthesia in NMRs for short procedures that may be painful, the authors noted that it should be used with caution. Finally, Ambar

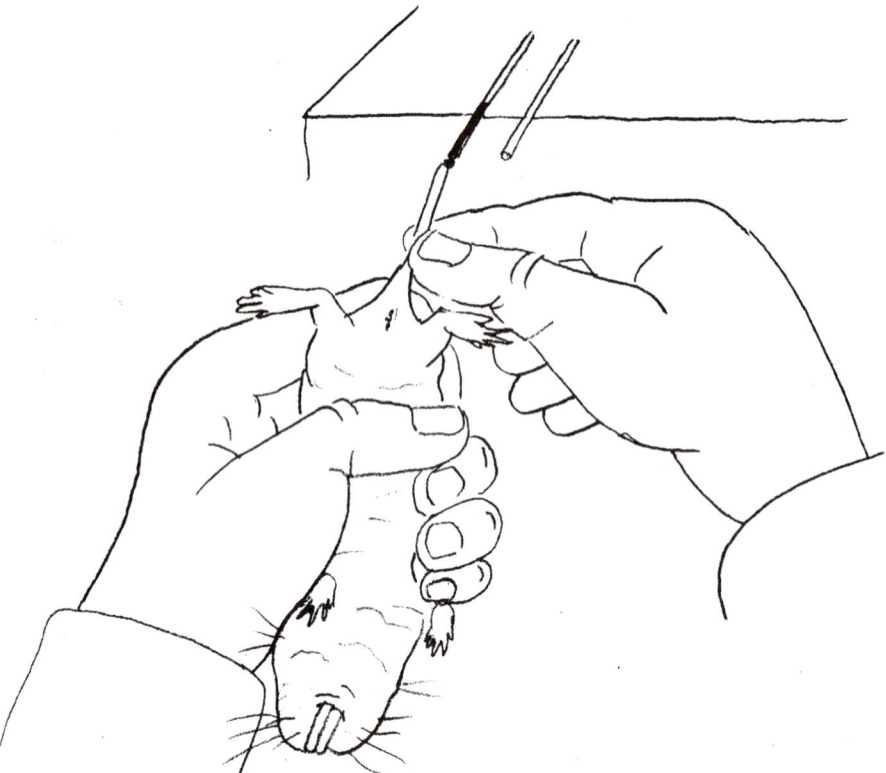

Figure 26.8 Blood sampling from the tail of an NMR. Drops of blood are collected into a microhematocrit tube from a small incision, by gently stroking the tail with forefinger and thumb.

et al. (2020) investigated i.m. administration of an alfaxalone–ketamine (AK) mix (4.0 mg/kg A; 20 mg/kg K). None of the animals showed any adverse responses to the anaesthesia. Overall, the results indicated that AK is a safe and effective method for brief, light anaesthesia in male naked mole-rats and deeper anaesthesia in females, for non-invasive or non-pain inducing procedures (as AK does not include an analgesic).

In the UK, the killing of animals protected by the Animals (Scientific Procedures) Act 1986 is regulated by Schedule 1 of the Act (see Chapter 17: Euthanasia and other fates for laboratory animals). Administration of CO_2 for euthanasia should be avoided in NMRs as they are naturally adapted to living in conditions where ambient CO_2 may reach high levels. Physical methods such as cervical dislocation are also more difficult in NMRs than in a mouse or rat due to the thickness of muscle and fat tissue around the neck. Intraperitoneal injection of pentobarbitone or overdose of a volatile anaesthetic followed by decapitation is arguably the least stressful and most rapid option for the animal.

Common welfare problems

Health (diseases/injuries)

Naked mole-rats are renowned for their longevity and lack of senescence, and generally remain free from health problems. However, as they do not drink free water, if they become unwell and stop eating, they can become dehydrated very quickly. NMRs can be rehydrated by administering up to 1 ml of saline or dextrose-saline solution subcutaneously in the neck or shoulder region twice a day. It is possible to add antibiotics to this solution to treat infection; however, extreme caution is needed when giving NMRs antibiotics as they may upset their gut microbiome. Removal of sick animals from their social group should be avoided if possible, because even short periods of isolation (of more than 24 hours) may make reintroduction difficult without triggering fighting when the individual is returned.

One of the more common health issues reported in NMRs are gastrointestinal problems, often resulting from *Escherichia coli* infections from soiled food or food washed with contaminated water. Animals become bloated with excess gas leading to a heavily distended abdominal region. It is possible to nurse NMRs through such periods of sickness by giving daily rehydration therapy as described in the preceding text. Jarvis (1991b) notes that secondary respiratory illness can follow gastrointestinal problems.

Another nutrition-related health issue that has been reported in several captive collections of NMRs is kidney calcification, thought to be due to provisioning with nutritional supplements (e.g. Pronutro) that provide too much vitamin D and/or minerals (Figure 26.9; Delaney et al. 2013, 2016a; Lewis & Buffenstein 2016). In the wild in their dark, subterranean environment, NMRs have no obvious sources of vitamin D and therefore likely to have an impoverished vitamin D status. Indeed, they have undetectable levels of the main circulating metabolite of vitamin D (25(OH) vitamin D),

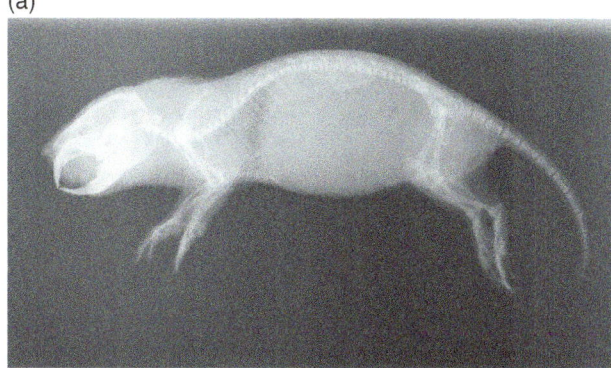

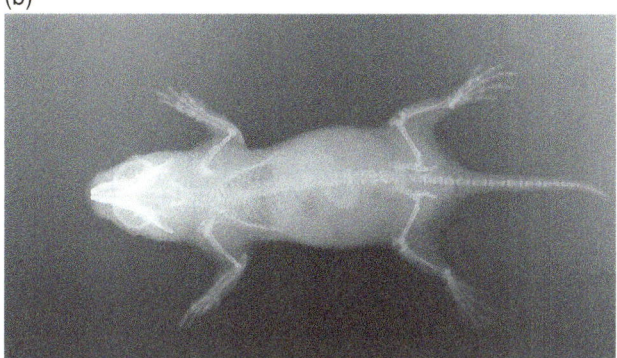

Figure 26.9 Ventral and lateral views showing X-ray dense calcified kidneys in an NMR from a captive colony in London, likely resulting from excessive nutritional supplementation.

although they are to maintain serum calcium levels (Buffenstein et al. 1994). Vitamin D intoxication has been investigated and described fully in NMRs by Buffenstein et al. (1995).

The most common health problems are fighting-related injuries and bite wounds, usually between females. Wounds can be washed clean and may be treated with gentian violet or veterinary antiseptic sprays or cream suitable for small mammals (and odourless). More importantly, the injured animal needs to be removed from the colony/aggressor and housed singly until recovered and behaving normally. The animal should then be paired with another for company, ideally of the opposite sex, from the same or a different colony. Opposite sexed pairs separated in this way will usually reproductively activate and start breeding to form a new colony.

While some laboratory rodents show high rates of cancer-related death, causing up to 90% mortality in mice (Lipman et al. 2004), only a handful of cases have been reported in captive colonies of NMRs (Delaney et al. 2016b; Taylor et al. 2017). While research is ongoing, a number of traits have been implicated in their resistance to cancer (Lewis & Buffenstein 2016; Tian et al. 2017), including the production of high-molecular-mass hyaluronan (Tian et al. 2013).

Like other rodents, NMRs have continuously growing incisors which grow at an average rate of 228.7 μm per day (approximately 0.2 mm) when impeded, or in occlusion. If a tooth breaks and growth is unimpeded, the rate increases to 624.7 μm per day (Berkovitz & Faulkes 2001). Naked mole-rats therefore need both tough food and substrate in the burrow that can be continuously gnawed to keep incisors at a natural length. Overgrown incisors can be trimmed with appropriate clippers.

Sudden and excessive urination throughout the burrow system has also been linked to fatalities in captive colonies of NMRs. The triggers for this remain unclear but may be due to environment factors such as disturbance or unfamiliar odours (C.G. Faulkes, unpublished observations; R. Buffenstein, personal communication). If unnoticed, in acrylic tubing the result is a build-up of urea and ammonia (which in the wild would soak away into the soil substrate), leading to chemical burns on the extremities and around the muzzle. Animals rapidly become sick and immobile and die. Fatalities may continue for several days even on removal from the affected burrow system. In the last such incident at Queen Mary, post-mortem histopathology proved inconclusive as to the exact cause of death.

Given their longevity and long health span, understanding the end-of-life pathology of NMRs has become of considerable interest. Age-related frailty seems to be limited to the last quartile of life, in animals aged 25 years or more (Lewis & Buffenstein 2016). In a retrospective study of a zoo population over a 15-year period including observations from 138 adult NMRs, Delaney et al. (2013) note that the most common cause of death or euthanasia were bite wounds or complications arising from these. At autopsy, commonly found histologic lesions and their prevalence were renal tubular mineralisation (82.6%), mentioned in the preceding text, hepatic hemosiderosis (64.5%), bites (63.8%), chronic progressive nephropathy (52.9%) and calcinosis cutis (10.1%). Three-quarters of animals had more than one of the aforementioned lesions. See Delaney et al. (2013); Lewis and Buffenstein (2016).

Signs of poor welfare

The most obvious signs of illness or poor welfare are animals becoming listless and not exhibiting their normal range of behaviours (described in the preceding text and in the Appendix). A loss of body weight can be an indication of problems, but it should be noted that breeding males naturally become thin with no apparent underlying health issues. Jarvis et al. (1991) followed five breeding males that mated the most often in their colonies and found that their weight loss levelled off at 17–30% below their greatest previous body mass. Bite wounds from fighting can sometimes be difficult to spot, but the accompanying swelling (particularly for wounds around the head and neck) is more obvious.

References

Ambar, N., Eshar, D., Shrader, T.C. et al. (2020) Anesthetic Effects of Intramuscular Alfaxalone–Ketamine in Naked Mole Rats (*Heterocephalus glaber*). *Journal of the American Association for Laboratory Animal Science*, 10.30802/AALAS-JAALAS-19-000170 [published online ahead of print].

Bennett, N.C. and Faulkes, C.G. (2000) *African Mole-Rats: Ecology and Eusociality*. Cambridge University Press, Cambridge.

Bennett, N.C. and Jarvis, J.U.M. (2004) *Cryptomys damarensis*. *Mammalian Species*, **756**, 1–5.

Berkovitz, B.K.B. and Faulkes, C.G. (2001) Eruption rates of the mandibular incisors of naked mole-rats (*Heterocephalus glaber*). *Journal of Zoology*, **255**, 461–466.

Bishop, W.W. (1962) The mammalian fauna and geomorphological relations of the Napak volcanics, Karamoja. *Uganda Geological Survey, Records 1957–1958*, pp. 1–18.

Bishop, W.W., Miller, J.A. and Fitch, F.J. (1969) New potassium–argon age determinations relevant to the Miocene fossil mammal sequence in East Africa. *American Journal of Science*, **267**, 669–699.

Brand, A., Smith, E.S., Lewin, G.R. et al. (2010) Functional neurokinin and NMDA receptor activity in an animal naturally lacking substance P: the naked mole-rat. *PLoS One*, **5**, e15162.

Braude, S. (1991). The behaviour and demographics of the naked mole-rat, *Heterocephalus glaber*. Unpublished Ph.D. Thesis, University of Michigan, USA.

Braude, S. (2000) Dispersal and new colony formation in wild naked mole-rats: Evidence against inbreeding as the system of mating. *Behavioural Ecology*, **11**, 7–12.

Brett, R.A. (1991a) Ecology of naked mole-rat colonies: Burrowing, food and limiting factors. In: *The Biology of the Naked Mole-Rat*. Eds Sherman, P.W., Jarvis, J.U.M. and Alexander, R.D., pp. 137–184. Princeton University Press, New Jersey.

Brett, R.A. (1991b) The population structure of naked mole-rat colonies. In: *The Biology of the Naked Mole-Rat*. Eds Sherman, P.W., Jarvis, J.U.M. and Alexander, R.D., pp. 97–136. Princeton University Press, New Jersey.

Buffenstein, R. (2005) The naked mole-rat: A new long-living model for human aging research. *The Journals of Gerontology. Series A, Biological Sciences and Medical Sciences*, **60**, 1369–1377.

Buffenstein, R. (2008) Negligible senescence in the longest living rodent, the naked mole-rat: insights from a successfully aging species. *Journal of Comparative Physiology B*, **178**, 439–445.

Buffenstein, R. and Jarvis, J.U.M. (2002) The naked mole rat – a new record for the oldest living rodent. *Science of Aging Knowledge Environment*, **21**, pe7.

Buffenstein, R. and Yahav, S. (1991) Is the naked mole-rat *Heterocephalus glaber* an endothermic yet poikilothermic mammal? *Journal of Thermal Biology*, **16**, 227–232.

Buffenstein, R., Jarvis, J., Opperman, L. et al. (1994) Subterranean mole-rats naturally have an impoverished calciol status, yet synthesize calciol metabolites and calbindins. *European Journal of Endocrinology*, **130**, 402–409.

Burda, H., Honeycutt, R.L., Begall, S. et al. (2000) Are naked and common mole-rats eusocial and if so, why? *Behavioral Ecology and Sociobiology*, **47**, 293–303.

Cain, B.W., Reynolds, T. and Sarko, D.K. (2019) Superficial, suprahyoid, and infrahyoid neck musculature in naked mole-rats (*Heterocephalus glaber*): Relative size and potential contributions to independent movement of the lower incisors. *Journal of Morphology*, **280**, 1185–1196.

Catania, K.C. and Remple, M.S. (2002) Somatosensory cortex dominated by the representation of teeth in the naked mole-rat brain. *Proceedings of the National Academy of Sciences of the United States of America*, **99**, 5692–5697.

Ciszek, D. (2000) New colony formation in the "highly inbred" eusocial naked mole-rat: outbreeding is preferred. *Behavioral Ecology*, **11**, 1–6.

Clarke, F.M. and Faulkes, C.G. (1997) Dominance and queen succession in eusocial colonies of the naked mole-rat (*Heterocephalus glaber*). *Proceedings of the Royal Society of London. Series B: Biological Sciences*, **264**, 993–1000.

Clarke, F.M. and Faulkes, C.G. (1998) Hormonal and behavioural correlates of male dominance and reproductive status in captive colonies of the naked mole-rat, *Heterocephalus glaber*. *Proceedings of the Royal Society of London. Series B: Biological Sciences*, **265**, 1391–1399.

Clarke, F.M. and Faulkes, C.G. (1999) Kin discrimination and female mate choice in the naked mole-rat, *Heterocephalus glaber*. *Proceedings of the Royal Society of London. Series B: Biological Sciences*, **266**, 1995–2002.

Clarke, F.M. and Faulkes, C.G. (2001) Intra-colony aggression in the naked mole-rat, *Heterocephalus glaber*. *Animal Behavior*, **61**, 311–324.

Davis-Walton, J. and Sherman, P.W. (1994) Sleep arrhythmia in the eusocial naked mole-rat. *Naturwissenschaften*, **81**, 272–275.

Debebe, T., Biagi, E., Soverini, M. et al. (2017) Unraveling the gut microbiome of the long-lived naked mole-rat. *Science Reports*, **7**, 9590.

Delaney, M.A., Nagy, L., Kinsel, M.J. et al. (2013) Spontaneous histologic lesions of the adult naked mole rat (*Heterocephalus glaber*): A retrospective survey of lesions in a zoo population. *Veterinary Pathology*, **50**, 607–621.

Delaney, M.A. Kinsel, M.J., Treuting, P.M. (2016a) Renal pathology in a nontraditional aging model: the naked mole-rat (*Heterocephalus glaber*). *Veterinary Pathology*, **53**, 493–503.

Delaney, M.A., Ward, J.M., Walsh, T.F. et al. (2016b) Initial case reports of cancer in naked mole-rats (*Heterocephalus glaber*). *Veterinary Pathology*, **53**, 691–696.

Eshar, D., Huckins, G.L., Shrader, T.C. et al. (2019) Comparison of intramuscular administration of alfaxalone-ketamine-dexmedetomidine and alfaxalone–butorphanol–midazolam in naked mole-rats (*Heterocephalus glaber*). *American Journal of Veterinary Research*, **80**, 1089–1098.

Faulkes, C.G., Abbott, D.H. and Jarvis, J.U.M. (1990) Social suppression of ovarian cyclicity in captive and wild colonies of naked mole-rats, *Heterocephalus glaber*. *Journal of Reproduction and Fertility*, **88**, 559–568.

Faulkes, C.G. and Abbott, D.H. (1991) Social control of reproduction in both breeding and non-breeding male naked mole-rats, *Heterocephalus glaber*. *Journal of Reproduction and Fertility*, **93**, 427–435.

Faulkes, C.G., Abbott, D.H., Liddell, C.E. et al. (1991a) Hormonal and behavioral aspects of reproductive suppression in female naked mole-rats. In: *The Biology of the Naked Mole-Rat*. Eds Sherman, P.W., Jarvis, J.U.M. and Alexander, R.D., pp. 426–444. Princeton University Press, New Jersey.

Faulkes, C.G., Abbott, D.H. and Jarvis, J.U.M. (1991b) Social suppression of reproduction in male naked mole-rats, *Heterocephalus glaber*. *Journal of Reproduction and Fertility*, **91**, 59–604.

Faulkes, C.G. and Abbott, D.H. (1993) Evidence that primer pheromones do not cause social suppression of reproduction in male and female naked mole-rats, *Heterocephalus glaber*. *Journal of Reproduction and Fertility*, **99**, 225–230.

Faulkes, C.G, Bennett, N.C., Bruford, M.W. et al. (1997a) Ecological constraints drive social evolution in the African mole-rats. *Proceedings of the Royal Society of London. Series B: Biological Sciences*, **264**, 1619–1627.

Faulkes, C.G., Abbott, D.H., O'Brien, H.P et al. (1997b) Micro- and macro-geographic genetic structure of colonies of naked mole-rats, *Heterocephalus glaber*. *Molecular Ecology*, **6**, 615–628.

Faulkes, C.G., Verheyen, E., Verheyen, W. et al. (2004) Phylogeographical patterns of genetic divergence and speciation in African mole-rats (Family: Bathyergidae). *Molecular Ecology*, **13**, 613–629.

Faulkes, C.G., Mgode, G.F., Le Comber, S.C. et al. (2010) Cladogenesis and endemism in Tanzanian mole-rats, genus *Fukomys*: (Rodentia Bathyergidae): A role for tectonics? *Biological Journal of the Linnean Society*, **100**, 337–352.

Faulkes, C.G., Bennett, N.C., Cotterill, F.P.D. et al. (2011) Phylogeography and cryptic diversity of the solitary-dwelling silvery mole-rat, genus *Heliophobius* (Family: Bathyergidae). *Journal of Zoology*, **285**, 324–338.

Faulkes, C.G. and Bennett, N.C. (2013) Plasticity and constraints on social evolution in African mole-rats: ultimate and proximate factors. *Philosophical Transactions of the Royal Society of London. Series B: Biological* Sciences, **368**, 20120347–20120347.

Faulkes, C.G., Mgode, G.F., Archer, E.K. et al. (2017) Relic populations of *Fukomys* mole-rats in Tanzania: description of two new species *F. livingstoni* sp. nov. and *F. hanangensis* sp. nov. *PeerJ*, **5**, e3214.

Faulkes, C.G., Thomas, R., Eykyn, T.R. and Aksentijevic, D. (2019) Cardiac metabolomic profile of the naked mole-rat–glycogen to the rescue. *Biology Letters*, **15**, 20190710.

Garcia Montero, A., Burda, H. and Begall, S. (2015) Chemical restraint of African mole-rats (*Fukomys* sp.) with a combination of ketamine and xylazine. *Veterinary Anaesthetics and Analgesia*, **42**, 187–191.

Gilbert, J.D., Rossiter, S.J. and Faulkes, C.G. (2020) The relationship between individual phenotype and the division of labour in naked mole-rats: It's complicated. *PeerJ*, **8**, e9891.

Goldman, S.L., Forger, N.G. and Goldman, B.D. (2006) Influence of gonadal sex hormones on behavioral components of the reproductive hierarchy in naked mole-rats. *Hormones and Behavior*, **50**, 77–84.

Grimes, K.M., Lindsey, M.L., Gelfond, J.A. et al. (2012) Getting to the heart of the matter: Age-related changes in diastolic heart function in the longest-lived rodent, the naked mole rat. *The Journals of Gerontology. Series A, Biological Sciences and Medical Sciences*, **67**, 384–394.

Hawkey, C.M. (1975) *Comparative Mammalian Haematology*. William Heinemann Medical Books, London.

Hess, J. (2004) A population genetic study of the eusocial naked mole-rat (*Heterocephalus glaber*). Unpublished PhD Thesis. University of Washington, Washington, DC, USA.

Hetling, J.R., Baig-Silva, M.S., Comer, C.M. et al. (2005) Features of visual function in the naked mole-rat. *Journal of Comparative Physiology*, **191**, 317–330.

Hickman, G.C. (1983) The swimming ability of the naked mole-rat, *Heterocephalus glaber*. *Mammalia*, **46**, 293–298.

Horvath, S., Haghani, A., Macoretta, N. et al. (2022) DNA methylation clocks tick in naked mole rats but queens age more slowly than non-breeders. *Nature Aging*, **2**, 46–59.

Huchon, D. and Douzery, E.J.P. (2001) From the Old World to the New World: A molecular chronicle of the phylogeny and biogeography of Hystricognath rodents. *Molecular Phylogenetics and Evolution* **20**, 238–251.

Huckins, G.L., Eshar, D., Shrader, T. et al. (2020) Anesthetic effect of dexmedetomidine-ketaminemidazolam combination administered intramuscularly to zoo-housed naked mole-rats (*Heterocephalus glaber*). *Journal of Zoo and Wildlife Medicine*, **51**, 59–66.

Ingram, C.M., Burda, H. and Honeycutt, R.L. (2004). Molecular phylogenetics and taxonomy of the African mole-rats, genus *Cryptomys* and the new genus *Coetomys* Gray, 1864. *Molecular Phylogenetics and Evolution* **31**, 997–1014.

Ingram, C.M., Troendle, N.J., Gill, C.A. et al. (2015) Challenging the inbreeding hypothesis in a eusocial mammal: Population genetics of the naked mole-rat, *Heterocephalus glaber*. *Molecular Ecology*, **24**, 4848–4865.

Jarvis, J.U.M. (1981) Eusociality in a mammal: Cooperative breeding in naked mole-rat colonies. *Science*, **212**, 571–573.

Jarvis, J.U.M. (1985) Ecological studies on *Heterocephalus glaber*, the naked mole-rat, in Kenya. *National Geographic Society Research Reports* **20**, 429–437.

Jarvis, J.U.M. (1991a) Reproduction of naked mole-rats. In: *The Biology of the Naked Mole-Rat*. Eds Sherman, P.W., Jarvis, J.U.M. and Alexander, R.D., pp. 384–425. Princeton University Press, New Jersey.

Jarvis, J.U.M. (1991b) Methods for capturing, transporting and maintaining naked mole-rats in captivity. In: *The Biology of the Naked Mole-Rat*. Eds Sherman, P.W., Jarvis, J.U.M. and Alexander, R.D., pp. 467–484. Princeton University Press, New Jersey.

Jarvis, J.U.M. and Bennett, N.C. (1991) Ecology and behaviour of the Family Bathyergidae. In: *The Biology of the Naked Mole-rat*. Eds Sherman, P.W., Jarvis, J.U.M. and Alexander, R.D., pp. 66–96. Princeton University Press, New Jersey.

Jarvis, J.U.M., O'Riain, M.J. and McDaid, E. (1991) Growth and factors affecting body size in naked mole-rats. In: *The Biology of the Naked Mole-Rat*. Eds Sherman, P.W., Jarvis, J.U.M. and Alexander, R.D., pp. 358–383. Princeton University Press, New Jersey.

Jarvis, J.U.M. and Bennett, N.C. (1993) Eusociality has evolved independently in two genera of bathyergid mole-rats – but occurs in no other subterranean mammal. *Behavioral Ecology and Sociobiology*, **33**, 353–360.

Jarvis, J.U.M., O'Riain, M.J., Bennett, N.C. et al. (1994) Mammalian eusociality: A family affair. *Trends in Ecology and Evolution*, **9**, 47–51.

Jarvis, J.U.M. and Sherman, P.W. (2002) *Heterocephalus glaber*. *Mammalian Species*, **706**, 1–9.

Johansen, K., Lykkeboe, G., Weber, R.E. et al. (1976). Blood respiratory properties in the naked mole rat (*Heterocephalus glaber*) a mammal of low body temperature. *Respiratory Physiology*, **28**, 303–314.

Katsushima, K., Nishida, C., Yosida, S. et al. (2010). A multiplex PCR assay for molecular sexing of the naked mole-rat (*Heterocephalus glaber*). *Molecular Ecology Resources*, **10**, 222–224.

Ke, Z., Vaidya, A., Ascher, J. et al. (2014) Novel husbandry techniques support survival of naked mole rat (*Heterocephalus glaber*) pups. *Journal of the American Association for Laboratory Animal Science*, **53**, 89–91.

Kim, E.B., Fang, X., Fushan, A.A. et al. (2011) Genome sequencing reveals insights into physiology and longevity of the naked mole rat. *Nature*, **479**, 223–227.

Lacey, E.A. Alexander, R.D., Braude, S.H. et al. (1991). An ethogram for the naked mole-rat: Non-vocal behaviors. In: *The Biology of the Naked Mole-Rat*. Eds Sherman, P.W., Jarvis, J.U.M. and Alexander, R.D., pp. 209–242. Princeton University Press, New Jersey.

Lacey, E.A. and Sherman, P.W. (1991) Social organization of naked mole-rat colonies: Evidence for divisions of labor. In: *The Biology of the Naked Mole-rat*. Eds Sherman, P.W., Jarvis, J.U.M. and Alexander, R.D., pp. 275–336. Princeton University Press, New Jersey.

Lacey, E.A. and Sherman, P.W. (1997) Cooperative breeding in naked mole-rats: implications for vertebrate and invertebrate sociality. In: *Cooperative Breeding in Mammals*. Eds Solomon, N.G. and French, J.A. pp. 267–301. Cambridge University Press, United Kingdom.

Lavocat, R. (1973) Les rongeurs du Miocene Afrique orientale. I. Miocene inferieur. *Mémoires et Travaux de l'Institut de Montpellier* **1**, 1–284.

Lee, B.P., Smith, M., Buffenstein, R. et al. (2020) Negligible senescence in naked mole-rats may be a consequence of well-maintained splicing regulation. *GeroScience*, **42**, 633–651.

Lewis, K.N., Mele, J., Hornsby, P.J. et al. (2012) Stress resistance in the naked mole-rat: the bare essentials – a mini-review. *Gerontology*, **58**, 453–462.

Lewis, K.N. and Buffenstein, R. (2016) *The Naked Mole-Rat*. In: *Handbook of the Biology of Aging*. 8th edn. Eds Kaeberlein, M.R. and Martin, G.M., pp. 179–204. Academic Press, New York.

Lipman, R., Galecki, A., Burke, D.T. et al. (2004) Genetic loci that influence cause of death in a heterogeneous mouse stock. *The Journals of Gerontology. Series A, Biological Sciences and Medical Sciences*, **59**, 977–983.

Lowe, R., Danson, A.F., Rakyan, V.K. et al. (2020) DNA methylation clocks as a predictor for ageing and age estimation in naked mole-rats, *Heterocephalus glaber*. *Aging* **12**, 4394.

Maina, J.N., Maloiy, G.M.O. and Makanya, A.N. (1992) Morphology and morphometry of the lungs of two East African mole rats, *Tachyoryctes splendens* and *Heterocephalus glaber* (Mammalia, Rodentia). *Zoomorphology*, **112**, 167–179.

McNab, B.K. (1966) The metabolism of fossorial rodents: a study of convergence. *Ecology*, **60**, 1010–1021.

Michener, C.D. (1969) Comparative social behaviour of bees. *Annual Review of Entomology*, **14**, 299–342.

Mooney, S.J., Filice, D.C.S., Douglas, N.R. et al. (2015) Task specialization and task switching in eusocial mammals. *Animal Behavior*, **109**, 227–233.

Nathaniel, T.I., Saras, A., Umesiri, F.E. et al. (2009) Tolerance to oxygen nutrient deprivation in the hippocampal slices of the naked mole rats. *Journal of Integrative Neuroscience*, **8**, 123–136.

Nemec, P., Burda, H. and Peichl, L. (2015) Subcortical visual system of the African mole-rat *Cryptomys anselli*: To see or not to see? *European Journal of Neuroscience*, **20**, 757–768.

O'Connor, T.P., Lee, A., Jarvis, J.U.M. et al. (2002) Prolonged longevity in naked mole-rats: Age-related changes in metabolism, body composition and gastrointestinal function. *Comparative Biochemistry and Physiology*, **133**, 835–842.

Omerbašić, D., Smith, E.S., Moroni, M. et al. (2016) Hypofunctional TrkA accounts for the absence of pain sensitization in the African naked mole-rat. *Cell Reports*, **17**, 748–758.

O'Riain, M.J., Jarvis, J.U.M. and Faulkes, C.G. (1996) A dispersive morph in the naked mole-rat. *Nature*, **380**, 619–621.

O'Riain, M.J. and Jarvis, J.U.M. (1998) The dynamics of growth in naked mole-rats – the effects of litter order and changes in social structure. *Journal of Zoology*, **246**, 49–60.

O'Riain, M.J., Jarvis, J.U.M., Alexander, R. et al. (2000) Morphological castes in a vertebrate. *Proceedings of the National Academy of Sciences of the United States of America*, **97**, 13194–13197.

O'Riain, M.J. and Faulkes, C.G. (2008) In: *African Mole-Rats: Eusociality, Relatedness and Ecological Constraints*. Eds Heinze, J. and Korb, J., pp. 205–220. Ecology of Social Evolution, Springer-Verlag, Berlin.

Park, T.J., Lu, Y., Juttner, R. et al. (2008) Selective inflammatory pain insensitivity in the African naked mole-rat (*Heterocephalus glaber*) *PLoS Biology*, **6**, 156–170.

Park, T.J., Reznick, J., Peterson, B.L. et al. (2017) Fructose-driven glycolysis supports anoxia resistance in the naked mole-rat. *Science*, **356**, 307–311.

Patterson, B.D.N. and Upham, S. (2014) A newly recognized family from the Horn of Africa, the Heterocephalidae (Rodentia: Ctenohystrica). *Zoological Journal of the Linnean Society*, **172**, 942–963.

Pepper, J.W., Braude, S.H., Lacey, E.A. et al. (1991) Vocalisations of the naked mole-rat. In: *The Biology of the Naked Mole-Rat*. Eds Sherman, P.W., Jarvis, J.U.M. and Alexander, R.D., pp. 243–274. Princeton University Press, New Jersey.

Porter, A. (1957) Morphology and affinities of entozoa and endophyta of the naked mole-rat. *Proceedings of the Zoological Society of London*, **128**, 515–517.

Reeve, H., Westneat, D.F., Noon, W.A. et al. (1990) DNA 'fingerprinting' reveals high levels of inbreeding in colonies of the eusocial naked mole-rat. *Proceedings of the National Academy of Sciences of the United States of America*, **87**, 2496–2500.

Reeve, H.K. and Sherman, P.W. (1991) Intracolonial aggression and nepotism by the breeding female naked mole-rat. In: *The Biology of the Naked Mole-Rat*. Eds Sherman, P.W., Jarvis, J.U.M. and Alexander, R.D., pp. 337–357. Princeton University Press, New Jersey.

Ross-Gillespie, A., O'Riain, M.J. and Keller, L.F. (2007) Viral epizootic reveals inbreeding depression in a habitually inbreeding mammal. *Evolution*, **61**, 2268–2273.

Ruby, J.G., Smith, M. and Buffenstein, R. (2018) Naked Mole-Rat mortality rates defy Gompertzian laws by not increasing with age. *Elife*, **7**, e31157.

Rüppell, E. (1842) *Heterocephalus* nov. gen. uber saugethiere aus der ordnung der nager (1834). *Museum Senckenbergianum Abhandlungen* No. 3, pp. 99.

Seki, F., Hikishima, K., Nambu, S. et al. (2013) Multidimensional MRI-CT atlas of the naked mole-rat brain (*Heterocephalus glaber*). *Frontiers of Neuroanatomy*, **7**, 45.

Seluanov, A., Hine, C., Azpurua, J. et al. (2009) Hypersensitivity to contact inhibition provides a clue to cancer resistance of naked mole-rat. *Proceedings of the National Academy of Sciences of the United States of America*, **106**, 19352–19357.

Sherman, P.W., Braude, S. and Jarvis, J.U.M. (1999) Litter sizes and mammary numbers of naked mole-rats: Breaking the one-half rule. *Journal of Mammalogy*, **80**, 720–733.

Sherman, P.W. and Jarvis, J.U.M. (2002) Extraordinary life spans of naked mole-rats (*Heterocephalus glaber*). *Journal of Zoology*, **258**, 307–311.

Smith, T.E., Faulkes, C.G. and Abbott, D.H. (1997) Combined olfactory contact with the parent colony and direct contact with nonbreeding animals does not maintain suppression of ovulation in female naked mole-rats. *Hormones and Behavior*, **31**, 277–288.

Smith, E.S., Omerbašić, D., Lechner, S.G. et al. (2011) The molecular basis of acid insensitivity in the African naked mole-rat. *Science*, **334**, 1557–1560.

Stoll, E.A., Karapavlovic, N., Woodmass, M. et al. (2016) Naked mole-rats maintain healthy skeletal muscle and Complex IV mitochondrial enzyme function into old age. *Aging*, **8**, 3468–3485.

Streicher, S., Boyles, J.G., Oosthuizen, M.K. et al. (2011) Body temperature patterns and rhythmicity in free-ranging subterranean Damaraland mole-rats, *Fukomys damarensis*. *PLoS One*, **6**, e26346.

Taylor, K.R., Milone, N.A. and Rodriguez, C.E. (2017) Four cases of spontaneous neoplasia in the naked mole-rat (*Heterocephalus glaber*), a putative cancer resistant species. *The Journals of Gerontology. Series A, Biological Sciences and Medical Sciences*, **72**, 38–43.

Tian, X., Azpurua, J., Hine, C. et al. (2013) High-molecular-mass hyaluronan mediates the cancer resistance of the naked mole rat. *Nature*, **499**, 346–349.

Tian, X., Seluanov, A. and Gorbunova, V. (2017) Molecular mechanisms determining lifespan in short- and long-lived species. *Trends in Endocrinology and Metabolism*, **28**, 722–734.

Urison, N.T. and Buffenstein, R. (1994) Kidney concentrating ability of a subterranean xeric rodent, the naked mole-rat (*Heterocephalus glaber*). *Journal of Comparative Physiology B*, **163**, 676–681.

Van Daele, P.A.A.G., Dammann. P., Kawalika, M. et al. (2004) Chromosomal diversity in *Cryptomys* mole-rats (Rodentia: Bathyergidae) in Zambia; with the description of new karyotypes. *Journal of Zoology*, **264**, 317–326.

Van Daele, P.A.A.G., Verheyen, E., Brunain, M. et al. (2007) Cytochrome b sequence analysis reveals differential molecular evolution in African mole-rats of the chromosomally hyperdiverse genus *Fukomys* (Bathyergidae, Rodentia) from the Zambezian region. *Molecular Phylogenetics and Evolution*, **45**, 142–157.

Van Daele, P.A.A.G., Blondé, P., Stjernstedt, R. et al. (2013) A new species of African Mole-rat (*Fukomys*, Bathyergidae, Rodentia) from the Zaire-Zambezi Watershed. *Zootaxa*, **3636**, 171–189.

Withers, P.C. and Jarvis, J.U.M. (1980) The effect of huddling on thermoregulation and oxygen consumption for the naked mole-rat. *Comparative Biochemistry and Physiology*, **66**, 215–219.

Xiao, J., Levitt, J.B. and Buffenstein, R. (2006) A stereotaxic atlas of the brain of the naked mole-rat (*Heterocephalus glaber*). *Neuroscience*, **141**, 1415–1435.

Xiao, J. (2007) A new coordinate system for rodent brain and variability in the brain weights and dimensions of different ages in the naked mole-rat. *Journal of Neuroscience Methods*, **162**, 162–170.

Appendix A
A naked mole-rat ethogram for non-vocal behaviours

This ethogram is summarised and adapted from the catalogue of behaviours grouped into 17 categories, first published by Lacey et al. (1991) in *The Biology of the Naked Mole-Rat*. Vocal behaviours are described elsewhere by Pepper et al. (1991), with accompanying sonograms.

1. Grooming related

Seven autogrooming behaviours are commonly observed, although at a comparatively low frequency

1.1 *Cleaning feet with incisors (fore or hind)*
1.2 *Cleaning incisors with forefeet*
1.3 *Wiping the face and muzzle with forefeet*

This behaviour is illustrated in Figure 26.A1.

1.4 *Scratching the body with hindfeet*

This can include the head and around the mouth, flank and axillary regions, often observed in the toilet chamber.

1.5 *Grooming tail with forefeet or incisors*
1.6 *Grooming genitalia*
1.7 *Sharpening/honing of incisors*

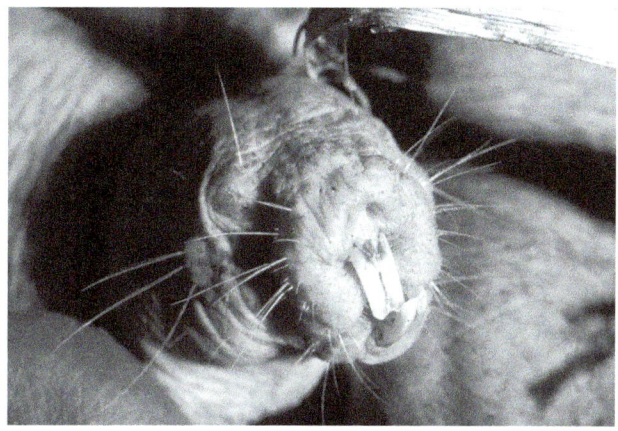

Figure 26.A2 NMR exhibiting behaviour 1.7, sharpening incisors. The upper incisors can be seen to be displaced from the lower pair, prior to rubbing upwards. Source: Photo: Neil Bromhall.

While the incisors on NMRs are ever growing, they are periodically sharpened by rubbing the ends of the upper and lower incisors together (Figure 26.A2).

1.8 *Allogrooming*

Allogrooming between adults is not normally observed, but can be seen between adults and pups as part of neonate tending behaviour.

2. Resting related

2.1 *Yawning*
2.2 *Sleeping/dozing*
2.3 *Reclining*

Dozing refers to sleeping while standing up, normally within the tunnels. Sleeping can also occur in tunnels while reclining, but is most commonly within the nest chamber, often in a large group of 'huddling' animals in close body contact (Figures 26.A3 and 26.A4). Individuals may be completely buried beneath others, but this is quite normal and no cause for concern. Reclining forms a major part (commonly around 60%) of the time budget for NMRs. Huddling has

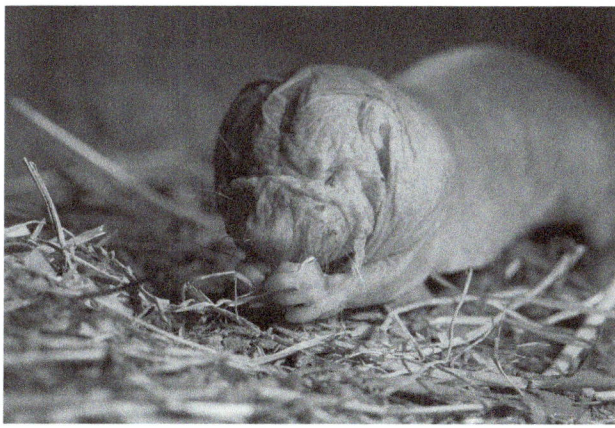

Figure 26.A1 NMR exhibiting behaviour 1.3, grooming/wiping the face and muzzle with forefeet. Source: Photo: Lorna Faulkes.

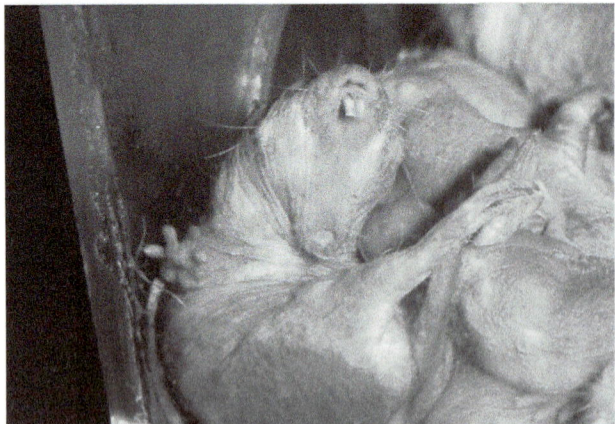

Figure 26.A3 NMR exhibiting yawning behaviour 2.1 in a nest chamber huddle. Source: Photo: Chris Faulkes (author).

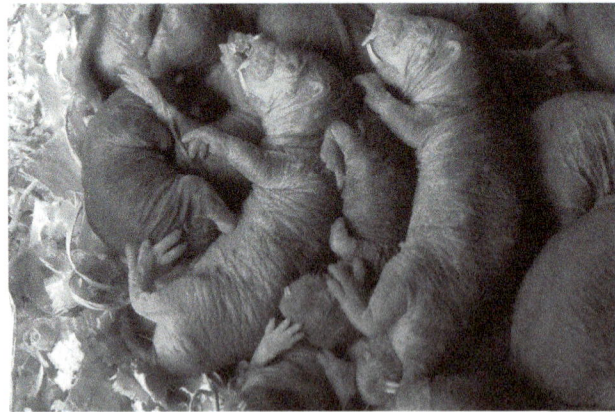

Figure 26.A4 NMRs exhibiting sleeping (behaviour 2.2), reclining (behaviour 2.3) and huddling in a nest chamber. Source: Photo: Chris Faulkes (author).

4. Feeding related

4.1 Brushing of food
4.2 Licking
4.3 Nibbling
4.4 Chewing

Brushing involves holding a smaller food item with the incisors while moving the forefeet up and down in a brushing motion before feeding, normally when the food is wet or has soil on the outside. Gnawing is mainly restricted to large food items, while nibbling occurs when eating smaller items that can be held in the forefeet (Figure 26.A5).

5. Elimination

5.1 Defaecating
5.2 Urinating
5.3 Urinating with crotch dragging
5.3 Urinating with scratching
5.5 Wallowing

Elimination normally occurs in the specific toilet chamber. Notable among elimination-related behaviours are urinating with scratching and crotch dragging. The former occurs when, following urination, an animal grooms itself by scratching with a hind foot into its open mouth and around the head and shoulders. Wallowing can also precede or follow scratching, and involves rubbing the shoulders and/or flanks against the sides of the toilet chamber and often also includes rolling over onto the back. Crotch dragging involves dragging of the anogenital region along the toilet chamber floor immediately following urination.

both thermoregulatory and energetic benefits for NMRs, and also reduces evaporative water loss from the skin (Withers & Jarvis 1980).

3. Thermoregulation

3.1 Crouching
3.2 Shivering
3.3 Basking at local heat sources

Thermoregulation is an important component of NMR behaviour as they are poikilothermic mammals, with body temperature varying with ambient temperature. Crouching involves an individual standing hunched while in physical contact with others in the colony, often in a tunnel. Shivering is also often seen when crouching. Basking occurs when an individual stands next to a localised heat source, such as a heat lamp.

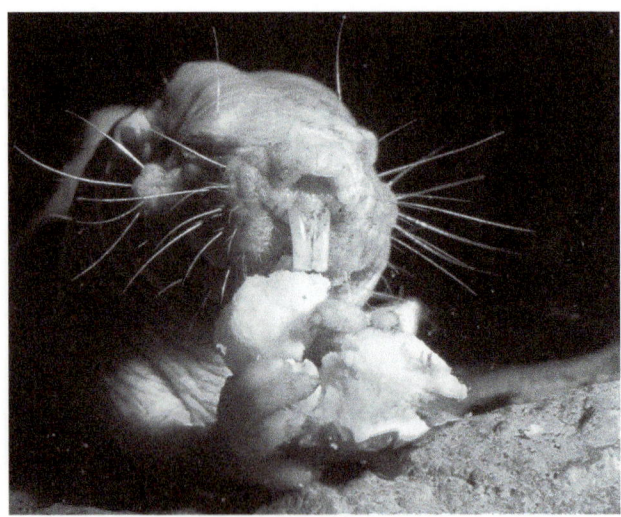

Figure 26.A5 NMR nibbling a food item (behaviour 4.3). Source: Photo: Neil Bromhall.

6. Coprophagy

6.1   Autocoprophagy
6.2   Allocoprophagy
6.3   Begging

Naked mole-rats produce both moist and soft light-coloured faeces and hard, dry and dark-coloured faeces. The first type is most often consumed in the act of coprophagy after the animal assumes a double-up posture (autocoprophagy). Allocoprophagy occurs when adult non-breeders provide faeces to pups, who may beg for faeces as they begin weaning. Begging has also been observed in breeding queens and often directed at breeding males (Lacey *et al.* 1991), but not seen among other adults. Begging is also associated with a specific vocalisation (Pepper *et al.* 1991). It is thought that coprophagy has nutritional benefits (as in lagomorphs, like rabbits), and allows transfer of the endosymbiotic gut microbiome from adults to pups.

7. Locomotion

7.1   Walking (forward or back)
7.2   Running (forward or back)
7.3   Splayed walking
7.4   Crouch advancing
7.5   Darting
7.6   Swimming
7.7   Passing
7.8   Turning

A characteristic of NMR locomotion is their ability to move forwards and backwards with apparently equal ease. However, detailed analysis has shown that average forwards locomotion was around 1.3 times faster than that of backwards locomotion when running (Debra Richardson, Monica Daley, Steve Portugal and Chris Faulkes unpublished data). It is possible that walking and running backwards could also be a defensive trait, enabling the animal to face a predator or intruder while retreating. With respect to some of the more unusual gaits observed, splayed walking occurs when an animal walks with the body held low and the legs extended sidewards, while crouch advancing most often occurs during disturbance to the colony when the animal advances a few steps at a time with the body held low. Darting is rapid and short movement forwards or backwards. The swimming ability of NMRs is unlikely to be observed in captivity, but has been described by Hickman (1983).

Passing behaviour can be from side to side, or more commonly over/under, either following a head to tail approach, or head to head. The latter encounters (unless done at high speed) are preceded by mutual facial sniffing, which implies recognition, and plays an important role in the maintenance of colony social structure (Figure 26.A6). A number of studies have shown that passing behaviour reflects dominance, with more dominant individuals more often than not passing over the top of subordinates (Clarke & Faulkes 1997, 1998, 2001).

Turning in tunnels is another characteristic behaviour of NMRs, especially when taking the form of a tight forward

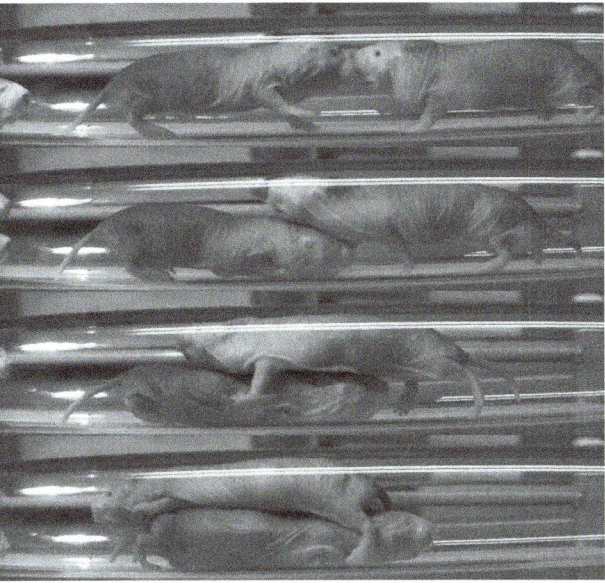

Figure 26.A6   Head-to-head meeting, sniffing and passing sequence.
Source: Photo: Chris Faulkes (author).

somersault with a twist to reverse direction. Turning can also be accomplished by reversing into a suitable space before moving forwards again in the desired direction.

8. Orientation

8.1   Sniffing
8.2   Head pressing
8.3   Exit darting
8.4   Tail sweeping

Touch, odour and hearing are the primary sensory modalities in NMRs. Of especial importance for tactile information are the teeth and sensory hairs which line the head, body and tail (Catania & Remple 2002). During tail sweeping, an animal moves its tail from side to side when moving through the tunnel system (forwards and backwards), and in doing so may gather spatial information through touch. Exit darting is darting behaviour as described in the previous section, but specific to chambers, and involves repeated forward darts and contact with the walls of the chamber until an exit tunnel is located. Head pressing occurs when a motionless animal stands with its head contacting the roof of a tunnel.

9. Transport

9.1   Mouth carrying
9.2   Dragging
9.3   Sweeping
9.4   Backward kicking

Transport-related behaviours form an important component of NMR worker behaviour and include the movement of various items derived from food and the substrate, or other debris. Both mouth carrying and dragging involve using the incisors to hold an item while moving it through the burrow. Sweeping is a frequently observed activity whereby items are kicked behind the animal with the hind feet while moving backwards down a tunnel. Backward kicking differs in that the animal lifts the hind legs together while kicking upward, but not moving backwards. Material may be moved vertically as well as horizontally.

10. Digging

10.1 Gnawing
10.2 Backshoveling
10.3 Foreleg digging

Digging behaviours are also frequently observed if suitable substrate is available, and 'digging chains' of animals will form to cooperatively move and pass material from the front individual to the back (Figure 26.A7). Sweeping (behaviour 9.3) and backward kicking (behaviour 9.4) are also deployed in this context. Following removal of soil by gnawing, backshoveling transfers material under the body and behind the animal using the forelegs. Foreleg digging is the alternate use of each forelimb to dig material loosened by gnawing, prior to removal by backshoveling.

11. Mating

11.1 Backing
11.2 Mounting
11.3 Copulating

Mating behaviours are not commonly observed due to the infrequency of oestrous behaviour arising from long interbirth intervals. Breeding queens initiate mating by backing up to breeding males, often while emitting a trilling vocalisation (Pepper *et al.* 1991), before being mounted from behind and brief (<15 seconds) copulation.

12. Parturition

Prior to parturition, the queen may show increased levels of activity, autogrooming and attention to her genital area. Pups are born head-first and the queen often adopts a doubled over 'sitting' position so that the mouth and muzzle are in close contact with the emerging pup.

13. Pup care

13.1 Pup carrying
13.2 Pup grooming
13.3 Pup nudging
13.4 Pushing
13.5 Nursing
13.6 Sweeping of pups

Neonate tending behaviours occur mainly up to weaning, normally during the first four weeks following birth, and can be carried out by both adult and juvenile colony members. Carrying and nudging can be seen in Figures 26.A8 and 26.A9. Nudging may be forceful, and together with

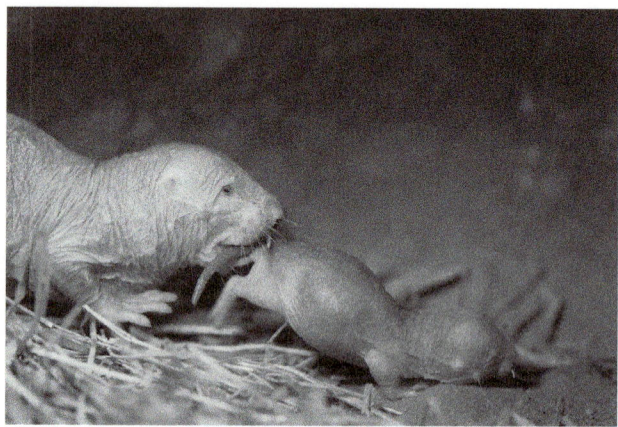

Figure 26.A8 A three-week-old pup being carried from a chamber. Source: Photo: Lorna Faulkes.

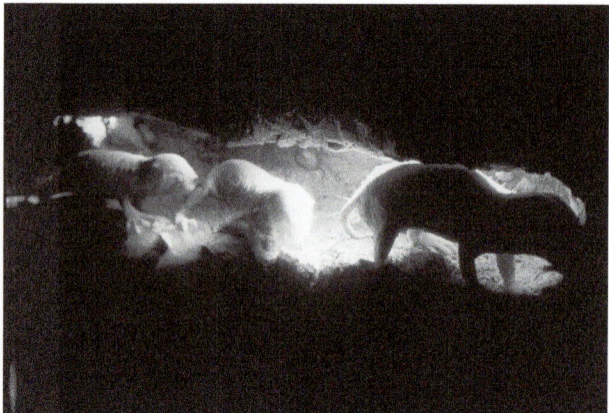

Figure 26.A7 Naked mole-rats in a digging chain. Source: Photo: Neil Bromhall.

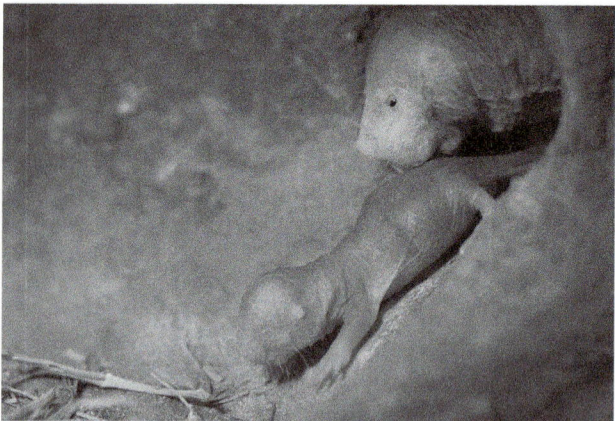

Figure 26.A9 Pup nudging by a non-breeding colony member. Source: Photo: Lorna Faulkes.

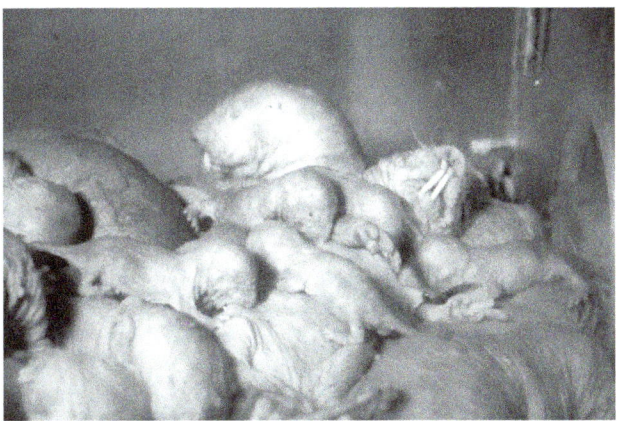

Figure 26.A10 A breeding queen reclining while nursing pups. Source: Photo: Chris Faulkes (author).

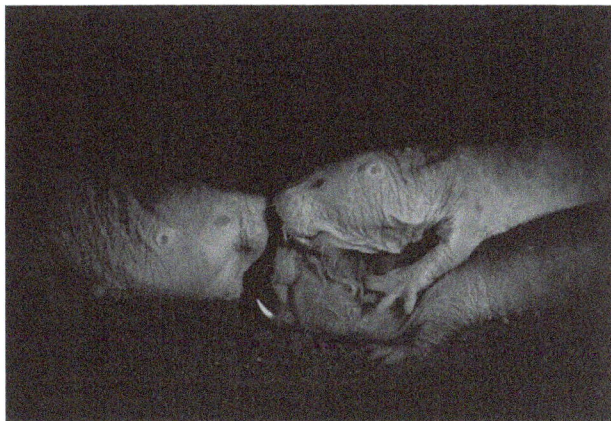

Figure 26.A11 Sniffing and nose pressing. Source: Photo: Lorna Faulkes.

pushing, can move pups some distance down tunnels. Although in some colonies, both male and female non-breeders can develop enlarged teats, only the breeding queen lactates and feeds her offspring (Figure 26.A10).

14. Juvenile specific

14.1 Wrestling
14.2 Dragging

Juvenile-specific behaviours are commonly seen from weaning over a period of several months and can involve pairs and small groups. Wrestling can include batting and incisor fencing (see Section 16), while dragging involves one juvenile grabbing another with its incisors and pulling it down to a tunnel.

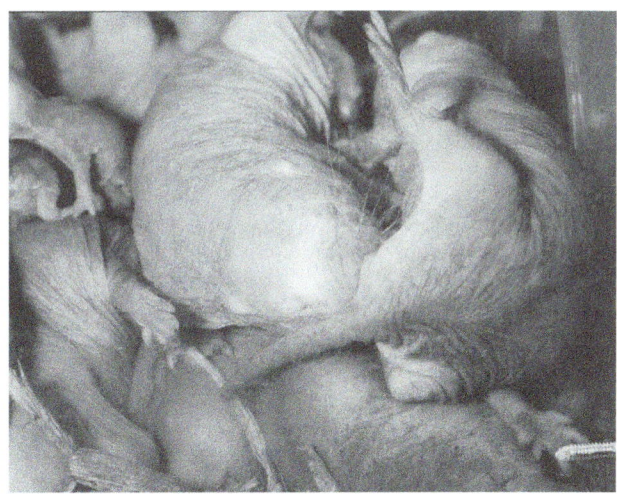

Figure 26.A12 Anogenital nuzzling and sniffing. Source: Photo: Chris Faulkes (author).

15. Interactive

15.1 Nose pressing
15.2 Nuzzling
15.3 Anogenital nuzzling and sniffing
15.4 Sniffing another animal
15.5 Head deflecting
15.6 Pawing

Mutual sniffing forms an important component of several of the interactive behaviours. Nose pressing is the brief pressing together of muzzles (Figure 26.A11), while nuzzling is when an animal rubs its muzzle against the body of another individual. Anogenital nuzzling mainly occurs between breeding queens and breeding males, but can occasionally be seen among non-breeding animals (Figure 26.A12). When head deflecting, one animal turns its head to the side and downwards leaving the muzzle of a second animal, close to the side of the head in the ear region (Figure 26.A13). Pawing occurs when an animal drags a forelimb repeatedly along the body of a second individual.

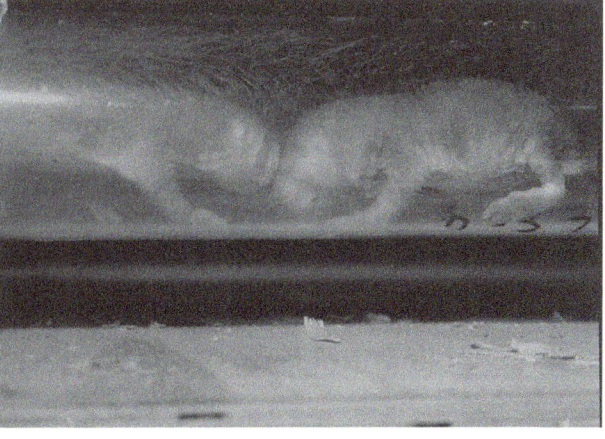

Figure 26.A13 Head deflecting. Source: Photo: Lorna Faulkes.

16. Aggressive/agonistic

16.1 *Open-mouth gaping*
16.2 *Incisor fencing*
16.3 *Batting*
16.4 *Biting*
16.5 *Shoving*
16.6 *Tugging*
16.7 *Tetany*

Open-mouth gaping occurs when two animals stand open mouthed facing each other with the top and bottom incisors separated (Figure 26.A14). A hissing sound is produced by the rapid inhalation and exhalation of air. Incisor fencing involves the locking together of incisors, often with pushing and pulling (Figure 26.A15), sometimes leading to biting (Figure 26.A16). Shoving is a behaviour almost always initiated by the queen and can involve the recipient animal being pushed up to 1 m down a tunnel (Reeve & Sherman 1991). Shoving is often accompanied by aggressive hissing from the

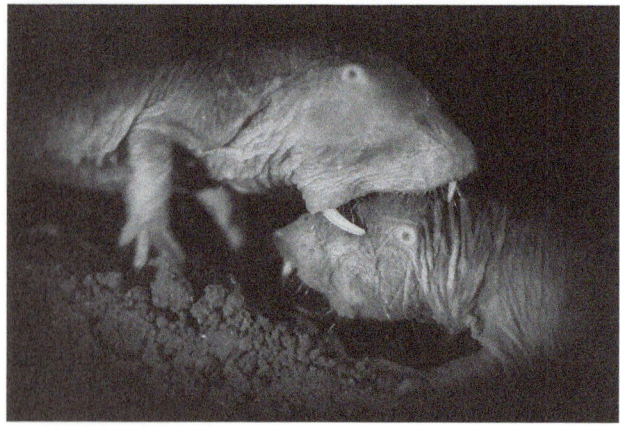

Figure 26.A16 Biting. Source: Photo: Lorna Faulkes.

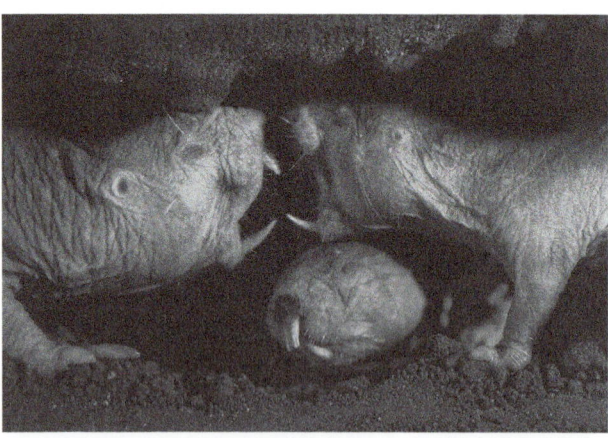

Figure 26.A14 Open-mouth gaping. Source: Photo: Lorna Faulkes.

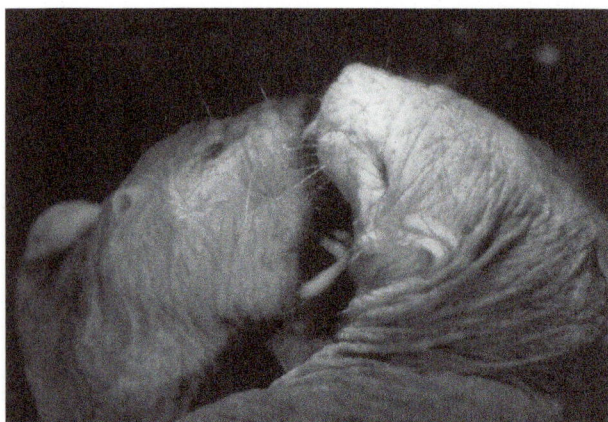

Figure 26.A15 Incisor fencing. Source: Photo: Neil Bromhall.

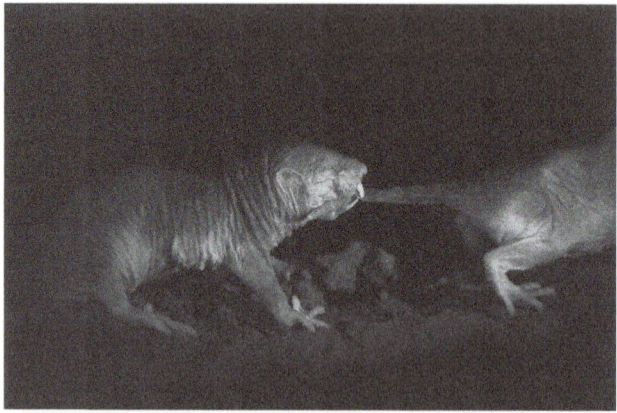

Figure 26.A17 Tail tugging. Source: Photo: Lorna Faulkes.

initiator. The association of shoving with reproductive status has led to the hypothesis that it may be an important social cue involved in reproductive suppression (Clarke & Faulkes 1997, 1998, 2001). Tugging is when an individual grasps the skin or tail of another in its incisors and pulls (Figure 26.A17). Tetany describes when an individual doubles up, lying still (sometimes for several minutes) and often with its legs in the air; this behaviour can follow being shoved by the queen.

17. Alarm

17.1 *Freezing*
17.2 *Scrambling*

Naked mole-rats are sensitive to loud noises and vibrations and may respond with alarm behaviours, freezing all motion or with a panicked scramble where many individuals dart off simultaneously in an uncoordinated fashion.

27

The guinea pig

Sylvia Kaiser, Christine Krüger and Norbert Sachser

Biological overview

The guinea pig (*Cavia aperea* f. *porcellus*) was domesticated about 3000–6000 years ago in the highlands of South America (Hückinghaus 1961; Gade 1967; Hyams 1972; Wing 1977; Herre & Röhrs 1990; Benecke 1994). The main aim of domestication was to provide the indigenous people with meat (Herre & Röhrs 1990) and guinea pigs are still one of the main sources of meat in some rural populations of South America. They have also, occasionally, been used for ritual healing (Gade 1967; Hyams 1972; Weir 1974; Wing 1977; Clutton-Brock 1989; Herre & Röhrs 1990; Benecke 1994). Guinea pigs in South America today are left to scavenge in and around the huts of the local indigenous people, and it may be assumed that a similar husbandry has always existed (Weir 1974; Stahnke & Hendrichs 1988). In the middle of the sixteenth century, the Spaniards discovered guinea pigs and introduced them into Europe. Within the European population, the animals rapidly became a popular pet (Gade 1967; Hyams 1972; Clutton-Brock 1989; Benecke 1994). Nowadays, guinea pigs are one of the most popular pets throughout the world, raised for companion uses and showing.

The wild ancestor *Cavia aperea*

According to anatomical and morphological studies, the domestic guinea pig derives from the subspecies *tschudii* of the wild cavy (*Cavia aperea*), which is among the most common and widespread rodents of South America (e.g., Rood 1972; Trillmich et al. 2004; Kruska & Steffen 2013). Please note, however, that some authors assign the ancestor *tschudii* to its own species, *Cavia tschudii* (Spotorno et al. 2004, 2007). The wild cavy and the domestic guinea pig (Figure 27.1) belong to the order Rodentia and to the family Caviidae. All cavy-like members of this family (about 14 species; Wilson & Reeder 2005) are medium-sized, tailless rodents that have four digits on the front feet and three digits on the hindfeet. All digits have claws. All forms – except the domestic guinea pig – have agouti dorsal pelage and a lighter underside (Rood 1972; Wagner 1976). The cavy-like members of the Caviidae are divided into four genera (*Cavia*, *Galea*, *Kerodon* and *Microcavia*), which are widely distributed throughout South America and inhabit a wide range of ecological niches (Mares & Ojeda 1982; Redford & Eisenberg 1992; Eisenberg & Redford 1999).1953

The wild cavy is an herbivorous, neotropical rodent that occurs from Colombia through Brazil into Argentina (Mares & Ojeda 1982; Stahnke & Hendrichs 1988; Redford & Eisenberg 1992). It is a crepuscular, non-climbing species, which does not dig burrows, but hides and moves through tunnels made in dense vegetation (Rood 1972; Stahnke & Hendrichs 1988; Guichón & Cassini 1998). The typical habitat of *C. aperea* contains a cover zone with high and dense vegetation, which the animals use as protection from predator attacks (Rood 1972), and an adjacent, more open zone of short vegetation where cavies forage (Cassini 1991; Cassini & Galante 1992; Guichón & Cassini 1998; Asher et al. 2008).

The wild cavies live in small harem groups consisting of one adult male and up to three females and their unweaned offspring (Rood 1972; Sachser et al. 1999; Asher et al. 2004, 2008). Males do not defend a territory, but they also do not accept other mature males near their females, resulting in little overlap between the home ranges of neighbouring males (Asher et al. 2004, 2008). Younger and lighter males show alternative strategies as roamers who regularly traverse females' home ranges or as satellites of males with stable home ranges (Asher et al. 2008; Adrian & Sachser 2011).

Under semi-natural and laboratory conditions, adult male *C. aperea* are highly incompatible in the presence of females, whereas female *C. aperea* organise themselves into linear dominance hierarchies. The male–male competition brings about a polygynous mating system (Sachser et al. 1999). Whenever a female comes into oestrus, only one male is present. This male thus mates with several females, whereas every female mates with a single male (Sachser 1998). Females play an active role in bringing about this species' social and mating system by displaying clear preferences for single males (Adrian et al. 2008). Moreover, the low relative testis weights and the small epididymis size of *Cavia apera*

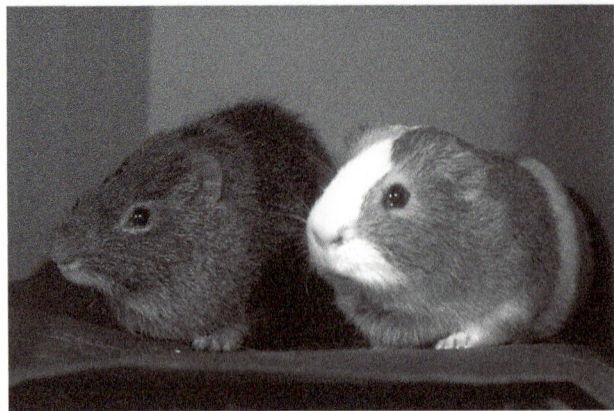

Figure 27.1 The wild cavy (*Cavia aperea*, left) and the domestic guinea pig (*Cavia aperea* f. *porcellus*, right). Source: Photo: Department of Behavioural Biology, Münster/M. Aulbur.

Table 27.1 Physiological and behavioural consequences of domestication: comparison between domestic (*Cavia aperea* f. *porcellus*) and wild guinea pigs (*Cavia aperea*) (− rare/low; + frequent/high).

		Domestic	Wild
Endocrine stress response	Adrenocortical system	−	+
	Adrenomedullary system	−	+
Behaviour	Attentive	−	+
	Vocal	+	−
	Courtship	+	−
	Sociopositive	+	−
	Aggressive	−	+

Source: For references and original data, see Künzl and Sachser (1999), Künzl et al. (2003) and Sachser (2001).

are within the typical range of species with a single-male mating system (Kenagy & Trombulak 1986; Sachser 1998; Sachser et al. 1999; Cooper et al. 2000).

Behavioural and physiological consequences of domestication

As described in the preceding text, the domestic guinea pigs derived from the wild cavy at least 3000 years ago. The process of domestication is always accompanied by distinct changes in morphology, physiology and behaviour (Haase & Donham 1980; Price 1984; Clutton-Brock 1989; Herre & Röhrs 1990; Künzl & Sachser 1999; Jensen 2006; Kaiser et al. 2015). As a consequence, wild and domestic animals require somewhat different conditions and resources to achieve good welfare although, in a biological sense, they still belong to the same species (Sachser 2001).

Behavioural studies indicate that the repertoire of behavioural patterns is similar in domesticated and wild guinea pigs. Thus, domestication has not resulted in the loss or addition of behavioural elements (Rood 1972; Künzl & Sachser 1999). Distinct differences have, however, developed in behavioural frequencies and thresholds (Künzl & Sachser 1999) (Table 27.1). Domestic guinea pigs display lower levels of intraspecific aggressive behaviour and higher levels of sociopositive behaviour (e.g. social grooming) than the wild ancestors. They also show more frequent overt courtship behaviour and have a lower threshold for vocalisation. Finally, domesticated guinea pigs are less attentive to their physical environment and show much less exploration behaviour than their ancestors (Künzl & Sachser 1999; Künzl et al. 2003; Kaiser et al. 2015).

These behavioural differences are associated with marked changes in social structure compared with the wild form. When domestic guinea pigs are kept in breeding groups of one adult male and several adult females, the mature sons and daughters will integrate rather peacefully into the social system of the groups and all animals will cohabitate in a non-aggressive and non-stressful way (Sachser 1998). When adult wild cavies are kept in breeding groups of one male and several females, a completely different picture emerges: the daughters integrate into the linear dominance hierarchy of the females. In contrast, the father and his sons often become incompatible when the sons attain sexual maturity. In most cases, the sons must then be taken out of the groups, otherwise the father will injure or kill them (Sachser 1998).

There are no indications that the learning abilities of the domestic guinea pig are impaired. For instance, in the Morris Water Maze (a frequently used test for the assessment of spatial learning in rodents) male and female domestic guinea pigs perform even better than their wild relatives (Lewejohann et al. 2010).

A series of experiments has been conducted to compare endocrine stress responses between wild and domestic guinea pigs (Table 27.1). Wild cavies respond with a significantly larger increase of their serum cortisol concentrations to environmental challenge than domestic guinea pigs. Furthermore, immediately after removing animals from their home cages catecholamine concentrations are distinctly higher in the wild than in the domesticated form. In addition, significantly lower cortisol levels in response to an adrenocorticotropic hormone (ACTH) challenge indicate that there is a generalised reduction in the stress response of the domestic guinea pig (Künzl & Sachser 1999; Künzl et al. 2003; Kaiser et al. 2015). This seems to be the physiological correlate of the reduced alertness, nervousness and sensitivity of the domesticated animals. While the reduced stress response obviously helps domestic animals to live in artificial housing conditions, it would be counter-selected for by natural selection in wild animals in their natural habitats (Künzl & Sachser 1999).

Biological data

Newborn guinea pigs (body mass of about 60–100 g; Table 27.2) are precocial, looking like small-sized adults. They are fully furred; their eyes are open and the secondary teeth have already replaced the primary teeth during foetal development. All teeth are open rooted and grow continuously throughout life. On the day of birth, young guinea pigs start to eat solid food and drink water, although lactation lasts for 3–4 weeks. Young males reach their sexual maturity within 2–3 months of age (body mass about 500 g), while young females may reach sexual maturity at less than 1 month of age (with a body mass of around 300 g) (Table 27.3).

Table 27.2 Biological data for the guinea pig.

Parameter	Normal value
Lifespan (years)	2–8
Birth weight (g)	60–100
Adult weight (g)	700–1300
Food consumption (g/100 g body weight per day)	6
Water consumption (ml/100 g body weight per day)	10–14.5
Rectal temperature (°C)	37.2–39.8
Heart rate (beats/minute)	150–400
Blood pressure (mmHg)	
Systolic	77–94
Diastolic	47–58
Respiratory rate (breaths/minute)	42–150
Tidal volume (ml)	1.0–5.3
Total blood volume (ml/kg)	69–75
Dental formula	$I^1_1 C^0_0 Pm^1_1 M^3_3$

Source: Reprinted from North (1999) with permission of Blackwell Publishing.

Table 27.3 Reproductive data for the guinea pig.

Reproductive parameter	
Sexual maturity	
Female	About 1 month of age
Male	2–3 months of age
Oestrous cycle	Polyoestrus, about 16 days
Gestation period	63–72 days
Lactation	About 21 days
Litter size	1–7

Guinea pigs are fully grown at the age of 8–12 months. They live up to an age of 8 years and reach a body mass of about 800 to more than 1000 g, which is distinctly higher than in the wild form. The males' body mass is 11% higher than the body mass of non-pregnant females. Adult guinea pigs measure up to 30 cm in length.

Wild cavies have an agouti dorsal pelage and a lighter underside (see the preceding text), but in the domestic guinea pig there is a wide variety of colours. The coat can be unicoloured or multicoloured. The most popular breed of guinea pigs in scientific research is the short-haired English, and the most common strain is the Dunkin–Hartley (albino outbred guinea pig of the English breed). Furthermore, several inbred guinea pig strains have been produced. If not bred on-site in the facility, animals are obtained from commercial breeders.

Female guinea pigs exhibit a post-partum oestrus which means they become receptive immediately after giving birth. If they do not become pregnant at this time, females show periodic oestrous cycles of about 16 days (Shi et al. 1999). It is well known that female guinea pigs have some behavioural changes during their oestrous cycle (Birke 1981). The young are born after a gestation period of around 67 days. Usually, one to four (up to a maximum of seven) young are born in one litter (Table 27.3) (Fey & Trillmich 2008; Sachser 1994a).

Guinea pigs are characterised by an ultradian rhythm, that is, alternating phases of activity and rest last for about 2–3 h. Thus, the activity is not dependent on the light–dark regime (Sachser et al. 1992).

Guinea pigs have dichromatic colour vision (possessing retinal cones with peak sensitivities of about 429 nm and 529 nm) with a spectral neutral point centred at about 480 nm (Jacobs & Deegan 1994). However, guinea pigs may have poor depth perception.

The peak auditory sensitivity is around 500 and 8000 Hz. However, guinea pigs are behaviourally responsive to frequencies of 125–32 000 Hertz (Harper 1976). The upper limit of their hearing is probably 40 000–50 000 Hz.

The olfactory sense is most important in social behaviour (Beauchamp et al. 1979, 1980, 1982; Martin & Beauchamp 1982). Male guinea pigs mark individual females as well as the environment with their perineal glands. Urine has a high communicative value for this species. Young guinea pigs, for example, discriminate between maternal urine and urine of an unknown lactating female (Jäckel & Trillmich 2003).

Social organisation

There is a long tradition of basic research concerning the social life of guinea pigs (Kunkel & Kunkel 1964; Rood 1972; Berryman & Fullerton 1976; Sachser 1986; Sachser 1994a, 1994b; Kaiser et al. 2003a; Hennessy & Morris 2005; Hennessy et al. 2006; Wallner et al. 2006; Bauer et al. 2008; Fey & Trillmich 2008; Sachser et al. 2013; Zimmermann et al. 2017). As for other species, the social interactions of guinea pigs are composed of agonistic behaviours and the development of dominance hierarchies, together with positive or sexual interactions, which may result in the establishment of social bonds. The overall structure of dominance relationships and social bonds constitute the animals' social organisation.

Low and high population density

At low population densities (for example, three males and three females) the social organisation is characterised mainly by a linear dominance hierarchy among the adult males. Subordinate males retreat whenever a higher-ranking conspecific approaches; this largely precludes threat displays and fights. Individuals of identical rank are never found. The highest-ranking male shows much more courtship behaviour towards each of the females than any other male, and he is probably the father of the offspring (Sachser 1986, 1994b). Among the females, there is also a linear rank order (Thyen & Hendrichs 1990). However, their agonistic interactions are less pronounced than those among males. Between the sexes fighting and threat displays do not occur.

When individual numbers increase, the social organisation also changes. Groups of 10–15 or more split into subunits, each consisting of one to four males and one to seven females (Figure 27.2). The highest-ranking male of each subunit, the alpha-male, establishes long-lasting social bonds towards all females of his subunit. The alphas guard and defend their females around oestrus, and they sire more than 85% of offspring, as shown by DNA fingerprinting (Sachser 1998). The lower-ranking males also have bonds with the females of their subunits, i.e., they interact predominantly with these animals. Alphas of different subunits respect each other's bonds, that is, they do not court other alphas' females even if these are receptive (Sachser 1986, 1994b).

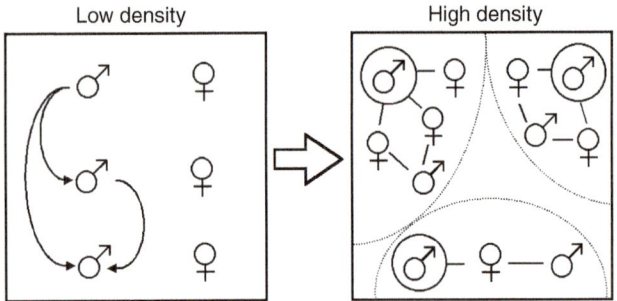

Figure 27.2 Social organisation in guinea pigs at high and low densities. Low density at the left side: arrows among males indicate direction of aggressive behaviours. High density at the right side: lines between males and females indicate individual social bonds. Alpha males (circled males) dominate non-alpha males (non-circled males). Dotted lines represent the borders of 'territories' (Sachser 1986). Reproduced from Sachser (1998) Naturwissenschaften, copyright with kind permission of Springer Science and Business Media.

Social organisation at high population densities is therefore characterised by the following: (1) the splitting of the whole group into subunits provides all individuals with social and spatial orientation; (2) escalated fighting is rare because alphas respect the male–female bonds of other alphas; (3) the individuals' different social positions are stable over months, and the basic patterns of social organisation are independent of individual animals. Thus, the change in social organisation from a strictly dominance-structured system to a system in which long-lasting bonds are predominant seems to be a mechanism for adjusting to increasing population density.

Physiological consequences of social stratification

When male guinea pigs living at different population densities are compared, those at high densities show increased activity of the sympathetic–adrenomedullary (SAM) system. In contrast, the activity of the hypothalamic pituitary–adrenocortical (HPA) system is not affected by population density. That is, a male living in a large colony does not have higher cortisol concentrations than a male living in a small group or with only one female. These endocrinological data support the behavioural findings that a change in density does not necessarily result in increased social stress for the individuals as long as a stable social environment is maintained by social mechanisms (Sachser 1990, 1994a).

At high and low population densities, males take different social positions, which are stable over months. Alphas, for example, always clearly dominate non-alphas of the same subunit. Alphas bite more often and are bitten less often than non-alphas, and display far more courtship and sexual behaviour than the lower-ranking males (Sachser 1990). Surprisingly, despite these clear differences in behaviour and status, alphas and non-alphas do not differ significantly in their activity of their HPA and SAM systems (Sachser 1987, 1994b; Sachser et al. 1998); that is, having low social status does not necessarily entail a higher degree of social stress than having high social status. This is probably because of the stable social relationships which result in predictable behaviour.

Social support

In a variety of animals, the presence of specific social partners can often inhibit or ameliorate the individual's neuroendocrine responses in stressful situations; i.e. the increase of the HPA and the SAM activities is reduced (Sachser et al. 1998; Kawachi & Berkman 2001; Hennessy et al. 2009). This class of effects, often referred to as social buffering of the stress response, is clearly seen in the context of the mother–infant relationship. The domestic guinea pig is one of the few animals in which social buffering effects on HPA activity have been found in both infants and adults.

Prior to weaning, guinea pig pups show evidence of a specific attachment to their mother, and the presence of the mother reduces or eliminates HPA responses in a novel environment (Hennessy & Ritchey 1987; Hennessy 1997, 1999; Hennessy et al. 2006). During the pre-weaning period, the presence of other animals, particularly adult females, has also been found to reduce HPA activity in pups, but not as consistently as the presence of the mother (Hennessy & Ritchey 1987; Ritchey & Hennessy 1987; Sachser et al. 1998; Graves & Hennessy 2000; Hennessy et al. 2002a, 2002b). The spatial environment also seems to influence the neuroendocrine and behavioural responses of guinea pig pups to a threatening situation. For example, the pups express more distress calls in an unfamiliar than in a familiar environment irrespective of whether their mothers are present or absent (Pettijohn 1979). Furthermore, cortisol concentrations in infant guinea pigs do not increase after separation from their mother when they stay in their familiar enclosure together with familiar group members (Wewers et al. 2003).

Adult males and females form attachment-like bonds with opposite-sex partners (see earlier in this chapter) (Sachser 1986). As regards female interactions with an individual colony-living male, females can be placed in three categories: (1) females bonded with the male and between which most amicable interactions take place; (2) females that live in the same colony, and with whom the male is familiar but has no social ties and (3) unfamiliar females which the male has never encountered before. Interestingly, the male's endocrine stress response – i.e. increase in HPA activity – when placed in an unfamiliar cage is sharply reduced if a female with whom he is bonded is present. In contrast, the presence of an unfamiliar female or of one with whom he is merely acquainted has little effect. Thus, the effect of various types of relationships differs remarkably, and substantial social support to the male is given only by the bonded partner (Sachser et al. 1998; Hennessy et al. 2006, 2009).

The presence of the bonded partner also leads to a sharp reduction in the acute stress response in female guinea pigs living in large mixed-sex colonies indicating that there is a two-way provision of social support between male and female bonded pairs. However, female guinea pigs show a different reaction to males in the presence of a familiar conspecific, who is not the bonded partner. In this case, their stress response is lower than in the absence of a familiar conspecific, so a familiar social partner can provide social support for females but not for males (Kaiser et al. 2003a).

Effects of social experiences on physiology and behaviour

A number of studies show that social experiences during early phases of life (Kaiser and Sachser 2005) and adolescence (Sachser *et al*. 2013, 2018) can have distinct effects on physiology and behaviour. Adolescence is a sensitive phase during which aggressiveness of males is shaped by social experiences and this can have important consequences for their husbandry. When two adult males reared in different large colonies are placed into an unfamiliar enclosure in the presence of an unfamiliar female, they quickly establish stable dominance relationships without displaying overt aggression. No significant changes in stress hormone concentrations are found, either in the dominant or in the subdominant male (Sachser & Lick 1991). However, this 'peaceful' stratification into different social positions requires that during adolescence the opponents have been involved in agonistic interactions with older dominant males, which is the case in individuals reared in colonies. In these encounters, the subdominant individuals acquire the social skills needed to adapt to conspecifics in a non-aggressive and non-stressful way (Sachser & Lick 1991; Sachser 1993; Sachser *et al*. 1994).

In contrast, a male that has grown up singly or with a female does not experience agonistic interactions during adolescence (since in this species no fighting and threat displays are found between the sexes) and thus does not learn these social skills. If two of these males confront one another in the presence of an unfamiliar female in an unfamiliar enclosure, high levels of aggressive behaviour occur, and escalated fighting is frequent which, if not stopped, may lead to severe injuries. During the first days of the confrontation, no stable dominance relationships are established but once this has occurred marked and persistent increases in pituitary–adrenocortical system activities occur in the subdominant males (Sachser & Lick 1991; Sachser *et al*. 1994).

The crucial role of social experiences has also been shown in a study taking a different approach (Sachser & Renninger 1993). Colony-reared males introduced singly into unfamiliar colonies of conspecifics easily adjust to this new social situation. They explore the new environment, but do not court any female, thereby avoiding attacks from the male residents, which have established bonds with the females. The colony-reared males gradually integrate into the social network of the established colonies and may even gain a higher social rank than they had in their native colonies. In contrast, individually reared males placed into a colony of conspecifics are frequently involved in threat displays and fights (Sachser & Lick 1991; Sachser & Renninger 1993) and may achieve significant body weight loss, even when not injured or attacked by the residents. The underlying neuroendocrine mechanisms of these shaping processes have been studied in detail in a series of experiments (see Lürzel *et al*. 2010, 2011a,b).

In contrast, female guinea pigs reared in colonies or in pairs can adapt to introduction into a group of unfamiliar conspecifics without the occurrence of overt aggression and high degrees of social stress. Thus, female guinea pigs are able to adapt to unfamiliar conspecifics independent of their social rearing conditions (Kaiser *et al*. 2003b).

Use in research

The guinea pig is commonly used in scientific research, in areas such as toxicology, allergies and respiratory diseases, nutritional research, auditory perception, product development and medical quality control.

General husbandry

Enclosures and environmental enrichment

Guinea pigs from commercial breeders are frequently used as specific pathogen free (SPF) animals. Such guinea pigs have to be housed under barrier conditions (e.g. separate positive-pressure rooms) to prevent introduction of pathogens. It is also possible to house guinea pigs in individually ventilated cages (IVCs) such as 1500 cm^2 or 2000 cm^2 cages for rats, but the space of the smaller ones does not comply with Appendix A of the *European Convention for the Protection of Vertebrate Animals used for Experimental and Other Scientific Purposes* (ETS 123; Council of Europe 2006) or Annex III of the European Directive 2010/63/EU (European Parliament and the Council of the European Union 2010). Moreover, the 2000 cm^2 cages are difficult to handle, and are therefore not in common use.

Guinea pigs can be kept in various types of pens or cages (Figure 27.3a,b,c). The authors also have experience with keeping guinea pigs in pens on the floor (Figure 27.3d) and can also recommend this type of housing. In this case, bedding (e.g., wood shavings) is necessary. However, certain floor covering materials such as flagstones can become contaminated with uroliths because adequate cleaning at regular intervals is difficult. For this reason, rooms should be emptied periodically for cleaning, descaling and disinfection.

It is important to provide enough space. High stocking densities can lead to endocrine stress reactions and high frequencies of aggression (see section in the preceding text: low and high population density). Appendix A of the ETS 123 and Annex III of Directive 2010/63/EU give guidelines for the accommodation and care of guinea pigs (Council of Europe 2006; European Parliament and the Council of the European Union 2010). These recommend a minimum enclosure size of 2500 cm^2 and a floor area per adult animal (>700 g body weight) of 900 cm^2. Sachser *et al*. (2004), however, suggest providing a floor area of about 2500 cm^2 per adult animal. According to the European documents, a minimum enclosure size of 1800 cm^2 for smaller animals (≤ 450 g body weight) is possible. However, the usual height of 20 cm in Makrolon type IV cages is not sufficient, since this impairs play behaviour ('frisky hops') of juveniles and prevents adult individuals from fully standing on their hindlegs. A minimum height of 23 cm is recommended by Appendix A, whereas Sachser *et al*. (2004) recommend 30 cm.

Specific forms of grid floors (e.g. in metabolic cages) can cause problems and therefore should be used only for short periods during experiments. Grid floors are often the cause of diseases (e.g. pododermatitis). Young animals' extremities are especially vulnerable if the mesh is too wide. On the other hand, openings have to be big enough to ensure the

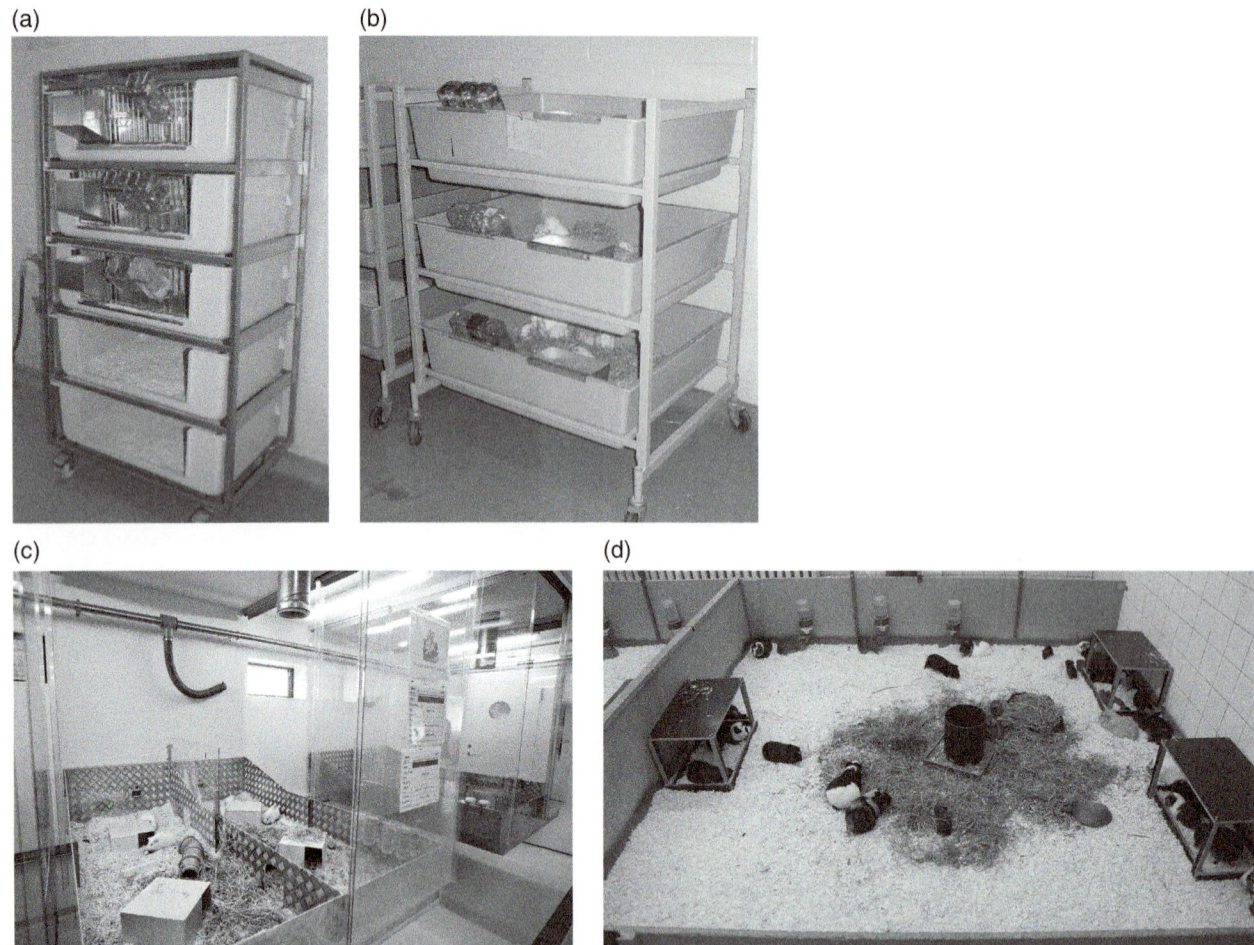

Figure 27.3 Different types of cages for housing of guinea pigs (a,b,c) as well as floor housing (d). Source: Photo 27.3a,b Christine Krüger (Author); Gero Hilken. Photo 27.3c Novo Nordisk A/S, Bagsværd, Denmark. Photo 27.3d Department of Behavioural Biology, Münster, Germany.

passage of faeces. If solid floors are not possible for experimental reasons, so that grids or wire mesh have to be used, then at least a solid or bedded area should be provided on which the animals can rest. Furthermore, it is important to check the grid floors closely to ensure that there is no risk of injury from loose or sharp projections. Pregnant and lactating females should always be kept on solid floors with bedding.

The most important environmental enrichment for the guinea pig is the social group. However, some physical enrichment should also be provided: e.g. in the enclosures, shelters should be provided in a sufficient number. Several enrichment items are commercially available such as polycarbonate huts. Plastic piping can also be used into which all animals can retreat. It is important, however, to provide sufficient ventilation holes. Piping should be short enough to prevent more than two animals using it simultaneously. If more animals can enter it, a number of animals may press into the piping and there is a risk that animals in the middle will be asphyxiated. Furthermore, it has been suggested to offer shaders which should be placed over the central portion of a cage. This will increase utilisation of cage space, since guinea pigs avoid exposed areas such as the centres of their enclosures (Byrd et al. 2016). Branches for gnawing are a very easy kind of enrichment. If necessary, they can be autoclaved before use. Hay provides a substrate and is a useful enrichment (see section on feeding).

Physical environment

Accommodation must provide draught-free ventilation. Relative humidity should be around 50–60%. The optimal temperature is around 18–22 °C (according to the European convention, Appendix A, 20–24 °C (Council of Europe 2006)). Guinea pigs are better able to withstand cold than heat. There are some indications that reproduction will decrease if temperature exceeds 30 °C.

Guinea pigs should be kept neither in constant light nor in constant darkness. A light–dark rhythm of about 12 h light and 12 h dark and also the natural light–dark rhythm are suitable (e.g. if the animals are living in outdoor pens). Guinea pigs should be protected against loud noise, which can cause panic reactions, leading to injuries.

Feeding/watering

Guinea pigs are herbivores. Their wild ancestors live on grass, roots and seeds. In the laboratory, guinea pigs are usually fed with commercial plant-based pellets. The food has to be stored in cool, dry conditions and be protected against contamination. It should be available *ad libitum*. It is essential that food is provided in such a way to ensure access by all animals. Pellets have to be small (with a diameter of about 3 mm), enabling the guinea pigs to take them directly by mouth. If suitable, it is also useful to feed fresh vegetables and small amounts of fruits, e.g. lettuce, carrots and apples. If possible, these food items should be introduced when guinea pigs are young. Once adults, the animals might take a long time to approach new food items. It is important to ensure the availability of vitamins, especially of vitamin C, since guinea pigs are unable to synthesise vitamin C. Signs of vitamin C deficiency include: poor skin, poor haircoat, weight loss, stiffness, difficulties in walking, and even paralysis and poor bone and tooth development. If the vitamin C content in the food is insufficient (it remains active in pellets for only 90 days), ascorbic acid can be added to the drinking water (0.5 g/l). This should be freshly made as dissolved vitamin C decomposes rapidly (e.g. Jansson *et al.* 2004).

Good-quality hay should always be available. Besides diet-related benefits (e.g. it may protect against digestive disturbances), hay is used for play as well as a material in which to burrow and hide. Due to the high proportion of fibre, hay also seems to prevent alopecia and teeth overgrowth (Wolf & Kamphues 2004; Wasel 2007). Since hay can represent an infection risk, heat treatment at 70 °C (autoclaving at higher temperatures may lead to injury due to hardening of the haulms) or the use of irradiated hay is recommended. Furthermore, guinea pigs can develop urinary stones from excessive calcium. Thus, food items containing a high amount of calcium such as alfalfa hay or dark leafy greens should be avoided.

Feeding dishes or food hoppers should be designed and positioned so as to prevent animals being able to defecate or urinate into them. Guinea pigs often spill food, and on grid floors (which should be avoided, see Housing section), the food will be wasted. Some suitable hoppers are available that reduce wastage. The water supply should be spatially separated from the feeding dish because guinea pigs tend to dribble water into the feeding dish, resulting in agglutinated pellets. Guinea pigs will rapidly learn to use drinking nipples attached to bottles or automatic systems and even prefer them to open dishes (Balsiger *et al.* 2017). Stainless steel sipper tubes and nipples should be used because the animals like to gnaw at them. There should always be more than one water access (bottle or nipple) because guinea pigs tend to spit food into the nipples and therefore could block them.

Bedding

The bedding material, e.g. wood fibres or granulate, has to be dry and absorbent. It should be free of toxic residue (e.g. timber preservative), parasites and infectious agents. Dust should be kept to a minimum. The interval between cleaning depends on the kind of cage or pen used. Normally, once a week is reasonable.

Table 27.4 Beneficial and detrimental housing conditions for guinea pigs. See also Sachser *et al.* (2004).

Housing condition	Recommended	To be avoided
Solitary		X
Pair: 1 male, 1 female	X	
Harems (1 male, several females)	X	
Female groups: 2 females	X	
>2 females	X	
Male groups: 2 males	X	
>2 males		X
Small mixed-sex groups	X	
Large mixed-sex groups	X	

Social housing

Table 27.4 summarises the housing conditions which can be recommended and those which should be avoided (see Sachser *et al.* 2004).

Solitary housing

Domestic guinea pigs still bear the heritage of their wild ancestors, the cavy (*Cavia aperea*). Thus, we should not expect that they are able to adjust to any artificial housing but instead require at least some essential features of the environment in which their wild ancestors evolved (Sachser 2001). Since the ancestor of the guinea pig is a socially living wild species, solitary housing is not appropriate for its domesticated counterpart and must be avoided!

Housing in pairs (one male, one female)

This housing condition is appropriate for guinea pigs. In this species, no fighting or threat displays are found between the sexes. Moreover, pair-reared males can cope with adversity in a much more effective way than solitary housed conspecifics.

Housing in harems

This housing system is also appropriate for guinea pigs. Agonistic interactions do occur between females, but such aggression is rare and of low intensity: escalated fights and bites almost never occur.

Female groups

Guinea pigs can be satisfactorily housed in all-female groups. The number is limited only by the enclosure size, since females can be housed without problems in large groups. It is true that in all-female groups, levels of aggression are slightly higher than in groups with one male and several females (Thyen & Hendrichs 1990) but aggression is usually rare and of low intensity. As in groups of one male and several females, escalated fights and bites almost never occur. Females living in large all-female groups do not experience high levels of stress.

Male groups

In groups consisting of two males, agonistic behaviour is rarely or never found. In contrast, in groups of more than two males, escalated agonistic interactions frequently occur beginning when the animals reach about 3–4 months. Additionally, animals that live in groups of two or four individuals show lower concentrations of the stress hormone cortisol than animals living in groups of six or twelve (Beer & Sachser 1992). Thus, there seems to be good welfare when guinea pigs are housed in groups of two males, while indicators of social stress regularly occur in larger groups. Where mixed-sex housing is not possible, we recommend keeping male guinea pigs in groups of two.

Males show courtship and sexual behaviour towards each other in the same way as males usually court females: pseudo-copulations occur including mounts and ejaculations. Specific males also display female-typical behaviour. These individuals, termed 'pseudofemales', not only tolerate the courtship and mounting by others, but also actively display defence urine-spraying, a behavioural pattern which is typical for females and usually serves to keep off courting males. The other males of the group behave towards these pseudofemales as towards real females and compete with each other for them. The pseudofemales do not take part in the aggressive conflicts. They rarely receive aggressive behaviour (Beer & Sachser 1992).

Mixed-sex groups of a few males and females

Housing guinea pigs in small mixed-sex groups can also be acceptable. However, the formation of such a group with animals of unknown social rearing experience should be avoided since it frequently leads to intensive threat and fighting behaviour, extreme stress responses and injuries (see paragraph on effects of social experiences on physiology and behaviour).

Mixed-sex groups of many males and females

Guinea pigs can also be housed in large mixed-sex colonies (see the preceding text). However, such a large mixed-sex group should have a varied age structure. The best system is to allow a small mixed-sex group to increase to the desired size. The assembly of a large group, using animals coming from pairs or solitary housing as well as with animals of unknown origin, should be avoided since it frequently leads to intensive threat and fighting behaviour, extreme stress responses and health problems.

Environmental changes

Guinea pigs react highly sensitively to changes of environment, so it is important to habituate them slowly to new conditions. The combination of several factors – each of which individually would have no negative effects – may result in strong stress responses and severe health problems. For example, simultaneous provision of a new cage and a new drinking bottle should be avoided. New drinking bottles should be offered together with the old one until the animals begin to drink from the new one. Furthermore, unfamiliar food should be mixed with the familiar food, and the portion of the old food should be reduced step-by-step. When transferring animals to a new cage, no other modifications, such as providing new food or removing a social partner, should be made simultaneously. The ability of an animal to adjust to a new situation can be assessed reliably from its drinking and feeding behaviour. If the animals are feeding and, particularly, drinking, then they can adapt to the new situation. In contrast, refusing water and food, scrubby fur and apathy point to extremely poor welfare (Broom & Johnson 1993).

Identification and sexing

Coloured animals can be identified individually by natural markings without problems. Albino animals can be coloured, e.g. with food colouring or a non-toxic marker on the fur. The dyes have to be renewed at regular intervals (3–4 weeks).

A frequently used method for permanent marking is ear tattooing. Another method is to implant microchips: Animals can be individually marked using small encapsulated radio frequency identification (RFID) microchips. The animals can be identified with suitable readers, but only at short distances. All methods of marking or tagging involve some degree of stress and consideration should be given to using the least invasive method that is compatible with the study.

Guinea pigs are easy to sex (Figure 27.4a,b). Male and female guinea pigs can be differentiated by gentle pressing around the genital area. The penis is easily extruded. In older animals, the testes are also apparent, but can be lifted through the open inguinal ring into the abdominal cavity. In females, this technique will expose the vaginal membrane which closes the vagina (except during oestrus and parturition).

Health monitoring

Guinea pigs should undergo regular health checks: appearance should be assessed (coat and skin state, teeth, claws, eyes, nose, anal and genital region) and the body weight

(a) 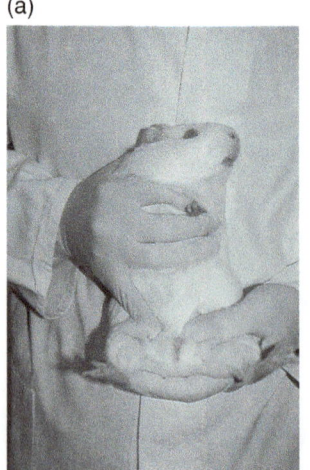 (b)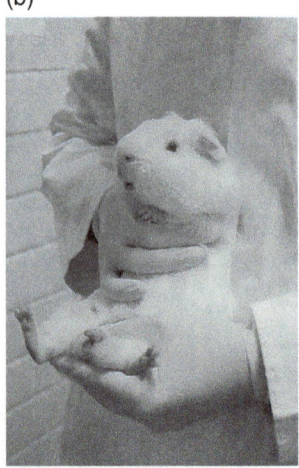

Figure 27.4 Sexing a guinea pig. In the female (a) the vaginal membrane will be exposed. In the male (b) the penis is easily extruded from the genital opening using gentle pressure. Source: Photos: Christine Krüger (Author); Gero Hilken.

should be measured regularly. Furthermore, behavioural abnormalities should be recorded and investigated. Incoming animals should be quarantined and screened for potential infections.

When laboratory guinea pigs are kept as SPF animals, care must be taken to maintain this status for microbiological standardisation. Therefore, besides well-organised housing, the colony should be involved in health-monitoring programmes. On the one hand, such programmes serve to prevent the facility from introducing pathogens by newly arrived animals; on the other hand, long-term colony health status will be monitored for accidental infections. Monitoring protocols, including the number of animals tested, can vary based upon the number of animals in the colony and the duration of their husbandry. Recommendations for reasonable monitoring design are provided by the Federation of European Laboratory Animal Science Associations (FELASA 2014) (Table 27.5).

Care of aged animals

Guinea pigs can live to about 8 years. As in many old animals, aged guinea pigs show a lower locomotor activity as well as lower frequencies of social interactions. Obesity can be a problem of old age. Ovarian cysts often occur in older females with or without symptoms like bilateral alopecia. Overall, there seem to be no specific age-related problems in guinea pigs. Since they are more prone to diseases, the regular health check should be carried out more frequently.

Table 27.5 Based on FELASA recommendations (2014) for the health monitoring of guinea pig colonies.

Disease	Test frequency
Viruses	
Guinea pig adenovirus	3 months
Guinea pig parainfluenza virus 3	3 months
Sendai virus	3 months
Guinea pig cytomegalovirus	Annually
Bacteria, mycoplasma and fungi	
Bordetella bronchiseptica	3 months
Corynebacterium kutscheri	3 months
Streptococci β-haemolytic (not group D)	3 months
Streptococcus pneumoniae	3 months
Clostridium piliforme	Annually
Encephalitozoon cuniculi	Annually
Salmonella spp.	Annually
Streptobacillus moniliformis	Annually
Parasites	
Ectoparasites	3 months
Endoparasites:	3 months
Additional agents (optional)	
Chlamydophila caviae	
Cilia-associated respiratory bacillus	
Dermatophytes	
Pasteurellaceae	
Pseudomonas aeruginosa	
Staphylococcus aureus	
Yersinia pseudotuberculosis	

Source: Based on FELASA (2014).

Laboratory procedures

Handling

Guinea pigs are usually docile and bite very rarely. They should be picked up carefully with both hands: one hand holding the shoulder and chest, and the other supporting the hindquarters. The latter is particularly important for pregnant females. After picking up, guinea pigs should be held against the handler's body (Figure 27.5a,b).

Sampling techniques

Blood collection

Choosing the right site for blood sampling depends on the size of the guinea pig and the required amount of blood. For a single blood collection, no more than 10% of the total blood volume (approximately 75 ml/kg of the body mass) should be taken and there should be a recovery period of at least two weeks. Weekly collected blood volumes should not exceed 7.5% and daily collected volumes should not exceed 1% of the total blood volume (Joint Working Group on Refinement (JWGR) 1993; Diehl *et al.* 2001). Since rodent blood tends to coagulate within the cannula, short needles are recommended (e.g. butterfly cannulas with the tubing cut off, or cannulae with the hub removed).

For collecting small amounts of blood, the ear vessels can be punctured (Figure 27.6a). In coloured animals, a cold point lamp behind the ear increases the visibility of the blood vessels. In albinos, this is not necessary. To increase blood flow, the veins can be compressed manually. After disinfecting the skin, the ear vessels are punctured with a sterile disposable cannula (e.g. 0.6 × 25 mm (23G)) and the blood can be collected directly or via capillaries.

The lateral saphenous vein is the preferred sampling site for larger blood volumes (Figure 27.6b,c). After shaving the fur from the back of the hindlimb and disinfecting the skin, one person restrains the guinea pig with one hindlimb

(a) 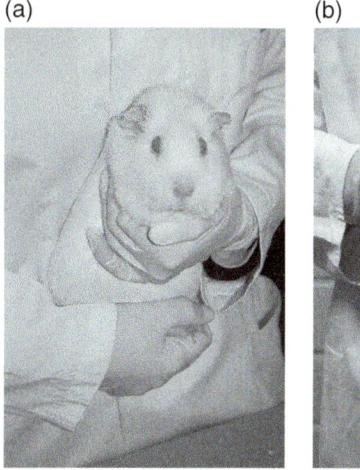 (b)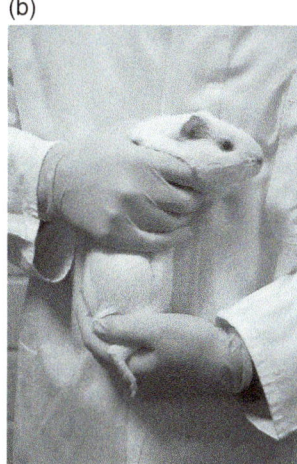

Figure 27.5 Methods of handling a guinea pig. Source: Photos: Christine Krüger (Author); Gero Hilken.

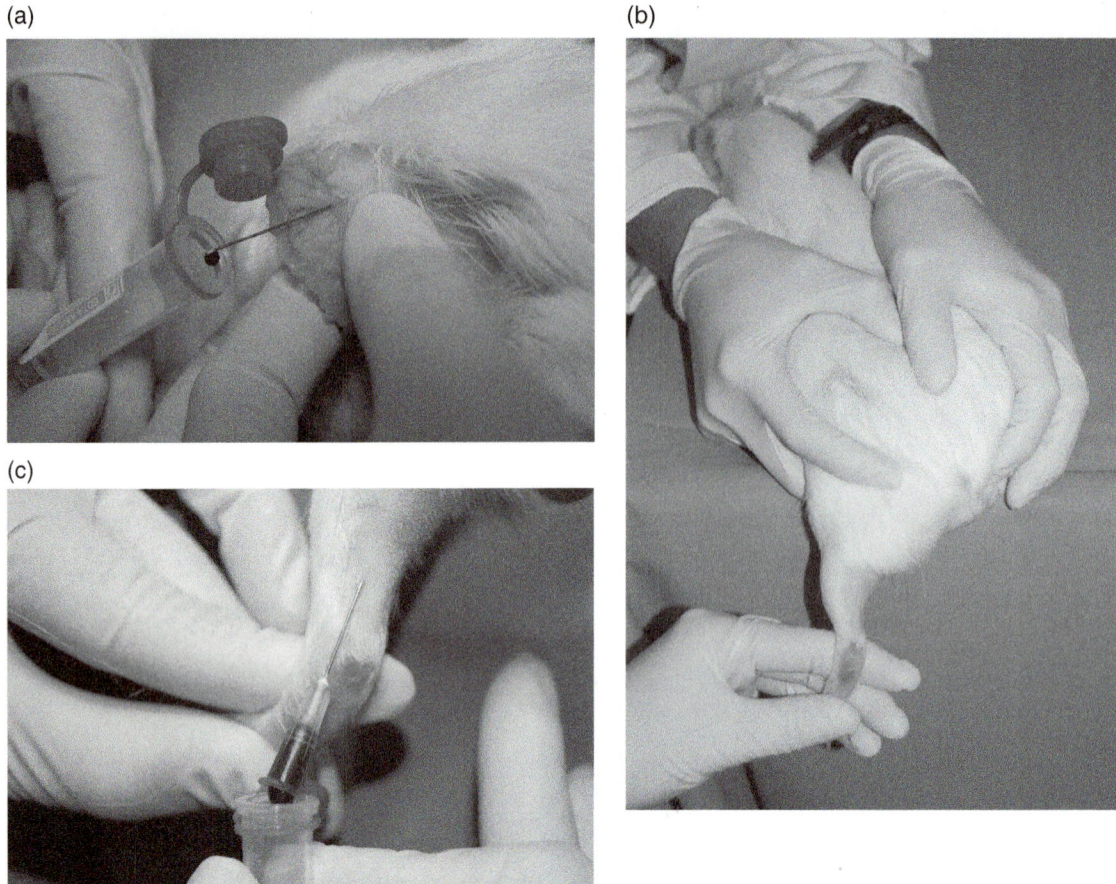

Figure 27.6 Blood sampling procedures. (a) Ear vessels. (b, c) Saphenous vein. Source: Photos: Christine Krüger (Author); Gero Hilken.

extended backwards. The vein runs laterally to the Achilles tendon, and the insertion site is close to the tendon in the middle third of the lower leg. Even if the vein is not visible, the needle (e.g. 0.7 × 30 mm (22G) or 0.6 × 25 mm, 23G) can be inserted at a 30–45° angle from distocaudal direction and blood can be collected in a vial.

To collect large volumes of blood, the jugular vein or the cranial vena cava can also be used as a survival method, although there is a risk of haemorrhage or cardiac tamponade. The procedure should be done under anaesthesia in dorsal recumbency. The puncture site is the thoracic inlet left or right of the sternum. A needle with a 2 ml syringe is inserted at a 45° angle while pulling back the plunger until blood appears in the syringe. After removal of the needle, pressure should be applied to the puncture site. Hillyer et al. (1997) described a method to collect blood from the jugular vein without anaesthesia by restraining the animal with the forelegs extended down over a table edge and head and neck extended up. This procedure appears to be very stressful and should be done by trained personnel only, since location of the vein is often difficult.

Cardiac puncture should only be performed as a terminal procedure under general anaesthesia because of a high risk of cardiac tamponade. The heart can be punctured laterally in the area where the heartbeat is palpated, or from the caudal direction with the insertion site behind the xiphoid. A syringe with mounted cannula should be used by moving it slowly forward under constant aspiration until blood appears.

The retro-bulbar sinus may be used for sampling under anaesthesia, but access to the sinus is more difficult than in rats and mice and may result in severe complications (e.g. exophthalmus). Moreover, the technique samples a mixture of blood and tissue fluid, rather than blood alone. The JWGR (1993) considered that this technique should only be carried out under terminal anaesthesia. A good summary of possible blood sampling methods in guinea pigs is given at the NCRs website[1] and in Birck et al. (2014).

Urine collection

Urine may be collected manually by applying gentle pressure over the caudal abdominal area. This method provides a cleaner sample than collecting urine in a metabolic cage, where faeces may contaminate the urine sample. Uncontaminated urine samples can be collected via cystocentesis. For this, the guinea pig should be prepared for surgery. Anaesthesia may be necessary for safe restraint and the bladder should be fixed manually while it is punctured with a fine needle through the abdominal wall.

---

[1] https://www.nc3rs.org.uk/blood-sampling-guinea-pig (accessed 15 July 2021)

A method to introduce a fine, flexible catheter into the urethra of male and female guinea pigs has been described, but there are risks of pathogen introduction into the bladder and mucosa injury, particularly in males (Wasel 2007; Ewringmann & Gloeckner 2012).

Administration of substances

Oral medications can be administered by adding small quantities of liquids or solids to the feed or drinking water. However, using this method it is not possible to determine or ensure the dose consumed. Furthermore, the intake may be influenced by drug-related changes of appearance or taste of feed or water. Liquids can be administered directly with a syringe, administering the substance carefully onto the back of the tongue. A rat dosing needle with rounded tip or a polyethylene catheter with outside diameter 1.0–1.3 mm can be used for this purpose. The syringe or catheter should be introduced via the interdental space. Care has to be taken that the animals have enough time to swallow during these procedures. For application of exact or larger doses of compounds, oral gavage via a gastric tube can be performed (Figure 27.7b). For this, another person has to restrain the animal and a mouth gag with a hole in its middle should be placed behind the incisors to prevent the animals from biting into the tube. Subsequently, the moistened tube can be inserted very carefully into the oesophagus. The procedure is complicated by the anatomical characteristic of a small palatal ostium, which may be injured during the procedure (Timm *et al.* 1987; Rosenthal *et al.* 2008). If coughing or dyspnoea occurs during administration of the compound, the procedure must be stopped immediately and the tube reinserted.

Parenteral administration may be done in several ways. Injection sites should be clipped and swabbed with a suitable antiseptic. Depending on the route of administration and the volume of the substance which is administered, it may be necessary to use multiple injection sites. Subcutaneous or intramuscular injections (Figure 27.7a) are both suitable methods, even though, depending on the agent to be administered, the subcutaneous method should be generally preferred. For administration of small volumes, intramuscular injections into the perilumbar or thigh muscles can be performed. If injecting into the posterior part of the thigh (*M. biceps femoris/M. semitendinosus*), the needle should not be introduced too deeply to avoid damage to the femur or *Nervus ischiadicus* (sciatic nerve) with associated bruising, periostitis or nerve irritation. It is safer to use the quadriceps muscle. No more than 0.1 ml (0.3 ml in exceptional cases) should be injected into one site (Hull 1995; Terril & Clemons 1998; North 1999) to minimise risks of muscle necrosis. Subcutaneous injections can be used for application of larger volumes (up to 3 ml per site) under the skin of the neck, back or flanks of the animal. For intradermal injections (maximum 0.1 ml), the usual sites are the flank or the dorsum. Larger volumes of up to 10 ml/kg body mass can be given by intraperitoneal injection, but care has to be taken to avoid injuries to the internal organs or injecting the substance into the caecum, where it may not be absorbed. If the substance is irritant, peritonitis or adhesions of the caecum can result. Although access to superficial veins is sometimes difficult in guinea pigs, intravascular administration is also possible. The auricular (ear) veins are the most suitable. Fine needles are recommended; veins may be dilated by warming before injection; and injection must be performed very slowly by a trained person. For trained persons, it is also possible to place a small intravenous catheter (e.g. 0.7 × 19 mm, 24G) into the cephalic or saphenous vein, anaesthesia should therefore be considered (see e.g. NC3Rs website[1]).

Anaesthesia and analgesia

Anaesthesia

Anaesthesia should be used for all procedures causing more pain or stress than the anaesthesia itself. Due to their high sensitivity to stress, an appropriate acclimation time of at least three days before carrying out any procedure is recommended

(a)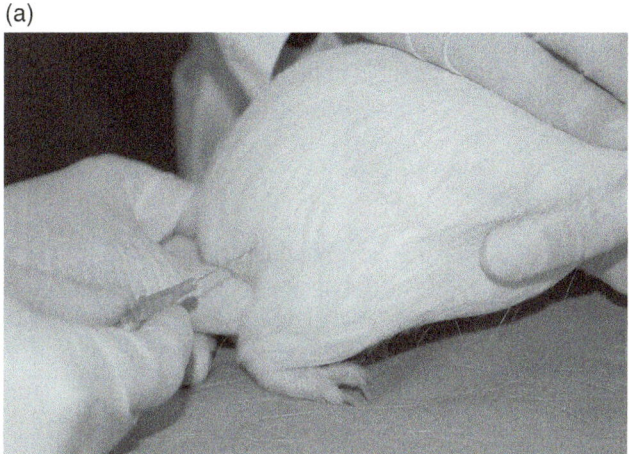

(b)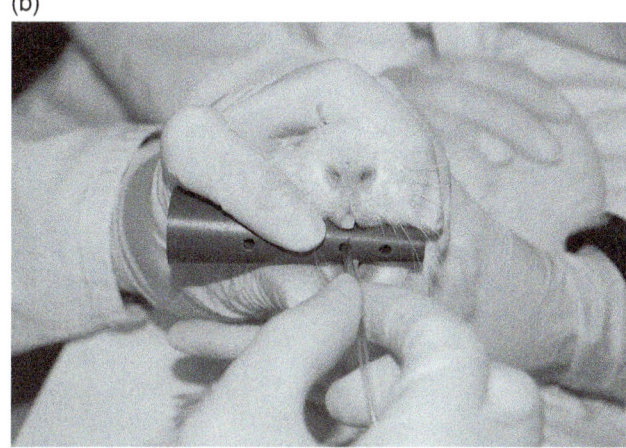

Figure 27.7 Administration techniques. (a) Intramuscular injection into the hindlimb of a guinea pig. (b) Oral gavage via gastric tube. A mouth gag prevents the guinea pig from biting into the tube. Source: Photos: Christine Krüger (Author); Gero Hilken.

for newly arrived animals (e.g. website of ULAM veterinary staff[2]). Guinea pigs, like other small rodents, have a high metabolic rate and oxygen consumption, so hypoglycaemia, dehydration, hypothermia and hypoxaemia can develop rapidly. For this reason and because of the risk of gastrointestinal stasis, animals should not be fasted except for experimental reasons. If fasting is necessary, fasting time should not exceed 4 h (Abou-Madi 2006); water should not be restricted. As guinea pigs can easily become hypoxic or even apnoeic, oxygen supplementation is recommended. To avoid hypothermia circulating warm water blankets, hot air warmers, heating pads or heat lamps may be used (please note: animals have to be protected appropriately from the heat source to avoid burns), only small areas of fur should be clipped for surgery, and warmed fluids can be given subcutaneously (10–20 ml/kg, different injection sites). Anticholinergics like atropine (0.05 mg/kg sc) and glycopyrrolate (0.01–0.02 mg/kg sc) (Mason 1997; Ewringmann & Glöckner 2012) can be recommended to avoid excessive salivation, bronchial secretion and vagally induced bradycardia. Ocular lubrication should be used during anaesthesia or sedation to prevent corneal drying. Due to the fact that guinea pigs frequently become hypothermic, hypotensive, and hypoxic under general anaesthesia, a close monitoring should be carried out during anaesthesia including heart and respiratory rate, temperature, and where possible, oxygen saturation and capnography (Schmitz et al. 2016).

Inhalation anaesthesia

Because of its potential to induce respiratory and cardiovascular depression as well as excessive salivation and secretion, it is preferable not to use inhalation anaesthetics alone. It is more reasonable to use a balanced technique that takes advantage of both sedative and analgesic effects of injectable compounds. The main advantages of inhalants are their good controllability and the rapid recovery of the animals (Ellen et al. 2016; Flecknell 2015; Henke & Erhardt 2012). Volatile anaesthetics like isoflurane and sevoflurane require an anaesthesia machine with oxygen source and vaporiser. Anaesthesia should be induced in an anaesthetic chamber and maintained via face mask. An anticholinergic premedication should be administered before inhalation anaesthesia to decrease secretion. Some authors practise endotracheal intubation of guinea pigs with a tube size of 1.5–3.5 mm (Blouin & Cormier 1987), but long and narrow approaches to the larynx and the palatal ostium makes this difficult. In addition, food remnants stored in the cheeks may lead to obstruction or aspiration pneumonia and should be removed with cotton swabs before intubation. Unless ventilatory support is required, intubating guinea pigs is an uncommon method and face masks are normally used instead.

Injectable anaesthesia

Various combinations of anaesthetics are widely used for injectable anaesthesia. Compared to inhalation anaesthesia, the precise control of depth of anaesthesia and attainment of a surgical stage is more difficult when using injectable agents. Exact dosing may be difficult due to variable gastrointestinal content and its effect on body weight. Sedative and analgesic agents may be used for premedication or in combinations to induce general anaesthesia. Various anaesthetics and their dosages are summarised in Table 27.6. Increased dosages often lead to a longer anaesthetic time. In general, anaesthetics should be administered intramuscularly because subcutaneous applications often prove insufficient. Where appropriate, depending on the anaesthetic agents used, reversal agents like naloxone and atipamezole should be given to promote rapid recovery (Henke & Erhardt 2012; Schmitz et al. 2016).

Local anaesthetics can be used to reduce the dose of general anaesthetics or for minor procedures in combination with some premedication. Usually, they are used as infiltrations, injected subcutaneously. Lidocaine 0.5–2% may be used in small volumes of 0.5–2 ml (4–5 mg/kg), diluted if necessary. Another option is bupivacaine (1 mg/kg), combinations are also possible (Ellen et al. 2016). For further advice, see Flecknell (2015).

Analgesia

To control pain during and after surgery, analgesics should be administered pre-emptively, intra- and/or post-operatively, depending on the type of anaesthesia and the severity of the intervention. Different types of analgesics like NSAIDs or opioids may be used as a single treatment or combined as multimodal pain therapy (Flecknell 2018; Mueller 2018). A list of analgesics and suggested dosages is provided in Table 27.7, although there are only few studies that evaluated the species-specific dosage and efficacy of analgesics in guinea pigs (Oliver et al. 2017; Smith et al. 2016).

Euthanasia

With *Annex IV* of the *Directive 2010/63/EU on the Protection of Animals Used for Scientific Purposes* (European Parliament and the Council of the European Union 2010), permitted killing methods have been specified in the EU for the first time. Other methods are only allowed to be used in unconscious animals or when scientifically justified as part of a project. Further and more detailed information on euthanasia methods are given by the *Guidelines on Euthanasia* of the American Veterinary Medical Association (AVMA 2013).

Annex IV of the Directive 2010/63/EU lists euthanasia methods permissible in Europe. Guinea pigs may be euthanised by anaesthetic overdose, carbon dioxide, concussion and inert gases (Ar, N_2). In general, an overdose of injectable anaesthetic is preferred; the most suitable agent being sodium pentobarbital, which may be applied intracardially (under anaesthesia), intrapulmonary (200–400 mg/kg, only under anaesthesia), or intraperitoneally (400–800 mg/kg). A combination product of three different anaesthetics (embutramide, mebenzonium iodide and tetracaine hydrochloride), T-61® or Tanax®, is approved exclusively for euthanasia in many countries. It should never be used without anaesthesia, as it induces respiratory paralysis. It can be administered intravenously, intracardially or

---

[2] https://az.research.umich.edu/animalcare/guidelines/guidelines-anesthesia-and-analgesia-guinea-pigs (accessed 15 July 2021)

Table 27.6 Sedative and anaesthetic agents for guinea pigs.

Anaesthetics	Dosage in mg/kg	Route	Comments	Reference
Diazepam/midazolam	2.5–5	im	Only sedation	Terril & Clemons 1998, Henke & Erhardt 2012
Xylazine	3–5	im/ip	Pre-anaesthetic, sedation	Terril & Clemons 1998
Medetomidine	0.15–0.5	im	Pre-anaesthetic, sedation	North 1999, Henke & Erhardt 2012
Ketamine + Xylazine	25–80 0.15–13	im/ip	Variable effect and duration, surgical anaesthesia possible	Radde et al. 1996, Terril & Clemons 1998, North 1999, Schmitz et al. 2016
Ketamine + Medetomidine	40–60 0.25–0.5	im/ip	Surgical anaesthesia	North 1999, Pfizer product information
Ketamine + Diazepam	44–125 0.1–5	im/ip		Radde et al. 1996, North 1999
Pentobarbital	15–35	ip	Lasts 2 h, no analgesia	Radde et al. 1996, Terril & Clemons 1998
Fentanyl + Midazolam + Medetomidine	0.025 1 0.2	im	Surgical anaesthesia	Henke & Erhardt 2012, Schmitz et al. 2016
Fentanyl + Midazolam + Xylazine	0.05 2 2	im	Surgical anaesthesia	Henke & Erhardt 2012
Reversal agents: Naloxone + Flumazenil + Atipamezole	0.03 0.1 1	sc		Henke & Erhardt 2012
Tiletamine + Zolazepam (Zoletil®)	10–80	im	Minor procedures, more effective when combined with xylazine	Terril & Clemons 1998, Jacobson 2001

Table 27.7 Analgesic drug dosages for guinea pigs (NSAIDs: non-steroidal anti-inflammatory drugs).

Analgesic	Dosage in mg/kg	Route	Reference
Opioids			
Buprenorphine	0.05–0.5 q 8–12 h	sc/im/ip	Terril & Clemons 1998, Dobromylskyj et al. 2000, Wasel 2007, GV-SOLAS 2015, Flecknell 2018
Butorphanol	1–5 Q 4–6 h	sc	GV-SOLAS 2015, Mueller 2018
Morphine	2–10 q 2–4 h	sc/im	Terril & Clemons 1998
Pethidine (meperidine)	10–20 q 2–4 h	im	Terril & Clemons 1998, Dobromylskyj et al. 2000
NSAIDs/mild analgesics			
Carprofen	4–5 q 12–24 h	sc	Henke et al. 2003, GV-SOLAS 2015, Flecknell 2017, Mueller 2018
Flunixin	2.5 q 12–24 h	sc/im	Mason 1997, Mueller 2018
Meloxicam	0.2–0.5 q 24 h	po/sc	Henke et al. 2003, GV-SOLAS 2015, Flecknell 2017
Metamizole (dipyrone)	80 q 4–6 h	po	GV-SOLAS 2015, Mueller 2018

intrapulmonary. Inhalant agents like carbon dioxide or volatile anaesthetics like isoflurane are also commonly used, but these substances are irritant and aversive to the animals and carbon dioxide is painful in higher concentrations. However, carbon dioxide is still widely used because it is a practical method for larger numbers of animals, and it may be indicated for studies in which no chemical residues should remain in tissues. Carbon dioxide is only acceptable and allowed, if a gradual fill method is used to avoid pain. According to AVMA (2013), a displacement rate of 10% to 30% of the chamber volume/minute is recommended. Isoflurane should also not be used in higher concentrations than for anaesthesia until unconsciousness is reached. AVMA (2013) does not recommend the use of nitrogen or argon, as hypoxia resulting from exposure to these gases is highly aversive at least to rats and mice. Decapitation by guillotine and exsanguination subsequent to stunning are possible methods, but require well-trained personnel and, in the case of decapitation, specialised guillotines. Under Directive 2010/63, decapitation is only permissible when no other methods can possibly be used. Cervical dislocation is not recommended for this species due to its short and strong neck; this method is, however, permissible for rodents in Europe, provided the animals weigh less than 1 kg and animals over 150 g are sedated prior to the carrying out of the procedure.

Welfare Assessment in guinea pigs

As for other mammals, the welfare of guinea pigs can be assessed from: (1) the guinea pig's general appearance; (2) body condition; (3) behaviour and (4) physiological parameters (e.g. Broom & Johnson 1993).

1. General appearance of the animals: Experienced animal technicians, who know the normal appearance and behaviour of the animals, are well suited to monitor welfare and health. The fur should be smooth and not ruffled or scruffy, the claws should be short, the eyes clear and lucent, not clotted and dull, and the nose and anal region should be clean. Abnormal respiratory rate and pattern can point to disease and/or pain.
2. Body weight records/body condition score: Body weight is a non-specific, but extremely reliable, indicator of welfare, but it should always be observed together with the body condition since body weight losses may be masked by certain conditions such as the growth of tumours. Body weights of infant guinea pigs should increase regularly. In contrast, the body weights of adult animals should remain relatively constant. If there are modifications to their environment, guinea pigs can lose body weight. If an adult guinea pig loses more than 10% of its body weight within 3 days, the former housing conditions should be restored immediately (Beer et al. 1994; Sachser et al. 2004). Loss of body weight can also be an indication for dental diseases. Weight increase in adults should be investigated as tumour growth or – in females – ovarian cysts may lead to unexpected increase in weight. Therefore, the additional monitoring of the body condition score is recommended (Ullman-Culleré & Charmaine Foltz 1999; Hickman & Swan 2010).
3. Behaviour: In general, normal frequencies of courtship, comfort, feeding, drinking and locomotor activity point to good welfare of the individuals. In juveniles, play behaviour ('frisky hops') should be displayed regularly. In contrast, high frequencies of aggression, apathy and absence or reduced frequencies of feeding, drinking and comfort behaviour indicate high degrees of stress. Such behavioural patterns are often paralleled by extreme neuroendocrine stress responses. Moreover, in guinea pigs there are specific vocalisations which signal stress: In juveniles the so-called 'distress call' occurs. It is a high-pitched whistle, which indicates excitement or anxiety. The distress call can be repeated several times in a bout of calls. Distress calls are most frequently encountered upon separation of the juveniles from their mothers. Frequent occurrence of the vocalisation 'chirp' is also a stress indicator. This call is emitted in situations of discomfort (Rood 1972). Chirps are a rapidly repeated series of high-pitched birdlike notes. The animal is in an alert posture and the body twitches at each note. Chirps may be given in a continuous series lasting for 10 or 15 minutes. Vocalisation in response to handling can indicate pain or stress. In guinea pigs, only few behaviours are pain-specific and can be used to assess pain in guinea pigs (e.g. *subtle body-movement*, Dunbar et al. 2016; Oliver et al. 2017; *change in posture*, Ellen et al. 2016). See also Chapter 6 – Brief introduction to welfare assessment.
4. Physiological parameters: Stress levels can be diagnosed reliably from endocrine parameters. In mammals, two stress axes exist: the hypothalamic-pituitary–adrenocortical (HPA) and the sympathetic–adrenomedullary (SAM) systems (von Holst 1998). These systems play a major role in adjusting an individual to its physical and social environment. The activation of each of these systems provides the organism with energy and shifts it into a state of heightened reactivity that is a prerequisite for responding to environmental changes in an appropriate way. Although the short-term or moderate activation of both systems represents an adaptive mechanism to cope with conflict situations, the long-term hyperactivation of both the HPA and the SAM systems is related to the aetiology of injury and even death (von Holst 1998). Serum glucocorticoid concentrations represent a good indication of the activity of the HPA system. Good indicators for the activity of the SAM system are e.g. the serum concentrations of catecholamines (epinephrine, norepinephrine) as well as the heart rate (Sachser 1994a; von Holst 1998). The most common method to assess stress in guinea pigs is to determine concentrations of serum cortisol (in guinea pigs, cortisol is the main glucocorticoid (Jones 1974; Fujieda et al. 1982)). Blood samples for this (about 20 µl blood) can be taken from the ear vessels (Sachser & Pröve 1984). Guinea pigs rarely struggle or vocalise during sampling with this procedure, and, since it is not necessary to anaesthetise the animals, later samples are not influenced by previous exposure to anaesthesia (Sachser 1994a). This sampling procedure is described in detail earlier in this chapter. Blood samples should be taken within a time span of 5 minutes as glucocorticoid concentrations do not increase until 5 minutes after exposure to a stressor. Furthermore, non-invasive techniques to assess indicators of stress have been developed. For example, glucocorticoids can be determined from saliva. In guinea pigs, saliva can be sampled very easily by putting a cotton swab into the mouth of the animal for several minutes. Aside from endocrine stress parameters, other indicators such as immune parameters can contribute to the diagnosis of stress and welfare in guinea pigs. Furthermore, measurements of haematological parameters as well as of blood biochemistry are helpful to indicate abnormal physiological states.

For haematological and biochemical data, see Tables 27.8 and 27.9.

Common welfare problems

Diseases

Details of diseases of guinea pigs are given among others in Owen (1992), Huerkamp et al. (1996), North (1999), Richardson (2000), Wasel (2007), Harkness and Wagner (2010), Ewringmann

Table 27.8 Guinea pig haematological data.

Haematological parameter	Normal value
Erythrocytes (10^6/mm^3)	4.4–8.2
Packed cell volume (haematocrit) (%)	37–48
Haemoglobin (g/dl)	11–15
Total leucocytes (10^6/mm^3)	4–18
Neutrophils (%)	17–44
Lymphocytes (%)	32–72
Eosinophils (%)	1–16
Monocytes (%)	1–12
Basophils (%)	0–3
Platelets (10^3/mm^3)	250–850
Total blood volume (ml/kg)	69–75

Source: Reprinted from North (1999) with permission of Blackwell Publishing.

Table 27.9 Guinea pig biochemical data.

Blood biochemistry parameter	Normal value
Serum blood glucose (mg/dl)	60–125
Blood urea nitrogen (mg/dl)	9–31.5
Total plasma protein (g/dl)	4.2–6.5
Albumin (g/dl)	1.8–3.9
Globulin (g/dl)	0.8–2.6
Creatinine (mg/dl)	0.6–2.2
Total bilirubin (mg/dl)	0.3–0.9
Cholesterol (mg/dl)	20–43
Serum calcium (mg/dl)	4.5–12
Serum phosphate (mg/dl)	3.0–7.6

Source: Reprinted from North (1999) with permission of Blackwell Publishing.

and Gloeckner (2012), Minarikova et al. (2015) and Shomer et al. (2015). Signs of diseases may be non-specific, including symptoms such as weight loss, lethargy or a rough coat. First indications of diseases are described in the section on welfare assessment. Routine checks should include observation of the behaviour, gait, urine and faeces. Animals should be regularly examined with special attention paid to their coat, eyes, nose, ears, mouth and teeth, as well as feet and nails.

Bacterial diseases, like salmonellosis, pneumonia and *Staphylococcus aureus* infections, viral diseases like adenovirus, parainfluenza virus and herpesvirus infections, as well as parasitic diseases like mite and lice infestations can cause problems in guinea pigs. Bordetella bronchiseptica can cause significant respiratory disease and can be carried by asymptomatic rabbits. Therefore, rabbits and guinea pigs should not be co-housed. Non-infectious diseases include dental diseases, behavioural problems, nutritional imbalances and deficiencies (e.g. hypovitaminosis C), and reproductive disorders. A relatively common health problem is the overgrowth of teeth, especially the molar teeth, which can cause tongue entrapment and dental root inflammation. Clinical signs include weight loss and salivation. It requires consistent and ongoing veterinary treatment to control the teeth overgrowth with the aspect of potential burden for the animals. In pregnant guinea pigs, especially in obese or anorexic females, toxaemia can occur during the last 2 weeks of gestation or 7–10 days after parturition. Dystocia often occurs in guinea pigs due to the large foetuses, particularly if females are bred either too young or too old for the first time. If they are older than 6–8 months, the pubic symphysis may not separate sufficiently, and obesity may furthermore obstruct the birth canal. Ovarian cysts often occur in older females with or without symptoms like abdominal swelling, bilateral alopecia or aggressive behaviour.

Tumours do not develop frequently and occur mainly in older animals. Lymphosarcoma and mammary gland tumours are the most common tumour diseases in guinea pigs and can occur both in females and males.

Table 27.10 summarises common diseases of guinea pigs. More detailed information can be taken from the cited authors as well as from North (1999).

Treatment of diseases is often difficult. Animals suffering from an infectious disease should be separated from the

Table 27.10 Common diseases of guinea pigs (Noonan 1994; Schaeffer & Donnelly 1997; Wasel 2007).

Organ system	Diseases
Skin	Dermatophytosis (mainly *Trichophyton mentagrophytes*)
	Ectoparasites (mites like *Trixacarus caviae*, *Chirodiscoides caviae*, lice like *Gliricola porcelli*, *Gyropus ovalis*)
	Pododermatitis
	Endocrine alopecia (gestational, ovarian cysts)
	Bite wounds
	Barbering
Gastrointestinal tract	Dental disease (tooth elongation and malocclusion; incisors as well as molar teeth)
	Antibiotic-associated enterotoxaemia
	Bacterial enteritis (*Salmonella* sp., *Clostridium* sp., *Escherichia coli*, *Yersinia pseudotuberculosis*, *Clostridium piliforme*, etc.)
	Parasitic diarrhoea (*Eimeria caviae*, *Paraspidodera uncinata*)
Respiratory tract	Bacterial pneumonia (*Bordetella bronchiseptica*, *Streptococcus pneumonia*, *Streptococcus zooepidemicus*, *Pasteurella multocida*, *Klebsiella pneumoniae*)
	Viral pneumonia (adenovirus)
Urogenital tract	Cystitis
	Urolithiasis
	Chronic interstitial nephritis (found in older animals)
	Ovarian cysts
	Endometritis
	Dystocia
	Pregnancy toxaemia
	Mastitis
Nervous system	Lymphocytic choriomeningitis (LCM virus), zoonotic disease!
	Torticollis (caused by progressive otitis media/interna, *Streptococcus pneumonia*, *Streptococcus zooepidemicus*, *Bordetella bronchiseptica*, etc.)

others. However, since separation from the social group is stressful, in all other cases it should be avoided. Housing conditions should be checked and optimised if necessary. The same papers cited in the preceding text as well as Smith and Burgmann (1997), Ewringmann and Gloeckner (2012) and Wasel (2007) give information on treatment and drug dosages. Some bacterial diseases may be treated with antibiotics; however, antibiotic sensitivity should be tested first. Unlike most other species, the gastrointestinal flora of guinea pigs is predominated by Gram-positive bacteria. Therefore, certain antibiotics including penicillin, ampicillin or lincomycin cause an alteration to Gram-negative bacteria like *Escherichia coli* or *Clostridium difficile*, often resulting in severe enterotoxaemia. Broad-spectrum antibiotics such as sulphonamide/trimethoprim or enrofloxacin should be used for therapy, but only if really necessary. Above all, attention should be paid to preventive measures.

Acknowledgements

Thanks go to Prof Dr Gero Hilken for substantial comments on aspects of care and use of guinea pigs in experimental animal sciences. Furthermore, we would like to thank the referees for their helpful comments.

References

Abou-Madi, N. (2006) Anesthesia and analgesia of small mammals. In: *Recent Advances in Veterinary Anesthesia and Analgesia: Companion Animals*. Eds Gleed, R.D. and Ludders, J.W. http://www.ivis.org/advances/Anesthesia_Gleed/toc.asp. International Veterinary Information Service, Ithaca NY.

Adrian, O., Dekomien, G., Epplen, J.T. and Sachser, N. (2008) Body weight and rearing conditions of males, female choice and paternities in a small mammal, *Cavia aperea*. *Ethology*, 114, 897–906.

Adrian, O. and Sachser, N. (2011) Diversity of social and mating systems in cavies: a review. *Journal of Mammalogy*, 92, 39–53.

American Veterinary Medical Association (AVMA) Panel on Euthanasia (2013) *Guidelines for the Euthanasia of Animals*; 2013 Edition. https://www.avma.org/KB/Policies/Documents/euthanasia.pdf (accessed 27 February 2019).

Asher, M., Lippmann, T., Epplen, J.T. *et al.* (2008) Large males dominate: ecology, social organization, and mating system of wild cavies, the ancestors of the guinea pig. *Behavioral Ecology and Sociobiology*, 62, 1509–1521.

Asher, M., Oliveira, E.S. and Sachser, N. (2004) Social system and spatial organization of wild guinea pigs (*Cavia aperea*) in a natural population. *Journal of Mammalogy*, 85, 788–796.

Balsiger, A., Clauss, M., Liesegang, A. *et al.* (2017) Guinea pig (*Cavia porcellus*) drinking preferences: do nippledrinkers compensate for behaviourally deficient diets? *Journal of Animal Physiology and Animal Nutrition*, 101, 1046–1056.

Bauer, B., Womastek, I., Dittami, J. and Huber, S. (2008) The effects of early environmental conditions on the reproductive and somatic development of juvenile guinea pigs (*Cavia aperea f. porcellus*). *General and Comparative Endocrinology*, 155, 680–685.

Beauchamp, G.K., Criss, B.R. and Wellington, J.L. (1979) Chemical communication in *Cavia*: responses of wild (*C. aperea*), domestic (*C. porcellus*) and F1 males to urine. *Animal Behaviour*, 27, 1066–1072.

Beauchamp, G.K., Martin, I.G., Wysocki, C.J. and Wellington, J.L. (1982) Chemoinvestigatory and sexual behaviour of male guinea pigs following vomeronasal organ removal. *Physiology and Behavior*, 29, 329–336.

Beauchamp, G.K., Wellington, J.L., Wysocki, C.J. *et al.* (1980) Chemical communication in the guinea pig: urinary components of low volatility and their access to the vomeronasal organ. In: *Chemical Signals: Vertebrates and Aquatic Invertebrates*. Eds Müller-Schwarze D. and Silverstein R., pp. 327–339. Plenum Press, New York.

Beer, R., Kaiser, S., Sachser, N. and Stanzel, K. (1994) *Merkblatt zur tierschutzgerechten Haltung von Versuchstieren: Meerschweinchen*. Tierärztliche Vereinigung für Tierschutz e.V., Bramsche.

Beer, R. and Sachser, N. (1992) Sozialstruktur und Wohlergehen in Männchengruppen des Hausmeerschweinchens. In: *Aktuelle Arbeiten zur artgemäßen Tierhaltung* 1991, KTBL-Schrift 351. Eds Kuratorium für Technik und Bauwesen in der Landwirtschaft e.V. & Deutsche Veterinärmedizinische Gesellschaft e.V., pp. 158–167. KTBL-Schriften-Vertrieb im Landwirtschaftsverlag GmbH, Darmstadt.

Benecke, N. (1994) *Der Mensch und seine Haustiere*. Konrad Theiss Verlag GmbH & Co, Stuttgart.

Berryman, J.C. and Fullerton, C. (1976) A developmental study of interactions between young and adult guinea pigs. *Behaviour*, 59, 22–39.

Birck, M.M., Tveden-Nyborg, P., Lindblad, M.M. and Lykkesfeldt, J. (2014) Non-terminal blood sampling techniques in guinea pigs. *Journal of Visualized Experiments*, 92, 51982.

Birke, L.I.A. (1981) Some behavioural changes associated with the guinea-pig oestrus cycle. *Zeitschrift für Tierpsychologie*, 55, 79–89.

Blouin, A. and Cormier, Y. (1987) Endotracheal intubation in guinea pigs by direct laryngoscopy. *Laboratory Animal Science*, 37, 244–245.

Broom, D.M. and Johnson, K.G. (1993) *Stress and Animal Welfare*. Chapman & Hall, London.

Byrd, C.P., Winnicker, C. and Gaskill, B.N. (2016) Instituting dark-colored cover to improve central space use within guinea pig enclosure. *Journal of Applied Animal Welfare Science*, 19, 408–413.

Cassini, M.H. (1991) Foraging under predation risk in the wild guinea pig *Cavia aperea*. *Oikos*, 62, 20–24.

Cassini, M.H. and Galante, M.L. (1992) Foraging under predation risk in the wild guinea pig: the effect of vegetation height on habitat utilization. *Annales Zoologici Fennici*, 29, 285–290.

Clutton-Brock, J. (1989) *A Natural History of Domesticated Mammals*. Cambridge University Press, Cambridge.

Cooper, T.G., Weydert, S., Yeung, C.H. *et al.* (2000) Maturation of epididymal spermatozoa in the non-domesticated guinea pigs *Cavia aperea* and *Galea musteloides*. *Journal of Andrology*, 21, 154–163.

Council of Europe (2006) Appendix A of *European Convention for the Protection of Vertebrate Animals Used for Experimental and Other Scientific Purposes (ETS 123)* http://www.arsal.ro/wp-content/uploads/2017/02/ETS-123-1.pdf (accessed 27 February 2019).

Diehl, K.-H., Hull, R., Morton, D. *et al.* (2001) A good practice guide to the administration of substances and removal of blood, including routes and volumes. *Journal of applied toxicology*, 21, 15–23.

Dobromylskyj, P., Flecknell, P.A., Lascelles, B.D. *et al.* (2000) Management of postoperative and other acute pain. In: *Pain Management in Animals*. Eds Flecknell, P.A. and Waterman-Pearson, A., pp. 81–145. W.B. Saunders, London.

Dunbar, M.L., David, E.M., Aline, M.R. and Lofgren, J.L. (2016) Validation of a behavioral ethogram for assessing postoperative pain in guinea pigs (*Cavia porcellus*). *Journal of the American Association for Laboratory Animal Science*, 55, 29–34.

Eisenberg, J.F. and Redford, K.H. (1999) *Mammals of the Neotropics*, Vol. 3, The Central Neotropics. University of Chicago Press, Chicago.

Ellen, Y, Flecknell, P. and Leach, M. (2016) Evaluation of using behavioural changes to assess post-operative pain in the guinea pig (*Cavia porcellus*). *PLoS ONE*, **11**(9), e0161941.

European Parliament and the Council of the European Union (2010) *Directive 2010/63/EU on the Protection of Animals Used for Scientific Purposes.* https://eur-lex.europa.eu/LexUriServ/LexUriServ.do?uri=OJ:L:2010:276:0033:0079:en:PDF (accessed 27 February 2019).

Ewringmann, A. and Gloeckner, B. (2012) *Leitsymptome bei Meerschweinchen, Chinchilla und Degu*. Enke Verlag, Stuttgart.

FELASA working group on revision of guidelines for health monitoring of rodents and rabbits (2014) FELASA recommendations for the health monitoring of mouse, rat, hamster, guinea pig and rabbit colonies in breeding and experimental units. *Laboratory Animals*, **48**, 178–192 lan.sagepub.com/content/48/3/178.full.pdf (accessed 27 February 2019).

Fey, K. and Trillmich, F. (2008) Sibling competition in guinea pigs (*Cavia aperea* f. *porcellus*): scrambling for mother 's teats is stressful. *Behavioral Ecology and Sociobiology*, **62**, 321–329.

Flecknell, P.A. (2015) *Laboratory Animal Anaesthesia*, 4th edn. Academic Press, London.

Flecknell, P. (2018) Rodent analgesia: assessment and therapeutics. *The Veterinary Journal*, **232**, 70–77.

Fujieda, K., Goff, A.K., Pugeat, M. and Strott, C.A. (1982) Regulation of the pituitary-adrenal axis and corticosteroid-binding globulin-cortisol interaction in the guinea pig. *Endocrinology*, **111**, 1944–1949.

Gade, D.W. (1967) The guinea pig in Andean folk culture. *Geographical Review*, **57**, 213–224

Gesellschaft für Versuchstierkunde (GV-SOLAS) Ausschuss für Anästhesie (2015) Schmerztherapie bei Versuchstieren. www.gv-solas.de/fileadmin/user_upload/pdf_publikation/Anaest._Analgesie/Schmerztherapie_Mai2015.pdf (accessed 27 February 2019).

Graves, F.C. and Hennessy, M.B. (2000) Comparison of the effects of the mother and an unfamiliar adult female on cortisol and behavioral responses of preweaning and postweaning guinea pigs. *Developmental Psychobiology*, **36**, 91–100.

Guichón, M.L. and Cassini, M.H. (1998) Role of diet selection in the use of habitat by pampas cavies *Cavia aperea pamparum* (Mammalia, Rodentia). *Mammalia*, **62**, 23–35.

Haase, E. and Donham, R.S. (1980) Hormones and domestication. In: *Avian Endocrinology*. Eds Epple, A. and Stetson, M.H., pp. 549–565. Academic Press, New York.

Harkness, J.E. and Wagner, J.E. (2010) *The Biology and Medicine of Rabbits and Rodents*. 5th edition. Eds Harkness, J.E., Turner, P.V., VandeWoude, S. and Whele, C.L. Wiley Blackwell, Oxford.

Harper, L.V. (1976) Behavior. In: *The Biology of the Guinea Pig*. Eds. Wagner, I.E. and Manning, P.J., pp. 31–52. Academic Press, New York.

Henke, J. and Erhardt, W. (2012) Speziesspezifische Anaesthesie, Nager. In: *Anästhesie & Analgesie beim Klein- und Heimtier*, 2nd edn. Eds Erhardt, W., Henke, J. and Haberstroh, J., pp. 703–725. Schattauer GmbH, Stuttgart.

Henke, J., Faltermeier, C. and Erhardt, W. (2003) Anaesthesie, Analgesie und Euthanasie bei kleinen Heimtieren. *Tierärztliche Praxis (K)*, **31**, 394–397.

Hennessy, M.B. (1997) Hypothalamic-pituitary-adrenal responses to brief social separation. *Neuroscience and Biobehavioral Reviews*, **21**, 11–29.

Hennessy, M.B. (1999) Social influences on endocrine activity in guinea pigs, with comparisons to findings in nonhuman primates. *Neuroscience and Biobehavioral Reviews*, **23**, 687–698.

Hennessy, M.B., Hornschuh, G., Kaiser, S. and Sachser, N. (2006) Cortisol responses and social buffering: a study throughout the life span. *Hormones and Behavior*, **49**, 383–390.

Hennessy, M.B., Kaiser, S. and Sachser, N. (2009) Social buffering of the stress response: diversity, mechanisms, and functions. *Frontiers in Neuroendocrinology*, **30**(4): 470–482.

Hennessy, M.B., Maken, D.S. and Graves, F.C. (2002a) Presence of mother and unfamiliar female alters levels of testosterone, progesterone, cortisol, adrenocorticotropin, and behavior in maturing guinea pigs. *Hormones and Behavior*, **42**, 42–52.

Hennessy, M.B. and Morris, A. (2005) Passive response of young guinea pigs during exposure to a novel environment: influences of social partners and age. *Developmental Psychobiology*, **46**, 86–96.

Hennessy, M.B., O'Leary, S.K., Hawke, J.L. and Wilson, S.E. (2002b) Social influences on cortisol and behavioral responses of preweaning, periadolescent, and adult guinea pigs. *Physiology and Behavior*, **76**, 305–314.

Hennessy, M.B. and Ritchey, R.L. (1987) Hormonal and behavioral attachment responses in infant guinea pigs. *Developmental Psychobiology*, **20**, 613–625.

Herre, W. and Röhrs, M. (1990) *Haustiere – zoologisch gesehen*. Gustav Fischer Verlag, Stuttgart.

Hickman, D.L. and Swan, M. (2010) Use of a body condition score technique to assess health status in a rat model of polycystic kidney disease. *Journal of the American Association for Laboratory Animal Science*, **49**, 155–159.

Hillyer, E.V., Quesenberry, K.E. and Donnelly, T.M. (1997) Biology, husbandry, and clinical techniques. In: *Ferrets, Rabbits, and Rodents*. Eds Hillyer, E.V. and Quesenberry, K.E., pp. 243–259. W.B. Saunders Company, Philadelphia.

Huerkamp, M.J., Murray, S.E. and Orosz, S.E. (1996) Guinea pigs. In: *Handbook of Rodent and Rabbit Medicine*. Eds Laber-Laird, K.E., Swindle M.M. and Flecknell, P.A., pp. 91–149. Pergamon Press, Oxford.

Hückinghaus, F. (1961) Zur Nomenklatur und Abstammung des Hausmeerschweinchens. *Zeitschrift für Säugetierkunde*, **26**, 108–111.

Hull, R.M. (1995) Guideline limit volumes for dosing animals in the preclinical stage of safety evaluation. *Human & Experimental Toxicology*, **14**, 305–307.

Hyams, E. (1972) *Animals in the Service of Man: 10 000 Years of Domestication*. J.M. Dent and Sons Ltd., London.

Jacobs, G.H. and Deegan, J.F. (1994) Spectral sensitivity, photopigments, and color vision in the guinea pig (*Cavia porcellus*). *Behavioral Neuroscience*, **108**, 993–1004.

Jacobson, C. (2001) A novel anaesthetic regimen for surgical procedures in guinea pigs. *Laboratory Animals*, **35**, 271–276.

Jäckel, M. and Trillmich, F. (2003) Olfactory individual recognition of mothers by young guinea-pigs (*Cavia porcellus*). *Ethology*, **109**, 197–208.

Jansson, P.J., Jung, H.R., Lindqvist, C. and Nordström, T. (2004) Oxidative decomposition of Vitamin C in drinking water. *Free Radical Research*, **38**, 855–860.

Jensen, P. (2006) Domestication – From behavior to genes and back again. *Applied Animal Behaviour Science*, **97**, 3–15.

Joint Working Group on Refinement (1993) Removal of blood from laboratory mammals and birds. First Report of the BVA/FRAME/RSPCA/UFAW Joint Working Group on Refinement. *Laboratory Animals*, **27**, 1–22.

Jones, C.T. (1974) Corticosteroid concentrations in the plasma of fetal and maternal guinea pigs during gestation. *Endocrinology*, **95**, 1129–1133.

Kaiser, S., Hennessy, M.B. and Sachser, N. (2015) Domestication affects the structure, development and stability of biobehavioural profiles. *Frontiers in Zoology*, **12**(Suppl. 1), S19.

Kaiser, S., Kirtzeck, M., Hornschuh, G. and Sachser, N. (2003a) Sex specific difference in social support – a study in female guinea pigs. *Physiology and Behavior*, **79**, 297–303.

Kaiser, S., Nübold, T., Rohlmann, I. and Sachser, N. (2003b) Pregnant female guinea pigs adapt easily to a new social environment irrespective of their rearing conditions. *Physiology and Behavior*, **80**, 147–153.

Kaiser, S. and Sachser, N. (2005) The effects of prenatal social stress on behaviour: mechanisms and function. *Neuroscience and Biobehavioral Reviews*, **29**, 283–294.

Kawachi, I. and Berkman, L.F. (2001) Social ties and mental health. *Journal of Urban Health*, **78**, 458–467.

Kenagy, G.J. and Trombulak, S.C. (1986) Size and function of mammalian testes in relation to body size. *Journal of Mammalogy*, **67**, 1–22.

Kruska, D.C.T. and Steffen, K. (2013) Comparative allometric investigations on the skulls of wild cavies (*Cavia aperea*) versus domesticated guinea pigs (*C. aperea* f. *porcellus*) with comments on the domestication of this species. *Mammalian Biology*, **78**, 178–186.

Kunkel, P. and Kunkel, I. (1964) Beiträge zur Ethologie des Hausmeerschweinchens. *Zeitschrift für Tierpsychologie*, **21**, 602–641.

Künzl, C., Kaiser, S., Meier, E. and Sachser, N. (2003) Is a wild mammal kept and reared in captivity still a wild animal? *Hormones and Behavior*, **43**, 187–196.

Künzl, C. and Sachser, N. (1999) The behavioural endocrinology of domestication: a comparison between the domestic guinea pig (*Cavia aperea* f. *porcellus*) and its wild ancestor the wild cavy (*Cavia aperea*). *Hormones and Behavior*, **35**, 28–37.

Lewejohann, L., Pickel, T., Sachser, N. and Kaiser, S. (2010) Wild genius – domestic fool? Spatial learning abilities of wild and domestic guinea pigs. *Frontiers in Zoology*, **7**, 9.

Lürzel, S., Kaiser, S. and Sachser, N. (2010) Social interaction, testosterone, and stress responsiveness during adolescence. *Physiology and Behavior*, **99**, 40–46.

Lürzel, S., Kaiser, S. and Sachser, N. (2011a) Social interaction decreases stress responsiveness during adolescence. *Psychoneuroendocrinology*, **36**, 1370–1377.

Lürzel, S., Kaiser, S., Krüger, C. and Sachser, N. (2011b) Inhibiting influence of testosterone on stress responsiveness during adolescence. *Hormones and Behaviour*, **60**, 691–698.

Mares, M.A. and Ojeda, R.A. (1982) Patterns of diversity and adaptation in South American hystricognath rodents. In: *Mammalian Biology in South America*. Eds Mares, M.A. and Genoways, H.H., pp. 393–432. Pymatuning Laboratory of Ecology, Special Publications No. 6., Pittsburgh, Pennsylvania.

Martin, I.G. and Beauchamp, G.K. (1982) Olfactory recognition of individuals by male cavies (*Cavia aperea*). *Journal of Chemical Ecology*, **8**, 1241–1249.

Mason, D.E. (1997) Anesthesia, analgesia, and sedation for small mammals. In: *Ferrets, Rabbits, and Rodents*. Eds Hillyer, E.V. and Quesenberry, K.E., pp. 378–391. W.B. Saunders Company, Philadelphia.

Minarikova, A., Hauptmann, K., Jeklova, E. et al. (2015) Diseases in pet guinea pigs: a retrospective study in 1000 animals. *Veterinary Record*, **177**, 200.

Mueller, K. (2018) Schmerztherapie bei Kaninchen, Meerschweinchen, Chinchillas und Frettchen – ein Update. *Der Praktische Tierarzt*, **99**, 348–360.

NCR3s https://www.nc3rs.org.uk/blood-sampling-guinea-pig (accessed 10 September 2019).

NCR3s https://www.nc3rs.org.uk/guinea-pig-blood-vessel-cannulation-surgical (accessed 10 September 2019).

Noonan, D. (1994) The guinea pig (*Cavia porcellus*). *ANZCCART News*, **7**, 1–8.

North, D. (1999) The guinea-pig. In: *The UFAW Handbook on the Care and Management of Laboratory Animals, Vol 1, Terrestrial Vertebrates*, 7th edn. Ed. Poole, T., pp. 367–388. Blackwell Publishing, Oxford.

Oliver, V.L., Athavale, S., Simon, K.E. et al. (2017) Evaluation of pain assessment techniques and analgesia efficacy in a female guinea pig (*Cavia porcellus*) model of surgical pain. *Journal of the American Association for Laboratory Animal Science*, **56**, 425–435.

Owen, D.G. (1992) *Parasites of Laboratory Animals*. Laboratory Animals Handbooks. Royal Society of Medicine Services, London.

Pettijohn, T.F. (1979) Attachment and separation distress in the infant guinea pig. *Developmental Psychobiology*, **12**, 73–81.

Price, E.O. (1984) Behavioral aspects of animal domestication. *The Quarterly Review of Biology*, **59**, 1–32.

Radde, G.R., Hinson, A., Crenshaw, D. and Toth, L.A. (1996) Evaluation of anaesthetic regimes in guinea pigs. *Laboratory Animals*, **30**, 220–227.

Redford, K.H. and Eisenberg, J.F. (1992) *Mammals of the Neotropics, Vol. 2, the Southern Cone*. University of Chicago Press, Chicago.

Richardson, V.C.G. (2000) *Diseases of Domestic Guinea Pigs*, 2nd edn. Blackwell Science Ltd, Oxford.

Ritchey, R.L. and Hennessy, M.B. (1987) Cortisol and behavioral responses to separation in mother and infant guinea pigs. *Behavioral and Neural Biology*, **48**, 1–12.

Rood, J.P. (1972) Ecological and behavioural comparisons of three genera of Argentine cavies. *Animal Behaviour Monographs*, **5**, 1–83.

Rosenthal, K., Forbes, N., Frye, F. and Lewbart, G. (2008) *Rapid Review of Exotic Animal Medicine and Husbandry*. London, CRC Press, https://doi.org/10.1201/b15200

Sachser, N. (1986) Different forms of social organization at high and low population densities in guinea pigs. *Behaviour*, **97**, 253–272.

Sachser, N. (1987) Short-term responses of plasma-norepinephrine, epinephrine, glucocorticoid and testosterone titers to social and non-social stressors in male guinea pigs of different social status. *Physiology and Behavior*, **39**, 11–20.

Sachser, N. (1990) Social organization, social status, behavioural strategies and endocrine responses in male guinea pigs. In: *Hormones, Brain and Behavior in Vertebrates. Comparative Physiology*, Vol. 9. Ed. Balthazart, J., pp. 176–187. Karger, Basel.

Sachser, N (1993) The ability to arrange with conspecifics depends on social experiences around puberty. *Physiology and Behavior*, **53**, 539–544.

Sachser, N. (1994a) *Sozialphysiologische Untersuchungen an Hausmeerschweinchen. Gruppenstrukturen, soziale Situation und Endokrinium, Wohlergehen*. Parey, Berlin.

Sachser, N. (1994b) Social stratification and health in non-human mammals – a case study in guinea pigs. In: *Social Stratification and Socioeconomic Inequality*, Vol. 2. Ed. Ellis, L., pp. 113–121. Praeger, Westport.

Sachser, N. (1998) Of domestic and wild guinea pigs: studies in sociophysiology, domestication, and social evolution. *Naturwissenschaften*, **85**, 307–317.

Sachser, N. (2001) What is important to achieve good welfare in animals? In: *Coping with Challenge: Welfare in Animals Including Humans*, Dahlem Workshop Report 87. Ed. Broom, D.M., pp. 31–48. Dahlem University Press, Berlin.

Sachser, N., Dürschlag, M. and Hirzel, D. (1998) Social relationships and the management of stress. *Psychoneuroendocrinology*, **23**, 891–904.

Sachser, N., Hennessy, M.B. and Kaiser, S. (2018) The adaptive shaping of social behavioural phenotypes during adolescence. *Biological Letters*, **14** (DOI: 10.1098/rsbl.2018.0536).

Sachser, N., Kaiser, S. and Hennessy, M.B. (2013) Behavioural profiles are shaped by social experience: When, how and why. *Philosophical Transactions of the Royal Society B Biological Sciences B*, **368**(1618) (DOI: 10.1098/rstb.2012.0344).

Sachser, N., Künzl, C. and Kaiser, S. (2004) The welfare of laboratory guinea pigs. In: *The Welfare of Laboratory Animals*. Ed. Kalista, E., pp. 181–209. Kluwer Academic Publishers, Dordrecht.

Sachser, N. and Lick, C. (1991) Social experience, behavior, and stress in guinea pigs. *Physiology and Behavior*, **50**, 83–90.

Sachser, N., Lick, C., Beer, R. and Weinandy, R. (1992) Tagesgang von Serum-Hormonkonzentrationen und ethologischen Parametern bei Hausmeerschweinchen. *Verhandlungen der Deutschen Zoologischen Gesellschaft*, **85**, 120.

Sachser, N., Lick, C. and Stanzel, K. (1994) The environment, hormones, and aggressive behaviour: a 5-year-study in guinea pigs. *Psychoneuroendocrinology*, **19**, 697–707.

Sachser, N. and Pröve, E. (1984) Short-term effects of residence on the testosterone responses to fighting in alpha male guinea pigs. *Aggressive Behaviour*, **10**, 285–292.

Sachser, N. and Renninger, S.-V. (1993) Coping with new social situations: the role of social rearing in guinea pigs. *Ethology Ecology Evolution*, **5**, 65–74.

Sachser, N., Schwarz-Weig, E., Keil, A. and Epplen, J.T. (1999) Behavioural strategies, testis size, and reproductive success in two caviomorph rodents with different mating systems. *Behaviour*, **136**, 1203–1217.

Schaeffer, D.O. and Donnelly, T.M. (1997) Disease problems of guinea pigs and chinchillas. In: *Ferrets, Rabbits, and Rodents*. Eds Hillyer, E.V. and Quesenberry, K.E., pp. 260–282. W.B. Saunders Company, Philadelphia.

Schmitz, S., Tacke, S., Guth, B. and Henke, J. (2016) Comparison of physiological parameters and anaesthesia specific observations during isoflurane, ketamine-xylazine or medetomidine-midazolam-fentanyl anaesthesia in male guinea pigs. *PloS one*, **11**(9), p.e0161258.

Shi, F.X., Ozawa, M., Komura, H. et al. (1999) Secretion of ovarian inhibin and its physiologic roles in the regulation of follicle-stimulating hormone secretion during the estrous cycle of the female guinea pig. *Biology of Reproduction*, **60**, 78–84.

Shomer, N.H., Holcombe, H. and Harkness, J.E. (2015) Biology and diseases of guinea pigs. In: *Laboratory Animal Medicine*, 3rd edn. Eds Fox, J.G., Anderson, L., Otto G. et al., pp. 247–283. Academic Press, New York.

Smith, D.A. and Burgmann, P.M. (1997) Formulary. In: *Ferrets, Rabbits, and Rodents*. Eds Hillyer, E.V. and Quesenberry, K.E., pp. 392–403. W.B. Saunders Company, Philadelphia

Smith, B.J., Wegenast, D.J., Hansen, R.J. et al. (2016) Pharmacokinetics and paw withdrawal pressure in female guinea pigs (*Cavia porcellus*) treated with sustained-release buprenorphine and buprenorphine hydrochloride. *Journal of the American Association for Laboratory Animal Science*, **55**, 789–793.

Spotorno, A.E., Manríquez, G., Fernández, L.A. et al. (2007) Domestication of guinea pigs from a Southern Peru-Northern Chile wild species and their middle pre-Columbian mummies. In: *The Quintessential Naturalist: Honoring the Life and Legacy of Oliver P. Pearson*. Eds Kelt, D.A., Lessa, E.P., Salazar-Bravo, J. and Patton, J.L., pp. 367–388. University of California Publications in Zoology 134.

Spotorno, A.E, Valladares, J.P., Marín, J.C. and Zeballos, H. (2004) Molecular diversity among domestic guinea-pigs (*Cavia porcellus*) and their close phylogenetic relationship with the Andean wild species *Cavia tschudii*. *Revista Chilena de Historia Natural*, **77**, 243–250.

Stahnke, A. and Hendrichs, H. (1988) Meerschweinchenverwandte Nagetiere. In: *Grzimeks Enzyklopädie Säugetiere*. Ed. Grzimek, B., pp. 314–357. Kindler Verlag, München.

Terril, L.A. and Clemons, D.J. (1998) *The Laboratory Guinea Pig*. CRC Press, Boca Raton.

Thyen, Y. and Hendrichs, H. (1990) Differences in behaviour and social organization of female guinea pigs as a function of the presence of a male. *Ethology*, **85**, 25–34.

Timm, K.I., Jahn, S.E. and Sedgwick, C.J. (1987) The palatal ostium of the guinea pig. *Laboratory Animal Science*, **37**, 801–802.

Trillmich, F., Kraus, C., Künkele, J. et al. (2004) Species-level differentiation of two cryptic species pairs of wild cavies, genera *Cavia* and *Galea*, with a discussion of the relationship between social systems and phylogeny in the Caviinae. *Canadian Journal of Zoology*, **82**, 516–524.

ULAM veterinary staff, Guidelines on anesthesia and analgesia in guinea pigs. (2021). https://az.research.umich.edu/animalcare/guidelines/guidelines-anesthesia-and-analgesia-guinea-pigs (accessed 18 October).

Ullman-Culleré, M.H. and Foltz, C.J. (1999) Body condition scoring: a rapid and accurate method for assessing health status in mice. *Laboratory Animal Science*, **49**, 319–323.

von Holst, D. (1998) The concept of stress and its relevance for animal behavior. In: *Advances in the Study of Behavior*. Eds Lehman, D.S., Hinde, R. and Shaw, E., pp. 1–131. Academic Press, New York.

Wagner, J.E. (1976) Introduction and taxonomy. In: *The Biology of the Guinea Pig*. Eds Wagner, J.E. and Manning, P.J., pp. 1–4. Academic Press, New York.

Wallner, B., Dittami, J. and Machatschke, I. (2006) Social stimuli cause changes of plasma oxytocin and behavior in guinea pigs. *Biological Research*, **39**, 251–258.

Wasel, E. (2007) Meerschweinchen. In: *Krankheiten der Heimtiere*. Eds Fehr, M., Sassenburg, L. and Zwart, P., pp. 49–86. Schlütersche Verlagsgesellschaft, Hannover.

Weir, B.J. (1974) Notes on the origin of the domestic guinea pig. *Symposium of the Zoological Society of London*, **34**, 437–446.

Wewers, D., Kaiser, S. and Sachser, N. (2003) Maternal separation in guinea pigs: a study in behavioural endocrinology. *Ethology*, **109**, 443–453.

Wilson, D.E. and Reeder, D.M. (2005) *Mammal Species of the World*. Vol 1, 3rd edn. The John Hopkins University Press, Baltimore.

Wing, E.S. (1977) Animal domestication in the Andes. In: *Origins of Agriculture*. Ed. Reed, C.A., pp. 837–859. Mouton Publishers, The Hague.

Wolf, P. and Kamphues, J. (2004) Ernaehrung der Heimtiere – Einfluss der Fuetterung auf das Zahnwachstum. *Kleintier konkret*, 21–24.

Zimmermann, T.D., Kaiser, S., Hennessy, M.B. and Sachser, N. (2017) Adaptive shaping of the behavioural and neuroendocrine phenotype during adolescence. *Proceedings of the Royal Society of London B*, **284**, 20162784.

28 The laboratory rabbit

Lena Lidfors and Therese Edström

Biological overview

General biology (natural history)

The rabbit belongs to the *Lagomorpha* order and the *Leporidae* family, and is a monogastric herbivore that has developed a special digestive strategy, caecotrophy, which makes it adapted to live on plants (Gidenne *et al.* 2010). The rabbit is descended from the European wild rabbit (*Oryctolagus cuniculus*) (Harcourt-Brown 2002), which appears to have had a widespread distribution across Europe before the last Pleistocene glaciations 1.8 million to 10,000 years ago (Flux 1994). After the last Ice Age (20,000 years ago), it was confined to the Iberian Peninsula and small areas of France and northwest Africa (Parker 1990; Wilson & Reeder 1993). The spread of the rabbit over the world has mainly been the result of man's activities (Flux 1994). Due to the adaptability of the species, the European rabbit exists in the wild on every continent except Asia and Antarctica (Parker 1990; Wilson & Reeder 1993).

In many places where rabbits have been introduced, the lack of predators has led to an explosion in the number of animals, leading them to become regarded as pests, i.e. Australia, New Zealand (Waikato Regional Council Fact Sheet 2015). In order for the Australian ecosystem to recover, rabbit populations need to be kept at low numbers (Cooke 2012). To find ways to diminish the high population of wild rabbits, their behaviour and reproduction have been investigated in detail.

The Phoenicians discovered rabbits on the Iberian Peninsula about 3000 years ago and brought some of them home to the Mediterranean area (Buseth & Saunders 2015). Romans gradually began to keep rabbits for meat and by the year CE 230 many rabbits lived in captivity in Italy (Buseth & Saunders 2015). Domestication started in the French monasteries around CE 500–1000, where several different breeds were developed (Buseth & Saunders 2015). These were further developed to create a large number of breeds for different purposes during the past century.

When the behaviour of European wild rabbits has been compared with domestic strains of rabbits kept in semi-natural enclosures, their behaviour has been found to be very similar in most aspects (reviewed by Bell 1984); however, there are some differences (Stodart & Myers 1964; Mykytowycz 1968; Kraft 1979). When European wild rabbits were brought into the laboratory, they failed to breed, and females born into the laboratory as a result of egg transfer from wild to domestic mothers retained their nervous disposition and failed to mature sexually (Adams 1982). European wild rabbits may be used for experimental research, but there are several problems in keeping and breeding them (Bell 1999), and they also may bring in several infectious agents that are normally excluded in barrier housing.

Size range and lifespan

The European wild rabbit has been reported to vary widely in both adult weight range and lifespan both within and between populations. From northern to southern Europe, the body weight (Rogers *et al.* 1994) and skull size (Sharples *et al.* 1996) are reduced. It has been suggested that this is due to phenotypic rather than genetic variation (Sharples *et al.* 1996). In a long-term study, the body weight of European wild rabbits in East Anglia, UK, was found to be 1.3–2.1 kg in males and 1.3–2.3 kg in females (Bell 1999).

The European wild rabbit has no dimorphism in adult body size (Webb 1993). The only difference in appearance between males and females is that bucks have a more rounded, broader appearance to the front of the head, whereas does have a more pointed head (Bell 1999). Domesticated rabbit breeds do not seem to have developed dimorphism in size either.

In the European wild rabbit, mortality in the wild is very high during the first year of life and can reach up to 90% (Nowak 1999), mainly due to myxomatosis and predation (Bell & Webb 1991; Rogers *et al.* 1994). In a long-term English study, maximum age of bucks was 8 years and of does 9 years (Bell 1999), whereas Gibb (1993) had rabbits living over 10 years in a study in New Zealand.

The UFAW Handbook on the Care and Management of Laboratory and Other Research Animals, Ninth Edition.
Edited by Huw Golledge and Claire Richardson.
© 2024 John Wiley & Sons Ltd. Published 2024 by John Wiley & Sons Ltd.

Social organisation of wild rabbits

European wild rabbits live in small, stable, territorial breeding groups (Gibb et al. 1978; Cowan 1987; Bell & Webb 1991). This is the social unit and consists of one to four males and one to nine females, but different breeding groups may comprise colonies of up to 70 rabbits (Meredith 2000). The breeding group defends its territory, a core area with a warren within a larger home-range, by patrolling the borders and scent-marking (Bell 1999). A warren is an area of soil or sand containing underground tunnels and nests made by the rabbits. Breeding groups can occupy either single warrens (Myers & Schneider 1964; Bell 1977) or multiple warrens (Wood 1980; Daly 1981; Cowan 1987). Each warren has several entrances that allow quick escape from predators (Cowan 1987). Neighbouring breeding groups can move out from their territories to forage in communal grazing areas at dawn and dusk (Bell 1980).

Dominance hierarchies forms within each sex for each breeding group, and they are stable over time (Bell 1983). Rabbits keeping a fixed distance from one another and exhibiting submissive behaviour maintain the hierarchy. Among free-living European wild rabbits observed 24 h non-stop, dominant males spent 16% of their time on aggressive interactions, whereas dominant females spent 7% and subordinate females spent 2% of their time involved in aggressive interactions (Mykytowycz & Rowley 1958). In the wild, does have been found to be more aggressive than bucks (Southern 1948; Myers & Poole 1961), and to fight as strongly (Lockley 1961) mainly over breeding nests (Cowan & Garson 1985), and they can be more aggressive towards juvenile does than towards juvenile bucks (Cowan 1987). When the number of wild rabbits living together increases, fighting increases dramatically (Myers 1966; Myers et al. 1971). Young bucks normally move to a new social group before starting their first breeding season, while young does stay on to breed in their natal group (Parer 1982; Webb et al. 1995).

In a study of New Zealand White (NZW) rabbits kept in a semi-natural enclosure, 20 different social behaviours and their changes with age were described (Lehmann 1991). Lehmann grouped the behaviours into indifferent contacts, amicable behaviour, subdominant behaviour, aggressive behaviour and fights. This shows that rabbits have a wide repertoire of behaviours that they are simply unable to perform in a cage, and that group-housed rabbits needs to be given space and furnishings that enable them to evade aggressive encounters. Lehmann (1991) found that aggressive behaviour was rare in the young NZW rabbits, but it may have occurred already at 30 days of age.

The rabbit has three specialised scent glands. These are located in the anal region, the groin and under the chin (Mykytowycz 1968). Rabbit territory is scent-marked by placing faeces in dunghills, and by pressing the under-chin against structures in the environment so that droplets from the rabbit's submandibular glands are excreted through pores of the skin (Mykytowycz 1968). Male rabbits scent-mark more intensively than females and dominant individuals more than subdominant animals; this is correlated with larger anal and submandibular glands in dominant males (Mykytowycz 1968). Bucks also scent-mark does and young rabbits of their breeding group by spraying urine on them (Mykytowycz 1968).

Does scent-mark their young, attack other young within the same breeding group, and may chase and even kill young from other breeding groups (Mykytowycz 1968). Does may attack even their own young if they have been smeared with foreign urine (Mykytowycz 1968).

Biological data

Basic biological data presented here may be of interest for research purposes as well as for checking animal health. Cardiovascular and respiratory functions are of great importance for anaesthesia and normal values are presented in Table 28.1. Haematology and blood chemistry parameters can be used to assess the homeostasis of the animals prior to surgery or dosing as well as after any experimental procedure. Normal haematology values are shown in Table 28.2 and normal values of clinical blood chemistry are shown in Table 28.3.

The body temperature of rabbits varies from 38.5 to 39.5 °C (Ruckebusch et al. 1991), but Flecknell & Thomas (2015) report 38°C. A calm and resting rabbit has a lower body temperature than the agitated animal. Rabbits' ears are richly vascularised and are used in regulating body temperature (Kawoto et al. 1989).

It is normal for the urine of rabbits to vary widely in colour, from different shades of yellow, light brown and even reddish; various degrees of turbidity are also normal because of the high concentration of calcium and mucus, among other reasons (Jenkins 2008). Red colouration of urine may result from porphyrins excreted by the kidneys depending

Table 28.1 Normal values of cardiovascular and respiratory functions in rabbits (Gillett 1994; Flecknell 2015) (*Flecknell & Thomas 2015).

Parameter	Values
Respiratory rate (breaths/min)	40–60 (55)*
Heart rate (beats/min)	200–300 (220)*
Tidal volume (ml/kg)	4–6
Arterial systolic pressure (mmHg)	90–130
Arterial diastolic pressure (mmHg)	80–90
Arterial blood pO_2 (kPa)	11–12.5
Arterial blood pCO_2 (kPa)	5–6.5
Arterial blood pH	7.35–7.45

Table 28.2 Normal values of haematology in rabbits (Jenkins 2008).

Parameter	Values
Erythrocytes (count) ($\times 10^6/mm^3$)	5.4–7.6
Haematocrit/packed cell volume (%)	33–50
Haemoglobin (g/dl)	10.0–17.4
Mean corpuscular volume (μm^3)	60–69
Mean corpuscular haemoglobin (pg)	19–22
Mean corpuscular haemoglobin concentration (%)	30–35
Leucocytes ($\times 10^3/mm^3$)	5.2–12.5
Lymphocytes (%)	30–85
Neutrophils (%)	20–75
Eosinophils (%)	1–4
Basophils (%)	1–7
Monocytes (%)	1–4
Platelets ($\times 10^3/mm^3$)	250–650

Table 28.3 Normal values of blood clinical chemistry in rabbits (Jenkins 2008).

Parameter	Values
Alanine aminotransferase (IU/l)	27.4–72.2
Aspartate aminotransferase (IU/l)	10.0–78.0
Creatine kinase (IU/l)	58.6–175.0
Bilirubin (mmol/l)	2.6–17.1
Blood urea nitrogen (mmol/l)	4.6–10.7
Creatinine (µmol/l)	74–171
Glucose (mmol/l)	5.5–8.2
Calcium (mmol/l)	2.2–3.9
Phosphorus (mmol/l)	1.0–2.2

on the diet, and this may be mistaken for blood (Jenkins 2008). The urine volume produced daily is 50–75 ml/kg and the urinary pH is 8–9 (Jenkins 2008). Rabbit urine is alkaline due to the herbivorous diet although lower urinary pH can result from high protein intake and catabolic states such as starvation and severe disease (Jenkins 2008).

Reproduction

In this section, we describe natural reproduction in European wild rabbits from different studies, and in the Breeding section further ahead, all aspects of breeding domesticated rabbits are presented.

The European wild rabbit is a seasonal breeder, with seasonality determined by the interaction of day length, climate, nutrition, population density, social status and other factors (Bell & Webb 1991; Bell 1999). In Australian wild rabbits, sexual maturity occurs at the age of 5–7 months in bucks and 9–12 months in does depending on climate (Myers *et al.* 1994). Before mating, an elaborate courtship takes place – the rabbits circle around each other, parade side by side, jump over each other and sniff the genital region (Lehmann 1991). When the doe allows mating, she raises the hindquarters (Bennett 2001). Mating takes only a few seconds, after which the buck falls to one side or backwards (Bennett 2001).

Gestation in European wild rabbits lasts 28–30 days (Bell 1999). Some days before the birth, the doe digs a short underground tunnel or 'stop' either within the main warren or separately from it and within this constructs a nest (Bell 1999). High-ranking does often give birth in a special breeding chamber dug as an extension to the warren, whereas some of the subordinate females are chased away from the warren and forced to give birth in isolated breeding 'stops' (Mykytowycz 1968). The survival rate of the young is much higher for high-ranking than the low-ranking females (Mykytowycz 1968). Does of both European wild rabbits and free-ranging NZW rabbits collect and carry grass to their burrows and shortly before giving birth pluck their own fur from the belly, sides and dewlap, which is placed on top of the grass (González-Mariscal *et al.* 1994; Bell 1999).

The size of the litter is five to six young for European wild rabbits (Vaughan *et al.* 2000). Once the young are born, the doe leaves the burrow and covers the entrance with soil, urine marks it and then leaves (Mykytowycz 1968). She returns to the burrow once daily, and then digs herself into the burrow and nurses her young for just a few minutes (Bell 1999). After 21 days, the doe ceases closing the burrow or breeding stop and the young come up to the surface (Bell 1999). In NZW does, the young are about 18 days old when she stops closing the entrance to the breeding stop and the young are nursed outside (Lehmann 1989).

At 4 weeks of age, the young are very mobile, and soon after emergence they leave their breeding stop and do not return to it again (Lloyd & McCowan 1968). They start seeking forage, but continue to suckle for several more weeks. The mothers are not preferred social partners for NZW young except during suckling attempts (Lehmann 1989). Milk production reaches a maximum about 2 weeks after giving birth, then declines during the fourth week, although lactation may continue for an additional 2–4 weeks (Hagen 1974). Lehmann (1989) also found that, in NZW rabbits, nursing was uncommon after 4 weeks and the doe littered again within a few days, although suckling attempts occurred up to 60 days. At 8 weeks of age, the young consume approximately 90% of their intake in the form of plant proteins (Hagen 1974).

Normal behaviour (wild and captive)

The rabbit has been reported to be crepuscular, i.e. mostly active during dawn and dusk (Cobb 2011). The old bucks emerge first, about 4 h before sunset (Mykytowycz & Rowley 1958), and at sunset 90% of the rabbits have emerged from the burrows up to the ground (Fraser 1992). The rabbits are above ground for 11–14 h of the diurnal cycle (Mykytowycz & Rowley 1958). When they are above ground, they spend about 44% of their time eating, 33% inactive, 13% moving and 10% on other activities including social interactions (Gibb 1993). Young NZW rabbits were active for an average of 30% of the daytime, during which, feeding on pellets occupied one-third of this time, grazing took one-third of this time and the remaining one-third was spent in exploring, gnawing, intensive locomotion, social interactions and, for the older rabbits, sexual behaviour (Lehmann 1989). The rabbit's choice of habitat depends on the opportunities to find shelter and protection; where the soil is loose it digs burrows, and where the soil is more compact it often seeks protection in dense vegetation (Kolb 1994).

Foraging is performed over an area known as the home-range; this is much larger than the 'territory' that breeding groups defend. The size of the home-range varies depending on food availability, number of rabbits in the group and other factors (Donnelly 1997). Wild rabbits have been found to gather in large colonies of up to hundreds of animals under good feeding conditions or at high population densities (Myers & Poole 1963). The home-range of European wild rabbits has been found to vary between studies from 0.4 to 2.0 ha (Cowan & Bell 1986), 0.8 ha (Vastrade 1987), 5 ha (Myers *et al.* 1994) and 0.7–2.5 ha (Devillard *et al.* 2008). In nature, rabbits mainly eat grass and herbs, but also fruit, roots, leaves and bark (Cheeke 1987). Rabbits need coarse fibre for their digestion, not just lush grass (Brooks 1997; Meredith 2000). The colon of the rabbit separates faecal waste from the B vitamin-rich faecal pellets, made up of microbes that the rabbit will ingest (Björnhag 1981). These smaller, soft and green-coated faecal pellets produced by the caecum 4–8 h after feed intake (Carpenter *et al.* 1995; Brooks 1997) are picked up directly from the anus, whereas the fibrous pellets are placed on specific latrines close to the territory borders (Donnelly 1997).

The rabbit is a prey animal with many enemies. When threatened, rabbits stamp with a hind foot that makes the other rabbits flee underground (Mykytowycz 1968; Black & Vanderwolf 1969). If caught by a predator, they may emit a high-pitched distress scream (Cowan & Bell 1986), which may cause the predator to release it. Green & Flinders (1981) found that the pygmy rabbit could emit alarm calls up to 6000 Hz. Apart from this and some low sounds during mating and mother–young care, rabbits are silent animals.

Rabbit movement consists of hopping, crawling and intensive locomotion (i.e., running, start-and-stop, jumping, double jumps and capriole) (Kraft 1979; Lehmann 1989). Hopping is used to travel longer distances; whereas crawling is performed when feeding on grass or exploring on the spot and during social encounters (Lehmann 1989). Rabbits rear when they are looking at their surroundings (Lockley 1961). The rabbit has a light and fragile skeleton that only makes up 7–8% of the body weight (Donnelly 1997).

Rabbits have good eyesight with a maximum field of vision of almost 360° (Peiffer et al. 1994). They have dichromatic (two-colour) vision where the retina mainly has green sensitive cones and a small area of blue sensitive cones (Lumpkin & Seidensticker 2011). They have a high density of rods, which help them to see well in lowlight conditions, such as dawn and dusk. However, they lack the tapetum lucidum which reflects light through the retina, and this prevents them to see light in low light conditions (Lumpkin & Seidensticker 2011). Rabbits have very poor depth perception making it difficult to see how far away things are and poor visual acuity making the vision a bit blurred (Lumpkin & Seidensticker 2011).

Rabbits have a very good sense of smell reflected in the large size of the olfactory lobes in the brain and in the 100 million olfactory receptor cells in the nose (Lumpkin & Seidensticker 2011). They use the interior lining of the nostrils to smell and have a vomeronasal organ, which consist of two small openings in the roof of the mouth with ducts that lead to receptors (Lumpkin & Seidensticker 2011). Domesticated European rabbits have 17,000 taste buds, and they show preference for sweet and salt, and dislike bitter and sour (Lumpkin & Seidensticker 2011). They can also discriminate between different sugars, and prefer maltose to sucrose and fructose (Lumpkin & Seidensticker 2011). When chewing on vegetation, the rabbit's salivary secretion break starch down into maltose, and they eat little fruit, which contains fructose (Lumpkin & Seidensticker 2011).

Rabbits have 20–25 whiskers on each side of the upper lip, and these are endowed with nerves at the base (Lumpkin & Seidensticker 2011). The whiskers help rabbits to orientate in the dark and to place their mouth correctly on vegetation before biting it off.

Rabbits have longer ears in warmer climate, which follow Allen's rule who has stated that mammals living in colder climates have relatively smaller ears and tails than do their relatives that live in warmer climates (Lumpkin & Seidensticker 2011). Rabbits have good hearing, and in colder climate the smaller ears are compensated by the fact that sound travel better in cold and wet air (Lumpkin & Seidensticker 2011).

Rabbits regularly perform comfort behaviours such as licking and scratching themselves, shaking the body, rubbing against objects and stretching their body.

Sources/supply of laboratory rabbits

Laboratories usually buy rabbits of defined health status from designated accredited breeders (Eveleigh & Pease 1976; Eveleigh et al. 1984). There has been a decline in the number of breeding units in Europe due to the diminishing use of rabbits in laboratory animal experimentation. There is an increased focus on the inclusion of the Three Rs in breeding colony management, which means often laboratory rabbits are bred to meet customer demand rather than bred in anticipation of demand. This has led to an overall reduction in the number of rabbits being bred. There has been progress in replacement of rabbits in several studies for example replacing the rabbit pyrogen test with an *invitro* method using a plasma-derived alternative (Valentini et al. 2019).

Use in research

Of the 9.5 million animals used for experimental and other scientific purposes in the 27 member states of the European Union in 2015–2017 (Report 2019 on the Usage of Animals for Scientific Purposes in the EU membership states 2015–2017), rabbits use counted around 350 thousand animals each year. The most commonly used species were mice (5.7 million), followed by rats (1.5 million) and fish (500 thousand zebra fish and 700 thousand other fish). In United States, it was the second (18.4%, 145,841 rabbits) most commonly used laboratory animal covered by the Animal Welfare Act in research (they do not report rodents) (USDA 2017).

The most common breed used for laboratory research is the NZW rabbits (DAD-IS 2018), which was originally bred for meat production (Bennett 2001). Other breeds used include the Dutch (Batchelor 1999). In the domesticated rabbit, differences in weight between breeds are large: from around 1 kg (Netherland Dwarfs) to 4 kg (NZW) and up to 10 kg (German Grey Rabbits) (Bennett 2001). There is large variation in the size and position of ears, body conformation and coat colour between breeds of rabbits (Bennett 2001). When kept as laboratory rabbits, NZWs tend to lay down excessive amounts of body fat in the abdominal cavity and around the chin when they grow older. This occurs irrespective of whether they are kept single-housed in a cage or group-housed in a pen (Batchelor 1999). This is more likely to occur if rabbits are fed *ad libitum* on pellets rather than hay.

Rabbits have traditionally been used for antibody production, development of new surgical techniques, physiology and toxicity studies when testing new drugs (Bősze & Houdebine 2006). Rabbits can be used for collecting more blood, cells and tissue, have a longer life span and their immune system genes are more like humans than rodents (Esteves et al. 2018). Rabbits have a more diverse genetic background than mice, which is an advantage when studying complex human disease models such as atherosclerosis (Bősze & Houdebine 2006).

Rabbits were used in research already by Pasteur (1885), who produced a vaccine against rabies by studying the tissue of infected rabbits. The first animal model of cancer caused by a mammalian virus used the cottontail rabbit papillomavirus (CRPV) (Shope & Hurst 1933). A pronuclear injection created the first transgenic rabbits (Brem *et al*. 1985). Much of what we know today about the structure, function and regulated expression of antibodies comes from studies of rabbits (Esteves *et al*. 2018). Even though there has been a decline in the use of polyclonal antibodies produced in rabbits, there is still a demand for these antibodies (Cooper & Paterson 2008). While rabbits are still being used in pyrogen testing of intravenous fluids and other technical products intended for patients, other test methods without live animals have been proved effective in replacing the use of rabbits in these tests (Hoffman *et al*. 2005; Valentini *et al*. 2019).

Rabbits have been used in the study of atherosclerosis after being fed high fat and high-cholesterol diets, which lead to the development of atherosclerotic lesions in the major arteries after approximately 2 months (Yanni 2004). The Watanabe heritable hyperlipidaemic (WHHL) rabbits, which carry a spontaneous mutation for hyperlipidaemia, is used as a model to study hypercholesterolaemia and atherosclerosis *in vivo* (Watanabe *et al*. 1985; Wetterholm *et al*. 2007). The myocardial infarction-prone Watanabe heritable hyperlipidaemic (WHHLMI) rabbits have been developed as a model to study human acute coronary syndromes (Shiomi & Jianglin 2008).

In safety studies, rabbits are used to detect teratogenic effects of candidate drugs because the embryological development of the rabbit foetus is well-known, the gestation period is short and rabbits produce a large number of offspring (Wooding & Burton 2008).

The use of rabbits in research have extended to many human diseases, for example syphilis, tuberculosis, HIV-AIDS, acute hepatic failure and diseases caused by noroviruses, ocular herpes and papillomaviruses (Esteves *et al*. 2018). Also, rabbit viral haemorrhagic disease and myxomatosis offers models to understand co-evolution between a vertebrate host and viral pathogens (Esteves *et al*. 2018).

General husbandry

Enclosures

During the last 10–20 years, the approach to housing rabbits has changed considerably, and group housing in floor pens has been introduced in many laboratories and countries (Figure 28.1). In the 2003 Guidelines for the Housing of Rabbits in Scientific Institutions in Australia (Animal Research Review Panel 2003), two key recommendations are that '*Rabbits should be housed in groups in pens*' and '*Rabbits should not be housed singly in conventional (un-enriched) cages except in exceptional circumstances …*'. European guidelines (Council of Europe 2006; European Commission 2007) also recommend that wherever it is possible, rabbits should be kept in pens. Housing in pens enables rabbits to express social behaviours and to exercise (Heath & Stott 1990; Batchelor 1991). The RSPCA/UFAW (Hawkins *et al*. 2008) resource recommends that young rabbits and older females should be housed in harmonious pairs or social groups

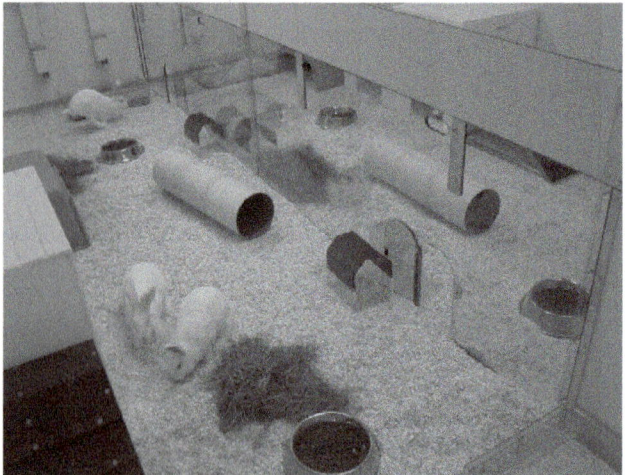

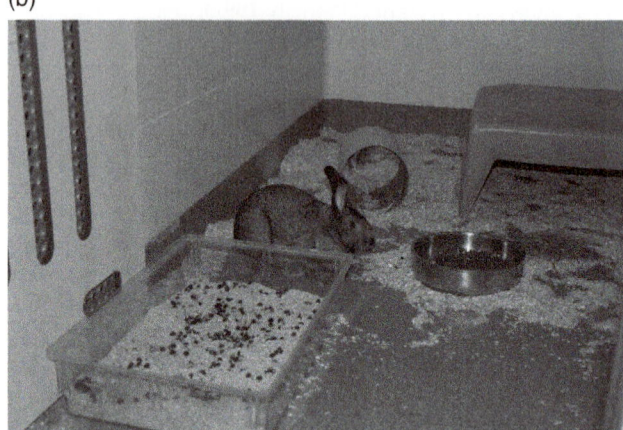

Figure 28.1 Group housing of NZW does in a floor pen (a) and floor housing of a male Chinchilla with a latrine area (b) (courtesy of Joanna Moore).

unless veterinary advice or study design recommends differently. Adult entire males, on the other hand, are recommended to be singly housed due to their territorial behaviour and the consequent risks of serious injury.

Floor pens should be large enough and include complexity (Baumans 1997) for the rabbits to be able to carry out basic behaviours such as locomotion, rearing, grooming and avoiding cage mates. European Commission (2007, Table B.1) recommends that rabbits should be provided with at least the same pen floor area as in cages, and an extra floor area of 3000 cm^2 per rabbit should be added for three to six rabbits and thereafter 2500 cm^2 for every additional rabbit over six. This is much less than recommended by Morton *et al*. (1993), who suggested that group houses should have a clear area of 20,000 cm^2 with an overall minimum floor area of 6000–8000 cm^2 per rabbit for groups up to six rabbits. One problem with using weight as a criterion for determining floor area is that young animals are more active and might need more space to carry out play behaviours (Stauffacher *et al*. 1994), as rabbits grow older they need space to avoid conflict. Swiss legislation from 1991 requires that each rabbit must be able to hop for several steps or to jump up and down onto a shelf; however, both would be ideal for floor-pen-housed rabbits. This may help to maintain a level of fitness and reduce the occurrence of disuse osteoporosis (Morton et al. 1993). European Commission (2007) recommends that rabbits younger than 10 weeks should be provided with a minimum enclosure size of 4000 cm^2 and a minimum floor area per animal of 800 cm^2 from weaning to 7 weeks and 1200 cm^2 from 7 to 10 weeks.

The height of floor pens should be 1.25 m, and enrichment objects should be placed so that they cannot be used for jumping over walls (Morton et al. 1993) or a cover should be put across the pen to prevent the rabbits jumping out. Table B.1 in European Commission (2007) recommends the same minimum height for pens as for cages, but this is too low to stop rabbits from jumping out of the pen. The pen should contain structures such as tunnels, fences and shelves that subdivide the space to provide visual barriers and so that the animals are able to initiate or avoid social contact. Examples of group housing of NZW does in a research laboratory are shown in Figure 28.1. It has been shown that trios are a stable compatible group number (Ferrante et al. 1992).

The floor should be solid and provided with enough bedding to allow digging or perforated, rather than grid or wire mesh (European Commission 2007). Wire floors should not be used unless a resting area is provided which is large enough to hold all rabbits at any one time (European Commission 2007). Morton et al. (1993) regarded dimple polycarbonate floors as the best type of floors in metal cages.

One concern when housing rabbits in floor pens is the occasional occurrence of spinal injury ('broken back'). If rabbits are sourced from breeders where they are cage-housed, it is recommended to introduce them to a slightly smaller pen at first (still compliant with Code of Practice), then open access to the larger area after 1–2 weeks. This prevents newly arrived rabbits becoming startled and suddenly running or jumping thus causing themselves injury before their muscles are toned by exercise. Providing a complex environment with plenty of hides and obstacles spread around the pen also reduces the straight-line distance and speed that a rabbit could run.

When rabbits are offered a latrine area, they will use it and show a preference to have a latrine area away from where they rest (Moore 2018). Rabbits have been seen to avoid sawdust based substrates (Turner et al. 1992), and in floor pens having an area where they can avoid sawdust may improve their well-being. A raised resting areas with a perforated base could be used to enable them to regulate their body temperature, and observations of rabbits confirm that they prefer this over resting in sawdust (Moore 2018).

Laboratory rabbits were traditionally housed individually in cages, depending on the research purpose. One reason for individual housing has been the problems with aggression that may arise in group housing, especially between males. Several different cage types made of metal, plastic and wire grid have been common until one or two decades ago (Stauffacher et al. 1994; Morton et al. 1993). They may still exist in some countries, however; cages must allow rabbits to sit upright without ears touching the cage ceiling. Cages with solid sides, back and top should be avoided as they tend to isolate the animals, and prevent them from seeing the source of disturbance, which may cause them to be startled, and in breeding units, lead to losses due to cannibalism (Stauffacher et al. 1994). It is, therefore, recommended that barred 'windows' occupy 30–50 % of the total wall area (Stauffacher et al. 1994). Clear Perspex can also be used to increase the visibility for the rabbit. Simple measures, such as turning racks of cages to face each other, allow rabbits to have sight of conspecifics, even while caged. There should still be some solid wall area so the rabbit can move from vision. Staff should be encouraged to knock before entering the rabbit room, or creating a noise to alert the rabbits of their presence in the room.

Appendix A of the European Convention for the protection of vertebrate animals used for experimental and other scientific purposes (Council of Europe 2006) recommends larger areas and heights than in the preceding Convention from 1986, and these have been adopted by the Commission (European Commission 2007). The minimum floor area and minimum height in cages and pens for rabbits over 10 weeks of age and for does with a litter is presented in Table 28.4. The weights are for the final body weight that any rabbit will reach in the housing. The minimum floor area is for one or two socially harmonious animals. In cages, a raised area should be provided. If there are scientific or veterinary justifications for not providing a raised area, then the floor area should be 33% larger for a single rabbit and 60% larger for two rabbits.

Improved cages have been developed and tested in parallel with the development of new regulations for housing rabbits. These cages generally have a larger floor area and greater height to enable more upright sitting, a shelf for rabbits to hop up onto or hide under, racks to make hay feeding easier and flexible cage racks so that several cages can be built together (Figure 28.2). Hawkins et al. (2008) provide practical suggestions on how to house and manage laboratory rabbits based on their needs. Caged rabbits use boxes and shelves as sources of enrichment and lookout posts (Hansen & Berthelsen 2000), and the presence of the shelf reduces restlessness, grooming, bar-gnawing and nervous responses when being captured (Berthelsen & Hansen 1999). When testing boxes for hiding as enrichments to caged male

Table 28.4 Recommendations for minimum enclosure dimensions and space allowance for one or two socially harmonious rabbits over 10 weeks of age or a doe plus litter with additional area for nest boxes, and optimum shelf size and height from the enclosure floor (Council of Europe 2006; European Commission 2007).

Final body weight (kg)	Minimum floor area (cm^2)	Minimum height (cm)	Addition for nest boxes (cm^2)	Optimum shelf size (cm)	Optimum height of shelf (cm)
<3	3500	45	1000	55 × 25	25
3–5	4200	45	1200	55 × 30	25
>5	5400	60	1400	60 × 35	30

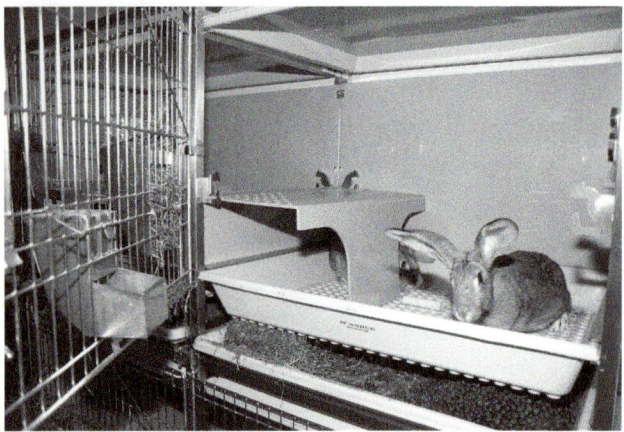

Figure 28.2 Caged rabbits can benefit from this cage, which links two cages to allow pair-housing (courtesy of Ann-Christine Nordkam).

rabbits, they turned them around and used them as latrine areas (Lidfors 1997). This supports the use of latrines also in caged rabbits. In UK, a couple of facilities have homemade adapted cage racks, which are joined vertically by 'ladders', allowing the rabbit to move up and down the rack, rather than across it. This promotes exercise and rabbits were noted to move up or down according to time of day.

Environmental provisions during transport

Very little research has been done into the effect of transport on rabbits. Batchelor (1999) found considerable differences in body weight in rabbits that were housed in group pens compared to solitary in cages after transportation. The loss of weight in rabbits after transport is mostly due to a loss of gastrointestinal contents, which account for about 10% of the total body weight (Swallow 1999). These losses are probably maximal after about 15 h of transport and similar to depriving animals of food and water for the same time (Swallow 1999). It can take up to 7 days to recover the loss in live weight (Swallow 1999). Research on the effect of providing male rabbits with or without hay and with change or no change in the feed after a 10 h transport by truck, plane and truck showed that the provision of hay significantly reduced the occurrence of diarrhoea (L. Lidfors unpublished observation).

The rabbits should be in good condition and good health before transport. Most rabbits must be transported from the breeder to the laboratory, and this may be done in an animal transport truck, railway or airplane. Transportation vehicles should be equipped to monitor temperature, and provided with ventilation that can cool the air during warm weather and provide heating during cold weather.

Rabbits are most often transported in containers made of rigid plastic with a wire mesh screen covering air vents (Swallow et al. 2005). This mesh may have a filter cover to protect the rabbit from the environment. Each transport box will have a viewing panel on the top so the rabbit can be observed. The containers have sawdust on the floor, and rabbits are usually individually kept to avoid injury (Swallow et al. 2005). The height of the container should be restricted to prevent back injury caused by the rabbit kicking out (Swallow et al. 2005). If the containers are constructed without a wire mesh liner, it must have wire screening cover on all air vents (Swallow et al. 2005). A source of water, for example a gel and feed, must be provided (Olfert et al. 1993; Batchelor 1999). See also Chapter 12: Transportation of laboratory animals.

After arrival at the new animal housing, the rabbits should be checked for any health problems and injuries, which could either be caused by the transport or have been acquired before the transport. Rabbits should be given time for acclimatisation after the transport before they are used for research. This depends on the potential stress that the animals have experienced during transport, which in turn depends on many factors such as the duration of the transport, the age of the animals and the change of the social environment (European Commission 2007). It is also important to match care routines with those of the supplier. Where this is not possible, it is important to be mindful of the dramatic change in environment for the rabbits, requiring adaptation to new routines. It is good practice also to match feeding with supplier, or at least make changes in feeding slowly over a week or so. This is because rabbits are hindgut fermenters, so the bacterial flora need time to adapt (Björnhag 1981).

Environmental enrichment

Abnormal behaviours in rabbits can be reduced by providing environmental enrichment in their cage or floor pen. Roughage, hay, hay blocks and chew sticks are recommended as suitable enrichment (Council of Europe 2006; European Commission 2007), forage is also a good source of enrichment, which can be easy to offer when rabbits are housed in floor pens. Morton et al. (1993) suggested the following enrichment for caged rabbits: straw, hay, hay blocks, hydroponic grass, pieces of wood or chew sticks, hay rack, small cardboard boxes, taking them out of the cage for handling/ petting or for exercise and relief of boredom, provision of bedding, vet beds for pregnant and nesting does (additionally to the required nest box, authors comment) and background noise. Gunn (1994) found that stereotypic behaviour in caged rabbits was reduced by the provision of hay, wooden sticks and wire balls. Singly housed male rabbits interacted most often with hay, less with hay blocks, even less with a plastic box and least with chewing sticks (Lidfors 1997), and showed the highest preference for hay, then hay blocks, chewing sticks and lastly a plastic box (Lidfors 1996). This shows that hay is very important for rabbits, and it should be regarded as a dietary requirement as rabbits need long fibre for digestion and caecal motility. Large cardboard boxes/tunnels are good enrichment item as the rabbit can climb on to it as a lookout area, walk through it, rip the card from it and rest in it.

The enrichment items used most often are those that the rabbits can chew on (Huls et al. 1991; Lidfors 1997; Berthelsen & Hansen 1999) and high-fibre objects are preferred, with hay or straw remaining effective enrichments for long periods (Brummer 1975; Lidfors 1997). If the supplementary hay is ground, it is ineffective at reducing problem behaviours, demonstrating a need for long fibre (Mulder et al. 1992), which is also a basic nutritional requirement. Hay and straw also cause less weight gain than proprietary fibre sticks or compressed grass cubes (Lidfors 1997). Studies on dietary enrichments, including the supply of fibrous food to reduce boredom, are hay (Berthelsen & Hansen 1999); grass cubes or hay in a bottle (Lidfors 1997) and fresh grass (Leslie *et al.* 2004). Abnormal maternal behaviours and trichophagia or fur-chewing (Brummer 1975; Mulder *et al.* 1992) are eliminated in caged rabbits when hay or straw is given (Beynen *et al.* 1992). Also, consider olfactory enrichment for rabbits, as this is an important sense and often overlooked. Tactile enrichment, such as bedding substrate to allow digging behaviour should also be considered.

In safety studies, hay may be a risk factor, and Poggiagliolmi *et al.* (2011), therefore, tested the effect of cardboard rolls, cardboard rings and rubber balls with a bell inside. The rabbits tested with these enrichments showed more general chewing behaviour and less sitting than the control rabbits. Mirrors placed in the living area of caged rabbits increase the time they spend there, and especially the time that they spend investigating their environment and feeding (Jones & Phillips 2005; Dalle Zotte *et al.* 2009). The mirrors probably stimulate activity by increasing the amount of movement perceived by the rabbit (Jones & Phillips 2005). If the racks are placed opposite to each other so that the rabbits can see other rabbits, that may also be a form of enrichment (Morton *et al.* 1993), but they still need a refuge where they can hide from the other rabbit if they need to.

Giving individually housed rabbits access to a refuge area with objects to play with was suggested by Verga *et al.* (2007). Seaman *et al.* (2008) tested how much individually housed rabbits would work (by pushing doors with increasing weights) to get access to a platform or limited social contact. They found that they were as motivated to get access to social contact as to food, and almost as motivated to be near a platform, but they rarely used those (Seaman *et al.* 2008).

When housing entire males for years due to breeding or other reasons, one way to enrich their environment could be to place them individually in an exercise arena at regular intervals. This allows them to move around on a larger floor surface, to investigate enrichment objects and to be exposed to odours from other males that have been exercised before them. Knutsson (2011) evaluated this for stud males kept at a pharmaceutical company and found that moving and sitting was more common in the exercise pens whereas lying and eating was more common in the home cages. There were no differences in behaviour when the rabbits were exercised once or three times per week (Knutsson 2011). When rabbits were exercised, the rabbits watching them from their home cage became more active. In rabbits exercised once per week, corticosterone from blood samples were elevated after exercise the first week compared to the week before exercise, but not during week 4 and 8 (Knutsson 2011). Exercised rabbits lost some weight compared to the non-exercised rabbits, and there were no general health problems (Knutsson 2011).

Another feature of an environmental enrichment plan is to include an element of predictability. This includes having regular hours for certain maintenance and care procedures, allowing the same staff to care for a group of animals to promote recognition of individual staff and using the same laboratory for interventions such as sampling, dosing, measuring, scanning. See also Chapter 10: Enrichment: animal welfare and scientific validity.

Feeding/watering

In the wild, rabbits usually graze during their active periods at dawn and dusk (Lockley 1961), or during early morning and at night (Cheeke 1987). Facility lighting can mimic natural dawn and dusk to promote normal feeding behaviour in rabbits (see section Light and noise). Krohn *et al.* (1999) compared feeding laboratory rabbits in the morning with in the afternoon and they found that abnormal behaviours were reduced in the rabbits fed at 14.00 h compared to the rabbits that were fed at 08.00 h.

Laboratory rabbits in cages are almost invariably not fed the diet of grass for which they are adapted. There is little evidence that they prefer a grass diet to one based on compound feed (Leslie *et al.* 2004). Despite this, it is often beneficial to supplement their ration of compound pellets with dietary enrichment, as well as providing adequate nutrients (National Research Council (NRC) 1977). In particular, fibre (Lehmann 1990) will increase the time spent procuring food and reduce abnormal behaviours such as chewing their cage (Leslie *et al.* 2004). The visual stimulus of a varied diet is particularly important (Ruckebusch *et al.* 1971). Hay should make up a larger part of the feed intake of adult rabbits, and at the same time be an important enrichment (see also Chapter 10: Enrichment: animal welfare and scientific validity).

Water should always be available *ad libitum* (Mader 1997). Rabbits fed on dry diets require approximately 120 ml water/kg body weight (Cheeke 1987), or 10% of the body weight per 24 h (Meredith 2000). More water is required for growing animals, pregnant and lactating females and for rabbits fed high-fibre diets (Cizek 1961). Use of bottles or drinker nozzles rather than bowls is useful to measure water intake. Lack of water intake is often an early indicator of rabbits not being well, whether caused by study procedures or other reasons.

Social housing

The major factors that need to be considered when group-housing rabbits are compatibility of individual animals, size of pens, stocking density, husbandry practices and environmental enrichment (Morton *et al.* 1993). Rabbits can be group-housed either in floor pens or in cages. In the latter case, weight and size limitations usually restrict this to pair-housing (Bigler & Oester 1994; Huls *et al.* 1991; Stauffacher 1993), but joining several cages together, that increase the floor area can allow for one or two more rabbits. This combines the benefits of cage housing (e.g. hygiene and experimental purposes, with animal welfare interests) and has been established in several countries (Stauffacher *et al.* 1994). While Stauffacher *et al.* (1994) report that groups of up to 20 laboratory rabbits have been successfully managed as stock and to produce polyclonal antibodies, for monitoring and observation reasons the number of rabbits kept in group pens should not exceed six to eight mature animals (Morton *et al.* 1993; Stauffacher *et al.* 1994). Practical experiences from vaccine studies, however, shows that up to 10 rabbits have been kept together without problems.

The degree of compatibility of grouped rabbits depends on factors such as strain, individual characteristics, sex, age and weight, size and structuring of pens, methods of husbandry and the interest and ability of the animal care staff (Bell & Bray 1984; Zain 1988; Morton *et al.* 1993; Stauffacher 1993). Some of the small strains of rabbits may show more aggression than the larger strains (Stauffacher *et al.* 1994), for example, Dutch rabbits are more aggressive than NZW, whereas Lops are more docile (Morton *et al.* 1993). Individual animals may be highly aggressive, and fights can occur unexpectedly, even in groups that have been stable for a long time and in which an apparently stable dominance hierarchy has formed (Morton *et al.* 1993). Incompatible rabbits fight when placed together in a group, and the greatest problems occur when placing adult males together (Morton *et al.* 1993). The best option is to form female groups from litter mates which have been kept together from weaning (Zain 1988). Groups of intact, mature females not intended for breeding can be kept together (Morton *et al.* 1993). Fighting can occur in groups of does, and a dominant female in oestrus can mount and damage the skin on the backs of other females and harass the group (Morton *et al.* 1993). Groups of rabbits need to be carefully selected and regularly monitored. It is important to check underneath each rabbit at least weekly to ensure there are no abdominal wounds that could be missed if the rabbits are only observed from above.

During resting, does, bucks and older young kept in mixed groups congregate and snuggle against each other or engage in mutual grooming (Stauffacher 1992). Does have demonstrated a weak preference for a large, enriched, solitary pen over a group pen, but a strong preference for a group pen over a smaller, barren, solitary pen (Held *et al.* 1995). From around 10 weeks of age, it may be necessary to house males individually to avoid fighting (Morton *et al.* 1993). Groups of males kept in proximity to females tend to fight and urinate more frequently (Portsmouth 1987). Castration of males kept for longer periods in the laboratory may be one solution to keeping them in groups, although this raises ethical issues, as discussed by Hawkins *et al.* (2008). The practical experience from castration of males is that aggression is reduced and stable for a long time afterwards (Lennart Lindberg, personal communication). Castration should be carried out only by qualified persons when the males reach sexual maturity and before they start to show aggressive behaviour, about 3-4 weeks after weaning (Morton *et al.* 1993; Stauffacher *et al.* 1994). The testicles move down during sexual maturation, but can be withdrawn again via the cremaster muscle. Another consideration is the type of research the animals will be used for, as castration influences the animal's physiology and behaviour.

When establishing new groups of rabbits in floor pens, the best option is to wean and mix at the same time around 6 weeks of age (Morton *et al.* 1993). The supplier should be asked which rabbits have been kept together since birth, as this works the best (Zain 1988; Stauffacher 1993). Smaller groups may be more stable (Love & Hammond 1991). Some animals do not appear to settle well in groups, either because they are too dominant and bully the others or are too timid and prone to be bullied (Morton *et al.* 1993). When grouping rabbits that have been caged for 6 months or more, it may be difficult to avoid fighting or self-inflicted injuries (Morton *et al.* 1993). However, individually caged adult female rabbits of strains that are known to be docile can be paired successfully, preferably in structured cages (Stauffacher 1993). It is very important to provide refuge and hiding places for subordinate animals (Morton *et al.* 1993), and sufficient access to feed to prevent domination by some rabbits. It has been suggested that grouping rabbits in trios may reduce conflict.

Identification and sexing

Young rabbits are weaned at 5–7 weeks. At this time, the young are also sexed and males and females placed in separate cages. This procedure requires some training. The male rabbit's penis can be extruded from the age of 2 months, which is considerably later than weaning age (Harkness & Wagner 1995).

Many breeders also perform identity marking at weaning using subcutaneously implanted microchips, or ear tattoos, tags, etc. As a general principle, the least invasive method, compatible with the end use, should be chosen. Other options for identification include numbering on one ear with a water-based non-toxic marker pen, but this require remarking every few days.

Physical environment (including climatic)

Temperature and humidity

European guidelines recommend a mean room temperature for rabbits of 18 °C with a range of 15–21 °C (Council of Europe 2006; European Commission 2007). In rabbits, the low critical temperature is −7 °C and the high critical temperature is 28 °C (Spector 1956). Wild rabbits avoid high temperatures and stay away from sunshine, and during the day they stay in the cooler burrows (Gibb *et al.* 1978). The ears of the rabbit are highly vascular and can function as radiators (Harkness & Wagner 1995).

The relative humidity in rabbit facilities should not be less than 45% (European Commission 2007).

Light and noise

Rabbit rooms are recommended to have a regular light–dark cycle and to be isolated from external lighting fluctuations (Batchelor 1999). The lights in many laboratories are usually put on a 12:12 h light–dark cycle. Some laboratory facilities have introduced artificial dawn and dusk periods, which usually last 30 minutes. Sudden illumination of active rabbits may cause them to leap and possibly fracture the spine (Adams 1982). If there is a need to observe rabbits during the period of activity, a partially reversed lighting schedule can be used, because rabbits are crepuscular in their activity pattern (Batchelor 1999). The normal rest period can be disrupted by noise or scheduled feeding in the laboratory (Jilge 1991).

According to Iwarsson *et al.* (1994) the optimal light intensity in rabbit rooms should be 200 lux at 1 m above the floor. However, if the illumination level is too high it can lead to retinal degeneration in some albino mammals, which may also apply to NZW rabbits (Batchelor 1999). Cages with solid sides reduce the amount of light, and cages higher up in the rack have a higher light intensity (Batchelor 1999). In floor pens, shelves and boxes may provide hiding places from high light intensity.

The rabbit's hearing threshold has been reported to be 75–50 000 Hz with the most sensitive hearing between 2000 and 9000 Hz (Iwarsson *et al.* 1994). The rabbit is, therefore, sensitive to high-pitched sounds (Milligan *et al.* 1993), and sudden noise may scare rabbits and lead to injuries. A common practice is to use background music to attempt to mask sudden sounds, and this is claimed by some to result in lower excitability (Batchelor 1999). A good practice is to knock on the door or speak gently when entering the rabbit room.

Ventilation

European guidelines recommend 15–20 air changes per hour (Council of Europe 2006; European Commission 2007). However, it is possible to have 8–10 air changes per hour if cleaning routines are of high standard and stocking density is low (Adams 1982). There should be no draughts or turbulence in the rabbit room. If the ventilation is not working properly, high levels of ammonia and carbon dioxide may become a problem for the rabbits.

Ammonium level in animal housing should not exceed 14 ppm according to Boden *et al.* (2015), and these editors of Black's Veterinary Dictionary claim that a hydrolysis occur in stale litter in rabbit hutches which release ammonium in sufficient quantities to affect rabbits seriously. High ammonium levels can inactivate the cilia in the airways. *Black's Veterinary Dictionary* (Boden *et al.* 2015) suggest that use of peat moss as litter in rabbit trays and on the floor may counteract the effect of this hydrolysis. In a study of individually caged NZW rabbits, the mean ammonium concentration was 1.64 ppm (range 0.25 to 3.06 ppm) and the mean emission factor was 0.718 mg/(min x rabbit) (Ooms *et al.* 2008). Ammonium emission was significantly higher on day 7 and 14 before cleaning compared to days 1 and 8 when cages were clean (Ooms *et al.* 2008).

The rabbit moults two to three times per year. Rabbit hair may also be released during handling which increases the risk of laboratory animal allergen exposure to staff. In order to reduce the risk for Laboratory Animal Allergy, it is recommended for staff to wear facemasks and gloves when handling rabbits.

Hygiene

Since rabbits have a sensitive digestive system with intensive interaction between the intestine and its microbiological flora, the hygiene of the cage or pen where the rabbit is held is important. Rabbits are coprophagic, but they ingest only a certain type of small soft faecal pellets (caecotrophs), made up of microflora remnants, rich in vitamins and proteins. The remaining, fibrous faeces may contain coccidia spores and pinworm eggs that can re-infect the animal and the heavy breeds may develop cutaneous infections on their hindlegs from soiled bedding or wire floors (Bergdall & Dysko 1994).

The frequency of cleaning out and disinfection of pen floors, cage waste pans or other areas where the faeces and urine of the animals may accumulate depends on the number of animals in each cage or pen, the sizes of the animals, their diet and on other physical and practical arrangements in the animal rooms such as the efficiency of the ventilation equipment. It is not possible to give specific recommendations because circumstances vary between laboratories. Latrine areas can be provided to rabbits, using old rat cage bases, which help keep pens cleaner and mimics what happens in the wild. The room air should be perceived as fresh and clean without any smell. If there is any doubt, ammonia levels in the air can be measured. The animals should have clean fur coats and be clinically healthy. Over-zealous cleaning of any animal environment could be stressful to the animals because of changes to the olfactory environment (Batchelor 1999).

Health monitoring and quarantine and barrier systems

High health standards result in good welfare and good science. Most breeders use barrier breeding systems with regular health monitoring. The biosafety strategy of breeders includes control of entry of staff and goods into the breeding rooms; procedures for sterilisation of goods such as bedding, diets and other materials; and regular education and awareness training for staff. Strict barrier regimes avoid introduction of animals from elsewhere, but rely on re-deriving rabbit pups from pregnant does by caesarean section, after which the young are hand-reared. Some breeders even have regularly scheduled refurbishments of their breeding units as a part of their biohazard management.

Animal health records should show the frequency and interval of different samples taken, the result of analysis and the methods used as well as which laboratory was used. In Europe, the Federation of European Laboratory Animal Science Associations (FELASA) has issued recommendations for health monitoring laboratory animals in different situations, at the breeding site and in the research laboratory (FELASA 2014).

When rabbits are introduced to a colony, quarantine can be used as a precaution if there is any doubt about their health status, but most health problems of laboratory animals are subclinical. Thus, it is unlikely that there will be clinical signs of disease during the period of quarantine. Regular animal health monitoring by the breeder and good relations with the breeder combined with certain in-house sampling of animals in long-term studies can be a pragmatic way of handling surveillance of rabbit health.

Care of aged animals

Laboratory rabbits seldom become older than 3–4 years, unless used for specific studies of age-related disease. The exemption is breeding does and bucks and rabbits used for antibody production, which may be up to three years or a bit older. Still, it is far from being an ageing animal. Pet rabbits have been reported to have an average life expectancy of 8 to 13 years (Buseth & Saunders 2015), but a survey showed that the average lifespan of pet rabbits was only 4.2 years due to poor husbandry (Schepers *et al.* 2009). Despite the reduction in life span, regular health checks should include body condition, checking teeth are not abnormal or overgrown, checking for any skin lesions, lumps, back problems, abnormal weight loss or gain and checking the claws (Buseth & Saunders 2015). Sharp spurs can develop on molar teeth, due to uneven wearing as the teeth grow – these can cause painful cuts and sores on tongue and cheeks, which leads to anorexia. Monitor rabbit body condition score (Rabbit Welfare Association UK[1]) as thin rabbits indicate a need to check the teeth and fat rabbits indicate a need to check the diet.

Breeding

Females can be mated for the first time at 4–5 months if they are of a small breed, at least 5 months if they are of a medium breed (for example NZW, according to Bennet, 2001) and 6–9 months if they are of a large breed (Harkness & Wagner 1995). Bucks are usually used for breeding for the first time at about 6 months of age (Harkness & Wagner 1995). The decision to use a female for breeding is based on her age, clinical condition, weight (3–4 kg for NZW) and observation of periodic congestion of the vulva (Harkness & Wagner 1995).

The doe has a cycle of 16–18 days during which she is receptive for 12–14 days followed by 2–4 days when she refuses to mate (Patton 1994). Does may vary in receptivity due to individual differences, sexual stimulation and environmental factors, such as nutrition, light and temperature (Cheeke et al. 1987). Sometimes, does refuse to mate with a certain buck, possibly because the buck adopts a poor mounting position or because of his aggressiveness (Patton 1994). When the doe is receptive, the vulva changes colour (Cheeke et al. 1987) and it changes to a darker pink or red and becomes swollen and moist (Patton 1994). In captivity, the male's courtship behaviour is often restricted to tail flagging, urination and licking the genitalia (Patton 1994). A jet of urine (enurination) may also be directed at a doe (Patton 1994).

For mating, the doe should be taken to the buck's living area to avoid problems, i.e., either the doe attacking the buck due to not being receptive or the buck showing more interest in exploring and marking the new territory (Patton 1994; Bennett 2001). If the doe is not receptive, she becomes aggressive and produces a special vocalisation (B.-Å. Sandeberg, personal communication). When a receptive doe has been placed in the buck's living area, she raises her hindquarters to allow copulation (see Reproduction section for more details). If copulation does not occur within 2 minutes, she should be removed as injuries and stress to both doe and buck may occur if they are left together too long, and bucks may become poor breeders if does repeatedly reject them (Patton 1994). Giving them more space during mating could be good due to their natural courtship behaviours (see Lehmann 1991). If bucks are used several times in a 24 h period, they are often rested on the next day, but they can also be used for multiple matings several days in a row and then be rested for several days (Patton 1994). A common practice is to keep one buck for every 10 does, but many breeding facilities use up to one buck per 25 does (Patton 1994).

Ovulation is induced by mating and occurs 8–10 h (Bennet 2001) or 10–13 h after coitus (Patton 1994); it may also be induced artificially by injecting luteinising hormone or human chorionic gonadotropin, electrical or mechanical stimulation or after contact with other does (Patton 1994). Some does may fail to ovulate after coitus, possibly because of a deficiency of luteinising hormone (Fox & Krinsky 1968). The number of ova released has been found to be positively correlated with body weight (Staples & Holtkamp 1966). High ambient temperature has been found to depress the conception rate (Sittman et al. 1964). The most important influence on litter size has been found to be the parity of the doe (Rollins et al. 1963). Breeding of rabbits are done all year round, but Sittman et al. (1964) demonstrated seasonal variation in litter size, with the highest born in February and the lowest in September.

Pregnancy can be determined by palpating the developing foetuses at 12–14 days of pregnancy (Cheeke et al. 1987) or by looking at swelling of the mammary glands in late gestation (Patton 1994). The doe should be housed individually and have access to a nest box where she can construct a nest in good time before giving birth. Canali et al. (1991) found that the better the construction of the nest, the higher the survival rate of the young.

Domesticated rabbits have a gestation length of 28–34 days, with most litters being born on day 31–32 (Cheeke et al. 1987; Bennett 2001). The birth of each young takes less than 30 minutes, but young may be born several hours or days apart (3 days for live young (Patton 1994)).

Rabbits are born with no, or only little, hair cover, and are deaf and blind (Batchelor 1999). Pannon White rabbits were found to weigh 39–70 g at birth and they gained 9.2–18.5 g per day during the first 21 days of life (Poigner et al. 2000). The size of the litter is four to twelve young for domesticated rabbits (Batchelor 1999). It is possible to cross-foster kits if the litter is very large. At birth, the young rabbits are very sensitive to cold but, as their fur starts to grow some days after birth, they become less sensitive (Bennett 2001). The eyes open at 10–11 days (Kersten et al. 1989; Batchelor 1999), and hearing develops at the same time.

The composition of the milk is very nutritious with 10% protein, 12% fat and 2% lactose (Harkness & Wagner 1995). Rabbit milk contains high levels of k-Casein denatured in the stomach, which result in the milk being trapped in the stomach and only reaching the intestine in small amounts (McClellan et al. 2008). In a study of Dutch Belted rabbits, the nursing took place in the early morning and lasted for 2.7–4.5 minutes (Zarrow et al. 1965).

The does may be stressed by having the kits so close, as they leave them in the nest for most of the 24 h in nature. Different methods to keep doe and kits separated have been developed by rabbit breeders. Baumann et al. (2005) used a cat-flap at the nest entrance to mimic the wild European rabbit's behaviour for domesticated breeding. In commercial rabbit breeding, the young are weaned and separated from the doe at 6–7 weeks of age (Hagen 1974; Bennett 2001).

Post-partum mating usually occurs 4–8 weeks after birth of a litter, when the young have been weaned (Patton 1994) but can be done as early as 11 days post-partum (B-Å Sandeberg,

---

[1] https://rabbitwelfare.co.uk/rabbit-health/further-reading/body-condition-score/ (Accessed April 28, 2022)

personal communication). Does will mate immediately following parturition, and if the young are removed, sexual receptivity continues for at least 36 days (Hagen 1974; Patton 1994). Females are most difficult to breed at the peak of lactation – approximately the third week (Cheeke et al. 1987), which may be a result of loss of body weight (Patton 1994).

Laboratory procedures

Handling

Handlers should keep in mind that rabbits, as prey animals, naturally try to flee if they perceive a threat. Rabbits can recognise individual humans by their voice. Rabbits are rarely aggressive if handled in a calm and steady manner without intimidating the rabbit by unfamiliar sounds or odours.

To pick up an animal, first speak to it and approach it quietly, then the scruff of the neck is grasped firmly with one hand (not including the ears); the animal is lifted, using the other hand to support the body, and placed on the other arm with its head in the opening between the elbow and the body of the handler (Figure 28.3). For transport over a short distance, this lets the animal rest in a normal posture on the forearm of the handler with its head hidden (Stein & Walshaw 1996). It is also possible to transport the rabbit a very short distance by holding the scruff of the neck with one hand and supporting the rabbits either by slipping a hand between the hind legs, or under the rump of the rabbit. Rabbits can be trained to be handled without the neck scruff grip, picking them up with a grip around the rib cage, supporting the rump and carrying them close to the body of the handler. While handling rabbits, it is advisable to wear long-sleeved garments because the claws of rabbits may scratch the skin of the handler's arms if they are unprotected by

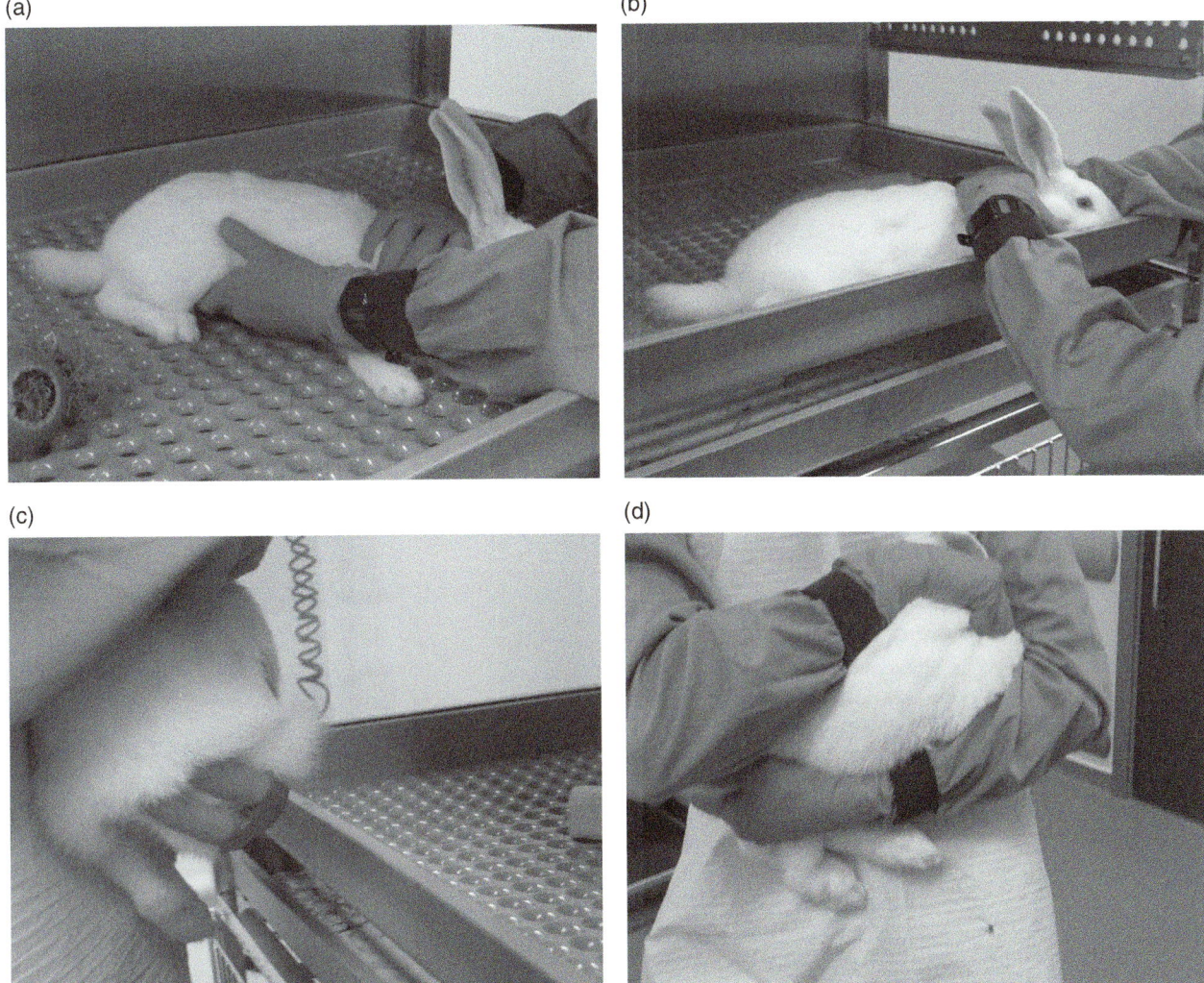

Figure 28.3 Lifting a rabbit out from its cage should be performed according to the following steps: (a) Place one hand on the scruff and the other between the hind limbs to lift and bring the rabbit to the front of the cage. (b) Place hands under the back feet and on the scruff to lift and bring the rabbit towards the handler. (c) Lift and tuck the head under one arm and the other hand bring the body of the rabbit close to the handler. (d) Tuck the head under one arm, and protect the back of the rabbit. Keep the other hand across the rear legs to prevent the rabbit kicking and scratching the handler (courtesy of Joanne Moore).

clothing (Suckow & Douglas 1997). Because rabbits have a fragile skeleton and strong hind leg muscles, struggling may cause fracture of the spinal vertebrae (Rothfritz et al. 1992) so it is important to protect the back of the rabbit when they are being carried or held for any length of time.

Rabbits should be placed on a firm, non-slip surface in order to carry out examination or procedures, as they may panic if they feel insecure and the use of a soft material, such as VetBed is advisable to improve comfort. Many procedures can be carried out single-handed by a skilled person but in case of doubt, or where rabbits are not well-habituated, an assistant should be used to hold the rabbit. Restraint should be gentle but firm enough to prevent excessive movement. Wrapping the rabbit up gently in a large towel may help with restraint alternatively, or placing the rabbit in a box of similar size to the animal's body.

Training/habituation for procedures

Rabbits can be accustomed to laboratory procedures just as any other animals. It has been shown that early handling of kits during the nursing period results in more exploratory animals that are less fearful and approach novel stimuli or an experimenters hand more often (Denenberg et al. 1973; Kersten et al. 1989; Csatádi et al. 2005; Zucca et al. 2012). Animals which are well-acquainted with their handlers and environment are less stressed in experimental situations and this improves the outcome of the scientific work (Toth & January 1990). Rabbits show reduced fearful behaviour with familiar handlers (Podberscek et al. 1991). Rabbits that have been handled will approach people sooner and for longer periods compared to unhandled rabbits (Verwer et al. 2009; Swennes et al. 2011). There is a lot of evidence of the benefit of early, gentle handling for how rabbits respond to human interaction (see also Chapter 15: The use of positive reinforcement training techniques to enhance the care and welfare of laboratory and research animals).

Rabbits can also be trained using positive reinforcement, or 'clicker', for example to come to the front of the cage, to sit quietly on weighing balance, to have its rectal temperature taken or to take liquid medication. Covering the rabbit's eyes with a soft cloth is also helpful in reducing anxiety when carrying out procedures such as blood sampling from the ear vessels, or prior to injection. Recommendations for habituation are, for example in floor pens, sitting with the rabbits and letting them come to the animal carer, or removing them from the cage regular so they are habituated to humans (Figure 28.4).

Monitoring methods

Rabbits are often used in immunisation studies involving blood sampling. General advice on blood sampling techniques can be found in Joint Working Group on Refinement (JWGR) (1993). Blood can be taken from the marginal ear vein (Figure 28.5), from the central artery of the ear or by cardiac puncture. Cardiac puncture is carried out with the animal in dorsal recumbence and only under anaesthesia (Batchelor 1999). After cardiac puncture, the animal should

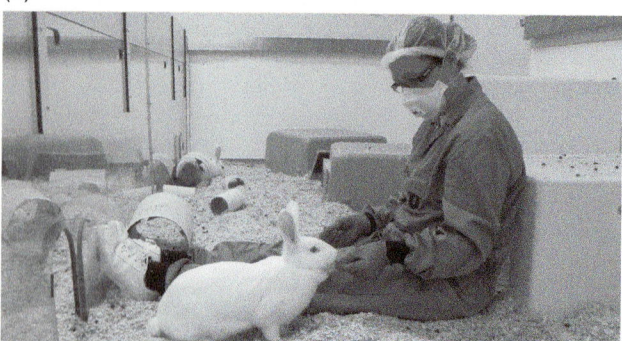
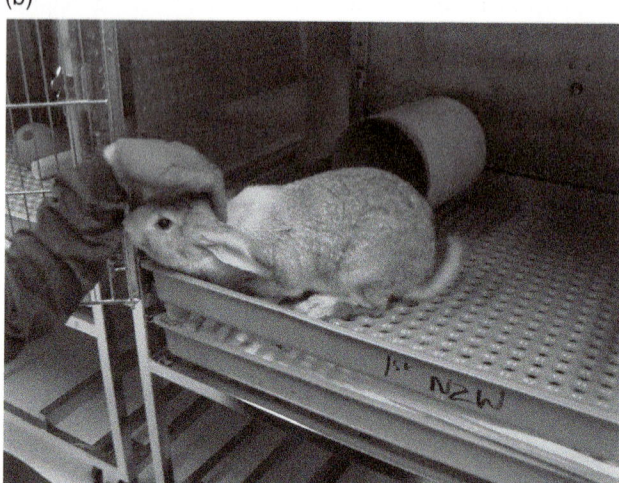

Figure 28.4 Habituation of rabbits to handlers by sitting down with NZW rabbits in floor housing (a) and by petting a male Chinchilla in a cage (b) (courtesy of Joanna Moore).

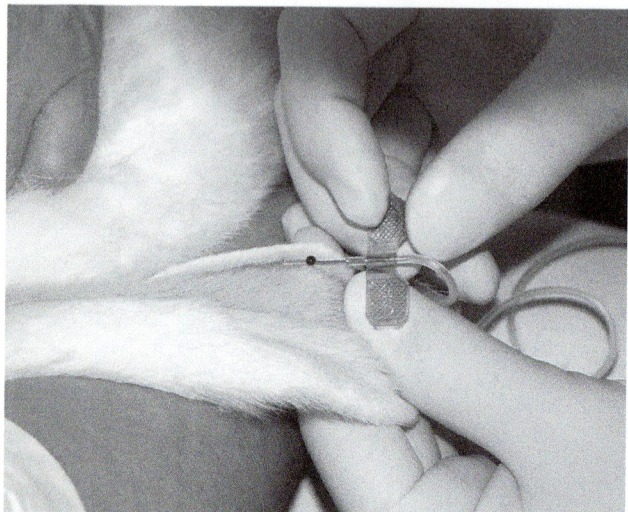

Figure 28.5 Collection of blood from the ear vein of a rabbit (courtesy of Ann-Christine Nordkam).

be immediately killed because of the risk of damage to the pericardium and subsequent heart tamponade. When using the marginal ear vein, application of a local anaesthetic ointment 15 minutes earlier facilitates the removal of blood from those animals which are distressed by the insertion of the needle into the ear vein.[2]

For collecting larger volumes of blood, the central ear artery is a better choice since the blood flow is stronger here, but care must be taken to ensure that the puncture site is compressed afterwards in order to stop the vessel from bleeding after sampling. This can be achieved using manual compression or a temporary compression bandage. Up to 15% of the total blood volume of the rabbit can be sampled in a single blood withdrawal, after which the rabbit needs a 4-week recovery period. In single blood withdrawals, there is risk of hypovolemic shock if surpassing 15% of the total circulating blood volume. In a multiple sampling situation, maximally 15–20% of the total circulating blood volume can be withdrawn in 24 h, after which the rabbits need at least 3 weeks' recovery. In case of multiple blood sampling, the red blood cells regeneration is the main issue. Rabbits have 44–70 ml of circulating blood per kg body weight (Diehl *et al.* 2001).

The body temperature of rabbits should be taken by a suitable thermometer that has been lubricated for ease of introduction into the anus (Batchelor 1999). The rabbit should be gently restrained, the tail lifted and the thermometer inserted without any force. The thermometer should be left *in situ* for 1–2 minutes.

Administration of drugs

General advice on the administration of drugs can be found in Joint Working Group on Refinement (2001). Rabbits are easily dosed subcutaneously under the skin of the neck and the upper back area. The drugs or compounds given should be pH neutral because rabbits tend to develop subcutaneous abscesses after injections of irritant substances. Intramuscular injections can be given in the hind leg, in the quadriceps muscle; they can also be given into the dorsal lumbar muscles but there is a risk of damage to the ischiatic nerve running down the back and lateral part of the hind leg. In general, intramuscular injections should be avoided because they are often painful for the animal and the rate of absorption is not much quicker than from subcutaneous sites.

It is relatively easy to perform intravenous injections with a needle or infusions using an indwelling catheter placed in the marginal ear vein, and this route has many advantages such as quick onset of action of the injected compound.

Intraperitoneal (IP) injections could also be used but there is a great variability in the rate of uptake after injecting IP since there is a likelihood that at least some of the material injected will enter the gut (caecum), fatty tissue or the urinary bladder rather than the abdominal cavity serosa. Rabbits which are not trained usually struggle when restrained with their belly upwards for receiving the IP injection, and this increases the risk of a less-than-perfect injection.

For enteral administration, gavage can be performed with a soft tube passed into the rabbit's stomach. This technique must be learnt under supervision of a person skilled in the procedure. Rabbits can be trained to ingest sweetened fluids from a syringe and it is possible to dose rabbits orally by this route, for example to provide post-surgical pain relief.

Anaesthesia/analgesia

Suitable anaesthetic and analgesic regimes should be chosen in co-operation with the laboratory animal veterinary surgeon. Depending on the equipment available, a regime based on injectables alone, called TIVA (Total Intravenous Anaesthesia) or a combination of injectable agents and gaseous anaesthesia may be used. Rabbits are sensitive to smells of anaesthetic gas, which renders induction of the anaesthesia difficult using gaseous agents (Svendsen 1994). Premedication with sedative, followed by induction with injectable agents, is preferable, followed by gaseous anaesthesia, which allows easy control of the depth and length of the anaesthesia (Svendsen 1994). Where a surgical procedure is intended, an analgesic should also be included in the premedication. When using only injectable agents, the use of a continuous infusion can be considered because it is easier to adjust the duration of anaesthesia to suit the length of the surgical procedure than with bolus administration (Svendsen 1994). In both TIVA and inhalational anaesthesia, intermittent positive pressure ventilation (IPPV) after endotracheal intubation is necessary (Hedenqvist *et al.* 2013). This skill needs practical training by an experienced supervisor. Physiological monitoring such as with a pulse oximeter or capnography is advisable when anaesthetising rabbits, as they are a relatively challenging species to anaesthetise safely. Further advice can be found in Flecknell (2015) or through the NC3Rs website; topic Anaesthesia[3].

Post-surgical care of rabbits includes administering analgesic medication, placing them in a recovery cage, the box they were placed in before surgery or the home cage which has been lined with a tray liner (Batchelor 1999). The liner may be folded over the animal to minimise hypothermia. Commercially available veterinary bedding may also be used. The liner or bedding should be removed about 30 minutes after the animal has regained consciousness and recumbence (Batchelor 1999). The effect of administered analgesia must be monitored and followed by additional drug administrations on demand or according to a protocol. Pain has negative effects on gut movement, reduces appetite and can lead to digestive imbalance (dysbiosis) in rabbits. As prey animals, rabbits may hide signs of pain from observers but use of CCTV or Webcam can be very useful to monitor the animals remotely. The 'Rabbit Grimace Scale' (Keating *et al.* 2012) is helpful in assessing pain. Other indications of pain include teeth grinding and hunched, immobile posture. Early awakening, animal eating and good pain control are essential for speedy recovery, and surgical success.

---

[2] https://www.nc3rs.org.uk/rabbit-marginal-ear-veinartery-non-surgical (Accessed 28 April, 2022)

[3] https://www.nc3rs.org.uk/3rs-resources/anaesthesia (Accessed 28 April, 2022)

If several group-housed animals have undergone surgery, the last animal must be completely conscious before all the animals are returned to the pen simultaneously (Batchelor 1999). If animals are returned to a group pen while still recovering consciousness, they may be subjected to aggression (Batchelor 1999). Incision sites should be covered with a clear plastic dressing spray.

Euthanasia/killing

Euthanasia is described as 'the good death' and as humanely killing animals for ethical or animal welfare reasons (AVMA Guidelines for the Euthanasia of Animals 2020). The EU directive 2010/63 requires that the killing of animals should only be done by persons trained and proven competent in the specific procedure. Killing is most commonly performed by intravenous injection of an overdose of anaesthetic agent, such as sodium pentobarbital or anaesthetic mixtures. Captive bolt followed by exsanguination is another method for euthanasia that can be used by experienced personnel if the use of chemical euthanasia is for some reason unsuitable or contraindicated. Physical dislocation of the neck followed by exsanguination is an option for rabbits under 1 kg body weight. In this case, animals over 150 grams must be sedated. Concussion and exsanguination can be done in rabbits under 5 kg body weight. Electrical stunning can also be used but this requires specialised equipment (Appendix IV, EU Directive 2010/63).

Common welfare problems

Health (diseases/injuries)

The clinical health of modern laboratory animals is rarely a major issue; more important are subclinical infections and the ways they may affect and alter research results. For example, it is quite possible for rabbits not to show clinically obvious signs or symptoms of disease unless they are negatively influenced by multiple agents or other stressors simultaneously (Nerem 1980). However, there are some differences between rabbits and more commonly used species – mice and rats. Health management of mice and rats is an issue mainly of maintaining freedom from pathogens of viral, bacterial and more rarely parasitic origin; rabbit health management is mainly concerned with maintaining freedom from parasites and to some degree from bacteria. All major breeders of laboratory rabbits use a health monitoring programme and these programmes comprise microbiological testing and some pathology surveillance. In Europe, the FELASA recommendations (2014) are widely accepted.

A healthy rabbit has alert and clear eyes and well-groomed fur. Even if the animal is well-accustomed to being handled by humans, it will jump in an effort to escape if startled by a handler. A daily health check should include observation of the animal's posture, its eyes and nose to look for discharge and the state of the fur. When rabbits are group-housed, a check for wounds inflicted by other animals should also be made at least once daily. The faeces and urine should also be checked for abnormalities. Normal faeces should consist of dry pellets of a uniform size and normal urine can vary in colour from yellow to dark red and is often cloudy due to the excretion of calcium.

The FELASA (2014) recommendations are based on the incidence of different infections and vary depending on the size and purpose of each colony. When the FELASA guidelines for health monitoring of laboratory rabbits are followed, the animal can be called a 'health defined rabbit'. There are similar terms of earlier origin that are sometimes used for the same purpose (SPF, specific pathogen free or VAF, virus antibody free animal). These different terms aim to provide information about the microbiological health status of the rabbits in a colony. Health monitoring results are always historical and documentation should be read carefully with attention to how often the samples are taken, which method of evaluation has been used and the rationale for why certain agents are or are not evaluated in the specific colony.

Infectious diseases

Bacterial agents

The main infective causes of respiratory inflammations are *Pasteurella multocida* and *Bordetella bronchiseptica*, which cause symptoms such as sneezing, coughing, nasal discharge and lethargy. Abscesses in subcutaneous tissues, behind the eye bulb or in internal organs, as well as inflammation of the mucous membranes of the eyes and middle ear are often caused by *Pasteurella multocida* and *Staphylococcus aureus*. Bacterial eye infections by *Moraxella catarrhalis* can also occur in laboratory rabbits.

Young rabbits are particularly susceptible to bacterial imbalances within the intestine leading to conditions such as mucoid enteritis. Depression, anorexia, diarrhoea and mucus in the stool are the main symptoms; the cause is multifactorial with the bacterium *Clostridium spiroforme* being one of the major factors (Peeters 1986). Bacterial enteritis associated with diarrhoea as main symptom may also be caused by *Escherichia coli* and other strains of clostridia. Nutritional imbalance, lack of dietary fibre and stress can predispose rabbits to enteritis.

Viral infections

Even though viral infections are not a major problem in barrier-bred laboratory rabbits, it is important to be aware of the potential of viral causes of disease. Mild diarrhoea may be caused by rotavirus and rabbit enteric coronavirus. Breeders and owners of pet rabbits fear rabbit viral haemorrhagic disease (RVHD). The symptoms of RVHD include lethargy, anorexia, diarrhoea and haemorrhage from body openings such as the nose and urogenital openings. This disease is unlikely to occur within a modern laboratory rabbit colony. Myxoma virus can be transferred to laboratory rabbits by vectors such as fleas and other insects. Because myxomatosis is common in wild rabbits, it is possible for laboratory rabbit colonies located in areas with large populations of wild rabbits to be infected.

Parasites

Endoparasites (parasites inside the body) are more common than ectoparasites in laboratory rabbits; among endoparasites, coccidiosis is the greatest problem. This disease is caused by different strains of *Eimeria*. For example, *E. stiedae* is a strain infecting the liver and causes a wide range of symptoms from slight growth retardation to death. Several *Eimeria* strains such as *E. perforans* and *E. magna* affect the intestine of rabbits. The symptoms of coccidiosis depend on the location and number of coccidia in the gut and on the susceptibility of the animal. It may be prudent to ask the breeder if they are using coccidiostatic medication in the diet. This may influence the change of diet and the rabbit health after transfer to the laboratory. Younger animals more often show symptoms such as weight loss and mild to severe intermittent diarrhoea, whereas older animals rarely show any signs at all (Peeters 1986).

Passalurus ambiguus, the rabbit's pinworm, can colonise the caecum and colon and its eggs are passed in the faeces but these infections seldom affect the animals to such a degree that signs can be seen.

Encephalitozoon cuniculi, an intracellular protozoan, gives rise to a disease called encephalitozoonosis or nosematosis. This disease is common in pet and wild rabbits and regularly occurs in laboratory rabbits. The parasite is transmitted by the urine of infected animals via the oral route to the intestine and tissues of susceptible rabbits. Clinical signs are not always apparent, but heavy infections damage the kidneys and the brain of infected animals.

The two most common ectoparasites of pet rabbits are ear mites and fur mites, although these are rare in laboratory rabbit colonies. *Psoroptes cuniculi*, the ear mite, causes wounds on and around the ears. The fur mite, *Cheyletiella parasitivorax*, along with other mites, fleas and lice of rabbits, can cause considerable suffering and may induce self-inflicted wounds. Itching and anaemia caused by these blood-sucking insects result in poor general condition in the rabbit.

Traumatic injuries

Among animals that are housed in pairs or groups, the most common cause of traumatic injury is fighting. Both sexually mature males and females that are not acquainted with each other can fight aggressively. The likelihood of fighting increases when groups of animals are housed in overcrowded pens with too few water bottles, food hoppers or no structures in the pen for them to escape and break eye contact. The wounds inflicted by fighting males can be severe and need suturing but may often be concealed by the fur of the animal if they are small.

The skeleton of rabbits is fragile in comparison to its muscular hind leg strength (Rothfritz *et al*. 1992), and rabbits which are not accustomed to handling by humans may struggle forcefully when picked up in the cage, resulting in vertebral fracture.

Diseases associated with housing, feeding and breeding regimes

The standards of housing, maintenance routines, hygiene measures and feeding and watering regimes all affect the health and well-being of rabbits. Animals held in floor pens or in solid-bottom cages need management and thorough cleaning and disinfection of the pen or cage in order to minimise the spread of intestinal parasites and bacteria. Keeping the litter dry prevents coccidia from multiplying and minimises the need for frequent changes, which may then be as low as once monthly. Perforated cage floors that allow droppings to fall onto a tray underneath or the use of a litter tray for the latrine areas in floor housing help reduce the number of coccidian spores and bacteria in the immediate environment of the animal.

If larger rabbit breeds are kept in poorly designed perforated or wire mesh floors, 'sore hocks' or pododermatitis can occur. Some individuals seem to be sensitive to wood shavings and other materials commonly used as bedding material in pens or solid-bottom cages. Inadequate hygiene is a predisposing factor. Symptoms include bleeding and chronic wounds on the hindfeet of affected animals. Softer bedding material and improved hygiene will be beneficial to these animals.

Dietary fibre concentration is critical for the intestinal flora and the intestinal morphology of rabbits (Tawfik *et al*. 1997). Young animals are most sensitive to imbalances caused by lack of fibre leading to dysbiosis, which may be life-threatening. Dietary fibre is essential to keep the animals gut function normal and to reduce obesity. This should be provided as hay and in fibre-enriched pellets.

Health problems may also arise from the feeding of modified laboratory diets during investigations, where the aim may be to produce metabolic changes in the rabbit. For example, diets containing high concentrations of fatty acids and cholesterol intended to produce atherosclerosis during long-term studies, may cause the deposition of fat in the liver and cholesterol in different parts of the body.

Behavioural/abnormal behaviour

Laboratory rabbits kept in small or barren cages may develop stereotypic behaviour, for example, wire-gnawing and excessive wall-pawing (Lehmann & Wieser 1985; Wieser 1986; Bigler & Lehmann 1991; Loeffler *et al*. 1991; Stauffacher 1992). Wall-pawing, which is derived from digging, may be constrained by the solid floor of the cage (Podberscek *et al*. 1991). Individually caged rabbits can show changes in their behaviours such as somersaulting, no full hops, less activity than group-penned rabbits, and less marking and investigatory behaviour than in group pens (Podberscek *et al*. 1991). Social isolation can induce physiological symptoms of stress, which may be relieved by the presence of conspecifics (Held *et al*. 1995). Stereotypic behaviour may indicate frustration, anxiety or boredom, and develop through a number of stages involving a progressive narrowing of the behavioural repertoire (Gunn 1994).

Singly housed laboratory rabbits in barren environments often show signs interpreted as boredom, such as hunched posture (Gunn & Morton 1995a, 1995b), inertia (Metz 1984), and a staring coat and dull eyes (Wallace *et al*. 1990). Chu *et al*. (2003) found that singly housed rabbits showed more abnormal behaviour and less movement than pair-housed rabbits. Prolonged inactivity associated with unresponsiveness may occur as well as, or in place of stereotypic behaviour, and is thought to be associated with changes in brain chemistry intended to help alleviate boredom (Broom 1988).

Under-grooming may lead to development of a staring coat (Gunn & Morton 1995a), whereas over-grooming may result in development of hair-balls in the stomach (gastric trichobezoars) which in turn may cause intestinal stasis (Jackson 1991) and, if uncorrected, lead to death (Wagner *et al.* 1974). Other behavioural problems include under-eating and over-eating, associated with weight loss and obesity, respectively (Gunn & Morton 1995a).

The freedom of movement of rabbits housed in cages is very limited; for example normal hopping and bipedal rearing/orienting posture is impossible. This causes changes in the muscles, joints and bones (Lehmann 1989; Stauffacher 1992); and changes in the bone structure particularly evident in the femur proximalis (thinner and less strong bone) and the vertebral column (Lehmann 1989; Drescher & Loeffler 1991a, 1991b). Growing rabbits kept in cages perform almost no hopping or intensive locomotion, for example associated with play, when compared to those reared in outdoor enclosures (Lehmann 1989). The most common movement pattern, crawling, occurs at a slightly lower frequency in the cages (Lehmann 1989). In cages, rabbits often perform interrupted jumps, where the hindlegs are only lifted slightly and then put down again, so that the musculoskeletal system is not used as in normal hopping (Lehmann 1989). Rabbits may also show abnormal postures because of spatial constraints, for example when lying stretched out during resting or when performing stretching behaviour (Gunn 1994).

Rabbits may also show restlessness, such as non-functional bouts of activity with disconnected elements of feeding, comfort, resting, alertness and withdrawal behaviour alternating with locomotion with social and temporal disorder in behaviour, and panic (Lehmann & Wieser 1985; Bigler & Lehmann 1991; Stauffacher 1992).

A variety of disturbances to sexual behaviour have been described, some of which may lead to low conception rates (30–70 %), for example, abnormal mating behaviour following placement of the doe into the buck's cage (Stauffacher 1992). If the cage had enough space for the mating ritual, then a more successful outcome may be achieved. The doe may show disturbed nesting behaviour and nesting stereotypies which may lead to rearing losses (Wieser 1986; Wullschleger 1987; Loeffler *et al.* 1991). This could be alleviated if she is offered straw as a nesting material (Blumetto *et al.* 2010) and a cat-flap at the nest entrance so she is able to escape from her young (Baumann *et al.* 2005). In addition, the doe may show disturbed nursing and cannibalism associated with restlessness, which may also increase rearing losses (Bigler 1986; Brummer 1986; Stauffacher 1992).

Signs of poor welfare

In rabbits, signs of poor welfare are the above-presented abnormal, stereotypic or apathetic behaviours. Wounds on group-housed rabbits may be caused by fights, which can occur suddenly during night time. It is important to separate a rabbit with wounds from the group to avoid further fighting. Body condition score rabbits routinely to assess well-being. This enables identification of rabbits who may be subordinate and bullied away from access to food/water. It also allows recognition of when rabbits are becoming obese due to lack of exercise, poor diet (usually, insufficient hay) or both, so that the management can be remedied.

Finding rabbits in pain may be difficult as prey animals try to hide that they are in a vulnerable position. Remote monitoring of rabbit behaviour and body postures by Webcam could help surveillance of rabbit well-being. Looking for signs such as the fur being dirty or a starry coat may indicate that the rabbit has not been grooming itself for some time. Obvious signs are reduced water intake and the rabbits not eating their feed, especially if they have restricted access. A hunched posture while sitting or moving and curled ear margins may be other signs of pain. Keating *et al.* (2012) when testing if EMLA cream during ear tattooing would lead to less pain in rabbits developed the Rabbit Grimace Scale (RbtGS). Hampshire & Robertson (2015) evaluated the RbtGS when observing rabbits after different laboratory procedures. The observer assesses the rabbit's orbital tightening, cheek flattening, nostril shape, whisker shape and position, and ear shape and position[4].

Acknowledgements

The authors want to thank AstraZeneca R&D Mölndal for letting Lena Lidfors carry out research on improving the housing of laboratory rabbits and for financing the time for Therese Edström to write this chapter. They also want to thank the Department of Animal Environment and Health for financing the time Lena Lidfors has used to write this chapter. They send a special thanks to Bengt-Åke Sandeberg at KB Lidköpings Rabbit Farm for sharing his knowledge on breeding laboratory rabbits with them. Special thanks are also sent to Joanna Moore at GSK Medicines Research Centre, Hertfordshire, UK and Ann-Christine Nordkam at Astra Zeneca Gothenburg, Sweden for sharing their photos in this chapter.

References

Adams, C.E. (1982). Artificial insemination in the rabbit: the technique and application to practice. *Journal of Applied Rabbit Research*, **4**, 10–13.

Animal Research Review Panel (2003). *Guidelines for the Housing of Rabbits in Scientific Institutions*. ARRP Guideline 18. Animal Welfare Unit, New South Wales Agriculture, Sydney, Australia. http://www.animalethics.org.au/__data/assets/pdf_file/0013/222511/housing-rabbits-scientific-institutions.pdf (Accessed 10 February 2020).

AVMA Guidelines for the euthanasia of animals: 2020 Edition (2020). American Veterinary Medical Association, 1931 N. Meacham Road, Schaumburg, IL 60173, USA. https://www.avma.org/sites/default/files/2020-02/Guidelines-on-Euthanasia-2020.pdf

Batchelor, G.R. (1991). Group housing on floor pens and environmental enrichment in sandy lop rabbits (I). *Animal Technology*, **42**, 109–120.

Batchelor, G.R. (1999). The laboratory rabbit. In: *The UFAW Handbook on the Care and Management of Laboratory Animals*, 7th edn. Ed. Poole, T., pp. 395–408. Blackwell Publishing, Oxford.

---

[4] https://nc3rs.org.uk/rabbit-grimace-scale (Accessed April 28, 2022)

Baumann, P., Oester, H. and Stauffacher, M. (2005). The use of a cat-flap at the nest entrance to mimic natural conditions in the breeding of fattening rabbits (*Oryctolagus cuniculus*). *Animal Welfare*, **14**, 135–142.

Bell, D.J. (1977). *Aspects of the Social Behaviour of Wild and Domesticated Rabbits Oryctolagus cuniculus L.* Unpublished PhD thesis, University of Wales.

Bell, D.J. (1980). Social olfaction in lagomorphs. In: *Symposia of the Zoological Society of London*, **45**, 141–164.

Bell, D.J. (1983). Mate choice in the European rabbit. In: *Mate Choice*. Ed. Bateson, P.P.G., pp. 211–223. Cambridge University Press, Cambridge.

Bell, D.J. (1984). The behaviour of rabbits: implications for their laboratory management. In: *Proceedings of UFAW/LASA Joint Symposium. Standards in Laboratory Animal Management, Part II*. pp. 151–162. Universities Federation for Animal Welfare, Potters Bar.

Bell, D.J. (1999). The European wild rabbit. In: *The UFAW Handbook on the Care and Management of Laboratory Animals*, 7th edn. Ed. Poole, T., pp. 389–394. Blackwell Publishing, Oxford.

Bell, D.J. and Bray, G.C. (1984). Effects of single- and mixed-sex caging on post-weaning development in the rabbit. *Laboratory Animals*, **18**, 267–270.

Bell, D.J. and Webb, N.J. (1991). Effects of climate on reproduction in the European wild rabbit *Oryctolagus cuniculus*. *Journal of Zoology*, **224**, 639–648.

Bennett, B. (2001). *Storey's Guide to Raising Rabbits*. Eds Burns, D. and Salter, M. Storey Communications Inc, USA.

Berthelsen, H. and Hansen, L.T. (1999). The effect of hay on the behaviour of caged rabbits (*Oryctolagus cuniculus*). *Animal Welfare*, **8**, 149–157.

Bergdall, V.K. and Dysko, R.C. (1994). Metabolic, traumatic and miscellaneous diseases in rabbits. In: *The Biology of the Laboratory Rabbit*, 2nd edn. Eds Manning, P.J., Ringler, D.H. and Newcomer, C.E., pp. 335–353. Academic Press, San Diego.

Beynen, A.C., Mulder, A., Nieuwenkamp, A.E. *et al.* (1992). Loose grass hay as a supplement to a pelleted diet reduces fur chewing in rabbits. *Journal of Animal Physiology and Animal Nutrition*, **68**, 226–234.

Bigler, L. (1986). *Mutter-Kind-Beziehung beim Hauskaninchen*. Lizentiatsarbeit, Universität Berne.

Bigler, L. and Lehmann, M. (1991). *Schlussbericht ueber die Pruefung der Tiergerechtheit eines Festwandkaefigs fuer Hauskaninchen-Zibben*. Report Swiss Federal Veterinary Office, Berne.

Bigler, L. and Oester, H. (1994). Paarhaltung nicht reproduzierender Zibben im Käfig. *Berliner und Münchener tierärztliche Wochenschrift*, **107**, 202–205.

Björnhag, G. (1981). Separation and retrograde transport in the large intestine of herbivores. *Livestock Production Science*, **8**, 351–360.

Black, S.L. and Vanderwolf, C.H. (1969). Thumping behavior in the rabbit. *Physiology & Behaviour*, **4**, 445–446.

Blumetto, O., Olivas, I., Torres, A.G. *et al.* (2010). Use of straw and wood shavings as nest material in primiparous does. *World Rabbit Science*, **18**, 237–242.

Boden, E. and Andrew, A. (2015). *Black's Veterinary Dictionary*, 22nd edn. Bloomsbury Information, 816 pp.

Brem, G., Brenig, B., Godman, H.M. *et al.* (1985). Production of transgenic mice, rabbits and pigs by microinjection into pronuclei. *Zuchthygiene*, **20**, 251–252.

Brooks, D.L. (1997). Nutrition and gastrointestinal physiology. In: *Ferrets, Rabbits and Rodents – Clinical Medicine and Surgery*. Eds Hillyer, E.W. and Quesenberry, K.E., pp. 169–175. WB Saunders, London.

Broom, D.M. (1988). The scientific assessment of animal welfare. *Applied Animal Behaviour Sciences*, **20**, 5–19.

Brummer, H. (1975). Trichophagia: a behavioural disorder in the domestic rabbit. *Deutsche Tierärztliche Wochenschrift*, **82**, 350–351.

Brummer, H. (1986). Symptome des Wohlbefindens und des Unwohlseins beim Kaninchen unter besonderer Beruecksichtigung der Ethopathien. In: *Wege zur Beurteilung tiergerechter Haltung bei Labor-, Zoo- und Haustieren*. Ed. Militzer, K., pp. 44–53. Parey Schriften Versuchstierkunde.

Buseth, M.E. and Saunders, R.A. (2015). *Rabbit Behaviour, Health and Care*. 225 pp. CABI, Malta.

Bősze, Z.S. and Houdebine, L.M. (2006). Application of rabbits in biomedical research: a review. *World Rabbit Science* **14**, 1–14.

Canali, E., Ferrante, V., Todeschini, R. *et al.* (1991). Rabbit nest construction and its relationship with litter development. *Applied Animal Behaviour Sciences*, **31**, 259–266.

Carpenter, J.W., Mashima, T.Y., Gentz, E.J. *et al.* (1995) Caring for rabbits: An overview and formulary. *Veterinary Medicine*, **90**, 340–364.

Cheeke, P.R. (1987). *Rabbit Feeding and Nutrition*. Academic Press, New York.

Cheeke, P.R., Patton, N.M., Lukefahr, S.D. *et al.* (1987). *Rabbit Production*, 6th edn. Interstate Printers and Publishers, Danville, Illinois.

Chu, L., Garner, J.P. and Mench, J.A. (2003). A behavioural comparison of New Zealand White rabbits (*Oryctolagus cuniculus*) housed individually or in pairs in conventional laboratory cages. *Applied Animal Behaviour Science*, **85**, 121–139.

Cizek, L.J. (1961). Relationship between food and water ingestion in the rabbit. *American Journal of Physiology*, **201**, 557–566.

Cobb, A.B. (2011). *Macmillan Science Library: Animal Sciences*, Vol. 1. Macmillan Reference USA. 2001–2006.

Cooke, B.D. (2012). Rabbits: manageable environmental pests or participants in new Australian ecosystems. *Wildlife Research*, **39**, 279–289.

Cooper, H.M. and Paterson, Y. (2008). Production of polyclonal antisera. In: *Current Protocols in Molecular Biology*. Ed. Ausubel, F.M., pp. 11.12.1–11.12.10. John Wiley & Sons, New York.

Council of Europe (2006). Appendix A of the European Convention for the protection of vertebrate animals used for experimental and other scientific purposes (ETS No. 123). Guidelines for accommodation and care of animals (Article 5 of the convention). Approved by the multilateral consultation https://www.coe.int/t/e/legal_affairs/legal_co-operation/biological_safety_and_use_of_animals/laboratory_animals/2006/Cons123(2006)3AppendixA_en.pdf (Accessed 7 July 2020).

Cowan, D.P. (1987). Aspects of the social organisation of the European wild rabbit (*Oryctolagus cuniculus*). *Ethology*, **75**, 197–210.

Cowan, D.P. and Bell, D.J. (1986). Leporid social behaviour and social organization. *Mammal Review*, **16**, 169–179.

Cowan, D.P. and Garson, P.J. (1985). Variations in the social structure of rabbit populations: causes and demographic consequences. In: *Behavioural Ecology: the Ecological Consequences of Adaptive Behaviour*. Eds Sibly, R.M. and Smith, R.H., pp. 537–555. Blackwell Publishing, Oxford.

Csatádi, K., Kustos, K., Eiben, C. *et al.* (2005). Even minimal human contact linked to nursing reduces fear responses toward humans in rabbits. *Applied Animal Behaviour Science*, **95**, 123–128.

DAD-IS (2018). Domestic Animal Diversity Information System. Global Rabbit Breeds by Country. FAO (Food and Agriculture Organization of the United Nations). Last edited 16 June 2020. Retrieved 7 July 2020. https://en.wikipedia.org/wiki/List_of_rabbit_breeds

Dalle Zotte, E., Princz, Z., Matics, Z.S. *et al.* (2009) Rabbit preference for cages and pens with or without mirrors. *Applied Animal Behaviour Science*, **116**, 273–278.

Daly, J.C. (1981). Effects of social organisation and environmental diversity on determining the genetic structure of a population of the wild rabbit (*Oryctolagus cuniculus*). *Evolution*, **35**, 689–706.

Denenberg, V.H., Wyly, M.V., Burns, J.K. *et al.* (1973). Behavioral effects of handling rabbits in infancy. *Physiology & Behavior*, **10**, 1001–1004.

Devillard, S., Aubineau, J., Berger, F. et al. (2008). Home range of the European rabbit (*Oryctolagus cuniculus*) in three contrasting French populations. *Mammalian Biology*, **73**, 128–137.

Diehl, K.H., Hull, R., Morton, D. et al. (2001). A good practice guide to the administration of substances and removal of blood, including routes and volumes. *Journal of Applied Toxicology: An International Journal*, **21**, 15–23.

Donnelly, T.M. (1997). Basic anatomy, physiology and husbandry. In: *Ferrets, Rabbits and Rodents – Clinical Medicine and Surgery*. Eds Hillyer, E.W. and Quesenberry, K.E., pp. 147–159. WB Saunders, London.

Drescher, B. and Loeffler, K. (1991a). Einfluss unterschiedlicher Haltungsverfahren und Bewegungsmöglichkeiten auf die Kompakta der Röhrenknochen von Versuchs – und Fleischkaninchen. *Tierärztliche Umschau*, **46**, 736–741.

Drescher, B. and Loeffler, K. (1991b). Einfluss unterschiedlicher Haltungsverfahren und Bewegungsmöglichkeiten auf die Kompakta der Röhrenknochen von Mastkaninchen. *Tierärztliche Umschau*, **47**, 175–179.

Esteves, P.J., Abrantes, J., Baldauf, H.-M. et al. (2018). The wide utility of rabbits as models of human diseases. *Experimental & Molecular Medicine*, **50**, 1–10.

European Commission (2007). Commission recommendations of 18 June 2007 on guidelines for the accommodation and care of animals used for experimental and other scientific purposes. Annex II to European Council Directive 86/609. See 2007/526/EC. https://eur-lex.europa.eu/LexUriServ/LexUriServ.do?uri=OJ:L:2007:197:0001:0089:EN:PDF (Accessed 7 July 2020).

Directive 2010/63/EU of the European Parliament and of the Council of 22 September 2010 on the protection of animals used for scientific purposes; The European Parliament and the Council of the European Union, Annex IV Methods of killing animals. https://eur-lex.europa.eu/legal-content/EN/TXT/?qid=1546895248778&uri=CELEX:32010L0063#d1e79-72-1 (Accessed 7 July 2020).

Eveleigh, J.R. and Pease, S.S. (1976). The establishment of a breeding nucleus of category 4. *Dutch Rabbits*, **10**, 297–303.

Eveleigh, J.R., Taylor, W.T.C. and Cheeseman, R.F. (1984). The production of specific pathogen free rabbits. *Animal Technology*, **35**, 1–12.

Flecknell, P. (2015). *Laboratory Animal Anaesthesia*. 4th edn. Academic press, USA.

Flecknell, P.A. and Thomas, A.A. (2015). 39 Comparative Anesthesia and Analgesia of Laboratory Animals. In: *Veterinary Anesthesia and Analgesia*. 5th edn. Eds Grimm, K.A., Lamont, L.A., Tranquilli, W.J. et al., pp. 754–763. Wiley Blackwell, USA.

Fraser, K.W. (1992). Emergence behaviour of rabbits, *Oryctolagus cuniculus*, in Central Otago, New Zealand. *Journal of Zoology*, **228**, 615–623.

FELASA Working Group on Revision of Guidelines for Health Monitoring of Rodents and Rabbits, Mähler, M., Berard, M., Feinstein, R. et al. (2014). FELASA recommendations for the health monitoring of mouse, rat, hamster, guinea pig and rabbit colonies in breeding and experimental units. *Laboratory Animals*, **48**, 178–192.

Ferrante, V., Verga, M., Canali, E. et al. (1992). Rabbits kept in cages and in floor pens: reactions in the open-field test. *The Journal of Applied Rabbit Research*, **15**, 700–707.

Flux, J.E.C. (1994). World distribution. In: *The European Rabbit – The History and Biology of a Successful Colonizer*. Eds Thompson, H.V. and King, C.M., pp. 8–21. Oxford University Press, Oxford.

Fox, P.R. and Krinsky, W.L. (1968). Ovulation in the rabbit related to dosage of human chorionic gonadotrophin and pregnant mare's serum. *Proceedings of the Social Experimental Biological Medicine*, **127**, 1222–1227.

Gibb, J.A. (1993). Sociality, time and space in a sparse population of rabbits (*Oryctolagus cuniculus*). *Journal of Zoology*, **229**, 581–607.

Gibb, J.A., Ward, C.P. and Ward, G.D. (1978). Natural control of a population of rabbit, *Oryctolagus cuniculus* L. for 10 years in the Kourarau enclosure North Island New Zealand. *New Zealand Department of Scientific and Industrial Research Bulletin*, **223**, 6–89.

Gidenne, T., Lebas, F. and Fortun-Lamothe, L. (2010). Feeding behavior of rabbits. In: *Nutrition of the rabbit*, Eds de Blas, C. and Wiseman, J., pp. 233–252. CABI, Wallingford UK.

Gillett, C.S. (1994). Selected drug dosages and clinical reference data. In: *The Biology of the Laboratory Rabbit*, 2nd edn. Eds Manning, P.J., Ringler, D.H. and Newcomer, C.E., pp. 496–492. Academic Press, San Diego.

González-Mariscal, G., Díaz-Sánchez, V., Melo, A.I. et al. (1994). Maternal behaviour in New Zealand White rabbits: quantification of somatic events, motor pattern, and steroid plasma levels. *Physiology and Behaviour*, **55**, 1081–1089.

Green, J. and Flinders, J. (1981). Alarm call of the Pygmy rabbit (*Brachylagus idahoensis*). *The Great Basin Naturalist*, **41**, 158–160.

Gunn, D. (1994). *Evaluation on Welfare in the Husbandry of Laboratory Rabbits*. PhD Thesis University of Birmingham.

Gunn, D. and Morton, D.B. (1995a). Rabbits. In: *Environmental Enrichment Information Resources for Laboratory Animals 1965-1995* (No. 2). Eds Smith, C.P. and Taylor, V., pp. 127–143. DIANE Publishing, USA.

Gunn, D. and Morton, D.B. (1995b). Inventory of the behaviour of New Zealand White rabbits in laboratory cages. *Applied Animal Behaviour Sciences*, **45**, 277–292.

Hagen, K.W. (1974). Colony husbandry. In: *The Biology of the Laboratory Rabbit*. Eds Weisbroth, S.H., Flatt, R.E. and Kraus, A.L., pp. 23–47. Academic Press Inc, New York.

Hampshire, V. and Robertson, S. (2015). Using the facial grimace scale to evaluate rabbit wellness in post-procedural monitoring. *Laboratory Animals*, **44**, 259–261.

Hansen, L.T. and Berthelsen, H. (2000). The effect of environmental enrichment on the behaviour of caged rabbits (*Oryctolagus cuniculus*). *Applied Animal Behaviour Sciences*, **68**, 163–178.

Harcourt-Brown, F. (2002). *Textbook of Rabbit Medicine*. Butterworth-Heineman, Oxford.

Harkness, J.E. and Wagner, J.E. (1995). *The Biology and Medicine of Rabbits and Rodents*, 4th edn. Williams and Wilkins, Baltimore.

Hawkins, P., Hubrecht, R., Buckwell, A. et al. (2008). Refining rabbit care. A resource for those working with rabbits in research. RSPCA-UFAW, UK.

Heath, M. and Stott, E. (1990). Housing rabbits the unconventional way. *Animal Technology*, **41**, 13–25.

Hedenqvist, P., Edner, A., Fahlman, Å. et al. (2013). Continuous intravenous anaesthesia with sufentanil and midazolam in medetomidine premedicated New Zealand White rabbits. *BMC Veterinary Research* **9**, 1–9.

Held, S.D.E., Turner, R.J. and Wootton, R.J. (1995). Choices of laboratory rabbits for individual or group-housing. *Applied Animal Behaviour Sciences*, **46**, 81–91.

Hoffman, S., Peterbauer, A., Schindler, S. et al. (2005). International validation of novel pyrogen tests based on human monocytoid cells. *Journal of Immunological Methods*, **298**, 161–173.

Huls, W.L., Brooks, D.L. and Bean-Knudsen, D. (1991). Responses of adult New Zealand White rabbits to enrichment objects and paired housing. *Laboratory Animal Science*, **41**, 609–612.

Iwarsson, K., Lindberg, L. and Waller, T. (1994). Common non-surgical techniques and procedures. In: *Handbook of Laboratory Animal Science*. Eds Svendsen, P. and Hau, J., pp. 229–272. CRC Press, Boca Raton.

Jackson, G. (1991). Intestinal stasis and rupture in rabbits. *Veterinary Record*, **129**, 287–289.

Jenkins, J.R. (2008). Rabbit diagnostic testing. *Journal of Exotic Pet Medicine*, **17**, 4–15.

Jilge, B. (1991). The rabbit: a diurnal or nocturnal animal? *Journal of Experimental Animal Science*, **34**, 170–183.

Jones, S.E. and Phillips, C.J.C. (2005). The effects of mirrors on the welfare of caged rabbits. *Animal Welfare*, **14**, 195–202.

Joint Working Group on Refinement (1993). Removal of blood from laboratory mammals and birds. First Report of the BVA/FRAME/RSPCA/UFAW Joint Working Group on Refinement. *Laboratory Animals*, **27**, 1–22.

Joint Working Group on Refinement (2001). Refining procedures for the administration of substances. Report of the BVAAWF/FRAME/RSPCA/UFAW Joint Working Group on Refinement. *Laboratory Animals*, **35**, 1–41.

Kawoto, F., Kouno, T. and Harada, Y. (1989). A scanning electron microscopic study of the arteriovenous anastomoses of rabbit ear using corrosive rein casts. *Kaibogaku Zasshi*, **64**, 185–195 (in Japanese with English abstract).

Keating, S.C.J., Thomas, A.A., Flecknell, P.A. et al. (2012). Evaluation of EMLA cream for preventing pain during tattooing of rabbits: changes in physiological, behavioural and facial expression responses. *PloS One*, **7(9)**, e44437.

Knutsson, M. (2011). *Exercise Pens as an Environmental Enrichment for Laboratory Rabbits*. Student report 2011:48 in Veterinary program, Swedish University of Agricultural Sciences, 32 pp.

Kraft, R. (1979). Vergleichende Verhaltensstudien an Wild- und Hauskaninchen. *Zeitschrift für Tierzuechtungsbiologie*, **95**, 165–179.

Kersten, A.M., Meijsser, F.M. and Metz, J.H. (1989). Effects of early handling on later open-field behaviour in rabbits. *Applied Animal Behaviour Sciences*, **24**, 157–167.

Kolb, H.H. (1994). The use of cover and burrows by a population of rabbits (Mammalia: *Oryctolagus cuniculus*) in eastern Scotland. *Journal of Zoology*, **233**, 9–17.

Krohn, T.C., Ritskes-Hoitinga, J., and Vendsen, P. (1999). The effects of feeding and housing on the behaviour of the laboratory rabbit. *Laboratory Animals*, **33**, 101–107.

Lehmann, M. (1989). *Das verhalten junger hauskaninchen unter verschieden umgebungsbedingungen*. PhD thesis, Universität Berne.

Lehmann, M. (1990). Activity requirement for young domestic rabbits: raw fibre consumption and animal welfare. *Schweiz Archiv Tierheilkeld*, **132**, 375–381.

Lehmann, M. (1991). Social behaviour in young domestic rabbits under semi-natural conditions. *Applied Animal Behaviour Science*, **32**, 269–292.

Lehmann, M. and Wieser, R.V. (1985). Indikatoren für mangeinde Tiergerechtheit sonie Verhaltensstorungen bei Hauskaninchen. *KTBL – Schrift*, **307**, 96–107.

Leslie, T.K., Dalton, L. and Phillips, C.J.C. (2004). Preference of domestic rabbits for grass or coarse mix feeds. *Animal Welfare*, **13**, 57–62.

Lidfors, L. (1996). Behaviour of male laboratory rabbits given environmental enrichment in a preference test and in an individual cage. In: *Proceedings of the 30th International Congress of the International Society for Applied Ethology*. Eds Duncan, I.J.H., Widowski, T.M. and Haley, D.B., p. 67. Guelph, Canada.

Lidfors, L. (1997). Behavioural effects of environmental enrichment for individually caged rabbits. *Applied Animal Behaviour Sciences*, **52**, 157–169.

Lloyd, H.G. and McCowan, D. (1968). Some observations on the breeding burrows of the wild rabbit on the island of Skokholm. *Journal of Zoology*, **156**, 540–549.

Lockley, R.M. (1961). Social structure and stress in the rabbit warren. *Journal of Animal Ecology*, **30**, 385–423.

Loeffler, K., Drescher, B. and Schulze, G. (1991). Einfluss unterschiedlicher Haltungsverfahren auf das Verhalten von Versuchs- und Fleischkaninchen. *Tieraerztliche Umschau*, **46**, 471–478.

Love, J.A. and Hammond, K. (1991). Group-housing rabbits. *Laboratory Animals*, **20**, 37–43.

Lumpkin, S. and Seidensticker, J. (2011). *Rabbits – The Animal Answer Guide*. The Johns Hopkins University Press, Baltimore.

Mader, D.R. (1997). Basic approach to veterinary care. In: *Ferrets, Rabbits and Rodents – Clinical Medicine and Surgery*. Eds Hillyer, E.W. and Quesenberry, K.E., pp. 160–168. WB Saunders, London.

McClellan, H., Miller, S. and Hartmann, P. (2008). Evolution of lactation: nutrition v. protection with special reference to five mammalian species. *Nutrition Research Reviews*, **21**, 97–116.

Meredith, A. (2000). General biology and husbandry. In: *Manual of Rabbit Medicine and Surgery*. Ed Flecknell, P., pp. 13–23. British Small Animal Veterinary Association, Gloucester.

Metz, J.H.M. (1984). Effects of early handling in the domestic rabbit. *Applied Animal Ethology*, **11**, 71–87.

Milligan, S.R., Sales, G.D. and Khirnykh, K. (1993). Sound levels in rooms housing laboratory animals: an uncontrolled daily variable. *Physiology and Behavior*, **53**, 1067–1076.

Moore, J. (2018). *Assessing Environmental Enrichment as a Means to Refine Laboratory Animal Housing with a Focus on the New Zealand White Rabbit*. PhD thesis, University of Lincoln, UK.

Morton, D.B., Jennings, M., Batchelor, G.R. et al. (1993). Refinement in rabbit husbandry. *Laboratory Animals*, **27**, 301–329.

Mulder, A., Nieuwenkamp, A.E., van der Palen, J.G. et al. (1992). Supplementary hay reduces fur-chewing in rabbits. *Tijdschrift fur Diergeneeskunde*, **117**, 655–658.

Myers, K. (1966). The effects of density on sociality and health in mammals. *Proceedings of the Ecological Society of Australia*, Volume I, CSIRO, pp. 40–64.

Myers, K., Hale, C.S., Mykytowycz, R. et al. (1971). The effects of varying density and space on sociality and health in animals. In: *Behaviour and Environment*. Ed. Esser, A.H., pp. 148–187. Plenum Press, New York.

Myers, K., Parer, I., Wood, D. et al. (1994). The rabbit in Australia. In: *The European Rabbit: The History and Biology of a Successful Coloniser*. Eds Thompson, H.V. and King, C.M., pp. 108–157. Oxford University Press, Oxford.

Myers, K. and Poole, W.E. (1961). A study of the biology of the wild rabbit, *Oryctolagus cuniculus* (L.), in confined populations II. The effects of season and population increase on behaviour. *CSIRO Wildlife Research*, **6**, 1–41.

Myers, K. and Poole, W.E. (1963). A study of the biology of the wild rabbit, *Oryctolagus cuniculus* (L.), in confined populations. V. Population dynamics. *CSIRO Wildlife Research*, **8**, 166–203.

Myers, K. and Schneider, E.C. (1964). Observations on reproduction, mortality and behaviour in a small, free-living population of wild rabbits. *CSIRO Wildlife Research*, **9**, 138–143.

Mykytowycz, R. (1968). Territorial marking by rabbits. *Scientific American*, **218**, 116–126.

Mykytowycz, R. and Rowley, I. (1958). Continuous observations of the activity of the wild rabbit, *Oryctolagus cuniculus* (L.) during 24-hour periods. *CSIRO Wildlife Research*, **3**, 26–31.

National Research Council (NRC) (1977). *Nutrient Requirements of Rabbits*. Second revised edition. National Academy of Sciences, Washington, D.C..

Nerem, R.M. (1980). Social environment as a factor in diet-induced atherosclerosis. *Science*, **208**, 1475–1476.

Nowak, R. (1999). *Walker's Mammals of the World*, 6th edn. The John's Hopkins University Press, Baltimore.

Olfert, E.D., Cross, B.M. and McWilliam, A.A. (1993). *Guide to the Care and Use of Experimental Animals*, Vol. 2, 2nd edn. Canadian Council on Animal Care, Ottawa, Ontario.

Ooms, T., Artwohl, J.E., Conroy, L.M. et al. (2008). Concentration and emission of airborne contaminants in a laboratory animal facility housing rabbits. *Journal of the American Association for Laboratory Animal Science*, **47**, 39–48.

Parer, I. (1982). Dispersal of the wild rabbit, *Oryctolagus cuniculus*, at Urana in New South Wales. *Australian Wildlife Research*, **9**, 427–441.

Parker, S. (1990). *Grzimek's Encyclopedia of Mammals*. McGraw-Hill Inc, New York.

Pasteur, L. (1885). Méthode pour prévenir la rage après morsure. *Comptes Rendus Hebdomadaires des Seances de l'Academie des Sciences*, **101**, 765–774.

Patton, N.M. (1994). Colony husbandry. In: *The Biology of the Laboratory Rabbit*, 2nd edn. Eds Manning, P.J., Ringler, D.H. and Newcomer, C.E., pp. 27–45. Academic Press, New York.

Peeters, J.E. (1986). Etiology and pathology of diarrhea in weanling rabbits. In: *Rabbit Production Systems including Welfare*, A seminar in the community program for the coordination of agricultural research, 6–7 November 1986, pp. 128–131.

Peiffer, R.L. Jr., Pohm-Thorsen, L. and Corcoran, K. (1994). Models in ophthalmology and vision research. In: *The Biology of the Laboratory Rabbit*, 2nd edn. Eds Manning, P.J., Ringler, D.H. and Newcomer, C.E., pp. 409–433. Academic Press, New York.

Podberscek, A.L., Blackshaw, J.K. and Beattie, A.W. (1991). The behaviour of group penned and individually caged laboratory rabbits. *Applied Animal Behaviour Science*, **28**, 353–363.

Poggiagliolmi, S., Crowell-Davis, S.L., Alworth, L.C. et al. (2011). Environmental enrichment of New Zealand White rabbits living in laboratory cages. *Journal of Veterinary Behavior*, **6**, 342–350.

Poigner, J., Szendrö, Z.S., Levai, A. et al. (2000). Effect of birth weight and litter size on growth and mortality in rabbits. *World Rabbit Science*, **8**, 17–22.

Portsmouth, J. (1987). *Commercial Rabbit Keeping*, 3rd edn. Nimrod Press Ltd, Alton.

Report from the Commission to the European Parliament and the Council – 2019 report on the statistics on the use of animals for scientific purposes in the Member States of the European Union in 2015-2017. Brussels, 5.2.2020. COM (2020) 16 final. Published 2020-02-05 by Directorate-General for Environment (European Commission). (https://eur-lex.europa.eu/legal-content/SV/TXT/HTML/?uri=CELEX:52020DC0016&from=EN).

Rogers, P.M., Arthur, C.P. and Soriguer, R.C. (1994). The rabbit in continental Europe. In: *The European Rabbit: The History and Biology of a Successful Coloniser*. Eds Thompson, H.V. and King, C.M., pp. 22–63. Oxford University Press, Oxford.

Rollins, W.D., Casady, R.B., Sittman, K. et al. (1963). Genetic variance components analysis of litter size and weaning weight of New Zealand White rabbits. *Journal of Animal Science*, **22**, 654–654.

Rothfritz, P., Loeffler, K. and Drescher, B. (1992). Einfluss unterschiedlicher Haltungsverfaren und Bewegungsmöglichkeiten auf die Spongiosastruktur der Rippen sowie Brust- und Lendenwirbel von Versuchs- und Fleischkaninchen. *Tierärztliche Umschau*, **47**, 758–768.

Ruckebusch, Y., Grivel, M.L. and Fargeas, M.J. (1971). Electrical activity of the intestine and feeding associated with a visual conditioning in the rabbit. *Physiology & Behavior*, **6**, 359–365.

Ruckebusch, Y., Phaneuf, L.P. and Dunlop, R. (1991). *Physiology of Small and Large Animals*. Dekker, Philadelphia.

Schepers, F., Koene, P. and Beerda, B. (2009). Welfare assessment in pet rabbits. *Animal Welfare*, **18**, 477–495.

Seaman, S.C., Waran, N.K., Mason, G. et al. (2008). Animal economics: assessing the motivation of female laboratory rabbits to reach a platform, social contact and food. *Animal Behaviour*, **75**, 31–42.

Sharples, C.M., Fa, J.E. and Bell, D.J. (1996). Geographical variation in size in the European rabbit Oryctolagus cuniculus (*Lagomorpha: Leporidae*) in Western Europe and North Africa. *Zoological Journal of the Linnean Society*, **117**, 141–158.

Shiomi, M. and Jianglin, F. (2008). Unstable coronary plaques and cardiac events in myocardial infarction-prone Watanabe heritable hyperlipidemic rabbits: questions and quandaries. *Current Opinion in Lipidology*, **19**, 631–636.

Shope, R. and Hurst, W. (1933). Infectious papillomatosis of rabbits with a note on the histopathology. *Journal of Experimental Medicine*, **58**, 607–624.

Sittman, D.B., Rollins, W.C., Sittman, K. et al. (1964). Seasonal variation in reproductive traits of New Zealand White rabbits. *Journal of Reproductive Fertility*, **8**, 29–37.

Staples, R.E. and Holtkamp, D.E. (1966). Influence of body weight upon corpus luteum formation and maintenance of pregnancy in the rabbit. *Journal of Reproductive Fertility*, **12**, 221–224.

Southern, H.N. (1948). Sexual and aggressive behaviour in the wild rabbit. *Behaviour*, **1**, 173–194.

Spector, W. (1956). *Handbook of Biological Data*. WB Saunders, Philadelphia.

Stauffacher, M. (1992). Group housing and enrichment cages for breeding, fattening and laboratory rabbits. *Animal Welfare*, **1**, 105–125.

Stauffacher, M. (1993). Tierschutzorientierte Labortierethologie in der Tiermedizin und in der Versuchstierkunde – ein Beitrag zum Refinement bei der haltung und im Umgang mit Versuchstieren. In: *Ersatz- und Ergänzungsmethoden zu Tierversuchen*, Vol. 2. Eds Schöffl, H., Spielmann, H., Gruber, F. et al., pp. 6–21. Springer, Wien.

Stauffacher, M., Bell, D.J. and Schulz, K.-D. (1994). Rabbits. In: *The Accommodation of Laboratory Animals in Accordance with Animal Welfare Requirements*. Ed. O'Donoghue, P.N., pp. 15–30. Proceedings the International Workshop Bundesgesundheitsant, Berlin 17–19 May 1993.

Stein, S. and Walshaw, S. (1996). Rabbits. In: *Rodent and Rabbit Medicine*. Eds Laber-Laird, K., Swindle, M.M. and Flecknell, P., pp. 183–211. Elsevier, Oxford.

Stodart, E. and Myers, K. (1964). A comparison of behaviour, reproduction and mortality of wild and domestic rabbits in confined populations. *C.S.I.R.O. Wildlife Research*, **9**, 144–159.

Suckow, M.A. and Douglas, F.A. (1997) The laboratory rabbit. In: *The Laboratory Animal Pocket Reference Series*. Ed. Suckow, M., pp. 71–74. CRC Press LLC, Boca Raton.

Svendsen, P. (1994) Laboratory animal anaesthesia. In: *Handbook of Laboratory Animal Science*. Eds Svendsen, P. and Hau, J., pp. 311–337. CRC Press, Boca Raton.

Swallow, J.J. (1999). Transporting animals. In: *The UFAW Handbook on the Care and Management of Laboratory Animals*, 7th edn. Ed. Poole, T., pp. 171–187. Blackwell Publishing, Oxford.

Swallow, J., Anderson, D., Buckwell, A.C. et al. (2005). Guidance on the transport of laboratory animals. *Laboratory Animals*, **39**, 1–39.

Swennes, A.G., Alworth, L.C., Harvet, A.B. et al. (2011). Human handling promotes compliant behaviour in adult laboratory rabbits. *Journal of the American Association for Laboratory Animal Science*, **50**, 41–45.

Tawfik, E.S., Sherif, S.Y., El-Hindawy, M. et al. (1997). The role of fibre in rabbit nutrition. *Der Tropenlan, Beitrage zur Tropischen Landwirtschaft und Veternarmedizin*, **98**, 73–81.

The American Rabbit Breeders Association (ARBA). https://www.arba.net (Accessed 11 February 2018)

Toth, L.A. and January, B. (1990). Physiological stabilisation of rabbits after shipping. *Laboratory Animal Science*, **40**, 384–387.

Turner, R.J., Selby, J.L., Held, S.D.E. et al. (1992). Preferred substances for penned laboratory rabbits. *Animal Technology*, **43**, 185–192.

United States Department of Agriculture Animal and Plant Health Inspection Service Annual Report Animal Usage (2017). https://www.aphis.usda.gov/animal_welfare/downloads/reports/Annual-Report-Animal-Usage-by-FY2017.pdf

Valentini, S., Santoro, G., Baffetta, F. et al. (2019). Monocyte-activation test to reliably measure the pyrogenic content of a vaccine: An in vitro pyrogen test to overcome in vivo limitations. *Vaccine*, **37**, 3754–3760.

Vastrade, M. (1987). Spacing behaviour of free-ranging domestic rabbits, *Oryctolagus cuniculus* L. *Applied Animal Behaviour Sciences*, **18**, 185–195.

Vaughan, T., Ryan, J. and Czaplewski, N. (2000). *Mammalogy*. Harcourt Inc, New York.

Verga, M., Luzi, F. and Carenzi, C. (2007). Effects of husbandry and management systems on physiology and behavior of farmed and laboratory rabbits. *Hormones & Behavior*, **52**, 122–129.

Verwer, C.M., Van der Ark, A., Van Amerogen, G. et al. (2009). Reducing variation in a rabbit vaccine safety study with particular emphasis on housing conditions and handling. *Laboratory Animals*, **43**, 155–164.

Wagner, J.L., Hackel, D.B. and Samsell, A.G. (1974). Spontaneous deaths in rabbits resulting from trichobezoars. *Laboratory Animal Science*, **24**, 826–830.

Waikato Regional Council biosecurity factsheet series. Updated June 2015 (4283-0515) https://www.waikatoregion.govt.nz/assets/PageFiles/3508/4283%20-%20Rabbits%20factsheet%202015_web.pdf

Wallace, J., Sanford, J., Smith, M.W. et al. (1990). The assessment and control of the severity of scientific procedures on laboratory animals. Report of the Laboratory Animal Science Association Working Party. *Laboratory Animals*, **24**, 97–130.

Watanabe, T., Hirata, M., Yoshikawa, Y. et al. (1985). Role of macrophages in atherosclerosis. Sequential observations of cholesterol-induced rabbit aortic lesion by the immunoperoxidase technique using monoclonal antimacrophage antibody. *Laboratory Investigation; A Journal of Technical Methods and Pathology*, **53**, 80–90.

Webb, N.J. (1993). Growth and mortality in juvenile European wild rabbits *Oryctolagus cuniculus*. *Journal of Zoology*, **230**, 665–677.

Webb, N.J., Ibrahim, K.M., Bell, D.J. et al. (1995). Natal dispersal and genetic structure in a population of the European wild rabbit (*Oryctolagus cuniculus*). *Molecular Ecology*, **4**, 239–247.

Wetterholm, R., Caidahl, K., Volkmann, R. et al. (2007). Imaging of atherosclerosis in WHHL rabbits using high-resolution ultrasound. *Ultrasound Medical Biology*, **33**, 720–726.

Wieser, R.V. (1986). *Funktionale analyse des verhalten als grundlage zur beurteilung der tiergerechtheit. Eine untersuchung zu normalverhalten und verhaltensstoerungen bei hauskaninchen-zibben*. PhD thesis, University of Berne.

Wilson, D. and Reeder, D. (1993). *Mammal Species of the World: A Taxonomic and Geographic Reference*. The Smithsonian Institution, Washington, DC.

Wood, D.H. (1980). The demography of a rabbit population in an arid region of New South Wales, Australia. *Journal of Animal Ecology*, **49**, 55–80.

Wooding, P. and Burton, G. (2008). *Comparative Placentation: Structures, Functions and Evolution*. SpringerLink, Heidelberg.

Wullschleger, M. (1987). Nestbeschaeftigung bei saeugenden Hauskaninchenzibben. *Revue Suisse de Zoologie*, **94**, 553–562.

Yanni, A.E. (2004). The laboratory rabbit: an animal model of atherosclerosis research. *Laboratory Animals*, **38**, 246–256.

Zain, K. (1988). *Effects of Early Social Environment on Physical and Behavioural Development in the Rabbit*. PhD thesis, University of East Anglia.

Zarrow, M.X., Denenberg, V.H. and Anderson, C.O. (1965). Rabbit: frequency of suckling in the pup. *Science*, **150**, 1835–1836.

Zucca, D., Redaelli, V., Marelli, S.P. et al. (2012). Effect of handling in pre-weaning rabbits. *World Rabbit Science*, **20**, 97–101.

Carnivora

29 The ferret

Maggie Lloyd

Introduction

Ferrets are primitive carnivores belonging to the family Mustelidae, and are related to stoats, weasels, badgers and mink. They are curious and playful animals, increasingly kept as pets, as well as being used as working or research animals.

Mustelids are among the most primitive of terrestrial carnivores. All mustelids secrete a strong-smelling musk from their anal glands especially when frightened, and ferrets are no exception. They have the Latin name *Mustela putorius furo*, which translates as 'smelly weasel thief'.

Phylogenetic studies suggest that the ferret may be a domesticated form of a North African lineage of the European polecat (*Mustela putorius*) (Sato et al. 2003), and they can interbreed with polecats. They can be distinguished as their masks are different and polecats have darker fur. Ferrets are more docile than polecats but have retained many of their natural behaviour patterns. Other ferret species (not discussed here) include the steppe polecat (*Mustela eversmanii*), native to Central and Eastern Europe and Central Asia, and the black-footed ferret (*Mustela nigripes*), an endangered species native to central North America. An alternative theory is that the ferret is related to the steppe polecat, which it resembles in skull morphology (Fox 2014).

The natural history of the domestic ferret is uncertain due to the lack of written records, but analysis of mitochondrial DNA suggests that ferrets have been domesticated for at least 2,500 years (Lloyd 1999; Sato et al. 2003; Fox 2014). Early Greek and Roman records describe an animal that appears to be the ferret, and pictures have been found in Egyptian tombs of ferret-like animals on leads, although no ferret remains have been found in the area. It is not certain why ferrets were originally domesticated, but likely explanations are for hunting small game such as rabbits, and for control of rodents and snakes. Their sleek, flexible bodies make them ideal for working in confined spaces, as they can move freely and turn around in narrow tunnels. They can be trained to work on leads and to come to call and have been used to lay cables – indeed they are still being used on occasion for this purpose (BBC News 1999). Ferrets have also been bred for their fur, which is known as fitch. Ferrets are still used for hunting today but increasingly they are kept simply as pets.

Different varieties of domestic ferret can be distinguished based on fur colouration. The most common or wild type variety is known as 'fitch' or 'polecat' (black guard hair, cream undercoat, black points, lighter facial fur with dark mask, dark brown or black eyes). This fur pattern is very similar to that of the wild European polecat. Other colours include cinnamon (beige guard hair, cream undercoat, no mask) and the albino or English ferret. Albinos have yellow or white fur and pink eyes. The albino variety is genetically recessive to the pigmented wild type.

Male ferrets are called hobs, and females are known as jills.

Biological overview

General biology

The general external morphology of the ferret resembles that of other members of the family Mustelidae, showing the typical characteristics of a sleek, flexible, elongated tubular body, relatively short legs, and small rounded ears. The heart is located more caudally in the body than in dogs and cats.

Both males and females show marked seasonal variations in coat and body weight (Lloyd 1999). Under natural lighting conditions, ferrets moult in the autumn and may develop seasonal alopecia, which becomes more prominent as they age. Alopecia is also a common presenting sign in several ferret diseases. The overall coat colour and pigment distribution are similar throughout the year, although the coat is shorter and darker in summer and longer and lighter in winter (Bixler & Ellis 2004). The coat in males is not usually fully replaced until the end of the breeding season. Females tend to moult after ovulation, especially the first one of the season, and this can sometimes result in marked alopecia. Moulting may be delayed during lactation.

Body weight can fluctuate by up to 40% between summer and winter, as animals lay down fat as the winter months approach.

See Table 29.1 for basic biological data for ferrets.

The UFAW Handbook on the Care and Management of Laboratory and Other Research Animals, Ninth Edition.
Edited by Huw Golledge and Claire Richardson.
© 2024 John Wiley & Sons Ltd. Published 2024 by John Wiley & Sons Ltd.

Table 29.1 Biological and breeding data.

Adult weight[1]		Puberty (months)	9–12
Male	1–2 kg	Age to breed (days)	
Female	600–900 g	Male	365
Food intake (g)	50–75	Female	275
Water intake (ml)	75–100	Gestation (days)	38–44 (average 42)
Chromosome number (diploid)	40	Length of breeding life (years)	2–5
Natural lifespan (years)	5–9	Litter size	1–18 (average 8)
Rectal temperature (°C)	37.8–40	Birth weight (g)	6–12
Heart rate/min	170–280	Weaning age (weeks)	6–8
Cardiac output (ml/min)	200–400	Eyes open (days)	34
Blood pressure (mmHg)		Onset of hearing (days)	32
Systole	110–140	Oestrous cycle	Induced ovulator
Diastole	31–35	**Biochemical data**	
Blood volume (ml/kg)	45–70	PCV (%)	42–61
Respiratory rate/min	25–40	Hb (g/dl)	12–18
Diploid number	40	Serum protein (g/dl)	3.5–7.4
Dental formula		Albumin (g/dl)	2.6–3.8
Permanent	$I^3_3 C^1_1 Pm^3_3 M^1_2$	Globulin (g/dl)	2.5–4.8
Deciduous	$I^4_3 C^1_1 Pm^3_3$	Glucose (mg/dl)	94–207
Vertebral formula	C7, T15, L5(6),	Blood urea nitrogen (mg/dl)	10–45
S3, Cy18		Creatinine (mg/dl)	0.2–0.9
Haematological data		Total bilirubin (mg/dl)	0–0.4
Red blood cells ($\times 10^6$/mm^3)	6.8–12.2	Cholesterol (mg/dl)	64–296
White blood cells ($\times 10^3$/mm^3)	4–19	Urine volume (ml/24 h)	26–28
Neutrophils (%)	11–84	Urine pH	6.5–7.5
Lymphocytes (%)	12–69		
Eosinophils (%)	0–7		
Monocytes (%)	0–8		
Basophils (%)	0–2		
Platelets ($\times 10^3$/mm^3)	297–910		

[1] Seasonal body weight fluctuations up to 40%.
Source: Bixler and Ellis (2004); Wolfensohn and Lloyd (2013).

Behaviour

Ferrets are highly intelligent, agile, lively, playful and curious. They do not develop a fear of humans or human environments, and their natural instinct is to explore (Porter & Brown 1997).

Ferrets are domesticated animals and are not generally found in the wild. What is known of their natural social organisation comes from studies of feral ferret populations and of the European polecat. These studies concluded that ferrets in a natural environment are largely solitary (Clapperton 2001). Hobs occupy large territories, which usually include those of several jills, with whom they mate. Young ferrets are born in the spring or summer, and initially accompany their mother on hunting expeditions. They may remain together as a group after weaning until they finally disperse in the spring following their birth and establish their own territories. However, domestic ferrets are sociable and gregarious, and seem to benefit from being kept in compatible groups in captivity, where interaction with other animals provides enrichment. Groups of jills without litters, young animals and castrated males (hobbles) should be kept together, although group housing is not advisable for adult hobs, jills with litters, and breeding females that are in oestrus or have been mated, which may need to be kept separately to prevent pseudopregnancy (Fox & Broome 2014). Singly housed animals benefit from regular interaction with their human caretakers to help prevent boredom.

Ferrets kept in standard laboratory housing spend up to 70% of the time sleeping, with short episodes of activity in between (Jha *et al.* 2006). When awake, ferrets are very lively and like to burrow, hide and explore. When given a complex, three-dimensional environment, ferrets will make good use of it (see Figure 29.1). Ferrets are tunnel dwellers, and particularly benefit from tubes and tunnels to explore (Fox & Broome 2014). Typically, they are very active for short periods then sleep soundly for several hours. They are more active at night. The remainder of their time is spent actively exploring the environment and playing and interacting with other ferrets. They spend much time burrowing through their bedding, which can lead to bouts of sneezing. Exercise periods often coincide with feeding time. They like to sleep in dark, enclosed areas such as wooden or cardboard boxes, and will even sleep in paper bags.

Young ferrets play constantly. Mock aggression, play chasing, wrestling and pouncing may be commonly observed. They will nip at anything and may bite when first handled, but become more docile if handled frequently.

Ferrets are able to vocalise and produce a number of different sounds. When playing, they may hiss and chuckle, and when frightened or threatened, they may scream. When foraging, they may produce a low-pitched grumble.

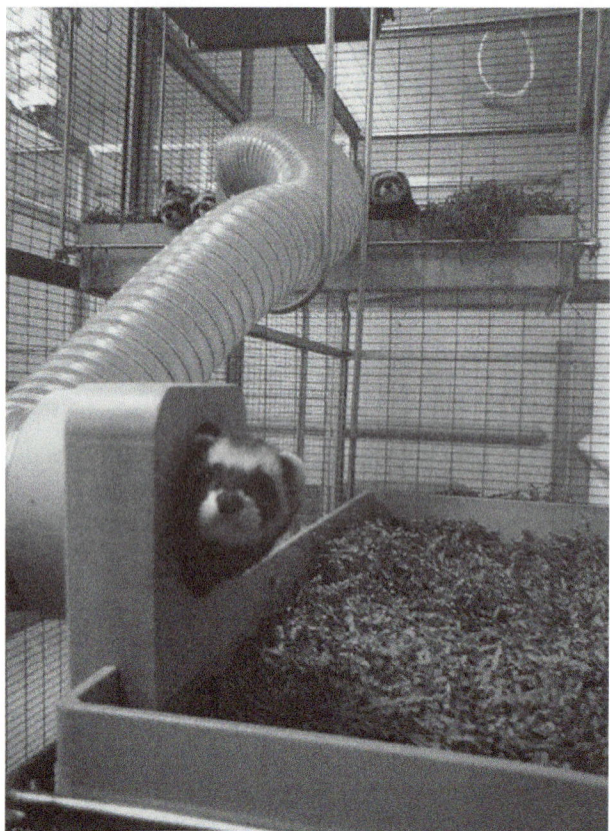

Figure 29.1 An enriched environment suitable for ferrets.
Source: Wolfensohn and Lloyd (2013), figure 12.02/with permission from John Wiley & Sons, Inc.

Ferrets have an undeserved reputation for being aggressive. Their play can be rough, dragging other ferrets by the neck and ears with lots of squealing, and they may mistake a tentatively approaching hand for food. However, ferrets respond well to frequent handling and rapidly become friendly. Properly handled ferrets are not aggressive.

Uses in the laboratory

The domestic ferret is an invaluable biomedical research model. Ferrets are used for a variety of disease models, due to the anatomical and physiological features they share with humans and their susceptibility to many human pathogens, including influenza virus and severe acute respiratory distress (SARS) associated coronavirus, including coronavirus disease 2019 (COVID-19) caused by severe acute respiratory syndrome coronavirus 2 (SARS-CoV-2) (Muñoz-Fontela et al. 2020). Ferrets are used in cardiovascular research (Morgan 2014), respiratory research, auditory research (Nodal & King 2014) and increasingly in neurological research (Sukhinin et al. 2016). Use of the ferret in immunological studies has been hampered by a lack of validated reagents, however these are being developed (Albrecht et al. 2018), making the ferret an increasingly valuable research model.

Husbandry and management

Housing

Ferrets are intelligent and playful animals that need a complex and stimulating environment. The curious nature of these animals leads them to test all avenues of escape and adventure. Ferrets can squeeze into very tight spaces, and any hole large enough to get a head through will allow the animal to escape, with potentially tragic consequences for the ferret itself or for neighbouring rodent or bird populations (Lewington 2000). Ferrets will chew items in their environment (Fox & Broome 2014) and any cage furniture should also take this inquisitiveness into account. Ferrets like to burrow and hide, and tubes, tunnels, boxes, paper bags and deep burrowing substrate can all help to provide an interesting and stimulating environment, which is essential for the well-being of ferrets. Any enrichment must be sufficiently durable that the animals cannot chew or swallow bits of them, which can lead to gastrointestinal foreign bodies. Chewing may also cause trauma to teeth and gums, which should be checked regularly for signs of injury (Fox & Broome 2014). See Figure 29.1.

Ferrets will urinate and defaecate in one corner of their enclosure, usually against a vertical surface, and they can be trained to use a litter box. Clay cat litter is not recommended however as ferrets dig and burrow into the substrate, which can dry the coat and cake the nostrils (Bixler & Ellis 2004).

Environment

Ferrets can tolerate a wide range of temperatures, although they have poorly developed sweat glands so they tolerate extreme heat poorly (Fox & Broome 2014). They are susceptible to heat exhaustion when exposed to temperatures above 32°C. Ferrets affected by heat stroke may be recumbent and unresponsive, with body temperatures over 40°C. The recommended temperature range is of 15–24 °C, and unweaned young should be kept above 15 °C. Approximately 10–15 air changes per hour are recommended (Home Office 2014), to reduce the musky odour and minimise the risk of respiratory diseases (Fox & Broome 2014).

Nutrition

A detailed discussion of ferret nutrition can be found in Fox et al. (2014). Ferrets are obligate carnivores with a short intestinal tract, and have evolved to eat frequent, small meals (Powers & Brown 2012). The gastrointestinal tract transit time is only 3–4 hours, so food needs to be easily digestible as there is little time for nutrients to be absorbed. Although the exact nutritional needs of ferrets have not been established, it is known that ferrets need a protein-rich diet and cannot readily utilise carbohydrates (Bell 1999; Fox et al. 2014). There is little need for dietary fibre, and microbes seem to play little or no part in digestion (Fox et al. 2014). Since they eat to calorie requirements, feeding foods rich in carbohydrates may lead to protein deficiency. Adult ferrets appear to need meat-based diets containing 30–40% protein, 18–20% fat and 2% fibre.

Dry diets may be soaked and fed as a stiff paste. Breeding and young animals may need higher protein and fat levels. Treats should be given in moderation and should themselves be nutritionally appropriate. Diets designed for dogs should not be fed to ferrets, as they may not contain sufficient protein and often contain high levels of vegetable matter. It has been suggested that inappropriate diets may be associated with the development of diseases such as eosinophilic gastroenteritis, urolithiasis and insulinoma, although this is not proven (Bixler & Ellis 2004).

Ferrets should be provided with access to fresh water at all times.

Reproduction and breeding

Ferrets are seasonal breeders. They become sexually mature in the spring following birth, at between 8 and 12 months of age. The breeding season is determined by photoperiod, responses being mediated via the pineal body; however, this can be altered by manipulating the light cycle. Males are light-negative: they begin coming into season as the day shortens, whereas females are light-positive, responding to increasing day length. In the Northern Hemisphere, males are in breeding condition between December and July, and females between March and September. The seasonal nature of breeding means that ferrets generally have one litter per year, in the late spring or early summer, and may sometimes have a second litter at the end of the summer, although first litters are generally superior in vigour to subsequent ones.

Care must be taken to provide an appropriate light cycle for breeding ferrets or problems may ensue. Mated and lactating females need to be maintained on long day cycles, otherwise they may fail to reproduce or maintain lactation. Year-round breeding can be achieved by careful manipulation of the light cycle. Having two ferret breeding rooms, one on Northern Hemisphere light cycles and one on southern hemisphere light cycles or one winter and one summer, allows for year-round breeding. Alternatively, males maintained in short photoperiods (8 hours) will remain in breeding condition for more than a year. Each male should have an annual period of rest for 5–6 weeks in a long photoperiod (14 hours) before returning to short days. Females can also be kept in short photoperiod, and moved into long photoperiod to bring them into season as required. Females begin their season after 6–8 weeks on long days.

Females in oestrus develop vulval swelling which peaks one month after the onset of oestrus. As an adaptation to solitary life, ferrets are induced ovulators, and jills remain in oestrus until either mated or until the days begin to shorten, when they enter a period of anoestrus. Oestrous females are exposed to high oestrogen levels, which if prolonged can lead to serious health problems. Active management of oestrus is needed for females which are not to be used for breeding (see section Common Diseases: hyperoestrogenism).

During the non-breeding season, the testes of the male recede into the body, becoming almost invisible under the heavy winter coat. About the time of the shortest day, they begin to move back into the scrotum. The males need to come into season about 4 weeks prior to the females to allow for sperm maturation. The male reaches his sexual peak in March or April as the females begin to come into season, remaining in breeding condition until the end of the summer, when the testes begin to withdraw back into the body cavity

The condition of the jill should always be checked prior to mating, and only animals in good condition should be mated. The birth process is particularly demanding on jills, and an unfit female is more likely to have problems during pregnancy and birth, and as a result produce small, weak young.

The female is responsive to the male when there are about 14–15 hours of daylight. She should be taken to the male and left with him for 2 days. The optimum time for conception is 14 days after vulval swelling appears. Mating is vigorous, prolonged and noisy. The male will grasp the jill by the scruff of the neck and drag her around for up to one hour before coitus, which can then take up to a further three hours. The skin on the back of the jill's neck is sufficiently thick to withstand biting by the male, but injuries may occur occasionally. Ovulation occurs 30–35 hours after mating. The vulval swelling recedes within a few days of mating.

After mating, jills should be housed away from stud males, to reduce the risk of disturbance to the jill leading to cannibalism of the young, and should not return to the same enclosure as unmated cage mates, as this can cause pseudopregnancy in the unmated females.

Pregnant females should be moved into their littering cages about 2–3 weeks prior to parturition and provided with a nest box containing suitable nesting material. Jills lose their winter coat and may look rather scruffy during gestation. It is important that they get adequate nutrition. They should be fed ad lib a diet of 35–40% protein and 18–20% fat during pregnancy, increasing the fat content to 30% during lactation. Jills are prone to pregnancy toxaemia (Ball 2006), and nutritional supplementation may be required.

Pregnant females become more aggressive as gestation progresses, and jills are very protective of their young.

Dystocia is common, and neonatal mortality can reach 8–10%, due to stillbirths, congenital defects and cannibalism (Lewington 2000). Cannibalism is common with larger litters and may also be an inherited trait. Hypothermia or bloat caused by poor hygiene or overeating may also lead to neonatal death. Mortality declines after 5 days, and deaths after this time may be due to maternal neglect or agalactia, often caused by a return to oestrus. With litters larger than 5, oestrus is usually suppressed, but with small litters the jill may return to oestrus before weaning. In this case, she should be mated again, as high oestrogen levels suppress the milk supply. The jill may also kill a small litter, allowing her to return into season.

Good management can reduce problems encountered in the periparturient period. The jill should be left undisturbed for several days post-partum, and given adequate nutrition, with increasing quantities of food offered from two to three days after birth. Calcium supplementation may be needed to prevent hypocalcaemia, which can occur at peak lactation 3–4 weeks after birth.

Gestation lasts for 40–42 days and, assuming an early mating, litters are born in early summer when the days are at their longest and warmest. Up to 18, young can be produced, the average litter being 8, each kit weighing around 6–12 g. All kits have white hair regardless of their eventual coat colour. Ferret milk contains 23.5% solids, composed of 34% fat, 25.5% protein and 16.2% carbohydrate (Lloyd 1999). Kits have voracious appetites, and they develop rapidly, doubling their birth weight in 5 days. The jill therefore needs to produce copious amounts of milk. Jills have eight nipples but can feed more kits if the milk supply is good.

Although their eyes are closed until around 34 days, kits start to become active from about 14 to 21 days. At this point, they start to eat solids, and the jill will take food to the kits. Growth is gradual up to weaning at about 6–8 weeks of age, when body weight reaches at least 200–250 g. At this point, kits fed ad lib eat approximately 30 g of solid food and drink about 125 ml daily. Kits can be weaned at the end of the summer and can build up their supply of body fat during the autumn for the coming winter. Adult weight is reached at approximately 16 weeks.

Breeding performance declines after approximately three years of age in males, or after three or four litters in females.

Care of aged animals

Ferrets can live to 5–9 years of age. Aged ferrets are not commonly used in the laboratory, although they may be used to study age-related susceptibility to influenza virus infection (Paquette et al. 2014). It is normal for the hair coat to become coarser as animals age, and the footpads may become hard and dry with corny growths. Older ferrets may become less playful and spend more time sleeping. Health problems are more likely to develop beyond 3–4 years of age, including neoplasia, cardiovascular conditions, dental problems and hairballs. Aged ferrets may develop arthritis or other joint problems, but this is rare. Such ferrets may need adjustments in the environment such as softer bedding and floor feeding. They benefit from regular health checks as they age, which may include taking blood samples to check for renal and other systemic diseases.

Handing and techniques

Identification

Ferrets can be identified using a number of different methods. Electronic microchips are probably the most reliable method, and these can be inserted at any age without sedation or anaesthesia. Collars can be used for short-term identification, but the narrow head of the ferret makes it difficult to keep them in place. Tattooing provides a permanent method of identification, and the best site is on the inside of the thigh. Anaesthesia is usually recommended for this. Ferrets have small pinnae which are not suitable for tattooing or ear tags. Albino ferrets may be identified using dyes, but these have to be renewed on a regular basis. Shaving patches over the back may also be used for short-term identification.

Handling

Ferrets are generally docile and easy to restrain, although they have poor eyesight and may bite anything that crosses their field of view. Ferrets handled frequently from a young age will become friendly and amenable, facilitating the performance of procedures. Ferrets may be picked up easily by

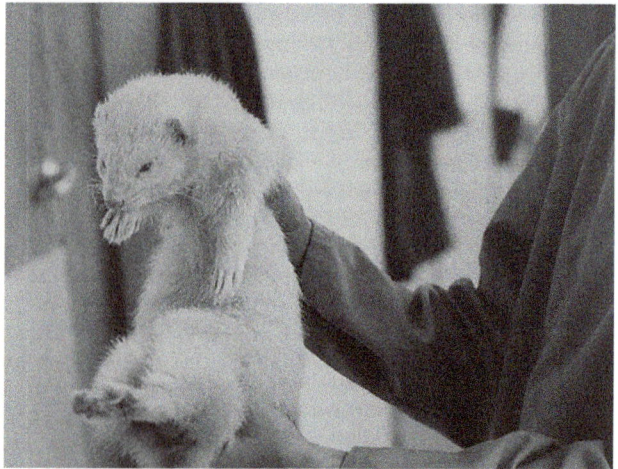

Figure 29.2 Handling the ferret. Source: Wolfensohn and Lloyd (2013), figure 12.03/with permission from John Wiley & Sons, Inc.

distracting them with one hand and then grasping them over the shoulders or under the ribcage with the other. The animal can then be lifted from the table and the hindquarters supported if necessary. Lively ferrets may need to be held by the scruff of the neck for additional restraint. Most animals will relax when lifted in this way. See Figure 29.2.

Minor techniques

Ferrets have very tough skin, and it can be hard to penetrate. A new, sharp needle should always be used when giving injections. Many procedures are best performed by two people, as it can be difficult to properly restrain a ferret with one hand and administer an injection with the other.

Blood sampling

Ferrets have a higher packed cell volume than other species, so relatively larger blood samples may be needed to collect sufficient plasma or serum for the proposed study. Several sites are available depending on the volume of blood required. Large volumes can be collected form the jugular vein or anterior vena cava. The cephalic, saphenous or ventral tail veins may be used for smaller volumes. Most ferrets can be manually restrained for blood sampling.

For the anterior vena cava, three people may be needed. The animal is placed in dorsal recumbency, and one person restrains the body and legs while a second holds the head with the neck extended. A third person draws the blood sample: first the notch where the first rib meets the manubrium is identified. A 25G needle is then inserted at a 45° angle to the skin, directed towards the opposite hind leg.

For jugular venepuncture, place the ferret in dorsal recumbency, and restrain it, as above. The neck should be shaved and pressure applied at the thoracic inlet to raise the vein. A 21G needle can then be inserted into the vein, angled towards the heart. Alternatively, the ferret can be wrapped firmly in a towel, with the forelimbs extended back along the thorax, and the head extended to provide access to the ventral neck area. See Figure 29.3.

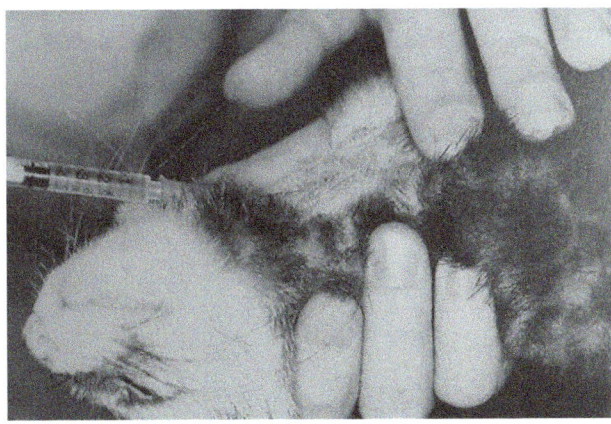

Figure 29.3 Jugular venepuncture in the ferret. Source: Wolfensohn and Lloyd (2013), figure 07.06 / with permission from John Wiley & Sons, Inc.

The lateral saphenous vein is found on the outside of the hind leg just above the ankle. The ferret is restrained in lateral recumbency and the outer surface of the leg shaved. The palm of one hand is used to support the pelvis while simultaneously raising the vein by applying pressure with the fingers above the stifle.

The ventral tail vein is accessed by placing the ferret on its back. The vein is located in the midline and can be accessed via the groove on the ventral surface of the proximal third of the tail. A needle is advanced slowly into the midline at a 45° angle close to the tail base until blood is observed in the hub of the needle.

Administration of substances

Subcutaneous injections: These can be given into the loose skin over the shoulders. The skin is very thick here and a 21G needle may be needed, to prevent the needle from bending.

Intramuscular injections: These can be given into the quadriceps on the front of the thigh or the hamstrings on the back of the thigh. Small volumes may be injected into the epaxial muscles either side of the spine. Intramuscular injections can be painful, and the injection volume should be kept to a minimum.

Intravenous injections: These can be made into the cephalic vein – these are usually made via an indwelling catheter, which may be placed under general anaesthesia. Catheters may also be inserted into the saphenous veins, but it is difficult to maintain catheters in this site.

Surgical techniques

In general, ferrets tolerate surgical procedures well (Bennett 2009). Animals should be checked before surgery to ensure they are healthy, and this may include appropriate pre-operative laboratory tests, such as a complete blood count and biochemistry profile.

Surgical procedures on ferrets can often be performed in a similar manner to those in other small domestic animals and small animal basic surgery textbooks can be a useful source of information. See also Lightfoot *et al.* (2012) for information about specific procedures in ferrets.

Ferrets have thick skin in some places, and thin skin in others, with thin abdominal musculature. For abdominal surgery, the skin and muscles are thin and there is little subcutaneous fat so great care must be taken when making an incision with a scalpel not to apply too much pressure. Ferrets often have an enlarged spleen, and care should be taken not to damage the spleen when incising into the cranial abdomen.

Ferrets are keen suture chewers and are unforgiving if sutures are uncomfortable, so care must be taken to ensure that the sutures are secure. Wounds in the neck appear to irritate more than abdominal ones, although ferrets are prone to the development of a serosanguinous discharge from abdominal wounds following surgery, which is normally self-limiting (Lloyd 1999). It is recommended that subcuticular sutures using fine synthetic absorbable suture materials are placed in the skin to reduce the likelihood of wound breakdown. Widespread bruising around incision sites is common and can last 5–7 days (Bennett 2009).

Antibiotic therapy should not normally be required after surgery provided aseptic techniques are employed.

Anaesthesia and analgesia

Pre-anaesthetic considerations

Anaesthesia in ferrets can be challenging, due to their small size and lack of accessible blood vessels. Stress and ill health increase the risk of problems. Therefore, only healthy animals should be anaesthetised, and good care taken before, during and after anaesthesia. Ensure there are no cardiovascular or respiratory problems and obtain an accurate weight to avoid over- or underestimation of the drug doses required.

Ferrets vomit readily and should be fasted for up to four hours prior to anaesthesia. Due to the short gut transit time of only 3–4 hours, longer periods of fasting may lead to hypoglycaemia. Free access to water should be given until immediately prior to induction.

Animal need to be calm before anaesthesia, so premedication may be appropriate. For short, non-painful procedures, a sedative alone may be sufficient. For major surgical procedures, combinations including an analgesic are recommended. Since the airways are small and easily blocked, drying agents may also be indicated. Table 29.2 gives suggested doses of sedatives and premedicants. Note that these doses are only intended as a guideline and there may be considerable variation between animals depending on their body weight, sex and general health (Hawkins & Pascoe 2012).

General anaesthesia

General anaesthesia may be induced in ferrets by injection or inhalation.

Intravenous injection can be difficult in the conscious animal, and therefore agents that can be administered by a different route are commonly used. In friendly or sedated ferrets, an intravenous cannula can be placed into the cephalic vein to facilitate the administration of anaesthetic agents or fluids. It may be necessary to make a tiny cut in the skin over the vein before inserting the cannula, otherwise the

Table 29.2 Sedatives and premedicants.

Drug	Dose	Comments
Midazolam[1] with ketamine[1]	0.2 mg/kg with 10 mg/kg im	Short-term sedation with relaxation
Medetomidine	0.01–0.2 mg/kg sc or im	Dose-dependent sedation. Reverse with atipamezole
Diazepam[1] or midazolam[1]	0.25–0.5 mg/kg iv	Reduces anxiety and produces relaxation. Can be hypotensive
Ketamine[1]	10–30 mg/kg im	Poor muscle relaxation if used alone
Acepromazine	0.1–0.2 mg/kg sc/im	Hypotensive
Acepromazine with buprenorphine[1]	0.1–0.2 mg/kg with 0.01–0.03 mg/kg im	For premedication
Atropine	0.05 mg/kg sc	Dries airway secretions

[1] Note: these are controlled drugs under the Misuse of Drugs Regulations in the UK. Special storage and record-keeping requirements may apply. Doses are intended as a guide only.
Source: Dose rates from Carpenter and Marion (2013); Hawkins and Pascoe (2012); Ko and Marini (2008); Lloyd (2002); Meredith (2015).

thick skin can make insertion difficult. Injectable agents should be dosed by weight, but account should be taken of the time of year, since in the winter ferrets accumulate fat and may require relatively more anaesthetic. Always administer oxygen, since many anaesthetics cause respiratory depression. Respiratory failure is a common cause of anaesthetic emergencies in ferrets. Suitable drug combinations for anaesthesia are given in Table 29.3.

Anaesthesia can be induced in friendly or sedated ferrets by intravenous injection of alphaxalone or propofol. Induction of anaesthesia is rapid; however, propofol can cause significant respiratory depression or even apnoea. Propofol also reduces myocardial contractility. Animals should be intubated and given oxygen during propofol anaesthesia (Ko & Marini 2008). Alternatively, intramuscular injection of ketamine in combination with xylazine, medetomidine, diazepam or acepromazine can produce 20–30 minutes of surgical anaesthesia.

Volatile anaesthetics can be used for both induction (after sedation if required) and maintenance. If using an induction chamber, do not use the same chamber that is used for rodents, since the smell of the ferret will cause distress to any rodents placed in the chamber subsequently. Isoflurane is recommended, and induction takes 1–2 minutes. Isoflurane is pungent, so ferrets may salivate during induction, and premedication with atropine may be needed. Anaesthesia can be maintained using a low resistance circuit, such as a T-piece. For short procedures, a face mask can be used for maintenance of anaesthesia, but for longer procedures, rapid endotracheal intubation is recommended using a 2.5–4 mm tube or a modified urinary catheter. Place the animal in sternal recumbency and have an assistant bend the head upwards as far as possible by placing thumb and forefinger in the corners of the mouth. Pull the tongue forwards and over the lower incisors to depress the mandible. Advance the lubricated tube into the mouth – a laryngoscope may be needed to visualise the larynx – and slide the tube gently through the glottis.

At the end of the procedure, allow the animal to breathe oxygen only for a few minutes. Animals usually recover consciousness in about 5 minutes.

Post-operative care and analgesia

Hypothermia under anaesthesia is common in ferrets, due to their small size and large surface area. Keep the animal warm throughout the procedure by wrapping it up and providing supplementary heating. Following surgery, keep the body temperature up until the animal has fully regained consciousness.

It is important to maintain fluid balance to prevent dehydration. The daily fluid requirement is approximately 75–100 ml/kg, and in addition any blood or fluid losses during surgery should be replaced. Warmed, isotonic fluids such as Hartmann's solution or normal saline can be given by

Table 29.3 Drug combinations suitable for anaesthesia in ferrets.

Drug	Dose	Comments
Isoflurane	3–4% induction 1.5–3% maintenance	Premedication recommended to smooth induction
Medetomidine with Ketamine[1]	0.08–0.1 mg/kg with 4–8 mg/kg	Mix in same syringe, administer im for 30–60 minutes surgical anaesthesia. Can reverse with atipamezole, 0.25–0.5 mg/kg im
Xylazine with Ketamine[1]	1–4 mg/kg with 10–25 mg/kg im	As above, but with more respiratory depression
Alphaxalone	8–12 mg/kg im or iv without premedication / 6–8 mg/kg im or iv with premedication	Premedicate with diazepam. Short anaesthesia with good relaxation. Slow induction if im. Incremental doses 6–8 mg/kg iv for prolonged anaesthesia
Ketamine[1] with Diazepam[1]	25 mg/kg with 2 mg/kg im	Surgical anaesthesia for approximately 30 minutes. Less respiratory depression than with α_2 agonists
Propofol	6–8 mg/kg iv without premedication, 1–3 mg/kg iv with premedication	Can be used for total intravenous anaesthesia.

[1] Note: these are controlled drugs under the Misuse of Drugs Regulations in the UK. Special storage and record-keeping requirements may apply.
Note: Doses are intended as a guide only and all doses may have to be modified if given after premedication. All the times are approximate.
Source: Dose rates from Carpenter and Marion (2013); Hawkins and Pascoe (2012); Ko and Marini (2008); Lloyd (2002); Meredith (2015).

slow intravenous injection during long procedures at a rate of 10 ml/kg/hr into the cephalic or saphenous veins. Fluids may also be given by subcutaneous injection.

Postoperatively the animal may have a depressed appetite, and solid food may be refused. Offer small amounts of liquid diet, soaked pelleted diet or give a convalescent diet for dogs and cats. Anorexic animals may need to be force-fed meat-based baby food or convalescent diet or given nutritional supplements until the appetite has returned to normal. After abdominal surgery, food should be given in small amounts until digestive functions have returned to normal.

Euthanasia

Euthanasia in ferrets is best achieved by administration of an overdose of barbiturate anaesthetic such as pentobarbitone, by intravenous or intraperitoneal injection (AVMA 2013). Prior sedation is recommended, e.g. with inhalation anaesthetic or medetomidine. Depending on the research project, it may be necessary to use a method which for example fixes the tissue, does not leave drug residue, or preserves brain tissue, in which case methods such as decapitation, inhalation anaesthesia followed by exsanguination or perfusion fixation under general anaesthesia may be used. Note that in some jurisdictions, these latter methods require licence authority.

Recognition and management of pain and distress

Evaluation of pain in ferrets can be difficult, because signs of pain are not obvious, and because they are asleep for much of the time. Assessment of pain and distress can only be done when the animals are awake, when evaluation of their behaviour can be undertaken.

Pain-related behaviours in ferrets can be very subtle, depending on the cause of the pain, and may only be noticed by those who are very familiar with the behaviour of the individual animal. Behaviours that may be observed by an animal in pain include diminished activity and exploratory behaviour, altered posture or gait, uncharacteristic aggression or apathy, vocalisation, hiding, lack of grooming, reduced food and water intake, salivation or bruxism (tooth grinding, especially in abdominal pain) or weight loss. Ferrets in severe pain may have a bushy tail due to piloerection (Bixler & Ellis 2004; van Oostrom et al. 2011).

Animals should be observed in their home cages for natural behaviour and signs of illness, before being removed from the cage to make an assessment of provoked behaviour. Normal ferrets exhibit exploratory behaviour: if this is absent, it may be a sign of illness. The gait of the animal can be observed for signs of hind-limb paresis and other musculoskeletal or neurological disturbances such as generalised tremor.

Grimace scales have successfully been developed for the assessment of pain in many animal species. Recently, a grimace scale has been developed for ferrets, based on evaluation of five facial action units (orbital tightening, nose bulging, cheek bulging, ear changes and whisker retraction). Preliminary studies suggest that the grimace score, and orbital tightening in particular, are potentially useful tools for pain assessment of ferrets (Reijgwart et al. 2017). However, because of the risk of false negatives, a negative grimace score should not be used as a reason not to provide pain relief.

Table 29.4 Analgesics.

Drug	Dose	Comments
Buprenorphine[1]	0.01–0.03 mg/kg sc or im	Repeat after 8–12 hours
Butorphanol[1]	0.05–0.4 mg/kg sc or im	Repeat after 4–6 hours
Morphine[1]	0.2–2 mg/kg sc or im	Repeat after 2–6 hours
Carprofen	2–5 mg/kg po or sc	Repeat after 12–24 hours
Meloxicam	0.1–0.3 mg/kg sc or po	Once daily
Ketoprofen	1–3 mg/kg sc	Once daily

[1] Note: these are controlled drugs under the Misuse of Drugs Regulations in the UK. Special storage and record-keeping requirements may apply. Note: all doses are intended as a guide only. Products listed in Tables 29.2–29.4 may not have product licences for use in ferrets. Source: Dose rates from Carpenter and Marion (2013); Hawkins and Pascoe (2012); Ko and Marini (2008); Lloyd (2002); Meredith (2015).

Analgesics should be administered routinely after surgery to avoid unnecessary pain, and in any circumstance where pain behaviours are observed. Doses of suitable analgesics are given in Table 29.4.

Common welfare problems

Disease control, vaccinations and routine health checks

A programme of routine preventive care is recommended, to allow for prevention and early detection of diseases. Young ferrets should be given a health check and first vaccination at 6–8 weeks of age, an annual check until 4–5 years old, then twice-yearly checks, since older animals are more prone to diseases. Ferrets acquired from dealers or other laboratories should be isolated for 40 days before introduction to a colony, to minimise the risk of introducing infections. Animals should be checked for the ear mite *Otodectes cynotis* on arrival and treated prior to entering the main colony.

A routine health check should include examination of the teeth, skin and hair coat, ears, and anal area for evidence of diarrhoea. The nails may also need trimming.

Ferrets may need to be vaccinated against canine distemper depending on the degree of biosecurity employed (Kubiak 2016).

Ferrets are not susceptible to feline panleukopenia, canine parvovirus, leptospirosis or mink enteritis.

Regular health screening of the colony may also be required. This should include screening for viruses (Distemper, coronavirus and Aleutian disease) and faecal screening for endoparasites and pathogens. Blood sampling for haematology, serology and biochemistry may also be needed.

Common diseases

Laboratory ferrets can develop non-specific conditions such as hairballs and dental disease, as well as specific infectious and non-infectious diseases.

Infectious diseases

Viral diseases

Canine distemper virus: Canine distemper is an incurable, fatal disease in ferrets. It is found regularly in unvaccinated domestic populations, so ferrets for use in the laboratory should be sourced from suppliers with a high health status. Routine vaccination using a live or recombinant vaccine and/or strict biosecurity precautions should be followed to prevent the disease being brought into a laboratory. No single distemper vaccine exists in the UK: all available vaccines are produced for domestic dogs and combine distemper components with other vaccines. Some available canine vaccines have been produced using viruses grown in ferret cell cultures – these are not recommended for use in ferrets, as there is a small risk that the virus will revert to virulence and cause disease. Inactivated vaccines do not provide adequate protection. Live vaccines derived from avian cell cultures may be effective and safe. It is advised that the manufacturer be contacted prior to using any vaccine in ferrets to confirm whether the vaccine is safe to be used (Kubiak 2016). Vaccination can confer lifelong immunity (Kuipel & Perpiñán 2014). Vaccination for distemper typically involves a single vaccination in animals more than 12 weeks old, though young animals in situations where exposure risk is high may be vaccinated earlier.

Transmission is by contact or droplet infection, with an incubation period of 10–12 days. Affected animals exhibit fever, loss of appetite and an initially serous then mucopurulent ocular and nasal discharge, which can stick the eyelids together. There may be photophobia and blepharospasm. A rash develops under the chin and in the inguinal area on day 10–12, and there may be keratitis of the footpads producing classical hardpad. The disease progresses to tracheitis, bronchitis and severe bronchopneumonia. Death usually follows on day 12–25 depending on the strain. If animals survive this phase, they develop a CNS phase within a few weeks, characterised by hyperexcitability, excess salivation, muscle tremor, convulsion, coma and death. Vomiting and diarrhoea are uncommon. Canine distemper virus causes suppression of cell-mediated immunity, predisposing to secondary bacterial infection.

There is no treatment, and affected animals should be euthanised.

Coronavirus: This is associated with epizootic catarrhal enteritis. This highly contagious disease can affect 100% of animals in a colony but death is uncommon (Kuipel & Perpiñán 2014). Affected animals develop green watery diarrhoea, vomiting, dehydration and very occasionally die (Bixler & Ellis 2004). Animals may appear clinically normal until stressed, at which point the symptoms may appear. The disease can lead to chronic malabsorption and ill health. Ferrets can become carriers and be a source of infection throughout their lives. Some animals may develop a condition similar to feline infectious peritonitis in cats. This is seen mainly in young ferrets and is caused by a related strain of virus. The clinical signs are vague and non-specific, including lethargy, anorexia and occasionally ataxia or seizures (Kuipel & Perpiñán 2014).

Aleutian disease: This is an uncommon disease caused by a parvovirus which may be found in pet ferrets with prevalences of 6–60% reported in different countries (Kuipel & Perpiñán 2014). Symptoms can be very variable. Infected animals may show no signs at all, or develop weight loss, ill thrift, melaena, inappetence, paresis, infertility or signs associated with immune complex deposition such as uveitis and glomerulonephritis. Clinical signs depend on the organs most affected. Frequently, there is central nervous involvement, with a non-suppurative encephalomyelitis. The virus can spread both vertically and horizontally, although the transmission rate appears to be low. Animals of any age may be affected, and the signs may develop over 24 hours or progress over several months. There is no treatment. Animals may respond to supportive therapy, corticosteroids and antibiotics although they will remain infected and present a risk to other animals. Culling of infected animals is recommended. Since the transmission rate is low, it is possible to test individual animals, and cull those testing positive.

Influenza: Ferrets are highly susceptible to both influenza virus types A and B, and it can pass from ferret to human and vice versa. The disease in adult ferrets is usually mild and self-limiting, but it can cause mortality in kits. The virus causes catarrhal inflammation in the upper respiratory tract leading to congestion, oedema and some necrosis in the nasal mucosa. Ferrets may exhibit high fever, sneezing and coughing, nasal discharge, respiratory distress and cyanosis. Young ferrets may also develop secondary bacterial infection.

Bacterial diseases

Helicobacter: *Helicobacter mustelae* is associated with the development of chronic gastritis and gastric ulcers in ferrets (Swennes & Fox 2014). Helicobacter is found in the pyloric area in up to 100% of animals, and although clinical disease is rare it can produce ulceration and death, particularly at times of stress. Affected animals may exibit bruxism due to abdominal pain and present with black, tarry stools due to intestinal bleeding. Large ulcers can erode into submucosal blood vessels causing rapid death. Ulcers cause anorexia and stress, leading to further development of the disease and a progressive deterioration in the animal's condition.

Clinical signs include lethargy, anorexia and weight loss, vomiting, ptyalism, and tooth grinding. Chronic cases may be dehydrated. There may also be melaena, peripheral lymphocytosis and regenerative anaemia. The presence of black tarry stools with tooth grinding are highly suggestive of gastroduodenal ulceration.

If the animal is not vomiting, frequent, small meals of a bland, highly digestible diet can encourage the animal to eat and break the cycle that allows ulcers to form. If the animal is vomiting, food should first be withheld for 6–12 hours until vomiting ceases. Parenteral fluids and electrolytes may be needed. *Helicobacter mustelae* can be treated using a combination of antimicrobials and bismuth subsalicylate for at least 14 days. It may take four weeks or more for ulcers to heal completely and recurrence is common.

Botulism: Ferrets are susceptible to botulism, a neuroparalytic disease caused by ingestion of pre-formed toxin produced by Clostridium botulinum contamination in spoiled meat. Although rare, the disease is usually fatal. Initial signs include blepharospasm, photophobia, lethargy and incontinence, leading to muscular stiffness, incoordination and ascending paralysis 12–96 hours after eating contaminated food (Swennes & Fox 2014). The animal eventually dies of anoxia due to paralysis of the respiratory muscle. To prevent this, remove any uneaten meat shortly after feeding, and take particular care when feeding raw meat.

Abscesses: Subcutaneous abscesses in group-housed ferrets are common and are often associated with infections in skin wounds resulting from neck biting during the early breeding season, or from other penetrating injuries. Abscesses tend to remain locally sequestered, and may manifest as large swellings that may involve the salivary glands and even erosion of bone at the base of the skull. Treatment involves ensuring there is adequate drainage – antibiotic treatment is rarely required (Swennes & Fox 2014).

Vaginitis and pyometra: Vaginitis and pyometra may occur in oestrous females, secondary to immune suppression. Jills produce a mucoserous discharge during oestrus which causes the perineal area to become wet, predisposing to infection. Vaginitis may also be caused by irritation from bedding adhering to the vulva. Pyometra leads to lethargy, and there may be a purulent discharge from the vagina and enlarged uterine horns. Treatment consists of removal of the source of irritation, and the use of broad-spectrum antibiotics.

Mastitis: Mastitis is quite common in ferrets, occurring immediately after parturition or at peak lactation. It can manifest as cellulitis, mammary abscesses, necrotic mastitis or chronic mastitis. Necrotic mastitis presents rapidly with large areas of liquefactive necrosis extending into surrounding tissues. Affected areas can become gangrenous within hours of infection and the jill can become very ill. Immediate surgical treatment may be required to remove the affected areas. In chronic mastitis, mammary tissue is gradually replaced by fibrous tissue and milk production falls, resulting in the loss of the litter and possibly the jill herself. Antibiotic therapy and surgical removal of the affected glands may be necessary. Mastitis is usually very infectious, and suckling kits can transfer infection from one gland to another. Affected jills should be isolated from the remainder of the colony to avoid spreading infection, and should not be used for breeding again. Kits should be left with their mother while she is undergoing treatment: fostering them may spread the infection to other jills, and removing the milk from affected glands aids recovery.

Parasites

External parasites: Ferrets are susceptible to infection with the ear mite *Otodectes cynotis*. Affected animals may be asymptomatic, or present with pruritus, rubbing the ears or head shaking, and thick, dark brown waxy debris in the ear canals. Secondary bacterial infection can lead to otitis media and a head tilt. The mites complete their 3-week life cycle within in the ear canal (Patterson *et al*. 2014). Adult mites, larvae and eggs are visible in the exudate under a microscope. Regular cleaning (usually under general anaesthesia) and treatment with parasiticides such as selamectin may be needed. The adult mite spreads by direct contact. All susceptible animals should be treated concurrently. Eradication of *Otodectes cynotis* from a ferret colony can be achieved by treatment of all individuals in the colony every three weeks for three or four treatments, using acaricides such as ivermectin or selamectin (authors).

Internal parasites: intestinal parasites are uncommon in laboratory ferrets. Ferrets may become infected with nematodes, e.g. *Toxascaris 29eonine* if they come into contact with infected dogs. Ferrets are susceptible to heartworm (*Dirofilaria immitis*), and affected animals may present with signs of heart failure or respiratory distress. Ferrets from infected colonies should be treated prophylactically. *Dirofilaria* is transmitted by mosquitoes, so control of this vector is an important part of the management strategy for this disease.

Intestinal protozoa such as *Giardia* and *Isospora* are occasionally observed in ferrets. Clinical signs from these infections are rare, although heavy infestations can lead to diarrhoea, rectal prolapse and occasionally death (Patterson *et al*. 2014).

Non-infectious diseases

Hyperoestrogenism

As induced ovulators, females may remain in oestrus unless mated. Exposure to high oestrogen levels for periods in excess of one month can cause severe health problems including weight loss, alopecia and bone marrow depression. All bone marrow blood cell series may be affected, causing leukopenia, thrombocytopaenia or anaemia. There may be pale mucous membranes, haemorrhages, a systolic murmur and secondary bacterial infections. Subdural haematomas may lead to posterior paralysis.

This condition can be life threatening. If animals remain in oestrus for more than two months, the reduction in platelet count may lead to haemorrhage and death (Lloyd 1999; Lewington 2000). Treatment depends on the severity of clinical signs.

Oestrus in female ferrets needs to be actively managed to prevent hyperoestrogenism, by inducing ovulation artificially, by spaying, or by the use of hormones to prevent or terminate oestrus. Females should not remain in heat for longer than one month. Ovariohysterectomy at 6–8 months of age is recommended for jills that are not to be bred. Ovulation can be induced by mating jills in oestrus with a vasectomised male. Hormone treatments can also be used to postpone oestrus until the following breeding season.

Adrenal-related endocrinopathy

Disease of the adrenal glands is common in neutered ferrets and may be linked to neutering, housing ferrets indoors and genetic background. There appears to be a correlation between age at neutering and age of onset of adrenal disease (Schoemaker *et al*. 2000). One or both adrenals may be affected. In the absence of gonadal hormones, the pituitary secretes excessive amounts of gonadotrophin releasing hormone GNRH, which acts on the adrenal glands and causes them to produce sex hormones (Schoemaker 2013). This leads to a range of signs including symmetrical hair loss, enlarged vulva in females and prostatic cysts with stranguria in males. Pruritus is frequently seen in ferrets with hyperandrogenism. The optimal treatment for hyperadrenocorticism in ferrets is a combination of surgery and placement of an implant containing deslorelin (Schoemaker 2013).

Cardiomyopathy

Cardiac diseases such as dilated cardiomyopathy, arrhythmias or valvular insufficiency are relatively common in older pet ferrets (Wagner 2014). Dilated cardiomyopathy occurs in older ferrets. Affected ferrets may exhibit weight loss, lethargy and hind-limb weakness. Signs of heart failure including tachypnoea and weak pulses may be observed, and muffled heart sounds or harsh lung sounds may be heard on auscultation (Bixler & Ellis 2004). Treatment is aimed at reducing left ventricular filling pressure and maintaining cardiac output (Wagner 2014). Oxygen, vasodilators, positive inotropes and diuretics may be beneficial, and thoracocentesis may be required to remove pleural fluid. A low salt diet and exercise restriction can be of benefit. Treatment failure is not uncommon.

Foreign bodies

Intestinal foreign bodies are common in ferrets, because they are inquisitive and playful. Gastric foreign bodies may cause lethargy, inappetence, diarrhoea with or without tarry stools, weakness and dehydration. Vomiting is uncommon, although nausea can lead to ptyalism and face rubbing. Foreign bodies lodged at the pylorus can ulcerate through the stomach wall. Intestinal foreign bodies may cause sudden collapse with a painful abdomen. Foreign bodies rarely pass unaided and removal under general anaesthesia is usually required. Prevention of a recurrence may be achieved by 'ferret-proofing' the environment carefully.

Posterior paresis

Hind-limb weakness is a common presenting sign in ferrets and may be associated with generalised systemic disease, neoplasia, intervertebral disc disease, trauma or viral diseases such as Aleutian disease. The animal presents with abducted, uncoordinated hindlimbs or a frog-legged appearance. The body may lose its curved appearance as the animal is unable to flex the spine as much as usual. The withdrawal and placing reflexes may be absent, and the animal may be incontinent. Often, the animal remains bright and alert and otherwise normal.

Specific treatment depends on the diagnosis. However, recurrence is common, and the prognosis is guarded.

Neoplasia

Neoplasia in ferrets is increasingly reported. Common neoplasms include insulinoma, lymphoma and adrenal neoplasia. It is quite common for two or more different neoplasms to be found in the same animal. Nearly half of all tumours reported have been malignant.

Insulinoma: Insulinomas are neoplasms of the pancreatic beta cells, which secrete excess insulin resulting in hypoglycaemia. This is the most common neoplasm of ferrets reported in the USA but is apparently rarely reported in Europe. It is commonly seen in animals of four to five years. Animals may present with weight loss, weakness, lethargy and decreased appetite. They may also collapse due to hypoglycaemic episodes. Immediate veterinary attention should be sought. Medical treatments can be used in older animals or those with intercurrent disease, although surgical removal is indicated in young animals (Lewington 2000).

Lymphosarcoma: This is relatively common in ferrets and is often multicentric, with masses in multiple organs and lymph nodes. The clinical signs depend upon the site of the lesion and are often non-specific. Affected animals may show weakness, weight loss, inappetence and lymphadenopathy, and symptoms may be slow to develop.

The choices for treatment are surgery, chemotherapy, radiotherapy or combinations of these. However, the prognosis is guarded since even if there appears to be only one organ affected, the disease is likely to be systemic.

Waardenburg syndrome and deafness

Waardenburg syndrome causes minor defects of the neural crest pathways of affected ferrets, and is related to certain colour and pattern combinations of the fur, which often indicate the presence of the condition. Deafness is the most common characteristic of the condition (usually, but not always, total deafness affecting both ears) and around three-quarters of all ferrets that carry the specific colour and pattern markings that signify the condition will be deaf.

The colour markings that accompany Waardenburg syndrome in the ferret consist of a small white stripe (known as a blaze) on the back of the head, or an all-white head right from the tip of the nose to the back of the head, known as a panda pattern. Ferrets with the condition may also have rather widely set eyes, and a slightly flattened appearance to the skull. In one study of 152 pet ferrets with a variety of colour marking patterns, 10 (7%) were unilaterally deaf and 34 (22%) were bilaterally deaf. None of the coloured animals *without* white markings were deaf. No gender differences were seen (Piazza *et al*. 2014; Strain 2015).

Acknowledgements

Thanks are due to Mike Plant, who co-wrote the previous edition of this chapter, which provided the basis for this version. I am also grateful to the Red Kite team for their helpful input during the preparation of this manuscript.

References

Albrecht, R.A., Liu, W-C., Sant, A.J. et al. (2018) Moving forward: recent developments for the ferret biomedical research model. *mBio* [online], **9**, e01113–18. Available from: doi: 10.1128/mBio.01113-18. [Viewed 9 November 2018].

American Veterinary Medical Association (2013) *The AVMA Guidelines for the Euthanasia of Animals*: 2013 Edition. Available from https://www.avma.org/KB/Policies/Documents/euthanasia.pdf [Viewed 23 January 2019].

Ball, R.S. (2006) Issues to consider for preparing ferrets as research subjects in the laboratory. *ILAR Journal*, **47(4)**, 348–357.

BBC News (1999) Ferrets save millennium concert. http://news.bbc.co.uk/1/hi/uk/582123.stm. 29 December 1999. Accessed 3 September 2019.

Bell, J. (1999) Ferret nutrition. *Veterinary Clinics of North America Small Animal Practice*, **2**, 169–192.

Bennett, R.A. (2009) Nonabdominal surgeries in ferrets. *Proceedings of CVC, Washington D.C. 1 April 2009.* Available from http://veterinarycalendar.dvm360.com/nonabdominal-surgeries-ferrets-proceedings [Viewed 7 Jan 2019].

Bixler, H. and Ellis, C. (2004) Ferret care and husbandry. *Veterinary Clinics Exotic Animal Practice*, **7**, 227–255.

Carpenter, J.A. and Marion, C.J. (Eds) (2013) *Exotic Animal Formulary*, 4th edn. Elsevier, St Louis.

Clapperton, B.K. (2001) Advances in New Zealand mammalogy 1990-2000: feral ferret. *Journal of the Royal Society of New Zealand*, **31**(1), 185–203.

Fox, J.G. (2014) Taxonomy, history, and use. In: *Biology and Diseases of the Ferret*, 3rd edn, Eds Fox, J.G and Marini, R.P., pp. 5–22. Wiley Blackwell, Chichester.

Fox, J.G. and Broome, R. (2014) Housing and management. In: *Biology and Diseases of the Ferret*, 3rd edn, Eds Fox, J.G and Marini, R.P.,) pp. 145–156. Wiley Blackwell, Chichester.

Fox, J.G., Schultz, C.S. and Vester Boler, B.M. (2014). Nutrition of the ferret. In: *Biology and Diseases of the Ferret*, 3rd edn, Eds Fox, J.G. and Marini, R.P., pp. 123–144. Wiley Blackwell, Chichester.

Hawkins, M.G. and Pascoe, P.J. (2012) Anesthesia, analgesia and sedation of small mammals. In: *Ferrets, Rabbits and Rodents: Clinical Medicine and Surgery*, 3rd edn, Eds Quesenberry, K.E. and Carpenter, J.W., pp. 429–451. Elsevier, St Louis.

Home Office (2014) *Code of Practice for the Housing and Care of Animals Bred, Supplied or Used for Scientific Purposes*. HMSO.

Jha, S.K., Coleman, T. and Frank, M.G., (2006) Sleep and sleep regulation in the ferret (Mustela putorius furo). *Behavioural Brain Research*, **172**, 106–113.

Ko, J. and Marini, R.P. (2008) Anesthesia and analgesia in ferrets. In: *Anesthesia and Analgesia in Laboratory Animals*, 2nd edn, Eds Fish, R., Danneman, P.J., Brown, M. and Karas, A.,) pp. 443–456. Elsevier, St Louis.

Kubiak, M., (2016). Exotic mammal vaccination. *Veterinary Times*, November 28, 2016. Available from https://www.vettimes.co.uk/article/exotic-mammal-vaccination/ [Viewed 13 December 2018].

Kuipel, M. and Perpiñán, D. (2014) Viral diseases of ferrets. In: *Biology and Diseases of the Ferret*. 3rd edn, Eds Fox, J.G. and Marini, R.P.,) pp. 439–518. Wiley Blackwell, Chichester.

Lewington, J.H. (2000) *Ferret Husbandry, Medicine and Surgery*. Butterworth Heinemann, Oxford.

Lightfoot, T., Rubinstein, J., Aiken, S. and Ludwig, L. (2012) Soft tissue surgery. In *Ferrets Rabbits and Rodents: Clinical Medicine and Surgery*, 3rd edn, Eds Quesenberry, K. and Carpenter, J. Elsevier, St Louis.

Lloyd, M. (1999) *Ferrets: Health Husbandry and Diseases*. Blackwell Science Publication, Oxford.

Lloyd, M. (2002) Veterinary care of ferrets 2. Common clinical conditions. *In Practice*, **24**, 136–145.

Meredith, A (Ed.) (2015) *BSAVA Small Animal Formulary. Part B: Exotic Pets.* BSAVA, Gloucester.

Morgan, J.P. (2014) Use of the ferret in cardiovascular research. In: *Biology and Diseases of the Ferret*, 3rd edn, Eds Fox, J.G and Marini, R.P., pp. 653–664. Wiley Blackwell, Chichester.

Muñoz-Fontela, C., Dowling, W.E., Funnell, S.G.P. *et al.* (2020). Animal models for COVID-19. *Nature* **586**, 509–515. https://doi.org/10.1038/s41586-020-2787-6 [Viewed 25 January 2022]

Nodal, F. and King, A.J. (2014). Hearing and auditory function in ferrets. In: *Biology and Diseases of the Ferret*, 3rd edn, Eds Fox, J.G. and Marini, R.P., pp. 685–710. Wiley Blackwell, Chichester.

Paquette, S.G., Huang, S.S.H, Banner, D. *et al.* (2014) Impaired heterologous immunity in aged ferrets during sequential influenza A H1N1 infection. *Virology*, **464–465**, 177–183. Available from doi: 10.1016/j.virol.2014.07.013. Epub 2014 Aug 1. [Viewed 4 September 2019].

Patterson, M.M., Fox, J.G. and Eberhard, M.L. (2014) Parasitic diseases. In: *Biology and Diseases of the Ferret*, 3rd edn, Eds Fox, J.G and Marini, R.P.,) pp. 553–572. Wiley Blackwell, Chichester.

Piazza, S., Abitbol, M., Gnirs, K. *et al.* (2014) Prevalence of deafness and association with coat variations in client-owned ferrets. *Journal of the American Veterinary Medical Association*, **244**(9), 1047–1052.

Porter, V. and Brown, N. (1997) *The Complete Book of Ferrets*. D & M Publications, Bedford.

Powers, L. and Brown, S. (2012) Basic anatomy, physiology and husbandry. In: *Ferrets, Rabbits and Rodents: Clinical Medicine and Surgery*, 3rd edn, Eds Quesenberry, K.E. and Carpenter, J.W., pp. 1–12. Elsevier, St Louis, Missouri.

Reijgwart, M., Schoemaker, N., Pascuzzo, R. *et al.* (2017) The composition and initial evaluation of a grimace scale in ferrets after surgical implantation of a telemetry probe. *PLoS ONE* [online], **12**(11). Available from https://doi.org/10.1371/journal.pone.0187986. [viewed 9 November 2018].

Sato, J., Hosoda, T., Wolsan, M. et al. (2003) Phylogenetic relationships and divergence times among mustelids (Mammalia: Carnivora) based on nucleotide sequences of the nuclear interphotoreceptor retinoid binding protein and mitochondrial cytochrome b genes. Zoological Science [online], **20**(2), 243–264. Available from *doi*:10.2108/zsj.20.243. PMID 12655187. [viewed 16 October 2018].

Schoemaker, N. (2013) Hyperadrenocorticism in ferrets. In: *Clinical Endocrinology of Companion Animals*. Ed. Rand J., pp. 86–94. Chichester: John Wiley & Sons.

Schoemaker, N., Schuurmans, M., Moorman, H. and Lumeij, J. (2000) Correlation between age at neutering and age at onset of hyperadrenocorticism in ferrets. *Journal of the American Veterinary Medical Association*, **216**(2), 195–197.

Strain, G. (2015) The genetics of deafness in domestic animals. *Frontiers in Veterinary Science* [online], **2**, 29. Available from http://doi.org/10.3389/fvets.2015.00029. [viewed 16 October 2018].

Sukhinin, D., Engel, A., Manger, P. and Hilgetag, C. (2016) Building the ferretome. *Frontiers in Neuroinformatics* [online], **10**, 16. Available from https://doi.org/10.3389/fninf.2016.00016. [viewed 16 October 2018].

Swennes, A.G. and Fox, J.G (2014) Bacterial and mycoplasmal diseases. In: *Biology and Diseases of the Ferret*, 3rd edn. Eds Fox, J.G and Marini, R.P., pp. 519–552. Wiley Blackwell, Chichester.

Van Oostrom, H., Schoemaker, N. and Uilenreef, J. (2011) Pain Management in Ferrets. *Veterinary Clinics of North America Exotic Animal Practice*, **14**(1), 105–116.

Wagner, R.A. (2014) Diseases of the cardiovascular system. In: *Biology and Diseases of the Ferret*, 3rd edn. Eds Fox, J.G and Marini, R.P., pp. 401–420. Wiley Blackwell, Chichester.

Wolfensohn, S.E. and Lloyd, M.H. (2013) *A Handbook of Laboratory Animal Management and Welfare*, 4th edn. Wiley-Blackwell.

30 The laboratory dog

Laura Scullion Hall and Jackie Boxall

Biological overview

General biology

Domestic dogs (*Canis lupus familiaris*) are gregarious, social carnivores widely kept as companion animals, and are also found in free-ranging colonies across the world. The dog was the first animal to be domesticated by humans; fossil records indicate that there have been domestic dogs in Europe for around 15,000 years (Thalmann *et al.* 2013). Dogs have associated with humans for at least 25,000 years, with multiple domestication events taking place and admixtures with the wolf population (Freedman *et al.* 2014).

All breeds of the domestic dog (*Canis lupus familiaris*) are thought to be descended from a now-extinct subspecies of the Eurasian grey wolf (*Canis lupus*) (Serpell 1995; Freedman *et al.* 2014). There is a great diversity in domestic dog breeds, with 361 breeds currently recognised by the Fédèration Cynologique Internationale (2019). Dogs have been subject to a high degree of selective breeding for traits relating to working ability and companionship, leading to traits such as cooperation and tolerance for living in close contact with humans and other dogs, rarely seen in other canids.

Dogs' patterns of activity vary throughout the day. They have a highly sensitive sense of smell, which may be used as their primary sense for exploring the world. Dogs also have sensitive hearing, particularly at high frequencies, making them more sensitive to sounds in the laboratory environment. Dogs' hearing is most sensitive between 1 and 20 kHz, in comparison to 1–5 kHz in humans, with the upper limit of dog hearing of 50 kHz in comparison to 20 kHz in humans. The dog bark peaks in the 500 Hz–16 kHz range, where hearing is 24 dB more sensitive than humans (Sales *et al.* 1997).

Touch is used to explore the environment, in particular social contact with conspecifics and humans. Touch can have an impact on both behaviour and physiology, which can be pleasant or unpleasant depending on the circumstances. Juvenile dogs will typically spend around 10% of their day resting in contact with pen mates, with adults performing this behaviour for 2% of the day (Hubrecht *et al.* 1992).

Vision is dichromatic, with the greatest sensitivity between 429 nm and 555 nm; objects are primarily seen in blues, yellows and greens (Nietz *et al.* 1989). Dogs have a high sensitivity for moving objects (Miklósi 2015). Visual discrimination is greatest when objects are moving and dogs can detect a change in movement that exists in a single dioptre of space within their eye. The field of vision is wide, allowing dogs to be aware of movement around them. Dogs are unable to focus on objects closer than 30–55 cm (Miller & Murphy 1995). *Canid* species prefer high vantage points, allowing them to monitor movement around them. At close distances, vision is less sensitive and dogs rely on touch and smell.

The beagle is the de facto dog breed used in laboratories worldwide. Beagles are scenthounds and have been selectively bred to perform hunting and scenting tasks. The beagle possesses many of the characteristics which have been cited as advantages of using the dog in scientific research for example its small size and pleasant temperament make it amenable to regular handling and conducting procedures. Its history as a pack-living, working dog also makes group housing amenable and the volume of historical data available is also important (Box & Spielmann 2005).

Size, range and lifespan

The median lifespan of all dog breeds is 10–15 years. There is a negative relationship found between body mass and longevity, with larger breeds having shorter lifespans than smaller breeds (Wolfensohn & Lloyd 2008). Due to the diversity of dog breeds, weight varies considerably between breeds, from 500 g for toy breeds, to over 140 kg for the largest (Young 1994; Guinness World Records 2018). The purpose-bred laboratory beagle typically weighs between 7 and 15 kg, with male dogs on average being heavier than female dogs. A range of standard data can be found in Table 30.1.

Table 30.1 Standard biological data in the laboratory beagle, adapted from Andersen (1970), Wolfensohn and Lloyd (2008) and Gad (2016).

Measure	Normal values
Adult weight (kg)	7–15
Life span (years)	12.5
Body temperature (°C)	37.8 (±0.13)
Heart rate (beats per minute)	124 (±20)
Mean arterial pressure (mmHg)	82 (±30)
Systolic blood pressure (mmHg)	121 (±40)
Diastolic blood pressure (mmHg)	65 (±27)
Arterial blood pH	7.44 (7.37–7.51)
PaO_2 (mmHg)	98.2 (±3.7)
$PaCO_2$ (mmHg)	39.4 (±1.8)
Tidal volume (ml/kg)	16 (±2)
Resting respiration rate	20/min
O_2 consumption	0.36 ml O_2/g/h/h[b]
Basal metabolism	2 cal/kg/h
Daily food consumption	25–40 g/kg body weight
Daily water consumption	70–80 ml/kg body weight

Social organisation

In the dog, we do not have information from a wild counterpart as all extant dogs are domesticated or feral. Instead, information is gained from the study of free-ranging dogs, pet and working dogs. Free-ranging dogs can be considered a close analogue of a wild counterpart. Free-ranging dogs will typically form fluid groups, composed of several stable breeding pairs (Spotte 2012). Dogs have complex repertoire of social behaviours and are able to form bonds with humans as well as conspecifics (Serpell 2016). Young dogs, aged 1–2 years, may gather together in mixed-sex bands (Miklósi 2014).

One of the defining features of the domestic dog is the ability to readily form relationships with humans, being found as companions or working dogs globally. Dogs have travelled with humans to all continents of the planet and are estimated to fulfil a number of working and companion roles (Semyonova 2003).

Dogs have a complex repertoire of social behaviours which are used to communicate with conspecifics. The laboratory environment may impede this behaviour. The importance of olfactory communication for dogs should not be underestimated. Dogs can detect odours in the range of parts per trillion to parts per quadrillion (in contrast, humans can detect odours in the range of parts per million, Ong et al. 2017) as well as sight and sound; therefore, care must be taken to ensure that dogs are able to make olfactory contact with each other and that smells associated with adverse events should be minimised. Dogs use scent to communicate information about their identity and social status. They examine the faeces, urine, anal, genital, ear and mouths of others for information (Fox 1971). Dogs also use scent to identify humans; staff should take care to avoid strong scents which may interfere with olfactory communication.

Dogs also communicate via a range of vocalisations. Barking may indicate arousal, fear or the appearance of a stranger. Other vocalisations such as whining and yowling may indicate high arousal negative states. Staff should be able to distinguish between vocalisations associated with play behaviour, affiliative behaviour and adverse social interactions in order to monitor colony harmony.

Standard biological data

A range of standard biological data on the laboratory beagle can be found in Andersen (1970), Wolfensohn and Lloyd (2008) and Gad (2016). Commercial breeders of dogs should have their own reference values and should be referred to whenever possible. Commonly used reference data are depicted in Table 30.1.

Reproduction

Dogs are a *monoestorus* species (Concannon 1991; Lamm & Makloski 2012). Some standard reproductive data can be found in Table 30.2. England and Allen (1998) provide a detailed review of fertility and obstetrics in the dog. National Research Council (1994) also has a chapter on Management of Breeding Colonies.

Normal behaviour

Dogs should display a relaxed demeanour in the home pen, including loose, relaxed, body posture, calm locomotion within the pen and interaction with pen mates and the surroundings, including making use of a range of effective enrichment items in the home pen. A lack of interaction with enrichment indicates that it is either unsuitable, uninteresting or there is a welfare concern for the dog. Dogs should be willing to approach unfamiliar staff, and should not display anxious behaviour in the presence of humans (e.g. jumping, barking, pacing). See also Chapter 10: Enrichment: animal welfare and scientific validity.

Staff interactions with dogs should be calm and not rely on the use of force. Dogs should freely exit the home pen for the purposes of husbandry, activity and procedures. A dog which must be physically removed from the home pen is fearful, requires additional training and is not suitable for use in experimental procedures. The importance of staff familiarity with individual dogs is critical here, any deviations from normal behaviour may be indicative of illness, adverse reactions to scientific procedures, poor welfare or conflicts with pen mates.

Table 30.2 Selected reproductive data in the laboratory beagle, adapted from Andersen (1970).

Measure		Normal values
Age at puberty (mo)	Male	7–8
	Female	8–14
Breeding age (mo)	Male	10–12
	Female	9–12
Gestation period (days)		57–69
Litter size range		1–11 (av. 5–6)
Oestrous interval (months)		7–8
Oestrus	Proestrus	5–15 days
	Oestrus	5–15 days
	Metoestrus	60–65 days
	Anoestrus	Variable

Beagles are a highly excitable breed (Fogel 1990). In studies of personality traits, they appear not to be prone to displaying aggressive behaviour and rate highly on 'agreeableness' (Kraeuter 2001). In combination with their small body size, these traits make them well-adapted for an environment which can involve intensive handling and group living and have contributed to the popularity of the beagle as a laboratory breed. While all dogs have keen olfactory capabilities, being bred as scenting hounds, beagles make greater use of olfaction in exploration and communication.

Sources of supply

Approximately 140,000 dogs are used in research globally per year (Prescott et al. 2004), although precise estimates are difficult to make. Although dogs have historically been the preferred non-rodent model in safety assessment, other large animals (e.g. mini-pigs) have gained popularity, and dog use has shown a trend towards decreasing use in some areas (e.g. Europe). The acceptable sources of dogs destined for use in scientific research varies considerably in international legislation. Within the EU, it is a legal requirement to obtain dogs from a designated or registered breeder, except for certain tightly regulated circumstances; however, legislative requirements vary between nations. For example, in the USA class A breeders provide purpose-bred dogs, while class B breeders provide random source dogs (e.g. including stray, surrendered or hobby bred dogs; National Research Council 2009) The beagle is the most common choice of breed, due to the volume of historical data available, and the physiological and behaviour characteristics of the breed.

Non-purpose-bred dogs may be used for a variety of reasons. In the EU, the use of random source dogs is prohibited except in special circumstances, for example a specific breed or genetic strain of dog being unavailable from commercial breeders. Elsewhere, legislation may not prohibit the use of random source dogs (e.g. USA, National Research Council 2009). However, there are many disadvantages to using random source dogs, including unknown health and disease status, poor adaptability to the laboratory environment, poorer welfare and unknown genetic background. Purpose-bred dogs have the advantages that they are sourced with genetic and health information, disease status, and may be better able to adapt to confinement, and handling.

There is an increasing trend towards rehoming laboratory dogs, and guidance has been produced to that end (Jennings et al. 2004; Home Office 2015). In the USA, there is a legislative requirement to consider rehoming of dogs following the end of their study use in several states. Some rehomed laboratory beagles are able to adapt to the domestic home environment (Döring et al. 2017); however, a behaviour assessment should be carried out to assess each dog's suitability. Training programmes can help dogs to adapt to new environments. Veterinary authority may be required in some countries (e.g., in the UK, Home Office 2015).

Use in the laboratory

The dog is a popular non-rodent species in safety assessment studies (Smith et al. 2002) with dog use dating back to the seventeenth century (Gad 2016). Dogs have been the preferred large animal species in preclinical studies, although there is a trend towards replacing dogs in large animal use with the minipig.

Safety assessment studies account for most dog use, at 60–85% of dog use. Within the EU, approximately 50% of dogs are used for regulatory safety assessment. Smith et al. (2002) provides detailed descriptions of studies using dogs, including steps which can be taken to minimise or optimise dog use.

Sequencing of the canine genome (Starkey et al. 2005) suggests that the dog is a good model for the study of human disease, while dogs also share 220 homologous hereditary diseases with uniform genetic mutations (Zurlo et al. 2011). Dogs are used as models in cardiovascular and nervous system research (Moscardo et al. 2009). A study commissioned by the International Life Sciences Institute (Olson et al. 2000) found that dog studies were considerably more predictive of human toxicity than rodent studies. Veterinary medicines, testing of medical devices and pet food products are also common uses of the dog in research (Zurlo et al. 2011). Dogs may also be used in the development of new methods of testing for chemical safety.

General husbandry

Husbandry practices have the potential to impact positively or negatively on dog welfare and, therefore, data quality. Although dog environments are growing more complex, many do not provide what is necessary for normal behaviour. It is, therefore, important to ensure that practices are based upon best available practice and should promote good welfare. Care and technical staff should be familiar to the dogs so as to be able to observe undisturbed behaviour. Unfamiliar visitors should be restricted from viewing the dogs where possible so as to minimise disturbance. Dogs use scent to identify humans and strong perfumes or scents should be avoided. Dogs should be trained to perform husbandry-related behaviours, including moving between pens, exercise areas, procedure areas or others as necessary, sitting or standing for health checks or being transported between areas of the site.

Husbandry is an opportunity to observe behaviour. A range of staff may be responsible for different parts of the study, such as husbandry, study-related procedures and oversight of the study design and so all should be adequately trained in recognising behavioural indicators of welfare. Note that although many indicators of poor welfare may be exhibited transiently by any dog (e.g. jumping, barking), persistent exhibition of undesirable behaviours should be investigated.

Staff and visitors should not reinforce inappropriate behaviours. Behaviours such as jumping or barking are reinforced through a variable schedule of reinforcement when dogs are petted or given attention. As a variable schedule of reinforcement makes a behaviour resistant to extinction, the behaviour is maintained even when only rarely reinforced. Desirable, calm behaviour should be encouraged when staff enter the animal room; excitable or fearful behaviour is likely to adversely impact study outcomes. See also Chapter 15: The use of positive reinforcement training techniques to enhance the care and welfare of laboratory and research animals.

Transport

General guidance

The transport of dogs can be considered in terms of transport by air, road and sea, or within and between buildings. General guidance on the transport of animals can be found in Chapter 12: Transportation of laboratory animals as well as Swallow et al. (2005), Council Regulation No. 1/2005 (European Union 2005) and the Live Animal Regulations (LAR) produced by IATA (International Air Transport Association 2018).

The experience of dogs during transport is influenced by factors such as the nature and duration of the journey, the containers, the experience and handling of staff, and the destination. Dogs should be fed a small meal and provided with water approximately two hours before dispatch. They should be exercised immediately before dispatch to encourage defecation.

The transportation of females in oestrus is not recommended. Bitches with unweaned pups, or weaned pups younger than eight weeks should not be transported. The risk of abortion or foetal injury increases in the last third of pregnancy and should be discouraged. Bitches should not be transported within seven days of parturition.

Transport by air, road and sea

In transport by air, dogs will usually be transported beneath the floor in the cargo section. By sea, dogs will usually be transported aboard ventilated vehicles which have a power source. Dogs will, therefore, often be unattended for significant periods during the journey.

Staff should be trained in protocols and restrictions relating to the loading and unloading of animals, and ensure adherence to national and international regulations and guidelines. Dogs should be provided with clean substrate to ensure comfort and hygiene during the journey. A check should be made every 2–3 h. Water should be offered during these checks. If food is offered, a 30-minute period should be offered before restarting the journey.

When transporting by road, vehicles equipped with temperature and mechanical ventilation controls should be used to ensure temperature control throughout the journey. Drivers should be trained to a high standard and be either trained in dog handling or accompanied by a trained dog handler. On arrival at the destination, dogs should be transferred to quarters quickly and with minimal delays. Fresh drinking water and bedding should be available, as should food of the same type as used in the dispatching facility to avoid digestive upsets. A competent person should conduct a health check upon arrival. It is good practice that groups of newly arrived dogs should be quarantined for a suitable period, and barriers should be in place to prevent cross-contamination with existing stock.

Transport of dogs within sites

The transportation of dogs within sites may require dogs to be moved within or between buildings. For transport within buildings, trained dogs can be walked on leads and harnesses. This requires that dogs are suitably accustomed to the surroundings and equipment and should never be forced or dragged. For very short distances, it may be possible to carry dogs (see later section on Handling and training); correct handling methods are needed to prevent injury to dog or handler. Otherwise, transit within buildings should use trolleys and carts. Dogs should be provided with substrate or rubberised, non-slip flooring and made comfortable. The wheels and hinges of carts should be oiled and well-maintained to avoid excessive noise. Dogs should never be left unattended while in trolleys or carts to avoid the risk of injury. Transit between buildings may require the use of suitable vehicles and purpose-built containers. The same standards should be adhered to as with transport by road.

Dogs must be suitably acclimatised to transport containers and handling. Handling should be sympathetic and staff should understand transport may cause stress which persists following arrival.

Effects of transport

Transport has a significant impact upon dog behaviour and physiology. The biggest impact is psychological, which results from exposure confinement, noise, unfamiliar surroundings and unfamiliar people Broom (2005), all of which can result in fear and anxiety. Staff should be mindful of the impact of transport when handling dogs during and after transport. There may be a range of disturbances to physiology including immune function, injury or incidences of disease.

Dogs must be permitted suitable time to adjust and to prevent adverse impact upon study outcomes (Boxall et al. 2004). It is recommended that a minimum of 14 days should be permitted for acclimatisation following long-distance transport. Following transport on a vehicle or between sites, dogs should be permitted at least seven days to adjust and recover. When moved within site, at least three days should be permitted. A change of home pen or animal room also causes stress and at least 24 h should be allowed for recovery.

A programme of husbandry and training should begin following arrival (e.g. Meunier 2006), and no more than 24 h later. This may mitigate the manifestation of unwanted behaviours and anxiety towards staff and surroundings.

Enclosures

The design of the home pen and animal room (the area which includes home pens, corridors and any indoor exercise areas) has a major impact on welfare (Scullion Hall et al. 2017). EU legislation (European Union 2010) mandates minimum pen sizes of 2 m^2 per dog (10–20 kg) for group-housed dogs and 4 m^2 for singly housed dogs. These pen sizes apply to both experimental animals and post-weaned breeding stock. In other legislation (e.g. National Research Council 2010), there is mandated a significantly smaller minimum enclosure size, e.g. 0.74 m^2 for dogs of a similar size. Such restriction of home pen or exercise space is likely to be detrimental to dog welfare, with free-ranging dogs having a home range of many hectares and travelling up to 30 km in a single foray

(Meek 1999). These smaller pen sizes are too small to permit a normal range of behaviours and should not be utilised except for brief time periods (e.g. metabolism studies, see section for details).

Detailed information on the provision of housing for both stock and study animals can be found in European legislation (European Union 2010).

The impact of housing systems and home pen design should be considered part of the experimental protocol, being weighed up in cost-benefit analyses (Sherwin 2007). Pen design should include consideration of visibility, choice of resting places or platforms, size, ease of entry for staff, ease of partitioning dogs and use of noise reducing materials (Hubrecht et al. 1992; Sales et al. 1997; Prescott et al. 2004). Lack of visibility can lead to allelomimetic barking (barking resulting in increasing barking by neighbouring dogs) which can result in considerable noise (Prescott et al. 2004), see later section on Environmental provisions and enrichment, as can the use of hard surfaces with no provision of soundproofing materials (e.g. foam ceiling boards). Home pens may be constructed from a range of materials; however, not all of these are suitable. These include concrete, stainless steel, galvanised metal or wood. Wood is not considered a hygienic construction material due to its porous nature. Modern home pens are typically constructed with opaque or transparent plastics and stainless steel. Plastics are warm and noise-absorbing, reducing the noise in the room. Stainless steel is easy to clean and preferable to galvanised metal as it is less likely to flake or be ingested by dogs. Flooring should be solid with in-built drainage for ease of cleaning. Mesh or grid floors are unsuitable for housing and should not be used. Epoxy or concrete may be used to provide solid flooring. Concrete is less preferable as the porous surface is not amenable to thorough cleaning. A substrate should be provided. Sawdust aids daily cleaning of pens but provides little comfort. Additional substrate such as shredded paper or cardboard should be provided in bedding areas. Canids typically defecate and urinate away from the sleeping area and the design of the home pen should be such that this is possible (Fox 1971).

The design of home pens should be flexible, allowing dogs a choice of location within the pen and the ability to withdraw from pen mates. Hatches allow dogs to move between pens and can also be used to separate dogs when necessary. Ledges at varying heights allow dogs further choice within the pen and increase the visibility of the animal room. A bedding area should be provided. Solid plastic beds are suitable and should not be overly chewed unless insufficient enrichment is provided. The provision of bedding materials such as fleece bedding, shredded paper or corrugated cardboard encourage nesting and exploratory behaviour and are typically well-utilised but care should be taken to ensure that dogs do not ingest bedding (e.g. by ensuring appropriate enrichment is available, see later section on Environmental provisions and enrichment). See Figure 30.1 for examples of modern home pen design.

A separate exercise area should be provided for all dogs. An indoor or outdoor exercise area may be preferable depending on the design of the facility; however, it offers the dogs a range of novel stimuli. Outdoor exercise areas have the additional benefit of changing weather, temperature and olfactory stimuli. Staff contact should be available through exercise times. Dogs are more active in the presence of staff and this provides an excellent opportunity to create positive associations with staff. Examples of indoor and outdoor exercise areas can be seen in Figure 30.2.

Environmental provisions and enrichment

Dedicated indoor and outdoor areas provide dogs with an environment which is separate from the home pen where they can access enrichment items not available in the home pen. Exercising dogs away from the home pen also prevents stress to those remaining in their home pen.

There is a large body of literature on the benefits of environmental enrichment for kennelled dogs' welfare (see Wells 2004b, for review). Minimum housing standards provide insufficient stimuli or space needed to display species-specific behaviours (Schipper et al. 2008). Providing increased social contact (e.g. Mertens & Unshelm 1996) and toys are most frequently recommended in the literature (e.g. Wells 2004a). Wells (2004a) found that providing kennelled dogs with increased opportunities to make social contact, with conspecifics and humans, may allow the dog to gain more control over its environment.

Positive changes in laboratory dogs' behaviour are seen following the introduction of feeding toy enrichment (Hall 2014). An area separate from the dog's home pen suitable for exercise is also recommended; exercise areas should include a variety of chews, toys and climbing equipment, allowing the expression of natural behaviour. Examples of enrichment items and exercise areas can be seen in Figure 30.2.

There are concerns that altering the environment of a laboratory animal will interact with the effects of the test substance and will invalidate comparisons with historical data Dean (1999). However, dogs kept in low-stimulus housing conditions may, for example, develop excessive fear or aggression, increased auto-grooming and vocalisations, increased passiveness, and show manipulation of enclosure barriers, repetitive locomotive behaviour (stereotypies) and coprophagy (Hetts et al. 1992; Hubrecht et al. 1992; Beerda et al. 1999). Most of these behaviours are also indicative of chronic stress (e.g. Beerda et al. 1999). Providing feeding enrichment toy can reduce the amount of time spent inactive, as well as the rate of stereotypies displayed over time (Schipper et al. 2008). See also Chapter 10: Enrichment: animal welfare and scientific validity.

Feeding and watering

The nutritional requirements of growing and adult dogs can be found in Table 30.3.

Natural and laboratory requirements

Dogs are opportunistic feeders, relying on scavenging as well as hunting in groups. Therefore, food should be considered as part of the environment as well as on a purely dietary basis. Most laboratory dogs are likely to be fed on a commercially

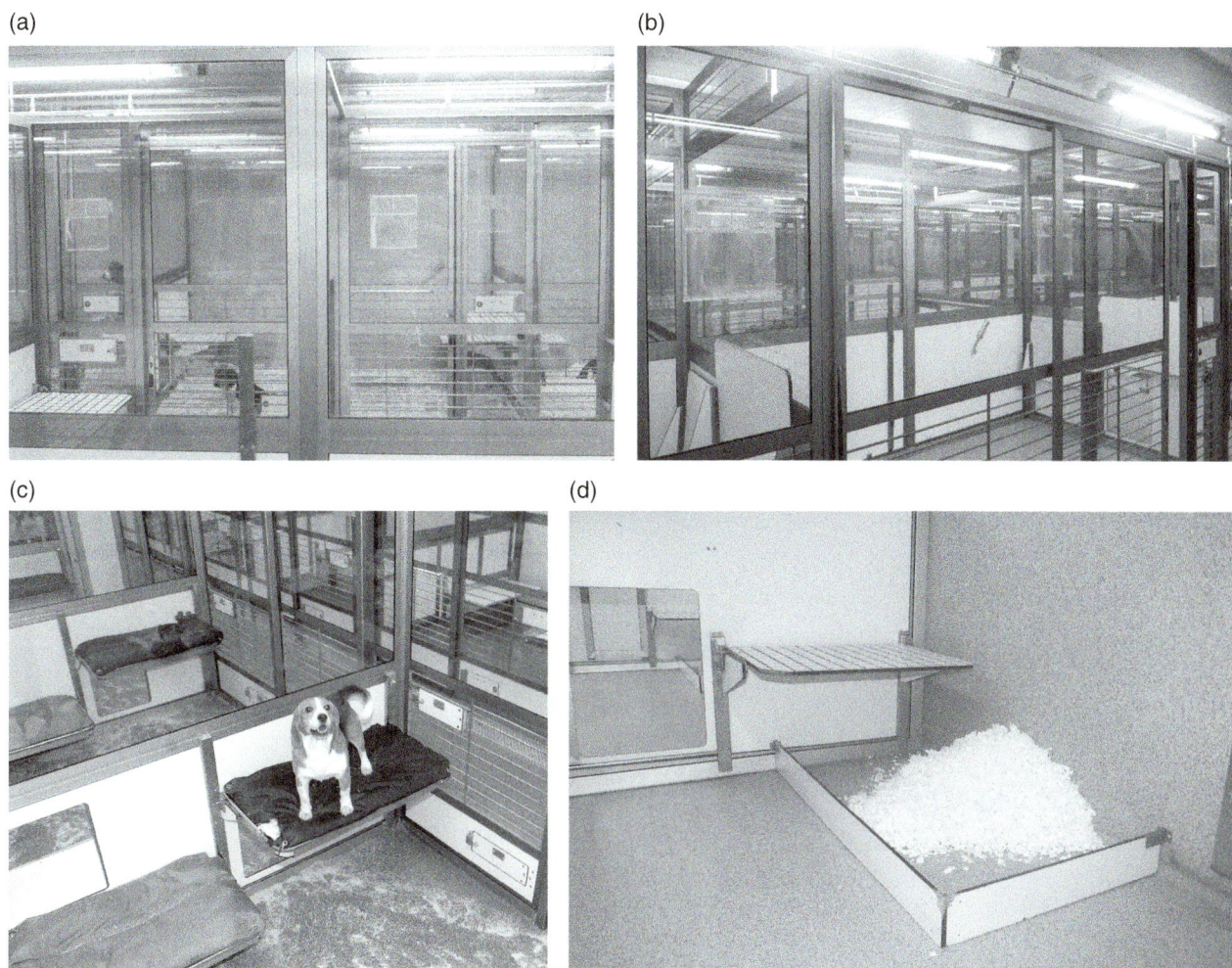

Figure 30.1 Design of modern home pens. Note the use of ledges, multiple exits and transparent materials. (a) The use of transparent materials and ledges provides increased visibility for dogs. (b) The layout of the animal room. (c) Platforms of varying heights permit choice within the home pen. (d) Textured bedding encourages environmental exploration while hatches permit movement between pens.

prepared standard dry diet which should be nutritionally adequate for the stage of life, uncontaminated and palatable. Dogs have a preference for meat-based diets over cereal-based diets; this should be taken into consideration when selecting a laboratory diet. Dogs are also likely to crave novelty and additions should be made to the standard diet, e.g. food treats which can be used in training or biscuits which can be given to dogs in the home pen. Variations in size, textures and odours provide novelty and are likely to stimulate interest in the environment. Changing the presentation of food is also likely to be enriching. Staff should recognise that aversion to the diet may occur if it is associated with adverse study outcomes and alternative diets should be available to prevent weight loss.

Dietary requirements

The energy requirements of dogs will depend upon the environmental conditions, as well as life stage and health status. During gestation, bitches will increase their body weight by around 20–25%, with most of this weight increase occurring after the 28th day (Romsos et al. 1981). Energy requirements increase by up to 50% with underweight bitches being more likely to produce stillborn pups. More information can be found in later section on Nutrition during pregnancy and lactation. Newborn pups require around 25 kcal/100 g body weight. Bitch milk meets the energy requirements of unweaned pups, providing about 1.45 kcal/g. Bitches produce up to 8% of their body weight in milk, peaking in week 4 post parturition. During lactation, nutritional demands increase substantially to peak when the pups are three to four weeks of age. The bitch will require up to four times her daily maintenance ration available throughout the day, and increased water intake is necessary to prevent dehydration. Growing pups require around twice the energy of adults of the same breed (National Research Council 2006). Growth curves can be found in Andersen (1970). Breeders should also provide growth curves for their colonies.

A reliable system should be used to monitor the weight of dogs to ensure that dogs are neither underweight nor obese. The body condition score (Laflamme 1997) provides a scoring system which rates body condition based on appearance and weight from 1 to 9. Healthy dogs should score 4–5 on this scale.

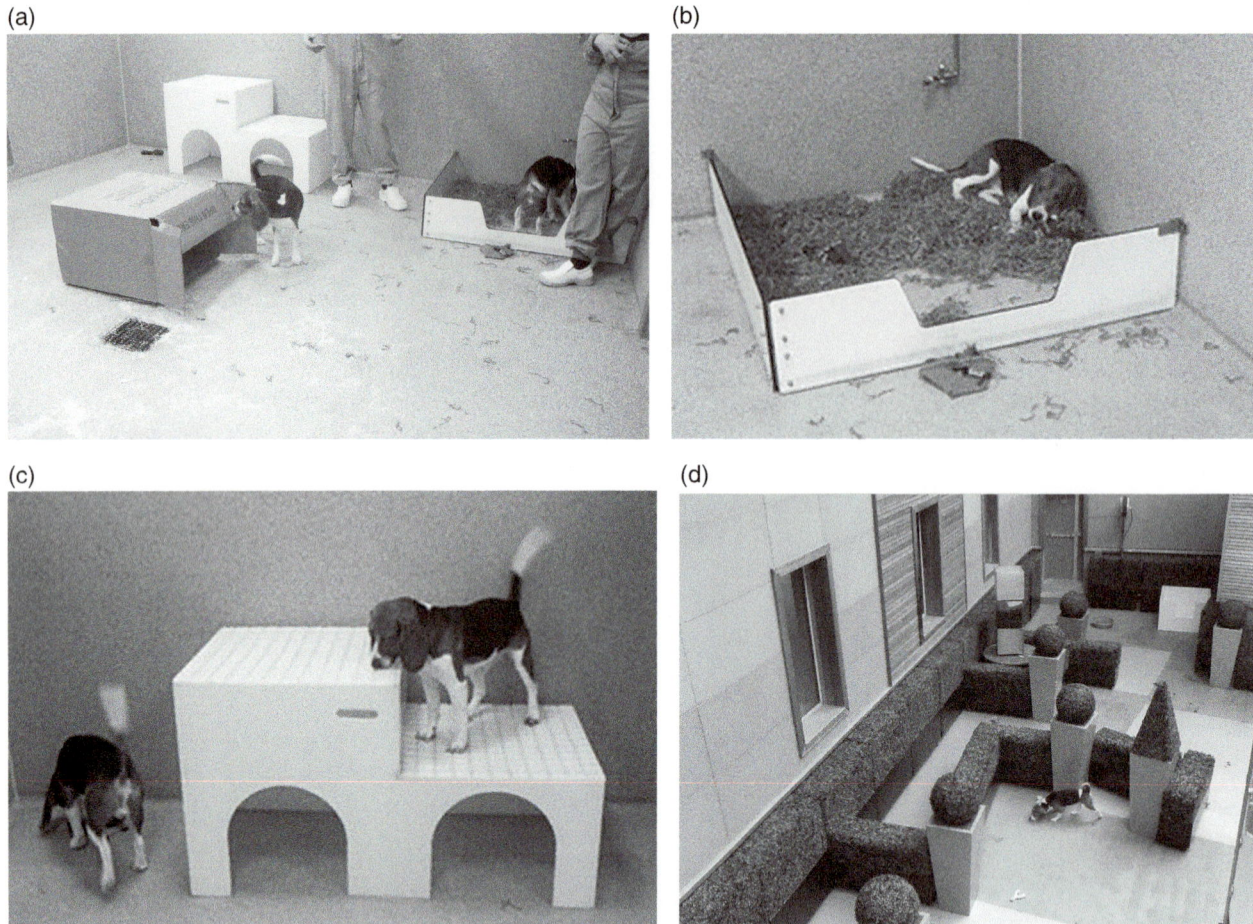

Figure 30.2 The design of external and internal exercise areas, noting features of good practice. (a) Internal exercise area. Note play equipment and use of cardboard as enrichment items. (b) Provision of toys and nesting material. (c) Provision of toys within the exercise area. (d) External exercise area. Note the range of items to encourage activity and exploration.

Laboratory diets will usually have been subjected to more rigorous testing than commercial pet food, including analysis sampled at each batch, and controlled levels of contaminants. Dry diets should be stored in opaque, air-tight containers in a cool and dry environment to prevent growth of mould or bacteria. Canned food is less susceptible to environmental contamination while sealed (avoiding freezing or high temperatures) but are susceptible to contamination once opened. Dogs fed on an exclusively dry diet are more likely to develop dental disease by around 2–3 years old. The provision of other food stuffs and some chewable enrichments may help to prevent dental disease.

Water

When water is freely available, healthy dogs easily regulate their intake to prevent dehydration (National Research Council 2006). Dehydrated dogs are capable of rehydrating quickly given free access to water. In dogs, water is lost predominantly through respiration or through excretion in urine and faeces. The recommended water intake is 70–80 ml/kg/day; therefore, a 10 kg dog should ingest between 700 and 800 ml per day. It is recommended that the intake of water should be double or triple the intake of dry matter (in grams) (Case et al. 2000), and dogs which are fed on an exclusively dry diet may require more water than those with access to wet food. The demand for water intake increases with increased environmental temperature, decreased humidity and increased exercise. Although clear guidelines are not available, it is usually recommended that water intake increase in line with increased food requirements for pregnant and lactating bitches, and for growing puppies (National Research Council 2006).

Water can be provided via an automated drinking system. This removes the need for water bowls which are soiled or spilled easily, and are labour-intensive for staff to maintain. Dogs quickly learn to use drinkers in the pen. The drinking system should be constructed from a high-quality stainless steel and valves should be checked twice daily to ensure that dogs' water intake is not restricted by blockages.

Presentation of food and water

When given choice, dogs eat 4–8 meals per day (Mugford & Thorne 1978), predominantly during daylight hours. Dogs do not have clear circadian rhythms, and metabolism may be driven by eating patterns (Piccione et al. 2005); therefore, dogs may show irregular patterns of activity during the night,

Table 30.3 The nutritional requirements of dogs for growing and adult dogs, adapted from National Research Council (2006).

Nutrient	Unit	Growth (14 wks+) amt./kg BW$^{0.75}$	Adult maintenance amt./kg BW$^{0.75}$
Fat	g	5.9	1.8
Linoleic acid	mg	0.8	0.36
α linoleic acid	g	0.05	0.014
Protein	g	12.2	3.28
Arginine	g	0.46	0.11
Histidine	g	0.17	0.062
Isoleucine	g	0.35	0.12
Leucine	g	0.57	0.22
Lysine	g	0.49	0.11
Methionine + cysteine	g	.37	0.21
Phenylalanine + tyrosine	g	0.7	0.24
Threonine	g	0.44	0.14
Tryptophan	g	0.13	0.046
Valine	g	0.39	0.16
Minerals			
Calcium	g	0.68	0.13
Phosphorus	g	0.68	0.10
Sodium	mg	100	26.2
Chloride	mg	200	40
Magnesium	mg	27.4	19.7
Iron	mg	6.1	1.0
Copper	mg	0.76	0.2
Manganese	mg	0.38	0.16
Zinc	mg	6.84	2.0
Iodine	μg	61.0	29.6
Selenium	μg	25.1	11.8
Vitamins			
A	RE	105	50
D3	IU	0.96	0.45
E	mg	2.1	1.0
K	mg	0.11	0.054
Thiamin (B1)	mg	0.096	0.074
Riboflavin (B2)	mg	0.37	0.171
Niacin (B3)	mg	1.18	0.57
Choline (B4)	mg	118	56
Pantothenic acid (B5)	mg	1.04	0.49
Pyridoxine (B6)	mg	0.10	0.049
Biotin (B7)	mg	–	8.9
Folic acid (B9)	21 mg	18.8	1.15
Cobalamin (B12)			2.4

including eating. Mugford and Thorne (1978) describe *ad libitum* feeding as providing dogs with a more naturalistic eating pattern. A stainless-steel food hopper mounted within the pen allows multiple dogs to access unrestricted food. However, around 30–40% of dogs will become obese on unrestricted feeding. Weight should be monitored regularly to ensure that all dogs are able to access food and, therefore, maintain body weight and restrictions made if necessary. Food hoppers should be regularly maintained and cleaned to remove soiled or caked food. Free-ranging dogs spend a considerable amount of time obtaining food, and providing free access may remove a significant source of enrichment in the environment. Providing food in feeding toys is a better alternative.

Restricted feeding, usually a single meal provided for 2–4 h, is typically used when study requirements necessitate monitoring of food intake or restricting for other reasons, such as fasting before sampling. Feeding typically takes place while dogs are singly housed in order to achieve accurate measurements of food consumption. Food should be provided in stainless-steel bowls which can be mounted on brackets within the pen. Modern pens have hatches which allow staff to remove these bowls without opening the pen door. If the remaining food does not require to be weighed, dry food can also be scattered across a clean pen floor. Dogs eat more slowly when singly housed so it is important to provide a sufficient period for dogs to eat.

Social housing

Dogs are a highly social species, and social housing should be the default for laboratory dogs. Dogs should only be single-housed under specific conditions (see section on Single-housing in this chapter for details) and with sufficient justification. There is a strong evidence-base to support the social housing of kennelled dogs in various circumstances (e.g. Hetts *et al.* 1992; Hubrecht *et al.* 1992; Hubrecht 1995a; Mertens & Unshelm 1996), and social enrichment should be the cornerstone of an enrichment programme. Social housing also provides olfactory enrichment which may encourage increased interaction with the environment or other enrichment items (Hubrecht *et al.* 1992). Single-housing, except for brief periods (e.g. for feeding or post-dose observations), is detrimental to dog welfare and the possible impact on study outcomes should be recognised. Within the European Union, single-housing for a period of greater than four hours in considered a regulated procedure because of its perceived negative impact upon welfare (see section on Single-housing). Pair- or group housing has been successfully used within good laboratory practice (GLP) studies, e.g. for regulatory studies.

The available space may limit the size of groupings; legislation or best practice guidance (e.g. European Union 2010) on space requirements should be followed to ensure adequate space for all animals. Housing in very large groups may lead to conflict, especially where resources such as space, bedding areas or toys are in limited supply. Dogs will naturally form small, fluid group when free-ranging and this composition should be taken into account when deciding upon stocking density.

Care should be taken to ensure that dogs are matched based on compatibility. Group- or pair-housing of incompatible individuals is likely to lead to aggression or competition over resources. Such interactions are likely to lead to poorer data outcomes. Dogs are frequently randomised into groups based on physical data such as weight, age and sibling status. Compatibility with other colony members should be included in this process. Staff should be familiar with their dogs, and relationships between individuals, to facilitate this process. Individual records may take note of compatible groupings so that this information can be maintained during the dog's lifetime. Groupings may be established at the breeding facility and information regarding compatibility should be transferred with the dogs. Dogs will typically be regrouped into smaller groups for study upon arrival in the facility, information from the breeder should be used here to ensure compatibility. In some countries, it is common for animal rooms to be fitted with video recording equipment; this permits the monitoring of social groupings. Given the impact of social interactions on welfare, the compatibility of groups should be used as a factor in study group randomisation. This prevents difficulties in re-assigning incompatible dogs once a study is underway.

Social housing is particularly important during puppyhood, with considerable deficits in social and physical development seen in puppies exposed to varying degrees of isolation (Fox & Stelzner 1966). Behavioural problems involving social conflict seen in puppyhood (e.g. inter-dog aggression, resource guarding) may persist into adulthood and so staff should be appropriately trained to deal with these issues, or independent consultation sought. Providing dogs with sufficient choice of location, ability to withdraw from others and sufficient enrichment for all animals will ameliorate many issues in later life.

Single-housing

Single-housing is a major welfare concern in the laboratory environment, and European legislation (European Union 2010) states that dogs shall not be single-housed for more than four hours at a time. Time periods great than this require authorisation. Dogs are a highly social species, and solitary housing may induce dogs to perform repetitive behaviours such as pacing, circling, tail chasing and flank sucking (Hubrecht 1993). These can lead to changes in physiology; thus, influencing experimental data (Beerda et al. 1997).

Single-housing disturbs both behaviour (Hetts et al. 1992; Hall 2014) and haemodynamic parameters (Klumpp et al. 2006). Singly housed dogs are more likely to be vigilant, restless, to engage in pacing behaviour and to vocalise. These behaviours can be associated with an increase in haemodynamic parameters (Hall 2014). EU legislation (European Union 2010) recognises the impact of single-housing as a regulated procedure and it should, therefore, be justified against the detrimental impact on welfare.

It may occasionally be necessary to singly house dogs for health or welfare reasons. Dogs recovering from anaesthesia or surgery, or undergoing veterinary care may require to be separated during recovery. The benefits of single-housing should be weighed against the costs to the animals. Pregnant bitches should be singly housed shortly before parturition and lactating bitches singly housed until pups are weaned, although bitches may exercise together once pups reach a suitable age to be separated from her for brief periods.

Single-housing for research reasons has become much rarer. In the past, it was common practice to singly house dogs during safety assessment studies, particularly following dosing or feeding or for instrumented dogs. It is now more common for dogs to be pair or group-housed for the majority of a study, with only short separations (of up to four hours) used when necessary. Food consumption data can be collected across the dose group and is commonly used in place of individual food consumption data.

Instrumented dogs may be fitted with jackets or devices which permit social housing. With sufficient training and acclimatisation, dogs can readily adapt to the presence of jackets which protect the device. Modern telemetric systems are compatible with social housing, allowing dogs to remain together during data collection (see section on Telemetry in this chapter) by operating across multiple frequencies or allowing devices to be switched off *in situ*. Other approaches can also permit social housing of dogs in situations which may previously have prevented it, including the use of a naive companion.

In the very few instances where single-housing is deemed necessary, pen design should be such that dogs can maintain visual and olfactory contact with conspecifics. Additional human contact and enrichment should also be provided where possible to ameliorate the effects of separation from pen mates.

Metabolism cages

The use of metabolism cages that are smaller than the minimum recommended pen size and which require single-housing is recognised in the EU as a regulated procedure because of the potential negative impact on welfare.

The following aspects of good practice should be followed to ensure that the negative welfare impact is minimised. For example, the metabolic cage should be large enough to allow the dog to stand, lie and stretch out freely. Gridded flooring materials should be designed such that they do not damage dogs' paws. Dogs should be able to see, smell and hear other dogs. Metabolism cages which can be wheeled into the animal room are available and allow the dog to maintain contact with other dogs. Group-housing of dogs in metabolism cages is also possible (Kendrick et al. 2020). Conversely, it may be possible to house a non-study animal close by the metabolism cage to provide some companionship or to conduct metabolism studies on pairs of dogs such that two dogs can be housed side by side. Additional staff contact should be implemented during time in the cage, and enrichment items should be available. The time required in the metabolism cage should be minimised as far as possible and balanced against the welfare harms caused. When repeated use of the metabolism cage is indicated, dogs should be allowed a two-week period of recovery between instances of confinement.

Identification

Dogs should be marked using the least painful manner possible. A subcutaneous microchip is the most common method of identification. In some jurisdictions, there are special requirements for marking dogs (European Union 2010).

Physical environment

Temperature

Adult dogs can adapt to a range of temperature variations given sufficient shelter, food and water; however, to avoid changes in energy use, a temperature range of 15 – 21 °C should be maintained. If dogs are to be exposed to temperatures below 10 °C, e.g. when they have access to outdoor runs, sufficient time should be permitted for dogs to adapt and sufficient shelter should be provided.

Puppies have a limited capacity to thermoregulate and so particular attention should be paid to the maintenance of temperature in breeding facilities and during the first 10 days of life. The ability to thermoregulate develops during the first three weeks of life, as does the ability to move independently which allows pups to move away from or towards sources of heat (Jones et al. 1982). A temperature range of 26 °C–30 °C should be maintained during this time. Pups should be warm to the touch and sleepy if their body temperature is correct. Pups which are cold or limp to touch, or which cry should be examined.

Ventilation and relative humidity

Facilities should aim to maintain relative humidity of 30% to 70% throughout the year to provide a comfortable range that does not adversely affect dogs' welfare. Ventilation in indoor areas should be maintained at 10–15 air changes per hour to minimise the effects of odours or ammonia on air quality (National Research Council 2010).

Lighting

Natural lighting with seasonal variation is acceptable for dogs. Where natural light does not provide, an appropriate light/dark cycle shall be provided to satisfy the biological requirements of the animals and to provide a satisfactory working environment e.g. a 10–12 h daylight period, with dawn dusk settings and provision of a low level night lighting e.g. (Prescott et al. 2004) and Annex III, European Union (2010).

Noise

Dogs communicate through a range of vocalisations including barking, growling and whining; however, noise most commonly results from barking. Barking can be a response to increased arousal, either through excitement (e.g. movement of other dogs through the animal room) or fear (e.g. stranger in the animal room). Dogs' hearing is more sensitive to noise than that of humans, especially in the higher frequencies which correspond to the peak energy of the bark (Sales et al. 1997). Noise can also be detrimental to humans. The levels of noise reached in the animal room can exceed 100 dB (Scullion Hall et al. 2017) which is above the threshold of potential hearing damage for humans and can interfere with communication between staff and dogs. Allelomimetic barking frequently occurs around exercise times, feeding, husbandry or procedures. The design of housing influences the rate of barking, which is lower when dogs are provided with a view of the animal room (aided by the use of transparent materials in pen construction) and a range of ledges which can be used to elevate the dog and provide a better view. Adequate training should prevent such occurrences and staff should view excessive barking as a sign, as well as cause of, poor welfare.

Hygiene

Pens should be cleaned throughout the day, with soiled substrate and faeces being removed regularly. Dogs tend to defecate shortly after eating, and cleaning at this time is most effective. Canids prefer to defecate away from the sleeping area and providing dogs with regular access to another area, or providing a large enough home pen, will prevent contamination of the sleeping area with faecal matter. This is less true in puppies so more regular cleaning will be needed. Cleaning should take place while the dogs are out of the pen, either during daily exercise, or by moving dogs to an adjacent pen. The use of a suitable substrate, such as sawdust or shredded paper, will aid the cleaning of pens and reduce the soiling of the dogs themselves. Pen washing should be conducted once per week and is most effective when a combination of pressure hoses, disinfectants and detergents is used. Dogs should always be removed from the animal room during wet cleaning to prevent stress resulting from noise and disturbance, or irritation from exposure to disinfectants and detergents.

Health monitoring, quarantine and barrier systems

Physical barriers and procedures should be used to govern the entry of animals, staff, visitors, consumables, including diet, bedding, and equipment into the unit to limit the risk of disease entry. Procedures may include prior knowledge and/or testing of the health status of new animals joining the colony and isolation of new animals from the existing population until the results of screening tests are available. A change of clothing including footwear for staff and visitors, coupled with handwashing or hand sanitation on entry and exit, and the wearing of gloves when handling the animals is recommended. A pest control scheme should be in operation on the perimeter of the building and in diet storage areas.

The Federation of European Laboratory Animal Science Associations (FELASA) working group on health monitoring (Rehbinder et al. 1998) outlines guidelines for health monitoring of dogs. All animals should be observed daily, and any signs of disease investigated. A minimum of 10 animals should be sampled every three months. If dogs are not vaccinated as part of the establishment, prophylactic regime viruses should be monitored by serology. Bacterial culture and parasitology should be performed on samples from the tonsils, combed samples of skin and hair, and faeces. For further details on the pathogens to be monitored, refer to Rehbinder et al. (1998) and Section on Health and disease in this chapter.

Care of aged animals

Many dogs will complete their study use and be euthanised before the age of 12 months. However, some dogs, such as those surgically prepared animals, donor colonies and breeding colonies, will live for up to five or six years of age. Davis (1996), Mosier (1989) and Willems et al. (2017) describe the effects of the ageing process on the body systems. In addition to regular health checks, caregivers should be trained in the specialised needs and health risks of older animals. Dental disease is common, and prophylactic dental descaling under general anaesthesia may be required but regular teeth brushing may reduce the need for intervention. Oral tumours are common in dogs over 10 years of age and, therefore, unlikely to be seen in laboratory populations.

Osteoarthritis may result in joint pain, lameness or reduced proprioception, affected animals should be provided with soft bedding. Respiratory disease e.g. obstructive lung disease and bronchitis, and cardiovascular disease e.g. chronic valvular fibrosis and coronary arteriosclerosis may result in breathlessness, coughing and exercise intolerance. Renal and hepatic disease can be diagnosed with routine haematological and biochemical screening, which may also assist in the diagnosis of endocrine disease and neoplasia. The incidence of sebaceous gland adenomas and sebaceous cysts increases in older animals.

Mammary tumours and pyometra are common in older bitches. Prostatic hypertrophy and testicular tumours occur commonly in males. The prevalence of anal adenomas increases in both males and females, with higher incidence in males. Chronic thyroiditis and hypothyroidism are common in older dogs, as are deficits in hearing and vision. Canine cognitive dysfunction can result in confusion and anxiety in some animals. See also Chapter 16: 3Rs considerations when using ageing animals in science.

Breeding

Identifying the fertile state

There are many detailed texts describing fertility and reproduction in the dog (Andersen 1970; England & Allen 2008; Concannon 1991; Feldman et al. 2014; Greer 2014). Bitches reach sexual maturity between 6 and 14 months of age, which correlates with approximately 80% of adult bodyweight, with peak fertility occurring at approximately two years of age and reducing from 6 to 7 years of age. Male dogs reach sexual maturity from 10 months of age with peak fertility also occurring at approximately two years of age (England et al. 2010). Reproductive information can be found in Table 30.2.

Bitches have a monoestrous reproductive cycle with an ovulatory clinical oestrous cycle occurring approximately twice a year (Thulin et al. 2018). The oestrous cycle is divided into four stages. Pro-oestrus (10 days) characterised by vulval swelling, a bloody vaginal discharge and high levels of oestrogen circulating in the blood. Oestrus, the bitch is receptive to the dog, with her rump raised and her tail carried to one side, and mating occurs. Metoestrous or luteal phase (pregnant or non-pregnant) lasts approximately 63 days (pregnant) and 66 days (non-pregnant state), with continued high levels of progesterone. Anoestrus lasts between 5 and 7 months and is characterised by both low oestrogen and progesterone levels.

A bitch will allow a dog to mate for several days both before and after ovulation, which in dogs is spontaneous. Both oocytes and spermatozoa can remain viable in the female reproductive tract for several days, enabling fertilisation to occur up to two to five days post ovulation (England et al. 2010). The result is a variable gestation period of 57–69 days post mating (Lamm & Makloski 2012). Gestation length can be more reliably predicted as 62–64 days from the pre-ovulatory surge of circulating luteinising hormone (Concannon et al. 1983).

The most common cause of infertility is the incorrect timing of mating. The optimal time is from the day of ovulation which is hard to predict, to four days post ovulation. Methods of prediction include the number of days from the start of pro-oestrus, the onset of oestrous behaviour, onset of valvular softening, measurement of hormone concentrations – oestrogen, luteinising hormone and progesterone (England et al. 2010). Vaginal cytology can be also used to predict the stage of the oestrous cycle (Concannon & DiGregorio 1986; Bowen 1998).

Pseudopregnancy. Due to persistence of a corpus luteum during metoestrus, most bitches will show slight enlargement of the mammary glands. In some bitches, the levels of prolactin are high, although not as high as in pregnancy levels, and mammary gland development is significant. Other signs of pseudopregnancy can include lactation, anorexia, anxiety, aggression, nest-building and nursing of toys and in some cases treatment with prolactin inhibitors e.g. cabergoline may be necessary (England et al. 2010).

Breeding systems

Observed Matings. The bitch is usually taken to the dog on day 10–12 after the first signs of proestrus, the behaviour of the bitch and stud will determine whether the bitch is receptive and whether mating or tying occurs (Prescott et al. 2004). The bitch is usually returned to her home pen and mating, with the same dog to ensure knowledge of parentage, may be repeated periodically for a further 10 days to increase the success rate for pregnancy. The bitch and male may be housed together during the oestrous period but 'tying' (in which the pair are locked together for up to 30 minutes due to the bulbus glandis of the male's penis swelling inside the bitch's vagina) may not always be observed, resulting in difficulty confirming a successful mating and predicting an accurate whelping date.

Harem System. Groups of usually 4–6, but can be up to 12, compatible breeding bitches are housed with a dog. Mating is less likely to be observed so pregnancy diagnosis is recommended, but this system is less time consuming to maintain, and care staff do not need to observe and monitor the bitches for signs of oestrus. The disadvantages of a harem system are the potential for aggression between bitches and reduced fertility of the stud male if several bitches are mated simultaneously (Prescott et al. 2004).

Artificial Insemination. Farstad (2010) provides detailed descriptions of artificial insemination in dogs, which can be useful when animals are in different facilities, cannot be moved or when it is inappropriate or impractical to introduce new breeding stock e.g. due to differences in health status. Bitches are housed in same sex groups and checked regularly for signs of oestrus. Appropriate timing for artificial insemination can be predicted by checking for softening of the vulva, which often occurs around the time of ovulation; by demonstrating the appropriate vaginal cytologic characteristics of advanced oestrus or by measuring the rise in blood progesterone levels, four days after the surge in luteinising hormone post ovulation. Ideally, two inseminations should occur before vaginal smears show reduced cornification (National Research Council 1994; Prescott et al. 2004).

Pregnancy and parturition

Methods of pregnancy diagnosis include palpation at three to five weeks into the pregnancy, abdominal ultrasound – the foetus can be detected from day 17 but delay until days 24–28 of pregnancy is recommended (Davidson & Baker 2009). Radiography can be useful, once the skeleton has calcified after day 41, to determine litter size and measurement of plasma relaxin levels from day 25 of gestation can reliably confirm pregnancy (Johnston et al. 2001; Farstad 2010; Lamm & Makloski 2012).

Two weeks prior to parturition, bitches should be moved to a whelping area, to be housed with other dogs (Prescott et al. 2004). Close to term, bitches seek a quiet are in which to whelp and may be restless (Johnson 1986; Johnston et al. 2001; Lamm & Makloski 2012). One to two days prior to parturition, bitches should be housed in single-housing with a nesting box and nesting material, a platform to allow the bitch respite from the pups, within sight and smell of other bitches (Prescott et al. 2004). Decreases in blood progesterone to levels less than 1 ng/mL 24 to 48 h prior to parturition (Johnston & Romagnoli 1991) can assist in predicting the time of whelping as can a transient decrease in body temperature for 8 h from 39 °C to 36 °C, which occurs 12–24 h prior to whelping (Concannon et al. 1977; Lamm & Makloski 2012). Relaxation of the pelvic and abdominal muscles and the perineal region can signal parturition is imminent (Forsberg 2010).

Smith (2012) and Jones et al. (1982) describe in detail the stages of normal parturition, complications that may arise and interventions that may be required. The three stages of whelping comprise:

Stage I: usually 6–12 h in duration but could be 36 h is characterised by reclusive or restless behaviour, nesting, panting, shivering and anorexia. During this stage, uterine contractions of increasing strength result in cervical dilation.
Stage II: can last 3–12 h, and should not extend longer than 42 h, during which obvious uterine contractions expel the pups through a fully dilated cervix, usually at an average rate of 1 pup per hour. Stimulation of respiration and removal of foetal membranes is achieved through licking of the pups by the bitch, and she also usually severs the umbilical cord. It is normal for a non-purulent green discharge to be passed during this period.
Stage III: involves expulsion of the placenta, usually within 15 minutes of delivery of the foetus.

Smith (2012) describes in depth the signs of dystocia and medical or surgical interventions which may be required. Dystocia signs include failure to deliver a foetus within 24 h of the onset of Stage I labour, 60 minutes of active labour with no foetus delivered, presence of a greenish-black discharge before any foetus has been passed, gestation greater than 70 days from the first mating.

Nutrition during pregnancy and lactation

Chandler (2015) and National Research Council (2006) detail the pregnant and lactating bitch's feeding requirements. Additional nutrition is required in the third trimester of pregnancy; supplementary protein (29% to 32% protein from an animal source) 18% fat, and 20% to 30% carbohydrates, plus trace nutrients, is recommended and can be provided by feeding breeding or puppy diets (Lamm & Makloski 2012). The bitch must not become obese, however, as this can predispose to dystocia and metabolic disorder (Johnson 1986). During lactation, nutritional demands increase substantially to peak when the pups are three to four weeks of age. The bitch will require up to four times her daily maintenance ration available throughout the day, and increased water intake is necessary to prevent dehydration.

Reproductive problems

Pseudopregnancy. Due to persistence of a corpus luteum during metoestrus, most bitches show slight enlargement of the mammary glands. In some bitches, the levels of prolactin are high, although not as high as in pregnancy levels, and mammary gland development is significant. Other signs of pseudopregnancy can include lactation, anorexia, anxiety, aggression, nest-building and nursing of toys and in some cases treatment with prolactin inhibitors e.g. cabergoline may be necessary (England et al. 2010).

Pregnancy toxaemia. Ketosis can develop due to inadequate intake of carbohydrate, particularly bitches with large litters (Johnston et al. 2001). Signs are non-specific but the condition can be life-threatening and is diagnosed by the presence of ketones in the urine. Diabetes mellitus can develop during pregnancy and can be diagnosed by the presence of glucose and ketones in the urine. Hypocalcaemia or eclampsia typically, but not always, occur after parturition, when lactation results in high demand for calcium. Signs again can be non-specific but can progress to muscle tremors, pyrexia and death (Lamm & Makloski 2012). Fontbonne (2007) and Okkens et al. (1992) describe causes of infertility in the bitch and dog.

Rearing the young

Prescott et al. (2004) and Lawler (2008) describe care of the bitch and puppies in the neonatal period. The temperature should be raised in the whelping area to 26 °C – 30 °C as pups lack the ability to maintain their body temperature until 3 weeks of age. The pups should be checked for congenital defects e.g. cleft palates, umbilical and inguinal hernias, hydrocephalus; and to ensure they consume sufficient colostrum within the first 72 h after delivery. The provision of a quiet environment for the dam is recommended and strict hygiene practices should be implemented to prevent the transmission of infectious disease. The pups should be weighed regularly and supportive feeding introduced every two to three hours, if bodyweight loss or poor weight gain is observed. Low body temperature can suppress gut motility; therefore, slow warming, and supportive fluid therapy may be necessary before supplementary feeding is introduced. Close observation should continue during the first week of life to ensure adequate feeding and to monitor health and growth. Cross-fostering, to another dam with pups of a similar age, can be considered if litter size is large, or milk supply is poor, with good success rates.

Physiological development

Losses may be as high as 15–30% in dogs; however, under controlled conditions in a commercial breeding facility, still-births should be less than 5% and neonatal losses between 5 and 7%. Increased rates of loss should be investigated by a veterinarian and contributory factors addressed. Records should be periodically reviewed for patterns in losses. Factors which increase the likelihood of losses include previous reproductive problems with the bitch and poor hygiene in the whelping area. Stillbirths can also be reduced by monitoring the health of the bitch throughout the gestation period and ensuring adequate nutrition.

Losses can be reduced through close management of whelping; gestation can be most accurately estimated by dating the mating period. Other methods of identifying conception include vaginal cytology, hormonal concentrations, ultrasound and body temperature. More details can be found in section on Pregnancy and parturition in this chapter. Close management of whelping may require resuscitation and stimulation of pups and managed delivery in cases of dystocia. Nulliparous bitches may require additional assistance, particularity in cleaning pups and encouraging them to suckle.

Pups are most vulnerable in the 36 h period following birth and close monitoring should continue during this time. Particular attention should be paid to cleanliness, air quality and temperature. Pups which are not warm and content should be investigated. Health checks should be conducted within 24 h of birth. Breeding facilities should have a clear euthanasia policy for pups with serious health issues.

Until the eyes open, olfaction and touch are the dominant senses. Puppies open their eyes between 10 and 14 days of age and ears open shortly after. New stimuli should be introduced as the senses develop to ensure pups are acclimatised to surroundings. Pups walk at around 21 days of age and begin to explore the environment and engage in play with their littermates. Pups begin eating solid food between 3 and 4 weeks of age.

Behavioural development

The impact of early life experiences on later welfare has a profound impact. There is a particular responsibility from breeding facilities due to the timing of sensitive periods in dog development. Typically, dogs are used in safety assessment at an age of nine months or younger so opportunities to influence behaviour and resilience in later life occur in the breeding facility before being transferred to a dog facility. Stressors associated with transport and acclimatisation to a new facility mean that early opportunities for desensitisation in the breeding facility are particularly important to future welfare.

At birth, dogs have limited sensory and motor abilities (Fox & Stelzner 1966). They are born with eyes and ears closed; however, they have olfactory abilities as well as developed tactile and thermal sensory capabilities (Jones 2007). Desensitisation to unfamiliar stimuli during the period in which the startle response emerges may also be beneficial to the pups' future responses to unfamiliar stimuli.

Exposure to age-appropriate, gentle stimulation can encourage maturation of the brain, heart and motor skills (Fox & Stelzner 1966). Animals with more developed nervous systems are more likely to be able to adapt to the environment or stressors, a quality which is necessary in laboratory animals. Pups which experience daily handling from birth are more emotionally stable, less likely to yelp or vocalise in a novel environment and more likely to explore it (Gazzano et al. 2008). In a review, Meunier (2006) suggested that the most important factors are to develop a programme which succeeds in reducing distress through the implementation of training, desensitisation and socialisation tailored to the individual future experiences of the dogs. Early training programmes from week 10 to 12 should introduce the examination table and health checks. Early acclimatisation to jackets and instrumentation for dogs likely to experience these during studies may prevent later issues. Although increasingly uncommon, breeding within the same site provides continuity of exposure to staff, handling and environment. The challenges are greater when dogs are transported from commercial breeders to experimental facilities.

Hand rearing

Lawler (2008) and Casal (2010) provide advice on hand rearing of pups by bottle or tube feeding. A warm proprietary milk substitute should be fed every 2 h: 12 ml/100 g per day. The time between feeds can be increased gradually, along with the volume fed: 14 ml/100 g/day in week two increasing to and 18 ml/100 g in week three. If tube feeding alone is used, no more than 4 ml/100 g should be fed at each meal. A warm mash of puppy food and water can be introduced from three weeks of age.

Weaning and rearing

Weaning most commonly takes place between 6 and 8 weeks of age and is best led by the bitch and pups. Sudden separation from the dam is likely to lead to distress in the pups and should be avoided. The beagle reaches sexual maturity at between 9 and 12 months. Growth and food consumption increase between 5 and 10 months, then begins to level off and dogs reach their adult body weight at approximately 10–12 months of age.

Chandler (2015), National Research Council (2006) and Debraekeleer et al. (2010) detail the nutritional requirements for growth. Puppies are supported by the lactating bitch until about three weeks of age when a high protein, high energy puppy diet can be introduced. After weaning, at six to eight weeks of age puppies should continue feeding on an appropriate puppy diet with a protein content of 22–32%, and containing the omega-3 fatty acid docosahexaenoic acid (DHA) for normal neural, retinal and auditory development (Bauer et al. 2006) and higher calcium and phosphorus content than for adult dogs (Chandler 2015).

Selection of breeding stock

Guidance on the management of breeding colonies is available from the National Research Council (1994). The selection of breeding stock is based on a number of physical characteristics including body size, reproductive history, previous reproductive issues, health status in the line and inbreeding co-efficient. The offspring of a primiparous bitch should not be bred from until the health of the line can be established. Breeding colonies are increasingly managed digitally and breeding stock selected by algorithms.

Particular attention should be paid to behaviour and temperament. Behaviour is both heritable and learned, meaning that undesirable traits in the dam and sire may be reproduced in the offspring. The sociability of laboratory beagles has a genetic component (Persson et al. 2016), and a validated, objective behavioural test should be utilised to identify suitable breeding stock. This should include factors such as response to novel environments and people, a calm and even temperament and ability to adapt to unfamiliar situations such as confinement. Dogs showing a tendency to reactivity, vigilance or restlessness are unlikely to adapt to the laboratory environment and should not be selected as breeding stock.

Oestrous control and impact on research

Oestrous control is not frequently practised in the laboratory beagle. Many safety studies are conducted in male animals only in the early stages, and only at later stages are female animals introduced to examine the impact of hormonal variation on outcomes. Oestrous control can be performed by the administration of exogenous progestins, delivered orally or by long-lasting subcutaneous injection. Oestrous control may have adverse impacts such as an increase in mammary nodules (Van Os *et al.* 1981) or cystic endometrial hyperplasia (Maenhoudt *et al.* 2014) and should be used with caution.

Laboratory procedures

Handling and training

Poor handling techniques lead to physical problems for the handler caused by carrying an unbalanced weight, or the risk of the dog jumping away from the handler, as well as inducing fear and anxiety in the dog. Good handling techniques should incorporate securing the dog so that its weight is supported. Scruffing or other rough handling techniques should never be used, and the dog's body should be kept close to the handler's body to prevent strain on the handler's back (if the trained dog needs to be carried at all). Staff should be given training in correct handling methods and should be observed conducting handling until competency is achieved. The correct methods for handling dogs are depicted in Figure 30.3.

Laboratory dogs experience frequent interactions with staff, during husbandry, restraint and regulated procedures, which have the potential to cause stress. Training dogs, using positive reinforcement training (PRT), to cooperate during husbandry and for routine procedures can improve animal welfare, increase cooperation with husbandry and procedures, reduce the effects of stress on experimental data and increase the efficiency of routine tasks (see also Chapter 15: The use of positive reinforcement training techniques to enhance the care and welfare of laboratory and research animals). Adequate staff time is needed to implement a training programme (Hall *et al.* 2015; Figure 30.4).

There is an overwhelming array of information on the training of dogs as pets and working dogs, and on the benefits of positive techniques. However, few of the available training guides can be applied to the laboratory environment, where the behaviours required and pressures on resources are different from other environments. Training programmes are most successful when the following principles are adhered to:

1. The training protocol is developed in conjunction with an accredited animal trainer.
2. Staff have a comprehensive understanding of animal behaviour, learning and the techniques used to modify behaviour.
3. All staff understand the need for the success of the programme.

(a) Carrying the dog supported with two hands.

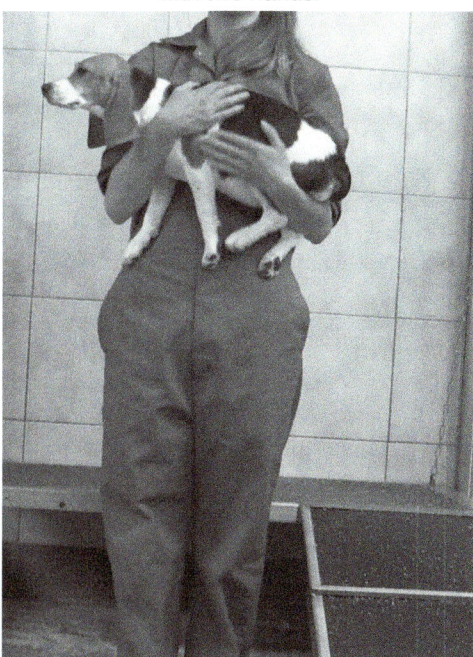

(b) Carrying the dog supported with one hand.

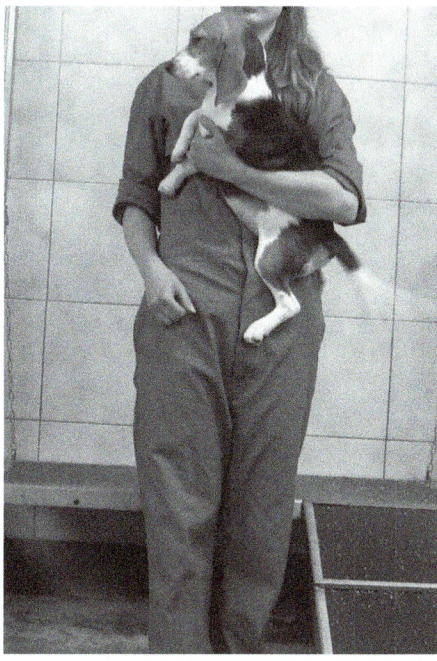

Figure 30.3 The correct methods for handling dogs. Note that the weight for the front and rear legs are always supported so that weight is evenly distributed, and the dog feels secure.

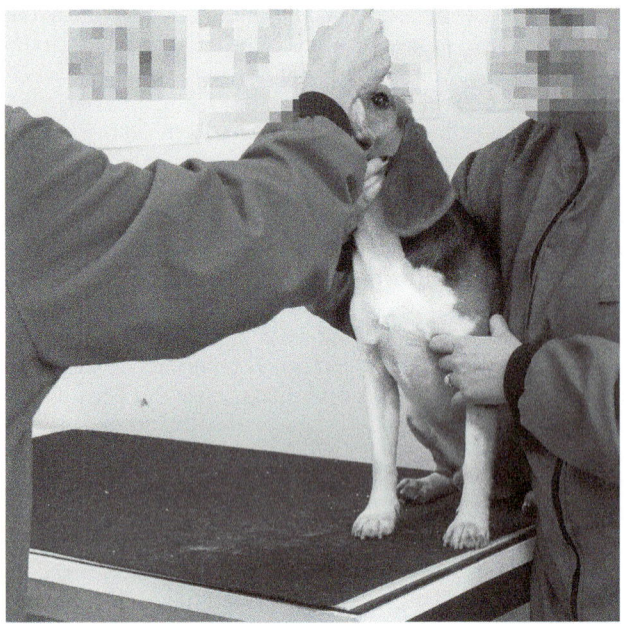

Figure 30.4 A dog is trained for restraint using shaping techniques.

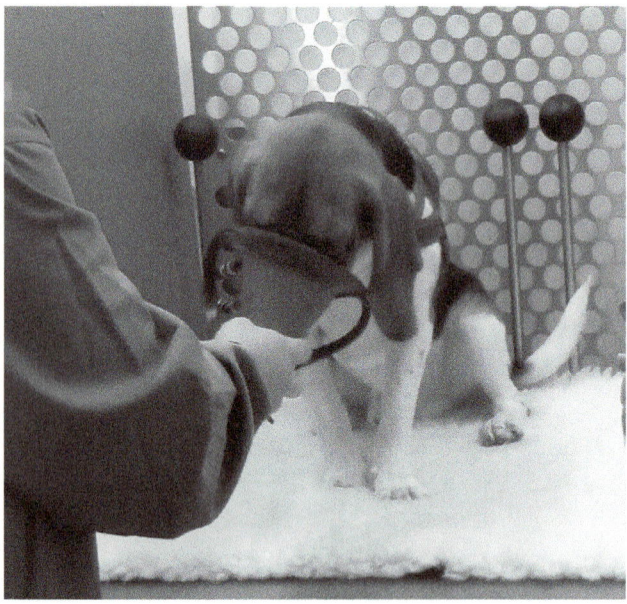

Figure 30.5 A trained dog places its muzzle into the inhalation mask during training.

4. A clear programme with defined techniques and stages of development is produced and adhered to (Hall & Robinson 2016).
5. Understanding and support of the programme at all levels of management.

Physical restraint

Restraint is used for a number of reasons, the most common for procedures and to protect staff from injury. Physical restraint is frequently stressful and can induce a state of distress in dogs (Hall 2014; Hall et al. 2015), particularly when animals are restrained for prolonged periods (Wolfe 1990; Stokes & Marsman 2014). However, restraint can, in some cases, be replaced by PRT, using techniques such as stationing and targeting, during the pre-study period to train the dogs to hold a position during procedures (Hall et al. 2015) (see also Chapter 15).

Physical restraint for longer periods of time for example for aerosol inhalation delivery (Authier et al. 2009) may require the use of restraint equipment. However, refinements should be sought. Dogs can be trained to accept harnesses, slings using PRT (see Figure 30.5). The resulting procedure reduces staff interaction and also results in less stress for the dogs, offsetting the increasing training period needed before the outset of the study.

Physiological monitoring

Recording body temperature

Rectal temperature is normally between 38 °C and 39 °C. Digital thermometers with a short recording time (e.g. 10–30s) are preferable. Ear thermometers are not recommended due to poor correlation between ear and core body temperature. Remote temperature measurement using a subcutaneously implanted microchip is possible but again the recorded value may not accurately reflect core body temperature.

Telemetry

The assessment of cardiovascular function (ECG, heart rate and blood pressure) in a non-rodent species is a requirement for new chemical entities (International Conference on Harmonization 2000, 2005). Although cardiovascular function is typically recorded in the dog during safety pharmacology telemetry studies, it is becoming increasingly common to integrate cardiovascular endpoints into toxicology studies and, therefore, provide important information regarding cardiac effects early in preclinical development (Prior et al. 2016).

The use of animals, restrained either by anaesthetic or slings (Hanton & Rabemampianina 2006; Moscardo et al. 2009) often results in high heart rates, reducing data quality and making detection of QT interval changes more difficult (Hanton & Rabemampianina 2006; McMahon et al. 2006). Unanaesthetised and unrestrained assessment of the QT interval via telemetry is considered the 'gold standard', and surgically implanted telemetry is now widely used in safety pharmacology. However, implantation of telemetry devices is cost-intensive and invasive, and, therefore, not practical for use in large numbers of animals. Jacketed external telemetry, in which the telemetry device is mounted in a jacket worn by the animal, has become increasingly popular as a less invasive alternative. It also has the benefits of being able to collect data at the high dose ranges used in toxicology studies, continuous data collection and acting as a prescreen to assess potential candidates prior to surgery to implement a telemetry device. Both implanted and jacketed telemetry have the advantage of collecting continuous data, with the potential to collect more critical cardiac safety-related information such as drug-induced QT interval prolongation (Chui et al. 2009).

External telemetry devices are usually attached to dogs for 24 h (Xing *et al.* 2015) using jackets equipped with pockets to contain the respective components (Morton *et al.* 2003). However, these jackets may cause stress due to their weight, size and shape. Furthermore, jacketed dogs in telemetry studies are frequently housed singly because of concerns about interference from other dogs and damage to equipment (Prior *et al.* 2016).

The quality of ECG data varies under different housing conditions (Klumpp *et al.* 2006). Dogs pair-housed with a familiar dog produce higher quality CV data, and the quality of data in social housed animals is accepted as being the same or better than from individually housed animals (Prior *et al.* 2016). Refinements such as a jacket design that minimises irritation, combined with acclimatisation and training, can prevent destruction of the jacket so encouraging social housing during data collection.

Collection of specimens

Blood samples

Guidance on blood sampling, needle size and blood volumes is available (Morton *et al.* 1993; National Centre for the Replacement and of Animals in Research[1]). Blood samples can be taken from the jugular or cephalic veins of dogs using a needle with an appropriate bore size (21G). Samples may be obtained more rapidly from the jugular vein and are, therefore, preferred. The saphenous vein is small and mobile but may be appropriate for single samples in some circumstances. Dogs should be trained to sit calmly on a table for blood sampling for a food reward. Sampling should be performed with light restraint from a familiar handler under aseptic conditions. The area should be clipped of fur and cleaned with a water-based antiseptic solution. The handler places their right arm over the shoulders of the dog, holding them close to the body. The sampler occludes the vessel, ensuring good visibility, and inserts the needle cranially into the vein. Following removal of the sample, gentle pressure is applied to the site for 30 seconds to prevent haemorrhage and haematoma formation (see Figure 30.6).

Hair removal cream and shaving should be avoided because of the potential for skin irritation in dogs and in other species. The application of local anaesthetic cream (e.g. EMLA, Astra), applied 45–60 minutes prior to sampling and be covered with an occlusive dressing, can reduce the discomfort of venepuncture (Flecknell *et al.* 1990). Temporary venous cannulation should be considered when repeated samples are required over short time periods. Dogs may be restrained in a sling or returned to the kennel with the cannula covered with a dressing. Surgical cannulation may be appropriate when prolonged venous access is required (see Wolfensohn & Lloyd 2008 for details).

[1] https://www.nc3rs.org.uk/dog-cephalic-vein-non-surgical#all (Accessed May 23, 2022)

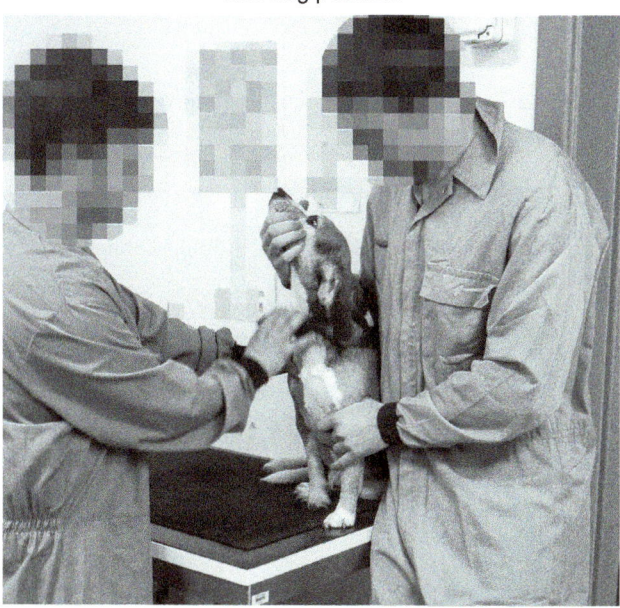

(a) A trained dog is restrained in the dosing or jugular bleeding position.

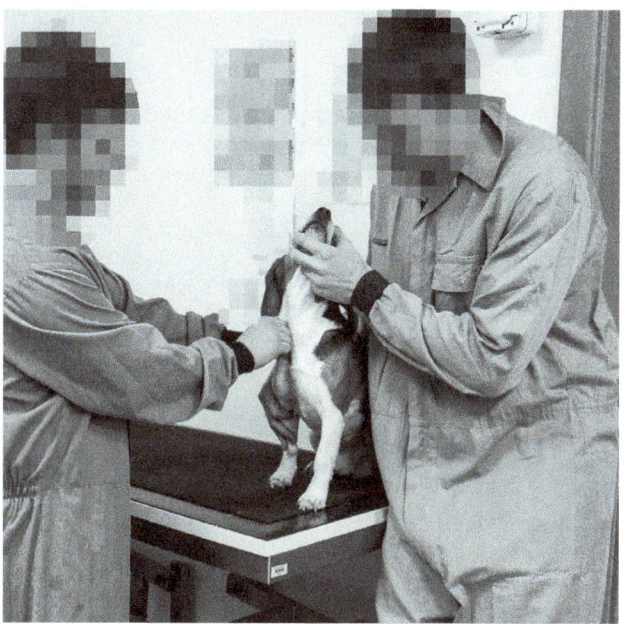

(b) The dog maintains the restraint position while the jugular vein is identified.

Figure 30.6 Methods for restraining dogs for the collection of blood samples.

Bone marrow

The procedure for taking fine needle aspirates or core bone marrow biopsies from the iliac crest is described in detail by Dunn *et al.* (1990). Sedation combined with local anaesthesia or general anaesthesia is recommended. Following full aseptic preparation and local anaesthetic infiltration, insertion of a 16 G 37 mm Klima needle stylet into the bone marrow and removal of the stylet, marrow samples can be aspirated and transferred to microscope slides prior to staining. The same site can be used to take bone marrow biopsies, using a 14 G 95 mm Jamshidi biopsy needle.

Urine

Urinary catheterisation is an invasive and potentially painful procedure, and repeated catheterisation is likely to result in trauma (Boothe 2000) and a higher prevalence of urinary tract infections (Bubenik et al. 2007). The procedure is far more difficult to conduct in female dogs than in males due to anatomical differences. Justification should be made for the use of catheterisation.

Urine is more commonly collected in safety assessment and DMPK studies in metabolism cages, in which all urine and faeces are collected over a given period of time, typically 24 h (see also section on Single-housing in this chapter). Dogs are likely to show signs of distress during use of the metabolism cage and so the procedure requires ethical justification. Dogs should be trained to adapt to confinement in the metabolism cage (see section on Handling and training in this chapter).

Faeces

Faeces can be collected from the pen floor or, when scientifically justified, from a metabolism cage

Abdominal organ biopsy

Vignoli et al. (2011) describes in detail imaging-guided sampling, including ultrasound, computed tomography (CT), magnetic resonance imaging (MRI) and fluoroscopy. Ultrasound-guided biopsy is the most commonly used technique for abdominal organs. Endoscopic biopsy or laparotomy are common techniques for intestinal biopsy. Laparoscopic-assisted gastrointestinal biopsies are becoming safe, effective alternatives to a laparotomy for full-thickness diagnostic samples of the stomach, small intestine, pancreas, liver, and lymph nodes (Mitterman et al. 2016).

Administration of substances

Guidance is available on the administration of substances (Diehl et al. 2001; Morton et al. 2001). Additional guidance on selecting dose ranges has also been produced by NC3Rs (Chapman et al. 2013). The route of administration is typically dictated by the route of administration in clinical practice; however, the least invasive method should be chosen where possible.

Intravenous route

The technique for intravenous dosing is similar to that described for venous sampling described in the preceding text and the reference papers in the preceding text. Morton et al. (1993) also provides detail on venous access and cannulation relevant to intravenous dosing. The cephalic and saphenous veins are most suitable for dosing in dogs and are easily accessible. Administration of substances by a rapid bolus or a longer infusion is possible.

Intramuscular route

Intramuscular injections seem to be more painful than other routes of administration and should only be used when other routes are not possible, and only small volumes are appropriate. The quadriceps muscles at the front of the thigh or, with care, the muscles running alongside the lumbar spine can be utilised.

Subcutaneous route

Subcutaneous injection is a common route of administration. The scruff of the neck is frequently used; a small fold of skin is raised, and a needle inserted parallel to the body. Injections can be painful, and there is the potential for irritation and necrosis. Multiple sites may be appropriate if dosing of larger volumes is required. Rotation of sites is advised if repeat dosing is necessary.

Intraperitoneal route

The intraperitoneal route is not commonly used or recommended in dogs.

Oral route

Oral doses are typically delivered by capsule or gavage. Oral gavage is a technique for delivering a substance directly into the stomach using a flexible tube which is inserted into the stomach via the oesophagus. Gavage is frequently used for oral administration of test compounds in research and toxicity testing.

In a standard one- or three-month toxicology study, dogs may experience daily oral gavage, while other study types may require multiple doses in a day. Its invasive and aversive nature is likely to have a negative impact on dog welfare (Wallace et al. 1990). Habituation to the procedure, or 'sham dosing' is commonly used to acclimatise dogs to the procedure but are not effective techniques and may increase the distress experienced by dogs (Hall et al. 2015) and so should not be used.

Dogs should be trained using PRT techniques used with the head raised in the sitting position with the feet on the table. Dogs should be gently held in this position at approximately waist height for the handler to permit comfortable restraint. Dogs should never be restrained on the floor or between the handler's legs. During training, dogs should be introduced to experimental staff and equipment. Introduction of the dosing tube should be paired with food rewards. A flavoured paste coated on the tube during training may encourage swallowing rather than regurgitation due to insertion of a foreign object into the oesophagus. A proficient technician should be able to complete the dosing procedure swiftly with minimal disturbance to the dog.

Inhalation

Inhalation doses are typically delivered over a period of time (e.g. one hour) through a mask which is fitting to the face, requiring the dog to be stationary for extended periods of time. Dogs can be trained to station on a bench, which usually has fleece bedding for comfort. A harness is used for safety rather than as the main form of restraint which reduces the number of staff needed to restrain each dog. Dogs are trained to place their muzzle in the inhalation mask using PRT which reduces the aversive nature of the procedure (see Figure 30.5). Dogs which are adequately trained may lie down during the procedure.

Anaesthesia, analgesia and post-operative care

Comprehensive information on canine anaesthesia, analgesia and post-operative care can be found in Duke-Novakovski *et al.* (2016) and Flecknell (2016). Specific guidance on pain management can be found in Flecknell *et al.* (2000) and Self (2019). See also Table 30.4.

Peri-anaesthetic care

Pre-anaesthetic checks: a full physical examination including body weight and condition score, cardiovascular and respiratory system examination should be performed, and basic haematological and biochemical tests and a blood coagulation profile should be considered. Fasting for at least six to eight hours is generally recommended to reduce the risk of vomiting, regurgitation and aspiration.

Pre-medication and sedation

Pre-medication reduces the dose of other anaesthetic agents required and contributes to preventive post-operative analgesia. Pre-medication can induce sedation, minimise anxiety prior to induction and facilitate a smother recovery. Agents can also be used to reduce the side effects of other drugs e.g. vomiting and bradycardia.

Murrell (2016) and Flecknell (2016) provide in-depth information on the properties of pre-medication and sedative agents and describe common combination protocols. Medetomidine or dexmedetomidine, alpha-2 agonists, produce a dose dependant sedation which can be completely reversed with atipamezole. The addition of an opioid, benzodiazepine, ketamine or other agents can increase the depth of sedation and provide analgesia. Acepromazine, a benzodiazepine, produces light sedation, the depth of which can be increased with the addition of an opioid which also provides analgesia.

Analgesia

Pain assessment and post-operative care. A universally accepted definition of pain: an unpleasant sensory and emotional experience associated with actual or potential tissue damage has been described (Merskey 1979). As the same sensory pathways are present in humans and sentient animals, we assume animals feel pain in the same way we do. Analgesia should be provided during painful procedures such as surgery. Roughan and Flecknell (2003), Morton *et al.* (1985) and Hawkins (2002) advocate the use of behaviour-based pain assessment. Several assessment scales are available; the Glasgow Pain Scale (Reid *et al.* 2013) is specific to dogs. Although they have limitations due the subjective nature of assessment, pain scales are valuable to assess and record the condition of the animal and the response to analgesia. The requirement for pain relief should be assessed according to the needs of the individual, and reassessed following therapy (Berry 2010).

Pain is likely to impact on scientific outcomes (Carbone 2011; Carbone & Austin 2016) and must be controlled for ethical and scientific reasons. It is necessary to use objective measures to assess pain in order to administer pain relief effectively (e.g. Flecknell *et al.* 2000; Holton *et al.* 2001). Flecknell *et al.* (2000) review the signs of pain in dogs which can include abnormal posture, guarding or tensing of the abdomen, 'praying' position (forequarters on the ground, hindquarters in the air), sitting or lying in an abnormal position or not resting in a normal position (e.g. sternal or curled up), abnormal gait, stiffness, limping or abnormal weight bearing on an injured limb, abnormal or no movement, thrashing, restless, vocalisation, screaming, whining or crying (intermittent, constant or when touched), looking, licking or chewing at the painful area. More severe pain may be recognised by persistent vocalisation such as howling, shivering or crouching (Prescott *et al.* 2004). Changes in facial expression are also useful in the identification of pain (Descovich *et al.* 2017).

A multimodal pre-emptive analgesia protocol, which uses a combination of different analgesic classes to target the different underlying pain mechanisms, is the ideal. By combining drugs, the actions of which are complementary, it is possible to lower the required dose of each individual drug, and address all areas of the pain pathway (Self 2019). Multimodal anaesthesia ideally includes the use of an opioid, an NSAID, local anaesthesia, alpha-2 agonists as required and non-pharmacological techniques e.g. acupuncture (Berry 2010), but the nature of the research may preclude inclusion of all the recommended components.

Nursing Care. Dogs should be closely monitored in the post-anaesthetic/post-operative period in addition to pain assessment, pulse rate and respiratory rate, body temperature, bodyweight, food and water intake and urine and faecal out should all be assessed and recorded. Dogs should continue to be provided with supplementary thermostatically controlled heat source in a warm room until fully recovered, soft bedding and palatable food to which they have been previously acclimatised. Single-housing of dogs should be avoided or minimised. Sutures or staples should be removed after 7–10 days, and exercise restricted until this time.

Anaesthesia

Canine anaesthesia is complex and should only be performed by trained and experienced personnel in a dedicated area. There is a wide range of anaesthetic sedative agents available, all of which will have a physiological effect. The choice of agents will depend on the scientific model, but the common aim is repeatable physiological stability with minimal side effects on the dog and the data collected. Balanced anaesthesia; an anaesthetic protocol which combines smaller doses of more than one anaesthetic drug can be used to minimise the side effects from a single drug.

During anaesthesia (regardless of the route) or during sedation, a supply of supplementary oxygen should be available via an appropriate anaesthetic machine and circuit; Baines, modified Baines or Magill circuits are most commonly used

Table 30.4 Sedatives, tranquillisers, analgesics and anaesthetics for laboratory dogs, adapted from Wolfensohn and Lloyd (2008) and Flecknell (2016).

Anaesthetics

Drug	Dose rate	Effect	Duration of Anaesthesia (min)	Sleep time (min)
Alphaxalone	2 mg/kg iv	Surgical anaesthesia	10–15	15–20
Ketamine/dexmedetomidine	2.5–7.5 mg/kg i.m. + 20ug/kg i.m.	Light to medium anaesthesia	30–45	60–120
Ketamine/medetomidine	5–7.5mg/kg im + 40 ug/kg im	Light to medium anaesthesia	30–45	60–120
Ketamine/xylazine	15 mg/kg iv–1 mg/kg im	Light to medium anaesthesia	30–60	60–120
Pentobarbital	20–30 mg/kg iv	Surgical anaesthesia	30–40	60–240
Propofol	6.5 mg/kg iv unpremedicated 4 mg/kg iv premedicated	Surgical anaesthesia	5–10	15–30
Thiopental	10–20 mg/kg iv	Surgical anaesthesia	5–10	20–30

Sedatives, tranquillisers and other pre-anaesthetic medications

Drug	Dose rate	Comments
Acepromazine	0.03–0.125 mg/kg im	Light to moderate sedation
Acepromazine/buprenorphine	0.07 mg/kg im + 0.009 mg/kg im	Heavy sedation, immobilisation, some analgesia
Atropine	0.05 mg/kg sc or im	Anticholinergic
Dexmedetomidine	up to 375ug/m2 body surface area i.v. or up to 500ug.m2 body surface area i.m.	Light to heavy sedation, mild to moderate analgesia
Glycopyrrolate	0.01 mg/kg iv	Anticholinergic
Medetomidine	0–80 ug/kg im, sc or iv	Light to heavy sedation, mild to moderate analgesia
Medetomidine + butorphanol	10–25 ug/kg im, sc+ 0.1–mg/kg im	Light to heavy sedation, mild to moderate analgesia
Xylazine	1 mg/kg im	Light to moderate sedation, mild to moderate analgesia

Analgesics

Opioid Analgesics

Drug	Dose rate	Comments
Buprenorphine	0.005–0.02 mg/kg sc, im or iv	Given every 6–12 h
Butorphanol	0.2–0.4 mg/kg sc or im	Given every 3–4 h
Fentanyl	0.5–5 mg/kg sc or im	Give every 4h
Morphine	0.5–5 mg/kg s.c.or i.m.	Give every 4h
Nalbuphine	0.5–2.0mg/kg s.c.or i.m.	Give every 3–4h
Pentazocine	2 mg/kg i.m. or i.v	Give every 4h
Pethidine	10 mg/kg im	Given every 2–3 h relief
Tramadol	2–5 mg/kg i.v. or s.c. 2–5mg/kg p.o.	give every 8h

Non-steroidal anti-inflammatories

Drug	Dose rate	Comments
Aspirin	10–25 mg/kg po	Give every 4h relief
Carprofen	4 mg/kg ivor sc 2-4 mg /kg twice daily p.o for 7 days 2 mg/kg p.o. after 7 days	Give every 24h for once daily dosing For twice daily dosing per os give every 12 hours
Ibuprofen	10mg/kg po	Give every 24
Ketoprofen	2 mg/kg sc, im or ivdaily for up to 3 days. 1 mg/kg per os daily for up to 5 days	Give every 24 h
Meloxicam	0.2 mg/kg scor p.o. once daily for the first day then 0.1 mg/kg s.c or p.o.	Give every 24h
Paracetamol	15mg/kg po	Give every 6–8 h
Tolfenamic acid	4 mg/kg s.c. for 2 days	Give every 12 h

for dogs, with an appropriate-sized face mask or an endo-tracheal tube. Alibhai (2016) and Flecknell (2016) describe components of anaesthetic machines and circuits.

Anaesthetic monitoring should include pain reflexes, eye position, respiratory rate and rhythm, pulse oximetry, capnography, electrocardiogram, temperature and can include blood pressure, central venous pressure and urine output (Flecknell 2016; Schauvliege 2016).

Maintenance of body temperature during anaesthesia is essential (Redondo et al. 2012). All anaesthetic drugs cause hypothermia by depression of the thermoregulatory centre of the brain with an effect on biological processes metabolic pathways coagulation, increases the potency of volatile anaesthetics (Regan & Eger 1967) and prolongs recovery time (Pottie et al. 2007). To combat hypothermia, the room temperature should be increased (23 °C) and excessive hair clipping and wetting of the hair and skin with disinfectants and alcohol should be avoided. The use of a thermostatically controlled supplementary heat mat, with an insulating layer between the animal and the mat to prevent thermal injury, or an active heat supply (e.g. Bair Hugger, Arizant Inc) is recommended during anaesthesia and on recovery. Warming of inspired gases can reduce heat loss via the respiratory system and intravenous fluids, and fluids used to flush body cavities should be warmed to 40 °C.

Fluids. Administration of warmed crystalloid fluids intravenously during anaesthesia is recommended to replace fluids lost during fasting and during the procedure, and to counteract the side effects of some anaesthetics, e.g. diuresis. The recommended rate of infusion is to start at 5 ml/kg/hr and reduce the rate by 25% per hour until to the recommended daily maintenance rate; 40 ml/kg/24 h has been reached (Davis et al. 2013). Fluids can be warmed in an incubator, at low temperatures in a microwave followed by agitation and temperature check or using a proprietary fluid warming device placed close to the patient (Aukbullary 2016).

General Anaesthesia. Flecknell (2016), Kaster (2016) (injectable agents) and Pang (2016) (inhalation agents) provide in-depth information on the properties of anaesthetic agents and dose rates are detailed in the table in the earlier part of this chapter. The dose of anaesthetic agents in Table 30.4 can be reduced by 30–50% following pre-medication.

Injectable agents. Venous administration of injectable anaesthetic agents is simple and is the most common route of administration in the dog, although some injectable agents or combinations e.g. ketamine/medetomidine may be administered intramuscularly. Intravenous administration is via an over-the-needle cannula introduced into the superficial cephalic vein in the forelegs or less commonly via the saphenous vein in the hindlimb. Preparation of the site: clipping to remove hair and cleaning with antiseptic is recommended and again, discomfort can be minimised by application of a local anaesthetic cream (e.g. EMLA, Aspen Pharma UK) 45–60 minutes prior to introduction of the cannula. Flushing with saline or heparinised saline helps maintain cannula patency. Following induction, anaesthesia can be maintained by repeated bolus administration of the agent, continuous infusion via an infusion pump or transferring to an inhaled volatile agent. Propofol is the most commonly used injectable agent, producing rapid induction, short duration anaesthesia and smooth recovery but it can induce apnoea and provides little analgesia. Other injectable agents include barbiturates e.g. thiopental alfaxalone and ketamine.

Inhalation agents. Induction of anaesthesia using volatile anaesthetic agents via a face mask is not recommended in the dog, but their use for maintenance of anaesthesia after induction with an injectable agent is common, often for prolonged duration. Intubation via an endotracheal tube is relatively simple in the dog, which is then connected to an anaesthetic machine appropriate circuit as described in the preceding text and in Flecknell (2016). Vapourisers, calibrated for the specific volatile agent, deliver the anaesthetic with an oxygen carrier supply and either active or passive scavenging of the expired gases is essential. The side effects of volatile anaesthetic agents are similar: pronounced cardiovascular and respiratory depression; and reduced renal and hepatic perfusion as a result of hypotension. Balanced anaesthetic protocols, which reduce the dose required for each component, can minimise the side effects. Isoflurane and sevoflurane are common agents used in the dog, with desflurane being introduced more recently. Flecknell (2016) and Pang (2016) describe the properties of these agents in more detail. Use of a mechanical ventilator may be appropriate, e.g. anaesthesia of long duration, to counteract respiratory depression and maintain blood oxygen and carbon dioxide levels within normal ranges, or procedures which involve a thoracotomy. More detailed information on ventilators is available (Hammond & Murison 2016; Flecknell 2016).

Euthanasia

Dogs should be euthanised in a calm familiar environment, away from the presence of other dogs, by a known caregiver (Prescott et al. 2004). The method of euthanasia should induce rapid loss of consciousness followed by respiratory and cardiac arrest, with minimal distress prior to loss of consciousness. The most commonly use method of euthanasia for dogs is an overdose of anaesthetic, delivered intravenously into the cephalic vein e.g. sodium pentobarbitone dose rate of 75–150 mg/kg and concentrations of 60–400 mg/ml. Due to its alkaline pH, pentobarbitone should only be administered intravenously. On some occasions, it may be necessary to sedate a dog prior to intravenous administration of a barbiturate. See above and Flecknell (2016) for sedative dose rates. Close et al. (1996) and Leary et al. (2013) describe appropriate alternative methods of euthanasia if required to meet the scientific objective. Following euthanasia, death must be confirmed by, for example, absence of respiration, heartbeat confirmed by auscultation with a stethoscope, femoral pulse or by onset of rigor mortis (Prescott et al. 2004). Alternative methods of confirmation may also be used (see Annex IV, European Union 2010).

Common welfare problems

Health and disease

Health checks and veterinary inspections should be conducted regularly. Health checks should be conducted on experimental and stock dogs once per week, and breeding bitches should be examined before each mating.

Additional checks should be scheduled when health issues may be expected, e.g. new arrivals into the unit or whelping bitches in a breeding unit. The 2008 Joint Working Group report on veterinary care (Voipio et al. 2008) provides guidance on veterinary care and competencies and responsibilities of veterinary staff.

Veterinary health checks can be conducted alongside regular health checks. Training the dogs to exit and re-enter the home pen independently to move to the procedure area will accustom dogs to the behaviours expected during experimental use and allow staff to pick up subtle changes in behaviour or health. On the examination table, dogs can be trained to raise a forelimb for examination and staff should check for abnormalities in movement and the feet, pads and nails. Nails may be trimmed if they are not naturally worn through exercise. Checks should also be made for dehydration, which is evident through the loss of elasticity in the skin of the scruff, for skin irritation or lesions, body weight and overall body condition score. Respiration rate and heart rate should also be recorded. Abdominal palpation should be conducted to detect abnormal masses or pain.

Common diseases and prophylaxis

Major canine infectious diseases include Distemper, Canine infectious hepatitis, parvovirus, leptospirosis and rabies. Vaccinations are available (see Table 30.5), and WSAVA Vaccination Guidelines Group (Day et al. 2016) provides advice on appropriate vaccination schedules. Rabies vaccination may be an import requirement for some countries. An appropriate prophylactic regime which combines vaccination with treatment of endo- and ectoparasites should be tailored to the specific risks of an institution. The prophylactic requirements of a breeding establishment will differ from that of a stable colony of dogs or an institution with regular introduction of new susceptible animals. Incidence of disease is usually low in a well-managed laboratory environment, but may include diarrhoea, usually multifactorial with involvement of one or more endemic enteric pathogens, skin disease, including otitis externa, associated with parasites or *Malassezia*, oral or cutaneous papillomatosis and minor skin wounds.

Two conditions which are endemic in some laboratory beagle populations are idiopathic epilepsy and polyarteritis, an inflammatory condition otherwise known as beagle pain syndrome. The clinical signs of polyarteritis include sudden onset pyrexia, subdued behaviour, hunched posture and stiff gait and neutrophilia and thrombocytosis. Treatment with steroid resolves the clinical signs but relapse is common.

Comprehensive information on infectious diseases of the dog and treatment can be found in Greene (2012). Tenant (2001) describes helminth diseases.

Behavioural problems

Behavioural indicators of poor welfare are likely to become evident when dogs' social or environmental needs are not met. The behavioural response may be adaptive (e.g. seeking contact with pen mates or staff following periods of restricted social contact) or maladaptive, e.g. stereotypic behaviour which becomes divorced from the original cause (see Chapter 6: Brief introduction to welfare assessment: a 'toolbox' of techniques).

Vigilant behaviour (a perpetually alert state in the absence of stimulus) is one of the most common behaviours that may be associated with a reduced welfare status (Hall 2014). Vigilance is particularly evident in single-housed dogs or before procedures. Other behaviours indicating increased arousal include pacing, jumping and standing with the forepaws against the walls of the enclosure. Dogs persistently showing these behaviours should be of concern and a scoring system can be used to identify dogs at risk (e.g. Hall et al. 2015).

Indicators of acute stress include the sudden raising of a forepaw, lip smacking or licking, and panting in the absence of excessive heat or exercise (e.g. Beerda et al. 1997). These behaviours will commonly be seen during times of disturbance in the animal room if dogs are stressed by such events, or in relation to events which involve staff such as handling or procedures.

An adequate training programme has been shown to reduce the incidence of such behaviours. Postural indicators of welfare may also be observed, with dogs which deviate from a calm, relaxed posture for prolonged periods being of concern. High posture is associated with vigilant behaviour, agonistic interactions with conspecifics and play behaviour. Staff knowledge is needed to correctly interpret behaviour. Low or crouched posture is rarely seen in the home pen but may be more likely to occur during handling or procedures. Such dogs are exhibiting fear or anxiety and should not be used in procedures until training has taken place (Hall 2014).

Preventing problems

There should be an effective policy for anticipating and addressing behavioural problems to prevent problems developing. Appropriate housing design (Scullion Hall et al. 2017), stock training programmes (Hall & Robinson 2016), procedural training (Hall et al. 2015) and predictability in routines (Bassett & Buchanan-Smith 2007) will help to prevent issues related to housing and handling. Staff should be suitably trained to carry out common tasks such as handling and husbandry in effective manners. Additional training should be undertaken to allow staff to implement training programmes.

An effective welfare monitoring protocol (see next section on Monitoring welfare in this chapter) will allow staff to detect changes in welfare rapidly and address the cause.

Monitoring welfare

Hall developed an integrative welfare assessment framework for the laboratory dog, allowing assessment of welfare through the monitoring of behaviour (Hall 2014; Hall et al. 2015). Staff should be skilled in observing behaviour both in the home pen and in relation to procedures.

Welfare should be monitored on an ongoing basis, as some negative welfare indicators (e.g. alert behaviour, interacting with the environment, high posture) may be seen in the normal behavioural repertoire in response to disturbance in the environment. Persistent signs should be investigated.

Table 30.5 Common diseases of the dog.

Disease	Causal agent	Symptoms	Notes
Viral diseases			
Infectious Canine Hepatitis	Canine Adenovirus 1(CAV-1)	Young dogs <1 year, moribund, death. Vomiting, abdominal pain, and diarrhoea +/_ haemorrhage, fever, cough, abdominal tenderness, nose bleeds, abdominal distension, CNS signs, corneal oedema ('Blue Eye'), watery ocular discharge.	Vaccine available
Canine Distemper Virus (CDV)	*Morbillivirus* (Paramyxovirus)	Up to 50% of infections may be subclinical. Mild form: Fever, upper respiratory tract infection, oculo-nasal discharge, cough. Severe generalised form, common in young unvaccinated puppies: conjunctivitis, cough, depression & anorexia, vomiting, diarrhoea, death. Vesicular & pustular dermatitis, nasal and digital hyperkaratosis. Neurological signs 1–3 weeks after recovery vary with area of brain affected. Include seizures, paresis.	Vaccine available.
Canine Infectious Respiratory Disease ('Kennel Cough', Infectious Canine Tracheobronchitis)	Canine parainfluenza virus (CpiV), Canine Adenovirus 2 (CAV-2) Canine Influenza virus (CIV) *Bordetella bronchiseptica*, *Mycoplasma sp* (CDV, Canine Herpes Virus (CHV), Canine reovirus, Canine respiratory coronavirus CRCoV, isolated from respiratory tract of dogs with CIRD but not primary pathogens)	Acute paroxysmal cough, tracheitis. Any one of the pathogens can cause CIRD, co-infection with more than one pathogen likely to occur.	Vaccine available for some agents.
Canine Herpes Virus (CHV)	Canine Herpes Virus CHV	New-born puppies in utero: transplacental infection, from dam or littermates. Infertility and abortion. Death of puppies 1–3 weeks. Depression, anorexia, weight loss, yellow-green faeces, persistent crying, abdominal discomfort.	Vaccine available (Dam).
Canine Corona Virus (CCoV)	Canine coronavirus (CcoV)	Enteric and Pantropic forms. Diarrhoea often in conjunction with Canine Parvo Virus.(CPV)	
Canine Parvo Virus Enteritis	Canine Parvo Virus 1 (CPV-1), Canine Parvo Virus -2 (CPV2)	Common cause of infectious diarrhoea. CPV-2 causes highly infectious and fatal diarrhoea. Enteric: Vomiting, diarrhoea, anorexia, rapid dehydration. Faeces often contain blood. High rectal temperature and leucopoenia. Death. Neurologic: usually secondary because of haemorrhage into CNS Myocarditis: infection in utero or infection of young pups. Dyspnoea and sudden death. Less common. CPV-1 can cause mild illness in pups < 8 weeks old.	Vaccine available
Canine rotavirus (CRV)	Reovirus	Pups <12 weeks with diarrhoea. Can cause diarrhoea in a mixed viral infection.	
Rabies	*Lyssavirus* genus Rhabdovirus family	Prodromal – anxiety, fever. Furious – excitable, photophobic, irritability, vicious, hide. Paralytic.	Vaccine available. Zoonosis
Bacterial diseases			
Leptospirosis	*Leptospira interrogans*	Fever, vomiting, dehydration, polydipsia, haemorrhages – petechial or ecchymotic, coughing, jaundice.	Vaccine available.
Canine Brucellosis	*Burcella canis*	Reproductive problems- abortion 45-60 days gestation. Epididymitis in male dogs.	Zoonosis

(Continued)

Table 30.5 (Continued)

Disease	Causal agent	Symptoms	Notes
Enteric bacterial infections			
Enteropathogenic *E. coli*	*E. Coli*	Chronic, watery diarrhoea	
Helicobacter	*Helicobacter sp.*	May cause disease in immunodeficient animals. Gastritis	Possible zoonosis
Campylobacter	*Campylobacter jejuni*	Dogs often asymptomatic carriers. Diarrhoea. Range of symptoms - loose faeces to watery diarrhoea, to bloody mucoid diarrhoea	Zoonosis
Salmonellosis	*Salmonella sp.*	Gastroenteritis, bacteraemia, endotoxaemia, organ localisation	Zoonosis
Shigellosis	*Shigella sp.*	Dogs relatively resistant to infection. Organism isolated from normal dogs.	Zoonosis
Yersinia enterocolitica	*Yersinia enterocolitica*	Diarrhoea, increased frequency of faeces, tenesmus, mucous and blood	Zoonosis
Tyzzer's disease	*Clostridium piliforme*	Rapid onset lethargy, depression, anorexia and abdominal discomfort followed by hypothermia, moribund and death within 24–48 h.	
Clostridial diarrhoea	*Clostridiumperfringens* and *Clostridium difficile*	Two of the most common bacteria in canine diarrhoea but are also present in the faeces of normal dogs. Symptoms vary from subclinical disease to potentially fatal haemorrhagic diarrhoea.	
Fungal diseases			
Dermatophytosis (Ringworm)	*Microsporum spp. (M. canis, M. gypseum)* *Trichophyton spp.* *Epidermophyton spp.*	Hair loss, scaling and crusting, pruritus.	Zoonosis
Malassezia dermatitis	*Malassezia spp.*	Localised or generalised skin disease. Moist areas interdigital skin, ventral neck, lips, axillae, groin, ear canals.	
Protozoal Diseases			
Leishmaniasis	*Leishmania spp.*	Can be subclinical. Skin lesions, local or generalised lymphadenopathy, loss of bodyweight, decreased appetite, lethargy, splenomegaly, polyuria and polydipsia, ocular lesions, lameness, vomiting and diarrhoea.	Possible zoonosis
Enteric Protozoal diseases			
Giardiasis	*Giardia spp.*	Diarrhoea & weight loss especially in younger or immunosuppressed animals.	Zoonosis.
Trichomoniasis	*Trichomonas spp.*	Present in diarrhoeic faeces, possible opportunistic pathogen.	
Coccidiosis	*Isospora spp. Neospora spp. Sarcocystis spp.*	Diarrhoea in immunocompetent animals in conjunction with other infectious agents.	
Toxoplasmosis	*Toxoplasma gondii*	Neuromuscular, respiratory or GI localised disease. Generalised infection – dogs <1 year. Fever, tonsillitis, dyspnoea, diarrhoea, and vomiting. Jaundice.	
Cryptosporidiosis	*Cryptosporidium spp.*	isolated from dogs with and without signs of GI disease. Diarrhoea and weight loss	Zoonosis
Helminths			
Ascariasis	*Toxocara canis*	Subclinical infection. Young animals can cause diarrhoea, vomiting, abdominal discomfort, poor growth.	Visceral Larva Migrans Zoonosis
Hookworm	*Ancylostoma caninum* *Uncinaria stenocephala,* *Ancylostoma braziliense and spp.*	Anaemia, poor growth, haemorrhagic diarrhoea. Mild diarrhoea.	Zoonosis Zoonosis

Table 30.5 (Continued)

Disease	Causal agent	Symptoms	Notes
Tapeworm	Dipylidium caninum	Anal irritation.	Zoonosis
	Taenia spp.	Rarely cause clinical signs. Heavy burdens may cause intestinal obstruction or mild diarrhoea.	Zoonosis
	T. pisiformis, T. multiceps, T. serialis, T. ovis	May cause hydatid cysts.	
	Echinococcus granulosus		
	E. Multilocularis		
Whipworms	Trichuris vulpis	Large bowel diarrhoea with fresh blood and mucous.	Possible zoonosis
Strongyloides	Strongyloides spp.	May cause haemorrhagic diarrhoea.	Zoonosis
Demodicosis			
	Demodex mites	Localised – lesions on the face, eyes and lips, onset at a few months of age. Generalised version: onset in dogs less than 18 months of age, widespread alopecia, superficial and deep pyoderma. Marked peripheral lymphadenopathy. Adult onset – dogs >4 years Demodectic pododermatitis usually associated with severe secondary pyoderma.	

Signs of poor welfare

The indicators of poor welfare discussed here should be used in conjunction with behavioural indicators of poor health and pain discussed previously. Physical indicators of poor welfare can be observed in the dog. Many of these indicators should be incorporated into regular checks which are conducted of stock, breeding or experimental animals in order to quickly address problems. Chronic and acute stress may manifest in increased plasma cortisol concentrations (Beerda et al. 1999), which in turn may influence immune function (e.g. Beden & Brain 1982). Dogs which experience poor welfare in relation to experimental procedures may demonstrate high heart rates and blood pressure, even at rest in the home pen (Hall 2014). Signs that may be indicative of reduced welfare may include vocalisations, body weight loss, reduced food consumption, vomiting, diarrhoea, subdued behaviour, restlessness, dehydration, abnormal vocalisation, and ataxia or convulsions (Robinson et al. 2009; Chapman et al. 2013).

Acknowledgements

The authors thank C. Jane Pomeroy and Judy McArthur-Clark for their contributions in the previous edition of this chapter, collaborators at AstraZeneca, Charles River Laboratories and GlaxoSmithKline for their contributions to the content of this chapter and anonymous reviewers for their comments which have improved the chapter.

References

Alibhai, H.I. (2016). The anaesthetic machine and vaporizers. In: *BSAVA Manual of Canine and Feline Anaesthesia and Analgesia*, pp. 24–44. BSAVA Library, Gloucester.

Andersen, A.C. (1970). *The Beagle as an Experimental Dog*. Iowa State University Press, Ames, LA.

Aukbullary, A. (2016). Fluid therapy and blood transfusion. In: *BSAVA Manual of Canine and Feline Anaesthesia and Analgesia*, pp. 77–96. BSAVA Library.

Authier, S., Legaspi, M., Gauvin, D. and Troncy, E. (2009). Respiratory safety pharmacology: positive control drug responses in Sprague–Dawley rats, beagle dogs and cynomolgus monkeys. *Regulatory Toxicology and Pharmacology*, 55, 229–235.

Bassett, L. and Buchanan-Smith, H.M. (2007). Effects of predictability on the welfare of captive animals. *Applied Animal Behaviour Science*, **102**, 223–245.

Bauer, J.E., Heinemann, K.M., Lees, G.E. and Waldron, M.K. (2006). Retinal functions of young dogs are improved and maternal plasma phospholipids are altered with diets containing long-chain n-3 polyunsaturated fatty acids during gestation, lactation, and after weaning. *The Journal of Nutrition*, **136**, 1991S–1994S.

Beden, S.N. and Brain, P.F. (1982). Studies on the effect of social stress on measures of disease resistance in laboratory mice. *Aggressive Behavior*, **8**, 126–129.

Beerda, B., Schilder, M., Bernadina, W. et al. (1999). Chronic stress in dogs subjected to social and spatial restriction. II. Hormonal and immunological responses. *Physiology and Behavior*, **66**, 243–254.

Beerda, B., Schilder, M., Van Hooff, J. and De Vries, H. (1997). Manifestations of chronic and acute stress in dogs. *Applied Animal Behaviour Science*, **52**, 307–319.

Berry, S. (2010). Analgesia in the peri-operative period. *Veterinary Clinics of North America: Small Animal Practice*, **45**, 1013–1027.

Boothe, H.W. (2000). Managing traumatic urethral injuries. *Clinical Techniques in Small Animal Practice*, **15**, 35–39.

Bowen, R. (1998). Cytologic changes through the canine estrous cycle. In: *Vaginal Cytology*. Colorado State University. Available at: http://www.vivo.colostate.edu/hbooks/pathphys/reprod/vc/index.html [Accessed 26 Mar 2020].

Box, R. and Spielmann, H. (2005). Use of the dog as non-rodent test species in the safety testing schedule associated with the registration of crop and plant protection products (pesticides): Present status. *Archives of Toxicology*, **79**, 615–626.

Boxall, J., Heath, S., Bate, S. and Brautigam, J. (2004). Modern concepts of socialisation for dogs: implications for their behaviour, welfare and use in scientific procedures. *ATLA*, **32**, 81–93.

Broom, D.M. (2005). The effects of land transport on animal welfare. *Revue scientifique et technique-Office international des ́epizooties*, **24**, 683.

Bubenik, L.J., Hosgood, G.L., Waldron, D.R. and Snow, L.A. (2007). Frequency of urinary tract infection in catheterized dogs and comparison of bacterial culture and susceptibility testing results for catheterized and non- catheterized dogs with urinary tract infections. *Journal of the American Veterinary Medical Association*, **231**, 893–899.

Carbone, L. (2011). Pain in laboratory animals: the ethical and regulatory imperatives. *PLoS One*, **6**, e21578.

Carbone, L. and Austin, J. (2016). Pain and laboratory animals: publication practices for better data reproducibility and better animal welfare. *PloS One*, **11**, e0155001.

Casal, M. (2010). Management and critical care of the neonate. In: *BSAVA Manual of Canine and Feline Reproduction and Neonatology*, pp. 135–146. BSAVA Library, Gloucester.

Case, L.P., Carey, D.P., Hirakawa, D.A. et al. (2000). *Canine and Feline Nutrition: A Resource for Companion Animal Professionals*. Mosby Elsevier, Missouri.

Chandler, M. (2015). Nutrition. In: *BSAVA Manual of Canine Practice*. BSAVA, Gloucester.

Chapman, K., Sewell, F., Allais, L. et al. (2013). A global pharmaceutical company initiative: An evidence-based approach to define the upper limit of body weight loss in short-term toxicity studies. *Regulatory Toxicology and Pharmacology*, **67**, 27–38.

Chui, R.W., Fosdick, A., Conner, R. et al. (2009). Assessment of two external telemetry systems (PhysioJacket and JET) in beagle dogs with telemetry implants. *Journal of Pharmacological and Toxicological Methods*, **60**, 58–68.

Close, M.B., Banister, K., Baumans, V. et al. (1996). Recommendations for euthanasia of experimental animals: Part. *Laboratory Animals*, **30**, 293–316.

Concannon, P., Powers, M., Holder, W. and Hansel, W. (1977). Pregnancy and parturition in the bitch. *Biology of Reproduction*, 16, 517.

Concannon, P., Whaley, S., Lein, D. and Wissler, R. (1983). Canine gestation length: variation related to time of mating and fertile life of sperm. *American Journal of Veterinary Research*, **44**, 1819–1821.

Concannon, P.W. (1991). Reproduction in the dog and cat. In: Reproduction in Domestic Animals, 4th edn., Ed. Cupps, P. Academic Press, New York.

Concannon, P.W. and DiGregorio, G.B.(1986). Canine vaginal cytology. In: *Small Animal Reproduction and Infertility: A Clinical Approach to Diagnosis and Treatment*, Ed. Burke, T.J. Lea and Febiger, Philadelphia.

Davidson, A.P. and Baker, T.W. (2009). Reproductive ultrasound of the bitch and queen. *Topics in Companion Animal Medicine*, **24**, 55–63.

Davis, H., Jensen, T., Johnson, A. et al. (2013). 2013 aaha/aafp fluid therapy guidelines for dogs and cats. *Journal of the American Animal Hospital Association*, **49**, 149–159.

Davis, M. (1996). *Canine and Feline Geriatrics*. Blackwell Science, Osney Mead, Oxford.

Day, M., Horzinek, M.C., Schultz, R.D. and Squires, R.A. (2016). Guidelines for the vaccination of dogs and cats compiled by the vaccination guidelines group VGG of the World Small Animal Veterinary Association (WSAVA). *Journal of Small Animal Practice*, **57**, E1–E45.

Dean, S. (1999). Environmental enrichment of laboratory animals used in regulatory toxicology studies. *Laboratory Animals*, **33**, 309–327.

Debraekeleer, J., Gross, K. and Zicker, S. (2010). Feeding growing puppies: post-weaning to adulthood. *Small Animal Clinical Nutrition*, 5th edn., pp. 311–319. Topeka, KS, Mark Morris Institute.

Descovich, K., Wathan, J., Leach, M.C. et al. (2017). Facial expression: An under-utilised tool for the assessment of welfare in mammals. *ALTEX*, **34**.

Döring, D., Nick, O., Bauer, A. et al. (2017). Behavior of laboratory dogs before and after rehoming in private homes. *ALTEX-Alternatives to Animal Experimentation*, **34**, 133–147.

Duke-Novakovski, T., Vries, M.D., Seymour, C. et al. (2016). *BSAVA Manual of Canine and Feline Anaesthesia and Analgesia*, Ed. 3. British Small Animal Veterinary Association.

Dunn, J. et al. (1990). Bone marrow aspiration and biopsy in dogs and cats. In *Practice*, **12**, 200–206.

England, G.C., Heimendahl, A.V. et al. (2010). *BSAVA Manual of Canine and Feline Reproduction and Neonatology*, Ed. 2, British Small Animal Veterinary Association, Gloucester.

England, G.C. and Allen, W.E. (1998). *Allen's Fertility and Obstetrics in the Dog*. Blackwell Science, Oxford.

European Union. (2010). Directive 2010/63/EU of the European Parliament and of the Council of 22 September 2010 on the protection of animals used for scientific purposes. *Official Journal of the European Union*, L 276/33.

Farstad, W.K. (2010). Artificial insemination in dogs. In: *BSAVA Manual of Canine and Feline Reproduction and Neonatology*, pp. 80–88. BSAVA Library, Gloucester.

Fédèration Cynologique Internationale (2019). Breeds recognised on a definitive basis. URL: http://www.fci.be/en/Nomenclature/Default.aspx.

Feldman, E.C., Nelson, R.W., Reusch, C. and Scott-Moncrieff, J.C. (2014). *Canine and Feline Endocrinology*. Elsevier health sciences, Oxford.

Flecknell, P. (2016). *Laboratory Animal Anaesthesia and Analgesia*. Academic Press, Oxford.

Flecknell, P., Liles, J. and Williamson, H. (1990). The use of lignocaine-prilocaine local anaesthetic cream for pain-free venepuncture in laboratory animals. *Laboratory Animals*, 24, 142–146.

Flecknell, P.A., Waterman-Pearson, A. et al. (2000). *Pain Management in Animals*. WB Saunders, Oxford.

Fogel, B. (1990). *The Dog's Mind: Understanding Your Dog's Behavior*. Macmillan, New York.

Fontbonne, A. (2007). *Approach to Infertility in the Bitch and in the Dog*. World Small Animal Veterinary Association World Congress Proceedings.

Forsberg, C.L. (2010). Pregnancy diagnosis, normal pregnancy and parturition in the bitch. In: *BSAVA Manual of Canine and Feline Reproduction and Neonatology*, pp. 89–97. BSAVA Library, Gloucester.

Fox, M. (1971). *Behaviour of Wolves, Dogs and Related Canids*. Dogwise Publishing: Wenatchee, WA.

Fox, M. and Stelzner, D. (1966). Behavioural effects of differential early experience in the dog. *Animal Behaviour*, **14**, 273–281.

Freedman, A.H., Gronau, I., Schweizer, R.M. et al. (2014). Genome sequencing highlights the dynamic early history of dogs. *PloS Genetics*, **10**, e1004016.

Gad, S.C. (2016). *Animal Models in Toxicology*. CRC Press, Boca Raton.

Gazzano, A., Mariti, C., Notari, L. et al. (2008). Effects of early gentling and early environment on emotional development of puppies. *Applied Animal Behaviour Science*, **110**, 294–304.

Greene, C.E. (2012) *Infectious Diseases of the Dog and Cat. Fourth Edition*. Elsevier Saunders, Missouri.

Greer, M.L. (2014). *Canine Reproduction and Neonatology*. Teton NewMedia, Jackson, WY.

Guinness World Records (2018). *Guinness World Records 2019*. Guinness World Records Limited, New York.

Hall, L. and Robinson, S. (2016). Implementing a successful positive reinforcement training protocol in laboratory-housed dogs. *Animal Technology and Welfare*, 15.

Hall, L.E. (2014). A practical framework for harmonising welfare and quality of data output in the laboratory-housed dog. Unpublished PhD Thesis, University of Stirling.

Hall, L.E., Robinson, S. and Buchanan-Smith, H.M. (2015). Refining dosing by oral gavage in the dog: A protocol to harmonise welfare. *Journal of Pharmacological and Toxicological Methods*, **72**, 35–46.

Hammond, R. and Murison, P.J. (2016). Automatic ventilators. In: *BSAVA Manual of Canine and Feline Anaesthesia and Analgesia*, pp. 65–76. BSAVA Library, Gloucester.

Hanton, G. and Rabemampianina, Y. (2006). The electrocardiogram of the beagle dog: reference values and effect of sex, genetic strain, body position and heart rate. *Laboratory Animals*, **40**, 123–136.

Hawkins, P. (2002). Recognizing and assessing pain, suffering and distress in laboratory animals: a survey of current practice in the UK with recommendations. *Laboratory Animals*, **36**, 378–395.

Hetts, S., Derrell Clark, J., Calpin, J.P. et al. (1992). Influence of housing conditions on beagle behaviour. *Applied Animal Behaviour Science*, **34**, 137–155.

Holton, L., Pawson, P., Nolan, A. et al. (2001). Development of a behaviour-based scale to measure acute pain in dogs. *Veterinary Record*, 148, 525–531.

Home Office (2015). *Advice Note: 03/2015 Animals (Scientific Procedures) Act 1986 Re-homing and setting free of animals. Animals in Science Regulation Unit*. Her Majesty's Stationary Office, London.

Hubrecht, R. (1993). A comparison of social and environmental enrichment methods for laboratory-housed dogs. *Applied Animal Behaviour Science*, **37**, 345–361.

Hubrecht, R. (1995a). Enrichment in puppyhood and its effects on later behaviour of dogs. *Laboratory Animal Science*, **45**, 70–75.

Hubrecht, R. (1995b). *The Welfare of Dogs in Human Care*. Cambridge University Press: Cambridge.

Hubrecht, R., Serpell, J. and Poole, T. (1992). Correlates of pen size and housing conditions on the behaviour of kennelled dogs. *Applied Animal Behaviour Science*, **34**, 365–383.

International Air Transport Association (2018). *Live Animal Regulations*, 44th edn. Available at: https://www.iata.org/en/programs/cargo/live-animals/ [Accessed 26 Mar 2020].

International Conference on Harmonization (2000). Guidance for Industry. S7A Safety Pharmacology Studies for Human Pharmaceuticals. URL: www.ich.org.

International Conference on Harmonization (2005). Guidance for Industry. S7B The Nonclinical Evaluation of the Potential for Delayed Ventricular Repolarisation (QT Interval Prolongation) by Human Pharmaceuticals. URL: www.ich.org.

Jennings, M., Howard, B., Farningham, D. et al. (2004). LASA Guidance on the Rehoming of Laboratory Dogs. A report based on a LASA working party and LASA meeting on rehoming laboratory animals. Available at: http://www.lasa.co.uk/wp-content/uploads/2018/05/LASA-Guidance-on-the-Rehoming-of-Laboratory-Dogs.pdf [Accessed 26 Mar 2020].

Johnson, C. (1986). Reproduction and periparturient care. *Veterinary Clinics of North America*, **16(3)**, 417–605.

Johnston, S. and Romagnoli, S. (1991). Canine reproduction. *Veterinary Clinics of North America*, **21(3)**, 421–640.

Johnston, S.D., Root Kustritz, M.V. and Olson, P.S. (2001). *Canine and Feline Theriogenology*. Saunders, Philadelphia.

Jones, A. (2007). Sensory development in puppies (Canis lupus f. familiaris): implications for improving canine welfare. *Animal Welfare*, 319–329.

Jones, D.E., Joshua, J.O. et al. (1982). Reproductive Clinical Problems in the Dog. John Wright & Sons, London.

Kaster, S. (2016). Injectable anaesthesia. In: BSAVA Manual of Canine and Feline Anaesthesia and Analgesia, pp. 77–96. BSAVA Library.

Kendrick, J., Stow, R., Ibbotson, N., et al. (2020). A novel welfare and scientific approach to conducting dog metabolism studies allowing dogs to be pair housed. *Laboratory animals*, **54(6)**, 588–598.

Klumpp, A., Trautmann, T., Markert, M. and Guth, B. (2006). Optimizing the experimental environment for dog telemetry studies. *Journal of Pharmacological and Toxicological Methods*, **54**, 141–149.

Kraeuter, K. (2001). *Training your beagle. Barron's Educational Series*. Simon & Schuster, New York.

Laflamme, D. (1997). Development and validation of a body condition score system for dogs: a clinical tool. *Canine Practice*, **22**, 10–15.

Lamm, C.G. and Makloski, C.L. (2012). Current advances in gestation and parturition in cats and dogs. *Veterinary Clinics: Small Animal Practice*, **42**, 445–456.

Lawler, D. (2008). Neonatal and pediatric care of the puppy and kitten. *Theriogenology*, 70, 384–392.

Leary, S.L., Underwood, W., Anthony, R. et al. (2013). *Avma Guidelines for the Euthanasia of Animals: 2013 edition*. American Veterinary Medical Association, Schaumburg, IL.

Maenhoudt, C., Santos, N. and Fontbonne, A. (2014). Suppression of fertility in adult dogs. *Reproduction in Domestic Animals*, **49**, 58–63.

McMahon, N., Schofield, J., Prior, H., Simpson, D., and Hammond, T. (2006). Optimisation of a non-invasive telemetry system for electrocardiogram assessments in dogs: a 3-years review. *The Society of Toxicology Annual Meeting*, 6–9th March 2006. San Diego, USA.

Meek, P.D. (1999). The movement, roaming behaviour and home range of free-roaming domestic dogs, Canis lupus familiaris, in coastal New South Wales. *Wildlife Research*, **26**, 847–855.

Miller, P.E. and Murphy C.J. (1995). Vision in dogs. *Journal of American Veterinary Medical Association*, **207(12)**, 1623–1634.

Merskey, H. (1979). Pain terms: a list with definitions and notes on usage. Recommended by the IASP subcommittee on taxonomy. *Pain*, **6**, 249–252.

Mertens, P.A. and Unshelm, J. (1996). Effects of group and individual housing on the behavior of kennelled dogs in animal shelters. *Anthrozoos*, **9**, 40–51.

Meunier, L.D. (2006). Selection, acclimation, training, and preparation of dogs for the research setting. *ILAR Journal*, **47**, 326–347.

Miklósi, A´. (2014). *Dog Behaviour, Evolution, and Cognition*. OUP: Oxford.

Mitterman, L., Bonczynski, J., Hearon, K. and Selmic, L.E. (2016). Comparison of perioperative and short-term post-operative complications of gastrointestinal biopsies via laparoscopic-assisted technique versus laparotomy. *The Canadian Veterinary Journal*, **57**, 395.

Morton, D. and Griffiths, P. (1985). Guidelines on the recognition of pain, distress and discomfort in experimental animals and an hypothesis for assessment. *Veterinary Record*, **116**, 431–436.

Morton, D., Abbot, R., Barclay, B. et al. (1993). Removal of blood from laboratory mammals and birds. First report of the BVA/FRAME/RSPCA/UFAW Joint Working Group on Refinement. *Laboratory Animals*, **27**, 1–22.

Morton, D., Hawkins, P., Bevan, R. et al. (2003). Refinements in telemetry procedures. Seventh report of the BVAAWF/FRAME/RSPCA/UFAW joint working group on refinement, part A. *Laboratory Animals*, **37**, 261–299.

Morton, D., Jennings, M., Buckwell, A. et al. (2001). Refining procedures for the administration of substances: Report of the BVAAWF/FRAME/RSPCA/UFAW Joint Working Group on refinement. *Laboratory Animals*, **35**, 1–41.

Moscardo, E., Fasdelli, N., Giarola, A. et al. (2009). An optimised neurobehavioural observation battery integrated with the assessment of cardiovascular function in the beagle dog. *Journal of Pharmacological and Toxicological Methods*, **60**, 198–209.

Mosier, J.E. (1989). Effect of aging on body systems of the dog. *Veterinary Clinics of North America: Small Animal Practice*, **19**, 1–12.

Mugford, R. and Thorne, C. (1978). Comparative studies of meal patterns in pet and laboratory-housed dogs and cats. In: Nutrition of the Dog and Cat: Proceedings of the International Symposium on the Nutrition of the Dog and Cat, Arranged by the Institute of Animal Nutrition in Conjunction with the 200-Year Anniversary of the Veterinary School, Hannover, 26 June 1978, Ed. Anderson, R.S. Pergamon Press, New York.

Murrell, J.C. (2016). Pre-anaesthetic medication and sedation. In: BSAVA Manual of Canine and Feline Anaesthesia and Analgesia, pp. 170–189. BSAVA Library, Gloucester.

National Research Council (1994). *Laboratory Animal Management: Dogs*. National Academies Press, Washington DC.

National Research Council (2006). *Nutrient Requirements of Dogs and Cats*. National Academies Press, Washington DC.

National Research Council (2009). *National Research Council (US) Committee on Scientific and Humane Issues in the Use of Random Source Dogs and Cats in Research*. National Academies Press, Washington, DC.

National Research Council (2010). *Guide for the Care and Use of Laboratory Animals*. National Academies Press, Washington DC.

Neitz, J., Geist, T. and Jacobs, G. (1989). Color vision in dog. *Visual Neuroscience*, **3**, 119–125. 10.1017/S0952523800004430.

Okkens, A., Bevers, M., Dieleman, S. et al. (1992). Fertility problems in the bitch. *Animal Reproduction Science*, **28**, 379–387.

Olson, H., Betton, G., Robinson, D. et al. (2000). Concordance of the toxicity of pharmaceuticals in humans and in animals. *Regulatory Toxicology and Pharmacology*, **32**, 56–67.

Ong, T.H., Mendum, T., Geurtsen, G. et al. (2017). Use of mass spectrometric vapor analysis to improve canine explosive detection efficiency. *Analytical Chemistry*, **89**, 6482–6490.

Pang, D.S. (2016). Inhalant anaesthetic agents. In: *BSAVA Manual of Canine and Feline Anaesthesia and Analgesia*, pp. 207–213. BSAVA Library.

Persson, M.E., Wright, D., Roth, L.S. et al. (2016). Genomic regions associated with interspecies communication in dogs contain genes related to human social disorders. *Scientific Reports*, **6**, 33439.

Piccione, G., Caola, G. and Refinetti, R. (2005). Daily rhythms of blood pressure, heart rate, and body temperature in fed and fasted male dogs. *Journal of Veterinary Medicine Series A*, **52**, 377–381.

Pottie, R., Dart, C., Perkins, N. and Hodgson, D. (2007). Effect of hypothermia on recovery from general anaesthesia in the dog. *Australian Veterinary Journal*, 85, 158–162.

Prescott, M., Morton, D.B., Anderson, D. et al. (2004). Refining dog husbandry and care: Eighth report of the BVAAWF/FRAME/RSPCA/ UFAW Joint Working Group on Refinement. *Laboratory Animals*, **38**, S1:1–S1:94.

Prior, H., Bottomley, A., Champ'eroux, P. et al. (2016). Social housing of non-rodents during cardiovascular recordings in safety pharmacology and toxicology studies. *Journal of Pharmacological and Toxicological Methods*, **81**, 75–87.

Redondo, J., Suesta, P., Serra, I. et al. (2012). Retrospective study of the prevalence of post-anaesthetic hypothermia in dogs. *Veterinary Record*, 171, 374–374.

Regan, M.J. and Eger, E.I. (1967). Effect of hypothermia in dogs on anesthetizing and apneic doses of inhalation agents: Determination of the anesthetic index (apnea/mac). *Anesthesiology*, **28**, 689–700.

Rehbinder, C., Baneux, P., Forbes, D. et al. (1998). FELASA recommendations for the health monitoring of breeding colonies and experimental units of cats, dogs and pigs: report of the federation of European laboratory animal science associations (FELASA) working group on animal health. *Laboratory Animals*, **32**, 1–17.

Reid, J., Scott, M., Nolan, A. and Wiseman-Orr, L. (2013). Pain assessment in animals. In *Practice*, **35**, 51–56.

National Centre for the Replacement, and of Animals in Research. Bloodsampling.URL:https://www.nc3rs.org.uk/blood-sampling-dog.

Tenant, B. (2001) The alimentary tract. *In BSAVA Manual of Infectious Diseases, pp.* 144–148. BSAVA Library, Gloucester.

Robinson, S., Chapman, K., Hudson, S. et al. (2009). Guidance on dose level selection for regulatory general toxicology studies for pharmaceuticals. NC3Rs/LASA, London.

Romsos, D.R., Palmer, H.J., Muiruri, K.L. and Bennink, M.R. (1981). Influence of a low carbohydrate diet on performance of pregnant and lactating dogs. The Journal of Nutrition, 111, 678–689.

Roughan, J.V. and Flecknell, P.A. (2003). Pain assessment and control in laboratory animals. *Laboratory Animals*, **37**, 172–172.

Sales, G., Hubrecht, R., Peyvandi, A. et al. (1997). Noise in dog kennelling: is barking a welfare problem for dogs? *Applied Animal Behaviour Science*, **52**, 321–329.

Schauvliege, S. (2016). Patient monitoring and monitoring equipment. In: *BSAVA Manual of Canine and Feline Anaesthesia and Analgesia*, pp. 77–96. BSAVA Library, Gloucester.

Schipper, L.L., Vinke, C.M., Schilder, M.B. and Spruijt, B.M. (2008). The effect of feeding enrichment toys on the behaviour of kennelled dogs (Canis familiaris). *Applied Animal Behaviour Science*, **114**, 182–195.

Scullion Hall, L.E., Robinson, S., Finch, J. and Buchanan-Smith, H.M. (2017). The influence of facility and home pen design on the welfare of the laboratory-housed dog. *Journal of Pharmacological and Toxicological Methods*, **83**, 21–29.

Self, I. (2019). *BSAVA Guide to Pain Management in Small Animal Practice*. British Small Animal Veterinary Association, Gloucester.

Semyonova, A. (2003). The social organization of the domestic dog; a longitudinal study of domestic canine behavior and the ontogeny of domestic canine social systems. The Carriage Horse Foundation, The Hague.

Serpell, J. (1995). *The Domestic Dog: Its Evolution, Behaviour and Interactions with People*. Cambridge University Press: Cambridge.

Serpell, J. (2016). *The Domestic Dog*. Cambridge University Press, Cambridge.

Sherwin, C. (2007). Animal welfare: reporting details is good science. *Nature*, **448**, 251.

Smith, D., Broadhead, C., Descotes, G. et al. (2002). Preclinical safety evaluation using non-rodent species: an industry/welfare project to minimize dog use. *ILAR Journal*, **43**, S39–S42.

Smith, F.O. (2012). Guide to emergency interception during parturition in the dog and cat. *Veterinary Clinics: Small Animal Practice*, **42**, 489–499.

Spotte, S. (2012). *Societies of Wolves and Free-Ranging Dogs*. Cambridge University Press, Cambridge.

Starkey, M.P., Scase, T.J., Mellersh, C.S. and Murphy, S. (2005). Dogs really are man's best friend – canine genomics has applications in veterinary and human medicine! *Briefings in Functional Genomics & Proteomics*, **4**, 112–128.

Stokes, W.S. and Marsman, D.S. (2014). Animal welfare considerations in biomedical research and testing. In: *Laboratory Animal Welfare*, pp. 115–140. Elsevier, London.

Swallow, J., Anderson, D., Buckwell, A.C. et al. (2005). Guidance on the transport of laboratory animals. *Laboratory Animals*, 39, 1–39.

Thalmann, O., Shapiro, B., Cui, P. et al. (2013). Complete mitochondrial genomes of ancient canids suggest a European origin of domestic dogs. *Science*, **342**, 871–874.

Van Os, J., Van Laar, P., Oldenkamp, E. and Verschoor, J. (1981). Oestrus control and the incidence of mammary nodules in bitches, a clinical study with two progestogens. *Veterinary Quarterly*, 3, 46–56.

Vignoli, M., Barberet, V., Chiers, K. et al. (2011). Evaluation of a manual biopsy device, the 'spirotome', on fresh canine organs: liver, spleen, and kidneys, and first clinical experiences in animals. *European Journal of Cancer Prevention*, 20, 140–145.

Voipio, H.M., Baneux, P., de Segura, I.A.G. et al. (2008). Guidelines for the veterinary care of laboratory animals: report of the FELASA/ECLAM/ESLAV Joint Working Group on Veterinary Care. *Laboratory Animals*, **42(1)**, 1–11.

Wallace, J., Sanford, J., Smith, M. and Spencer, K. (1990). The assessment and control of the severity of scientific procedures on laboratory animals: Report of the Laboratory Animal Science Association working party (Assessment and control of severity). *Laboratory Animals*, **24**, 97–130.

Thulin, J.D., Bergdall, V.K. and Bradfield, J.F. (2018). Facilitating the research process: Limiting regulatory burden and leveraging performance standards–management of animal care and use programs in research, education, and testing. In: *Management of Animal Care and Use Programs in Research, Education, and Testing, 2nd edn*. Eds. Weichbrod, R., Thompson, G., Norton, J. CRC Press, Boca Raton.

Wells, D. (2004a). The influence of toys on the behaviour and welfare of kennelled dogs. *Animal Welfare*, **13**, 367–373.

Wells, D. (2004b). A review of environmental enrichment for kennelled dogs, Canis familiaris. *Applied Animal Behaviour Science*, **85**, 307–317.

Willems, A., Paepe, D., Marynissen, S. *et al*. (2017). Results of screening of apparently healthy senior and geriatric dogs. *Journal of Veterinary Internal Medicine*, **31**, 81–92.

Wolfe, T. (1990). Policy, program and people: the three P's to well-being. In: *Canine Research Environment*. Eds Mensch, J.A. and Krulisch, L. Scientists Center for Animal Welfare: Bethesda.

Wolfensohn, S. and Lloyd, M. (2008). *Handbook of Laboratory Animal Management and Welfare*. John Wiley & Sons, Oxford.

Xing, G., Lu, J., Hu, M. *et al*. (2015). Effects of group housing on ECG assessment in conscious cynomolgus monkeys. *Journal of Pharmacological and Toxicological Methods*, **75**, 44–51.

Young, M.C. (1994). *The Guinness Book of Records 1995*. Facts on File, New York.

Zurlo, J., Bayne, K., Cimino Brown, D. *et al*. (2011). Critical evaluation of the use of dogs in biomedical research and testing. *ALTEX*, **4**, 355.

31 The domestic cat

Emma Desforges

Biological overview

General biology

Most cats used within the laboratory setting are domestic short-haired cats *Felis silvestris catus*, the same species that is commonly kept as a companion animal and which exists in substantial numbers in a feral state. Cats are intelligent, highly specialised mammals that have evolved a range of morphological adaptations and sensory abilities to suit their exclusively carnivorous lifestyle and dietary needs (reviewed by Bradshaw 1992). A cat's perception of the world is therefore different from ours. Hunting by sight at night means they see in lower light intensities than we can and are particularly sensitive to rapid movement. They are not, however, able to see in fine detail or to discriminate clearly between shades of colour (Bradshaw 1992). They also hunt by sound and are very sensitive to the ultrasonic frequencies that rodents use to communicate. Their sensitive sense of smell helps them to locate prey although, in the final stages of a kill, touch is the dominant sense. Smell is also used to select food while an accessory olfactory system (the vomeronasal organ) is used in social communication. Sebaceous glands are located throughout the body, especially on the head and the peri-anal area, and between the digits. Scratching, which deposits scent from the interdigital glands, is a marking behaviour which leaves visual and olfactory signals, and helps to maintain the claws in good shape (Rochlitz 2005). The deposition of urine and faeces, and rubbing of the body against objects, may also be used in olfactory signalling. Allo-rubbing, where cats rub their face and body against each other and intertwine their tails, serves to exchange scent profiles between cats. Standard biological data are listed in Table 31.1. The International Cat Care[1] website is a reliable source of information on domestic cats.

Breeds, strains and genetics

The genetics of domestic cats and their wild progenitors, *Felis silvestris* (European wildcat), *F. s. lybica* (Near Eastern/north African wildcat), *F. s. ornata* (central Asian wildcat), *F. s. cafra* (southern African wildcat) and *F. s. bieti* (Chinese desert cat), indicate that each wild group represents a distinctive subspecies of *Felis silvestris* (Driscoll *et al.* 2007). Of these, two *lybica* lineages in the Near Eastern and Egyptian domestication centres have contributed to the maternal genetic ancestry of the domesticated cat (Ottoni *et al.* 2017). Cat taming began in the Fertile Crescent of the Near East and North Africa, coinciding with the development of agricultural villages where cats fed on the rodents that infested the grain stores of the first farmers. The first evidence of cat remains buried together with human remains was found in Cyprus, and determined to be 9,500 years old (Vigne *et al.* 2004). The second domestication event occurred in ancient Egypt around the fourth millennium BCE (Van Neer *et al.* 2014). Cats dispersed to almost every habitable area along the trade routes in the Old World, developing regional variations (Lipinski *et al.* 2008).

Cats were not subject to strong selective pressure during domestication, probably due to their natural ability to control rodent pests, limiting differences to feral *Felis silvestris* subspecies with which they can interbreed (Bradshaw & Hall 1999). Recent selective pressure in cat breeding has mainly focused on aesthetic qualities.

Pedigreed cats present a small subset of domestic cats that have been intensively selected and inbred to fix distinct traits found at low-to-moderate levels in the random-bred cat population. The concept of cat breeds dates from the nineteenth century. Today, more than 70 cat breeds with different head shapes, body conformations or coat types are recognised by different cat registries (Cat Fanciers' Association[2], Fédération Internationale Féline[3], The International Cat Association[4]), with most breeds being developed in the past 50–75 years.

Inherited diseases can affect all domestic cats. Comprehensive genetic screening is available for measuring genetic diversity,

---

[1] www.icatcare.org (accessed 31 October 2019)

[2] The Cat Fanciers Association http://www.cfa.org/ (accessed 31 October 2019)

[3] Fédération Internationale Féline A leading international cat fancier site http://fifeweb.org/index.php (accessed 31 October 2019)

[4] The International Cat Association (TICA), the world's largest genetic registry of pedigreed and domestic cats. https://www.tica.org/ (accessed 31 October 2019)

The UFAW Handbook on the Care and Management of Laboratory and Other Research Animals, Ninth Edition.
Edited by Huw Golledge and Claire Richardson.
© 2024 John Wiley & Sons Ltd. Published 2024 by John Wiley & Sons Ltd.

Table 31.1 Standard biological data.

Parameter	Value
Average life expectancy (years)	12–14 (+20 yrs has been recorded)
Body weight:	
Adult (kg)	4.5
Birth (g)	90–100
Body condition score (9-point scale)	5 (ideal)
Body temperature (°C)	38.1–39.2
Resting heart rate (bpm)	120–140
Resting respiratory rate (breaths/min)	16–40
Urine volume (ml/kg/bwt/day)	10–20
Urine specific gravity	1.020–1.040
Dental formulae:	
Deciduous (upper/lower)	2(I3/3 C1/1 Pm3/2) = 26
Permanent (upper/lower)	2(I3/3 C1/1 Pm3/2 M1/1) = 30
Age at eruption of permanent dentition (months)	3–6
Oestrus cycle (days)	3–20
Gestation (days)	60–66
Litter size (average)	4
Lactation (weeks)	7
Age at weaning (weeks)	4–7

[1]Banfield Pet Hospital State of Pet health 2013 Report. https://www.banfield.com/Banfield/media/PDF/Downloads/soph/Banfield-State-of-Pet-Health-Report_2013.pdf (accessed 31 October 2019)
[2]WSAVA Global Nutrition Committee 2013 Feline Body Condition Score. https://www.wsava.org/sites/default/files/Body%20condition%20score%20chart%20cats.pdf (accessed 31 October 2019)
[3]Merck Sharp & Dohme Corporation 2019 MSD Veterinary Manual Professional Edition. www.msdvetmanual.com/ (accessed 31 October 2019)
Source: Derived from Banfield Pet Health[1], WSAVA[2] 2013; O'Neill et al. 2015; MSD[3].

genetic blood type, known risk variants associated with genetic disease and trait variants such as coat colour, coat type and morphology in domestic cats, e.g. Wisdom™ Health, Vancouver, WA, USA. Coat colour mutations typically affect pigmentation only; however, a partial FeLV (feline leukaemia virus), insertion in the KIT gene, resulting in a dominant white phenotype with uniform white coat and blue iris colour, is associated with hearing impairment that is more common in cats with two copies of the mutation (David et al. 2014). A catalogue of inherited diseases and traits is available via Online Mendelian Inheritance in Animals, OMIA[5] and descriptions of the health and welfare impact of various genetic conditions is available at the UFAW website.[6]

More recently, development of interspecies hybrid cats, by crossing the domestic cat to various different wild cat species, has gained popularity. Of these, one of the first and today the most common breed with wild ancestry is the Bengal cat, an interspecies hybrid between several domestic cat breeds and the Asian leopard cat (*Prionailurus bengalensis*) (Johnson 1991). Hybrid cats are generally considered domestic cats after they are four generations removed from their wild cat ancestor.

Social organisation

Cats can adapt to a wide range of population densities. Feral cat populations and home range varies greatly depending on resource, habitat and prey availability (Bengsen et al. 2016). The size of each male home range is determined by both food supply and social considerations including availability of breeding females, whether females are solitary or social and the degree of competition for females. Male home ranges encompass the territories of several breeding females. The home ranges of females are determined by the needs for shelter and food, both for themselves and for any dependent young. Where cats have to support themselves solely by hunting, they are often solitary as their prey is unlikely to be sufficiently abundant to sustain a social group. If food is more common but patchily distributed, then the home ranges of cats may overlap though they would rarely hunt in the same area at the same time.

Social groups exist where food is locally concentrated, usually as a result of human activities (Bonanni et al. 2007). These groups are basically matrilineal, consisting of females, usually related, and their offspring (including immature males). The size of the groups is very variable and seems to be determined largely by food availability, mortality among kittens from a range of infectious diseases and extermination by humans. Females are tolerant of other members in the group but defend their communal core area (containing their den and major source of food) aggressively against intruders. Their aggression intensifies if there are young kittens in the group. This exclusion of outsiders makes it difficult for females to move between groups. Males tend to disperse away from their mother's home range when they are 2 or 3 years old. Initially, they avoid contact with all other cats but as they mature and become stronger they will challenge other males for access to females. Mature males are only loosely associated with any group but in areas where most females are group-living, a particular male may concentrate his mating efforts within a single group. Further information on cat behaviour and social organisation can be found in Beaver (2003); American Association of Feline Practitioners[7] and Turner and Bateson (2013).

Reproduction

General advice can be found in Beaver (2003) and Noakes et al. (2018).

Female cats (queens) are induced ovulators with ovulation occurring around 24 hrs after copulation. Under optimum conditions, females become sexually mature at around 9 months (range 4–18 months) and males (toms) are sexually mature by 8 months, though some may be fertile earlier.

[5]Online Mendelian Inheritance in Animals, University of Sydney, 2018 www.omia.org (accessed 31 October 2019)
[6]Genetic Welfare Problems of Companion Animals: An information resource for prospective pet owners https://www.ufaw.org.uk/cats/cats (accessed 31 October 2019)

[7]American Association of Feline Practitioners 2004 AAFP Feline Behavior Guidelines https://catvets.com/guidelines/practice-guidelines/behavior-guidelines (accessed 31 October 2019)

Females are seasonally polyoestrous with oestrous cycles lasting between 18 and 24 days with oestrus lasting about 4 days if mating occurs but otherwise between 5 and 10 days.

Cats are normally seasonal breeders in temperate climates, but females can breed all year round if they are kept indoors with no exposure to sunlight and with a 12/12-hour light/dark regime. Toms are most sexually active in spring though they can sire kittens at any time of the year.

Successful pregnancies last about 63 days (range 58–72 days) and sterile copulation may result in pseudopregnancy which lasts about 36 days. Females are capable of coming into oestrus 3–4 weeks after a litter is weaned. The average litter size is 4 (typical range, 3–10) with maximum litter size usually reached by the third litter. Females are optimally fertile between the ages of 1 and 8; subsequently, their oestrous cycles may become irregular, and litters are fewer and smaller. Although sperm quality declines with age, males can remain fertile into their twenties.

Sources of supply

Each region will have specific regulatory requirements for the supply and breeding of animals for laboratory use. Unless it is an experimental requirement to do otherwise, cats should be sourced from approved breeding establishments as behavioural, health and genetic status of individuals should be known. Early communication with suppliers will ensure the cats are appropriate for the research requirements, and cats should be behaviourally prepared for the future facility (e.g. by habituation to handling and husbandry procedures). Cats raised under good welfare conditions may still have behavioural and handling problems. Behavioural and clinical issues, especially genetic, should be reported back to the supplier to enable continuous improvement in breeding stock.

Some facilities may be able to become a breeding establishment to replenish internal stock (as long as there are adequate facilities, trained staff and necessary permissions in place).

Many laboratories use specific pathogen free (SPF) cats which will be sourced from recognised SPF suppliers. These cats should be free from viral and chlamydial upper respiratory disease, FeLV, FIV (feline immunodeficiency virus), coronavirus and both ectoparasites and endoparasites. A full and recent health monitoring report should be requested and assessed to understand the historical infectious condition of the sourcing colony. Cats should be quarantined for at least 3 weeks before joining a new colony and for 6 weeks if from a random source or where disease status is unknown.

Travel causes stressors that can compromise the cat's welfare and physiological parameters. Such stressors include carrier confinement, loud and unpredictable noise, unfamiliar smells, interactions with strangers and other animals, handling and change of environment. Direct transportation routes should be prioritised over indirect routes to minimise travel delays which may add journey time and compromise welfare. Cats should ideally be accompanied to ensure their safety and welfare; if cats are to travel unaccompanied, across borders, or by air, sea or rail, special regulations will apply, and each country and carrier will have its own regulations regarding animal transport (see also Chapter 12: Transportation of laboratory animals).

Cats carried in SPF conditions will need to be protected from infection during transit including compliance to specific containers and ventilation. Cats travelling by air will require containers approved by the International Air Transport Association (IATA) who revise their regulations annually. Temperatures during travel and at the final destination should be considered to ensure transport carriers can accommodate temperature extremes, avoid fluctuation in temperatures and to avoid heat stress. Travel during cooler temperatures and avoiding the hottest part of the day is ideal, especially when travelling from a cooler to a warmer climate. Risk of heat stress in increased in ill, obese, brachycephalic, kitten or geriatric cats. Air journeys of over 10 h duration appear to be especially stressful (Bradshaw & Holloran 2005). Conditioning the cat to the carrier and appropriate carrier type has been shown to reduce cat stress during transportation (Pratsch et al. 2018). A behavioural protocol for conditioning laboratory cats to handling and transport has been described (Gruen et al. 2013).

Use in research

The laboratory cat has historically been considered a valuable model for research in human disease including immunodeficiency, neurological, sensory and toxicological studies. Research pertaining to the cat, such as veterinary, nutritional, behavioural and human–animal interaction studies, occurs within and outside of traditional laboratory settings. In the UK, cats (dogs, horses and primates) are considered a specially protected species requiring licence holders to demonstrate that no other species are suitable for the intended research. While all laboratory animals deserve continuous improvement and refinement to maximise their welfare, the scientific use of cats and other animals which are considered sentient or typically kept as pets can be especially emotive. As such, public expectations are that the welfare of the laboratory cat should be optimal and associated outputs of research benefit society.

General Husbandry

Husbandry systems should use best health care practices, which emphasise good welfare to meet the animals' social, physiological and ethological needs. Use of husbandry standard operating procedures (SOPs) will help ensure consistency in care provision.

Government regulations and scientific guidance documents detailing minimum standards for the care and accommodation of animals exist, e.g. European Commission (2007); National Research Council (NRC) (2011) and United States Department of Agriculture (2013) and, in the UK, Home Office 2014[8].

---

[8]Home Office (2014) Code of Practice for the Housing and Care of Animals Bred, Supplied or Used for Scientific Purposes https://www.gov.uk/government/publications/code-of-practice-for-the-housing-and-care-of-animals-in-designated-breeding-and-supplying-establishments (accessed 31 October 2019)

Housing

The quality of the living environment can have a major impact on the cat's welfare. Housing systems should provide safe, comfortable, cat-friendly conditions which allow opportunities for environmental choice, sensory stimulation, physical and mental exercise.

Cats can be housed outdoors or indoors. Considerations of environmental control, costs and disease transmission mean most colonies are kept in closed indoor accommodation. To minimise the risk of environmental injury, the setting must be safe, secure and free from hazards and harmful substances. All areas must be structurally sound, constructed from robust materials and in good decorative condition and repair. Surfaces should be smooth with no sharp edges, durable and impervious to aid cleaning.

Outdoor exposure can provide an environmental enrichment opportunity (Figure 31.1). If provided, this should be a contained facility which ensures protection from predation, feral cats, extreme weather and ingestion of foreign material, e.g. bird droppings. Access to indoor housing which meets minimum standards must be provided.

Individual housing

Single housing of cats may be permitted in certain circumstances such as post-/pre-parturition females; reproductively entire ('stud') males that are chronically intolerant of other cats; sick, injured or quarantined individuals; or as a necessary part of a specific research programme. Enrichment and human interactions should be enhanced, and time spent in individual housing should be limited to the minimum period necessary. Large, single housing such as the lodges described by Loveridge et al. (1995) provide individually housed cats with an enriched environment, freedom of choice, mental and physical stimulation (Figure 31.2). Glass allows visual stimulation by those on either side, by human and cat activity within the colony, and by activity in the grounds outside the colony building; however, privacy provision should be made to allow the cat to retreat out of sight. Controlled, individual access (e.g. microchip cat flaps) to provisions such as food or litter trays enables collection of individual data from cats housed in their normal social setting without the need for single housing. Users should explore the possibilities of these techniques before resorting to individual housing methods which may severely compromise the welfare of cats.

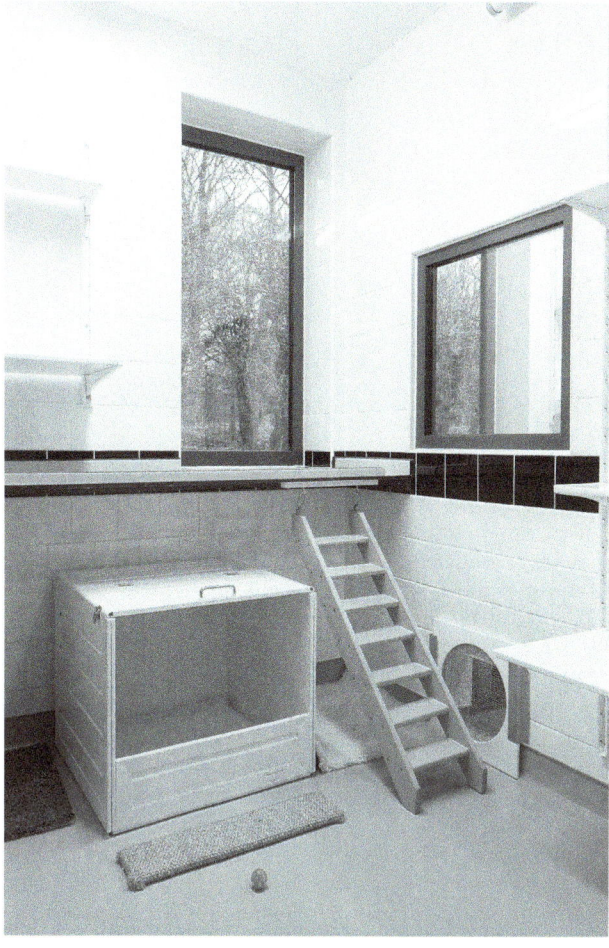

Figure 31.2 Separate rooms such as lodges can be used for individual data collection or as separate accommodation away from the rest of the colony to help protect the queen and young kittens. Source: Mars, Incorporated.

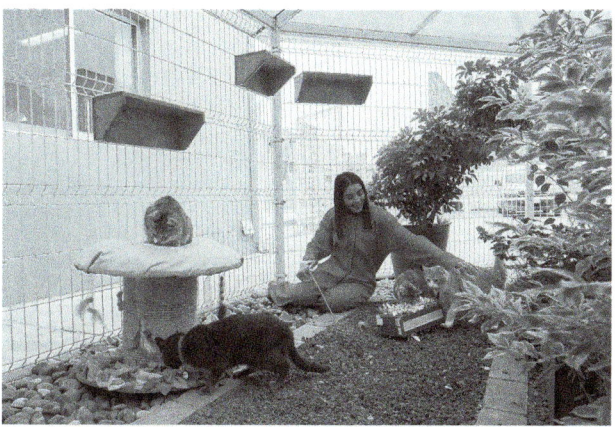

Figure 31.1 Outdoor exposure can provide an environmental enrichment opportunity. Source: Mars, Incorporated.

The most specialised or extreme form of single housing is the open floor system such as a metabolism cage which is used, for example, to facilitate collection and assessment of urine and/or faeces. Open flooring systems are not recommended for cats as they can cause pain, injury or disease and provide a barren environment, devoid of comfort and facilities which provide physical and mental stimulation. These cages are usually made of metal (often stainless steel) with wire mesh flooring. Stressors with this system include unfamiliar setting, lack of space for normal movement for species-typical behaviours, prevention of the normal behaviours of digging and burial of eliminations and enforced social isolation especially if normally socially housed. If used, these cages should be made as appealing as possible with the addition of resting boards, hiding areas, toys and sensory stimulation of other cats and should be used for the minimum time possible. Minimum space provision should allow the cat to stretch fully horizontally and vertically, to

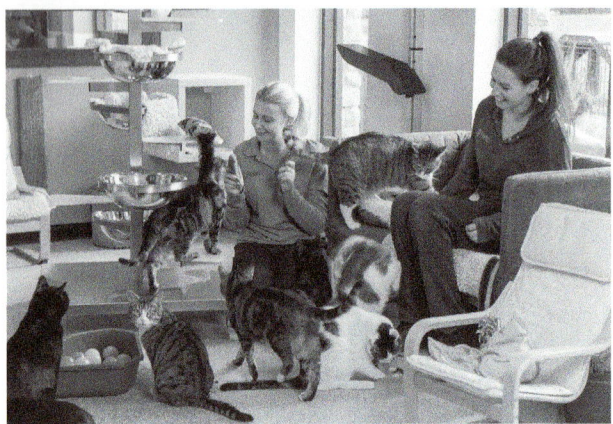

Figure 31.3 Consistent and predictable social interaction with humans and cats is beneficial. Source: Mars, Incorporated.

lie down and turn around. Acclimatisation to the cages and refinements to the macro-environment (lighting, noise levels) should be considered to improve welfare (Stella et al. 2014).

Cats previously housed in a social setting can usually be returned to familiar social groups in between research studies or for a period each day. As a minimum, single-housed cats should have the choice to spend time outside of the individual housing each day for human and cat social interaction (Figure 31.3). The introduction or re-introduction of cats to established groups should be carefully facilitated and monitored to avoid and manage problems of incompatibility and disrupted social dynamics. Studies of stray cats housed communally at a shelter have shown that most overt aggression occurs within the first 4 days and that mutual toleration is established after 2 weeks (Bradshaw 1992). However, although many of these cats appear to have behaviourally habituated to confinement at this stage, cats still show abnormally high urinary cortisol levels up to 5 weeks after entry to a quarantine cattery (Rochlitz et al. 1998). Increasing availability of social resources and hiding opportunities can help reduce agonistic behaviours and social stress during re-introduction (Crowell-Davis et al. 1997).

Group housing

Colony density and space recommendations should be followed. Minimum space requirements for post-weaned cats housed for scientific purposes as floor area have been specified as 1.5 m², shelf provision of 0.5 m² and 2.0 m height with each additional cat allocated 0.75 m² floor space and 0.25 m² shelf space (European Commission 2007); however, smaller space provision is specified in other jurisdictions, e.g. USDA (2013). Cats in social settings require sufficient space between each other to maintain group stability, yet allow adequate social distancing for individual behaviours and to reduce competition for resource and aggressive interactions. Usually, cats will avoid physical confrontation by using behaviours to maintain distance, such as olfactory marking, posturing and vocalisation. A distance of 1–3 m has been suggested as desirable proximity between indoor cats (Barry & Crowell-Davis 1999).

Ideally, a group size of 10–12 cats should not be exceeded (Rochlitz 2005; Griffin & Hume 2006); however, larger group sizes can successfully live together where there is adequate space and resource provisions for hiding, feeding and elimination. Female cats and neutered cats of both sexes are generally sociable. Benefits of smaller groups of cats include reducing the risk of conflict, infectious disease transmission and to allow effective monitoring. Housing cats at high densities increases the likelihood of stress (Bernstein & Strack 1996; Kessler & Turner 1997). Individual cat backgrounds, personalities, degrees of socialisation, relatedness, familiarity, gender, age, body weight, availability and preference of enrichment all contribute to group cohesion (Crowell-Davis et al. 2004; Bonanni et al. 2007; Damsceno & Genaro 2014). Social housing provides opportunities for complex social interactions and can increase mental and physical stimulation; however, group composition should be kept fairly constant to avoid disrupting established group dynamics. Social cohesion is maintained through behaviours such as allo-rubbing, which involves tactile communication and the mixing and exchange of scent, such that all individuals in the group have a shared scent profile. Cohesion can be negatively impacted by the frequent addition of new cats into a group, which can disrupt relationships and introduce new olfactory profiles.

Behaviours such as resting together, allo-grooming, nose touch and body rubbing are examples of affiliative behaviours observed in colony environments and are indicative of positive social bonds between individuals and occur more often in related cats, than cats that have lived their entire lives together in the same home (Bradshaw & Hall 1999). Monitoring of group dynamics can help early identification of group instability. Cats which fail to adapt to a particular social group, for example those which avoid contact with all other group members, should be rehoused either with a smaller group or singly or considered for homing.

When cats are housed in groups, attention should be paid to the availability of resources. Limited floor space owing to the need for fundamental provisions such as litter trays, water, food and beds can subsequently affect the amount of available space for other behaviours and social interactions. Resource quantities, locations and availability are essential in managing agonistic behaviours and social stress which can be achieved by providing resources in several areas and in isolation of one another (Crowell-Davis et al. 1997). A minimum of 0.5 m between various functional provisions and at least one litter box of 300 x 400 mm for every two cats has been recommended (European Commission 2007) for reasons of cleanliness, to minimise social conflict and impact food intake (Bourgeois et al. 2004). Cats can develop individual preferences for litter tray type (open or closed) and substrate which should be accommodated.

Given that provisions are predominantly located at floor level, space provision per cat must be sufficient to allow for this proximity; however, distribution of resources across a range of accessible heights can allow each cat to access resources with a degree of privacy, without competition and out of direct visual contact with other cats (Overall & Dyer 2005; Heath & Wilson 2014). Increasing functional space can be easily achieved by adding walkways (Figure 31.4), shelving or climbing towers (Figure 31.5).

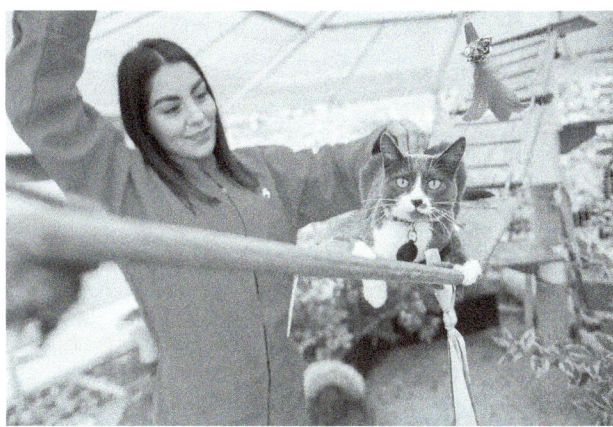

Figure 31.4 Increasing functional space can be easily achieved by adding walkways. Source: Mars, Incorporated.

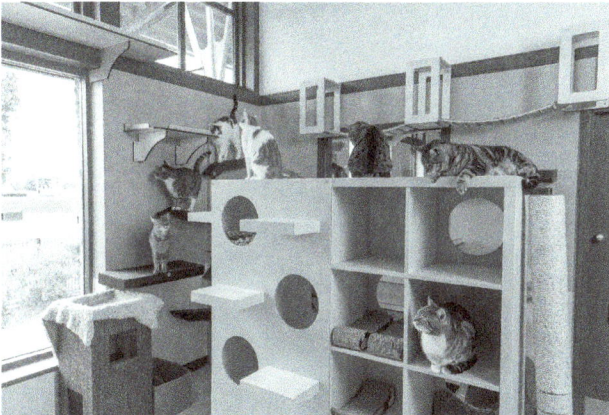

Figure 31.5 Increasing functional space can be easily achieved by adding walkways and shelving. Source: Mars, Incorporated.

Environmental provisions and enrichment

The individual response to confinement varies widely and is based on many factors including the quality of the confined space and the cat's previous experience. Optimal housing conditions can positively impact the cat's physiological and psychological well-being as well as reducing variability in research outcomes (Russell & Burch 1959; Poole 1997; Balcombe et al. 2004) and it is generally accepted that the quality of the space is as, if not more, important than the quantity (Rochlitz 2000; Stella et al. 2017). See also Chapter 10: Environmental enrichment: animal welfare and scientific validity. As a minimum, species appropriate enrichment which allows the cat opportunities to perform behaviours consistent with their telos (Broom & Johnson 1993; Rollin 2015) and opportunities for physical, social and environmental control should be provided.

Good laboratory housing for cats should include a range of shelving at different heights, and a choice of resting and hiding places. Timid cats and those less well integrated into the social group will occupy the higher shelves (Rochlitz et al. 1998), particularly those in corners as they provide the best vantage points and protect the cat from being approached from behind. Cats spend a large portion of their day either resting or sleeping, so it is important that there are plenty of rest areas with comfortable surfaces.

Hiding is a coping behaviour that cats often show in response to stimuli or changes in their environment (Rochlitz 2005). It is commonly seen when cats want to avoid interactions with other cats or people, and in response to other potentially stressful situations. Hiding enrichment such as a cardboard box can encourage more relaxed behaviours and approachability to humans (Kry & Casey 2007). Visual barriers can be useful, to enable cats to get out of sight of others and also to break up the three-dimensional space into sections or compartments, making it more complex, giving the cat more choice and reducing conspecific agonistic interactions (Rochlitz 2005; Desforges et al. 2016).

Enrichment aids should be selected to suit the age, personality and response of the individual (Figure 31.6) and can be tactile, structural, auditory, olfactory, visual, social, human–animal and cognitive. Cats show most interest in toys that mimic prey, but toys need to be changed frequently and offered in randomised rotation to sustain long-term interest. Olfactory enrichment is relatively underused in animal housing. Surfaces for the deposition of olfactory and visual signals, for claw abrasion, such as scratch posts, rush matting, pieces of carpet, wood and scented cloth should be provided (Figure 31.7). It is vital that the purpose of enrichment is understood to ensure intended goals are met and there is a clear improvement in welfare. Examples of essential enrichment and function are listed in Table 31.2. Further environmental and enrichment guidelines have been described by Ellis et al. (2013), and Overall and Dyer (2005).

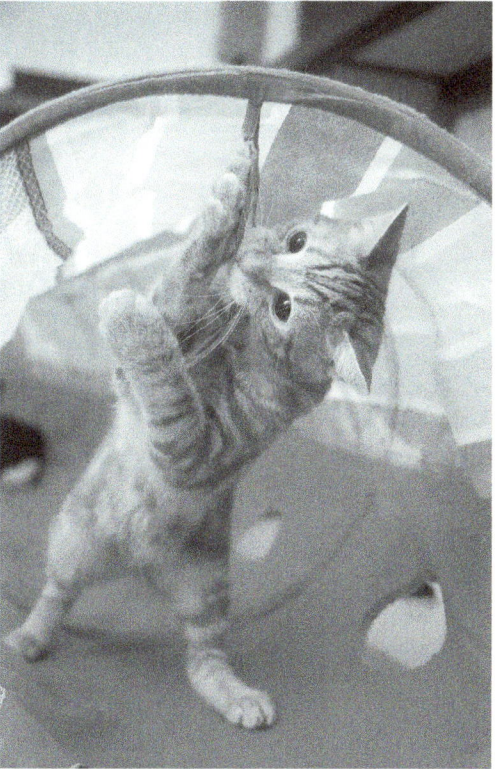

Figure 31.6 Enrichment should be optimised for the cat's age. Source: Mars, Incorporated.

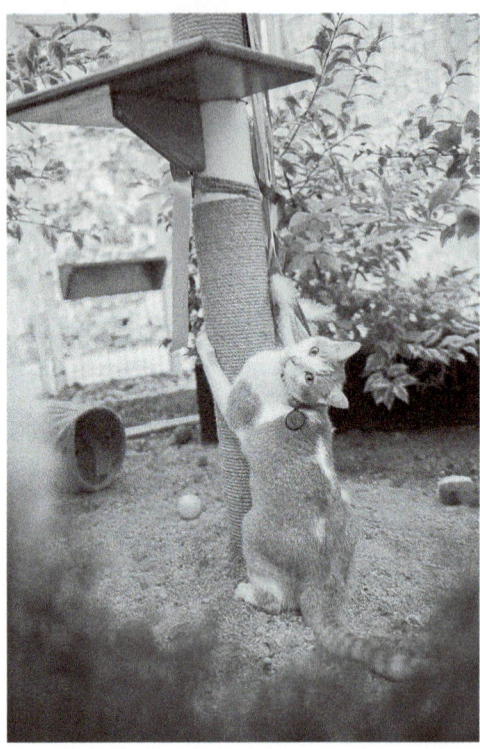

Figure 31.7 Scratch posts are important for the deposition of olfactory and claw abrasion. Source: Mars, Incorporated.

Feeding and watering

The nutritional requirements, physiology and metabolism of domestic cats are highly adapted to the predatory lifestyle of their wild predecessors, and they are therefore still considered obligate carnivores (Morris 2002; Zoran & Buffington 2011).

Wild or feral cats must eat most parts of their prey, including muscle tissue (meat), bones, fat, viscera and other tissues, to meet their specific nutrient requirements. Cats are generally solitary hunters and tend to take prey that is considerably smaller than themselves, typically small vertebrates and insects (Plantinga *et al.* 2011). Although their natural feeding behaviour is to eat small meals throughout the day, cats are opportunistic feeders and will adjust their patterns of activity to suit the frequency with which food becomes available. Confined adult cats at maintenance can adapt to being fed once or twice a day but growing kittens and lactating queens require more frequent feeds. Confined cats given food *ad libitum* will generally eat small quantities at frequent intervals; however, some cats will need a restricted amount to prevent excessive consumption. They can be highly selective feeders and require their food and water to be highly palatable and fresh. Odour and texture may play an important part in diet selection. Careful observation is required to establish individual preferences and the correct level of feeding. Most cats seem to be able to monitor, and therefore adjust, their own calorie and macronutrient intake to match their requirements quite accurately (Hewson-Hughes *et al.* 2016).

Most confined cats are fed solely on commercially prepared, complete and balanced wet or dry cat foods. These diets have been designed to supply all the essential nutrients and energy needed, and have been tested for nutritional adequacy, digestibility and palatability. When feeding complete diets, supplements should be avoided as they can result in nutritional imbalances. Wet foods provided in cans, pouches or trays are heat-sterilised and, as such, a safe product with a very long storage life requiring no special storage conditions. The moisture (water) content of these foods can be as much as 80%. High-quality complete dry food (5–10% moisture) made specifically for cats can also be used as the sole source of nutrition. Dry food can be kept for many months provided it is stored in dry, cool conditions.

Table 31.2 Essential enrichment and function.

Environmental provision	Goal of enrichment	Consideration
Bedding	Comfort, resting, hiding	One bed per cat will avoid competition for resting areas
Elevated shelving and multi-levelled furniture, e.g. towers, cat trees	Climbing, hiding, additional space, environmental control, vantage points, visual barrier	Ensure cats are able to safely retreat off high areas and cannot access hazards Essential to help cats cope with and alleviate social stress by hiding or fleeing to elevated locations
Boxes, plastic cubes, Feline Forts®, cardboard boxes	Hiding, destructive play	One box per cat to allow a safe retreat for concealment
Scratch posts, e.g. sisal rope, cardboard scratchers, carpet	Scratching, claw abrasion, olfactory signalling	Can be wall mounted horizontally or vertically. Consider floor-based provision for less mobile, young or elderly cats. Good practice is to provide one scratch post per cat (plus an additional one for choice) positioned in different locations
Herbs, catnip, odour cloths, external exposure	Olfactory stimulation. Can also be used for acclimatisation	Items should be approved as not hazardous or poisonous before use. Consideration to the effect of catnip may be required
Soft brush	Grooming, olfactory signalling	Brushes can be fixed to allow facial marking. Consider placement for accessibility
Windows, bubbles, TV, cat specific technology	Visual stimulation	Cats should be monitored for signs of frustration if unable to interact with the source of the stimulation

Table 31.2 (Continued)

Environmental provision	Goal of enrichment	Consideration
Natural sounds, e.g. bird song	Auditory stimulation Can also be used for acclimatisation	Noise should be provided quietly and periodically. Cats should be given the opportunity to avoid sound
Toys, e.g. ping pong balls, soft toys, brain games, wands, feathers	Chasing, pouncing, capturing, biting and scratching with the hind legs	Toys need assessment for supervised or unsupervised use. Variation in toy provision can reduce familiarity. Hiding toys can increase exploratory play. Toy type should be selected based on cat's life stage and environmental limitations, e.g. ball in a cage may cause frustration
Human interaction	Stimulation, affection, bonding, care	Interaction should be consistent, predictable and individualised to each cat's personality
Running space, exercise wheels	Exercise	Exercise can be encouraged through social play. Cats should be monitored for stereotypic behaviour

Offering some dry food maintains oral hygiene in cats. Its natural abrasive action helps to prevent build-up of plaque and reduces the risk of gum disease. Another advantage is that it can be left out longer than canned food, which allows the cats to adopt a more natural feeding pattern of many small meals throughout both the day and night. However, in general, most cats find dry foods less palatable than wet foods.

Diets can also be made directly from raw ingredients. The US NRC (National Research Council 2006) gives nutritional guidelines for cats, often both minimum requirements and maximum tolerable levels, and lists the composition of a wide range of ingredients from which diets can be formulated to meet the cat's nutritional requirements. Further information can be found in Hand *et al.* (2010).

Food should be kept fresh and ideally split over several, small meals per day. Removing food for a period each day can renew the cats' interest. Feed enrichment items can be an efficient strategy to promote natural hunting and play behaviours in domestic cats (Dantas-Divers *et al.* 2011; Damasceno & Genaro 2014). Dry food hidden in puzzle boxes can extend the handling time of the food if the cat has to work to extract individual pieces. (Figure 31.8). Food items should be stored off the floor in vermin-proof containers and in non-extreme temperatures.

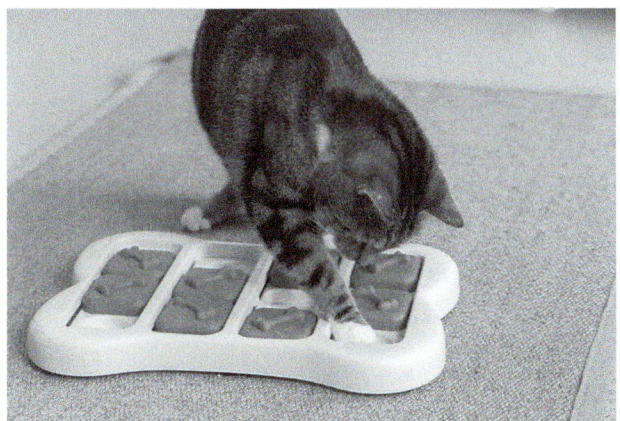

Figure 31.8 Food ration offered in a puzzle can provide a rewarding challenge. Source: Mars, Incorporated.

The time of feeding and food availability can increase agonistic interactions between cats because of arousal and competition relating to feeding strategy (Knowles *et al.* 2004; Bonanni *et al.* 2007; Finkler *et al.* 2011), though interactions can often be ritualised (Crowell-Davis *et al.* 2004). Kasanen *et al.* (2010) described the behavioural need for a carnivore to perform species-specific feeding behaviours such as foraging and hunting, which may not be fulfilled in artificial feeding environments and may contribute to agonistic behaviour around feed times within the research environment. Feeding cats in individual cages will ensure each cat obtains adequate time and opportunity for eating and allows monitoring of individuals' diet intake and refusal.

The requirement for fresh, clean water is at least as important as that for other nutrients. An average water consumption is 60 ml/kg/day; however, the water content of the diet affects the amount of water cats will drink. As many cats will only drink fresh water and therefore may voluntarily drink very limited amounts, supplying parts of their ration in the form of moist food will increase moisture intake considerably. This practice can be beneficial for at least some cats in diluting the urine and thereby help prevent kidney and lower urinary tract diseases, including stone formation (Hand *et al.* 2010).

Clean, fresh water should always be available and, ideally, replenished constantly from a chlorinated mains supply. Where cats are group housed, a minimum of two water supplies should be available. Some cats prefer to drink from a moving water source, e.g. tap or water fountain.

Dietary requirements

Dietary requirements will change with life stage, physiological and health status, and activity level, as does the way in which the food should be presented. The NRC (2006) has estimated energy and nutrient requirements across various life stages. Other sources, such as Hand *et al.* (2010), take into account evolving husbandry and health issues that can affect these.

The daily energy intake recommendations especially are guidelines only and adjustments will be needed on an individual basis regarding the amount of food provided to maintain a healthy body mass and body condition regardless of life stage. Influencing factors include, but are not limited to, age, sex, season/temperature, activity level, fur characteristics, neutering and health status.

Table 31.3 Estimated daily metabolisable energy requirements (kcal per day) for adult cats from two different sources.

Adult body weight (kg)	Metabolisable energy (total kcal per day)	
	NRC 2006	Bermingham et al. 2010
2	159	127
3	209	169
4	253	208
5	294	244
6	332	277
7	368	310
8	403	340

Adult cats

Estimated daily metabolisable energy (ME) daily requirements for adult cats can be calculated using an exponential equation provided by NRC (2006):

$$ME(kcal/day) = 100 * BW^{0.67}$$; where BW = body weight in kg

ME for the normal range of body weights observed in cats is provided in Table 31.3, using the National Research Council (2006) equation above and, alternatively, by the equation supplied by Bermingham et al. (2010):

$$ME(kcal/day) = 77.6 * BW^{0.711}$$; where BW = body weight in kg

This latter study was a meta-analysis conducted on a larger data set provided by 115 cat studies, in which some of the influencing factors mentioned in the preceding text were taken into account.

Due to physiological and behavioural changes, both male and female neutered cats can increase food intake and/or decrease activity levels compared to reproductively intact counterparts, and more careful monitoring of feed intake may be needed to avoid excessive weight gain and obesity (Larsen 2017). A 10% reduction in energy supplied to avoid weight gain following neutering has been suggested (Bermingham et al. 2010; Mitsuhashi et al. 2011).

Pregnant and lactating queens

Pregnant and lactating queens should be fed a specially formulated diet, e.g. kitten food, which meets specific nutritional requirements to support the queen's basic needs, foetal development, milk production and nutrients in the milk. The diet should be provided *ad libitum*. The National Research Council (2006) recommends the following equation to calculate energy requirements for gestation:

$$ME(kcal/day) = 140 * BW^{0.67}$$; where BW = body weight in kg

Cats typically increase their food intake and body weight from the first day of pregnancy and, on average, gain about 40% of their pre-mating weight during pregnancy (reviewed in Hand et al. 2010). Weight gain will, however, vary with the size of the litter, which can be accounted for with the following equation:

Weight gain (g) = 888.9 + 106.5 N; where N is the number of kittens in the litter

Some of the weight queens accumulate will be lost at parturition, while the rest provide an energy reserve for lactation (Loveridge 1986). Especially in the first 4 weeks of the 7–9-week-long lactation period, queens can expend more energy than they can take in, again depending on the size of the litter and therefore the amount of milk produced. Even following the lactation peak at approximately week 3–4, queens will continue to need extra energy while they suckle and rebuild body reserves. Thus, the National Research Council (2006) recommendation for ME in lactating cats is based on the maintenance requirement increased by factors determined by the number of kittens in the litter and the stage of lactation:

$$ME(kcal/day) = maintenance + [K * BW * L]$$; where BW = body weight in kg, K = factor for the number of kittens in the litter: 18 for <3, 60 for 3–4, and 70 for >4 kittens, and L = factor for lactation week 1 to 7: 0.9, 0.9, 1.2, 1.2, 1.1, 1.0, and 0.8, respectively.

Growing kittens

Nutrition is one of the major determinants of kittens' growth rate, along with genetic factors, the kitten's sex and high-quality husbandry practices, including adequate hygienic conditions, parasite treatment and vaccination to ensure freedom from disease (Hand et al. 2010). Optimal nutrition of the queen during pregnancy and lactation will give kittens the best start in life. During a kitten's first few weeks, it is entirely dependent on its mother's milk to achieve the desired growth rate of nearly 100 g a week. If the queen's milk is insufficient, or kittens are being hand reared, specially manufactured milk replacers should be given at frequent intervals. Milk replacers mimic the composition of queen's milk, are highly digestible and may include a probiotic to help establish a healthy gut microbiome.

Although deciduous teeth appear about 14 days after birth, very young kittens are not very interested in solid food until about 3–4 weeks, at which time they will start eating the solid food that their mother is eating. By week 6, kittens should be given finely chopped, wet or moistened dry food. Commercial food specifically formulated for kittens is available; these have a higher concentration of energy, protein, minerals and other nutrients than food formulated for adult cats to support muscle, skeletal and other tissues' growth and development. The amount of food kittens can ingest at one meal is limited and, ideally, they should be fed *ad libitum* or at the minimum 4–5 meals per day initially with the frequency gradually reduced to 2–3 at 6 months. National Research Council (2006) recommends a factorial equation to estimate the ME requirements for kittens:

$$ME(kcal/day) = 100 * BW_a^{0.67} * 6.7 * [e^{(-0.189p)} - 0.66]$$; where $p = BW_a/BW_m$, BW_a = actual body weight at time of evaluation, BW_m = expected mature body weight, and e = base of natural log ~ 2.718.

However, recording and maintaining a stable growth curve is a valuable, alternative tool to monitor healthy weight development in growing kittens. An average 100 g and a minimum of 50 g weight gain per week from birth until approximately week 24–28 for females and week 28–32 for males is considered optimal. Weaned kittens do not need milk and may become less able to digest lactose as their gut matures. At 6 months of age, most kittens have gained 75% of their final adult weight and can be given food formulated for adult cats.

Older cats

Most colony cats are retired when they are around 8–9 years old. If older cats are kept or studies require geriatric cats, some changes in feeding regimens may be required. Some of the challenges observed as cats age are changes in body weight, body condition score and muscle mass, as well as coat condition, the senses of sight and smell, and behaviour, many of these caused by changes in activity levels, digestion and possibly by developing disease conditions. For older, over-weight cats, feeding less energy-dense diets frequently rather than *ad libitum* allows food intake to be monitored more closely. Maintaining a lean body condition will assist mobility and other health issues. Most geriatric cats require small but regular feeds, with about one in three cats requiring a high-energy, highly palatable and digestible diet as they age to prevent weight or muscle loss due to reductions in their ability to digest fat and/or protein (Laflamme & Gunn-Moore 2014). It may be necessary to offer finely chopped, wet or moistened dry food if they have poor dentition. The latter will also supply additional water, which can be beneficial as they are inclined to become dehydrated due to a reduced sensitivity to thirst and ability to concentrate urine if kidney health issues develop (Hand *et al.* 2010). Regular health checks can identify a need for dietary or medical intervention.

Identification and sexing

The identification method should be reliable and cause the minimum pain and discomfort to the animal. In small colonies, cats can be identified by their markings and other characteristics. In larger colonies, microchip implants provide a secure, safe and permanent method of identifying individuals. Insertion of microchips is less painful than tattooing. Collars can be used but their fit needs to be checked regularly and they are unsuitable for very young kittens. Cats can be sexed at birth from the anogenital distance (about 6 mm in females and 13 mm in males).

Physical environment

The physical environment should be regularly monitored and adjusted for comfort. Cats may be maintained within a wide temperature range provided that their welfare is not compromised and temperature extremes are avoided. Establishing a temperature and humidity range avoids climatic fluctuations and can reduce experimental variation; a temperature range between 15 °C and 21 °C has been suggested by the UK Home Office (2014). Climatic changes should be made gradually to allow the cat sufficient time to adjust. Cats with opportunity for outdoor exposure should have access to an indoor temperature-controlled area.

Good ventilation is important to dilute and remove airborne pathogens, odour and to disperse heat produced by animals and equipment. A ventilation rate of 10 to 15 air changes per hour of fresh or conditioned air has been suggested as adequate (Home Office 2014; European Commission 2007). Re-circulation of untreated air should be avoided.

A natural 24-hour light-dark cycle is acceptable. Supplementary artificial lighting can be used where the light part of the photoperiod (10–12 hours daily) is required. Lighting levels should be adequate to allow completion of husbandry practices, but cats should not be exclusively exposed to intense artificial lighting. If natural light is totally excluded, total darkness should be avoided through provision of low-level night lighting (5–10 lux) to allow cats to retain some vision and to take account of their startle reflex.

Intermittent, unpredictable and loud noises can be stressful for cats. The hearing range of cats is 0.07–91 kHz, with peak sensitivity 1–40 kHz and extends beyond the range of human hearing in terms of frequency and sensitivity. Noise disturbance can be reduced by locating housing away from high noise areas within the hearing range of the cat, e.g. ultrasound, as well as using sound-absorbing building materials or the use of background sound. Alarm systems are generally loud and unpredictable and safe alternatives should be considered to minimise disturbance to the cat, e.g. voice alarm evacuation systems.

Hygiene

The combination of good facility design and an effective cleaning regimen will minimise disease transmission and ensure a clean living environment for cats. The frequency and extent of cleaning will depend on the facility materials, housing management model and cat health status.

A spot clean model can be completed in individual and group housing settings, where cats are of the same health status. Spot cleaning involves the targeted cleaning of specific and localised dirty areas with detergent and disinfectant. Spot cleaning can be daily or less frequently in a stable colony. As a daily minimum, bedding should be changed if dirty; litter trays should be checked and cleaned with detergent and disinfectant if excessively soiled. Cats should have a safe area to retreat and hide during the spot cleaning; however, some cats may find the additional human interaction enriching. Spot cleaning is generally accepted to be a less stressful cleaning method than a daily deep clean.

A deep clean model may be required when cat populations change. Deep cleaning involves the removal of cats from the living space to clean all walls, surfaces and furniture with detergent and disinfectant and replacing all bedding and litter. Pressure washers, steam cleaning and hosing can be used on impervious materials and where adequate drainage exists. Cats have a complex sensory system relying on chemical and olfactory communication such as urine spraying and pheromonal marking which is used to establish boundaries and maximise their sense of security and comfort. Frequent removal of this chemical marking through deep cleaning could be stressful to cats through interference with their cat's olfactory and chemical signalling and therefore this method should not be performed more than necessary especially in an established cat colony. Keeping furniture and cleaning equipment cat room specific can help with room and odour familiarisation and predictability.

Cleaning agents must be safe for human and cat exposure and meet the cleaning objective. Areas should be dry before allowing cats' access. Cats are particularly sensitive to phenolic and quaternary ammonium compounds (Bates & Edwards 2015). In cases of disease outbreak or changes in barrier status, professional medical decontamination may be required. Further details on safe and effective disinfection for feline environments are described by Addie et al. (2015).

Every care should be taken to avoid any wild, stray or pet animals entering the animal facility. Particular care needs to be taken with drains and other services that penetrate the fabric of the building to minimise any potential route into the cat housing.

Health monitoring

Cats should be handled frequently and checked daily for signs of ill health. Every week, they should have a specific health check (ears, eyes, nose, genitalia and general body condition), be groomed, weighed and body condition scored (Figure 31.9). For feline-friendly handling guidelines, see Rodan et al. (2011).

Dental examinations and haematology and biochemistry screens should be performed at least once a year, and more often in younger or older cats. Colonies should be screened for viruses, bacteria and parasites. Viral screening should occur on an epidemiological basis. Assuming a low incidence of disease, a large number of cats may need to be screened to find a problem. Any unexpected death should be thoroughly investigated.

The probability of cats contracting an infectious disease depends on a number of factors, including: age, genetic predisposition, nutritional status, levels of stress, concurrent illness, level of infectious disease challenge and virulence of the infectious organism. Disease transmission can be limited further by housing all cats according to their susceptibility and across several individual buildings to minimise the potential for disease to spread throughout a colony (Hawthorne et al. 1995). Preferably each susceptibility group should be handled by different personnel, otherwise the sequence in which they are handled should be on a susceptibility basis from most to least susceptible, e.g. early weaned kittens, queens with kittens, older cats, quarantine cats and sick cats. Further details are given by Mostl et al. (2013).

Isolation, quarantine and barrier systems

Isolation and quarantine facilities should be a self-contained facility located away from the main colony, ideally, with a separate air ventilation system. The type of air filtration, e.g. high efficiency particulate air (HEPA) will be defined by the required hygiene status. Ventilation systems can be used to create differential air pressures by maintaining areas with a higher hygiene status at a higher pressure.

An isolation facility would be required should a cat from the existing colony require separation due to signs of infectious disease. A quarantine facility would be required for entry of new, external cats before integration into the existing colony, or where an existing cat has been to an external facility of unknown or different health status, e.g. for off-site veterinary treatment. An isolation and quarantine facility could be a single facility; however, it should not be used concurrently for separate purposes and should be cleaned and decontaminated between use.

A barrier system should be applied to minimise the transmission of infectious agents between facilities of different health status. The extent of barrier entry procedures will vary depending on the desired barrier goal. Further details are given by National Research Council (2011).

Breeding

Condition of adults

Selection criteria for breeding should include phenotype, reproductive performance, temperament and health. Genetic breeding analysis through DNA screening can provide insights into genetic disease and traits. The benefits of breeding from healthy, confident, well socialised, unrelated parents will help preserve the quality of a cat colony. Breeding females should be good mothers and have produced good-sized litters with an even sex ratio and good-sized offspring.

Cats reach sexual maturity at around 4–12 months of age, but this can be influenced by external factors, e.g. season and climate. Queens that begin to cycle and are not bred are likely to develop uterine pathology that decreases reproductive performance. Therefore, if the colony has reproduction as a goal, queens should be placed into a harem in their first year.

Retirement age of breeding populations will vary depending on behaviour, health and productivity. Cats used for breeding typically live longer within a research setting, and consideration should be given to specific behavioural and housing needs of this population, within the mating system

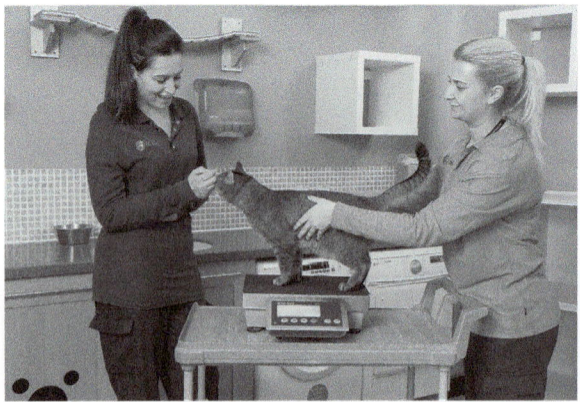

Figure 31.9 Health assessments such as weight and body condition scoring can be completed during routine handling and are essential to ensure the well-being of individuals. Source: Mars, Incorporated.

used. An example of good practice is to neuter and retire queens from breeding at 5 years of age and limit litters to one per year; toms can continue until up to 10 years of age.

Identifying the fertile state

Anoestrous females will respond aggressively to any sexual approach by a male. Females in pro-oestrus show subtle changes in their behaviour; they tend to be rather restless and rub up against objects. They allow males to approach but prolonged contact is not tolerated. Over the next 24 h, the females rub their head and flank against objects with increasing intensity, they roll on the floor, stretch, purr and rhythmically open and close their paws, flexing their claws. At this stage, they will tolerate grooming by the male but not mounting. Full sexual receptivity is indicated by females adopting the lordosis position; the female crouches with her head close to the ground, her hind legs treading and partly extended, and her tail laterally displaced to expose the perineum (UK Cat Behaviour Working Group 1995).

Mating systems

In the harem or group mating system, ideally one male cat is kept with a group of females. The dominant male will usually mate with more than 80% of the females. A potential difficulty with this system is that the exact date of mating is not always known, and pregnancy is determined by a combination of palpation, x-ray, ultrasound or the female gaining weight. The female is then moved to kittening accommodation 10–14 days before birth is due to allow her to habituate to the new surroundings.

Despite being territorial, familiar toms can be housed in small groups if there is adequate space and hiding opportunities. Aggressive interactions can be minimised by avoiding visual and auditory contact with oestrous queens; however Natoli and De Vito (1991) observed that following an initial aggressive inter-tom interaction, toms did not fight around the queen in oestrus. If queens and toms are housed in a non-harem status, matings can be orchestrated in a neutral space.

An alternative system is to house females together in groups and to accommodate the males in individual housing. When signs of oestrus are observed, the female is taken to the male. The advantage of this system is that parentage and date of mating are known; however, disadvantages include the need to singly house males with relatively little social contact with other cats and males need to be replaced regularly to avoid inbreeding.

Artificial insemination

Feline-assisted reproduction is not routinely used; however, recent advances have been made. The success of artificial insemination is dependent on the technique used and has been described further by Johnson (2018).

Conception and pregnancy

Ovulation occurs after copulation and is likely triggered by vaginal stimulation by the tom or by artificial means. Post copulation both cats wash their urogenital area, the female continues to roll for about 30 minutes before they mate again. Multiple copulations are normally required to trigger ovulation. Females may mate many times and with different males. Pregnancy can be reliably diagnosed by palpation at 21–28 days, by ultrasound after 21 days and by radiography after 40–45 days. Pregnancy can be assessed by monitoring weight gain.

Nesting and parturition

Cats do not usually build nests but make use of whatever protective shelter is available; they will usually make use of boxes, newspaper, cardboard or other forms of bedding if provided. They like to choose where to give birth, and may visit suitable sites several times before coming to a decision. Some cats prefer dark, quiet places; a box provided in the breeding area will generally be used. Following parturition, if space permits, the queen may move the nest site and kittens several times, possibly to prevent predators and tomcats from finding the kittens.

Group-housed pregnant cats are moved to separate accommodation (Figure 31.2) about 14 days before parturition to protect the new-born kittens from cannibalism or being taken by another female. Feral queens living in social groups do use communal dens and collaborate to nurse each other's offspring; in large groups mothers and daughters tend to cooperate but in small groups all adult females may nurse each other's offspring (Bradshaw 1992).

Before giving birth, the queen cleans herself thoroughly, particularly her ventrum around the nipples, and her anogenital area. Parturition is usually straightforward. The kittens are born at 2–30-minute intervals. After the birth, the queen removes the amniotic sac from around the kitten, severs the umbilical cord, eats the placenta and licks the kitten clean which stimulates its breathing. After delivery of the last kitten, the queen then encircles her litter and encourages them to suckle by nuzzling and licking them. Kittens find the nipple and suckle spontaneously using innate reflexes, olfaction and touch. Suckling must be established promptly as neonatal kittens cannot withstand even short periods without food and need to acquire maternal antibodies from the milk. The mother will remain in contact with the kittens for at least the first 24 h. For the first month, the queen spends about 70% of her time in the nest caring for her kittens, initiating feeding bouts, grooming and stimulating their perineal area to encourage urination and defecation (this must be done until they are about 7 weeks old).

Weaning and rearing

The queen begins weaning by spending more time away from her kittens and by adopting postures which make her nipples inaccessible. Weaning can be encouraged by providing shelving to which queens can retreat and by removing queens for increasingly longer periods. The kittens are encouraged to eat solid food from approximately 3 weeks of age, which helps to reduce their dependence on mothers' milk. Weaning is usually complete at 8 weeks of age. In breeding colonies, weaned kittens are usually housed separately from their mothers.

Housing kittens aged 8–18 weeks together widens their social experience and increases their sociability to other cats.

Young toms can be allowed supervised socialisation with groups of kittens. This provides stimulation and activity for the tom and teaches kittens how to interact with adults. Older kittens are usually grouped with others of a similar age.

Kitten development

Sensory systems are not fully operational in the new-born kitten. They are born blind, virtually deaf and completely dependent. They have a fully developed sense of touch, and can detect and respond to temperature gradients. Olfaction is fully developed by 3 weeks and hearing by 4 weeks. Kittens' eyes open at about 6 days. They can follow visual cues by 3–4 weeks and visual acuity is fully developed by about 16 weeks. Internal control of body temperature is not fully developed until 7 weeks.

Motor skills develop in parallel with sensory abilities. New-born kittens move by writhing against a surface. By 3 weeks, they can stand though their balance is poor, and by 5 weeks they are attempting complex movements. Motor control is fully developed by 11 weeks. Predatory behaviour is observed in cats with no experience of prey, but they require experience to become efficient hunters. Feral kittens learn by interacting with prey brought to the nest by their mothers. Domesticated kittens learn by interacting with toys, litter mates and their mothers (Figure 31.10).

In the first 2 weeks, kittens mainly sleep and eat. The sensitive and optimal period for socialisation to people lies between the end of the second and seventh weeks (Karsh & Turner 1988), and it is generally accepted that the period of socialisation of kittens to other cats also occurs during this time (Rochlitz 2005). Kittens should be given plenty of opportunity to socialise with other cats and humans, to play and experience colony routines (Figure 31.11). Older kittens should continue to be given a wide range of experiences as this will help them to accept novel events as adults (Figure 31.12). Cats that are handled from birth show more rapid physical development and, as adults, are more responsive to humans and to novel events (McCune 1992). Early socialisation is a critical time in the development of kittens and, if handled sensitively, will produce cats that are more tractable and pleasant to work with. Fear of humans can be

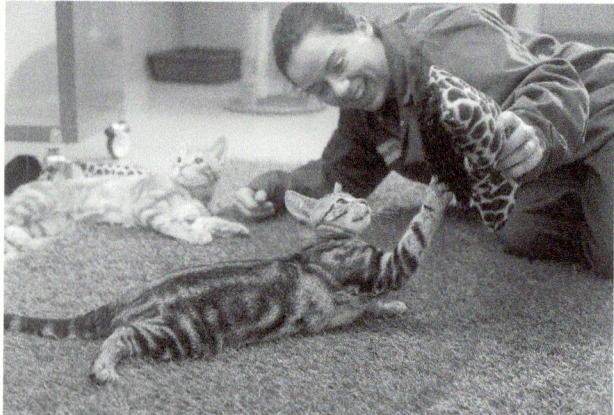

Figure 31.11 Quality handling and socialisation helps build confidence in kittens. Source: Mars, Incorporated.

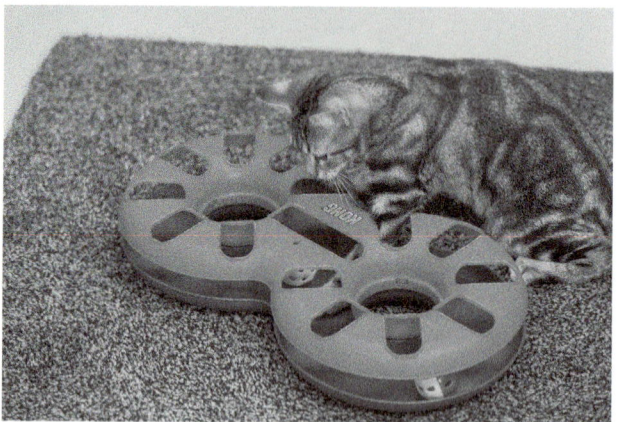

Figure 31.12 Older kittens should be given a wide range of experiences to help acceptance of novel events as adults. Source: Mars, Incorporated.

reduced when kittens are provided with enhanced socialisation between the second and ninth week of life (Casey & Bradshaw 2008). Their friendliness to people is affected by the quality and quantity of handling they receive (reviewed in McCune et al. 1995) but is also dependent on their parent's temperament (McCune 1995a). Kittens from confident fathers are more confident themselves and cope better when faced with unfamiliar situations such as being handled by strangers or being caged (McCune 1992) and the same is likely true of females. Consequently, it is important to consider temperament when selecting individuals for a breeding programme.

Reproductive problems

Major causes of infertility in both toms and queens include inbreeding, poor husbandry, disease, anatomical or reproductive defects and social stress. Investigation should first eliminate any non-reproductive disorders by a thorough physical, haematological and biochemical examination, followed by a thorough evaluation of the reproductive system and semen. Prolonged anoestrus is usually a management problem. The cats' general health and nutrition should be

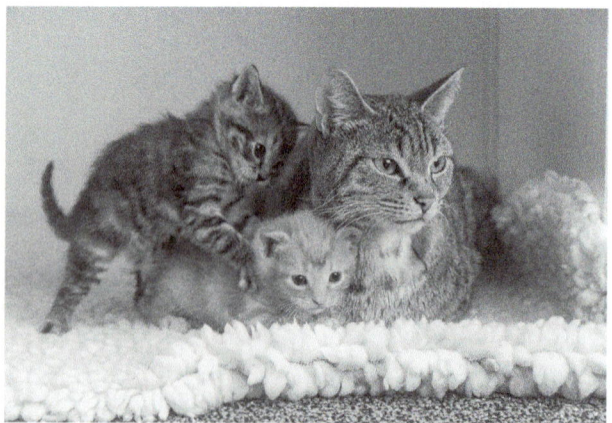

Figure 31.10 Kittens learn by interacting with litter mates and their mothers. Source: Mars, Incorporated.

optimised, and they should be exposed to 14–16 h of light per day and to reproductively active cats. Some queens cycle but do not show any oestrous behaviour (silent heat); however, they may breed if housed with a male. Failure to mate may be caused by inexperience. Virgins should be partnered with an amenable, experienced mate. Immature toms can lack libido, but may respond after visual exposure to breeding males. Toms should be mated in familiar surroundings otherwise they may concentrate on territory marking instead of mating. Mating may fail because the cats are incompatible; have mating preferences or some physical incompatibility may prevent intromission. Failure of the queen to conceive following mating is occasionally caused by vaginal or, more commonly, by uterine disease. Ovulation may fail because of inadequate vaginal stimulation or hormonal insufficiencies. Toms may fail to inseminate and their fertility declines if they are mated too frequently. Failure to carry a pregnancy to term has been associated with environmental stress, dietary insufficiencies or failure of extra-ovarian progesterone.

Effects of neutering

Neutering eliminates sexual behaviour in males and females, and maternal behaviour in females. It reduces the incidence of behaviours such as urine marking in both sexes, and increases tolerance towards cats from outside the social group (Bradshaw 1992).

Neutering predisposes to obesity by causing a reduction in energy expenditure, with the risk increased if the cat is confined in a small enclosure and is inactive. Allaway *et al.* (2017), found that early-age neutering may enable a more gradual weight gain through growth when food intake is regulated to maintain an ideal BCS. An association between ovariohysterectomy and mammary carcinoma has been reported with female cats showing a significantly reduced risk of developing a feline mammary carcinoma if spayed prior to 1 year of age compared with intact cats (Overley *et al.* 2005). Early-age neutering (between 6 and 14 weeks) is generally accepted to provide behavioural, physical and welfare benefits compared to traditional age neutering, discussed further by Joyce and Yates (2011).

Laboratory procedures

Handling and restraint

Laboratory cats must undergo handling and restraint for health examinations, veterinary and research procedures. Good handling techniques help cats feel comfortable, secure and a familiar handler reduces the cat's desire to struggle (Lockart *et al.* 2013). Inadequate handling and restraint can cause the cat stress, result in incomplete examination and sample collection, and human injury. See also Chapter 15: The use of positive reinforcement training techniques to enhance the care and welfare of laboratory and research animals.

Grown cats can be picked up with one hand under the chest, just behind the front paws, and the other under the hindquarters (Wills 1993). Once picked up, the cat will probably be most comfortable sitting in the crook of the handler's arm, with its forepaws either leaning against the handler's shoulder or held in the handler's other hand. Most of the cat's weight should be taken on the handler's arms. Young kittens should be picked up with one hand under the chest and the other under the hind legs. A young kitten will be small enough to sit on a palm as long as the handler supports its head with the other hand.

Procedures are easier with two experienced handlers; one restrains the cat while the other performs the procedure. The more relaxed the handlers and the cat are, the easier and less distressing the procedure. The amount and type of restraint will vary between the cat and the degree of restraint necessary for the procedure. Full-body restraint requires placing cats on their side and immobilising their head, body and limbs. Passive restraint is preferable and involves handling the cat in a normal upright position with minimal contact (Figure 31.13). Cats display significantly less negative behavioural and physiological responses and take less time to place in position when handled in a passive restraint method compared to a full-body restraint (Moody *et al.* 2018).

Chemical restraint may be required to increase safety and reduce stress for the cat and handler when a cat shows severe signs of fear or aggression. Procedure length can also be reduced with chemical restraint and diminishes the effect of stimulating the fight or flight response on blood values.

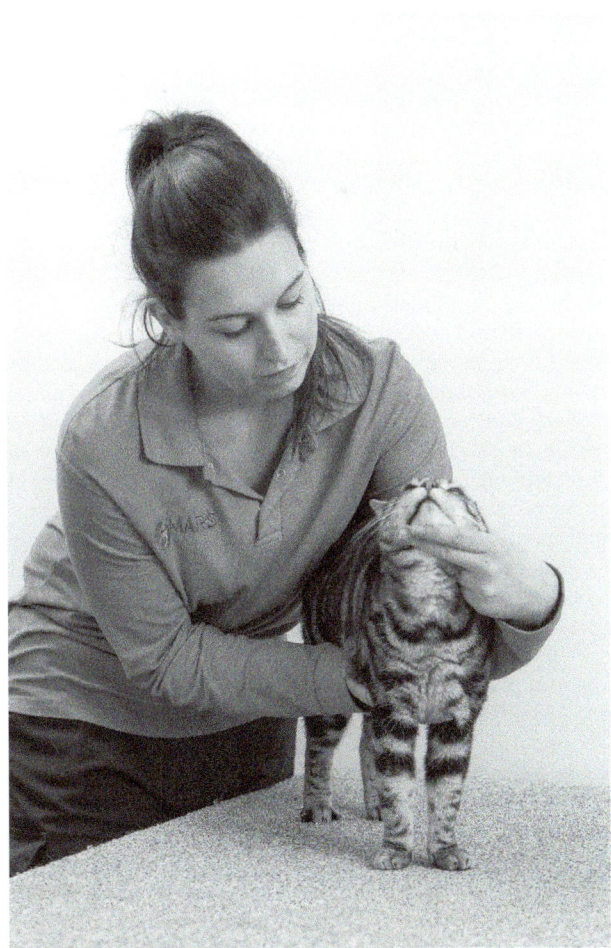

Figure 31.13 Passive restraint involves handling the cat in a normal upright position with minimal contact. Source: Mars, Incorporated.

Reversible agents administered by intramuscular or subcutaneous routes are preferable as they require minimal restraint.

Scruffing is a restraint technique whereby the handler grasps the skin at the back of the cat's neck, and when used with further full-body restraint, can render the cat immobile. Scruffing between cats is a behaviour which can occur when a kitten is transported by the queen or during mating. These situations are far-removed from the act of human scruffing, which is considered to cause stress and discomfort to the cat. Gentle scruffing could be beneficial in emergency situations or where human/cat safety is compromised and cats should not be lifted or suspended by scruffing alone. Gentler forms of restraint (e.g. passive) are more positively accepted by the cat, time efficient and generally safer for personnel (Moody et al. 2018). International Cat Care have a position statement on the use of scruffing[9].

A handling technique called 'clipnosis' or 'clipthesia' has been described (Pozza et al. 2008), which is used to immobilise cats for nail clipping, blood sampling and other minor procedures. The application of a clip or clips gently grasps the skin along the dorsal midline of the neck and cranial thorax to render the cat immobile. The pressure applied by the clip varies between clip type, and care should be taken to avoid contusion or ischaemia. Although the technique's effectiveness varies between individuals, it appears to be useful for providing gentle restraint in most cats. Based on their behavioural responses, the application of the clips does not appear to be aversive to most cats; however, there is not uniform agreement that clipnosis is an acceptable form of restraint. For feline-friendly handling guidelines, see Rodan et al. (2011). Further restraint techniques have been described by Herron and Shreyer (2014).

Training/habituation for procedures

An effective acclimatisation programme is essential in preparing cats and staff to the procedural experiences and social interactions to which they will be exposed, as well as minimising experimental variability. Staff must be adequately trained and familiar with experimental requirements to ensure the acclimatisation programme mimics the procedure, without exposing the cat to unnecessary stress. Training intensity should be individualised to the cat's temperament and based on breed and individual-specific behaviours. Close observations of the cat's behavioural responses should be noted to monitor the cat's welfare and training techniques adapted accordingly.

Positive reinforcement training (PRT) is a reward-based training method which can be used to increase acceptance of procedural and husbandry techniques (See also Chapter 15). The method rewards desired behaviours with a positive reinforcer (such as food or praise), immediately after the cat displays the desired behaviour. The process is repeated to encourage the cat to increase the frequency of the behaviour and is generally rewarding for both cat and trainer. PRT reduces the need for physical restraint or other interventions so is consequently less stressful for the cat (Bradshaw & Ellis 2016).

Training plans should have a degree of predictability and provide the cat an element of environmental control thus reducing the physiological response to stressors (Weinberg & Levine 1980). However, highly predictable environments may in themselves be stressful for the animal (Bassett & Buchanan-Smith 2007).

Monitoring methods

To maximise welfare and data quality, monitoring methods should be as non-invasive as possible.

Temperature, pulse and respiration

Most cats can simply be held while their rectal temperature is taken. Additional restraint may be needed in cats that object. Pulse and respiration can increase during stress and pain. Palpation of the peripheral pulse via the femoral artery can provide information about heart rate and rhythm as well as pulse quality. Respiration rate can be monitored easily by visual assessment or auscultation. Capnography, blood gas analysis, electrocardiography and pulse oximetry are additional tools for respiratory and cardiovascular monitoring.

Blood pressure

Monitoring of blood pressure can be required during anaesthesia, cardiovascular compromise or disease diagnosis. Arterial measurements can be taken directly using an arterial catheter, or indirectly using Doppler or oscillometric methods. Practical recommendations on the measurement of indirect blood pressure in cats have been described by International Catcare[10].

Activity monitoring

Accelerometers are a relatively novel tool which can be used to collect cat movement data when attached to cat's collars or harness (Figure 31.14). Activity data may allow for objective measurement of behaviour and mobility changes (Gruen et al. 2017).

Collection of specimens

Blood

The jugular vein should ideally be used for single blood samples to preserve peripheral veins; however, the antebrachial cephalic veins in the foreleg can be used for samples of 1–2 ml. For smaller samples, blood can be collected directly by letting it drop out through the needle into the collection vessel rather than being drawn out by syringe. Catheter placement is recommended for serial samples and can be less stressful than

---

[9]International Cat Care's position statement on the use of scruffing https://icatcare.org/our-campaigns/scruffing-position-statement/ (accessed 31 October 2019)

[10]International Cat Care: Hypertension in cats https://icatcare.org/advice/hypertension-high-blood-pressure/ (accessed 31 October 19)

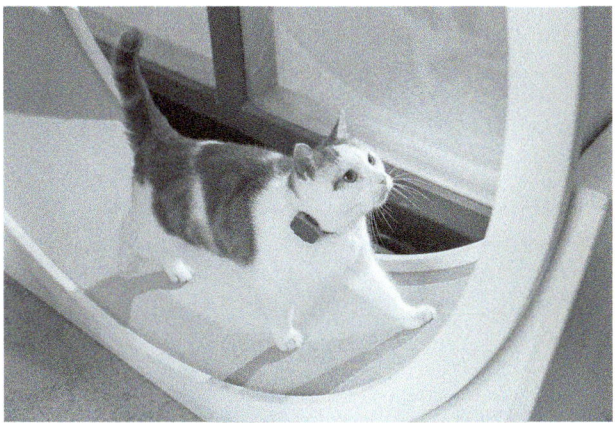

Figure 31.14 Accelerometers attached to a cat's collar may allow for objective measurement of activity data. Source: Mars, Incorporated.

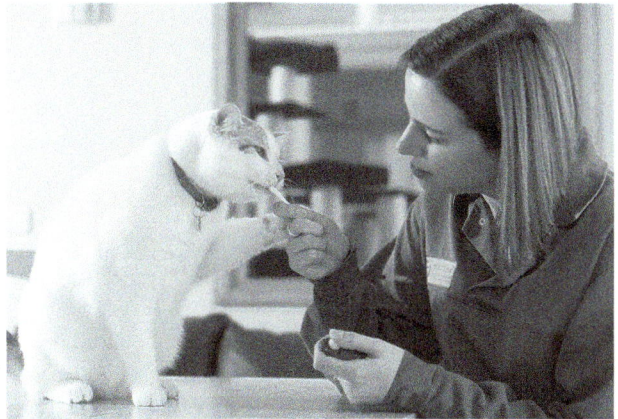

Figure 31.15 Cats can be trained for collection of saliva. Source: Mars, Incorporated.

multiple venepunctures and can reduce stress hyperglycaemia. Local anaesthetic (LA) creams applied to the skin 30–60 min before sample collection can help reduce discomfort associated with venepuncture. Covering the LA with cohesive bandage will discourage cats from ingesting LA cream.

For accurate haematological reference ranges, the laboratory performing the blood analysis should be consulted, as the cat's age, breed and analysis procedure can affect the test specificity and sensitivity. Local regulatory requirements will specify limits to blood volume withdrawal. See Joint Working Group on Refinement (JWGR) (1993) for general guidance.

Urine and faeces

Hydrophobic sand (a biodegradable material with a non-toxic urine-repelling coating) can replace normal litter substrate during the collection period and still allows for normal elimination behaviour of digging and burial. Most cats can be trained to urinate in a clean tray by decreasing the amount of litter until the tray is empty; however, this method does not allow for normal elimination behaviours and may take longer to habituate to. Gradual weaning to new collection protocols will increase acceptance of a new litter provision. A non-invasive collection system whereby urine can be continuously monitored has been described by Markwell and Smith (1993). The outlet of the tray can be connected to a collection vessel outside the individual housing, enabling urine to be collected separately from faeces.

Users should explore the possibilities of these techniques before resorting to invasive collection methods which may severely compromise the welfare of cats. See also section on individual housing.

Other methods for urine collection (cystocentesis, catheterisation, manual transabdominal expression) are unnecessarily invasive, interfere with the cat's normal urination pattern and may be traumatic, particularly when testing is repeated or long term.

Milk

Milk can be manually expressed with some difficulty from lactating queens by gentle massaging of the teats. Oxytocin administered subcutaneously, intramuscularly or transdermally may or may not be used to stimulate milk flow. The queen should ideally remain in the same location as the kittens during collection in order to provide reassurance to both queen and kittens. Samples from each teat are likely to be small (<1 ml) and pressure should not be applied if no milk sample is obtained.

Saliva

Saliva collected via a buccal swab is a less invasive sample collection method than blood collection, especially in young kittens and aggressive cats. Small saliva specimens can be collected using commercially available cotton wool swabs inserted into the cheek pouches and under the tongue of the cats.

Cats can be trained for collection of larger volumes of saliva, using PRT to encourage the cat to chew a cotton bud (Figure 31.15). Once saturated, the cotton bud(s) can be expressed into a collection vessel. The procedure can be repeated for around 10 minutes or before if the cat loses interest.

Administration of substances

Dosing and injection procedures

Most cats will detect drugs mixed in their food and may refuse to eat. To give a tablet, grasp the cat's head from above, at the points where the jaws meet, with forefinger and thumb, tip the head back and press in with thumb and finger (Figure 31.16). Push on the lower jaw with the index finger of the other hand to open the animal's mouth and drop the tablet far back on the middle of the tongue. Push it quickly and gently so it moves over the back of the tongue. Close the mouth and gently stroke the throat to encourage swallowing. Large tablets should be broken into smaller, manageable pieces. When giving liquid medicines, let the liquid run down the tongue drop by drop, allowing the cat to swallow after every two to three drops.

Cats need to be restrained for the application of eye and ear drops. To give ear drops, hold the cat's head to one side and insert the drops to the front of the ear canal, externally

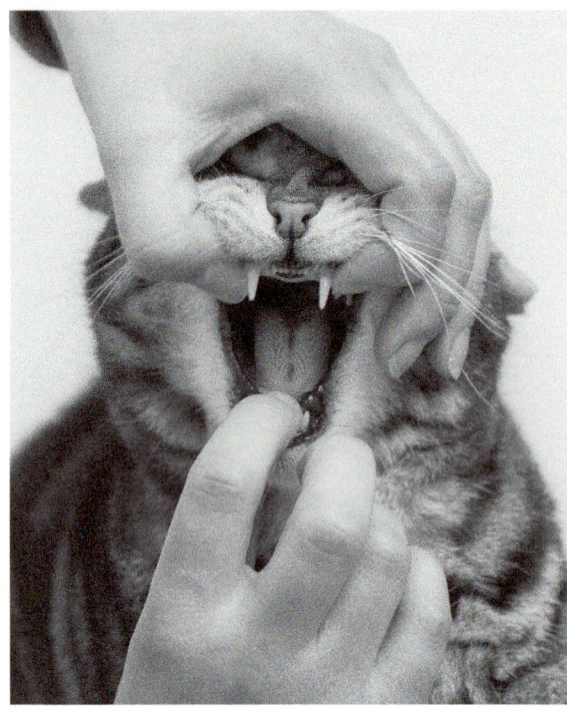

Figure 31.16 Oral dosing technique. Source: Mars, Incorporated.

massaging the ear canal to help the drops penetrate. To give eye drops, hold the cat's head back and open the eye with forefinger and thumb to apply eye drops to the inner corner of the eye. Keep the head back for a while to allow the drops to cover the eye's surface.

Injections are given when the cat is restrained. Subcutaneous injections are usually given into the scruff of the neck, intramuscular injections into the muscle (quadriceps) overlying the femur of the hind leg or, for small volumes, into the paralumbar (epaxial) muscles. Absorption can be accelerated by gentle massage. Cats which require routine subcutaneous injections (e.g. diabetics) can be trained to accept injection without restraint by associating the procedure with a highly palatable food treat.

General advice on the administration of substances can be found in Joint Working Group on Refinement (2001).

Anaesthesia/analgesia

General advice can be found in Feline Anaesthesia and Pain Management (Steagall 2017). Drug regulatory licences will vary between regions and local formulary and data sheets should be consulted for dosage, combination and route of administration, e.g. BSAVA Small Animal Formulary (Ramsey 2017).

Pre-anaesthesia

Fasting is routinely recommended before general anaesthesia to decrease the risk of aspiration. Fasting times are controversial, but it is now accepted that adult cats do not require prolonged fasting (8–12 hours). Fasting for approximately 4–6 hours is suggested. Longer fasting periods have been associated with increased incidence of reflux and gastric acidity. A thorough physical examination prior to any anaesthesia should be performed on each individual cat to detect any potential signs that could require a tailored anaesthetic protocol.

Premedication with a sedative and an analgesic is advisable, even in placid cats. A multimodal anaesthetic approach is currently recommended to help reduce stress during induction, reduce dose of inductive agents, recovery is smoother and analgesia is more effective.

Pain

Pain can be difficult to recognise in cats, as their behavioural responses may not be as overt as in other species. Behaviours indicating pain can be subtle, easily overlooked and there may be individual variation. Several studies have examined the behavioural indicators of pain; these indicators include the inhibition or loss of normal behaviour (such as decreased grooming or failure to eat), the expression of abnormal behaviours such as altered posture or aggression (Waran et al. 2007), and increased touch sensitivity (Taylor & Robertson 2004). Chronic long-term pain, such as that caused by degenerative joint disease, is likely to have a more significant impact on the welfare of cats than is currently recognised. Typical signs of chronic pain include reduced activity, hiding, decreased interest and decreased response to surroundings; there may be inappetence leading to weight loss. Proper assessment of pain in cats will require the development and validation of behaviour-based, multidimensional pain measurement tools. Different tools have been reviewed (Merola & Mills 2016) and are under development (Reid et al. 2017) but there are currently no tools valid for the assessment of both sensorial and emotional aspects of pain applicable to a wide range of situations. A combination of the different tools available is recommended to ensure appropriate pain assessment in cats.

Analgesia

Safe and effective methods of analgesia are now available. Pain should be prevented whenever possible. Pain can be managed more effectively if analgesia is given before the pain occurs, and it is recommended to provide analgesia as part of the premedication protocol. Some analgesics, such as opioids, will not only provide analgesia during surgery and post-operatively, but also help reduce doses of other anaesthetic agents. If a procedure or a disease is known to cause pain in other species, or it seems probable that it might be painful, then analgesia must be given. Animals should be regularly monitored for signs of pain, and additional doses of analgesia provided where necessary.

Pharmacological analgesia is mainly achieved by the following drug groups:

- Opioids
- NSAIDs (non-steroidal anti-inflammatory drugs)
- LAs

Prolonged, effective analgesia is best achieved by using a combination of these drugs with non-pharmaceutical techniques (described in post-anaesthesia section).

Anaesthesia

For procedures lasting 20 minutes or less, or for minor surgery (e.g. suturing small skin wounds), cats are often given intravenous general anaesthetics or heavy sedation with analgesia (e.g. xylazine, dexmedetomidine or ketamine and opioids). It is recommended to always have an intravenous catheter placed, even if no fluid therapy is administered, for easy vein access in case of complications. For longer procedures or major surgery, general anaesthesia is usually induced with intravenous agents (e.g. propofol) and then maintained with a volatile anaesthetic. The preferred route for intravenous administration is into the cephalic vein in the fore leg (using a 0.6 mm or 0.5 mm (23–25G), 16 mm needle). If this is not possible, the injection can be made into the saphenous vein. In order to reduce risk of vascular damage, it is suggested to place an intravenous catheter prior to the anaesthetic administration.

For intubation, a selection of endotracheal tubes, from 3.0–6.0 mm, should be available. Cats have a very sensitive laryngeal reflex. To prevent laryngeal spasm, the larynx is sprayed with 2% lidocaine and the endotracheal tube is lubricated with lidocaine gel. The formulation of some LA sprays can cause laryngeal oedema in cats, and the spray should be checked to ensure it is safe for use in cats. Consideration should be given in allowing enough time for the lidocaine spray application to have effect before intubation (between 60 and 90 seconds). A semi-rigid wire in the lumen of the endotracheal tube or a laryngoscope can facilitate tracheal intubation. The end of the tube should not pass further than the point of the shoulder.

Intravenous agents and dosages

The most common agent used for intravenous induction of anaesthesia in cats is propofol, 10 mg/ml emulsion (2–5 mg/kg IV for a pre-medicated cat).

Inhaled agents

Most common inhalation agents include:

- Isoflurane: the minimum alveolar concentration required to maintain surgical anaesthesia in 50% of cats is 1.6% (BSAVA Small Animal Formulary 2017).
- Sevoflurane: the minimum alveolar concentration required to maintain surgical anaesthesia in 50% of cats is 2.5% (BSAVA Small Animal Formulary 2017).

Nitrous oxide (N_2O) can be used in combination with oxygen (minimum of 30%) to carry volatile anaesthetic agents. N_2O reduces the concentration if inhalant required to maintain anaesthesia.

Anaesthetic protocol – best practice

A best practice protocol for routine surgery should include: a sedative (e.g. dexmedetomidine or acepromazine), an opioid (e.g. buprenorphine, or butorphanol), an induction agent (e.g. propofol) and a local anaesthetic into the wound (e.g. lidocaine). Depending on the surgery, an NSAID administration could be given pre- or intra-operatively. The anaesthesia should be monitored at all times by measuring vital signs (e.g. heart rate, respiration rate, temperature, blood pressure, oxygen saturation and pCO_2).

Post-anaesthesia

A variety of non-pharmaceutical techniques can be used to create the optimum conditions in the cat's external and internal environments. Cats should be allowed to recover from anaesthesia in a quiet warm room. Thermoregulation may be compromised after anaesthesia and rectal temperature should be checked regularly. They should be nursed on soft bedding and kept clean and comfortable. A semi-enclosed box or high-sided soft bed where the cat can feel secure and still be monitored can be useful. Cats that are used to contact with humans can be given plenty of reassuring verbal and physical contact. Frightening noise and smells should be excluded from the recovery area. Any painful tissues should be immobilised using splints or bandages. The cat should be carefully monitored throughout the post-anaesthesia recovery period, as it is during this time that complications are most likely to occur (Robertson et al. 2018). Provision of food and water post-anaesthesia should be monitored to ensure the swallowing reflex is functioning.

Euthanasia

Euthanasia should be performed in a dignified manner, minimising any mental or physical suffering to the cat. The method of choice is injection of an anaesthetic agent sufficient to cause rapid unconsciousness and a certain death. A common method is to give a high overdose (about 200 mg/kg) of pentobarbital by intravenous injection. This results in an immediate loss of consciousness, rapidly followed by deep narcosis and respiratory and cardiac arrest. The cat dies within a few seconds apparently without pain or distress. If a cat is difficult to handle or is stressed, it may benefit from being sedated before being euthanised; in these cases, the standard anaesthetic protocol and dosage can be followed. In the UK, death must always be confirmed by the permanent cessation of circulation, the onset of rigor mortis or various other methods[11]. See also Chapter 17: Euthanasia and other fates for laboratory animals.

Common welfare problems

Disease

This section summarises the diseases that most commonly threaten laboratory cats. More detailed reviews are provided by Chandler et al. (2007); Sherding (2008); King and Boag (2007); Miller and Zawistowski (2013). Cats can carry zoonotic diseases that may be a risk to people (reviewed by Greene & Levy 2006).

---

[11]Home Office. 2014. Guidance on the Operation of the Animals (Scientific Procedures) Act 1986. London, UK: Home Office. https://www.gov.uk/government/publications/operation-of-aspa (accessed 31 October 2019)

Prophylaxis

Cats are susceptible to a number of viral, bacterial and parasitic diseases. Colony cats can be vaccinated as early as 4–6 weeks of age against feline viral rhinotracheitis, feline calicivirus and feline infectious enteritis (Day et al. 2016). Rabies vaccine is required in some countries. Closed colonies are unlikely to be exposed to FeLV and FIV. Cats entering the colony should be treated to eliminate all internal and external parasites; in a closed colony reinfestation is unlikely and the higher risk comes from personnel or new arrivals. For new animals entering the colony, a quarantine of at least three weeks is recommended. In cases of serology testing, cats may be required to be SPF, unvaccinated and free of various feline pathogens. Antibody titre in these cats should be routinely monitored.

Signs of disease

A cat's behaviour and appearance reflect its state of health. A healthy cat will have an alert bearing and move easily and confidently about its accommodation. It will be interested in its surroundings and its food, and groom frequently. It will have clean ears, eyes, mouth and skin. Animals that show any deviations from these signs should be observed and examined carefully to investigate the cause. Any cat exhibiting sneezing, watery lacrimation, purulent discharges from eyes, nose or ears, excessive salivation, respiratory signs, vomiting or diarrhoea should be isolated immediately.

Viral diseases

Feline immunodeficiency virus (FIV)

FIV is a lentivirus that shares many characteristics of other lentiviruses, such as human immunodeficiency virus. FIV is transmitted primarily by parenteral inoculation of virus present in saliva or blood, via bite and fight wounds. This accounts for the higher prevalence of the virus in adult male cats. Occasional transmission of virus *in utero* and post parturition via the milk may occur. FIV infection progresses through several stages: an acute phase; a clinically asymptomatic phase of variable duration and a terminal phase of infection often referred to as feline acquired immunodeficiency syndrome (Sellon & Hartmann 2006). The hallmark of FIV pathogenesis is progressive disruption of normal immune function. During the last stages of infection, clinical signs are often a reflection of opportunistic infections, neoplasia, myelosuppression and neurological disease. However, with proper care some FIV-infected cats can live for many years with a good quality of life, and may die in old age from causes unrelated to FIV infection. Diagnosis of FIV infection is made most commonly by detection of FIV-specific antibodies in blood by either enzyme-linked immunosorbent assay (ELISA) or rapid immunomigration-type assays (Sellon & Hartmann 2006).

FIV vaccines are available commercially; because the vaccine contains whole virus, cats respond to vaccination by producing antibodies that are indistinguishable from those produced during natural infection; however, recently validated polymerase chain reaction (PCR) diagnostics can differentiate infected vs vaccinated animals.

Feline leukaemia virus (FeLV)

FeLV is a retrovirus and member of the Oncornavirus subfamily and causes clinical illness related to the haemopoeitic and immune systems and neoplasia. FeLV spreads between susceptible cats primarily via saliva, where virus concentration is higher than in plasma.

Vertical transmission can also occur: kittens can be infected transplacentally or when the queen licks and nurses them. Susceptibility to infection is highest in young kittens. The outcome of FeLV infection mainly depends on immune status and age of the cat, but is also affected by virus pathogenicity, infection pressure and virus concentration. Guidelines for testing cats for FeLV have been published (Day et al. 2016). While persistently viraemic cats have a decreased life expectancy, treatments for the many clinical syndromes that accompany infection are available. FeLV vaccines are available but only FeLV-negative cats should be vaccinated. FeLV testing must be performed to ensure negative results prior to vaccination. In 1991, an increased incidence of tumours in cats that developed at injection sites was first reported in the United States. This observation was connected to an increased use of rabies and FeLV vaccinations. As a consequence, these tumours were first called feline 'vaccine-associated sarcomas'. However, the subsequent finding that other, non-vaccinal injectables can also cause this type of tumour has led to reclassification of these neoplasms as feline injection-site sarcomas (FiSSs). Guidelines are available to prevent and manage FiSSs in cats (Hartmann et al. 2015).

Feline infectious peritonitis (FIP)

Feline coronavirus (FCoV) exists as two pathotypes, and FCoV spike gene mutations are considered responsible for the pathotypic switch in feline infectious peritonitis (FIP) pathogenesis (Felten et al. 2017). According to the internal mutation hypothesis, FIP virus emerges from feline enteric coronavirus (FECV) by spontaneous mutations within an infected cat. FCoV is particularly prevalent in multi-cat households or where cats are kept in crowded conditions.

Transmission is primarily indirect through contact with virus-containing faeces or fomites, for example contaminated litter trays. Two basic forms of FIP, effusive (wet) and non-effusive (dry), are recognised. Approximately half the cats with FIP are less than 2 years of age, although all age groups can be affected (Addie & Jarrett 2006). The risk factors for FIP development are age and crowding, with young cats in crowded catteries being most at risk. It is considered that good husbandry and low stress levels are particularly important in controlling FIP mutations. When establishing a colony, a decision must be made on whether to focus on FIP or the coronavirus family. If it is the broader family, then the goal should be to maintain the cats free of antibodies to coronaviruses. This would require a different level of surveillance and then the use of vaccines. An intranasal vaccine, given to cats over 16 weeks of age, has been developed but it is not effective if the cat has already been exposed to the virus. Definitive diagnosis of FIP is by post-mortem examination or by using DNA sequencing to detect FIP virus peritoneal fluid or tissue biopsy. Serology and RT-PCR assay results cannot differentiate between FECV and FIP (Miller & Zawistowski 2013).

Feline panleukopenia (FPV)

Feline panleukopenia is a parvovirus; it is shed in all body secretions during acute stages of disease, but mainly in the vomitus and faeces. It has a short shedding period but long survival in the environment (Greene & Addie 2006), where it is resistant to heat and to many disinfectants. FPV is a highly infectious disease with a high mortality rate. The virus is usually transmitted by indirect contact of susceptible animals with contaminated premises; *in utero* transmission does occur, and may cause early foetal death and resorption or result in the birth of live kittens with varying degrees of neurological damage. Subclinical cases of infection, more common in older cats, may go unrecognised, while severe clinical illness is the rule in young kittens; sudden death may occur. A presumptive diagnosis is usually made based on clinical signs and the presence of leukopenia. With appropriate symptomatic therapy and nursing care, cats may recover from infection. Vaccination has been very effective at reducing the incidence of this disease and guidelines are available (Day *et al*. 2016).

Feline viral upper respiratory infection (cat 'flu')

Between 85% and 90% of cases are caused by either feline herpesvirus (which causes feline viral rhinotracheitis) or feline calicivirus. Feline herpesvirus (FHV) generally causes more severe disease than feline calicivirus (FCV). The viruses are shed mainly in ocular, nasal and dosing secretions, and transmission is largely by direct contact from infected to susceptible cat. After FHV infection, virtually all recovered cats become latently infected carriers, with intermittent episodes of virus shedding, particularly after periods of stress. Most cats can shed FCV for more than 30 days post recovery, and some cats will shed it for life (carrier state).

Primary bacterial pathogens affecting the feline respiratory tract

Bordetella bronchiseptica is also recognised as a primary pathogen to the feline respiratory tract, although its precise contribution to disease in the field is not yet fully established (Gaskell *et al*. 2006). Only intranasal vaccines are available for cats and is only recommended if there is evidence of clinical Bordetella infection in the colony (Day *et al*. 2016).

Chlamydophila felis, formerly known as *Chlamydia psittaci*, is a primary cause of conjunctivitis in cats housed in catteries. Ophthalmic ointments containing chloramphenicol are usually an effective treatment. Vaccines are available and recommended if there is presence of disease within the colony.

Mycoplasma spp. are bacteria occasionally associated with ocular and respiratory symptoms in cats. Some species are non-pathogenic and some cats are sub clinically infected. Diagnosis can be achieved by culturing ocular or nasal swabs on a special media. Treatment with systemic antibiotics following sensitivity tests on the culture are recommended and are usually effective.

Injuries

Potential injuries in a laboratory setting include accidental ingestion of hazardous, non-food materials such as chemicals or toys and trauma as a result of inter-cat aggression. See 'hygiene' section for methods to minimise the risk of environmental injury. Opportunities to reduce conspecific aggression are described in 'group housing'.

Stress and Abnormal behaviour

Abnormal behaviours can be a good indicator of stress in cats; however, behavioural inhibition is also a common response of cats with chronic stress and is easy to miss unless detailed observation is made of the cat (McCune 1992). If the stress experienced is brief, mild and infrequent, it is unlikely to impact significantly on the cat's overall well-being and ability to cope. However, if a negative experience is severe, prolonged or repeated, suffering can occur. Specific problems associated with confinement include boredom, aggression, fearfulness, behavioural inhibition, depression-like inactivity, escape behaviour, hiding, poor reproductive success, anorexia, weight loss, tail chasing, stereotypies, fabric eating, inappropriate elimination and self-injurious behaviours (reviewed in McCune 1995b). Behaviours should be contextualised, for example, an undesirable behaviour such as urine spraying may be deemed a more acceptable behaviour for a human-owned cat with free access to outdoors; however, this behaviour can be problematic in a laboratory setting. Prevention of stress in the confined cat may be achieved by selective breeding of the most suitable individuals; an investment of time and effort in the early development phase of kittens and maintaining a varied and stimulating environment which offers the cat choices. All these approaches have been discussed in this chapter.

Stress responses and thresholds will vary between individual cats and their relationship with their environment. As such, the subjective state of the cat should be measured from the individual's perspective (Scott *et al*. 2007). Regular physiological and behavioural observations can help identify emotional state, early signs of stress and compromised welfare. Feline specific ethograms have been described by Bradshaw *et al*. (1995) and Stanton *et al*. (2015). A Cat Stress Score has been developed by Kessler and Turner (1997).

Feline pheromones

Pheromones are chemicals contained in bodily fluids such as urine, sweat and mucus, which can be used to chemically signal between cats (Ley 2016). A range of pheromones have been isolated from feline facial secretions (Mills 2005), and two fractions are available commercially; F3 as an environmental spray or diffuser and F4 as a human topical hand spray.

The F3 fraction is believed to help reduce stress associated with environmental changes such as adaptation to new environments, transportation and unpredictable noise (DePorter 2016). It has been shown to have a beneficial effect in the treatment of behavioural problems such as urine spraying (Mills *et al*. 2011) and territorial scratching. Application in a laboratory setting could be to support integration of feline populations to each other or to a new environment.

The F4 fraction is believed to facilitate social interactions between people and cats by improving familiarity. It may be useful in situations whereby cats require introduction to unfamiliar people such as during a veterinary examination.

Monitoring welfare

Cumulative experience and Quality of Life (QoL)

Scientific requirements can affect the welfare of an animal over its lifetime. Procedural severity, intensity, duration, frequency and type as well as all aspects of health, welfare and care can be considered as cumulative experiences. Measures to determine the effect of cumulative experiences could present opportunities to predict, identify and minimise potential causes of suffering in individuals. Examples of methods to classify and report severity experienced by animals used in scientific procedures have been described by Honess & Wolfensohn (2010); Smith *et al.* (2018).

QoL measures are widely used in human medicine and this concept is starting to be adapted to assess the emotional state of companion animals (Kiddie & Collins 2014). Objective assessment of resource and animal-based measures can indicate whether physical, environmental, nutritional, behavioural and social needs are met to provide a holistic QoL assessment. A validated tool for use by caregivers to monitor a cat's QoL over time or to compare QoL between different housing and husbandry management practices would be beneficial in a confined setting, where the cat is less likely to have opportunities to perform species-typical behaviours and form stable social groupings. Such a tool could also support a cumulative experience assessment. A feline health-related quality-of-life tool exists (Noble *et al.* 2019); however, at the time of writing there is no published, validated feline QoL tool which encompasses multiple welfare aspects (such as health, environmental and management).

Quality of staff

As caregivers, laboratory staff have a responsibility to promote, demonstrate and be accountable for a culture of care within their facility and wider communities; ensuring animals are treated with respect. See also RSPCA & LASA[12]; Klein and Bayne (2007). Competent, trained staff are an essential pre-requisite for enabling quality science, who comply with ethical and legal requirements and safeguard the welfare of animals. Humane training and care will deliver more confident, cooperative and manageable animals who are better for research purposes (Poole 1997). Staff should be encouraged to continue professional development, education and training in cats and laboratory animal science to ensure the science is of the highest quality and the individual cat's physiological and psychological needs are met. See also Chapter 14: Attaining competence in the care of animals used in research.

Care of aged animals

A range of physiological and behavioural conditions are recognised in older cats. Common medical conditions associated with ageing include renal disease, dental disease, hyperthyroidism, diabetes mellitus and osteoarthritis. Sensory loss of hearing and eyesight may be evident and signs of cognitive dysfunction may include disorientation, altered interaction with others, sleep problems, increased vocalisation, house soiling and reduction of appetite. Resting and sleeping can be increased, and coat condition may deteriorate due to lack of grooming.

It is essential that care staff recognise pain and signs of ageing in order to modify the environment and husbandry methods. The environment should be more suited to the older cat by providing lower and accessible resources such as comfortable resting, litter and scratch areas. Age-appropriate play and increased social contact will stimulate and maintain mental processes. Increased health checks and grooming can aid early identification of illness. Meals should be little and often, tailored for digestibility, palatability, nutritional requirement and dentition. See also Chapter 16: 3Rs considerations when using ageing animals in science.

Homing

Cats no longer required for research purposes can be assessed for suitability for homing into a domestic setting. Cats can adapt very well to a home environment and become highly valued family members (DiGangi *et al.* 2006). To maximise homing success, a homing programme can be initiated to acclimatise the cat to home life experiences. Homed cats should be indoor-only cats or very gradually introduced to the outdoors. Cats with severe health or behavioural issues should be assessed before being considered as a suitable candidate for homing. An alternative retirement solution to homing can be a separate facility which is optimally designed for the life stage and lifestyle of the cats.

Acknowledgements

The author would like to thank Dr Heidi Anderson, Dr Anne-Marie Bakke, Dr Adria Martorell and Dr John Rawlings for their technical contributions. This chapter was revised from The Domestic Cat by Dr Sandra McCune in *The UFAW Handbook on the Care and Management of Laboratory Animals*, eighth edition.

---

[12]RSPCA and LASA, 2015, Guiding Principles on Good Practice for Animal Welfare and Ethical Review Bodies. A report by the RSPCA Research Animals Department and LASA Education, Training and Ethics Section. (M. Jennings ed.) http://www.lasa.co.uk/PDF/AWERB_Guiding_Principles_2015_final.pdf (accessed 31 October 2019)

References

Addie, D.D., Boucraut-Baralon, C., Egberink, H. *et al.* (2015) Disinfectant choices in veterinary practices, shelters and households: ABCD guidelines on safe and effective disinfection for feline environments. *Journal of Feline Medicine and Surgery*, **17**, 594–605.

Addie, D. and Jarrett, O. (2006) Feline coronavirus infections. In: *Infectious Diseases of the Dog and Cat*, 3rd edn. Ed. Greene, C., pp. 88–102. Elsevier Inc, St. Louis, Missouri.

Allaway, D., Gilham, M., Colyer, A. et al. (2017) The impact of time of neutering on weight gain and energy intake in female kittens. *Journal of Nutritional Science*, **6**, e19, 1–4.

Balcombe, J.P., Barnard, N.D. and Sandusky, C. (2004) Laboratory routines cause animal stress. *Contemporary Topics in Laboratory Animal Science*, **43**, 42–51.

Barry, K.J. and Crowell-Davis, S.L. (1999) Gender differences in the social behavior of the neutered indoor-only domestic cat. *Applied Animal Behaviour Science*, **64**, 193–211.

Bassett, L. and Buchanan-Smith, H.M. (2007) Effects of predictability on the welfare of captive animals. *Applied Animal Behaviour Science*, **102**, 223–245.

Bates, N. and Edwards, N. (2015) Benzalkonium chloride exposure in cats: a retrospective analysis of 245 cases reported to the Veterinary Poisons Information Service (VPIS). *Veterinary Record*, **176**, 229–229.

Beaver, B.V. (2003) *Feline Behaviour: A Guide for Veterinarians*, 2nd edn. Saunders, St. Louis, Missouri.

Bengsen, A., Algar, D., Ballard, G. et al. (2016) Feral cat home-range size varies predictably with landscape productivity and population density. *Journal of Zoology*, **298**, 112–120.

Bermingham, E.N., Thomas, D.G., Morris, P.J. et al. (2010) Energy requirements of adult cats. *The British Journal of Nutrition*, **103**, 1083–1093.

Bernstein, P.L. and Strack, M. (1996) A game of cat and house: spatial patterns and behavior of 14 domestic cats (*Felis catus*) in the home. *Anthrozoos*, **9**, 25–39.

Bonanni, R., Cafazzo, S., Fantini, C. et al. (2007) Feeding-order in an urban feral domestic cat colony: relationship to dominance rank, sex and age. *Animal Behaviour*, **74**, 1369–1379.

Bourgeois, H., Elliot, D., Marniquet, P. et al. (2004) *Dietary Preferences of Dogs and Cats*. Focus Special Edition Royal Canin Paris.

Bradshaw, J.W.S. (1992) *The Behaviour of the Domestic Cat*. CAB International, Wallingford.

Bradshaw, J.W.S., Brown, S.L., Cook, S.E. et al. (1995) An ethogram for behavioural studies of the domestic cat (*Felis silvestris catus L.*). Universities Federation for Animal Welfare (UFAW), UK.

Bradshaw, J.W.S. and Ellis, S.E. (2016) *The Trainable Cat*. Basic Books, New York.

Bradshaw, J.W.S. and Hall, S.L. (1999) Affiliative behaviour of related and unrelated pairs of cats in catteries: a preliminary report. *Applied Animal Behaviour Science*, **63**, 251–255.

Bradshaw, J.W.S. and Holloran, D. (2005) Effects of air transportation on behavioural signs of stress in cats. *BSAVA Congress 2005: Scientific proceedings: 48th Annual Congress*, 7th–10th April 2005, ICC/NIA Birmingham UK.

Broom, D.M. and Johnson, K.G. (1993) *Stress and Animal Welfare*, 1st edn. Chapman & Hall, London.

British Small Animal Veterinary Association (2017) *Small Animal Formulary Part A: Canine and Feline, British Small Animal Veterinary Association*, 9th edn, Ed. Ian Ramsey. BSAVA, Gloucester.

Casey, R.A. and Bradshaw, J.W.S. (2008) The effects of additional socialisation for kittens in a rescue centre on their behaviour and suitability as a pet. *Applied Animal Behaviour Science*, **114**, 196–205.

Chandler, E.A., Gaskell, C.J. and Gaskell, R.M. (2007) *Feline Medicine and Therapeutics*, 3rd edn. Blackwell Publishing, Oxford.

Crowell-Davis, S.L., Barry, K. and Wolfe, R. (1997) Social behavior and aggressive problems of cats. *The Veterinary Clinics of North America: Small Animal Practice*, **27**, 549–568.

Crowell-Davis, S.L., Curtis, T.M. and Knowles, R.J. (2004) Social organization in the cat: a modern understanding. *Journal of Feline Medicine and Surgery*, **6**, 19–28.

Damasceno, J. and Genaro, G. (2014) Dynamics of the access of captive domestic cats to a feed environmental enrichment item. *Applied Animal Behaviour Science*, **151**, 67–74.

Dantas-Divers, L.M.S., Crowell-Davis, S. L., Alford, K. et al. (2011) Agonistic behavior and environmental enrichment of cats communally housed in a shelter. *Journal of the American Veterinary Medical Association*, **239**, 796–802.

David, V.A., Menotti-Raymond, M., Wallace, A.C. et al. (2014) Endogenous retrovirus insertion in the KIT oncogene determines white and white spotting in domestic cats. *G3 (Bethesda, Md.)*, **4**, 1881–1891.

Day, M.J., Horzinek, M.C., Schultz, R.D. et al. (2016) WSAVA Guidelines for the vaccination of dogs and cats. *The Journal of Small Animal Practice*, **57**, 4–8.

DePorter, T.L. (2016) Use of pheromones in feline practice (chapter 18). In: *Feline Behavioral Health and Welfare*. Eds Rodan, I. and Heath, S., pp. 235–244. W.B. Saunders, St. Louis.

Desforges, E.J., Moesta, A. and Farnworth, M.J. (2016) Effect of a shelf-furnished screen on space utilisation and social behaviour of indoor group-housed cats. *Applied Animal Behaviour Science*, **178**, 60–68.

DiGangi, B.A., Crawford, P.C. and Levy, J.K. (2006) Outcome of cats adopted from a biomedical research programme. *Journal of Applied Animal Welfare Science*, **9**, 143–163.

Driscoll, C.A., Menotti-Raymond, M., Roca, A.L. et al. (2007) The Near Eastern origin of cat domestication. *Science (New York, N.Y.)*, **317**, 519–523.

Ellis, S.L., Rodan, I., Carney, H.C. et al. (2013) AAFP and ISFM feline environmental needs guidelines. *Journal of Feline Medicine and Surgery*, **15**, 219–230.

European Commission (2007) Commission recommendations of 18 June 2007 on guidelines for the accommodation and care of animals used for experimental and other scientific purposes. Annex II to European Council Directive 86/609. See 2007/526/EC.

Felten, S., Leutenegger, C.M., Balzer, H.J. et al. (2017) Sensitivity and specificity of a real-time reverse transcriptase polymerase chain reaction detecting feline coronavirus mutations in effusion and serum/plasma of cats to diagnose feline infectious peritonitis. *BMC Veterinary Research*, **13**, 228.

Finkler, H., Gunther, I. and Terkel, J. (2011) Behavioral differences between urban feeding groups of neutered and sexually intact free-roaming cats following a trap-neuter-return procedure. *Journal of the American Veterinary Medical Association*, **238**, 1141–1149.

Gaskell, R.M., Dawson, S. and Radford, A. (2006) Feline respiratory disease. In: *Infectious Diseases of the Dog and Cat*, 3rd edn. Ed. Greene, C., pp. 145–153. Elsevier Inc, St. Louis, Missouri.

Greene, C.E. and Addie, D. (2006) Feline parvovirus infection. In: *Infectious Diseases of the Dog and Cat*, 3rd edn. Ed. Greene C.E., pp. 78–87. Elsevier Inc, St. Louis, Missouri.

Greene, C.E. and Levy, J.K. (2006) Immunocompromised people and shared human and animal infections: zoonoses, sapronoses, and anthroponoses. *Infectious Diseases of the Dog and Cat*, 3rd edn. Ed. Greene, C., pp. 1051–1068. Elsevier Inc, St. Louis, Missouri.

Griffin, B. and Hume, K.R. (2006) Recognition and Management of Stress in Housed Cats (chapter 76). In: *Consultations in Feline Internal Medicine*, 5th edn. Ed. August, J.R., pp. 717–734. W.B. Saunders, Saint Louis.

Gruen, M.E., Alfaro-Cordoba, M., Thomson, A.E. et al. (2017) The use of functional data analysis to evaluate activity in a spontaneous model of degenerative joint disease associated pain in cats. *PLoS One*, **12**, e0169576.

Gruen, M.E., Thomson, A.E., Clary, G.P. et al. (2013) Conditioning laboratory cats to handling and transport. *Laboratory Animals*, 385.

Hand, M.S., Thatcher, C.D., Remillard, R.L. et al. (2010) *Small Animal Clinical Nutrition*, 5th edn. Mark Morris Institute, Topeka, KS, USA.

Hartmann, K., Day, M.J., Thiry, E. et al. (2015) Feline injection-site sarcoma: ABCD guidelines on prevention and management. *Journal of Feline Medicine and Surgery*, **17**, 606–613.

Hawthorne, A.J., Loveridge, G.G. and Horrocks, L.J. (1995) Housing design and husbandry management to minimise transmission of disease in multi-cat facilities. In: *Cats on the Capital. Proceedings of 1995 Symposium on Feline Infectious Disease*, pp. 97–107. American Association of Feline Practitioners Academy of Feline Medicine, Washington, DC.

Heath, S. and Wilson, C. (2014) Canine and feline enrichment in the home and kennel: a guide for practitioners. *The Veterinary Clinics of North America. Small Animal Practice*, **44**, 427–449.

Herron, M.E. and Shreyer, T. (2014) The pet-friendly veterinary practice: A guide for practitioners. *Veterinary Clinics of North America: Small Animal Practice*, **44**, 451–481.

Hewson-Hughes, A.K., Colyer, A., Simpson, S.J. et al. (2016) Balancing macronutrient intake in a mammalian carnivore: disentangling the influences of flavour and nutrition. *Royal Society Open Science*, **3**, 160081.

Home Office (2014) *Code of Practice for the Housing and Care of Animals Bred, Supplied or Used for Scientific Purposes*. OGL, London, UK.

Johnson, A.K. (2018) Assisted reproduction in the female cat. *Veterinary Clinics of North America: Small Animal Practice*, **48**, 523–531.

Johnson, G. (1991) *The Bengal Cat*. Greenwell Springs, LA: Gogees Cattery.

Joint Working Group on Refinement (1993) Removal of blood from laboratory mammals and birds. First report of the BVA/FRAME/RSPCA/UFAW Joint Working Group on Refinement. *Laboratory Animals*, **27**, 1–22.

Joint Working Group on Refinement (2001) Refining procedures for the administration of substances. Report of the BVAAWF/FRAME/RSPCA/UFAW Joint Working Group on Refinement. *Laboratory Animals*, **35**, 1–41.

Joyce, A. and Yates, D. (2011) Help stop teenage pregnancy!: Early-age neutering in cats. *Journal of Feline Medicine & Surgery*, **13**, 3–10.

Karsh, E.B. and Turner, D.C. (1988) The human-cat relationship. In: *The Domestic Cat: the Biology of its Behaviour*, pp. 159–177. Cambridge University Press, Cambridge.

Kasanen, I.H.E., Sørensen, D.B., Forkman, B. et al. (2010) Ethics of feeding: The omnivore dilemma. *Animal Welfare*, **19**, 37–44.

Kessler, M.R. and Turner, D.C. (1997) Stress and adaptation of cats (*Felis silvestris catus*) housed singly, in pairs and in groups in boarding catteries. *Animal Welfare*, **6**, 243–254.

Kiddie, J.L. and Collins, L.M. (2014) Development and validation of a quality of life assessment tool for use in kennelled dogs (*Canis familiaris*). *Applied Animal Behaviour Science*, **158**, 57–68.

King, L.G. and Boag, A. (2007) *Manual of Canine and Feline Emergency and Critical Care*, 2nd edn. British Small Animal Veterinary Association, Gloucester.

Klein, H.J. and Bayne, K.A. (2007) Establishing a culture of care, conscience, and responsibility: addressing the improvement of scientific discovery and animal welfare through science-based performance standards. *ILAR Journal*, **48**, 3–11.

Knowles, R.J., Curtis, T.M. and Crowell-Davis, S.L. (2004) Correlation of dominance as determined by agonistic interactions with feeding order in cats. *American Journal of Veterinary Research*, **65**, 1548–1556.

Kry, K. and Casey, R. (2007) The effect of hiding enrichment on stress levels and behaviour of domestic cats (*Felis sylvestris catus*) in a shelter setting and the implications for adoption potential. *Animal Welfare*, **16**, 375–383.

Laflamme, D. and Gunn-Moore, D. (2014) Nutrition of aging cats. *Veterinary Clinics of North America: Small Animal Practice*, **44**, 761–774.

Larsen, J.A. (2017) Risk of obesity in the neutered cat. *Journal of Feline Medicine and Surgery*, **19**, 779–783.

Ley, J.M. (2016) Feline communication (chapter 3). In: *Feline Behavioral Health and Welfare*. Eds Rodan, I. and Heath, S.W.B., pp. 24–33. Saunders, St. Louis.

Lipinski, M.J., Froenicke, L., Baysac, K.C. et al. (2008) The ascent of cat breeds: genetic evaluations of breeds and worldwide randombred populations. *Genomics*, **91**, 12–21.

Loveridge, G.G. (1986) Body weight changes and energy intakes of cats during gestation and lactation. *Animal Technology and Welfare*, **37**, 7–15,.

Loveridge, G.G., Horrocks, L.J. and Hawthorne, A.J. (1995) Environmentally enriched housing for cats when housed singly. *Animal Welfare*, **4(2)**, 135–141.

Markwell, P.J. and Smith, B.H.E. (1993) An effective urine pH monitoring system for cats. *Animal Technology*, **44**, 239–245.

McCune, S. (1992) *Temperament and the Welfare of Caged Cats*. University of Cambridge, Cambridge, UK.

McCune, S. (1995a) The impact of paternity and early socialisation on the development of cats' behaviour to people and novel objects. *Applied Animal Behaviour Science*, **45**, 111–126.

McCune, S. (1995b) Environmental enrichment for the laboratory cat. *Environmental Enrichment Information Resources for Laboratory Animals: Birds, Cats, Dogs, Farm Animals, Ferrets, Rabbits, and Rodents*, AWIC Resources Series No. 2, Animal Welfare Information Centre/Universities Federation for Animal Welfare, Maryland.

McCune, S., McPherson, J.A. and Bradshaw, J.W.S. (1995) Avoiding problems: the importance of socialization. In: *The Waltham Book of Human–Animal Interaction: Benefits and Responsibilities of Pet Ownership*. Ed. Robinson, I., pp. 71–86. Pergamon Press, Oxford.

Merola, I. and Mills, D.S. (2016) Systematic review of the behavioural assessment of pain in cats. *Journal of Feline Medicine and Surgery*, **18**, 60–76.

Miller, L. and Zawistowski, S. (Eds) (2013) *Shelter Medicine for Veterinarians and Staff*. Wiley, UK.

Mills, D. (2005) Pheromonatherapy: theory and applications. In: *Practice*, 2005, v.27, no.7, pp. 368–373.

Mills, D.S., Redgate, S.E. and Landsberg, G.M. (2011) A meta-analysis of studies of treatments for feline urine spraying. *PLoS One*, **6**, e18448.

Mitsuhashi, Y., Chamberlin, A.J., Bigley, K.E. et al. (2011) Maintenance energy requirement determination of cats after spaying. *British Journal of Nutrition*, **106**(S1), S135–S138.

Moody, C., Picketts, V.A., Mason, G. et al. (2018) Can you handle it? Validating negative responses to restraint in cats. *Applied Animal Behaviour Science*, **204**, 94–100.

Morris, J.G. (2002) Idiosyncratic nutrient requirements of cats appear to be diet-induced evolutionary adaptations. *Nutrition Research Reviews*, **15**, 153–168.

Mostl, K., Egberink, H., Addie, D. et al. (2013) Prevention of infectious diseases in cat shelters: ABCD guidelines. *Journal of Feline Medicine and Surgery*, **15**, 546–554.

National Research Council (2006) *Nutrient Requirements of Dogs and Cats*. The National Academies Press, Washington, DC.

National Research Council, U.S. (2011) *Guide for the Care and Use of Laboratory Animals*. National Academies Press, Washington, DC.

Natoli, E. and De Vito, E. (1991) Agonistic behaviour, dominance rank and copulatory success in a large multi-male feral cat, *Felis catus* L., colony in central Rome. *Animal Behaviour*, **42**, 227–241.

Noakes, D.E., Parkinson, T.J. and England, G.C.W. (Eds) (2018) *Veterinary Reproduction & Obstetrics*, 10th edn. Saunders Ltd, Edinburgh, Scotland.

Noble, C.E., Wiseman-Orr, L.M., Scott, M.E. et al. (2019) Development, initial validation and reliability testing of a web-based, generic feline health-related quality-of-life instrument. *Journal of Feline Medicine and Surgery*, **21(2)**, 84–94.

O'Neill, D.G., Church, D.B., McGreevy, P.D. et al. (2015) Longevity and mortality of cats attending primary care veterinary practices in England. *Journal of Feline Medicine and Surgery*, **17**, 125–133.

Ottoni, C., Van Neer, W., De Cupere, B. et al. (2017) The palaeogenetics of cat dispersal in the ancient world. *Nature Ecology & Evolution*, **1**, 0139.

Overall, K.L. and Dyer, D. (2005) Enrichment strategies for laboratory animals from the viewpoint of clinical veterinary behavioral medicine: emphasis on cats and dogs. *ILAR Journal*, **46**, 202–216.

Overley, B., Shofer, F.S., Goldschmidt, M.H. *et al.* (2005) Association between Ovariohysterectomy and Feline Mammary Carcinoma. *Journal of Veterinary Internal Medicine*, **19**, 560–563.

Plantinga, E.A., Bosch, G. and Hendriks, W.H. (2011) Estimation of the dietary nutrient profile of free-roaming feral cats: possible implications for nutrition of domestic cats. *The British Journal of Nutrition*, **106**(Suppl. 1), S35–48.

Poole, T. (1997) Happy animals make good science. *Laboratory Animals*, **31**, 116–124.

Pozza, M.E., Stella, J.L., Chappuis-Gagnon, A. *et al.* (2008) Pinch-induced behavioral inhibition ('clipnosis') in domestic cats. *Journal of Feline Medicine and Surgery*, **10**, 82–87.

Pratsch, L., Mohr, N., Palme, R. *et al.* (2018) Carrier training cats reduces stress on transport to a veterinary practice. *Applied Animal Behaviour Science*, **206**, 64–74.

Ramsey, I.K. (Ed.) (2017) *BSAVA Small Animal Formulary, Part A: Canine and Feline*, 9th edn. BSAVA.

Reid, J., Scott, E.M., Calvo, G. *et al.* (2017). Definitive Glasgow acute pain scale for cats: validation and intervention level. *Veterinary Record*, **180**, 449–449.

Robertson, S.A., Gogolski, S.M., Pascoe, P. *et al.* (2018) AAFP Feline Anesthesia Guidelines. *Journal of Feline Medicine and Surgery*, **20**(7), 602–634. doi: 10.1177/1098612X18781391.

Rochlitz, I. (2000) Recommendations for the housing and care of domestic cats in laboratories. *Laboratory Animals*, **34**, 1–9.

Rochlitz, I. (2005) A review of the housing requirements of domestic cats (*Felis silvestris catus*) kept in the home. *Applied Animal Behaviour Science*, **93**, 97–109.

Rochlitz, I., Podberscek, A.L. and Broom, D. (1998) Welfare of cats in quarantine cattery. *Veterinary Record*, **143**(2), 35–39.

Rodan, I., Sundahl, E., Carney, H. *et al.* (2011) AAFP and ISFM Feline-Friendly Handling Guidelines. *Journal of Feline Medicine and Surgery*, **13**, 364–375.

Rollin, B.E. (2015) Telos, conservation of welfare, and ethical issues in genetic engineering of animals, *Current Topics in Behavioral Neurosciences*, pp. 99–116.

Russell, W.M.S. and Burch, R.L. (1959) *The Principles of Humane Experimental Technique*. Methuen, London, UK.

Scott, M.E., Nolan, A., Reid, J. *et al.* (2007) Can we really measure animal quality of life? Methodologies for measuring quality of life in people and other animals. *Animal Welfare*, **16**(S), 17–24.

Sellon, R.K. and Hartmann, K. (2006) Feline immunodeficiency virus infection. In: *Infectious Diseases of the Dog and Cat*, 3rd edn, Ed. Greene, C., pp. 131–143. Elsevier Inc, St. Louis, Missouri.

Sherding, R.G. (2008) *The Cat: Diseases and Clinical Management*, 3rd edn. Saunders, Philadelphia.

Smith, D., Anderson, D., Degryse, A.D. *et al.* (2018) Classification and reporting of severity experienced by animals used in scientific procedures: FELASA/ECLAM/ESLAV Working Group report. *Laboratory Animals*, **52**, 5–57.

Stanton, L.A., Sullivan, M.S. and Fazio, J.M. (2015) A standardized ethogram for the felidae: A tool for behavioral researchers. *Applied Animal Behaviour Science*, **173**, 3–16.

Steagall, P.V.M. (2017) *Feline Anesthesia and Pain Management*. Wiley Blackwell, Chichester, West Sussex.

Stella, J., Croney, C. and Buffington, T. (2014) Environmental factors that affect the behavior and welfare of domestic cats (*Felis silvestris catus*) housed in cages. *Applied Animal Behaviour Science*, **160**, 94–105.

Stella, J.L., Croney, C.C. and Buffington, T.C. (2017) Behavior and welfare of domestic cats housed in cages larger than U.S. norm. *Journal of Applied Animal Welfare Science*, **20**(3), 296–312.

Taylor, P.A. and Robertson, S.A. (2004) Pain management in cats past, present and future. Part 1. The cat is unique. *Journal of Feline Medicine and Surgery*, **6**, 313–320.

Turner, D. and Bateson, P. (Eds.) (2013) *The Domestic Cat: The Biology of its Behaviour*. Cambridge University Press, Cambridge, UK.

UK Cat Behaviour Working Group (1995) An Ethogram for Behavioural Studies of the Domestic Cat (*Felis silvestris catus* L.). Universities Federation for Animal Welfare, Potters Bar.

United States Department of Agriculture (USDA) (2013) Code of Federal Regulations, Title 9 volume 1, chapter I, subchapter A: Animal Welfare, United States. Department of Agriculture, United States, North America.

Van Neer, W., Linseele, V., Friedman, R. *et al.* (2014) More evidence for cat taming at the Predynastic elite cemetery of Hierakonpolis (Upper Egypt). *Journal of Archaeological Science*, **45**, 103–111.

Vigne, J.D., Guilaine, J., Debue, K. *et al.* (2004) Early taming of the cat in Cyprus. *Science*, **304**(5668), 259.

Waran, N., Best, L., Williams, V. *et al.* (2007) A preliminary study of behaviour-based indicators of pain in cats. *Animal Welfare*, **16**, 105–108.

Weinberg, J. and Levine, S. (1980) Psychobiology of coping in animals: The effects of predictability. In: *Coping and Health*. Eds Levine, S. and Ursin, H., pp. 39–59. Springer US, Boston, MA.

Wills, J. (1993) Handling. In: *Handbook of Feline Medicine*. Eds Wills, J. and Wolf, A., pp. 1–11. Pergamon Press, Oxford.

Zoran, D.L. and Buffington, T.C.A. (2011) Timely topics in nutrition: effects of nutrition choices and lifestyle changes on the well-being of cats, a carnivore that has moved indoors. *Journal of the American Veterinary Medical Association*, **239**, 596–606.

Ungulates

32 Pigs and minipigs

Adrian Zeltner and Henrik Duelund Pedersen

Biological overview

General biology

Pigs are found in almost every part of the world. Within the order Artiodactyla (even-toed ungulates), the Suiformes, encompassing pigs, peccaries and hippopotamuses form a suborder of animals with a single stomach. There are two families: Tayassuidae (Central and South American pigs) and Suidae (true pigs). Within the Suidae are the genera: *Potamochoerus* (bush pigs), *Phacochoerus* (wart hogs), *Hylochoerus* (forest hogs), *Babirusa* (Celebes hogs) and *Sus* (European pigs).

All modern domestic pigs are varieties of the species *Sus scrofa*. They are omnivorous mammals with a high degree of adaptability and intelligence, a lively temperament and high fecundity. The anatomy and physiology of pigs is thoroughly covered in a range of veterinary textbooks, most comprehensively in Pond and Mersmann (2001). Most of the information is also applicable to miniature pigs (minipigs), which are often used in biomedical research as an alternative to larger breeds. Minipigs are smaller than large domestic pigs, but there is close resemblance with regard to proportions and functions. Texts covering various aspects of minipigs are Glodek and Oldigs (1981), Svendsen (1998), McAnulty *et al.* (2012), Pedersen and Mikkelsen (2019), etc.

Size range and lifespan

The typical body masses of farm and miniature pigs (Göttingen strain) at various ages is presented in Table 32.1. The growth curve of farm pigs rises steeply in the first months and flattens out later (Figure 32.1), whereas in minipigs it is more linear, with full mature weight reached at approximately 2 years of age (Brandt *et al.* 1997; Koehn *et al.* 2008). Farm pigs reach their adult body mass of 180–250 kg, or sometimes more, at an age of 3 years. According to information compiled by Swindle (2016), among the miniature pig breeds the Göttingen Minipigs is the lightest, reaching 35–45 kg at the age of 2 years. In order of increasing adult mass, other breeds are the Yucatan micro, Sinclair, Yucatan and Hanford. The average life expectancy is 10–20 years.

Senses communication and cognition

Little is known about the visual capacity of the pig. The studies that have addressed pigs' ability to distinguish size and shape have found large individual variation. Gieling *et al.* (2011) concluded that contrasts are difficult to distinguish, as are smaller symbols at close range. Pig colour vision is still a source of debate. Most probably, pigs can discriminate blue from other colours by hue and exhibit red–green colour blindness but do not perceive contrasts well. Tanida *et al.* (1991) and Neitza *et al.* (1989) examined pig eyes with electroretinogram (ERG) flicker photometry. They revealed an average maximum sensitivity (λmax) at 439 nm and 556 nm (blue to green), thus a retinal basis for dichromatic colour vision. Tanida also found that visual as well as auditory cues are more important than olfactory cues in distinguishing between people (Tanida & Nagano 1998). On the other hand, Kittawornrat and Zimmerman (2010) concluded that pigs have some ability to discriminate among colours but not much information is available on the impact of colour on pig behaviour. Tanida *et al.* (1996) reported a general preference for illuminated areas rather than dark spaces, but Taylor *et al.* (2006) found that pigs prefer dimmer places. In nature, they are most active at dusk and dawn, which might be related to relative safety from predators during this period. The preference for lit areas would explain the findings of Grandin (1982) that it is easier to move pigs to illuminated areas, especially in unfamiliar surroundings. The general principle, then, is to have the place where you want the pigs move to illuminated, but not to shine the light directly into the eyes of the animals. Their field of vision is typical for a prey animal. The panoramic range of vision is 310°, but binocular vision accounts only for a relatively small angle of 35–50° of this (Prince 1977). Binocular vision is sacrificed for the benefit of a large field of monocular vision to remain alert to and detect any danger.

The UFAW Handbook on the Care and Management of Laboratory and Other Research Animals, Ninth Edition.
Edited by Huw Golledge and Claire Richardson.
© 2024 John Wiley & Sons Ltd. Published 2024 by John Wiley & Sons Ltd.

Table 32.1 Typical body masses (kg) of female breeding stock of farm pigs (ad libitum feeding, figures assembled from several sources) and Göttingen Minipigs (restricted feeding, figures from the breeding herd at Dalmose/Denmark).

Age	Farm pigs	Göttingen Minipigs
Newborn	1.3	0.45
4 weeks (weaning)	7.5	3,5
3 months	33	7
6 months	90	14
1 year	150	26
2 years	200	45

The pig's hearing range is from 42 Hz to 40.5 kHz with the highest sensitivity at 8 kHz. It exceeds the human hearing range in the ultrasound range (Heffner & Heffner 1990). Regarding sound localisation, pigs are more accurate than many carnivores with a threshold of 4.6°, not far behind humans (1.2°) (Heffner & Heffner 1992). Sounds that cannot be heard by the human ear can affect pig behaviour. Practical experience shows that pigs quickly accustom themselves to a wide variety of sounds, even at high levels, but react to sudden noises or changes. However, sudden as well as constant loud noise is aversive to pigs and should therefore be avoided. Noise levels in buildings where pigs are housed should be kept below 85 dB (Broucek 2014). It is not quite clear if playing music has a beneficial effect on behaviour or welfare of pigs. This area seems to be notably under-investigated. Pigs have a rich repertoire of vocal signals; there might be up to 20 different signals. We do not yet fully understand their vocalisation; the pig's vocal ethogram is not fully mapped, but some are easily recognisable. A warning call is similar to a dog's bark and if a pig 'barks' in fear, the rest of the group will immediately repeat the sound and either run or freeze and listen intently. Pigs make grunts of greeting and have squeals which indicate submission. The grunt is one of the most common sounds, given in response to familiar sounds or while looking for food (rooting). A short grunt is given when the pig is excited, while a long grunt is a contact call and normally associated with pleasurable stimuli. When pigs are aroused, or anticipating they may squeal, and they may scream when hurt. Squealing also occurs when they are unhappy with a situation. Sows and piglets have a distinctive 'vocabulary' of their own.

Olfaction is the principal sense in pig communication, although visual and auditory signals are of importance as well. Pigs have a very acute sense of smell, which is developed early in the life, and the sensitivity matches that of a dog (Hafez & Signoret 1962; Søndergaard 2010). It is important for survival and pigs use a wide range of olfactory cues in their natural behaviour. They use this type of information as the predominant basis for individual recognition and it plays a special role in reproductive behaviour.

There are nearly 20,000 taste buds on the pig tongue; that is, 3 times more than a human tongue and 10 times more than that of a dog (Chamorro et al. 1994). The taste buds have receptors for sweet, umami, sour, bitter and salty, just as in humans (Roura 2003). Sugars stimulate sweet taste in pigs and enhance

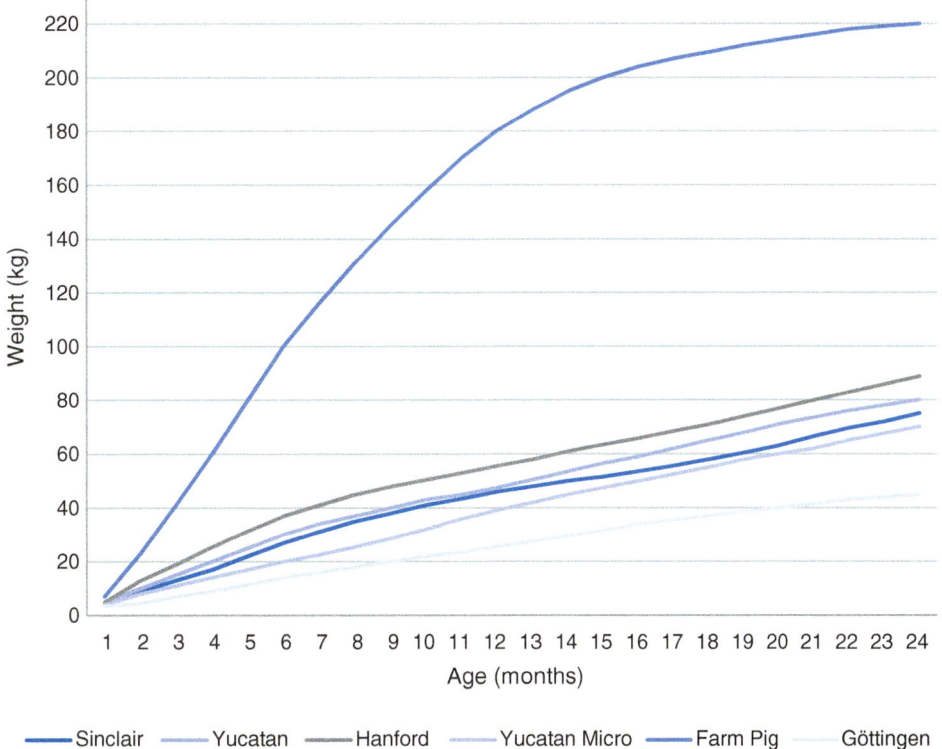

Figure 32.1 Growth curves for farm pigs and various minipigs. Source: Data for farm pigs from several sources, Göttingen Minipigs from the breeding herd at Dalmose/Denmark, others from Sinclair website[1]

[1] http://www.sinclairbioresources.com/resources/book-of-normals/download-the-sinclair-book-of-normals/ (accessed 15 May 2019)

voluntary intake. Natural carbohydrate sweeteners are similar in potency for pigs as in humans, but artificial sweeteners are far less, or not potent at all for pigs (Glaser *et al.* 2000). In a classical double choice study, McLaughlin *et al.* (1983) studied 96 different flavours divided into 8 basic groups. Pigs showed preferences for 30 flavours over the 96 flavours tested. Highest preferences were recorded for cheesy, fruity, meaty and sweet flavours. Sour taste is of particular relevance in pigs, not surprising as a lot of natural food resources in the wild are rich in organic acids. Therefore, a lot of different fruits, especially apples, are excellent treats and rewards and ripe banana is a well-liked flavour by pigs. In some cases, however, a certain amount of neophobia needs to be conquered before they accept tastes other than their normal diet.

The pig snout disc is also a powerful, yet very sensitive, tactile organ. It has as many nerve endings as a human fingertip. It is used to dig up and examine food, and to explore the environment. Tactile communication is used by the boar during sexual behaviour to stimulate the sow, as well as by the piglets during nursing to trigger milk ejection.

Pigs have good cognitive abilities. It is known that the pig's ability to learn from experience, memorise and combine new memories is outstanding, especially when food-related, and they can be easily trained to perform operant tasks to gain rewards (Kornum and Knudsen 2011; Murphy *et al.* 2013; Haagensen *et al.* 2013). Cerbulis (1994) found that pigs were indeed capable of complex learning in tasks requiring discriminative responses to different gestural and verbal symbols regarding a variety of objects and actions. Consideration, however, must be given to the visual capacity of the pig. Pigs can also learn from other pigs and can differentiate between individuals not only when they are present but also just by scent, calls or image (McLeman *et al.* 2008). Pigs do not always use all their advanced cognitive abilities but rely on simple clues and rules of thumb in many situations.

Social organisation

Pigs are social animals. In the wild, they live in family groups usually comprising related females and their offspring. Young males typically band together once they are sexually mature and form their own groups. Mature boars leave these bachelor groups to lead solitary lives once they become sexually active.

Even in a domesticated setting, there is clear evidence of pig bonding and grouping, and in groups, pigs develop stable hierarchies of a simple linear type that are maintained through the avoidance and submissive behaviour of lower-ranking individuals (Curtis *et al.* 2001). The largest animals are not necessarily the dominant ones (Ewbank & Messe 1971), but Francis *et al.* (1996) suggests that mixing pigs heterogeneously by weight will reduce hierarchical conflict and decrease the intensity of fighting by clear weight differentiation. If new pigs are introduced into a group, there will be fierce fighting, mainly expressed by butting and biting the neck and ears, but the level of aggression drops dramatically after about one hour (Symoens & Van Den Brande 1969). Odour masking by applying pheromones and/or artificial compounds to all pigs when mixing has little, if any effect in limiting aggression and increasing hierarchical stability (Gonyou, 1997; Friend *et al.* 1983). Unless they are used for breeding, boars can be kept in groups. In production, boars are grouped as early as possible, usually at weaning (4–5 weeks of age) and kept together until they are shipped to the recipient unit. Aggression among boars is rarely a problem in such a group, even if they are temporarily parted, but they will mount each other. Pigs do not engage in allogrooming and there are no reports of strong individual affiliation. On the other hand, pigs in a group tend to coordinate and synchronise behaviour in space and time. Despite their tendency to synchronise, pigs differ a lot individually in their behaviour. Most probably, the personalities of pigs consist of several dimensions, similar to those shown in humans, other primates and dogs (Špinka 2009).

Humans are important components in the social environment of domesticated pigs, and handling affects the welfare of the pigs. In commercial breeding situations, they often have minimal human interaction, although there is rather more at minipig breeders. It is not only the quantity of the interaction that is important, quality has an enormous influence on well-being and emotional state of the pigs. Negative, aversive handling leads to fear of humans with all its implications. On the other hand, regular positive, friendly interaction reduces fear and leads to relaxed animals that are easy to handle. It cannot be stressed enough that it is imperative to socialise as much as possible with pigs in the acclimation phase of the study to ensure easy handling, low stress and better results.

Wild and feral pigs have home ranges which vary in size. Scientists do not agree on the specific area required by pigs, but it appears that pigs will occupy whatever space is provided for them, since exploratory behaviour is almost as important as foraging. If food availability is not an issue, then the space will be utilised for exploration and for avoiding dominant individuals.

Within a litter of newborn piglets, a social hierarchy is established within 3–4 days after birth. From then on, each piglet suckles its individual teat, with dominant piglets usually gaining the more productive anterior teats. When piglets from different litters are mixed after weaning, they establish a new dominance hierarchy. Usually, ranking is established through aggressive interaction, but may take place without overt aggression. Dominant–subordinate relationships remain mainly unchanged as long as the group stays together. Subordinates that have been separated from a group for some time will be attacked after reintroduction, whereas reintroduction of dominant animals does not often result in aggression.

Reproduction

Domestic pigs are prolific and reproduce at all times of the year. They are polyestrous and the uterus consists of two long convoluted horns. The oestrous cycle averages 21 (17–25) days. The first oestrous is at the age of 6 to 7 months for domestic pigs and 4 to 6 months for Göttingen Minipigs. The presence of boars plays an important role in stimulating the onset of the cycle. Initial signs of heat (pro-oestrus) are seen 2–3 days before the beginning of oestrus. Oestrus is characterised by the standing reflex (lordosis), a rigid stance, when pressure is applied on the rump. Oestrus lasts for 2.5 (1–5) days, and within another 2–3 days the symptoms gradually subside (post- or metoestrus). Ovulation occurs early in the second half of standing oestrus (Figure 32.2) and extends over 1–4 h. Signs of oestrus include swelling and reddening

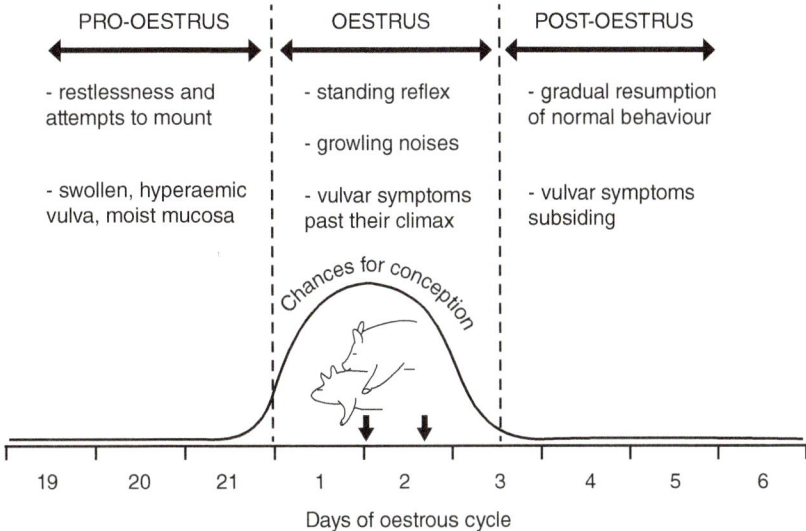

Figure 32.2 Oestrous symptoms and the best time for having sows mated or inseminated (arrows). The oestrous cycle of approximately 21 days is divided up into 2–3 days of pro-oestrus, 2–3 days of 'standing' oestrus, 2–3 days of post-oestrus and the inter-oestrous period. In the absence of a boar, the standing reflex will be elicited 12 h later than indicated in the diagram.

of the vulva, restlessness, increased interest in other animals, especially males, mounting of other animals, occasionally growling sounds and, eventually, display of the standing reflex in the presence of a male or if mounted by another female. Appetite is generally decreased during this period.

Mating is preceded by foreplay: the male circling, sniffing and nudging the female and attempting to mount. This courtship behaviour plays an important role in inducing the standing reflex. If the sow displays the standing reflex, intromission occurs and the corkscrew-shaped tip of the penis is locked into the cervix of the sow. Copulation lasts 3–10 minutes and the semen is deposited in the uterus. Intrauterine sperm transport is rapid, and fertilisation occurs in the ampullar segment of the oviduct. Embryos enter the uterus 2–3 days after fertilisation at the four-cell stage. Six days after fertilisation, the blastocysts hatch from the zona pellucida, start migrating throughout both uterine horns and are eventually evenly distributed. Attachment to the endometrium begins 2 weeks after conception. There are no specialised areas of contact (*placenta diffusa*) and, compared with primates, attachment is rather superficial (epitheliochorial). This is the reason that antibodies are not transferred to the foetus during pregnancy, making colostrum ingestion after parturition crucial. The average length of the gestation period is 115 days, plus or minus 3 days. Small litters are typically carried a day or two longer than larger ones. The embryology of the pig is described in detail in Patten (1948) and Marrable (1971). Corresponding information on minipigs may be found in Glodek and Oldigs (1981).

In well-managed herds of domestic breeds, the typical pregnancy rates are 80–90% with an average of 12 piglets weaned per litter. In Göttingen Minipigs, the litter size is 4–5 for primiparous and 8 on average for pluriparous sows. Typical reproductive parameters are summarised in Table 32.2.

Sows produce milk rich in dry matter, containing about 9% fat, 6% protein, 5% lactose and 0.7% minerals. Colostrum

Table 32.2 Typical reproductive data for adult farm pigs (data from various sources) and miniature pigs (Göttingen strain, data from Ellegaard Göttingen Minipigs, Dalmose, Denmark).

Parameter	Farm pig	Minipig (Göttingen strain)
Age at puberty (months)	7	4–5
Minimum breeding age (months)	8	7
Length of oestrous cycle (days)	21	20
Duration of oestrus (days)	2.5	3
Gestation period (days)	115	115
Average litter size	12	8
Birth weight/piglet (g)	1300	450

contains close to 20% protein, comprising mainly gamma-globulins that act as antibodies. These need to be imbibed by the piglets within the first few hours after parturition to cross the wall of the alimentary tract and provide passive immunity. Milk production of suckling sows increases up to the third week of lactation and declines gradually thereafter. The daily milk production of a sow suckling 10 piglets is about 8 l. Data on milk production in minipigs are not available. The natural suckling period may extend to 10 weeks, and in extreme cases up to 17 weeks. In commercial production units, piglets are usually weaned at around 4 weeks, but sometimes at 5 or 6 weeks of age. Suckling sows usually do not come into oestrus. The first post-partum oestrus, which is accompanied by ovulation, is usually recorded 4–8 days after weaning. In primiparous sows and under unfavourable environmental conditions, the return to oestrus may be delayed. Oestrus symptoms that are observed about 3 days after parturition in many animals are not associated with ovulation.

Standard biological data

Published information on biological parameters of the pig is inconsistent. Reference values for cardiovascular, respiratory, haematological and clinical chemical parameters vary within a wide range. Some variation may be explained by genetic differences; however, age, reproductive status and a variety of environmental factors such as husbandry system, microbiological status and conditions under which the information was obtained have a much greater impact. Differences between various pig breeds and among farm pigs and miniature pigs at a comparable stage of development are comparatively minor. Differences between adult miniature pigs and weight-matched farm piglets, however, may be substantial because of the difference in the physiological state of maturity. Likewise, biological parameters for vital functions are greatly affected by handling/restraining (chemical or physical) to obtain the respective data. Data originating from anaesthetised animals do not necessarily agree with those of conscious animals, depending on the anaesthetic used. Factors that may be responsible for variability include immobilisation, transportation or fasting of the animals, sampling site and method (venepuncture or permanently indwelling catheter). Specific data for different minipig strains are usually available from the breeders. Extensive tables with background data for Göttingen Minipigs have been published (Pedersen & Mikkelsen 2019).

Table 32.3 provides some values for vital functions and Table 32.4 provides physiological means and ranges of relevant blood parameters typical for farm and miniature pigs.

Table 32.3 Typical resting values for some vital functions for farm and miniature pigs (data assembled from several sources).

Respiration rate (breaths/min)	18–25
Heart rate (beats/min)	60–100
Mean arterial blood pressure (mmHg)	90–100
Rectal temperature (°C)	37.5–39.5

Table 32.4 Physiological values of some haematological and clinical chemical parameters for adult farm and miniature pigs (values assembled from various sources).

Parameter	Mean	Range
Blood volume (ml/kg)	65	55–75
Erythrocyte count (10^9/ml)	7	5–9
Haematocrit (%)	33	30–50
Haemoglobin (mg/ml)	125	90–180
Leucocyte count (10^6/ml)	13	12–17
Neutrophils (%)	48	40–55
Eosinophils (%)	1.5	0–4
Basophils (%)	0.5	0–1
Monocytes (%)	3.5	1–7
Lymphocytes (%)	50	35–60
Thrombocytes (10^6/ml)	450	200–500
Total protein (g/dl)	7	6–9
Albumin (g/dl)	4	3–5
Aspartate aminotransferase (AST) (U/l)	38	20–200
Creatine kinase (CK) (U/l)	450	100–3000
Alkaline phosphatase (AP) (U/l)	60	30–130

Breeds, strains and genetics

There are close to 100 known breeds of pigs, mostly reared for pork and bacon production. Breeding stock have been selected with an emphasis on growth rate, feed conversion and lean content, as well as fecundity and mothering ability. The most common domestic breeds are Yorkshire and Landrace (white), Pietrain and Hampshire (spotted or belted) and Duroc (red). In commercial pork production, hybrid crosses of two, three or more breeds are common.

Miniature pig breeds were established for the purpose of biomedical research. They are smaller than farm pigs but resemble them in proportion and physiology. Many of the present breeds of miniature pigs have their origin in the Minnesota (Hormel) minipig, which was developed in 1949 at the Hormel Institute in Austin, USA. Miniature pigs derived from this population are Göttingen Minipigs, developed in the years up to 1969, the NIH (Beltsville) minipig and the Sinclair minipig. Others are the Pitman-Moore and the Hanford (derived from the Pitman-Moore). A Mexican feral pig was used in research in 1960 and later referred to as Yucatan mini- and micropig. In Japan, the Ohmini breed was established and the cross with Göttingen Minipigs produced the Clawn minipig. The NIBS minipig was created by mating Göttingen Minipigs with Pitman-Moore and Chinese native (Nunoya et al. 2007). The Bama minipig is a popular minipig for research in China. In addition, several other breeds have been established.

Colonies bred for biomedical research may be random-bred, outbred or (partially) inbred. In commercial pig farming, random breeding and crossing are typical. Purpose-bred minipigs for biomedical research typically originate from colonies with outbred genetics. It is advisable to choose a large breeder to obtain genetically defined and well characterised minipigs for biomedical research.

Pigs have 18 autosomal chromosome pairs plus the X and Y chromosomes. A map of the entire genome of several breeds, including Göttingen Minipigs, has been established (Swine Genome Sequencing Consortium (SGSC) 2009; Vamathevan et al. 2013). This will facilitate research on locating genes associated with traits of economic or disease importance and has opened the possibility to produce transgenic animal models. The similarity of the human and porcine genome maps suggests that there will be further development of the pig as a model for human diseases and in xenotransplantation research.

Sources of supply

Pigs from 'non-purpose-bred' colonies are typically of farmed strains, often hybrids, whose breeding has been focused on production, muscle mass and fat percentage rather than family genetics. In these populations, individual genetic and phenotypic variation can be high, especially from producer to producer, and such animals may not be suited for large experiments for that reason. Purpose-bred pigs and minipigs for biomedical research typically originate from a closed colony with outbred genetics and a high health status. These populations require genetic management to ensure continued genetic variability. Monitoring may involve biomedical, immunologic or DNA markers or quantitative genetic analysis of physiological variables. Some minipigs are partially inbred as a result of selection for a specific phenotype, such as expression for major histocompatibility complex (MHC) homozygosis (e.g. the NIH minipig).

Pigs and minipigs may be sourced from breeders with different health status, such as conventional, minimal disease (MD), specific pathogen free (SPF) and microbiologically defined. MD, SPF and microbiologically defined pigs are produced under barrier protection with increasing security (Table 32.5). Breeders with a sizeable production can supply large, uniform and genetically stable groups worldwide. Conventional pigs are kept in a less rigidly controlled environment without a regular health monitoring schedule and thus have a more unknown microbiological and genetic status.

Uses in the laboratory

Pigs and minipigs are valuable models in various areas of biomedical research, including physiology, pharmacology, toxicology, radiology, surgery and organ transplantation, traumatology, pathology, embryology and paediatrics. Characteristics that make them particularly suitable for research include:

- Many similarities with humans, in particular regarding skin, skeleton and joints, teeth, gastrointestinal tract, pancreas, liver and kidney, cardiovascular system, lung, immune system and physiological state of the newborn
- The ease and safety of handling and housing under confined conditions
- A convenient body size for most clinical and surgical experiments or trials involving repeated collection of blood samples, biopsies, etc.
- The availability of reproductive technologies, including collection, storage and manipulation of gametes
- Relatively low price of acquisition and maintenance

And for minipigs, further advantages include:

- Highly standardised animals are available (genetically and microbiologically)
- Available worldwide in large uniform groups (e.g. Göttingen Minipigs)
- Small body size, allowing chronic studies while still having animals that are easy to handle and house
- More and more available background data, including on the background pathology for regulated toxicology studies
- Fully accepted by FDA, EMA and other regulatory authorities

General husbandry

Housing

Female wild pigs form groups (sounders) and roam in forests with no permanent retreat except when they build a nest to raise a litter. Wild boars are solitary once they become sexually active. Their domesticated descendants are kept indoors during the winter months in cold climates; however, year-round indoor housing is common practice to protect the herd from parasites and epidemics. This, however, can conflict with the pig's natural qualities of alertness and curiosity and restricts activity. In regions with mild climatic conditions (e.g. UK and France), the use of huts or kennels on pasture for breeding sows has gained popularity.

Detailed information on the housing of farm pigs may be found in husbandry texts (see Further reading section). In a typical commercial piggery, separate quarters are provided for:

1. young stock from weaning to breeding age (growing quarters);
2. weaned sows and gilts that are to be mated and are, therefore, kept in close proximity to a boar (mating quarters);
3. pregnant sows (gestation quarters);
4. parturient and nursing sows (farrowing quarters).

Young stock, gilts and pregnant sows are usually housed in groups. During the first 4 weeks and at an advanced stage of gestation, sows should be able to enter a protected area, especially when feeding, otherwise fighting and crushing against rails can lead to abortion. Farrowing sows have traditionally been caged in special farrowing crates (Figure 32.3a). The crates are equipped with rails to prevent the sows from lying on and crushing their young. They also provide hygienic conditions and protect the stock person from sow aggression while managing the litter. Farrowing crates, however, seriously compromise sow welfare by restricting nest-building behaviour and other periparturient behavioural patterns and are, therefore, much disputed and banned in some countries. For European breeders that have specialised in the production of laboratory animals, farrowing crates are not acceptable as they operate under Directive 2010/63/EU. A special designed farrowing pen is in place and the welfare of the sow and piglets is enormously increased (Figure 32.3b). The sow has enough space to turn around and to establish a dunging area. The floor is for a big part solid and bedding as well as nest-building material is provided. The pen has

Table 32.5 Conditions for accommodation of various categories of pigs for experimental purposes (Hansen 1997).

Condition	Conventional	MD or SPF	Microbiologically defined
Caesarean originated	−	+	+
Quarantine regulation	−	+	+
Change of dress	−	+	+
Shower in	−	+	+
Decontamination of:			
Diet	−	−	+
Equipment	−	−	+
Water	−	−	+
Absolute filter ventilation	−	−	+
Health monitored	−	+	+

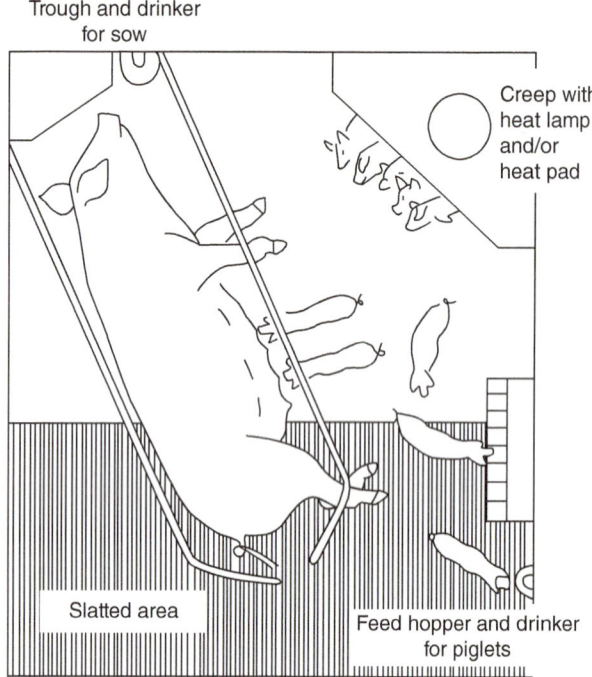

Figure 32.3a Top view of a traditional farrowing crate. The sow is confined in a narrow space and can only stand or lie down.

anti-crushing rails, and a separate heated creep area is installed for the protection of the piglets. There is a heat pad and/or creep area with overhead heat lamp to provide them with a suitable microclimate. If no heat source is available, ample straw bedding must be provided to enable the piglets to burrow into it, huddling together for warmth.

In laboratory settings, farrowing is generally only planned as part of juvenile or reproduction toxicity studies. In such cases, an ordinary pen can often be converted to a farrowing pen with a reasonable welfare status and without too much effort (Figure 32.3c).

In research facilities, pigs and minipigs should be housed in pens with a solid floor. Please check local regulations for minimum sizes of the pens. It is not recommended to house pigs with different health status in the same building or in the vicinity of each other as the status of the cleaner pigs might be compromised. For experimental purposes, pigs can occasionally be housed in special crates or cages for short periods. Several manufacturers supply special miniature pig cages, including metabolism cages that permit collection of urine and faeces. Dog facilities can usually be modified to house young pigs or minipigs. Most contract research organisations (CROs) have pens that can be used for minipigs as well as dogs for added flexibility. Partitions between pens should be 1.10–1.20 m high; a trapdoor between the pens will give the option to combine pens. The division between the pens should be of solid material in the back of the pen to allow for privacy. The front part of the division and the door can be constructed of vertical bars (Figure 32.4) to allow for visual, olfactory and snout contact. Cages should be large enough for the confined animal to have separate sleeping and dunging areas. Minimum floor space recommended by various sources varies considerably. Directive 2010/63/EU calls for a minimum pen size of 2 m^2, and guidelines from its Annex III for minimum floor space per animal are provided in Table 32.6. These represent a compromise between the requirements of the animals and practical and economic considerations of space limitation. More confined enclosures may be justified for limited periods to serve special experimental conditions, for example, when monitoring individual feed consumption, or taking serial samples.

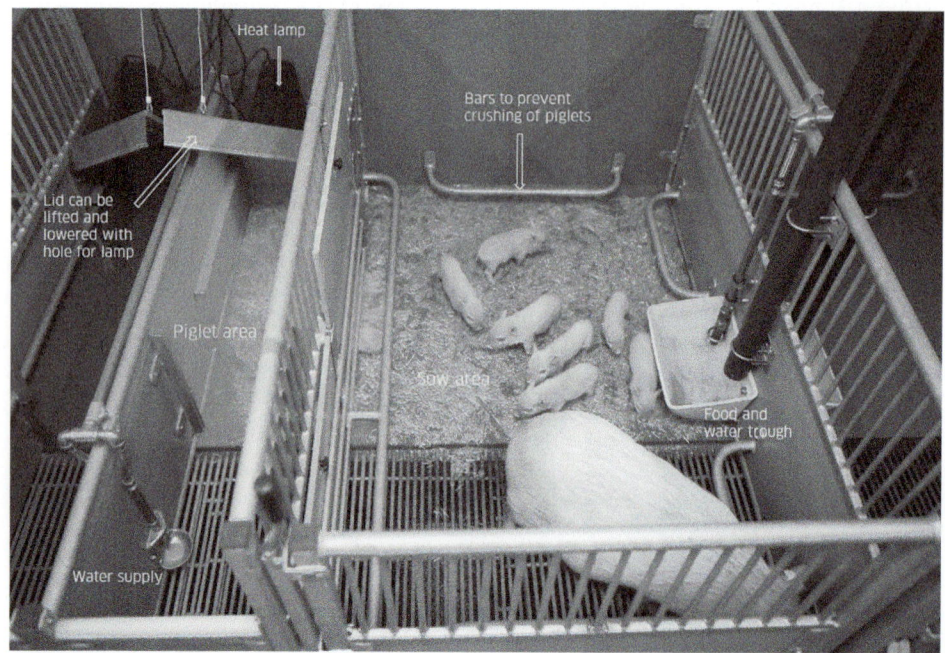

Figure 32.3b A farrowing pen at the breeder with the main welfare aspects taken care of Ellegaard Göttingen Minipigs, Denmark.

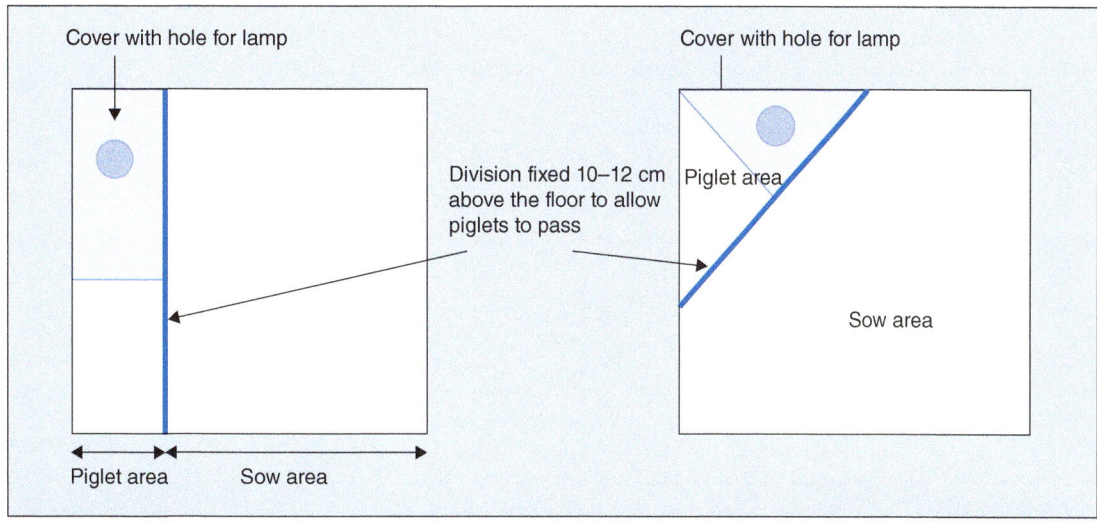

Figure 32.3c Suggestions for turning a normal pen into a farrowing pen. The minimum size of pen in Europe is 2 m². Source: Based on Directive 2010/63/EU.

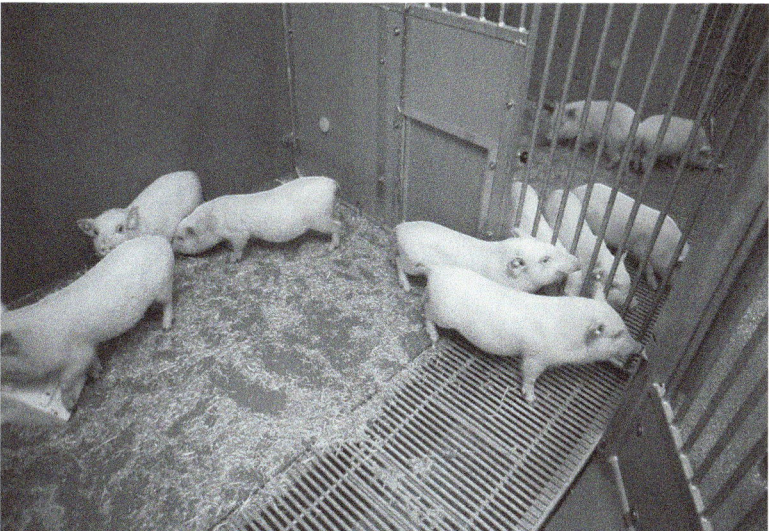

Figure 32.4 A pen for young minipigs with slatted floor in the front for defecation and solid floor in the back for eating, sleeping and playing. The gaps in the slatted floor should be narrow to provide a good foothold also for the small claws of young animals and minipigs. The division is partly solid for privacy and partly with bars for interaction with neighbouring pigs.

Table 32.6 Recommended minimum enclosure dimensions and space allowances for the accommodation of farm and miniature pigs. Modified from 2010/63/EU

Live weight (kg)	Minimum enclosure size (m²)	Minimum floor area (m²/animal)	Minimum lying in thermoneutral conditions (m²/animal)
Up to 5	2.0	0.2	0.10
>5–10	2.0	0.25	0.11
>10–20	2.0	0.35	0.18
>20–30	2.0	0.50	0.24
>30–50	2.0	0.70	0.33
>50–70	3.0	0.80	0.41
>70–100	3.0	1.0	0.53

Physical environment and hygiene

With their scanty hair covering and lack of sweat glands, provision of the right thermal environment is important, as pigs have a poor capacity for thermoregulation, which furthermore is underdeveloped at birth. A particularly efficient heating and ventilation system is required when pigs are kept on perforated floors. Optimum environmental temperatures vary with age. Newborns need temperatures around 34 °C. The temperature may be lowered by 1 °C for every day of the first week and by 1 °C each week for the second, third and fourth weeks of age. Adult animals housed singly and without bedding feel comfortable at 20 °C or more. With an insulated floor and abundant bedding, they will tolerate temperatures as low as 10 °C without ill effect, especially in a group-housing system where they are able to huddle. In order to satisfy the special temperature needs of the young without exposing the mother to heat stress, farrowing pens should be provided with a heated creep area (Figure 32.3). In hot climates, the lack of shade and of wallows or sprinklers may lead to sunburn or heat stroke.

The ideal relative humidity for pigs is around 60–70%. It should not range beyond extremes of 50% or 90%. Ventilation is critical to keep the concentration of potentially harmful gases low, especially in densely stocked quarters. Air speed must not exceed 0.2–0.3 m/s for adult animals and 0.1 m/s for piglets.

Pens should be cleaned out frequently, and on concrete floors dry bedding is most desirable. The daily excretions of an adult farm pig amount to 0.5–3.0 kg faeces (water content 55–75%) and up to 6 liter of urine. Göttingen Minipigs of 15 kg excrete around 700–1300 ml urine (females considerably more than males) and 200 g of faeces. Once a fortnight, pens should be emptied for thorough cleaning and disinfection. Floors, walls and caging utensils should be soaked and scrubbed or washed down with a high-velocity water jet and treated with a disinfectant. The animals should be returned to the dry pen.

Environmental provisions

Like their wild ancestors, domestic pigs and minipigs are sociable, lively and exploratory animals. While wild boar spend about 50% of their time resting and sleeping, domestic pigs do it for 70–80% of their time; during the remaining time, they like to romp, wallow and root in soil or bedding. Pigs are naturally very clean, choosing specific sites for defecation and urination, and keeping their sleeping area dry. If the pen design allows for a functional division of the available area, they will use specific dunging areas for elimination. In commercial pig farming, however, animals are commonly kept in less welfare-friendly conditions sometimes single stalls or crowded pens, on slatted floors with no bedding. Single stalls are now illegal in Europe except for defined periods in some countries (4 weeks after mating and during farrowing and lactation). Commercial pig farming environments are often deficient in external stimuli and objects to keep them occupied. Tethering of sows used to be common but is now banned. Pigs, being curious and agile animals, suffer from boredom if not given the opportunity to perform a range of activities (Wemelsfelder 2005). Common enrichment items include the provision of hanging chains or objects in the pens. Straw provides comfortable bedding, keeps the animals occupied with rooting and chewing activities, and serves as low-calorie fodder, providing a feeling of satiation without leading to obesity. Therefore, clean, dry straw contributes substantially to the well-being of pigs (Day et al. 2002). Unless experimental conditions require otherwise, the best way of accommodating pigs or minipigs is by housing them in groups of up to 10 in spacious pens with straw-covered floors. Further enrichment might include the provision of toys, training operant tasks, or letting them loose in the corridor or specially designed activity rooms so that they can explore new areas and things. In several countries, rules and regulations are laid down to improve husbandry conditions for pigs, and providing bedding material might be mandatory (e.g. European Council 1991; European Commission 1997; EFSA 2007; New Zealand National Animal Welfare Advisory Committee 2005).

Social grouping

Socialisation within groups and the establishment of a social hierarchy are behavioural traits typical of free-ranging pigs. These behavioural patterns should be considered when housing pigs in pens. Isolated housing of individuals should be avoided as far as possible, with the exception of breeding boars and farrowing sows. The AAALAC Guide states that single housing of social species should be the exception (NRC 2011). If it is necessary to single house pigs, it should be assured that they have visual, olfactory, and tactile (snout) contact to other pigs. As they lack social interaction with other pigs, human contact can be a substitute. When animals are grouped and feed is restricted, feeding space should be sufficient to permit all animals to feed at the same time. Ideally, partitions should be provided, enabling weaker animals to evade aggression from others. If group size exceeds 10, agonistic behaviour tends to be increased because no lasting hierarchy is established. This is not always the case, however, because in addition to the amount of space, the quality of space is also important (pen divisions, availability of substrates, feeding places, etc.). If possible, stable groups should remain together. When animals are mixed from different pens, fighting can be minimised by grouping them just before feeding or sleeping time, preferably in a new, unfamiliar pen. It also helps to give extra space initially so there is a chance to escape. It is also advisable to form new groups according to the temperament and social status of the individuals. Trying out a few combinations might be necessary. Grouping pigs heterogeneously by weight may reduce hierarchical conflict and fighting (Francis et al. 1996), whereas odour masking has little effect (Gonyou 1997).

Adult boars tend to live a solitary life when given the opportunity. Therefore, for them, individual housing might be appropriate. Nonetheless, it is possible to group-house boars provided that they have been reared together or given the opportunity to get accustomed to each other under unconfined conditions, such as on pasture or in a yard. At times, it is not possible, even with the greatest effort, to form a stable group; in such cases, individual housing is appropriate. The level of aggressiveness in males is reduced greatly if they are castrated at an early age (barrows) and they might even be housed together with a group of females (Braun & Wetzel 2018).

Presentation of food and water

Pigs are generally fed once or twice a day. Dry pelleted rations may be presented on the clean floor as long as there is a sufficient distance from the dunging area. More commonly, the feed is presented in a trough or bowl of non-corrosive material installed at, or close to, ground level. Trough space per animal should be 20–40 cm depending on body size. The feed may be dry or mixed with water or whey to make a gruel or soup. Troughs need to be cleaned daily. Stale feed may lead to digestive disorders; diet that has not been consumed should be removed after two hours. As adult pigs tend to put on excessive fat, transponder systems with computer-controlled feeding stations have been designed. One of these stations will serve 40–50 animals. A hayrack with freshly cut green fodder, hay or straw is valuable from a nutritional and behavioural point of view.

Clean drinking water should always be available, so automatic drinkers (nipple or bowl type) are recommended. Nipples should be installed at an adjustable height of 15–50 cm, so that they are at the shoulder height of the animals, preferably in the front of the pen, otherwise, in the pen area where the animals are expected to defecate and urinate. Farrowing pens should be equipped with an extra easy-to-operate automatic drinker for the piglets (Figure 32.3).

Health monitoring, quarantine and barrier systems

Existing systems for disease control in pigs are generally aimed at improving the economy of farming operations. Minimal disease (MD) or specific pathogen free (SPF) animals may be infected with pathogens which, although of little economic relevance, could interfere with experiments by changing physiological responses through immunosuppression, contamination of biological products, anaesthetic death, etc. Therefore, pigs bred for biomedical research should ideally originate from a caesarean-derived colony, be kept in a protected environment (see sources of supply) and have a regular health monitoring programme, as is common practice in laboratory rodent colonies. Staff should not have contact with other pigs, and all materials, including feed, bedding and equipment, should be of controlled origin and might need to be decontaminated before introducing to the pigs.

The Scandinavian Federation for Laboratory Animal Science (Scand-LAS) has published guidelines for health monitoring of pigs (Hem *et al.* 1994), and the Federation of European Laboratory Animal Science Associations (FELASA) has published similar guidelines (Rehbinder *et al.* 1998).

Transport

Transportation is stressful for pigs (Saco *et al.* 2003; Piñero *et al.* 2007). Hot, humid conditions should be avoided, as should extremely low temperatures and draught.

Large pigs are generally transported by truck or trailer. A space of 0.5 m²/100 kg body mass should be allowed. Floors must not be slippery and should be fitted with battens or covered with a deep layer of sand. Large loading surfaces should be subdivided by partitions. When driving or loading animals, it is important to understand that they are bewildered and anxious, rather than stubborn. Therefore, be patient, determined and firm, but never rough. Pigs are apprehensive of sloping surfaces, especially if these are unstable or slippery, and do not like entering dark or brightly lit areas.

Minipigs and young farm pigs may be transported in portable dog kennels or custom-made durable crates or boxes. Ample straw or shavings must be provided to furnish soft bedding and absorb moisture. There should be openings for fresh air and enough space for all animals to lie down comfortably. Feed should be made available on longer journeys, and water should be available throughout the trip. Additional information may be obtained from the latest issue of Live Animals Regulations by the International Air Transport Association (IATA)[2]. See also Chapter 12: Transportation of laboratory animals.

Microbiologically defined or SPF pigs or minipigs should preferably be transported in air-conditioned vans equipped with filtered ventilation to prevent infection.

Within the laboratory, smaller animals can be carried on the arm, larger animals may either be walked from one place to another or transported in a trolley; the sides of this should be high enough to prevent the animals from jumping out, but not too high to make it impractical to lift them in and out. When driving pigs, a group always handles better than single individuals. Training the animals by letting them run up and down the aisle will reduce their fear of moving and gives them extra exercise and enrichment (Abbott *et al.* 1997).

Identification and sexing

Ear tags are required by law in many countries. Ear notching (Figure 32.5) is a method to permanently identifying pigs at birth; tattoos can be applied as well but it can be a challenge with pigmented animals. Electronic identification systems are also available, consisting of transponders that are attached to the ear or injected into the tissue at the base of the ear. Stationary or portable readers can be used to read the transponders. The least invasive method of marking should always be used. Identification methods are likely to be painful and warrant administration of analgesia (Leslie *et al.* 2010).

For temporary marking, special colour markers or sprays with water-soluble dye are available.

Sexing of pigs presents no problem as they have clearly discernible sex organs from birth.

Breeding

Condition of adults

In contrast to their feral ancestors, reproductive activity in the domestic pig is not seasonal. Normally, sows ovulate every 21 days. Males are always ready to mate. Ovulation is accompanied by characteristic oestrous symptoms climaxing in the standing reflex.

As previously mentioned, well-managed pig herds achieve farrowing rates of 80–90%. The average gestation period in pigs and Göttingen Minipigs is 115 days (see Reproduction).

Artificial insemination has become standard in pig farming and can also be used with minipigs. Semen collection and insemination are easy to conduct, and, with experienced personnel, success rates are comparable with natural mating. Semen can be stored in a commercially available diluent at 15–18 °C for 3–4 days. Conception rate and litter size after insemination with cryopreserved semen is usually unsatisfactory.

There are reasonable success rates for transfer of pre-implantation embryos, usually flushed from super-ovulated donors around day 7 after conception (Bruessow *et al.* 2000). Existing techniques for cryopreservation of embryos are

---

[2]http://www.iata.org (accessed 15 May 2019)

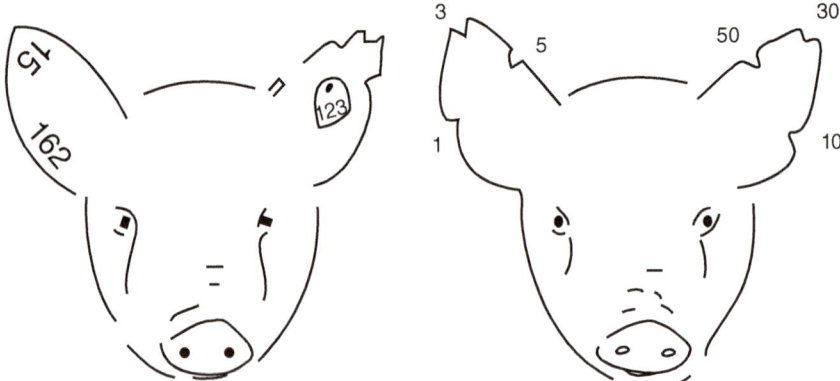

Figure 32.5 Pigs are commonly identified by ear tattoo, ear tag or notches in the ears (notching key used for Göttingen Minipigs worldwide on the right). The latter method has the advantage that it can be read from a distance.

unsatisfactory and, at present, embryo transfer must be looked upon as a technique for special situations and experimental purposes.

The traditional method of pregnancy detection is to carefully observe the sows for oestrous signs around the 3rd and 6th week (one and two cycles) after insemination. Ultrasound scanning will deliver confirmation of pregnancy. Approximately 1 week before they are due to farrow, sows should be moved to the farrowing quarters (Figure 32.3).

During the 2–3 days prior to farrowing, feed supply to the sow should be reduced to half. The diet should contain components rich in crude fibre. Water is supplied *ad libitum*. These measures help to reduce the incidence of constipation and parturient infection of uterus and mammary glands, commonly termed metritis–mastitis–agalactia (MMA) or post-partum dysgalactia (PPD) syndrome.

About 1 day before parturition, sows will display nest-building behaviour when given the opportunity. In nature, they will carry grass and other nesting material in their mouth to a shallow pit and, with snout and forelimbs, arrange it in a cup-shaped nest of more than 2 m^2. The young are born into the nest. Nest-building is a very strong behavioural need for sows and therefore it is important to provide nest-building material when they are housed indoors. Sows penned in a conventional farrowing crate will start getting restless, repeatedly change their posture, paw and root the floor, gnaw and tear on the confining rails or boards and defecate frequently. This is interpreted as redirected nest-building behaviour and reflects frustration.

Signs of approaching parturition are enlargement of the vulva and swelling of the mammary glands with the presence of colostrum, restlessness and nest-building behaviour. Eventually, the sow lies down on her side and the piglets are delivered at intervals of 10–30 minutes, the placenta being expelled within 2–3 h after the birth of the last piglet. Although birth is usually trouble free, supervising parturition can minimise piglet losses. It may be necessary to free newborn pigs from the enveloping membranes, remove mucus from mouth and nose to help them start breathing, help weaker ones to reach the udder or the heated creep area. As a rule, intervention should be limited to a minimum. Occasionally, savaging of piglets becomes a problem. In these cases, piglets should be removed from the sow and placed back under supervision as soon as she has finished farrowing. Parturition may be induced prematurely to facilitate supervision and cross-fostering of piglets ('batch-farrowing'). Induction can be achieved by injecting prostaglandin F$_2\alpha$ or one of its analogues. Normally, delivery commences 24–30 h after prostaglandin injection. Parturition should never be induced before 111–112 days after the last mating, otherwise premature piglets will be born that have reduced chances of survival. Individual variation in response to the prostaglandin treatment can be further reduced by following the prostaglandin injection, about 20 h later, with a long-acting oxytocin preparation.

The young

Pigs produce precocial offspring born with all sense organs functioning. The newborn immediately start seeking the udder and generally achieve their first successful suckle within about 45 minutes. Baby pigs need antibody-containing colostrum within the first few hours. The energy reserves of newborn piglets are limited, and they rely heavily on a warm, protected environment and frequent milk feeds. Young piglets suckle at less than 1 h intervals; later, the frequency declines. Soon after birth, piglets fight fiercely until a teat order is established. The teat order is established by about 4 days after parturition and is adhered to until weaning.

When nursing, the sow lies down on her side calling her litter with a series of grunts. The piglets start nosing the udder vigorously until the milk let-down reflex is elicited. After 15–20 seconds, during which the sow gives a series of low grunts in quick succession, the milk flow ceases. Young piglets fall asleep at the udder; as they grow older, they move back to the creep area. Neonatal mortality averages 10–15%, 80% of which occurs within the first week. Most losses occur during the first 24 h after birth, especially if the individual birth mass is low and litter size exceeds the number of functional teats. The primary causes of death are crushing by the mother (almost half of the losses), chilling and starvation.

Cross-fostering piglets from one sow to another (e.g. in the case of extranumerary piglets, agalactia or loss of a sow) is not a major problem and works best within the first 2 days after birth among sows that have farrowed within a day or so of each other. Unsuckled mammary glands dry up after about 3 days. When adjusting unequally sized litters, a measure facilitated by batch-farrowing, the most vigorous members of a litter should be fostered, especially if the offspring of the host are older and stronger. When cross-fostering older piglets, it is important to camouflage their individual scent and mix the foster piglets with the original litter for 2–3 h before presenting them to the new mother.

Before 48 hours after birth, the piglets need to receive an iron product to prevent anaemia. Iron is typically given by IM injection in the neck muscle. Piglets are born with a very limited store of iron and the iron content of the sow's milk is low.

After parturition, the amount of feed provided to the sow must be gradually increased to reach *ad libitum* levels within one or two weeks.

Piglets are usually weaned at about 4 weeks of age. At this stage, farm pigs weigh 7–8 kg, minipigs 3–4 kg; these are strong enough and are able, from an immunological point of view, to cope alone.

The accommodation after weaning must give protection from draught; temperatures should be around 24° and relative humidity should not exceed 60–70%.

Breeding programmes

The selection of breeding stock must comply with the breeding goal in question, and this may differ for farm and research pigs. Miniature pigs have been selected for low body mass (Koehn *et al.* 2008). The original breeding policy for Göttingen Minipigs has been described in Glodek and Oldigs (1981) and Glodek *et al.* (1977). Special breeding programmes, such as selection for larger ear veins (to enable better access to the blood system) are used at Dalmose, Denmark, where Göttingen Minipigs are being bred. Attempts to select strains for hereditary diseases, such as diabetes mellitus, arteriosclerosis, cutaneous melanoma and congenital ventricular septum defect, to generate genetic models of human disease, tend to fail because most defects have a multifactorial genetic background (Hand *et al.* 1987).

Genetically modified models have been developed and, as methods have become easy to implement, it is assumed that they will play a greater role in the future.

Feeding

Natural and laboratory diets

Wild and domesticated pigs are truly omnivorous, consuming and digesting anything from grass to highly concentrated food of plant or animal origin. Their ability to break down and utilise raw fibre, however, is limited. Although a large proportion of the nutrient requirements can be provided by good pasture, it is more common to keep domestic pigs indoors throughout the year and feed them on concentrates. These usually consist of ground cereals supplemented with protein (fish meal, soybean meal, milk by-products), essential amino acids (mostly L-lysine, D-methionine, L-threonine, L-tryptophan), vitamins (A, D_2, D_3, E, several B vitamins) and minerals. Standard diets may be obtained from commercial producers as meal or in pelleted form. They may be fed as complete rations, or in combination with several kinds of roughage or by-products such as brewers' grains or whey. If roughage is supplied, it may consist of grass, alfalfa, clover, hay, silage or root and tuber crops.

Meal or pelleted feed may be offered dry or mixed with water or whey to make a mash. For young stock and animals kept on a maintenance diet, a single feed per day suffices; lactating animals should be fed more than once. Where computer-controlled feed dispensers are available, transponders, usually attached to the ear, make sure each individual receives the appropriate amount.

Laboratory diets for pigs and minipigs are based on natural ingredients and are usually fixed-formula diets. They are available from specialised commercial producers as diets for growth or maintenance. Some producers offer expanded diets that have been heat-treated with steam. This process is claimed to give a better availability of nutrients, a low microbial count and good acceptability by the animals. Laboratory diets should be batch controlled for nutrient content and contaminants, as variation in nutrients may produce unexpected experimental results. Contaminants such as heavy metals, fungal toxins or pesticides may also seriously impair the health status of animals and interact with drugs.

Before introduction into an SPF environment, diets may be sterilised by autoclaving or irradiation. In general, expanded diets have a low microbial count, and may be introduced into a barrier after decontamination of the feed containers.

Water

Since most diets are offered in a dry form, clean drinking water must be constantly available, even though pigs drink mainly after eating. The average daily water demand of adult pigs varies between 80 and 120 ml/kg/day. The individual demand is quite variable and considerably higher for lactating sows. Under high temperature conditions, the demand may be substantially increased. Therefore, functioning automatic drinkers are the best solution. Usually, but not always, water from the public supply is of good quality. If necessary, water may be decontaminated with chlorine or ultraviolet light.

Dietary requirements

Nutrient requirements for animals of different ages and reproductive status differ, especially regarding protein, energy and crude fibre content. Under farming conditions, generally three types of rations are supplied: (1) creep feed for suckling and newly weaned piglets (at least 20% crude protein, not more than 7–8% crude fibre); (2) production rations for growing, late pregnant or nursing animals (16–18% crude protein, not more than 7–8% crude fibre); (3) maintenance rations for mature animals (12% crude protein, 14% crude fibre). The lipid content of most rations is in the range 3–3.5%. Changes from one type of ration to another should occur gradually. Dietary requirements for pigs are given in detail by the National Research Council (NRC 1998). Even though these are minimum requirements to prevent deficiencies, the NRC guidelines are based on maximum growth and, when keeping mature animals on a maintenance ration, it may lead to obesity. Table 32.7 lists lower energy requirements for pigs of 21–120 kg. Since sows that are hungry tend to be restless and aggressive, it is advisable to feed rations with high crude fibre content or include good-quality hay or straw with the ration. Gastric emptying time and gastrointestinal transit time will increase if fibre levels are high (Bollen *et al.* 2010).

If pigs are fed in groups, diet should be spread out and it is important that all animals are able to eat, otherwise slow

Table 32.7 Basic nutrient requirements of farm pigs (NRC 1998 and other sources) and miniature pigs (GV-SOLAS 1999b) at various ages and reproductive states.

Category	Metabolisable energy (MJ/day)	Crude protein (%)	Maximum crude fibre (%)
Piglet			
3–5 kg	2–5	25	2
6–10 kg	6–8	22	6
11–20 kg	10–13	20	6
21–50 kg	18–24	18	6
51–120 kg	25–40	14	7
Adult maintenance	16–28**	12	14
Minipig (20–40 kg)			
Breeding	12–19	12–15	6–8
Maintenance	4–6	12	14

* $0.44 \times BM^{0.75}$.

eaters and weaker animals will not get their share, while others grow fat. If this is the case, it might be necessary to feed the animals individually. By monitoring the appetite and condition of the animals, individual requirements must be recognised and met by adjusting the amount of feed accordingly.

More detailed information on the nutrition of domestic pigs is provided in standard texts (NRC 1998; Lewis & Southern 2000; Lindberg & Ogle 2001; Kirchgessner et al. 2008; Jeroch et al. 2008).

The nutritional requirements of miniature pigs closely resemble those of farm pigs. The daily energy requirement for maintenance is about 0.4 MJ/kg body weight $^{0.75}$; during the growth phase it approaches 1.2 MJ/kg body weight$^{0.75}$. Most publications relating to swine nutrition are focused on efficient growth and economy. Maximum growth is not considered the optimum in scientific research, it is more important to control weight gain, especially with minipigs as they are prone to obesity. Restricted feeding is necessary to maintain normal physiological conditions. When a restricted feeding regime is applied, it is important to assure that the animals still get all the nutrients, minerals and vitamins they require; therefore, certified minipig diet should be used. Various commercial producers have developed special minipig diets for growth and maintenance. Composition varies from brand to brand, but also within brands as they are produced with natural ingredients. Common to all is a high fibre, low fat content (Ritskes-Hoitinga & Bollen 1997). Breeders will also provide specific information on this topic that is relevant for their respective strains.

Laboratory procedures

Acclimation

Pigs that are not used to being handled are shy and excitable. When anxious or confined, they tend to panic. They scream, struggle and may even succumb to circulatory collapse. Force or subjugation will aggravate the situation, where patience, treats and a calm voice will render a pig tame and co-operative. Proper acclimation including socialisation is very important. There should be an adequate acclimation period, the length of which depends on company policy and type of study. Acclimation should not be regarded as idle time. During acclimation, the switches for easy handling and a successful study can already be set. It pays to make good use of the acclimation period (Tsutsumi et al. 2001). Leaving an animal alone in this time is not acclimation. Pigs are motivated to have visual and physical contacts with humans and refusal to have physical interaction and/or eye contact is aversive for most pigs (Terlouw & Porcher 2005).

After delivery, pigs should be left for a day to settle in and become familiar with their new environment. The next day, socialising with the animals can start. Feeding time provides a good opportunity, as this is a situation where they naturally get a reward. Pigs are prey animals, so most likely they will be shy and wary, maybe even frightened. It is important to understand the 'flight zone' that pigs have. This could be considered personal space and if a person enters this zone, the animal will escape or try to do so. An animal's flight zone will vary depending on how calm or how tame it is. The flight zone gets bigger when an animal becomes excited. The flight zone is also larger when you approach 'head on'. The first efforts should be on reducing this flight zone or, in other words, gaining trust. Moving slowly around pigs and avoiding abrupt movements is less frightening. Squatting down is less intimidating, especially for minipigs, and talking in a low, pleasant voice is encouraging. Food pellets or treats will help to lure the pigs to come closer. Pigs are curious and inquisitive – let the pigs come to you rather than the opposite. It may take a while to gain enough trust so that the animal can be touched.

If there is a formal training programme for the animals, start as soon as the pigs are not afraid anymore and eat the treats they are offered. This might not occur at the same time for all animals in the group. Even if there is no training schedule, it is advisable to desensitise the pigs to the upcoming procedures. The general principles of animal training should be applied: reward desired behaviour only and reward for a purpose. See also Chapter 15: The use of positive reinforcement training techniques to enhance the care and welfare of laboratory and research animals. There should be a pleasant, undisturbed atmosphere when working with pigs and the hearing and visual capacities of pigs should be accounted for. Pigs should be handled with confidence and certainty but be gentle and caring at the same time. Pigs need assurance and clear guidance, and in this sense staff training is just as important as the animal training.

It is advisable to keep records of the progress with socialisation in the acclimation phase. This will allow to optimise resources in spending more time with the animals that are a bit behind, not as relaxed and friendly.

Handling and restraining

Restriction of movement can be considered as restraint. For pigs, less is often more and if a base of trust has been established during acclimation, handling will be much easier. Pigs can be gently cornered, possibly with a board, for brief and minimally aversive treatment, or they can be trained to walk up a ramp into a box to give the technician a more comfortable working position. Depending on the size, pigs can easily be picked up and carried on the arm. Holding on to a hind leg will control movement, then putting the other hand under the

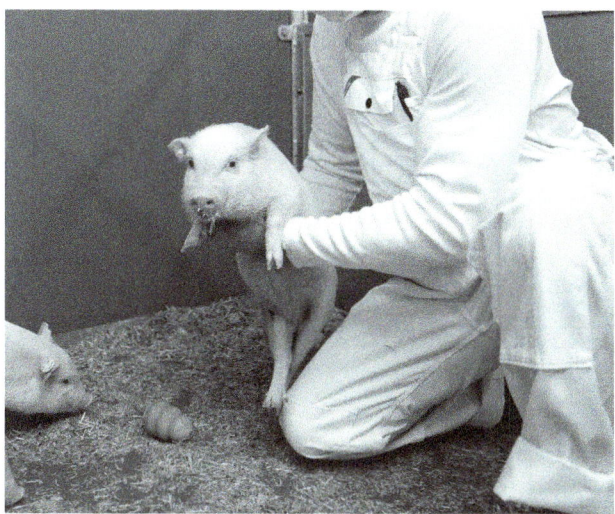

Figure 32.6 Picking up a pig: Put a hand under the thorax and lift the front legs off the floor first.

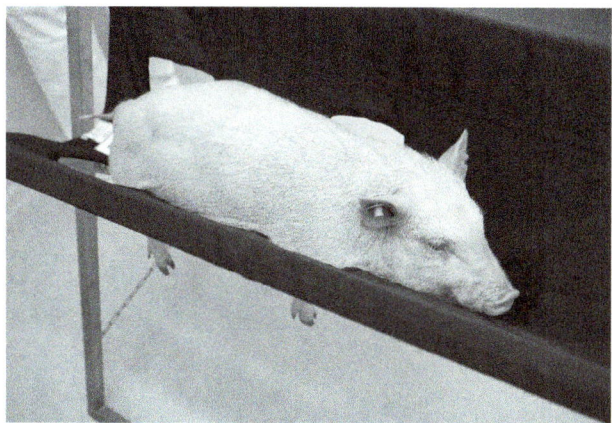

Figure 32.8 A minipig placed in a sling for longer procedures.

thorax the pig can be lifted, front first (Figure 32.6). Do not lift them up by the hind legs only as this can cause injury. Hold the pig close to your body, forelegs over your arm and hold it loosely if the pig is not struggling (Figure 32.7). Holding a pig on the arm is fine for short procedures; for slightly longer procedures, the handler can sit down on a chair with the pig on the arm. If restraining for longer procedures is required, the use of hammock-like sling with holes for the legs is advisable (Figure 32.8). Pigs are quite content to be in a sling; however, it is best to train this form of restraint in the acclimation period. It is possible to take a blood sample from a pig in the sling (but small pigs are often restrained in a V-trough on their back for blood sampling; please refer to the section on collection of specimens, blood). For an oral gavage, pigs up to 20 kg can be restrained in an upright position by a sitting technician (Figure 32.9). With increasing size, restraining gets more and more difficult and certain procedures cannot be performed anymore if the animals are conscious. The use of minipigs prolongs the time where they can be restrained effectively. The best way, though time consuming, is for the handler to establish a relationship with the animal that will enable him or her to train the pig to accept regular routine procedures such as injections or blood sampling, using appropriate positive reinforcement.

When moving individual pigs or groups of pigs, light boards or hurdles are useful. Single animals may also be driven by walking behind them, directing them with hand movements or paddle. Pigs are quick to learn and easy to train to step onto a scale or enter a restraint box. Rewards will help, but force and punishment are counterproductive.

Physiological monitoring

Recording body temperature, cardiac and pulmonary functions

Body temperature in pigs is measured by inserting a thermometer 5–6 cm deep into the rectum or vagina. The heart rate may be taken by placing the palm of the hand (or a stethoscope) against the thoracic wall under the left elbow, and the pulse by palpating the inside of the thigh where the femoral artery is close to the skin. Alternatively, an artery on the rostral rim of the ear or the coccygeal artery on the underside of the tail may be palpated (Figure 32.10). Careful auscultation of heart and lung must be carried out with a stethoscope as described in Straw *et al.* (2006). Blood pressure may be obtained by applying the inflatable cuff method of Riva-Rocci, using the coccygeal artery at the base of the tail or on the legs (Figure 32.11). Direct measurement of arterial and venous pressures requires introduction of catheters or probes into blood vessels (Marshall *et al.* 1972; Neundorf & Seidel 1977). To obtain an electrocardiogram, the electrodes of the recording unit may be attached to the extremities or to the trunk of the animal in a triangle with the heart in its centre: with one electrode behind the right ear, one on the sacrum and one on the xiphoid process – as shown in Figure 32.12. This latter way of placing the electrodes is recommended, as it results in higher wave amplitudes in minipigs (Nahas *et al.* 2002). The animals must be kept off the ground and should, therefore, be placed in a sling (see Figure 32.12) or on a non-conducting surface. A long-term electrocardiogram recording system for miniature pigs has been described by Suzuki *et al.* (1998). Further procedural information on a range of electrophysiological, haemodynamic and other procedures can be found in Swindle (2016).

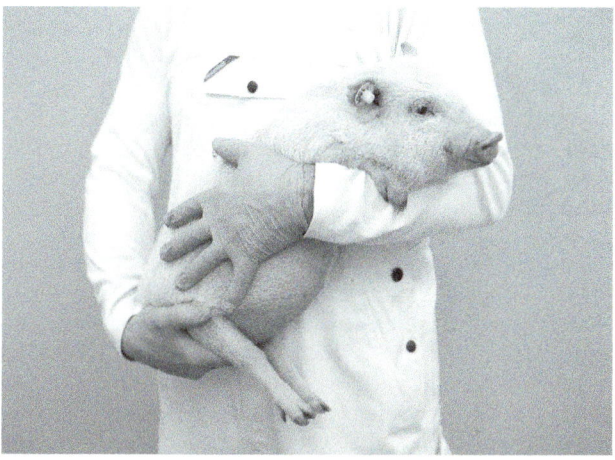

Figure 32.7 Holding and carrying a pig on the arm: Front legs over the arm and support the caudal part with the other hand.

584 Pigs and minipigs

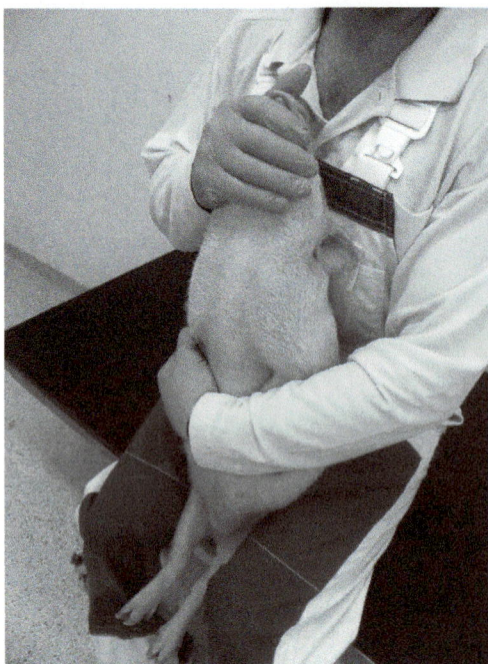
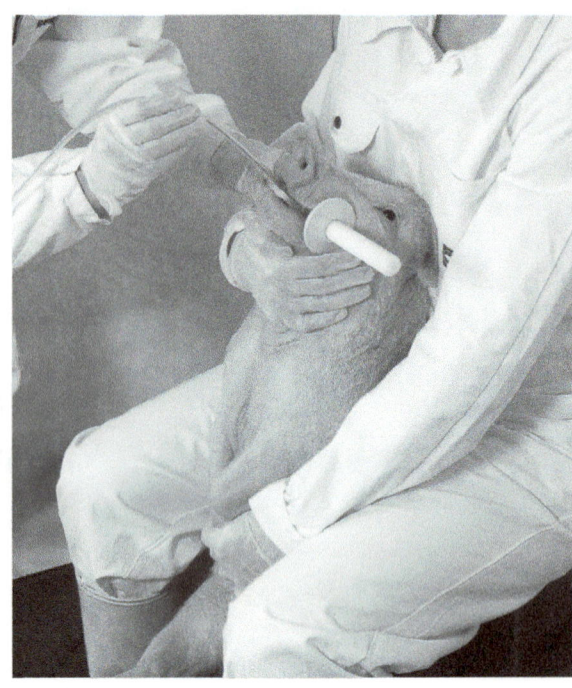

Figure 32.9 Restraining a pig by a sitting technician for blood sampling and oral gavage (right).

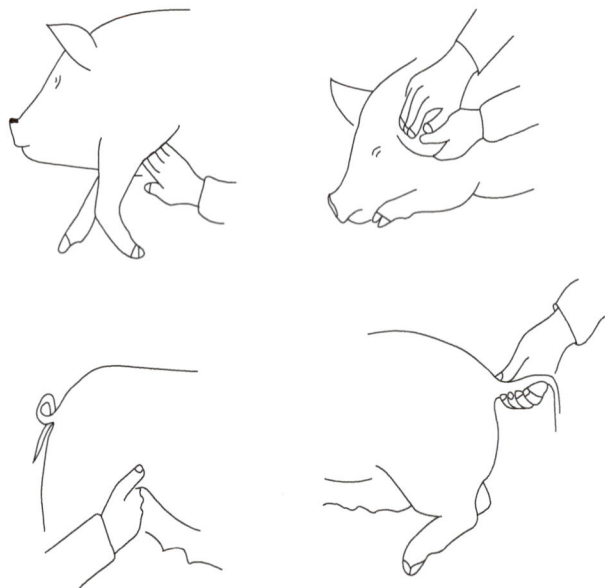

Figure 32.10 Pulse rate may be monitored by placing the palm of the hand under the left elbow or by palpitating auricular, femoral or coccygeal vessels.

Collection of specimens

Blood

General advice on blood collection and volumes can be found in Joint Working Group on Refinement (JWGR) (1993) and Diel et al. (2001). In the pig, there are not many easily accessible blood vessels. Depending on the quantity desired, several approaches may be taken. To obtain just a few drops or up to 1 ml of blood, it is easiest to nick an ear vein with the tip of a scalpel blade. As the ears are very sensitive to pain it will be difficult to repeat this procedure several times. Larger volumes are drawn from the cranial vena cava, the brachiocephalic or the external jugular vein. The external and internal jugular veins run from the head towards the heart on both sides of the trachea and join to form the brachiocephalic veins. These are joined into the cranial vena cava, which leads to the right atrium. To draw blood from these veins, animals weighing up to 25 kg are held in a supine position, preferably in a V-trough, head and neck straightened out and front limbs drawn backwards (Figure 32.13). It is easier and better from an animal welfare point of view to restrain pigs above 10 kg in a sling for blood sampling. The head is placed at the short end and lifted by a technician to give access to the vessels in the neck (Figure 32.14). A 20G hypodermic needle (0.9 × 40 mm) is appropriate in pigs up to 25 kg, larger animals may require a longer needle. The insertion is cranial to the sternum slightly lateral to the midline. While advancing the needle in a caudal-dorso-medial direction, a vacuum is maintained in the syringe so blood starts streaming in as soon as the vessel is punctured. The use of vacutainers facilitates the operation. To find the external jugular vein further up the neck, the jugular fossa may be used for orientation. In heavier landrace pigs, the same procedure is followed while they are standing up with the head pulled forward and slightly upward by an upper jaw snare. A snare is not generally used with laboratory pigs and should not be used with minipigs. Arterial blood may be collected from the brachiocephalic artery (Neundorf & Seidel 1977).

Excitement before or during the collection of blood can induce contraction of the spleen, resulting in an increase in packed cell volume of more than 10%. It is also likely to result in a neuro-endocrine response. Therefore, indwelling catheters are often used for repeated blood collection. Adult pigs, that have big enough ear veins, may be fitted with ear vein catheters extending to the jugular vein and

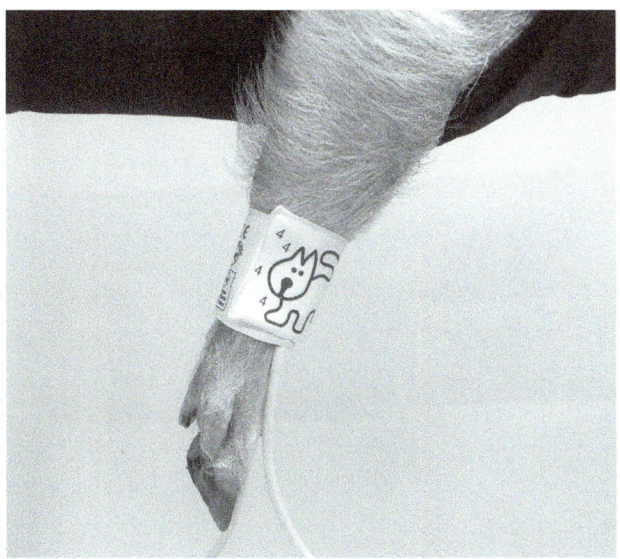 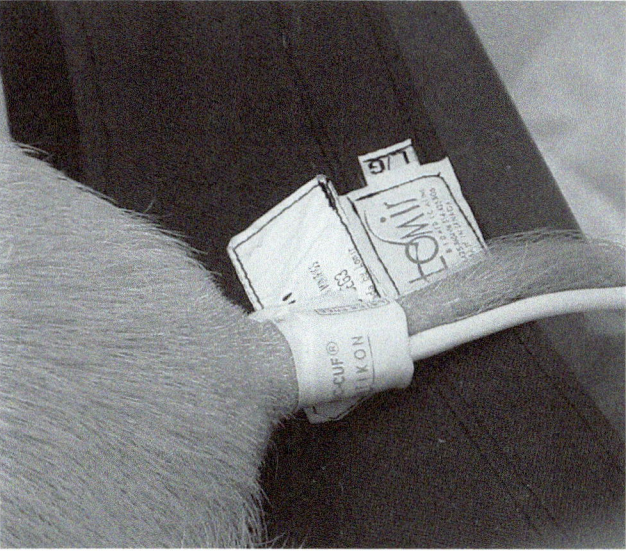

Figure 32.11 Pig in a sling with cuff around leg and tail for non-invasive measuring of blood pressure.

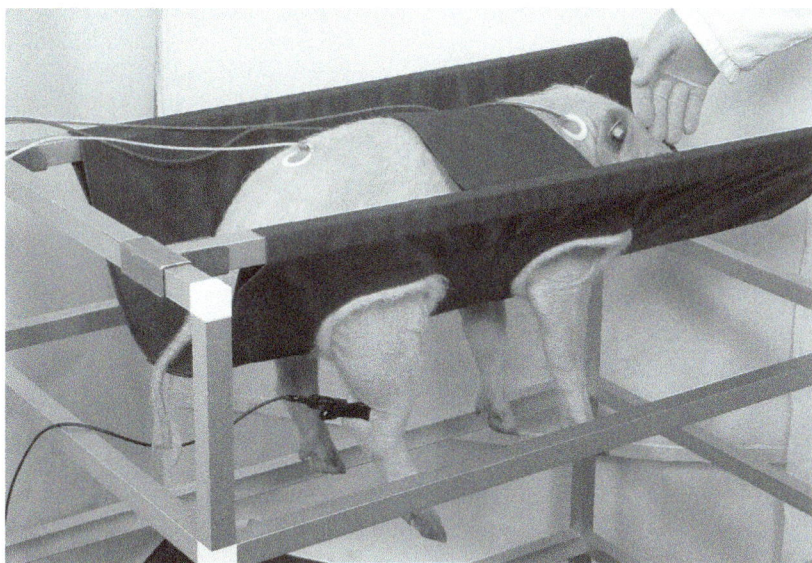

Figure 32.12 Minipigs in the sling for ECG recording. The lead placement is described in the preceding text.

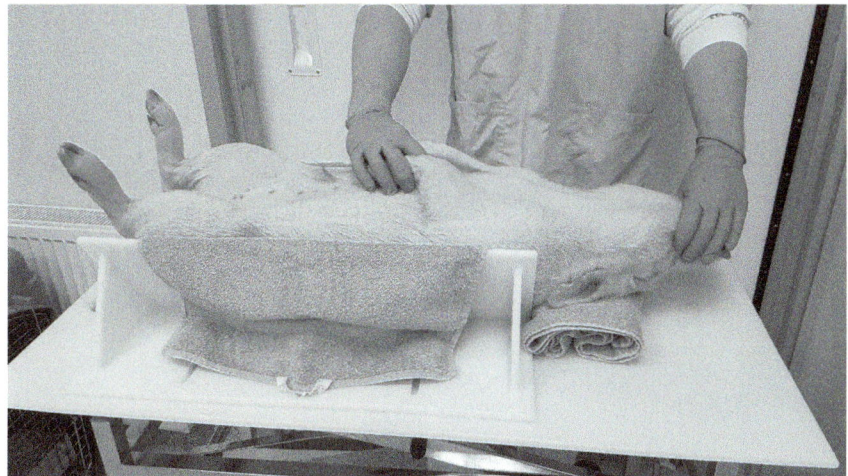

Figure 32.13 A minipig restrained in a V-bench for blood sampling from the large veins in the neck. Depending on the temperament of the animal and the amount of training the handler and the pig have received, more than one person may be necessary to hold the animal.

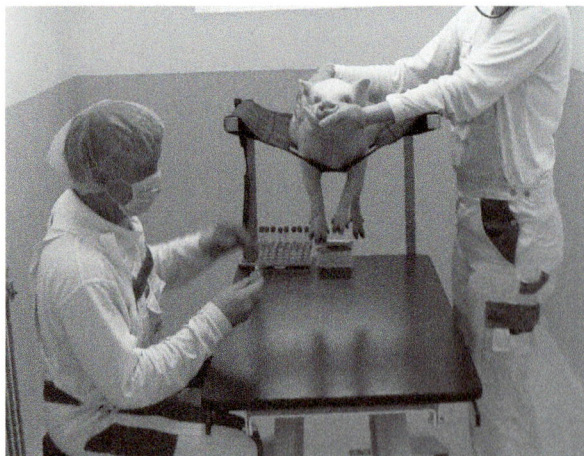
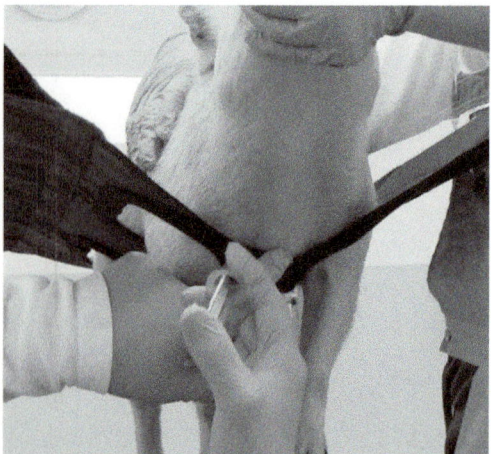

Figure 32.14 Blood sampling with the pig in a sling.

vena cava cranialis. While the pig is anaesthetised, the marginal (*V. auricularis lateralis*) or central (*V. auricularis intermedia*) ear vein is penetrated and a 3–4 fr catheter can be implanted by Seldinger technique (Seldinger 1953).

In small pigs, with small ear veins, it is best to resort to jugular catheters. These may be fitted by non-surgical means as described by Carroll *et al.* (1999) for young pigs and Damm *et al.* (2000) for adult animals. Catheters up to 7 fr can be inserted by Seldinger technique in the jugular vein using triangulation as landmark (Flournoy & Mani 2009). Adapted methods can be applied to catheterise the saphenous vein. For long-term catheterisation, a surgical approach is preferable. The catheter may be secured by a retention cuff when exteriorised, or a vascular access port (VAP) can be attached to the catheter and placed subcutaneously. Recently, also rat Vascular Access Buttons (VAB) have been successfully implanted in minipigs. These procedures have been described in various literature (Baille *et al.* 1986; Palmisano *et al.* 1989; Swindle 2016). The vessel of interest is dissected, and a silicon or PU catheter is inserted and fixed to the vessel. The distal end is tunnelled to an appropriate site where a subcutaneous pocket is formed. The catheter is connected to the VAP, and all incisions are closed. This provides a fully integrated system and the pigs can be group-housed as there are no external parts. The port can be accessed through the skin with a needle for withdrawal or infusion. In the case of VAB, there is a protected exterior part that allows needle free and painless accesses to the vascular system.

Catheterised animals must be kept in a clean environment and the catheter exteriorisation site should checked regularly. After sampling, catheters must be rinsed with sterile saline and locked with an appropriate lock solution. Lock solutions are commercially available but heparinised saline, up to 500 U/ml, is most commonly used. Alternatives are taurolidine citrate, glycerol, sodium citrate, glucose or sucrose. Provided strict hygienic principles are followed, catheters may remain functional for many weeks. Bilateral jugular catheterisation, even if resulting in complete occlusion of both veins, is well tolerated by the animals. Instead of the jugular, the cephalic vein may be used by making an incision in the sagittal plane halfway between shoulder joint and *manubrium sterni*.

Arterial catheters may be inserted in the carotid artery, which is easily localised dorsal to the jugular vein by digital palpation of the pulse.

Porcine erythrocytes are fragile and excessive turbulence and agitation during blood collecting and processing will bring about haemolysis. Coagulation of porcine blood is rapid and, to avoid clotting, the collecting vials must contain an anti-coagulant (Straw *et al.* 2006).

Urine

The easiest way to obtain urine from a pig is to keep it in a metabolism cage; however, this is a restricted environment for the pig. Collecting urine during spontaneous micturition is best done after making the animals get up from a resting position, as they will usually urinate soon afterwards. Collection directly from the urinary bladder may be carried out in the female by introducing a catheter into the urethral orifice with the aid of a vaginal speculum under general anaesthesia. In the male, the urethral approach is not feasible and urine specimens can only be obtained by turning the animal on its back and piercing the abdominal wall cranial to the pubic arch with a long cannula. For repeated collection, a flexible catheter can be introduced via an incision in the suprapubic area (Marshall *et al.* 1972).

Faeces

Specimens may be collected by introducing one or two gloved fingers into the rectum. The faecal sample is grasped with one hand, while the other hand pulls down the plastic glove, everts it and ties the top of the glove to a knot, thus sealing the sample. The use of positive reinforcement techniques might be an option in some studies. If large amounts of faeces are to be collected, animals must be placed in a metabolism cage.

Milk

Milk may be stripped from the teat of a lactating sow. If the sows are trained, they will readily present their udder for massage and stripping. In some cases, oxytocin might need to be administered (5 IE im for a minipig sow).

Biopsies

Biopsies have been taken from the testes, skin, liver and other organs, usually under full anaesthesia or after tranquillisation and local anaesthesia.

Other specimens

To obtain information on the collection of specimens not covered in this chapter, such as CSF, bile, bone marrow, stomach or intestinal contents, skin scrapings, biopsies or entire organs, the following sources may be consulted: Mount and Ingram (1971); Marshall *et al.* (1972); Neundorf & Seidel (1977); Glodek and Oldigs (1981); Swindle (2016); Bollen *et al.* (2010). A system for continual perfusion or dialysis of internal organs in freely moving miniature pigs has been described by Jarry *et al.* (1990) and van Kleef (1996).

Administration of substances

General advice on the administration of substances is provided in JWGR (2001) and Diel *et al.* (2001).

Tablets, pills and capsules

Administration of drugs often involves restraint of the animals. Tablets, pills or capsules may be deposited deep in the mouth with the aid of a balling gun. When offered concealed in a morsel of tasty feed, they may be taken voluntarily. In order to circumvent the first pass effect, rectal suppositories may be inserted.

Liquids

Sweet tasting liquids may be ingested voluntarily if offered with the aid of a syringe. Small amounts can be mixed with juice or yoghurt. For large amounts, animals must be restrained, and a mouth gag made of wood or non-toxic hard plastic, with a hole in the centre, is wedged between the jaws. This is typically stressful for the pig. Handlers should be well-trained to restrain pigs appropriately and perform the procedure quickly and smoothly to minimise stress (Morton *et al.* 2001). A lubricated stomach tube (4–10 mm outside diameter) with rounded tip is introduced through the hole into the oesophagus. To be sure, the end of the tube is placed in the ventricle, the insertion length is the distance from the last rib to the snout of the pig. There is a diverticulum at the beginning of the oesophagus and if there is resistance while feeding the tube, it is likely that the tip ended there. Retract the tube and try again. It will be easier if the swallowing reflex can be initiated. If the tube finds its way to the trachea, the pig will cough and fight immensely. If the whole length can be inserted, it is very likely that the tube is in the stomach; to be sure, vacuum can be applied, or the distal end can be placed in a bowl of water and checked that it does not bubble.

Injections

The routes of injection are:

- *Intradermal* (id, intracutaneous). These injections usually involve small volumes (50–200 µl) and are administered to the corium layer of the skin on the ear, behind the ear or in flank of the animal with a fine (0.5 mm/25G) hypodermic needle. Pigs should be sedated for this procedure. Alternatively, a jet injector can be used (Ploemen *et al.* 2014).
- *Subcutaneous* (sc). In animals up to 25 kg, such injections are most conveniently administered by lifting them up, gripping the skin fold between flank and hind leg and introducing the needle (0.9 mm) between the two layers of skin. Larger animals can be trained to stay still, or they can be distracted with food for this injection. Dziuk (1991) reports that 'with a little patience and some dexterity' it is possible, even in unrestrained pigs, to place an injection under the thin, loose and relatively insensitive skin area of the chest just behind the elbow. Another site that can be used is just caudal to the base of the ear in a perpendicular or angled direction (Figure 32.15). For pharmacological testing, this site represents the human anatomy best, as it leads to injection into fat as an sc injection typically does in man. As in humans, the skin in pigs is firmly attached to the underlying tissue and sc injections can therefore be done into subcutaneous fat. To be sure of the proper site and depth, the area

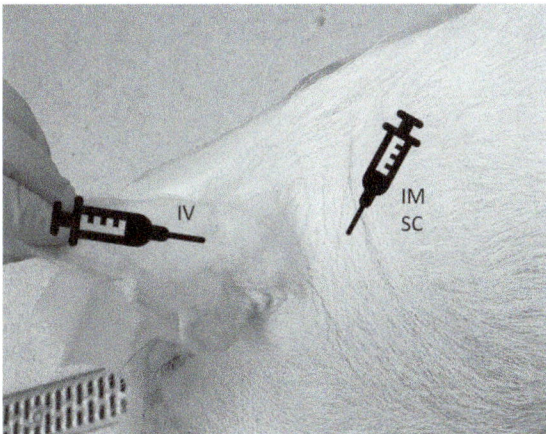
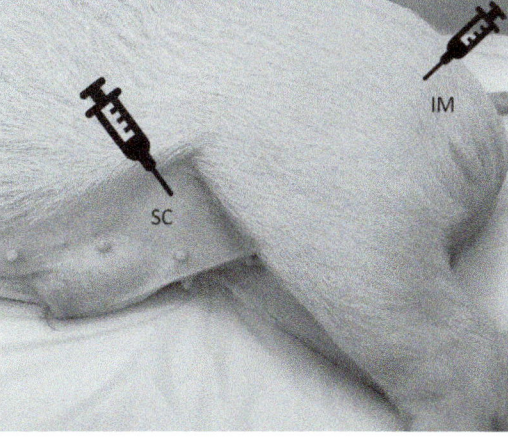

Figure 32.15 Typical injection sites: intramuscular, intravenous and subcutaneous.

can be scanned by ultrasound and marked with a pen. The needle must either be short or have a stopper mounted in order not to risk injecting into the underlying muscle instead.

- *Intramuscular* (im). Usually, these injections are administered by inserting the needle (0.9 mm) 1 or 2 cm caudal to the base of the ear in a ventromedial direction. Alternatively, the musculature of the dorsal neck or the thigh may be used (Figure 32.15). The volume administered should be small.
- *Intraperitoneal* (ip). Intraperitoneal injections are not very common in pigs; however, they can be successfully accomplished on anaesthetised animals. Usually, ip injections are applied to animals light enough to be picked up. To reduce the risk of penetrating intestines, the use of a Veress needle is recommended. If this is not available, a large bore needle can be used to penetrate the skin when it is pulled up. Proper placement of the needle tip is tested by injecting saline first and immediately withdrawing it again. If the liquid is clear or withdrawal is impossible, the position is most likely fine. If the liquid is cloudy or faecal matter can be seen, intestines might have been penetrated.
- *Intravenous* (iv). Few superficial veins in a pig are easily accessible. The ear vein is the most commonly used site. The saphenous/tarsal vein is an alternative, but the skin on older animals can be very tough to penetrate at this site. It might be necessary to sedate the animal or use topical anaesthetic agents, such as lidocaine or EMLA, for this procedure. The use of an over-the-needle catheter can be useful for multiple dosing and infusions. It can be left in place for up to three days. The use of a mandrin (stylet within the catheter) to prevent coagulation is an option, otherwise the use of a lock solution is appropriate. Good stasis will facilitate the penetration of the veins, especially concerning the ear vein, and for this a rubber band tied with an artery clamp is helpful. Needle size for minipigs starts at 23G; bigger diameters can be chosen for larger vessels. Consideration should be given to the properties of the compound and vehicle (in terms of pH, osmolality, viscosity, protein content, etc.) in deciding whether a peripheral vein is the right route of dosing or whether catheterisation of a large vessel is more appropriate.

Injection volumes considered to be good practice and maximum acceptable doses are summarised in Table 32.8. The figures refer to aqueous solutions, not to solvents such as dimethyl sulfoxide (DMSO), carboxymethylcellulose (CMC) or oily suspensions. If the administration of larger volumes is unavoidable, multiple injection sites may be indicated. It should be kept in mind that injections might cause pain and tissue damage and should, where possible, be replaced by other routes of administration. In the case of antibiotics, administration *per oral* is usually possible.

For continuous drug administration, permanently indwelling catheters or ambulatory infusion pumps positioned, for example, in a pocket of a specially tailored vest, might be employed. An alternative approach is to implant an osmotic pump or small programmable infusion pumps (Tan *et al.* 2011). For shorter infusions, pigs might be placed in a sling and the catheters connected to a free-standing pump.

Anaesthesia and analgesia

Sedation

Pigs that are to be anaesthetised should be deprived of feed, but not water, for at least 12 h. To minimise stress, it is advisable to sedate them by administering an intramuscular injection of a tranquillising agent in familiar surroundings. The use of flexible tubing between the syringe and the hypodermic needle gives flexibility during injection if the animal moves. The most commonly applied tranquillising drug for farm pigs is azaperone (1–4 mg/kg) sometimes combined with midazolam (0.5–1 mg/kg) or ketamine (5–20 mg/kg). Azaperone has been widely used in the past to sedate pigs, but some major manufactures in Europe have ceased production and it is increasingly difficult to obtain the drug. Animals should be left alone for 5–15 minutes, preferably in dark surroundings, for the sedative to take full action. The animals will remain sensitive to acoustic stimuli and the body temperature will drop.

For minipigs, a moderate sedation can be achieved with midazolam, 0.5 mg/kg im. This sedation lasts for around 30 min. and is useful for non-invasive procedures like echocardiography or similar. They are still responsive to some stimuli but, if handled carefully and gently, they are easy to manipulate without getting excited. A variety of other sedation protocols can be found in Swindle (2016) or Lumb & Jones (2007).

Surgical anaesthesia

No single anaesthetic product satisfies all possible requirements (i.e. sedation, hypnosis, analgesia and muscular relaxation). Therefore, depending on the type and duration of the surgical intervention, combinations of various agents may be indicated. Minor surgery may be performed by combining sedation with local anaesthesia using, for example, procaine or lidocaine. For longer interventions it is recommended to induce with an im injection which might be enough for tracheal intubation, followed by inhalation anaesthesia. If the anaesthetic depth does not allow intubation, an indwelling catheter can be placed in the lateral ear vein for an intravenous injection to deepen anaesthesia or run CRI (continuous rate infusion) anaesthesia. Anaesthesia should always be supplemented with oxygen.

Table 32.8 Good practice dose volumes for injecting miniature pigs of 25–40 kg body mass (GV-SOLAS, 2017, Diehl *et al.* 2001). For lighter pigs, smaller volumes are recommended; however, for heavier pigs approximately similar volumes are appropriate.

Dose volumes	ml/injection site			ml/kg body weight			
				ip		iv	
	id	sc	im			Bolus	Slow injection
Recommended	0.1	10	5	1	1		2
Maximum	0.2	20	10	20	2		5

Injectable anaesthesia

Ketamine is commonly used with pigs. As ketamine tends to increase muscle tone and exerts little visceral analgesia; it is usually combined with other agents such as azaperone, acepromazine, diazepam, midazolam, fentanyl, butorphanol, telazol, medetomidine or xylazine. According to Green and Benson (2002), the group of tranquillisers that is most effective in pigs is the butyrophenone class. Alpha-2-agonist sedatives are useful, especially in combination with other agents, but relatively high doses must be used (e.g. 2.2 mg/kg xylazine). Various laboratories have established protocols of their own depending on the purpose of study. A protocol found to be effective, safe and both clinically and economically sound (Erhardt et al. 2004) consists of an intramuscular injection of a mixture of azaperone (2 mg/kg), ketamine (15 mg/kg) and atropine (0.02 mg/kg) followed, 10 minutes later, by an intravenous injection of propofol (4 mg/kg); for extension of anaesthesia, additional amounts of propofol may be infused and an analgesic has to be administered. The amount required may vary considerably.

In minipigs, a combination of medetomidine (0.08 mg/kg), ketamine (10 mg/kg) and butorphanol (0.22 mg/kg) is often used for induction and the animals can be intubated on this mix alone. The most common injectable anaesthesia is a mixture of telazol, ketamine, xylazine and butorphanol. Telazol is an equal blend of tiletamine and zolazepam. The respective doses are 1.25 mg/kg, except for butorphanol at 0.25 mg/kg. It is a very powerful cocktail and the minipigs have a fast loss of consciousness. Advantages are a low injectable volume and very stable cardiovascular and respiratory parameters. It provides safe anaesthesia for 60–90 min and has all the ingredients for minor surgeries to be performed on this injection alone.

Propofol has a fast onset and is metabolised rapidly. It is usually injected as a single bolus for induction of general deep anaesthesia to enable intubation. General anaesthesia can be continued with propofol as CRI. Propofol has no analgesic properties and can only be dosed iv. A side effect of fast injection can be a temporary respiratory depression, so animals should be carefully observed for apnoea.

Inhalation anaesthesia

Anaesthesia may be accomplished with the aid of an inhalation drug, but surgical interventions should not be carried out under inhalation anaesthesia alone. Inhalation anaesthetics have no analgesic properties; therefore, a separate analgesic protocol needs to be in place. Depending on the expected pain, a multi modal approach with local anaesthetic, non-steroidal anti-inflammatory drugs (NSAIDs) and opioids should be considered. For inhalation anaesthesia, sevoflurane or isoflurane are recommended. As induction, well-socialised animals rapidly pass into deep anaesthesia without excitation if they inhale 5% Sevoflurane in oxygen via a face mask. Prior sedation might be necessary if they are not socialised. Once intubated, surgical anaesthesia can be maintained at a concentration of 1–2% for Isoflurane and at 3–4% for Sevoflurane. MAC values in pigs have been reported to be 1.6–2.2 % (Malavasi et al. 2008) for Isoflurane and 2.5–4.4 % for Sevoflurane (Otsuki et al. 2010). Great variations are found in literature regarding MAC, but it is evident that other anaesthetic compounds reduce the need for volatile gases. Anaesthetics can be delivered in oxygen or in an oxygen : air mix. The need for anaesthetic varies a great deal, depending on a lot of factors. If injectable anaesthetics have been used as induction, the amount of inhaled agent may be greatly reduced initially. It is advised to monitor the depth of anaesthesia carefully and continuously and adjust the dose accordingly. A further reduction in agent concentration may be accomplished by replacing pure oxygen with a mixture of one-half to two-thirds nitrous oxide (Smith et al. 1997). With some susceptible breeds (Pietrain, Poland China and their crossbred offspring), the use of fluranes is not advised as they can induce malignant hyperthermia syndrome; this is characterised by a rapid increase in body temperature, hyperventilation, muscle rigidity and sudden death. This heritable condition is transmitted by a single dominant gene, and it is associated with general susceptibility to stress. Breeding programmes are conducted, aimed at eliminating the trait from the population. In Göttingen Minipigs, the condition is not seen, as the responsible gene is not present.

Finding face masks for pigs that fit snugly and have little dead space can be challenging. Shape and size of the pigs' heads vary depending on breed and age. Sometimes, commercially available dog masks, consisting of a plexiglass dome fitted with a rubber diaphragm with a central opening for the snout, may be suitable. Some leakage may occur and for personal safety an air extraction system should be in place when using volatile gases. Custom-made masks have been designed for inhalation studies but are difficult to come by.

Endotracheal intubation requires experience, as pigs cannot open the mouth very wide, have a long pharynx and a narrow and angled larynx. They need to be sedated and anaesthetised either via a mask or by injection. Treatment with atropine might be advised, depending on anaesthetic regime and strain. Preoxygenation by mask or nasal tube is highly recommended to increase the oxygen reserves in the FRC (functional residual capacity). Pigs are placed in lateral or ventral recumbency, the neck is extended and the mouth is opened as wide as possible so that the larynx can be seen with the aid of a laryngoscope. The epiglottis might be engaged on the soft palette and can be released with the help of a long pin or the blade of the laryngoscope to see the larynx. The tongue is pulled forward and pressed down with the long spatula of the laryngoscope. The arytenoid cartilage and the voice cords should be visible and should get a dose of lidocaine spray to prevent laryngospasm when intubating. An endotracheal tube of appropriate size should be carefully inserted into the trachea with a twisting movement. Once proper position in the trachea is confirmed, the cuff can be inflated to a maximum pressure of 25 cm H_2O. It is advised to use a manometer, as it is very easy to overinflate and cause trauma to the trachea. The tube is fixed to the upper jaw with a gauze bandage or a soft string. Depending on the body weight, the outer diameter of the tube should be between 9 and 12 mm. For miniature pigs, normal oral paediatric endotracheal tubes of 5–10 mm outer diameter are suitable. Detailed descriptions of the procedure may be found in Lumb & Jones (2007), Svendsen & Rasmussen (1998), Erhardt et al. (2004) and Swindle (2016).

As an alternative to endotracheal intubation, a laryngeal mask airway (LMA), designed for use in humans, may be inserted into the hypopharynx of a pig. Once inflated, it will provide an airtight seal around the laryngeal inlet and proved to be efficient in both spontaneously breathing (Wemyss-Holden et al. 1999) and mechanically ventilated pigs (Goldmann et al. 2005; Fulkerson et al. 2007). The system is proved to be convenient and efficient even when applied by relatively inexperienced personnel. It is important to make sure the epiglottis is not pressed down to the trachea and prevents respiration.

Epidural anaesthesia

If surgery is to be performed caudal to the umbilicus, epidural anaesthesia may be applied. Animals are tranquillised and procaine or lidocaine infused into the spinal canal by inserting a long 20–22G hypodermic needle through the lumbosacral aperture as described elsewhere (Neundorf & Seidel 1977; Bolin et al. 1992; Swindle 2016).

Peri- and post-operative care

Most precautions taken to maintain anaesthetised animals in a state of near homeostasis are the same for most mammals. Pigs, lacking a dense hair coat, are particularly prone to hypothermia. To aid in body heat retention, it helps to drape them and/or place them on a heating pad both during anaesthesia and the recovery phase. At induction, they should be lifted off a cold floor and onto a warm pad as soon as possible. Recuperating pigs should have a warm recovery room with heat lamps and floor heating, or at least be bedded on a layer of straw and covered with a blanket or clean dry straw. During extended interventions, additional care might be warranted, including administration of parenteral fluids for maintenance of water and electrolyte balance. Anaesthesia should be carefully monitored that should as a minimum include: anaesthetic depth, respiration, heart rate, body temperature and SpO_2. Depth of anaesthesia can be determined by checking reflexes and jaw tone. Palpebral reflex is tested by touching the periphery of the eye with a clean, blunt instrument, inter-digital by applying a clamp between the claws and tail flick by pinching the area below the tail with forceps. Depending on the type of surgery, monitoring of blood pressure, blood gases, ECG or EEC might be required as well. Appropriate ways of accomplishing this can be found in Swindle (2016).

An effective analgesic regime, appropriate for the procedure, must be in place and a multi modal approach is recommended. Intra- and post-operative analgesia may be provided by using local anaesthesia, NSAIDs such as carprofen or meloxicam, and/or opiates like fentanyl, remifentanil or buprenorphine. Ketamine has some analgesic properties; its effects on the NMDA receptors suggest effective reduction of hyperalgesia following tissue trauma (Stubhaug et al. 2008; Boo Hwi Hong et al. 2011). It is reported that α2-agonists do not provide very effective analgesia in pigs.

The effect of analgesics depends on the substance used. For post-operative analgesia, long-lasting products like buprenorphine (8 h), NSAIDs (often 24 h) or fentanyl patches (72 h) should be used to be able to leave the pigs undisturbed for longer periods. The route of dosing must be considered as well; carprofen can be administered as a tasty chewable tablet and meloxicam is available as an oral suspension. Both are voluntarily ingested by pigs; thus, injection can be avoided. The use of a fentanyl (an opiate) patch, attached to the shaven skin behind the ear, has been found to be useful (Malavasi et al. 2005; Stubhan et al. 2008). As there is considerable individual variation in analgesic requirement, it important to assess analgesic effects frequently and adjust dose and frequency accordingly.

Pain assessment is a complex task, and it requires often a good knowledge of the species as well as the individual. Most significant is the absence of normal behaviour if pigs are in pain, e.g. inactivity, reluctance to move or get up, hanging posture, altered gait and so on. Reduced food intake is an indicator, but females in oestrus are generally not that interested in food. The position of the tail is a very good indicator of general well-being. However, in some breeds or if the tail is docked it is not very helpful. See also section: Signs of poor health. Viscardi et al. (2017) have developed a pig grimace scale for pain assessment which might help.

Emergencies

Most anaesthetic agents cause mild respiratory and cardiac depression, except ketamine which has the opposite effect. Adding ketamine to the anaesthetic protocol will reduce these cardiorespiratory effects. If respiration fails, animals that are intubated must be bagged or connected to a ventilator with pre-adjusted settings appropriate to the patient. It may be necessary to intubate them at this point. If they are not, or cannot be intubated, place them in lateral recumbency, and compress the thorax rhythmically with both hands 10–20 times per minute and reduce anaesthesia if available. Oxygen should always be offered. As long as the heart is beating, artificial respiration should be maintained as the animal has a good chance of recovery. Artificial respiration should be interrupted, from time to time, to reactivate the respiratory centre. In some cases, intravenous application of emergency drugs such as lidocaine (arrythmias), dopamine (hypotension), Atropine (bradycardia) or, as a last resort, adrenaline (cardiac arrest) may be indicated.

Detailed treatises covering anaesthesia and analgesia in the pig are to be found in Riebold (1995); Thurmon & Benson (1996); Svendsen & Rasmussen (1998); Erhardt et al. (2004); Lumb & Jones (2007); Swindle (2016) and Flecknell (2015).

Euthanasia

Euthanasia should be accomplished by methods that induce rapid unconsciousness and death of the animal without pain or distress. See Chapter 17: Euthanasia and other fates for laboratory animals. In the EU, this is governed by Directive 2010/63/EU. Generally, an anaesthetic overdose (e.g. more than 150 mg/kg pentobarbital iv, ic) after sedation is preferable to physical methods such as a penetrating captive bolt. Use of a captive bolt requires subsequent 'sticking' or 'bleeding' to cause death by loss of blood. This is done by using a knife, not less than 120 mm long cranial to the sternum, to sever *all* major blood vessels leading to the head In exceptional cases, a free bullet may be used, but only in field conditions by experienced marksmen. Other methods allowed by the above legislation are the use of inert gases and electrical stunning. In anaesthetised animals, an overdose of anaesthetic compound is acceptable under Directive 2010/63/EU. In all cases, the killing of animals shall be completed by one of the following methods:

a. confirmation of permanent cessation of the circulation;
b. destruction of the brain;
c. dislocation of the neck;
d. exsanguination; or
e. confirmation of the onset of rigour mortis.

Common welfare problems

Disease

Prophylaxis

Pathogenic microbes travel with airborne particles or droplets, but more commonly they are transmitted via animal vectors. The most important of these are infected pigs. Other vectors include domestic animals, such as cats and dogs, vermin, such as rats and mice, birds, insects and, most frequently, humans. Therefore, good barrier systems should ideally be employed. Principles and procedures of such systems are described in the section on health monitoring, quarantine and barrier systems. When the establishment of a barrier system is not feasible, precautions must be taken to minimise the risk of infectious disease. A few basic principles to be considered are the provision of appropriate housing, husbandry and feeding conditions, a good sanitation programme and, as far as possible, prevention of the introduction of infectious agents.

Before moving animals into quarters formerly occupied by others, the rooms must be thoroughly cleaned and scrubbed with antiseptic solution, preferably with a high-pressure jet and hot water or steam. Complete units should be evacuated, cleaned and restocked (all-in, all-out). Animals should be treated for internal and external parasites before being introduced to sanitised housing, especially when they have previously been run on pastures or dirt lots. Animal traffic and visits by people who have been in contact with other pigs within the last 48 h should not be permitted. Foot dips and changing of clothes should be mandatory. Health control specialists advocate that a shower be taken before entering a unit. The origin and quality of biological material (feed, bedding, experimental materials) and equipment should be controlled to prevent the introduction of infectious agents. A rodent and insect barrier should be part of the disease-control programme.

Depending on the source of the pigs and the diseases prevalent in the area, vaccination protocols could be warranted. It should be kept in mind that vaccination will protect against disease but will not usually prevent the transmission of pathogens. Furthermore, vaccinated pigs will be seropositive, which may interfere with health monitoring. Prophylactic antibiotic treatment may control bacterial propagation and enable the host to develop immunity, but will not eliminate the pathogen. In many cases, administration of pro-biotics (yoghurt or commercially available paste of highly concentrated lactobacillus) is a great help for newly delivered pigs to cope with the microbiological environment of the new place. Animals to be introduced into the herd should originate from suppliers providing a high standard of hygiene (preferably with MD or SPF status) and a defined disease-control system. It is good practice to quarantine new arrivals for at least 3, preferably 6, weeks before integrating them into the herd. The first 3 weeks are a period of isolation, the animals are being monitored, wormed, vaccinated, etc.; during the following 3 weeks, animals from the herd are to be integrated in are introduced so they may adapt immunologically.

Signs of poor health

General symptoms indicating poor health in adult pigs are emaciation; listlessness and lack of appetite; increased body temperature; discoloration (cyanosis) of skin areas; stiffness of limbs; diarrhoea; snuffling and coughing; in certain conditions hyperactivity, excitability, frequent change of posture and convulsions. Typical symptoms of diseased young piglets are wasting; listlessness; rough coat; abnormal posture and behaviour; diarrhoea; sneezing, coughing and laboured breathing ('pumping'); swollen joints; increased body temperature and skin conditions. Depending on the strain of pig or minipig, the position of the tail is a very good indicator of the general well-being as well. Göttingen Minipigs for example have a straight tail that hangs down in a neutral position, is wagging when happy, up when alert and between the legs when unwell, scared submissive or unsure.

In addition, there will generally be specific symptoms indicative of the particular ailment involved.

Common diseases

In commercial pig husbandry, usually large numbers of animals are kept under confined conditions, facilitating rapid spreading of infectious diseases.

The most important infectious diseases to be aware of are covered by the FELASA guidelines for health monitoring (Rehbinder *et al.* 1998). The screening programmes used by large commercial breeders can be more extensive than those described in the guideline and can point to other diseases that can also be of relevance (see for instance the health reports published on www.minipigs.dk).

Useful handbooks covering diseases in pigs are Taylor (1999), Prange (2004), Waldmann and Wendt (2004), and Straw *et al.* (2006).

Suboptimal housing conditions can result in disease. For instance, it is important to have dry, clean areas in the pens to avoid dermal problems; well-socialised groups to avoid fighting-related wounds; optimal temperature and air change to avoid respiratory problems; and optimal diet and feeding guidelines to avoid over-/under-weight and diseases such as gastric ulceration. Finally, as mentioned above, it is important to have clean and disinfected pens when receiving new animals – or the animals will be at increased risk of developing diarrhoea shortly after arrival. Such a diarrhoea problem can also result from cross-contamination if pigs with another – typically lower – status are housed next to ones with a high health status. And although a short period of diarrhoea may seem harmless, it can have a significant impact on animals for a long period, as reflected in, for instance, the levels of acute phase proteins (Christoffersen *et al*. 2015).

Abnormal behaviour

Prevailing husbandry conditions for many farmed pigs are notoriously deficient in providing a complex enriched environment (see the section titled 'Environmental provisions') and high-quality individual attention (see the section titled 'Handling'). Under conditions with increasing herd size and growing economic pressures, farms are increasingly reduced to anonymous production units. More acceptable production systems, with far better animal welfare, are provided by breeders of laboratory pigs. In the EU, they operate under the legislation for the protection of animals used for scientific purposes (Directive 2010/63/EU), which is far more stringent and has a greater focus on welfare than the respective legislation for farm animals.

Apart from getting a healthier and better characterised pig by choosing a well-established breeder of laboratory pigs, the animals are also raised under better conditions.

Unfavourable conditions facilitate behavioural aberrations which are not acceptable for laboratory pigs. The most common stereotypic, redirected behaviours and other abnormal behaviours observed are:

1. Bar biting. The animals take horizontal bars in their mouth and either bite on it with a chewing motion or just hold it in their mouth for extended periods. This behaviour is commonly observed in sows kept in single crates on concrete floors without bedding and is an expression of boredom and frustration but can also indicate chronic hunger.
2. Vacuum chewing. Animals chew with an empty mouth, froth dripping from the lips and the corners of the mouth. Sometimes, the chewing motion is interrupted by gaping. As in the case of bar biting, this behaviour is associated with isolation and boredom.
3. Dog-sitting. Animals spend extended periods in a dog-sitting posture with a sad and distracted look on their faces; it suggests depression. This behaviour is usually associated with stimulus-poor situations under conditions of single housing and cold floors.
4. Cannibalism. This usually begins with a non-injurious sucking and nibbling of the ears, legs and, most commonly, the tail of another animal. Typically, the tail is taken into the mouth crosswise and bitten playfully; first gently, then harder until blood is drawn. Now all other animals join in and the injured animal becomes the object of a hunt. Once the tail is bitten off, the ears and other parts of the body are mutilated. Eventually, the victim becomes apathetic and will usually succumb to bacterial infection. This behaviour is often observed in crowded conditions without any enrichment or bedding.
5. Piglet savaging. This abnormality is usually limited to sows giving birth for the first time. Sometimes, newborns are killed immediately after birth. This might be related to pain and anxiety associated with parturition. Occasionally, a sow savages her young after initially accepting them. In some cases, this occurs following severe disturbance and turmoil. The occasional consumption of dead piglets by the mother is not directly associated with killing.

With the possible exception of piglet savaging, all the abnormal behaviours mentioned are related to environmental deficiencies such as lack of space, exercise and distraction (see section titled 'Environmental provisions'), unsuitable floor construction, microclimate or ventilation, insufficient access to feed and water, no means of social interaction, large group size, high stocking density and lack of ability to evade aggressive pen members.

Reproductive problems

Reproductive problems are not common in pigs and minipigs. If they occur, it is usually due to shortcomings in housing, feeding, health status or management. Pigs may produce more than two litters per year and have been selected for centuries to have a high rate of reproduction. Oestrus detection may pose a problem when applying artificial insemination, especially in the absence of a teaser boar. Newly mated sows are sensitive to environmental changes around the time of implantation. During that time, shipping or changes in diet should be avoided, otherwise embryo survival is impaired, and sows will return to oestrus. In some herds, puerperal infection is an issue and may assume epidemic dimensions. The so-called MMA syndrome is a combination of metritis, mastitis and, as a sequel of the latter, agalactia. Rigorous hygiene programmes and antibiotic therapy may help to alleviate the problem. Abortion and stillbirths may occur and are usually caused by infections such as parvovirus.

Further reading

Further information of relevance for pig experimenters can be to be found in specialised texts covering the fields of porcine anatomy (Sack 1982), physiology (Pond & Mersmann 2001; McGlone & Pond 2002), nutrition (Kyriazakis & Whittemore 2006), husbandry and breeding (Glodek 1992; EFSA 2007), behaviour and welfare (Report of the Scientific Veterinary Committee1997; Kaliste 2004; Broom & Fraser 2007) and experimentation (Stanton & Mersman 1986; Tumbleson 1986; Tumbleson & Schook 1996; Bollen *et al*. 2010; Swindle 2016; Swindle *et al*. 2012). Texts focusing specifically on miniature pigs are Glodek and Oldigs (1981), Fisher (1993), and 'The Minipig in Biomedical Research' (McAnulty *et al*. 2012). In addition, attention should be given to websites such as those offered by breeders on handling of miniature pigs, anaesthesia and surgical techniques and to the RETHINK Project (Curtis 2010) on the use of minipigs in toxicity testing.

Acknowledgements

We acknowledge Prof Dr Wolfgang Holtz from Göttingen University in Germany for his work on this chapter in the previous edition – it has provided a solid base for us to work on.

References

Abbott, T.A., Hunter E.J., Guise H.J. and Penny R.H.C. (1997) The effect of experience of handling on pigs' willingness to move. *Applied Animal Behaviour Science*, 54, 371–375.

Baille, M., Wixson, S. and Landi, M. (1986) Vascular-access-port implantation for serial blood sampling in conscious swine. *Laboratory Animal Science*, 36, 431–433.

Bolin, S.R., Runnels, L.J. and Bane, D.P. (1992) Chemical restraint and anaesthesia. In: *Diseases of Swine*, 7th edn. Eds Leman, A.D., Straw, B.E., Mengeling, W.L. *et al.*, pp. 933–942. Iowa State University Press, Ames, Iowa.

Bollen, P.J.A., Hansen, A.K. and Rasmussen, H.J. (2010) *The Laboratory Swine*, 2nd edn. CRC Press, Boca Raton.

Brandt, H., Moellers, B. and Glodek, P. (1997) Prospects for a genetically very small minipig. In: *The Minipig in Toxicology*. Ed. Svendsen, O., pp. 93–96. Satellite Symposium to Eurotox, Aarhus, Denmark.

Braun, C. and Wetzel, M. (2018) Experience with mixed groups of intact female and castrated male Göttingen Minipigs for pharmacokinetic studies in drug discovery research – summary of behavioral observations and collected back-ground data *Ellegaard Newsletter*, 52, 2018. www.minipigs.dk

Broom, D.M. and Fraser, A.F. (2007) *Domestic Animal Behaviour and Welfare*. Oxford University Press, Oxford.

Bruessow, K.P., Torner, H., Kanitz, W. *et al.* (2000) in vitro technologies related to pig embryo transfer. *Reproduction, Nutrition and Development*, 40, 469–480.

Broucek, J. (2014) Effect of noise on performance, stress and behaviour of animals. *Slovak Journal of Animal Science*, 47, 2014(2), 111–123.

Carroll, J.A., Daniel, J.A., Keisler, D.H. *et al.* (1999) Non-surgical catheterization of the jugular vein in young pigs. *Laboratory Animals*, 33, 129–134.

Cerbulis, I.G. (1994) Cognitive abilities of the domestic pig (*Sus scrofa*). PhD Diss. The Ohio State Univ., Columbus.

Chamorro, C.A., Paz, P., Fernandez, J.G. and Anel, L. (1994). Scanning electron microscopy of the wild boar and pig lingual papillae. *Histology and Histopathology*, 94, 657–667.

Christoffersen, B.O., Jensen, S.J., Ludvigsen, T.P. *et al.* (2015) Age- and sex-associated effects on acute-phase proteins in Göttingen Minipigs. *Comp Med*, 65, 333–341.

Curtis, M.J. (2010) Special issue: The Rethink project. *Journal of Pharmacological and Toxicological Methods*, 62(3), 157.

Curtis, S.E., Edwards, S.A. and Gonyou, H.W. (2001) *Ethology and Psychology, Biology of the Domestic Pig*. Eds Pond, W.G. and H.J. Mersmann. Cornell University Press, Ithaca and London.

Damm, B.I., Pedersen, J.L., Ladewig, J. *et al.* (2000) A simplified technique for non-surgical catheterization of the vena cava cranialis in pigs and an evaluation of the method. *Laboratory Animals*, 34, 182–188.

Day, J.E.L., Burfoot, A., Docking, C.M. *et al.* (2002) The effects of prior experience of straw and the level of straw provision on the behavior of growing pigs. *Applied Animal Behaviour Science*, 76, 189–202.

Diel, K.H., Hull, R., Morton, D. *et al.* (2001) A good practice guide to the administration of substances and removal of blood, including routes and volumes. *Journal of Applied Toxicology*, 21, 15–23.

Dziuk, P. (1991) Subcutaneous and intramuscular injection. In: *Handbook of Methods for Study of Reproductive Physiology in Domestic Animals Section 9B, 1 Pig*. Eds Dziuk, P. and Wheeler, M. Dept. of Animal Science, Urbana.

Ewbank, R. and Meese, G.B. (1971) Aggressive behavior in groups of domesticated pigs on removal and return of individuals. *Animal Production*, 13, 685–693.

European Commission (1997) The Welfare of Intensively Kept Pigs. Report of the Scientific Veterinary Committee: Adopted 30 September 1997. https://ec.europa.eu/food/sites/food/files/animals/docs/aw_arch_1997_intensively_kept_pigs_en.pdf (accessed 9 August 2019).

European Council (1991) COUNCIL DIRECTIVE 19 November 1991 laying down minimum standards for the protection of pigs (91/630/EEC). http://eur-lex.europa.eu/LexUriServ/LexUriServ.do?uri=CELEX:31991L0630:EN:HTML (accessed 9 August 2019).

European Food Safety Authority (EFSA) (2007) Scientific report on animal health and welfare aspects of different housing and husbandry systems for adult breeding boars, pregnant, farrowing sows and unweaned piglets. *Annex to the EFSA Journal*, 572, 1–13 https://efsa.onlinelibrary.wiley.com/doi/epdf/10.2903/j.efsa.2007.572(accessed 9 August 2019).

Erhardt, W., Henke, J. and Haberstroh, J. (2004) *Anästhesie und Analgesie beim Klein- und Heimtier*. Schattauer Verlag, Stuttgart.

Fisher, T.F. (1993) Miniature swine in biomedical research – applications and husbandry considerations. *Laboratory Animals*, 22, 47–50.

Flecknell, P.A. (2015) *Laboratory Animal Anaesthesia*, 4th edn. Academic Press, London, https://doi.org/10.1016/C2013-0-13494-0

Flournoy, W.S. and Mani, S. (2009) Percutaneous external jugular vein catheterization in piglets using triangular technique. *Laboratory Animals 2009*, 43, 344–349.

Francis, D.A., Christison, G.I. and Cymbaluk, N.F. (1996) Uniform or heterogeneous weight groups as factors in mixing weanling pigs. *Canadian Journal of Animal Science*, 76, 171–176.

Friend, T.H., Knabe, D.A. and Tanksley, T.D. Jr. (1983). Behavior and performance of pigs grouped by three different methods at weaning. *Journal of Animal Science*, 57, 1406–1411.

Fulkerson, P.J. and Gustafson, S.B. (2007) Use of laryngeal mask airway compared to endotracheal tube with positive-pressure ventilation in anesthetized swine. *Veterinary Anaesthesia and Analgesia*, 2007, 34, 284–288.

Gieling, E.T., Nordquist, R.E. and van der Staay, F.J. (2011) Assessing learning and memory in pigs. *Animal Cognition*, 14, 151–173.

Glaser, D., Wanner, M., Tinti, J.M. and Nofre, C. (2000) Gustatory responses of pigs to various natural and artificial compounds known to be sweet in man. *Food Chemistry*, 68, 375–385.

Glodek, P. (1992) *Schweinezucht*. Eugen Ulmer Verlag, Stuttgart.

Glodek, P., Bruns, E., Oldigs, B. *et al.* (1977) Das Goettinger Miniaturschwein – ein Laboratoriumstier mit weltweiter Bedeutung. *Zuechtungskunde*, 49, 21–32.

Glodek, P. and Oldigs, B. (1981) *Das Goettinger Miniaturschwein*. Paul Parey Verlag, Berlin.

Goldmann, K., Kalinowski, M. and Kraft, S. (2005) Airway management under general anaesthesia in pigs using the LMA-ProSeal: a pilot study. *Veterinary Anaesthesia and Analgesia*, 32, 308–313.

Gonyou, H.W. (1997) Can odours be used to reduce aggression in pigs? (1997) *Annual Research Report*, Prairie Swine Centre, Saskatoon.

Grandin, T. (1982) Pig behaviour studies applied to slaughter-plant design. *Applied Animal Ethology*, 9(2), December 1982, 141–151.

Green, S.A. and Benson, G.J. (2002) Porcine Anaesthesia. In: *Veterinary Anaesthesia and Pain Management Secrets*, Vol. 45. Ed. Green, S.A., pp. 273–275. Hanley and Belfus, Philadelphia.

GV-SOLAS (German Society for Laboratory Animal Science) (2017) Ausschuss fuer Tierschutzbeauftragte: Empfohlene maximale Injektionsvolumina bei Versuchstieren. http://www.gv-solas.de/fileadmin/user_upload/pdf_publikation/Tierschutzbeauftragte/2017Fachinformation_Injektionsvolumina.pdf (accessed 5 September 2019).

GV-SOLAS (German Society for Laboratory Animal Science) (1999b) Ausschuss der Ernaehrung der Versuchstiere:http://www.gv-solas.de/fileadmin/user_upload/pdf_publikation/Ernaerung/ern_fuetterung_minipig.pdf (accessed 6 September 2019).

Haagensen, A.M.J., Klein, A.B., Ettrup, A. *et al.* (2013). Cognitive performance of Göttingen Minipigs is affected by diet in a spatial hole-board discrimination test. *PLoS One*, 8, e79429.

Hafez, E.S.E. and Signoret, J.P. (1962) *The Behaviour of Swine. The Behaviour of Domestic Animals*. Ed. Hafez, E.S.E. Williams & Wilkins, Baltimore.

Hand, M.S., Surwit, R.D., Rodin, J. et al. (1987) Failure of genetically selected miniature swine to model NIDDM. *Diabetes*, **36**, 284–287.

Hansen, A.K. (1997) Health status of experimental pigs. *Pharmacology and Toxicology*, **80**(Suppl. 2), 10–15.

Heffner, H.E. and Heffner, R.S. (1990) Hearing in domestic pigs. *Hearing Research*, **48**(1990), 231–240.

Heffner, H.E. and Heffner, R.S. (1992) Auditory Perception. *Farm Animals and the Environment*. Eds C. Philips and D. Piggins. C.A.B. International, Wallingford, UK.

Hem, A., Hansen, A.K., Rehbinder, C. et al. (1994) Recommendations for health monitoring of pig, cat, dog and gerbil breeding colonies. Report of the Scandinavian Federation for Laboratory Animal Science (Scand-LAS) Working Group of Animal Health. *Scandinavian Journal of Laboratory Animal Science*, **21**, 97–115.

Hong, B.H., Lee, W.Y., Kim, Y.H. et al. (2011) Effects of intraoperative low dose ketamine on remifentanil induced hyperalgesia in gynecologic surgery with sevoflurane anesthesia. *Korean Journal of Anesthesiology*, 2011 September, **61**(3), 238–243.

Jarry, H., Einspanier, A., Kanngiesser, L. et al. (1990) Release and effects of oxytocin on estradiol and progesterone secretion in porcine corpora lutea as measured by an in vivo microdialysis system. *Endocrinology*, **126**, 2352–2358.

Jeroch, H., Drochner, W. and Simon, O. (2008) *Ernährung landwirtschaftlicher Nutztiere*. Uni Taschenbuecher fuer die Wissenschaft, Ulmer Verlag, Stuttgart.

Joint Working Group on Refinement (1993) Removal of blood from laboratory mammals and birds. First Report of the BVA/FRAME/RSPCA/UFAW Joint Working Group on Refinement. *Laboratory Animals*, **27**, 1–22.

Joint Working Group on Refinement (2001) Refining procedures for the administration of substances. Report of the BVAAWF/FRAME/RSPCA/UFAW Joint Working Group on Refinement. *Laboratory Animals*, **35**, 1–41.

Kaliste, E. (2004) *The Welfare of Laboratory Animals*. Kluwer Academic Publishers, New York.

Kirchgessner, A., Roth, F.X., Schwarz, F.J. et al. (2008) *Tierernaehrung*, 12th edn. DLG-Verlag, Frankfurt.

Kittawornrat, A. and Zimmerman, J.J. (2010) *Toward a Better Understanding of Pig Behavior and Pig Welfare*. Animal Health Research Reviews, **12**(1), 25–32.

Koehn, F., Sharifi, A.R., Taeubert, H. et al. (2008) Breeding for low body weight in Goettingen minipigs. *Journal of Animal Breeding and Genetics*, **125**, 20–28.

Kornum, B.R. and Knudsen, G.M. (2011). Cognitive testing of pigs (Sus scrofa) in translational biobehavioral research. *Neuroscience & Biobehavioral Reviews*, **35**, 437–451.

Kyriazakis, I. and Whittemore, C.T. (2006) *Whittemore's Science and Practice of Pig Production*, 2nd edn. Blackwell Publishing, Oxford.

Lewis, A.J. and Southern, L.E. (2000) *Swine Nutrition*. CRC Press, Cleveland.

Lindberg, J.E. and Ogle, B. (2001) *Digestive Physiology of Pigs*. CABI Publishers, New York.

Leslie, E., Hernández-Jover, M., Newman, R. and Holyoake, P. (2010) Assessment of acute pain experienced by piglets from ear tagging, ear notching and intraperitoneal injectable transponders. *Applied Animal Behaviour Science*, **127**(3–4), 86–95.

Lumb & Jones (2007) *Veterinary Anesthesia and Analgesia*, 4th edn. Blackwell Publishing, Oxford.

Malavasi, L.M., Augustsson, H., Jensen-Waern, M. et al. (2005) The effect of transdermal delivery of fentanyl on activity in growing pigs. *Acta Veterinaria Scandinavica*, **46**, 149–157.

Malavasi, L.M., Jensen-Waern, M., Augustsson, H. and Nyman, G. (2008) Changes in minimal alveolar concentration of isoflurane following treatment with medetomidine and tiletamine/zolazepam, epidural morphine or systemic buprenorphine in pigs. *Laboratory Animals*, **42**, 62–70.

Marrable, A.W. (1971) *The Embryonic Pig*. Pitman Medical, London.

Marshall, M., Lydtin, H., Krawitz, W. et al. (1972) Das Miniaturschwein als Versuchstier in der experimentellen Medizin. *Research in Experimental Medicine*, **157**, 300–316.

McAnulty, P.A. et al. (2012) *The Minipig in Biomedical Research*. CRC Press, Boca Raton, London, New York.

McLaughlin, C.L., Baile, C.A., Buckholtz, L.L. and Freeman, S.K. (1983) Preferred flavours and performance of weanling pigs. *Journal of Animal Science*, 1983, **56**, 1287–1293.

McLeman, M.A., Mendl, M.T., Jones, R.B. and Wathes, C.M. (2008) Social discrimination of familiar conspecifics by juvenile pigs, Sus scrofa: development of a non-invasive method to study transmission of unimodal and bimodal cues between live stimuli. *Applied Animal Behaviour Science*, **115**, 123–137.

McGlone, J. and Pond, W.G. (2002) *Pig Production: Biological Principles and Applications*. Cengage Learning, Boston.

Morton, D.B., Jennings, M., Buckwell, A. et al. (2001) Refining procedures for the administration of substances. *Laboratory Animals*, January 1, 2001, **35**, 1–41.

Mount, L.E. and Ingram, D.L. (1971) *The Pig as Laboratory Animal*. Academic Press, London.

Murphy, E., Nordquist, R.E. and Van der Staay, F.J. (2013) Responses of conventional pigs and Göttingen miniature pigs in an active choice judgement bias task. *Applied Animal Behaviour Science*, **148**, 64–76.

Nahas, K., Baneux, P. and Detweiler, D. (2002). Electrocardiographic monitoring in the Göttingen Minipigs. *Comp Med*, **52**, 258–264.

Neitz, J., and Jacobs, G.H. (1989) Spectral sensitivity of cones in an ungulate. *Visual Neuroscience. Volume 2*, **02**, 97–100.

National Research Council (1998) *Nutrient Requirements of Swine*, 10th edn. National Academic Press, Washington, DC.

National Research Council (2011) *Guide for the Care and Use of Laboratory Animals*. The National Academies Press, Washington.

Neundorf, R. and Seidel, H. (1977) *Schweinekrankheiten*. Gustav Fischer Verlag, Jena.

New Zealand National Animal Welfare Advisory Committee (2005). *Animal Welfare (Pigs) Code of Welfare 2018*. https://www.mpi.govt.nz/protection-and-response/animal-welfare/codes-of-welfare/ (accessed 7 February 2022).

Otsuki, D.A., Fantoni, D.T., Holms, C. et al. (2010) Minimum alveolar concentration and hemodynamic effects of two different preparations of Sevoflurane in pigs. *Clinics*, **65**(5), 531–537.

Palmisano, B.W., Clifford, P.S. and Coon, R.L. (1989) Chronic vascular catheters in growing piglets. *Journal of Developmental Physiology (Eynsham)*, **12**, 363–367.

Patten, B.M. (1948) *Embryology of the Pig*. Blakiston, Philadelphia.

Pedersen, H.D. and Mikkelsen, L.F. (2019) Göttingen Minipigs as large animal model in toxicology. *Biomarkers in Toxicology, Second Edition*. https://doi.org/10.1016/B978-0-12-814655-2.00003-7

Piñeiro, M., Piñeiro, C., Carpintero, R. et al. (2007) Characterisation of the pig acute phase protein response to road transport. *The Veterinary Journal*, **173**(3), 669–674.

Ploemen, I., Hirschberg, H.K., Zeltner, A. et al. (2014) Minipigs as an Animal Model for Dermal Vaccine Delivery. *Comp Med*. **64**(1), 50–54.

Pond, W.G. and Mersmann, H.J. (2001) Biology of the domestic pig. *Comstock Publishing Associates*, Ithaca.

Prange, H. (2004) *Gesundheitsmanagement in der Schweinehaltung*. Eugen Ulmer Verlag, Stuttgart.

Prince, J.H. (1977) The eye and vision. In: *Dukes' Physiology of Domestic Animals*. Ed. Swenson, M.J., pp. 696–712. Cornell University Press, Ithaca, London.

Rehbinder, C., Baneux, P., Forbes, D. et al. (1998) FELASA recommendations for the health monitoring of breeding colonies and experimental units of cats, dogs and pigs. Report of the Federation of European Laboratory Animal Science Associations (FELASA) *Laboratory Animals*, **32**, 1–17.

Report of the Scientific Veterinary Committee (1997) The Welfare of Intensively Kept Pigs. https://ec.europa.eu/food/sites/food/

files/animals/docs/aw_arch_1997_intensively_kept_pigs_en.pdf (accessed 5 September 2019).

Riebold, T.W. (1995) *Large Animal Anaesthesia: Principles and Techniques*, 2nd edn. Iowa State University Press, Ames.

Ritskes-Hoitinga, J. and Bollen, P. (1997) Nutrition of minipigs: facts, assumptions and mysteries. *Pharmacology & Toxicology*, **80**(Suppl. II).

Roura, E. (2003) Recent Studies on the Biology of Taste and Olfaction in Mammals. New Approaches in Pig Nutrition. https://pdfs.semanticscholar.org/40e3/5c964c86595be5292c3db445c9390785f3c7.pdf (accessed 5 September 2019).

Sack, W.O. (1982) *Essentials of Pig Anatomy*. Veterinary Textbook Ithaca.

Saco, Y., Docampo, M.J., Fàbrega, E. et al. (2003) Effect of transport stress on serum haptoglobin and pig-MAP in pigs *Animal Welfare*, **12**(3), 403–409.

Seldinger, S.I. (1953) Catheter replacement of the needle in percutaneous arteriography. a new technique. *Acta Radiologica*, 1953; **39**, 368–376.

Smith, A.C., Ehler, W. and Swindle, M.M. (1997) Anaesthesia and Analgesia in Swine. In: *Anaesthesia and Analgesia in Laboratory Animals*. Eds Kohn, D.H., Wixson, S.K., White, W.J. et al., pp. 313–336. Academic Press, New York.

Špinka, M. (2009) Behaviour of pigs. In: *The Ethology of Domestic Animals*, 2nd edn. Ed. Jensen P., p. 177. CAB International, Wallingford, UK.

Søndergaard, L.V. et al. (2010) Determination of Odour Detection Threshold in the Göttingen Minipigs. *Chem. Senses* **35**, 727–734.

Stanton, H.C. and Mersmann, J.H. (1986) *Swine in Cardiovascular Research*, Vol. 1 and 2. CRC Press, Boca Raton.

Straw, B.E., Zimmerman, J.J., D'Allaire, S. et al. (2006) *Diseases of Swine*, 9th edn. Blackwell Publishing, Oxford.

Stubhan, M., Markert, M., Mayer, K. et al. (2008) Evaluation of cardiovascular and ECG parameters in the normal, freely moving Göttingen Minipigs. *Journal of Pharmacological and Toxicological Methods*, **57**, 202–211.

Stubhaug, A., Breivik H., Eide P.H., Kreunen M., Foss A. (2008) Mapping of punctuate hyperalgesia around a surgical incision demonstrates that ketamine is a powerful suppressor of central sensitization to pain following surgery. *Wiley Online Library* https://doi.org/10.1111/j.1399-6576.1997.tb04854.x

Suzuki, A., Tsutsumi, H., Kusakabe, K. et al. (1998) Establishment of a 24-hour electrocardiogram recording system using a Holter recorder for miniature swine. *Laboratory Animals*, **32** 165–172.

Svendsen, O. (1998) The minipig in toxicology. Proceedings of the Satellite Symposium to Eurotox, Aarhus, Denmark, 24–25 June 1997. *Scandinavian Journal of Laboratory Animal Science*, **25**(Suppl. 1), 1–243.

Svendsen, P. and Rasmussen, A. (1998) Anaesthesia of minipigs and basic surgical techniques. *Scandinavian Journal of Laboratory Animal Science*, **25**(Suppl. 1), 31–43.

Swine Genome Sequencing Consortium (SGSC) (2009) https://www.animalgenome.org/pig/genome/db/ (accessed 5 September 2019).

Swindle, M.M. (2016) *Swine in the Laboratory*, 3rd edn. CRC Press, Boca Raton.

Swindle, M.M., Maikin, A., Herron, A.J. et al. (2012) Swine as models in biomedical research and toxicology testing. *Veterinary Pathology*, **49**(2), 344–356.

Symoens, J. and Van Den Brande, M. (1969) Prevention and cure of aggressiveness in pigs using the sedative azaperone. *Veterinary Record*, **85**, 64–67.

Tan, T., Watts, S.W. and Davis, P.D. (2011) Drug delivery: enabling technology for drug discovery and development. iPRECO Micro Infusion Pump: programmable, refillable, and implantable. *Frontiers in Pharmacology*, **29**, 2: 44. doi: 10.3389

Tanida, H., Senda, K., Suzuki, S. et al. (1991) Color discrimination in weanling pigs. *Animal. Science and Technology*, **62**, 1029–1034.

Tanida, H. and Nagano, Y. (1998) The ability of miniature pigs to discriminate between a stranger and their familiar handler. *Applied Animal Behaviour Science*, **56**, 149–159.

Tanida H., Miura A., Tanaka, T. and Yoshimoto T. (1996) Behavioral responses of piglets to darkness and shadows. *Applied Animal Behaviour Science*, **49**, 173–183.

Taylor, D.J. (1999) *Pig Diseases*, 8th edn. D.J. Taylor, Glasgow.

Taylor, T., Prescotta, N., Perry, G. et al. (2006) *Applied Animal Behaviour Science*, **96**, 19–31.

Terlouw, E.M.C. and Porcher, J. (2005) Repeated handling of pigs during rearing. II. Effect of reactivity to humans on aggression during mixing and on meat quality. *Journal of Animal Science*, **83**, 1664–1672.

Nunoya, T., Shibuya, K., Saitoh, T. et al. (2007) Use of Miniature Pig for Biomedical Research, with reference to Toxicology. *Journal of Toxicologic Pathology*, **20**, 125–132.

Thurmon, J.C. and Benson, G.J. (1996) *Lumb and Jones Veterinary Anaesthesia*, 3rd edn. Williams and Wilkins, Baltimore.

Tsutsumi, H., Morikawa, N., Niki, R. and Tanigawa, M. (2001) Acclimatization and response of minipigs toward humans. *Laboratory Animals* 2001, **35**(3), 236–242.

Tumbleson, M.E. (1986) *Swine in Biomedical Research*, Vol. 1–3. Plenum Press, New York.

Tumbleson, M.E. and Schook, L.B. (1996) *Advances in Swine in Biomedical Research*, Vol. 1 and 2. Plenum Press, New York.

Vamathevan, J.J. et al. (2013) Minipig and beagle animal model genomes aid species selection in pharmaceutical discovery and development. *Toxicology and Applied Pharmacology*, **270**, 149–157.

van Kleef, D.J. (1996) A new system for continuous intravenous infusion in pigs. *Laboratory Animals*, **30**, 75–78.

Viscardi, A.V., Hunniford M., Lawlis P. et al. (2017) Development of a Piglet grimace scale to evaluate Piglet Pain Using Facial Expressions Following castration and Tail Docking: a Pilot study, doi: 10.3389/fvets.2017.00051

Waldmann, K.-H. and Wendt, M. (2004) *Lehrbuch der Schweinekrankheiten*, 4th edn. Parey Verlag, Berlin.

Wemelsfelder, F. (2005) Animal boredom: understanding the tedium of confined lives. In: *Mental Health and Well-Being in Animals*. Ed. McMillan, F.D., pp. 79–84. Blackwell Publishing Ames, Iowa.

Wemyss-Holden, S.A., Porter, K.J., Baxter, P. et al. (1999) The laryngeal mask airway in experimental pig anaesthesia. *Laboratory Animals*, **33**, 30–34.

33 Cattle

Ute Weyer and Shellene Hurley

Introduction

The use of cattle in research is not limited to investigating agricultural practices and management procedures. In recent years, cattle have gained importance in many areas of research such as molecular biology, genetic engineering, biotechnology and clinical research, and their increased use is reflected in a wide range of available literature. Increasing concern for the welfare of this species has led to the need for a greater understanding of their biology and behaviour leading to improved husbandry and management practices. Due to their extensive commercial use, farmers, consultants, agriculturalists, animal scientists, veterinarians and stock-people are well-versed in the welfare codes, relevant legislation, farm assurance standards and the practical application of these to the care of cattle. These practices are relevant and can be applied to some extent in a research environment and cattle diseases, nutrition and requirements are well-described.

Biological overview

General biology (natural history)

Cattle belong to the genus *Bos* within the family Bovidae (suborder Ruminantia, order Artiodactyla). Most breeds can be placed within two groups derived from the non-humped *Bos Taurus* and the humped Zebu, *Bos Indicus*. Cattle were first domesticated from local aurochs in the near East some 10,000 years ago and genetic data indicates that modern cattle originate from as few as 80 progenitors (Bollongino et al. 2012). More recently, since 2009, the genome sequence of taurine cattle has been fully mapped (Elisk et al. 2009).

From ancient times, up to the present, cattle have been used for the production of milk and meat, and for draught purposes. In addition, cattle hide is used for the production of leather and their faeces (dung) as agricultural fertiliser. In some regions, such as parts of India, cattle also have a significant religious meaning. The majority of cattle breeds naturally grow horns, although a few breeds grow smaller horns or have no horns (polled breeds). Cattle are even-toed, hoofed, ungulate ruminant mammals that do not have upper incisor teeth, instead having a hard upper palate consisting of a cartilaginous dental pad. The tongue is used to pull off tufts of vegetation. The digestive system is compartmented with a forestomach, referred to as the 'rumen and reticulum', followed by the omasum and the true stomach or abomasum. This complex system of digestion enables them to digest a great variety of phorates.

Size range and lifespan

At the beginning of the 2000s, there were more than 1000 cattle breeds in existence (Hall 2002). Some have been developed for the efficient production of high volumes of milk, others primarily for the production of meat and a small number are essentially draught animals. More traditional breeds are less specialised, and dual-purpose and even triple-purpose breeds and types are recognised. There is an increasing interest in protecting more traditional and local breeds, for example through organisations such as the *Rare Breeds Survival Trust*[1] in the UK and overseas through FAO.

Adult size and weights vary significant between breed and sex. Small breeds such as Dexter range between 250 kg and 450 kg whereas large, heavy beef cattle such as Charolais or Belgian Blue can reach weights of up to 1200 kg. The standard biological data for cattle, including size range and lifespan, are shown in Table 33.1 and further information can be found in Underwood et al. (2015).

Biological data

Haematological and clinical reference data for cattle are widely available and include overviews of normal values, ranges and influence on the haemogram of many metabolic,

---

[1] https://www.rbst.org.uk/ (Accessed 25 March, 2022)

Table 33.1 Biological data for cattle.

Parameter	Typical value
Age adult weight attained (years)	3–4
Adult weights (depending on breed)	
Males (kg)	600–1000
Females (kg)	400–800
Total lifespan (years)	15–20
Body temperature (°C)	38.5±1.0
Pulse rate (beats/minute)	50–70
Respiration rate (breaths/minute)	15–30
Blood volume (ml/kg body weight)	57–62

nutritional and other variables (Weiss & Wardrop 2010). Many veterinary diagnostic laboratories have haematological reference data and profiles, along with acceptable tolerance ranges. These references should be consulted when analysing haematological and biochemistry data as part of the research and/or health protocol.

Behaviour and senses

Cattle evolved as prey animals (Phillips 2002). They are herd-living animals with a hierarchal organisation, usually following the same leading cow, which, however, is not necessarily the most dominant in the herd (Phillips 1993). In free-living semi-wild cattle dominance, relationships are very firm, with few aggressive conflicts (Reinhardt et al. 1986) although minor expressions of dominance such as head-butting and pushing each other are commonly seen. Social standing depends on age and sex, with older animals usually being dominant over younger ones and males being dominant over females. Cattle are predominantly diurnal, with crepuscular peaks for the grazing activity (Phillips 1993).

Cattle acquire 50% of their total sensory information from vision (Phillips 2002). They have panoramic vision of around 330 degrees, due to laterally positioned eyes, which provides good predator awareness (Phillips 1993). Experiments have suggested that cattle can only discriminate long wavelengths of light (coloured red) from short (blue) or medium (green) wavelengths, and not short from medium wavelengths (Phillips & Lomas 2001). Cattle hearing ranges from 23 Hz to 35 kHz, with a well-defined point of best sensitivity at 8 kHz (Heffner & Heffner 1983) and this 'best frequency' is usually reserved for alarm calls which in cattle reach 8 kHz (Phillips 1993). The sense of smell (olfaction) is important for social organisation, recognition and reproduction, including the bonding of dam and calf (Padodara & Jacob 2014). Cattle have chemo-receptors located in the epithelium of the nostrils and also possess a second olfactory organ (Jacob's Organ or vomeronasal organ) located in the upper palate, which is more sensitive to the detection of pheromones. The characteristic 'Flehmen' behaviour whereby the animal holds its head upwards with the upper lip curled upwards is thought to aid odour detection by facilitating air flow over the roof of the mouth (Philips 1993).

Reproduction

Cows are continual polyoestrus with an average cycle of 21 days. Puberty occurs when the animal reaches around 45% of its adult body weight. When on heat (oestrus), they tend to show characteristic behaviours such as standing to be mounted, vocalisation (bellowing) and increased general activity (restlessness). A clear, viscous discharge may be seen issuing from the vulva. Each oestrus lasts approximately 12–16 hours, with a range of 6–24 hours (Smith et al. 2019). Ovulation usually occurs 12–18 hours after onset of oestrus, and groups of cows must be observed several times a day if all the heat periods are to be detected.

Under normal conditions, cattle are capable of producing, on average, one calf per year (Table 33.2 for reproductive data) and most management systems are based on this. Farmers tend to limit the number of males which are allowed to grow to sexual maturity, and the traditional domesticated cattle breeding herd is (or was) a group of females with one attendant bull. Due to the ease and efficiency of artificial insemination in bovines, commercial dairy cattle groups are sometimes totally female.

The simplest way of producing a calf crop is to run a known fertile bull with a group of cows and/or heifers. However, this practice has now become relatively rare in the beef or cattle industry and is mostly replaced by artificial insemination. The cows are usually synchronised by means of prostaglandins prior to artificial insemination (AI) to determine the parturition date. This is described in detail by Hafez and Hafez 2016 and Van der Werf and Pryce (2019). AI is usually achieved by inserting a long sterile plastic pipette into the vagina and depositing semen either on to the cervix, or better still, into the cervical canal. This is a skilled job done by trained farm staff and/or technicians, generally using semen that has been stored in liquid nitrogen. In many countries, there are licensed commercial and/or governmental agencies that undertake a travelling cattle AI service.

The advantage of this synchronisation technique is that a number of inseminations can be carried out at one time, and it also means that the synchronised group will usually all calve down at approximately the same time which is usually advantageous when planning a research project.

Table 33.2 Reproductive data for cattle.

Parameter	Typical value
Onset of puberty	45% mature weight; 12–15 months, depending on growth rate
Length of reproductive life	12–15 years
Type of oestrus cycle	Polyoestrus
Duration of oestrus (heat)	12–14 h (shorter duration in the winter)
Frequency	Every 20–21 days
Seasonality	Oestrus occurs all the year round, but most strongly in the summer; herds running all the year with a bull tend to calve in the spring
Length of gestation	Approx. 280 days (about 7 days less for twins)
Number of calves born	1 to 2; very occasionally, 3 or more; twinning rate about 2–3%
Average calf weight at birth	23 to 45 kg; much breed variation; males tend to be slightly heavier than females of the same breed/type
First post-partum oestrus	30–60 days after parturition

Pregnancy determination can be carried out by methods such as measurements of milk progesterone or glycoprotein, and more commonly by transrectal examination with the aid of ultrasonic scanning (for more information, see NADIS Animal Health Skills[2]). The gestation period for a cow is about 283 days, varying from 279 to 287 days dependant on breed, age and size (semen from short gestation bulls is available). The size and weight of newborn calves varies with breed, sex of calf, but typically lie between 23 kg and 45 kg. As the pregnancy progresses, there is an increase in the size of the abdomen and after about the sixth month, an increase in the size of the mammary gland. These changes are more readily detected in heifers than cows. The signs of imminent parturition are as follows:

1. Behavioural changes such as restlessness, seeking solitary areas, vocalisation, tail-raising;
2. Increasing distension of the udder and stiffening of the teats;
3. Slackening of the pelvic ligaments each side of the tail, which may appear some 3–4 days before calving;
4. The vulva may become swollen;
5. Drops of honey-coloured colostrum (first milk) may appear some 6–8 h before the birth;
6. Abdominal discomfort with possible straining.

Most cows and heifers deliver their offspring without difficulty and should, wherever possible, be allowed to calve without human interference, but should be observed to ensure there are no issues of progress and/or calf presentation. Risk factors for complications at birth (dystocia) are multi-factorial and can depend, for example, on breed, age, body score or calf size (Mee 2008). Parturition can be induced in cattle, in the last 2–3 weeks of their pregnancies, by the injection of short acting corticosteroids and/or prostaglandin $F_2\alpha$; however, this is not common and is restricted on welfare grounds by legislation in some countries. The calves produced under these induction regimes may initially need greater care from animal care staff and the earlier the stage of gestation, the greater the need for such care. There is also a tendency for induced cows to retain their placentas (Hartigan 1995).

Cattle close to parturition (on the basis of the udder and/or vulva showing signs of calving) are typically separated out to form a smaller 'transition' or 'springer' group. Parturition should be allowed to take place either outside, weather conditions permitting, in a conveniently located calving paddock or inside, in a clean draught-free loose box. The animal should have sufficient space to turn round easily, stand up and lie down at will. The loose box should have a well-bedded non-slip floor; water should be provided and there should be a good source of artificial light. Once abdominal contractions (second-stage labour) have started, the calf should be born in under 4 h and expulsion of the placenta (afterbirth) is usually completed within 30 minutes to 12 h after parturition. Calves born to dairy cows are usually separated from their mothers during the first couple of days. It is, however, important to ensure that the calf has suckled during the first 12 hours post-partum in order to receive colostrum which is essential for the health and survival of the calf.

Sources and supply

Cattle are not listed in Annex 1 of the EU Directive 2010/63/EU, which describes animals that can only be used in research if bred for the purpose of such procedures. Under this regulation, cattle can therefore be sourced from any suitable supplier:

1. by purchase, at any age, from a public market;
2. by purchase, at any age, direct from an established breeder, rearer or contract supplier who has genetically defined animals, which are known to be healthy and disease free and who allows their premises to be inspected and, where appropriate, selected animals to be blood tested and/or vaccinated or treated prior to transport to the research establishment;
3. by breeding at the research establishment.

Cattle bred at a research establishment have the advantages that they are of known health and rearing history and have usually been handled from an early age. Unfortunately, this approach demands substantial resources of land, buildings and staff, and is often only practical at the larger institutes.

Most research establishments purchase their animals from an established breeder, rearer or contract supplier. Depending on the nature of the scientific investigation, the cattle may be examined/sampled on the farm of origin to assess suitability and health status and, if necessary, are vaccinated against respiratory disease (particularly if they are going to be mixed with other cattle). It is also important to ensure that the supplier has implemented robust welfare and quality assurance systems. After transportation to the research establishment, they will probably be placed in quarantine for further tests, etc., if required, and to allow a period of acclimatisation. If dietary changes are necessary, these should be gradual, and it is recommended to keep cattle on their original diet initially while slowly phasing in the new feed. Whatever the source, the overall strategy should be to ensure that the biosecurity of the institute is maintained, and that the condition/health status of the cattle is suitable for the management system in which they will be kept and the experiments to which they will be subjected.

Transport

Cattle transportation is covered by laws and regulations that vary between different countries, for example in Europe, the Welfare of Animals during Transport Council Regulation (EC 1/2005). Transport must also comply with relevant legislation surrounding import/export testing or TB control measures stipulated in each country. In the UK, the Department for Environment, Food & Rural Affairs (Defra) regulates the movement of cattle and the control of notifiable diseases such as TB. In addition, the European Commission launched a three-year pilot project in 2015 with the aim of improving animal welfare during transport with the outcome guidelines and fact sheets published in 2019[3].

---

[2] https://www.nadis.org.uk/ Service (Accessed 25 March, 2022)

[3] http://animaltransportguides.eu/wp-content/uploads/2016/05/D3-Cattle-Revised-Final-2018.pdf (Accessed 25 March, 2022)

For long journeys (more than 8 hours), cattle should be transported in specially designed animal transport lorries, which should be climate-controlled if transporting cattle in high temperatures (30 °C and above) and a valid transporter authorisation is required in most counties. Stock trailers towed behind a van or tractor can be used for short local journeys and within the institute. Trailers and lorries should be designed, constructed and maintained so that they are easily cleaned and disinfected in order to maintain and do not injure the animals transported within them. Care must be taken in loading and unloading animals from these transport vehicles; non-slip loading and unloading ramps must be used in areas that are secure and safe. For in-depth information on cattle transportation, see Temple Grandin (2016) and see also Chapter 12: Transportation of laboratory animals.

General husbandry

Animals that are healthy, thriving and contented and which are kindly handled are most likely to yield valid and useful data. Cattle are no exception to this – they give the best experimental results when humane husbandry is provided and are treated with care and consideration. Cattle respond well to gentle treatment and can be readily trained to co-operate in many scientific procedures (see Chapter 15: The use of positive reinforcement training techniques to enhance the care and welfare of laboratory research animals).

Enclosures

The housing requirements of research cattle (e.g. pens, paddocks, outdoor grazing) depends on their age, sex and reproductive status. Whenever possible, feeders, waterers and flooring surfaces or walking areas should be provided to accommodate natural feeding, drinking and movement patterns. The research requirements (e.g. invasiveness of daily monitoring and/or biosecurity requirements) may also have an impact on the nature of the housing provided. Indoor facilities and even some outdoor paddocks can be equipped with closed-circuit television to record animal behaviour and monitor animal health.

Cattle kept for research purposes will most likely be accommodated in one of the following:

- Small paddocks close to the laboratories.
- Open-sided buildings with deep litter bedding material or slatted-floors. The building may contain cubicles (known as 'free stall' or 'cubicle' systems) or have a bedded area with aisle in front of the feeder.
- Enclosed buildings, for example loose boxes or enclosed sheds. The study of infectious diseases may require barriered buildings that are bird and/or insect proof. For contagious disease studies, a sophisticated containment building with negative pressure air regimes and waste containment equipment may be required.

The accommodation must be well ventilated (naturally or artificially) to prevent the build-up of waste gases from anaerobic decomposition of waste products (e.g. ammonia) and dust created by feed and bedding, eliminate condensation from creating a damp environment, and maintenance of temperature control. Poor ventilation may lead to respiratory disease, especially in young cattle. Ventilation requirements for facilities will vary based on the type of accommodation, number and size of animals present, as well as the relative temperature and humidity. For example, in cold weather the ventilation rate required to keep humidity between 50 and 65% may be too high for the heat released from the animals to maintain the temperature within the building at an acceptable level (Benson & Rollin 2008). A clean, dry, comfortable (as indicated by dry lying time) bedding area is essential. The choice of bedding will depend on the design of the building, the availability of suitable material and the nature of the experiment. The facility should be built and maintained so there is a low risk of injury to the health of animals and workers.

Many animal facilities have solid concrete floors for ease of disinfection. This is usually easy to keep clean, but if it is too smooth, the cattle may slip and injure themselves; if too rough, it may be uncomfortable and can damage the udder, legs and feet of the animals. In order to increase animal comfort and add traction, whenever possible, concrete floors should be covered with either a deep layer of bedding over a thin scattering of sand.

In loose box systems or creep boxes for calving animals and youngstock, deep litter is one of the best types of bedding using a thick layer of straw and/or shavings and/or sawdust can be used. As cattle defecate indiscriminately, the soiled bedding must be removed and/or fresh bedding added on top each day to keep the bed surface dry and clean. Dairy animals should have no contact between udders and dung (faeces). If well managed, deep litter bedding provides comfort and some warmth (from bacterial action occurring deep in the bed). Further details on housing, flooring, description of designs (with diagrams), ventilation, and parlour design can be found in Phillips (2018).

As a general rule, the enclosure must provide enough floor space for lying, grooming and normal animal to animal interactions. The animals should, if appropriate to the experiment, have continuous access to individual or communal dry bedded-down lying area. Many countries require minimum pen sizes for the accommodation of research cattle, often depending on numbers and size/live weight. The rules governing research animals is country dependent, so it is important to investigate and follow the current codes and legal requirements for the country and region. Appendix 1 in Animal Behaviour Editorial (2019) provides a comprehensive International list of sources of legislation and regulations regarding animal use and procurement of animals. Additional guidelines may be found in the UK's *Code of Practice for the Housing and Care of Animals Bred, Supplied or Used for Scientific Purposes* (Home Office 2014), the American *Guide for the Care and Use of Laboratory Animals* (Institute of Laboratory Animal Resources 2011), and the European Commission recommendations (European Commission 2007).

As discussed previously, cattle are herd animals so wherever possible, they should be housed in sight of each other and have direct contact with other cattle (age and gender restrictions may apply). Rault (2012) reviewed the protective (buffering) effects of social support against stressful challenges and concluded that social support may be the foundation for positive welfare and emotional experiences. Bayne *et al*. (2015) states that abnormal behaviours can be exacerbated by many non-social factors, such as floor, feeder and waterer space; enclosure configuration (e.g. lack of 'escape' areas for subordinate animals), and lack of general environmental stimulation. Single/individual housing of cattle should be considered as a harm to the animal that must be justified and avoided as far as possible. If research requires either single or small group sizes, then enhanced environmental enrichment will be critical for the welfare of the animal.

Accommodation for cattle after calving may require access to a milking facility to alleviate pressure of milk within the udder (e.g. a high milk yield animal where production is higher than the calves' demand or where the calf was removed). Proper milking technique and well-maintained equipment are essential to prevent introducing health and welfare issues (e.g. mastitis, discussed in the following text). There are many types of milking equipment systems available that vary in complexity from milking parlours where multiple animals are milked simultaneously (milk is collected in a large tank) to small self-contained portable milking units (milk is collected into a bucket). Biggs (2009) gives an overview of the milking machine and milking routine, including appropriate hygiene to prevent mastitis and Reinemann (2013) gives an engineer's perspective on milking machines and parlours.

Environmental enrichment

Accommodation without access to the natural environment will often have artificial ventilation and lighting. In this setting, the 'occupation' of grazing has been removed and although the physical needs of the animal are being met, the animals may be under-stimulated and develop abnormal behaviours. Newberry (1995) defined environmental enrichment as an improvement in the biological functioning of captive animals resulting from modifications to their environment. Baumans and Van Loo (2013) stated that refinement of the animal's environment can be focused on both the social environment (social partners, including human beings), and the physical environment, consisting of sensory stimuli (auditory, visual, olfactory and tactile) and nutritional aspects (supply and type of food).

Enrichment that builds on the evolved natural characteristics of an animal is ideal; however, for research animals kept in conditions that restrict or do not permit natural behaviours, it is more useful to emphasise the functionality and adaptiveness of behaviour as 'enrichment attempts will fail if the environmental modifications have little functional significance to the animals, are not sufficiently focused to meet a specific goal or are based on an incorrect hypothesis regarding the causation and mechanisms underlying a problem' (Newberry 1995). As an alternative to grazing, cattle may benefit from increased food variety to stimulate searching and handling behaviour. In a review of the effects of social, occupational, physical, sensory, and nutritional enrichment on dairy cows and calves in closed housing, with no access to grazing, Mandel *et al*. (2016) found that enrichment methods that build on natural behaviours, such as providing cows with a secluded area to calve, brushes to rub (groom) when trees are not available or feeding calves with milk through a nipple, rather than a bucket have the potential to advance the animals' welfare. Less biologically relevant enrichment such as classical music and the small of lavender for auditory and olfactory stimulation, respectively, did not have a clear effect on the well-being of cattle.

Environmental enrichment for individually housed pre-weaned dairy calves was investigated by Pempek *et al*. (2017) by adding 'furniture' to calf hutches. The calves were given access to two artificial teats, a stationary brush, a calf 'lollie' and a rubber chain link for manipulation. Calves used all of the items depending on the time of day, but they spent the most time using the brush. Calves with environmental enrichment spent almost 50% more time engaged in locomotor play. A correlation between play and positive emotional state, as well as an increase in adaptiveness during periods of change or stress has been found (Špinka *et al*. 2001; Boissy *et al*. 2007; Held & Špinka 2011).

Feeding/watering

Modern feeding systems for cattle are designed to first meet the nutritional needs of the cow's ruminal micro-organisms and then to supply the requirements of the cow with metabolisable energy and protein from the products of ruminal and post-ruminal digestion (for more information, see Cronjé 2000). Agriculturalists, farm animal nutritionists, veterinarians and numerous computer programs may be used to determine the best cattle feeding regimes, usually based on the live weight, body condition, activity and physiological needs of the animal (e.g. growth rate, stage of pregnancy or lactation).

The main parts of the daily ration of a ruminant consist of:

- Bulky feeds – supplying sufficient functional fibre (essential for healthy ruminal micro-organisms), energy and some protein
- Concentrated feeds – supplying extra protein and/or energy, additional vitamins and minerals
- Water

Total mixed rations (TMRs) are commonly offered to housed cattle and are made by weighing and blending all feedstuffs into a single diet containing the required level of nutrients (energy, protein, minerals and vitamins) needed by the animal. The TMR is 'cut' (mixed) to an appropriate fibre length to ensure good rumen function and health. Additional information on cattle nutrition can be found in NRC (2016), Underwood *et al*. (2015), Webster (2011) and Phillips (2010).

Feed is usually presented to cattle in raised troughs and/or 'hay' racks. For larger groups, if space permits, ring feeders may be used with the benefit of a greater number of animals able to feed simultaneously. Due to space limitations, troughs and racks are often found along the side of the pen. All troughs and racks should be designed, constructed and sited so that they are not readily contaminated with faeces and are easily cleaned. The trough should be positioned at an appropriate height for the age and breed of the animal and in a location that will not cause injury due to sharp edges or projections. Ideally, there should be enough trough space for animals to have access to feed at all times. Requirements and guidance for minimum trough space per animal are location dependent and should be consulted. Recommendations may be found in the UK's *Code of Practice for the Housing and Care of Animals Bred, Supplied or Used for Scientific Purposes* (Home Office 2014) and the American *Guide for the Care and Use of Laboratory Animals* (Institute of Laboratory Animal Resources 2011).

Ad libitum, clean, fresh water must be provided. Ideally, water will be provided in a large volume (cattle may consume 30 to 50 litres a day) with a calm surface (e.g. water trough). If cattle have the ability to drink water quickly (a rate of up to 20 litres per minute), their overall water consumption increases (Cockcroft 2015). Lactating animals will have a higher daily water intake requirement (additionally about five times the volume of milk produced) and should drink immediately following milking. Water can be provided in troughs, bowls or buckets. The more traditional troughs or bowls can be piped so they are automatically kept at a constant water level. Push-system bowls ('nose drinkers') have the water pumped into the bowl when a pressure plate is activated by the animal's nose when it leans in drink. Water metres can readily be fitted to piped supplies to monitor consumption, but not to buckets. Water buckets are often used for calves, despite being more labour intensive. The bucket should be fitted to prevent it being knocked-over and elevated to prevent faecal contamination. Ideally, water should be placed near a floor drain so that spilt water does not increase humidity within the building, become a slip hazard and/or wet the bedding.

Whatever the system or means by which cattle are fed and watered, the end results can be judged by the body condition, live weight, health and production (if applicable) of the animals. Live weight and body condition should be monitored at frequent and regular intervals and any loss of condition must be assessed and, if necessary, action must be taken to overcome the cause. Sometimes, all that is needed is a gradual increase in the quantity and/or quality of the feed provided. Behavioural changes (e.g. vocalisation) may also be associated with feed deficit.

There are a variety of ways to measure live weight and body condition score (BCS). Wangchuk *et al.* (2018) compared five methods of determining live weight (including two types of weigh tape and three formula/calculations) to a calibrated weighbridge and concluded that Schaefer's formula was the most reliable indicator of live weight. Schaefer's formula: $W = (L \times G^2)/300$, where W is body weight in pounds (lbs), L is length of the animal from point of shoulder to pin bone in inches, and G is the chest girth of the animal in inches. The final weight was converted into kg.

BCS may be determined by automated systems and are used on dairy farms (Hansen *et al.* 2018). This option has the advantage of being unobtrusive and will provide continuous welfare monitoring of the cattle. Alternatively, the more traditional use of drawings or pictures may be used. A scale of 1–10 (or 1–5 with half points) are often used with different scoring systems for beef and dairy breeds. Additional information on optimal BCSs depending on breed and life stage can be found in Bazeley and Hayton (2007) and publications from animal producer organisations (e.g. Agriculture and Horticulture Development Board (AHDB) 2020 Body Condition Scoring) and government guidance (e.g. Defra Body condition guides 2011).

Social housing

Cattle are a herd-living species. Housing cattle in small groups has been shown to be beneficial to the health and welfare of cattle (FASS 2010; Proudfoot *et al.* 2012; Rault 2012). The appropriate size of the group will be dictated by the accommodation space and the animal's age, sex and reproductive status. A social environment has a positive effect on individual adjustments to the environment through social facilitation or learning. When all physical and visual contact between calves is suppressed, stress behaviours increase (Keeling & Gonyou 2005).

Identification and sexing

Many countries have statutory requirements that all cattle should be permanently, individually and uniquely marked. They can be permanently marked by having tattooed numbers or 'tamper-proof' numbered tags placed in their ears. It should be noted that 'tamper-proof' tags, once correctly placed fully into position, cannot be removed without either mutilating the ear and/or damaging the tag. Identification of animals from a distance may be accomplished by placing large coloured and/or plastic tags in the ears, collars around the neck, freeze-branding (the intense cold of the freeze-branding process permanently damages the pigment-forming cells and white hairs grow in the treated areas) or non-pigmented areas of the skin dyed by application of hair dyes (must be renewed as the hairs grow and are replaced). The marking system chosen should be the least invasive method, consistent with the husbandry system and the aims of the research. No matter what type of individual identification is used, it is good practice (in some countries, a legal requirement) to have a database containing information on individual animals. The data retained should trace key life events and list any medical interventions and/or research procedures.

Physical environment

Webster (2011) stated that the four most important environmental requirements of farm animals are comfort, security, hygiene and freedom to perform behaviours intended to achieve these things (i.e. 'choice'). Housing comfort includes temperature, relative humidity and ventilation. The ideal parameters are dependent on the construction and design of the building as well as the animal's age, breed and status (e.g. neonatal and post-operative animals will require a higher temperature). Recommendations may be found in the UK's *Code of Practice for the Housing and Care of Animals Bred, Supplied or Used for Scientific Purposes* (Home Office 2014) and the American *Guide for the Care and Use of Laboratory Animals* (Institute of Laboratory Animal Resources 2011).

Hygiene (best practice for health and welfare; any welfare hygiene conflicts)

A clean, dry lying area is essential for the health and welfare of cattle. Dung (faeces) management and bedding must be sufficiently well-managed to protect milking animal's udder as well as to prevent build-up of gas (ammonia), which would otherwise have a negative impact on the health of the animals. To address the correlation between a dirty environment and udder health, several hygiene scoring systems have been developed for dairy cows (e.g. University of Wisconsin-Madison in the USA, and AHDB in the UK), in which the legs, udders and flank/upper leg are scored from 1 to 4 (1 being clean and 3–4 needing intervention). Cockcroft (2015) discusses the use of hygiene score cards to determine the dirtiness of the environment through regular health and management audits. Although designed for the dairy industry, this regular audit approach is also applicable for a research facility. The score requiring intervention and environmental adjustment would likely be lower in a research facility to maintain a higher standard of hygiene and health than required in the cattle production industry.

In a research setting, additional environmental enrichment is encouraged; however, when choosing what environmental enrichment to use, it is important that it is possible to clean and disinfect it. Research requirements may make certain types of environmental enrichment impractical (Mandel et al. 2016).

Health monitoring, quarantine and biosecurity

It is advisable that each institute develops an internal cattle health management plan that is compatible with the intended use of the animals and addresses a specific dietary, veterinary and welfare management (for further information on health screening, see FELASA Working Group Report on Farm Animals, In Prep). In general, the health plan is a system for recording, managing through prevention and treatment, and monitoring any changes within groups/individual animals. The data collected from regular audits should be analysed periodically (minimum of annually) and changes made when problems are identified.

The Cattle Health Plan should include incidence and prevention plan for:

- Infectious disease (e.g. respiratory disease, scours)
- Reproductive performance, if breeding animals are present
- Mastitis
- Lameness
- Nutrition and/or metabolic disease

The prevention plan may contain routine prophylactic use of vaccines, regular treatment for parasites and drying-off for mastitis control. The health plan should be agreed with the veterinarian and should determine local disease incidence, potential for exposure, and research cross-reactions and the required research exclusions. One of the major health risks is the introduction of new animals into an establishment and/or the mixing of different groups within the same establishment. These moves should be planned and, if possible, animals screened to ensure they are of similar health and vaccination status.

If possible, all animals entering the establishment should be pre-screened for diseases common to the region of origin (e.g. Johnes, brucellosis, bovine tuberculosis (TB) Bovine Viral Diarrhoea (BVD), respiratory diseases, parasites, foot conditions and Bovine Leukosis Virus (BLV)). Animals should be placed into a vermin and bird proof quarantine/containment facility that can be easily disinfected. Ideally, the quarantine facility should be separate from the main animal buildings and should have its own food and bedding stores as well as its own handling facilities. It should be surrounded by its own double, stock-proof fence. The manure from the quarantined cattle should be kept adjacent to the quarantine quarters. The quarantine area should have its own separate drainage and waste product disposal system. For additional information on farm animal biosecurity, see Dewulf and Van Immerseel (2018); Anderson and Rings (2009); Belk et al. (2007); Gibson and Andrews (2000); and Smith et al. (2019).

All animals undergoing procedures will require additional health monitoring. Scoring systems should be agreed on and any changes recorded. Guidelines should be provided regarding actions to be taken (e.g. Endpoints established to prevent unnecessary suffering). The records should be kept of all procedures, veterinary treatments and operations. Any animal mortality should be examined post-mortem, the reasons for their deaths determined and recorded, and any potential preventions added to the cattle health plan.

Care of aged animals

In long-term cattle projects, attention should be paid to the animal's feet and diet. Commercial diets are usually designed to feed growing beef cattle and/or productive dairy cows, while cattle that have reached maturity need a diet which maintains their live weight and body condition, while providing them with suitable amounts of vitamins and minerals.

Checking the teeth, body condition and live weight regularly in aged animals will allow the assessment of the suitability of the diet and best source of nutrition to be provided. If the teeth are worn-down, missing or broken, then they will need an easy-to-chew supplemental feeding programme. If the research programme permits, access to suitable *ad lib* minerals and vitamin blocks/licks may also help maintain a good body condition.

Some issues relating to aged cattle:

- Arthritis may be detected by extended lying time and/or walking stiffly.
- Urolithiasis in entire and castrated males may be observed by loss of body condition and straining to urinate. There is often also a decrease in urine volume (drops instead of a stream).
- Reproductive issues in aged animals are more likely (e.g. metabolic issues), so appropriate body condition is essential. Cows may need appropriate extra (transition) nutritional assistance prior to calving, and bulls will need good footing for mounting.

- Endpoints must be pre-determined and include lameness (stiffness), live weight/size and/or body condition as cumulative factors to ensure an aged animal is to be euthanised to prevent unnecessary suffering.

Laboratory procedures

Handling

Handling of cattle should be undertaken by suitably well-trained staff who are aware of the risks (Coleman & Hemsworth 2014). Age- and breed-appropriate specialised equipment (e.g. squeeze crushes, chutes/race) should be used to avoid causing fear and distress in the animal. All staff should strive to instil in the animals a sense of security and use a calm and consistent approach. This will allow animals to become accustomed to normal sights and sounds, as well as potentially stressful routine procedures (e.g. foot trimming).

Mature bulls should never be handled by one person alone; they are often large, quick in action and may be aggressive. Accommodation for this type of animal should be designed with safe refuges for staff. Cows with young calves at foot can sometimes be very protective towards their young and must also be managed with care.

Within a research establishment, cattle can be moved in small groups by being quietly driven by one or two handlers. It must be made obvious to the animals which way they are expected to go by the correct deployment of handlers and barriers and by opening and closing gates in the correct sequence.

In an emergency, it may be necessary to restrain cattle by holding them with a finger and thumb in the nostril pressing on the nasal septum or by grasping them in the same place using a metal pincer device ('bulldog'). A looped cotton rope tightened round the abdomen just in front of the hind legs (in females, place the rope in front of the udder) generally prevents cattle kicking with the hindlegs, and thus can make it easier to examine and/or manipulate the hind end of the animal. It must be emphasised that it should not be necessary, except in an emergency, to use these physical means of restraint when carrying out routine procedures on trained cattle and also that staff should be trained in the safe and humane use of the techniques used. For further information on cattle handling, see Grandin (2016); Humane Slaughter Association (2013); Albright and Fulwider (2007); Ewbank and Parker (2007); Holmes (1991).

Stressors

Common stressors may include routine procedures such as dehorning, foot trimming and loading onto a transport vehicle. Rushen et al. (1999) studied the behavioural and physiologic responses of cattle to stress, concluding that even brief periods of social isolation in unfamiliar surrounds increase heart rate, endocrine activity and vocalisation. As previously discussed, a dampening of the stress response in cattle may be obtained by providing cattle with appropriate social group support (Rault 2012; Proudfoot et al. 2012).

Training/habituation for procedures

Most cattle can be trained to tolerate many minor routine experimental procedures, such as blood sampling and injections with the minimum of physical restraint (Dickfos 1991). Examples of cattle trainability in other environments include 'Show' cows and calves being halter-trained to be led around the show ring in front of judges or to come in to be milked when an automobile horn connected to a timer and the electric fence is sounded (Houpt 2011).

Monitoring methods

Hawkins et al. (2011) produced a guide to defining and implementing protocols for the welfare assessment of laboratory animals. Accurate monitoring methods are required for refinement of husbandry and procedures. For physiologic monitoring, the body temperature of cattle is readily taken by carefully inserting a lubricated blunt-ended clinical or digital thermometer into the rectum. The thermometer must be touching the rectal wall. Alternatively, there are sensor and tracking systems available that attach to a collar around the neck, ear, leg, tail or a microchip (injected or ingested). Potential data collected includes the animal's activity levels, health and other key behaviours such as reproduction activity. Neethirajan (2017) reviewed the use of biosensors in animal health monitoring. Other useful measurements that can be obtained through examination are live weight and BCS, respiration rate and effort, the presence or absence of nasal discharge, mobility score, rumen fill and rumination rate.

Collection of samples/specimens

Blood

Blood can be readily obtained from the jugular vein (large external vessel in neck) in cattle of all ages and/or coccygeal vein (underside of the tail) of adult cattle. As long as the animals are used to being handled, a very sharp and appropriately sized bleeding needle and syringe (or vacutainer) is used. If contamination is present on the neck, the skin over the jugular vein site should be clipped, cleaned and, if thought necessary, disinfected.

Milk

If using a portable milking machine, a mixed sample from all four teats (quarters) of the udder can be obtained from the milking-machine bucket. An individual sample from a teat (quarter sample) can be collected by first cleaning and disinfecting the teat end and then squeezing out, by a stripping action of the first finger and thumb, the contents of the lumen of the teat into its own small collecting vial. To reduce contamination, it is usual to discard the first five squirts from the teat and then collect the sample into the vial. The end of the teat should then be disinfected with a suitable teat dip and the cow allowed (or persuaded) to stand for 30 minutes in order for the teat sphincter to close properly.

Faeces

These can be collected from the floor behind tied-up cattle or from a special bag fitting over the hindquarters, or removed manually from the rectum.

Ruminal contents

Ruminal contents may be sampled to assess microbiome and volatile fatty acids. A rounded-end 'stomach' tube is passed via the mouth and oesophagus into the rumen. The ruminal contents are then drawn out by a hand-operated pump, or large veterinary 'syringe' attached to the stomach tube. There are further details of experimental techniques used with cattle (Underwood et al. 2015).

Administration of substances

General advice on the administration of substances can be found in Joint Working Group on Refinement (2001).

Dosing and injection procedures

Some medicines may be given in the food. This is an effective way to dose a large group of animals, but the amount each receives will be variable. If accurate dosing is required, then one of the following methods may have to be used:

- Making the dose up as a drench (usually with water) and dosing by means of a specially designed drenching 'gun' or, where very large volumes are required, by stomach tube or pump;
- Putting the substance into cellulose-based capsules and placing them far back in the mouth of the animal by means of a specially designed balling gun.

Many medicines are precisely and easily given by injection via the appropriate intravenous, intramuscular, subcutaneous or intraperitoneal routes. For details of the various techniques available, see Blowey (2016), Fowler (2008) and Battaglia (2007).

Anaesthesia and analgesia

Cattle are very suitable subjects for regional analgesia, for example paravertebral blocks, caudal epidurals or perineural blocks. They can be given general anaesthetics but must first be starved of concentrate feed overnight and forage should be removed a few hours prior to induction. Cattle should have a cuffed tube placed in the trachea to allow the administration of gaseous anaesthetic and to stop inhalation of regurgitated rumen contents. The front end should be propped upright on their sternums so that dangerous levels of gas do not accumulate in the rumen interfering with venous return. Alternatively, local analgesics can be injected at or close to the operation site and further information can be found in Clarke et al. (2014); Fubini and Ducharme (2017); Abrahamsen (2008); Riebold (2007).

Euthanasia

The appropriate method of euthanasia will depend on research demands, age, temperament of the animal, environment (e.g. indoor housing vs. grazing) and the availability of restraint. Injectable (e.g., intravenous), firearms, and captive bolt devices may all be used. Permitted euthanasia (humane killing) methods for research animals may vary depending on location. The person doing the killing may be required to be licensed or approved by a government authority. Anyone euthanising an animal must be familiar with the legal requirements, as well as experienced in the method being used.

The best method will be fastest with the least amount of stress on the animal. In the UK, an Animal Procedures Committee (APC) review (2006) determined that humane killing methods can be defined as 'methods in which there is a judgement that (i) they do not cause poor welfare prior to death, because death is instantaneous or (ii) the procedure has no negative effects, or in which poor welfare is caused for a few seconds only'. Guidance on choosing the most appropriate form of euthanasia can be found in AVMA (2013) and in the United Kingdom, ASPA (1986), while specific details of cattle euthanasia techniques and recommendations (including appropriate calibre of bullet and placement) can be found in Shearer et al. (2018) and Humane Slaughter Association (2013a and 2013b).

Common welfare problems

Health (diseases/injuries)

Healthy cattle usually graze for about 8 hours a day and ruminate for a further 6–7 hours. They should chew their cud without difficulty and have a normal rumen turnover rate of about 3 times in 2 minutes. They should have a rumen fill (concavity of left paralumbar fossa) and a body condition score appropriate for their breed, age and sex. Cattle spend about half of every 24-hour period lying down. They should be free from lameness, excessive salivation, nasal, eye and vulva discharges; they should only cough occasionally. Cattle should urinate and defaecate without any signs of distress, and the consistency of their faeces should be appropriate to the nature of the bulky part of their daily ration. If, for example, they are eating grass their faeces should be fairly loose, whereas when fed on hay their faeces should be firm. Their respiration and pulse rate and their body temperature should be within the normal range.

The more obvious signs of ill health in cattle are the following:

- Loss of appetite
- Arched back/hair raised/dry and/or dull coat
- Separation from the group or herd
- Fall in milk yield
- Loss of body condition
- Cessation of rumination
- Rise in body temperature
- Lameness, salivation, excessive coughing
- Sudden change in consistency of faeces

All staff should be aware of the common local diseases, as well as the notifiable diseases of the region. There may be duty in law for keepers of cattle to know about the common symptoms of these notifiable diseases, and to report to the appropriate government authorities when they suspect that their animals may be suffering from them. Some of the more common diseases that impact on the welfare of cattle in a laboratory setting are discussed below. A more comprehensive list of cattle diseases and a description of their most common symptoms can be found in Peek and Divers (2018); Scott (2018); Chase et al. (2017); Cockcroft (2015); Underwood et al. (2015); Scott et al. (2011); Webster (2011); Watson (2009) and Smith et al. (2019).

Ectoparasites

Lice can be a problem in housed cattle. They can be treated with an appropriate non-toxic injectable or pour-on insecticide. Ticks are important as transmitters of viral and rickettsial diseases. Cattle kept outside in some tick-infested areas may have to be regularly treated.

Endoparasites

Gastrointestinal parasites may cause diarrhoea, debility and loss in young cattle grazing outside. The parasites may be treated with an anthelmintic (i.e. wormer). Many oral and pour-on preparations are available. Unfortunately, there is an increasing problem with certain parasitic worm populations showing a resistance to many of the medications currently used. Veterinary advice should always be sought when setting up a control and treatment programme in the health plan.

Liver fluke causes a persistent wasting disease but can be treated. Control programmes are mainly based on eradicating the intermediate hosts (a snail) by draining the cattle-grazing areas, fencing waterways and the use of molluscicides.

Lungworm causes coughing and debility in young animals. A vaccine is available, and a control and treatment programme should be instigated based on regular dosing with a suitable wormer, pasture control of the parasite and, where appropriate, the use of a vaccine.

Eye infection/injury

Cattle with watering eyes that stains their face may be suffering from injury and/or infection which caused a corneal abrasion. The eye is often light sensitive and as a result the animal will squint and be reluctant to fully open the eye(s). If left untreated, corneal ulceration and/or bacterial infection may occur. Veterinary advice will be needed to determine the extent of corneal damage and if any additional treatment and/or pain management is needed. Preventative measures include: reducing flies in the environment to prevent infectious spread across a group of animals and ensuring that dust from chopped straw/hay and feeding racks are not the cause of eye injury.

Mobility and lameness

Lameness is a description of a behaviour caused by many issues in cattle (e.g. injury, overgrown feet and specific bacterial infections). Individual cases should be treated, and if the problem is common within a group, veterinary advice will be needed. Preventive measures include attention to floor surfaces, routine trimming of feet and the regular use of footbaths. Lameness scoring systems are an important part of cattle health and management. There are different scoring methods that use different techniques, scales and parameters. Van Hertem et al. (2014) and Hansen et al. (2018) used 3D video recording to monitor and detect lameness. Wood et al. (2015) used infrared thermometry to document temperature increases in claws where lesions were present. The study concluded that lesions may have been present for as long as 6 weeks prior to the observation of behavioural changes associated with lameness being detected. The traditional manual scoring systems vary by organisation and are generally on a 5- or 10-point scale with 0 being normal to 5 or 10, respectively, being unable to stand on all four legs (Webster 2011). A comparison of the two manual scoring systems and further information on how to undertake lameness scoring can be found in Edwards-Callaway et al. (2017).

Mastitis

Mastitis is caused by a variety of bacteria, but in many instances there may be predisposing management, building and environmental factors. Individual cases can be treated with antibiotics, but preventive programmes should first be set up (attention to environments and buildings; hygiene at milking time; ensuring the milking machine is working correctly; post-milking teat dipping; the rational use of intra-mammary antibiotic treatments; the possible use of vaccines) after taking veterinary advice. For more information on mastitis causes, treatments, and preventions, see Biggs (2009).

Teat scoring systems are an important part of cattle health and management. Organisations (e.g. AHDB, NADIS) have developed guidance for scoring the teat end of lactating animals being milked. The University of Wisconsin-Madison offers pictorial guidance on their website and a phone app for data collection[4]. The scoring system is on a 4-point scale, with 0 being the 'perfect' teat end to scores of 3 or 4 with rough keratin protrusions and damaged sphincter. Scores over 3 have an increased potential of infection due to the damaged teat end.

Metabolic diseases

These are caused by the breakdown of internal metabolic processes, and their development is influenced by environmental stress, the nutritional state of the animal and the production demands being made of it. To ensure that an appropriate diet is fed and to eliminate the risk of metabolic disease caused by sudden dietary changes, a preventative programme can be set up by consulting a veterinarian and/or cattle nutritionist.

Pneumonia

There are many causes of pneumonia in cattle, both bacterial and viral, and it is particularly prevalent and severe in young cattle when they are mixed from various sources. There can be a wide range of bacteria and viruses involved and vaccines are available, although to be effective, they need to be combined with suitable management and husbandry practices (e.g. vaccination prior to mixing; logical antibiotic treatment of individual clinical cases; buildings designed to allow suitable ventilation). Calf scoring systems are an important part of cattle health and management. The University of Wisconsin-Madison offers pictorial guidance on their website and a phone app for data collection[4]. The calf health scoring chart may assist in identifying calves that require immediate veterinary treatment.

Ringworm

This specific fungal infection is indicated by round, raised whitish lesions on the skin of young cattle. Vaccines and treatment regimes are available, but even untreated animals usually recover. The disease is transmissible to humans.

Scours (diarrhoea)

Many diseases may produce scour in adult cattle and calves. In adult cattle, a common cause of diarrhoea is diet-related (nutritional scour, see section 'Metabolic disease' in the preceding text). Although nutritional scour may occur in calves (for example, during weaning), the majority of calf scour is caused by exposure to infectious organisms in the environment. The most common causes include rotavirus, coliform bacteria, coccidiosis, *Cryptosporidium*, end parasites, BVD and Johne's disease. Rapid identification of loose faecal consistency and the administration of electrolytes to prevent mortality from dehydration is important. For young calves, clean environment and feeding equipment, correct feeding management and sufficient good-quality colostrum given soon after birth will often considerably reduce the occurrence of the problem.

Behaviour/abnormal behaviour

Cattle kept outdoors on pasture with the ability to browse, graze and ruminate at 'natural' intervals are less likely to show abnormal behaviours (Bergeron *et al.* 2006). This may be a result of ruminants spending a large part of their day (e.g. 8 hours or more) grazing. In essence, the natural grazing behaviour of cattle allows them to be 'gainfully occupied' for most of the day and reduces the likelihood of developing abnormal stereotypy behaviour (compulsive licking, tongue sucking, tongue rolling and horizontal bar grasping). Bayne *et al.* (2015) discuss these types of behavioural problems often seen in farm animal research animals and potential environment enrichment (e.g. exercise, grooming devices and adequate roughage).

Persistent frustration is a key component to abnormal behaviour in cattle (Mandel *et al.* 2016) and a typical example would be calves provided with milk from buckets redirecting oral behaviour towards pen mates and animals forced to stand for prolonged periods of time stamping their feet. Rushen *et al.* (2008) discuss abnormal behaviours associated with pain, which include head rubbing following dehorning or tail licking after tail-docking. A decrease in frequency or magnitude of 'normal' behaviours may also be considered abnormal, which includes lethargy due to ill health and less time standing and/or eating due to lameness.

Signs of poor welfare

Pain and nociception (response to painful/harmful stimuli) in cattle are a major welfare concern and are well-described in a wide range of veterinary and cattle management literature. Pain behaviour of cattle is often subtle and non-specific as cattle evolved as prey animals and the demonstration of pain is disadvantageous (Phillips 2002). There are also certain behavioural changes that are caused by disease or injury that can be indicative of pain (Eskebo & Gunnarson 2018):

- Dullness or depression
- Inappetence
- Groaning, teeth grinding (bruxism)
- Restlessness or reluctance to move
- Lameness
- Rolling, kicking, circling

Cattle also develop learned avoidance behaviour after repeated painful stimuli. Research is under way trying to improve our ability to recognise pain behaviour in cattle by applying grimace scales (Gleerup *et al.* 2015); however, grimace scales may give false negatives and should not be used alone to make clinical decisions about individual animals.

Behaviour is often considered abnormal when the function is not known to the observer. The challenge is how to distinguish between behaviour that is rare and that which is due to poor welfare. Rushen *et al.* (2008) discussed the use of performance of certain behaviours by the animal to make inferences about the actual state of welfare of the animal (e.g. aggression, fear and signalling behaviour). In a survey of research, Mason and Latham (2004) concluded that there was a link between stereotypies and poor welfare, but there are many unknown aspects to the development of stereotypic behaviour that may lead to the misinterpretation of an animal's behaviour.

References

Abrahamsen, E.J. (2008) Ruminant field anesthesia. *Veterinary Clinics of North America: Food Animal Practice*, **24**, 429–441. doi: https://doi.org/10.1016/j.cvfa.2008.07.001.

Agriculture and Horticulture Development Board (AHDB). (2020) Body Condition Scoring (BCS). Online from AHDB.org.uk. (Accessed 25 March, 2022). Body condition scoring flow chart: BodyConditionFlowChart_WEB.pdf (windows.net).

Albright, J.L. and Fulwider, W.K. (2007) Dairy cattle behaviour, facilities, handling, transport, automation and well-being. In: *Livestock Handling and Transport*, 3rd edn. Ed. Grandin, T., pp. 109–133. CAB International, Wallingford.

American Veterinary Medical Association (AVMA). (2013) AVMA guidelines on Euthanasia. (Accessed 25 March, 2022) Online at: https://www.avma.org/KB/Policies/Documents/euthanasia.pdf

Animal Procedures Committee (APC). (2006) Review of Schedule 1 of the Animals (Scientific Procedures) Act 1986: Appropriate Methods of Humane Killing. (Accessed 25 March, 2022). Online at

---

[4]https://www.vetmed.wisc.edu/fapm/svm-dairy-apps (Accessed 25 March, 2022)

https://assets.publishing.service.gov.uk/government/uploads/system/uploads/attachment_data/file/231253/0041.pdf

Anderson, D.E. and Rings, M. (2009) *Current Veterinary Therapy 5: Food Animal Practice*. Saunders Elsevier, St. Louis.

Animal Behaviour Editorial. (2019) Guidelines for the treatment of animals in behavioural research and teaching. *Animal Behaviour*, **147**, I–X. doi: https://doi.org/10.1016/j.anbehav.2018.12.015.

Animals (Scientific Procedures) Act (ASPA). (1986) Schedule 1. Appropriate Methods of Humane Killing. London: H.M.S.O. (Accessed 25 March, 2022) URL: https://www.legislation.gov.uk/ukpga/1986/14/schedule/1

Battaglia, R.A. (2007) *Handbook of Livestock Management*. Pearson Education/Prentice Hall, Upper Saddle River (Nueva Jersey, Estados Unidos); Columbus (Ohio, Estados Unidos).

Baumans, V. and Van Loo, P.L.P. (2013) How to improve housing conditions of laboratory animals: The possibilities of environmental refinement. *The Veterinary Journal*, **195**, 24–32. doi: https://doi.org/10.1016/j.tvjl.2012.09.023.

Bayne, K., A.L., Beaver, B.V., Mench, J.A. and Winnicker, C. (2015) Laboratory animal behavior. In: *Laboratory Animal Medicine*, 3rd edn., pp. 1617–1651. Academic Press, London.

Bazeley, K. and Hayton, K. (2007) *Practical Cattle Farming*. Crowood Press, Ramsbury, Wiltshire.

Belk, K.E., Scanga, J.A. and Grandin, T. (2007) Biosecurity for animal health and food safety. In: *Livestock Handling and Transport*, 3rd edn. Ed. Grandin, T., pp. 354–369. CAB International, Wallingford.

Benson, G.J. and Rollin, B.E. (2008) *The Well-Being of Farm Animals: Challenges and Solutions*. John Wiley & Sons, Hoboken.

Bergeron, R., Badnell-Waters, A.J., Lambton, S. and Mason, G. (2008) Stereotypic oral behaviour in captive ungulates: Foraging, diet and gastrointestinal function. In: *Stereotypic Animal Behaviour: Fundamentals and Applications to Welfare*. Eds Mason, G. and Rushen, J. CABI Publ, Wallingford, UK; Cambridge, MA.

Biggs, A. (2009) *Mastitis in Cattle*. Crowood Press, Ramsbury.

Blowey, R.W. (2016) *The Veterinary Book for Dairy Farmers*, 4th edn. Old Pond Publishing Ltd., Ipswich, UK.

Boissy, A., Manteuffel, G., Jensen, M.B. et al. (2007) Assessment of positive emotions in animals to improve their welfare. *Physiology and Behavior*, **92**, 375–397. doi: https://doi.org/10.1016/j.physbeh.2007.02.003.

Bollongino, R., Burger, J., Powell, A. et al. (2012). Modern taurine cattle descended from small number of Near-Eastern founders. *Molecular Biology and Evolution*, **29**(9), 2101–2104. DOI:10.1093/molbev/mss092

Chase, C., Lutz, K., McKenzie, E. and Tibary, A. (2017) *Blackwell's Five-Minute Veterinary Consult Ruminant*. Wiley-Blackwell. Oxford, UK. Published online at: http://www.fiveminutevet.com/ruminant

Clarke, K.W., Trim, C.M. and Hall, L.W. (2014) *Veterinary Anaesthesia*. Elsevier, Edinburgh.

Cockcroft, P.D. (2015) *Bovine Medicine*, 3rd edn. Wiley/Blackwell, Chichester, West Sussex.

Coleman, G.J. and Hemsworth, P.H. (2014) Training to improve stockperson beliefs and behaviour towards livestock enhances welfare and productivity. *Revue scientifique et technique (International Office of Epizootics)*, **33**, 131–137.

Cronjé, P.B. (2000) *Ruminant Physiology: Digestion, Metabolism, Growth and Reproduction*. CABI Publ, New York. (Online version accessed 25 March, 2022). URL: https://animal-ration.ru/wp-content/uploads/2018/11/Ruminant_phisiology_digestion_metabolism_growth_a.pdf#page=18

Council Regulation (EC) No 1/2005 of 22 December 2004 on the protection of animals during transport and related operations and amending Directives 64/432/EEC and 93/119/EC and Regulation (EC) No 1255/97. (Accessed 25 March, 2022) URL: https://eur-lex.europa.eu/legal-content/EN/TXT/?uri=celex%3A32005R0001

Department for Environment, Food and Rural Affairs (DEFRA). (2011) Condition scoring of dairy cows. Online from.gov.uk. (Accessed 25 March, 2022). Dairy:https://assets.publishing.service.gov.uk/government/uploads/system/uploads/attachment_data/file/69371/pb6492-cattle-scoring-diary020130.pdf; Beef:https://assets.publishing.service.gov.uk/government/uploads/system/uploads/attachment_data/file/69370/pb6491-cattle-scoring-020130.pdf

Dewulf, J. and Van Immerseel, F. (2018) *Biosecurity in Animal Production and Veterinary Medicine: From Principles to Practice*. CABI Publ, Belgium, The Netherlands and Luxembourg.

Dickfos, J.A. (1991) Training Cattle for Scientific Experiments, Commonwealth, Scientific Industrial Research Organization. Division of Tropical Animal, Production Australia.

DIRECTIVE 2010/63/EU OF THE EUROPEAN PARLIAMENT AND OF THE COUNCIL of 22 September 2010 on the protection of animals used for scientific purposes, article 10 and Annex 1.

Edwards-Callaway, L.N., Calvo-Lorenzo, M.S., Scanga, J.A. and Grandin, T. (2017) Mobility scoring of finished cattle. *Veterinary Clinics of North America: Food Animal Practice*, **33**, 235–250. doi: https://doi.org/10.1016/j.cvfa.2017.02.006.

Elsik, C.G., Tellam, R.L. and Worley, K.C. (2009) The Bovine genome sequencing and analysis consortium. *Science*, 24th April 2009, **324**(5926), 522–528.

Eskebo, I. and Gunnarson, St. (2018) *Farm Animal Behaviour*, 2 edn. CAB International, Wallingford, UK.

European Commission (2007) Commission recommendations of 18 June 2007 on guidelines for the accommodation and care of animals used for experimental and other scientific purposes. Annex II to European Council Directive 86/609. See 2007/526/EC.

Ewbank, R. and Parker, M. (2007) Handling cattle raised in close association with people. In: *Livestock Handling and Transport*, 3rd edn. Ed. Grandin, T., pp. 76–89. CAB International, Wallingford, UK.

Federation of Animal Science Societies (FASS). (2010) *Guide for the Care and Use of Agricultural Animals in Agricultural Research and Teaching*. 3rd edn. Champaign, IL, FASS, Savoy.

Federation for Laboratory Animal Science Associations (FELASA). In prep. Recommendations of best practices for the health monitoring of ruminants and pigs used in biomedical research (Website accessed 25 March, 2022). URL: http://www.felasa.eu/

Food and Agricultural Organization for the United States (2010) *Statistical Yearbook of the Food and Agricultural Organization for the United States*.

Fowler, M.E. (2008) *Restraint and Handling of Wild and Domestic Animals*. Wiley-Blackwell, Oxford, UK.

Fubini, S.L. and Ducharme, N.G. (2017) *Farm Animal Surgery*. Elsevier, Inc, St. Louis, Missouri.

Gleerup, K.C.B., Andersen, P.H., Munksgaard, L. and Forkman, B. (2015) Pain evaluation in dairy cattle. *Applied Animal Behaviour Science*, **171**, 25–32.

Gibson, L.A.S. and Andrews, A.H. (2000) Disease security. In: *The Health of Dairy Cattle*. Ed. Andrews, A.H., pp. 328–350. Blackwell Publishing, Oxford, UK.

Grandin, T. (2016) *Livestock Handling and Transport*. CAB International, Wallingford, UK.

Hafez, B. and Hafez E.S.E. (2016) *Reproduction in Farm Animals*, 7th edn. Wiley-Blackwell. Philadelphia, Pennsylvania. Online at: Front Matter – Reproduction in Farm Animals – Wiley Online Library (last accessed 25 March, 2022).

Hall, J.J. (2002) Behaviour of cattle. In: *The Ethology of Domestic Animals, An Introductory Text*. Ed. Jensen, P., pp. 131–143. CAB International, Wallingford, UK.

Hansen, M.F., Smith, M.L., Smith, L.N. et al. (2018) Automated monitoring of dairy cow body condition, mobility and weight using a single 3D video capture device. *Computers in Industry*, **98**, 14–22. doi: 10.1016/j.compind.2018.02.011.

Hartigan, P.J. (1995) Cattle breeding and fertility. In: *Animal Breeding and Fertility*. Ed. Meredith, M.J., pp. 1–75. Blackwell Publishing, Oxford, UK.

Hawkins, P., Morton, D., Burman, O. *et al.* (2011) A guide to defining and implementing protocols for the welfare assessment of laboratory animals: Eleventh report of the BVAAWF/FRAME/RSPCA/UFAW Joint Working Group on Refinement.

Held, S.D.E. and Špinka, M. (2011) Animal play and animal welfare. *Animal Behaviour*, **81**, 891–899. doi: https://doi.org/10.1016/j.anbehav.2011.01.007.

Heffner, R.S., and Heffner, H.E. (1983). Hearing in large mammals: Horses (Equus caballus) and cattle (Bos taurus). *Behavioral Neuroscience*, **97(2)**, 299–309.

Holmes, R.J. (1991) Cattle. In: *Practical Animal Handling*. Eds Anderson, R.S. and Edney, A.T.B., pp. 15–38. Pergamon Press, Oxford, UK.

Home Office (2014) *Animals (Scientific Procedures) Act 1986: Code of Practice for the Housing and Care of Animals Used in Scientific Procedures*. HMSO, London, UK.

Houpt, K.A. (2011) *Domestic Animal Behavior for Veterinarians and Animal Scientists*. Wiley-Blackwell, Ames, Iowa.

Humane Slaughter Association (2013a) Humane Killing of Livestock Using Firearms, HSA, Wheathampstead (Accessed 25 March, 2022) URL: https://www.hsa.org.uk/downloads/publications/hsa-humane-killing-of-livestock-using-firearms.pdf

Humane Slaughter Association (2013b) Captive-Bolt Stunning of Livestock, HSA, Wheathampstead (Accessed 25 March, 2022) URL: https://www.hsa.org.uk/downloads/publications/captiveboltstunningdownload.pdf

Humane Slaughter Association (2013) Humane Handling of Livestock. HSA, Wheathampstead (Accessed 25 March, 2022) URL: https://www.hsa.org.uk/downloads/publications/humanehandlingdownload.pdf

Institute of Laboratory Animal Resources (2011) *Guide for the Care and Use of Laboratory Animals*. National Academy Press, Washington, DC.

Joint Working Group on Refinement (2001) Refining procedures for the administration of substances. Report of the BVAAWF/FRAME/RSPCA/UFAW Joint Working Group on Refinement. *Laboratory Animals*, **35**, 1–41.

Keeling, L.J. and Gonyou, H.W. (2005) *Social Behaviour in Farm Animals*. CABI Publishing, Wallingford, UK.

Mandel, R., Whay, H.R., Klement, E. and Nicol, C.J. (2016) Invited review: Environmental enrichment of dairy cows and calves in indoor housing. *Journal of Dairy Science*, **99**, 1695–1715. doi: https://doi.org/10.3168/jds.2015-9875.

Mason, G.J. and Latham, N.R. (2004) Can't stop, won't stop: Is stereotype a reliable animal welfare indicator? *Animal Welfare*, **13**, S57–S69.

Mee, J.F. (2008) Prevalence and risk factors for dystocia in dairy cattle: A review. *The Veterinary Journal*, **176**, 93–101. doi: https://doi.org/10.1016/j.tvjl.2007.12.032.

National Animal Disease Information Service (NADIS) Animal Health Skills. (Accessed 25 March, 2022) URL: www.nadis.org.uk

National Research Centre (NRC) and Committee on Nutrient Requirements of Beef. (2016) Nutrient requirements of beef cattle.

Neethirajan, S. (2017) Recent advances in wearable sensors for animal health management. *Sensing and Bio-Sensing Research*, **12**, 15–29. doi: https://doi.org/10.1016/j.sbsr.2016.11.004.

Newberry, R.C. (1995) Environmental enrichment: Increasing the biological relevance of captive environments. *Applied Animal Behaviour Science*, **44**, 229–243. doi: https://doi.org/10.1016/0168-1591(95)00616-Z.

Padodara, R.J. and Jacob, N. (2014, Feb). Olfactory sense in different animals. *The Indian Journal of Veterinary Science*, **2(1)**, 1–14.

Peek, S.F. and Divers, T.J. (2018) *Rebhun's Diseases of Dairy Cattle*, 3rd edn. Saunders, Elsevier.

Pempek, J.A., Eastridge, M.L. and Proudfoot, K.L. (2017) The effect of a furnished individual hutch pre-weaning on calf behavior, response to novelty, and growth. *Journal of Dairy Science*, **100**, 4807–4817. doi: https://doi.org/10.3168/jds.2016-12180.

Phillips, C.J.C. (2018) *Principles of Cattle Production*. CABI.

Phillips, C.J.C. (2002) *Cattle Behaviour and Welfare*, 2nd edn. Blackwell, Oxford, UK.

Phillips, C.J.C. and Lomas, C.A. (2001) The perception of colour by cattle and its influence on behavior. *Journal of Dairy Science*, **84(4)**, 807–813.

Phillips, C.J.C (1993) *Cattle Behaviour*. Farming Press Books, Wharfdale Rd, Ipswich, U.K.

Proudfoot, K.L., Weary, D.M. and von Keyserling, M.A.G. (2012) Linking the social environment to illness in farm animals. *Applied Animal Behaviour Science*, **138**, 203–215. doi: https://doi.org/10.1016/j.applanim.2012.02.008.

Rare Breed Survival Trust (Accessed 25 March, 2022) URL: https://www.rbst.org.uk/

Rault, J.L. (2012) Friends with benefits: Social support and its relevance for farm animal welfare. *Applied Animal Behaviour Science*, **136**, 1–14. Doi: https://doi.org/10.1016/j.applanim.2011.10.002.

Reinemann, D. (2013) *Handbook of Farm, Dairy and Food Machinery Engineering*. Ed. Kutz, M. Academic Press, London, UK.

Reinhardt, C., Reinhardt, A. and Reinhardt, V. (1986) Social behaviour and reproductive performance in semi-wild Scottish Highland cattle. *Applied Animal Behaviour Science*, **15(2)**, pp. 125–136.

Riebold, T.W. (2007) Ruminants. In: *Lumb and Jones' Veterinary Anesthesia and Analgesia*, 4th edn. Eds Tranquilli, W.J., Thurmon, J.C. and Grim, K.A., pp. 731–736. Blackwell Publishing, Oxford, UK.

Rushen, J., Boissy, A., Terlouw, E.M. and de Passille, A.M. (1999) Opioid peptides and behavioral and physiological responses of dairy cows to social isolation in unfamiliar surroundings. *Journal of Animal Science*, **77**, 2918–2924.

Rushen, J., Passillé, A.M.D., Keyserlingk, M.A.V. and Weary, D.M. (2008) *The Welfare of Cattle*. Springer, Dordrecht.

Scott, P.R., Penny, C.D. and Macrae, A.I. (2011) *Cattle Medicine*. Manson Publishing, London.

Scott, D.W. (2018) *Color Atlas of Farm Animal Dermatology*. 2nd edn. Wiley-Blackwell, Ames, Iowa. Published online at: Frontmatter - Color Atlas of Farm Animal Dermatology - Wiley Online Library

Shearer, J.K., Griffin, D. and Cotton, S.E. (2018) Humane euthanasia and carcass disposal. *Veterinary Clinics of North America: Food Animal Practice*, **34**, 355–374. doi: https://doi.org/10.1016/j.cvfa.2018.03.004.

Smith, B.P., Man Metre, D.C., and Pusterla, N. (2019) *Large Animal Internal Medicine*. Elsevier Mosby, St Louis, Missouri.

Špinka, M., Newberry, R.C. and Bekoff, M. (2001) Mammalian play: Training for the unexpected. *The Quarterly Review of Biology*, **76**, 141–168. doi: 10.1086/393866.

Underwood, W.J., Blauwiekel, R., Delano, M.L. *et al.* (2015) Biology and diseases of ruminants (sheep, goats, and cattle). In: *Laboratory Animal Medicine*, 3rd edn. Academic Press, London, UK.

Van der Werf, J. and Pryce, J.E. (2019) *Advances In Breeding Of Dairy Cattle*. Burleigh Dodds Science Pu, [S.l.].

Van Hertem, T., Viazzi, S., Steensels, M. *et al.* (2014) Automatic lameness detection based on consecutive 3D-video recordings. *Biosystems Engineering*, **119**, 108–116. doi: https://doi.org/10.1016/j.biosystemseng.2014.01.009.

Watson, C. (2009) *The Cattle Keeper's Veterinary Handbook*. The Crowood Press, Ramsbury, Marlborough, Wiltshire.

Wangchuk, K., Wangdi, J and Mindu, M. (2018) Comparison and reliability of techniques to estimate live cattle body weight. *Journal of Applied Animal Research*, **46(1)**, 349–352. doi: 10.1080/09712119.2017.1302876.

Webster, J. (2011) *Management and Welfare of Farm Animals*. Wiley-Blackwell, Oxford.

Weiss, D.J. and Wardrop, K.J. (Eds) (2010) *Schalm's Veterinary Hematology*. Wiley-Blackwell, Philadelphia, Pennsylvania.

Wood, S., Lin, Y., Knowles, T.G. and Main, D.C.J. (2015) Infrared thermometry for lesion monitoring in cattle lameness. *Veterinary Record*, **176**, 308. doi: 10.1136/vr.102571.

34 Sheep and goats

Colin L. Gilbert and Cathy M. Dwyer

Biological overview

Introduction

Sheep and goats, often referred to as small ruminants, are highly adaptable and social ungulate (hoofed) species which originally evolved to occupy upland (sheep) and mountain (goats) areas. As ruminants, they are efficient users of herbage (grass and forages), which can be converted to energy and proteins through the action of gut microbes and rumenal fermentation. Sheep and goats can survive in harsh climates on poor grazing and their adaptability means that they have colonised a wide variety of habitats, from desert areas to the sub-Arctic and Antarctic, and can be found in mountain, island and coastal areas worldwide. They have adapted to forage on a wide range of food stuffs in addition to herbage, including cacti, fruit, trees, bushes, shrubs and even seaweed. Sheep and goats are predated animals unless protected in domestic management, hunted by wolves, bears, lynx and other predators, including man, and this has shaped many aspects of their behaviour, particularly their social behaviour, reproductive strategies and responses to stress (Dwyer 2004).

Sheep and goats were among the first species to have been domesticated by man and have provided meat, milk, fibre, manure for fuel and fertiliser and even portage for about 10,000 years. Their adaptability and hardiness mean that they are used extensively in countries with poor grazing and harsh climates, and small ruminants play a vital role in feeding many of the world's poorest peoples in Africa, Asia and the Middle East, where they are believed to have been first domesticated. These species had many characteristics that favoured domestication, such as flocking, promiscuous reproductive behaviour, large, mobile and well-developed young, and are relatively more docile and tolerant of stress compared to other ungulate species, such as deer or gazelle. These traits have been exploited by man in their management and have therefore been retained or even enhanced through domestication. Sheep and goats are relatively defenceless in the presence of predators, and tend to group or flock together and run when confronted by predators. This tendency is used in management either by use of dogs in sheep husbandry, or to facilitate movement and management of groups of sheep or goats. In many areas of the world, sheep are managed in very extensive environments, with very infrequent contact with or exposure to humans. Under these conditions, humans are often perceived as predators by these animals, and close contact will elicit flight or fear reactions, which can be counterproductive in a laboratory setting. However, sheep and especially goats are also kept in shepherded flocks or herds in other agricultural settings, and can become readily accustomed to close contact with humans when this is associated with provision of food and other positive experiences. It is, therefore, perfectly possible to acclimatise sheep and goats to frequent close contact with humans, particularly if the animals encounter positive human contact at an early age (Nowak & Boivin 2015), which can facilitate handling for use in the laboratory. Although sheep and goats prefer social contact and the presence of conspecifics, they can become accustomed to single housing particularly if visual and auditory contact with other animals can be maintained. Like many animals, sheep and goats are also neophobic, and will thus find novel environments stressful. Habituation or accommodation to the environment and handling should always be the first objective of all laboratory users of small ruminants for medium- to long-term experiments. Benefits will accrue to animal handlers, the quality of data and most importantly to the animals themselves.

Natural behaviour

Social organisation

Under natural conditions, both species will form sexually segregated (except during mating) social groups which are matrilineal, that is composed of related animals that are grand-mothers, mothers and daughters. The social group is an important part of anti-predator behaviour in both species.

The UFAW Handbook on the Care and Management of Laboratory and Other Research Animals, Ninth Edition.
Edited by Huw Golledge and Claire Richardson.
© 2024 John Wiley & Sons Ltd. Published 2024 by John Wiley & Sons Ltd.

This means that, even in the absence of predators, sheep and goats prefer the company of conspecifics and can become extremely distressed if they are isolated. The preferred size of social groups is influenced by the environment, breed and physiological state. In open areas, group sizes can be large (30–50 individuals) whereas in hill, mountain or wooded areas, sheep and goats aggregate into smaller social groups, particularly when the environment is more constrained with respect to nutrient or forage availability. More domesticated or lowland breeds, which may have been indirectly selected by man for greater gregariousness and tolerance for closer spatial proximity, will form larger sub-groups with closer nearer neighbour distances than breeds adapted for the hill environment (Dwyer & Lawrence 1999). When females are lactating, they are considerably less gregarious, and will be tolerant of separation from other ewes or does as long as their lambs/kids are present. The males, and particularly older males of wild species are sometimes found singly, and males are in general less fearful than females in both species (Vandenheede & Bouissou 1993). In general, however, both species require another 3–4 individuals for the social group to feel like a 'flock' and for the animals to feel comfortable (Penning et al. 1993).

Sheep and goats have well-developed individual recognition abilities (Peirce et al. 2000, and see the following text), which are an important part of maintaining stable social groups. Although outright aggression is not particularly common in either species (except in males during the breeding season), some animals will be dominant over others. Dominance is maintained via subtle behavioural responses such as eye contact, resting the chin on the back of subordinate animals and displacement from preferred lying or feeding locations. This can mean that when resources are limited, subordinate animals may be more likely to lose condition and to be exposed to thermal extremes. Individual animals will also maintain contact with preferred social partners, which means that, although social grooming is not common, resting with and foraging with particular individuals may be important to social cohesion. Social recognition is maintained through visual and olfactory cues. When new animals are introduced, or if groups of animals are mixed, social disruption and occasional bouts of fighting can occur. It is important when planning experiments that these facets of social behaviour are borne in mind to reduce variability in data within and between pens of animals.

Feeding behaviour

It is important that rumenal health is considered in the management of both species. In general, sheep are considered to be predominantly grazing animals, although they will also browse (foraging on shrubs and tree leaves for example), whereas goats are mainly browsers, which also graze. Goats are generally more inquisitive and adventurous in their feeding habits than sheep, are able to easily adopt a bi-pedal stance when feeding and are known to climb trees. Goats are also more tolerant of bitter flavours than sheep. Their relatively non-specific feeding behaviour also means that goats are often willing to sample non-food items and may be vulnerable to poisoning.

Both species will spend around 8 hours a day feeding, although this can increase to 12 hours if food is scarce (Lynch et al. 1992). For both species, there is a requirement to find time to ruminate, where food is regurgitated and re-chewed to allow the cellulose walls of plant cells to be broken for rumenal fermentation to proceed efficiently. Providing opportunities to ruminate must be part of the normal management of goats and sheep. During rumination, animals enter a 'relaxed' state, usually while lying, which analysis of EEG patterns suggests might be akin to non-REM sleep in non-ruminants (Perentos et al. 2015).

Sheep and goats show a pronounced diurnal rhythm in their feeding behaviour in an unconstrained setting. Animals camp on higher ground overnight, and gradually descend in daylight to reach preferred grazing areas. This is followed by a period of ruminating before animals' return, while grazing, to their night areas. Goats also show a diurnal rhythm in diet selection, with browsing preferred during the morning, and grazing in the afternoon. Feeding overnight is relatively rare. This means that animals need to be provided with enough feeder space to all feed at the same time; otherwise, some animals may need to feed at non-preferred times, which may affect data variability within a social group. There is also evidence that sheep show seasonal as well as circadian movement patterns, which are affected by environment (Wyse et al. 2018).

Following and allo-mimetic (synchronous) behaviour is very pronounced in sheep, but also present in goats. The more independent animals in the social group, which are often not the most dominant, usually start any movement and other animals follow. In a managed setting, this can be exploited to bring about desired changes in location.

Reproductive behaviour

Temperate breeds of sheep and goats are seasonally polyoestrous, with shortening day length inducing oestrous cyclical activity in females. Some breeds have a longer receptive period and thus can be bred over a longer time course. Tropically adapted breeds of both species are less seasonal and can reproduce all year around. In general, the breeding season is driven by the receptivity of the females, while males, although they do show seasonal changes in testicular size and other male characteristics, are usually willing to breed whenever oestrous females are present.

Male reproductive behaviour: Males compete for access to oestrous females, and only the most dominant or preferred males mate. Aggression between adult males of both species occurs if cues from oestrous females are present. Rams fight by butting and chasing, whereas bucks rear up on their hindlegs to rise above opponents, and clash heads on the descent. Horns are common in males of both species, where they function predominantly as a symbol of male fitness rather than weapons, but rams and bucks can be potentially dangerous animals. Care must be taken when handling adult males of either species during the breeding period, and to prevent subordinate males being injured or even killed during fights. Outside of the breeding season, males may be kept together in social groups without any serious risk of fighting, as long as adequate resources are present to limit competition.

Rams and bucks detect oestrus using pheromonal cues, court oestrous females prior to mating and will follow and guard receptive females. Males and females can be paired together in pens, particularly if the date of conception is important, allowing animals to move undisturbed through courtship, proceptive and receptive behaviours that culminate in mating. Alternatively, males can mate a small number of ewes in a single sire mating group, particularly if known parentage is important, or in a larger multi-sire group as is sometimes used in agricultural practice. In general, the latter is associated with a higher conception rate as all oestrous females are more likely to be detected and mated by the males.

Female reproductive behaviour: Pregnancy in sheep is 145±5 days and in goats 150 days. Litter sizes of 1–3 lambs or kids are most common, with twins being most frequent in domesticated animals. There are, however, breed differences in litter size with hill or mountain animals tending to have smaller litters (commonly 1 or 2), and some sheep breeds, such as Romanov or Finn, having larger litters with four or even five lambs possible within a single litter. When given the opportunity, pre-parturient females of both species choose to move away from the social group to secluded places in which to give birth (Dwyer & Lawrence 2005). Even in managed settings, females choose a birth site before they begin to show signs of imminent birth, and many choose cubicles, fencelines or elevated areas if available. Labour lasts for between 15 minutes and 2 hours, and birth can usually occur without the need for human intervention provided the mothers are able to deliver in a quiet and undisturbed environment and the lamb or kid is presented normally (forwards, with the nose lying along the forelegs).

Sheep and goats do not normally show maternal behaviour towards lambs and kids respectively until they give birth, although some stealing of the newborn young of other ewes can occur in experienced mothers towards the end of their pregnancies. When they give birth, maternal behaviour and selective bonding are triggered by feedback to the brain from receptors in the vagina and cervix activated during labour contractions and the expulsion of the foetus. Lambs delivered from pregnant ewes by caesarean section or following an epidural anaesthetic block are often not mothered. Maternal behaviour in sheep and goats is characterised by a period of intensive licking or grooming of the offspring, accompanied by frequent low-pitched vocalisations or 'rumbles'. These behaviours serve to dry and stimulate the neonate, and provide reassurance and a focus for the udder-seeking responses of the newborn. Newborn lambs or kids are precocious, and are able to stand within 5–20 minutes of birth, and seek the udder and suckle within 30 minutes to an hour of birth. Rapid ingestion of colostrum is important for offspring survival and any neonate that has not fed within 2 hours of birth should be assisted to suckle from the mother or artificially fed with colostrum. Large single lambs, which may have experienced a prolonged delivery and triplet lambs, or those from larger litters, are often slower to stand and suck and may require more assistance.

Birth also triggers selective bonding behaviour with offspring in both sheep and goats, whereby the mother rapidly learns to recognise the odour signatures of its individual lambs or kids and will subsequently refuse sucking attempts from offspring other than its own. In sheep, this process of selective bonding generally occurs within 1 hour post-partum, although with Saanen goats as little as 15 minutes may be sufficient. Primiparous ewes and does take longer to bond with their offspring, often 4 h or more (Kendrick 1994), since maternal experience is required to alter the brain to respond to the vaginal and cervical dilatation during birth.

The process of taking care of and interacting with the neonate promotes changes in olfactory processing structures that underlie the bonding process. Thus, bonding between first-time mothers and their young relies almost exclusively on physical interactions between mother and offspring and removal of the offspring for even short lengths of time or contaminating them with strange odours (including human ones) may result in the mother rejecting her own young. This is often seen as disturbed maternal behaviours such as butting or moving away as the neonate attempts to find the udder and suck (Dwyer & Lawrence 1998). Successful mothers can recognise their own offspring at close quarters (primarily by olfactory cues) within a few hours of birth, and restrict maternal care to them. Within 12–24 hours of birth, mothers can recognise their own offspring from a distance of several metres or more, initially by sight and then by auditory cues.

Sheep are described as 'followers' in their maternal care, which means that the lamb will follow the mother closely from birth, and ewe and lambs both become distressed if separated. Goats, by contrast, are considered to have a 'hiding' period immediately after birth, as do some other ungulate species such as cattle or deer. In this strategy, the offspring are left hidden in long grass or undergrowth while the mother returns to the social group. Mothers return to their hidden offspring to suckle them until they are old enough to integrate into the natal herd. Lambs and kids learn to discriminate their own dam through frequent sucking contacts, and can reliably recognise their own dam by 24–48 hours after birth (Lickliter 1984; Nowak *et al.* 1989), although this may take longer in lambs from larger litters.

Perceptual and cognitive abilities of sheep and goats

It is entirely wrong to equate the strong retention of flight instincts in these species with a lack of intelligence. Indeed, behavioural and neurobiological studies of the perceptual and cognitive abilities of sheep and goats have revealed that they make sophisticated use of both visual and olfactory cues from their environment to enable them to rapidly learn to recognise individual offspring, flock members and humans as well as palatable and unpalatable foods. Their ability to do this almost rivals that is seen in higher primates including man; and one obvious conclusion that must be drawn from such studies is that, if they need to be able to recognise a number of specific individuals and objects and, if their brains are specialised for carrying out this process, then their social requirements and interactions must be far more complex than a cursory view of their behaviour within a flock might suggest. Research has also shown that sheep and goats have individual personality traits. Therefore, as intelligent, sentient species, the use of sheep and goats in experimental procedures should be undertaken thoughtfully and only when specific need arises.

There has been a tendency to overlook the possibility that sheep and goats, or for that matter other domestic ungulates, use vision to learn about and interact with their environment. While they lack an accommodation reflex, their visual acuity in the frontal eye field is very good and probably lies somewhere between that of a cat and a monkey (Piggins 1992). They are capable of recognising individuals from visual cues from the face region and are able to visually discriminate between different types of grass, clover and concentrates (Kendrick 1992; Kendrick et al. 2001; Tate et al. 2006). Indeed, sheep can identify and remember at least 50 different sheep and 10 different human faces, even after long periods of absence (Peirce et al. 2000; Kendrick et al. 2001). Both sheep and goats can be trained to perform operant tasks (e.g. choices indicated by pressing panels with their nose); to discriminate between different faces (human or sheep/goat) or other visual stimuli (Baldwin 1979, 1981; Tate et al. 2006) or to choose between faces or geometrical stimuli in a Y-maze (Kendrick et al. 1995, 1996; Tate et al. 2006). Animals can be easily trained to use this apparatus either for food, water or social rewards.

Faces clearly have an important emotional significance for sheep and goats. Studies have shown that when sheep are exposed to social isolation stress, the sight of pictures of familiar sheep can alleviate behavioural, autonomic and endocrine indices of stress and reduce activation of brain centres controlling stress and fear responses (Da Costa et al. 2004). Showing animals video sequences depicting other sheep can also evoke profound interest and relieve stress (Elliker 2006). Recent work has also shown that sheep and goats can detect and respond to human face expressions (smiling and angry), preferring calm faces over angry faces, and also respond to emotional cues in conspecific faces (fearful/stressed vs calm) (Kendrick 2004; Elliker 2006; Tate et al. 2006; Bellegarde et al. 2017; Nawroth et al. 2018). Further, there is some evidence that they may be able to form and use mental images of faces (Tate et al. 2006).

Both sheep and goats also have a remarkably acute sense of smell and can discriminate between a large number of biological and chemical odours in operant experiments (Baldwin & Meese 1977). However, in spite of possessing a highly developed sense of smell, they do not appear to need it for food recognition or even individual recognition in most cases, although it is entirely possible that olfactory cues might complement visual ones to speed up recognition or improve its accuracy. The main exception to the predominance of vision over olfaction is the selective olfactory recognition of offspring which develops in both species very quickly after they have given birth and which seems to be essential since accurate visual and vocal discrimination of offspring develops much more slowly (Kendrick et al. 1996). Another context in which olfactory cues are important appears to be synchronisation of oestrus which occurs in response to odours from the fleece of a male – the so-called 'ram effect'.

The hearing sensitivities of sheep and goats are broadly similar to those of humans with the exception that they can hear frequencies above the human upper limit of hearing (ultrasound). However, their ability to localise sounds is relatively poor compared to that of some other mammals (Heffner & Heffner 1992) and may reflect their greater reliance on vision. Sheep also only have a limited vocal repertoire which essentially falls into three different types. These include a high-pitched or protest bleat which can be used to signify anything from slight agitation or mild impatience to extreme fear; a low-pitched more rumbling bleat used specifically by maternal ewes to call their lambs; and a similar type of low-pitched vocalisation sometimes used by rams engaged in courtship with ewes. Maternal ewes and does learn to recognise their lambs' or kids' voices, and vice versa (Shillito & Alexander 1975; Briefer et al. 2012), and appear to remember the call of their offspring even after weaning. Goats have also been shown to use different sensory modes in the recognition of familiar animals, showing evidence of recognition on the basis of calls (Pitcher et al. 2017). However, the ability of sheep to recognise individual members of the flock from their high-pitched bleats has yet to be demonstrated convincingly (Kendrick et al. 1995; Elliker 2006), although sound spectrograms show clear individual differences in sheep voices. It seems fair to conclude at this stage that the main function of the high-pitched bleats is for an individual to express some degree of concern or impatience and, in certain circumstances, to warn other flock members of some impending danger.

The cognitive abilities of sheep and goats enable them to cope successfully with changing environments. Goats appear to have better abstract learning and categorisation abilities compared to sheep, for example goats can understand concepts such as learning sets based on categorisation of visual objects, identification of similarity and 'oddity'. Sheep can show categorisation, such as between different plant species, but have more limited abilities to use inferential learning about rewards in specific tests compared to goats (Nawroth et al. 2014). These differences may be related to their feeding habits, as goats select of browse in more patchy and resource limited environments, which may require better learning and discriminatory abilities than for sheep grazing a more evenly resourced sward. There are other examples of sheep learning about their physical environment. They are capable of discerning that there is a physical barrier between them and a human no matter what form that barrier may take (wire fence, chain fence, gate, etc.). Even with a single-stranded electric fence, a sheep appears to know that what keeps it in will also keep humans out. Sheep will often tolerate the presence of humans at much smaller distances to themselves when there is an intervening fence and will often not show an alerting response when a human approaches the fence. Sheep also modify their flight behaviour depending on the types of approaches made by humans (standing, running or crawling) and whether they are accompanied by a dog or not, which might be related to their perception of the risks posed by the human. Learning skills of sheep are also dependent, to some extent, on the type of objects that they are being trained to visually discriminate. When they are trained to discriminate between unfamiliar geometrical symbols, they are relatively slow at learning (Baldwin 1981; Kendrick et al. 1996). However, if they are required to discriminate between familiar types of real object, such as faces, they can learn very rapidly (Kendrick et al. 1996; Peirce et al. 2000), and have been shown to recognise and remember at least 50 different sheep and 10 different human faces for up to 2 years. Hence if speed of learning is an important issue, it is important to use familiar types of objects. Although goats have also been shown to discriminate between conspecifics, and to pay attention to the emotional content of specific goat faces (Bellegarde et al. 2017), their ability to recognise different categories of humans has not yet been tested. However, both sheep and goats respond to the gaze of humans, and alter their behaviour depending on the attentive state of humans, including understanding pointing (Nawroth et al. 2015) although they were better at following the gaze of a conspecific than a human.

Developmental influences are also important for learning and preferences. The development of offspring can be influenced before birth, for example if the mother experiences stress or undernutrition (Sinclair et al. 2016). In both sheep and goats, where a selective and initially exclusive bond exists between mother and offspring, the mother is an enormously influential role model. There is evidence, for example, that dietary preferences learned from the mother can be retained for periods in excess of 3 years. Moreover, work on the effects of cross-fostering between sheep and goats, or between different breeds of sheep, has shown that maternal rather than genetic influences dictate social, foraging and sexual preferences in adulthood and that maternal influence appears to be practically irreversible in this respect (Kendrick et al. 1998; Dwyer & Lawrence 2000). Therefore, it is preferable to rear infant kids and lambs with a mother since this close emotional mother–infant relationship is of great importance to their normal social and emotional development. In addition, trying to make an animal do something that conflicts with what it has learned from its mother (e.g. diet choice or attitudes towards humans) is always going to be difficult. Lambs learn to avoid humans from the actions of their mothers within a few days of birth and this attitude can be extremely difficult to overcome, even with the best possible interactions between them and humans. The emotional connection to the mother as a primary caregiver seems to be exclusive and lambs will not form a second relationship with a human in the presence of the mother, although gentle hand-rearing without the mother can have long-term benefits in terms of reduced fearfulness of humans. For experimental purposes that require close interactions between sheep and humans, it is preferable to ensure that a positive initial attitude to humans is passed on from mother to offspring by creating this attitude in the mother first, by pairing interactions with rewards and avoiding negative contacts such as restraint or use of fear-inducing stimuli. With goats, this is not so much of a problem since most breeds are tolerant of, and even interact with, humans. Nonetheless, even with this species, positive human interactions with the mothers may result in easier interactions with their young. Young lambs have also been shown to be capable of observational learning from conspecifics when reared in a group of peers, such as learning how to use a milk feeder, which can allow vertical transmission of information within the social group.

Standard biological data

Standard biological data for sheep and goats are shown in Table 34.1 and comprehensive haematological and biochemical data for these species may be found in Wolfensohn and Lloyd (2013) and Aitken (2007).

Table 34.1 Some standard biological data for sheep and goats.

Parameters	Sheep	Goats
Normal temperature (°C)	38.5–39.5	38.5–39.5
Chromosome number	54	60
Life span (years)	10–15	10–15
Heart rate (beats/minute)	65–110	70–120
Resting respiratory rate (breaths/minute)	15–20	15–25
Dental formula	$I^0_3 \, C^0_1 \, P^3_3 \, M^3_3$	$I^0_3 \, C^0_1 \, P^3_3 \, M^3_3$

Choice of breed

Theoretically, almost any breed of sheep or goat should readily adapt to most experimental conditions provided that they are treated correctly. However, a number of criteria should be assessed when deciding which breed is suitable for a particular research project. There are more than 1000 sheep breeds and more than 200 breeds of goats, with many localised to specific countries or conditions. Animals have been selected for milk, meat or fibre production, although some breeds are dual purpose, and thus the experimental purpose may dictate which are the most appropriate breeds. Sheep breeds also vary in their mature body weight, from meat sheep breeds such as Suffolk or Texel which can exceed 80 kg, to hill-adapted breeds of 50–60 kg, or feral Soay sheep which may only reach 15–29 kg. Similarly, Saanen and Anglo-Nubian goat breeds are usually considerably larger than British Alpine or Bagot. Larger animals will require more space and more food, and may be harder to handle for some experimental manipulations. Tropically adapted breeds and some temperate breeds such as Dorset are relatively aseasonal, and if lambs are required year-round these breeds may be suitable. In addition, the fecundity of the ewe can vary from hill breeds which typically have one or two lambs, to Booroola Merino, Finn or Romanov which may have much larger litters that can be useful for some experiments.

Some researchers find horns useful for attaching equipment although the horns should never be used as a means of catching or restraint. Horns can also be hazardous to both handlers and other animals, and this should be part of the decision-making process. Horned and polled goats should not be co-housed. Although goats can be disbudded as kids, if horns are not needed then choosing a polled breed is a more ethical approach. To remove horn buds in goats safely, kids should be between 3 and 7 days of age. Adequate anaesthesia and analgesia are essential during removal and providing the right balance of drugs for different circumstances requires experience. Sensory innervation to the horns varies between species. The use of a hot disbudding iron in goats can easily result in brain damage as the thin cranial vault offers little thermal protection to neural tissues. In the UK, disbudding goat kids may only be performed by a veterinary surgeon.

Other special considerations for breed choice might include growth rate, carcase quality, wool or coat colour. Some sheep breeds can be wool-shedding (e.g. Wiltshire Horn, Lleyn or Dorper Merino) and this can reduce or obviate the need to shear the sheep.

Generally, different breeds also have different temperaments, with heavier meat sheep being less reactive and less flighty than hill or more primitive breeds, which may make them easier to handle and acclimatise to experimental equipment. However, learning ability may also be different in these breeds, and proper habituation and handling can accustom all breeds to experimental designs.

Source of animals

Ideally, an on-site breeding flock/herd should be maintained. This allows for continuity of supply, standardisation of genetic, nutritional and experiential background and maintenance of a health barrier (see the following text). It can also allow for gentling of animals at an early stage to mitigate the impact of stress on experimental procedures. If maintaining flocks on-site is impractical, then animals may be bought in, bearing in mind that known single sources of supply are generally better and more accountable than open markets, and that availability of animals is likely to be seasonal.

Uses in the laboratory

Current areas of research that routinely use sheep and goats as experimental animals include studies into the seasonal control of reproductive activity, parturition, neonatal care and reproduction in general, lactation, growth, ruminant metabolism and physiology, and behavioural and neurobiological studies of cognitive and motivational processes. They have also been used as large-scale producers of antibodies in blood and trialled for synthesising bioactive compounds in milk through transgenic manipulation. Other studies include those related directly to disease conditions which cause harm to sheep (such as foot and mouth disease and bluetongue), and zoonoses such as the transmissible spongiform encephalopathies (TSEs). Models of human disease include bone metabolism studies and polycystic ovarian disease. Perhaps the most famous research animal is Dolly the sheep, the first example of a cloned mammal created from a somatic cell fused with a de-nucleated ovum.

General husbandry

Enclosures, pasture and shelters

Well-fleeced sheep are very tolerant of low temperatures providing that the fleece is dry. Hill breeds of sheep are more tolerant of poor weather than lowland breeds, but even the hardiest animals require some protection from wind and rain. Goats are also fairly tolerant to cold weather provided they are dry, but prefer warmer climates and should have access to shelter at all times. Shelters can take the form of small huts in pastures during the summer (with the entrance way sheltered from prevailing winds), but these can be inadequate in the winter for goats. Particularly for goats, entrances to shelters should be wide enough to allow animals to enter unimpeded by those wishing to guard the entrance. A dry lying area should always be made available. Both sheep and goats benefit from access to shade during the summer to prevent heat stress. Goats have a tendency to eat their shade, which may constitute an enrichment in the short term but can then contribute to both overheating and poisoning, so should be monitored carefully. Animals at pasture need to be protected from predators and harassment by dogs.

Group housing

Where possible, sheep and goats should be kept in groups of 3–4 or more animals. Species and sexes are normally kept separately, and frequent mixing with other animals can be stressful for both species. An open-plan floor area which can be partitioned off with hurdles under a high roof provides a versatile solution to varying group sizes (Figure 34.1). The use of straw bales can complement the hurdles. In this system, a floor of rammed chalk or similar is ideal to provide natural drainage on top of which a deep litter bed of straw can be laid. Impervious floors such as concrete are an alternative and can be more easily decontaminated between groups, but must be sloped to prevent pooling of liquids. The system depends absolutely on sufficient straw or other suitable bedding material laid often enough to provide a dry top layer. Inadequate drainage leads to waterlogged pens, damp fleeces and skins and potential feet problems, a humid atmosphere, condensation, chilling of animals and compromised well-being. An increase in respiratory disease may also result.

Sheep have been shown to have a preference for straw bedding over other flooring types, particularly when shorn (Færevik et al. 2005), and sufficient bedded space is required for all animals to lie simultaneously. Goats, however, prefer to lie on hard rocky and elevated surfaces when managed in mountainous environments, and have a marked preference for lying on harder rather than bedded surfaces. Goats can jump and climb very well so, in addition to bedded space, enough raised areas should be provided to prevent dominant animals impeding access to others.

Some older group housing systems use wooden, plastic or metal slats through which urine and faeces fall to a collecting pit below, the advantage being that animals are dry underfoot. However, slats are less comfortable than a straw bed, are expensive to maintain and, if allowed to deteriorate (or not sufficiently well constructed in the first place), can result in severe leg injuries when feet and legs become trapped (especially fine-boned breeds). For this reason, and due to the belly draughts which rise through the slats, these systems are unsuitable for goats and for parturient animals. Indeed, guidance within the Council of Europe ETS 123 revised appendix A (Council of Europe 2006) states that the entire enclosure for both sheep and goats should have a 'solid floor with appropriate bedding provided'.

Both sheep and goats rely on friction from walking on hard surfaces to maintain their hoof shape. Where only soft bedding is provided, this can lead over time to deformed or overgrown hooves and lameness. As hoof-trimming may be associated with pain, and is not considered an appropriate treatment for footrot (Green and Clifton 2018), ensuring a hard walking surface is best practice for foot care of both sheep and goats.

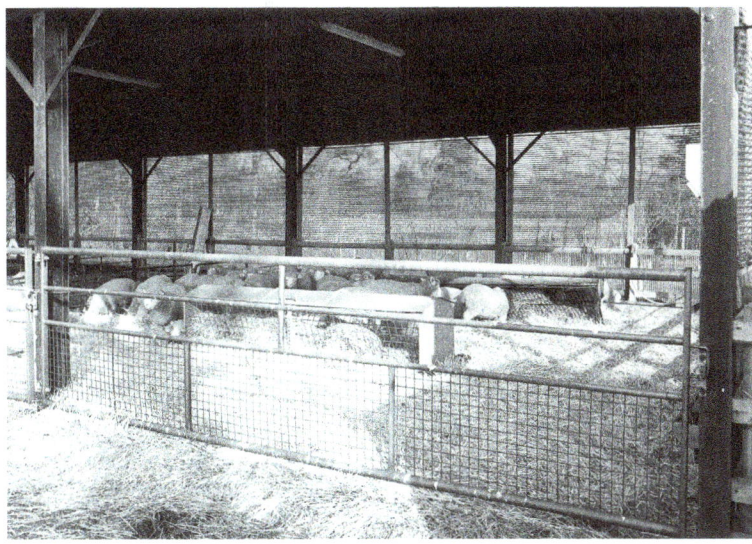

Figure 34.1 An open-plan barn accommodating sheep during the winter. Notice: (1) a layer of straw thick enough to present a dry top layer to the animals; (2) front gates large enough for tractor access; (3) strip lighting to allow thorough inspection of animals whenever needed; (4) netting at the rear of the barn cuts the force of prevailing wind and rain without reducing ventilation; (5) hay racks (on wheels) of sufficient length to allow all animals simultaneous access, fitted with lids to prevent soiling of the feed.

Good ventilation is the key to successful housing of sheep and goats. Inadequate air movement produces similar problems to those encountered with poor drainage. In high-ceilinged barns, the walls need not be solid to the eaves and the upper part may consist of hit and miss boarding or heavy-duty netting in temperate climates to reduce the effect of prevailing winds. Netting is very versatile if kept on a roller blind apparatus, so that it can be easily lifted clear during fine weather. In buildings with low ceilings or solid sides, adequate ventilation will require the provision of ceiling-mounted extractor fans (with a reliable power supply) and wall air inlets above animal height. High-roofed buildings should have a gap running along the roof apex to allow warm, humid air to escape. This is helped by providing insulation on the underside of a sloping roof, particularly if the roof is metal, preventing the warm air from cooling and falling back, forming condensation and a stagnant atmosphere.

Group housing of laboratory sheep and goats depends absolutely on a reliable method of identification (see later in this chapter). Adequate trough space must be supplied to allow all animals to feed together when concentrates are offered (Table 34.2). Less space may be needed when food is offered *ad libitum*, but close observation is required to ensure that no bullying occurs at the food rack, especially if a fine mesh is used for the rack (see section on feeding for more details), or if the animals have horns.

Individual penning

Experimental demands may require sheep or goats to be housed individually. Researchers must always critically review the need for single housing before imposing it. Animals with long-term surgical preparations may need to be singly housed to prevent damage to implants from curious penmates. Sexually active males may require single penning to avoid fighting. Singly penned sheep and goats should always be able to see and hear companions. Prior to any experimental procedure, animals require a period of acclimatisation to a new environment, routines and staff. Goats tend to adapt more rapidly to penning than do sheep and generally show fewer escape behaviours when being caught and handled.

Table 34.2 shows minimum space allowances under European Union recommendations for laboratory sheep and goats. Floors for permanent indoor single housing of sheep

Table 34.2 Recommended minimum pen dimensions for sheep and goats being used for scientific procedures. From Appendix A of the European Convention for the protection of vertebrate animals used for experimental and other scientific purposes (ETS 123). Source: Modified from Council of Europe (2006).

Animal weight (kg)	Minimum individual enclosure size (m^2)	Minimum floor area/animal (m^2)	Minimum partition height (m)*	Minimum length of ad libitum feeding space (m/animal)	Minimum length of restricted feeding space (m/animal)
<20	1.0	0.7	1.0	0.1	0.25
20–35	1.5	1.0	1.2	0.1	0.3
35–60	2.0	1.5	1.2	0.12	0.4
>60	3.0	1.8	1.5	0.12	0.5

* May need to be higher for adult goats.

and goats should normally be of an impervious material such as concrete or tiles, with at least a 1 in 15 slope to provide drainage. Floor texture needs to achieve a compromise between minimal abrasion to exposed skin and good grip to hooves. Warmth from radiant heat or underfloor heating may be of value for young, sick or infirm animals, or in a surgical recovery area especially for goats or shorn sheep. Gentle underfloor heating can also help to maintain a dry floor and reduce humidity in buildings of low volume, but is costly both to instal and maintain. Straw bedding or wood shavings may be provided, although shavings achieve little more than to absorb urine and do not otherwise add to comfort. Bedding in individual pens needs to be changed very regularly, preferably daily.

Pen walls can be solid and impervious to fluids to animal head height, above which a barred arrangement may continue, or barred to floor level to keep animals in but allowing easy observation by staff and visual contact between animals. Horizontal bars near floor level are dangerous as limbs may poke underneath when animals lie down and then break when they attempt to rise. All pens must be free from projections such as bolts or sharp metal edges. Concentrate food may be provided in free-standing plastic bins or troughs. Built-in metal troughs tend to be cumbersome, are difficult to clean *in situ*, hard to replace when they rust or rot and can cause pain when kicked by either sheep or handler. Removable hayracks can be hung from partitions. Water may be provided in automatic drinkers or in bowls that hang from the gate, filled by hoses. The latter are preferable in being easy to remove when necessary for cleaning, or to deprive animals of water prior to surgery; and when in use, give the animal technician an immediate indication of individual water intake. Individual drinkers of whatever type should be cleaned and checked daily and under normal circumstances should never be allowed to become empty. In exposed locations, the pipes may need frost protection. A typical individual sheep or goat pen is shown in Figure 34.2.

Occasionally, it is necessary to hold sheep in metabolism cages or slings. The former are used when collection of urine and faeces is required and the latter for behavioural testing, visual discrimination experiments or similar. Due to their restrictive nature, both of these methods should only be used when a clear scientific need arises for which normal penning would be inadequate. When using metabolism crates a minimum of a week of acclimatisation is recommended prior to experimentation and in slings, the same period is necessary with animals only spending 6–8 h per day in slings, under constant supervision. Both systems should use animals already familiarised to human contact and a laboratory environment.

In order to induce out-of-season breeding or to study other light-related phenomena, controlled lighting rooms may be required, but a light-tight space must not be achieved at the expense of good ventilation. In a large laboratory, it may be useful to set aside a separate area or building for special care and quarantine of sick, injured or convalescent animals.

Environmental enrichment

Careful consideration should be given to opportunities to provide environmental enrichment for animals. Social companionship is very important for both species, so allowing

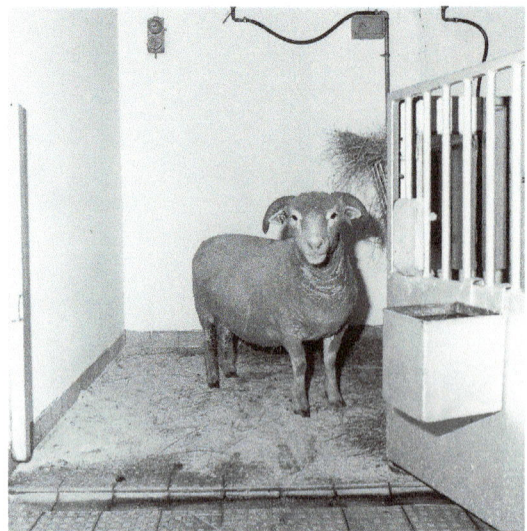

Figure 34.2 A pen for individual housing of sheep or goats in a research environment. Notice: (1) a water bowl, mineral lick and hay rack are all provided but easily removable, the free-standing plastic food trough has been removed; (2) the floor consists of a textured tile which is non-abrasive but gives good grip even when wet, a covering of sawdust helps to maintain dryness; (3) the floor slopes gently to a drain in front of the gate; (4) the bars in the gate allow singly penned animals to see adjacent companions; (5) a convenient electricity supply is provided. Although convenient, single pens are relatively barren environments for long-term holding of a social species.

the company of others, even if only visual, auditory or olfactory contact, will help to reduce stress. For goats, it is important to remember that as mountain-dwelling animals, vertical or 3-dimensional space can be important, so shelves to climb on can be useful. As ruminants, both species need regular access to forage, browse and/or fibre. For penned animals, ensuring daily exercise allows animals to express exploratory behaviour.

Identification

A reliable and easily read method of identification is vital for animals kept in groups. Ear-tagging with electronic radio-frequency identification (RFID) chips is now mandatory in the EU and is a popular and generally effective identification method, but two ear tags should be used to mitigate against the likelihood of one being lost. Poorly designed tags with sharp edges or protruding surfaces, or poor practice in placing the tags, can lead to tags catching in fencing and to ear tags being torn out, causing pain and potential infection. Likewise, ear notching or cutting causes pain and routes for infection and should not be used. Plastic numbered collars, necklaces and coloured tapes wound around the horns are all other potentially cheap and suitable methods to identify individuals. A non-toxic spray applied to the flanks allows animals to be identified over a considerable distance but must be regularly renewed and is lost at shearing. An RFID in a rumenal bolus or subcutaneous implant is becoming more popular, especially for valuable individuals.

Health monitoring and quarantine and barrier systems

Sheep and goats intended for research are no less susceptible to disease than stock in commercial flocks. Maintenance of a high health status among research animals is an important ethical responsibility for research groups and will also improve data quality through minimising intercurrent, and possibly subclinical disease, during procedures and reducing between-animal variation. Strategies to exclude disease include: membership of national disease eradication or notification schemes; local barriers such as quarantining and well-maintained fencing; and use of disease prevention measures such as vaccinations and strict worming policies. Veterinary advice should be taken on these matters, bearing in mind the geographical location and standard practice routines built into the annual cycles of flock management. It is also important to maintain disease prevention routines when an animal leaves the stock pool and enters a laboratory.

Quarantine policy

Keeping stock healthy is more difficult to achieve in open than closed flocks (those with a non-buying-in policy). Veterinary advice should be sought in advance of acquiring new animals. Any bought-in stock must be quarantined for at least 4 weeks on a pasture or in a building well away (more than 100 m) from other stock. Bought-in animals should come with a comprehensive clinical history of the flock from which they originate. On arrival, the animals should be carefully and individually examined for signs of ill-health (see later) by a veterinary surgeon and animals suspected of having particular problems rejected. Further investigation may include serological testing for diseases such as border disease, chlamydophila or toxoplasmosis using blood samples taken after 2 weeks of quarantine to allow for seroconversion to diseases experienced immediately prior to purchase. During quarantine, routine measures such as vaccinations, treatment against parasitic worms and ectoparasites should be undertaken as necessary to correct for any imbalance between the health status of incoming animals and that of the resident stock. Visitors to the quarantine area should be discouraged, and suitable personal protective equipment provided. In contact, equipment should be new or thoroughly disinfected before use. Despite these precautions, it is still possible to transfer disease between flocks. A closed flock is therefore highly desirable.

Transport and movement

Never begin to move animals from place to place until there are adequate staff who are fully prepared. Well-handled goats and sheep can be trained to walk on a halter, and this can be the simplest means to move individuals over short distances. Both sheep and goats can also be trained to follow a handler, sometimes by the use of food rewards, or the evolved following behaviour can be employed to bring about movements through the use of a trained animal. However, the vast majority of sheep and goats are moved by making use of their 'flight zone' or distance, whereby human movement into this space causes the animal to move away. Low stress-handling techniques should always be employed by working at the outer edges of the flight zone such that the animal moves away at a slow and steady pace. Sudden and rapid movements into the flight zone by an impatient handler can cause panic, which may result in self-inflicted injury to animals or handlers. As social animals, both species move more easily from place to place in groups. All routes except the desired route should be closed and then the animals should be allowed to go at a steady walk with gentle encouragement from behind, or in front if trained to move in this way. Single animals are very difficult to move by this method and should be loaded by ramp into a wheeled crate. A confined and roofed transporter is best for this purpose as it prevents a frightened animal from accelerating into an obstruction. For moving flocks over longer distances, specialised animal wagons are required and national regulations regarding animal transport apply. Loading ramps must have barriered sides and ridged walkways. All transporters and transport procedures should comply with current animal transport legislation requirements.

Breeding

If well-fed, sheep and goats reach puberty at around 5 months of age and females begin to cycle in the autumn due to reducing day length. The inter-oestrous period is 16.5 days in the sheep and 21 days in the goat. Ewe lambs and kids may be large enough to be mated in the autumn of their first year if born early in the season with no subsequent growth check (achieving 75% or more of final adult weight). It is preferable not to breed from the smaller ewe lambs or from goats until the following season when they will be at least 1 year old. Early breeding is becoming a more common farming practice, especially with faster growing breeds, although litter sizes and neonatal survival may be reduced in young females. The rearing conditions used for prospective working rams are also important since there is evidence that rearing rams together from weaning in single sex groups with no access to females can lead to high incidence of homosexual rather than heterosexual preferences. It is, therefore, better to let the ram lambs run with the ewes for as long as possible while the ewes and any ewe lambs remain in anoestrus. A good introduction to reproduction in the sheep and goat is provided by Evans & Maxwell (1988).

To ensure a compact lambing period, ewes or does may be synchronised in oestrus. This can occur naturally by the sudden introduction of a male (the 'ram effect'), sometimes using a teaser (vasectomised) ram, or by the use of progesterone-containing vaginal sponges or controlled internal drug release (CIDR) devices and injections of gonadotropin-releasing hormone (GnRH) analogues or pregnant mare serum gonadotrophin. Melatonin implants may also be used to advance the onset of the breeding season. A disadvantage of synchronising oestrus is that more males are needed. For example, a good-quality fertile ram may be able to serve up to 50 unsynchronised ewes, but only 10–12 ewes in a synchronised flock.

Both rams and ewes may require supplementary feeds in the pre-mating period. This will build up body condition in rams to maintain them through to the end of mating and improve ovulation rate in females (a practice known as 'flushing' through providing a rising plane of nutrition). A body condition score of 3 (Figure 34.3) is ideal for a ewe at mating.

Behavioural changes in oestrous ewes are often difficult to detect under farm conditions, so rams or teasers usually wear coloured crayons on their brisket which leave a mark on the ewe's rump following service. Some goats show inappetence, a drop in milk yield, restlessness and increased vocalisation during oestrus but these signs are not reliable, and willingness to accept the buck is the only sure indicator. Female sheep and goats can display a number of proceptive (invitational) and receptive behaviours, such as head turning, tail fanning and interest in the male, in response to the courtship responses of males (low-pitched rumble bleats, chin-resting on the back of the ewe, kicking with a foreleg and flehmen). Under experimental conditions, these behaviours have been quantified to produce an overall receptivity index (Fabre-Nys & Venier 1987).

Although the normal reproductive pattern of sheep and goats leads to the production of one set of offspring in the spring of each year, some breeds, such as the Dorset or the Finnish Landrace, are capable of producing offspring more frequently than this, with three lambing periods in two years, or five in three years sometimes achieved in commercial 'accelerated lambing' systems. However, this requires early weaning of the lambs, places pressure on husbandry systems and maternal physiology and has been associated with higher lamb mortality and reduced ewe longevity. In benign conditions and when well-fed, goats can also have more oestrous cycles and can therefore produce offspring over a longer season.

Pregnancy is indicated by non-return to oestrus, and may be confirmed using blood or milk progesterone assays in goats, or through the use of ultrasound scanning, which carries the additional advantage of determining the number of offspring. A skilled interpreter of ultrasound images can identify a pregnancy at 30 days but more usually ewes are scanned at 50–90 days post-mating. Recent advances in scanning mean that foetuses can be aged to within 5 days of gestational age, which can be very beneficial for management of lambing.

The gestation period is normally 145 days in the sheep and 150 days in the goat with 5 days variation in either direction being normal. Signs of imminent parturition include: seeking isolation from the main group, restlessness including circling and pawing the ground, mammary development, the ability of handlers to express milk from the teats, lifting of the head with licking of the lips and, finally, immediately before birth, powerful abdominal contractions. The experimental conditions may interfere with the expression of some of these behaviours and potentially delay or slow up parturition. If some control over parturition is required for experimental reasons, then an intravenous injection of dexamethasone (0.25 mg/kg) can be given between days 140 and 142 of gestation and ewes will give birth around 48 h later (usually between 40 and 54 h). Intramuscular administration of dexamethasone is not nearly as reliable in this respect. Earlier induction of parturition is not recommended as lambs will be progressively weaker with more respiratory problems, and higher mortality.

Clear and simple guides to obstetrics in sheep are provided by Eales and Small (2004) and Winter and Hill (2003). Knowing when to intervene in lambing or kidding requires considerable experience, and the novice should never be put in a position of supervising lambings without skilled back-up. As a general rule of thumb, ewes or nannies which do not produce young within 1 hour after the appearance of fluid-filled membranes or a rush of fluid from the vulva may need assistance. Earlier intervention may be required if the animals become weak or unwell, or if the lamb or kid is not presented in a forwards position with the forelegs extended and the nose lying along the legs. Ewes or nannies which show just a head or one limb protruding from the vulva need assistance immediately. A number of diseases causing abortion are zoonotic, and human contact with parturient ewes should be strictly controlled; in particular, pregnant women should avoid all contact with lambing ewes, placentae, recently lambed ewes and lambs or any materials that have been contaminated with foetal fluids.

Normally, ewes and does will stand following birth, begin intensive licking of their offspring and emit frequent low-pitched vocalisation. It is normal for the mothers to consume the foetal membranes. Although some movement away from the neonate may occur initially in females giving birth for the first time, frequent or sustained aggression, avoidance or

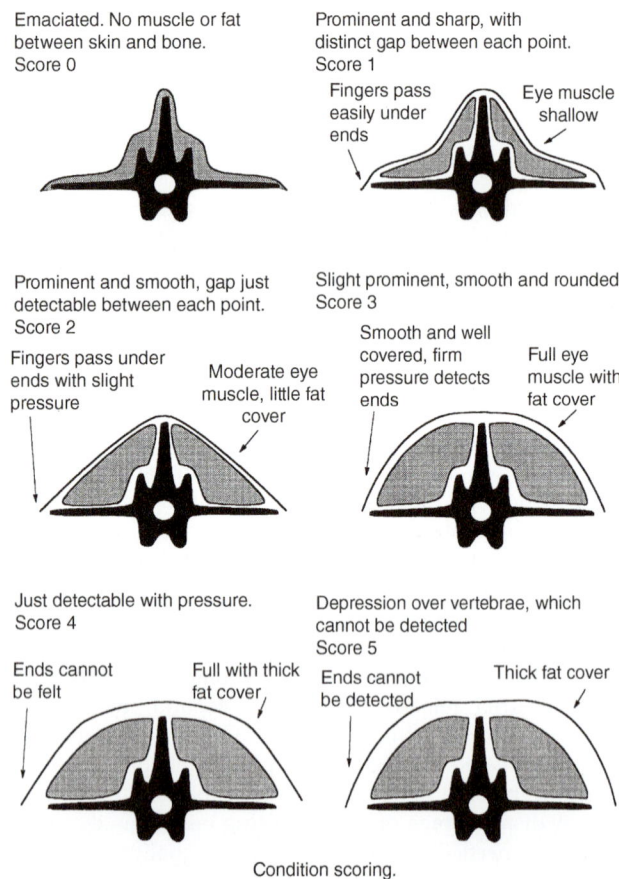

Condition scoring.
Find the last rib and feel the spine over the loin.

Figure 34.3 Drawings of transverse sections through the lumbar spine of sheep with different body scores. Source: Reproduced with permission from Hindson (1989).

lack of interest in the newborn is abnormal and mothers and offspring may need particular attention to ensure that bonding occurs in these cases. Following birth, the ewe's udder should be checked to ensure that milk is normal and abundant. The majority of lambs and kids are able to stand within 10–20 minutes of birth and should be able to find their own way to the udder, and suck within 30 minutes to an hour of birth. Neonates which have not sucked successfully from their mothers within two hours of birth may need assistance to locate the teat and to suckle. Weak newborn animals also need special attention, particularly warmth, dryness and food. Assessing lamb temperature, for example by using a rectal thermometer, is an important part of the care of very weak lambs as lambs whose temperatures have fallen to 35 °C require immediate warming through the use of a hot box or similar. Initial feeds must be given as colostrum (or a colostrum replacer) at 50 ml/kg within 6 h of birth, repeated at 6–8-hourly intervals for the first day if artificial rearing is needed. Colostrum from donor ewes can be frozen and stored for up to 12 months. Stomach tubing may be necessary for neonates that will not suck but should be performed only by a competent person, ensuring that equipment is cleaned and sterilised before and after use. In severe, hypothermic cases, an intraperitoneal injection of a calculated dose of warm sterile isotonic fluid containing glucose may be lifesaving. Dams and offspring should only be separated if this is essential for their well-being as hand rearing is time consuming and affects behaviour when lambs reach adulthood.

Maternal behaviour and selective bonding

Mothers and offspring require about 4–6 hours of close contact for ewes to learn to recognise their offspring and a secure bond to be formed. During this period, separation should be avoided if at all possible, and care taken not to contaminate the coat of the young animal with the smell of other animals as bonds are based on olfactory cues. Once the bond is secure, mothers and offspring can be safely separated for short periods, if required for experimental purposes, without the bond being weakened, although both partners will find this extremely stressful. As these bonds are selective, maternal ewes or nannies may violently reject the offspring of another animal if it attempts to suckle, and therefore care must be taken to prevent injury to vulnerable newborns. While selective bonding may ensure the offspring an exclusive milk supply and, for that matter, an individual role model, this has caused farmers problems for hundreds of years when they want to foster orphan or triplet/quadruplet lambs. Where large numbers of animals are giving birth in the same period, then 'wet fostering' becomes possible since both maternal ewes and nannies will accept other young prior to forming a selective bond with their own. Wet fostering involves covering the foster lamb or kid in the amniotic fluids of the parturient mother and presenting this at the same time as the mother gives birth to her own singleton newborn. This method is generally successful particularly if the foster animal is young and keen to suck from the foster mother. Fostering can also be achieved where the ewe or nanny has delivered a dead offspring which it has licked. This animal can be skinned and the skin placed over the foster lamb or kid for a period of time until the mother accepts the new offspring. Other methods have sometimes been used, such as restraint of the mother to allow the lamb or kid to suckle, or attempting to mask the scent of the foster lamb or kid with another novel odour, but are generally less successful. Manually stimulating the vagina and cervix of a post-partum mother for 2 minutes even up to 3 days after she has given birth can also be used to mimic the natural birth process and induce the mother to form a new selective bond with the foster neonate.

With the exception of wet fostering or vaginocervical stimulation, fostering can be difficult, unsuccessful, involve welfare issues relating to prolonged restraint and can often result in higher foster lamb/kid mortality. Ensuring a quiet, well-managed lambing/kidding environment, where mothers are able to bond successfully with their own offspring, should help to ensure these manipulations are rarely needed. If given proper feeding and care, many mothers can also successfully rear three lambs which will reduce the need to foster surplus lambs.

Weaning and rearing

It is essential that lambs and kids receive adequate quantities of colostrum after birth, to provide passive immunity, nutrition and to promote the proper development of the gut. Once lambs and kids have received colostrum, it is possible to rear them artificially 'on the bottle' using milk replacer powders, introducing solids from 7 days of age. Ideally, neonates should be kept in a peer group and allowed *ad libitum* access to milk via an artificial feeder to allow more natural sucking patterns and to prevent over consumption in a short period of time. If lambs or kids can only be bottle fed, they should be gradually weaned off milk no later than 6 weeks of age to avoid problems of abomasal bloat, from too rapid ingestion of milk substitute during a small number of feeds.

Lambs and kids reared naturally normally start the process of eating solid foods themselves at 3 weeks of age, with the rumen starting to function around 4 weeks of age. Young lambs and kids can be offered specialised creep feed from 2 weeks old, in addition to the milk from their mothers. This creep feed should be given in a feeder which does not allow the mothers access. While it is possible to leave offspring with their mothers indefinitely, it is usual to wean lambs and kids completely onto solid food at around 16 weeks of age. This allows the mother to recover fully prior to the next breeding season. If a schedule of enforced weaning is not used, especially with prolific breeds, the body condition of the mothers can deteriorate as a result of persistent suckling by the offspring. In frequent-breeding systems, where an earlier than usual return to sexual receptivity and pregnancy is required, early weaning at 6–8 weeks is necessary as lactating ewes rarely exhibit oestrous cycles.

Gradual weaning is best carried out by separating a group of lambs/kids from their mothers at the same time, for example by separating into adjacent pens or fields for a period of time before the mothers are completely removed. It is best to relocate the ewes/nannies rather than take the offspring to new accommodation, because the young then remain familiar with their surroundings and can easily find water and feed hoppers. When weaning is complete, the ewes/does should be removed to a location out of earshot and regular checks should be made to ensure that none of them develop mastitis. The lambs/kids can be fed on creep feed and hay or grass during this time and, if necessary, can be re-introduced to the flock after 3–4 weeks, at which time their mothers will not accept any suckling attempts.

Feeding

The correct feeding of sheep and goats for maximum productivity and health is a large and complex field beyond the scope of this article. Morand-Fehr (2005) and Fthenakis et al (2012) provide reviews on this topic for goats and sheep respectively and numerous publications are available from agricultural advisory services and colleges (e.g. Feeding the ewe manual[1], Improving ewe nutrition for Better Returns[2]). Sheep and goats are ruminant animals which possess a digestive system and physiology that is highly specialised and adapted to the extraction and metabolism of usable nutrients from plants, and in particular the cellulose in plant cell walls. The rumen is little more than a fermentation vat where a delicate mix of micro-organisms is provided with the right conditions and substrates from which to produce short chain fatty acids from cellulose; the adapted biochemical systems of the adult ruminant are able to use these as an energy source or as a substrate from which to manufacture glucose. Rapid changes to diet, particularly a sudden excess of nutrient-rich food, are likely to upset the fermentation process with potentially disastrous and fatal consequences. It therefore follows that dietary stability should be a prime feature of any feeding regime, and any changes in either quality or quantity must be introduced gradually with careful monitoring.

In the wild, the natural food of the sheep is grass, whereas goats tend to browse on the leaves of bushes and trees. The inquisitive feeding habit of goats is well known, and care must be taken to keep poisonous plants, for example, yew trees, and dangerous objects, such as electric cables, out of reach of a goat even at full stretch. Presentation of strictly limited quantities of safe hedge trimmings or freshly fallen branches with leaves can be a treat for goats, and can add to environmental enrichment.

Providing adequate nutrition is essential for the health and welfare of sheep and goats at any time but this is particularly important for animals that are to reproduce. To ensure that animals are adequately fed, and are neither under or over fed, they should be body condition scored regularly to ensure that body fat remains relatively constant throughout the year. Sheep with a thick fleece are impossible to condition score properly without being caught and palpated. Body condition can be scored by manual palpation of the lumbar spine, feeling for the transverse processes and the level of fat cover (see Figure 34.3). Goats may also be scored by feeling the size of the fat pad at the sternum and feeling for fat cover over the ribs. Body condition for both species is usually scored on a 5-point scale, where 1 indicates emaciation and 5 implies obesity. Ideally, animals should remain between 2.5 and 4.0 throughout the year, with low scores indicating inadequate nutrition, poor dentition or concurrent health conditions, and high scores being risk factors for metabolic disorders and dystocia.

At different periods of the reproductive cycle, nutritional requirements are higher. Ewes from mid-pregnancy (especially late gestation) and during lactation need a higher energy intake, and diets may need to be adjusted to give more energy per unit of bulk to supply sufficient nutrition at the limit of appetite. A guide to the feeding of pregnant ewes can be found here[3].

Sheep and goats kept indoors can be fed fresh cut grass (but not lawn mowings which rapidly ferment), but more usually are given hay, which is readily but slowly broken down in the rumen and helps to maintain rumenal stability. Mouldy or rotten hay will be rejected. Goats tend to be more selective than sheep when offered hay, and will eat the leafy parts and seed heads at the expense of the stalks. Silage is an acceptable alternative to hay for sheep and goats, but is less palatable to some animals, which can affect intake. Silage is heavy and more difficult to manhandle in a laboratory environment and it is hard to keep fresh when only a small number of animals are being fed from a large bale. Poor-quality silage carries a risk of listeriosis but will often be rejected.

The design of fodder racks is an important consideration, particularly with goats. Goats are agile climbers and will readily stand on their hindlegs to pull down fodder. They will also climb onto racks if allowed to, and subsequent contamination of feed with urine and faeces will cause much wastage. Feed racks should therefore be designed with a cover.

A fine mesh (1.5 cm square) for hay racks is preferable since it slows intake and thus increases feeding time to more closely match time spent grazing. This increase in time spent acquiring food may also be considered as a welfare refinement, especially for singly housed animals. It also reduces waste. Sufficient rack space is essential to avoid bullying, ideally allowing all animals to feed at the same time.

Other bulk foods used for sheep include good-quality barley straw, chopped maize and roots such as mangolds. These foods are only generally suitable as part of a balanced diet that also includes forage and concentrates. Bulky foods are useful to control obesity when animals have limited opportunities for exercise. Sugar beets may be used as a treat for penned animals. Roots may be inedible to animals with poor front teeth and may accelerate tooth wear if fed for long periods.

Concentrate foods are widely available as proprietary products with 'guaranteed' nutritional content shown on the food bag label. The actual constituents of these diets may vary seasonally. Vitamins and other ingredients may 'go off' in the bag so freshness and a dry cool food storage area are

---

[1] http://beefandlamb.ahdb.org.uk/wp-content/uploads/2018/03/Feeding-the-ewe.pdf (accessed 30 May 2019)

[2] https://beefandlamb.ahdb.org.uk/wp-content/uploads/2016/04/BRP-Improving-ewe-nutrition-manual-12-050416.pdf (accessed 30 May 2019)

[3] https://www.qmscotland.co.uk/sites/default/files/ewe_timeline_0.pdf (accessed 30 May 2019)

important. Always observe any 'use by' dates and keep the storage area free from vermin. Animals kept indoors for prolonged periods should be supplied with licks to provide supplementary metal ions and minerals. Particular attention should be paid to copper, selenium and cobalt levels, and to vitamin D in animals with no access to natural daylight. Copper and selenium, in excessive quantities, are toxic to sheep and goats. Licks and concentrate feeds should always be specific for the species concerned as some foods for e.g. cattle and pigs may contain inappropriate amounts of copper. It is important to check the overall likely intake from all feed sources to avoid excesses.

The diets for lambs and kids need special attention, particularly when they are newly weaned. A careful balance needs to be drawn between providing sufficient nutrient-rich food for rapid growth and avoiding over-feeding which can lead to diarrhoea and acidosis.

Given the variables outlined above, it will be clear that there are no universally reliable rules by which to calculate how much food to offer any one animal. A starting point might be that individually housed ewes at maintenance only will receive 1.5–2.5 kg of fresh good-quality hay and 0–150 g of 16% protein concentrate food daily, depending on condition score. All animals should have constant access to clean fresh water.

Laboratory procedures

Handling and training

The key to catching and handling sheep and goats in a confined space is to move calmly and confidently. Once acclimatised to humans, the animals should be handled with the minimum frequency that is compatible with experimental success. The increasing use of telemetry for physiological monitoring and even blood sampling which requires minimal restraint and creates animals who are their own 'mobile labs' is to be greatly encouraged.

Nervous animals may need two catchers in a large pen. Guide the animal into a high-walled corner with no protrusions. Reduce freedom of movement gradually until the animal can be grasped firmly with one hand under the chin and the other used to draw the body against the handler's legs. Resist the temptation to make a wild lunge if an animal tries to escape, but rather let it go and begin again. Do not grab or hold animals by the horns, fleece, ears or tail, as they will struggle and injure themselves. Restraint by the fleece can lead to tissue damage which may impact on experimental studies. Horns may also be broken off which can cause pain and considerable bleeding. Goats are so inquisitive that they often approach handlers (especially those with a food bucket) and can be caught easily. Once the head is held, the body of a sheep or goat can be pressed gently against a wall with one knee against the lumbar vertebrae in front of the stifle and the animal thus restrained by one person.

Some procedures may require an animal to be cast (tipped over onto its rump). To cast a sheep or goat first turn the head round horizontally using mild-to-moderate force until the neck is bent and the head faces towards the tail. Then apply moderate downward pressure on the rump, back and turn the animal away from the head around a bent knee, and the animal should fall to the ground. The head and shoulders may then be lifted and held between the handler's knees with the animal on its back (Figure 34.4).

Beware rams and billy goats! These animals are larger than ewes and nannies and may elect to charge rather than run, especially when sexually active. Horned males are potentially dangerous.

Sheep and goats which have been treated gently by diligent staff using positive reinforcement techniques respond well to regular handling and this facilitates efficient and stress-free completion of tasks. Nervous or newly acquired animals require particular patience which will eventually benefit all. Guides to shepherding sheep and handling goats are provided by Holmes (1991) and Mews and Mowlem (1991).

Recording body temperatures

Measurement of an animal's temperature is usually done using a lubricated clinical thermometer inserted into the rectum.

Administration of substances

Any procedure must only be undertaken following appropriate training. If done for experimental purposes, this may need to follow a formal certification process.

Oral

Liquids can be given to sheep and goats using a strong smooth-sided bottle or dosing gun introduced gently into the diastema (the gap rostral to the premolars). A calibrated dosing gun may also be used. Plastic syringes are easily chewed and destroyed. The head should be held steadily and tilted slightly upward. Liquids should be dribbled in slowly and animals allowed to swallow. The process must be stopped at the first sign of choking. This method always results in some spillage. Stomach tubing requires a mouth gag and is a skilled procedure. Some substances may be delivered in accurate dosages using rumenal boluses.

Injections

Subcutaneous injections should be given under the loose skin above or behind the scapulae. Short needles (less than 25 mm with a diameter 0.4–1.2 mm, 23–18 G (the larger size for oily liquids)) are suitable. Intramuscular injections may be given into the gluteal muscles caudal to the tuber coxae, the quadriceps muscle groups in front of the femur or the muscle bellies dorsal to the neck vertebrae in the midpoint of the neck; 25 mm needles of 0.8–1.2 mm diameter (21–18 G) are suitable. Injections into the muscle behind the femur should be avoided as there is a risk of damaging the sciatic nerve. Intravenous injections may be given and intermittent blood samples withdrawn using a 0.8 mm, 21 G (small volume) to 1.6 mm 16 G (large volume) needle inserted into the jugular vein. Vacutainer systems can be a convenient

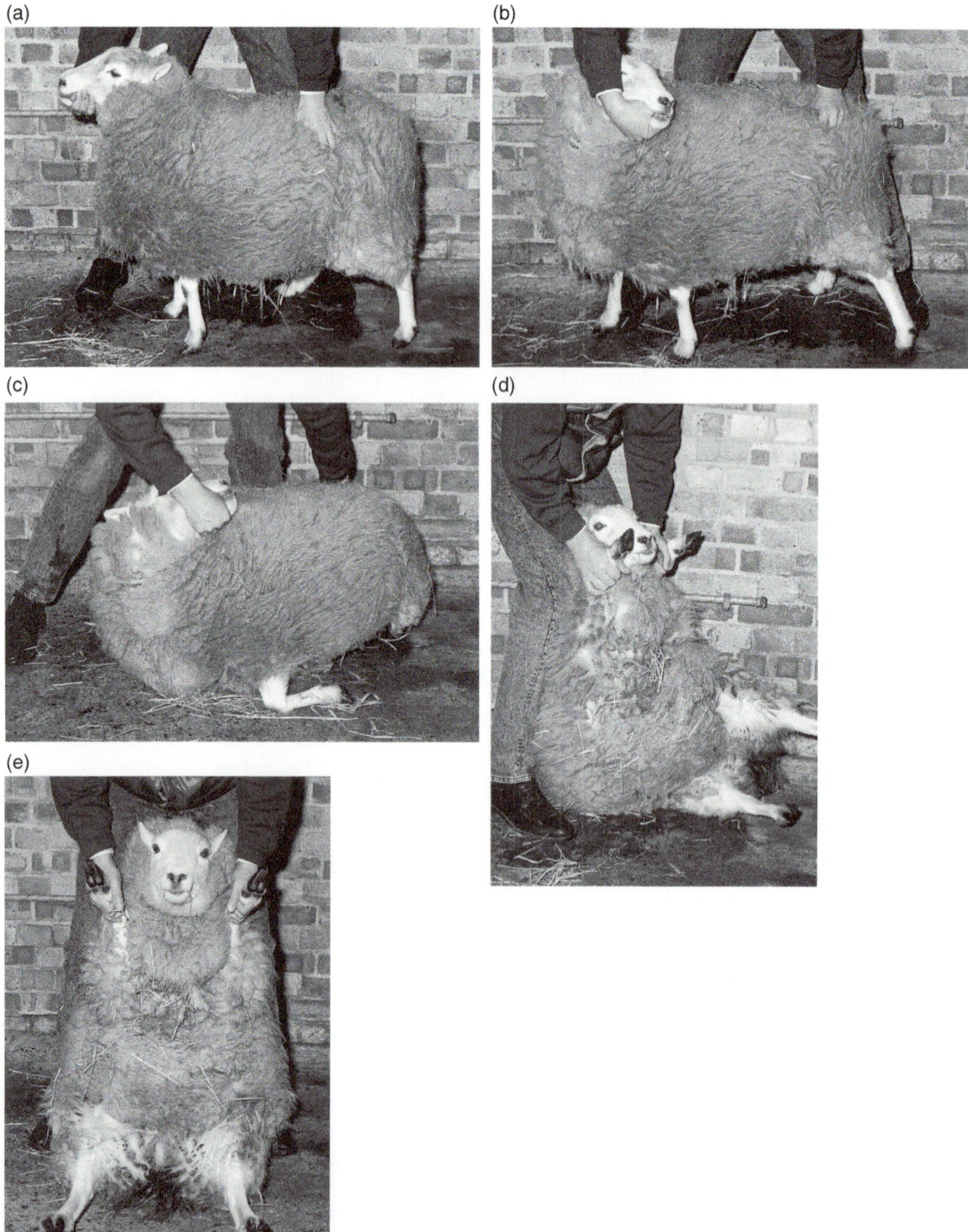

Figure 34.4 Restraining and casting sheep. (a) Restraint. The animal's head is held by the lower jaw, with the thumb passing through the diastema (a natural gap in the dental arcades behind the incisors and before the premolars). The body is restrained against the handler's knee and firm pressure from the hand in opposing sublumbar fossae (the depressions in the flanks behind the ribcage and in front of the hip bones). For additional control, the animal may be backed into a corner or gently pressed against a wall with a knee in one sublumbar fossa. (b) Casting. The animal's head is turned away from the handler in a horizontal plane so that it points towards the tail, using moderate force. The hindquarters are kept under control using the knees and the spare hand without pulling on the wool. (c) The animal is pushed backwards using the hand controlling the head, and rotating the body in a horizontal plane around the knee in the sublumbar fossa, using downwards pressure with the hand placed on the animal's flanks. The sheep will collapse to the ground. It is important that this stage is performed quickly to prevent the animal from adjusting the position of its feet, which will enable it to remain standing. Practice is required. (d) The grip is transferred to the forelegs (moving the hand that was on the flanks first) and lifting the ewe's forequarters. The animal is lifted using the knees and not the back. (e) The animal is held resting on its tail with the shoulders gripped between the handler's knees. Inspections of the animal's feet and undersurface are now possible.

alternative to syringes for taking blood samples, and also allow immediate mixing with anti-coagulants if required.

If repeated access to the blood stream is required, an indwelling cannula should be placed in the jugular vein using a sterile technique under local anaesthesia. The best method is that described by Seldinger (1953) and Harrison (1995), which involves passing a wire through a needle and into the vein, which, after withdrawal of the needle, acts as a guide over which a nylon, vinyl or silastic cannula may be passed and sutured in placed. See Joint Working Group on Refinement (JWGR) (1993) for guidance on limits to blood volume that can be acceptably withdrawn. Ambulatory devices have been developed to allow remote collection of blood samples where the effect of handling may confound experimental studies (Goddard et al. 1988).

Anaesthesia and surgery

Anaesthesia of sheep and goats, including premedication and peri-operative analgesia has been described by Flecknell (2009). Rumenal fermentation is accelerated by rapidly digestible foods, which should be temporarily withdrawn before surgery to avoid rumenal tympany. Prolonged food deprivation before surgery will have a metabolic and welfare impact. Regurgitation of gas and fluids under anaesthesia may still occur, risking airway integrity, especially if animals need to be positioned for surgery such that natural drainage of the pharynx is difficult.

A cuffed endotracheal tube must always be used when sheep or goats are kept under general anaesthesia, to prevent rumenal fluids or saliva (which is copiously secreted) from entering the trachea. A laryngoscope is necessary during intubation to visualise the larynx over the large dorsum of the tongue. After intubation, a slight incline to the surgical table allows the head to be lower than the body and will help secretions to drain from the mouth. Pressure on the diaphragm and the great veins due to the weight of the rumen contents or from the accumulation of rumenal gas (bloat) is a hazard of all ruminant anaesthesia. It may be helpful to pass a stomach tube into the rumen to reduce this risk during long operations. Surgical preparations commonly used in research are described by Harrison (1995). Techniques for placement of probes or cannulae into specific areas of the central nervous system and making electrophysiological recordings or measuring *in vivo* transmitter release have been described (Fabre-Nys *et al*. 1991; Kendrick 1991; Kendrick & Baldwin 1991).

After surgery, animals should be continuously monitored and provided with fluid therapy if needed and analgesia. The endotracheal tube must be removed when the swallowing reflex returns. The restoration of normal standing, eating and drinking should be recorded.

Euthanasia

Sheep and goats may be humanely killed using an intravenous injection of pentobarbital (150 mg or more/kg body weight). If suitable equipment and expertise is available, then shooting a captive bolt directly into the brain is an acceptable alternative, bearing in mind that the approach must be from directly above or behind the skull, not between the eyes (Humane Slaughter Association 2006). In either case, once unconscious, great vessels should be severed. The booklet *The Casualty Sheep* (Sheep Veterinary Society 1994) provides further details of all methods of euthanasia, and see also Chapter 17: Euthanasia and other fates for laboratory animals. The use of firearms for this purpose is restricted to authorised people.

Common health and welfare problems

Assessing the health and welfare of any animal must be based upon a sound knowledge and experience of what is normal. In a laboratory setting, where the environment may be very different from that in which sheep and goats evolved, attempts should be made to allow the animals to display normal behaviours, to prevent the development of abnormal, agitated or stereotypical behaviours. Signs of ill-health might include an elevated temperature (over 40 °C is a cause for concern), reduction in appetite, changes in behaviour, either becoming excessively withdrawn or overly active, colour change of the mucous membranes (pale pink is normal), a cessation of rumination, abnormal discharges from mouth, nose, eyes, ears, anus or genitalia, losses of patches of fleece and lameness. Sheep and goats lagging behind the flock when driven should be caught and examined. Animals in pain or distress may be reluctant to rise, display an abnormal posture and often grind their teeth noisily. Although harsh and laboured breathing is an indication of respiratory disease, moderate hyperventilation can be deceiving in the sheep as healthy animals tend to breathe more rapidly than other species, especially when being handled. Likewise, the heart rate may be considerably elevated in a normal but nervous animal.

Welfare assessment

The welfare of experimental animals should be checked at least daily, focusing on whether animals are alert, interested and engaged with the environment, social companions and eating normally. Animals that appear withdrawn, disinterested in the environment or excessively agitated should always be given additional attention to determine the causes of these behavioural changes. Animals should also be assessed regularly for weight and body condition score, coat or fleece appearance and cleanliness, particularly in the anogenital region, and for the presence of lameness, overgrown hooves or swellings or callus on the joints. These can indicate that the environment is sub-optimal and help to detect the presence of subclinical disease, allowing the earlier treatment of welfare problems. Specific welfare assessment protocols for farmed sheep and goats have been developed[4,5] and can be adapted for use in a laboratory setting.

---

[4]https://www.researchgate.net/publication/275887069_AWIN_Welfare_Assessment_Protocol_for_Sheep (accessed 30 May 2019)

[5]http://www.academia.edu/13468105/AWIN_welfare_assessment_protocol_for_goats (accessed 30 May 2019)

Common diseases

Sheep and goats are susceptible to a wide range of diseases. Many of the more common diseases are preventable using vaccination (for example clostridiosis, pasteurellosis, contagious pustular dermatitis (orf), and infectious abortion caused by *Chlamydophila* and *Toxoplasma*) or prophylaxis (for parasitic infestations including coccidiosis). Wherever a particular disease is known to occur, preventive steps should be taken in preference to treatment after the disease appears. The growing incidence of resistance to antibiotics and anthelmintics makes preventive strategies of good husbandry, pasture management and vaccination all the more important. Contagious pustular dermatitis and chlamydophila abortion are among the more worrying zoonoses transmissible to humans. Other potential zoonoses include toxoplasmosis, louping ill, listeriosis, campylobacteriosis, leptospirosis, Q fever and salmonellosis.

The following brief outline of the more common clinical signs and diseases of sheep and goats is intended only to introduce the reader to the complexity of the subject. For a general introduction to sheep management and disease, Henderson (1990) is useful, while Aitken (2007) is the standard reference work in the UK. Amateur diagnosis and treatments should never be attempted: a veterinary surgeon should be consulted.

Weight loss

Weight loss in a group of animals is usually due to poor diet, poor teeth or parasitism by intestinal nematodes or liver flukes. Nutritional deficiencies may occur as a result of diets with insufficient carbohydrates, proteins, minerals such as cobalt, or vitamins, or a combination of these. Weight loss may, of course, also occur if the diet has an adequate composition but is fed in inadequate amounts. The dietary requirements of growth and pregnancy must be considered. Weight loss in individuals may be the result of any chronic condition; for example, lameness, abscessation, maedi-visna, Johne's disease, caseous lymphadenitis, ovine pulmonary adenomatosis or tumours.

Diarrhoea

Diarrhoea is usually a consequence of over-feeding, intestinal parasitism or coccidiosis. Diarrhoea in pre-weaned lambs is frequently associated with bacterial infections and can result in a rapid deterioration in condition due primarily to dehydration. Bacterial infections are less commonly a primary cause in adult sheep. It is important to encourage fluid intake while awaiting a diagnosis.

Nervous signs

Nervous signs and ataxia owing to disease processes are relatively common in sheep and goats of any age. A wide variety of causes exist, such as thiamine deficiency, copper deficiency, scrapie, listeriosis, plant or chemical poisoning, brain space-occupying lesions due to tapeworm cysts, abscesses or tumours, louping ill or metabolic disorders. Some conditions may progress to convulsions or coma (see later). Accurate and early diagnosis is essential.

Intestinal worms and liver flukes

Most adult sheep and goats carry a limited mixed burden of these parasites, which with proper treatment and management are not clinically significant. More severe endoparasitism in flocks can be seen as loss of condition/reduced weight gain, diarrhoea, anaemia and hepatitis in the case of live flukes. Clinical disease is more often seen in young stock. In all cases, to minimise the impact of endoparasitism on animal health it is necessary to pay careful attention to pasture maintenance. Significant numbers of infective nematode larvae can develop, even on fields used only for occasional grazing, if the adult stock are inadequately wormed, pasture access is not properly rotated or stocking density is too high when animals are allowed access. This can make small paddocks adjacent to research facilities which are used for animal exercise potentially dangerous locations for unprotected grazing animals. Nematode resistance to wormers (anthelmintics) is an increasing problem worldwide, and appears to be particularly prevalent in goats. A strategic control programme should be developed (Gascoigne *et al*. 2018). Boggy areas of pasture should be drained to discourage the snails that act as intermediate hosts for liver flukes.

Foot care

Animals housed indoors for prolonged periods with limited exercise tend to develop overgrown hooves. Overgrown hooves can lead to lameness, bad posture, cracking of the hoof wall and damaged white line areas of the hoof. Animals at pasture are susceptible to damaged feet produced by poached soils, sharp stones and the like. All sheep and goats kept for research should therefore be turned regularly (see the section on handling for techniques) the feet cleaned and hoof walls pared as necessary by a skilled person. It is important to disinfect equipment between animals to reduce the spread of bacteria which lead to footrot. Beware overparing and causing damage to the sensitive structures of the hoof, as this can lead to permanent lameness. Standing sheep and goats with clean feet three to four times a year in shallow non-irritant footbaths containing 10% zinc sulphate solution (followed by a period on concrete to allow the chemicals to dry) helps to maintain strong disease-free hooves. The likelihood of wet and damaged pastures precipitating foot problems is particularly high in areas of high rainfall, and strong consideration should be given to housing animals indoors over winter in such locations.

If access to the outside is intended to be for exercise only on a daily basis, and space is limited, a concrete floored yard may be better than a pasture. These are washable, will help to stop hooves becoming overgrown and will not retain a significant worm burden. Pasture is of course preferable but needs more work and a bigger area to keep a given number of animals healthy and contented. Further information on foot care can be found in Winter (2004), and advice on treating interdigital dermatitis and footrot (*Dichelobacter nodosus*) infections in Green and Clifton (2018).

Shearing and fleece care

Sheep are normally shorn annually in the late spring. Animals with surgical preparations, such as rumen fistulae, cranial implants or blood vessel loops, should be shorn separately from the main flock and with great care. Policies of regular control measures should be put in place to control or prevent skin parasites, especially sheep scab (caused by a *Psoroptes* mange mite), and blowfly larvae (maggots) which are prevalent during the summer. As with worming and foot care, animals under experiment or permanently housed indoors should not be excluded from routine skincare treatments. Housed sheep and goats are particularly susceptible to infestations by lice.

Ageing and normal life span

A normal life span is around 10–12 years for sheep and 12–15 for goats. Key determinants for retaining sheep and goats in commercial flocks are fertility, udder quality, condition of the feet and lost or worn teeth. Breeding stock are examined annually before the mating season and these defects may be criteria for culling. Research animals often have value other than as breeding stock and may be retained into old age. However, issues such as chronically bad hoof conformation and poor digestion owing to loss of teeth should still be regularly monitored, and avoided through good foot care and careful nutrition, respectively. Other age-related welfare problems include scrapie, arthritis and ovine pulmonary adenocarcinoma (Jaagsiekte) in sheep and caprine arthritis/encephalitis in goats. Dolly the sheep lived for less than 7 years, having developed both Jaagsiekte and arthritis.

Special health problems

Occasionally, sheep and goats will present with veterinary problems with a rapid onset that are immediately life-threatening or very serious.

1. Rumenal bloat. A grossly dilated abdomen is seen, accompanied by rapid shallow breathing and eventual collapse.
2. Urolithiasis. This is particularly common in young male kids and rams. A rigid stance and inability to urinate freely are characteristic. Sometimes, urine can escape in small quantities which stains the coat around the penile sheath. Excessive straining may cause a rectal prolapse and if this is seen in a male animal, urolithiasis should always be suspected.
3. Poisoning or metabolic disorders caused by ion imbalance. These diseases may be difficult to distinguish. Signs including hyperexcitability or deep depression, tremors and convulsions may all be seen in one or more individuals.
4. Diseases caused by clostridial organisms. Very high rectal temperatures (42 °C or more) and rapid deterioration in condition are seen, leading to recumbency and death.
5. Obstetrical problems.
6. Acute mastitis. Signs are a discoloured udder, thin, blood-coloured milk, high temperature and a very sick animal.
7. Pregnancy toxaemia. Poor energy balance in late pregnancy can lead rapidly to neurological signs and collapse.
8. Acute pneumonia. Often occurs following stress, with *Mannheimia* (formerly, *Pasteurella*) species predominating. Animals have a high temperature and severe respiratory distress. This can be confused with heat stress following transport in a poorly ventilated vehicle.

Extreme clinical signs of these types should be recognisable to technicians and help sought immediately.

Conclusions

In general, sheep and goats are adaptable, resilient and resourceful species which, when handled well from an early age, can readily cope with a laboratory environment. A thorough understanding of sheep and goat behaviour is essential to provide these animals with an optimal environment, and to ensure that behavioural needs for social companionship, environmental complexity and varied foraging opportunities are met. Both species form close social bonds, firstly with their mothers, and thereafter with peers and maintaining some social contact is important for their well-being. Although animals that are rarely handled, or only managed with fear-inducing stimuli to encourage flight, can be fearful and panic when confronted with novelty or social isolation, both species have a significant capacity to learn about places, objects and people. Training animals to cooperate with experimental requirements and novel environments, for example through the use of food or other positive stimuli, can be rewarding and will reduce stress for both animals and handlers alike, as well as providing better quality data.

Acknowledgement

This chapter has been revised and updated from the 8th edition chapter of the same name by Colin Gilbert and Keith Kendrick. The authors would like to thank Drs Pete Goddard, Lindsay Hamilton and Jane Robinson for their helpful comments and amendments to the text.

References

Aitken, I.D. (2007) *Diseases of Sheep*. Blackwell Publishing, Oxford.

Baldwin, B.A. (1979) Operant studies on shape discrimination in goats. *Physiology and Behaviour*, **23**, 455–459.

Baldwin, B.A. (1981) Shape discrimination in sheep and calves. *Animal Behaviour*, **29**, 830–834.

Baldwin, B.A. and Meese, G.B. (1977) The ability of sheep to distinguish between conspecifics by means of olfaction. *Physiology and Behaviour*, **18**, 803–808.

Bellegarde, L., Haskell, M.J., Duvaux-Ponter, C., Weiss, A., Boissy, A. and Erhard, H. (2017) Face-based perception of emotions in dairy goats. *Applied Animal Behaviour Science* **193**, 51–59. https://doi.org/10.1016/j.applanim.2017.03.014

Briefer, E.F., de la Torre, M.P. and McElligott, A.G. (2012) Mother goats do not forget their kids' calls. *Proceedings of the Royal Society B-Biological Sciences*, **279**, 3749–3755.

Council of Europe (2006) Multilateral Consultation of Parties to the European Convention for the Protection of Vertebrate Animals used for Experimental and other Scientific Purposes (ETS 123) Appendix A. *Cons 123 (2006)* 3. https://www.coe.int/t/e/legal_affairs/legal_co-operation/biological_safety_and_use_of_animals/Laboratory_animals/Revision%20of%20Appendix%20A.asp (accessed 19 June 2019).

Da Costa, A.P., Leigh, A.E., Man, M-S. et al. (2004) Face pictures reduce behavioural, autonomic, endocrine and neural indices of stress and fear in sheep. *Proceedings of the Royal Society Biology B*, **271**, 2077–2084.

Dwyer, C.M. (2004) How has the risk of predation shaped the behavioural responses of sheep to fear and distress? *Animal Welfare*, **13**, 269–281.

Dwyer, C.M. and Lawrence, A.B. (1998) Variability in the in expression of maternal behaviour in primiparous sheep: effects of genotype and litter size. *Applied Animal Behaviour Science*, **58**, 311–330.

Dwyer, C.M. and Lawrence, A.B. (1999) Ewe–ewe and ewe–lamb behaviour in a hill and a lowland breed of sheep: A study using embryo transfer. *Applied Animal Behaviour Science*, **61**, 319–334.

Dwyer, C.M. and Lawrence, A.B. (2000) Effects of maternal genotype and behaviour on the behavioural development of their offspring in sheep. *Behaviour*, **137**, 1629–1654.

Dwyer, C.M. and Lawrence, A.B. (2005) A review of the behavioural and physiological adaptations of extensively managed breeds of sheep that favour lamb survival. *Applied Animal Behaviour Science*, **92**, 235–260.

Eales, A. and Small, J. (2004) *Practical Lambing – A Guide to Veterinary Care at Lambing*. Blackwell Publishing, Oxford.

Elliker, K. (2006) *Recognition of Emotion in Sheep*. PhD Thesis, University of Cambridge.

Evans, G. and Maxwell, W.M.C. (1988) *Salamon's Artificial Insemination of Sheep and Goats*. Butterworth, Sydney.

Fabre-Nys, C., Blache, D. and Lavenet, C. (1991) A method for accurate implantation in the sheep brain. In: *Neuroendocrine Research Methods: Implantation and Transfection Procedures*. Ed. Greenstein, B., pp. 295–314. Harwood, Chur.

Fabre-Nys, C. and Venier, G. (1987) Development and use of a method for quantifying female sexual behaviour through the breeding season in two breeds of sheep. *Animal Reproduction Science*, **21**, 37–51.

Færevik, G., Andersen, I.L. and Bøe, K.E. (2005) Preferences of sheep for different types of pen flooring. *Applied Animal Behaviour Science*, **90**, 265–276.

Flecknell, P.A. (2009) *Laboratory Animal Anaesthesia*, 3rd edn. Academic Press, London.

Fthenakis, G.C., Arsenos, G., Brozos, C. et al. (2012) Health management of ewes during pregnancy. *Animal Reproduction Science*, **130**, 198–212.

Gascoigne, E., Morgan, E.R., Lovatt, F. and Vineer, H.R. (2018) Controlling nematode infections in sheep: application of HACCP. *In Practice* **40**, 334–347.

Goddard, P.J., Gaskin, G.J. and Macdonald, A.J., (1988) Automatic blood sampling equipment for use in studies of animal physiology. *Animal Science*, **66**, 769–775.

Green, L. and Clifton, R. (2018) Diagnosing and managing footrot in sheep: an update. *In Practice* **40**, 17–26.

Harrison, F. (1995) *Surgical Techniques in Experimental Farm Animals*. Oxford University Press, Oxford.

Henderson, D.C. (1990) *The Veterinary Book for Sheep Farmers*. Old Pond Publishing, Ipswich.

Heffner, H.E. and Heffner, R.S. (1992) Auditory perception. In: *Farm Animals and the Environment*. Eds Phillips, C. and Piggins, D., pp. 159–184. CAB International, Wallingford.

Hindson, J. (1989) Examinations of the sheep flock before tupping. *In Practice*, **11**, 149–155.

Holmes, R.J. (1991) Sheep. In: *Practical Animal Handling*. Eds Anderson, R.S. and Edney, A.T.B., pp. 39–49. Pergamon Press, Oxford.

Humane Slaughter Association (2006) *Captive-bolt Stunning of Livestock*, 4th edn. Humane Slaughter Association, Wheathampstead.

Joint Working Group on Refinement (1993) Removal of blood from laboratory mammals and birds. First Report of the BVA/FRAME/RSPCA/UFAW Joint Working Group on Refinement. *Laboratory Animals*, **27**, 1–22.

Kendrick, K.M. (1991) Microdialysis in large unrestrained animals: neuroendocrine and behavioural studies of acetylcholine, amino acid, monoamine and neuropeptide release in the sheep. In: *Microdialysis in the Neurosciences*. Eds Robinson, T.E. and Justice, J.B., Jr., pp. 327–348. Elsevier, Amsterdam.

Kendrick, K.M. (1992) Cognition. In: *Farm Animals and the Environment*. Eds Phillips, C. and Piggins, D., pp. 209–234. CAB International, Wallingford.

Kendrick, K.M. (1994) Neurobiological correlates of visual and olfactory recognition in sheep. *Behavioural Processes*, **33**, 89–112.

Kendrick, K.M. (2004) Faces in the flock: implications for understanding animal minds. *New Scientist*, **182**, 48–49.

Kendrick, K.M., Atkins, K., Hinton, M.R. et al. (1995) Facial and vocal discrimination in sheep. *Animal Behaviour*, **49**, 1665–1676.

Kendrick, K.M., Atkins, K., Hinton, M.R. et al. (1996) Are faces special for sheep? Evidence from facial and object discrimination learning tests showing effects of inversion and social familiarity. *Behavioural Processes*, **38**, 19–35.

Kendrick, K.M. and Baldwin, B.A. (1991) Single-unit recording in conscious sheep. In: *Methods in Neurosciences: Electrophysiology and Microinjection*, Vol 4. Ed. Conn, P.M., pp. 3–14. Academic Press, San Diego.

Kendrick, K.M., Da Costa, A.P., Hinton, M.R. et al. (2001) Sheep don't forget a face. *Nature*, **414**, 165–166.

Kendrick, K.M., Hinton, M.R., Atkins, K. et al. (1998) Mothers make sexual preferences. *Nature*, **395**, 229–230.

Lickliter, R.E. (1984) Mother-infant spatial relationships in goats. *Applied Animal Behaviour Science*, **13**, 93–100.

Lynch, J.J., Hinch, G.N. and Adams, D.B. (1992) *The Behaviour of Sheep: Biological Principles and Implications for Production*. Melbourne: CSIRO.

Mews, A.R. and Mowlem, A. (1991) Goats. In: *Practical Animal Handling*. Eds Anderson, R.S. and Edney, A.T.B., pp. 51–55. Pergamon Press, Oxford.

Morand-Fehr, P. (2005) Recent developments in goat nutrition and application: a review. *Small Ruminant Research*, **60**, 25–43.

Nawroth, C., von Borell, E. and Langbein, J. (2014) Exclusion Performance in Dwarf Goats (*Capra aegagrus hircus*) and Sheep (*Ovis orientalis aries*). *PLoS One*, **9**, e93534.

Nawroth, C., von Borell, E. and Langbein, J. (2015) Object permanence in the dwarf goat (*Capra aegagrus hircus*): Perseveration errors and the tracking of complex movements of hidden objects. *Applied Animal Behaviour Science*, **167**, 20–26.

Nawroth, C., Albuquerque, N., Savalli, C. et al. (2018) Goats prefer positive human emotional facial expressions. *Royal Society Open Science*, **5**, article 180491.

Nowak, R., Poindron, P. and Putu, I.G. (1989) Development of mother discrimination by single and multiple newborn lambs. *Developmental Psychobiology*, **22**, 833–845.

Nowak, R. and Boivin, X. (2015) Filial attachment in sheep: similarities and differences between ewe–lamb and human–lamb relationships. *Applied Animal Behaviour Science*, **164**, 12–28.

Peirce, J.W., Leigh, A.E. and Kendrick, K.M. (2000) Configurational coding, familiarity and the right hemisphere advantage for face recognition in sheep. *Neuropsychologia*, **38**, 475–483.

Penning, P.D., Parsons, A.J., Newman, J.A. et al. (1993) The effects of group size on grazing time in sheep. *Applied Animal Behaviour Science*, **37**, 101–109.

Perentos, N., Martins, A.Q., Watson, T.C. *et al.* (2015) Translational neurophysiology in sheep: measuring sleep and neurological dysfunction in CLN% Batten disease affected sheep. *Brain*, **138**, 862–874.

Piggins, D. (1992) Visual perception. In: *Farm Animals and the Environment*. Eds Phillips, C. and Piggins, D., pp. 131–158. CAB International, Wallingford.

Pitcher, B.J., Briefer, E.F., Baciadonna, L. and McElligott, A.G. (2017) Cross-modal recognition of familiar conspecifics in goats. *Royal Society Open Science* 4, article 160346.

Seldinger, S.I. (1953) Catheter replacement of the needle in percutaneous arteriography. *Acta Radiologica*, **39**, 368–376.

Sheep Veterinary Society (1994) *The Casualty Sheep*. British Veterinary Association Animal Welfare Foundation, Swindon Press, Swindon.

Shillito, E. and Alexander, G. (1975) Mutual recognition amongst ewes and lambs of four breeds of sheep (*Ovis aries*). *Applied Animal Ethology*, **1**, 151–165.

Sinclair, K.D., Rutherford, K.M.D., Wallace, J.M. *et al.* (2016) Epigenetics and developmental programming of welfare and production traits in farm animals. *Reproduction, Fertility and Development*, **28**, 1443–1478.

Tate, A.J., Fischer, H., Leigh, A.E. *et al.* (2006) Behavioural and neurophysiological evidence for face identity and face emotion processing in animals. *Philosophical Transactions of the Royal Society London B-Biological Sciences*, **361**, 2155–2172.

Vandenheede, M. and Bouissou, M.F. (1993) Sex differences in fear reactions in sheep. *Applied Animal Behaviour Science*, **37**, 39–55.

Wolfensohn, S. and Lloyd, M. (2013) *Handbook of Laboratory Animal Management and Welfare*. 4th Edition, Blackwell Publishing, Oxford.

Winter, A.C. (2004) *Lameness in Sheep*. The Crowood Press, Marlborough.

Winter, A.C. and Hill, C.W. (2003) *A Manual of Lambing Techniques*. The Crowood Press, Marlborough.

Wyse, C.A., Zhang, X., McLaughlin, M. *et al.* (2018) Circadian rhythms of melatonin and behaviour in juvenile sheep in field conditions: Effects of photoperiod, environment and weaning. *Physiology & Behavior*, **194**, 362–370.

35 The Horse

Updated by Heather Ewence and Fleur Whitlock

Biological Overview

Introduction

The horse was domesticated around 2500 BC. Its relatively compliant behaviour, together with its speed, agility and strength, gave it a unique role among domesticated animals. Because it could be trained to harness or saddle, the horse provided humans with a means of transport and traction for work, war or recreation.

With the increasing use of the internal combustion engine in the early part of the twentieth century, the number of horses declined and with it, equine research. However, over the past 50 years, horse numbers have steadily increased because of the renewed interest in using horses for recreational purposes. The equine industry contributes to economies worldwide and continues to expand. This growing commerce has led to greater equine research into diverse areas such as nutrition, reproduction, sports injuries, infectious diseases, biosecurity and welfare. Although the ultimate beneficiary of this research is the horse, horses are also used in research for human benefit including the production of hyperimmune antiserum and also for the production of conjugated oestrogens for use in human medicine. There are numerous resources on equine husbandry and management, but the majority of these are centred on the use of horses as a ridden animal. There are limited resources to learn more about horses use in research.

Social organisation

Horses are herd animals and in the feral state live in small family groups, which historically were thought to have a clearly defined hierarchy. Ongoing work in this sector has shown that the dominant rank or pecking order that was initially observed and based on domestic fowl (Schjelderup-Ebbe 1922) has not been clearly substantiated in horses (ISES 2019). In natural conditions, established equine groups tend to consist of a stallion, several mares and their offspring (Keiper 1986). It has been proposed that within social groups of horses, hierarchy within a group can be influenced by weight, height or sex, but studies provide conflicting results (Houpt *et al.* 1978; Van Dierendonck *et al.* 1994; Giles *et al.* 2015). The one factor that has been positively validated is that age is correlated with rank, and it was suggested that this finding may be related to the older animals being more resourceful (Keiper & Receveur 1992). See Figure 35.1 for an example of a herd of ponies.

Biological data

Normal biological values are summarised in Table 35.1. The first, second and third permanent incisors erupt at 2.5, 3.5 and 4.5 years, respectively. All permanent teeth (incisors, premolar and molars) are present by 4.5 years (Muylle 2005). A horse's height is traditionally measured in hands, one hand being equal to 4 inches (1 inch = 2.54 cm). The measurement is taken from the ground level to the highest point on the horse's withers (Kleijn & Sloet van Oldruitenborgh-Oosterbaan 2009). Horses range in height from about 60 cm (6 hands) to more than 173 cm (>17 hands). They very often remain fit and active into their twenties, and some will live in excess of 30 years.

Because of the stay apparatus of the hindlimbs, adult horses can rest and sleep while standing, but rapid eye movement (REM) sleep can only occur when the horse is in sternal or lateral recumbency (Bertone 2015). The time spent in this stage is less than in humans; horses seem to spend only 15% (about 30 min/day) of their total sleep time in REM sleep (Aleman *et al.* 2008). Lateral recumbency is commonly adopted, but sternal recumbency has also been observed. They enjoy rolling, especially in mud and dust, and stabled horses will frequently roll in their beds if still warm and sweaty from exercise.

Horses change their coat twice yearly in the spring and autumn (Figure 35.2). The winter coat usually provides

---

The UFAW Handbook on the Care and Management of Laboratory and Other Research Animals, Ninth Edition.
Edited by Huw Golledge and Claire Richardson.
© 2024 John Wiley & Sons Ltd. Published 2024 by John Wiley & Sons Ltd.

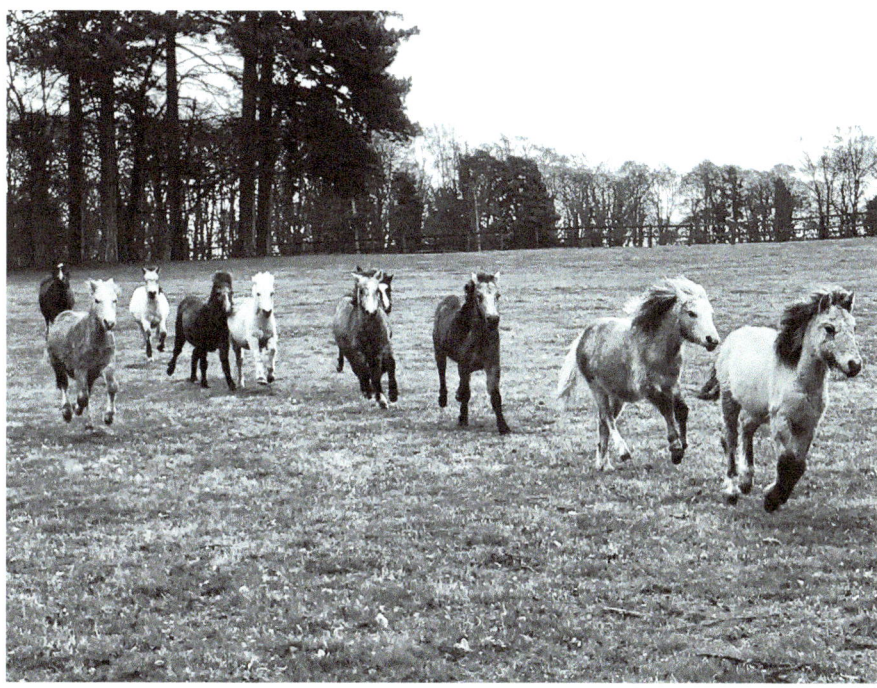

Figure 35.1 A herd of ponies.

Table 35.1 Normal biological values for horses.

Parameter	Value
Rectal temperature (°C)	38 ± 0.5
Resting pulse (beats/min)	25–45
Respiratory rate (breaths/min)	8–12
Permanent teeth	$I^3_3 \, C^{*1}_1 \, P^{3or4\dagger}_3 \, M^3_3$
Deciduous teeth	$I^3_3 \, C^0_0 \, P^3_3 \, M^0_0$

*Rare or rudimentary in mares.
†First premolar (wolf tooth) is vestige and remnant of a tooth well developed in ancestors of the horse. Often shed, but if retained and thought to be associated with biting problems, it is usually removed by a veterinarian.

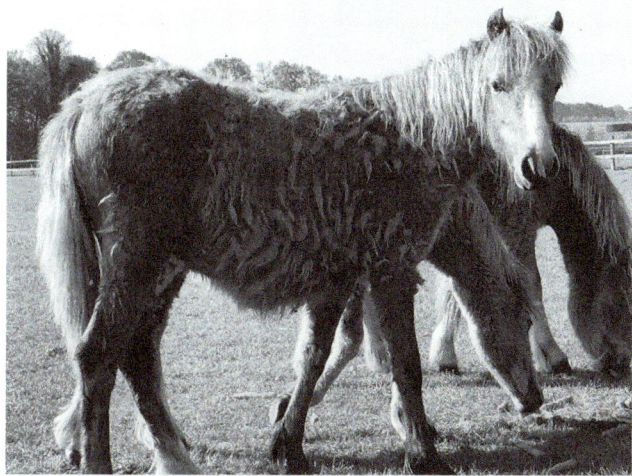

Figure 35.2 An example of shedding of a winter coat in a yearling.

sufficient protection from inclement weather for most native breed horses not in work in northern temperate areas, though field shelters or wind breaks should be available. If living out, the winter coat should not be groomed as this would remove secretions, which assist in keeping the animal warm and dry (DEFRA 2018). In more extreme climates, horses are usually housed during the winter months, for example, a less hardy breed, an older horse or a mare due to foal, though they can be turned out, suitably rugged if required, into paddocks every day during the winter months. A full winter coat may also result in excessive sweating during ridden work, and therefore, it is customary to clip the winter coat off and rug the horse, if the horse is a ridden animal.

Reproduction

Mares first show signs of oestrus at puberty (about 18–24 months of age) and continue to cycle until 20–30 years old. The majority (80%) of mares are seasonally polyoestrous with regular cycles during the breeding season (spring–summer) and a period of sexual quiescence in the winter months. Daylight length (photoperiod) is the most important regulating factor, increasing daylight length in the spring in temperate regions being the main stimulus for the initiation of ovarian activity. However, even at the equator, where day length is approximately 12 h throughout the year, mares show a definite seasonal pattern to oestrus. Good nutrition and housing to protect mares from harsh weather conditions will increase the likelihood that they cycle and ovulate normally at the beginning of the breeding season (van Niekerk 1992). The breeding season, under natural conditions, for example, in pony herds, is usually later than that artificially imposed on Thoroughbreds, where 1 January in the Northern Hemisphere, or 1 August in the Southern Hemisphere, is the official birthday of all Thoroughbred racehorses. The exact dates enable standardisation within the industry, and the concept of producing foals as near as possible to these dates is aimed for thus ensuring equal eligibility in age-graded racing, for example, a two-year-old horse born in the earlier part of the year will tend to be more mature than one born later.

Spermatogenesis starts during the second year of life in colts receiving adequate nutrition, and the testes are usually functional by 2 years of age. Colts of less than 2 years of age have lower sperm production rates than older stallions, and rates in the non-breeding season are about 75% of that in the breeding season (Thompson 1992).

Behaviour

Normal behaviour

Healthy equids are active and alert. When stabled, they commonly nicker or whinny to their attendant, particularly at feeding time. They are usually keen to eat, and some will paw or kick at the stable door whilst waiting to be fed. Some horses will also weave (see Abnormal behaviour section) whilst waiting for feed.

Horses urinate about six times daily and defecate approximately every 2 h. Attendants should check faecal consistency and quantity automatically as they clean the stable, as any changes from the normal pattern could be indicative of illness. They should also note the state of the bedding: evidence of excess activity could indicate distress, for example, due to colic (signs indicative of abdominal pain, see Common diseases section). Alternatively, the bed may be relatively undisturbed, indicating that the horse had not lain down in sternal or lateral recumbency to rest.

When at pasture, horses usually graze as a group and an animal separated from the group may be unwell. When resting, at least one number of the group often remains standing whilst the remainder rest in sternal or, if warm and sunny, in lateral recumbency (Figure 35.3). Before getting up, horses frequently roll. Once up, they will often stretch and shake themselves before moving off to start grazing. When in groups at pasture, the affiliations between pairs of horses will become obvious, as they usually graze together and mutually groom. Attendants should be aware of these relationships so that they are allowed to continue during the winter housing period: accidental splitting up of these affiliations can be stressful and so should be avoided.

Social facilitation (same, or similar, behaviour initiated as a response to the occurrence of an action by another animal within the social group) is common both within and between groups, and the pattern of behaviour involved includes resting, grazing, walking, rolling, eliminative behaviour (defecation and urination) and sucking. Mutual grooming (Figure 35.4), although potentially a response to the irritation caused by ectoparasites (see Common diseases section) or coat shedding, is also an important form of social contact (Tyler 1972; Crowell-Davis 1986). It has been proposed by Hogan et al. (1988) that increased social grooming may be significant in helping individuals reduce stress levels naturally.

It is thought that play in young animals may contribute to individuals developing skills that are needed in maturity and helps promote well-being (Figure 35.5). Traditionally, play was thought to be a reliable indicator of good welfare (Mills & Nankervis 1999; Goodwin & Hughes 2005), but later studies found that the demonstration of play could also be associated with chronic stress and that adult horse play was not a reliable welfare indicator (Hausberger et al. 2012). Social play behaviour patterns appear to be expressed mainly during the juvenile phase of development (Byers 1998). The opportunity for animals to socialise in a herd and have freedom of movement provide a chance for them to initiate play behaviours, which include play fighting, neck wrestling, mounting, rearing and chasing (Goodwin et al. 2002). Environmental factors can influence play, for example, hot

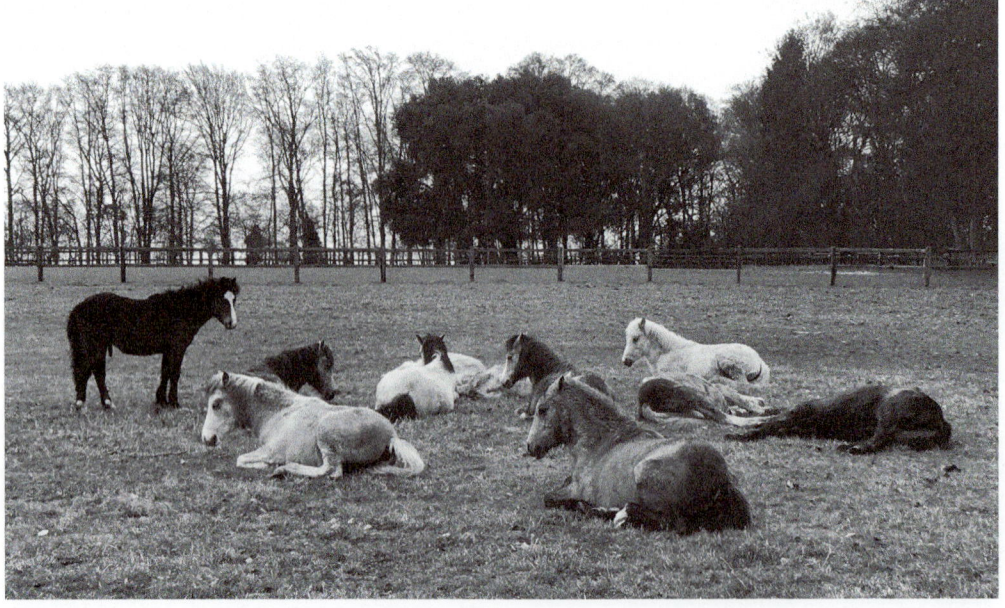

Figure 35.3 A resting herd.

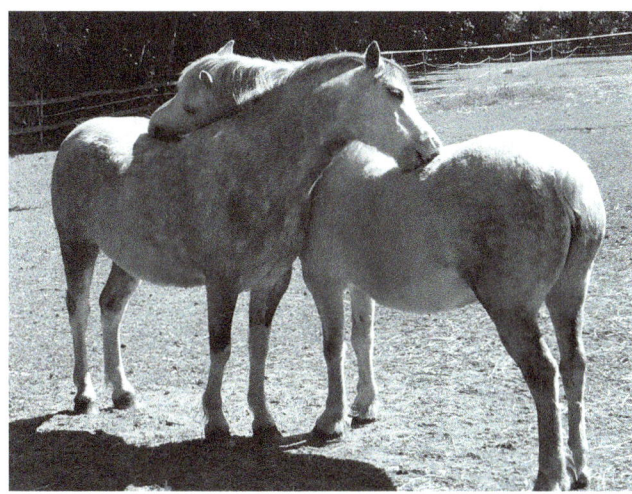

Figure 35.4 Mutual grooming.

at feeding times, subordinate horses may be denied access to food (Houpt 1991).

Abnormal behaviour including stereotypies

Ideally, management systems for equines should accommodate their freedom to express natural behaviour, in particular the need to graze, exercise and socialise. They are flight animals and, hence, easily startled, and this should also be taken into account (Council Directive 2010/63/EU 2010). One of the most effective management strategies for reducing abnormal behaviour is to increase turnout time as restricted access to natural foraging behaviour can impact welfare. Stereotypies are repetitive abnormal behaviours. McGreevy Cripps *et al.* (1995) found that horses that were kept stabled for a large percentage of a 24-h period had the highest occurrence of stereotypic behaviours. Endorphins are released from the central nervous system during stereotypic behaviour, possibly encouraging the horse to persist in the behaviour.

Weaving/box (stall) walking

Weaving describes behaviour where the horse sways from side to side on its forelimbs. Box or stall walking is expressed by the animal where it endlessly walks round its box. Both are typical examples of behavioural stereotypies. They are usually the consequence of the stress or thwarted motivation for locomotory behaviour, experienced by an open-country animal being kept isolated in a restricted area such as a stall or loose box (Houpt 1992). Amelioration can be achieved by providing the horse with sufficient windows or openings to enable it to see its companions and its immediate environment at all times. Placing mirrors in the stables of weavers significantly reduces this abnormal behaviour. The mirror is believed to mimic visual contact providing environmental distraction (McAfee *et al.* 2002).

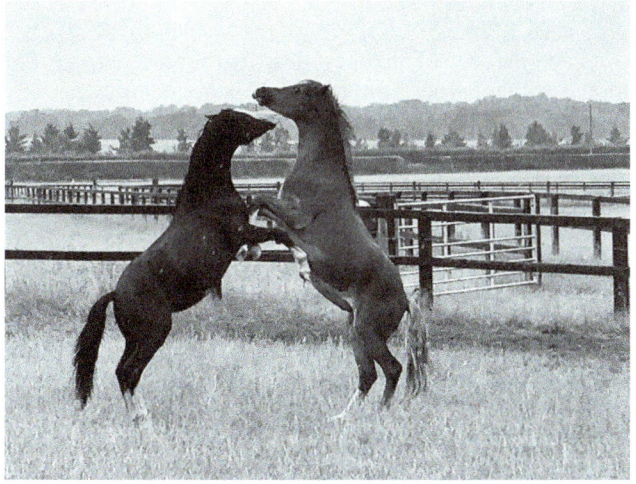

Figure 35.5 Play behaviours being demonstrated by yearlings in the field.

Biting and kicking

Biting and kicking, or threatening to do so, are the horse's main ways of showing aggression. Normally, this is reserved for other horses, especially at feeding time or to newcomers to a group. It is important to note that horses use kicking as a defensive mechanism and can be an instinctive response if they feel threatened. Horses are known to have about a wide lateral range of vision with small areas of blind spots in front of their nose and just behind their tails (Hanggi & Ingersol 2012). Unless a horse is startled, they can accommodate by moving their head to gain a better perspective. A quiet manner while using your voice to let them know you are approaching them, where possible, diagonally at their shoulder will avoid startling them. With time, patience, experienced handling and expert advice, most horses can be trained to trust their handlers.

Wood chewing

Low-roughage diets in horses can encourage wood chewing; this can be rectified by providing more hay in the diet, but it may also be necessary to apply a bitter wood treatment as a

climates diminish the inclination to instigate play and windy conditions reduce play as horses' awareness of potential dangers is reduced and the demand for seeking shelter is more important.

The individually stabled horse can be denied these social interactions, and this may contribute to the development of abnormal behaviours such as box walking, weaving, crib-biting and wind-sucking. However, there are various enrichments that can be provided to horses, for example, daily grooming by knowledgeable and sympathetic stable attendants may provide some compensation to horses for the reduced social interaction with their own species, but are not complete substitutes.

When kept at pasture or housed in groups, the group size is often larger than in a typical horse herd and is not a family group, but consists of horses introduced as adults. This results in social reorganisation and, on occasion, in fighting when the groups are first formed or when they are crowded together. Injuries are likely if there is no room to escape, and deterrent to chewed areas to discourage further wood chewing in the short term.

Crib-biting/wind-sucking

Crib-biting and wind-sucking are common oral stereotypic behaviours, and both are perceived as detrimental to the horses' health.

Crib-biting is an oral stereotypy, where a fixed object is grasped with the incisors, and the lower neck muscles contract to retract the larynx caudally; air is drawn into the cranial oesophagus, which produces the characteristic grunt (Nicol et al. 2002). There is a view that this type of behaviour could be harmful (McGreevy, Cripps et al. 1995). In wind-sucking, the same posture and grunt are adopted but without grasping a fixed object. The exact causes behind these two stereotypies remain unclear. Heritability, management, feeding practices, social contact, crowding and many more have all been suggested as being responsible for their development or have been shown to increase the risk of them happening. A permanent cure is yet to be found, and attempts to prevent it occurring have included surgery, acupuncture, environmental enrichment and others (McGreevy & Nicol 1998).

Recognition of pain and distress

Early detection of poor welfare in the form of pain and/or distress is essential to minimise the possibility of excessive suffering in horses used for research. Welfare should be routinely monitored, typically using score sheets which record several parameters including basic measures such as bodyweight and behaviour as well as specific indicators of pain and distress. For experimental procedures, humane end points should be established prior to the study to allow timely intervention (treatment of excessive suffering or euthanasia if it cannot be treated) if levels of suffering exceed these pre-defined levels.

Being prey animals, signs of pain and distress can be very subtle in horses (de Grauw & van Loon 2016). Depending on the cause of the pain or discomfort, signs may be specific such as limping due to lameness or rolling due to colic. However, signs may be less obvious and non-specific such as hanging back from the rest of the group, mild lethargy or 'sham' eating (where an animal pretends to eat but actually is not). Knowledge of individual horse's behaviours in the herd will assist in accurate and fast recognition of abnormalities. Any concerns should trigger further investigations, including a physical examination. Recognition of pain and distress is paramount to ensure optimal welfare. If a horse demonstrates undue suffering that is unresponsive to medical intervention or carries a hopeless prognosis, a good case stands for euthanasia of the horse. Constant, objective assessments are ethically necessary to guarantee animal welfare.

Welfare scales can be a useful way of assessing and monitoring the severity of pain. van Loon and Van Dierendonck (2018) have reviewed the utility of several pain scales including, singular, composite and facial-expression-based scales in horses. More generally, Dalla Costa et al. (2016) describe the development and implementation of the AWIN (Animal Welfare Indicators) protocol in horses. The AWIN is a multi-factor assessment protocol designed for horses on-farm, which may also be useful for the assessment of horse welfare in a research setting.

For further information on the general principles of welfare assessment, see also Chapter 6 – Brief introduction to welfare assessment: A toolbox of techniques.

Uses of horses in research

When used as research subjects, the Replacement, Reduction and Refinement (3Rs), in particular reduction and refinement, should be applied wherever possible (see Chapter 2), ensuring that the minimum number of animals is used and that their welfare is maximised by treating horses in the most humane way compatible with achieving the aims of the research. Equine care and welfare should also be based on the 'Five Freedoms' or 'Five Domains' that will ensure that both the mental and physical needs of the horse are met (see Figure 35.6).

Whilst the Five Freedoms describe a basic concept of animal welfare where the emphasis is largely on ensuring that animals are free from negative welfare, the newer concept of the five domains (Mellor 2017) describes four functional domains: nutrition, environment, health and behaviour that contribute to the fifth domain of mental state. The five domains model makes it clearer that positive experiences as well as the absence of negative experiences are a key component of good welfare, emphasising the necessity of giving horses opportunities to have such positive experiences whilst also minimising pain, suffering or distress.

The majority of equids used in research are acquired from outside sources. However, there is occasionally a need to breed them within an institute, for example, when parasite-free foals and weanlings, or horses with a specific blood type are required. Sound, ex-racehorses (Thoroughbreds) are a good source of animals for use in exercise physiology

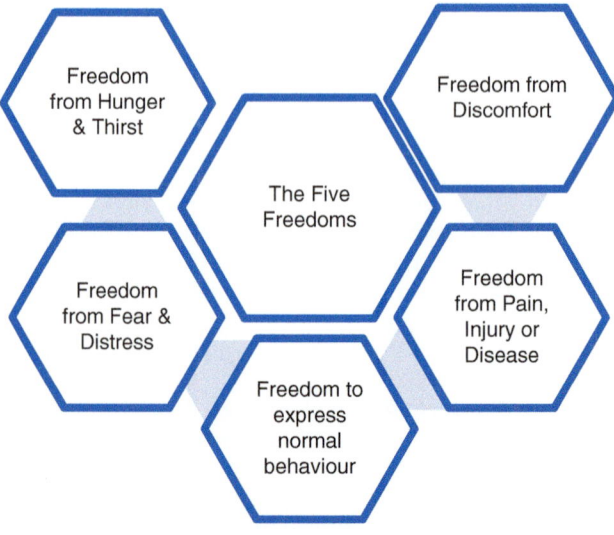

Figure 35.6 The Five Freedoms.

research, as they are adjusted to stable routines and training procedures. Having been handled frequently since the early stages of life, they are usually amenable to most minimally invasive procedures such as the collection of blood samples.

Horses are frequently used in behavioural studies, in reproductive physiology, pharmaceutical, infectious diseases and nutritional research. The Welsh Mountain pony is a well-established breed used in research. These ponies are small, hardy and overall have a very good and easy temperament, adapting quickly to new routines and procedures. If they can be sourced from their natural habitat at a young age, it can be hoped that they will typically be naïve to equine influenza and strangles (*Streptococcus equi*). This is due to their isolation from fully domesticated horses that are exposed to endemic infections within the general population. When testing to confirm their prior infectious disease exposures, at six months of age, any maternally derived antibody should have waned, so if antibodies were present in a serological blood sample, this would most likely be secondary to natural infection.

Horses are normally obtained directly from breeders or dealers; they may have had minimal exposure to humans and will require a quarantine and an acclimatisation period. This includes regular handling and training to ensure that they accept being restrained during common procedures and routine husbandry measures such as farriery and worming.

Blood and serum production horses are usually former recreational horses, which may not be able to work at the level expected of them because of an irreversible injury such as a tendon strain or joint damage. They should, however, be healthy and capable of light exercise without discomfort.

When working with equids in research, good clinical practice (GCP) should be encouraged alongside the rigorous application of the 3Rs, ensuring that the highest quality data are obtained from each animal. GCP is a concept that was initiated in 1996 by a scheme based on the principles of the International Cooperation on Harmonisation of Technical Requirements for Registration of Veterinary Medicinal Products. The program is aimed at unifying standards internationally in the design and management of clinical studies that are carried out involving veterinary products in the target species (European Medicines Agency 2016). It enables the study animals to be safeguarded and standard methods to be put into place to ensure that reliable data are captured and produced.

Reuse or Rehoming

At the end of a study period, there will be a process where either a request is made for reusing an animal in a newly proposed study or a horse may be rehomed or euthanised. All options should undergo a review, whereby each individual animal is discussed by an Animal Welfare and Ethical Review Body.

In the UK, guidance states that an animal may only be rehomed if '. . . it is in the best interests of the welfare of the individual animal and when it poses no danger to public or animal health, or to the environment' (Home Office 2015). Permission from the Home Office must be obtained before a horse is rehomed after being used in a scientific procedure.

New owners are often identified through existing networks with the suitability of the prospective new owner assessed when they visit to view the animals.

During the visit, the following areas should ideally be discussed and assessed:

- Level of experience and detail of any previous equine ownership
- The suitability of the animal, age, temperament, behaviour, training record and health record
- How the animal will be transported to its new home
- Socialisation program, e.g. access to other ponies or animals as companions
- The suitability of the new home – the facilities for the short term (e.g. small area until the pony is familiar with new people and surroundings) and for the longer term (availability of grazing/turn out, quality of paddocks, fencing and shelter)
- How will veterinary cover be met

A home visit/assessment will be arranged if deemed necessary.

The new owner is made fully aware of their responsibility for the animal's health and well-being. They are also made aware of their legal responsibility to change ownership details on the passport, of which evidence will be required. Once satisfied that the person is suitable, the animal should undergo a health check by a veterinary surgeon to certify its good health status at the time of the rehoming and a collection date organised. Contact with the new owner should be considered approximately 4 weeks after the animal's departure for an update on its progress. Ordinarily animals with medical conditions, abnormal conformation, handling or behavioural issues should not be considered for rehoming.

In the UK, an animal that has been used for scientific procedures must not be subject to reuse in further procedures unless the study classification is within mild to moderate limits (as documented in the project licence). Typically, animals that have already been subject to severe procedures should not be reused (Home Office 2014b). A veterinary surgeon with in-depth knowledge of the animal needs to have confirmed, by examination, that the health and well-being has been restored sufficiently following previous procedures. Most establishments recommend at least a 6-week period of rest prior to reuse. Whilst determining the actual severity classification, it is imperative to focus on the impact of the procedures that have been carried out on each animal. Each of the methods used will have had an impact that can vary between individual animals. In the UK and European legislation, there are three levels of severity that are recognised: mild, moderate and severe. Mild procedures are those whereby any pain or suffering experienced is only slight or momentary and the animal returns to its normal state of health quickly. Moderate procedures are those likely to cause short-term moderate pain, suffering or distress or long-lasting mild pain, suffering or distress as well as procedures that are likely to cause moderate impairment of the well-being or general condition of the animals. Such procedures can have a significant impact on the animal and have the potential to produce signs of discomfort, weight loss and uncharacteristic behaviours, but tend not to affect appetite or thirst. A severe classification is fairly uncommon; this is where an animal is likely to experience severe pain, suffering or distress or long-lasting moderate pain, suffering or distress, as well as procedures that are likely to cause severe impairment of the well-being or general condition of the animals.

Husbandry of the horse

Housing

Traditionally, the horse has been housed individually in loose boxes or communally. A modern variation on the individual loose box is the American barn style of housing (Figure 35.7), which comprises rows of individual loose boxes under a single roof. Unlike the traditional loose box where the partitions between the boxes are usually solid from floor to ceiling, the upper half of the boxes in the American barn are not usually solid and comprise vertical bars or metal mesh. Horses can also be kept loose in groups, in barns similar to those used for cattle. The advantages and disadvantages of the various types of housing are summarised in Table 35.2 (Mills & Clarke 2007).

Statutory recommended minimum floor areas for individually housed horses are illustrated in Table 35.3. These are minimum recommended dimensions in the UK. Also see the Home Office Code of Practice for the housing and care of animals used in scientific procedures (2014a) for further guidance. European and US guidelines for accommodation and care of animals used for experimental and other scientific purposes are also available – refer to Annex III of European Union Directive 2010/63/EU and the Guide for the Care and

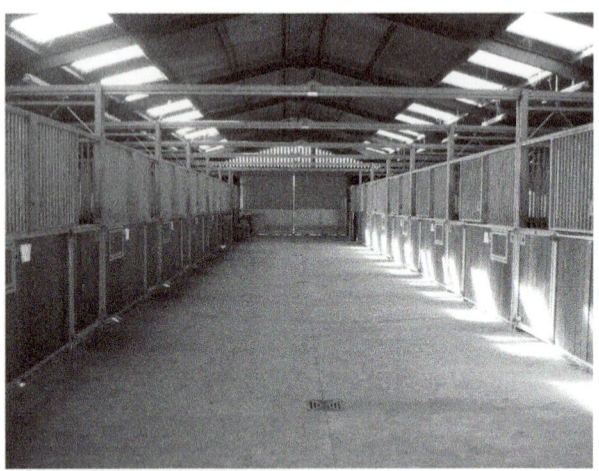

Figure 35.7 American barn.

Table 35.3 Dimensions recommended for housing horses in loose boxes (DEFRA 2017). Note that housing may be subject to statutory requirements in some countries.

Height of horse at withers	Minimum floor area when housed individually
Ponies	3.05 m × 3.05 m (10 ft × 10 ft)
Large ponies (13.2 hh+)	3.05 m × 3.65 m (10 ft × 12 ft)
Horses (>14.2 hh)	3.65 m × 3.65 m (12 ft × 12 ft)
Large horses (>17 hh)	3.65 m × 4.25 m (12 ft × 14 ft)
Foaling box	4.25 m × 4.25 m (14 ft × 14 ft)

(hh = hands).

Table 35.2 Types of housing suitable for horses and their advantages and disadvantages.

Type of housing	Advantages	Disadvantages
Loose (individual) box	Some degree of freedom of movement Individual airspace, if floor to ceiling walls Visual contact if top half door open Can provide thermal comfort and good ventilation	Solitary confinement Reduced visual contact Labour intensive as require daily cleaning, results in extensive use of bedding material
American style barns	Some degree of freedom of movement Easier working conditions for staff as stable yard undercover Visual and some social contact (through bars)	Shared airspace Direct horse-to-horse contact possible, aiding infection spread Ventilation is often inadequate Labour intensive as require daily cleaning, results in extensive use of bedding material
Loose yarding/undercover pens	Freedom of movement Full socialisation possible Less labour intensive as can deep litter bedding	Shared airspace Direct horse-to-horse contact possible, aiding infection spread Aggression especially at feeding may lead to injuries Timid horses may be denied food
Pasture with field shelter access	More in line with natural environment Full freedom of movement Full socialisation possible	Some less hardy horses may not be able to be kept at pasture 24/7 in the winter months Aggression especially at feeding may lead to injuries Timid horses may be denied food Direct horse-to-horse contact possible, aiding infection spread

Use of Agricultural Animals in Research and Teaching (American Society of Animal Science 2020), respectively.

Three-sided field shelters (Figure 35.8) should be provided for horses and ponies at pasture, and the shelter size will depend on the number and size of animals in the group. For a straight shelter of 12 ft in length, it is advisable to allow 10–12 ft in width for one horse and an added 5 ft in width for each additional horse (BHS 2005). The shelter should face the sun and be bedded in cold climates and should face away from the sun in hot climates. At a minimum, shelter should provide shade from the sun and wind. In wet climates, it must be on a well-drained surface (DEFRA 2017). Feeding racks should be situated outside the shelters in a protected position. Four-sided windbreaks (Figure 35.9) or natural hedging sufficient to supply shelter from driving weather and the prevailing wind can be used for native ponies kept outside.

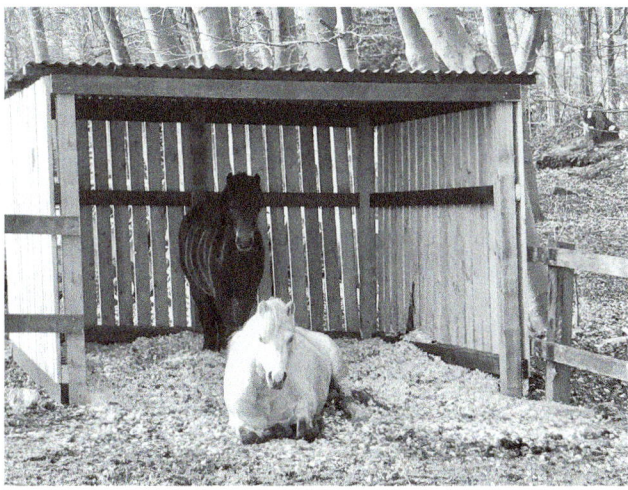

Figure 35.8 Example of a field shelter.

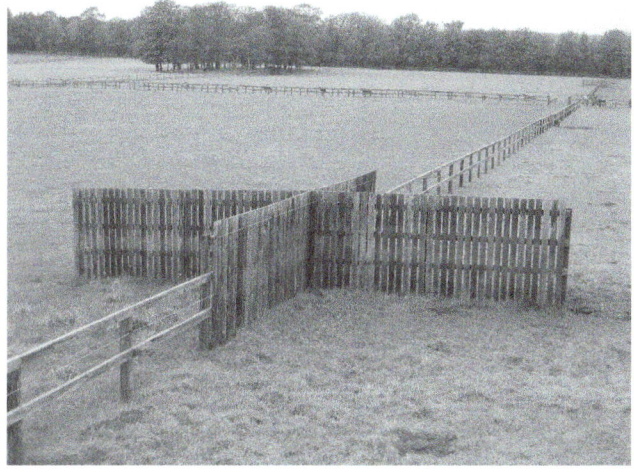

Figure 35.9 Four-sided windbreak to shelter animals kept outside.

Optimising air quality in stables

When bedding management is good, a minimum of four air changes per hour, under still air conditions, is required to ensure optimal ventilation for stabled horses (Webster et al. 1987). Well-designed loose boxes, with the top half of the stable door open, provide this. In very cold weather, it is better to provide the horse with extra rugs if required and to resist the temptation to shut the top door, as the number of air changes per hour will drop to dangerously low levels. Ventilation rates in barns are usually poorer (Mills & Clarke 2007), but can be improved by either providing draught-free inlets (at least $0.3\ m^2$) on the outside wall of each box, or by using spaced vertical boarding (Yorkshire boarding) along the walls starting 2 m above the ground.

Modifying source materials, such as hay and bedding, is another important means of optimising air quality. Some degree of fungal contamination is present in all hays (Dauvillier et al. 2019). Steaming or totally immersing the hay in water will reduce the respirable challenge (Moore-Colyer et al. 2014). Complete immersion of hay for up to 30 min should sufficiently reduce dust (Clements & Pirie 2007). Soaking hay for long periods of time in warm weather is not advised as such conditions are favourable for bacterial and mould proliferation.

Less dusty alternatives to hay include haylage and silage, both of which must be packed airtight at harvesting and used within a few days of opening, as they will decompose when exposed to the air (Dalefield 2017). These alternatives are to be recommended if hay quality is poor and for routine use in animals with respiratory disease. Feeding forage from floor level is the most natural way for the horse to eat (DEFRA 2017), encouraging good natural posture.

The other major source of fungal spores is bedding. Horses prefer straw bedding, and it may act as a stimulant for investigatory behaviour, providing environmental enrichment, particularly if fresh straw is left in sections from a bale. Horses must be closely monitored, as they can be prone to eating straw beds, with the potential for adverse consequences (Cohen & Peloso 1995; Luthersson et al. 2009). Alternatives to straw bedding, such as wood shavings, peat moss and shredded paper are less dusty alternatives but may be poorer in terms of enrichment (Goodwin et al. 2002). Whilst these are practically free of contaminants and dust when fresh, they too can become heavily contaminated in poorly ventilated stables and in deep litter systems. Commercially available non-biological bedding material such as rubber matting is clean, thermally efficient and dust free.

The risk of stabled horses developing allergic respiratory disease and the recovery time from all causes of respiratory diseases (see Common diseases section) can be reduced by ensuring that ventilation is optimal, by feeding good-quality dust-free hay, silage or haylage, by managing bedding well (daily removal of dropped roughage, faeces and urine-soiled bedding) and by avoiding 'dust raising' procedures, for example, shaking out fresh straw bedding while the horse is in the stable and grooming the horse in the stable (Clements & Pirie 2007; Couëtil et al. 2016).

Environmental enrichment

Environmental enrichment can improve animal welfare and also plays a key role in the quality of experimental data obtained from animal research (see Chapter 10 – Enrichment: Animal welfare and experimental outcomes). Wherever possible, environmental enrichment should be provided to horses used for research purposes.

As a herbivore, the horse is accustomed to continuous feeding, and in the feral state, horses spend most of their time grazing or browsing, particularly in the winter months when grazing is scarce and of poor nutritive value (Tyler 1972). The horse's digestive anatomy and physiology have evolved to digest small amounts at regular intervals, so one of the ways to mimic the horse's natural foraging behaviour is to introduce feeding methods that slow down intake alongside existing practices. The use of hay nets has been shown to increase feeding time compared to when fed off the floor (Glunk *et al.* 2014). Ideally, the use of small holed nets or double netting hay is preferable (trickle net slow feeding), combined with being able to provide more than one source of forage at any one time. It should be noted that some horses can become frustrated when trying to access forage with the trickle net slow feeding system, and this can potentially have a negative impact, so close monitoring of intake and behaviour is always advised.

If turnout is available, then the introduction of items within the field that encourages the animal to interact with the environment is recommended, especially if grazing is restricted as it may contribute to more play, movement and resting periods. Although there appears to be limited scientific evidence, the introduction of wilted stinging nettles in lines can help mimic foraging behaviour. Placement of obstacles such as logs (if practical), scratching posts, or mats can provide interesting objects for interaction. Allowing a water source where animals can play with fruit, such as apple bobbing (Figure 35.10), can stimulate and limit boredom.

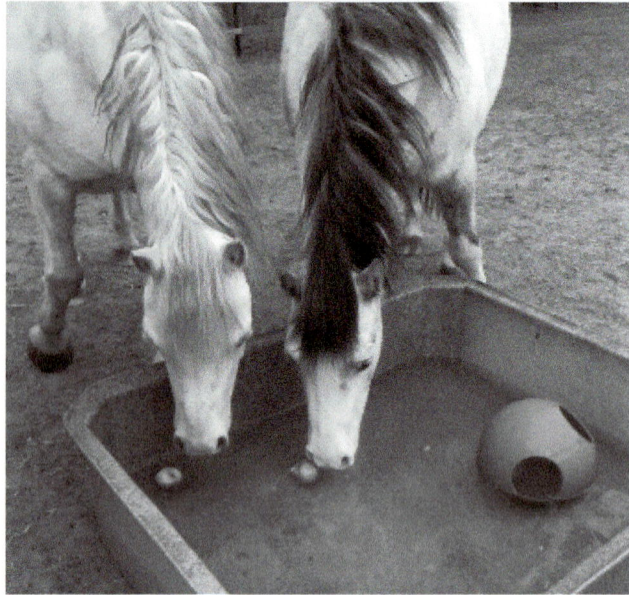

Figure 35.10 Field-based environmental enrichment.

There are several types of trickle or ball feeders on the equestrian market that can provide an affordable and durable enrichment source, allowing the horse to interact and explore how to push the ball around, releasing small amounts of edible treats, such as high-fibre cubes or hay (see Figure 35.11). This activity provides mental stimulation and relief from boredom, encouraging movement and play activity.

There are toys that are ball shaped, made of soft, pliable material but retain their shape if punctured, that are designed for one or multiple animals to engage with.

Sensory enrichment is essential to the horse's welfare, so when horses are kept in situations that require containment within an artificially lit area, replication of daylight and

(a)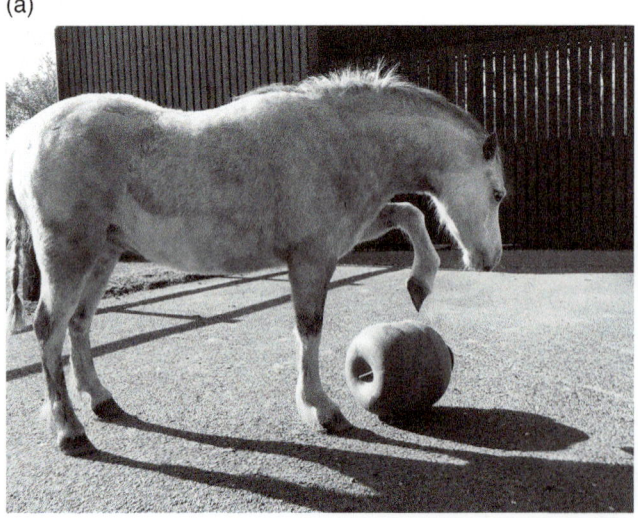

(b)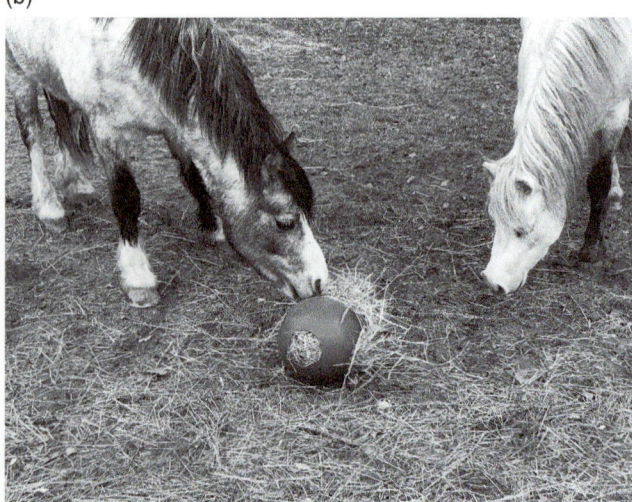

Figure 35.11 (a and b) Examples of trickle cube/hay feeders.

moonlight should also be considered. Horses are well adapted at being able to navigate their surroundings at any time and light fundamentally controls the mare's reproductive cycle. The value of providing music is debated, but it appears that there is no difference in response to various selections of music (Houpt et al. 2000). Interestingly, it is suggested that the genre of music has a more significant impact on the attendants' work satisfaction, ultimately affecting their approaches to the animal during handling. Sense of touch is the primary means by which humans and horses communicate. Grooming can provide attendants a chance to thoroughly check health and general well-being of the animal. If the horses have to be kept in any form of containment, then rubber scratching mats placed around the room or a stiff brush head attached to a surface will not only enable interaction with their environment but also allow them to express mutual grooming behaviour.

Nutrition

The individually stabled horse

It has been shown that visual contact and the smell or noise of adjacent horses encourages horses to eat (Sweeting et al. 1985; Houpt 1991). The provision of a small window or grille in the partition between loose boxes and the repositioning of the manger may be sufficient to encourage shy feeders to eat. If a horse is in regular strenuous ridden work, as it becomes fitter, it may not finish its early morning feed, so the size of the individual concentrate meal should be adjusted down to what the horse is willing to consume at that meal; an extra feed can be included later in the day to meet energy requirements. Turning stabled horses in work out in a paddock or sand arena for a short period daily is invariably beneficial for the overall well-being of the horse and is to be encouraged.

Groups of horses

The main problem of group feeding is ensuring that the more timid horses in the group get sufficient feed. If at pasture, feed racks or troughs should be situated on a well-drained surface, sufficient in number and located in a sheltered position, avoiding field shelters or confined areas due to the increased risk of injury from fighting (Figure 35.12). Group housing may aggravate the situation because of the greater restriction in space. Group-managed horses should be examined carefully daily, as long winter coats may mask weight loss.

Feeding

The horse is a non-ruminant herbivore with significant microbial fermentation occurring in the caecum and colon. The stomach is only about 8% of the capacity of the total digestive tract and is relatively small in relation to body size. In contrast, the hindgut comprises 62% of the capacity of the total digestive tract. The sacculations of the colon are thought likely to reduce the rate of passage of digesta, leading to enhanced microbial fermentation and digestion (Hintz & Cymbaluk 1994). By individually stabling horses, their movements are restricted and optimisation is reduced. Managing these horses, if they are in work and on a diet high in concentrates but low in roughage, is challenging. There is an increased possibility of both gastrointestinal (e.g. colic) and behavioural problems arising from individual housing and intermittent feeding.

Feeding practices should aim to provide adequate roughage (fibre) to ensure gut health and foraging behaviours are met, adequate amounts of feed to meet energy requirements and optimal balanced amounts of essential nutrients (Geor & Harris 2014). All feed types must be carefully sourced and stored. Food source availability should be provided at similar intervals to that of a horse kept under grazing conditions, therefore ideally continuously, with forage being the predominant food source (Geor 2017). Feeding choice and regime in individual or groups of horses will depend on multiple factors, and this can be split into animal factors such as current health, individual metabolic activity, previous and current dietary history, current weight, breed, life stage, activity level and environmental factors such as available facilities, food source availability, number in group, climate, season and ambient temperature (Geor 2017). All groups of horses should have a documented feed plan, feeds including roughages should ideally be weighed prior to administration

(a) 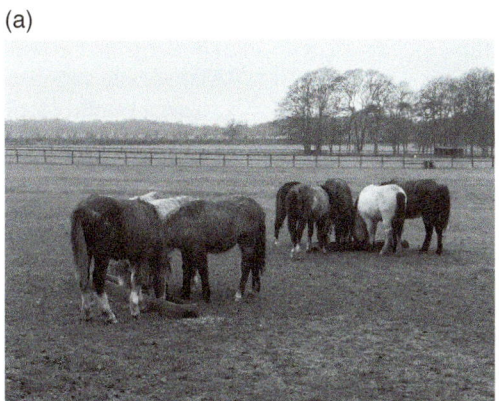 (b)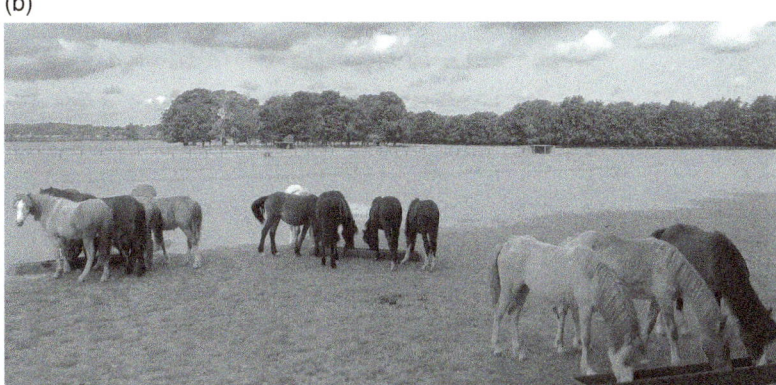

Figure 35.12 (a and b) Supplementary group feeding at pasture.

to ensure correct amounts are given and feed plans should have continual reassessment. Any changes to a feed plan, including introduction of new feeds, changing food sources, or hay batches should be done gradually, as there is an increased risk of colic in the 2-week period after a change is made (Geor 2017).

Energy requirements

The energy requirements of individual or groups of horses vary according to the factors described in the feeding section above. Exact calculations, such as digestible energy (DE) requirements, act as an estimate of the amount of energy required to be fed. Horses should be regularly evaluated in regard to their weight and body condition, with rations then adjusted accordingly (Geor & Harris 2014). Exact energy requirements can be calculated using specific computer programs or a form can be used to collect all the necessary data to formulate a diet, such as the form described by Geor (2017).

Requirements increase for horses in light to intensive work (Pratt-Phillips & Lawrence 2014). These increases, including those required as a result of growth, pregnancy and lactation, are usually met by roughages and the introduction of concentrates into the diet (Lawrence 2013). Requirements during lactation depend on milk yield, but can be double those required for maintenance. Horses in heavy training may require more energy than they can consume on a conventional diet. Increasing the energy density of the diet has been achieved by the addition of carbohydrate and fat, with these being practically added through the addition of concentrates and oils. Although dietary protein is important for tissue maintenance, it is regarded as a minor energy source and supplementing with protein as a means of increasing energy is not as efficient when compared to supplementing with carbohydrate and fat (Pratt-Phillips & Lawrence 2014). There is no evidence of any benefits of vitamin supplementation above the required levels (Pratt-Phillips & Lawrence 2014). For more detailed information on the nutritional needs of growing, breeding and exercising horses, the reader is referred to excellent reviews by Ott (1992) and Geor et al. (2013).

Cold weather increases DE requirements. These requirements are best met by feeding good-quality hay (at least 50% of the ration), *ad libitum*. This encourages high voluntary intake of a feed with good energy content and a high heat increment (HI). HI is the heat of nutrition, metabolism, digestion and muscular activity involved during digestion (Ellis 2013). In hot weather, the diet should not include excessive levels of feeds with a high HI such as hay, as this would aggravate heat stress. The HI of grains or fat is lower than that of fibrous feeds.

Water requirements

Whether stabled or at pasture, horses should have constant access to clean water. When housed in groups, the water supply should be sufficiently large to allow several horses to drink at one time. Cattle troughs are quite satisfactory for this purpose. Care should be taken to ensure that there are no sharp edges, which could cause injury. When on a predominantly hay diet, stabled horses require 5 l of water per 100 kg live-weight per day; when on a hay and grain diet, 3 l of water per 100 kg live-weight per day should suffice (Cymbaluk & Christison 1990). Voluntary water intake is reduced in cold weather, so it is important that horses kept outside are provided with highly digestible feeds in order to minimise the risk of intestinal impaction secondary to reduced water intake. In cold weather, water temperature should be 2–10 °C in order to optimise intake (Cymbaluk & Christison 1990). Water can be supplied in plastic buckets or via automatic drinkers. The former, though more laborious, are to be preferred, as monitoring of water intake is possible. Water buckets should be scrubbed out daily, and troughs should be regularly cleaned and well maintained.

Pasture management

It is recommended that each horse requires approximately 0.5–1.0 hectares (1.25–2.5 acres) of grazing of a suitable quality if no supplementary feeding is provided. This size recommendation can be affected by a number of factors such as size of animal, length of time spent stabled, time of year, pasture quality and number of animals on the pasture (DEFRA 2017). Pasture should not be overstocked, and attempts should be made to ensure that young horses get the cleanest and best pasture in an attempt to reduce worm burdens (endoparasites) in this high-risk group. Estimation of pasture forage intake (grass) for each horse is hard to quantify, and amounts of grass present in the field will vary with time of year.

Fencing should be robust and well maintained, with no sharp edges, and height of fences is dependent on the size of horses. For most horses, fences should be around 1.25 m (4 ft), and for stallions, fence heights should be at least 1.38 m (4ft 6 in) (DEFRA 2017).

Large paddocks should be subdivided so that they can be more easily managed, and special electric fencing material is available for doing this cost effectively. Broad electric tape that is easily visible should be used when first introducing the horses to this area.

Faeces should be removed from the pasture twice weekly, particularly in warm moist periods when conditions are optimal for endoparasite larval development on pasture. Machines are available, which will both collect faeces and debris and harrow the pasture. Mixed grazing with cattle (or sheep) will reduce pasture infectivity from endoparasites, as the main equine parasites are host specific. Pasture quality and palatability are also improved by mixed grazing, as ruminants will graze areas rejected by horses.

There are numerous types of poisonous plants that may be present in paddocks, and these will vary between countries (Figure 35.13). It is recommended that readers should familiarise themselves with the variety of species relevant within their locality. It is important that efforts are made to reduce the risks of poisoning by implementing good pasture management practices. The use of herbicides and the manual removal of the plants and their roots are good practical measures that can be utilised. It is important to remember that there are multiple factors influencing plant toxicity levels such as the stage of growth of the plant, the quantity of plant that an animal is exposed to, the age and health of the animals grazing, boredom and inclination of the animals to graze undesirable areas, season of growth and numerous environmental influences.

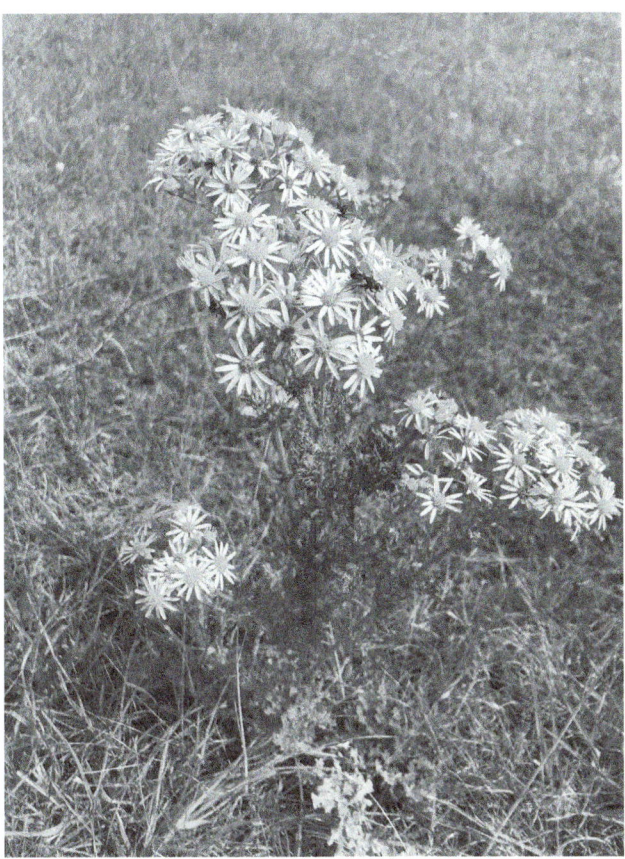

Figure 35.13 An example of the poisonous plant Ragwort (Senecio jacobaea), which has widespread distribution and can cause liver disease in horses.

Roughages

Additional roughage may not be required in many climates; however, seasonal administration may be necessary, such as in the winter, when grass growth has stopped. The hay requirements of horses will vary depending on previously discussed factors but range between 0.8% and 5.2% of body weight (National Research Council 2007). Horses in intensive work that are fed large quantities of concentrate may only consume the lower amount of roughage. In this situation, the main function of the hay is mechanical to ensure normal gut function. Although it could be replaced by other sources of long fibre such as chaffed straw, hay occupies the horses' attention, which is an important consideration in avoiding behavioural problems in stabled horses, and low-roughage diets are associated with issues such as colic and gastric ulcers. Where hay provides most of the dietary intake (e.g. adult horses on maintenance rations and ponies during the winter months), any alternatives must provide both fibre and nutrients. A minimum required amount of fibre in a horse's diet is thought to be 1 kg of roughage per 100 kg body weight (Geor 2017).

Silage, especially big bale silage, is now more readily available; if harvested at the correct stage of growth and stored properly, it should be superior to hay as it is not field cured for long periods. The risk of botulism can be minimised by ensuring that the storage bags are airtight, that there is no smell of ammonia when they are opened, that the pH is less than 5 and that there is no contamination with soil. It is also important that the dry matter content is not too low, to avoid horses in hard work having to consume inappropriately large quantities. Haylage, high dry matter silage, is another excellent product available for horses. Both silage and haylage are excellent alternatives to hay for horses with respiratory allergies; however, they have a higher sugar content, which must be taken into account when formulating the diet, and a diet containing sugar would not be advisable for any horse at the risk of excessive weight gain or laminitis.

Roughages should ideally be fed from the floor, which is more wasteful but more natural. By lowering the head the tracheal mucociliary clearance is accelerated, which contributes to avoiding lower respiratory tract disease (Raidal et al.1996). Alternatively, they can be fed in wall-mounted racks or in hay nets. Racks and hay nets should be at an appropriate height (head height) so that there is no risk of a hoof becoming entrapped. Hay nets should not be available for foals because of the risk of injury.

In comparison with good or average hay, straws have low densities of energy, protein and minerals. Wheat and rye straw are not suitable for feeding to horses because of their high lignin content, which makes them indigestible, but spring sown oat or barley straw, which have been under sown with grass, can be added to diets to provide good doers with a feed source to provide satiety with minimal energy. But additional feed sources are needed to provide protein, energy and minerals, and care must be taken as consuming straw has been correlated with impaction colic (Cohen & Peloso 1995; Luthersson et al. 2009).

Grass cubes, manufactured from chopped and ground grass (Figure 35.14), usually provide sufficient protein and calcium and could be fed exclusively to horses. However, these products and other 'complete cubed' diets have a major disadvantage in that they are usually consumed quickly and thus encourage the development of behavioural problems

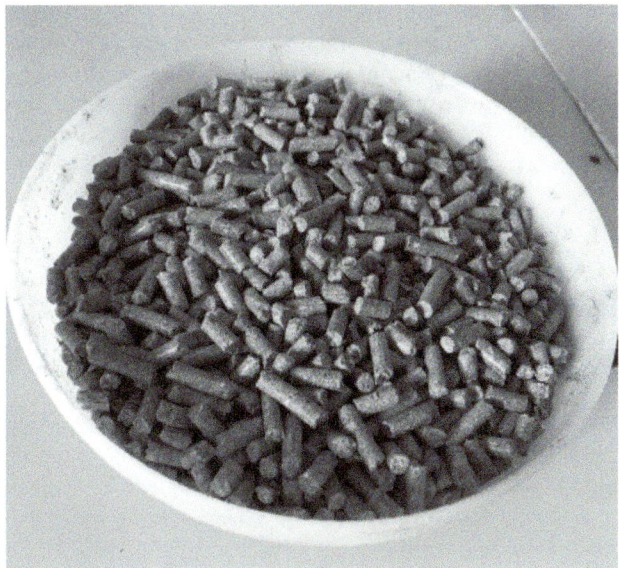

Figure 35.14 Grass cubes.

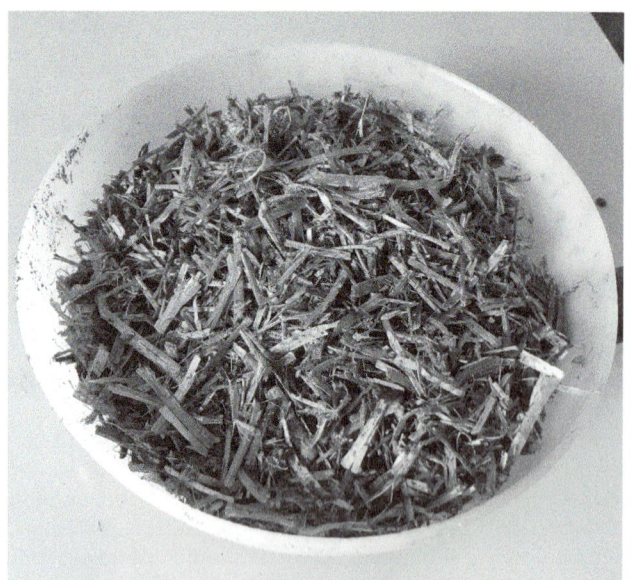

Figure 35.15 Chaff.

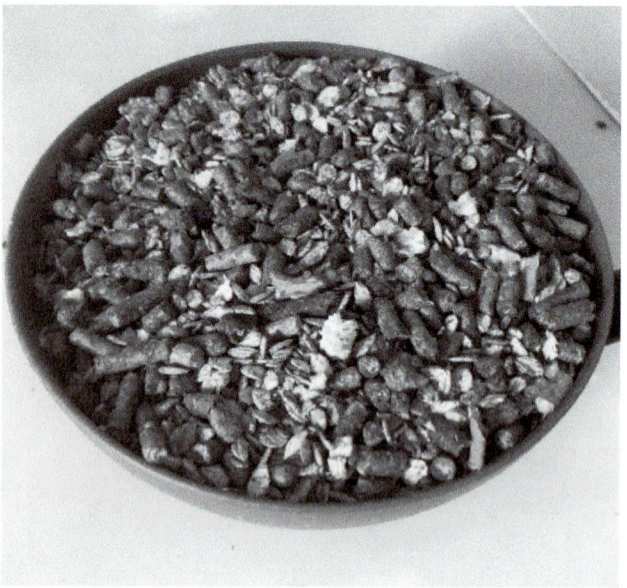

Figure 35.16 An example of a mixed compound feed.

in stabled horses and dental abnormalities as a result of changing the masticatory motion of a horse (Bonin *et al.* 2007). Older animals with poor dentition that may struggle to eat hay may benefit from a hay replacer, a high-fibre feed that can be used as a substitute for hay and is fed after soaking.

Good-quality chaffed hay (Figure 35.15) or straw can be fed in place of hay on a weight for weight basis, but should not be chosen as complete alternative to hay/haylage/silage. Care must be taken in choice of product as many may also contain molasses, and this sugar addition may be detrimental to particular animals. Chaff is frequently mixed with the grain ration to discourage too rapid consumption of the feed.

Concentrates

High-starch/sugar grain-based concentrates include oats, barley and maize. Barley and maize have higher energy density than oats. In view of this, when they are substituted for oats, it should be on a basis of energy and not volume. Their digestibility can be enhanced through further processing such as milling, grinding and heat treatment. Oats can be fed whole, crimped, rolled or ground. Maize can be fed whole, cracked, flaked or ground, but processing is probably only advantageous for very young animals, those with poor chewing habits or poor teeth. Barley should be processed (steam or dry rolled) in order to expose the barley kernel. It is suggested that a maximum of 2 g starch/kg body weight should be fed at one time, as higher amounts may have negative effects on the digestive tract (Geor 2017).

Compound feeds are now much more conventional to feeding horses than grains alone; there are numerous proprietary horse feeds available, in the form of pellets or as coarse mixtures (Figure 35.16). These are specially formulated to meet the needs of horses and ponies of different ages and at varying activity levels and are very simple to use, with a clear ingredients list and recommended feeding amounts.

When wanting to feed a horse more energy, it is always best to try to increase the amount of fats and oils fed, rather than carbohydrate (starch/sugar). Some compound feeds require soaking prior to feeding. Dried sugar beet pulp, as pellets or shredded, can be usefully added to the concentrate ration but must be thoroughly soaked before use or else there is the risk of oesophageal obstruction (choke) (see Common diseases section). Wheat bran and dried brewers grains can also be fed, but both have high phosphorus levels and should be used with discretion.

Despite vitamin supplementation being heavily promoted commercially, their efficacy in exercising horses is controversial. Salt is probably the cheapest and most useful supplement for all horses and is commercially available in the form of mineralised salt blocks. These provide salt and essential trace elements and should be provided all year round.

The concentrate ration is usually fed in mangers, which can be at chest height or on the ground. However, there is greater risk of fouling if mangers are at ground level. They should be kept clean, and rejected food, rain water and debris should be removed before fresh feed is put in.

Identification

Horses usually differ sufficiently in their colour, markings and conformation for individuals to be recognised, even within a breed. Under current European Union legislation, all horses, ponies and donkeys must have a horse passport, which is a permanent record of age, breed, sex and colour distribution, together with the position of whorls (areas where the hairs are radially arranged). Microchipping became a compulsory requirement in England from 2020 (DEFRA, Equine Identification (England) Regulations 2018). Freeze-branding is not a recommended procedure, and ear tags and tattooing are not suitable for horses.

Exercise

Horses and ponies not in work, but kept at pasture or loose yarded when housed, will usually get sufficient exercise for their needs. The individually stabled horse in work will benefit from being kept loose in a paddock or arena for as much time as practicable. However, there are situations where specific provision must be made for some form of daily exercise: for example, for horses used for serum and/or blood production and which are individually housed during the winter months and horses or ponies being raised parasite-free and thus denied access to pasture. For these animals, it is just as important that exercise and social interaction are part of the daily routine, and they can be turned out in small groups into winter grass paddocks, sand or peat arenas for at least an hour daily. This will allow them to have complete freedom of movement and to interact socially with each other, although care must be taken to ensure compatible grouping if injuries are to be avoided.

Other forms of non-ridden exercise are lungeing, where the horse is exercised on grass or other suitable surface on a circle at the end of a long lead, or the use of horse walker machines (Figure 35.17). Lungeing is labour intensive, whereas horse walkers allow several horses to be exercised at once. Both, however, are poor substitutes for the freedom provided when the horse is turned out loose.

Weight monitoring

The evaluation of weight and what constitutes an 'ideal weight' is inevitably reliant on multiple factors and can be subjective, but consistency in methods of measurements will help ensure the accuracy of weight monitoring. Different methods can be used to establish an animal's weight. Calibrated weigh scales provide the most accurate results but are not always a feasible option (Figure 35.18).

Weight tapes that can be placed around the girth area can provide an approximate weight. It is also possible to gauge a weight using a formula from different measurements taken using the weight tape. One method for horses over 12 months of age is to measure the heart girth circumference and the

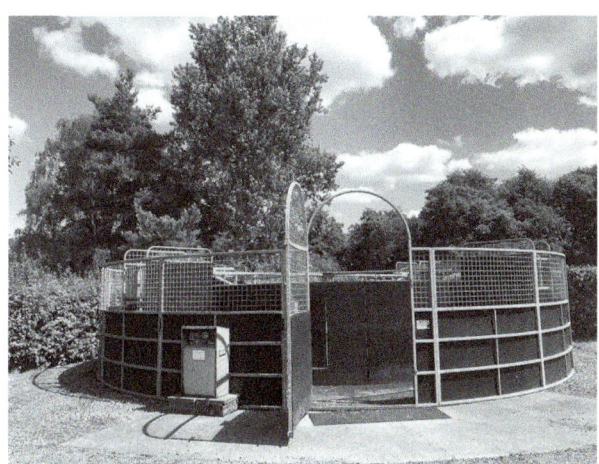

Figure 35.17 A horse walker machine.

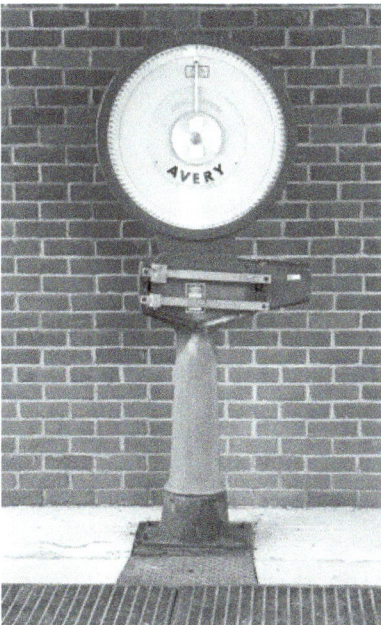

Figure 35.18 A horse weighbridge.

body length (which is taken from the point of shoulder to the point of buttocks), apply the following formula:

(heart girth circumference × heart girth circumference) × body length and then divide that total by 330 to provide an estimated body weight in pounds.

Body condition scoring was initially developed as a method of quantifying the body fat being carried by animals within the food chain. In the early 1980s, Henneke *et al.* (1983) established a numerical scale ranging from 1, whereby the horse is classed as poor and extremely emaciated, to 9, where a horse is described as extremely fat. This method was universally adopted and was subsequently adapted by Kohnke (1992) and used in subsequent work by Dugdale *et al.* (2010) who suggested that although useful, it appeared to be less accurate when assessing obese horses and ponies. There are a number of different scoring systems available, but comparisons can be difficult due to the subjective nature of observations.

Routine weight monitoring should be performed for all animals on a regular basis, with comparisons made between each animal's weight evaluation. Having a documented, up-to-date weight for each animal in combination with a body condition score and observational records will help monitor fluctuations, address the animal's physical and mental welfare status and also ensure accurate dosage of any administered medications. Under- and overweight animals both pose a welfare issue. An underweight animal may be suffering from an underlying disease, with weight loss being an early indicator. Overweight animals are at an increased risk of multiple diseases including laminitis or hyperlipaemia (see Common diseases section) (Johnson *et al.* 2009). In particular, ponies and other breeds such as cobs are 'good doers', meaning that they gain weight easily and require very careful management of their weight.

Hoof care

The growth rate of horses' hooves depends on age, season and nutritional status and is normally faster in young horses and in the spring. The average rate of growth is about 10 mm/month (Butler 1992). The feet should be carefully inspected daily, and trimming should be done as regularly and as often as is necessary, by trained personnel, ideally a qualified farrier (Figure 35.19) (O'Grady 2009). Although a 6-week interval is the average for many horses, it can vary from 2 weeks to 2 months. An overgrown hoof can result in numerous health issues and is a welfare issue (see Figure 35.20).

Horses in work may require shoeing, as they invariably have to exercise on hard surfaces. However, serum-producing horses and ponies rarely require shoeing and, if being kept in groups, should never have hind shoes on because of the risk of causing serious injury from kicks. Foals should start to have their feet trimmed when about 1 month old, or earlier if they have limb deformities, many of which can be corrected by foot trimming and exercise alone. During dry weather, horses at pasture may develop vertical cracks in the feet and require regular foot rasping or even the application of a shoe to limit damage. Stabled horses should have their feet cleaned and examined at least once daily.

Dental care

Horses have hypsodont (long-crowned) teeth, which continually erupt at about 2–3 mm/year. The diet horses consume results in wear of the teeth, with eruption counteracting this wear. At a certain point in later life, wear will exceed eruption, with this having an influence on limiting a horse's life expectancy. Equine dental anatomy includes deciduous and permanent dentition (St Clair 1975).

There are many developmental and acquired dental abnormalities that can occur such as malocclusions, focal dental overgrowths, sharp enamel points and diastema (gaps between teeth) with resultant periodontal (gum) disease, to name a few. Abnormalities can be prevented or addressed with regular examinations and corrective dental procedures. A routine oral examination should be performed under sedation to ensure that abnormalities are diagnosed early and effectively. Rasping is a routine requirement for horses over the age of about 2 years old (or younger if required) and has been carried out for hundreds of years (Ralston et al. 2001). Rasping primarily addresses sharp enamel points of cheek

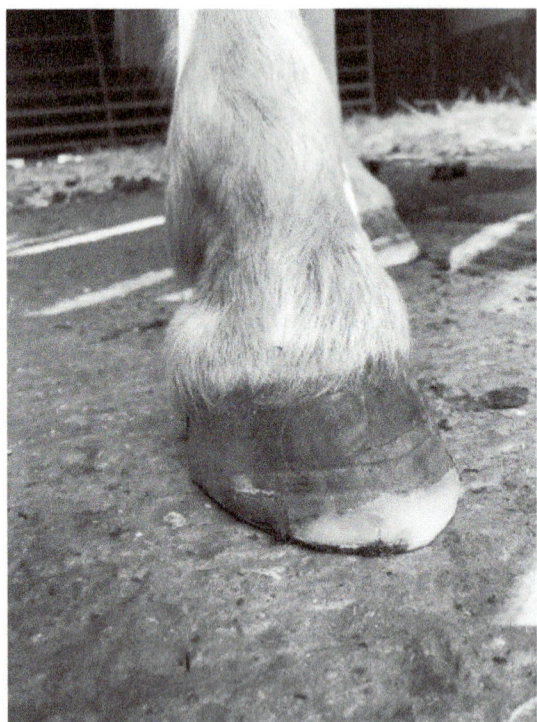

Figure 35.19 The same hoof, after trimming by a farrier.

(a) 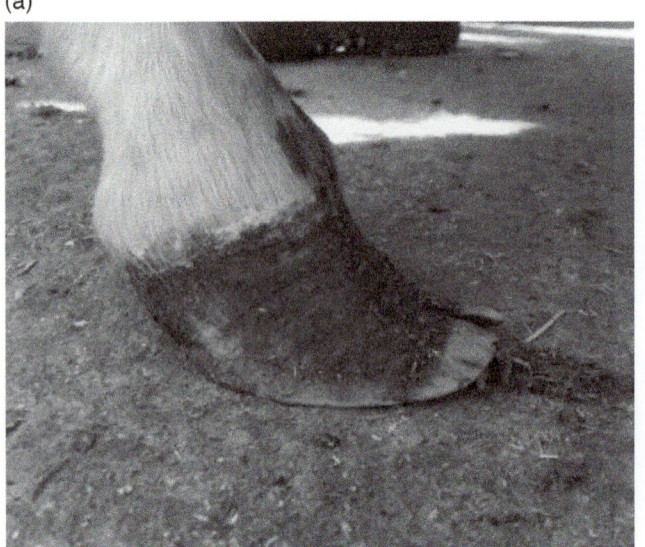 (b)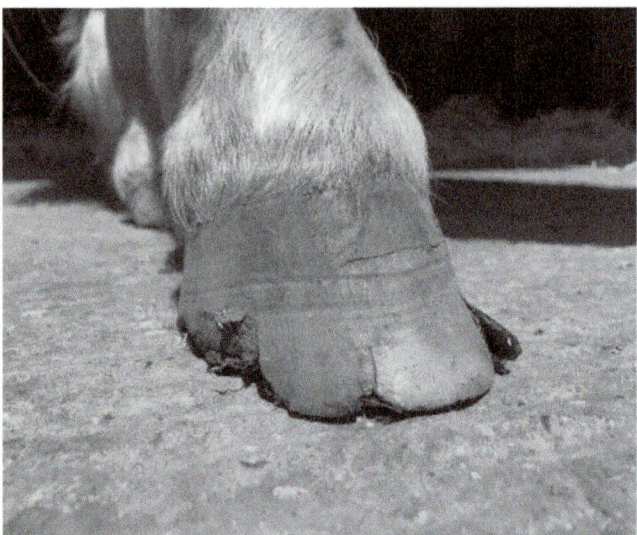

Figure 35.20 (a and b) Dorsal flare occurs when the hoof has been allowed to go too long without trimming.

teeth (premolars and molars) to alleviate secondary soft tissue damage. Rasping can also improve masticatory function by addressing abnormalities such as occlusal overgrowths. Dental examinations and corrective procedures should only be performed by suitably trained personnel, such as a veterinary surgeon. Frequency of examinations will be established by the treating clinician, but are usually required once a year as a minimum.

Prevention of parasites (endoparasites)

Having a multi-staged approach to parasite control is an integral part of horse husbandry (Nielsen *et al.* 2012). Certain endoparasites live inside the horse during phases of their lifecycles and all grazing horses will have a burden of internal parasites (Nielsen & Reinemeyer 2018). Detrimental effects on horses as a result of a high parasite burden are numerous and depend on the parasite involved. Gastrointestinal signs such as diarrhoea and weight loss are the most common outcomes of infection; however, coughing, ill-thrift, liver disease or death are also potential outcomes (Sanchez 2018). Parasites include roundworms, tapeworms and bots (larvae of the bot fly, *Gasterophilus* spp.). Some roundworms are specific to unweaned foals and yearlings, for example, threadworms (*Strongyloides westeri*) and ascarids (*Parascaris equorum*). However, roundworms, such as large and small strongyles, are found in horses of all ages and are potentially very pathogenic. Small strongyles (cyathostomins/small redworms) have the potential to cause severe damage to the gut wall in the emergence of an encysted larval stage that lies dormant in the gut wall as part of the parasites lifecycle and emerges en masse in late winter or early spring (causing the disease larval cyathostominosis) (Lyons *et al.* 2000). Large strongyles (*Strongylus* sp.) have a migratory stage through gastrointestinal vessels, causing arteritis and thrombus formation, damaging vital organs. With the introduction of broad-spectrum anthelmintics over the last three decades, the prevalence of large strongyles has declined dramatically (Fritzen *et al.* 2010). Ascarids are a particular concern in youngstock, with ill-thrift or even intestinal blockage possible. Tapeworms are another potential endoparasite, and burdens can cause colic (abdominal pain) and impactions. Pin worm (*Oxyuris equi*) infections are possible and cause irritation from female worms laying eggs on the perineum, with resultant itchiness of a horse's tail and perineum. Diagnosis is through microscopic evaluation of tape impressions taken from around the anus, and treatment is with licensed oral wormers with coverage for pin worm. Lungworm (*Dictyocaulus arnfieldi*) is most likely to be diagnosed in horses grazed with donkeys, and donkeys may be infected with no clinical signs. Diagnosis and treatment should be sought from a veterinarian. Finally, liver fluke (*Fasciola hepatica*) is a potential parasite, commonly found in wet, warm locations, with the potential to cause liver damage and weight loss.

Traditional control programmes based on treatments every few months are now insufficient, and an integrated approach to control is necessary (Peregrine *et al.* 2014). Diagnosis of roundworms is achieved through performing individual faecal worm egg counts (laboratory faecal analysis technique that counts the number of parasite eggs in a faecal sample). Treatment of roundworms is by administration of licensed oral antiparasitics (wormers). Intelligent/targeted administration of such wormers is advised, as there is documented resistance increasing with their every use (Fritzen *et al.* 2010). None of the available equine anthelmintics are effective against the full spectrum of endoparasites infecting horses, but each class of anthelmintic has a specific unique indication (Table 35.4). The manufacturers' datasheets should be read carefully prior to selection of an anthelmintic. There are a number of wormers licensed including fenbendazole, pyrantel, ivermectin and moxidectin. There is now documented cyathostome resistance to fenbendazole (Sallé *et al.* 2017). Testing for tapeworm is through a blood test to detect immunological response to a burden, but results provide information on the preceding 6 months rather than at the specific sampling time point. A saliva test has been recently

Table 35.4 Broad-spectrum anthelmintics commonly used in the horse and efficacy spectrum.

Chemical group	Lumen adults/Larvae	Encysted larvae[a]	Arterial/tissue larvae[b]	Tapeworms
Benzimidazoles				
Fenbendazole	√/√	√[c]	√[c]	X
Oxibendazole	√/√	X	X	X
Mebendazole	√/X	X	X	X
Macrocyclic lactones				
Ivermectin	√/√	X	√	X
Moxidectin	√/√	√	√	X
Tetrahydropyrimidines				
Pyrantel	√/√	X	X	√[d]

√, Activity; X, no activity.
[a] Cyathosomes (small strongyles).
[b] Large strongyles.
[c] Larvicidal dose rate.
[d] Double routine dose rate.

Table 35.5 An example of an annual worm plan for a specific premises.

Season	Approach
Spring	Faecal-worm-egg-count all horses individually. Treat any horses with a count greater than a specific threshold. Also treat for tapeworm if required.
Summer	Faecal-worm-egg-count all horses individually. Treat any horses with a count greater than a specific threshold.
Autumn	Faecal-worm-egg-count all horses individually. Treat any horses with a count greater than a specific threshold. Also treat for tapeworm if required.
Winter	Worm all horses on the premises with a wormer that treats encysted red worms regardless of faecal worm egg count values.

developed and is thought to be more reflective of an immune response to a more current burden of a horse (Lightbody et al. 2018). Treatment for tapeworm is through administration of an oral wormer called 'praziquantel'. Tapeworm treatments should be given twice yearly, during the wetter months, i.e. in the autumn and again 6 months later in the spring.

A worming plan should be tailor made for a premises, with assistance from a veterinary surgeon, taking into account factors such as ages, breeds, use and pasture management to name a few (see Table 35.5). A plan should also utilise additional preventative measures such as removal of faecal matter from paddocks, co-grazing with livestock and pasture rotation. All newcomers should have faecal worm egg counts, and they should receive a wormer if they have no prior worming history. Mares should be treated in the last month of pregnancy to limit contamination of the pastures used by them and their foals: datasheets should be consulted for safety when administering to pregnant or lactating mares or foals. Foals should be introduced into the worm control programme when about 6 weeks of age, and both they and their dams should be treated regularly throughout the rearing period. Specific treatments for bots, tapeworms, and migrating large strongyle worm larvae should be given at the appropriate time of the year for the climatic region. In general terms, in northern temperate regions, treatment for mucosal cyathostome larvae, tissue stages of large strongyles and bots is given in the autumn and/or winter months. In the warmer southern regions, treatment for these parasites may extend into the late spring and may require to be done twice yearly.

Transportation

Horses and ponies are usually transported in purpose-built motorised horse boxes or trailers, though they may also be transported in modified cattle lorries. Halter trained adult horses should be fitted with a strong, properly fitting headcollar (halter) and are usually loosely tethered. If shod, their lower limbs should be protected from tread injuries by the application of either woollen bandages (stable bandages) on top of cotton wool or a similar material or purpose-made padded leggings, from below the knee or hock to the coronet. Kneecaps will protect them from injury should they stumble and fall during loading and unloading, and poll guards, hock guards and tail guards are other protective items of clothing that may be used. When transporting mares and foals, each mare and foal usually occupy the area needed for two adult horses. The mare is usually loosely tethered, the foal not. Foals adapt remarkably well to being transported so long as they are in close proximity to their dam and they frequently suck during travel. Short rest periods (10 min for every hour of the journey) should be provided during longer journeys. Unbroken ponies are best transported loose in small groups (Figure 35.21).

Patience and care are needed when loading and unloading both experienced travellers and unbroken animals if injuries are to be avoided. The ramps of the vehicles should have a non-slip surface and sidewings to ensure that the horse walks down the middle of the ramp: as horses have an aversion to stepping on such surfaces, the floor of the box should be covered with straw or other suitable material. Studies have been undertaken to try to clarify the effects of tethering a horse to be forward- or rear-facing during travel. Studies have found that that there is some benefit from rear-facing travel for some horses (Clark et al. 1993; Smith et al. 1994; Waran et al. 1996). Later studies found that neither forward- nor rear-facing orientation when travelling had a greater benefit (Collins et al. 2000; Toscano & Friend 2001). Most commercial trailers are designed for forward-facing travel.

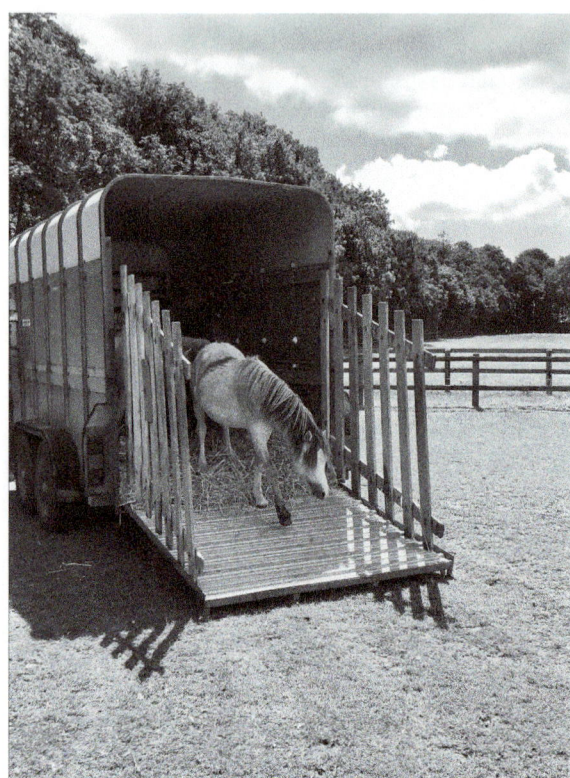

Figure 35.21 Horses being travelled loose in a trailer.

Biosecurity

Equine infectious diseases are endemic (always present at an expected level) in most horse populations. There are many different potential infectious agents, and these will vary between countries. Protocols must be in place to avoid the introduction of such infectious diseases into a herd. Equine research may involve the development of vaccines for horses, and if an animal destined for such testing was naturally infected prior to commencement of the study, it would render them unsuitable for inclusion in that study. There are multiple measures that can be instigated to mitigate the risk of such scenarios, as outlined below.

Vaccination

There are numerous vaccinations available for horses, and those administered will depend on a country's disease status. The administration of vaccines will also depend on the research programme the horse is entering; for example, previous vaccination may be contraindicated in horses being used in vaccine research. Vaccination against tetanus is essential in all countries (see Common diseases section).

Management of new arrivals

Facilities should have protocols in place for the arrival of newcomers. All newcomers should be isolated for a minimum quarantine period of 3–4 weeks in facilities enabling no contact, including no shared airspace, with the resident population. New arrivals should be handled by separate staff who do not handle the resident population. If this is not possible, new arrivals should be dealt with last, and protective clothing including gloves should be used. New arrivals should be closely monitored during the quarantine period, including temperature monitoring if possible. If there appear to be any signs of infectious disease, veterinary advice should be immediately sought and further sampling undertaken. Examples of additional testing by veterinary surgeons may include the taking of nasopharyngeal swab samples (large cotton bud inserted through the nose into the back of the throat), to enable the testing for respiratory tract infectious agents and blood samples to test for previous exposure to infections.

Prior to their arrival, newcomers may be screened to rule out previous exposure to specific infectious diseases. This is especially important if the animal is destined for infectious disease or vaccine research, and study inclusion criteria require there to have been no prior evidence of exposure to a specific infectious agent. As soon as possible after the arrival of newcomers, a full clinical examination and routine infectious disease laboratory screening tests should be conducted. Endemic infectious diseases commonly tested for in the UK include Equine Herpes Virus-1/-4, Equine Influenza, and *Streptococcus equi*.

Management of the herd

Personnel who manage the herd should ideally not have contact with any other horses on other premises, to maintain a closed herd status. If any infectious diseases are suspected within the herd, rapid diagnosis is required to ensure effective implementation of preventative measures, to avoid spread among the groups. This can include isolation of affected individuals. Where horses are used to living in a herd, another horse may be required to be isolated with the infected individual.

Breeding

Overview

General reproductive features of the mare (average values) are summarised in Table 35.6.

Stallions are typically used to detect oestrus in mares, though some mares will indicate receptivity to geldings grazing with them. 'Teasers' (entire males that are of a suitable temperament) need to be enthusiastic and vocal so they can be used effectively in place of valuable stallions.

Oestrus in the mare is usually 3–7 days in length and is the period of her cycle where she is receptive to the stallion. The optimal time to be bred is as close to ovulation (release of the egg for fertilisation) as possible; this usually happens 24–48 h prior to the end of oestrus. The mare in oestrus adopts a urination posture where the hindlegs are extended backward and the tail is raised. Small amounts of urine are expelled, and the clitoris is exposed in a rhythmic fashion ('winking'). The intensity of the signs of oestrus varies considerably between animals. They increase progressively during oestrus and are maximal as ovulation approaches; some mares are very reluctant to be separated from the stallion at this time. In contrast, the mare in dioestrus is not receptive and can show hostility to the stallion by biting, kicking and laying her ears back. Mares that are overly protective of their foals, even when in oestrus, will sometimes display hostility to the stallion, particularly if their foal is within earshot.

Teasing can either be done on an individual or group basis. With the former, the mare is separated from the stallion by a padded, solid barrier. The barrier should be about the same height as the withers, so that limited physical contact is possible. With the latter, the stallion can be led past the paddocks where the mares are grazing. Alternatively, the stallion can be placed in a small pen near the paddock. Mating ('covering') is usually carried out with the mare and stallion suitably restrained. Both should be bridled, and covering should be

Table 35.6 Reproductive features of the mare.

Parameter	Value
Onset of puberty (months)	18–24
Oestrus cycle (days)	
In spring	25 (range 9–50)
In late spring/summer	20.9
Duration of oestrus (days)	5–7
Duration of dioestrus (days)	14–16
Ovulation (days before end of oestrus)	1–2
Foal heat (first oestrus post-partum) (days)	9 (range 5–18)
Gestation length (days)	340 (range 320–360)

done in an enclosed area with a good surface so that neither the mare nor the stallion is likely to slip. Hind shoes should always be removed from the mare. When using valuable stallions, it is customary to fit felt boots to the hindfeet of the mare to prevent injury to the stallion. A nose twitch may be applied for additional restraint if necessary. As the results of teasing are not always conclusive, the optimum time for mating can be determined by veterinary examinations per rectum where the ovaries, uterus and cervix are palpated, and/or by scanning using ultrasonography and by vaginal examination using a speculum where the colour and state of relaxation of the cervix are determined.

Pregnancy can be confirmed using several techniques. Ultrasound echography, using an ultrasound probe carried into the rectum and directed over the uterus, can be used to detect pregnancy as early as 14–16 days post-conception (Simpson et al. 1982). Repeated scans are essential, as early pregnancy failures can occur. Scanning should be used in conjunction with the other methods of pregnancy diagnosis, for example, manual palpation, per rectum, of the uterus. The changes experienced with manual palpation are described in a review by Sharp (1992). This examination should only be performed by trained, suitably qualified personnel. Biochemical tests for pregnancy are available commercially if the technology and/or expertise for ultrasound and palpation techniques are not available. The most useful test is the measurement of equine chorionic gonadotrophin in the plasma. This test can only be done after day 40 of pregnancy and is not effective after day 120 and false results can also occur.

Management of the in-foal mare

In-foal mares should lead as natural a life as possible. In temperate areas, they are usually at pasture by day and housed by night. In warmer climates, they can remain at pasture 24 h per day. Shelter from sun and insects may be required. Their nutritional needs will increase as the pregnancy progresses and increasing amounts of concentrates are usually fed to meet these, particularly in the latter third of pregnancy. However, they should not be allowed to become fat as overfat pony mares, in particular, run the risk of developing hyperlipaemia in late pregnancy (see Common diseases section) if their management is suddenly changed; for example, a sudden fall in energy intake. They should be up to date with their tetanus and influenza vaccinations. Mares should also be vaccinated against equine herpesvirus 1 and 4 (EHV-1 and EHV-4) according to the manufacturer's recommendation, to help reduce clinical signs or viral shedding in cases of respiratory disease and abortion caused by this virus. Routine anthelmintic treatments should also be given (see Prevention of parasites section). The average gestation length of mares tends to be around 340 days, and the range of normal gestations is considered to be 320–360 days (Rossdale 1993).

Preparation for foaling

In temperate climates, mares are normally foaled indoors where they can be observed frequently and easily and given assistance if needed. Pony mares and mares in warmer climates are often left to foal outside. They should still be closely observed as parturition approaches, and lights can be used to provide some illumination of the foaling paddocks. Mares foaling inside should be provided with as large a loose box as possible (a minimum of 4.25 m × 4.25 m (14 ft × 14 ft)): it should have a deep, clean straw bed and the bedding should be extended and banked up along each wall to provide further protection. Hay should be fed off the ground and mangers, and water buckets are better at chest height. Small red light bulbs (10 W) will provide sufficient light for observation without disturbing the mare. Closed circuit television can be used to observe when the mare or mares are due to foal at the same time. Foaling alarms are available commercially and can work as an aid to alert the staff when birth is imminent.

Parturition

Mares usually tend to foal at night and seem to be able to delay foaling until conditions are right for them, for example, when the stable yard is quiet (Bain & Howey 1975; Newcombe et al. 1998).

They seem to prefer to foal unobserved: hence, any lighting should be dim. Signs of impending parturition are not consistent and can only serve as a rough guide. Udder development starts 3–6 weeks pre-foaling, and distension of the udder with colostrum occurs in the last 2–3 days. When colostrum begins to ooze from the teats and forms honey-coloured wax-like beads at the teat orifice ('waxing'), foaling is imminent. Mares can deviate from the predicted foaling date by 1–2 weeks or more. This is quite normal and does not require veterinary intervention: each pregnancy is a unique combination of maternal and foetal traits and will be terminated at the appropriate time (Sharp 1992). The various stages of parturition and their main presenting signs are given in Table 35.7.

Foaling is a normal physiological process, and attendants should be sufficiently acquainted with the normal pattern of foaling and resist the temptation to interfere unnecessarily. However, as parturition is very rapid in the mare compared with other domestic animals, experienced veterinary help should be readily available and immediately sought should it not proceed normally. Swift intervention is necessary if premature separation of the allantochorion is likely, as may occur if delivery is delayed. Any traction applied to the foal should coincide with the mare's own efforts at expulsion. The amniotic sac may be manually ruptured if it has failed to do so after the foal is delivered. The mare should be left undisturbed and allowed to rest after foaling. The umbilical cord should be left to break naturally to allow passage of placental blood to the foal; this could take several minutes. Excessive human activity will stimulate the mare to rise too soon, and in nervous primiparous mares, this could interfere with the normal bonding between the mare and her foal. The establishment of the bond between the mare and her foal is triggered by hormonal changes, which may be based on olfaction, as the mare licks the newborn for a few hours after parturition.

The normal healthy foal is in sternal recumbency within 1–2 min of delivery, and a suck reflex is present within 2–20 min. On average, a healthy foal will take up to 1 h to stand and up to 2 h to suck. By 12 h of age, it is able to walk, trot and gallop.

Table 35.7 Stages of parturition in the mare and their main presenting signs.

	Stage		
	1	2	3
	Up to time of rupture of allantochorionic membranes	Delivery of foal	Expulsion of placenta
Duration	Approx. 1 h	<30 min	Approximately 1 h
Activity	Uterine contractions begin; foal rotates head and forelimbs into dorsal position; allantochorion ruptures releasing fluid; amniotic membranes and forelimbs appear in birth canal	Foal completes its rotation, assumes diving position and passes through the birth canal	Continuing uterine contractions to expel the placenta
Behavioural signs	Mare increasingly restless; box walking; rolling/gazing at flanks; patchy sweating; often runs milk	Powerful abdominal contractions, usually when in lateral recumbency; may get up and down, adjusting position before the final push to give birth; profuse sweating	Mild colic signs and some straining; may move into sternal recumbency prior to expelling the placenta

Post-foaling procedures

In the immediate post-partum period, the foal's navel should be dressed with 2% potassium iodide solution to reduce the chance of bacterial infection; this should continue twice daily until the navel is dry (about 48 h). It is important that the foal suckles as soon as possible (within 2 h) as absorption of protective immunoglobulins present in the colostrum is maximal at birth, marginal by 15 h and has ceased by 24 h post-partum. Factors that may affect colostrum uptake, resulting in failure of passive transfer of immunoglobulins, include premature lactation of the mare, maiden mares not allowing the foal to drink and weak or compromised foals unable to nurse effectively (Jeffcott 1974). Primiparous mares, in particular, may not accept their foals and may not allow them to suckle, either because of udder distension or possibly because of an association with pain at parturition. Occasionally, these mares will attack their foals in addition to refusing to let them suckle. Assuming that no mastitis is present, they should be held by an attendant, with or without prior sedation, whilst another attendant helps the foal to suck.

The mare should be provided with a warm bran mash as laxative and her water buckets kept full. Tetanus antitoxin must be given to both mare and foal if the mare is unvaccinated. The mare should be checked for foaling injuries, which should be stitched and repaired as necessary by a veterinary surgeon. The foetal membranes should be examined to ensure that they are complete and intact. Retained placenta is a serious complication in mares, and a veterinary surgeon must be consulted if this is suspected. If the foal is straining and having difficulty in passing meconium (the first faeces), proprietary enemas should be given *per rectum*. The foal's blood immunoglobulin G levels should be tested at 24 h old to confirm whether adequate passive transfer of immunoglobulins has occurred. Any foal with failure of passive transfer should receive a plasma transfusion, to reduce the risk of future infections as a result of poor immunity. If the weather is suitable, the foal should be haltered and led out to pasture with the mare: if not, the mare and foal should be turned into a covered arena for exercise.

If for any reason a foal has not received colostrum within a few hours of birth, for example, the mare dies at foaling or the mare does not accept the foal, the foal should be given colostrum by stomach tube as soon as possible after birth. Most breeding studs keep deep-frozen supplies of mare colostrum for such emergencies. Rearing is best done using a foster mother, though foals can be reared artificially using commercially available mare milk replacers. Foals reared artificially may not grow as well as those raised by the mare and so every effort should be made to find a foster mother. Mare's milk is lower in both protein and fat content than cow's milk, but higher in lactose. The milk replacer should be fed at a temperature of approximately 37.5 °C. All utensils must be thoroughly washed and sterilised before and after use. The teat should be introduced carefully to the side of the foal's mouth, and care must be taken to ensure that milk is not inhaled. The foal must, therefore, be given frequent opportunities to rest during feeding.

For the first few days following parturition, mares are extremely protective of their offspring. Stabled mares will rapidly circle their foals and even threaten their attendants. When outside, they will drive away other mares and foals, even if they have previously had a close relationship with another mare. This protectiveness may be related to the fact that the young foal takes about a week to visually recognise its mother (Houpt 1992). A human–foal bond can be usefully established during the first few days of life and is best done by an attendant with whom the mare is familiar and trusts.

Management of youngstock

Foal behaviour

Foals nurse about four times per hour in the first week of life: the duration of nursing increases as the foal becomes older, but the frequency of nursing decreases. If separated from their mother, even briefly, or if frightened, they will immediately nurse. Foals spend 70–80% of their time resting when very young. When they get up to nurse, they generally stretch their limbs and arch their neck and back before going to the mare to feed. Since so much time is spent resting, usually lying down, it is important that young foals are not left outside in inclement weather, as they would then only rest standing. A healthy foal is normally very active and within a few days of birth will be confidently galloping and bucking round its mother. As they get older, they soon start to play with their mother and, if allowed to do so, play with other foals in the group.

Foals less than 4 weeks of age will often nibble at their mother's freshly passed faeces: this is normal behaviour thought to be important in the establishment of bowel flora and presents no hazard to the foal (Carson & Wood-Gush 1983). The first faeces passed by foals, the meconium, are frequently difficult to pass. However, once the foal has nursed, the laxative effect of the colostrum usually ensures no further problems. A transient diarrhoea often occurs in the foal at the time of the foal heat, the mare's first oestrus after foaling; this usually resolves without treatment.

Early handling and training

When first approached by humans, young foals will be nervous, try to evade being caught and may start snapping (also referred to as 'champing' or mouthing). This is a submissive gesture and usually indicates fear: the foal's ears turn back slightly, the neck is stretched out, the corner of the mouth is drawn back and the jaws start to move vertically in a rhythmical fashion. This gesture is adopted by young animals when approaching older ones, including their mothers. A short time spent every day quietly talking to young foals and gently scratching their crest and along their spine will help them to relax and accept being handled. Their hooves should be picked up daily so that they habituate to the procedure. This will minimise problems with the farrier at a later stage. They should also accept being cleaned with a soft cloth all over their body in preparation for grooming when older. Special lightweight foal headcollars (foal slips) should be put on daily from birth onwards before the mare and foal go to pasture and the foal taught to be led. A foal is usually led from its left side and close to its mother's left shoulder. A long piece of rope should be looped through the ring on the foal slip: if the foal should escape the handler, the rope will then pull free and not get entangled round the foal's legs.

Verbal commands should precede the physical commands so that, eventually, the voice alone is sufficient. Foals should be rewarded by scratching the withers rather than patting anywhere. If they misbehave and kick or try to kick, they should be discouraged immediately. Other behaviour management techniques should be explored as an alternative to punishment. Colt foals, in particular, will strike out with the front feet; this should be discouraged promptly. It is better to spend time disciplining and teaching a foal 'manners' when it is small and manageable than to leave this initial training until it is 500 kg and unmanageable.

Weaning

As some mares will be in foal again within a few months of parturition, it is customary to wean the foals when they are about 4–5 months of age. By this age, the foals are already physically fairly independent of their dams, will be grazing like adult horses and have usually been introduced to concentrate feeding ahead of the anticipated weaning date. Thus, they have little, if any, setback. The time of weaning is a period of peak growth and a time when stereotypical behaviours can become apparent. Post-weaning concentrates can be introduced 4–6 weeks prior to the foal being separated from its dam.

At weaning, it is important that the mare is moved out of sight and earshot of the foal. The foal is usually kept in a loose box with the top door shut until it has settled down, which is usually within a few hours of separation. Being able to see other foals will minimise stress at this time. Weanlings are usually turned out into a securely fenced paddock with the other weanlings within 24 h of being separated from their mothers. If other foals are not available, quiet mares or geldings can serve as suitable companions. Alternatively, the mares may be moved from the paddocks one by one over a period of time leaving the foals with their usual companions.

Mares usually settle down quickly after the foals have been weaned. Their udders are usually distended for a few days but soon start to dry off. It is customary to cut back the amount of concentrate feed and ensure the mare can take exercise until the udder has 'dried off'. The milk should not be stripped off during this phase as it can encourage continued lactation.

Management of stallions

Stallions, like brood mares, should be allowed to lead as natural a life as possible. Pony stallions may be left to run out with their mares, if pregnancy is desired. However, because of the risk of injury and the greater value of the animal, stallions are often individually stabled, and when turned out to graze, this is also on an individual basis, but it is beneficial for stallions to see other horses. The fencing surrounding stallion paddocks must be robust and sufficiently high to deter them from jumping out. They need to be fit for the breeding season if they have many mares to cover: regular exercise (ridden or in-hand) is required in the preceding months. They can be more unpredictable than mares or geldings, and it is important that they have experienced handlers.

Research procedures

Health monitoring and record keeping

An annual health plan will vary depending on the facilities and research being performed. Such an annual plan includes timings for dentistry, farriery, parasitic prevention and field rotations, to name a few. All horses used in research are closely monitored at all times. Records should be kept of all routine care, veterinary treatment and study details. Health and welfare meetings should take place regularly at the institution, and committees should review the overall animal care, paying particular attention to animal welfare, ethical review and the principles of 3Rs of animal research (Flecknell 2002, see also Chapter 2: The three Rs). Such committees ensure the health and welfare of horses used in research and the optimum quality of research produced, including dissemination of findings (see Chapter 18 – Ethics review of animal research).

Handling and training

The adult horse is potentially dangerous because of its size, strength and agility, together with its ability to bite and to kick with both front and hindlegs. Therefore, it is essential that it is handled and trained by experienced people. The very young foal should be introduced to normal stable procedures and trained to accept simple procedures by its handler as soon after birth as possible (see Foal behaviour section). If more invasive procedures (e.g. the collection of blood samples) are necessary, it is important that the foal is restrained by experienced, strong handlers and that the person collecting the sample is adept at venepuncture. This will minimise stress and with time and subsequent exposure to the procedure, the foal will usually accept it. Training a horse to be ridden does not normally begin until it is 3–4 years old, except in the case of the racing Thoroughbred. This is skilled work and should only be done by people with training and experience. Additionally, horses should be trained to accept the bit and should be taught to exercise on the lunge. If not required to be ridden, the basic training such as acceptance of normal husbandry procedures and being restrained in or out of stocks (Figure 35.22) for different procedures should continue. The horse should always be rewarded when it has behaved well during procedures (for more information, see Chapter 15 – The use of positive reinforcement training techniques to enhance the care and welfare of laboratory and research animals). For safety reasons, during all the procedures described below, the horse should have an experienced

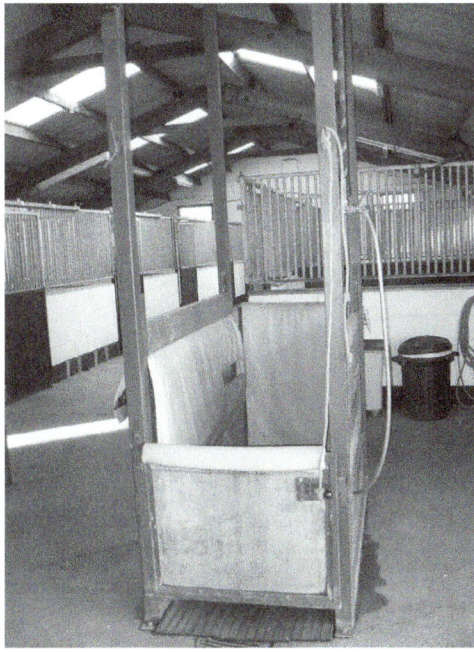

Figure 35.22 Rear view of type of stocks used for restraining horses for veterinary examinations and procedures. The boards on the sides can be removed if access is needed.

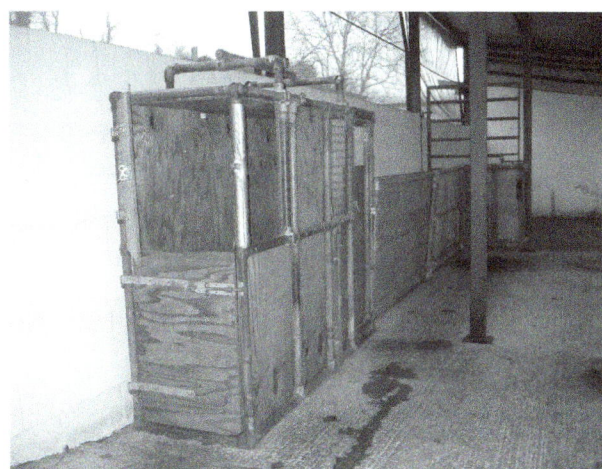

Figure 35.23 System of race and crush for handling large numbers of ponies.

handler present to restrain it if and when it is necessary. The person carrying out the procedures should have been correctly trained and be experienced in the techniques.

For large numbers of ponies, a system of race and crush is advisable to use to facilitate the handling and the procedures (Figure 35.23). Animals should be slowly introduced to this system from a young age. They are restrained in the crush, and procedures like measuring body temperature, taking faecal samples and bleeding can be easily performed.

Most horses and ponies will accept being restrained for various procedures if they have been well handled since birth. The voice should be used to calm them, and they should be approached, in a firm and confident manner, from the shoulder area. In a study conducted by Birke et al. (2011) using naïve, feral ponies, it was found that the speed and manner in which a handler approaches an animal can have a significant effect in prompting a flight response. A quiet, relaxed approach is suggested as the best method for minimising stress, reducing risk of injury and providing a useful management application. A headcollar, with or without a bit attachment, should then be put on and a long lead, preferably with a quick release catch, attached to the centre back loop of the headcollar. Short-term, relatively painless procedures, such as the collection of venous blood samples, usually do not require additional control in a horse accustomed to the procedure. If more control is needed, then grasping a fold of skin in the neck with one or both hands and twisting it (neck twitch) is usually sufficient to keep the horse still until the sample is collected. Grasping the ear in the form of an ear twitch is not to be recommended and could make the horse head shy. For more fractious animals, a twitch can be applied to the upper lip (Figure 35.24), although specific training should be considered as a long-term alternative. Twitches should only be applied by staff experienced in their use and should only be used for a short period of time.

Young foals should be restrained by one arm around the front of the chest and the other around the back of the hindquarters and held against a wall in the loose box: they should not be held round the chest/abdomen.

All the physical methods of restraint are suitable for short-term procedures in most horses. The horse should always be

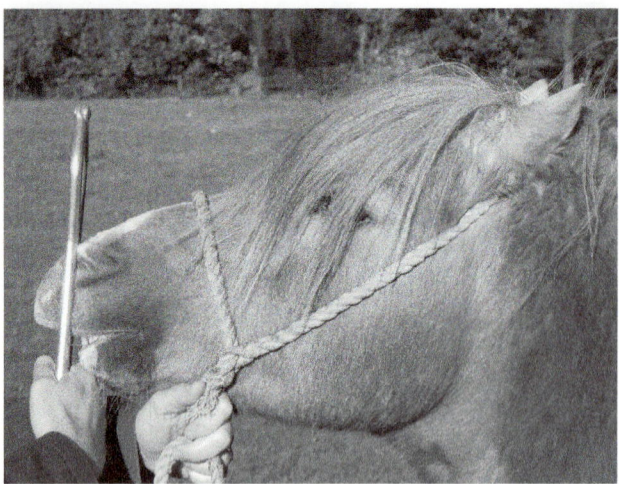

Figure 35.24 Nose twitch for restraining. Other types of twitches with rope or chain loop can also be used.

rewarded with a rub of the withers after all procedures and on occasions, with a small handful of feed, particularly when it is being trained, but care should be taken to avoid undesired resultant biting behaviour as a potential consequence of hand feeding.

Special frames (stocks) designed to restrain horses for veterinary examinations are particularly useful during time consuming or invasive procedures (Figures 35.22 and 35.23). Stocks should have no sharp projections. The horizontal bars should be well rounded and the floor surface non-slip when wet or dry. Some means of quick side release should be available should a horse slip and go down. Chemical restraint, such as the administration of sedatives, is often advisable for longer term, more invasive procedures.

Chemical restraint

Sedation

Sedation may be necessary for numerous research and veterinary procedures. The horse should still be standing, but will be relaxed, with its head dropped, with reduced reactions to stimuli. If a horse is very fractious or excited prior to the administration of sedative drugs, they may have a reduced effect. Sedation is generally administered by the intravenous route (see Intravenous section for technique). Intramuscular or oral administration of certain products is possible and may be necessary in animals not amenable to intravenous injections, but they will have a delayed onset following administration and may also have a prolonged duration of action (Michou & Leece 2012). Any sedated horse can still be dangerous, losing their inhibitions and reacting without warning, so care must always be taken, with slow movements by handlers and close monitoring of sedated horses.

Before any central nervous depressant drug is administered, a full clinical examination should be carried out, in order to detect any pre-existing condition that may be exacerbated by the use of the drug or may potentiate the side effects of the drug. The patient should be kept in quiet surroundings before drug administration and while sedation is allowed to develop. Prior to administration of any drug, the manufacturer's datasheet should always be consulted for dosage, route of administration, contraindications and possible side effects.

Sedative drugs are usually administered in combination to enable administration of lower doses, therefore avoiding side effects. Commonly used sedatives include alpha-2 agonists (e.g. detomidine or romifidine) in combination with an opioid (e.g. butorphanol). Horses under sedation will develop ataxia (wobbly gait), and therefore, care should be taken if they are required to walk anywhere. There are numerous possible side effects in horses from their use, particularly in relation to the alpha-2 agonists causing a reduction in gastrointestinal motility. Horses receiving large doses or prolonged duration of administration for longer procedures will require very close monitoring after.

Acepromazine (ACP) may be used, particularly in its oral formulation, for procedures such as farriery. However, care must be taken as sedation level may be mild and horses will still respond to visual and aural stimuli and so arousal during sedation is possible. Other more serious side effects from ACP use are priapism and paraphimosis, which are of particular concern in breeding stallions, so ACP use is avoided in them (Driessen et al. 2010).

General anaesthesia

General anaesthesia in the horse carries a greater risk than for other domestic animals (Jones 2001) and should only be undertaken by a veterinarian assisted by trained staff. Major complications include the possibility of cardiac arrest or ischaemic muscle necrosis associated with the prolonged pressure of recumbency (Dugdale & Taylor 2016). The introduction of safer, effective and more reliable drugs allows many procedures, which previously required general anaesthesia, to be done in the standing horse, using a combination of sedatives and analgesics together with local or regional anaesthesia. Sedatives (such as the combination of an alpha 2 agonist and an opioid) must be given to achieve sedation prior to the administration of the general anaesthetic induction agent (such as ketamine or sodium thiopental). Monitoring during general anaesthesia is required at all times given the risks from such a procedure and should be performed by suitably qualified personnel. The use of an intravenous catheter is essential in case of emergencies during anaesthesia and to reduce the risk of accidental perivascular administration of drugs such as sodium thiopental, which would cause tissue damage and sloughing. Induction of anaesthesia is normally done in a padded induction and recovery room; the anaesthetised horse is then transported to an adjacent operating theatre where there is specialist equipment for the monitoring and maintenance of long-term anaesthesia through the use of inhaled anaesthetics and specialist monitoring equipment. However, short-term anaesthesia using intravenously administered drugs is possible under field conditions and is acceptable for short, minor surgical procedures (McFadzean & Love 2017). A well-bedded pen with straw bales lining the walls would be a suitable place to carry out the procedure.

Analgesics

Analgesics most commonly used in horses are non-steroidal anti-inflammatories (NSAIDs) such as flunixin or phenylbutazone. NSAIDs can be administered by numerous different routes, depending on the drug and formulation, and these include oral, intravenous and intramuscular, with careful evaluation of the relevant datasheet prior to administration to determine the correct administration route for a particular formulation. Prolonged usage or high doses of NSAIDs can cause side effects such as gastric or colonic ulceration, so administration of NSAIDs requires care (Knych 2017). Other classes of analgesics include opioids, with these potentially being under legislative restriction, as in many countries they are controlled drugs requiring judicious use. Side effects from their use include a reduction in gastrointestinal motility. For more detailed information, the reader is referred to Bowen et al. (2020).

Physiological monitoring

Physical examination

A full physical examination includes evaluation of demeanour (attitude and interaction with herd), appetite, body condition, heart rate, respiratory rate and effort, submandibular lymph node size, evidence of any nasal discharge (including if unilateral/bilateral or serous/mucoid/mucopurulent) and ocular discharge. Recording of body temperatures are taken per rectum under suitable restraint. Ideally, rectal temperatures should be taken at around the same time during the day in order to minimise variation in the data collected due to normal circadian rhythms. The digital thermometer should be dipped in lubricant gel before being gently and carefully inserted into the anus, taking care to respond to any sudden movement by the animal in order to avoid damage to the rectum. The thermometer should remain inserted with the tip touching the rectal wall until the temperature is registered, when it can be carefully removed, cleaned and accurately read. If the thermometer has been inserted into faecal material, a false reading may be obtained.

Collection of blood samples

Blood is normally collected from the jugular vein, which is readily visible when the vein is raised by manual pressure in the jugular groove (Figure 35.25). Horses accustomed to the procedure require minimal restraint. Foals should be handled by experienced attendants in order to obtain a sample. If large volumes of blood are to be collected, large-gauge needles or sterile indwelling catheters are to be recommended. If frequent blood sampling is required, for example, in a pharmacokinetic study, it may be better to insert an indwelling catheter under local anaesthesia and suture it in place. The catheter is kept patent by regular flushing with sterile heparinised saline. With care, good technique and adequate supervision, these can be left *in situ* for several days. The catheter site must be closely evaluated daily to ensure that there is no heat, pain or swelling; if this occurs, the catheter must be removed, as there is the potential of a catheter site reaction or infection. Catheterisation is a specialist procedure that

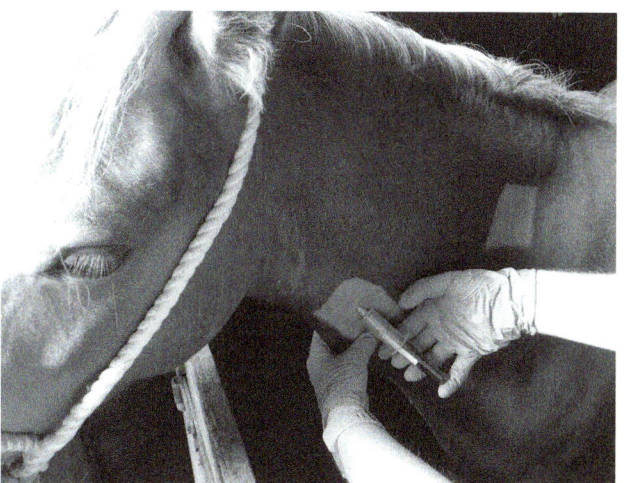

Figure 35.25 Blood sampling procedure.

must be performed in a sterile manner by suitably trained and qualified personnel. The decision to catheterise or not will depend on the number of samples, the temperament of the horse and how it tolerates repeated injections (see also Joint Working Group on Refinement (JWGR) 1993).

Nasopharyngeal swabbing

The required animal should ideally be restrained in stocks for this procedure. The thickness and shape of the cotton of the swab should be adequate to pass easily into the nasal passages. Continuous swabbing of the nasal passages can cause distress and potentially irritation of the nasal mucosa. To alleviate potential irritation of nasal passages when requiring collection each day, the swabs need to be alternated between the right and left nostril where practicable. Distance of insertion can be established by measuring a swab against the horse's face, from the medial meatus of the eye to the nose (see Figure 35.26). The swab should be removed from its packaging and gently inserted into the nasal cavity (see Figure 35.27), directing it away from the 'false' nostril (dorsal meatus) and towards the midline without using force if there is resistance to progress. Normally, a swab collection should take no more than 5 s. If the head cannot be held sufficiently steady, then a twitch should be applied. Once the swab sample has been taken, it should be placed into a tube containing the required transport medium and gently rotated up and down.

Genital swabs

Swabs are routinely collected from breeding mares and stallions to check for the presence of infection, specifically venereal pathogens, prior to mating (Metcalf 2011). Clitoral and endometrial swabs may be required. Endometrial swabs require the aid of a speculum to dilate the vagina; the swab is passed into and through the cervix, at the correct stage of the cycle to ensure a more open cervix, and rubbed against the mucosa of the uterus. Mares should be restrained in stocks prior to carrying out these procedures. The sites for examination in the stallion are the urethral fossa, the sheath, the urethra and pre-ejaculatory fluid. Further information

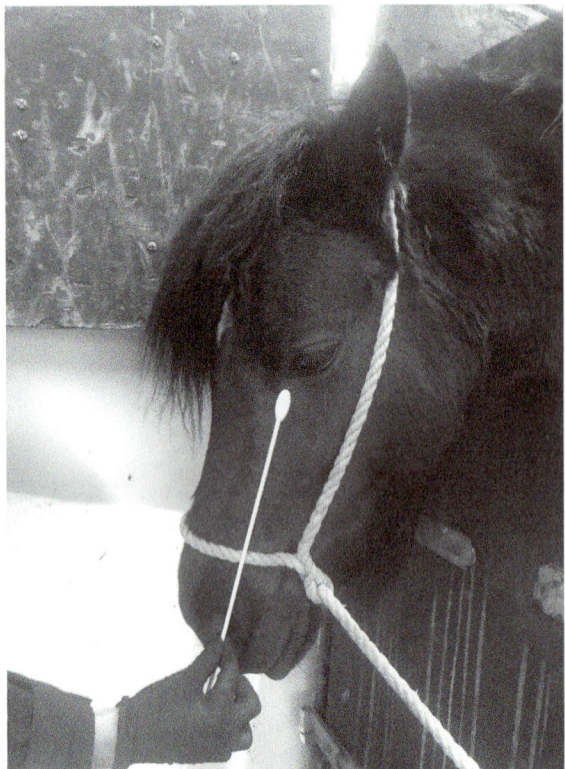

Figure 35.26 Measuring distance of insertion for a nasopharyngeal swab.

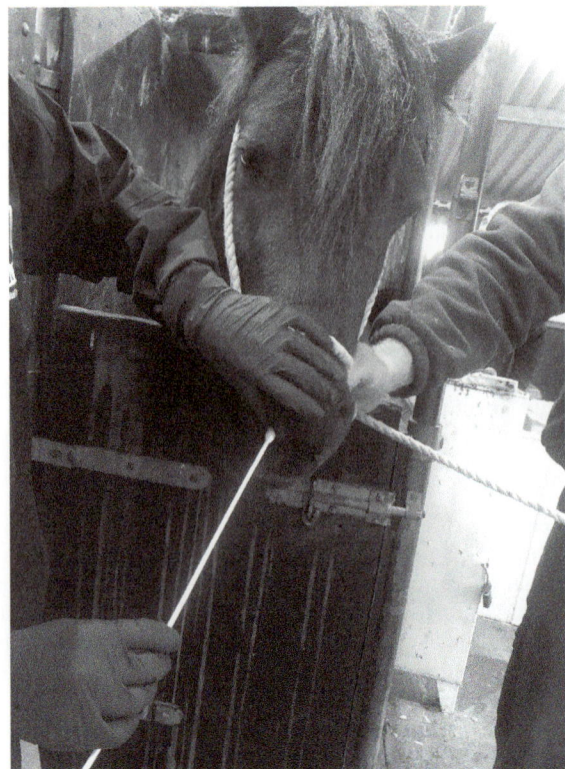

Figure 35.27 Inserting a nasopharyngeal swab into the nasal cavity.

regarding pre-breeding screening tests can be found in the Horserace Betting Levy Board Codes of Practice (HBLB 2019).

Urine sampling

Catheterisation of the bladder can be performed in males and females. Free catch samples are also possible (Figure 35.28).

Faecal sampling

If collection from the floor will not suffice or is not possible, faecal samples are best collected carefully per rectum: lubrication should be used, as horses have tight anal sphincters and care must be taken to not cause any damage to the rectum as such damage could be fatal. Extra restraint may be necessary, such as utilisation of stocks.

Administration of substances

Oral (paste/suspensions/granules/powders)

If they are palatable, administration of medicines in the feed is easy and involves no restraint of the horse, if the horse is kept individually. If the horse is in a herd group, oral formulations should be made into a paste and administered directly into the oral cavity by use of an oral syringe (Figure 35.29). If very large volumes of fluid must be

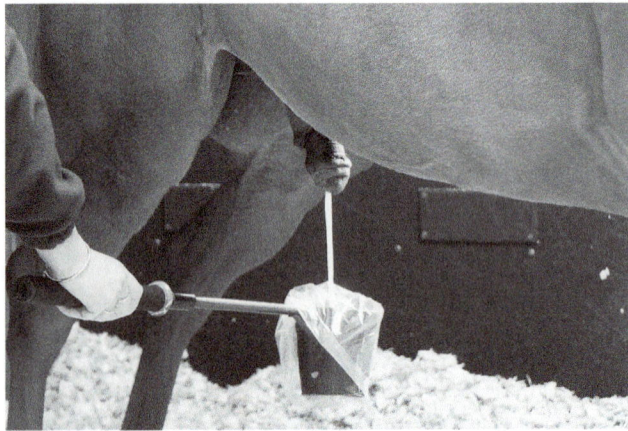

Figure 35.28 Free catch sample for urine collection.

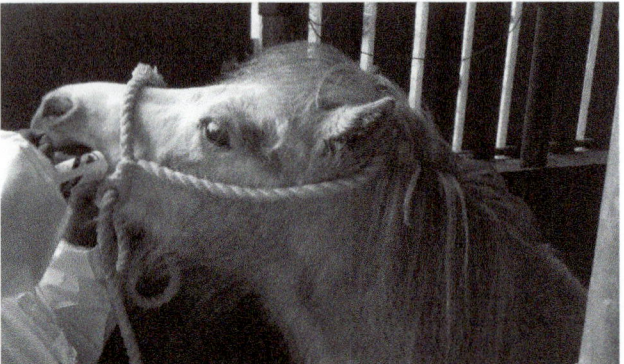

Figure 35.29 Administration of oral paste medication.

administered, this should be done using a nasogastric tube, by operators correctly trained in the procedure, in order to avoid accidental introduction of fluid into the lungs. This procedure may require prior sedation.

Intravenous

Products should first be confirmed to be safe for intravenous injection. Inadvertent intravenous administration of the wrong product could result in death. Intravenous access is achieved through use of the jugular vein, located in the jugular groove. Intravenous injection should only be performed by suitably trained/qualified personnel as inadvertent injection of the carotid artery is possible, which could result in death.

Intramuscular

The muscles of the neck (Figure 35.30), pectoral or gluteal muscles can be used for intramuscular injections. When several days' treatment is necessary, the injection site should be varied as sites can get sore. Occasionally, horses will develop stiffness/soreness following intramuscular injection into the neck, despite it being correctly sited: care should be taken to ensure that horses can reach their water buckets and feed mangers during this time. Complications post injection are possible and can include soreness, swelling or abscess formation. Severe site reactions should be investigated further by a veterinary surgeon. Injection into the pectorals may lead to dependent swellings, and occasionally, the horse is stiff when asked to move forward. The gluteal area is well muscled, has a good blood supply and is a good site for intramuscular injection of large volumes, despite the extra risk of kicks to the operator. Prior to injection, syringes should always be drawn back on when in the muscle, to ensure that needles are not inadvertently in a blood vessel, as many intramuscular products cannot be administered intravenously. Intramuscular injection should only be performed by suitably trained/ qualified personnel aware of the locations for injection, technique, safety for horse and personnel and potential side effects.

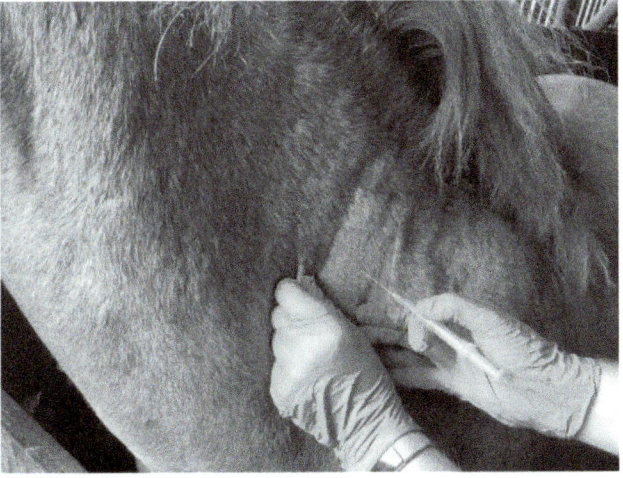

Figure 35.30 Administration of an intramuscular drug.

Subcutaneous

Through this route, products are administered under the skin. Not many products are administered through this route in the horse.

Intraocular

Administration of drugs into the eye may be necessary, for example, if a horse has a corneal ulcer. Care must be taken to not damage the cornea. The eye is held open with one gloved hand, and the eye medication is administered onto the surface of the eye. Applying the product at the medial canthus of the eye, into the ventral conjunctival sac, with the third eyelid across, protecting from inadvertent corneal damage, is the safest method. A horse may require further restraint through stocks or a twitch. Sedation may be necessary, but in such cases, due to the requirement of frequent applications, an indwelling ocular device called a 'sub-palpebral lavage system' would be applied by a veterinary surgeon, to facilitate administration.

Challenge with infectious agents

Challenge material should be transported in the correct manner, under controlled conditions. At the test site, operators must adhere to challenge safety regulations, including the wearing of a facemask to prevent inhalation of aerosolised microorganisms. The horse should be suitably restrained in the crush using a head collar and a twitch or sedation may be required to facilitate administration of the inoculum. The identification of the animal must be confirmed prior to challenge. Horses must be acclimatised to their new surroundings and the procedure prior to challenge. They usually remain quiet during the challenge procedure and are monitored throughout.

Challenge with a nasal tube

Measure the distance that the tube should be inserted by placing the end of the tubing half way between the eye and the nostril. Mark the tube with a marker pen at the nostril; this is the distance to insert into the nose, i.e. just at the border of the nasal passage and the nasopharynx. Approximately 15 ml of air should be drawn up into the syringe; then, the required volume of challenge material needs to be taken up into a sterile syringe with plastic tubing and nozzle already attached. Insert the nozzle up the required nostril until the mark on the tube is reached. Avoid entering the false nostril by keeping the direction of the tubing medial and ventral. Depress syringe plunger to spray inoculum around the nasal cavity using excess air in syringe to blow through and deliver the full inoculum. Finally, check all inoculum has been delivered. If some inoculum is remaining, remove the syringe, draw up 15 ml of air into the syringe and repeat.

Challenge by nebulisation

Carefully place the nebuliser over the horse's nose and mouth with the bottom exit valve open, so the horse can breathe normally. Push up until the nostrils are covered and

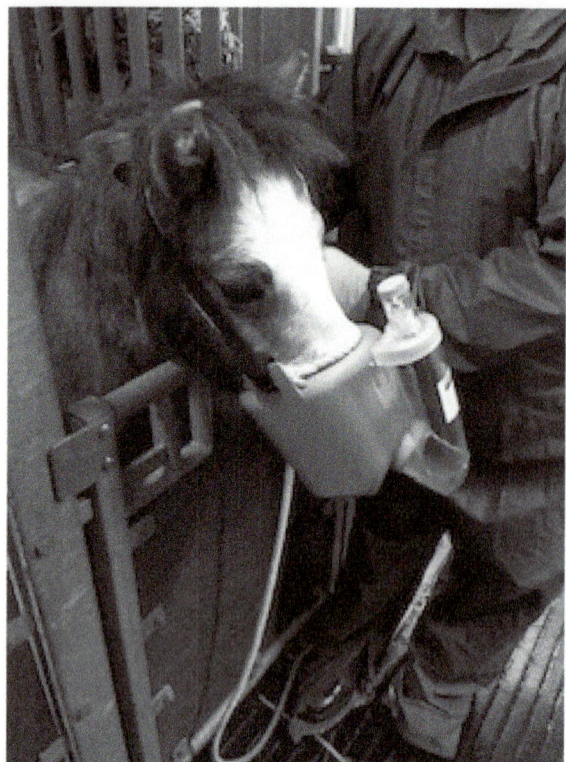

Figure 35.31 Challenge by nebulisation.

a seal is made around the nose and mouth (Figure 35.31). While the horse is getting used to the mask and breathing normally, shut the bottom valve by twisting the exit valve and commence treatment. Although the mask material is soft and flexible, the front aerosol chamber and battery controller is hard plastic; therefore, users should be mindful of the risk posed by the horse shaking its head with the nebuliser fitted. Fill the medication cup with the challenge dose/medication (up to 10 ml). Switch on the controller and nebulisation will begin after a few seconds. You will see the aerosol chamber fill with aerosol and empty when the horse inhales. Turn the controller off manually once the medication cup and aerosol chamber are empty. Horses should be habitualised to the nebuliser prior to challenge.

Euthanasia

Chemical euthanasia or penetrative captive bolt or gunshot are the most commonly utilised euthanasia methods. Chemical euthanasia drug availability and product type will depend on location. The majority of available chemical agents involve the overdose of a barbiturate. An example of an agent is a combination product containing a barbiturate (quinalbarbitone) and a local anaesthetic (cinchocaine hydrochloride) (Somulose, Dechra, UK). This is an optimal combination, with the barbiturate inducing a rapid loss of consciousness and cessation of respiration, while the local anaesthetic causes cardiac arrest. Other agents such as pentobarbitone only contain a barbiturate and, therefore, rely on cardiac arrest occurring secondary to profound hypoxia. A catheter should first be placed into the jugular vein as quantities of drugs administered are large volumes, given in one dose, with catheters ensuring safety for the horse and the operator (Cooney et al. 2012). A low dose of sedative may be administered prior to the euthanasia agent. All chemical methods of euthanasia render the carcass unsuitable for pet food manufacture. A free-bullet humane killer and a penetrative captive bolt are fast and efficient methods, in the hands of an experienced and appropriately trained and licensed person. Each method should only be performed by experienced personnel, and extreme care should be taken for personnel safety. Following application of the euthanasia method, death must be confirmed to ensure that the animal does not recover consciousness.

In a research environment, if euthanasia is the end point of the study, when two animals are left, it is often preferable that both animals are euthanised at the same time. For further reading on euthanasia of horses, see Knottenbelt (1995), the AVMA Guidelines for the Euthanasia of Animals (Leary et al. 2020) and Chapter 17 – Euthanasia and other fates for laboratory animals.

Management of horses in a containment facility

Infectious disease research may require the use of a containment facility designed to provide an environment to ensure all pathogens are contained within it. Challenge of animals with infectious material requires a level of containment appropriate to the pathogen concerned. Exemplary animal husbandry approaches are necessary to ensure minimal discomfort and stress to the animals involved in these studies.

Rooms within such facilities are sizeable, with handling systems to facilitate research procedures. Husbandry of animals in such environments is tailored to ensure optimal conditions for the horses involved, with continual monitoring and re-evaluation. Husbandry practices for each facility will be custom designed by the experienced personnel involved. Practices should include the use environmental enrichment, as discussed in the environmental enrichment section. An example of a room in a facility is shown in Figure 35.32.

Common diseases

Some of the more common diseases relevant to horses entering or participating in research programmes are listed in the following paragraphs and organised by body system affected. It is important that stable staff are aware of the main clinical signs of the more common diseases so that veterinary advice is sought promptly. More information can be found in *The Equine Manual* (Higgins & Snyder 2006).

Gastrointestinal system

Colic

Colic is the term used to describe pain arising from the gastrointestinal tract. All cases of colic should be regarded as potentially serious, and it is essential that a diagnosis is made swiftly and the appropriate treatment initiated (Southwood 2012). Cases of colic can be related to the effects of intestinal parasites, diet and feeding practices, changes in routine or sudden changes in weather. Some cases will have no obvious predisposing factor. Signs will vary according to

(a) 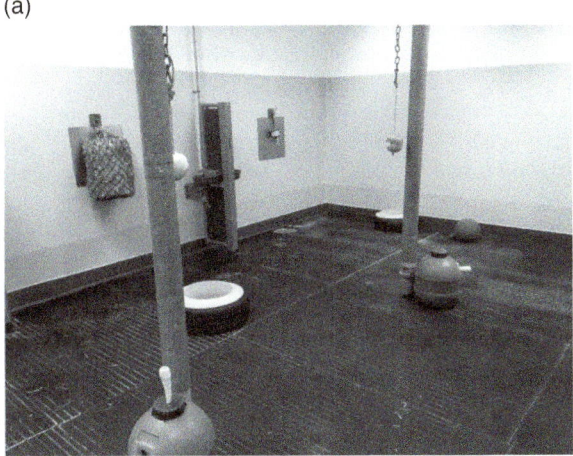 (b)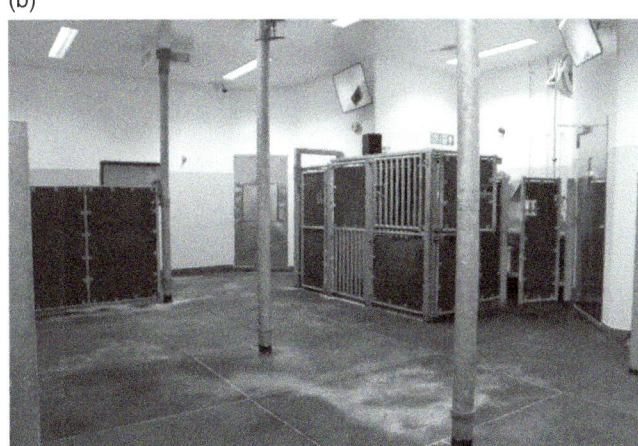

Figure 35.32 A room in a containment facility.

the type of colic, for example, whether impactive or spasmodic, and will also vary in intensity. Signs vary from mild, more subtle presentations such as depression, inappetence, scant faeces, restlessness, recumbency and flank watching, to severe signs such as rolling, scraping the floor with a foreleg, patchy sweating and kicking at the abdomen. Affected horses should be housed in a large loose box or cattle pen with a deep bed, the sides of which should be banked up along the walls. There should be no sharp projections and food should be withheld. Veterinary examination should be sought immediately, with a full veterinary work up performed including a full history, physical examination and rectal examination. Depending on findings, nasogastric intubation and diagnostic samples such as blood and peritoneal fluid may be taken. Information from these analyses is put together to reach a suspect or confirmed diagnosis (Archer 2017). Some diagnoses may require surgical correction. If diagnostics indicate that there is no requirement for immediate surgical intervention, medical treatment may be attempted, and this consists of the control of pain with NSAIDs or using compounds such as sedatives alone or in combination with synthetic opioids such as butorphanol, together with any specific therapy indicated by the cause of the colic. It is important to monitor cases frequently and record the vital signs (normal values in Table 35.1), so any deterioration can be detected in the early stages. The underlying causes, for example, endoparasitism or nutritional upset, should then be rectified to prevent further colic episodes.

Internal parasites

See Prevention of parasites (endoparasites) section for information on parasites and their prevention.

Oesophageal obstruction (choke)

Choke occurs when a blockage of food is present in a horse's oesophagus. This results in clinical signs of making multiple attempts to swallow, repeated neck extension, hypersalivation and bilateral nasal discharge. The majority of cases will resolve spontaneously after 30 min, and food and water should be withheld until the choke is resolved. If the case is unresolved, veterinary assistance should be sought. Potential secondary complications include aspiration pneumonia. Predisposing factors include feeding large sized or unsoaked food or poor dentition.

Ophthalmic

Ocular issues in horses are common, given the protrusion of their eyes. Any case that presents with signs of an ocular issue such as reddened conjunctiva, swollen eye, closed or partially closed eye, cloudy eye or ocular discharge, should have a veterinary examination. Conjunctivitis (Figure 35.33) is inflammation of the conjunctiva and can be primary or secondary to multiple causes such as ocular trauma or corneal ulceration (Brooks 2010). Primary conjunctivitis from a bacterial cause will require ocular administration of a broad-spectrum antibiotic. Other cases of conjunctivitis may be secondary to a corneal ulcer, with these requiring

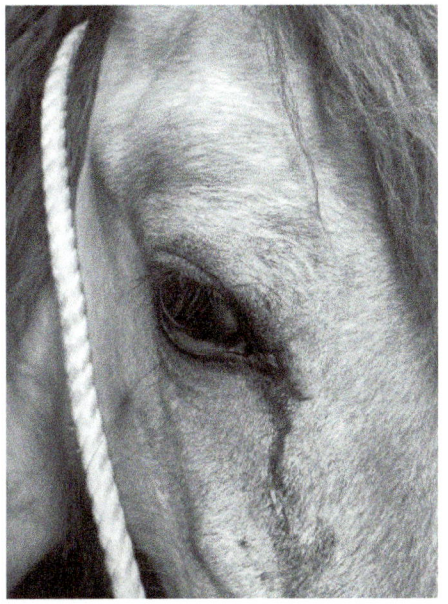

Figure 35.33 A case of conjunctivitis.

immediate treatment. Initial cause of an ulcer may be a result of trauma, but bacterial, fungal and viral corneal infections are possible as primary or secondary causes or an immune-mediated condition may be present (Hartley 2015). Finally, uveitis, or 'moon blindness' can cause severe ocular pain. This autoimmune condition can be chronic, is painful and could lead to blindness, so immediate vigorous veterinary treatment is required.

Respiratory system

Infectious causes of respiratory disease can spread rapidly through a population of horses, particularly when they share airspace and/or have direct horse-to-horse contact. Infectious respiratory diseases can also spread between horses, indirectly, via personnel and equipment. There are many preventative measures that can be taken to mitigate the risk of horses contracting infectious respiratory diseases including quarantine of new horses, laboratory screening new horses for infectious diseases prior to entering the resident herd and strict hygiene between groups of horses including hand washing and use of separate equipment. Vaccines are also available and should be used in conjunction with these other preventative measures. See Biosecurity section for further information. Potential infectious diseases will be country specific, and the most common infections will be discussed.

Viral causes

Infections with equine influenza or EHV-1 or EHV-4 are the more common causes of acute upper respiratory tract disease. Influenza occurs in susceptible horses of all ages, whereas herpesvirus infection is more common in young horses (Davis et al. 2014). Clinical signs of both can be similar and may include coughing, nasal discharge, inappetence, pyrexia and lethargy. Infection with EHV-1 may also cause neurological signs or abortion. Treatment includes rest, good nursing and may include antibiotics if secondary bacterial infection is involved. Prevention of influenza and EHV is possible by vaccination, though EHV vaccines are not universally available. Vaccination does not provide complete protection, so protocols for the prevention of infection are paramount, including those for new arrivals. To diagnose a suspect infectious disease case, a veterinary examination should be immediately sought, to enable a diagnosis to be reached and correct, effective preventative measures put in place.

Bacterial causes

Strangles is a bacterial infection of the upper respiratory tract caused by *Streptococcus equi*. The infection is often introduced when young horses and ponies from varying sources are bought in. Recovered animals may remain carriers for long periods of time, with no obvious clinical signs, and they are an important source of infection for in-contact animals hence the importance of isolation and a thorough clinical examination, including laboratory testing, of all newcomers. The main clinical signs of infection are loss of appetite, pyrexia, depression, serous or purulent nasal discharge and swelling and abscessation of the lymph nodes of the head and neck (Boyle et al. 2018). It is generally best to allow the infection to run its course as antibiotics will slow resolution of clinical signs. Good nursing is essential, and lancing and draining lymph node abscesses should be done by a veterinary surgeon as necessary.

Following a disease outbreak, because the organism is able to survive for weeks in pus, disinfection of stabling, feeding and watering equipment, and tack and grooming equipment is essential. Vaccines are available in some countries, but they do not completely prevent infection and have a short duration of action. Prevention of the introduction of carriers to a yard is essential to limit the spread of the infection, and there is a blood test available to screen horses for prior exposure to the bacteria, which is essential for new arrivals (Robinson et al. 2013). Other infectious bacterial causes include *Streptococcus zooepidemicus*, an opportunistic pathogen found in the nasopharynx. Clinical signs include nasal discharge, abscessation and coughing. Treatment may involve the judicious use of antibiotics.

Non-infectious

Allergic respiratory disease is an important and frequent cause of disease, particularly in stabled horses. A major drawback of all housing for horses is the potential for respiratory disease. The stabled horse is exposed to a variety of airborne contaminants (viruses, bacteria, fungal and actinomycete spores, dust mites, dust, dirt, noxious gases such as ammonia, and plant material). There are a few respiratory diseases that can affect horses, and these can be influenced by husbandry practices.

Recurrent airway obstruction (RAO) – referred to in the past as 'chronic obstructive pulmonary disease' – is a pulmonary (lower airway) hypersensitivity to inhaled allergens present in hay and straw (Couëtil et al. 2016). Horses affected can be any age, but the disease is more commonly diagnosed in middle-aged to old animals (7 years old or more). The allergens are the spores of fungi and actinomycetes, and these are the major constituents of respirable dust in stables. They are usually less than 5 μm in diameter and remain antigenic even when pathogens are no longer viable. Management is through optimal husbandry, but a veterinary examination may be necessary as additional medication may be required in some cases.

Another lower airway disease, distinct from RAO, but influenced by husbandry measures, is inflammatory airway disease (IAD), and it can affect horses of any age. In young horses, it is usually associated with bacterial infection; however, non-infectious IAD can occur in horses of all ages and ways of life (Allen & Franklin 2007). The specific cause of IAD is still unclear, and it is likely that several factors are involved. The section on optimising air quality in stables section in this chapter discusses these optimal husbandry practices further.

Musculoskeletal

Laminitis ('founder')

Laminitis is a common cause of lameness and disability in horses and ponies. It can affect both forefeet, both hindfeet, all of the feet or just one foot. The disease is metabolic in origin and is associated with numerous different risk factors such as: overfeeding of grain and concentrates to stabled horses; overfat, underexercised ponies grazing lush pasture; or elderly horses suffering from hormonal conditions such as equine metabolic syndrome or pituitary pars intermedia dysfunction (Cushing's disease). It can also be a complication of corticosteroid therapy, a sequel to systemic infections such as endometritis and enteritis or a sequel to stress. The extreme pain seen in the acute stage of the disease is caused by ischaemia of digital dermal tissue. Affected animals may throw their weight back on their heels or may rock back onto their hind feet if only both forefeet are affected, which is the most common presentation and are very reluctant to move. If permanent damage is to be avoided, veterinary assistance should be sought as soon as the lameness is noticed. Diagnosis may be by clinical signs alone, but utilising radiographs in the sub-acute and chronic stages provides invaluable information to assist treatment such as farriery. If a systemic illness such as endometritis is involved, then this must be treated immediately. Drugs to reduce hypertension and anxiety, such as ACP may be given. Analgesics such as NSAIDs are required, together with movement restriction, diet restriction, nursing and optimal farriery. Affected animals must be confined in a well-bedded loose box and provided with hoof support. Future prevention is by sensible feeding and grazing management and diagnosing and treating any other contributing factors (Menzies-Gow 2018).

Fracture

Acute, non-weight bearing lameness can be a result of a fracture. Veterinary assistance should be sought immediately as a non-weight bearing horse is an emergency. Unfortunately, numerous fractures are unable to be fixed as horses are not candidates for advanced surgeries as they cannot be maintained in recumbency. Therefore, cases may require euthanasia (Walmsley 1999).

Subsolar (foot) abscess

Subsolar abscesses are a build-up of purulent (pus) exudate within the hoof wall, and they often develop secondary to a defect in the white line of the hoof (where the sole of the hoof meets the wall of the hoof). They are the most common cause of acute non-weight bearing lameness in horses and require immediate treatment by a farrier or a veterinarian. Multiple factors may cause their development, and these include horse factors such as hoof quality, care and trauma (e.g. penetrating hoof wound) and environmental factors such as wet conditions and particular ground surface materials (Milner 2011).

Integument (skin)

Wounds   Horses are prone to traumatic injury as a result of the environment they live in and from other herd members. They have a relatively vulnerable anatomy increasing their risk for developing wounds, particular on the lower limbs. Small superficial wounds may not require treatment, but all wounds should be closely evaluated to establish if there is any damage to surrounding structures, including the possibility of joint involvement (with such cases being potentially life threatening and requiring immediate veterinary intervention). Veterinary advice should be sought to establish if further treatments are required such as suturing, antibiotics, bandaging or movement restriction (Caston 2012).

Skin infections   The more common skin infections are summarised in Table 35.8.

Miscellaneous

Amyloidosis   Although a rare clinical entity in the general horse population, amyloidosis is a frequent *post-mortem* finding in horses used for hyperimmune serum production, the liver and the spleen being the more commonly affected organs. Severe, serious liver (hepatic) disease is a potential cause of death in such horses, so on welfare and economic grounds, regular monitoring for evidence of any liver damage should be conducted. This may include blood

Table 35.8   Common skin infections of horses.

Common name/incidence	Cause	Lesions/signs	Treatment and control
Ringworm; more common in young horses/mixing of horses	*Trichophyton* and *Microsporum* species of fungi	Small tufts of hair agglutinated with serum, common in harness-abraded areas (tack can act as a fomite for spread)	Topical or systemic treatments available. Will self-cure in most cases with time. Disinfection of buildings, trailers, tack, clothing and grooming equipment. Potential for human infection (zoonotic)
Rain scald (body) and mud fever (legs); pastured ponies and horses in the winter months	*Dermatophilus congolensis* (bacterial infection)	Tufts of hair over crusts of exudate; pus underneath. Usually bilateral and symmetrical on back	House affected animals or provide with waterproof rugs if to remain at pasture. Clean area with topical antiseptics, e.g. dilute chlorhexidine. Mud fever on legs may benefit from clipping hair away
Sweet itch/summer itch; cases in summer	Hypersensitivity to midge saliva	Lesions at base of mane and tail head. Intense rubbing of affected areas (Marsella 2013)	Topical insect repellents. Fly rugs. House at dawn/dusk when midges are feeding
Pediculosis; all horses and ponies susceptible mainly in winter/late spring	Sucking and biting lice	Intense rubbing of infected areas (chest/hindlegs/neck). Weight loss/ill-thrift if extreme burden	Control with pour-on synthetic pyrethroid; repeat every 14 days until cured

samples to measure the levels of a liver enzyme, gamma-glutamyl transferase (GGT). Studies in hyperimmune serum-producing horses over a 5-year period have shown that GGT levels increase within 6–7 years of first starting the immunisation procedure and that constantly high values seemed to correlate with advanced liver amyloidosis (Abdelkader *et al.* 1991).

Equine pituitary pars intermedia dysfunction Equine pituitary pars intermedia dysfunction, sometimes referred to as 'Cushings', is a common progressive hormonal disorder of older horses (aged ≥15 years). Neuron degeneration causes an excessive production of hormones from the pituitary gland in the brain. The exact consequences of this hormone overproduction are not fully understood; however, clinical signs include laminitis, lethargy, muscle wastage, weight loss, changes in coat length or texture, delayed coat shedding and recurrent infections. Suspicious cases should be examined by a veterinary surgeon and diagnostic tests performed, oral medication is required to treat the condition and treatment is lifelong from diagnosis (McGowan *et al.* 2013).

Hyperlipaemia This is a disorder of lipid metabolism particularly seen in pony breeds, especially Shetland ponies. It is characterised by gross lipaemia (abnormally high concentration of lipids in the blood), elevated plasma triglyceride concentrations and fatty infiltration of body tissues leading to organ failure, especially of the liver and kidneys (Durham & Thiemann 2015). The most common clinical signs are anorexia and lethargy, and the mortality rate is high. Stress and obesity are important risk factors, and cases are commonly secondary to another underlying disease. Stressors include transportation, inclement weather and changes in management. The majority of affected ponies are in good or fat condition, and pregnant mares seem to be particularly susceptible. Diagnosis can be confirmed by measuring plasma triglyceride concentrations. Treatment involves identifying and treating any underlying disease predisposing to hyperlipaemia. High-energy diets should be fed, as the animals are in negative energy balance. Hyperlipaemia is very serious, and treatment should be directed by a veterinary surgeon.

Tetanus (lock jaw) The causal agent is *Clostridium tetani*, a Gram-positive spore-forming bacillus present in soil and as a commensal in the gastrointestinal tract. The spores can survive for years in the environment. The disease is mainly seen following skin puncture wounds, as the anaerobic conditions in devitalised tissue provide the ideal environment for the spores to generate and release a neurotoxin (MacKay 2014). Clinical signs are extreme and include difficulty eating, muscle stiffness or spasms, protrusion of the third eye lid, collapse and death. Treatment is often difficult and unsuccessful. It is imperative to vaccinate horses against the disease and in countries where vaccination is common the disease is rare. It is essential that tetanus antitoxin is administered following injury if the horse's vaccination history is unknown. Mares are usually given a booster vaccination 1 month prior to the anticipated date of foaling: their foals are then passively protected from infection via antibodies in the colostrum for about 3 months, after which they can start their active immunisation programme. Foals born to unvaccinated mares should be given tetanus antitoxin at birth and 6 weeks later. The timing of the start of a foal's active immunisation programme will depend on the vaccine being used. The manufacturer's datasheet should be consulted for the optimum time to start. After the initial vaccine course, booster vaccinations are usually given every 2–3 years.

Acknowledgement

This chapter is updated, but based on the chapter previously written by Elizabeth Abbott published in the seventh edition of the handbook and the updated chapter by Fernando Montesso in the eighth edition of the handbook. Their substantial contribution is gratefully acknowledged.

Further reading

Useful sources of general information on equine behaviour, care and breeding can be found in Houpt (2018); Warren Evans (1992) Mills and Nankervis (1999) and Higgins and Snyder (2006). Specific information on the care of horses used in research can be found in the Guide for the Care and Use of Agricultural Animals in Research and Teaching (American Society of Animal Science 2020).

References

Abdelkader, S.V., Gudding, R.J. and Nordstoga, K. (1991) Clinical chemical constituents in relation to liver amyloidosis in serum producing horses. *Journal of Comparative Pathology*, **105**, 203–211.

Allen, K. and Franklin, S. (2007) RAO and IAD: respiratory disease in horses revisited. *In Practice*, **29**, 76–82.

Aleman, M., Williams, D.C. and Holliday, T. (2008) Sleep and sleep disorders in horses. *Proceedings of the American Association of Equine Practitioners*, **54**, 180–185.

American Society of Animal Science (2020). *Guide for the Care and Use of Agricultural Animals in Research and Teaching*, 4th edn. https://www.asas.org/docs/default-source/default-document-library/agguide_4th.pdf?sfvrsn=56b44ed1_2 (accessed October 25, 2023).

Archer, D.C. (2017) Equine colic: putting the puzzle together. *Veterinary Record*, **181**, 289–290.

Bain, A.M. and Howey, W.P. (1975) Observations on the time of foaling in Thoroughbred mares, *Australian Journal of Reproduction and Fertility, Supplement*, **23**, 545–546.

Bertone, J.J. (2015) Sleep and sleep disorders in horses. In: *Equine Neurology*, Eds. Furr, M. and Reed, S. Wiley, Ames, Iowa.

Birke, L., Hockenhull, J., Creighton, E., *et al.* (2011) Horses' responses to variation in human approach. *Applied Animal Behavioural Science*, **134**, 56–63.

Bonin, S.J., Clayton, H.M., Lanovaz, J.L. and Johnston, T. (2007) Comparison of mandibular motion in horses chewing hay and pellets. *Equine Veterinary Journal*, **39**, 258–262.

Bowen, I.M., Redpath, A., Dugdale, A., *et al.* (2020), BEVA primary care clinical guidelines: Analgesia. *Equine Veterinary Journal*, 52: 13–27.

Boyle, A.G., Timoney, J.F., Newton, J.R. *et al.* (2018) Streptococcus equi infections in horses: guidelines for treatment, control, and prevention of strangles-revised consensus statement. *Journal of Veterinary Internal Medicine*, **32**, 633–647.

British Horse Society (BHS) (2005) Guidelines for the keeping of horses: stable sizes, pasture acreages and fencing. BHS welfare department: http://www.bhs.org.uk/~/media/BHS/Files/PDF%20Documents/Guide%20for%20the%20Keeping%20of%20Horses.ashx (accessed 30 July 2019).

Brooks, D.E. (2010) *Equine Veterinary Education*, **22**, 382–386.

Butler, K.D. (1992) Foot care. In: *Horse Breeding and Management*, Ed. Warren Evans, J., pp. 177–205. Elsevier, London.

Byers, J.A. (1998) Biological effects of locomotor play: getting into shape, or something more specific? In: *Animal Play – Evolutionary, Comparative and Ecological Perspectives*, Eds. Bekoff, M. and Byers, J.A., pp. 205–220. Cambridge University Press, Cambridge.

Carson, K. and Wood-Gush, D.G.M. (1983) Equine behaviour: I. A review of the literature on social and dam – foal behavior. *Applied Animal Ethology*, **10**, 165–178.

Caston, S.S. (2012) Wound Care in Horses. *Veterinary Clinics of North America: Equine Practice*, **28**, 83–100.

Clark, D.K., Friend, T.H. and Dellmeier, G. (1993) The effect of orientation during trailer transport on heart rate, cortisol, and balance in horses. *Applied Animal Behaviour Science*, **38**, 179–189.

Clements, J.M. and Pirie, R.S. (2007) Respirable dust concentrations in equine stables. Part 2: the benefits of soaking hay and optimising the environment in a neighbouring stable. *Research in Veterinary Science*. **83**, 263–268.

Cohen, N.D. and Peloso, J.G. (1995) Risk factors for history of previous colic and for chronic, intermittent colic in a population of horses. *Journal of the American Veterinary Medical Association*, **208**, pp. 607–703.

Collins, M.N., Friend, T.H., Jousan, F.D. *et al.* (2000) *Applied Animal Behaviour Science*, **67**, 169–179.

Cooney, K.A., Chappell, J.R., Callan, R.J. and Connally, B.A. (2012) *Veterinary Euthanasia Techniques: A Practical Guide.* John Wiley & Sons, Chicester, UK.

Couëtil, L.L., Cardwell, J.M., Gerber, V. *et al.* (2016). Inflammatory airway disease of horses – revised consensus statement. *Journal of Veterinary Internal Medicine*, **30**, 503–515.

Crowell-Davis, S.L. (1986) Developmental behaviour. In: *Veterinary Clinics of North America: Equine Practice*, **2**, 573–590.

Cymbaluk, N.F. and Christison, G.I. (1990) Environmental effects on thermoregulation and nutrition of horses. *Veterinary Clinics of North America: Equine Practice*, **6**, 355–372.

Dalefield, R. (2017) Agricultural and feed-related toxicants. In: *Veterinary Toxicology for Australia and New Zealand*, pp. 343–360. Elsevier, Amsterdam.

Dalla Costa, E., Dai, F., Lebelt, D., *et al.* (2016). Welfare assessment of horses: the AWIN approach. *Animal Welfare*, **25**(4), 481–488.

Dauvillier, J, Woort, F. and van Erck-Westergren, E. (2019) Fungi in respiratory samples of horses with inflammatory airway disease. *Journal of Veterinary Internal Medicine*, **33**, 968–975.

Davis, E.G., Freeman, D.E. and Hardy, J. (2014) Respiratory infections. In: *Equine Infectious Diseases*, 2nd edn, Eds. Sellon, D.C. and Long, M., pp. 1–21. W.B. Saunders, St Louis, Missouri.

DEFRA (2017) Code of Practice for the Welfare of Horses, Ponies, Donkeys and their Hybrids, Crown. Update available at https://assets.publishing.service.gov.uk/government/uploads/system/uploads/attachment_data/file/700200/horses-welfare-codes-of-practice-april2018.pdf/ (accessed 22 March 2019).

DEFRA (2018) Equine Identification (England) Regulations 2018. Available at https://www.legislation.gov.uk/uksi/2018/761/memorandum/contents (accessed 23 March 2019).

de Grauw, J.C. and van Loon, J.P. (2016) Systematic pain assessment in horses. *The Veterinary Journal*, 209, 14–22.

Driessen, B., Zarucco, L., Kalir, B. and Bertolotti, L. (2010) Contemporary use of acepromazine in the anaesthetic management of male horses and ponies: a retrospective study and opinion poll. *Equine Veterinary Journal*, 43, 88–98.

Dugdale, A.H.A., Curtis, G.C., Cripps, P.J., *et al.* (2010) Effect of dietary restriction on body condition, composition and welfare of overweight and obese pony mares. *Equine Veterinary Journal*, 42, 600–610.

Dugdale, A.H. and Taylor, P.M. (2016) Equine anaesthesia-associated mortality: where are we now? *Veterinary Anaesthesia and Analgesia*, 43, 242–255.

Durham, A.E. and Thiemann, A.K. (2015) Nutritional management of hyperlipaemia, *Equine Veterinary Education*, 27, 482–488.

Ellis, A.D. (2013) Energy systems and requirements. In: *Equine Applied and Clinical Nutrition*, Eds. Gear, R.J., Harris, P.A. and Coenen, M., pp. 96–112. Saunders, Edinburgh.

European Medicines Agency (2016) Guideline for good clinical practice – E6 (R2) *ICH Harmonised Tripartite Guideline*, pp. 1–70.

European Parliament and the Council of the European Union. (2010) Directive 2010/63/EU of the European Parliament and of the Council of 22 September 2010 on the protection of animals used for scientific purposes. *Official Journal of the European Union L 276*, 53, 33–79. https://eur-lex.europa.eu/LexUriServ/LexUriServ.do?uri=OJ:L:2010:276:0033:0079:en:PDF (accessed 3rd March 2022).

Flecknell, P. (2002) Replacement, Reduction, Refinement, *ALTEX – Alternatives to animal experimentation*, **19**, 73–78. Available at: https://www.altex.org/index.php/altex/article/view/1106 (accessed 25 July 2019).

Fritzen, B., Rohn, K., Schnieder, T. *et al.* (2010) Endoparasite control management on horse farms – lessons from worm prevalence and questionnaire data. *Equine Veterinary Journal*, **42**, 79–83.

Geor, R.J., Harris, P.A. and Coenen, M. (2013) *Equine Applied and Clinical Nutrition*, Eds. Gear, R.J., Harris, P.A. and Coenen, M., pp. i–iii. Saunders, Edinburgh.

Geor, RJ and Harris, P.A (2014) Nutrition for the equine athlete: above and beyond nutrients alone. In: *Equine Sports Medicine and Surgery (Second Edition)*, pp. 819–834. Saunders, Philadelphia.

Geor, R.J. (2017) Internal medicine and clinical nutrition. In: *Equine Internal Medicine*, 4th edn, pp. 191–217. Saunders, Edinburgh.

Glunk, E.C., Hathaway, M.R., Weber, W.J. *et al.* (2014) The effect of hay net design on rate of forage consumption when feeding adult horses. *Journal of Equine Veterinary Science*, **34**, 986–999.

Giles, S.L., Nicol, C.J., Harris, P.A. and Rands, S.A. (2015) Dominance rank is associated with body condition in outdoor-living domestic horses (*Equus caballus*). *Applied Animal Behavioural Science*, **166**, 71–79.

Goodwin, D., Davidson, H.P. and Harris, P. (2002) Foraging enrichment for stabled horses: effects on behaviour and selection. *Equine Veterinary Journal*, **34**, 686–691.

Goodwin, D. and Hughes, C.F. (2005) Equine play behaviour. In: *The Domestic Horse: The Evolution, Development and Management of its Behaviour*, Eds. Mills, D.S. and McDonnell, S.M., pp. 150–157. Cambridge University Press, Cambridge.

Hanggi, E.B., & Ingersoll, J.F. (2012). Lateral vision in horses: A behavioral investigation. *Behavioural Processes*, **91**(1), 70–76.

Hartley, C. (2015) Differential diagnosis and management of corneal ulceration in horses, part 2. *In Practice*, **37**, 23–30.

Hausberger, M., Fureix, C., Bourjade, M., *et al.* (2012) On the significance of adult play: what does social play tell us about adult horse welfare? *Die Naturwissenschaften*, **99**, 291–302.

Henneke, D.R., Potter, G.D., Kreider, J.L. and Yeates, B.F. (1983) Relationship between condition score, physical measurements and body fat percentage in mares. *Equine Veterinary Journal*, **15**, 371–372.

Higgins, A.J. and Snyder, J.R. (2006) *The Equine Manual*. Saunders Elsevier, Philadelphia

Hintz, H.F. and Cymbaluk, N.R. (1994) Nutrition of the horse. *Annual Reviews of Nutrition*, **14**, 243–267.

Home Office (2014a) Home Office Code of Practice for the housing and care of animals used in scientific procedures, HMSO London. 2014 update available at https://assets.publishing.service.gov.uk/government/uploads/system/uploads/attachment_data/file/388895/COPAnimalsFullPrint.pdf/ (accessed 22 March 2019).

Home Office (2014b) Guidance on the Operation of the Animals (Scientific Procedures) Act 1986. https://assets.publishing.service.gov.uk/government/uploads/system/uploads/attachment_data/file/662364/Guidance_on_the_Operation_of_ASPA.pdf (accessed August 2022).

Home Office (2015) Advice Note: 03/2015 Animals (Scientific Procedures) Act 1986 Re-homing and setting free of animals. https://assets.publishing.service.gov.uk/government/uploads/system/uploads/attachment_data/file/660241/Advice_Note_Rehoming_setting_free.pdf (accessed August 2022).

Horserace Betting Levy Board Codes of Practice (2019) https://codes.hblb.org.uk/index.php/page/19 (accessed 11 July 2019).

Houpt, K.A. (1991) Animal behaviour and animal welfare. *Journal of the American Veterinary Medical Association*, **198**, 1355–1360.

Houpt, K.A. (1992) Horse behaviour. In: *Horse Breeding and Management*. Ed. Warren Evans, J., pp. 63–83. Elsevier, London.

Houpt, K.A. (2018) *Domestic Animal Behaviour for Veterinarians and Animal Scientists*, 5th edition. Wiley-Blackwell, Ames, Iowa.

Houpt, K.A., Law, K. and Martinisi, V. (1978) Dominance hierarchies in domestic horses. *Applied Animal Ethology*, **4**, 273–283.

Houpt, K.A., Marrow, M. and Seeliger, M. (2000) A preliminary study of the effect of music on equine behaviour. *Journal of Equine Veterinary Science*, **20**, 691–737.

International Society for Equitation Science (ISES). (2019) Position statement on the use/misuse of leadership and dominance concepts in horse training. https://equitationscience.com/equitation/position-statement-on-the-use-misuse-of-leadership-and-dominance-concepts-in-horse-training (accessed 25 July 2019).

Jeffcott, L.B. (1974) Some practical aspects of the transfer of passive immunity to newborn foals. *Equine Veterinary Journal*, **6**, 503–509.

Johnson, P.J., Wiedmeyer C.E., Messer N.T. and Ganjam V.K. (2009) Medical implications of obesity in horses–lessons for human obesity. *Journal of Diabetes Science and Technology*, **3**, 163–174.

Jones, R.S. (2001) Editorial II. *British Journal of Anaesthesia*, **87**, 813–815.

Joint Working Group on Refinement (1993) First Report of the BVA/FRAME/RSPCA/UFAW Joint Working Group on Refinement. *Laboratory Animals*, **27**, 1–22.

Keiper, R.R. (1986) Social structure. *Veterinary Clinics of North America: Equine Practice*, **2**, 465–484.

Keiper, R. and Receveur, H. (1992) Social interactions of free-ranging Przewalski horses in semi-reserves in The Netherlands. *Applied Animal Behavioural Science*, **33**, 303–318.

Kleijn, W.M. and Sloet van Oldruitenborgh-Oosterbaan, M.M. (2009) Measuring the height at the withers of ponies at a competition and at home using a laser device. *The Veterinary Journal*, **182**, 193–197.

Knottenbelt, D. (1995) Euthanasia of horses – alternatives to the bullet. *In Practice*, **17**, 464–465.

Knych, H.K. (2017) Nonsteroidal anti-inflammatory drug use in horses. *Veterinary Clinics of North America: Equine Practice*, **33**, 1–15.

Kohnke, J. (1992) *Feeding and Nutrition: The Making of a Champion*, pp. 163–166. Birubi Pacific, Australia.

Lawrence, L.M. (2013) Feeding stallions and broodmares. In: *Equine Applied and Clinical Nutrition*, pp. 231–242. Saunders.

https://www.avma.org/sites/default/files/2020-02/Guidelines-on-Euthanasia-2020.pdf (accessed 26 October, 2023)

Leary, S. Underwood, W., Anthony, R. et al. (2020) *AVMA Guidelines for the Euthanasia of Animals: 2020 Edition*. American Veterinary Medical Association.

Lightbody, K.L., Matthews, J.B., Kemp-Symonds, J.G., et al. (2018) Use of a saliva-based diagnostic test to identify tapeworm infection in horses in the UK. *Equine Veterinary Journal*, **50**, 213–219.

Luthersson, N., Nielsen, K.H., Harris, P. and Parkin, T.D. (2009) Risk factors associated with equine gastric ulceration syndrome (EGUS) in 201 horses in Denmark. *Equine Veterinary Journal*, **41**, 625–630.

Lyons, E.T., Drudge, J.H. and Tolliver, S.C. (2000) Larval cyathostomiasis. *Veterinary Clinics of North America: Equine Practice*, **16**, 501–513.

MacKay, R.J. (2014) Tetanus. In: *Equine Infectious Diseases*, 2nd edn, Eds. Sellon, D.C. and Long, M., pp. 368–372. W.B. Saunders, St Louis, Missouri.

McAfee, L.M., Mills, D.S. and Cooper, J.J. (2002) The use of mirrors for the control of stereotypic weaving behaviour in the stabled horse. *Applied Animal Behaviour Science*, **78**, 159–173.

McFadzean, W. and Love, E. (2017) How to do equine anaesthesia in the field. *In Practice*, **39**, 452–461.

McGowan, T.W., Pinchbeck, G.P. and McGowan, C.M. (2013) Prevalence, risk factors and clinical signs predictive for equine pituitary pars intermedia dysfunction in aged horses. *Equine Veterinary Journal*, **45**, 74–79.

McGreevy, P.D., Cripps, P.J., French, N.P., et al. (1995) Management factors associated with stereotypic and redirected behaviour in the Thoroughbred horse. *Equine Veterinary Journal*, **27**, 86–91.

McGreevy, P.D. and Nicol, C.J. (1998) Prevention of crib-biting: a review. *Equine Veterinary Journal Supplement*, **27**, 35–38.

McGreevy, P.D., Richardson, J.D., Nicol, C.J. et al. (1995) Radiographic and endoscopic study of horses performing and oral based stereotypy. *Equine Veterinary Journal*, **27**, 92–95.

Menzies-Gow, N. (2018) Laminitis in horses. *In Practice*, **40**, 411–419.

Mellor, D.J. (2017). Operational details of the five domains model and its key applications to the assessment and management of animal welfare. *Animals*, **7**, 60.

Metcalf, E.S. (2011) Venereal disease. In: *Equine Reproduction*, 2nd edn, Eds. McKinnon, A.O., Squires, E.L.M., Vaala, W.E. and Varner, D.D., pp. 1250–1258. Wiley-Blackwell, Chichester, UK.

Michou, J. and Leece, E. (2012) Sedation and analgesia in the standing horse 1. Drugs used for sedation and systemic analgesia. *In Practice*, **34**, 524–531.

Mills, D.S. and Clarke, A. (2007) Housing, management and welfare. In: *The Welfare of Horses*. Ed. Warran, N., pp. 77–97. Springer, Dordrecht, The Netherlands.

Mills, D.S. and Nankervis, K.J. (1999) *Equine Behaviour: Principles and Practice*. Blackwell Publishing, Oxford.

Milner, P.I. (2011) Diagnosis and management of solar penetrations. *Equine Veterinary Education*, **23**, 142–147.

Moore-Colyer, M.J., Lumbis, K., Longland, A. and Harris, P. (2014) The effect of five different wetting treatments on the nutrient content and microbial concentration in hay for horses. *PloS one*, **9**, 1–14.

Muylle, S. (2005) Chapter 5 – Aging. In: *Equine Dentistry*, 2nd edn, Eds. Baker, G. and Easley, J., pp. 55–66. W.B. Saunders, Philadelphia.

National Research Council (2007) *Nutrient Requirements of Horses*, 6th edn. National Academies Press, Washington DC.

Newcombe, J.R. and Nout, Y.S. (1998) Apparent effect of management on the hour of parturition in mares. *The Veterinary Record*, **142**, 221–222.

Nicol, C.J., Davidson, H.P.D., Harris, P.A. et al. (2002) Study of crib-biting and gastric inflammation and ulceration in young horses. *The Veterinary Record*, **151**, 658–662.

Nielsen, M.K. and Reinemeyer, C.R. (2018) Biology and life cycles of equine parasites. In: *Handbook of Equine Parasite Control*, 2nd edn. John Wiley & Sons, Hoboken, NJ.

Nielsen, M.K., Mittel, L., Grice, A., *et al.* (2012) AAEP Parasite Control Guidelines. *AAEP Proceedings*, pp. 1–24.

O'Grady, S.E. (2009) Guidelines for trimming the equine foot: A review. *Proceedings American Association of Equine Practitioners*, **55**, 218–225

Ott, E.A. (1992) Nutrition. In: *Horse Breeding and Management*. Ed. Warren Evans, J., pp. 337–368. Elsevier, London.

Peregrine, A.S., Molento, M.B., Kaplan, R.M. and Nielsen, M.K. (2014) Anthelmintic resistance in important parasites of horses: does it really matter? *Veterinary Parasitology*, **201**, 1–8.

Pratt-Phillips, S.E. and Lawrence, L.M. (2014) Nutrition of the performance horse. In: *The Athletic Horse (Second Edition)*, Eds. Hodgson, D.R., McKeever, K.H. and McGowan, C.M., pp. 34–55. Saunders, St Louis, Missouri.

Raidal, S.E., Love, D.N. and Bailey, G.D. (1996) Effects of posture and accumulated airway secretions on tracheal mucociliary transport in the horse. *Australian Veterinary Journal*, **73**, 45–49.

Ralston, S.L., Foster, D.L., Divers, T. and Hintz, H.F. (2001) Effect of dental correction on feed digestibility in horses. *Equine Veterinary Journal*, **33**, 390–393.

Robinson, C., Steward, K.F., Potts, N., *et al.* (2013) Combining two serological assays optimises sensitivity and specificity for the identification of *Streptococcus equi* subsp. equi exposure. *The Veterinary Journal*, **197**, 188–191.

Rossdale, P.D. (1993) Clinical view of disturbances in equine foetal maturation. *Equine Veterinary Journal*, **14**, 3–7.

Sanchez, C.L. (2018) Chapter 12 – Disorders of the gastrointestinal system. In: *Equine Internal Medicine*, 4th edn, Eds. Reed, S.M., Bayly, W.M. and Sellon, D.C., pp. 709–842. W.B. Saunders, St Louis, Missouri.

Sallé, G., Cortet, J., Bois, I. *et al.* (2017) Risk factor analysis of equine strongyle resistance to anthelmintics. *International Journal for Parasitology: Drugs and Drug Resistance*, **7**, 407–415.

Schjelderup-Ebbe, T. (1922) Beiträge zur Sozialpsychologie des Haushuhns [Observation on the social psychology of domestic fowls]. *Zeitschrift für Psychologie und Physiologie der Sinnesorgane. Abt. 1. Zeitschrift für Psychologie*, **88**, 225–252.

Sharp, D.C. (1992) Pregnant mare and Jenny. In: *Horse Breeding and Management*. Ed. Warren Evans, J., pp. 299–323. Elsevier, London.

Simpson, D.J., Greenwood, R.E.S., Ricketts, S.W., *et al.* (1982) Use of ultrasound echography for early diagnosis of single and twin pregnancy in the mare. *Journal of Reproduction and Fertility Supplement*, **32**, 431–439.

Smith, B.L., Jones, J.H., Carlson, G.P. *et al.* (1994) Body position and direction preferences in horses during road transport. *Equine Veterinary Journal*, **26**, 374–377.

Southwood, L. (2012) *Practical Guide to Equine Colic*. John Wiley & Sons, Ames, Iowa.

St Clair, L.E. (1975) Teeth. In: *Sisson and Grossman's the Anatomy of the Domestic Animals*, 5th edn, Vol. 1, Ed. Getty, R., pp. 460–470. WB Saunders, Philadelphia.

Sweeting, M.P., Houpt, C.E. and Houpt, K.A. (1985) Social facilitation of feeding and time budgets in stabled ponies. *Journal of Animal Science*, **60**, 369–374.

Toscano, M.J. and Friend, T.H. (2001) A note on the effects of forward and rear-facing orientations on movement of horses during transport. *Applied Animal Behaviour Science*, **73**, 281–287.

Thompson, D.L. (1992) Reproductive physiology of the stallions and jack. In: *Horse Breeding and Management*. Ed. Warren Evans, J., pp. 237–261. Elsevier, London.

Tyler, S.J. (1972) The behaviour and social organization of the New Forest Ponies. *Animal Behaviour Monograph*, **5**, 5–196.

Van Dierendonck, M.C., De Vries, H. and Schilder, M.B.H. (1994) An analysis of dominance, its behavioural parameters and possible determinants in a herd of Icelandic horses in captivity. *Netherlands Journal of Zoology*, **45**, 362–385.

Van Loon, J.P.A.M. and Van Dierendonck, M.C. (2018). Objective pain assessment in horses (2014–2018). *The Veterinary Journal*, **242**, 1–7.

van NieKerk, C.H. (1992) Non pregnant mare and jenny. In: *Horse Breeding and Management*. Ed. Warren Evans, J., pp. 263–297. Elsevier, London.

Walmsley, J. (1999) Emergency management of fractures in horses. *In Practice*, **21**, 122–127.

Waran, N.K., Robertson, V., Cuddeford, D. *et al.* (1996) Effects of transporting horses facing either forwards or backwards on their behaviour and heart rate. *The Veterinary Record*, **139**, 7–11.

Warren Evans, J. (ed) (1992) *Horse Breeding and Management*. Elsevier, London.

Webster, A.J.F., Clarke, A.F., Madelin, T.M. *et al.* (1987) Air hygiene in stables. 1: Effects of stable design, ventilation and management on the concentration of respirable dust. *Equine Veterinary Journal*, **19**, 448–453.

Non-Human Primates

36 The mouse lemurs

Jennifer Wittkowski, Annette Klein, Annika Kollikowski, Marina Scheumann, Daniel Schmidtke, Elke Zimmermann† and Ute Radespiel

General biology

Taxonomy

Mouse lemurs (*Microcebus* spp.) form one genus within the family of the Cheirogaleidae that belongs to the 100% endemic lemurs (infraorder: Lemuriformes) of Madagascar and, thereby, to the primate suborder Strepsirrhini. Until the early 1990s, only two species of mouse lemurs were scientifically recognised, the grey mouse lemur (*Microcebus murinus*, J.F. Miller) from western and southern Madagascar and the rufous mouse lemur (*M. rufus*, E. Geoffroy) from the East (reviewed in Groves 2016). Facilitated by rapid developments in molecular techniques, 23 new mouse lemur species from various places across the island were described between 1994 and 2020, making *Microcebus* the second most speciose genus among lemurs. Mouse lemurs are cryptic species (Zimmermann & Radespiel 2014), and species descriptions were, therefore, mainly based on phylogenetic analyses of mitochondrial sequence data that were complemented by some phenotypic data, mostly on colouration and morphometric body dimensions, such as body length, tail length, lower leg length, hind foot length, head length and width, ear length and width, and body mass (Schmid & Kappeler 1994; Zimmermann *et al.* 1998; Rasoloarison *et al.* 2000; Yoder *et al.* 2000; Kappeler *et al.* 2005; Andriantompohavana *et al.* 2006; Louis *et al.* 2006; Olivieri *et al.* 2007; Louis *et al.* 2008; Radespiel *et al.* 2008; Radespiel *et al.* 2012; Rasoloarison *et al.* 2013; Hotaling *et al.* 2016). Mouse lemur species can differ considerably in their body dimensions. In the wild, average adult body mass can range from 30 ± 3.2 g (mean ± SD, *M. berthae*, Atsalis *et al.* 1996) to 78 ± 12.8 g (mean ± SD, *M. marohita*, Rasoloarison *et al.* 2013) and average tail lengths from 115 ± 5.2 mm (mean ± SD, *M. lehilahytsara*, Randrianambinina 2001) to 161 ± 8.8 mm (mean ± SD, *M. danfossi*, Olivieri *et al.* 2007). Due to their small body size and their unspecialised lifestyle, mouse lemurs are often regarded as a good model for the ancestral primate condition (e.g. Cartmill 1972; Martin 1990) but see also Andrews *et al.* (2016).

Ecology

Mouse lemurs are nocturnal and the smallest-bodied primates (Mittermeier *et al.* 2010; Fleagle 2014). As quadrupedal runners and leapers (Martin 1990), they inhabit various types of tropical forests on the island of Madagascar, from xerophytic (i.e., dry adapted) or spiny forests in the south and southwest to dry deciduous forests of the west and north to the low-, mid- and high-altitude rainforest of the east, north and the Sambirano region (Mittermeier *et al.* 2010; Rasoazanabary & Godfrey 2016). Some species are also found in forest fragments (Ganzhorn *et al.* 2013; Lehman *et al.* 2016; Steffens & Lehman 2016) and heavily anthropogenically disturbed forests (e.g. Ganzhorn *et al.* 2013). So far, it is unknown whether they can establish self-sustaining populations in such disturbed environments.

The best studied mouse lemur species, both in nature and in captivity, is the grey mouse lemur (*M. murinus*). It is also the species most commonly used in laboratory research (see section on Uses in research later in this chapter). This species has the broadest geographical distribution among mouse lemurs, from the northwest to the southeast, spanning various forest types from dry deciduous to riparian (i.e. along riverbanks) and littoral forests and is, thus, described as an ecological generalist (Pechouskova *et al.* 2015). It partially overlaps in distribution in the northwest and west with some of the rufous-coloured mouse lemur species and in the south and southeast (see Figure 36.1) with another grey-coloured species (*M. griseorufus*). All species besides *M. murinus*, such as the Goodman's mouse lemur (*M. lehilahytsara*), the golden-brown mouse lemur (*M. ravelobensis*) or the Berthae's mouse lemur (*M. berthae*), display a more local or regional range and are, thus, regarded as ecological specialists (Pechouskova *et al.* 2015; Radespiel 2016). All mouse lemur species that have so far been studied in the wild are flexible omnivores (Rasoazanabary & Godfrey 2016), eating a variety of food items such as gum from gum trees (e.g. Fabaceae, Combretaceae) and certain forms of lianas, nectar from flowers, flowers, fruits, young leaves or even seeds and mushrooms (Martin 1973;

---

†Deceased

The UFAW Handbook on the Care and Management of Laboratory and Other Research Animals, Ninth Edition.
Edited by Huw Golledge and Claire Richardson.
© 2024 John Wiley & Sons Ltd. Published 2024 by John Wiley & Sons Ltd.

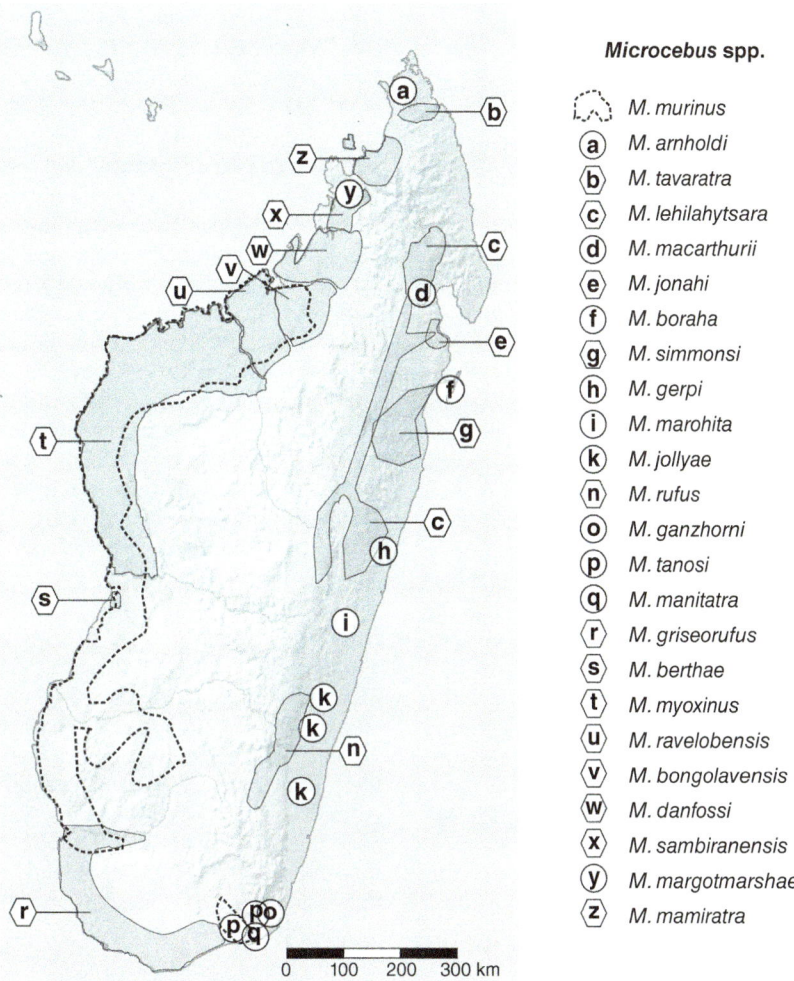

Figure 36.1 Distribution map of *Microcebus* spp. Distributions are either shown as polygons (abbreviated by letter in hexagon) or as local spots (encircled letter) if the full spatial distribution is not available. The distribution of *M. murinus* overlaps with that of several other species and is therefore depicted with a dashed line.

Hladik *et al.* 1980; Radespiel *et al.* 2006; Thorén *et al.* 2011; Lehman *et al.* 2016). They also lick sap-based secretions of moth-bugs (Flavidae) larvae, catch arthropods and small vertebrates, such as birds and reptiles, or eat eggs. There is a strong seasonality in ambient temperature and rainfall across Madagascar throughout the year, with a humid and warm rainy season in austral summer and a cooler dry season in austral winter, coinciding with a seasonally varying abundance of essential resources, such as food and sleeping sites. The annual variation in these resources shapes sleeping site usage and foraging activity, and reproduction. During the cooler dry season, some mouse lemur species show lower foraging activity and seasonal torpor to cope with periods of food scarcity (Ortmann *et al.* 1997; Schmid 2000; Schülke & Ostner 2007; Thorén *et al.* 2011; Zhang *et al.* 2015; Blanco *et al.* 2017), reducing energy expenditure by about 10%. The lack of torpor in captivity does not seem to affect longevity, which is a maximum of 8 years in the wild for *M. murinus* (Zimmermann *et al.* 2016) and 9 years for the brown mouse lemur (*M. rufus*, Zohdy 2012), but can be well beyond 10 years and, in rare cases, even up to 15 or 18 years under captive conditions (Weigl 2005; Zimmermann *et al.* 2016). A survival analysis for the grey mouse lemur in a population in northwest Madagascar showed that the median overall survival time in nature is only 10 months, meaning that most mouse lemurs die during their first two years of life (Lutermann *et al.* 2006). Correspondingly, the generation time of grey mouse lemurs, defined as the average age of parents, was estimated as 2.5 years based on parentage data from the same wild population (Radespiel *et al.* 2019). Due to their small body size, mouse lemurs face an enormous predation risk (by raptors, snakes and carnivores) for a nonhuman primate (Scheumann *et al.* 2007a; Fichtel 2016). The predation rate per year was estimated to be at least 25% of the population (Goodman *et al.* 1993). Sleeping sites are crucial for survival and reproduction in mouse lemurs, as they provide protection from predation and buffer strong differences in ambient temperature (Radespiel *et al.* 2003a). Field research has shown that in mouse lemurs, tree holes in dead or living trees, nests in lianas, tangles in the vegetation or even large dead leaves are used as sleeping sites. In *M. murinus* in northwestern Madagascar, sex-specific differences in sleeping site usage were found, with females using safer and thermally better insulated tree holes than males, which also change sleeping sites more frequently (Radespiel *et al.* 1998). Seasonal changes in sleeping site usage were also reported, with a higher usage of open sleeping sites during the warmer austral summer.

Reproduction

Mouse lemurs are seasonal breeders with an onset of reproduction that varies between different species (depending on an interplay between phylogeny, climate and habitat type), but mainly starts during the long-day period (Evasoa et al. 2018). The reproductive season starts with testicular growth in males. It precedes female oestrus by about a month, and large testes together with an extensive search for receptive females maximise male mating success during the very short receptive oestrus periods (Eberle & Kappeler 2004a, 2004b). Over the course of the year, mouse lemur testicles strongly fluctuate in size and, thus, in volume (Schmelting et al. 2000; Schmelting et al. 2007; see also section on Breeding later in this chapter and Figure 36.2). Additionally, plasma testosterone levels fluctuate corresponding to testicular growth (Perret 1985). An increasing photoperiod, i.e. increasing day length, induces annual reproductive activation in females of *M. murinus*. Females can have two to four oestrus cycles per season, with reproduction starting at a mean age of 349 days. Receptivity usually occurs on the first to third day of vaginal opening (Glatston 1979; Wrogemann et al. 2001), i.e. during oestrus. Females use multimodal oestrus advertisement signals (a combination of olfactory and acoustic signals) to indicate oestrus and receptivity to potential mates (Buesching et al. 1998). Females can mate with more than one male during one receptive period and cases of multiple paternity have been observed (Radespiel et al. 2002; Eberle & Kappeler 2004a; Eberle et al. 2007; Huchard et al. 2012). Overall, reproductive strategies of the sexes are mixed and there is evidence for male contest competition (male–male fighting in proximity to oestrus females), male mate guarding behaviour, sperm competition and female mate choice (i.e. females can and do reject males due to female dominance) (Radespiel et al. 2001; Radespiel et al. 2002; Eberle & Kappeler 2004a; Eberle & Kappeler 2004b; Eberle et al. 2007; Schwensow et al. 2008).

Gestation length is around 60 days (depending on the species, Wrogemann et al. 2001). After this time, usually one to three, more rarely four, infants are born (Wrogemann et al. 2001; Eberle & Kappeler 2006). *M. murinus* performs cooperative breeding. Each female grooms and nurses their own and related offspring and in case a mother dies, they can also adopt a dependent infant (Eberle & Kappeler 2006). However, they can distinguish their own offspring from others. If the breeding group changes the nesting site from one day to the next, they only carry their own offspring to the new nesting site (Eberle & Kappeler 2006). Around seven weeks after birth, the offspring become independent and are weaned (Glatston 1979; Kuhn 1989; Perret 1992). Both males and females become sexually mature and sexually active during the reproductive season following their own birth at an age of about eight months (Glatston 1979). However, sexual maturation precedes social maturation and one-year-old adults still differ in play, marking, aggression and social tolerance from older animals (Hohenbrink et al. 2015b).

Sociality

More than 20 years ago, mouse lemurs were described as solitary (Kappeler & Ganzhorn 1993; van Schaik & Kappeler 1993). However, intensive and ongoing field research has shown that their social structure and organisation are much more complex. All mouse lemur species studied so far forage solitarily, but nevertheless form flexible, individualised and complex social networks. Their composition and stability are most likely linked to the distribution and availability of food resources and sleeping sites, population density, sex ratio, climatic conditions, predation, as well as feeding strategies (Radespiel 2006; Schülke & Ostner 2007; Dausmann 2014; Kessler et al. 2016; Agnani et al. 2018). Males and females can be found sleeping alone, in pairs, in female or male groups, or in

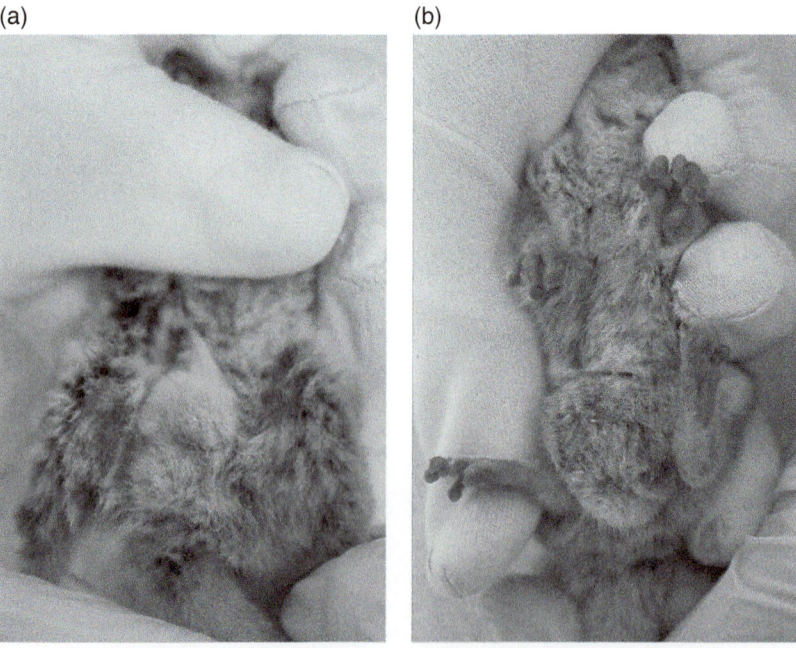

Figure 36.2 (a) Small testes during non-reproductive season; (b) Large testes during reproductive season.

multi-female-multi-male groups and typical grouping patterns differ considerably between species (Kessler et al. 2016). Kin selection seems to favour female philopatry, cooperative breeding in matrilines and cooperative infant care. Young males usually tend to disperse before their first mating season (Radespiel et al. 2003b; Schliehe-Diecks et al. 2012). A variety of acoustic, visual and chemical signals govern social life in these dispersed social networks (see also later section on Senses and communication in this chapter). Sleeping groups are mostly composed of maternally related individuals who roam solitarily at nighttime (Radespiel 2000; Braune et al. 2005; Schülke & Ostner 2005), with home ranges overlapping substantially between members of sleeping groups and between sexes. The size of a home range is linked to the distribution of resources necessary for survival and may double or triple in males during the breeding season (Radespiel 2000). Males are usually polygynous, mate with more than one female, guard the mated female for some time, and induce sperm plugs (Eberle & Kappeler 2004a) limiting sperm competition. Females may also mate with more than one male, resulting in multiple paternities in litters (Radespiel et al. 2002) and may also execute mate choice (Craul et al. 2004). Females of the grey mouse lemur are usually dominant over males (Radespiel & Zimmermann 2001), but there is high variation in this trait across individuals and species (Hohenbrink et al. 2016; Evasoa et al. 2019).

Senses and communication

Due to the nocturnal lifestyle of mouse lemurs, it is assumed that they mainly use their olfactory and auditory senses for communication and foraging (Braune et al. 2005; Unsworth et al. 2017). However, ongoing research demonstrates that vision also plays an important role. (Siemers et al. 2007; Piep et al. 2008) Mouse lemurs have binocular vision with overlapping visual fields (Cooper 1986; Fleagle 2013). As an adaptation to their nocturnal lifestyle, the eyes are large and equipped with a light-reflecting *tapetum lucidum* (Fleagle 2013). Experimental studies show that mouse lemurs can discriminate between different shapes of pictures (Joly et al. 2014; Picq et al. 2015; Schmidtke et al. 2018a) and that they use visual cues for food detection (Siemers et al. 2007; Piep et al. 2008; Valenta et al. 2013) as well as predator recognition (Rahlfs & Fichtel 2010). Photoreceptors also play an important role to regulate seasonal and daily activity pattern (Perret et al. 2010). To date, it is not clear to which extent mouse lemurs perceive colour. Even though both M/L opsin and S opsin are expressed, the S cone density is very low in the central visual field, suggesting monochromatic vision (Dkhissi-Benyahya et al. 2001; Peichl et al. 2001). However, modelling seed dispersal by mouse lemurs shows that they prefer fruits with higher chromatic (blue-yellow) contrast, supporting dichromatic vision (Valenta et al. 2013). Concerning conspecific communication, only a few visual signals, such as a swaying posture and tail-lashing, have been reported (Glatston 1979). Due to the poorly developed facial musculature, only limited facial expression can be produced (e.g. threat-face; Glatston 1979). Thus, vision might be more important in foraging than in social communication.

Mouse lemurs have a wet nose, a large olfactory epithelium, a functional vomeronasal organ and a large olfactory bulb (Fleagle 2013). The grey mouse lemur is also the primate species with the largest known repertoire of vomeronasal receptors (ca. 200 V1Rs and 2 V2Rs; Hohenbrink et al. 2012; Hohenbrink et al. 2013). These receptors seem to be already present in infants (Hohenbrink et al. 2014). The vomeronasal organ is suggested to play a major role in sexual communication, as marking behaviour of males in response to urine from oestrus and pre-oestrus females (Araújo 2003) as well as socio-sexual behaviour and aggression towards conspecifics (Aujard 1997) was drastically reduced in VNO-ectomised compared to intact animals. Enhanced excretion of whey acidic proteins (WFDC12) in the urine of male mouse lemurs during the mating season, significantly different volatile urinary profiles and the discriminatory capabilities shown by recent operant conditioning experiments suggest that these chemical signals may play a role in sexual selection and species recognition (Unsworth et al. 2017; Kollikowski et al. 2019; Caspers et al. 2020). Olfactory signals have been shown to influence the hormonal level of sex hormones in the receiver and may lead to sexual inhibition (Schilling & Perret 1987). Urinary cues are also reported to manipulate the sex ratio at birth (Perret 1990). Mouse lemurs show a variety of olfactory behaviours (e.g. urine-washing, substrate rubbing and anogenital rubbing) to distribute scent marks and urine (Glatston 1979; Hohenbrink et al. 2015a; Hohenbrink et al. 2015b). Besides intra- and interspecific communication, olfaction also plays an important role in predator recognition (Sündermann et al. 2008; Kappel et al. 2011) and foraging (Joly et al. 2004; Siemers et al. 2007; Piep et al. 2008).

Mouse lemurs can produce a variety of different calls in the audible and ultrasonic range (the vocal production range spans 400 Hz to 30 kHz of the fundamental frequency; 10 call types are described, e.g. Scheumann et al. 2007b; Zimmermann 2010; Leliveld et al. 2011; Zimmermann 2018) and perceive acoustic information from 800 Hz to 50 kHz (Niaussat and Petter 1980; Schopf et al. 2014). With ageing, a decline in the auditory sensitivity in the low-frequency range was reported (shift to 2 kHz, Schopf et al. 2014). Playback experiments showed that acoustic perception is important for prey detection (Goerlitz & Siemers 2007) and social communication (Braune et al. 2005; Kessler et al. 2012). The acoustically most complex call type is the *trill* which is uttered during various social interactions, such as mating (Buesching et al. 1998), mother–infant reunions (Scheumann et al. 2017) and sleeping group formation (Braune et al. 2005). The acoustic structure of *trills* carries indexical cues encoding species (Zimmermann et al. 2000; Zimmermann 2013; Zimmermann 2016; Hending et al. 2017; Hasiniaina et al. 2020), kinship (Zimmermann & Hafen 2001; Kessler et al. 2012; Kessler et al. 2018), familiarity (dialects: Hafen et al. 1998), individual identity (Zimmermann & Lerch 1993; Leliveld et al. 2011) and hormonal status (Zimmermann 1996). Neurophysiological aspects of vocal communication similar to humans can also be observed in mouse lemurs, such as the Lombard effect (Schopf et al. 2016), the lateralised processing of conspecific vocalisations (Scheumann & Zimmermann 2008; Leliveld et al. 2010) and features of babbling (Zimmermann 1991; Zimmermann 1992; Scheumann et al. 2017).

Sources and conservation

The largest threats for mouse lemurs, as for any other lemur species, are the continuous forest loss and fragmentation in Madagascar that impacts mouse lemurs due to their arboreal lifestyle and their local to regional distributions (see earlier sections on Taxonomy and Ecology, as well as Figure 36.1). Fragmented populations have been shown to have already lost genetic diversity, and connectivity between subpopulations cannot always be maintained (e.g. Olivieri et al. 2008). Furthermore, mouse lemurs are opportunistically hunted for food (e.g. Borgerson 2016). Consequently, of all 25 mouse lemur species described to date (October 2020), 24 are listed on the Red List by the IUCN[1]. Of these, 21 (87.5%) were categorised as threatened (vulnerable = 7, endangered = 10, critically endangered = 4). Of the remaining three species, two are currently listed as 'Least Concern' (M. murinus and M. griseorufus) and one as 'Data-deficient' (M. boraha).

Out of the 25 described mouse lemur species, only 2, M. murinus and M. lehilahytsara, are kept and successfully bred in captivity. Breeding colonies of M. murinus were first established and maintained in Europe as early as the 1960s (Petter-Rousseaux 1970; Martin 1972a). However, the exact geographical origin of founders is not well-documented and has only been specified as west ('Marosalaza', Petter-Rousseaux 1980), southwest (Perret 1986), or south (Martin 1972a; Martin 1972b). The largest extant European breeding colonies exist in Brunoy (France), Montpellier (France), and in Hannover (Germany) and smaller collections can be found in zoos or other research facilities worldwide (Fischer & Austad 2011). Only two M. lehilahytsara breeding colonies exist: one in Hannover (Germany) founded in 1996 (Wrogemann & Zimmermann 2001) and one at Zurich Zoo (Switzerland) founded in 2005 (Jürges et al. 2013). Both go back to founders that were obtained from the area around Andasibe, eastern Madagascar. Since 2005, no further animals have been taken from the wild and sent abroad.

Uses in research

Captive mouse lemurs as research subjects

Mouse lemurs, especially the grey mouse lemur (M. murinus), have a long history as subjects in laboratory research that dates back to the 1960s (Petter-Rousseaux 1970; Martin 1972a), when the first breeding colonies of M. murinus were established. The economic advantages of mouse lemurs over other nonhuman primates in laboratory research are obvious. Being the smallest primates in the world, they can be kept cost-effectively in large numbers. A recent article on mouse lemurs as genetic models in biomedical research estimates their generation costs to be at least one order of magnitude lower than for marmosets or macaques (Ezran et al. 2017). Mouse lemurs can be easily handled, for example, for routine medical check-ups and retain high fecundity in captivity. Furthermore, if desired, the reproduction cycle of seasonally breeding mouse lemurs can be artificially reduced in captivity by shortening the season length via light entrainment (Perret & Aujard 2001b).

The use of captive mouse lemurs as model species can roughly be divided into two large categories (1) behavioural and evolutionary research and (2) biomedical research. Behavioural and evolutionary research using captive mouse lemurs often complements field studies and comprises a diverse range of topics. Socio-ecological and ecophysiological studies, for example, investigated social dominance (e.g. Radespiel & Zimmermann 2001), communication (e.g. Scheumann et al. 2017), prey catching (e.g. Piep et al. 2008), grasping (e.g. Scheumann et al. 2011; Thomas et al. 2016; Peckre et al. 2019), thermoregulation (e.g. Perret & Aujard 2001a; Terrien et al. 2010; Biggar et al. 2015; Faherty et al. 2017), as well as chronobiology and reproduction (e.g. Perret & Aujard 2001b; Wrogemann et al. 2001). Comparative and functional anatomical studies included research on sensory organs and pathways (e.g. Hohenbrink et al. 2013; Peichl et al. 2019; Saraf et al. 2019), general brain architecture (e.g. Pellegrino et al. 2018; Nadkarni et al. 2019) and the testicular epithelium (Aslam et al. 2002). Comparative cognitive studies compared visuo-spatial paired-associates learning (Schmidtke et al. 2018a), navigation (Teichroeb & Vining 2019) and instrumental problem-solving (Kittler et al. 2018) capabilities of captive mouse lemurs to those of other species. Finally, the full genome of the grey mouse lemur has recently been sequenced and annotated, laying the ground for comparative genetic work (Horvath & Willard 2007; Larsen et al. 2017a). The attention mouse lemurs attract as evolutionary models relates to the independent evolution of the Malagasy primates over the last 60–70 million years (Karanth et al. 2005). Despite a high degree of radiation and specialisation that occurred during this time (Yoder et al. 2000), mouse lemurs are often described as having retained anatomical, physiological and behavioural traits of the ancestral primate condition, such as lissencephalic brains (Dhenain et al. 2003), functional vomeronasal organs (Schilling et al. 1990; Hohenbrink et al. 2013), nocturnal lifestyles, nest-building, and an infant parking system (Kappeler 1998). Thus, mouse lemurs allow scientists to probe into the origins of primate evolution. Initially, mouse lemurs and other strepsirrhines were also considered as having only 'basal' (i.e. lower) cognitive capabilities compared to Old and New World monkeys (e.g. Jolly 1966). This view, however, has repeatedly been challenged by demonstrating complex cognitive abilities in mouse lemurs, such as cognitive flexibility (Joly et al. 2004; Joly et al. 2014), spatial mapping of objects on different scales (Picq & Dhenain 1998; Joly & Zimmermann 2011; Schmidtke et al. 2018a) and instrumental problem solving (Kittler et al. 2018). The value of mouse lemurs as nonhuman primate models for large-sample studies with potentially high translational power for human medicine was recognised from the very beginning of their captive breeding (Martin 1972a). While behavioural and evolutionary research dominated the early decades of laboratory-based research on mouse lemurs, there was a significant increase in biomedical research using these nonhuman primates that can be traced back to a series of neuroanatomical and cognitive studies from the 1990s. These studies described biochemical and structural alterations of the brain, such as amyloid-β accumulations and plaque formation (Bons et al. 1992; Bons et al. 1994; Mestre-Francés et al. 2000), abnormally aggregated and hyperphosphorylated Tau (Bons et al. 1992; Delacourte et al. 1995) and cerebral atrophy (Bons et al. 1992; Dhenain et al. 2000; Fritz et al. 2020) in a subpopulation of aged grey mouse lemurs. In addition, age-related decline in sociality and working memory have simultaneously been reported (Picq 1992; Picq 1993). Numerous studies followed, using mouse lemurs as natural nonhuman primate models of both normal and pathological brain ageing, describing high, age-related phenotypic variation in brain-structure

---

[1] https://www.iucnredlist.org/ (accessed 13 October 2020)

and cytochemistry (for an overview see Bons et al. 2006; Lacreuse et al. 2020) as well as in behaviour and cognition (for a concise review on general mouse lemur cognition, see Picq 2016) and investigating possible connections between the two. Due to the similarities of the described proteopathies and human Alzheimer's disease, one clear focus of biomedical research in mouse lemurs since the 1990s was and still is on mechanisms and possible interventions of neurodegenerative diseases, such as Alzheimer's (Bons et al. 2006; Larsen et al. 2017b; Rahman et al. 2017) and Parkinson's disease (Mestre-Francés et al. 2018; Lasbleiz et al. 2019). Acute neurological mouse lemur models include models of prion transmission (Bons et al. 1999; Bons et al. 2002) and toxicity (Torrent et al. 2010) as well as spinal cord injury (Le Corre et al. 2018; Poulen & Perrin 2018). Apart from investigations of phenotypic variation in young and aged mouse lemurs and its relation to brain morphology and function, a recent research initiative set out to explore possible links between nutritive (Dal-Pan et al. 2011; Vinot et al. 2011; Royo et al. 2018) and metabolic factors (Djelti et al. 2017) and phenotypic variation. Initial results show that a diet that is rich in ω3 polyunsaturated fatty acids or a general caloric restriction, when started at a young age, has beneficial effects on spatial memory (Dal-Pan et al. 2011; Vinot et al. 2011). Caloric restriction has additionally been found to have a positive effect on longevity (Pifferi et al. 2018). As mentioned before, a chromosome-level reference assembly of the mouse lemur genome has recently been published (Larsen et al. 2017a), allowing the investigation and identification of genetic risk factors in mouse lemur diseases and their comparison to genetic diseases in humans (e.g. Schmidtke et al. 2018b).

General husbandry

The husbandry of primates is regulated on an international, continental and national scale. For most European countries, the directives of the European Commission (Directive 2010/63/EU) are applicable. Mouse lemurs are not explicitly mentioned in these directives, which is why the recommendations for husbandry described in the following text are based on more than 20 years of experience in keeping mouse lemurs (*M. murinus* and *M. lehilahytsara*) in Germany (Hannover and Göttingen). The trade, and thus also the exchange of mouse lemurs between colonies, is regulated by the Convention on International Trade in Endangered Species of Wild Fauna and Flora (CITES).

Housing, food and water

Since mouse lemurs, such as *M. murinus* and *M. lehilahytsara*, which are described here in particular, show a high degree of social flexibility (see also earlier section on Sociality in this chapter), they can be housed alone, in pairs, or in mixed-sex groups, as well as in same-sex groups of three to four individuals. The social compatibility within groups, however, must be monitored daily. During pregnancy or in the event of illness, an animal should be separated, but always while maintaining visible or auditory contact to conspecifics housed within the same room. In the Hannover colony, about 80 mouse lemurs are maintained in close-mesh wire cages (e.g. Ebeco Marmoset 0.65 m × 0.80 m × 1.55 m (W×D×H); one cage per animal; Figure 36.3) which can be connected to or separated from each other by opening or closing a connecting door (Figure 36.3a). Numerous climbing opportunities as well as hiding places should be offered (see also section on Environmental provisions later in this chapter). A variety of fresh fruit and vegetables in daily alternation with a portion of enriched pap (e.g. from cereals, cream, wheat germ oil, soya flour, vitamin drops, boiled eggs and bananas) is recommended. In addition, animal protein sources, such as locusts or meal worms, should be offered regularly, e.g. one to two times a week (see also Hülskötter et al. 2017). To avoid competition, at least as many feeding places as individuals per cage unit are required. Water must be provided *ad libitum* from bottles with sipper tubes.

Environmental provisions and enrichment

The enrichment provided in the cage should be adapted to the ecological requirements of the animals. Wooden boxes (20 cm × 11 cm × 11 cm) with an opening towards the cage can imitate tree holes and are suitable as hiding and sleeping places (Figure 36.3 + 36.3b). One of the wooden walls of the box can be replaced by a Plexiglas pane, which allows observation of the animals in the box. This can also be slid upwards so that it is possible to reach into the box. To prevent permanent penetration of light into the sleeping box, the Plexiglas pane should be opaquely covered (e.g. by a fixed piece of cardboard) at times when no observations are taking place (Figure 36.3b). The boxes are also useful for separation and transportation of animals (e.g. for medical treatment or experiments). At least one box per individual should be available to limit potential conflicts for a sleeping site. Due to the animals' ability to move vertically, cages should be enriched with vertical and horizontal climbing opportunities, such as tree branches, hanging pipes, and swings or hammocks of coconut rope and jute fabric (Figure 36.3 + 36.3c). Additionally, various food toys (e.g. licking boards, containers with openings to grasp for treats (Figure 36.3), chewing sticks) can be offered as behavioural enrichment. See also Chapter 10: Environmental enrichment: animal welfare and scientific validity. Unbleached and unprinted paper can be used as ground cover (Figure 36.3). This facilitates the cleaning of the cage and can, moreover, be used by the animals as nesting material.

Physical environment

In the Hannover colony, the indoor climate is fully controlled with a room temperature varying between 22 °C and 27 °C and a relative humidity ranging from 55% to 65%. In order to ensure successful reproduction of the animals, a seasonal adjustment of day length is mandatory, i.e. a long-day period mimicking the conditions during the mating season, with 14 hours of light and 10 hours of darkness (February to September) and a short-day period simulating the non-mating season, with 10 hours of light and 14 hours of darkness (October to January). To be able to work comfortably

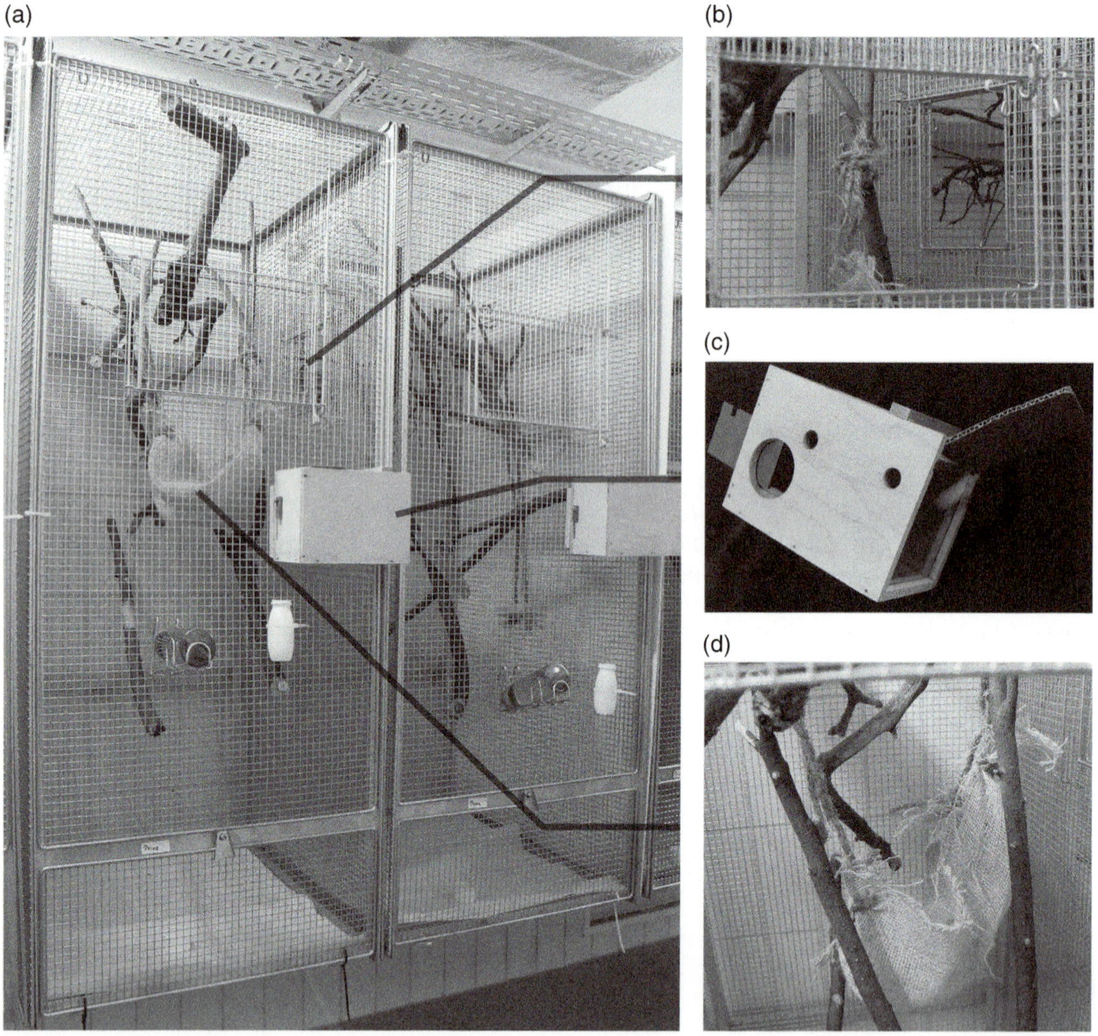

Figure 36.3 Two connected cages equipped with environmental enrichment (tree branches, swings, hammock, treat containers); (a) Connecting door; (b) Sleeping box with Plexiglas pane; (c) Hammock; (d).

with the animals during their activity phase, a reversed light cycle can be used (dark phase during the day; light phase at night). In this case, darkness means red light with less than 0.3 lux (equivalent to moonlight). It should be noted that in captivity daily torpor (defined by a core temperature below 33 °C) can be induced by reduced food supply as well as by photoperiod (short-day period) and temperature (temperatures below 18 °C), which may affect the results of experiments (Genin & Perret 2000; Séguy & Perret 2005).

Identification

For lifelong identification, each mouse lemur needs to be permanently marked, for example, with a small, subcutaneously injected RFID transponder (transponder approximately 9 mm long, as commonly used for mice, e.g. Planet ID GmbH, Essen, Germany), implanted under the skin at the neck or in the inguinal skinfold between the leg and body wall near the knee. Implantation should take place at the time of weaning from the mother at the latest. Although this is the most common method for small primates such as mouse lemurs, it should be noted that RFID transponders can lead to partial erasure of MRI images. For more spontaneous, visual identification and observations within a group, non-invasive markings such as fur shavings (e.g. on the tail or back) can be used.

Breeding

For successful breeding, there are different husbandry strategies. Firstly, it is possible to pair one male with one female to ascertain complete pedigree information. If this option is chosen, it is useful to socialise the mating partners for some time beforehand. However, if socialisation is not harmonious, the male can also be paired with the female during oestrus only. A certain risk of this approach is that fertilisation success depends on only one male and could fail, if this male is infertile or if the female rejects him. Secondly, it is possible to group one oestrus female together with several males. In this case, paternity must be genetically determined subsequently to ascertain complete pedigree information. In addition, there is a certain risk of fight-related injuries due to strong competition between males in the mating context. Also, grouping females with one or more males did not result in a different likelihood of pregnancies (49.3% pregnancies in pairs vs. 41.4% pregnancies in larger groups; Zimmermann and Radespiel 2003).

As previously mentioned, males show seasonal testicular growth. Figure 36.2 shows the obvious difference in testis size between the non-reproductive (a) and reproductive season (b). In order to identify the right time for pairing males and females and to be able to calculate the birth date as accurately as possible, it is recommended to carry out regular (3x/week) macroscopic cycle controls with each female during the reproductive season. The characteristic phases of an oestrus cycle are listed in Table 36.1 (modified from Glatston 1979; Stanger et al. 1995; Buesching et al. 1998). Dioestrus, prooestrus and oestrus are also shown in Figure 36.4. Male and female should be socialised at the latest when the characteristic vaginal swelling of the prooestrus becomes visible. The first day of oestrus (vaginal opening) should be taken to calculate the anticipated birth date. Daily cytological evaluation of the vaginal lavages (see section on Handling and health monitoring later in this chapter) provides information about the duration of oestrus. In addition, spermatozoa may also be detected after mating. If a vaginal plug is present, vaginal washing should not be performed so as not to destroy it. Approximately two weeks before birth, pregnancy can be clearly detected by a substantial gain in weight and by palpation. We recommend defining a period of 'maternal leave' for pregnant females starting about 14 days before the calculated date of birth. This means that the female should be exposed to as few stress factors as possible during this time period. For example, the animal may be excluded from weekly handling and should only be examined if necessary. Behavioural experiments should also not be carried out with the pregnant female during this period and up until about four weeks after birth. To avoid food stress and to cover additional nutritional needs during late pregnancy and lactation, females should be given a more lavish diet (double portion) and daily animal protein sources from two weeks prior to birth until four weeks after birth. If still housed together with a male, the male is typically separated from the female during this time and, if possible,

Table 36.1 Macro- and microscopic properties (vaginal cytology) during the course of an oestrus cycle.

Phase of oestrus cycle	Macroscopic properties	Microscopic properties
Dioestrus	White genital region Flat and sealed	No vaginal lavages possible
Prooestrus	Pink vagina First swollen but closed, then open and very swollen	Few leucocytes Round epithelial cells increased in size, more angular, with small dark nuclei
Oestrus	Pink or white vagina Wide open and very swollen	No leucocytes Epithelial cells large, angular and keratinised Nuclei disappearing
Metoestrus	White vagina Still open, swelling diminishing or already disappeared	Keratinised epithelial cells arranged in dense clumps Leucocytes reappear

Source: Modified after Buesching et al. (1998), Glatston (1979), Stanger et al. (1995).

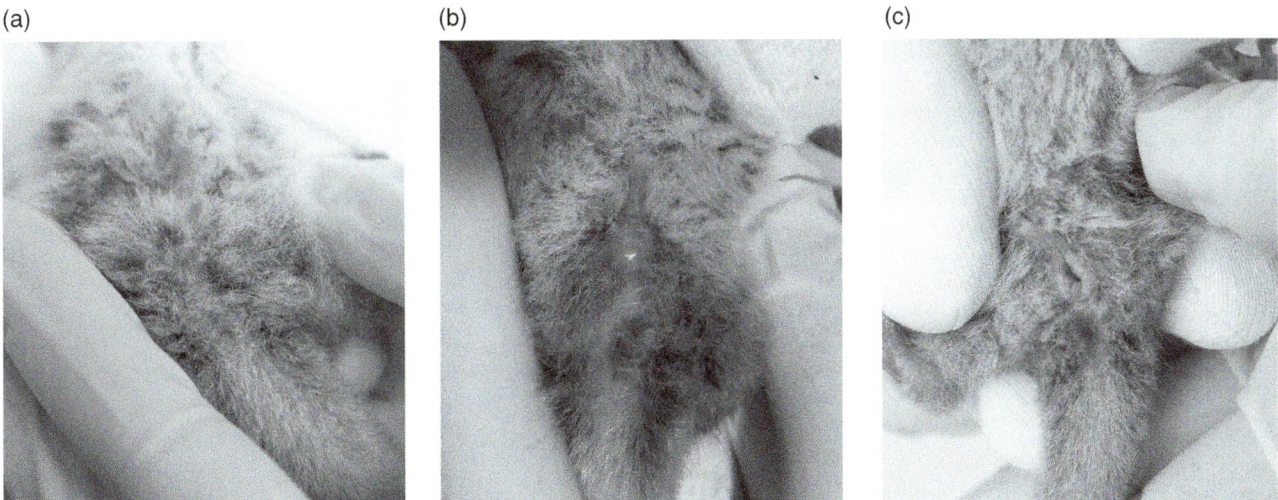

Figure 36.4 (a) Dioestrus (flat and sealed genital region); (b) Prooestrus (swollen vagina); (c) Oestrus (open and swollen vagina).

socialised with other males. If the cage contains a floor with wire mesh, a mat of easy-to-clean material should be placed on the floor of the cage a few days before the date of birth. If the mother does not give birth in the sleeping box, this prevents the newborn infants from slipping through the mesh. During their first week of life, mother and infants should be disturbed as rarely as possible. One look into the nestbox per day is enough to see if mother and babies are well. On about the fifth day after birth, it is recommended that the infants are handled for the first time. From then on, infant handling should be carried out twice a week to record developmental stages, growth, and health status. Infant handling should always be performed with disposable gloves. From the time of weaning (approximately seven weeks after birth) onwards, the young animals receive their own food portion. The available space should then be increased (one cage compartment per animal, as previously described in the section on housing in this chapter). Before the onset of the next reproductive season, young males need to be separated from their mothers and sisters in order to avoid inbreeding. Female offspring, on the other hand, can be housed with their mothers for any length of time. Occasionally, mothers have insufficient milk for their infants or the weight discrepancy between siblings is high (e.g. Glatston 1979; Kuhn 1989; unpublished data). In such a case, a supplementary feeding procedure can be successfully applied. Infants can be fed with a baby formula for human infants (e.g. follow-on formula after the sixth month; fat 3.5 g/100 ml, protein 1.4 g/100 ml, carbohydrate 8.1 g/100 ml; Hipp 2, Hipp GmbH & Co. Vertrieb KG, Pfaffenhofen, Germany) approximately four times a day. The baby formula is prepared in accordance with the standard recommendations of the manufacturer. It is dropped on the mouth of the infant using a 1 ml syringe and infants start to lick the baby formula (amount ingested ranging between 0.1 and 3 g depending on age). Afterwards, the infant's belly should be massaged to stimulate defaecation. During the feeding procedure, the mother is separated and distracted with a cricket. After supplementary feeding, the infant is placed back in the nestbox and the mother released to the infant. At approximately four weeks of age, the baby formula should be complemented with 2 g of banana milk pudding for human infants (e.g. milk pudding with banana; fat 10.8%, protein 12.4%, carbohydrate 70.7%; Milupa Nutricia GmbH, Frankfurt am Main, Germany) which infants start to lick out of a bowl, which can be placed into the nestbox. Six female Goodman's mouse lemur infants (*M. lehilahytsara*) have been raised successfully using this procedure (Figure 36.5). Two of these females successfully raised their own infants and all of the animals reached an age of more than 10 years (min. = 10; max. = 15). The same procedure was also used successfully for one *M. murinus* infant in the Hannover colony. In other colonies (compare, e.g., Glatston 1979; Kuhn 1989), hand-rearing of *M. murinus* infants has also proved successful.

Biological data

The biological data presented will focus on *M. murinus* and *M. lehilahytsara* in captive conditions, since they are the only two *Microcebus* spp. maintained in captivity.

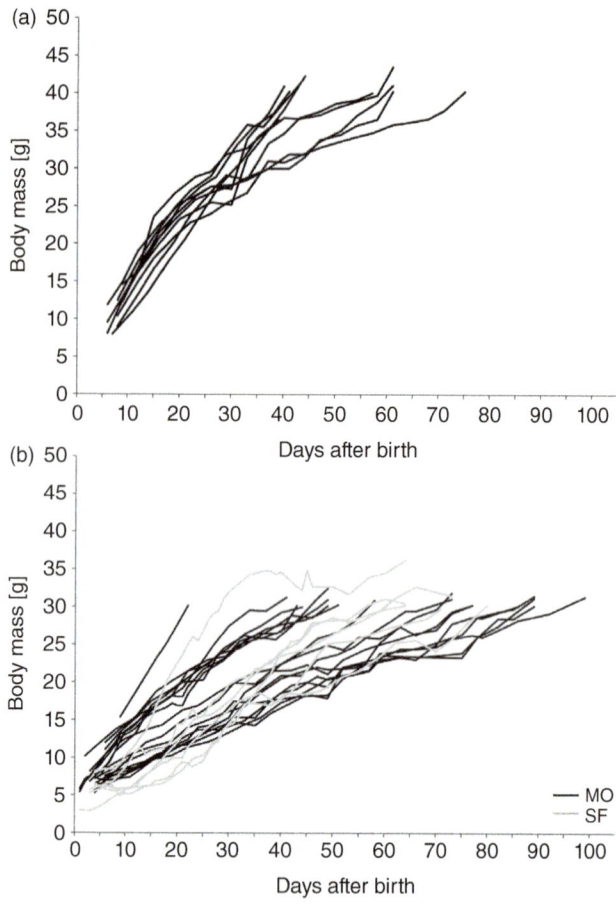

Figure 36.5 Body mass development in (a) *M. murinus* and (b) *M. lehilahytsara* from the weight at the day of first handling up to the weight at the time around weaning (*M. murinus* N = 10; 6♂♂; 4♀♀; *M. lehilahytsara* N = 24; 8♂♂; 16♀♀). Grey lines represent supplementary-fed (SF) animals, black lines represent animals reared by their mother only (MO).

Body mass

Body mass is subject to seasonal changes. A short photoperiod leads to an increase in body mass due to an increase in energy intake followed by a decrease in energy expenditure. This results in fat storage in the subcutaneous tissue, especially in the tail (Genin & Perret 2000; Perret & Aujard 2001b). Food intake and water loss subsequently decline, and locomotor activity is reduced. Accordingly, body mass was significantly higher during the long-day period than during short days in the Hannover colony (Table 36.2, data from the mouse lemur colony, Hannover, 2017–2018).

Body temperature

For *M. murinus*, the average core body temperature under short-day conditions varies between 35.3 °C ± 0.3 °C (mean ± SD) during the light phase (day) and 36.9 °C ± 0.2 °C (mean ± SD) during the dark phase (night) (Séguy & Perret 2005). During activity, body temperature can even rise to 37.6 °C under long-day conditions (Aujard & Vasseur 2001). In these studies, core body temperature of male individuals was obtained via a telemetric transmitter implanted in the abdominal cavity. Assessment of rectal temperatures, however, is a more feasible approach for routine health monitoring of captive mouse lemurs. Reference data for rectal temperatures of a larger sample size of both sexes of *M. murinus* and *M. lehilahytsara* over the course of one year are illustrated in Figure 36.6. *Microcebus* spp. are capable of hypometabolism (compare Schülke & Ostner 2007), which means a suppressed metabolic state with decreased metabolic rates and core body temperature as well as lower respiratory and heart rate. If this state lasts more than 24 hours, it is called hibernation, whereas shorter periods are referred to as daily torpor (Ganzhorn *et al.* 2003). Interestingly, species differences as well as seasonal fluctuations, i.e. a noticeable reduction in body temperature during short days and higher body temperature in *M. lehilahytsara* than in *M. murinus*, were observed even under constant ambient temperature (22–27 °C) and balanced diet (Figure 36.6, data from the mouse lemur colony Hannover).

Infant development

In *M. murinus*, the mean body mass of infants at their day of birth is 5.8 g and increases to 36.6 g at the time of weaning (Table 36.2). Infant body mass does not differ significantly

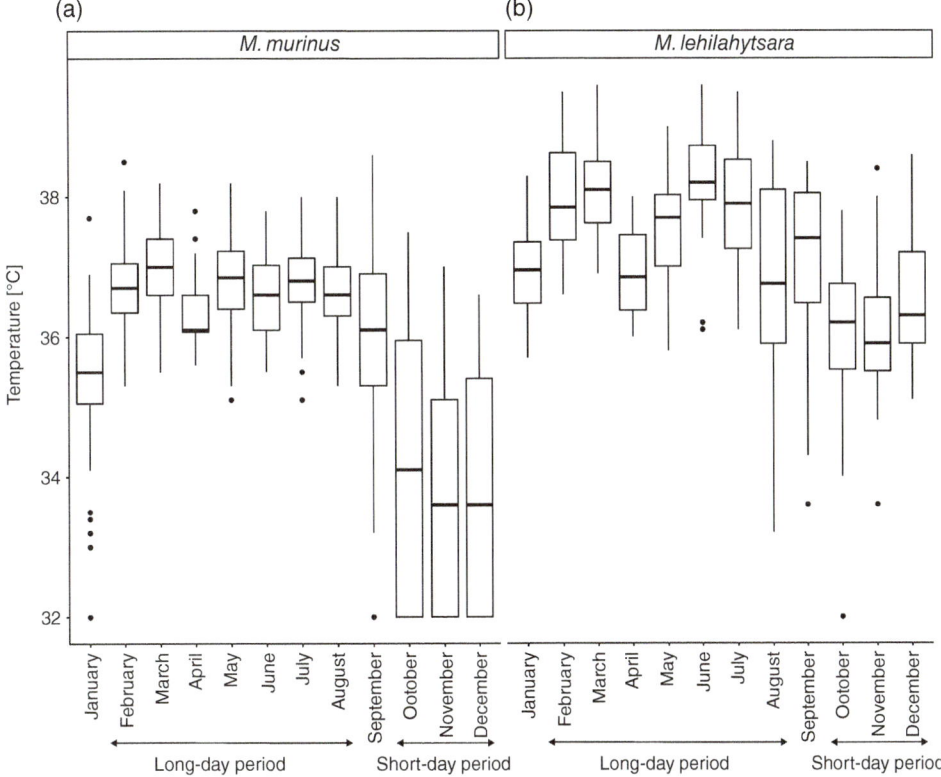

Figure 36.6 Monthly variations in rectal temperature of (a) *M. murinus* (N=40; 20♂♂, 20♀♀) and (b) *M. lehilahytsara* (N=20; 10♂♂, 10♀♀). The lower threshold for common clinical thermometers is 32 °C. No torpid state was observed despite low rectal temperatures.

Table 36.2 Body mass of the mouse lemurs in the Hannover colony in g. Displayed are mean (min – max), N = sample size, * = Kuhn (1989).

Adult body mass			
	Long-day period	Short-day period	Difference between seasons (t-test)
Microcebus murinus (N = 67)	75.8 (64.1–88.1)	92.6 (77.8–110.9)	t = −21.96; p < 0.001
M. lehilahytsara (N = 24)	54.3 (42.7–70.7)	72.8 (56.7–92.7)	t = −14.67; p < 0.001
Infant body mass development			
	Day of birth	four to seven days	Time of weaning
M. murinus	5.8 (3.1–7.8) (N = 11)*	10.5 (6–14.9) (N = 40)	36.6 (21.3–45.6) (N = 40)
M. lehilahytsara	NA	8.7 (5.3–12.1) (N = 36)	25.4 (14.3–36.8) (N =36)

between sexes (Zimmermann et al. 2016). For M. lehilahytsara, the information on body mass on the day of birth is missing. At four to seven days of age, the mean body mass is 8.7 g and increases to 25.4 g at the time of weaning (Table 36.2). Again, there is no significant difference between the sexes in this species (Zimmermann et al. 2016). The individual body mass development from the day of the first handling (day five to eight) up to the time around weaning for M. murinus (a) and M. lehilahytsara (b) is shown in Figure 36.5. Canine teeth and incisors erupt within the first week after birth, first molars around the time of weaning (around seven weeks after birth). Second dentition is completed at three months of age (unpublished data; Perret 1992).

Laboratory procedures

Handling and health monitoring

As with all animals kept for experimental purposes, a daily health check by the animal keepers is mandatory. Due to the nocturnality, small body size and the dense fur of the animals, many smaller injuries, swellings or other pathological abnormalities are not immediately recognisable when animals are moving through the cage. Therefore, it is important that every animal undergoes a manual health check on a regular basis (e.g. once a week). For this purpose, the animal is taken out of the cage during daylight and the general condition of the animal is examined by an animal keeper or veterinarian. Anomalies are recorded and the appropriate measures are taken, if necessary (see also section on Common welfare problems later in this chapter). The weight of the animal is checked and documented in order to draw conclusions about possible health problems, food competition within the social group or possible pregnancies. If necessary, the amount of food can be adjusted accordingly. Furthermore, on this occasion, the control of the oestrus cycle can be carried out during the mating season: After visual inspection (see Figure 36.4 and Table 36.1) and in case of a vaginal opening, vaginal lavages are performed (for cytological evaluation and to detect any existing spermatozoa) following the protocols established in small laboratory rodents (e.g. Cora et al. 2015). For this purpose, 0.1 ml saline solution is drawn into a disposable pipette. The pipette tip is gently inserted into the vaginal opening and saline is flushed into and back out of the vagina two to three times. A drop of the solution containing cells from the vaginal canal is then placed on a microscope slide and examined microscopically with 10x magnification. In order to minimise the frequency of handling for the individual animal, data or samples required for scientific purposes may also be collected during health checks, provided that experiments are authorised accordingly. These can be, for example, morphometric data, such as testicular size and tail circumference, or blood, urine and faecal samples.

Sampling

Faecal and urine samples can be collected directly during handling procedures. Alternatively, the mouse lemur can be confined to a modified sleeping box with a perforated aluminium floor attached to a collection device (analogous to a metabolism cage). Blood sample volumes are limited by the small body mass of Microcebus species. The total circulating blood volume (CBV) of mouse lemurs is estimated conservatively as 6% of the animal's body mass (the percentage is lower in obese individuals compared to those of normal weight). In accordance with guidelines for other small laboratory mammals (NIH Animal Research Advisory Committee Guidelines, GV-Solas, National Centre for the Replacement, Refinement & Reduction of Animals in Research), 10% of the CBV can be safely withdrawn every two to four weeks, 7.5% every seven days and 1% every 24 hours. For a mouse lemur of 60 g body mass (3.6 ml CBV), this would mean a maximum of 360 µl, 270 µl and 36 µl respectively. Blood samples can be taken via venipuncture from the saphenous vein of the hind leg (vena saphena parva (caudal) or vena saphena magna (medial)) or from the cephalic vein of the forearm (vena cephalica antebrachii). The tail vein is not recommended due to adipose tissue and seasonal fattening. Bloodsucking bugs (Dipetalogaster maximus) have also been used experimentally as an alternative, less-invasive blood sampling technique (Thomsen & Voigt 2006).

Administration of substances

Oral administration of substances can be performed either directly or admixed in food items (e.g. injected into locusts). Substances can also be safely injected subcutaneously in the flank area in conscious animals that are manually restrained. Intramuscular injections may be given in the thigh. However, caution needs to be taken when administering irritating substances with a low pH-value, as they are painful and may lead to tissue damage and necrosis. Intramuscular administration is only recommended for small volumes (max. 0.05 ml/site; Turner et al. 2011). Intravenous access has not been described in mouse lemurs and injections into the peritoneal cavity are, therefore, used more frequently. Intraperitoneal injections can be conducted in conscious animals that are firmly restrained, and irritating substances should be diluted.

Anaesthesia and analgesia

The small size of mouse lemurs requires special consideration with regard to standard veterinary anaesthetic equipment and techniques. Short procedures can be conducted under injectable anaesthetics and a variety of drugs and drug combinations have been used in mouse lemurs in captivity and under field conditions (summarised in Kästner et al. 2016). However, the ability to maintain and adjust anaesthesia using repeated injections of anaesthetic drugs is limited and inhalation anaesthesia (e.g. isoflurane or sevoflurane) is therefore recommended for medium- to long-term procedures. Anaesthetic systems designed for small laboratory rodents can easily be adapted for mouse lemurs. Induction of anaesthesia can be achieved using injectable agents followed by maintenance with inhalation agents or by inhalation performed by mask or chamber induction. To reduce handling stress, chamber induction is preferred in non-habituated animals and induction in the mouse lemur's familiar sleeping box can minimise stress responses. Mouse lemur anaesthesia, including drugs and dosages, is described and discussed in detail in Kästner et al. (2016).

Analgesics should be used pre- or perioperatively for all surgical procedures. Buprenorphine should be used for more invasive interventions, whereas Meloxicam is suitable for smaller surgical procedures, fight-related injuries, as well as inflamed wounds (for dosages and application, see Table 36.3). Duration of pain management depends on the surgical procedure and/or extent of injury and should be monitored and adjusted accordingly.

Euthanasia

Euthanasia needs to comply with national and international regulations, e.g. the European Directive (2010/63/EU), Annex IV or the AVMA (American Veterinary Medicine Association) Guidelines (Leary et al. 2020). See also Chapter 17: Euthanasia and other fates for laboratory animals. An overdose of anaesthetic (e.g. pentobarbital, or ketamine/xylazine followed by T61) is recommended for euthanasia in primates. In mouse lemurs, large volumes (minimum threefold overdose) can be injected intraperitoneally. An intracardial or intrapulmonary injection of T 61® should only be performed if the animal is under deep general anaesthesia.

Common welfare problems – selected diseases and injuries

Fight-related injuries

Fight-related injuries are more common during the reproductive season than the non-reproductive season and especially when social groups are first established. To reduce or prevent such injuries, the animals should be selected carefully (e.g. grouped by weight) and the newly established groups should be monitored for repeated fighting for several days. Providing more food than usual can help to reduce fighting. Fight-related injuries most commonly occur on the tail, the lower back and the ears, with severity ranging from superficial bite marks to deep wounds with substantial tissue loss. Superficial wounds usually heal best without further treatment. All wounds should be cleaned and debrided as needed and the surrounding hair should be clipped. Bite wounds should not be sutured due to the

Table 36.3 Information on drug application and medical treatment in mouse lemurs is limited. A list of drugs used in *Microcebus* species is given below.

Drug	Dosage	Indication	Route of administration	Reference
Buprenorphine	0.01–0.05 mg/kg	Analgesia, perioperative pain management	im or sc	(Le Corre et al. 2018) (personal experience)
Meloxicam	0.2 mg/kg	Analgesic and anti-inflammatory properties, pre-/ perioperative pain management, acute injuries, chronic arthropathies	sc or po	(Lovegrove et al. 2014; Cichon et al. 2017) (personal experience)
Enrofloxacin	5–10 mg/kg	Antibiotic, bacterial infections	sc or po	(Cichon et al. 2017; Le Corre et al. 2018) (personal experience)
Procaine benzylpenicillin		Antibiotic, bacterial infections	im	(Lovegrove et al. 2014)
Amoxicillin (Duphamox®)		Antibiotic, bacterial infections	im or sc	(Lovegrove et al. 2014)
Amoxicillin, Clavulanic Acid (Synulox®)	11 mg/kg	Antibiotic, bacterial infections	sc or po	Montpellier, personal communication
Chloramphenicol eye ointment (Ophtalon®)	3x/day	Antibiotic, bacterial eye infections	Topical	Montpellier, personal communication
Dexamethasone, Framycetin eye ointment (Fradexam®)		Antibiotic and anti-inflammatory properties, eye infections without corneal lesions	Topical	Montpellier, personal communication
Sucralfate	30–50 mg/kg 2x/day	Gastrointestinal ulcers	po	Personal experience
Brinzolamide eye ointment (Azopt®)	2x/day	Reduction of intraocular pressure	Topical	Personal experience
Benazepril	0.5 mg/kg	Congestive cardiac failure	po	Personal experience
Dimeticone (Polydimethylsiloxane)	70 mg/kg 3–6x/day	Gastrointestinal tympany	po	Personal experience
Embutramide, Mebezonium iodide, Tetracaine hydrochloride (T 61®)	1 ml/kg	Euthanasia	Intracardiac or intrapulmonary	Personal experience
Miconazole nitrate, Polymyxin B sulphate, Prednisolone acetate (Surolan®)	2x/day applied thinly	Antimycotic, antibiotic and anti-inflammatory properties, dermatitis	Topical	Personal experience

high risk of infection. Amputation of severely injured tails can be necessary. Depending on the origin and extent of injury, conflict rates within the social group, and the necessary medical interventions, it can be advisable to isolate injured individuals temporarily. To prevent the injured animal from licking or biting a wound, a pet cone (plastic or soft fabric collar) can be made. The fit of the collar needs to be checked regularly to avoid sores. For protection of tail injuries, a plastic tube (e.g. the central piece of a 2 ml or 5 ml syringe) can be fixed to the animal's tail using medical tape (examples given in Figure 36.7). Some animals might be irritated by the clinking sound the tube makes on the grid of the cage. In cases where an animal does not tolerate the tube, a normal bandage can be provided, but needs to be changed more frequently and provides less protection.

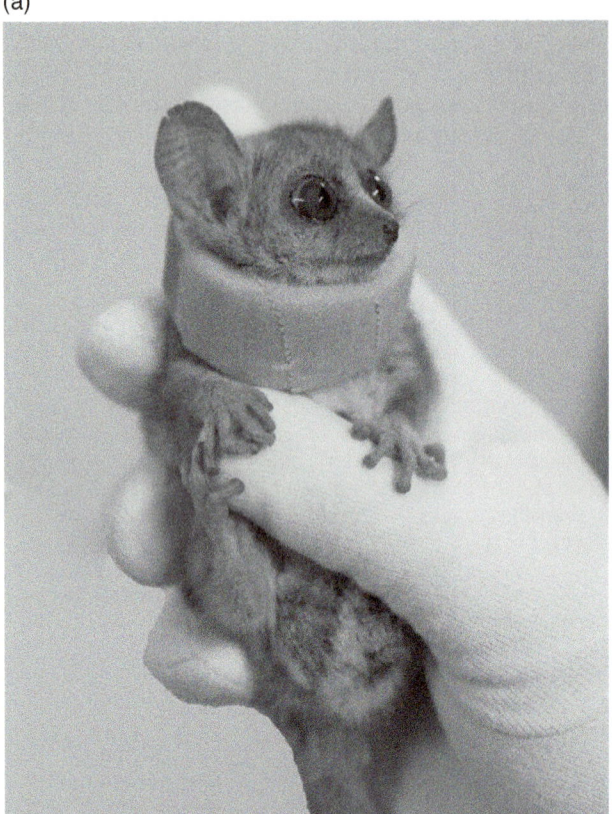

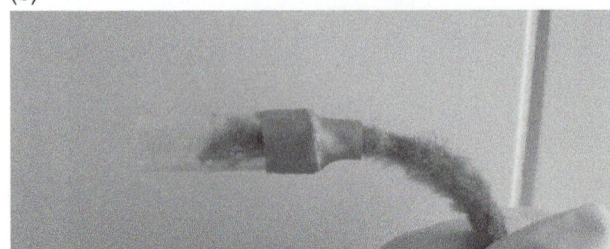

Figure 36.7 (a) Pet cone made of soft fabric collar; (b) Plastic tube fixed to the tail.

Ocular pathologies

The most common ocular findings in mouse lemurs are cataracts and nuclear sclerosis (NS), which both occur more frequently with increasing age (Beltran et al. 2007; Dubicanac et al. 2017). Both alterations manifest in a visual cloudiness of the lens but can be distinguished via funduscopic investigation. In cataracts, the opacity of the lens blocks the view of the retina. In NS, the ocular fundus is still visible. Mature cataracts can result in complete blindness of the affected individual, which needs to be considered with regard to animal husbandry measures (e.g. social grouping, enrichment, cage relocation). However, mouse lemurs adapt very well to this slowly progressing condition, although blindness may affect the circadian activity rhythm of the animal. In association with cataracts, some animals also show iris synechia or pupil seclusion. These diseases affect the iris muscle and can lead to an increase in intraocular pressure (Dubicanac et al. 2017). Intraocular pressure (physiological value 20.3 ± 2.8 mm Hg; mean ± SD) can be measured via tonometry (Dubicanac et al. 2016). Other rare ocular findings described in mouse lemurs are exophthalmos, phthisis bulbi, hyphaema, ectopia lentis, corectopia, trichiasis, staphyloma, cornea dystrophy and degeneration, corneal lipid infiltration, chorioretinitis, and scleral and corneal xanthomatous inflammation (Alleaume et al. 2017; Dubicanac et al. 2017, Robert Schopler, personal communication).

Neoplasia

Neoplasia in mouse lemurs are described for animals with a minimum age of five years (Remick et al. 2009; Liptovszky et al. 2011). The most common types are lymphoma, leukaemia and (adeno-) carcinoma (Remick et al. 2009). The organ systems most affected are the haematopoietic system, the reproductive system, the digestive system and the integumentary system (Remick et al. 2009). Surgical removal may be feasible for solid tumours.

Viral and bacterial diseases

There are no published reports of viral infections in captive mouse lemurs. However, a screening of wild *M. rufus* in Ranomafana National Park in Madagascar revealed five viral groups commonly associated with diarrhoeal disease in humans (adenovirus, enterovirus, rotavirus and norovirus (genogroups GI and GII; Zohdy et al. 2015)).

A *Listeria monocytogenes* outbreak was reported in a captive population of *M. murinus* (Hülskötter et al. 2017). Infected animals were in good nutritional state but deceased acutely after showing heavy breathing and multiple neurological deficits, like paraplegia, missing flight reflexes and apathy. Necropsy revealed hyperaemia of meningeal vessels and swelling of the liver with multifocal reddish to yellow or white areas (up to 3 mm in diameter). An infection with *L. monocytogenes* could be confirmed by immunohistochemistry and microbiological analyses based on culture methods. The route of infection could not be specified, but food contamination seems most likely. One case of *Yersinia pseudotuberculosis* in *M. murinus* was described post-mortem in the colony at Zurich Zoo, Switzerland (Bauert et al. 2007). It was assumed that the animal had been infected by contaminated food items.

Renal diseases

High morbidity and elevated mortality of mouse lemurs aged three to five years was observed in a mouse lemur colony in Brunoy (France) in the 1970s. Necropsy revealed *inter alia* pathologically altered kidneys due to chronic nephrosis with nephritis. A link to elevated glucocorticoid levels due to stress factors in laboratory-housed mouse lemurs was suggested (Perret 1982).

Obesity

Seasonal fattening during short-day periods in mouse lemurs occurs physiologically as described and mouse lemurs seem to be protected against glucose intolerance during fattening (Terrien et al. 2018). Furthermore, a major inflammatory response is absent, suggesting that pathological stages are not reached during the massive seasonal body weight gain and loss (Giroud et al. 2009; Terrien et al. 2018). However, fatty accumulations in the liver are described as a common pathological finding in the short-day period (Perret 1982) and uncontrollable diabetes occurs (Perret 1982). Moreover, in the second half of the short-day period, when animals lose weight again, mouse lemurs show increased fasting insulin levels and no protection against glucose intolerance anymore (Terrien et al. 2018). Moderate caloric restriction during the short-day period increases torpor frequency but does not result in oxidative stress (Giroud et al. 2009). It should therefore be used during short-day periods to prevent animals from obesity-associated diseases.

Idiopathic peripheral vestibular disease

Two cases of idiopathic peripheral vestibular disease were observed in the Hannover colony (unpublished data). Both individuals were aged females that presented a peracute onset of the typical symptoms of head tilt and ataxia (no nystagmus or strabismus was observed; however, both animals had mature cataracts). Supportive care (e.g. fluids, antinausea drugs) may help initial recovery, but a residual head tilt may persist.

Vasculitis

One case of an idiopathic granulomatous generalised vasculitis in a mouse lemur was described for a six-year-old male that showed acute onset of inappetence in combination with weight loss and haematuria (Cichon et al. 2017). In the genital region, the coat was blood-smeared, and, despite immediate medical treatment, the animal was found dead two days later. The pathogenesis remained unclear, but an autoimmune or allergic disorder is discussed (Cichon et al. 2017).

Spontaneous spongiform brainstem degeneration

One case of spontaneous spongiform brainstem degeneration was described for a female grey mouse lemur that died on postnatal day 125 (Schmidtke et al. 2018b). The animal showed severe growth retardation, neurological abnormalities, impaired development of motor skills and incipient bilateral cataracts as well as a missing optokinetic nystagmus. Several genes showed mutations and are discussed regarding a potential relation to the observed pathology.

Developmental delay and changes in fur colouration

A temporal change in fur colouration was observed in one female infant following neonatal diarrhoea (yellow pasty faeces) starting around day 7 postpartum. The previously normal body mass development stagnated, and the individual fell behind the siblings in body size and weight. The animal received supplementary feeding, to compensate for nutritional deficits in the course of the observed diarrhoeal disease (see section on Breeding earlier in this chapter), and regained the developmental level of the other infants at the age of three months. Interestingly, the fur colour changed in this individual and turned light grey to white during the period of developmental delay. The coat furthermore became dull, with hair loss and pronounced alopecia on the face. Changes in fur texture and colouration were reverted when she became an adult. Today (in 2020), this animal is 10 years old.

Abnormal behaviour

Stereotypies, or abnormal repetitive behaviours, can be used as welfare indicators. They mostly occur in the context of stressful situations (e.g. after treatment) or may be an expression of pain (Mills et al. 2006). Stereotypies include circling, excessive grooming and self-biting. See also Chapter 6: Brief introduction to welfare assessment: a 'toolbox' of techniques. Self-mutilation ranges from sucking on tail/fingers to severe self-biting of the tail or limbs, often following a previous injury. Therefore, animals should be prevented from accessing wounds (see the preceding text). Social housing after or sometimes during healing of self-inflicted wounds can help to prevent further automutilation. A case of adult cannibalism has been observed in the wild, with the cause of death of the cannibalised animal being unknown (Haemaelaeinen 2012). Partial eating of dead infants or dead adult conspecifics, has been documented in captivity in both, *M. murinus* as well as in *M. lehilahytsara*, that had been housed together for several years (unpublished data).

Acknowledgements

The authors would like to thank the animal keepers Achim Sauer, Wolfgang Mehl, Lisabelle Früh, Iris Grages, Johanna Samtlebe, Mandy Ruddat and Mariette Boeck, as well as the veterinarians Annette Klaus and Marko Dubicanac. We are also grateful to the technical employees Brigitte Lohmeier, Elisabeth Engelke, Birgit Haßfurther and Sönke von den Berg for technical support. Furthermore, we acknowledge Nadine Mestre-Francés and the veterinarian Jaques Damien Arnaud for sharing information about medical treatments at their mouse lemur colony in Montpellier, France. Finally, we thank the editor and two anonymous reviewers for their constructive comments on the first draft of this manuscript.

References

Agnani, P., Kauffmann, C., Hayes, L.D. and Schradin, C. (2018) Intraspecific variation in social organization of strepsirrhines. *American Journal of Primatology*, **80**, e22758. doi: 10.1002/ajp.22758.

Alleaume, C., Mrini, M.E., Laloy, E. et al. (2017) Scleral and corneal xanthomatous inflammation in a gray mouse lemur (*Microcebus murinus*). *Veterinary Ophthalmology*, **20**, 177–180. doi: 10.1111/vop.12374.

Andrews, C.A., Ramberloarivony, H., Génin, F. and Masters, J.C. (2016) Why cheirogaleids are bad models for primates ancestors: a phylogenetic reconstruction. In: *The Dwarf and Mouse Lemurs of Madagascar*. Eds Lehman, S.M., Radespiel, P.D. and Zimmermann, E., p. 19. Cambridge University Press, Cambridge, UK.

Andriantompohavana, R., Zaonarivelo, J.R., Engberg, S.W. et al. (2006) Mouse lemurs of northwestern Madagascar with a description of a new species at Lokobe Special Reserve. *Occasional Papers Museum Texas Tech University*, **259**, 1–23. doi: 10.5962/bhl.title.156966.

Araújo, A. (2003) Male behavioral response to the urine odor of females in lesser mouse lemur (*Microcebus murinus* Miller, 1777) (Cheirogaleidae, Primates). *Revista Brasileira de Zoociências*, **5**.

Aslam, H., Schneiders, A., Perret, M. et al. (2002) Quantitative assessment of testicular germ cell production and kinematic and morphometric parameters of ejaculated spermatozoa in the grey mouse lemur, Microcebus murinus. *Reproduction*, **123**, 323–332. doi: 10.1530/rep.0.1230323.

Atsalis, S., Schmid, J. and Kappeler, P.M. (1996) Metrical comparisons of three species of mouse lemur. *Journal of Human Evolution*, **1**, 61–68. doi: 10.1006/jhev.1996.0049.

Aujard, F. (1997) Effect of vomeronasal organ removal on male sociosexual responses to female in a prosimian primate (Microcebus murinus). *Physiology & Behavior*, **62**, 1003–1008.

Aujard, F. and Vasseur, F. (2001) Effect of ambient temperature on the body temperature rhythm of male gray mouse lemurs (*Microcebus murinus*). *International Journal of Primatology*, **22**, 43–56. doi: 10.1023/A:1026461914534.

Bauert, M., Furrer, S., Zingg, R. and Steinmetz, H. (2007) Three years of experience running the Masoala Rainforest ecosystem at Zurich Zoo, Switzerland. *International Zoo Yearbook*, **41**, 203–216. doi: 10.1111/j.1748-1090.2007.00012.x.

Beltran, W.A., Vanore, M., Ollivet, F. et al. (2007) Ocular findings in two colonies of gray mouse lemurs (*Microcebus murinus*). *Veterinary Ophthalmology*, **10**, 43–49.

Biggar, K.K., Wu, C.-W., Tessier, S.N. et al. (2015) Primate torpor: regulation of stress-activated protein kinases during daily torpor in the gray mouse lemur, *Microcebus murinus*. *Genomics, Proteomics & Bioinformatics*, **13**, 81–90.

Blanco, M.B., Andriantsalohimisantatra, A.A., Rivoharison, T.V. and Andriambeloson, J.B. (2017) Evidence of prolonged torpor in Goodman's mouse lemurs at Ankafobe Forest, central Madagascar. *Primates*, **58**, 31–37. doi: 10.1007/s10329-016-0586-3.

Bons, N., Lehmann, S., Nishida, N. et al. (2002) BSE infection of the small short-lived primate *Microcebus murinus*. *Comptes Rendus Biologies*, **325**, 67–74. doi: 10.1016/S1631-0691(02)01390-2.

Bons, N., Mestre-Frances, N., Belli, P. et al. (1999) Natural and experimental oral infection of nonhuman primates by bovine spongiform encephalopathy agents. *Proceedings of the National Academy of Sciences*, **96**, 4046–4051. doi: 10.1073/pnas.96.7.4046.

Bons, N., Mestre, N. and Petter, A. (1992) Senile plaques and neurofibrillary changes in the brain of an aged lemurian primate, *Microcebus murinus*. *Neurobiology of aging*, **13**, 99–105. doi: 10.1016/0197-4580(92)90016-Q.

Bons, N., Mestre, N., Ritchie, K. et al. (1994) Identification of amyloid beta protein in the brain of the small, short-lived lemurian primate *Microcebus murinus*. *Neurobiology of Aging*, **15**, 215–220. doi: 10.1016/0197-4580(94)90115-5.

Bons, N., Rieger, F., Prudhomme, D. et al. (2006) *Microcebus murinus*: a useful primate model for human cerebral aging and Alzheimer's disease? *Genes, Brain & Behavior*, **5**, 120–130. doi: 10.1111/j.1601-183X.2005.00149.x.

Borgerson, C. (2016) Optimizing conservation policy: the importance of seasonal variation in hunting and meat consumption on the Masoala peninsula of Madagascar. *Oryx*, **50**, 405–418. doi: 10.1017/S0030605315000307.

Braune, P., Schmidt, S. and Zimmermann, E. (2005) Spacing and group coordination in a nocturnal primate, the golden brown mouse lemur (*Microcebus ravelobensis*): the role of olfactory and acoustic signals. *Behavioral Ecology and Sociobiology*, **58**, 587–596. doi: 10.1007/s00265-005-0944-4.

Buesching, C., Heistermann, M., Hodges, J. and Zimmermann, E. (1998) Multimodal oestrus advertisement in a small nocturnal prosimian, *Microcebus murinus*. *Folia Primatologica*, **69**, 295–308. doi: 10.1159/000052718.

Cartmill, M. (1972) Arboreal adaptations and the origin of the order primates. In *The Functional and Evolutionary Biology of Primates*. Ed. Tuttle, R., pp. 97–122, Aldine/Atherton, Chicago, USA.

Caspers, J., Radespiel, U., Zimmermann, E. and Schulz, S. (2020) Volatile urinary signals of two nocturnal primates. *Microcebus murinus* and *M. lehilahytsara*. *Frontiers in Ecology and Evolution*, **8**. doi: 10.3389/fevo.2020.00158.

Cichon, N., Lampe, K., Bremmer, F. et al. (2017) Unique case of granulomatous arteritis in a grey mouse lemur (*Microcebus murinus*)–first case description. *Primate Biology*, **4**, 71–75. doi: 10.5194/pb-4-71-2017.

Cooper, H. (1986) The accessory optic system in a prosimian primate (*Microcebus murinus*): Evidence for a direct retinal projection to the medial terminal nucleus. *Journal of Comparative Neurology*, **249**, 28–47.

Cora, M.C., Kooistra, L. and Travlos, G. (2015) Vaginal cytology of the laboratory rat and mouse: review and criteria for the staging of the estrous cycle using stained vaginal smears. *Toxicologic pathology*, **43**, 776–793. doi: 10.1177/0192623315570339.

Craul, M., Zimmermann, E. and Radespiel, U. (2004) First experimental evidence for female mate choice in a nocturnal primate. *Primates*, **45**, 271–274. doi: 10.1007/s10329-004-0097-5.

Dal-Pan, A., Pifferi, F., Marchal, J. et al. (2011) Cognitive performances are selectively enhanced during chronic caloric restriction or resveratrol supplementation in a primate. *PLoS One*, **6**, e16581. doi: 10.1371/journal.pone.0016581.

Dausmann, K. (2014) Flexible patterns in energy savings: heterothermy in primates. *Journal of Zoology*, **292**, 101–111. doi: 10.1111/jzo.12104.

Delacourte, A., Sautiere, P.-E., Wattez, A. et al. (1995) Biochemical characterization of Tau proteins during cerebral aging of the lemurian primate *Microcebus murinus*. *Comptes rendus de l'Academie des sciences. Serie III, Sciences de la vie*, **318**, 85–89.

Dhenain, M., Chenu, E., Hisley, C.K. et al. (2003) Regional atrophy in the brain of lissencephalic mouse lemur primates: Measurement by automatic histogram-based segmentation of MR images. *Magnetic Resonance in Medicine*, **50**, 984–992. doi: 10.1002/mrm.10612.

Dhenain, M., Michot, J.L., Privat, N. et al. (2000) MRI description of cerebral atrophy in mouse lemur primates. *Neurobiology of aging*, **21**, 81–88. doi: 10.1016/S0197-4580(00)00098-1.

Djelti, F., Dhenain, M., Terrien, J. et al. (2017) Impaired fasting blood glucose is associated to cognitive impairment and cerebral atrophy in middle-aged non-human primates. *Aging*, **9**, 173. doi: 10.18632/aging.101148.

Dkhissi-Benyahya, O., Szel, A., DeGrip, W.J. and Cooper, H.M. (2001) Short and mid-wavelength cone distribution in a nocturnal strepsirrhine primate (*Microcebus murinus*). *Journal of Comparative Neurology*, **438**, 490–504.

Dubicanac, M., Joly, M., Strüve, J. et al. (2016) Intraocular pressure in the smallest primate aging model: the gray mouse lemur. *Veterinary Ophthalmology*, 1–9. doi: 10.1111/vop.12434.

Dubicanac, M., Radespiel, U. and Zimmermann, E. (2017) A review on ocular findings in mouse lemurs: potential links to age and genetic background. *Primate Biology*, **4**, 215–228. doi: 10.5194/pb-4-215-2017.

Eberle, M. and Kappeler, P.M. (2004a) Selected polyandry: female choice and inter-sexual conflict in a small nocturnal solitary primate (*Microcebus murinus*). *Behavioral Ecology & Sociobiology*, **57**, 91–100. doi: 10.1007/s00265-004-0823-4.

Eberle, M. and Kappeler, P. M. (2004b) Sex in the dark: determinants and consequences of mixed male mating tactics in *Microcebus murinus*, a small solitary nocturnal primate. *Behavioral Ecology & Sociobiology*, **57**, 77–90. doi: 10.1007/s00265-004-0826-1.

Eberle, M. and Kappeler, P.M. (2006) Family insurance: kin selection and cooperative breeding in a solitary primate (*Microcebus murinus*). *Behavioral Ecology & Sociobiology*, **60**, 582–588. doi: 10.1007/s00265-006-0203-3.

Eberle, M., Perret, M. and Kappeler, P.M. (2007) Sperm competition and optimal timing of matings in *Microcebus murinus*. *International Journal of Primatology*, **28**, 1267–1278. doi: 10.1007/s10764-007-9220-y.

Evasoa, M.R., Radespiel, U., Hasiniaina, A.F. et al. (2018) Variation in reproduction of the smallest-bodied primate radiation, the mouse lemurs (*Microcebus* spp.): a synopsis. *American Journal of Primatology*, e22874. doi: 10.1002/ajp.22874.

Evasoa, M.R., Zimmermann, E., Hasiniaina, A.F. et al. (2019) Sources of variation in social tolerance in mouse lemurs (*Microcebus* spp.). *BMC Ecology*, **19**, 20. doi: 10.1186/s12898-019-0236-x.

Ezran, C., Karanewsky, C.J., Pendleton, J.L. et al. (2017) The mouse lemur, a genetic model organism for primate biology, behavior, and health. *Genetics*, **206**, 651–664. doi: 10.1534/genetics.116.199448.

Faherty, S.L., Campbell, C.R., Hilbig, S.A. and Yoder, A.D. (2017) The effect of body mass and diet composition on torpor patterns in a Malagasy primate (*Microcebus murinus*). *Journal of Comparative Physiology B*, **187**, 677–688.

Fichtel, C. (2016) Predation in the dark: antipredator strategies of Cheirogaleidae and other nocturnal primates. In: *The Dwarf and Mouse Lemurs of Madagascar*. Eds Lehman, S.M., Radespiel, P.D. and Zimmermann, E., p. 15. Cambridge University Press, Cambridge, UK.

Fischer, K.E. and Austad, S.N. (2011) The development of small primate models for aging research. *ILAR Journal*, **52**, 78–88. doi: 10.1093/ilar.52.1.78.

Fleagle, J.G. (2013) *Primate Adaptation and Evolution*. Academic Press, San Diego, USA.

Fleagle, J. G. (2014) Identifying primate species: Introduction. *Evolutionary Anthropology*, **23**, 1–1. doi: 10.1002/evan.21398.

Fritz, R.G., Zimmermann, E., Picq, J.-L. et al. (2020) Sex-specific patterns of age-related cerebral atrophy in a nonhuman primate *Microcebus murinus*. *Neurobiology of Aging*, **91**, 148–159. doi: 10.1016/j.neurobiolaging.2020.02.027.

Ganzhorn, J.U., Hapke, A., Lahann, P. et al. (2013) Population genetics, parasitism, and long-term population dynamics of *Microcebus murinus* in littoral forest fragments of south-eastern Madagascar. In: *Leaping Ahead: Advances in Prosimian Biology*. Eds Masters, J., Gamba, M. & Génin, F., pp. 61–69. Springer, New York, USA.

Ganzhorn, J.U., Klaus, S., Ortmann, S. and Schmid, J. (2003) Adaptations to seasonality: some primate and nonprimate examples. In *Primate Life Histories and Socioecology*, pp. 132–148, The University of Chicago Press, Chicago, USA.

Genin, F. and Perret, M. (2000) Photoperiod-induced changes in energy balance in gray mouse lemurs. *Physiology & Behavior*, **71**, 315–321. doi: 10.1016/S0031-9384(00)00335-8.

Giroud, S., Perret, M., Gilbert, C. et al. (2009) Dietary palmitate and linoleate oxidations, oxidative stress, and DNA damage differ according to season in mouse lemurs exposed to a chronic food deprivation. *American Journal of Physiology-Regulatory, Integrative and Comparative Physiology*, **297**, R950–R959. doi: 10.1152/ajpregu.00214.2009.

Glatston, A.R. (1979) Reproduction and behaviour of the lesser mouse lemur (*Microcebus murinus*, Miller 1777) in captivity. London, University of London.

Goerlitz, H.R. and Siemers, B.M. (2007) Sensory ecology of prey rustling sounds: acoustical features and their classification by wild grey mouse lemurs. *Functional Ecology*, **21**, 143–153. doi: 10.1111/j.1365-2435.2006.01212.x.

Goodman, S. M., O'Connor, S. and Langrand, O. (1993) A review of predation on Lemurs: Implications for the evolution of social behavior in small, nocturnal primates. In *Lemur Social Systems and Their Ecological Basis*. Eds Kappeler, P.M. and Ganzhorn, J.U., pp. 51–66. Plenum Press, New York, USA.

Groves, C. (2016) The taxonomy of Cheirogaleidae: an ever-expanding species list. In: *The Dwarf and Mouse Lemurs of Madagascar*. Eds Lehman, S.M., Radespiel, P.D. and Zimmermann, E., p. 33, Cambridge University Press, Cambridge, UK.

Haemaelaeinen, A. (2012) A case of adult cannibalism in the gray mouse lemur, *Microcebus murinus*. *American Journal of Primatology*, **74**, 783–787. doi: 10.1002/ajp.22034.

Hafen, T., Neveu, H., Rumpler, Y. et al. (1998) Acoustically dimorphic advertisement calls separate morphologically and genetically homogenous populations of the grey mouse lemur (*Microcebus murinus*). *Folia Primatologica*, **69**, 342–356. doi: 10.1159/000052723.

Hasiniaina, A.F., Radespiel, U., Kessler, S.E. et al. (2020) Evolutionary significance of the variation in acoustic communication of a cryptic nocturnal primate radiation (*Microcebus* spp.). *Ecology and evolution*, **10**, 3784–3797.

Hending, D., Holderied, M. and McCabe, G. (2017) The use of Vocalizations of the Sambirano Mouse Lemur (*Microcebus sambiranensis*) in an Acoustic Survey of Habitat Preference. *International Journal of Primatology*, **38**, 732–750. doi: 10.1007/s10764-017-9977-6.

Hladik, C.M., Charles-Dominique, P. and Petter, J.J. (1980) Feeding strategies of five nocturnal prosimians in the dry forest of the west coast of Madagascar. In: *Nocturnal Malagasy Primates. Ecology, Physiology, and Behavior*. Eds Charles-Dominique, P., Cooper, H.M., Hladik, A. et al., pp. 41–73. Academic Press, New York, USA.

Hohenbrink, P., Dempewolf, S., Zimmermann, E. et al. (2014) Functional promiscuity in a mammalian chemosensory system: extensive expression of vomeronasal receptors in the main olfactory epithelium of mouse lemurs. *Frontiers in Neuroanatomy*, **8**. doi: 10.3389/fnana.2014.00102.

Hohenbrink, P., Mundy, N.I., Zimmermann, E. and Radespiel, U. (2013) First evidence for functional vomeronasal 2 receptor genes in primates. *Biology Letters*, **9**, 20121006. doi: 10.1098/rsbl.2012.1006.

Hohenbrink, P., Radespiel, U. and Mundy, N.I. (2012) Pervasive and ongoing positive selection in the vomeronasal-1 receptor (V1R) repertoire of mouse lemurs. *Molecular Biology and Evolution*, **29**, 3807–3816. doi: 10.1093/molbev/mss188.

Hohenbrink, S., Koberstein-Schwarz, M., Zimmermann, E. and Radespiel, U. (2015a) Shades of gray mouse lemurs: ontogeny of female dominance and dominance-related behaviors in a nocturnal primate. *American Journal of Primatology*, **77**, 1158–1169. doi: 10.1002/ajp.22452.

Hohenbrink, S., Schaarschmidt, F., Bünemann, K. et al. (2016) Female dominance in two basal primates, *Microcebus murinus* and *Microcebus lehilahytsara*: variation and determinants. *Animal Behaviour*, **122**, 145–156.

Hohenbrink, S., Zimmermann, E. and Radespiel, U. (2015b) Need for speed: Sexual maturation precedes social maturation in gray mouse lemurs. *American Journal of Primatology*, **77**, 1049–1059. doi: 10.1002/ajp.22440.

Horvath, J.E. and Willard, H.F. (2007) Primate comparative genomics: lemur biology and evolution. *Trends in Genetics*, **23**, 173–182.

Hotaling, S., Foley, M.E., Lawrence, N.M. *et al.* (2016) Species discovery and validation in a cryptic radiation of endangered primates: coalescent-based species delimitation in Madagascar's mouse lemurs. *Molecular Ecology*, **25**, 2029–2045. doi: 10.1111/mec.13604.

Huchard, E., Canale, C.I., Le Gros, C. *et al.* (2012) Convenience polyandry or convenience polygyny? Costly sex under female control in a promiscuous primate. *Proceedings of the Royal Society B: Biological Sciences*, **279**, 1371–1379.

Hülskötter, K., Schmidtke, D., Dubicanac, M. *et al.* (2017) Spontaneous listeriosis in grey mouse lemurs (*Microcebus murinus*), but not in Goodman's mouse lemurs (*Microcebus lehilahytsara*) of the same colony. *Veterinary Microbiology*, **208**, 94–96. doi: 10.1016/j.vetmic.2017.07.023.

Jolly, A. (1966) Lemur social behavior and primate intelligence. *Science*, **153**, 501–506. doi: 10.1126/science.153.3735.501.

Joly, M., Ammersdörfer, S., Schmidtke, D. and Zimmermann, E. (2014) Touchscreen-based cognitive tasks reveal age-related impairment in a primate aging model, the grey mouse lemur (*Microcebus murinus*). *PLoS One*, **9**, e109393. doi: 10.1371/journal.pone.0109393.

Joly, M., Michel, B., Deputte, B. *et al.* (2004) Odor discrimination assessment with an automated olfactometric method in a prosimian primate, *Microcebus murinus*. *Physiology & Behavior*, **82**, 325–329. doi: 10.1016/j.physbeh.2004.03.019.

Joly, M. and Zimmermann, E. (2011) Do solitary foraging nocturnal mammals plan their routes? *Biology Letters*, **7**, 638–640. doi: 10.1098/rsbl.2011.0258.

Jürges, V., Kitzler, J., Zingg, R. and Radespiel, U. (2013) First Insights into the Social Organisation of Goodman's Mouse Lemur (*Microcebus lehilahytsara*) – Testing Predictions from Socio-Ecological Hypotheses in the Masoala Hall of Zurich Zoo. *Folia Primatologica*, **84**, 32–48. doi: 10.1159/000345917.

Kappel, P., Hohenbrink, S. and Radespiel, U. (2011) Experimental evidence for olfactory predator recognition in wild mouse lemurs. *American Journal of Primatology*, **73**, 928–938. doi: 10.1002/ajp.20963.

Kappeler, P.M. (1998) Nests, tree holes, and the evolution of primate life histories. *American Journal of Primatology*, **46**, 7–33. doi: 10.1002/(sici)1098-2345(1998)46:1<7::aid-ajp3>3.0.co;2-#.

Kappeler, P.M. and Ganzhorn, J.U. (1993) The evolution of primate communities and societies in Madagascar. *Evolutionary Anthropology: Issues, News, and Reviews*, **2**, 159–171.

Kappeler, P.M., Rasoloarison, R.M., Razafimanantsoa, L. *et al.* (2005) Morphology, behaviour and molecular evolution of giant mouse lemurs (*Mirza* spp.) Gray, 1870, with description of a new species. *Primate Report*, **71**, 3–26.

Karanth, K.P., Delefosse, T., Rakotosamimanana, B. *et al.* (2005) Ancient DNA from giant extinct lemurs confirms single origin of Malagasy primates. *Proceedings of the National Academy of Sciences of the United States of America*, **102**, 5090–5095. doi: 10.1073/pnas.0408354102.

Kästner, S.B., Tünsmeyer, J. and Schütter, A.F. (2016) How to anesthetize mouse lemurs. In *The Dwarf and Mouse Lemurs of Madagascar: Biology, Behavior and Conservation Biogeography of the Cheirogaleidae*. Eds Lehman, S.M., Radespiel, U. and Zimmermann, E., pp. 135–160, Cambridge University Press, Cambridge, UK.

Kessler, S.E., Radespiel, U., Hasiniaina, A.I. *et al.* (2018) Does the grey mouse lemur use agonistic vocalisations to recognise kin? *Contributions to Zoology*, **87**, 261–274.

Kessler, S.E., Radespiel, U., Nash, L.T. and Zimmermann, E. (2016) Modeling the origins of primates sociality: social flexibility and kinship in mouse lemurs (*Microcebus* spp.). In: *The Dwarf and Mouse Lemurs of Madagascar*. Eds Lehman, S.M., Radespiel, U. and Zimmermann, E., pp. 422–445, Cambridge University Press, Cambridge, UK.

Kessler, S.E., Scheumann, M., Nash, L.T. and Zimmermann, E. (2012) Paternal kin recognition in the high frequency/ultrasonic range in a solitary foraging mammal. *BMC Ecology*, **12**, 26. doi: 10.1186/1472-6785-12-26.

Kittler, K., Kappeler, P.M. and Fichtel, C. (2018) Instrumental problem-solving abilities in three lemur species (*Microcebus murinus*, *Varecia variegata*, and *Lemur catta*). *Journal of Comparative Psychology*, **132**, 306. doi: 10.1037/com0000113.

Kollikowski, A., Zimmermann, E. and Radespiel, U. (2019) First experimental evidence for olfactory species discrimination in two nocturnal primate species (*Microcebus lehilahytsara* and *M. murinus*). *Scientific Reports*, **9**, 1–12.

Kuhn, M. (1989) Verhaltensbiologische Untersuchungen zur Ontogenese von Mausmakis (*Microcebus murinus*, Miller 1777) mit besonderer Berücksichtigung der akustischen Kommunikation. Stuttgart-Hohenheim, Universität Hohenheim.

Lacreuse, A., Raz, N., Schmidtke, D. *et al.* (2020) Age-related decline in executive function as a hallmark of cognitive aging in primates: an overview of cognitive and neurobiological studies. *Philosophical Transactions of The Royal Society B Biological Sciences*, **375**, 1811. doi: 10.1098/rstb.2019.0618.

Larsen, P.A., Harris, R.A., Liu, Y. *et al.* (2017a) Hybrid de novo genome assembly and centromere characterization of the gray mouse lemur (*Microcebus murinus*). *BMC Biology*, **15**, 110. doi: 10.1186/s12915-017-0439-6.

Larsen, P.A., Lutz, M.W., Hunnicutt, K.E. *et al.* (2017b) The Alu neurodegeneration hypothesis: a primate-specific mechanism for neuronal transcription noise, mitochondrial dysfunction, and manifestation of neurodegenerative disease. *Alzheimer's & Dementia*, **13**, 828–838. doi: 10.1016/j.jalz.2017.01.017.

Lasbleiz, C., Mestre-Francés, N., Devau, G. *et al.* (2019) Combining Gene Transfer and Nonhuman Primates to Better Understand and Treat Parkinson's Disease. *Frontiers in Molecular Neuroscience*, **12**, 10. doi: 10.3389/fnmol.2019.00010.

Le Corre, M., Noristani, H.N., Mestre-Frances, N. *et al.* (2018) A novel translational model of spinal cord injury in nonhuman primate. *Neurotherapeutics*, **15**, 751–769. doi: 10.1007/s13311-017-0589-9.

Leary, S., Underwood, W., Anthony, R. *et al.* (2020) *AVMA Guidelines for the Euthanasia of Animal: 2020 Edition*. AVMA American Veterinary Medical Association: Schaumburg, IL, USA.

Lehman, S.M., Radespiel, U. and Zimmermann, E. (2016) Conservation biology of the Cheirogaleidae: future research directions. In: *The Dwarf and Mouse Lemurs of Madagascar: Biology, Behavior and Conservation Biogeography of the Cheirogaleidae*. Eds Lehman, S.M., Radespiel, U. and Zimmermann, E., pp. 520–540, Cambridge University Press, Cambridge, UK.

Leliveld, L.M., Scheumann, M. and Zimmermann, E. (2010) Effects of caller characteristics on auditory laterality in an early primate (*Microcebus murinus*). *PLoS One*, **5**, e9031. doi: 10.1371/journal.pone.0009031.

Leliveld, L.M.C., Scheumann, M. and Zimmermann, E. (2011) Acoustic correlates of individuality in the vocal repertoire of a nocturnal primate (*Microcebus murinus*). *Journal of the Acoustical Society of America*, **129**, 2278–2288. doi: 10.1121/1.3559680.

Liptovszky, M., Perge, E., Molnár, V. and Sós, E. (2011) Osteoblastic osteosarcoma in a grey mouse lemur (*Microcebus murinus*). *Acta Veterinaria Hungarica*, **59**, 433–437. doi: 10.1556/AVet.2011.030.

Louis, E.E., Coles, M.S., Andriantompohavana, R. *et al.* (2006) Revision of the mouse lemurs (*Microcebus*) of eastern Madagascar. *International Journal of Primatology*, **27**, 347–389. doi: 10.1007/s10764-006-9036-1.

Louis, E.E., Engberg, S.E., McGuire, S.M. *et al.* (2008) Revision of the mouse lemurs, *Microcebus* (Primates, Lemuriformes), of northern and northwestern Madagascar with descriptions of two new species at Montagne d'Ambre National Park and Antafondro Classified Forest. *Primate Conservation*, **23**, 19–39. doi: 10.1896/052.023.0103.

Lovegrove, B.G., Canale, C., Levesque, D. *et al.* (2014) Are tropical small mammals vulnerable to Arrhenius effects and climate change? *Physiological and Biochemical Zoology*, **87**, 30–45. doi: 10.1086/673313.

Lutermann, H., Schmelting, B., Radespiel, U. *et al.* (2006) The role of survival for the evolution of female philopatry in a solitary forager, the grey mouse lemur (*Microcebus murinus*). *Proceedings of the Royal Society B*, **273**, 2527–2533. doi: 10.1098/rspb.2006.3603.

Martin, R.D. (1972a) A laboratory breeding colony of the lesser mouse lemur. In *Breeding Primates*. Ed. Beveridge, W.I.B., pp. 161–171. Karger, Basel, CHE.

Martin, R.D. (1972b) A preliminary field-study of the lesser mouse lemur (*Microcebus murinus* J.F. Miller 1777). *Zeitschrift fuer Tierpsychologie*, **9**, 43–89.

Martin, R.D. (1973) A review of the behaviour and ecology of the lesser mouse lemur (*Microcebus murinus*). In *Comparative Ecology and Behaviour of Primates*, Eds Michael, R.P. and Crook, J.H., pp. 1–68. Academic Press, London, UK.

Martin, R.D. (1990) *Primate Origins and Evolution: A Phylogenetic Reconstruction*. Chapman and Hall, London, UK.

Mestre-Francés, N., Keller, E., Calenda, A. *et al*. (2000) Immunohistochemical analysis of cerebral cortical and vascular lesions in the primate *Microcebus murinus* reveal distinct amyloid ⊠1–42 and ⊠1–40 immunoreactivity profiles. *Neurobiology of Disease*, **7**, 1–8. doi: 10.1006/nbdi.1999.0270.

Mestre-Francés, N., Serratrice, N., Gennetier, A. *et al*. (2018) Exogenous LRRK2G2019S induces parkinsonian-like pathology in a nonhuman primate. *JCI Insight*, **3**. doi: 10.1172/jci.insight.98202.

Mills, D., Luescher, A., Mason, G. and Rushen, J. (2006) Veterinary and pharmacological approaches to abnormal repetitive behaviour. In: *Stereotypic Animal Behaviour: Fundamentals and Applications to Welfare*, 2nd edn, Eds Mason, G. and Rushen, J. pp. 325–356, Cromwell Press, Trowbridge, UK.

Mittermeier, R.A., Hawkins, F., Louis, E.E. *et al*. (2010) *Lemurs of Madagascar*. Conservation International, Washington, D.C., USA.

Nadkarni, N.A., Bougacha, S., Garin, C. *et al*. (2019) A 3D population-based brain atlas of the mouse lemur primate with examples of applications in aging studies and comparative anatomy. *NeuroImage*, **185**, 85–95.

Niaussat, M.M. and Petter, J.J. (1980) Etude de la sensibilité auditive d'un lémurien malgache: *Microcebus murinus* (J.-F. Miller, 1777). *Mammalia*, **44**, 553–558. doi: 10.1515/mamm.1980.44.4.553.

Olivieri, G., Zimmermann, E., Randrianambinina, B. *et al*. (2007) The ever-increasing diversity in mouse lemurs: three new species in north and northwestern Madagascar. *Molecular phylogenetics and evolution*, **43**, 309–327. doi: 10.1016/j.ympev.2006.10.026.

Olivieri, G.L., Sousa, V., Chikhi, L. and Radespiel, U. (2008) From genetic diversity and structure to conservation: genetic signature of recent population declines in three mouse lemur species (*Microcebus* spp.). *Biological Conservation*, **141**, 1257–1271. doi: 10.1016/j.biocon.2008.02.025.

Ortmann, S., Heldmaier, G., Schmid, J. and Ganzhorn, J. U. (1997) Spontaneous daily torpor in Malagasy mouse lemurs. *The Science of Nature*, **84**, 28–32. doi: 10.1007/s001140050344.

Pechouskova, E., Dammhahn, M., Brameier, M. *et al*. (2015) MHC class II variation in a rare and ecological specialist mouse lemur reveals lower allelic richness and contrasting selection patterns compared to a generalist and widespread sympatric congener. *Immunogenetics*, **67**, 229–245. doi: 10.1007/s00251-015-0827-4.

Peckre, L.R., Fabre, A.-C., Hambuckers, J. *et al*. (2019) Food properties influence grasping strategies in strepsirrhines. *Biological Journal of the Linnean Society*. doi: 10.1093/biolinnean/bly215.

Peichl, L., Kaiser, A., Rakotondraparany, F. *et al*. (2019) Diversity of photoreceptor arrangements in nocturnal, cathemeral and diurnal Malagasy lemurs. *Journal of Comparative Neurology*, **527**, 13–37. doi: 10.1002/cne.24167.

Peichl, L., Rakotondraparany, F. and Kappeler, P. (2001) Photoreceptor types and distributions in nocturnal and diurnal Malagasy primates. *Investigative Ophthalmology & Visual Science*, **42**, S48–S48.

Pellegrino, G., Trubert, C., Terrien, J. *et al*. (2018) A comparative study of the neural stem cell niche in the adult hypothalamus of human, mouse, rat and gray mouse lemur (*Microcebus murinus*). *Journal of Comparative Neurology*, **526**, 1419–1443.

Perret, M. (1982) Stress-effects in *Microcebus murinus*. *Folia Primatologica*, **39**, 63–114. doi: 10.1159/000156069.

Perret, M. (1985) Influence of social factors on seasonal variations in plasma testosterone levels of *Microcebus murinus*. *Zeitschrift fuer Tierpsychologie*, **69**, 265–280. doi: 10.1111/j.1439-0310.1985.tb00152.x.

Perret, M. (1986) Social influences on oestrous cycle length and plasma progesterone concentrations in the female lesser mouse lemur (*Microcebus murinus*). *Reproduction*, **77**, 303–311. doi: 10.1530/jrf.0.0770303.

Perret, M. (1990) Influence of Social-Factors on Sex-Ratio at Birth, Maternal Investment and Young Survival in a Prosimian Primate. *Behavioral Ecology and Sociobiology*, **27**, 447–454. doi: 10.1007/BF00164072.

Perret, M. (1992) Environmental and social determinants of sexual function in the male lesser mouse lemur (*Microcebus murinus*). *Folia Primatologica*, **59**, 1–25. doi: 10.1159/000156637.

Perret, M. and Aujard, F. (2001a) Daily hypothermia and torpor in a tropical primate: synchronization by 24-h light–dark cycle. *American Journal of Physiology-Regulatory, Integrative and Comparative Physiology*, **281**, R1925–R1933. doi: 10.1152/ajpregu.2001.281.6.R1925.

Perret, M. and Aujard, F. (2001b) Regulation by photoperiod of seasonal changes in body mass and reproductive function in gray mouse lemurs (*Microcebus murinus*): differential responses by sex. *International Journal of Primatology*, **22**, 5–24. doi: 10.1023/A:1026457813626.

Perret, M., Gomez, D., Barbosa, A. *et al*. (2010) Increased late night response to light controls the circadian pacemaker in a nocturnal primate. *Journal of Biological Rhythms*, **25**, 186–196.

Petter-Rousseaux, A. (1970) Observations sur l'influence de la photopériode sur l'activité sexuelle chez *Microcebus murinus* (Miller, 1777) en captivité. Annales de Biologie Animale Biochimie Biophysique. EDP Sciences.

Petter-Rousseaux, A. (1980) Seasonal activity rhythms, reproduction, and body weight variations in five sympatric nocturnal prosimians, in simulated light and climatic conditions. In: *Nocturnal Malagasy Primates – Ecology, Physiology, and Behavior*. Eds Charles-Dominique, P., Cooper, H.M., Hladik, A. *et al*., pp. 137–152, Academic Press, London, UK.

Picq, J.-L. (1992) Aging and social behaviour in captivity in *Microcebus murinus*. *Folia Primatologica*, **59**, 217–220. doi: 10.1159/000156664.

Picq, J.-L. (1993) Radial maze performance in young and aged grey mouse lemurs (*Microcebus murinus*). *Primates*, **34**, 223–226. doi: 10.1007/BF02381394.

Picq, J.-L. (2016) The gray mouse lemur (*Microcebus murinus*): A novel cognitive primate brain aging model. In: *The Dwarf and Mouse Lemurs of Madagascar: Biology, Behavior and Conservation Biogeography of the Cheirogaleidae*. Eds Lehman, S.M., Radespiel, U. and Zimmermann, E., pp. 381–404. Cambridge University Press, Cambridge, UK.

Picq, J.-L. and Dhenain, M. (1998) Reaction to new objects and spatial changes in young and aged grey mouse lemurs (*Microcebus murinus*). *The Quarterly Journal of Experimental Psychology Section B*, **51**, 337–348. doi: 10.1080/02724995.1998.11733503.

Picq, J.-L., Villain, N., Gary, C. *et al*. (2015) Jumping Stand Apparatus Reveals Rapidly Specific Age-Related Cognitive Impairments in Mouse Lemur Primates. *PLoS One*, **10**. doi: 10.1371/journal.pone.0146238.

Piep, M., Radespiel, U., Zimmermann, E. *et al*. (2008) The sensory basis of prey detection in captive-born grey mouse lemurs. *Microcebus Murinus*, **75**, 871–878.

Pifferi, F., Terrien, J., Marchal, J. *et al*. (2018) Caloric restriction increases lifespan but affects brain integrity in grey mouse lemur primates. *Communications Biology*, **1**, 30. doi: 10.1038/s42003-018-0024-8.

Poulen, G. and Perrin, F.E. (2018) *Microcebus murinus*: A novel promising non-human primate model of spinal cord injury. *Neural Regeneration Research*, **13**, 421. doi: 10.4103/1673-5374.228721.

Radespiel, U. (2000) Sociality in the gray mouse lemur (*Microcebus murinus*) in northwestern Madagascar. *American Journal of Primatology*, **51**, 21–40. doi: 10.1002/(SICI)1098-2345(200005)51:1<21::AID-AJP3>3.0.CO;2-C.

Radespiel, U. (2006) Ecological diversity and seasonal adaptations of mouse lemurs (*Microcebus* spp.). In: *Lemurs: Ecology and Adaptation*. Eds Gould, L. and Sauther, M.L., pp. 211–233. Springer, New York, USA.

Radespiel, U. (2016) Can behavioural ecology help to understand the divergent geographic range sizes of mouse lemurs? In *The Dwarf and Mouse Lemurs of Madagascar*. Eds Lehman, S.M., Radespiel, P.D. and Zimmermann, E., p. 22, Cambridge University Press, Cambridge, UK.

Radespiel, U., Cepok, S., Zietemann, V. and Zimmermann, E. (1998) Sex-specific usage patterns of sleeping sites in grey mouse lemurs (*Microcebus murinus*) in Northwestern Madagascar. *American Journal of Primatology*, **46**, 77–84. doi: 10.1002/(SICI)1098-2345(1998)46:1<77::AID-AJP6>3.0.CO;2-S.

Radespiel, U., Dal Secco, V., Drögemüller, C. et al. (2002) Sexual selection, multiple mating and paternity in grey mouse lemurs, *Microcebus murinus*. *Animal Behaviour*, **63**, 259–268. doi: 10.1006/anbe.2001.1924.

Radespiel, U., Ehresmann, P. and Zimmermann, E. (2001) Contest versus scramble competition for mates: the composition and spatial structure of a population of gray mouse lemurs (*Microcebus murinus*) in north-west Madagascar. *Primates*, **42**, 207. doi: 10.1007/BF02629637.

Radespiel, U., Ehresmann, P. and Zimmermann, E. (2003a) Species-specific usage of sleeping sites in two sympatric mouse lemur species (*Microcebus murinus* and *M. ravelobensis*) in northwestern Madagascar. *American Journal of Primatology*, **59**, 139–151. doi: 10.1002/ajp.10071.

Radespiel, U., Lutermann, H., Schmelting, B. et al. (2003b) Patterns and dynamics of sex-biased dispersal in a nocturnal primate, the grey mouse lemur, *Microcebus murinus*. *Animal Behaviour*, **65**, 709–719. doi: 10.1006/anbe.2003.2121.

Radespiel, U., Lutermann, H., Schmelting, B. and Zimmermann, E. (2019) An empirical estimate of the generation time of mouse lemurs. *American Journal of Primatology*, **81**, e23062.

Radespiel, U., Olivieri, G., Rasolofoson, D.W. et al. (2008) Exceptional diversity of mouse lemurs (*Microcebus* spp.) in the Makira region with the description of one new species. *American Journal of Primatology*, **70**, 1033–1046. doi: 10.1002/ajp.20592.

Radespiel, U., Ratsimbazafy, J.H., Rasoloharijaona, S. et al. (2012) First indications of a highland specialist among mouse lemurs (*Microcebus* spp.) and evidence for a new mouse lemur species from eastern Madagascar. *Primates*, **53**, 157–170. doi: 10.1007/s10329-011-0290-2.

Radespiel, U., Reimann, W., Rahelinirina, M. and Zimmermann, E. (2006) Feeding ecology of sympatric mouse lemur species in northwestern Madagascar. *International Journal of Primatology*, **27**, 311–321. doi: 10.1007/s10764-005-9005-0.

Radespiel, U. and Zimmermann, E. (2001) Female dominance in captive gray mouse lemurs (*Microcebus murinus*). *American Journal of Primatology*, **54**, 181–192. doi: 10.1002/ajp.1029.

Rahlfs, M. and Fichtel, C. (2010) Anti-predator behaviour in a nocturnal primate, the grey mouse lemur (*Microcebus murinus*). *Ethology*, **116**, 429–439. doi: 10.1111/j.1439-0310.2010.01756.x.

Rahman, A., Lamberty, Y., Schenker, E. et al. (2017) Effects of acute administration of donepezil or memantine on sleep-deprivation-induced spatial memory deficit in young and aged non-human primate grey mouse lemurs (*Microcebus murinus*). *PLoS One*, **12**, e0184822. doi: 10.1371/journal.pone.0184822.

Randrianambinina, B. (2001) Contribution à l'étude comparative de l'écoéthologie de deux microcèbes rouges de Madagascar *Microcebus ravelobensis* (Zimmermann et al., 1998) *Microcebus rufus* (Lesson, 1840). Antananarivo, Madagascar, Université d'Antananarivo.

Rasoazanabary, E. and Godfrey, L.R. (2016) Living in riverin and xerci forests: *Microcebus griseorufus* at beza Mahafaly, southwestern Madagascar. In: *The Dwarf and Mouse Lemurs of Madagascar*. Eds Lehman, S.M., Radespiel, P.D. and Zimmermann, E., p. 26. Cambridge University Press, Cambridge, UK.

Rasoloarison, R.M., Goodman, S.M. and Ganzhorn, J.U. (2000) Taxonomic revision of mouse lemurs (*Microcebus*) in the western portions of Madagascar. *International Journal of Primatology*, **21**, 963–1019. doi: 10.1023/A:1005511129475.

Rasoloarison, R.M., Weisrock, D.W., Yoder, A.D. et al. (2013) Two new species of mouse lemurs (Cheirogaleidae: *Microcebus*) from eastern Madagascar. *International Journal of Primatology*, **34**, 455–469. doi: 10.1007/s10764-013-9672-1.

Remick, A., Van Wettere, A. and Williams, C. (2009) Neoplasia in prosimians: case series from a captive prosimian population and literature review. *Veterinary Pathology*, **46**, 746–772. doi: 10.1354/vp.08-VP-0154-R-FL.

Royo, J., Villain, N., Champeval, D. et al. (2018) Effects of n-3 polyunsaturated fatty acid supplementation on cognitive functions, electrocortical activity and neurogenesis in a non-human primate, the grey mouse lemur (*Microcebus murinus*). *Behavioural Brain Research*, **347**, 394–407. doi: 10.1016/j.bbr.2018.02.029.

Saraf, M.P., Balaram, P., Pifferi, F. et al. (2019) The sensory thalamus and visual midbrain in mouse lemurs. *Journal of Comparative Neurology*, **527**, 2599–2611.

Scheumann, M., Joly-Radko, M., Leliveld, L. and Zimmermann, E. (2011) Does body posture influence hand preference in an ancestral primate model? *BMC Evolutionary Biology*, **11**, 52. doi: 10.1186/1471-2148-11-52.

Scheumann, M., Linn, S. and Zimmermann, E. (2017) Vocal greeting during mother–infant reunions in a nocturnal primate, the gray mouse lemur (*Microcebus murinus*). *Scientific Reports*, **7**, 10321. doi: 10.1038/s41598-017-10417-8.

Scheumann, M., Rabesandratana, A. and Zimmermann, E. (2007a) Predation, communication, and cognition in lemurs. In: *Primate Anti-Predator Strategies*. Eds Gursky, S.L. and Nekaris, K.A.I., pp. 100–126. Springer, Oxford, UK.

Scheumann, M. and Zimmermann, E. (2008) Sex-specific asymmetries in communication sound perception are not related to hand preference in an early primate. *BMC Biology*, **6**, 3. doi: 10.1186/1741-7007-6-3.

Scheumann, M., Zimmermann, E. and Deichsel, G. (2007b) Context-specific calls signal infants' needs in a strepsirrhine primate, the gray mouse lemur (*Microcebus murinus*). *Developmental Psychobiology*, **49**, 708–718. doi: 10.1002/dev.20234.

Schilling, A. and Perret, M. (1987) Chemical signals and reproductive capacity in a male prosimian primate (*Microcebus murinus*). *Chemical Senses*, **12**, 143–158. doi: 10.1093/chemse/12.1.143.

Schilling, A., Serviere, J., Gendrot, G. and Perret, M. (1990) Vomeronasal activation by urine in the primate *Microcebus murinus*: A 2 DG study. *Experimental Brain Research*, **81**, 609–618. doi: 10.1007/BF02423511.

Schliehe-Diecks, S., Eberle, M., Kappeler, P.M. (2012) Walk the line – dispersal movements of gray mouse lemurs (*Microcebus murinus*). *Behavioral Ecology & Sociobiology*, **66**, 1175–1185. doi: 10.1007/s00265-012-1371-y.

Schmelting, B., Ehresmann, P., Lutermann, H. et al. (2000) Reproduction of two sympatrically living mouse lemur species (*Microcebus murinus, M. ravelobensis*) in North-Western Madagascar. First results of a long-term study. *Folia Primatologica*, **71**, 241–242.

Schmelting, B., Zimmermann, E., Berke, O. et al. (2007) Experience-dependent recapture rates and reproductive success in male grey mouse lemurs (*Microcebus murinus*). *American Journal of Physical Anthropology*, **133**, 743–752. doi: 10.1002/ajpa.20566.

Schmid, J. (2000) Torpor in the tropics: the case of the gray mouse lemur (*Microcebus murinus*). *Basic and Applied Ecology*, **1**, 133–139. doi: 10.1078/1439-1791-00019.

Schmid, J. and Kappeler, P.M. (1994) Sympatric mouse lemurs (*Microcebus* spp.) in western Madagascar. *Folia Primatologica*, **63**, 162–170. doi: 10.1159/000156812.

Schmidtke, D., Ammersdörfer, S., Joly, M. and Zimmermann, E. (2018a) First comparative approach to touchscreen-based visual object–location paired-associates learning in humans (*Homo sapiens*) and a nonhuman primate (*Microcebus murinus*). *Journal of Comparative Psychology*, **132**, 315–325. doi: 10.1037/com0000116.

Schmidtke, D., Lempp, C., Dubicanac, M. et al. (2018b) Spontaneous spongiform brainstem degeneration in a young mouse lemur (*Microcebus murinus*) with conspicuous behavioral, motor, growth, and ocular pathologies. *Comparative Medicine*, **68**, 489–495. doi: 10.30802/AALAS-CM-18-000019.

Schopf, C., Schmidt, S. and Zimmermann, E. (2016) Moderate evidence for a Lombard effect in a phylogenetically basal primate. *PeerJ*, **4**. doi: 10.7717/peerj.2328.

Schopf, C., Zimmermann, E., Tunsmeyer, J. et al. (2014) Hearing and age-related changes in the gray mouse lemur. *Journal of the Association for Research in Otolaryngology: JARO*, **15**, 993–1005. doi: 10.1007/s10162-014-0478-4.

Schülke, O. and Ostner, J. (2005) Big times for dwarfs: social organization, sexual selection, and cooperation in the Cheirogaleidae. *Evolutionary Anthropology*, **14**, 170–185. doi: 10.1002/evan.20081.

Schülke, O. and Ostner, J. (2007) Physiological ecology of cheirogaleid primates: variation in hibernation and torpor. *Acta Ethologica*, **10**, 13–21. doi: 10.1007/s10211-006-0023-5.

Schwensow, N., Eberle, M. and Sommer, S. (2008) Compatibility counts: MHC-associated mate choice in a wild promiscuous primate. *Proceedings of the Royal Society B – Biological Sciences*, **275**, 555–564. doi: 10.1098/rspb.2007.1433.

Séguy, M. and Perret, M. (2005) Factors affecting the daily rhythm of body temperature of captive mouse lemurs (*Microcebus murinus*). *Journal of Comparative Physiology B*, **175**, 107–115. doi: 10.1007/s00360-004-0467-8.

Siemers, B.M., Goerlitz, H.R., Robsomanitrandrasana, E. et al. (2007) Sensory basis of food detection in wild *Microcebus murinus*. *International Journal of Primatology*, **28**, 291–304. doi: 10.1007/s10764-007-9135-7.

Stanger, K.F., Coffman, B.S. and Izard, M.K. (1995) Reproduction in Coquerel's dwarf lemur (*Mirza coquereli*). *American Journal of Primatology*, **36**, 223–237. doi: 10.1002/ajp.1350360306.

Steffens, T.S. and Lehman, S.M. (2016) Factors determining *Microcebus* abundance in a fragmented landscape in Ankarafantsika National Park, Madagascar. In: *The Dwarf and Mouse Lemurs of Madagascar*. Eds Lehman, S.M., Radespiel, P.D. and Zimmermann, E., pp. 477–497. Cambridge University Press, Cambridge, UK.

Sündermann, D., Scheumann, M. and Zimmermann, E. (2008) Olfactory predator recognition in predator-naïve gray mouse lemurs (*Microcebus murinus*). *Journal of Comparative Psychology*, **122**, 146–155. doi: 10.1037/0735-7036.122.2.146.

Teichroeb, J.A. and Vining, A.Q. (2019) Navigation strategies in three nocturnal lemur species: diet predicts heuristic use and degree of exploratory behavior. *Animal Cognition*, **22**, 343–354. doi: 10.1007/s10071-019-01247-4.

Terrien, J., Gaudubois, M., Champeval, D. et al. (2018) Metabolic and genomic adaptations to winter fattening in a primate species, the grey mouse lemur (*Microcebus murinus*). *International Journal of Obesity*, **42**, 221. doi: 10.1038/ijo.2017.195.

Terrien, J., Perret, M. and Aujard, F. (2010) Gender markedly modulates behavioral thermoregulation in a non-human primate species, the mouse lemur (*Microcebus murinus*). *Physiology & Behavior*, **101**, 469–473. doi: https://doi.org/10.1016/j.physbeh.2010.07.012.

Thomas, P., Pouydebat, E., Brazidec, M.L. et al. (2016) Determinants of pull strength in captive grey mouse lemurs. *Journal of Zoology*, **298**, 77–81. doi: 10.1111/jzo.12292.

Thomsen, R. and Voigt, C.C. (2006) Non-invasive blood sampling from primates using laboratory-bred blood-sucking bugs (*Dipetalogaster maximus*; Reduviidae, Heteroptera). *Primates*, **47**, 397–400. doi: 10.1007/s10329-006-0194-8.

Thorén, S., Quietzsch, F., Schwochow, D. et al. (2011) Seasonal changes in feeding ecology and activity patterns of two sympatric mouse lemur species, the gray mouse lemur (*Microcebus murinus*) and the golden-brown mouse lemur (*M. ravelobensis*), in northwestern Madagascar. *International Journal of Primatology*, **32**, 566–586. doi: 10.1007/s10764-010-9488-1.

Torrent, J., Soukkarieh, C., Lenaers, G. et al. (2010) *Microcebus murinus* retina: a new model to assess prion-related neurotoxicity in primates. *Neurobiology of Disease*, **39**, 211–220. doi: 10.1016/j.nbd.2010.04.010.

Turner, P.V., Brabb, T., Pekow, C. and Vasbinder, M.A. (2011) Administration of substances to laboratory animals: routes of administration and factors to consider. *Journal of the American Association for Laboratory Animal Science*, **50**, 600–613.

Unsworth, J., Loxley, G.M., Davidson, A. et al. (2017) Characterisation of urinary WFDC12 in small nocturnal basal primates, mouse lemurs (*Microcebus* spp.). *Scientific Reports*, **7**. doi: 10.1038/srep42940.

Valenta, K., Burke, R.J., Styler, S.A. et al. (2013) Colour and odour drive fruit selection and seed dispersal by mouse lemurs. *Scientific Reports*, **3**, 2424. doi: doi:10.1038/srep02424.

van Schaik, C.P. and Kappeler, P.M. (1993) Life history, activity period and lemur social systems. In: *Lemur Social Systems and Their Ecological Basis*. Eds Kappeler, P.M. and Ganzhorn, J.U., pp. 241–260. Plenum Press, New York.

Vinot, N., Jouin, M., Lhomme-Duchadeuil, A. et al. (2011) Omega-3 fatty acids from fish oil lower anxiety, improve cognitive functions and reduce spontaneous locomotor activity in a non-human primate. *PLoS One*, **6**, e20491. doi: 10.1371/journal.pone.0020491.

Weigl, R. (2005) *Longevity of Mammals in Captivity; from the Living Collections of the World*. Schweizerbart Science Publishers, Stuttgart.

Wrogemann, D., Radespiel, U. and Zimmermann, E. (2001) Comparison of reproductive characteristics and changes in body weight between captive populations of rufous and gray mouse lemurs. *International Journal of Primatology*, **22**, 91–108. doi: 10.1023/A:1026418132281.

Wrogemann, D. and Zimmermann, E. (2001) Aspects of reproduction in the eastern rufous mouse lemur (*Microcebus rufus*) and their implications for captive management. *Zoo Biology*, **20**, 157–167. doi: 10.1002/zoo.1017.

Yoder, A.D., Rasoloarison, R.M., Goodman, S.M. et al. (2000) Remarkable species diversity in Malagasy mouse lemurs (Primates, *Microcebus*). *Proceedings of the National Academy of Sciences*, **97**, 11325–11330. doi: 10.1073/pnas.200121897.

Zhang, J., Tessier, S.N., Biggar, K.K. et al. (2015) Regulation of torpor in the gray mouse lemur: transcriptional and translational controls and role of AMPK signaling. *Genomics, Proteomics & Bioinformatics*, **13**, 103–110. doi: 10.1016/j.gpb.2015.03.003.

Zimmermann, E. (1991) Ontogeny of acoustic communication in prosimian primates. In: *Primatology Today*. Eds Ehara, A., Takenaka, O. and Iwamoto, M., pp. 337–340, Elsevier, Amsterdam, NL.

Zimmermann, E. (1992) Vocal communication by non-human primates. In: *The Cambridge Encyclopedia of Human Evolution*. Eds Jones, S., Martin, R. and Pilbeam, D., pp. 124–127. Cambridge University Press, Cambridge, UK.

Zimmermann, E. (1996) Castration affects the emission of an ultrasonic vocalization in a nocturnal primate, the grey mouse lemur (*Microcebus murinus*). *Physiology & Behavior*, **60**, 693–697. doi: 10.1016/0031-9384(96)81674-X.

Zimmermann, E. (2010) Vocal expression of emotion in a nocturnal prosimian primate group, mouse lemurs. In: *Handbook of Mammalian Vocalization: An Integrative Neuroscience Approach*. Ed. Brudzynski, S.M., pp. 215–225. Academic Press, Oxford.

Zimmermann, E. (2013) Primate serenades: call variation, species diversity, and adaptation in nocturnal strepsirrhines. In: *Leaping*

Ahead: Advances in Prosimian Biology. Eds Masters, J., Gamba, M. and Génin, F., pp. 287–295, Springer, New York, USA.

Zimmermann, E. (2016) Acoustic divergence in communication of cheirogaleids with special emphasis to mouse lemurs. In: *The Dwarf and Mouse Lemurs of Madagascar: Biology, Behavior and Conservation Biogeography of the Cheirogaleidae* Eds Lehman, S.M., Radespiel, U. and Zimmermann, E., pp. 405–421. Cambridge University Press, Cambridge, UK.

Zimmermann, E. (2018) High frequency/ultrasonic Communication in Basal Primates, the Mouse and Dwarf Lemurs of Madagascar. In: *Handbook of Ultrasonic Vocalization: A Window into the Emotional Brain.* Ed. Brudzynski, S.M., pp. 521–533. Academic Press, London.

Zimmermann, E., Cepok, S., Rakotoarison, N. *et al.* (1998) Sympatric mouse lemurs in north-west Madagascar: a new rufous mouse lemur species (*Microcebus ravelobensis*). *Folia Primatologica,* **69**, 106–114. doi: 10.1159/000021571.

Zimmermann, E. and Hafen, T.G. (2001) Colony specificity in a social call of mouse lemurs (*Microcebus* ssp.). *American Journal of Primatology,* **54**, 129–141. doi: 10.1002/ajp.1018.

Zimmermann, E. and Lerch, C. (1993) The complex acoustic design of an advertisement call in male mouse lemurs (*Microcebus murinus*, Prosimii, Primates) and sources of its variation. *Ethology,* **93**, 211–224. doi: 10.1111/j.1439-0310.1993.tb00990.x.

Zimmermann, E. and Radespiel, U. (2003) The influence of familiarity, age, experience and female mate choice on pregnancies in captive grey mouse lemurs. *Behaviour,* **140**, 301–318.

Zimmermann, E. and Radespiel, U. (2014) Species concepts, diversity, and evolution in primates: lessons to be learned from mouse lemurs. *Evolutionary Anthropology,* **23**, 11–14. doi: 10.1002/evan.21388.

Zimmermann, E., Radespiel, U., Mestre-Francés, N. and Verdier, J.-M. (2016) Life history variation in mouse lemurs (*Microcebus murinus, M. lehilahytsara*): the effect of environmental and phylogenetic determinants. In: *The Dwarf and Mouse Lemurs of Madagascar – Biology, Behavior and Conservation Biogeography of the Cheirogaleidae.* Eds Lehman, S.M., Radespiel, U. and Zimmermann, E., pp. 174–194. Cambridge University Press, Cambridge, UK.

Zimmermann, E., Vorobieva, E., Wrogemann, D. & Hafen, T. (2000) Use of vocal fingerprinting for specific discrimination of gray (*Microcebus murinus*) and rufous mouse lemurs (*Microcebus rufus*). *International Journal of Primatology,* **21**, 837–852. doi: 10.1023/A:1005594625841.

Zohdy, S. (2012) Senescence ecology: aging in a population of wild brown mouse lemurs (*Microcebus rufus*). Faculty of Biological and Environmental Sciences. Helsinki, University of Helsinki.

Zohdy, S., Grossman, M.K., Fried, I.R. *et al.* (2015) Diversity and prevalence of diarrhea-associated viruses in the lemur community and associated human population of Ranomafana National Park, Madagascar. *International Journal of Primatology,* **36**, 143–153. doi: 10.1007/s10764-015-9817-5.

37

Marmosets and tamarins

Hannah M. Buchanan-Smith

Biological overview

General biology

The New World monkeys of the family Callitrichidae has seven genera, and include the marmosets, tamarins and lion tamarins. Figure 37.1 illustrates the species most frequently held in captivity. There is little sexual dimorphism, and they are adapted to give birth to twins that all group members help to rear (Figure 37.1b). Species show a range of interesting pelage forms and colourations; some have ear tufts, others white crests on their heads or a large moustache, and some sport a golden fringe about the face. Why many of these small primates, which are vulnerable to predation by birds, snakes and mammals, are brightly coloured rather than cryptic is poorly understood.

Justification of the use of callitrichids in research should adhere to the Three Rs principle, and be based upon their suitability as models. Their small size, combined with their breeding success when housed in an appropriate environment, and easy handling make them a comparatively inexpensive primate to maintain in laboratories. However, without a good understanding of the natural history and basic adaptations of a species, it is not possible to provide appropriate environmental conditions, which ultimately impacts animal welfare and the quality of science conducted upon them (Buchanan-Smith 2010; Buchanan-Smith *et al*. in press).

Marmoset species

Taxonomy of animals changes with increased knowledge of geography, and advances in molecular genetic and chromosome research. Rylands and Mittermeier (2013) and Rylands *et al*. (2016) provide the most up-to-date description of our current taxonomic understanding of New World primates and is adopted here (Table 37.1).

There are 22 species of marmosets in four genera; six species from the Atlantic Forest (*Callithrix*), 13 from the Amazon Forest (*Mico*), two species of pygmy marmoset (*Cebuella pygmaea*) and one species of dwarf marmoset (*Callibella humilis*), also from Amazonia (Rylands & Mittermeier 2009; Boubli *et al*. 2018). The common marmoset, *Callithrix jacchus*, is the most extensively used callitrichid monkey in laboratory research with two whole books dedicated to them (Marini *et al*. 2019; National Academies of Sciences, Engineering, and Medicine 2019), and is therefore discussed in more detail. A behavioural and vocal ethogram is available for this species (Stevenson & Rylands 1988) and should be consulted. There is also an interactive website[1] with information, photographs, vocalisations and videos on *C. jacchus* behaviour and how best to provide care in captivity.

C. jacchus have large white ear tufts, a brindled black, brown and dark yellow pelage on their back and alternating wide dark and narrow pale bands on the tail. Young animals lack the adult body markings. This arboreal (tree-dwelling) species lives in north-eastern Brazil, occupying a wide variety of habitats such as the lower strata of gallery forests, secondary forests, dry scrub forests of Caatinga, swamps and tree plantations (Stevenson & Rylands 1988; Schiel & Souto 2017). All marmosets have specialised teeth for gouging trees, by using the lower teeth as a cutting-scoop (Coimbra-Filho & Mittermeier 1976; Forsythe & Ford 2011; Casteleyn *et al*. 2012). This enables them to consume the exudates, in the form of gum, from trees which are only secreted by trees as a response to damage created by the marmosets gnawing (see Figure 37.1c). Gum provides energy and some minerals, most importantly calcium, but it is not a complete food (Power & Koutsos 2019). Gum is also difficult to digest and species that depend upon it have digestive tract adaptations (Power & Koutsos 2019). *C. jacchus* spend up to 15–29% of their daily activity feeding on tree exudate (Maier *et al*. 1982; Alonso & Langguth 1989). In addition, marmosets eat fruits, flowers, insects and other small animals such as spiders, lizards, frogs and snails (Stevenson & Rylands 1988; Rylands & de Faria 1993; Arruda *et al*. 2019). In dry Caatinga, a harsh environment, they also eat cacti fruit. As cacti are protected with spines, Abreu *et al*. (2017) argue that factors influencing successful consumption are fine manual dexterity and cognitive ability.

When foraging for insects, *C. jacchus* use a foraging strategy known as 'saltatory search' or a 'stop and go' strategy

---
[1] https://www.marmosetcare.com (accessed February 2022)

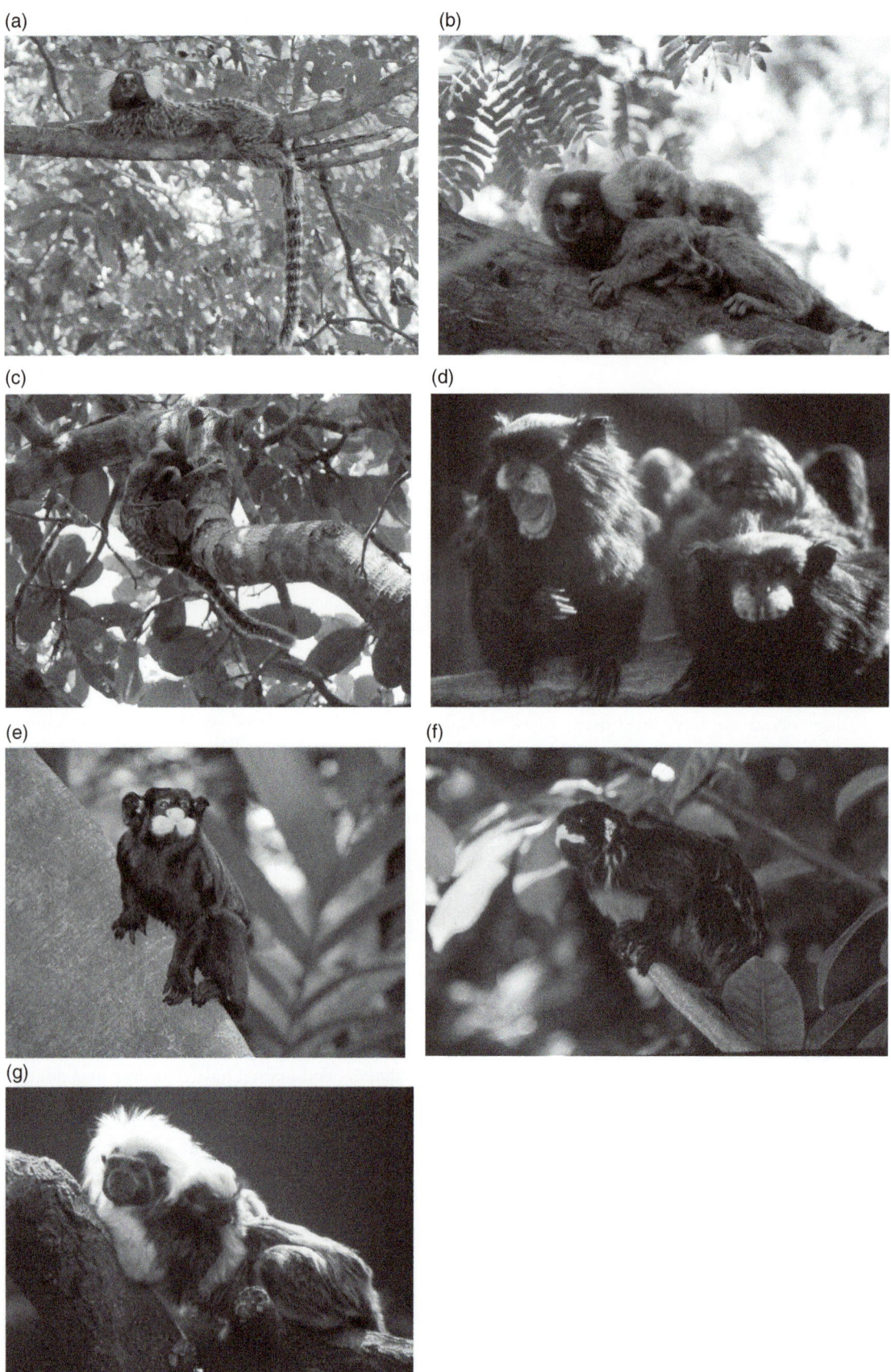

Figure 37.1 Photographs of species of callitrichids most commonly used in the laboratory: (a) *Callithrix jacchus* (common marmoset) (b) *C. jacchus* juvenile carrying twin infants (c) *C. jacchus* gouging for gum, (d) *Leontocebus fuscicollis* (Spix's saddle-back tamarin); (e) *Saguinus mystax* (black-chested moustached tamarin); (f) *Saguinus labiatus* (red-bellied tamarin); (g) *Saguinus oedipus* (cotton-top tamarin). Source: All photos: Hannah Buchanan-Smith, except (e), courtesy of Julia Diegmann.

Table 37.1 Latin name, common name, and conservation status of members the family Callitrichidae (from Rylands & Mittermeier 2009; Rylands & Mittermeier 2013; Rylands et al. 2016).

Latin name	Common name (English)	Conservation status[1]
Cebuella pygmaea	Western pygmy marmoset	LC
Cebuella niveiventris	Eastern pygmy marmoset	LC
Callibella humilis	Black-crowned dwarf marmoset	LC
Callithrix aurita[2]	Buffy-tufted-ear marmoset	VU
Callithrix flaviceps[2]	Buffy-headed marmoset	EN
Callithrix geoffroyi	Geoffroy's tufted-ear marmoset	LC
Callithrix jacchus	Common marmoset	LC (decreasing)
Callithrix kuhlii	Wied's black-tufted-ear marmoset	NT (decreasing)
Callithrix penicillata	Black-tufted-ear marmoset	LC (decreasing)
Mico acariensis	Rio Acarí marmoset	DD
Mico argentatus	Silvery marmoset	LC (decreasing)
Mico melanurus	Black-tailed marmoset	LC
Mico chrysoleucos	Golden-white tassel-ear marmoset	LC (decreasing)
Mico emiliae	Snethlage's marmoset	LC
Mico rondoni	Rondônia marmoset	
Mico humeralifer	Black and white tassel-ear marmoset	DD
Mico intermedius	Aripuanã marmoset	LC (decreasing)
Mico leucippe	Golden-white bare-ear marmoset	VU (decreasing)
Mico marcai[3]	Marca's marmoset	DD (decreasing)
Mico mauesi	Maués marmoset	LC (stable)
Mico nigriceps	Black-headed marmoset	DD
Mico saterei	Sateré marmoset	LC (decreasing)
Leontocebus fuscus	Lesson's saddle-back tamarin	LC (decreasing)[3]
Leontocebus nigricollis	Black-mantled tamarin	LC (decreasing)[3]
Leontocebus leucogenys	Andean saddle-back tamarin[5]	
Leontocebus illigeri	Illiger's saddle-back tamarin[5]	
Leontocebus lagonotus	Red-mantled saddle-back tamarin	LC (decreasing)[3]
Leontocebus tripartitus	Golden-mantled saddle-back tamarin	NT (decreasing)[3]
Leontocebus fuscicollis	Spix's saddle-back tamarin	LC (decreasing)[3]
Leontocebus nigrifrons	Geoffroy's saddle-back tamarin[4,5]	
Leontocebus cruzlimai	Cruz Lima's saddle-back tamarin[4,5]	
Leontocebus weddelli	Weddell's saddle-back tamarin[4,5,6]	
Saguinus mystax	Black-chested moustached tamarin	LC (decreasing)
Saguinus labiatus	Red-bellied tamarin	LC (decreasing)
Saguinus imperator	Emperor tamarin	LC (decreasing)
Saguinus inustus	Mottle-face tamarin	LC (stable)
Saguinus midas	Golden-handed tamarin	LC (stable)
Saguinus niger	Black-handed tamarin	VU (decreasing)
Saguinus ursulus	Eastern black-handed tamarin	
Saguinus bicolor[2]	Brazilian bare-faced tamarin	EN (decreasing)
Saguinus martinsi[2]	Martin's bare-face tamarin	LC
Saguinus geoffroyi[2]	Geoffroy's tamarin	LC (decreasing)
Saguinus leucopus[2]	Silvery-brown bare-face tamarin	EN (decreasing)
Saguinus oedipus[2]	Cotton-top tamarin	CR (decreasing)
Leontopithecus caissara[2]	Black-faced lion tamarin	CR (decreasing)
Leontopithecus chrysomelas[2]	Golden-headed lion tamarin	EN (decreasing)
Leontopithecus chrysopygus[2]	Black lion tamarin	EN (decreasing)
Leontopithecus rosalia[2]	Golden lion tamarin	EN (stable)
Callimico goeldii[2]	Goeldi's monkey	VU

[1] CR = critically endangered; EN = endangered; VU = vulnerable; NT = near threatened; LC = least concern; DD = data deficient (see IUCN[2], 2019 for full definitions). Indications of population trends refer to number of mature individuals, as indicated on the IUCN website. Some species are not listed.
[2] Included in CITES (Convention on International Trade in Endangered Species of wild Fauna and Flora) Appendix I which lists species that are the most endangered. All other primate species are in CITES Appendix II which lists species that are not necessarily now threatened with extinction but that may become so unless trade is closely controlled.
[3] *Mico manicorensis* (van Roosmalen et al. 2000) was found to be a synonym of *Mico marcai* by Garbino (2014).
[4] Listed as *Saguinus* (not *Leontocebus*) in the IUCN Red List.
[5] Listed as subspecies of *Saguinus fuscicollis* on the IUCN Red List.
[6] The IUCN Red List recognises the form *melanoleucus* as a full species, but it has now been shown to be a subspecies of *Leontocebus weddelli* (see Rylands et al. 2016).

[2] https://www.iucnredlist.org/ (accessed July 2019)

(Souto et al. 2007). This foraging strategy may be particularly adapted to detecting prey that are cryptic or widely distributed (Andersson 1981). Although primarily arboreal, *C. jacchus* will descend to the ground to cross forest clearings and pick up fallen fruits (Stevenson & Rylands 1988). Arruda et al. (2019) note that *C. jacchus* have a preference to be alone when they feed – on average they are 2 m apart. This has implications for food provision in captivity.

Several factors affect the home range size of wild marmoset groups; *C. jacchus* ranges vary from 0.5 to 6.9 ha (reviewed by Arruda et al. 2019). Species more dependent on exudates in their diet (*C. jacchus*, *C. penicillata*, *Cebuella*) generally have smaller home ranges than less gummivorous marmosets, although *C. aurita* and *C. flaviceps*, which also have a high proportion of gum in their diets have larger ranges of 11.5 ha and 35.5 ha, respectively (see Arruda et al. 2019). The availability of sleeping trees and food resources, and group size will also influence home range size. Although *C. jacchus* is classified as Least Concern by the International Union for the Conservation of Nature (IUCN 2019), their populations are declining due to habitat destruction and hunting for pets (Bezerra et al. 2018). Schiel and Souto (2017) and Arruda et al. (2019) provide detailed accounts of *C. jacchus* natural history.

Tamarin species

There are 22 species of tamarin in the Amazon Rainforest and the forests of northern Colombia and Panama. Until recently, all tamarins were placed in one genus (*Saguinus*), but Rylands et al. (2016) argue that the *nigricollis* group be recognised as a distinct genus, *Leontocebus* (Table 37.1). There are four species of lion tamarins (*Leontopithecus*) in the Atlantic Forest of south-east Brazil (Rylands & Mittermeier 2009; Rylands et al. 2016). Although known as lion tamarins, they are phylogenetically and genetically more closely related to marmosets (Rosenberger & Coimbra-Filho 1984; Buckner et al. 2015).

The red-bellied tamarin (*S. labiatus*), the black-chested moustached tamarin (*S. mystax*), and Spix's saddle-back tamarin (*Leontocebus fuscicollis*) are the most frequently used in laboratory testing and experimentation (Rensing & Oerke 2005). The cotton-top tamarin (*S. oedipus*) was used as a model for human inflammatory bowel disease (e.g. Clapp 1993) but no longer as it is critically endangered. However, it is frequently held in captivity, and a range of non-regulated research is conducted upon them. These four tamarin species are therefore described in more detail.

Tamarins inhabit primarily tropical lowland humid forests, although some extend into highland forests, and most species adapt well to secondary forests (Snowdon & Soini 1988). Tamarins are insectivore-frugivores and as such their dentition is not adapted for gnawing like the marmosets, and although they may consume tree exudates they lack the necessary digestive system adaptations to exploit its nutritional value fully. There are differences in foraging strategies among tamarins. Three distinct insect foraging patterns have been described (Garber 1993). The first pattern is shown by *S. oedipus* and *S. geoffroyi* who hunt for insects on thin flexible branches in the low shrub layer of the forest understorey. The second is shown by *S. labiatus*, *S. mystax*, *S. imperator* and possibly *S. midas* who have a similar insect foraging style to the marmosets, exploiting insects on leaves and branches in the lower and middle levels of the forest. Visual scanning plays an important role in the detection of their prey. The third pattern is shown by *L. fuscicollis* and possibly *L. nigricollis* and *S. bicolor*. These species are predominantly manipulative, specific site foragers, concentrating their feeding efforts on relatively large cryptic prey (Garber 1993). For example, orthopteran insects, have been found to make up 61–67% of the volume of the stomach ingesta in *L. fuscicollis* (Garber 1993). In addition, ripe fruits account for 20–65% of total feeding time in those species of tamarin studied in the wild (Garber 1993). Plant exudates and nectar are also consumed, the latter principally in the dry season (Garber 1993).

Tamarins, like marmosets, are arboreal, but they are more reluctant to go to the ground (Prescott & Buchanan-Smith 2004). The home ranges vary from 8–120 ha (*L. fuscicollis*: 16–120 ha, *S. mystax*: 30–40 ha, *S. labiatus*: 23–41 ha, *S. oedipus*: 8–10 ha). Their home ranges overlap with neighbouring groups from 13 to 83% (reviewed in Garber 1993). Classification by the IUCN is Least Concern for *L. fuscicollis*, *S. labiatus* and *S. mystax* but it is noted that the population trends for all three species are decreasing (Table 37.1). *S. oedipus* in critically endangered.

Goeldi's monkey

The jet black Goeldi's monkey (*Callimico goeldi*) also belongs to the Callitrichidae, but differs from marmosets and tamarins in several ways. For example, these monkeys have 36 teeth (marmosets and tamarins have 32), and like *Callibella* (van Roosmalen & van Roosmalen 2003) they give birth to just one infant, while the norm in the wild of other members of the family is twins. Their conservation status is vulnerable. Phylogenetically, they are in the marmoset clade (Buckner et al. 2015) but, as they are not used in laboratory research and testing, they are not discussed further.

Body mass and lifespan

The Amazonian pygmy marmoset (*Cebuella*) is the smallest higher primate with both males and females weighing around 128 g (Ford 1994), *Callibella* weighs 150–185 g (van Roosmalen & van Roosmalen 2003), while wild-caught *Mico* and *Callithrix* are heavier, weighing 182–357 g (Ford 1994). In the wild, male and female *C. jacchus* weigh approximately 317 g and 322 g, respectively (Araújo et al. 2000), but captive individuals have weighed as much as 600 g (Poole et al. 1999; and see Prescott & Buchanan-Smith 2004). *C. jacchus* reach puberty before 1 year of age and are skeletally and sexually mature by 2 years (Yamamoto 1993; Tardif et al. 2006). *Saguinus* and *Leontocebus* are slightly heavier; the average adult body weight for both males and females is 387–560 g (Ford 1994) and can be up to 700 g for captive-bred *S. oedipus* (Savage et al. 1993). *Leontopithecus rosalia* weigh from 361 to 794 g (Ford & Davis 1992).

It is not known exactly how long callitrichids live in the wild, but in captivity both males and females have lived over 21 years (Nishijima et al. 2012). The lifespan of *C. jacchus* in captivity is affected by a range of factors but if they survive to weaning it is usually around 5–7 years for dams in US and

UK breeding colonies (summarised by Ash & Buchanan-Smith 2014), and just over 9 years in a Japanese colony (Nishijima et al. 2012). While the reproductive burden on females has been cited as the cause for lower expected lifespan than for males, there is no clear relationship between litter size and dam longevity. Interbirth intervals, dam weight and age at first reproduction have also been analysed in relation to longevity, with mixed results (summarised in Ash & Buchanan-Smith 2014). The age of sexual maturity depends upon sex and species, but is usually 12–24 months (Yamamoto 1993).

Social organisation and reproduction

In the wild, groups of C. jacchus usually contain between 3 and 15 individuals (Hubrecht 1984; Scanlon et al. 1989; Digby & Barreto 1993; Pontes & Da Cruz 1995; Schiel & Souto 2017; Arruda et al. 2019). Groups are relatively stable (Ferrari & Lopes Ferrari 1989), although there are immigrations, emigrations, births and disappearances (Arruda et al. 2005, 2019). Females cycle throughout the year and males copulate with females, including during pregnancy. They ovulate soon after parturition, and can conceive again shortly after birth, when they are still lactating.

In captivity, C. jacchus groups are most stable when they consist of a monogamously breeding pair (e.g. Gerber et al. 2002a, 2002b), and sexual behaviour is inhibited in subordinate females by pheromones, visual stimuli and aggression from the breeding female (e.g. Saltzman et al. 1997). Occasionally, polygynous mating has been observed in captivity, but the groups are less stable than those that consist of monogamous pairs (Rothe & Koenig 1991). In wild populations, the mating system is best described as flexible. Monogamous groups have been frequently documented (Albuquerque et al. 2001; Yamamoto et al. 2009). There have also been numerous cases of two reproductive females in one group (e.g. Digby & Ferrari 1994; Roda & Mendes Pontes 1998; Arruda et al. 2005; de Sousa et al. 2005). Sometimes breeding between females is alternated or one set of offspring does not survive, sometimes due to infanticide by the other breeding female (Digby 1995; Roda & Mendes Pontes 1998; summarised in Arruda et al. 2019).

There is also flexibility in tamarin social organisation. While monogamous pairs are the most stable in captivity, Garber et al. (2016) provide genetic evidence that social polyandry may best characterise wild groups of L. fuscicollis. Comparative data on key reproductive parameters for C. jacchus and L. fuscicollis and S. oedipus are shown in Table 37.2. Although some species breed seasonally in the wild (e.g. S. oedipus) (Neyman 1977), tamarins and marmosets breed all year round in captivity.

Callitrichidae have no menopause, and females will continue to breed throughout their lives. Twin offspring are the norm in the wild (Figure 37.1b), and in addition to the mother, the father and other group members help rear the young by carrying, except for Callibella (van Roosmalen & van Roosmalen 2003). The co-operative rearing system may benefit helpers in several ways, including learning parental skills, improved survivorship through increased group size, increased chances of inheriting the natal territory and increased inclusive fitness (see Arruda et al. 2019). Parents and helpers may also provision the young with solid food, a behaviour that may be passive (all species studied) or active as recorded in S. oedipus, C. pygmaea, C. flaviceps, L. rosalia and L. chrysomelas (see Feistner & Price 1991).

A fascinating twist that may underpin the evolution of co-operative rearing is genetic chimerism (when an animal has genetically distinct cells that come from different zygotes and are created by fertilised eggs or embryos fusing together) the patterns of relatedness between twins, and between other family members change. This chimerism applies to marmosets and tamarins with multiple births because in the womb, placentas grow quickly and fuse, creating a network of blood vessels through which cells can travel from one twin to the other (Ross et al. 2007). Ross et al. claim that chimeras may exist in almost any part of the body – blood, hair, liver and even in sperm and eggs, but more recently they have been found only in hematopoietic cell lineages (i.e. those that give rise to other blood cells) (Sweeney et al. 2012). If they did occur in sperm, one brother may contribute the genetic makeup of his twin brother's offspring, effectively fathering nephews or nieces! Our understanding and the full implications of this phenomenon have yet to be explored, but in addition to the scientific interest in its role in the evolution of the co-operative rearing system, it may have implications for managing studbooks for optimal outbreeding, and in the selection of individuals for experimental protocols given the potential impact on variability of results.

Biological data

Kramer and Burns (2019) provide a thorough overview of basic biological data (including reproductive, physiological, normative haematological and blood chemistry values) in C. jacchus, and Rensing and Oerke (2005) in a range of callitrichids. Table 37.3 provides a summary of key data for C. jacchus. Infant weights vary depending upon litter size, with mean values of 34.7 g +/− 3.81 (n=5), 30.24 +/− 3.33 (n=59) and 27.73 +/− 2.03 (n=30) for singletons, twins and triplets respectively (Tardif & Bales 2004). Growth rates of infants can be divided into an early stage of rapid growth, with a weight gain of around 1.15 g/day for all infants regardless of litter

Table 37.2 Comparative reproductive data for C. jacchus, L. fuscicollis and S. oedipus (Savage 1995; Fortman et al. 2002; Rensing & Oerke 2005; Kramer & Burns 2019).

	C. jacchus	L. fuscicollis	S. oedipus
Sexual maturity (months)	24	26	24
Oestrous cycle length (days)	28	26	21
Gestation (days)	144	150–155	180–185
Post-partum ovulation (days)	10	17–18	17–18

Table 37.3 Summary of key biological data for *C. jacchus* (Ludlage & Mansfield 2003; Rensing & Oerke 2005; Wolfensohn & Honess 2005; Kuehnel et al. 2012; Kramer & Burns 2019 which includes other *C. jacchus* data).

Biological data	Normal values (if range provided, mean in brackets)
Rectal temperature (°C)	38.6 (day)
	36.8 (night)
Heart rate (beats per minute)	230–312 (sedation)
	348 +/− 51 (restrained)
	230 +/− 26 (unrestrained)
Mean arterial pressure (mmHg)	95–107 (day, using a range of methods)
Under sedation	50–95 (night)
Blood volume (ml/kg)	60–70
Haematological data	*Normal values*
Red blood cells (RBC) (×10³/mm³)	♂ 3.4–7.2 (5.7); ♀ 4.2–9.6 (5.7)
Packed cell volume (PCV) (%)	45–52
Haemoglobin (Hb) (g/dL)	♂ 10.9–19.3 (16.1); ♀ 11.1–17.8 (15.0)
White blood cells (WBC) (×10³/mm³)	♂ 2.7–17.5 (8.1); ♀ 4.5–18.7 (7.4)
Neutrophils (%)	♂ 17–80 (43); ♀ 32–85 (54)
Lymphocytes (%)	♂ 14–82 (51); ♀ 13–63 (40)
Eosinophils (%)	♂ 0–5 (0.4); ♀ 0–3 (0.5)
Monocytes (%)	♂ 0–16 (3.3); ♀ 0–9 (3.6)
Basophils (%)	♂ 0–5 (0.8); ♀ 0–8 (1.5)
Platelets (G/L × 10³/mm³)	17.6–788.6 (402.5)
Biochemical data	*Normal values (mean follows range)*
Serum protein (g/dl)	6.6–7.1
Albumen (g/dl)	3.8
Globulin (g/dl)	2.7–3.9
Glucose (mg/dl)	♂ 74–323 (172); ♀ 97–294 (192)
Blood urea nitrogen (mg/dl)	♂ 11–43 (22); ♀ 14–34 (22)
Creatinine (mg/dl)	♂ 0.1–1.1 (0.6); ♀ 0–0.9 (0.6)
Gamma glutamyl transferase (IU/l)	0.2–13.5 (2.8)
Total bilirubin (mg/dl)	♂ 0.02–4.41 (0.48); ♀ 0–0.95 (0.25)

size, followed by a slower, later growth rate which is more variable but averages at 0.81 g/day (Tardif & Bales 2004). Factors affecting growth rates of infants and their adult weight are numerous and interrelated. They include maternal age and weight, and also litter size (Tardif & Bales 2004).

Twins have the best survival rate (12% mortality, n=821 litters; Ash and Buchanan-Smith 2014). Large litters (>2 infants) accounted for about half the births in UK colonies and they result in high mortality (28% for triplets, n=783 litters, 43% for quadruplets, n=45, and 65% for quintuplets n=4; Ash & Buchanan-Smith 2014). A meta-analysis of data from five colonies in the Americas (n=625 dams) reported a mean of 50% loss between number of infants produced, and weaned at 3 months (Smucny et al. 2004). Litter size and infant weight are strongly correlated, and triplets and quadruplets, especially if very small (<20 g) have significantly lower survival compared to twins and very large (>35 g) infants which are often singletons (Jaquish et al. 1991, 1997). Infant weight has also been shown to be related to abuse (defined as physical injury by other members of the group); abused infants have lower birth weights than non-abused infants (Tardif et al. 1998).

Normal behaviour (wild and captive)

All animals should be allowed to express their natural patterns of behaviour in the captive environment. For callitrichids, this includes a range of locomotor and positional behaviours in relation to foraging strategies (e.g. gnawing for tree exudate (see Figure 37.1c), food capture and processing), social activities (e.g. resting, grooming, playing), the opportunity to explore novelty (either new environments or objects) and having safe and comfortable places to sleep. The type of cage (construction materials and dimensions) and furnishings (substrate types, orientation and its placement) should be designed to allow and encourage species-specific postures, behaviours and space-use preferences (Buchanan-Smith 2010). Videos of wild *C. jacchus* behaviours and postures can be viewed at marmosetcare.com[1].

Detailed descriptions of the development of young callitrichids are available for *C. jacchus* (Stevenson 1976) and *S. oedipus* (Cleveland & Snowdon 1984). Yamamoto (1993) compares behavioural ontogeny across genera. Until infants are 3 weeks old, they are carried all of the time, usually by all group members, but often exclusively by the mother in *Leontopithecus*. By week 4, the infants are showing interest in their environments and beginning to explore, to touch, lick and smell objects, and they leave the carriers' backs for increasing periods of time. If startled, young will try to climb back onto carriers for protection. The first social interactions occur while the infants are still on their carriers' backs but after week 8 (week 12 in *Leontopithecus*) they are only carried occasionally. Weaning from lactation occurs from weeks 8–15, although infants taste solid food earlier. Infant development is affected by enrichment (an artificial gum tree, additional shelves, a hanging cloth and a variety of manipulable objects on rotation), with the appearance of certain behaviours (chewing wood, begging towards animal care staff, solitary play, exploration and scent marking) occurring earlier in enriched environments (Ventura & Buchanan-Smith 2003). The neurobehavioural development of *C. jacchus* has been reviewed by Schultz-Darken et al. (2016), together with an evaluation of the various methods used to evaluate sensory-motor as well as socio-emotional spheres of *C. jacchus* development.

Senses and communication

Like other simians, vision is the dominant sensory modality of callitrichids. As both predators and prey, they use sight to detect prey items and potential threats. Their vigilance in captivity likely reflects that care staff may be seen as threats, and alertness has been found to increase after stressful events (Bassett et al. 2003). Callitrichids have binocular vision, with overlapping visual fields, and good visual acuity allowing them to manoeuvre themselves safely through complex three-dimensional worlds, judging depth and distance, and to respond to visual stimuli, be they potential threats, conspecifics or prey items, such as insects. Marmosets perform headcocking where they move their heads in the lateral direction. Young *C. jacchus* headcock more than older marmosets, and often this is in the context of novelty (Stevenson & Rylands 1988). Tamarins perform a behaviour termed head flicking by Snowdon and Soini (1988) but it should not be confused with headcocking – head flicking is directed towards conspecifics as a hostile display. *Leontopithecus* will sometimes bob up and down when staring threateningly (Kleiman *et al*. 1988).

While the Old World monkeys and apes have colour vision that is similar to our own (trichromacy, based on three classes of cone receptors) (Jacobs 1996), callitrichids are polymorphic and show a wide variety of colour vision phenotypes. Females have either trichromatic or dichromatic vision (based on two classes of cone receptors, like humans with red-green 'colour blindness') (Jacobs *et al*. 1993). However, all males are dichromatic. Trichromatic colour vision has been shown to be useful for selecting ripe fruits from unripe and semi-ripe ones, and may also be advantageous for the detection of insect prey and predators (Regan *et al*. 2001; Smith *et al*. 2003; Buchanan-Smith 2005; Jacobs 2007). Individuals with dichromatic vision may not be able to differentiate well between yellows, greens, browns and reds, and camouflaged prey makes up a greater proportion of their diets (Smith *et al*. 2012). The polymorphic colour vision has implications for choice of colour stimuli in experiments (Waitt & Buchanan-Smith 2006) and for choosing target colours for positive reinforcement training (Buchanan-Smith 2005).

All callitrichids have a well-developed sense of smell, possess specialised scent organs, and have a rich repertoire of chemosignalling behaviours (e.g. Epple *et al*. 1993). The most conspicuous of these are scent-marking patterns involving the circumgenital and subrapubic glands. Scent marking itself and the chemical signals deposited are important in many areas of their behavioural biology. They contain information on individual identity, rank and reproductive status, and play a role in reproductive suppression of subordinate females. It may also aid territorial defence, intergroup spacing and provide cues as to mate quality (Epple *et al*. 1993). The rate of scent marking in wild *C. jacchus* ranges from 0.19 to 0.45 scent marks/hour (Lazaro-Perea *et al*. 1999), much lower than is seen in captive conditions, where it exceeds 40 scent marks/hour post-stressor (Bassett *et al*. 2003). Adults scent mark more frequently than young in captivity (de Sousa *et al*. 2006).

Their acute sense of smell, together with taste, assists in food identification and selection. Callitrichids have a very varied diet (e.g. Smith *et al*. 2003 found that two mixed species groups of *Saguinus* consumed fruits from 833 plants of 167 species in 87 genera and 50 families during 164 days of observation!). Providing a variety of nutritional and appetising food is likely to be beneficial for their psychological well-being and is often used as enrichment, but may lead to nutrition-related illnesses in the long term (Plesker & Schuhmacher 2006) (see Feeding/watering).

Callitrichids have a range of high-pitched vocalisations. Several vocal ethograms have been published including that of *C. jacchus* (Stevenson & Rylands 1988; also available at marmosetcare.com[1]); *S. oedipus* (Cleveland & Snowdon 1982); *Leontopithecus* (Kleiman *et al*. 1988); and *Cebuella* (Soini 1988). The long calls, which serve many possible functions, including group defence against intruders, maintenance of group cohesion (e.g. reuniting separated group members) and mate attraction, have been studied extensively (Pook 1977; Cleveland & Snowdon 1982; Snowdon 1993). Vocalisations are also important indicators in welfare assessment (Jones 1997). Callitrichids can hear higher frequencies than humans (see Heffner 2004 for a review; Osmanski & Wang 2011). Ultrasonic frequencies present in the captive environment, such as a dripping tap, trolley wheels or computer monitors, may adversely affect welfare (Clough 1982; Brudzynski 2018).

Vocalisations have rarely been used as an enrichment technique, but can be very effective in promoting good welfare if used appropriately. Daily playback of affiliative chirp vocalisations at above average-rate influenced colony-housed monkeys to engage in more affiliative behaviours outside playback hours, relative to the control of silent playback (Watson *et al*. 2014). Music, however, is not recommended as it is more likely to be perceived as noise (Buchanan-Smith 2010). When given a choice among different music type and silence, marmosets and tamarins prefer silence (McDermott & Hauser 2007).

The sensory receptors in the epithelial and connective tissues of callitrichids respond to changes in temperature, touch, pressure and pain. These sensations then guide them in their behaviour. For example, Rumble and colleagues (2005) found that *C. jacchus* choose warmer, 'softer' wooden and plastic nest boxes over metal nest boxes. Providing different textures appears to be very rewarding for them (e.g. when given a fleece-like hammock, they will often roll around in it). Tactile contact, through huddling and grooming, develops and maintains affiliative bonds, and may help individuals to cope with stressors (Schaffner & Smith 2005). Grooming plays a role in keeping a healthy skin and coat. Tactile contact when young may be particularly critical and it is known that repeated early parental deprivation of infant *C. jacchus* can have long-term effects on their behaviour and physiology (Dettling *et al*. 2002a, 2002b).

Sources and supply

There are breeding programmes set up for all callitrichids used commonly in biological and biomedical research. These breeding programmes are often in-house, obviating the need for potentially stressful transport, quarantine and adaptation to a new colony. Breeding in-house also allows socialisation and training specific to their intended future use to begin early. However, some facilities may be too small, or lack expertise required for breeding, and therefore the primates must be transported to them. In these cases, legislation following the international trade in and transport of primates should be followed (see Health monitoring, transport, quarantine and barrier systems).

Use in research

Callitrichids are used in a wide range of studies, including: behavioural, reproductive physiology, neuroscience, obesity, ageing, infectious disease, drug development and safety assessment (Abbott *et al*. 2003; Mansfield 2003; Colman *et al*. 2021). *S. oedipus* were used to study colon adenocarcinoma as these animals spontaneously develop colitis and/or colon cancer (Saunders *et al.* 1999). There are specific chapters on the research applications of *C. jacchus* in Marini *et al.* (2019), including their genome, and the creation of genetically modified marmosets, ageing, visual neuroscience, Parkinson's disease, autoimmune encephalomyelitis, auditory research, behavioural neuroscience and psychiatric research, endocrine research, as well as toxicity testing and nonclinical safety assessment studies. The National Academies of Sciences, Engineering, and Medicine (2019) focus on their use is gene-editing-based biomedical research.

Laboratory husbandry, management and breeding

Enclosures

Callitrichids need sufficient space to exhibit species-typical locomotor patterns, and to use the vertical dimension, as in the wild they are arboreal and rarely come to the ground. In two-tier cages, monkeys in lower tiers are, by design, denied the use of the vertical dimension. Although few differences have been found in the behaviour of *C. jacchus* housed in upper- and lower-tier cages measuring 55 cm wide × 95 cm high × 110 cm deep (Buchanan-Smith *et al.* 2002; Badihi 2006), others have reported some differences. Activity is higher in upper-tier *C. jacchus* (Scott 1991) and *S. oedipus* (Box & Rohrhuber 1993) than lower tier, with the tamarins also spending more time in close physical contact. In addition, the behaviour of *C. jacchus* pairs improves (increases in calm locomotion and inactive rest behaviours and lower levels of agitated locomotion, inactive alert behaviours and watch observer) when they have access to a double enclosure incorporating both upper and lower tiers (Badihi 2006). Numerous other researchers have found behaviour indicative of improved welfare (such as increased play and exploration, and decreased stress-related behaviours) to be present in larger cages (e.g. *S. oedipus*, Box & Rohrhuber 1993; *C. jacchus*, Schoenfeld 1989; Kitchen & Martin 1996; Gaspari *et al.* 2000). Given these findings, it is not advisable that callitrichids are housed in small two-tier cages which compromise welfare.

Furthermore, light intensity in the lower tiers is reduced in comparison to the upper tiers (Scott 1991; Schapiro *et al.* 2000). Light intensity is known to impact behaviour and to improve reproduction. For example, Hampton and colleagues (1966) found that *S. oedipus* had markedly reduced activity when the light was dimmed, and Buchanan-Smith and Badihi (2012) found improvements in the behaviour of *C. jacchus* (e.g. increased levels of calm locomotion and social play in youngsters) at higher light intensities. Indeed, if given a choice, marmosets will turn on supplementary light in their enclosures (Buchanan-Smith & Badihi 2012). There has also been one report that reproduction in *C. jacchus* decreases at the very low light intensity of 20 lux (Heger *et al.* 1986).

Cages in laboratories generally consist of mobile enclosures (cages mounted on wheels), that can be autoclaved (Figure 37.2). The cages are often made of stainless steel, yet wooden cages provide a quieter environment, and although the wood can be protected from gnawing by wire mesh, they will require more frequent replacement. Ensuring the space is fully utilisable is of critical importance, and thus providing

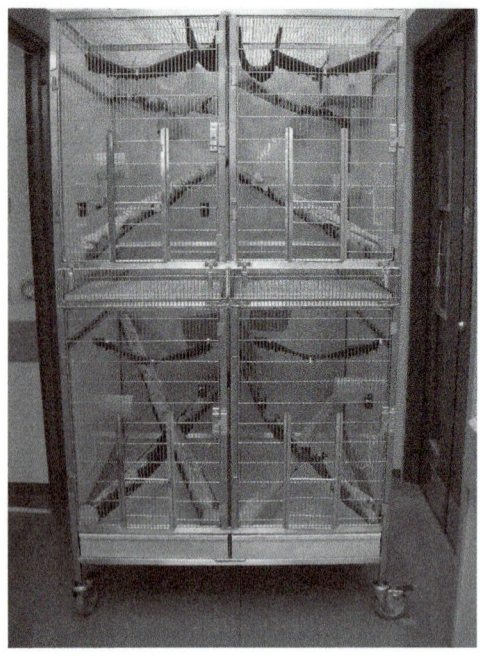

Figure 37.2 Cages on wheels can be easily washed in a conventional rack washer for washing with minimal dismantling. Note the plastic shelves at the front of the cage, and wooden shelves around the cage at various levels, which provide marmosets with good grip and a comfortable place to sit. The branches allow natural gnawing behaviour. The Perspex turrets allow the monkeys to extend their visual field. The nest box is plastic, ventilated and with a wooden base to provide warmth and comfort. A forage tray is provided (top left quadrant) to promote foraging behaviours. Ropes and rope ladders give movement. Such cages are able to house marmosets in small family groups providing social stimulation. Source: Colin Windle, University of Cambridge, UK.

mesh or some climbing structures on solid walls is important. This also applies to the ceiling material, so that the monkeys can hang down and play. A mesh ceiling also allows a greater variety of enrichment to be attached, for example, using cable ties or karabiner-type clips. Enclosures that have slide dividers can be very useful as they allow animals to be temporarily separated (for example, for veterinary treatment or experiments) while maintaining the familiarity within the cage and close contact with the group.

Solid cage floors with sawdust/wood shavings/wood chips are recommended, as callitrichids will often drop food, but later forage through the substrate for it. Care must be taken to ensure these do not harbour pathogens that might be transmitted between cages. A biofloor, which consists of a 25 cm covering of woodchips over a filterpad, with a concrete floor and drain, functions as a biological system to prevent build-up of pathogens or parasite infestation (Carroll 2002). Bakker *et al.* (2015) assessed the effects of indoor-outdoor housing with deep litter on *C. jacchus*, and concluded that the veterinary risk was minimal to none. Faeces need to be spot cleaned, but urine drains away. The biofloor requires total replacement every 3–4 years and provides excellent continuity of familiar scents for the monkeys and minimises the disruption of regular cleaning.

Specifying cage sizes is controversial, given the financial implications. Marmosets and tamarins have been treated the same, as cage size specifications are usually based upon their body weight (<1 kg; Buchanan-Smith *et al.* 2004; Prescott & Buchanan-Smith 2004). Poole and co-authors (1994) specified a minimum of 1 m² floor area for two animals and 0.25 m² for each additional animal, excluding carried infants (i.e. a floor area of 2 m² for a group of eight). The minimum cage height they specified was 1.5 m. However, marmosets and tamarins differ in some critical ways that impact on their welfare and captive conditions (Prescott & Buchanan-Smith 2004). Tamarins are slightly heavier, have larger home ranges (up to 50–100 ha), and longer daily path lengths related to a more frugivorous diet and less dependence on gum feeding. Tamarins have an even greater tendency than marmosets to avoid the ground where they behave nervously. Furthermore, tamarins seem to be more susceptible to developing locomotor stereotypies and to self-injure than marmosets (reviewed in Prescott & Buchanan-Smith 2004). Prescott and Buchanan-Smith (2004) have argued that based on this suite of characteristics, tamarin species should have larger minimum cage sizes in the laboratory than *C. jacchus*. Council of Europe Convention ETS 123 (Appendix A 2006) and the European Commission (2007) have taken this into account specifying a floor area of 0.5 m² for marmosets and 1.5 m² for tamarins (for 1–2 animals over 5 months), with a minimum height of 1.5 m, and the top of the enclosure should be at least 1.8 m from the floor. Each additional monkey over 5 months requires an extra 0.2 m³. The *Guide for the Care and Use of Laboratory Animals* (NRC 2011), which recommends minimum space in the US, still permits two-tier enclosures and specifies a height of 0.76 m, a floor area of 0.2 m²/animal for both marmosets and tamarins. Photographs of typical housing in the US are provided in Layne-Colon *et al.* (2019) together with descriptions of *C. jacchus* housing and husbandry.

Although prescribed minimum cage sizes have increased in Europe, as noted above, those exceeding current minimum size have been found to improve welfare (e.g. *S. oedipus*, Box & Rohrhuber 1993; *C. jacchus*, Schoenfeld 1989; Kitchen & Martin 1996; Gaspari *et al.* 2000). An example of a larger walk-in cage is shown in Figure 37.3. The opportunities to engage in locomotion are far greater, and the monkeys are known to engage in more solitary play and exploration (Badihi *et al.* 2007). However, care should be taken to ensure continuity for animals who are given larger enclosures, as if animals have to be moved to smaller enclosures there are severe welfare consequences (Schoenfeld 1989; Badihi *et al.* 2007).

Callitrichids scent mark territories and are aggressive to neighbouring groups, so physical or close (<1 m) visual contact between captive groups should be avoided. At the very least, the monkeys should be given choice to avoid visual contact with group mates and neighbouring groups should they wish to, and stability within a colony room should be maintained, so individuals may become familiar with each other. Providing choice to be in visual contact or not can be done by providing visual barriers, such as hanging screens within the cage (McKenzie *et al.* 1986). An alternative is to allow monkeys an opportunity to peep through a small hole at a neighbouring group (Moore *et al.* 1991). As the neighbours do not know they are being watched, it is unlikely to have any detrimental effects on them.

Turrets or verandas/balcony boxes have been used in several colonies, with mixed success. These are small mesh or Perspex additions to the enclosures that permit the monkeys to extend their visual field. Initial use may cause disturbances as animals unfamiliar with each other are able to directly threaten each other visually and vocally. If mesh, they should not be placed too close so monkeys can physically touch each other. They may have some benefits in increasing predictability of negative events (see Bassett & Buchanan-Smith 2007), as the marmosets will have a better view of what care staff are doing (in relation to cleaning, capture for procedures, etc.). Reliably signalling startling events, such as enclosure entry, has positive effects in other primate species (Rimpley & Buchanan-Smith 2013)

Empirical studies have shown that access to outdoor environments has a positive effect the welfare of primates in captivity (e.g. Novak & Suomi 1988) and the International Primatological Society (IPS) guidelines (2007) recommend a combination of indoor and outdoor housing, including exercise areas, where possible. Bakker *et al.* (2015) have shown that there is no significant health risks for *C. jacchus* in outdoor enclosures. Seasonal fluctuations in light and climate may contribute positively to the animals' welfare and allow animals a choice to experience a wider range of sensory stimulation such as sunshine and greater opportunities for exploration and manipulation (e.g. Novak & Suomi 1988; Pereira *et al.* 1989; Buchanan-Smith 1998; Pines *et al.* 2007). Free access to warm indoor or sheltered facilities is critical whenever outdoor enclosures are used. *C. jacchus* prefer to spend time outside than in a large indoor enriched enclosure when given access from their home cage (Pines *et al.* 2007) and they engage in more positive welfare behaviours outdoors (including increased play, allogrooming, exploration, rest relaxed and calm locomotion and decreased stress-related scratching and scent marking) than when housed indoors (Badihi 2006). Care must be taken to minimise the risk of disease transmission from outside vectors, including vaccination against *Yersinia* spp (Bakker *et al.* 2015). Outdoor housing can be connected to the indoor enclosures using flexible ducting obviating the need for capture and allowing rotational access (Badihi 2006). Additional points concerning outside enclosures are reviewed in Layne-Colon *et al.* (2019).

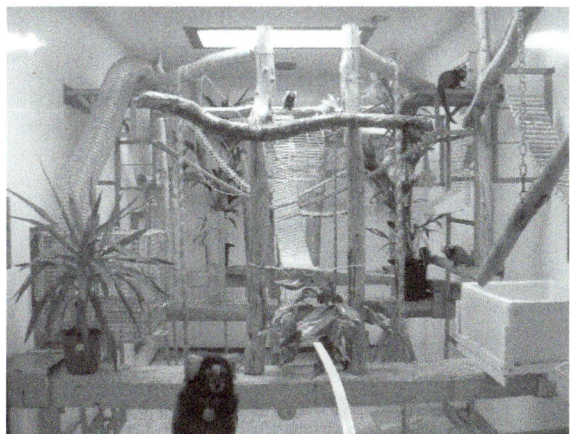

Figure 37.3 An example of a large walk-in enclosure for marmosets. Source: Keith Morris.

Environmental provisions

A number of key aspects of the environment promote good welfare. These include the ability to express natural behaviour, and unpredictable positive environmental changes which can elicit an adaptive response from the animal, the opportunities for animals to choose and to facilitate change in the environment, and the perception of control (Sambrook & Buchanan-Smith 1997; IPS 2007; JWGR 2009; and reviewed in Rennie & Buchanan-Smith 2006b).

All callitrichids have claw-like nails to facilitate grip and all cage furnishings should take grip into account (e.g. rough surfaces), allowing a range of different postures using grip and building muscle (see Figure 37.1c). Locomotion is primarily quadrupedal, but vertical clinging and leaping is seen in several species. Positioning of vertical supports is particularly important for *L. fuscicollis* which locomote extensively by vertical clinging and leaping. To allow full resting, huddling and grooming postures, flat surfaces which several individuals may occupy simultaneously should be provided. These may contain holes, to provide extra grip, and to prevent any puddles of urine from forming.

In the wild, most callitrichids sleep huddled together in tree forks or in dense tangles of vines and leaves and a secure place for sleeping is important in captivity. *Leontopithecus* are unusual in that they primarily use holes in tree trunks and branches as sleeping sites; therefore, providing nesting 'holes' in captivity is appropriate. Nest boxes should be provided as they provide comfort and security, as evidenced by reduced vigilance (*S. labiatus*) (Caine et al. 1992). The finding that *C. jacchus* prefer wooden and plastic nest boxes over metal ones (Rumble et al. 2005) may be related to comfort and temperature. Nest boxes should be placed high in the enclosure and well ventilated so that moisture from breathing does not condense and so there is no risk of suffocation. They also serve as a hiding place. They are not recommended as capture boxes, as they may lead to an association with potentially stressful events.

Feeding/watering

Nutritional status influences growth, reproduction and longevity, as well as resistance to disease and environmental stressors (Knapka et al. 1995). Callitrichids have a very varied natural diet, that they have to work hard to get; getting access to food (e.g. gnawing at trees to get exudates in marmosets, or removing inedible outer skin of fruits) and using memory (spatial, temporal and seasonal) for returning to fruiting trees. In the wild, they rarely encounter food in great abundance, and often they must search for it, with foraging occupying up to 50–60% of waking time, throughout the day (Garber 1984; Yoneda 1984). Providing a varied, appetitive and nutritionally balanced diet, and ensuring that foraging takes up a significant proportion of the day as it does in the wild, is critical. Food should therefore be made more difficult to find and process, and be provided at several times over the course of the day, taking their natural activity patterns into account. As insect foraging occupies much time in the wild, providing insects, or moving food, such as on a conveyor belt outside the cage, can be enriching (Buchanan-Smith 2010). It is especially important to feed in the early morning, and early afternoon as they would in the wild.

Cafeteria-style diets in which commercially available pellets containing the required nutritional constituents are augmented with a range of additional food items, such as fresh or dried fruit, vegetables, seeds, nuts and animal protein (e.g. insects, mealworms, hard-boiled eggs and boiled chicken) are often considered to cater well for psychological well-being, being varied and palatable. However, such a diet may lead to nutritional imbalance as pellets are generally not appetitive and callitrichids often avoid them in preference to the other food being offered. One solution to maintain the variability, but reduce nutritional imbalance is to soak the pellets in milk or flavoured juice to soften them and make them more palatable. Another solution is to use agar-based purified diets which are more appetising to marmosets, and have been used successfully (Layne & Power 2003). The National Research Council (NRC) (2003) provides a thorough review of nutrient requirements for primates, and Rensing and Oerke (2005) summarise the key points for callitrichid nutrition. Vitamin D3 is a critical supplement for callitrichids who cannot synthesise it without access to ultraviolet light. Feed supplements, such as yoghurt, are often provided to females in late pregnancy and who are lactating, but there is no evidence that this benefits their offspring. Infants from mothers fed a higher protein diet did not have higher survival, nor growth. Indeed, at 42 days the mean infant body weight of supplemented mothers was less than that of infants of non-supplemented mothers (Layne & Power 2003). Power and Koutsos (2019) provide a comprehensive overview of *C. jacchus* nutrition and dietary husbandry.

Care should be taken on placement of food dishes. In *S. oedipus*, group members carrying infants were reluctant to approach food dishes placed near floor level. This was remedied by placing food dishes at least 1 m from floor level, whereupon group members carrying infants readily approached food dishes and fed (Snowdon & Savage 1989). Furthermore, by providing a meal in two or more sets of dishes in larger groups, competition between group members may be reduced, and each individual is more likely to get a more varied diet and an equal share of the preferred food items (Price & McGrew 1990). As noted previously, wild *C. jacchus* prefer to be alone (on average 2 m apart) when feeding (Arruda et al. 2019), so placing dishes at a distance from each other is important.

Food choice and presentation should take their natural feeding adaptations into account. For example, *Leontopithecus* and some *Saguinus* species are described as being extractive foragers, and feeding devices fashioned to stimulate these particular foraging skills can be used (e.g. hiding food in bromeliads such as pineapple tops). Insects should be included as part of the diet if possible. Given the dental and intestinal adaptation to gum feeding, it is recommended that marmosets are given gum in such a way to encourage gnawing. It is easy to buy commercial gum arabic that can be syringed onto branches in the enclosure and requires little time to prepare or administer (Kelly 1993).

Fruit is often chopped to ensure an even distribution among group members, but leaving skin on bananas, oranges and other fruits increases animal processing time (although fruit should be washed prior to presentation to remove pesticides). Spearing whole fruits on bamboo encourages callitrichids to hang upside down and spend time picking off bits of apple or orange (see marmosetcare.com[1]) in a similar fashion to how they would forage naturally. A similar technique is to suspend plastic film cases filled with small food pieces on string from the top of the cage.

These foraging techniques are preferable to scattering food items in the wood shavings or other floor coverings, as callitrichids do not go to the ground regularly in the wild, or if they do they are especially cautious as they may be more vulnerable to predation. However, foraging boxes containing a mixture of sawdust with dried fruits, such as raisins, bananas or mealworms, attached higher in the enclosure work well. Fresh water should be available *ad libitum*, preferably from an automated watering system, as normal laboratory water bottles are potentially a source of infections.

Social housing

Housing callitrichids in harmonious social groups is fundamental to their welfare as it allows them to carry out species-specific behaviours and buffers the effects of stressful situations (Schaffner & Smith 2005). Callitrichids (with the exception of *Callibella*) have a co-operative rearing system where the mother generally gives birth to usually twin offspring, and the father and other group members care for the young by carrying, food sharing and perhaps by looking out for predators (e.g. Cleveland & Snowdon 1984; Price 1992). There are many published reports that if offspring are removed from their group before they have had experience with rearing infants, they have a much lower likelihood of raising offspring themselves (*L. fuscicollis*, Epple 1978; *L. rosalia*, Hoage 1977; *S. oedipus*, Cleveland & Snowdon 1984; Snowdon *et al.* 1985; Tardif *et al.* 1984a; *C. jacchus*, Tardif *et al.* 1984a). It is recommended that callitrichids should have experience with at least two sets of rearing episodes; otherwise, they will not make good parents themselves (Snowdon & Savage 1989). This applies to sons as well as daughters, because fathers as well as mothers care for the young and may be even more important for tamarins than for marmosets (Tardif *et al.* 1984a). Schultz-Darken *et al.* (2019) provide additional details on consideration for social housing, and the importance of monitoring group dynamics especially after the loss of a member of the breeding pair.

Optimal housing in captivity is in large family groups (up to 8–12 individuals if space allows), giving the offspring the opportunity for good social development. Offspring should not be removed until they are sexually mature. Pairing unfamiliar male and female callitrichids is usually a smooth process, but certain guidelines should be followed carefully (see JWGR 2009). With particular reference to callitrichids, the newly formed pair should be some distance away from the family as reproductive suppression through olfactory cues may still occur. If individuals have to be housed in pairs for experimental reasons, housing familiar siblings or vasectomised male or contracepted female pairs increases the likelihood of compatibility. Unrelated same-sex pairs of *C. jacchus* are often difficult to pair, unless one individual is younger (Majolo *et al.* 2003). Housing unrelated same-sex pairs in same-sexed rooms may increase stability, compared to mixed sex rooms. However, as unrelated same-sex pairs often do not affiliate, they are not recommended (Majolo *et al.* 2003). Disturbance within a colony room should be kept to a very minimum, as the presence of unfamiliar individuals may cause anxiety and even redirected aggression towards group mates. If a parent dies, it is possible to introduce a step-parent, but care should be taken, and the step-parent should be allowed to interact with his/her intended pair mate in the absence of other family members, who may mob the unfamiliar group member (Tardif *et al.* 2003).

Single housing of callitrichids is never recommended unless it is unavoidable for justifiable veterinary or human health reasons. It should be kept to a minimum time and the monkey should be able to see, hear and smell familiar compatible group mates. Although weaning to large same-sex 'gang groups' was once used, primarily for ease of management (Buchanan-Smith 2006), this practice is not recommended as it is an unnatural social grouping, and can lead to serious fighting.

Identification and sexing

International guidelines (IPS 2007) recommend that all primates have permanent identification to ensure accuracy as staff change and to permit matching with medical and research records. Accurate labelling on cages aids identification. The best permanent method to identify a primate is using a microchip (Rennie & Buchanan-Smith 2006c; JWGR 2009). The microchip is implanted subcutaneously and holds a unique code which must be read using a scanner. Monkeys previously required sedation before the microchip was inserted under the skin using a specially designed hypodermic needle, usually supplied ready loaded with a microchip. However, the chips are now so small that sedation is generally not required. For callitrichids, the chip is placed under the interscapular skin or the base of the tail (Casteleyn & Bakker 2019) and can be done at 3–6 months of age in *C. jacchus* (Layne-Colon *et al.* 2019). The scanner wand needs to be 5–10 cm away from the chip (Poole *et al.* 1999) for reading. Callitrichids can easily be trained to stay still while the microchip is scanned (Savastano *et al.* 2003). Microchips have been known to migrate under the skin leading to a potential reduction in efficiency of identification.

Although individuals of the same species may all look similar to the untrained observer, careful observation soon allows individuals to be identified by facial characteristics, size differences and markings. However, in large groups, or in facilities where a large number of callitrichids are kept, and there are regular staff changes, an easy method of accurately identifying individuals is strongly recommended (Fortman *et al.* 2002; Rennie & Buchanan-Smith 2006c). In addition to the benefits of immediate identification to assist with behavioural welfare assessment, it encourages naming individuals which facilitates positive staff-animal relationships to develop (Rennie & Buchanan-Smith 2006a). There are many different methods of temporary identification, including hair dyes, fur clipping (often done on the tail) and high-quality stainless steel ball chain collars with identity tags (Rennie & Buchanan-Smith 2006c). Tags/discs can be coloured and numbered. Dyes must be chosen so as not to cause irritation, especially to youngsters, and care taken to avoid injury with clipping. These methods may last less than a month, but dye can be re-applied without the need for capture and handling (Halloren et al. 1989). Collars and tags cannot be used until the animal has stopped growing. Collars and tags must be kept clean, and callitrichids may be trained to accept collar and tag cleaning without restraint.

Sexing of adult callitrichids is easy as males have prominent scrotal sacs, although females also have a pale glandular area around the genitalia, and this should not be confused. Sexing young infants is more difficult, but the key differences are illustrated in Figure 37.4. Casteleyn and Bakker (2019) state that manipulation of neonatal and young animals is needed to confirm the scrotum (an irregular fold of skin) and round preputial opening and glans penis (male) or the slit like vaginal opening (female).

Record-keeping

In order to provide the best care, each monkey should have an individual file or 'passport'. This should include details of their biography (date of birth, sire, dam, etc.) and their prior experiences (e.g. transport history, social groups, training, husbandry system, type of environmental enrichment, research project history and medical history) (see JWGR 2009). This information will assist with analyses of primate care, use and breeding, and to review the adequacy of systems in order to develop good practice (JWGR 2009).

Physical environment and hygiene

As callitrichids are tropical primates, they require an ambient temperature of around 23 °C (range of 23–28 °C) (Council of Europe 2006). In the US, the *Guide for the Care and Use of Laboratory Animals* (NRC 2011) recommends range of 18–29 °C for primates. However, the thermal neutral zone of *C. jacchus* is estimated as 27–33 °C (Power 1991 cited in Power & Koutsos 2019); below this temperature, they will need to raise their metabolic rates. Hence *C. jacchus* are normally kept at the higher end of the regulatory range (i.e. 27–29 °C). *S. oedipus* may be metabolically stressed at <32 °C (Stonerook et al. 1994, cited in Layne-Colon et al. 2019). Despite recommended indoor temperature ranges, callitrichids will choose to go outside, often in much cooler temperatures, especially if the sun is shining and they have shelter from the wind (Badihi 2006).

Humidity of 40–70% is recommended by Council of Europe (2006), which notes that prolonged exposure below this range may result in respiratory disorders, and they will tolerate levels >70%. A broad range of 30–70% for relative humidity is specified by the guidelines. Callitrichids respond adversely to noise (e.g. construction noise). The level of background noise should be kept low and if it is absolutely necessary to exceed 65dBA, it should only be for short periods. As previously mentioned, background sound does not promote welfare (McDermott & Hauser 2007). A photoperiod of no less than 12 hours of light in recommended by the Council of Europe (2006).

Callitrichids should be kept in hygienic conditions, with regular cleaning to remove stale food, and excreta. Scent marking leads to sticky substrates that can lead to oily coats. A complete cage clean, by autoclave, or by scrubbing using a hot water, domestic detergent and bleach, together with thorough rinsing, should only occur at 1–2-month intervals. Because of the role of scent marking in territorial behaviour, in modulating reproductive physiology and their importance in social interactions, familiar scents should not be totally removed from the captive environments during cleaning. Alternating cleaning and sanitation of enclosures and substrates and enrichment devices will have beneficial effects by maintaining familiarity and reducing over-stimulated scent marking (Prescott 2006).

Health monitoring, transport, quarantine and barrier systems

It is important that callitrichids are checked at least twice daily for changes in behaviour, inactivity, nasal discharge and signs of diarrhoea. Deviations from normality should be

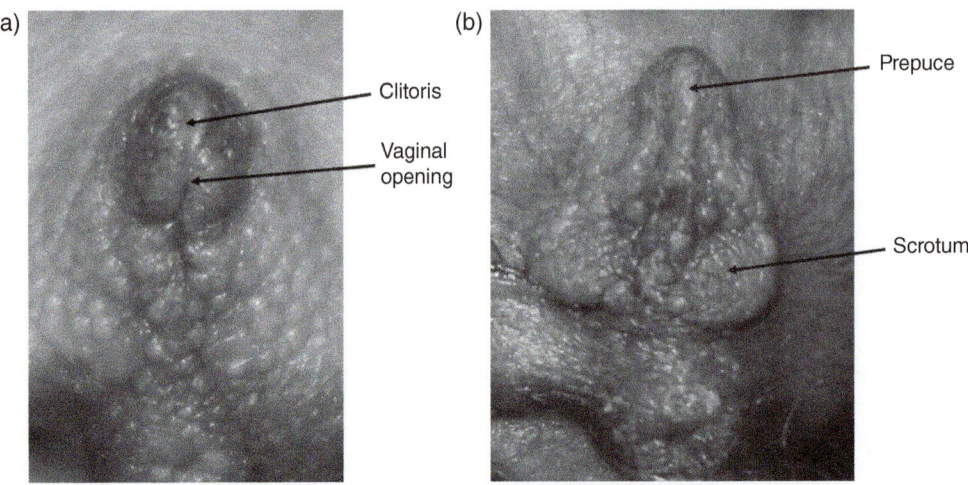

Figure 37.4 The external genitalia of (a) female and (b) male infant common marmosets. Source: Hannah Buchanan-Smith.

marked on a standardised scale to ensure records are accurately kept. Burns and Wachtman (2019) provide a body condition scoring scale for *C. jacchus*, and Tardif and Ross (2019) provide normal weight gain trajectories. Veterinary advice should be sought if non-normal patterns persist, or if the monkeys are listless, remain in their nest boxes or do not eat.

Although callitrichids are commonly bred in-house (Rennie & Buchanan-Smith 2005), occasionally relocation is required. A number of publications provide useful information on transport and should be consulted (Wolfensohn & Honess 2005; Joint Working Group on Refinement (JWGR) 2009). Trade and international travel of primates is regulated. Details can be found in the Convention on International Trade in Endangered Species of Wild Flora and Fauna (CITES), the World Organization for Animal Health (OIE: Office International des Epizooties), the US Centers for Disease Control and Prevention (CDC), the Lacey Act (US), the Endangered Species Act (US) and the International Air Transport Association (IATA). Marini (2019) provides an overview of the regulations and guidance pertaining to marmoset acquisition and transport.

If transport between facilities is required, callitrichids should be placed in a ventilated wooden box (a softer quieter environment than metal) with some soft substrate (Poole *et al.* 1999). There should be moist food available (e.g. fruit and vegetables) and a window to allow monitoring and to supplement food and water on longer journeys. Familiar conspecifics should be transported together. Transporting females in late pregnancy poses a serious welfare risk. Moreover, females with young infants may attack them, so transportation is not advised. In addition, the separation of offspring under 5 months from their parents is not acceptable during transport (Poole *et al.* 1999).

Marini (2019) summarises key considerations for quarantine, as the Public Health Service of the United States has granted to the CDC the regulatory authority for the prevention of communicable diseases. These specify a minimum quarantine of 31 days in a CDC-approved quarantine facility is required. The animal passport should be available to the new facility before the monkeys arrive and every effort should be made to achieve continuity (or in some cases improvement) of care and also help to ensure rapid acclimatisation to the new facility (JWGR 2009). Food should initially be identical or similar to that of the source colony, and changes introduced slowly (Tardif *et al.* 2003).

The transport to the facility will have caused stress, and extra care must be taken upon arrival to ensure the monkeys are not dehydrated. It is also important to ensure continuity of water supply as some animals may not learn a new method of acquiring water (Tardif *et al.* 2003). Quarantine must report within 24 hours any primate disease suspected of being yellow fever, monkey pox or filovirus (reviewed in Marini 2019). During quarantine, the monkeys should receive a thorough health check, including haematology, biochemistry and tuberculin testing (TB) (Poole *et al.* 1999).

There are no national or international standards of personal protective equipment (PPE) for humans interacting with callitrichids, although facilities usually develop their own. The health status/infectious state of the callitrichid dictates the level of PPE, but there are also a number of other considerations, including level of physical contact and staff experience. Callitrichids are susceptible to measles so staff and visitors should provide evidence they are immune to minimise risk of transmission, and free of tuberculosis. Staff should wear protective clothing, including face masks and gloves if they display any sign of a cough. Particular care should be taken to prevent contact with any human with cold sores, due to the *Herpes* virus that can prove fatal for callitrichids Mätz-Rensing and Bleyer (2019) provide a comprehensive review of viral diseases of *C. jacchus*.

Care of aged animals

We should consider the welfare of animals throughout their whole lifespan, and indeed the Refinement R of the three Rs includes this in the definition (Buchanan-Smith *et al.* 2005). Brando and Buchanan-Smith (2018) take the concept further to discuss the considerations that need to be taken into account at different stages of the lifecycle and in relation to different environmental factors to promote good welfare. Senescence is one of these key stages, as primates can experience disease and incapacity in similar way to humans. Waitt *et al.* (2010) review the range of environmental factors to consider in enclosure design. These include accessibility, furnishings and thermoregulation. As general principles, the environments of primates should be designed to encourage them to move around to minimise physical deterioration.

Marmosets are being used increasingly in ageing research (see Ross 2019). As marmosets age, they may display signs of pain and discomfort and care staff should monitor them carefully to ensure they are eating and remain hydrated, and be trained to handle and evaluate markers accurately (Ross 2019). Marmosets may lose their teeth when ageing so provision of accessible food (type and consistency, access of location, etc.) is important. Humane endpoints must be identified so suffering is minimised.

Breeding and rearing

As noted in the preceding text, setting up new breeding pairs is usually a smooth process, but certain guidelines should be followed carefully (see JWGR 2009). Comparative reproductive data are provided in Table 37.2. The method of pregnancy testing is generally by abdominal palpation, and pregnancy can be detected from 5 weeks post-conception (Kirkwood & Stathatos 1992), although as this can be disruptive and is not recommended on a regular basis. Weight gain and abdominal distension are clear signs of pregnancy in later stages. Ultrasound and urinary hormone measurement may also be used; callitrichids can be trained to accept ultrasound (Savastano *et al.* 2003). Marmosets and tamarins usually give birth at night (between 20.00 h and 07.00 h); if the female shows signs of labour during the day, veterinary intervention may be required. During birth, the group members gather around the mother and may share in eating the placenta (Stevenson 1976; Price 1990).

Although adapted to give birth to twins, *C. jacchus* are increasingly producing triplets (or even quadruplets) in captivity (e.g. Ash & Buchanan-Smith 2014). Dam age, parturition number and dam body weight at conception predicts litter size although the mechanism is not understood (Tardif & Jaquish 1997). There is conflicting evidence as to whether the litter size of the dam at her birth also predicts the size of her litters (Rutherford et al. 2014; Bakker et al. 2018). The increase in triplet and quadruplet births in captivity is problematic for both dam and infant mortality. Large litter size can lead to problems during pregnancy and birth complications (such as transverse presentation of the foetus, lameness in the pregnant female, hydrocephalus or a dead embryo blocking the cervix) (Poole et al. 1999).

Although, occasionally, the family will rear triplets without human intervention, this is often not the case, and the weakest may fall to the floor. A range of practices have been developed to reduce infant mortality (see below). Infants who have fallen to the floor, and have not been picked up by group members, should be examined carefully for injury and disease. The decision to hand-rear should not be made lightly as there are potential problems associated with this (Kirkwood & Stathatos 1992), and hand-reared individuals are unlikely to be suitable breeders or good models for scientific research. If individuals are hand-reared, they must be reintroduced into a conspecific group as soon as possible to minimise the serious adverse effects of separation from their natal groups.

Reproductive success and infant mortality vary quite substantially between facilities, suggesting there are numerous factors associated with successful breeding, including genetic factors, early rearing history of parents, temperament, housing, husbandry, including rearing management practices and diet. *C. jacchus* are successfully bred in many facilities, sometimes with mortality rates of less than 20% (Prescott & Buchanan-Smith 2004). Ash and Buchanan-Smith (2014) summarise reproductive success across a range of studies, the largest of which is a meta-analysis of data from five colonies in the Americas (n = 625 dams) reported a mean of 50% loss between number of infants produced, and weaned at 3 months (Smucny et al. 2004). Tamarins are more difficult to breed (Tardif et al. 1984b), but there is a strong link between quality of captive conditions and breeding success; when they are housed in large complex enclosures and with a group composition resembling those in the wild, they have greater success (reviewed in Prescott & Buchanan-Smith 2004). *C. jacchus* that first breed at a later age (>4 years) have better survivorship than those first reproducing when younger (<2.5 years) (Jaquish et al. 1991; Smucny et al. 2004).

Options to reduce mortality for larger litters include complete or partial hand-rearing, rotational hand-rearing, supplementary feeding and fostering (see Schultz-Darken et al. 2019 for a description of these practices). The practice of rotational hand-rearing, when two infants are reared by the family group and one is human reared rotationally, is successful in reducing mortality. However, it requires the animal care staff to disturb the group on a regular basis, to replace and remove an infant, and each offspring will be subjected to period of separation, which is known to influence behaviour and physiology (Dettling et al. 2002a, 2002b). The impact of this practice on future reproductive success, and on the suitability as models for scientific research has not been determined but it is likely to have an adverse effect due to isolation leading to separation anxiety (Buchanan-Smith 2006). Supplementary feeding (when all infants are removed together, and fed) has proved very successful and has no adverse effect on behaviour, or judgement bias (Ash & Buchanan-Smith 2016) as they are never isolated, but remain together with other litter mates. Another practice for successfully rearing triplets may be to provide supplementary feeding to the infants while they remain in the family group, or to cross-foster and supplementary feed the infants to surrogate *C. jacchus* parents, who are well-experienced but without their own offspring (e.g. because they are on contraception).

Laboratory procedures

Handling

Marmosets and tamarins generally do not like being handled, although with extensive gentle handling and desensitising (with small pieces of treat foods such as gum arabic, grape, raisin or marshmallow) some will tolerate it and a latex gloved hand can be used. However, to avoid handling they can be trained using positive reinforcement techniques (see Chapter 15: The use of positive reinforcement training techniques to enhance the care and welfare of laboratory and research animals) to co-operate with routine husbandry procedures such as capture, weighing, veterinary procedures, oral administration or palpation, or to provide samples for analysis (such as saliva or urine). If there is good reason why they need to be handled, a firm but gentle approach is critical. When possible, callitrichids should be trained, using positive reinforcement techniques, to enter a transport box or Perspex cylinder, and capture by gloved hand from the box will be substantially easier than capture from within the home cage. A detailed illustrated account of how to train marmosets to enter a transport box is provided by Prescott et al. (2005). Chasing individuals into nest boxes for capture is not recommended as the nest box should be seen as a safe place to rest, and not associated with any potential stressor (Rennie & Buchanan-Smith 2006c). Removal of a callitrichid from the transport box is best done by opening the door slowly and grasping the monkey around the shoulders as he/she exits. If heavy, the weight of the body should be supported with the other hand and the monkey should remain in an upright position so it can look around, as he/she will likely feel less vulnerable than in a supine position. Movements should be slow, and voices muted. When catching by hand the weight of the glove used must be carefully gauged to ensure that excessive pressure is not applied to the animal and that the handler is sufficiently well-protected (Sainsbury et al. 1989). Callitrichids may bite the glove, and this has been known to cause dental problems (e.g. broken teeth). They should not be left in a transport box for any longer than is absolutely necessary. The monkeys should be returned to their home cage as soon as possible following handling.

If monkeys are caught within the home cage, the handler should approach calmly and wait until they are stationary, and then grip the part of the tail nearest the body while the other hand is placed around the shoulders. This approach is not recommended unless monkeys have been very well habituated to it. If they are removed from wire mesh, great care must be taken to remove their tight grip from the mesh as injuries can occur to their claws. Capture by net is not recommended as it causes fear and distress, can result in injury when the animals are chased around and entanglement during removal from the net. Great care should be taken not to allow individuals to escape as this creates disruption as individuals in other cages in the colony room may attempt to bite them (and have been known to bite off digits). Swift return to the cage should be a priority; if animals are trained, they can be enticed back into their home cages with food rewards. However, if they are not, a net may be required as a last resort, but is very disturbing to all individuals in the room.

Training/habituation for procedures

Although all methods of restraint can be highly stressful, much of this stress can be eliminated if the method is used sensitively (Fortman et al. 2002), and if the callitrichids are desensitised to the procedure, by pairing it with food rewards, and by making the procedure predictable, so they are familiar with what is going to happen.

There is now very good evidence that callitrichids can be trained for a variety of tasks related to husbandry, veterinary treatment, scientific studies and tests of cognitive ability with no need for food or water management (e.g. McKinley et al. 2003; Savastano et al. 2003; Scott et al. 2003; Smith et al. 2004 and see Prescott et al. 2005). The benefits of training laboratory-housed primates are summarised by Westlund (2015), together with advice on use of different techniques. Cognitive testing within the home cage is preferred, for welfare and scientific reasons (Scott et al. 2003). Temperature is an important indicator of health, and callitrichids can be trained to accept a tympanic thermometer without restraint (Savastano et al. 2003). Temperature can also be read remotely in telemetric microchips (reviewed in Rennie & Buchanan-Smith 2006c).

C. jacchus have been trained to stand on a balance for weighing in the home cage (McKinley et al. 2003). The initial time investment is not high for this training (between 2 and 12, 10-minute training sessions per pair, with a mean of 6 sessions, see Figure 37.5). If the marmosets were already taking food from the trainer's hand, it took a mean of just two, 10-minute sessions per pair. A comparison with the standard weighing procedure showed that this initial time investment can be quickly recouped. One of the many advantages of training for in-home cage weighing is that it avoids the need for capture and restraint. Poole and colleagues (1999) have suggested that even the weights of carried young can be measured in this way, by weighing the carrier with and without a single youngster on his/her back. Schultz-Darken and co-workers (2004) have described habituation of C. jacchus to sling harness restraint for neuroendocrine experiments, and Ferris and colleagues (2001) described habituation for functional magnetic imaging experiments. Restraint devices for sample collection are described later in this chapter.

Monitoring methods

Surgically implanted telemetric devices have been used successfully in nonhuman primates to collect cardiovascular, blood pressure, temperature, motor, vocalisation, locomotion and pH data, and to record electrocardiograms (ECG), electromyograms (EMG), electroencephalograms (EEG) and electrocorticograms (ECoG) (Kinter & Johnson 1999). There are advantages and disadvantages to the non-invasive externally worn telemetry devices, and partially and fully surgically implanted devices (reviewed in Rennie & Buchanan-Smith 2006c). Hawkins (2014) explains how many of the harms to animals can be overcome by thoughtful experimental design and refinements to surgical procedures and husbandry practices. Fully implanted devices allow multiple subjects to be housed in pairs or groups; working instrumentation has been successfully maintained in C. jacchus for up to 2 years (Crofts et al. 2001), and used to monitor responses to a range of environments and events (e.g. Gerber et al. 2002a). External devices have not yet been used in marmosets (Korte & Everitt 2019).

Urine samples allow analyses of accumulation of metabolites, are easy to collect and provide sufficient volume. Marmosets can be trained, in a short period of time, to urinate into a collection vial on request (McKinley et al. 2003), or using a similar technique to provide a sample scent mark for analysis (Schultz-Darken 2003). Other methods of urine collection that do not necessitate social isolation have also been documented (Anzenberger & Gossweiler 1993; Smith et al. 2004). Steroid and protein metabolites can also be measured in faeces, but lag times must be well understood. Saliva has also been validated for cortisol in C. jacchus (Cross et al. 2004; Ash et al. 2018). The ease with which it is collected from known individuals, and the fact that it allows measurement of currently circulating cortisol, and may be collected at very regular intervals may make it the preferred method of cortisol analysis to determine acute stress levels. However, Davenport et al. (2006) showed that cortisol in hair is a reliable indicator of chronic stress in macaques. In marmosets, this could be a promising measure for chronic stress.

Training callitrichids to accept venipuncture has not been achieved, partially because their small size makes it difficult to access blood vessels, and because of the precision required. However, with training and desensitisation, the stress of capture and restraint can be minimised and thus the

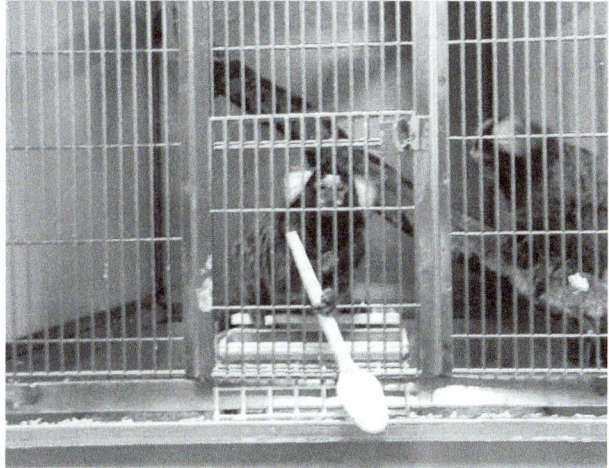

Figure 37.5 A marmoset holding a target (plastic spoon), while sitting on scales for in-home cage weighing. Source: Jean McKinley.

overall stress of routine procedures can also be reduced (Greig et al. 2006). Restraint devices offer some benefits over conventional handling techniques. First, they allow the procedure to be carried out by just a single person whereas sometimes two or three technicians are involved in manual restraint, one to restrain and the other(s) to carry out the procedure (e.g. Hearn 1977; Buchanan-Smith, personal observation). Second, with the restraint device, the animal's movement is quite restricted, for a short period, and the chance of a haematoma and bruising is decreased. There is good back support, and the marmoset is held in an upright position allowing him/her to look around. Third, most marmosets habituate to the device; they appear comfortable and without obvious signs of stress. They accept a food reward following the procedure (Greig et al. 2006), and indeed food rewards should be offered following all procedures to desensitise them. Figure 37.6 shows C. jacchus in a restraint device.

It is important to consider the timing and quantity of blood sampling given the small size of callitrichids. Korte and Everitt (2019) estimate that C. jacchus has a circulating mean blood volume between 19.5 and 31.2 mL (65 mL/kg) based upon 300–480 g body weight. Blood sampling requires a short, 0.4–0.5 mm diameter (25–27 g) needle, with a small 1–2.5 ml syringe (Poole et al. 1999; Burns & Wachtman 2019). Single blood samples of up to 0.5 ml/100 g body weight can be taken safely (Poole et al. 1999). If repeated sampling is required, no more than 15% of total blood volume should be taken per month (Diehl et al. 2001), approximating to 3.7 ml per month for a 350 g marmoset (Poole et al. 1999). However, this must be monitored closely to check for normal cell composition and haemoglobin concentration, and iron supplements should be given (Poole et al. 1999).

Greig and co-workers (2006) describe the procedure for blood collection from the femoral vein. The leg should be held straight by curling fingers around the length of the leg to ensure that the animal cannot bend at the knee or kick. The thumb provides extra restraint and support to the syringe. The syringe needle should be inserted at an angle of approximately 15° into the groove midway down the leg, the thumb can be used as a guide. The vein or the groove is not always visible in heavier animals so the midpoint should be used. The syringe plunger should be slowly pulled back just after insertion of the needle point, to ensure that it has entered the vein. If correctly inserted, blood should flow back into the syringe, if not then the needle should be inserted further until blood is seen entering the needle hub. There should be no further insertion of the needle at this point. The plunger should be pulled slowly until the appropriate volume is acquired. Schultz-Darken (2003) also provides details of blood sampling from a restraint device, and advice on an intravenous femoral catheter for repeated blood sampling and a jugular vein catheter for longer-term sampling over several hours.

A restraint device can also be used for collection of semen from mated females (details in Greig et al. 2006), and is seen as a refinement over other methods of sperm collection such as electro-ejaculation. Schultz-Darken (2003) describes a procedure for collecting semen using vibratory stimulation while the male marmoset is restrained.

Administration of substances

The substance to be administered and the route of its administration are determined to a great extent by the objectives of the experimental procedure concerned. A thorough review of refinement techniques for administration of substances has been provided by the BVAAWF/FRAME/RSPCA/UFAW working party (JWGR 2001). Korte and Everitt (2019) summarise administration of substances for toxicology and safety assessment in C. jacchus, including inhalation studies. Oral administration by gavage requires careful restraint because poor placement of the tube (into the trachea rather than the oesophagus or the top of the stomach) has the potential to harm or kill the subject animal, and marmoset teeth are delicate and easily damaged. A small soft plastic tube can be used to keep the mouth open. It is preferable to incorporate substances into treat feeds (such as marshmallows) or favoured fluids, a method considered to have minimal impact on the animal (JWGR 2001). If the callitrichid will not eat, the solution can be fed into the mouth with syringe. Subcutaneous injections are best administered into the loose skin above the shoulders, and the upper thigh is suitable for intramuscular injection (Poole et al. 1999). Intravenous injections should be performed into the saphenous or lateral tail vein which can be catheterised (Marini & Haupt 2019).

Anaesthesia/analgesia

There is a lack of information on the pharmacokinetics of agents used in sedation, anaesthesia and analgesia in callitrichids (C. jacchus, Marini & Haupt 2019). These authors

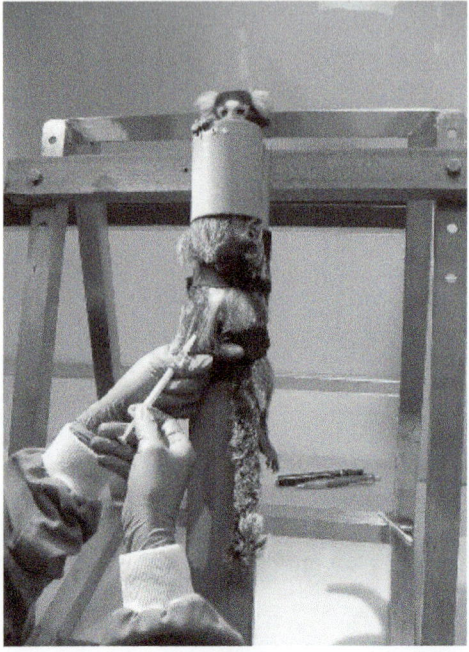

Figure 37.6 A marmoset in a restraint device, showing the plastic tube and Velcro straps, having a blood sample taken from the femoral vein. Source: Photo by Keith Morris, from Greig et al. (2006).

summarise the challenges, and points to consider, as well as reviewing the literature. Ketamine (a dissociative anaesthetic) is unfortunately still the most commonly used anaesthetic agent for marmosets and tamarins. Ketamine has many undesirable consequences when used alone, which include 'hypersalivation, myoclonus, poor muscle relaxation, spontaneous movement, prolonged recovery with higher doses, and, potentially, emergence delirium' (Marin & Haupt 2019, page 177). If administered intramuscularly, it may also cause myotoxicity in marmosets. Dosage depends upon depth of anaesthesia required, and the condition of the monkey, concurrently administered medication and clinical history (Marini & Haupt 2019). Poole and colleagues (1999) recommend 5–15 mg/kg by intramuscular injection for mild restraint such as fitting identity collars, although muscle relaxation is often poor. Rensing and Oerke (2005 and Rensing, personal communication), recommend up to 50 mg/kg for surgical procedures (combined with a potent analgesic) with a maximum of 25 mg/animal due to myotoxicity. To improve muscle relaxation, Poole and colleagues (1999) recommend a combination of ketamine and xylazine at a dose rate of 10–15 mg/kg ketamine and 1.5 mg/kg xylazine. Further, they and Rensing (personal communication) recommend a ketamine/medetomidine mixture (3 mg/kg ketamine with 0.05 mg/kg medetomidine given intramuscularly) as this has the advantage of being reversed by administration of atipamezole intravenously or intramuscularly. In order to maintain general anaesthesia, inhalation of the narcotic gaseous anaesthetic isoflurane or sevoflurane can be used, delivered via a modified endotracheal tube (2.0 mm) or with a face mask (Rensing & Oerke 2005; Marini & Haupt 2019).

Rensing and Oerke (2005) recommend Saffan® (new trade name is Alfaxan-CD RTU), of which the active constituents are alfaxalone, as a safer alternative to ketamine (dose rate: 18 mg/kg) to induce anaesthesia. Bakker *et al.* (2013) concur that for *C. jacchus*, alfaxalone (dose of 12 mg/kg) has no side effects yet provides comparable immobilisation to ketamine at 50 mg/kg. Bakker *et al.* (2013) consider length of procedures as a determinant of choice of anaesthetic. Doses may need to be incremented to maintain effect.

For longer surgery, Rensing and Oerke (2005) note that a combination of Saffan® (8 mg/kg) and diazepam (0.25 mg/animal) is reliable in *C. jacchus*; and ketamine (25 mg/kg) and midazolam (25 mg/kg) can be used for *S. oedipus*. Bakker *et al* (2018) found that buprenorphine caused a high incidence of complications. It is important to maintain body temperature during anaesthesia and surgery. This can be achieved using heat lamps or heat pads, or using an operating table with a built-in thermoregulator in the table surface. It is critical to monitor anaesthesia carefully to prevent deaths and ensure safe recovery. For general advice, see Flecknell (2015), and for *C. jacchus*, see Marini and Haupt (2019).

Euthanasia

Euthanasia is required if animals are found to experience an unacceptable level of pain or distress (specified humane endpoints), when the project requires pathology or histology examination of organs or tissues, or at the end of an experiment if they cannot be re-used (as outlined in the project licence). See also Chapter 17: Euthanasia and other fates for laboratory animals. For anaesthetised marmosets and tamarins, intravenous or intracardial injection of pentobarbital (also known as *sodium pentobarbital*, a barbiturate formulated for euthanasia, 70–100 mg/kg) is the only acceptable method for euthanasia (Poole *et al.* 1999; Rennie & Buchanan-Smith 2006c; IPS 2007). Too high a dose of pentobarbital can cause tissue artefacts on histology (Grieves *et al.* 2008).

Common welfare problems, and indicators of positive welfare

Health

If kept permanently indoors, immunoprophylaxis is generally not required for animals if housing and husbandry are appropriate and they are provided with nutritionally balanced diets. If callitrichids have access to outside runs, they will require protection against *Yersinia* and *Salmonella* bacteria and other infections which can be carried in bird droppings (Poole *et al.* 1999; Bakker *et al.* 2007, 2015).

Signs of illness include changes in activity, often listlessness including lack of alertness, a reduction in body weight, poor coat condition, diarrhoea and withdrawal from group mates. In relation to body weight, in a study of the effects of chronic psychosocial stress in *C. jacchus*, Johnson and colleagues (1996) observed a 10% drop in body weight in individuals taken from stable pairings and placed in isolation and considered this to be indicative of considerable social stress. This was accompanied by an increase in locomotion and cringing behaviours and in crying vocalisations. Burns and Wachtman (2019) state that any weight loss or gain of 10% or more should be entered on the records and diagnostic tests performed. Fluctuating body weight (in contrast to a stable body weight) in adults is also a useful indicator of poor welfare.

Callitrichids can be infected with a range of parasites, gut bacterial and viral infections some of which are zoonotic, as well as non-infectious diseases. Details can be found in Bennett *et al.* (1998), Potkay (1992), Rensing and Oerke (2005), Marini (2019), Kramer (2019) and Burns and Wachtman (2019) who provide symptoms and treatment.

Chronic lymphocytic enterocolitis (CLE), also known as wasting marmoset syndrome used to be a common killer of captive marmosets, and while still present in some colonies, is no longer quite as frequently observed. Symptoms are progressive weight loss despite of normal food intake and a deteriorating general condition, chronic diarrhoea, tail alopecia, muscle atrophy, anaemia and chronic colitis. Its aetiology is still poorly understood but it may be associated with stress, malnutrition (too much fruit, protein deficiency), parasitic, bacterial, viral infections or colitis (Sainsbury *et al.* 1987; Rensing & Oerke 2005). Unfortunately, no treatment is known. These marmosets are mostly euthanised to prevent suffering. Hemosiderosis (a deposit of iron pigment haemosiderin in the liver) has been found in marmosets with CLE (Miller *et al.* 1997). Welfare problems associated with reproduction have been described in the preceding text.

Behavioural indicators of good and poor welfare

Behaviour, postures and vocalisations are the most immediate way to determine good and poor welfare, and it is critical that staff are trained to accurately recognise and assess key indicators, not only to recognise pain and distress, but also to recognise happy healthy animals. It is important that staff are familiar with natural behaviour as a reference point. Significant increases or decreases in natural behaviour should be noted (i.e. abnormally high or low) as should the performance of unnatural behaviours. Although there has been a focus on poor welfare indicators in the literature, promotion of positive welfare is increasingly recognised (e.g. Yeates & Main 2008; Mellor & Beausoleil 2015).

Environmental enrichment promotes positive welfare. Buchanan-Smith (2010) describes example techniques in the physical, social, food, cognitive/occupational and sensory enrichment categories. A callitrichid monkey could be assessed as having good welfare if he/she appears relaxed (in his/her social group and in the presence of humans) and engages in calm allogrooming, play and exploration. He or she should interact with other group members affiliatively and in social support. A few non-injurious aggressive threats and physical contact may be expected from time to time. In *C. jacchus*, increases in calm locomotion (relaxed gait) and exploration, and decreased scent marking, scratching, agitated locomotion (but not in play context) and inactive non-alert behaviour are seen when conditions are improved (e.g. access from laboratory cages to outdoor runs) (Badihi 2006). Vocalisations correlated with positive welfare include whirr/ trills and chirp (Watson & Buchanan-Smith 2011).

In contrast, scent marking, scratching, inactive alert (vigilance) and locomotion are known to increase following stressful events (Cilia & Piper 1997; Bassett *et al.* 2003) and these increases are key indicators of reduced welfare, although the reliability of self-scratching as an indicator is debated (National Academies of Sciences, Engineering, and Medicine 2019). Inappropriate social behaviour, such as excessive grooming or infanticide, are causes for concern. Abnormal unnatural behaviours exhibited by callitrichids include locomotor stereotypies such as circling and weaving (Hubrecht 1995), head bobbing and self-injurious behaviour (Box & Rohrhuber 1993).

Tail-raised present is displayed in marmosets when threatened (Figure 37.1d), and other postures and facial expressions (e.g. movements of the ear tufts and baring of the teeth in open-mouth displays) serve as communication and can be used to monitor welfare (Stevenson & Poole 1976; Stevenson & Rylands 1988; Watson & Buchanan-Smith 2011). The chatter, loud shrill, ek, cough, tsik, see, seep and squeals indicate negative welfare (e.g. Watson & Buchanan-Smith 2011). If these behaviours and vocalisations are directed towards care staff on a regular basis, the staff are probably being viewed as predators, and efforts should be made to improve the human–monkey relationship, as this is arguably one of the most critical factors influencing welfare (Rennie & Buchanan-Smith 2006a). Many of these behavioural and vocal welfare indicators are illustrated on marmosetcare.com[1].

Hand-rearing may lead to a variety of behavioural abnormalities (Kirkwood & Stathatos 1992), and single housing may lead to locomotor stereotypies (Hubrecht 1995). Prescott and Buchanan-Smith (2004) argue that *Saguinus* may be more predisposed to develop such abnormal behaviour than marmosets; head bobbing and self-inflicted trauma has been reported in *S. oedipus* (Box & Rohrhuber 1993; Savage 1995) and *S. labiatus* (Buchanan-Smith, personal observation). However, if physical and social housing conditions are good, callitrichids rarely behave abnormally. Providing appropriate conditions to allow callitrichids to thrive should be our goal, for ethical reasons as well as for good science.

Acknowledgements

The author would like to thank the many people who have discussed issues concerning keeping marmosets and tamarins in captivity, but in particular Hilary Box, Robert Hubrecht, Mark Prescott, Herbert Brok, Jaco Bakker, Susanne Rensing, Jean McKinley, Inbal Badihi, Verity Bowell, Lois Bassett and Keith Morris. The author is most grateful to Anthony Rylands who provided the most up-to-date advice on taxonomy, and to the referees and editors whose comments improved the chapter.

References

Abbott, D.H., Barnett, D.K., Colman, R.J. *et al.* (2003) Aspects of common marmoset basic biology and life history important for biomedical research. *Comparative Medicine*, **53**, 339–350.

Abreu, F., de la Fuente, M.F.C., Schiel, N. *et al.* (2016). Feeding ecology and behavioral adjustments: Flexibility of a small Neotropical primate (*Callithrix jacchus*) to survive in a semiarid environment. *Mammal Research*, **61**, 221–229.

Albuquerque, A.C.S.R., Sousa, M.B.C., Santos, H.M. *et al.* (2001) Behavioral and hormonal analysis of social relationships between oldest females in a wild monogamous group of common marmosets (*Callithrix jacchus*). *International Journal of Primatology*, **22**, 631–645.

Alonso, C. and Langguth, A. (1989) Ecology and behavior of *Callithrix jacchus* (Primates: Callitrichidae) living on an Atlantic Forest island. *Revista Nordestina de Biologia*, **6**, 105–137.

Andersson, M. (1981) On optimal predator search. *Theoretical Population Biology*, **19**, 58–86.

Anzenberger, G. and Gossweiler, H. (1993) How to obtain individual urine samples from undisturbed marmoset families. *American Journal of Primatology*, **31**, 223–230.

Araújo, A., Arruda, M.F., Alencar, A.I. *et al.* (2000) Body weight of wild and captive common marmosets (*Callithrix jacchus*). *International Journal of Primatology*, **21**, 317–324.

Arruda, M.F., Araújo, A., Sousa, M.B.C. *et al.* (2005) Two breeding females within free-living groups may not always indicate polygyny: alternative subordinate female strategies in common marmosets (*Callithrix jacchus*). *Folia Primatologica*, **76**, 10–20.

Arruda, M.F., Yamamoto, M.E., Pessoa, D.M.A. *et al.* (2019) Taxonomy and natural history. In: *The Common Marmoset in Captivity and Biomedical Research.* Eds Marini, R.P., Wachtman, L.M., Tardif, S.D. *et al.*, pp. 3–15. Academic Press, London.

Ash, H. and Buchanan-Smith, H.M. (2014) Long-term data on reproductive output and longevity in captive female common marmosets (*Callithrix jacchus*). *American Journal of Primatology*, **76**, 1062–1073.

Ash, H. and Buchanan-Smith, H.M. (2016) The long-term impact of infant rearing background on the affective state of adult common marmosets (*Callithrix jacchus*). *Applied Animal Behaviour Science*, **174**, 128–136.

Ash, H., Smith, T.E., Knight, S. et al. (2018) Measuring physiological stress in the common marmoset (*Callithrix jacchus*): Validation of a salivary cortisol collection and assay technique. *Physiology & Behavior*, **185**, 14–22.

Badihi, I. (2006) The effect of complexity, choice and control on the behaviour and the welfare of captive common marmosets (*Callithrix jacchus*). PhD thesis, University of Stirling, Scotland, https://dspace.stir.ac.uk/bitstream/1893/120/1/Badihi%20PhD.pdf (accessed February 2022).

Badihi, I., Morris, K. and Buchanan-Smith, H.M. (2007) The effects of increased space, complexity, and choice, together with their loss, on the behavior of a family group of *Callithrix jacchus*: A case study. *Laboratory Primate Newsletter*, **46**, 1–5.

Bakker, J., Kondova, I., de Groot, C. et al. (2007) A report on Yersinia-related mortality in a colony of New World monkeys. *Laboratory Primate Newsletter*, **46**, 11–15

Bakker, J., Uilenreef, J.J., Pelt, E.R. et al. (2013) Comparison of three different sedative-anaesthetic protocols (ketamine, ketamine-medetomidine and alphaxalone) in common marmosets (*Callithrix jacchus*). *BMC Veterinary Research*, **9**, 113.

Bakker, J., Ouwerling, B., Heidtm P.J. et al. (2015) Advantages and risks of husbandry and housing changes to improve animal well-being in a breeding colony of common marmosets (*Callithrix jacchus*). *Journal of the American Association of Laboratory Animal Science*, **54**, 273e9

Bakker, J., Louwerse, A.L., Remarque, E.J. et al. (2018) Defining predictive factors for reproductive output in captive common marmosets (*Callithrix jacchus*). *American Journal of Primatology*, **80**, e22926.

Bassett, L. and Buchanan-Smith, H.M. (2007) Effects of predictability on the welfare of captive primates. In: *Animal Behaviour, Conservation and Enrichment*. Ed. Swaisgood, R.R. *Applied Animal Behaviour Science*, **102**, 223–245.

Bassett, L., Buchanan-Smith, H.M., McKinley, J. et al. (2003) Effects of training on stress-related behavior of the common marmoset (*Callithrix jacchus*) in relation to coping with routine husbandry procedures. *Journal of Applied Animal Welfare Science*, **6**, 221–233.

Bennett, B.T., Abee, C.R, and Henrickson, R. (Eds) (1998) *Nonhuman Primates in Biomedical Research*, Vol. II (Diseases). Academic Press, San Diego.

Bezerra, B., Bicca-Marques, J., Miranda, J. et al. (2018) *Callithrix jacchus*. *The IUCN Red List of Threatened Species*: e.T41518A17936001

Boubli, J.P., Silva, M.N.F. da, Rylands, A.B. et al. (2018) How many pygmy marmoset (*Cebuella* Gray, 1870) species are there? A taxonomic re-appraisal based on new molecular evidence. *Molecular Phylogenetics and Evolution*, **120**, 170–182.

Box, H.O. and Rohrhuber, B. (1993) Differences in behaviour among adult male, female pairs of cotton-top tamarins (*Saguinus oedipus*) in different conditions of housing. *Animal Technology*, **44**, 19–30.

Brando, S. and Buchanan-Smith, H.M. (2018) The 24/7 approach to promoting optimal welfare for captive wild animals. *Behavioural Processes*, **156**, 83–95.

Brudzynski, S.M. (Ed.) (2018) *Handbook of Ultrasonic Vocalization: A Window into the Emotional Brain*, Vol. 25. Academic Press, London

Buchanan-Smith, H.M. (1998) Enrichment of marmosets and tamarins – considerations for the care of captive callitrichids. In: *Guidelines for Environmental Enrichment*. Ed. Field, D.A., pp. 183–201. Top Copy, Bristol.

Buchanan-Smith, H.M. (2005) Recent advances in color vision research. *American Journal of Primatology*, **67**, 393–398.

Buchanan-Smith, H.M. (2006) Primates in laboratories: standardisation, harmonisation, variation and Science. *ALTEX – Alternatives to Animal Experimentation*, **23**, 115–119.

Buchanan-Smith, H.M. (2010). Environmental enrichment for primates in laboratories. *Advances in Science and Research*, **5**, 41–56.

Buchanan-Smith, H.M. and Badihi, I. (2012) The psychology of control: Effects of control over supplementary light on welfare of marmosets. *Applied Animal Behaviour Science*, **137**, 166–174.

Buchanan-Smith, H.M., Prescott, M.J. and Cross, N.J. (2004) What factors should determine cage sizes for primates in the laboratory? *Animal Welfare*, **13**, S197–S201.

Buchanan-Smith, H.M., Rennie, A., Vitale, A. et al. (2005) Harmonising the definition of refinement. *Animal Welfare*, **14**, 379–384.

Buchanan-Smith, H.M., Shand, C. and Morris, K. (2002) Cage use and feeding height preferences of captive common marmosets (*Callithrix jacchus*) in two-tier cages. *Journal of Applied Animal Welfare Science*, **5**, 139–149.

Buchanan-Smith, H.M., Tasker, L., Ash, H. et al. (in press) Welfare of primates in laboratories: Opportunities for Refinement. In: *Nonhuman Primate Welfare: From History, Science, and Ethics to Practice*. Eds Robinson, L.M. and Weiss, A. Springer, Switzerland.

Buckner, J.C., Alfaro, J.W.L., Rylands, A.B. et al. (2015) Biogeography of the marmosets and tamarins (Callitrichidae). *Molecular Phylogenetics and Evolution*, **82**, 413–425.

Burns, M. and Wachtman, L. (2019) Physical examination, diagnosis, and common clinical procedures. In: *The Common Marmoset in Captivity and Biomedical Research*. Eds Marini, R.P., Wachtman, L.M., Tardif, S.D. et al., pp. 145–175. Academic Press, London.

Caine, N.G., Potter, M.P. and Mayer, K.E. (1992) Sleeping site selection by captive tamarins (*Saguinus labiatus*). *Ethology*, **90**, 63–71.

Carroll, B. (Ed.) (2002) *EAZA Husbandry Guidelines for the Callitrichidae*. Bristol Zoo Gardens, Bristol.

Casteleyn, C., Bakker, J., Breugelmans, S. et al. (2012) Anatomical description and morphometry of the skeleton of the common marmoset (*Callithrix jacchus*). *Laboratory Animals*, **46**, 152–63

Casteleyn, C. and Bakker, J. (2019) The Anatomy of the Common Marmoset. In: *The Common Marmoset in Captivity and Biomedical Research*. Eds Marini, R.P., Wachtman, L.M., Tardif, S.D. et al., pp. 17–41. Academic Press, London.

Cilia, J. and Piper, D.C. (1997) Marmoset conspecific confrontation: An ethologically-based model of anxiety. *Pharmacology Biochemistry and Behavior*, **58**, 85–91.

Clapp, N.K. (1993) *A Primate Model for the Study of Colitis and Colonic Carcinoma: The Cotton-Top Tamarin (Saguinus oedipus)*. CRC Press, Boca Raton, Florida.

Cleveland, J. and Snowdon, C.T. (1982) The complex vocal repertoire of the adult cotton-top tamarin (*Saguinus oedipus oedipus*). *Zeitschrift Fuer Tierpsychologie*, **58**, 231–270.

Cleveland, J. and Snowdon, C.T. (1984) Social development during the first twenty weeks in the cotton-top tamarin (*Saguinus o. oedipus*). *Animal Behaviour*, **32**, 432–444.

Clough, G. (1982) Environmental effects on animals used in biomedical research. *Biological Reviews of the Cambridge Philosophical Society*, **57**, 487–523.

Coimbra-Filho, A.F. and Mittermeier, R.A. (1976) Exudate-eating and tree-gouging in marmosets. *Nature*, **262**, 630.

Colman, R.J., Capuano, S., Bakker, J. et al. (2021) Marmosets: welfare, ethical use, and IACUC/regulatory considerations. *Toxicology*, 1–12 [online].

Council of Europe (2006) *Multilateral Consultation of Parties to the European Convention for the Protection of Vertebrate Animals used for Experimental and other Scientific Purposes (ETS 123) Appendix A. Cons 123 (2006) 3*. Available from URL: https://rm.coe.int/CoERMPublicCommonSearchServices/DisplayDCTMContent?documentId=090000168007a445 (accessed February 2022).

Crofts, H.S., Wilson, S., Muggleton, N.G. et al. (2001) Investigation of the sleep electrocorticogram of the common marmoset (*Callithrix jacchus*) using radiotelemetry. *Clinical Neurophysiology*, **112**, 2265–2273.

Cross, N., Pines, M.K. and Rogers, L.J. (2004) Saliva sampling to assess cortisol levels in unrestrained common marmosets and the effect of behavioral stress. *American Journal of Primatology*, **62**, 107–114.

Davenport, M.D., Tiefenbacher, S., Lutz, C.K. et al. (2006) Analysis of endogenous cortisol concentrations in the hair of rhesus macaques. *General and Comparative Endocrinology*, **147**, 255–261.

Dettling, A.C., Feldon, J. and Pryce, C.R. (2002a) Repeated parental deprivation in the infant common marmoset (*Callithrix jacchus*, Primates) and analysis of its effects on early development. *Biological Psychiatry*, **52**, 1037–1046.

Dettling, A.C., Feldon, J. and Pryce, C.R. (2002b) Early deprivation and behavioral and physiological responses to social separation/novelty in the marmoset. *Pharmacology, Biochemistry and Behavior*, **73**, 259–269.

Diehl, K.H., Hull, R., Morton, D. et al. (2001) A good practice guide to the administration of substances and removal of blood, including routes and volumes. *Journal of Applied Toxicology*, **21**, 15–23.

Digby, L. (1995) Infant care, infanticide, and female reproductive strategies in polygynous groups of common marmosets (*Callithrix jacchus*). *Behavioral Ecology and Sociobiology*, **37**, 51–61.

Digby, L.J. and Barreto, C.E. (1993) Social organization in a wild population of *Callithrix jacchus*. I. Group composition and dynamics. *Folia Primatologica*, **61**, 123–134.

Digby, L.J. and Ferrari, S.F. (1994) Multiple breeding females in free-ranging groups of *Callithrix jacchus*. *International Journal of Primatology*, **15**, 389–397.

Epple, G. (1978) Reproductive and social behavior of marmosets with special reference to captive breeding. *Primates in Medicine*, **10**, 50–62.

Epple, G., Belcher, A.M., Kuederling, I. et al. (1993) Making sense out of scents: species differences in scent glands, scent-marking behaviour, and scent-mark composition in the Callitrichidae. In: *Marmosets and Tamarins: Systematics, Behaviour, and Ecology*. Ed. Rylands A.B., pp. 123–151. Oxford University Press, Oxford.

European Commission (2007) Commission recommendations of 18 June 2007 on guidelines for the accommodation and care of animals used for experimental and other scientific purposes. Annex II to European Council Directive 86/609 See 2007/526/EC. https://eur-lex.europa.eu/LexUriServ/LexUriServ.do?uri=OJ:L:2007:197:0001:0089:EN:PDF (accessed February 2022).

Feistner, A.T.C. and Price, E.C. (1991) Food offering in New World primates: two species added. *Folia Primatologica*, **57**, 165–168.

Ferrari, S.F. and Lopes Ferrari, M.A. (1989) A re-evaluation of the social organization of the Callitrichidae, with reference to the ecological differences between genera. *Folia Primatologica*, **52**, 132–147.

Ferris, C.F., Snowdon, C.T., King, J.A. et al. (2001) Functional imaging of brain activity in conscious monkeys responding to sexually arousing cues. *NeuroReport*, **12**, 2231–2236.

Flecknell, P.A. (2015) *Laboratory Animal Anaesthesia*, 4th edn. Academic Press, London.

Ford, S.M. (1994) Evolution of sexual dimorphism in body weight in platyrrhines. *American Journal of Primatology*, **34**, 221–244.

Ford, S.M. and Davis, L.C. (1992) Systematics and body size: implications for feeding adaptations in New World monkeys. *American Journal of Physical Anthropology*, **88**, 415–468.

Forsythe, E.C. and Ford, S.M. (2011) Craniofacial adaptations to tree-gouging among marmosets. *The Anatomical Record*, **294**, 2131–2139.

Fortman, J.D., Hewett, T.A. and Taylor-Bennet, B. (2002) *The Laboratory Non-human Primate*. CRC Press Ltd, Florida.

Garber, P.A. (1984) Use of habitat and positional behavior in a Neotropical primate, *Saguinus oedipus*. In: *Adaptations for Foraging in Nonhuman Primates*. Eds Rodman P.S. and Cant J.G.H., pp. 112–133. Columbia University Press, New York.

Garber, P.A. (1993) Feeding ecology and behaviour of the genus *Saguinus*. In: *Marmosets and Tamarins: Systematics, Behaviour, and Ecology*. Ed. Rylands A.B., pp. 273–295. Oxford University Press, Oxford.

Garber, P.A., Porter, L.M., Spross, J. et al. (2016) Tamarins: Insights into monogamous and non-monogamous single female social and breeding systems. *American Journal of Primatology*, **78**, 298–314.

Garbino, G.S.T. (2014) The taxonomic status of *Mico marcai* (Alperin 1993) and *Mico manicorensis* (van Roosmalen et al. 2000) (Cebidae, Callitrichinae) from southwestern Brazilian Amazonia. *International Journal of Primatology*, **35**, 529–546.

Gaspari, F., Perretta, G. and Schino, G. (2000) Effects of different housing systems on the behaviour of the common marmoset (*Callithrix jacchus*). *Folia Primatologica*, **71**, 291 (abstract).

Gerber, P., Schnell, C.R. and Anzenberger, G. (2002a) Behavioral and cardiophysiological responses of common marmosets (*Callithrix jacchus*) to social and environmental changes. *Primates*, **43**, 201–216.

Gerber, P., Schnell, C.R. and Anzenberger, G. (2002b) Comparison of a beholder's response to confrontations involving its pairmate or two unfamiliar conspecifics in common marmosets (*Callithrix jacchus*). *Evolutionary Anthropology*, **11**, 117–121.

Greig, I., Morris, K.D., Mathiesen, E. et al. (2006) An improved restraint device for infections and collection of samples from marmosets. *Laboratory Primate Newsletter*, **45**, 1–5.

Grieves, J.L., Dick, E.J. Jr., Schlabritz-Loutsevich, N.E. et al. (2008) Barbiturate euthanasia solution-induced tissue artefact in nonhuman primates. *Journal of Medical Primatology* **37**, 154–61

Hawkins, P. (2014) Refining housing, husbandry and care for animals used in studies involving biotelemetry. *Animals*, **4**, 361–373

Halloren, E., Price, E.C. and McGrew, W.C. (1989) Technique for non-invasive marking of infant primates. *Laboratory Primate Newsletter*, **28**, 13–15.

Hampton, J.K., Hampton, S.H. and Landwehr, B.T. (1966) Observations on a successful breeding colony of the marmoset, *Oedipomidas oedipus*. *Folia Primatologica*, **4**, 265–287.

Hearn, J.P. (1977) Restraining device for small monkeys. *Laboratory Animals*, **11**, 261–262.

Heffner, R.S. (2004) Primate hearing from a mammalian perspective. *Anatomical Record*, **281A**, 1111–1122.

Heger, W., Merker, H.J. and Neubert, D. (1986) Low light intensity decreases the fertility of *Callithrix jacchus*. *Primate Report*, **14**, 260 (abstract).

Hoage, R.J. (1977) Parental care in *Leontopithecus rosalia rosalia*: sex and age differences in carrying behavior and the role of prior experience. In: *The Biology and Conservation of the Callitrichidae*. Ed. Kleiman, D.G., pp. 293–305. Smithsonian Institution Press, Washington, DC.

Hubrecht, R.C. (1984) Field observations on group size and composition of the common marmoset (*Callithrix jacchus jacchus*), at Tapacura, Brazil. *Primates*, **25**, 13–21.

Hubrecht, R. (1995) *Report on a UK survey of Housing Husbandry and Welfare provision for Animals used in Toxicology studies by the Toxicology and Welfare Working Group (abstract)* The Implications of Non-Invasive and Remote Monitoring Techniques for Non-Human Primate Research and Husbandry: EUPREN/EMRG Meeting, Göttingen.

International Primatological Society (2007) International Primatological Society Captive Care Committee. *International Guidelines for the Acquisition, Care and Breeding of Nonhuman Primates*, http://internationalprimatologicalsociety.org/wp-content/uploads/2021/10/IPS-International-Guidelines-for-the-Acquisition-Care-and-Breeding-of-Nonhuman-Primates-Second-Edition.pdf (accessed February 2022).

International Union for the Conservation of Nature and Natural Resources (2019) *IUCN Red List of Threatened Species. Version 2019.1.* www.iucnredlist.org (accessed March 2019).

Jacobs, G.H. (1996) Primate photopigments and primate color vision. *Proceedings of the National Academy of Sciences of the USA*, **93**, 577–581.

Jacobs, G.H. (2007) New world monkeys and color. *International Journal of Primatology*, **28**, 729–759.

Jacobs, G.H., Neitz, J. and Neitz, M. (1993) Genetic basis of polymorphism in the color vision of platyrrhine monkeys. *Vision Research*, **33**, 269–274.

Jaquish, C., Gage, T.B. and Tardif, S.D. (1991) Reproductive factors affecting survivorship in captive Callitrichidae. *American Journal of Physical Anthropology*, **84**, 291–305.

Jaquish, C., Tardif, S.D. and Cheverud, J.M. (1997) Interactions between infant growth and survival: Evidence for selection on age-specific body weight in captive common marmosets (*Callithrix jacchus*). *American Journal of Primatology*, **42**, 269–280.

Johnson, E.O., Kamilaris, T.C., Carter, A.E. *et al.* (1996) The biobehavioral consequences of psychogenic stress in a small, social primate (*Callithrix jacchus jacchus*). *Biological Psychiatry*, **40**, 317–337.

Jones, B.S. (1997) Quantitative analysis of marmoset vocal communication. In: *Handbook: Marmosets and Tamarins in Biological and Biomedical Research*. Eds Pryce, C., Scott, L. and C. Schnell, C., pp. 145–151. DSSD Imagery, Salisbury.

Joint Working Group on Refinement (2001) Refining procedures for the administration of substances. Report of the BVAAWF/FRAME/RSPCA/UFAW Joint Working Group on Refinement. *Laboratory Animals*, **35**, 1–41.

Joint Working Group on Refinement (2009) Refinements in husbandry, care and common procedures for non-human primates. Ninth report of the BVAAWF/FRAME/RSPCA/UFAW Joint Working Group on Refinement. *Laboratory Animals*, **43**, S1:1–S1:47.

Kelly, K. (1993) Environmental enrichment for captive wildlife through the simulation of gum feeding. *Animal Welfare Information Center Newsletter*, **4**, 5–10.

Kinter, L.B. and Johnson, D.K. (1999) Remote monitoring of experimental endpoints in animals using radiotelemetry and bioimpedance technologies. In: *Humane Endpoints in Animal Experiments for Biomedical Research*. Eds Hendriksen, C.F.M. and Morton, D.B., pp. 58–65. Proceedings of the International Conference. Royal Society of Medicine Press, London.

Kirkwood, J.K. and Stathatos, K. (1992) *Biology, Rearing, and Care of Young Primates*. Oxford University Press, Oxford.

Kitchen, A.M. and Martin, A.A. (1996) The effects of cage size and complexity on the behaviour of captive common marmosets, *Callithrix jacchus*. *Laboratory Animals*, **30**, 317–326.

Kleiman, D.G., Hoage, R.J. and Green, K.M. (1988) The lion tamarins, genus *Leontopithecus*. In: *Ecology and Behavior of Neotropical Primates*, Vol. 2. Eds Mittermeier, R.A., Rylands, A.B., Coimbra-Filho, A.F. *et al.*, pp. 299–347. World Wildlife Fund, Washington, DC.

Knapka, J.J., Barnard, D.E., Bayne, K.A.L. *et al.* (1995) Nutrition. In: *Nonhuman Primates in Biomedical Research*. Eds Bennett, B.T., Abee, C.R. and Henrickson, R., pp. 211–248. Academic Press, San Diego.

Korte, S. and Everitt, J. (2019) The use of the marmoset in toxicity testing and nonclinical safety assessment studies. In: *The Common Marmoset in Captivity and Biomedical Research*. Eds Marini, R.P., Wachtman, L.M., Tardif, S.D. *et al.*, pp. 493–513. Academic Press, London.

Kramer, J.A. (2019) Diseases of the gastrointestinal system. In: *The Common Marmoset in Captivity and Biomedical Research*. Eds Marini, R.P., Wachtman, L.M., Tardif, S.D. *et al.*, pp. 213–230. Academic Press, London.

Kramer, R., and Burns, M. (2019) Normal clinical and biological parameters of the common marmoset (*Callithrix jacchus*). In: *The Common Marmoset in Captivity and Biomedical Research*. Eds Marini, R.P., Wachtman, L.M., Tardif, S.D. *et al.*, pp. 93–107. Academic Press, London.

Kuehnel, F., Grohmann, J., Buchwald, U. *et al.* (2012) Parameters of haematology, clinical chemistry and lipid metabolism in the common marmoset and alterations under stress conditions. *Journal of Medical Primatology*, **41**, 241e50.

Layne, D.G. and Power, R.A. (2003) Husbandry, handling, and nutrition for marmosets. *Comparative Medicine*, **53**, 351–359.

Layne-Colon, D., Goodroe, A. and Burns, M. (2019) Husbandry and housing of common marmosets. In: *The Common Marmoset in Captivity and Biomedical Research*. Eds Marini, R.P., Wachtman, L.M., Tardif, S.D. *et al.*, pp. 77–91. Academic Press, London.

Lazaro-Perea, C., Snowdon, C.T. and Arruda, M.F. (1999) Scentmarking behavior in wild groups of common marmosets (*Callithrix jacchus*). *Behavioral Ecology and Sociobiology*, **46**, 313–324.

Ludlage, E. and Mansfield, K. (2003) Clinical care and diseases of the common marmoset (*Callithrix jacchus*). *Comparative Medicine*, **53**, 369–382.

McKenzie, S.M., Chamove, A.S. and Feistner, A.T.C. (1986) Floorcoverings and hanging screens alter arboreal monkey behavior. *Zoo Biology*, **5**, 339–348.

Maier, W., Alonso, C. and Langguth, A. (1982) Field observations on *Callithrix jacchus jacchus*. L. *Zeitschrift Fuer Saeugetierkunde*, **47**, 334–346.

Majolo, B., Buchanan-Smith, H.M. and Morris, K. (2003) Factors affecting the successful pairing of unfamiliar common marmoset (*Callithrix jacchus*) females: preliminary results. *Animal Welfare*, **12**, 327–337.

Mansfield, K. (2003) Marmoset models commonly used in biomedical research. *Comparative Medicine*, **53**, 383–392.

Marini, R.P. (2019) Regulatory considerations. In: *The Common Marmoset in Captivity and Biomedical Research*. Eds Marini, R.P., Wachtman, L.M., Tardif, S.D. *et al.*, pp. 133–142. Academic Press, London

Marini, R.P. and Haupt, J. (2019) Anesthesia and Select Surgical Procedures. In: *The Common Marmoset in Captivity and Biomedical Research*. Eds Marini, R.P., Wachtman, L.M., Tardif, S.D. *et al.*, pp. 177–194. Academic Press, London.

Marini, R.P., Wachtman, L.M., Tardif, S.D. *et al.* (Eds.). (2019) *The Common Marmoset in Captivity and Biomedical Research*. Academic Press, London.

Mätz-Rensing, K. and Bleyer, M. (2019) Viral Diseases of Common Marmosets. In: *The Common Marmoset in Captivity and Biomedical Research*. Eds Marini, R.P., Wachtman, L.M., Tardif, S.D. *et al.*, pp. 251–264. Academic Press, London

McDermott, J., and Hauser, M.D. (2007) Nonhuman primates prefer slow tempos but dislike music overall. *Cognition*, **104**, 654–668

McKinley, J., Buchanan-Smith, H.M., Bassett, L. *et al.* (2003) Training common marmosets (*Callithrix jacchus*) to co-operate during routine laboratory procedures: ease of training and time investment. *Journal of Applied Animal Welfare Science*, **6**, 209–220.

Mellor, D.J. and Beausoleil, N.J. (2015) Extending the 'Five Domains' model for animal welfare assessment to incorporate positive welfare states. *Animal Welfare*, **24**, 241–253.

Miller, G.F., Barnard, D.E., Woodward, R.A. *et al.* (1997) Hepatic hemosiderosis in common marmosets, *Callithrix jacchus*: effect of diet on incidence and severity. *Laboratory Animal Science*, **47**, 138–142.

Moore, K., Cleland, J. and McGrew, W.C. (1991) Visual encounters between families of cotton-top tamarins, *Saguinus oedipus*. *Primates*, **32**, 23–33.

National Academies of Sciences, Engineering, and Medicine (2019) *Care, Use, and Welfare of Marmosets as Animal Models for Gene Editing-Based Biomedical Research: Proceedings of a Workshop*. The National Academies Press, Washington, DC.

National Research Council, Committee on Animal Nutrition (2003) *Nutrient Requirements of Non-human Primates*. National Academy of Science, Washington, DC.

National Research Council (2011) *Guide for the Care and Use of Laboratory Animals*. National Academies Press, Washington, DC.

Neyman, P.F. (1977) Aspects of the ecology and social organization of free-ranging cotton-top tamarins (*Saguinus oedipus*) and the conservation status of the species. In: *The Biology and Conservation of the Callitrichidae*. Ed. Kleiman, D.G. pp. 39–71. Smithsonian Institution Press, Washington, DC.

Nishijima, K., Saitoh, R., Tanaka, S. *et al.* (2012). Life span of common marmoset (*Callithrix jacchus*) at CLEA Japan breeding colony. *Biogerontology*, **13**, 439–443.

Novak, M.A. and Suomi, S.J. (1988) Psychological well-being of primates in captivity. *American Psychologist*, **43**, 765–773.

Osmanski, M.S. and Wang, X. (2011). Measurement of absolute auditory thresholds in the common marmoset (*Callithrix jacchus*). *Hearing Research*, **277**, 127–33

Pereira, M.E., Macedonia, J.M., Haring, D.M. et al. (1989) Maintenance of primates in captivity for research: the need for naturalistic environments. In: *Housing, Care and Psychological Wellbeing of Captive and Laboratory Primates*. Ed. Segal, E.F., pp. 40–60. Noyes Publications, New Jersey.

Pines, M.K., Kaplan, G. and Rogers, L.J. (2007) A note on indoor and outdoor housing preferences of common marmosets (*Callithrix jacchus*). *Applied Animal Behaviour Science*, **108**, 348–353.

Plesker, R. and Schuhmacher, A. (2006) Feeding fruits and vegetables to nonhuman primates can lead to nutritional deficiencies. *Laboratory Primate Newsletter*, **45**, 1–5.

Pontes, M.A.R. and da Cruz, M.M.A.O. (1995) Home range intergroup transfers, and reproductive status of common marmosets *Callithrix jacchus* in a forest fragment in north-eastern Brazil. *Primates*, **36**, 335–347.

Pook, A.G. (1977) A comparative study of the use of contact calls in *Saguinus fuscicollis* and *Callithrix jacchus*. In: *The Biology and Conservation of the Callitrichidae*. Ed. Kleiman, D.G., pp. 271–280. Smithsonian Institution Press, Washington, DC.

Poole, T.B., Costa, P., Netto, W.J. et al. (1994) Non-human primates. In: *The Accommodation of Laboratory Animals in Accordance With Animal Welfare Requirements*. Ed. O'Donoghue, P.N., pp. 81–86. Proceedings of an International Workshop Held at the Bundesgesundheitsamt, Berlin (The Berlin Workshop). Bundesministerium für Ernährung, Landwirtschaft und Forsten, Bonn, Germany.

Poole, T., Hubrecht, R. and Kirkwood, J.K. (1999) Marmosets and tamarins. In: *The UFAW Handbook on the Care and Management of Laboratory Animals*, 7th edn. Ed. Poole, T., pp. 559–573. Blackwell Publishing, Oxford.

Potkay, S. (1992) Diseases of the Callitrichidae: a review. *Journal of Medical Primatology*, **21**, 189–236.

Power, M.L. and Koutsos, L. (2019) Marmoset nutrition and dietary husbandry. In: *The Common Marmoset in Captivity and Biomedical Research*. Eds Marini, R.P., Wachtman, L.M., Tardif, S.D. et al., pp. 63–76. Academic Press, London.

Prescott, M. (2006) Primate sensory capabilities and communication signals: implications for care and use in the laboratory. NC3Rs, London, https://www.nc3rs.org.uk/sites/default/files/documents/Guidelines/Papers/Prescott%20article%20on%20senses%20and%20communication.pdf (accessed February 2022).

Prescott, M.J., Bowell, V.A. and Buchanan-Smith, H.M. (2005) Training of laboratory-housed non-human primates, part 2: Resources for developing and implementing training programmes. *Animal Technology and Welfare*, **4**, 133–148.

Prescott, M.J. and Buchanan-Smith, H.M. (2004) Cage sizes for tamarins in the laboratory. *Animal Welfare*, **13**, 151–158.

Price, E.C. (1990) Parturition and perinatal behaviour in captive cotton-top tamarins (*Saguinus oedipus*). *Primates*, **31**, 523–535.

Price, E.C. (1992) The benefits of helpers: Effects of group and litter size on infant care in tamarins (*Saguinus oedipus*). *American Journal of Primatology*, **26**, 179–190.

Price, E.C. and McGrew, W.C. (1990) Cotton-top tamarins (*Saguinus o. oedipus*) in a semi-naturalistic captive colony. *American Journal of Primatology*, **20**, 1–12.

Regan, B.C., Julliot, C., Simmen, B. et al. (2001) Fruits, foliage and the evolution of primate colour vision. *Philosophical Transactions of the Royal Society of London*, **B356**, 229–283.

Rennie, A. and Buchanan-Smith, H.M. (2005) Report on the extent and character of primate use in scientific procedures across Europe in 2001. *Laboratory Primate Newsletter*, **44**, 6–12.

Rennie, A.E. and Buchanan-Smith, H.M. (2006a) Refinement of the use of non-human primates in scientific research. Part I: The influence of humans. *Animal Welfare*, **15**, 203–213.

Rennie A.E. and Buchanan-Smith, H.M. (2006b) Refinement of the use of non-human primates in scientific research. Part II: Housing, husbandry and acquisition. *Animal Welfare*, **15**, 215–238.

Rennie A.E. and Buchanan-Smith, H.M. (2006c) Refinement of the use of non-human primates in scientific research. Part III: Refinement of procedures. *Animal Welfare*, **15**, 239–261.

Rensing, S. and Oerke, A.K. (2005) Husbandry and management of New World species: Marmosets and tamarins. In: *The Laboratory Primate*. Ed. Wolfe-Coote, S., pp. 145–162. Elsevier Academic Press, San Diego.

Rimpley, K., and Buchanan-Smith, H.M. (2013) Reliably signalling a startling husbandry event improves welfare of zoo-housed capuchins (*Sapajus apella*). *Applied Animal Behaviour Science*, **147**, 205–213.

Roda, S.A. and Mendes Pontes, A.R. (1998) Polygyny and infanticide in common marmosets in a fragment of the Atlantic Forest of Brazil. *Folia Primatologica*, **69**, 372–376.

Rosenberger, A.L. and Coimbra-Filho, A.F. (1984) Morphology, taxonomic status and affinities of the lion tamarins, *Leontopithecus* (Callitrichidae, Cebidae). *Folia Primatologica*, **42**, 149–179.

Ross, C.N. (2019) Marmosets in aging research. In: *The Common Marmoset in Captivity and Biomedical Research*. Eds Marini, R.P., Wachtman, L.M., Tardif, S.D. et al., pp. 355–376. Academic Press, London.

Ross, C.N., French, J.A. and Ortí G. (2007) Germ-line chimerism and paternal care in marmosets (*Callithrix kuhlii*). *Proceedings of the National Academy of Sciences*, **104**, 6278–6282.

Rothe, H. and Koenig, A. (1991) Variability of social organization in captive common marmosets (*Callithrix jacchus*). *Folia Primatologica*, **57**, 28–33.

Rumble, R., Saville, M., Simmons, L. et al. (2005) The preference of the common marmoset for nest boxes made from three different materials: wood, plastic, metal. *Animal Technology and Welfare*, **4**, 185–187.

Rutherford, J.N., Colon, D.G.L., Ross, C.N. et al. (2014). Developmental origins of pregnancy loss in the adult female common marmoset monkey (*Callithrix jacchus*). *PLoS One*, **9**, e96845.

Rylands, A.B. and de Faria, D.S. (1993) Habitats, feeding ecology, and home range size in the genus *Callithrix*. In: *Marmosets and Tamarins: Systematics, Behaviour, and Ecology*. Ed. Rylands A.B., pp. 262–272. Oxford University Press, Oxford.

Rylands, A.B. and Mittermeier, R.A. (2009) The diversity of the New World primates (Platyrrhini): An annotated taxonomy. In: *South American Primates Comparative Perspectives in the Study of Behavior, Ecology, and Conservation*. Eds Garber, P.A., Estrada, A., Bicca-Marques, J.C. et al., pp. 23–54. Springer, Chicago.

Rylands, A.B. and Mittermeier, R.A. (2013) Family Callitrichidae (marmosets and tamarins). In: *Handbook of the Mammals of the World. Vol. 3. Primates*, Eds Mittermeier, R.A., Rylands, A.B., Wilson, D.E., pp 262–346. Lynx Edicions, Barcelona.

Rylands, A.B., Heymann, E.W., Lynch Alfaro, J. et al. (2016) Taxonomic review of the New World tamarins (Primates: Callitrichidae). *Zoological Journal of the Linnean Society*, **177**, 1003–1028.

Sainsbury, A.W., Eaton, B.D. and Cooper, J.E. (1989) Restraint and anaesthesia of primates. *Veterinary Record*, **125**, 640–644.

Sainsbury, A.W., Kirkwood, J.K. and Appleby, E.C. (1987) Chronic colitis in common marmosets (*Callithrix jacchus*) and cotton-top tamarins (*Saguinus oedipus*). *Veterinary Record*, **121**, 329–330.

Saltzman, W., Schultz-Darken, N.J. and Abbott, D.H. (1997) Familial influences on ovulatory function in common marmosets (*Callithrix jacchus*). *American Journal of Primatology*, **41**, 159–177.

Sambrook, T.D. and Buchanan-Smith, H.M. (1997) Control and complexity in novel object enrichment. *Animal Welfare*, **6**, 207–216.

Saunders, K.E., Shen, Z., Dewhirst, F.E. et al. (1999) Novel intestinal *Helicobacter* species isolated from cotton-top tamarins (*Saguinus oedipus*) with chronic colitis. *Journal of Clinical Microbiology*, **37**, 146–151.

Savage, A. (1995) Cotton-top Tamarin SSP© Husbandry Manual, V, 1–15. Roger Williams Park Zoo.

Savage, A., Giraldo, L.H., Blumer, E.S. et al. (1993) Field techniques for monitoring cotton-top tamarins (*Saguinus oedipus oedipus*) in Colombia. *American Journal of Primatology*, **31**, 189–196.

Savastano, G., Hanson, A. and McCann, C. (2003) The development of an operant conditioning training program for New World primates at the Bronx Zoo. *Journal of Applied Animal Welfare Science*, **6**, 247–261.

Scanlon, C.E., Chalmers, N.R. and Monteiro da Cruz, M.A.O. (1989) Home range use and the exploitation of gum in the marmoset *Callithrix jacchus jacchus*. *International Journal of Primatology*, **10**, 123–136.

Schaffner, C.M. and Smith, T.E. (2005) Familiarity may buffer the adverse effects of relocation on marmosets (*Callithrix kuhlii*): preliminary evidence. *Zoo Biology*, **24**, 93–100.

Schapiro, S.J., Stavisky, R. and Hook, M. (2000) The lower-row cage may be dark, but behavior does not appear to be affected. *Laboratory Primate Newsletter*, **39**, 4–6.

Schiel, N. and Souto, A. (2017) The common marmoset: an overview of its natural history, ecology and behavior. *Developmental Neurobiology*, **77**, 244–262.

Schoenfeld, D. (1989) Effects of environmental impoverishment on the social behavior of marmosets (*Callithrix jacchus*). *American Journal of Primatology*, Suppl. **1**, 45–51.

Scott, L. (1991) Environmental enrichment for single housed common marmosets. In: *Primate Responses to Environmental Change*. Ed. Box, H.O., pp. 265–274. Chapman and Hall, London.

Scott, L., Pearce, P., Fairhall, S. et al. (2003) Training nonhuman primates to cooperate with scientific procedures in applied biomedical research. *Journal of Applied Animal Welfare Science*, **6**, 199–207.

Schultz-Darken, N.J. (2003) Sample collection and restraint techniques used for common marmosets (*Callithrix jacchus*). *Comparative Medicine*, **53**, 360–363.

Schultz-Darken, N.J., Pape, R.M., Tannenbaum, P.L. et al. (2004) Novel restraint system for neuroendocrine studies of socially living common marmoset monkeys. *Laboratory Animals*, **38**, 393–405.

Schultz-Darken, N., Braun, K.M. and Emborg, M.E. (2016) Neurobehavioral development of common marmoset monkeys. *Developmental Psychobiology*, **58**, 141–158.

Schultz-Darken, N., Ace, L. and Ash, H. (2019) Behavior and behavioral management. In: *The Common Marmoset in Captivity and Biomedical Research*. Eds Marini, R.P., Wachtman, L.M., Tardif, S.D. et al., pp. 109–117. Academic Press, London.

Smith, A.C., Buchanan-Smith, H.M., Surridge, A.K. et al. (2003) The effect of colour vision status on the detection and selection of fruits by tamarins (*Saguinus* spp.). *Journal of Experimental Biology*, **206**, 3159–3165.

Smith, A.C., Surridge, A.K., Prescott, M.J. et al. (2012). Effect of colour vision status on insect prey capture efficiency of captive and wild tamarins (*Saguinus* spp.). *Animal Behaviour*, **83**, 479–486.

Smith, T.E., McCallister, J.M., Gordon, S.J. et al. (2004) Quantitative data on training New World primates to urinate. *American Journal of Primatology*, **64**, 83–93.

Smucny, D.A., Abbott, D.H., Mansfield, K.G. et al. (2004) Reproductive output, maternal age, and survivorship in captive common marmoset females (*Callithrix jacchus*). *American Journal of Primatology*, **64**, 107–121.

Snowdon, C.T. (1993) A vocal taxonomy of the callitrichids. In: *Marmosets and Tamarins: Systematics, Behaviour, and Ecology*. Ed. Rylands A.B., pp. 78–94. Oxford University Press, Oxford.

Snowdon, C.T. and Savage, A. (1989) Psychological well-being of captive primates: General considerations and examples from callitrichids. In: *Housing, Care and Psychological Wellbeing of Captive and Laboratory Primates*. Ed. Segal, E.F., pp. 75–88. Noyes Publications, New Jersey.

Snowdon, C.T., Savage, A. and McConnell, P.B. (1985) A breeding colony of cotton-top tamarins (*Saguinus oedipus*). *Laboratory Animal Science*, **35**, 477–480.

Snowdon, C.T. and Soini, P. (1988) The tamarins, genus *Saguinus*. In: *Ecology and Behavior of Neotropical Primates*, Vol. 2. Eds Mittermeier, R.A., Rylands, A.B., Coimbra-Filho, A.F. et al., pp. 223–298. World Wildlife Fund, Washington, DC.

Soini, P. (1988) The pygmy marmoset, genus *Cebuella*. In: *Ecology and Behavior of Neotropical Primates*, Vol. 2. Eds Mittermeier, R.A., Rylands, A.B., Coimbra-Filho, A.F. et al., pp. 79–129. World Wildlife Fund, Washington, DC.

de Sousa, M.B.C., Albuquerque, A.C.S.R., Albuquerque, F.S. et al. (2005) Behavioral strategies and hormonal profiles of dominant and subordinate common marmoset (*Callithrix jacchus*) females in wild monogamous groups. *American Journal of Primatology*, **67**, 37–50.

de Sousa, M.B.C., Nogueira Moura, S.L. and Menezes, A.A.L. (2006) Circadian variation with a diurnal bimodal profile on scentmarking behavior in captive common marmosets (*Callithrix jacchus*). *International Journal of Primatology*, **27**, 263–272.

Souto, A., Bezerra, B.M., Schiel, N. et al. (2007) Saltatory search in free-living *Callithrix jacchus*: Environmental and age influences. *International Journal of Primatology*, **28**, 881–893.

Stevenson, M.F. (1976) Birth and perinatal behaviour in family groups of the common marmoset (*Callithrix jacchus jacchus*), compared to other primates. *Journal of Human Evolution*, **5**, 365–381.

Stevenson, M.F. and Poole, T.B. (1976) An ethogram of the common marmoset *(Callithrix jacchus jacchus)*: General behavioural repertoire. *Animal Behaviour*, **24**, 428–451.

Stevenson, M.F. and Rylands, A.B. (1988) The marmosets, genus *Callithrix*. In: *Ecology and Behavior of Neotropical Primates*, Vol. 2. Eds Mittermeier, R.A., Rylands, A.B., Coimbra-Filho, A.F. et al., pp. 131–222. World Wildlife Fund, Washington, DC.

Sweeney, C.G., Curran, E., Westmoreland, S.V. et al. (2012). Quantitative molecular assessment of chimerism across tissues in marmosets and tamarins. *BMC Genomics*, **13**, 98.

Tardif, S.D. and Bales, K.L. (2004) Relations among birth condition, maternal condition, and postnatal growth in captive common marmoset monkeys (*Callithrix jacchus*). *American Journal of Primatology*, **62**, 83–94.

Tardif, S., Bales, K., Williams, L. et al. (2006) Preparing New World monkeys for laboratory research. *ILAR Journal*, **47**, 307–315.

Tardif, S.D. and Jaquish, C.E. (1997) Number of ovulations in the marmoset monkey (*Callithrix jacchus*): Relation to body weight, age and repeatability. *American Journal of Primatology*, **42**, 323–329.

Tardif, S.D., Jaquish, C., Layne, D. et al. (1998) Growth variation in common marmoset monkeys (*Callithrix jacchus*) fed a purified diet: relation to care-giving and weaning behaviors. *Laboratory Animal Science*, **48**, 264–269.

Tardif, S.D., Richter, C.B. and Carson, R.L. (1984a) Effects of sibling rearing experience on future reproductive success in two species of Callitrichidae. *American Journal of Primatology*, **6**, 377–380.

Tardif, S.D., Richter, C.B. and Carson, R.L. (1984b) Reproductive performance of three species of Callitrichidae. *Laboratory Animal Science*, **34**, 272–275.

Tardif, S.D. and Ross, C.N. (2019) Reproduction, Growth, and Development. In: *The Common Marmoset in Captivity and Biomedical Research*. Eds Marini, R.P., Wachtman, L.M., Tardif, S.D. et al., pp. 119–132. Academic Press, London.

Tardif, S.D., Smucny, D.A., Abbott, D.H. et al. (2003) Reproduction in captive common marmosets (*Callithrix jacchus*). *Comparative Medicine*, **53**, 364–368.

van Roosmalen, M.G.M. and van Roosmalen, T. (2003) The description of a new marmoset genus, *Callibella* (Callitrichidae, Primates), including its molecular phylogenetic status. *Neotropical Primates*, **11**, 1–10.

van Roosmalen, M., van Roosmalen, T., Mittermeier, R.A. et al. (2000) Two new species of marmoset, genus Callithrix Erxleben, 1777

(Callitrichidae, Primates) from the Tapajós/Madeira interfluvium, south central Amazonia, Brazil. *Neotropical Primates*, **8**, 2–18.

Ventura, R. and Buchanan-Smith, H.M. (2003) Physical environment effects on infant care and infant development in captive common marmosets *Callithrix jacchus*. *International Journal of Primatology*, **24**, 399–413.

Waitt, C. and Buchanan-Smith, H.M. (2006) Perceptual considerations in the use of colored artificial visual stimuli to study nonhuman primate behavior. *American Journal of Primatology*, **68**, 1054–1067.

Waitt, C.D., Bushmitz, M. and Honess, P.E. (2010) Designing environments for aged primates. *Laboratory Primate Newsletter*, **49**, 5–9.

Watson, C.F.I. and Buchanan-Smith, H.M. (2011) Marmoset Care website. http://marmosetcare.com/ hosted by the University of Stirling.

Watson, C.F.I, Buchanan-Smith, H.M. and Caldwell, C.A. (2014) Call playback artificially generates a temporary cultural style of high affiliation in marmosets. *Animal Behaviour*, **93**, 163–171.

Westlund, K. (2015) Training laboratory primates–benefits and techniques. *Primate Biology*, **2**, 119–132.

Wolfensohn, S. and Honess, P. (2005) *Handbook of Primate Husbandry and Welfare*. Blackwell Publishing, Oxford.

Yamamoto, M.E. (1993) From dependence to sexual maturity: The behavioural ontogeny of Callitrichidae. In: *Marmosets and Tamarins: Systematics, Behaviour, and Ecology*. Ed. Rylands, A.B., pp. 235–254. Oxford University Press, Oxford.

Yamamoto, M.E., Arruda, M.F., Alencar, A.I. *et al.* (2009) Mating systems and female–female competition in the common marmoset, *Callithrix jacchus*. In: *The Smallest Anthropoids*, Eds Ford, S.M., Porter, L.M. and Davis, L.C., pp. 119–133. Springer, Boston, MA.

Yeates, J.W. and Main, D.C. (2008) Assessment of positive welfare: a review. *The Veterinary Journal*, **175**, 293–300.

Yoneda, M. (1984) Ecological study of the saddle backed tamarin (*Saguinus fuscicollis*) in northern Bolivia. *Primates*, **25**, 1–12.

38 Capuchin monkeys

James R. Anderson, Elisabetta Visalberghi and Arianna Manciocco

Biological overview

Capuchin monkeys are robust, medium-size neotropical primates, highly dexterous and with a prehensile tail used to grasp objects or branches and to support limited weight (only youngsters can suspend themselves). Until quite recently, most studies on capuchins referred to the following species: white-fronted capuchin (*Cebus albifrons*), black-capped, brown or tufted capuchin (*C. apella*), white-faced or white-throated capuchin (*C. capucinus*), weeper or wedge-capped capuchin (*C. olivaceus*), yellow-breasted capuchin (*C. xanthosternos*), the Ka'apor capuchin (*C. kaapori*), the black-striped or bearded capuchin (*C. libidinosus*), and the black or black horned capuchin (*C. nigritus*). The taxonomy of the genus *Cebus* has undergone major revision (see overview in Fragaszy *et al.* 2004) and molecular and morphological data have revealed that capuchin monkeys, formerly identified as the single genus *Cebus*, belong to two distinct genera, with the robust (tufted) forms (including *libidinosus*, *xanthosternos*, *apella* and several other species) now recognised as the genus *Sapajus*, and the gracile forms (including *albifrons*, *capucinus*, *olivaceus and several other species*) retained as the genus *Cebus* (Lynch Alfaro *et al.* 2012a, 2012b).

In most captive colonies, the geographical origin of the founder tufted capuchins is unknown, and it is likely that interbreeding of *C. apella*, *C. libidinosus* and *C. nigritus* has occurred. In many cases, instead of ascribing individuals to a particular *Sapajus* species, we recommend referring to them as *Sapajus* spp. Thus, most information about capuchins behavioural biology and husbandry comes from *Sapajus spp*. In this chapter, we will refer to *Sapajus* spp. whenever accurate species identification according to the most recent taxonomy is lacking, and occasionally we will mention the species according to the old taxonomy as used in the cited study.

Capuchins are successful and adaptable, with representatives widely distributed throughout Central and South America. Though most species are not endangered, some are, critically so (e.g. *S. xanthosternos*, *S. flavius*, *C. kaapori*; for updated information, search in the web for the most recent IUCN Red List).

Social organisation

Capuchins live in groups, typically ranging in size from around 12 to 35 individuals (Fragaszy *et al.* 2004). Although group size is variable across populations and species, groups typically contain at least one adult male and several adult females, juveniles and infants. Males usually emigrate from their natal group, and they may emigrate more than once in their lifetime. Newly immigrant males that attain alpha status may kill infants sired by the previous alpha or other resident males (Janson *et al.* 2012; Perry 2012).

Although some aspects of social organisation may vary across species, a linear dominance hierarchy is generally present (Fragaszy *et al.* 2004). However, given that social relations are characterised by a high degree of inter-individual tolerance and low rates of aggression, it can be difficult to identify dominance ranks precisely beyond the usually clearly defined alpha male. Sometimes, one individual can become the target of harassment or aggression by several other members of the group, thus becoming a scapegoat. In the wild, such a subordinate would be better able to avoid others by staying on the periphery of the group, possibly even leaving the group altogether, although fatal coalitionary attacks have been reported (Gros-Louis *et al.* 2003). Agonistic interactions do not usually escalate to involve two competing factions, but instead consist of one or more individuals pitted against another individual. Agonistic coalitions may reflect kinship or rank relations (Ferreira *et al.* 2006; Schino *et al.* 2009a). The extent of post-conflict reconciliation in the different species remains to be clarified, but the behaviour may be more common in captivity (*C. capucinus*: Leca *et al.* 2002).

Grooming is the most common affiliative behaviour. Female capuchins exchange grooming reciprocally and preferentially groom with kin (Perry *et al.* 2008; Schino *et al.* 2009a, 2009b). The extent to which they prefer to groom up the dominance hierarchy appears to be variable (Schino *et al.* 2009a; Tiddi *et al.* 2012).

Habitats and feeding habits

Capuchins live in a wide variety of habitats from sea level to above 2,500 m altitude, and mostly but not exclusively in forests (Fragaszy *et al.* 2004). Primarily arboreal, they spend most of their time in trees, especially in middle layers of the canopy, but depending on local habitat conditions they can spend almost 30% of their time on terrestrial substrates (Koops *et al.* 2014). Some groups inhabit forest patches surrounded by large open areas and secondary vegetation, and some are commensal with humans, living close to urban areas and coming into daily contact with people (Sabbatini *et al.* 2006).

Capuchins are omnivores. They eat mostly fruits, but include varying proportions of other vegetable items (shoots, flowers, buds, leaves, etc.), invertebrates (molluscs, insects, worms, etc.) and vertebrates (for example, birds and their eggs, snakes, lizards, small mammals) in their diet. Some groups also exploit human garbage and/or crops (e.g., de Souza Lins & Ferreira 2019). Capuchins are 'extractive' foragers, meaning that they exploit hidden and encased foods. Their foraging style includes 'strenuous' foraging actions, which may be combined: dig, rip, bite, bang, grab, break, carry, tap, roll, scrape and chase. 'Quiet' foraging actions, which may also be combined, include pick, visually examine, lick, mouth, sniff, manually examine, sift, take, feel, scoop, turn over, masticate, open by peeling (Fragaszy *et al.* 2004).

One particular combination of strenuous foraging activities typifies wild capuchins: breaking open hard-shelled fruits or nuts. For example, *S. apella* pluck hard-shelled fruits by biting through the stem, and then repeatedly banging the fruit against the tree trunk or a branch until cracks appear on the fruit. They then peel the cracked rind with their teeth and then bang the nut again until the husk breaks and the kernels can be extracted (Gunst *et al.* 2010). Combined foraging actions are also evident in searching for edible items among the debris to be found in palm fronds, in breaking off palm leaves and peeling off the stems, and in accessing the kernel of cashew nuts (Visalberghi *et al.* 2016). Tool-assisted extractive foraging, long known in captive groups, has been recently described in wild *Sapajus* populations (for recent descriptions of the use of percussors to access encased food (Figure 38.1) and of sticks as digging and probing tools, see Falótico & Ottoni 2014, and Falótico *et al.* 2018).

Biological data

Table 38.1 shows information on several aspects of growth and development of *Sapajus spp*. We provide data on this genus because it is by far the most commonly studied in captivity; furthermore, studies in captivity have not yet investigated differences among different *Sapajus* species. For data on body mass in wild bearded capuchins, see Fragaszy *et al.* (2016). Blood biochemistry, haematological and serum protein parameters are reported in Fragaszy *et al.* (2004) and Wirz *et al.* (2008).

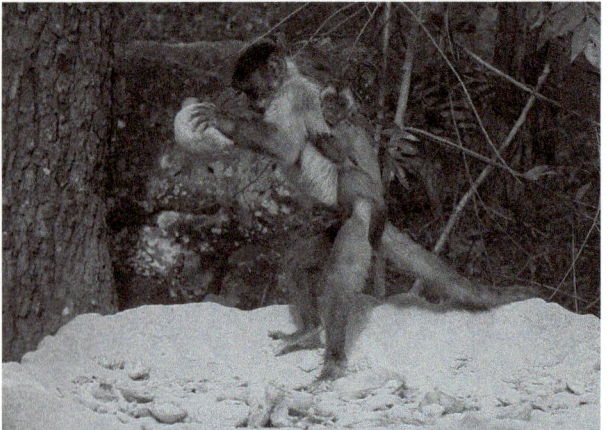

Figure 38.1 A wild adult female *Sapajus libidinosus* uses a stone tool to crack open a hard palm nut. Note the infant holding the fur of her mother during the lift. Source: E. Visalberghi.

Table 38.1 Reproduction, growth and development of *Cebus apella*.

Gestation	Captive capuchins, 160 days (Fragaszy & Adams-Curtis 1998)
Birth seasonality	Not marked. Peak birth period may coincide with increased availability of food (Di Bitetti & Janson 2000)
Interbirth interval	Captive capuchins, 20.6 months (Fragaszy & Adams-Curtis 1998)
	Wild capuchins, 19.4 months (Di Bitetti & Janson 2001); 22 months (Robinson, 1988)
Birth weight	170–260 grams (Fragaszy & Adams-Curtis 1998)
	220–270 grams[1]
Ovarian cycle	20.8+/− 1.2 days[2]
External signs of oestrus	Female proceptive behaviour
Age at sexual maturity	Males are fertile: 4–5 years (Fragaszy & Adams-Curtis 1998)
	Females give birth: 3;10 years (earliest) (Zunino 1990); 5;7 years (average) (Fragaszy & Adams-Curtis 1998)
Age at weaning	416 days (Fragaszy & Bard 1997)
Adult weight	Males: 3.3±0.5 kg; (max. >6 kg)
	Females: 2.4±0.4 kg; (max. 4 kg)
	Growth curves for males and females from birth to over 20 years are available in Carosi *et al.* (2005)
Dental formula	2/2 1/1 3/3 3/3 = 36 (Napier & Napier 1967)
Age at gingival eruption	First molar 1.2 years; second molar 2.2 years (Galliari 1985)
Longevity	Maximum 53 years[3]

[1]Data from the Primate Center of the Istituto di Scienze e Tecnologie della Cognizione in Rome concerning living newborns.
[2]Data based on measurements of hormonal levels (Linn *et al.* 1995; Nagle & Denari 1983; Carosi *et al.* 1999).
[3]Bartus (pers. comm.)

Information on reproductive biology (including hormonal profiles) is reported in Carosi et al. (2005), Carnegie et al. (2005a, b and 2011). Data concerning capuchins' anatomy in relation to other primate species is available in Ankel-Simons (2007) and Martin (1990).

In addition, some behavioural features make capuchins unique among New World monkeys. They have a similar variety of facial displays to Old World monkeys, with displays emerging at different points in development (Visalberghi et al. 2006; De Marco & Visalberghi 2007). Lip-smacking (an affiliative display) appears near the end of the first month; the open-mouth threat face is the last to emerge, between 4.5 and 10 months of age. Capuchins also possess a rich vocal repertoire that warrants systematic study for full understanding, and great manual dexterity that includes precision grips and diverse tool-using behaviours (Fragaszy et al. 2004; Truppa et al. 2018).

Captive capuchins' sexual behaviour is highly elaborate. *Sapajus* spp. females in oestrus actively solicit males, who may be at least initially reluctant (Carosi & Visalberghi 2002; Carosi et al. 2005). Females' soliciting behaviour includes facial expressions such as eyebrow raise, vocalisations, gestures such as head tilting and chest rubbing, and active following. This female 'proceptivity' is pronounced, and though the component behaviours may be used in other social contexts, when the female persistently shows them in combination it signals that she is in the periovulatory phase. Although copulation is mostly dorso-ventral, ventro-ventral posturing with mutual gaze also occurs. The sexual behaviour of wild and captive *Sapajus* species is broadly similar (Fragaszy et al. 2004); however, minor features may differ, and it is unclear whether the differences are at group or species level. Field data exist for *C. capucinus* (Manson et al. 1997; Carnegie et al. 2005a). In this species, chemical communication has a greater role, as indicated by males' interest in females' urine. Wild capuchins generally avoid breeding with close kin; when it does happen, there may be fitness costs (Godoy et al. 2016). Efforts should be made to minimise deleterious effects of inbreeding in captive groups, for example, by managing groups in ways that simulate natural emigration and immigration patterns, or by contraceptive methods.

It is easy to mistake male and female newborns and infants because the external sex organ of the female resembles that of the male in size, general shape and mobility (Figure 38.2); only close examination allows detection in females of a fissure instead of an orifice. For good illustrations of the genitalia of both sexes, see Fragaszy et al. (2004).

Like most other New World primates, capuchins show sex-linked colour vision polymorphism. Some females have trichromatic vision, whereas all males and other females have dichromatic vision (Fragaszy et al. 2004). Several studies have attempted to link this polymorphism to differences in wild monkeys' foraging strategies or efficiency. Wild *C. capucinus* trichromats have an advantage for feeding on reddish fruits (Melin et al. 2017). However, a study on captive *C. apella* reported an advantage of dichromacy compared to trichromacy for detecting camouflaged stimuli (Saito et al. 2005). Issues surrounding colour vision polymorphism have yet to be settled, but individual differences within a given captive group should be taken into account when choosing enrichment devices, feeding techniques and experimental testing.

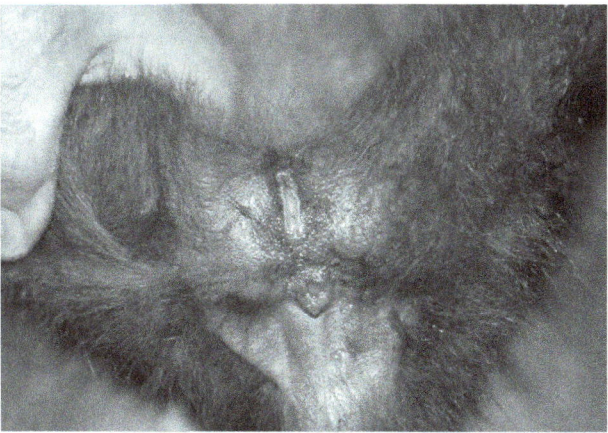

Figure 38.2 Clitoris of 1-day-old female *Sapajus spp*. In females, the tip of the genitalia has a fissure, whereas in males there is an orifice. Source: E. Visalberghi.

Sources of supply

Capuchins are widely distributed in the wild and breed well in captive conditions. They are quite hardy and resistant to disease (see the following text), although intestinal parasites (worms) may be present. Laboratories and zoos often have a surplus of animals, leading to the use of birth control methods. Surgical (vasectomy, hysterectomy) and chemical procedures (oestrogen and progestin) are commonly used. Laboratories that possess more than one group can pursue birth control and breeding on demand. Maintaining future production is still possible by (a) housing fertile males with infertile females (or vice versa) in the same group or (b) pairing one fertile male with one fertile female (during the periovulatory period) in neutral housing. The European Directive 2010/63 indicates that all monkeys used for research should be the offspring of captive monkeys kept in a certified breeding facility.

Uses in research

Due to their fascinating biological and behavioural features, capuchins have become very popular in behavioural studies both in the wild and captivity. This popularity seems likely to increase, with the first *in vivo* brain imaging study a notable development (e.g., Phillips et al. 2007). They are also used in biomedical studies, including for example research on ageing, pharmacology, dentistry, reproductive biology and neuroscience. Capuchins were used as 'simian helpers' to paraplegics, but welfare implications and limited effectiveness ended these initiatives.

Capuchins are especially interesting for their cognitive abilities (Fragaszy et al. 2004). Their psychological traits are currently studied from many perspectives including tool use (Spagnoletti et al. 2011; Falótico & Ottoni 2014), visual perception and visuo-spatial learning (De Lillo et al. 2011; Parrish et al. 2016), visual search, memory and metacognition (Kishimoto et al. 2019; Beran & Parrish 2012; Vining & Marsh 2015), planning (Prétôt & Brosnan 2019) cooperation, exchange and symbolic representation (Addessi et al. 2007, 2014), quantity judgements (Addessi *et al.* 2007; Beran *et al.* 2007), use of social and non-social cues for finding food (Hattori *et al.* 2007; Sabbatini & Visalberghi 2008), face processing (Dufour *et al.* 2006; Pokorny & de Waal 2009), self-control (Addessi *et al.* 2013) and personality (Uher *et al.* 2013; Wilson *et al.* 2014).

Although fieldwork has been done on several *Sapajus* and *Cebus* species, the laboratory population consists almost entirely of *Sapajus* spp., while zoos host also *C. capucinus*, *C. albifrons*, and *S. xanthosternos*. It should be noted that capuchins have potentially long lives, with captive individuals able to live for more than 50 years (Hakeem *et al.* 1996). Any plan to use capuchins in research should take this extended longevity into consideration.

General husbandry

Many of the safety- and hygiene-related requirements for the transportation, housing and handling of capuchins are identical to those that apply when dealing with other nonhuman primate species[1]. In this chapter, we focus particularly on aspects of welfare that might concern capuchins more specifically, given their distinctive biological and behavioural profiles. As a complementary source of relevant information, we recommend the *EAZA Best Practice Guidelines for Capuchin Monkeys* (2019).

From a welfare point of view, the planning of potentially stressful events that occur during routine husbandry (e.g. cleaning, moving animals, veterinary checks) and the choice of appropriate indicators to assess levels of stress should take into account individual variability. Ferreira *et al.* (2018) found that individual capuchins differ behaviourally and physiologically in the way they cope with aversive conditions. In particular, friendly, curious and active individuals have lower faecal glucocorticoid metabolites and lower levels of stress-related behaviours (e.g. alertness, bouncing, rocking, self-scratching); these features allow them to cope with stressful situations.

Although they may spend much time on the ground, capuchins are primarily arboreal, and they employ their semi-prehensile tail during above ground locomotion and posturing. The height of cages or enclosures should reflect these adaptations, for example, by providing perches above human eye level. Annex III of the European Directive 2010/63 does not provide specific recommendations for capuchins, but states that nonhuman primate enclosures should permit as wide a behavioural repertoire as possible, and that monkeys should be housed in complex environments where they can walk, run, climb, jump and feel secure. In general, space requirements are determined not only by group size, but also factors such as sex/age ratio, structure and furnishing of the environment, including potential escape routes (Olsson & Westlund 2007). For example, the Istituto di Scienze e Tecnologie della Cognizione del Consiglio Nazionale delle Ricerche in Rome houses groups of 5–10 *Sapajus* spp. in enriched enclosures of different sizes (outdoors, 106–374 m³; indoors, 25 m³). In the Strasbourg Primate Centre, different groups of 14+ *Sapajus* spp. and *C. capucinus* thrived in complex indoor/outdoor facilities of approximately 180 m² (height 3 m). In a study that involved an approximately 50% reduction in their normal indoor area, capuchins responded by avoiding social encounters and by increasing self-grooming (van Wolkenten *et al.* 2006).

Environmental provisions

Promoting the physiological and psychological well-being of captive primates is important for ethical and scientific as well as legal reasons (Broom 2009; Lundmark *et al.* 2014). Of course, it is neither feasible nor desirable for a laboratory or zoo to attempt to meticulously reproduce all aspects of natural settings (Veissier & Boissy 2007); appropriate compromise should be the goal. This entails focusing on features of the environment that elicit a similar range of social and non-social activities to that seen in the wild. For example, it is important to give sufficiently varied foods containing appropriate proportions of proteins, carbohydrates, vitamins, minerals, etc., and to do so in ways that encourage the kinds of manipulatory, locomotor and temporal patterns of feeding-related activities seen in wild primates. In view of their highly developed manipulatory propensities, broad repertoire of object-oriented actions and their sustained curiosity in objects, providing capuchins with a stimulating environment is not only a requisite of good husbandry, but also relatively easy and gratifying to do. Many potential enrichment techniques exist, ranging from increasing the diversity and processing requirements of food (to simulate aspects of foraging), to improving furnishing of the cage or enclosure (to widen locomotor possibilities and provide cover), and providing stimulating sensory events. Presenting various objects to explore, play with or destroy can do the latter. Enrichment devices differ in their impact on animal behaviour and their ability to reduce abnormal behaviour(s) (Lutz & Novak 2005; See also Chapter 10: Environmental enrichment: animal welfare and scientific validity). Therefore, incisive environmental enrichment plans should include the monitoring and recording of actual use of devices across the time and their behavioural and physiological effects. A long-overlooked source of enrichment is positive interaction with keepers (Reinhardt 2003). From a refinement perspective, the introduction into husbandry routines of predictable signs of aversive and positive events, and the possibility for monkeys to choose and exert some control over their own environment have a beneficial impact on well-being (Chamove & Anderson 1989; Rimpley & Buchanan-Smith 2013). Below, we make recommendations based upon species-typical behaviour in the wild and outcomes of enrichment studies in captivity.

One important goal of the care and management of captive primates is to reduce excessive inactivity in their daily lives, i.e. to reduce boredom and its negative consequences such as lethargy and abnormal behaviours (Dawson 2009) The following aspects are addressed from this perspective in the rest of this chapter: the social and physical environments, and routine capture and handling techniques.

Free-ranging capuchins are arboreal, move around on surfaces, which are vertical and horizontal, but mostly oblique and flexible, such as tree branches. Therefore, captive capuchins should be provided with oblique structures in addition

---

[1] http://pin.primate.wisc.edu/research/vet/ (accessed 2 September 2019)

to the more conventional vertical and horizontal ones. Panels, hanging screens, branches, slides, swings, ropes, crates, frames, poles, PVC pipes and plastic mats are all potentially valuable structures for promoting physical exercise, for better exploiting available cage space and providing appropriate substrates for resting and sleeping. Some can simulate vegetation and allow monkeys to avoid others if they so choose, as well as providing shade and shelter (if outdoors). Visalberghi and Albani (2014) have produced a video, available on request, that shows the use of caves to rest, play, sleep and shelter from inclement weather and heat.

An effective way of increasing use of available cage space is to make the floor more attractive. Plants may be a feasible addition to large enclosures (Figure 38.3), although in relatively small spaces capuchins eventually destroy all or most of them, except for stinging nettles, ivy or toxic varieties (e.g. Solanaceae). Vegetation is more likely to survive in spacious enclosures, especially if it is already well-established before the capuchins arrive. Many laboratories and zoos use deep litter, such as woodchips and/or bark. The best litters encourage locomotion and foraging activities and sometimes play; they also afford some protection if an animal falls from an elevated position. Early concerns regarding possible hygienic disadvantages of using deep litter have so far proved to be unfounded; litter may be safely left for several weeks without hosing or disinfecting. However, the removal of heavily soiled parts of the litter or rotten food is advisable, especially if there is the chance that rodents might be attracted.

Some regular husbandry procedures can also reduce boredom. For example, periodically switching groups between enclosures provides each with new visual and olfactory input, and promotes exploration and locomotion of the surroundings. The installation of visual barriers that partially limit the view of adjacent monkey groups or of zoo visitors also increases choice and hence a sense of control that improves well-being. The challenges present in cognitive tests can also have enriching effects (Whitehouse *et al.* 2013; Ruby & Buchanan-Smith 2015).

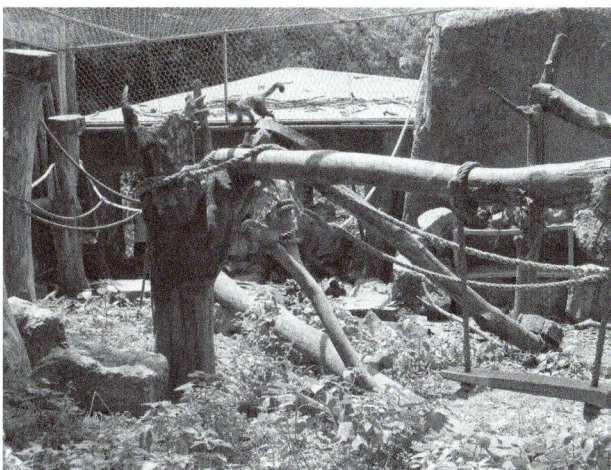

Figure 38.3 Outdoor enclosure in the Primate Center of the Istituto di Scienze e Tecnologie della Cognizione hosted by the Bioparco of Rome (Italy). Members of the public (in the background) can observe the capuchin monkeys; the latter are also used for research.
Source: V. Truppa.

Environmental provisions (inanimate objects)

Capuchins will readily manipulate and do their best to break open almost any object given. (They can learn to open cage doors or partitions that are secured only by simple latches or dog clips, so padlocks are advised.) Tennis balls, plastic and cardboard boxes, wooden blocks, rubber tubing, plastic mirrors are all examples of good, readily available and affordable enrichment objects, although their use as such must be weighed against possible disadvantages such as blocked drains, time required by caretakers to remove debris, etc. They must be checked carefully and all potentially dangerous parts (protruding wires, nails, sharp edges, etc.) removed. Sturdier enrichment objects and devices are generally preferable in laboratory environments. The most effective strategy for maintaining the monkeys' interest is to replace or rotate objects every few days. Capuchins do not readily enter deep water, but a plastic container filled with shallow water undoubtedly stimulates exploratory and playful activities, especially in hot weather.

In summary, there are many different ways in which the physical environment can be enriched. The choices need not be mutually exclusive. For example, simple objects can be baited with food treats to elicit a range of feeding techniques. Monkeys devote much time to sifting and searching through deep litters that contain buried food. Finally, structures and objects with holes or openings containing treats (syrup, honey, raisins, etc.) encourage extractive techniques, including tool use.

In the wild, capuchin monkeys have been observed rubbing leaves, fruits, ants and millipedes into their fur. Capuchins appear highly motivated and rub these items on their fur. This behaviour, referred to as 'anointing', is common also in captivity (Lynch Alfaro *et al.* 2014); all capuchin species anoint themselves, and in at least some species (e.g., *Cebus capucinus*) they may anoint other individuals as well. We have seen onions, citrus fruits, garlic, aromatic herbs and peat used for this purpose. Anointing is a response to specific chemical stimuli and may serve different purposes, such as self-medication (e.g., to reduce ectoparasite loads and infections) and as insect repellent (reviewed in Lynch Alfaro *et al.* 2012c). Given the high motivation of capuchins for this activity, we recommend that trial and error be used to identify which items appropriately elicit fur-rubbing, and that the capuchins are allowed to perform this behaviour periodically. It should be noted that both wild and captive capuchin monkeys also frequently rub their bodies with urine, which they collect on the hands and feet and tip of the tail. Although various thermoregulatory, social signalling and territorial hypotheses have been tested, the main functions of 'urine washing' remain to be identified, as it is affected by multiple factors including oestrus, weather and time of day (Roeder & Anderson 1991; Campos *et al.* 2007; Miller *et al.* 2008; Schino *et al.* 2011).

Social grouping

The optimal social grouping for captive capuchins is undoubtedly one that would contain similar proportions of age- and sex-classes as seen in natural conditions. However, given that capuchins' social structure is quite variable, this principle can be implemented with some flexibility, depending on space limitations and on the purposes for which the monkeys are maintained. In any case, except under truly exceptional circumstances, capuchin monkeys must be kept socially, as social companions are greatly valued (Dettmer & Fragaszy 2000) and excellent sources of interactive and ever-changing stimulation (Visalberghi & Anderson 1993).

As already mentioned, in some groups the lowest-ranking individual can become the target of repeated aggression. This is obviously a stressful situation for the victim, and in extreme cases its removal may be the best solution. However, potential drawbacks of removal that should be considered include the resulting isolation and possible problematic reintegration for a socially rejected individual. Furthermore, there is no guarantee that the remaining group members will not start to target another individual. The physical and psychological health of the victimised individual should be carefully monitored, and food supplements provided if necessary. We are not aware of cases of sustained harassment of subordinates resulting in death; indeed, not only physical but also social wounds usually heal with time. For example, in the Rome colony a female who was a scapegoat at 3 years of age rose to become the dominant female of her group a few years later. It should be ensured that subordinates have adequate access to resources, including shelter. Enclosures should be designed such that subordinates cannot easily be trapped or cornered during aggression. It should also be noted that haematological, physiological and immunological parameters of severely bullied or otherwise stressed animals might be outside the normal range of values.

If two or more groups are housed in the same facility, care should be taken to prevent direct physical contact between them. A single wire mesh partition is not sufficient for separating neighbouring groups; fingers, toes and tips of tails can easily be grabbed or bitten off. Groups in visual or auditory contact may react to each other, sometimes with negative consequences. The housing can be improved, giving the occupants more control over their social environment, by providing visual barriers that partially block visual access to neighbours. Several zoos successfully keep capuchins in mixed-species exhibits (Buchanan-Smith *et al.* 2013; Daoudi *et al.* 2017, see Figure 38.4); compatible mixed-species groups can be enriching not only for the species involved but also for visitors.

It is advisable to allow animals some choice regarding whom to be with within the group, and whether to be in visual contact with a neighbouring group (Fragaszy 2005; International Primatological Society 2007). This can be achieved by providing 'privacy' panels or other structures inside the cage(s), or housing groups in interconnecting rooms or cages, preferably with more than one connecting door or hatch between them.

Experimental testing sometimes requires working with a single subject at a time, leading to the question of how to separate the subject from the group while minimising stress. A good solution is to have the test apparatus in or alongside a cage or room connected to the colony quarters by sliding doors. We strongly recommend the use of horizontally or upward-sliding doors instead of the traditional downward-sliding guillotine door, to reduce the risk of injury to monkeys.

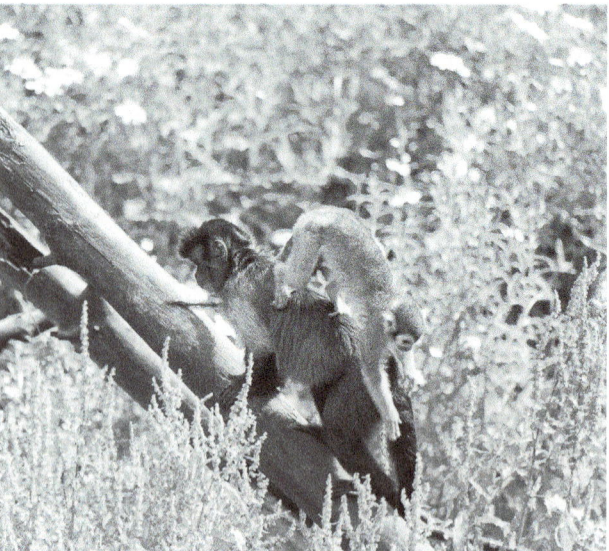

Figure 38.4 Capuchin monkeys and squirrel monkeys live in compatible mixed-species groups at Living Links, Edinburgh Zoo. Source: K. Grounds.

For most individuals, gradual habituation to increasingly long periods (up to 20–40 min) of separation associated with positive reinforcement, inherent interest of the tasks (using only positive reinforcement, never punishment) and subsequent reunion are sufficient to overcome the initial reluctance to be separated. See also Chapter 15: The use of positive reinforcement training techniques to enhance the care and welfare of laboratory and research animals.

As a general rule, a well-established stable group will pose fewer problems than the process of forming a new group or of introducing unfamiliar individuals into an established group. Below, we focus on the latter two scenarios, and draw upon personal experiences and the literature to suggest some procedures, as well as some pitfalls to avoid. It should be noted that most of our knowledge on how to form or modify capuchin groups comes not from systematic experimental manipulations but from experience of husbandry challenges faced occasionally by laboratories and zoos. Overall, group formation is a stressful procedure both for the animals and the caregivers, and although cumulative experience may help to reduce the risks of failure, the outcome can never be predicted with absolute certainty (see Visalberghi & Anderson 1993; Fragaszy 2005).

Introduction and re-introduction

Since an individually housed monkey is *de facto* living in impoverished conditions and therefore psychologically deprived, all efforts should be made towards compatible social housing. Sometimes, this may be feasible even shortly after major veterinary treatment (for an example with a newborn infant, see Anderson *et al.* 1995). Hand-reared (ages ranging from 5 to 9 mos.) and mother-reared (8–12 mos.) infants were successfully introduced to a group when full integration was preceded by a period of visual contact that allowed mutual familiarisation at a safe distance (Riviello 1992). For integrating single adult females, initial visual contact was followed by periods in which the female was together with the dominant male and then together with him and each of the other group members, before being housed permanently with the entire group (Anderson et al. 1991; Ludes & Anderson 1995). In the most extensive report on introduction and integration of strangers into captive groups of tufted capuchins, Fragaszy et al. (1994) describe the successful introduction of 2–4 individuals (adult males, females and juveniles) into three established groups of 6–9 capuchins. This report provides several behavioural categories that can be usefully employed for both monitoring and predicting the success of introductions. First, newcomers were familiarised with the resident group's living quarters, and only then were residents and newcomers mixed. No serious aggression-related injuries occurred during the introductions or in the following months. When one or more individuals persistently chased a new female, partial separations were used to form mixed subgroups of newcomers and residents for overnight housing.

One adult male capuchin (more than 10 years old), previously kept in a zoo, was successfully introduced to a group in which the dominant male was only 4 years old. The procedure included a quicker progression through stages similar to those described above for adult females, and with contact between the newcomer and the dominant resident male left until last. Strikingly, these two males immediately came into contact and performed joint threats, towards no particular target. They quickly developed a positive relationship, the newcomer being alpha male. Although all introductions are likely to involve some degree of stress, in none of the above cases did the introduced monkey need to be removed from the group due to aggression or stress-related ill-health. Two introduction scenarios did result in severe aggression: unfamiliar adult males going into a group with no resident adult male, and males familiar with each other going into a group containing an elderly resident male (Cooper et al. 2001). In contrast, moving two males familiar with each other into a group with no resident male was peaceful.

Overall, the risks associated with introductions appear greatly outweighed by the disadvantages of solitary housing. No foolproof recipe is yet available for group formation or introduction procedures, but the chances of success can be increased by having a good knowledge of the animals involved, careful monitoring before and after the introduction, and by taking into account factors such as sex, age and experience of the newcomers (Visalberghi & Anderson 1993). Given the reports of male-perpetrated infanticide in the wild (see Social organisation in the preceding text), introduction of a fully adult male into a group containing neonates should be considered risky. Also, introducing an adult female into a group containing more than one adult male may lead to a violent attempt by a subordinate to overthrow the dominant male, especially if the latter is old.

Identification

Observation of morphological characteristics and behavioural traits is a valid, cheap and non-invasive method for recognising and acquiring useful knowledge about capuchins.

The European Union requires that captive monkeys are permanently marked. Permanent individual identification can be achieved in different ways. Tattooing with an electric pen and ink is a commonly used method, and we are aware of no ill effects. Identification collars are not advised, as capuchins will try their best to destroy them. Implanted microchips are increasingly popular for identifying captive New World primates (see Savastano et al. 2003), including some pet capuchins (we do not recommend capuchins as pets). Microchips are also useful for automated recording of individual performance in cognitive testing (Fagot & Paleressompoulle 2009). However, the use of microchips is not problem-free; cost, equipment incompatibility, and possible migration of the microchip are all potential compromising factors (Rennie & Buchanan-Smith 2006).

The physical environment

Capuchins are quite hardy animals provided that they have constant access to heated indoor quarters. They may occasionally venture outdoors in temperatures close to freezing; however, they do not appear to enjoy walking on frozen surfaces. The US *Guide for the care and use of laboratory animals* (2011) recommends maintaining an indoor temperature of 18 °C to 19 °C for 'nonhuman primates'. From our own experience, we have found that for capuchins a temperature of around 23 °C, humidity of 50–60% and a ventilation rate of at least 4–5 air changes per hour are satisfactory. Although no scientific data are available, gradual light changes to simulate natural changes at dawn and dusk may be beneficial. Natural light from windows or skylights will provide low levels of light at night, similar to the situation in the wild. The auditory environment can also affect welfare of captive primates, depending on species and types of noise. Excessive noise should be avoided.

Quarantine

Quarantine procedures are broadly similar to those recommended for other primates (e.g., National Research Council 2017). Duration ranges from 40 to 90 days, during which time repeated tuberculin skin tests, serology and stool analyses are performed. Prophylactic treatment varies across institutions; for groups with access to outdoor areas, we recommend vaccination against tetanus. A zoo-housed colony was successfully protected against rabies using a human non-vaccinated exposure protocol consisting of periodic intramuscular doses of killed rabies (between possible post-exposure days 2–33) and a single dose of human rabies immune globulin (at possible post-exposure day 5) (Kenny et al. 2001).

At present, most captive nonhuman primates used in research or hosted in zoos are offspring of those already kept in captivity. They should be screened periodically to monitor their health status and before shipment to other facilities they undergo standard protocols (Hsu & Jia 2003). Such procedures reduce morbidity and mortality rates, and are advantageous to both animal welfare and the quality of research (Roberts & Andrews 2008).

Breeding

Pregnancy and newborns

We do not recommend separating pregnant females from their group, even though dead neonates are occasionally recovered. We attach greater importance to preserving the complex network of intra-group social relations than to episodic breeding success if the latter implies stress due to lengthy separation and later reintegration of the mother-infant pair into the group. Most capuchin populations show a seasonal pattern of births (Di Bitetti & Janson 2000); in captivity, most births occur at night (Fragazsy & Adam-Curtis 1998).

As in other primates, maternal performance may differ between primiparous and multiparous mothers, and the former may show less competence and occasionally abandon their infants (Di Bitetti & Janson 2001). Conceivably, delivery for primiparous females is relatively long and/or tiring, and the infant may be compromised after a lengthy delivery. Some females with inadequate early social experience might kill their newborn. If an abandoned or abused neonate is recovered in time, fostering by a lactating female or hand rearing are viable options (see Hand rearing in the following text). However, after initial problems, capuchin females may become competent mothers with subsequent offspring (Honeysett 2006). Age, previous experience of hormonal changes and interaction with infants, higher social status of the mother and the presence of other females with infants may contribute to the improvement.

In an analysis of breeding records of four American and European colonies of tufted capuchins, 2.4% of pregnancies resulted in twin births, a higher incidence than previously estimated, and not dissimilar to human twinning rates (Leighty et al. 2004). If twins survived the first day of post-natal life (45% did not, compared to 16% of singletons), then subsequent survival was similar to that of singletons. Three complete sets of twins out of 10 sets recorded survived beyond 30 days, while another 3 infants whose twin died survived beyond the first month. Twins were successfully weaned also in wild populations (EthoCebus Project, unpublished data).

Infant transfer is common in capuchins. Young infants, even newborns, may be held or transported (and, rarely, nursed) by individuals other than their mother. Adult male white-faced and tufted capuchins may carry infants for long periods. This is usually safe, but it may carry risks if the infant is very young or when the mother does not retrieve it. The infant may take the initiative in transferring from the mother onto a nearby individual, or the latter may solicit the transfer by adopting an inviting posture. The non-maternal carrier is rarely aggressive, but infants up to about 8 weeks run the risk of dehydration/starvation if they are unable to transfer back to the mother, so surveillance is recommended. Some mothers do not attempt to get their infant back, sometimes, but not always, because of the mother's subordinate status. In such cases intervention may become necessary. This can involve either bringing the mother and the carrier into close proximity, for example, by offering a non-transportable treat such as juice, or by restraining them in a restricted space. If these procedures fail, the carrier may need to be captured and the infant returned to its mother, with follow-up monitoring for adequacy of maternal care. Sometimes during this procedure, the carrier (even the mother) will forcefully dislodge the infant by rough pulling or even biting. Care should be taken to keep the capture process calm so as not to endanger the infant.

Hand rearing

Viable infants abandoned at birth can successfully be hand-reared and then introduced into a social group (Visalberghi & Riviello 1987), either their original one or another. Based on our experience, it is better to reintroduce the infant as soon as possible (2–3 months of age) to minimise attachment to humans and maximise positive social interactions with group members. Commercially available human infant milk formulas generally work well for common laboratory primate species. However, Milligan (2010) reports that capuchin milk is lower in lactose and higher in fat and protein than human milk. Following an initial few feeds, consisting of warmed rehydration fluid or 5% glucose, we recommend bottle-feeding newborns every 3 hours with powdered baby milk. The interval between feedings can be gradually increased, especially during the night. The concentration of the milk substitute can also be progressively increased, until full strength is reached by 24–36 hours. Usually, the infant vocalises when hungry. The hole in the nipple should be small enough to prevent excessively fast ingestion. The monkey stops drinking when satiated and it is advisable to keep it upright for a few minutes to facilitate burping and avoid regurgitation. Based on the development of feeding behaviour seen in the wild, we recommend giving small pieces of solid foods (e.g., pellets, banana or apple) to infant capuchins as early as 3–4 weeks. Not much is consumed at this age, but the animals lick or mouth it.

Infants grow rapidly, gaining about 100 g per month for the first 10 months. By 1 year of age, they will have reached more than 50% of the mother's non-pregnant body weight (Fragazsy & Adams-Curtis 1998). Like other New World monkeys, capuchins require vitamin D3 for adequate skeletal growth, especially if the monkeys have no access to unfiltered sunlight. Vitamin D3 is available in pelleted diets and vitamin/mineral supplements.

Feeding

Commercially available New World monkey food supplemented with fresh vegetables and fruits satisfies the general requirements of captive capuchins (Fragaszy 2005; see also National Research Council of the National Academies 2003). Live insects represent an excellent dietary supplement; wild capuchins consume invertebrates even when fruit is abundant, although they spend more time processing protected invertebrates when fruit and caterpillars are less abundant (Mosdossy et al. 2015). Commercial pellets appear nutritionally ideal, but they are not among capuchins' preferred foods (Addessi et al. 2005) despite containing all the requirements for physical health. Furthermore, given wild capuchins' wide variety of foods and feeding techniques (see Habitats and feeding habits in the preceding text), it is highly recommended to attempt to simulate some aspects of this diversity. For example, capuchins like to break open and peel fruits, so it is rarely necessary to peel and chop fruits into fine pieces. Whole fruits allow them to spend more time in species-typical feeding behaviour. Food can be placed in locations to encourage arboreality and increase search time; for example, if the top of the cage or enclosure is of wire mesh, foods big enough not to drop directly through the holes can be spread there to encourage a variety of food-gathering techniques. Food can also be hidden in a variety of ways and locations so as to stimulate searching. Specially constructed containers containing straw or woodchips and food treats can be used to elicit a range of species-typical foraging activities. Extensive, visually guided picking activities including fine precision grips are easily elicited by synthetic 'grass' secured to a board outside the cage and baited with grains or other small edible items. Variability can also be made a feature of the timing of feeding, although whether this has observable beneficial effects for capuchins requires confirmation.

Raw and unprocessed foods are an obvious way of challenging capuchins' natural extractive propensities. Unshelled nuts can be made even more of a challenge to manual or tool-assisted cracking techniques by increasing the resistance of their shells (Visalberghi & Vitale 1990). Every region has products suitable for capuchin 'treatment': corn on the cob, unshelled beans and nuts, coconuts and unhusked cereals are good examples, and all are excellent supplements to the staple balanced diet. Raw eggs are a preferred treat, although there may be an associated risk of salmonellosis, and of restricted biotin uptake due to the uncooked avidin. Especially when commercial food is not given, mealworms, cheese, yoghurt, etc., and cooked fish should be added to the regime to provide animal proteins, along with dried fruits. Obese capuchins are rare, even among those known to eat rich, processed human food; therefore, some food can be given almost *ad libitum*. It is advisable to provide a highly preferred mixture (cottage cheese, eggs, cereals, etc.) a few times a week and to use this occasion to administer unpalatable medicines (see the following text).

Care of aged capuchins

The welfare of elderly capuchins (older than 30 years of age) requires special care and monitoring by veterinarians. Nutritional supplements and vitamins should be prescribed as appropriate. Loss of hair and increased susceptibility to temperature conditions requires heated zones in winter and shady areas in summer. Declining locomotory abilities necessitate gentle husbandry procedures and cage furnishings that take this into account. Old capuchins do not jump and climb as younger ones; therefore branches, platforms and covered areas should be located within easy reach. Also, as access to food may be difficult due to competition, care should be taken over food distribution. Finally, their willingness to participate in behavioural/cognitive tests should always be rewarded, to enrich their daily life.

Laboratory procedures

Handling and training

The traditional way of capturing group-living capuchins is with a net, and/or protective gloves. The chasing involved in this method is extremely stressful, and the method is not without risk of injury to the animal(s). Whereas capuchins can be easily trained by positive reinforcement to move from one place to another, it is difficult and very time consuming to train them for capture and venepuncture (Dettmer et al. 1996). The expertise of the person doing the capture is paramount. Since stress increases over time, rapid, efficient netting may be preferable to a prolonged wait for a frightened animal to enter the tunnel (e.g. Linn et al. 1995). Nets should have padded rims to prevent injury to the animal (especially to its teeth) during capture. Capture-related stress can be reduced by giving piece of banana or grape containing a few drops of diazepam (0.5–1.0 mg/kg, Carpenter 2013). After receiving the anxiolytic administration, monkeys might lose their normal sense of balance; thus they should be monitored and their movements limited to avoid injury (e.g., falling from elevated structures).

Capture may be made less stressful by habituating the monkeys to sights and sounds associated with capture from an early age. Even so, capture typically results in the colony being highly aroused for some time afterward, although providing distracting foraging opportunities immediately after the event can lower this. We have noticed that events typically occurring on capture days often become associated with the stressful experience. For example, the arrival of the veterinarian, or the sight or noise of capture equipment (gloves, tunnel-cages, etc.), gives rise to tension and/or fear. Therefore, it may be advisable for those whose research activity involves direct observation of spontaneous behaviour not to be involved in capture. Stressful events can be combined with positive situations (e.g., offering highly preferred food) and persons involved in stressful procedures should spend time with the subjects to reduce arousal responses. Capuchins have extremely powerful jaws and can inflict serious bite wounds, so personnel should guard against being bitten (or scratched), for example, by wearing protective gloves.

Transport boxes are commonly used to take individual monkeys from their home cage to an experimental room, for example, to administer Wisconsin General Test Apparatus- or video-based tasks. Initial coaxing of the animal to enter the box may require any of a number of stratagems of varying forcefulness, ranging from attracting the monkey into the box using treats to chasing it in by blocking all escape routes except the entrance to the box. Capuchins can distinguish between different tones of voice and possibly words; this can be used in training. However, positive reinforcement is essential. Once the transport procedure becomes routine, monkeys often start to enter the transport cage spontaneously, sometimes even in absence of food reward. Indeed, it is common for a reliable order to emerge, often dominance-related, in which group members vie to be given access to the test apparatus.

Physiological monitoring

In zoos and laboratories, positive reinforcement training (see Chapter 15: The use of positive reinforcement training techniques to enhance the care and welfare of laboratory and research animals) is becoming popular as an alternative to capturing monkeys for collecting samples including saliva, vaginal swabs or blood (Prescott et al. 2005). However, there are still very few examples with capuchins; it is possible that capuchins are harder to train than macaques for such procedures (see Fragaszy et al. 2004). The measurement of nasal temperature variations by use of thermo-imaging has still to be validated on capuchins. Drug treatments can also be administered to co-operative animals by means of positive reinforcement training, thus circumventing the problem of rejection of food or liquid laced with the substance to be administered. Females can be trained to sit on a plastic bin for increasingly long periods and to urinate while seated. It took less than 1 month to fully train a female to urinate on the bin within a few minutes of taking up position. However, such training does not succeed with all individuals.

Administration of substances

Oral doses can readily be given either concealed in highly preferred food (see the preceding text), or administered directly into the mouth with a syringe (without the needle!) in fruit juice.

Intravenous injections should be given in either the femoral or saphenous veins, although the latter may be more difficult.

Anaesthesia

Short-term sedation can be induced with ketamine (10 mg. per kg.). To treat a sick infant every 2–3 days, we first lightly anaesthetised the mother with intramuscular ketamine 10 mg/kg. Inhalation anaesthetics and endotracheal techniques are indicated for surgical procedures. Specialised information on anaesthesia and analgesia can be found in Sedgwick (1986), Sainsbury (1991) and Popilskis and Kohn (1997); Popilskis and Kohn (1997) also address intra-operative monitoring and support, and special anaesthetic considerations, although no specific recommendations are made for capuchin monkeys.

Care must be taken to ensure that a captured animal is unable to reach the needle of a syringe. Capuchins are extremely swift and capable of exploiting any possibility to prevent capture, injections and so on, unless specifically trained. Training, however, may require patience. Dettmer et al. (1996) reported that repeated capture and venepuncture procedures in C. apella resulted in raised cortisol levels, before a reduction in week 7 brought them back down to week 1 levels. After this phase, however, behaviourally habituated animals no longer showed this physiological stress response to venepuncture, whereas non-habituated animals did.

The post-anaesthesia recovery period should follow standard monitoring and hygiene-related protocols, ensuring adequate warmth, freedom from potential injury, and return to the social group as soon as possible.

Euthanasia

If euthanasia is necessary, the animal should be anaesthetised and then injected intravenously with an overdose of pentobarbitone.

Common welfare problems

Health

Diseases and treatments

As in other primates, behavioural changes may be the last signs of underlying illness to appear; so regular careful monitoring (including weighing) is advised. Regular health check must include full body system review and should be performed by a qualified veterinarian. Lehner (1984) and Sainsbury (1991) give summaries of diseases to which capuchins and other members of the Cebidae are susceptible. These include the common human cold and other viral diseases (e.g., measles, chicken pox). Tuberculosis appears to be the most important of the bacterial diseases, although capuchins are quite resistant and diagnosis may be difficult. Among parasitic diseases, malarial infection (*Plasmodium brazilianum*) and haemo-flagellate infection (*Trypanosoma cruzi*) have sometimes been fatal. Lehner (1984) describes the various signs of these diseases and others, such as rickettsial and viral, along with treatments and prognoses. Two specimens of the genus *Cebus* and two of the genus *Sapajus* were found naturally infected by *Plasmodium simium*, providing a valuable case for malaria epidemiology among nonhuman primates (de Alvarenga et al. 2015). Many capuchin parasites are transmitted through the consumption of invertebrate intermediate hosts, making diet a critical component of capuchin-parasite ecology (Parr et al. 2013); *Filariopsis sp.*, *Strongyloides* sp. and the Hymenolepididae are among the more common parasites detected in wild capuchins (Agostini et al. 2018). Rondón et al. (2017) investigate the prevalence of parasites (i.e., the number of infected individuals divided by the total of examined individuals) in three Neotropical primate species, including untufted capuchins, living in a fragmented forest of Colombia in relation to seasonality.

With regard to the zoonotic infections, leptospirosis was reported in a colony of capuchins rescued from homes and housed in a wildlife rehabilitation centre in Colombia; rodent infestation was identified as the cause of the epidemic (Szonyi et al. 2011). Rabies antibodies in Brazilian free-ranging capuchin monkeys were also found (Machado et al. 2012).

Herpes B virus infection can cause fatal disease in humans and in capuchin monkeys, (see Coulibaly et al. 2004 for a case of persistent but asymptomatic infection). Herpes B lesions in nonhuman primates are usually on the mucosa of the buccal cavity or on the tongue. For this reason, monitoring of the oral cavity during periodic veterinary checks should be carried out, observing recommended safety standards for operators.

Conservation programmes should take into account the fact that, in anthropogenic-modified environments, the bi-directionality of disease transmission represents a particularly important challenge for capuchins' health (McKinney 2011). Three cases of tetanus have occurred in Italian colonies; two of them were successfully treated. The monkeys (all adults) were found rigid and presented marked locomotor impairment and 'lockjaw'. One died after several hours; the others were treated like humans with the same disease. Medical care consisted of immunoglobulin, diazepam, antibiotics and rehydration therapy with physiological solution, with vitamins administered in doses appropriate for the monkeys' body weights.

They were kept in a warm, dimly lit environment and fed by hand four times a day. Treatment lasted between 20 and 30 days, after which the monkeys slowly recovered and were able to return to their group (L. De Marco & F. Faiola, personal communication). A 32-year-old *C. capucinus* was successfully treated for *Toxoplasma* meningitis using clindamycin and trimethoprim-sulfamethoxazole (Fiorello *et al.* 2006).

Diarrhoea may occur in response to stress, inappropriate diet, or infection. Sainsbury (1991) indicates fenbendazole, mebendazole and ivermectin for the treatment of nematode parasites, and dichlorophen and niclosamide for the treatment of cestodes; these treatments are not always successful. Lee *et al.* (1996) administered albendazole for 2 weeks, successfully eliminating nematode larvae in the faeces and adult worms in the lungs. Nagle and Denari (1983) describe the treatment of respiratory tract infections and diarrhoea in recently captured capuchins using penicillin, chloramphenicol and electrolytes with 5% dextrose solution. They state that thiabendazole is effective against nematodes. Wolff (1990) provides an extensive table of internal and external parasites of cebid monkeys, along with host location, disease signs, and diagnostic and treatment procedures. Periodontal diseases and dental fractures are common in captive capuchins. Examples, and recommended procedures including scaling and polishing are described in Fecchio *et al.* (2008). Information on miscellaneous health problems including fractures and soft tissue injuries can be found in Sainsbury (1991).

Apes and macaques are reported to be highly susceptible to SARS-CoV-2 (Damas *et al.* 2020), but data for most non-human primates are lacking. Susceptibility to SARS-CoV-2 depends on how the virus binds to ACE2 (the cellular receptor protein angiotensin-converting enzyme-2) and variations at these critical residues modulate infection susceptibility. By analyzing the ACE2 of several nonhuman primates, Melin *et al.* (2020) found that whereas apes and catarrhines monkeys exhibit the same set of twelve key amino acid residues as human ACE2, platyrrhines (which include the capuchin monkeys), some tarsiers, lemurs and lorisoids, differ at critical contact residues. The authors hypothesize that the lower binding affinity of these species makes them less susceptible to SARS-CoV-2.

Signs of poor welfare

Effective management requires recognising behaviours that might indicate poor welfare. Stereotypic acts such as head twirling, pirouetting and pacing are relatively common in confined housing, but not necessarily signs of actual poor welfare. Others such as self-biting and severe hair-pulling do suggest unacceptably poor psychological well-being. Abnormal behaviours should be systematically monitored to assess whether they can be mitigated by, e.g., physical enrichment, visual contacts and/or social interactions with compatible companions or keepers. Many factors influence how individuals behave and respond to stressful conditions, including their life experiences, age-sex class, temperament and social status (e.g., Nagy-Reis *et al.* 2019). Furthermore, captive capuchins housed in the same environment typically behave and react to stress differently, and their responses are related to individuals' physiological profiles (Ferreira *et al.* 2018).

References

Addessi, E., Stammati, M., Sabbatini, G. *et al.* (2005) How tufted capuchin monkeys (*Cebus apella*) rank monkey chow in relation to other foods. *Animal Welfare*, **14**, 215–222.

Addessi, E., Crescimene, L. and Visalberghi, E. (2007) Food and token quantity discrimination in capuchin monkeys (*Cebus apella*). *Animal Cognition*, **11**, 275–282.

Addessi, E., Paglieri, F., Beran, M.J. *et al.* (2013) Delay choice versus delay maintenance: different measures of delayed gratification in capuchin monkeys (*Cebus apella*). *Journal of Comparative Psychology*, **127**, 392–398.

Addessi, E., Bellagamba, F., Delfino, A. *et al.* (2014) Waiting by mistake: symbolic representation of rewards modulates intertemporal choice in capuchin monkeys, preschool children and adult humans. *Cognition*, **130**, 428–441.

Agostini, I., Vanderhoeven, E., Beldomenico, P.M. *et al.* (2018) First coprological survey of helminths in a wild population of black capuchin monkeys (*Sapajus nigritus*) in northeastern Argentina. *Mastozool Neotropical*, **18**(2.0), 11 https://doi.org/10.31687/saremMN.18.25.2.0.11.

Alfaro, J.W.L., Boubli, J.P., Olson, L.E. *et al.* (2012b) Explosive Pleistocene range expansion leads to widespread Amazonian sympatry between robust and gracile capuchin monkeys. *Journal of Biogeography*, **39**, 272–288.

Alfaro, J.W.L., Izar, P. and Ferreira, R.G. (2014) Capuchin monkey research priorities and urgent issues. *American Journal of Primatology*, **76**, 705–720.

Alfaro, J.W.L., Matthews, L., Boyette, A.H. *et al.* (2012c) Anointing variation across wild capuchin populations: a review of material preferences, bout frequency and anointing sociality in *Cebus* and *Sapajus*. *American Journal of Primatology*, **74**, 299–314.

Alfaro, J.W.L., Silva Jr, J.D.S.E. and Rylands, A.B. (2012a) How different are robust and gracile capuchin monkeys? An argument for the use of *Sapajus* and *Cebus*. *American Journal of Primatology*, **74**, 273–286.

Anderson J.R., Andre A. and Wolf P. (1995) Successful mother- and group rearing of a newborn capuchin monkey (*Cebus apella*) following emergency major surgery. *Animal Welfare*, **4**, 171–182.

Anderson J.R., Combette C. and Roeder J.-J. (1991) Integration of a tame adult female capuchin monkey (*Cebus apella*) into a captive group. *Primate Report*, **31**, 87–94.

Ankel-Simons, F. (2007) *Primate Anatomy: An Introduction*. New York: Academic Press.

Beran, M.J., Evans, T.A., Leighty, K.A. *et al.* (2007) Summation and quantità judgments of sequentially presented sets by capuchin monkeys (*Cebus apella*). *American Journal of Primatology*, **70**, 191–194.

Beran, M.J. and Parrish, A.E. (2012) Sequential responding and planning in capuchin monkeys (*Cebus apella*). *Animal Cognition*, **15**, 1085–1094.

Broom, D.M. (2009) Animal welfare and legislation. *Food safety assurance and veterinary public health*, **5**, 339–350.

Buchanan-Smith, H.M., Griciute, J., Daoudi, S. *et al.* (2013) Interspecific interactions and welfare implications in mixed species communities of capuchin (*Sapajus apella*) and squirrel monkeys (*Saimiri sciureus*) over 3 years. *Applied Animal Behaviour Science*, **147**, 324–333.

Campos, F., Manson, J.H. and Perry, S. (2007) Urine washing and sniffing in wild white-faced capuchins (*Cebus capucinus*): testing functional hypotheses. *International Journal of Primatology*, **28**, 55–72.

Carnegie S.D., Fedigan L.M. and Melin, A.D. (2011) Reproductive seasonality in female capuchins (*Cebus capucinus*) in Santa Rosa (Area de Conservación Guanacaste), Costa Rica. *International Journal of Primatology*, **32**, 1076–1090.

Carnegie, S.D., Fedigan, L.M. and Ziegler, T.E. (2005a) Behavioral indicators of ovarian phase in white-faced capuchins (*Cebus capucinus*). *American Journal of Primatology*, **67**, 51–68.

Carnegie, S.D., Fedigan, L.M. and Ziegler, T.E. (2005b) Post-conceptive mating in white-faced capuchins, *Cebus capucinus*: hormonal and sociosexual patterns of cycling, noncycling and pregnant females. In: *New Perspectives in the Study of Mesoamerican Primates: Distribution, Ecology, Behavior, and Evolution*, Eds P.E. Garber et al., pp. 387–409. Springer: New York.

Carosi, M., Heistermann, M. and Visalberghi, E. (1999) Display of proceptive behaviors in relation to urinary and fecal progestin levels over the ovarian cycle in female tufted capuchin monkeys. *Hormones and Behavior*, 36, 252–265.

Carosi, M., Linn, G.R. and Visalberghi, E. (2005) The sexual behavior and breeding system of tufted capuchin monkeys (*Cebus apella*). *Advances in the Study of Behavior*, 35, 105–149.

Carosi, M. and Visalberghi, E. (2002) Analysis of tufted capuchin (*Cebus apella*) courtship and sexual behavior repertoire: Changes throughout the female cycle and female interindividual differences. *American Journal of Physical Anthropology*, 118, 11–24.

Carpenter, J.W. (2013) Exotic animal formulary. *Journal of Exotic Pet Medicine*, 22, 308–309.

Chamove, A.S. and Anderson, J.R. (1989) Examining environmental enrichment. In: *Housing, Care and Psychological Wellbeing of Captive and Laboratory Primates*, Ed. E.F. Segal, pp. 183–202. Noyes Publications: Park Ridge, NJ.

Cooper, M.A., Bernstein, I.S., Fragaszy, D.M. et al. (2001) Integration of new males into four social groups of tufted capuchins (*Cebus apella*). *International Journal of Primatology*, 22, 663–683.

Coulibaly, C., Hack, R., Seidl, J. et al. (2004) A natural asymptomatic herpes B virus infection in a colony of laboratory brown capuchin monkeys (*Cebus apella*). *Laboratory Animals*, 38, 432–438.

Daoudi, S., Badihi, G. and Buchanan-Smith, H.M. (2017) Is mixed-species living cognitively enriching? Enclosure use and welfare in two captive groups of tufted capuchins (*Sapajus apella*) and squirrel monkeys (*Saimiri sciureus*), *Animal Behavior and Cognition*, 4, 51–69.

Damas, J., Hughes, G. M., Keough, K. C. et al. (2020) Broad host range of SARS-CoV-2 predicted by comparative and structural analysis of ACE2 in vertebrates. *Proceedings of the National Academy of Sciences*, 117, 22311–22322.

Dawson, C. (2009). Environmental enrichment for mammals in captivity focusing primarily on primates. *The Plymouth Student Scientist*, 2, 184–194.

de Alvarenga, D.A.M., de Pina-Costa, A., de Sousa, T.N. et al. (2015) Simian malaria in the Brazilian Atlantic forest: first description of natural infection of capuchin monkeys (Cebinae subfamily) by *Plasmodium simium*. *Malaria Journal*, 14, 81 https://doi.org/10.1186/s12936-015-0606-6.

De Lillo, C., Palombo, M., Spinozzi, G. et al. (2011) Attention allocation modulates the processing of hierarchical visual patterns: a comparative analysis of capuchin monkeys (*Cebus apella*) and humans. *Journal of Experimental Psychology: Animal Behavior Processes*, 37, 341–352.

De Marco, A. and Visalberghi, E. (2007) Facial displays in young tufted capuchin monkeys (*Cebus apella*): appearance, meaning, context and target. *Folia Primatologica*, 78, 118–137.

de Souza Lins, P.G.A. and Ferreira, R.G. (2019) Competition during sugarcane crop raiding by blond capuchin monkeys (*Sapajus flavius*). *Primates*, 60, 81–91.

Dettmer, E. and Fragaszy, D. (2000) Determining the value of social companionship to captive capuchin monkeys (*Cebus apella*). *Journal of Applied Animal Welfare Science*, 3, 293–304.

Dettmer, E.R., Phillips, K.A., Rager, D.R. et al. (1996) Behavioral and cortisol responses to repeated capture and venipuncture in *Cebus apella*. *American Journal of Primatology*, 38, 357–362.

Di Bitetti, M.S. and Janson, C.H. (2000) When will the stork arrive? Patterns of birth seasonality in Neotropical Primates. *American Journal of Primatology*, 50, 109–130.

Di Bitetti, M.S. and Janson, C.H. (2001) Reproductive socioecology of tufted capuchins (*Cebus apella nigritus*) in northeastern Argentina. *International Journal of Primatology*, 22, 127–142.

Dufour, V., Pascalis, O. and Petit, O. (2006) Face processing limitation to own species in primates: a comparative study in brown capuchins, Tonkean macaques and humans. *Behavioural Processes*, 73, 107–113.

EAZA [European Association of Zoos and Aquaria] (2019) *EAZA Best Practice Guidelines: Capuchin Monkeys* (Sapajus *and* Cebus *sp.*) EAZA, Amsterdam.

European Directive 2010/63 (2010) European directive 2010/63 of the European Parliament and of the Council of 22 September 2010 on the protection of animals used for scientific purposes. *Official Journal of the European Union*, 276/33, https://eur-lex.europa.eu/LexUriServ/LexUriServ.do?uri=OJ:L:2010:276:0033:0079:en:PDF (accessed 10 May 2019).

Fagot, J. and Paleressompoulle, D. (2009) Automatic testing of cognitive performance in baboons maintained in social groups. *Behavior Research Methods*, 41, 396–404.

Falótico, T., Coutinho, P.H.M., Bueno, C.Q. et al. (2018) Stone tool use by wild capuchin monkeys (*Sapajus libidinosus*) at Serra das Confusões National Park, Brazil. *Primates*, 59, 385–394.

Falótico, T. and Ottoni, E.B. (2014) Sexual bias in probe tool manufacture and use by wild bearded capuchin monkeys. *Behavioural Processes*, 108, 117–122.

Fecchio, R.S., Gomes, M.S., Rossi, J.L. Jr. et al. (2008) Oral diseases in captive capuchin monkeys. *Exotic DVM*, 10, 29–34.

Ferreira, V.H.B., Da Silva, C.P.C., Fonseca, E.D.P. et al. (2018) Hormonal correlates of behavioural profiles and coping strategies in captive capuchin monkeys (*Sapajus libidinosus*). *Applied Animal Behaviour Science*, 207, 108–115.

Ferreira, R.G., Izar, P. and Lee, P.C. (2006) Exchange, affiliation, and protective interventions in semifree-ranging brown capuchin monkeys (*Cebus apella*). *American Journal of Primatology*, 68, 765–766.

Fiorello, C.V., Heard, D.J., Barnes Heller, H.L. et al. (2006) Medical management of *Toxoplasma* meningitis in a white-throated capuchin (*Cebus capucinus*). *Journal of Zoo and Wildlife Medicine*, 37, 409–412.

Fragaszy, D.M. (2005) Capuchin monkeys: enrichment for nonhuman primates. Department of Health and Human Services; NIH, Office of Laboratory Animal Welfare (OLAW). US Department of Agriculture, Animal Care.

Fragaszy, D.M. and Adams-Curtis, L.E. (1998) Growth and reproduction in captive capuchins (*Cebus apella*). *American Journal of Primatology*, 44, 197–213.

Fragaszy, D.M., Baer, J. and Adams-Curtis, L. (1994) Introduction and integration of strangers into captive groups of tufted capuchin monkeys (*Cebus apella*). *International Journal of Primatology*, 15, 399–420.

Fragaszy, D.M., Izar, P., Liu, Q. et al. (2016). Body mass in wild bearded capuchins, (*Sapajus libidinosus*): ontogeny and sexual dimorphism. *American Journal of Primatology*, 78, 473–484.

Fragaszy, D.M., Visalberghi, E. and Fedigan, L.M. (2004) *The Complete Capuchin*. Cambridge University Press, Cambridge.

Galliari C.A. (1985). Dental eruption in captive-born *Cebus apella*: from birth to 30 months old. *Primates*, 26, 506–510.

Godoy, I., Vigilant, L. and Perry, S.E. (2016) Inbreeding risk, avoidance and costs in a group-living primate, *Cebus capucinus*. *Behavioral Ecology and Sociobiology*, 70, 1601–1611.

Gros-Louis, J., Perry, S. and Manson, J.H. (2003) Violent coalitionary attacks and intraspecific killing in wild white-faced capuchin monkeys (*Cebus capucinus*). *Primates*, 44, 341–346.

Gunst, N., Boinski, S. and Fragaszy, D.M. (2010) Development of skilled detection and extraction of embedded prey by wild brown capuchin monkeys (*Cebus apella apella*). *Journal of Comparative Psychology*, 124, 194–204.

Hakeem, A., Sandoval, G.R., Jones, M. et al. (1996) Brain and life span in primates. In: *Handbook of the Psychology of Aging*, 4th edn. Eds J.E. Birren and K.W. Schaie, pp. 78–104. Academic Press, San Diego.

Hattori, Y., Kuroshima, H. and Fujita, K. (2007) I know you are not looking at me: capuchin monkeys' (*Cebus apella*) sensitivity to human attentional states. *Animal Cognition*, 10, 141–148.

Honeysett, J. (2006) Husbandry manual for brown capuchin/black-capped capuchin *Cebus apella* (Cebidae). *Sydney Institute of TAFE, Australia*.

Hsu, C.K. and Jia, R. (2003) Chinese macaques – East meets West. In: *International Perspectives: The Future of Nonhuman Primate Resources*, pp. 197–199. National Academies Press, Washington.

International Primatological Society (2007) *IPS International Guidelines for the Acquisition, Care and Breeding of Nonhuman Primates*, 2nd edn. www.internationalprimatologicalsociety.org (accessed 24 June 2019).

Janson, C., Baldovino, M.C. and Di Bitetti, M. (2012) The group life cycle and demography of brown capuchin monkeys (*Cebus [apella] nigritus*) in Iguazú National Park, Argentina. In: *Long-Term Field Studies of Primates*. Eds Kappeler, P. and Watts, D., pp. 185–214. Springer, Heidelberg.

Kenny, D.E., Knightly, F., Baier, J. *et al.* (2001) Exposure of hooded capuchin monkeys (*Cebus apella cay*) to a rabid bat at a zoological park. *Journal of Zoo and Wildlife Medicine*, **32**, 123–126.

Kishimoto, R., Iwasaki, S. and Fujita, K. (2019) Do capuchins (*Sapajus apella*) know how well they will remember? Analysis of delay length-dependency with memory strategies. *Journal of Comparative Psychology*. DOI: 10.1037/com0000164.

Koops, K., Visalberghi, E. and van Schaik, C. (2014) The Ecology of primate material culture. *Biological Letters*, **10**, 20140508. http://dx.doi.org/10.1098/rsbl.2014.0508.

Leca, J.-B., Fornasieri, I. and Petit, O. (2002) Aggression and reconciliation in *Cebus capucinus*. *International Journal of Primatology*, **23**, 979–998.

Lee, G.Y., Boyce, W.M. and Orr, K. (1996) Diagnosis and treatment of lungworm (*Filariopsis arator*; Metastrongyloidea: Filaroididae) infection in white-faced capuchins (*Cebus capucinus*). *Journal of Zoo and Wildlife Medicine*, 197–200.

Lehner, N.D.M. (1984) Biology and diseases of Cebidae. In: *Laboratory Animal Medicine*, Eds J.F. Fox, B.J. Cohen and F. Loew, pp. 321–353. Academic Press, Orlando.

Leighty, K.A., Byrne, G., Fragaszy, D.M. *et al.* (2004) Twinning in tufted capuchins (*Cebus apella*): rate, survivorship, and weight gain. *Folia Primatologica*, **75**, 14–18.

Linn, G.S., Mase, D., Lafrancois, D. *et al.* (1995) Social and menstrual cycle phase influences on the behavior of group housed *Cebus apella*. *American Journal of Primatology*, **35**, 41–57.

Ludes, E. and Anderson, J.R. (1995) Introduction d'une nouvelle femelle singe capucin (*Cebus apella*) dans un groupe en captivité. *Mammalia*, **59**, 303–313.

Lundmark, F., Berg, C., Schmid, O. *et al.* (2014) Intentions and values in animal welfare legislation and standards. *Journal of Agricultural and Environmental Ethics*, **27**, 991–1017.

Lutz, C.K. and Novak, M.A. (2005). Environmental enrichment for nonhuman primates: theory and application. *ILAR Journal*, **46**, 178–191.

Machado, G.P., de Paula Antunes, J.M.A., Uieda, W. *et al.* (2012) Exposure to rabies virus in a population of free-ranging capuchin monkeys (*Cebus apella nigritus*) in a fragmented, environmentally protected area in southeastern Brazil. *Primates*, **53**, 227–231.

Manson, J.H., Perry, S. and Parish, A.R. (1997) Nonconceptive sexual behavior in bonobos and capuchins. *International Journal of Primatology*, **18**, 767–786.

Martin, R.D. (1990) *Primate Origins and Evolution. A Phylogenetic Reconstruction*. Chapman and Hill Ltd, London.

McKinney, T. (2011) The effects of provisioning and crop raiding on the diet and foraging activities of human commensal white faced capuchins (*Cebus capucinus*). *American Journal of Primatology*, **73**, 439–448.

Melin, A. D., Janiak, M. C., Marrone, F. *et al.* (2020). Comparative ACE2 variation and primate COVID-19 risk. *Communications Biology*, **3**, 641. https://doi.org/10.1038/s42003-020-01370-w

Melin, A.D., Chiou, K.L., Walco, E.R. *et al.* (2017) Trichromacy increases fruit intake rates of wild capuchins (*Cebus capucinus imitator*). *Proceedings of the National Academy of Sciences*, **114**, 10402–10407.

Melin, A., Fedigan, L.M., Hiramatsu, C. *et al.* (2007) Effects of colour vision phenotype on insect capture by a free-ranging population of white-faced capuchins, *Cebus capucinus*. *Animal Behaviour*, **73**, 205–214.

Miller, K.E., Laszlo, K. and Suomi, S.J. (2008) Why do captive tufted capuchins (*Cebus apella*) urine wash? *American Journal of Primatology*, **70**, 119–126.

Milligan, L.A. (2010) Milk composition of captive tufted capuchins (*Cebus apella*). *American Journal of Primatology*, **72**, 81–86.

Mosdossy, K.N., Melin, A.D. and Fedigan, L.M. (2015) Quantifying seasonal fallback on invertebrates, pith, and bromeliad leaves by white-faced capuchin monkeys (*Cebus capucinus*) in a tropical dry forest. *American Journal of Physical Anthropology*, **158**, 67–77.

Nagle, C.A. and Denari, J.H. (1983) The Cebus monkey (*Cebus apella*). In: *Reproduction in New World Primates*. Ed. Hearn, J., pp. 41–67. MTP Press, Hingham.

Nagy-Reis, M.B., Mendonça-Furtado, O. and Resende, B. (2019) Do social factors related to allostatic load affect stereotypy susceptibility? Management implications for captive social animals. *Animal Welfare*, **28**, 183–190.

Napier, J.R. and Napier, P.H. (1967) *A Handbook of Living Primates: Morphology, Ecology and Behaviour of Nonhuman Primates*. Academic Press, New York and London.

National Research Council of the National Academies (2003) *Nutrient Requirements of Nonhuman Primates, Second Revised Edition*. National Academies Press, Washington, DC.

National Research Council (2011) *Guide for the Care and Use of Laboratory Animals*, 8th edn. The National Academies Press, Washington, DC.

National Research Council (2017) *NIH Policy Manual 3044-1: Nonhuman Primate Quarantine*. National Academies Press, Washington, DC.

Olsson, A.I. and Westlund, K. (2007) More than numbers matter: the effect of social factors on behavior and welfare of laboratory rodents and nonhuman primates. *Applied Animal Behaviour Science*, **103**, 229–254.

Parr, N.A., Fedigan, L.M. and Kutz, S.J. (2013) A coprological survey of parasites in white-faced capuchins (*Cebus capucinus*) from Sector Santa Rosa, ACG, Costa Rica. *Folia Primatologica*, **84**, 102–114.

Parrish, A., Agrillo, C., Perdue, B.M. *et al.* (2016) The elusive illusion: do children (*Homo sapiens*) and capuchin monkeys (*Cebus apella*) see the solitaire illusion? *Journal of Experimental Child Psychology*, **142**, 83–95.

Perry, S. (2012) The behavior of wild white-faced capuchins: demography, life history, social relationships, and communication. *Advances in the Study of Behavior*, **44**, 135–181.

Perry, S., Manson, J.H., Muniz, L. *et al* (2008) Kin-biased social behaviour in wild adult female white-faced capuchins, *Cebus capucinus*. *Animal Behaviour*, **76**, 187–199.

Phillips, K.A., Sherwood, C.C. and Lilak, A.L. (2007) Corpus callosum morphology in capuchin monkeys is influenced by sex and handedness. *PLoS ONE*, **8**, e792.

Pokorny, J.J. and de Waal, F. (2009) Face recognition in capuchin monkeys (*Cebus apella*). *Journal of Comparative Psychology*, **123**, 151–160.

Popilskis, S.J. and Kohn, D.F. (1997) Anesthesia and analgesia in nonhuman primates. In: *Anesthesia and Analgesia in Laboratory Animals*, pp. 233–255. Academic Press, New York.

Prescott, M.J., Bowell, V.A. and Buchanan-Smith, H.M. (2005) Training laboratory-housed non-human primates, part 2: Resources for developing and implementing training programmes. *Animal Technology and Welfare*, **4**, 133–148.

Prétôt, L. and Brosnan, S.F. (2019) Capuchin monkeys (*Cebus [Sapajus] apella*) show planning in a manual maze task. *Journal of Comparative Psychology*, **133**, 81–91.

Reinhardt, V. (2003) Compassion for animals in the laboratory: Impairment or refinement of research methodology? *Journal of Applied Animal Welfare Science*, **6**, 123–130.

Rennie, A.E. and Buchanan-Smith, H.M. (2006) Refinement of the use of non-human primates in scientific research. Part III: refinement of procedures. *Animal Welfare*, **15**, 239–261.

Rimpley, K. and Buchanan-Smith H.M. (2013) Reliably signalling a startling husbandry event improves welfare of zoo-housed capuchins (*Sapajus apella*). *Applied Animal Behaviour Science*, **147**, 205–213.

Riviello, M.C. (1992) Introduction of two infant capuchin monkeys (*Cebus apella*) in a captive group: analysis of their behavior. *Laboratory Primate Newsletter*, **31**, 17–18.

Roberts, J.A. and Andrews, K. (2008) Nonhuman primate quarantine: its evolution and practice. *ILAR Journal*, **49**, 145–156.

Roeder, J.-J. and Anderson, J.R. (1991) Urine washing in brown capuchin monkeys (*Cebus apella*): testing social and non-social hypotheses. *American Journal of Primatology*, **24**, 55–60.

Rondón, S., Ortiz, M., León, C. *et al.* (2017) Seasonality, richness and prevalence of intestinal parasites of three Neotropical primates (*Alouatta seniculus*, *Ateles hybridus* and *Cebus versicolor*) in a fragmented forest in Colombia. *International Journal for Parasitology: Parasites and Wildlife*, **6**, 202–208.

Ruby, S. and Buchanan-Smith, H.M. (2015) The effects of individual cubicle research on the social interactions and individual behavior of brown capuchin monkeys (*Sapajus apella*). *American Journal of Primatology*, **77**, 1097–1108.

Sabbatini, G., Stammati, M., Tavares, M.C.H. *et al.* (2006) Interactions between humans and capuchin monkeys (*Cebus libidinosus*) in the Parque Nacional de Brasilia, Brazil. *Applied Animal Behaviour Science*, **97**, 272–283.

Sabbatini, G. and Visalberghi, E. (2008) Inferences about the location of food in capuchin monkeys (*Cebus apella*) in two sensory modalities. *Journal of Comparative Psychology*, **122**, 156–166.

Sainsbury, A.W. (1991) Primates. In: *Manual of Exotic Pets*, 3rd edn. Eds P.H. Benyon and J.E. Cooper, pp. 111–121. British Small Animal Veterinary Association, Cheltenham.

Saito, A., Mikami, A., Kawamura, S. *et al.* (2005) Advantage of dichromats over trichromats in discrimination of color-camouflaged stimuli in non-human primates. *American Journal of Primatology*, **67**, 425–436.

Savastano, G., Hanson, A. and McCann, C. (2003) The development of an operant conditioning training program for New World primates at the Bronx Zoo. *Journal of Applied Animal Welfare Science*, **6**, 247–261.

Schino G., Di Giuseppe F., Visalberghi E. (2009a) Grooming, rank, and agonistic support in tufted capuchin monkeys. *American Journal of Primatology*, **71**, 101–105.

Schino G., Di Giuseppe F., Visalberghi E. (2009b) The time frame of partner choice in the grooming reciprocation of *Cebus apella*. *Ethology*, **115**, 70–76.

Schino, G., Palumbo, M. and Visalberghi, E. (2011) Factors affecting urine washing behavior in tufted capuchins (*Cebus apella*). *International Journal of Primatology*, **32**, 801–810.

Sedgwick, C.J. (1986). Scaling and anesthesia for primates. In: *Primates: The Road to Self-Sustaining Populations*. Ed. K. Benirschke, pp. 815–822. Springer-Verlag, New York.

Spagnoletti, N., Visalberghi, E., Ottoni, E. *et al.* (2011) Stone tool use by adult wild bearded capuchin monkeys (*Cebus libidinosus*). Frequency, efficiency and tool selectivity. *Journal of Human Evolution*, **61**, 97–107.

Szonyi, B., Agudelo-Flórez, P., Ramírez, M. *et al.* (2011) An outbreak of severe leptospirosis in capuchin (*Cebus*) monkeys. *The Veterinary Journal*, **188**, 237–239.

Tiddi, B., Aureli, F. and Schino, G. (2012) Grooming up the hierarchy: the exchange of grooming and rank-related benefits in a New World primate. *PLoS ONE*, **7**, e36641.

Truppa, V., Carducci, P. and Sabbatici, G. (2018) Object grasping and manipulation in capuchin monkeys (genera *Cebus* and *Sapajus*). *Biological Journal of the Linnean Society*, bly131, https://doi.org/10.1093/biolinnean/bly131.

Uher, J., Addessi, E. and Visalberghi, E. (2013) Contextualised behavioural measurements of personality differences obtained in behavioural tests and social observations in adult capuchin monkeys (*Cebus apella*). *Journal of Research in Personality*, **47**, 427–444.

Van Wolkenten, M.L., Davis, J.M., Gong, M.L. *et al.* (2006) Coping with acute crowding by *Cebus apella*. *International Journal of Primatology*, **27**, 1241–1256.

Veissier, I. and Boissy, A. (2007) Stress and welfare: two complementary concepts that are intrinsically related to the animal's point of view. *Physiology & Behavior*, **92**, 429–433.

Vining, A.Q. and Marsh, H.L. (2015) Information seeking in capuchins (*Cebus apella*): a rudimentary form of metacognition? *Animal Cognition*, **18**, 667–681.

Visalberghi, E. and Albani, A. (2014) The bearded capuchin monkeys of Fazenda Boa Vista. (DVD available upon request).

Visalberghi, E., Albani, A., Ventricelli, M. *et al.* (2016). Factors affecting cashew processing by wild bearded capuchin monkeys (*Sapajus libidinosus*, Kerr 1792). *American Journal of Primatology*, **78**, 799–815.

Visalberghi, E. and Anderson, J.R. (1993) Reasons and risks associated with manipulating captive primates' social environments. *Animal Welfare*, **2**, 3–15.

Visalberghi, E. and Riviello, M.C. (1987) The integration into a social group of a hand reared brown capuchin *Cebus apella*. *International Zoo Yearbook*, **26**, 232–236.

Visalberghi, E. and Vitale, A. (1990) Coated nuts as an enrichment device to elicit tool use in *Cebus*. *Zoo Biology*, **9**, 65–71.

Visalberghi, E., Valenzano, D. and Preuschoft, S. (2006) Facial displays in tufted capuchins (*Cebus apella*). *International Journal of Primatology*, **27**, 1689–1707.

Whitehouse, J., Micheletta, J., Powell, L.E. *et al.* (2013) The impact of cognitive testing on the welfare of group housed primates. *PLoS ONE*, **8**, e78308. https://doi.org/10.1371/journal.pone.0078308

Wilson, V., Lefevre, C.E., Morton, F.B. *et al.* (2014) Personality and facial morphology: links to assertiveness and neuroticism in capuchins (*Sapajus [Cebus] apella*). *Personality and Individual Differences*, **58**, 89–94.

Wirz, A., Truppa, V. and Riviello, M.C. (2008) Hematological and plasma biochemical values for captive tufted capuchin monkeys (*Cebus apella*). *American Journal of Primatology*, **70**, 463–472.

Wolff, P.L. (1990) The parasites of New World monkeys: a review. *Proceedings, American Association of Zoo Veterinarians*, 87–94.

Zunino, G.E. (1990) Reproducción y mortalidad de *Saimiri boliviensis* y *Cebus apella* en cautiverio. *Boletín Primatológico Latinoamericano*, **2**, 23–28.

39 Old world monkeys

Jaco Bakker, Annet L. Louwerse, Marit K. Vernes and Jan A.M. Langermans

Biological overview

General biology

Non-human primates (NHP) are divided into two groups: the Old World monkeys (OWM) (*Catarrhini*) that live in Africa and Asia, and the New World monkeys (NWM) (*Platyrrhini*) that live in South America (Figure 39.1). OWM are divided in several families, including *Cercopithecidae*, that includes more than 130 species. The living conditions in the wild range from fully terrestrial, such as most baboons, to arboreal such as colobus monkeys in a variety of climates ranging from sub-Saharan Africa to the colder regions in northern Japan. The *Cercopithecidae* are divided into two subfamilies – the *Cercopithecine* and the *Colobinae*. The *Cercopithicines* are omnivorous and have cheek pouches whereas *Colobines* are folivorous, lack cheek pouches and have more complex digestive systems. The genera in the *Cercopithecine* subfamily fall more or less into two groups: the African long-tailed monkeys (such as vervets, guenons, talapoins, and patas monkeys), and the macaques, baboons, and mangabeys. The genera of the *Colobine* subfamily are the colobine monkeys, langurs and other leaf eaters.

Cercopithecids have downward facing nostrils with a narrow nasal septum. Most have opposable thumbs, except for the genus *Colobus*, and flat nails. All *cercopithecids* have long to vestigial non-prehensile tails. They all have, in some degree, sciatic protuberances that are covered with keratinised skin patches (Casteleyn & Bakker 2021). Their facial muscles are well-developed allowing a wide range of facial expressions that are important in their social behaviour. Most live in groups that can be of varying size and among individuals a large array of complex social interactions can be observed. They are mostly diurnal.

This chapter focuses on selected species from the *Cercopithecine* subfamily which are commonly used in research, that is *Macaca mulatta* (rhesus monkey), *Macaca fascicularis* (long-tailed macaque, crab-eating macaque, or cynomolgus monkey), *Chlorocebus* sp. (formerly *Cercopithecus* sp.; Groves 2001; also called the 'African green monkey' or the 'vervet monkey') and *Papio* species (baboons).

Biological data

The use of OWM in biomedical research requires that both breeders and scientists involved in the research understand the biology and behaviour of the species with which they work. The literature on OWM biology, physiology, anatomy, ecology and behaviour is extensive from both field and laboratory studies (e.g. Roder & Timmermans 2002; Casteleyn & Bakker 2021; Overduin-de Vries *et al*. 2016; Fehlmann *et al*. 2017; Joly *et al*. 2017; Bono *et al*. 2018). OWM are highly social animals living in small to large groups. There are both costs and benefits from living in a group (Majolo *et al*. 2008). The potential negative consequences of group living such as competition for food or mates, or increased likelihood of parasitism or predation, are offset by co-operation resulting in the improved survival of individuals with shared genes (Krebs *et al*. 1993). This is achieved by living with close relatives, described as kin-bonded groups, which in OWM are typically female kin-bonded groups with the distribution of males superimposed on to that of the females.

Rhesus and cynomolgus macaques

Rhesus macaques are found in large parts of Asia, and their distribution ranges from Pakistan through India, Bangladesh, Myanmar, Thailand and Northern China in a diverse range of habitats. In densely populated areas, they can be found living closely with the human population where they can become a nuisance due to raiding of crops or stealing food from markets. They have light-brown hair, are of sturdily build and have a relatively short tail (Casteleyn & Bakker 2021). They show strong sexual dimorphism: adult males are large, can weigh approximately 8–15 kg and have pronounced canines, whereas adult females are smaller, weigh approximately 5–8 kg and lack the large canines. The median lifespan of rhesus macaques in the wild is < 15 years, but in captivity this can be much longer (Colman *et al*. 2009). Rhesus macaques are omnivores with a diverse diet, including seeds, roots, bark, fruits, plants and small insects.

Rhesus macaques are seasonal breeders. On average, the mating season starts in September and ends in January. With

---

The UFAW Handbook on the Care and Management of Laboratory and Other Research Animals, Ninth Edition.
Edited by Huw Golledge and Claire Richardson.
© 2024 John Wiley & Sons Ltd. Published 2024 by John Wiley & Sons Ltd.

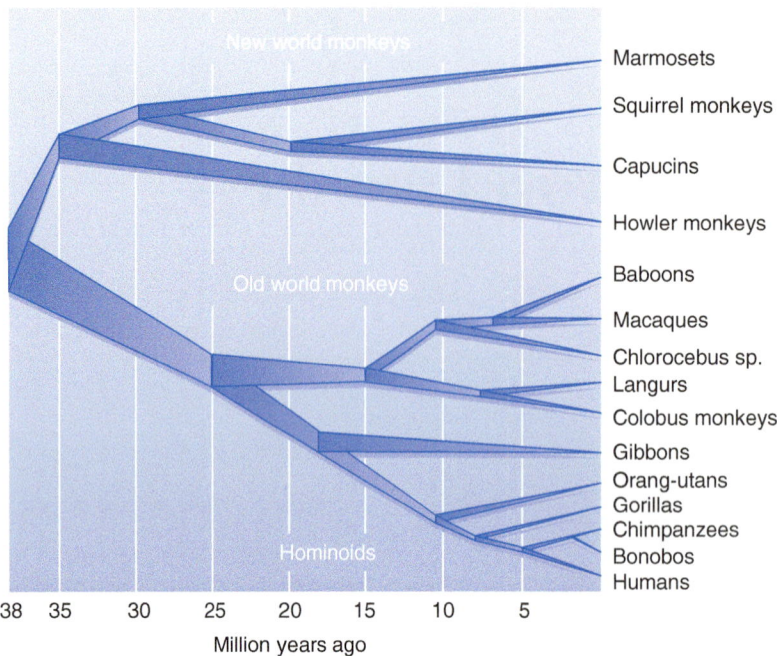

Figure 39.1 Phylogenetic tree of non-human primate evolution.

a gestation period of approximately 165 days, this leads to a birth season from March to July. During the mating season, a high-ranking male can form a consort with a fertile female, thus preventing other males to sire offspring.

Cynomolgus macaques are found in Southeast Asia (e.g. Indonesia, Philippines, Thailand, Cambodia, Vietnam, Laos and Myanmar). They live in tropical forest, preferably in the vicinity of water and are excellent swimmers. Compared to rhesus macaques, they have dark-greyish hair with thinner fur that does not shed. Newborns have black fur that during the first 6 months of their life gradually changes into the adult colour. Cynomolgus macaques have a tail that is longer than their body. Their posture resembles that of rhesus macaques, but they are smaller. Like rhesus macaques, they show sexual dimorphism, males being 5–9 kg with cheek whiskers whereas females weigh 3–6 kg and have both cheek whiskers and characteristic moustaches. The median lifespan of cynomolgus macaques in the wild is < 15 years, but in captivity can even reach 30 years. Cynomolgus macaques eat a variety of food, such as fruits, leaves, mushrooms, insects, fish and crabs.

In contrast to rhesus macaques, cynomolgus macaques are not seasonal breeders. The alpha male monopolises fertile females and sires the majority of offspring. When a new, non-related male takes over the alpha position in the group, he may kill newborn babies that he did not father (infanticide). Like in rhesus macaques, the gestation period is approximately 165 days.

Both rhesus and cynomolgus macaques are despotic species and live in large matrilineal multi-male, multi-female groups, composed of a number of females and their offspring (matrilines) and one or a few non-related adult males (of which one is the dominant (alpha) male). The number of adult females is larger than the number of adult males. The social groups are female-bonded, which means that females remain in their natal group throughout their whole life, whereas juvenile males (3–5 years old) disperse in small all-male groups (bachelor groups) to roam around and eventually integrate into new group. In this way, inbreeding is avoided.

Female dominance hierarchies are matrilinear – the high rank of a mother is passed on to her offspring, with the youngest infant being dominant over the older siblings (youngest ascendency). In this way, females from high-ranking families can defend their rank position against other group members. However, illness of a high-ranking animal or loss of female family members can result in extreme aggression as subordinate animals try to become higher-ranking. This can result in serious injuries, which in extreme cases can be fatal. To maintain a stable group in captivity, sufficient numbers of high-ranking related females must be kept present in the group in order to protect their position against the subordinate group members.

Dominance hierarchies of (sub)adult males are mainly determined by age. The older a male is, the stronger he becomes (a combination of age, bodyweight and character) which results in a higher position.

Rhesus and cynomolgus macaques communicate through vocalisation and behaviour (including body posture, and facial expressions). For example, baring teeth and giving ground indicate that an animal is submissive to the individual that receives these behaviours. Staring at an opponent, sometimes in combination with an open mouth, is aggressive (threatening) behaviour. Ears wide away from the head implies aggressive behaviour whereas raising of eyebrows (frowning or 'lifts') and lip smacking are friendly or affiliative behaviours (Lindburg 1971). When affiliative behaviours are shown, the ears are pressed flat against the head. The often observed grooming behaviour has no relation to the presence of parasites but serves to strengthen social bonding (Matheson & Bernstein 2000).

Baboons and Vervet monkeys

Other species of OWM used for research purposes are primarily baboons (genus *Papio*) and Vervet monkeys (genus *Chlorocebus*), although in Europe their use is limited.

Baboons are often just referred to as '*Papio sp.*'. It should be realised that five different species of baboons are distinguished, although there is a large overlap in genetics and behaviour (Rogers *et al.* 2019). Baboons are widespread throughout equatorial Africa and are primarily terrestrial, although olive baboons (*P. anubis*) are also found in tropical forests. The olive baboon is the most wide-ranging of all baboon species. All have dog-like muzzles, relatively short tails, large ischial callosities and cheek pouches. Baboons are omnivores, eating, for example, roots, fruits, grasses, insects, birds, and vertebrates, including other smaller NHP such as vervets. In areas where they overlap with humans, they are known to raid crops and feed on garbage. The hamadryas baboon (*P. hamadryas*) and Guinea baboon (*P. papio*) live in a harem structure in one male units, the other species live in multi-male, multi-female groups with strict dominance hierarchies based on matriline. They are sexually dimorphic, the males being up to twice as large as the females. Depending on the species, baboons vary in weight, size and coat. Weights range from 13 to 26 kg for a male Guinea baboon (*P. papio*), which is the smallest baboon species to > 40 kg for the largest baboon species, the Chacma baboon (*P. ursinus*). The coat ranges from greenish-grey to yellow-brownish/brown. In the wild, they become up to 30 years old, but they can reach an age of over 40 years in captivity. They breed throughout the year. Females show pronounced sexual swelling in the perineal area during oestrus and are fertile around 4 years of age. The gestation period is around 180 days. Female baboons are known to develop spontaneous endometriosis. Therefore, baboons are used as animal model that accurately represent the cellular and molecular changes associated with the initiation and progression of human endometriosis, which have significant potential to facilitate the development of better methods for the early detection and treatment of human endometriosis (Kondova 2021).

Vervets, also referred to as 'African green monkeys', are widely distributed in Africa. There are (at least) six different subspecies recognised but they are usually all referred to as '*Chlorocebus*' (formerly, *Cercopithicus*). There are five major subspecies, that is, *Chlorocebus aethiops* (Grivet), *C. aethiops pygerythrus* (vervet), *C. aethiops sabaeus* (Callithrix or sabaeus), *C. tantalus* (tantalus) and *C. cynosuros* (Malbrouck). The sixth subspecies, *C. djamdjamensis* (Bale mountains vervet) lives in a small area in Ethiopia. Most of the animals used in biomedical research are descendants of a small group of animals that was introduced to the Caribbean islands of St. Kitts, Nevis and Barbados some centuries ago. Males have a blue scrotal area contrasting with a red penis, weighing between 3 and 8 kg, whereas females are smaller and weigh around 2.5–5.5 kg. In the wild, they are often predated upon but in captivity they can reach ages of 20–30 years (Colman 2018). Vervets are prone to hypertension and blood pressure variations can be observed between individual animals (Rhoads *et al.* 2017). They live in multi-male/multi-female groups where females stay in their natal groups and males leave at sexual maturity, that is, at the age of 5 year. They have a linear matrilinear-based dominance hierarchy. Male dominance depends on physical strength and support of female coalitions. Dominant males display a characteristic behaviour towards subordinates by encircling them, lifting their tail and exposing their brightly coloured area around the anus and genitals to the subordinate male. Vervets are in general seasonal breeders, the season depending on the geographical location. Menstruation is often only detectable by vaginal swab and there is no cyclic perineal swelling. Females usually give birth for the first time when they are around 5 years of age. The gestation period is approximately 165 days. Babies have black coats and a pink face that will gradually change during the first three months into adult colours.

A summary of specific biological data is provided in Table 39.1.

Management of macaque breeding groups in captivity

In captivity, breeding groups should resemble the natural situation. For rhesus and cynomolgus macaques, these groups should preferably consist of a few larger families with several generations of related females and their offspring plus an unrelated adult male. Female macaques are fertile around 3 years of age. The menstrual cycle lasts around 28 days. Ovulation usually occurs 12–14 days after start of the menstruation. A male macaque is fertile around 3–4 years of age (Table 39.1). Around this age, the young, sub-adult males can be taken from their natal group and housed in small all-male groups. These males can become future alpha males. However, only after full development of secondary gender characteristics around the age of 6–7 are they able to take over the position as alpha male. In the breeding group, most (but not always all) of the offspring is fathered by the alpha male. To prevent inbreeding, the alpha male is taken from the group and replaced by another adult male when his daughters become fertile, that is, approximately 4 years after introduction into the group. Introduction of a new, unrelated adult male into a group is complex and can be accompanied by conflicts and fights resulting in (serious) injuries. Introductions should be supervised by experienced behavioural specialists. In general, it is less problematic when an adult, experienced male is introduced. Interaction with and acceptance by the females play an essential role in this introduction (Rox *et al.* 2021).

For rhesus macaques, matings occur during autumn-early winter resulting in most births during late spring–early summer. During the mating season, the skin of the face and genitals of the female become characteristically red when they ovulate (sex skin) (Casteleyn & Bakker 2021). Cynomolgus macaques have no mating season. In cynomolgus macaques, sex skin is mainly peri-anal. Rhesus macaques are so-called 'multi-mounters', not every mating results in ejaculation. In contrast, cynomolgus macaques are single-mounters and almost every mating results in ejaculation. After mating, the male and the fertile female stay together (consort formation) for a period of several hours to occasionally several days. This increases the chance that the alpha male is the father of the offspring.

Table 39.1 Biological and reproduction data.

	Rhesus macaque (Macaca mulatta)	Cynomolgus macaque (Macaca fascicularis)	Baboon (Papio sp.)	Vervet monkey (Chlorocebus sp.)
Biological data*				
Adult weight (kg)	Male 8–15 Female 5–10	Male 5–10 Female 3–8	Male 20–45 Female 10–25	Male 3–8 Female 2–5
Diploid number	42	42	42	60
Food intake (kJ/kg/day)	420 for maintenance, 523–628 for production, 840 for neonates			
Water intake	*Ad libitum*, 40–80 ml/kg daily***			
Median lifespan in captivity (years)**	20–30	20–30	20–30	11–20
Temperature (°C)	36–40	37–40	36–39	34–36#
Heart rate/min	120–180	240	75–200	100 ± 31
Blood pressure systole (mmHg)	125	125	135.	100–172#
Blood pressure diastole (mmHg)	75	75	80	
Blood volume (ml/kg)	55–80	50–96	62–65	
Respiratory rate/min	39 ± 7	39 ± 7	33 ± 7	29–34
Reproduction data				
Age at puberty	Male 3–4 years Female 2.5–3 years	Male 3–4 years Female 2.5–3 years	Male 3–6 years Female 3–4 years	Male 3–5 years Female 3–4 years
Age to breed	Male 4–6 years (full adult > 7) Female 3–5 years	Male 4–6 years (full adult > 7) Female 3–5 years	Male 7–8 years (full adult > 7) Female 4–5 years	Male 5–6 years Female 4–6 years
Gestation (days)	average 165 (146–180)	average 165 (153–179)	average 180 (164–186)	Average 165 (157–168)
Litter size (in general)	1	1	1	1
Birth weight (kg)	0.4–0.55	0.33–0.35	0.87–0.94	0.30–0.40
Average menstrual cycle (days)	28	29	33	31
Mating season	From September to January	All year around	All year around	Depending on geographical location

* Biological data for weight and lifespan differ for animals: in the wild they are lighter and become less old. Indicated ranges are from wild to animals in captivity. For baboons, weight differs per species.
** In captivity, lifespan is in general longer than in the wild. In the wild, vervets are often predated upon.
#Systolic blood pressure < 120 mm Hg is considered normotensive, > 140 hypertensive (Rhoads *et al.* 2017).
*** NRC (2003a).
#Vervets show heterothermic responses depending on season and stressors (Lubbe *et al.* 2014).

Bimanual palpation of the uterus per rectum, laparoscopy, chorionic gonadotropin level assessment in blood or urine and ultrasound are reliable methods for pregnancy diagnosis in animals, depending upon the stage of gestation (DiGiacomo & Shaughnessy 1972; Kumar *et al.* 2011).

Gestation is approximately 165 days and single births are normal. Twins are rare (1 in every 1000 births). Birth weight is between 300 and 600 g and for the first week after birth the baby remains constantly attached to the mother (Table 39.1). During the following two months, this contact quickly reduces to half the time. After one year, there is limited body contact between the young animal and its mother because by then there is usually a new baby. However, the close bond between a mother and her offspring remains. Sometimes, a newborn baby is not accepted by the mother. If this is the case, it may be possible to encourage adoption by a mother whose baby has recently died and is still lactating, but this is not often very successful. Babies can be hand-raised, but these infants will later lack the social skills that are needed when socially housed (Ljungberg & Westlund 2000).

There are considerable differences in weaning policies around the world. Weaning is usually performed to form peer groups of animals of the same age to facilitate group formation for research and commercial purposes. Some centres do not wean and leave animals in their natal groups as long as possible. According to European Directive 2010/63/EU (2010), babies should not be separated from their mother before they are at least 8 months of age. Weaning should not be considered earlier because nutritional dependency of the young animals on their mother is 8–12 months. The National Centre for the 3Rs (NC3Rs) advises not to wean before the animals are 10–14 months of age (Prescott *et al.* 2012). When young males are left in their natal group and are only removed when they would migrate in a natural situation, that is at the age of 3–4 years, they become more successful alpha males later in life (Rox *et al.* 2019). Although conflicts between males younger than 3–4 years and the alpha male might sometimes occur, this is in general not a major issue in a stable group setting. Maintaining animals in their natal groups as long as possible will provide them with more social skills and coping strategies to manage challenging situations later in life.

Birth control

There are various birth-control methods that can be used in OWM (Wallace *et al.* 2016). Hormonal, surgical and separation methods are available, but all have different behavioural and welfare implications. Males can be vasectomised or castrated under general anaesthesia. Castration results in hormonal changes resulting in diminished aggression and body hair. Castration is usually not preferred when animals may be included in research protocols. In contrast to castration, vasectomy does not result in behavioural changes as hormone production stays intact and undisturbed. Both castration and vasectomy are safe and reliable, but are definitive. Female animals can receive contraceptives, for example, by subcutaneous placement of a hormone implant, that are also used for human contraception (McDonald *et al.* 2021). The implant can be removed to restore fertility.

Marking

In both breeding groups and research, it is essential that animals can be identified. Identification must be permanent, not have an impact on normal behaviour and not result in more than momentary pain or discomfort for the animal. Microchips are the most common method. Application is relatively painless and fast. An alternative method is a tattoo with a unique number. A tattoo makes it possible to identify an animal from a certain distance. Tattooing must be done under anaesthesia with additional analgesia. Tattoos are commonly placed on the chest or upper median leg. Dye marking of fur can be used as a short-time non-permanent marker. The advantage is that one can link the dye location with the dominance rank position, which will help to distinguish families, and makes behavioural observations easier.

Transportation

Primates may be transported from the breeding colony to the research facility and may also be transported within the research facility. Transport over longer distances has been shown to have a negative impact on welfare of the animals (Wolfensohn 1997; Honess *et al.* 2004) and should be limited. See also Chapter 12: Transportation of laboratory animals. During long/mid-long-distance travels, unsedated animals must be housed in individual transport boxes and provided with sufficient water and food. Animals should only be transported by licensed transporters.

Transport of animals over short distances, for example, from one animal room to another or from a breeding pen to an experimental cage in the same facility, is preferably done without sedation. Animals can be trained to enter special transport boxes. Alternatively, animals can be sedated and transported to the new cage.

Re-housing of OWM always has a temporary negative impact on welfare of the animals due to induction of stress. After re-housing, sufficient time must be taken before the animals are included in research projects (acclimatization time). This should be at least 1 month (Honess *et al.* 2004) but preferably longer to allow the animals to become sufficiently adapted.

Use in Research

There is a particular societal concern and uncertainty over the acceptability of using NHP in research, principally because of their evolutionary proximity to human beings. It is also considered by some that they may have a greater capacity for suffering than other animals because of their more developed cognitive abilities. It is therefore particularly necessary when considering the use of NHP in research to consider the ethical issues as well as the merely practical ones. All OWM used for scientific purposes in Europe must come from purpose-bred colonies. Within the EU, from 10 November 2022 all OWM used must be at least second-generation animals born in captivity (F2 generation).

The total number of NHP used in research worldwide is not known exactly but estimated at between 1,00,000 and 2,00,000 per annum, with the majority being OWM (Carlsson *et al.* 2004). OWM are primarily used within the areas of regulatory toxicology, infectious diseases and neuroscience, but they are also used in various other translational research areas such as vision research, transplantation, and metabolic disorders (Harding 2017; Scheer 2017; Chen & Langermans 2021). OWM in research should preferably be genetically characterised. High-quality animal husbandry and optimal welfare conditions must be in place. It should be realised that variations in genetics, origin, rearing conditions and housing can have an impact on experimental results (Harding 2017) and if possible the genetic background of the animals should be included in research papers (Kilkenny *et al.* 2010). For example, for collagen induced arthritis (CIA) models, only animals which lack the MHC class I resistance marker Mamu-B26 as identified by genotyping results in a CIA-incidence of 95 % (Vierboom *et al.* 2007).

In general, the use of OWM used in Europe has been slightly declining or stabilising over the past years (Scheer 2017). In contrast, the use of NHP by the largest users of OWM, China and the USA is increasing (Cyranoski 2016; Grimm 2018). New scientific developments may lead to a further increase particularly with the development of gene-editing techniques, such as Crispr-Cas9 (Moran *et al.* 2015; Liu *et al.* 2016; Willyard 2016; Liu *et al.* 2018). Outbreaks of new diseases can also result in an increased demand for OWM as demonstrated by the SARS-CoV-2 pandemic where OWM have an essential role in vaccine development and pathogenesis studies (Rockx *et al.* 2020; Hild *et al.* 2021; Muñoz-Fontela *et al.* 2022).

Welfare assessment

Traditionally, animal welfare is focused on the exclusion of negative welfare aspects, such as pain and distress. It is now generally recognised that welfare also depends on the possibility for the animals to cope both mentally and physically with the environment in which they live. As such, the routine assessment of an animal's welfare should also include the animal's behaviour. Behaviour and changes in behaviour are the easiest, most accessible, and reliable indicator to judge animal welfare, but requires specialist knowledge of the involved species. To assess welfare, based on changes in normal behaviour, the normal behavioural pattern of the individual (and species) must be known in detail. Daily observations and registration of activity, vocalisation, use of environment and social behaviour are important tools. Use of ethograms and daily observation sheets are essential tools to assess welfare aspects. In addition, daily observation sheets can include additional clinical aspects, such as faeces consistency and appetite. Facial expressions (grimace scale) can also be used to analyse the emotional and physiological state of the animals (Descovich et al. 2017), but this is more complicated.

By combining various parameters of welfare aspects in a so-called 'animal welfare assessment grid' (AWAG), the total discomfort an animal has experienced over its life-time can be assessed (Honess & Wolfensohn 2010; Descovich et al. 2017; Descovich et al. 2019). In this way, these grids can be used to make informed decisions on re-use, rehoming, or euthanasia. Although mostly used for OWM in research, adapted grids can be used to assess welfare and management strategies for breeding colonies as well (Justice et al. 2017).

Cortisol levels can be used to determine stress level and can be measured in plasma, urine, faeces and saliva, but lag times must be well understood. Cortisol levels in saliva, faeces, urine and plasma represent a snapshot in time and may transiently be elevated or decreased with stress, activity, or illness. As an alternative to measure acute cortisol levels, hair cortisol is a reliable indicator of the long-term effects of various stressors on health disorders in OWM. The use of hair cortisol has possibilities for characterising chronic stress and evaluating husbandry management in captive populations including events like relocation (Davenport et al. 2006; Dettmer et al. 2012; Novak et al. 2013). Cortisol data must be carefully interpreted in the context of the situation. Whereas increased levels of cortisol can reflect increased stress (acute or chronic), they can in some cases also be associated with positive affective states (Ralph Tilbrook 2016).

Most laboratory NHP are housed for life in the breeding colonies of primate centres or are euthanised at the end of a study. However, sometimes it is possible to rehome NHP to specialised sanctuaries after their use in research. Rehoming and relocation of OWM is not a trivial issue and can only be done when a good quality of life for the animals is guaranteed. Reliable welfare assessment procedures form a major part to decide if an animal can be rehomed. The suitability for an animal to be rehomed needs to include the complete life history of the individual animal and its character. The balance between potential negative welfare aspects (e.g. introduction to a new group of conspecifics, a new environment and a new staff) and the quality of life after relocation must be considered in the decision to rehome animals.

Housing, husbandry, and enrichment

A good guideline for housing requirements for OWM as laboratory animals is provided by appendix A of EU Directive 2010/63 (2010), and these are a mandatory minimum requirement for EU member countries. This document describes general issues regarding the housing of these animals, such as ventilation, temperature, humidity, light and noise, but also specific issues such as minimum cage dimensions (Table 39.2). Also, NC3Rs provides guidelines for housing of macaques (NC3Rs 2017).

OWM are social animals, and individual housing is likely to result in failure to cope, which can lead to the development of abnormal behaviour, increased stress levels and affect research outcomes. Animals should only be single housed temporarily and only if there are compelling reasons, such as very specific (short-term) experimental actions. Reducing the incidence of aggressive encounters by resorting to long-term single housing of animals is not acceptable; the environment and group composition needs to be actively managed to ensure maintenance of social stability. A key component in a successful strategy is to start with the right compatible grouping, which may require coordination and effective communication with the source breeding facility. Because social housing is essential, it is sometimes necessary to introduce unknown animals to each other, for example, when an animal in pair-housing dies, when animals start to

Table 39.2 Housing Requirements Research Facility.

	Macaques (Macaca mulatta and fascicularis)	Vervet monkeys (Chlorocebus sp.)	Baboon (Papio sp.)
Housing requirements			
Minimum size enclosure (m^2)	2.0	2.0	7.0 (4.0 if < 4 years)
Minimum volume enclosure (m^3)	3.6	3.6	12.6 (7.2 if < 4 years)
Minimum volume per animal (m^3) research	1.8 (1.0 if < 3 years)	1.8 (1.0 if < 3 years)	6.0 (3.0 if < 4 years)
Minimum cage height for research (m)	1.8	1.8	1.8
Minimum volume per animal (m^3) breeding	3.5	3.5	12.0
Minimum cage height for breeding	2.0	2.0	2.0
Temperature (research facility) (°C)	16–25 (Mm) 21–28 (Mf)	16–25	16–28
Humidity (research facility)	40–70%	40–70%	40–70%

fight and need to be separated or when new animals arrive at the facility. Introduction of unfamiliar animals must be done by staff with extensive behavioural knowledge and the experience to estimate the course of introduction. The duration of the stay of the animals is relevant: the longer they stay in the experimental setting the more important it is to house them in an environment that satisfies their needs.

The best enrichment for OWM is therefore social enrichment, that is, group housing. Although group housing resembling natural conditions would be best, this is usually not possible in research settings. In general, in research facilities animals are housed in same-sex groups. Animals should be at least pair-housed, but when possible larger groups are even more enriching.

Cages are usually constructed of metal with wire mesh walls, or metal bars. Metal is easy to clean but materials that are warmer to the touch, chewable and which provide a quieter environment than the clanking of metal cages are preferable. Structural division of space in primate enclosures is important, with some form of visual barrier. Both space and complexity of the cages must be adequate to prevent intimidation by cage mates. It is essential that animals should be able to utilise as much of the enclosure as possible and have high perches. Environmental enrichment must be in place. Foraging is a natural and desirable behaviour which should occupy a significant part of daily activity budget, reducing boredom and the incidence of stereotypic behaviours. Therefore, a substrate such as woodchips or sawdust should be provided in which forage can be scattered. Hay, straw or other material such as shredded paper may be provided for additional environmental enrichment, adding complexity. It is also important that visual barriers and escape routes are included to allow the animals to be out of sight of each other and to get away from the dominant individual. Separation of animals should be possible. Therefore, cages should have a separate location, such as a balcony box, where the animals can be trained individually.

As described earlier, OWM are omnivores although the different species can have different preferences (national research council, 2003). In captivity, the main source of food is commercially available pellets, that contain all necessary nutrients. Analysis of wild primate activity budgets have shown that more time is given to foraging than to any other activity (Lindburg 1991), and arguably food gathering is the most profoundly affected activity of a captive existence. Therefore, it is advisable to have several feeding times during the day in which fruits, vegetables and grains can be offered. It is advisable to limit the amount of sugar-rich food. To further stimulate foraging behaviour, herbs and grains can be distributed in the bedding. Regular tap water is provided *ad libitum* with drinking bottles or automatic drinking systems, unless there are compelling reasons to restrict access. If water restriction is required by researchers (e.g. to motivate animals to perform complex tasks, such as in neurophysiological studies) consideration should be given to reducing the restriction by training and providing different rewards and reward schedules (Gray *et al.* 2019).

OWM that are kept in the laboratory should have a 12 h/12 h light/dark cycle, preferably with simulated dawn and dusk lighting. If possible, rooms should have windows to have access to natural light. However, if this is not possible, electric light with a comparable light spectrum as the sun can be used.

General housing conditions are summarised in Table 39.2.

Environmental enrichment is essential for captive OWM to meet their ethological and psychological needs and it should provide the animals with the opportunity to carry out a sufficiently varied daily programme of activity (Lutz & Novak 2005; Coleman & Novak 2017). Optimal enrichment programmes must be able to reduce stress, to minimise abnormal behaviour and to ensure physical health. See also Chapter 10: Environmental enrichment: animal welfare and scientific validity. The principle of good welfare is that each animal should have the opportunity to display its species-specific behaviour. In addition to social enrichment, environmental enrichment can consist of food or non-food enrichment, both used to stimulate natural behaviours. The availability of well-aimed enrichment items may prevent development of abnormal or stereotypic behaviour. Examples of enrichment items and regimes are described by Vernes and Louwerse (2010). When using a radio, it should be taken into account that the music serves as background noise, preventing startled reactions when other sounds are present. OWM are naturally inquisitive. To stimulate investigative play and social behaviours, different toys and objects can be provided, such as mirrors, teethers, rattles and food puzzles, or old books and magazines that the animals can tear and shred. To maintain interest, items must be changed and rotated regularly. Enrichment items must be regularly evaluated to confirm that they are used and effective in their serving their purpose. Care must be taken that enrichment items are safe, provided in a responsible way and are cleaned regularly. To prevent obesity or development of diabetes because of overfeeding, one should realise that food enrichment could be a source of high caloric food. Environmental enrichment, or the lack of it and any potential effect on the quality of the research, should be considered in the ethical reviews.

Environment and hygiene

Housing of OWM and research activities can have an impact on the environment. This includes protection of the environment against pathogens and genetically modified organisms (GMO). Care must be taken that all activities meet the requirements of local legislation.

OWM can be carriers of zoonotic pathogens (see the following text). Contact with faeces, body fluids such as blood and urine and with cleaning water against bare skin or mucous membranes must be prevented. Protective clothing should be worn when handling the animals or cleaning the holding rooms and cages.

Laboratory procedures

Handling

Training animals with positive reinforcement training (PRT) to co-operate with scientific, veterinary and husbandry procedures helps to reduce the stress that may be caused to both the animal and the laboratory staff. PRT has significant benefits for animal welfare, science and staff, especially when combined with appropriate socialisation, habituation and desensitisation. PRT can be used to train OWM, even when living in large social groups. However, staff must first be trained to communicate and interact positively with OWM through recognition and interpretation of primate communication, and to help the primates to respond positively to humans through habituation and socialisation. Establishment of a positive relationship between humans and the animals is a first step to reduce stress during daily routine procedures. This can easily be reached by, for example, handfeeding of the animals and keeping a relaxed and positive approach in a consistent way. All staff–animal interactions should be based on an understanding of species-typical behaviour patterns and communication systems, such that these are interpreted correctly and responded to appropriately. OWM are not domesticated animals and contact with humans can be stressful, especially where the OWM are not in control of the level and intensity of that contact, which is a particular problem in the laboratory. Habituating and socialising captive primates to the presence (sight, sound, smell) and behaviour of humans as early as possible in their lives is essential. This reduces fear or distress animals may experience when confronted with new situations. It can also facilitate handling, restraint and training of animals, and may reduce the experienced stress level and even the need for sedation (Reinhardt et al. 1995; Reinhardt 2003; Honess & Marin 2006b; Rennie & Buchanan-Smith 2006). This is additional to the training required for primates to carry out specific tasks in some areas of research. It allows staff to observe behaviour patterns which are relatively unaffected by their own presence, and this helps them to assess the welfare of the animals more effectively.

Training methods should primarily be based on PRT, which rewards desired behaviour, although a careful combination of positive reinforcement and negative reinforcement training can be an alternative method when there is a time constraint (Wergard et al. 2015). See also Chapter 15: The use of PRT techniques to enhance the care and welfare of laboratory and research animals. Training is recommended as essential practice to improve the care and use of OWM and various techniques for optimal training procedures have been described (Schapiro et al. 2003; Westlund 2015; Prescott 2016).

For some experimental procedures, conscious free-roaming animals are required. The use of a 'restraint' cage in which the back is pulled gently forward (squeeze cage) can be used to manipulate an animal, for example, to allow injections. However, this procedure is quite stressful and should therefore be used as little as possible, or at least as gentle as possible. Animals can be trained to present body parts for injection or blood sampling to avoid the need to use a squeeze-back mechanism (Sauceda & Schmidt 2000; Reinhardt 2003). Primate chairs are regularly used to support primates in a sitting position when it is deemed necessary to restrain conscious primates for prolonged periods, such as for electrophysiological recording within the central nervous system (CNS) or chronic infusion when they may be required to remain in one position for several hours. An overview of various approaches has been provided by McMillan et al. (2017). The use of pole-and-collar systems to transfer the animal into a primate chair or transport device is very stressful for the animals and in some countries not allowed. If possible, it should be avoided. Animals can be trained using PRT to voluntarily enter a primate chair or transport device (Mason et al. 2019).

Manual restraint should be avoided as much as possible. When conscious animals must be manually handled, the upper arms of the monkey just above the elbow should be grasped and then held behind its back so that its elbows almost touch.

Netting should only be used when there are no other possibilities or when animals escape from their enclosure and cannot be caught in any other way.

Administration of substances

The drug to be administered and its administration route are determined to a great extent by the objectives of the procedure concerned. If possible, animals should be trained to co-operate with the procedures by PRT. Recommendations for maximum dosing volumes for the various routes are listed in Turner et al. (2011). Post-administration monitoring can be needed.

Oral dosing can be accomplished by incorporating drugs into a favourite food item. However, OWM are adept at picking out the drug or eating around it. Depending on the compound, drugs can be more readily accepted when mixed into syrup. OWM can quite easily be trained to take syrup from a syringe. This oral dosing method has minimal impact on the animal. Unpalatable drugs can be given to a sedated monkey through an orogastric tube.

Subcutaneous (SC) injections are best administered under the dorsal cervical area into the loose skin above the shoulders. Intramuscular (IM) injections are usually given into the quadriceps muscle mass on the anterior thigh, into the left or right quadriceps femoris. Care must be taken that compounds are not injected directly into the circulation. Intravenous (IV) injections should be performed into the cephalic or saphenous vein. These are preferred over the femoral vein as the neighbouring femoral artery can be injected accidentally. Surgical implantation of a vascular access port (VAP) is an alternative for long-term IV dosing. The port is implanted subcutaneously, usually high on the back between the shoulder blades or in a limb. OWM can be trained with PRT to present their port for injections or sampling. The vascular system can also be accessed through a tether system consisting of a backpack pump allowing continuous infusion.

Administration into or sampling of cerebrospinal fluid (CSF) can be performed by lumbar (Turner et al. 2011) or suboccipital-intrathecal injection or puncture (Clingerman et al. 2010).

Sampling methods

A mature healthy animal has an estimated average blood volume of 7% of the body weight in grams. A typical rule of thumb is that for each blood withdrawal, 10% of the blood volume can be taken from an OWM with minimal adverse effects with a maximum withdrawal of 15% of total blood volume per month. Blood samples can easily be obtained from percutaneous venipuncture of the femoral vein (or artery) of monkeys using a vacutainer blood collection system. The skin of the femoral triangle must be shaved and cleaned subsequently with a disinfectant. The needle should be introduced just medial to the femoral pulse to obtain a sample from the vein because the anatomy is such that the vein is most medial, then the artery and then the nerve. After the sample is taken, firm pressure needs to be applied to the sample site to minimise haemorrhage risk. Other collection sites include the cephalic and saphenous veins. When numerous blood samples are required over a long period (weeks-months), placement of a VAP is preferable to multiple venipunctures. The VAP can be maintained for many months as long as sterile techniques are strictly adhered to and an anticoagulant is used to fill the VAP after each use (Graham et al. 2009; Mutch et al. 2018).

Urine samples can be collected by cystocentesis, placement of a urinary catheter or free-catch. Unfortunately, most animals urinate during the restraint procedure which results in an empty bladder. When performing cystocentesis, it must be ensured that the urine bladder is filled with urine by ultrasonography or manual palpation. After disinfecting the abdomen, the needle should enter perpendicular to the abdomen just cranial to the pubic bone to withdraw the urine. Placing a urinary catheter is challenging in females as the female urethra opens ventrally into the vagina. This opening, the ostium urethrae externum, forms the border between the actual vagina and the vestibulum vaginae (Casteleyn & Bakker 2021). For males, the urinary bladder can be reliably and reproducibly catheterised with minimal complications (Wickham et al. 2011). This may even be performed without sedation on thoroughly conditioned animals. A metabolism cage or a collection pan under the cage, that has a wire grid which separates urine and faeces, can be used to collect urine (free-catch). A major disadvantage of free-catch urine is the need for social isolation when urine from a particular individual animal is needed. When regular urine samples are needed for a longer time period, training the animals to provide urine should be considered.

Sperm samples are used for both research and colony management, such as determination of viruses or screening of male fertility. To obtain semen or sperm samples, various methods of electro ejaculation are used (Settlage & Hendrickx 1974; Gould & Mann 1988; Ma et al. 2016). In general, these have to be performed under anaesthesia. Where possible, the use of non-invasive methods, such as masturbatory ejaculates, should be used (Thomsen 2014).

Surgically implanted telemetric devices can be used in OWM to collect cardiovascular, blood pressure, temperature and locomotion data or to record electrocardiograms, electromyograms and electroencephalograms (Kinter & Johnson 1998). Telemetry benefits both science and animal welfare because it can sample data from free ranging and awake animals and provide indicators of animal well-being and can be used for earlier recognition of humane endpoints. However, telemetry can require invasive procedures such as implantation surgery, single housing or use of jackets, which can cause pain and distress. Telemetry is often considered as refinement, but care must be taken that the benefits outweigh any potential discomfort by the technique used (Rennie & Buchanan-Smith 2006). After implantation of telemetry devices, animals need to be allowed to recover separately during the immediate post-operative period, but surgically treated animals can be pair- or group-housed soon after recovery.

Infrared thermography can sometimes be used to assess body temperature in a non-invasive way (Laffins et al. 2017).

Anaesthesia and analgesia

Ketamine hydrochloride is the most frequently used chemical restraint for OWM. After IM injection of 10 mg/kg, peak effects are reached in 5–10 minutes and duration of sedation is approximately 30 minutes. However, the disadvantages of ketamine are poor muscle relaxation, grasping movements of limbs and hands, and a marked increase in salivation. In addition, ketamine has been associated with muscle damage in NHP. Therefore, ketamine is combined with medetomidine (with medetomidine reversed with atipamezole afterwards). This regime usually provides about 30–45 minutes of anaesthesia. Concurrent use of medetomidine reduces the amount of ketamine required (to 5 mg/kg), induces additional analgesia, causes less damage to muscle tissue at injection sites compared to ketamine alone as well as limits increased muscle tone and salivation. An important advantage is the quick recovery to normal function following reversal of medetomidine with the specific antagonist atipamezole.

Ketamine administered as anaesthetic induction allows placement of a tracheal tube followed by inhalation anaesthesia or propofol IV (5–10 mg/kg, intermittent bolus administration) to maintain anaesthesia. To prevent the occurrence of laryngospasm with intubation, the larynx is sprayed with a local anaesthetic, such as lidocaine spray. The advantages of propofol are the rapid return of consciousness after ending propofol administration, minimal residual effects on the CNS and a decreased incidence of post-operative nausea and vomiting (Short & Bufalari 1999; Stoelting & Miller 2000). Isoflurane and sevoflurane are most commonly used in OWM as inhalation anaesthetics.

During surgeries, it is recommended to monitor vital parameters such as rectal body temperature, blood haemoglobin oxygen saturation level (SpO_2) and end-tidal carbon dioxide levels. A heating blanket or patient warming system can be used to maintain core body temperature during surgeries. Warmed intravenous fluids are also helpful to maintain body temperature and to maintain physiological stability. This will assist the quality of the animal's recovery.

Animals should be allowed to recover in proximity to others from their social group, not in social isolation. Care must be taken that the animals cannot hurt themselves during the recovery period. If surgery involves producing neurological lesions, the home area may need to be adapted to take account of any possible long-term side effects. If single housing following surgery is needed, individual animals should have visual, auditory and, if possible, tactile contact with other monkeys.

Analgesics must be given for all procedures that are known to cause pain in humans, pre- and post-operatively. Analgesia can be provided with opioids or non-steroidal anti-inflammatory drugs (NSAID). Selection of the appropriate regime (dosage and frequency of administration and choice of analgesic) will depend on the expected pain level. Combinations of analgesics (opioids and NSAIDs) are standard (multimodal analgesia).

Euthanasia

Euthanasia is required if animals are found to experience an unacceptable level of pain, stress, or distress (specified humane endpoints) or when the project requires pathology or histology examination of organs or tissues, or when an animal has reached the end of the study. On a deeply sedated animal (e.g. ketamine 15 mg/kg IM), an intravenous or intracardial injection of pentobarbital 70–100 mg/kg is the only acceptable method for the euthanasia. It should be taken into account that an overdose of pentobarbital causes tissue artefacts on histology (Grieves et al. 2008). Animals must not be euthanised in their home cage or in presence of their cage- and roommates.

After euthanasia and necropsy, tissues can be stored in biobanks. Establishing NHP biobanks and data exchange networks is one means of coordinating, optimising, reducing and refining primate use. In the USA, Primate Info Net achieves this objective and in Europe, a biobank set up by EUPRIM-Net is offered through various primate centres.

Common welfare and health issues

Welfare

Common welfare problems include injuries due to suboptimal housing conditions, social incompatibility and the presence of stereotypic and/or self-injurious behaviours. Housing in incompatible pairs or groups can result in conflicts and lead to physical injuries or psychological stress. Incompatible housing conditions can even add more stress than single housing, for example when an individual is being chased around on a regular basis or when animals do not sleep together. To explore the compatibility of a pair or a group, behavioural observations should be made after group formation and whenever signals of agitation are present. Behavioural observations should always be carried out at various times throughout the day. When animals are injured due to social incompatibility, it is important to immediately observe the behaviour of the pair or group. This should include observations on aggressive and submissive behaviour, and determination of possible change in dominance hierarchy. Observations should also include sharing of food, grooming and other affiliative behaviours. Social interactions should be observed throughout the day. The use of a camera system can give insight in the behaviour of the animals without a bias due to human presence and disturbance. If this is not possible, the animals must be very well-habituated to the observer. Based on the observations, further actions can be taken if needed to optimise the housing conditions or group composition. For instance, if a dominant individual refrains from further aggression after a submissive animal shows submissive behaviours, it can be decided to maintain the same social structure.

When an animal needs to be taken out of the social group for a longer time period, the rank of the individual should be taken into account to decide if and when the animal can be reintroduced. In case of dominant individuals, one needs to be sure that the individual is not weakened to prevent hierarchy challenges and additional injuries.

The presence of stereotypic and self-injurious behaviour is a negative welfare indicator and must be immediately addressed. The intensity of the issue should be examined, and the triggers identified. A camera system can be very helpful in determining these aspects. When individuals show these behaviours throughout the day, without any identifiable cause, rearrangements in the housing situation and extra enrichment opportunities might be the solution. When an animal only shows these behaviours in the presence of humans, time should be invested in more and better habituation to people, in order to reduce these behaviours. When none of the measures to limit serious stereotypic behaviour or self-injury are successful, euthanasia should be taken into consideration.

Health

The first step in assessment of the monkey's health status is to observe the animal in its home cage and evaluate its appearance, behaviour, and general demeanour. Experience is required to be able to judge whether the animal is exhibiting a normal behavioural repertoire (NC3R 2017). Individual OWM exhibit individual behavioural patterns.

A sedated physical examination gives attention to evidence of diarrhoea, nasal or ocular discharge, condition of the respiratory and cardiovascular system, major organs inside the abdomen, condition of the skin and haircoat, lymph nodes and inspection of the dentistry. Body condition Score (BCS) should be assessed. BCS uses palpation of key anatomic features such as hips, spine, pelvis, thorax and abdomen (Clingerman & Summers 2005; Clingerman & Summers 2012) (Figure 39.2). Blood samples can be taken for haematology and clinical chemistry (Table 39.3).

Haematological and biochemical reference values depend in part on age, origin of the animals and method of analysis as described for various OWM (Schuurman et al. 2004; Schuurman & Smith 2005; Wolfensohn & Peters 2005; Liddie et al. 2010). Although these values can be well used as a guide, it must be realised that there might be differences in values for animals from different origin. Standard reference values must be validated for each colony and the equipment for analysis.

Injuries

The most common non-infectious health problems of OWM are injuries caused by aggressive encounters. Use of a subcuticular suturing pattern is recommended when closing incisions as monkeys are known to pull sutures out. Adequate perioperative analgesia is mandatory. In general, OWM remove bandaging themselves or it is removed by cage mates. Care must be taken to avoid conflicts that may be caused by weakening due to long absence of a reintroduced animal.

Animals can also become injured when cages are poorly maintained. A good maintenance program for the housing facility is therefore essential.

Infectious diseases

A short summary of infectious problems in OWM is provided in the following text. More details can be found in various reports (Owen 1992; Wolfe-Coote 2005; Balansard et al. 2019).

All described infectious diseases are zoonotic. Macaques are the natural host for herpes B virus. B-virus infection is characterised by lifelong infection with intermittent reactivation and

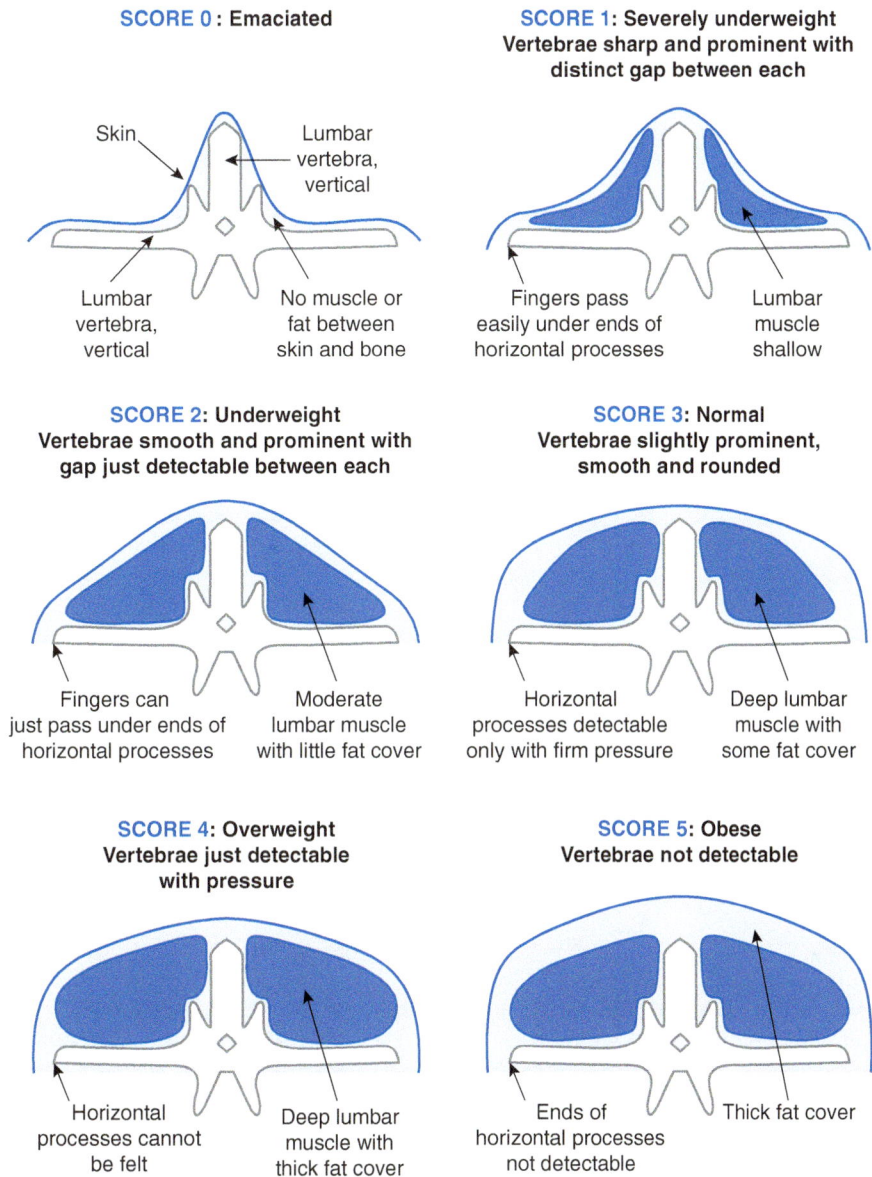

Figure 39.2 Condition score vertebrae (adapted from Wolfensohn, *The UFAW Handbook on the Care and Management of Laboratory and Other Research Animals, Eight Edition*).

shedding of the virus in saliva or genital secretions, particularly during periods of stress or immunosuppression. Infection can be transmitted via bites, scratches, sexual contact or contact with faeces, urine and other bodily fluids containing blood from an infected animal. Viraemia is intermittent and does not always coincide with the presence of clinical signs of infection. Infection is usually asymptomatic, but clinical signs include conjunctivitis, and vesicular lesions on the oral or genital mucosa. Animals are considered Herpes B positive when they have a positive antibody test or when they are housed together with seropositive animals. During periods of latency, antibody titers may decrease to a level below the detection limits of serological assays. Therefore, serial testing of an animal is advised. PCR on tissue from the buccal cavity can provide additional information, provided that the virus is being shed at the time of sampling. Transmission to humans is usually through bites and scratches from infected animals or through urinal or faecal splash into the eye. Human infection is rare but if untreated can be lethal.

Infections with immunosuppressive retroviruses [i.e., Simian Immunodeficiency virus (SIV), simian type D retrovirus (SRV) and simian T lymphotropic virus (STLV)] appear to have minor or no clinical signs in OWM. However, since these viruses affect the immune system, it is essential that the viral status of the animals is known. Transmission of immunosuppressive retroviruses occurs through direct contact between infected and susceptible animals, or indirectly through contact with contaminated bedding or equipment. Transplacental transmission is possible in females that are viraemic during pregnancy. SIV is not naturally present in wild populations of Asian macaques but can be present in African monkey, that is, vervets and baboons.

Table 39.3 Haematological and biochemical reference values for Macaques*.

Haematological reference values	Macaca mulatta	Macaca fascicularis
RBC ($\times 10^{12}$/L)	4.7–6.5	4.7–7.5
Hb (mmol/L)	7.0–9.2	6.5–8.8
WBC ($\times 10^9$/L)	3.4–21.0	4.3–24.2
Neutrophils (%)	14.1–90.5	44.8–95.0
Lymphocytes (%)	4.5–78.0	5–44
Eosinophils (%)	0–3.7	0–3.2
Monocytes (%)	0–8.2	1.5–10.9
Basophils (%)	0–0.7	0–0.04
Platelets ($\times 10^9$/L)	132–578	189–544
Biochemical reference values		
Serum protein (g/L)	58.2–74.6	58.9–81.5
Albumin (g/L)	35.6–48.5	3.8
Glucose (mmol/L)	1.9–6.0	0.22–7.0
Ureum (mmol/L)	4.2–10.5	2.9–11.0
Creatinine (umol/L)	31.5–68.4	22.1–104
Total bilirubin (umol/L)	0.07–3.3	0.0–3.1
Cholesterol (mmol/L)	1.7–5.7	0.8–5.5
ASAT (U/L)	10.8–73.4	11.6–62.6
ALAT (U/L)	8.0–59.9	0.0–102.2
LDH (U/L)	115–866	114.9–1150.7
Iron (umol/L)	6.4–32.9	9.1–36.4

* Data obtained from standard colony at the Biomedical Primate Research Centre (BPRC, Rijswijk, The Netherlands).

Simian Foamy Viruses are highly prevalent in OWM, approaching 100% prevalence in many populations. They are non-pathogenic but can interfere with studies requiring the growth or maintenance of cell cultures and transplant studies because of their cytolytic effects.

Measles belong to the infections that are highly dangerous for OWM colonies. Measles infections in colonies of macaques are generally the result of transmission from care staff to animal. Transmission occurs by aerosols or direct contact with secretions. Clinical signs in OWM generally appear approximately a week after infection and are similar to those seen in humans. The predominant signs being a papular skin rash, conjunctivitis, blepharitis, nasal and ocular discharge, and malaise. Sometimes, the infection will progress to depression, anorexia and even death (Willy et al. 1999). A major problem is the long-lasting immunosuppression that is induced by measles infection. Preventive measures are avoiding exposure to potentially infected humans or vaccination of the animals. Available human combinated vaccines against measles, mumps and rubella can be used.

Due to their zoonotic and anthroponotic potential, *Mycobacterium tuberculosis* and *M. bovis* are always of great concern (Panarella & Bimes 2010; Matz-Rensing et al. 2015). These infections induce serious diseases in OWM, resulting in death. The primary route of transmission is through the respiratory tract. The clinical symptoms of tuberculosis are usually not striking until the disease is in an advanced stage. The most common observed signs are coughing, dyspnoea, lethargy, and weight loss. Both latent and active infection can occur. In general, yearly screening is done by an intradermal tuberculin skin test (TST), commonly in the skin of the eyelid close to its margin using Mammalian Old Tuberculin (MOT) or *M. bovis* Purified Protein Derivative (PPD). Also, more specific tests can be used, such as enzyme-linked immunosorbent assay (ELISA) tests to detect antibodies or interferon-gamma release assays (IGRA) (Vervenne et al. 2004; Lyashchenko et al. 2007; Ravindran et al. 2014). Given the complexity in diagnosing Mycobacterial infection, all positive TST results should be investigated further. False positive results can be obtained in animals infected with other mycobacteria, such as *M. avium*. Thoracic radiography is not the first choice as pulmonary lesions are not specific for tuberculosis and may not be apparent very early in the course of the disease (Skoura et al. 2015). Staff working with OWM should be screened regularly for the disease.

Diarrhoea is a critical problem for breeders of captive NHP as it results in significant levels of morbidity and death annually. Diarrhoea is thought to be caused by a combination of factors such as infectious organisms, environment, genetics, husbandry, stress and nutrition. However, idiopathic chronic diarrhoea is often reported. Stress after relocation or due to changes in social hierarchy can cause subclinical infections to become clinical. Some organisms can cause explosive outbreaks of disease and death if not controlled immediately. *Escherichia coli*, *Shigella sp*, *Campylobacter* sp. and *Yersinia sp.* are common bacterial pathogens, and protozoa such as *Entamoeba histolytica*, *E. dispar*, *Balantidium coli* and *Giardia sp.* or *Cryptosporidium parvum* or helminth parasites may also pose a risk to develop diarrhoea. Due to the intermittent or low-level excretion of some organisms, regular faecal screening and timely treatment reduce the level of infection. This must be combined with strict hygiene and good husbandry to prevent transmission between OWM and with caretakers. Supportive treatment, like fluid and electrolyte replacement, are essential in cases of severe diarrhoea. Pest control policies for insects, rodents, birds, and other wildlife are important biosecurity measures in preventing the transmission of these organisms to OWM colonies. Protozoa, in low numbers, can be considered part of the normal gut flora, causing no adverse effect but in higher numbers, particularly in immunocompromised individuals intermittent to severe diarrhoea may be seen. Therefore, in apparently healthy animals, treatment is usually not required or recommended but in debilitated animals, treatment is indicated.

Various helminth species including Strongyloides and Trichuris can affect OWM. *Trichuris trichiura* is a common intestinal nematode parasite of OWM, infecting the large intestine and cecum. Pathogenesis commonly involves anaphylactic-type reactions and ischemic necrosis, both limited to tissue where adult worms reside. Signs range from subclinical to profuse watery diarrhoea, lethargy, weight loss and dehydration. Infection is detected by examination of faecal samples for parasite eggs. Because of its ability to persist in the external environment and the direct faecal–oral route of transmission, treatment, and control of *T. trichiura* by hygiene measures and antihelminthic treatment is essential.

Special consideration should be given to *Echinococcus multilocularis*. Echinococcus is only considered a risk if primates have access to outdoor enclosures, allowing possible contact with infected foxes in areas where this parasite is endemic. However, Echinococcosis can occur a long time after import from an endemic area. Serological, PCR screening and ultrasonography is possible (Rehmann *et al.* 2005).

Lung mites (*Pneumonyssus simicola*) can sometimes be diagnosed in macaques imported from regions of the world where the mites are still endemic. A single treatment with ivermectin is sufficient to kill the mites (Joseph *et al.* 1984).

Endocrine disorders

NHP can become ill due to a variety of endocrine disorders. However, naturally occurring endocrinologic disorders in NHP are rare (Bakker & de la Garza, 2022). In most cases, no clinical signs are noted and on gross pathology, the endocrine organs are unremarkable. The diagnosis is frequently made as incidental findings after standard histological examination.

The most reported, naturally occurring pancreatic disorder in OWM is diabetes mellitus (DM). Especially, cynomolgus macaques are known to develop spontaneous DM (Wagner *et al.* 2006; Hansen & Tigno 2007; Harwood *et al.* 2012). The majority of OWM diabetes cases are Type 2 DM (T2DM), which is characterised by normal glucose tolerance followed by insulin resistance (IR), a compensatory increase in insulin secretion, and deterioration of carbohydrate metabolism. T2DM is associated with increased age, with its onset mostly during middle age. Approximately 30% of cynomolgus macaques >15 years of age have basal and/or postprandial hyperinsulinemia and may also exhibit impaired glucose tolerance. The development of T2DM shows few symptoms in its earliest stages. In overweight macaques, a long-term pre-diabetic state is demarcated by increased insulin levels and enhanced beta cell responsiveness. Other types of DM are rare in macaques. Type 1 DM is sometimes diagnosed in infant and sub-adult animals. Gestational diabetes, characterised by elevated glucose and insulin levels during pregnancy, is usually a mild disease requiring no human intervention. In most cases, the animal reverts to normoglycemia postpartum.

Animals drinking the urine of the DM animal is suggestive of the presence of DM. Clinically, macaques with DM exhibit polydipsia, polyuria, weight loss, polyphagia, and lethargy. Regardless of type of diabetes, fasting serum hyperglycaemia is the most common diagnostic tool. Elevated blood glucose values under anaesthesia may be dismissed as an artefact of capture, restraint or anaesthesia. Laboratory tests should include a complete blood count, serum chemistry, fructosamine and haemoglobin A1c (HbA1c). For macaques, normal fasting serum glucose levels of 2.7–4.1 mmol/L are described as normal, and a fasting serum glucose level > 5.6 mmol/L as hyperglycaemia. Because of the inconsistent findings of glucose, due to food intake and stress, elevated levels of HbA1c and fructosamine play an important role as an indicator of T2DM. Reference values for fructosamine in rhesus macaques are 157–230 µmol/L (Williams-Fritze *et al.* 2011). Measurement of both fructosamine and glucose levels allows diagnosis of DM earlier in the course of the disease. Intravenous glucose tolerance testing (IV-GGT) is used as an early screening test and to monitor progression of disease (Staup *et al.* 2016; Liddie *et al.* 2019).

Primate diets, with few exceptions, contain high levels of carbohydrates, particularly the simple sugars that diabetics must avoid. It is important that animals that are diagnosed or suspected of diabetes have diets modified to reduce simple sugars.

Endometriosis

Endometriosis is a condition in which endometrial cell types are developing outside the uterine cavity. This is a condition which occurs naturally in OWM. Baboons have been described to develop spontaneous endometriosis with lesions that resemble human endometriosis (Folse & Stout 1978), endometriosis is also observed in other NHP species (Mattison *et al.* 2007; Nishimoto-Kakiuchi *et al.* 2018). Treatment could be the provision of NSAID during menstrual period, hormone contraception implants or hysterectomy.

Skin and hair abnormalities

In OWM, some endocrine disorders result in alterations to skin and hair coat (Bakker & de la Garza, 2022).

Alopecia, the partial or complete absence of hair on areas of the body where it normally grows, is a common problem with a poorly understood ethology in OWM (Novak & Meyer 2009; Kroeker *et al.* 2014). Alopecia can be the result of normal seasonal or hormonal variation. Macaques' hair coats can demonstrate natural seasonal variation that may be associated with levels of circulating sex hormones or pregnancy and resolves spontaneously. Males and females are affected equally. Captive monkeys can show forms of pelage loss that are absent in wild or free-living conspecifics, which results from excessive hair-pulling or over-grooming by cage mates. This behaviour appears to be associated with stress in captivity and is controllable to some extent with environmental enrichment (Lutz *et al.* 2016; Novak *et al.* 2017; Lutz *et al.* 2019).

Alopecia scoring can be managed using photographic images (Figure 39.3), cage-side observations and/or being recorded during routine physical examinations (Honess *et al.* 2005; Bellanca *et al.* 2014).

Nutritional aspects

To maintain physiological processes, a balanced diet is essential. Standard commercial primate diets are complete diets: they are formulated to meet the nutritional requirements of OWM. Combinations of vegetables, mixtures of grains and (limited) fruits can be provided additionally. However, it must be taken into account that stressed, ill, pregnant or lactating animals have greater needs. Amounts provided also depend on the use of additional food enrichment and treats for training. Care must be taken that such supplements do not negatively affect the nutrient balance needed. Overviews of required mineral concentrations and vitamin levels are described in, for example, Lewis *et al.* (2005); Wolfensohn & Honess (2005); NRC (2003b). Deficiencies in minerals or vitamins have a negative impact on animal health and can result in clinical and

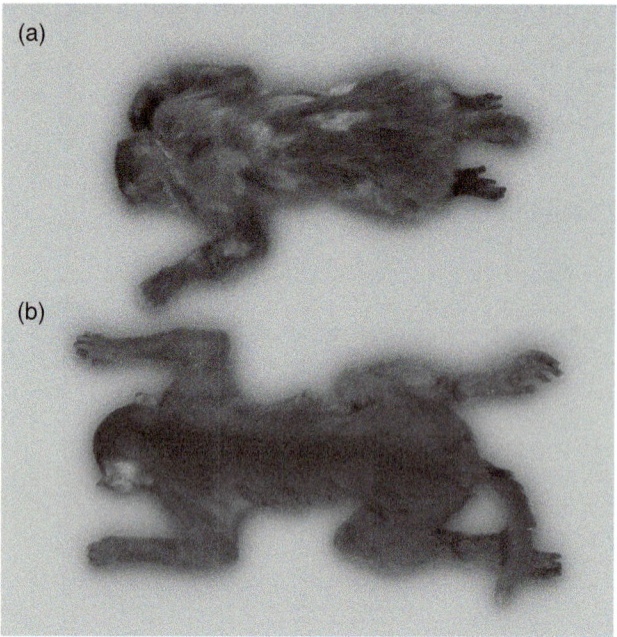

Figure 39.3 Alopecia (a) and normal (b) fur in rhesus macaques.

pathological abnormalities. A detailed overview is described in Lewis et al. (2005). A short summary is provided in Table 39.4.

Acute gastric dilatation (bloating)

Life-threatening bloat occurs sporadically nowadays in captive OWM. The cause is unknown, but it probably is multifactorial Anamnese includes food restriction, accidental overfeeding, and prior anaesthesia. Monkeys can be found dead or to have clinical signs of colic, abdominal distention, and dyspnea. Aetiologic factors include intragastric fermentation associated with Clostridium perfringens and abnormal gastric function (Pond et al. 1982). Gas inside the stomach should be removed immediately through an orogastric tube and in case of shock, shock must be treated accordingly.

Obesity

Commercial diets are generally designed as complete feeding. Regulation of supplemental feeding is recommended to avoid overfeeding as this increases the risk result on obesity and the occurrence of diabetes. It is apparent that some animals are more prone to obesity than others. This might be an individual genetic predisposition, as in humans but the genetic components are unknown. OWM social hierarchy may contribute to obesity in high-ranking animals, as well as lack of physical exercise.

Assessing the obesity level by BCS seems unreliable, and relative adiposity is best measured for rhesus macaques with WHI3.0 (weight/height^3) and for cynomolgus macaques WHI2.7 (weight/height$^{2.7}$), as these WHI measures are independent of height and are highly correlated with abdominal circumference, skinfold thicknesses and BCS. WHI measures are considered better than the BMI (Sterck et al. 2019).

Table 39.4 Clinical symptoms associated with nutrient deficiencies.

Nutrient deficiency	Clinical and pathological symptoms
Vitamin A	Weakness, diarrhoea, growth cessation, respiratory infections, ophthalmic pathology/blindness
Vitamin C	Skeletal scurvy, nutritional osteodystrophy, immunosuppression, weakness, lethargy weight loss, anaemia, teeth, gingiva problems
Vitamin D*	Osteomalacia, rickets, hypocalcaemia
Vitamin E (alpha- tocopherol)**	(Haemolytic) anaemia, cardiomyopathy, reproductive difficulties, degeneration of skeletal muscle
Iron	Anaemia

* Exposure to UBV (daylight or artificial) has beneficial effects on Vitamin D metabolism.
** Impaired vitamin E levels are considered to be a result of a complex nutritional deficiency involving vitamin E, selenium and proteins.

Intoxications

When animals present with clinical signs that cannot be linked to a disease or when they die suddenly, intoxication should be part of a differential diagnosis. Although intoxicatons are rare, they have been reported. Potential intoxications can be caused by e.g. zinc resulting in toxicosis induced by frequent licking of galvanised steel of the cages or by phytotoxins ingestion from the environment when animals have access to outdoor facilities. An overview of intoxications of nonhuman primates can be found in e.g. Bakker and Bomzon (2022).

Acknowledgement

We wish to acknowledge Sarah Wolfensohn, the author of the 8th edition chapter. This earlier chapter has been invaluable and the basis for the writing of the current chapter.

References

Bakker, J. and de la Garza M.A. (2022) Naturally occurring endocrine disorders in non-human primates: A comprehensive review. *Animals*, **12**, 407. doi.org/10.3390/ani12040407

Bakker, J. and Bomzon, A. (2022) A literature review of unintentional intoxications of nonhuman primates. *Animals*, **12**, 854. doi:10.3390/ani12070854

Balansard, I., Cleverley, L., Cutler, K.L. et al. (2019) Revised recommendations for health monitoring of non-human primate colonies (2018): FELASA Working Group Report. *Laboratory Animals*, 23677219844541. doi: 10.1177/0023677219844541.

Bellanca, R.U., Lee, G. H., Vogel, K. et al. (2014) A simple alopecia scoring system for use in colony management of laboratory-housed primates. *Journal of Medical Primatolology*, **43**, 153–161. doi: 10.1111/jmp.12107.

Bono, A.E.J., Whiten, A., van Schaik, C. et al. (2018) Payoff- and sex-biased social learning interact in a wild primate population. *Current Biology*, **28**, 2800–2805 e4. doi: 10.1016/j.cub.2018.06.015.

Carlsson, H.E., Schapiro, S.J., Farah, I. et al. (2004) Use of primates in research: a global overview. *American Journal of Primatology*, **63**, 225–237. doi: 10.1002/ajp.20054.

Casteleyn, C. and Bakker, J. (2021). Anatomy of the Rhesus monkey (Macaca mulatta): The essentials for the biomedical researcher. In *Updates on Veterinary Anatomy and Physiology*. Eds C. Rutland and S. El-Gendy. IntechOpen. doi.org/10.5772/intechopen.9906

Chen, H. and Langermans, J. (eds.) (2021) *Nonhuman Primate Models in Preclinical Research. Volume 1: Basics and Regulatory Principles*. Nova Science Publishers, New York. ISBN 978-1-53619-922-2.

Clingerman, K.J., Spray, S., Flynn, C. et al. (2010) A technique for intracisternal collection and administration in a rhesus macaque. *Laboratory Animals (NY)*, **39**, 307–311. doi: 10.1038/laban1010-307.

Clingerman, K.J. and Summers, L. (2005) Development of a body condition scoring system for nonhuman primates using Macaca mulatta as a model. *Laboratory Animals (NY)*, **34**, 31–36. doi: 10.1038/laban0505-31.

Clingerman, K.J. and Summers, L. (2012) Validation of a body condition scoring system in rhesus macaques (Macaca mulatta): Inter- and intrarater variability. *Journal of the American Association for Laboratory Animal Science*, **51**, 31–36.

Coleman, K. and Novak, M.A. (2017) Environmental Enrichment in the 21st Century. *ILAR Journal*, **58**, 295–307. doi: 10.1093/ilar/ilx008.

Colman, R.J. (2018) Non-human primates as a model for aging. *Biochimica et Biophysica Acta Molecular Basis of Disease*, **1864**, 2733–2741. doi: 10.1016/j.bbadis.2017.07.008.

Colman, R.J., Anderson, R.M., Johnson, S.C. et al. (2009) Caloric restriction delays disease onset and mortality in rhesus monkeys. *Science*, **325**, 201–204. doi: 10.1126/science.1173635.

Cyranoski, D. (2016) Monkey kingdom. *Nature*, **532**, 300–302. doi: 10.1038/532300a.

Davenport, M.D., Tiefenbacher, S., Lutz, C.K. et al. (2006) Analysis of endogenous cortisol concentrations in the hair of rhesus macaques. *General and Comparative Endocrinology*, **147**, 255–261. doi: 10.1016/j.ygcen.2006.01.005.

Descovich, K.A., Richmond, S.E., Leach, M.C. et al. (2019) Opportunities for refinement in neuroscience: Indicators of wellness and post-operative pain in laboratory macaques. *Alternatives to Animal Experimentation*. doi: 10.14573/altex.1811061.

Descovich, K.A., Wathan, J., Leach, M.C. et al. (2017) Facial expression: An under-utilised tool for the assessment of welfare in mammals. *Alternatives to Animal Experimentation*, **34**, 409–429. doi: 10.14573/altex.1607161.

Dettmer, A.M., Novak, M.A., Suomi, S.J. et al. (2012) Physiological and behavioral adaptation to relocation stress in differentially reared rhesus monkeys: hair cortisol as a biomarker for anxiety-related responses. *Psychoneuroendocrinology*, **37**, 191–199. doi: 10.1016/j.psyneuen.2011.06.003.

DiGiacomo, R.F. and Shaughnessy, P.W. (1972) Estimation of gestational age and birth weight in the rhesus monkey (Macaca mulatta). *American Journal to Obstetrics and Gynecoogyl*, **112**, 619–628. doi: 10.1016/0002-9378(72)90786-7.

Fehlmann, G., O'Riain, M.J., Kerr-Smith, C. et al. (2017) Extreme behavioural shifts by baboons exploiting risky, resource-rich, human-modified environments. *Scientific Reports*, **7**, 15057. doi: 10.1038/s41598-017-14871-2.

Folse, D.S. and Stout, L.C. (1978) Endometriosis in a baboon (Papio doguera). *Laboratory Animal Science*, **28**, 217–219.

Gould, K.G. and Mann, D.R. (1988) Comparison of electrostimulation methods for semen recovery in the rhesus monkey (Macaca mulatta). *Journal of Medical Primatolology*, **17**, 95–103.

Graham, M.L., Rieke, E.F., Dunning, M. et al. (2009) A novel alternative placement site and technique for totally implantable vascular access ports in non-human primates. *Journal of Medical Primatolology*, **38**, 204–212. doi: 10.1111/j.1600-0684.2009.00340.x.

Gray, H., Thiele, A. and Rowe, C. (2019) Using preferred fluids and different reward schedules to motivate rhesus macaques (Macaca mulatta) in cognitive tasks. *Laboratory Animals*, **53**, 372–382. doi: 10.1177/0023677218801390.

Grieves, J.L., Dick, E.J., Jr., Schlabritz-Loutsevich, N.E. et al. (2008) Barbiturate euthanasia solution-induced tissue artifact in nonhuman primates. *Journal of Medical Primatolology*, **37**, 154–161. doi: 10.1111/j.1600-0684.2007.00271.x.

Grimm, D. (2018) U.S. labs using a record number of monkeys. *Science*, **362**, 630. doi: 10.1126/science.362.6415.630.

Groves, C.P. (2001) *Primate Taxonomy*. Smithsonian Series in Comparative Evolutionary Biology., Smithsonian Institution Press, Washington D.C.

Hansen, B.G. and Tigno, X. (2007) The rhesus monkey (Macaca mulatta) manifests all features of human type 2 diabetes. In *Animal Models of Diabetes: Frontiers in Research*, 2nd edn, Ed. Shafrir, E., pp. 251–270, CRC Press, Boca Raton, USA.

Harding, J.D. (2017) Nonhuman primates and translational research: Progress, opportunities, and challenges. *ILAR Journal*, **58**, 141–150. doi: 10.1093/ilar/ilx033.

Harwood, H.J., Jr., Listrani, P. and Wagner, J.D. (2012) Nonhuman primates and other animal models in diabetes research. *Journal of Diabetes Science and Technology*, **6**, 503–514. doi: 10.1177/193229681200600304.

Hild, S.A., Chang, M.C., Murphy, S.J. et al (2021) Nonhuman primate models for SARS-CoV-2 research: Infrastructure needs for pandemic preparedness. *Lab Animal*, **50**, 140–141.

Honess, P., Gimpel, J., Wolfensohn, S. et al. (2005) Alopecia scoring: the quantitative assessment of hair loss in captive macaques. *Alternatives to Laboratory Animals*, **33**, 193–206. doi: 10.1177/026119290503300308.

Honess, P. and Wolfensohn, S. (2010) The extended welfare assessment grid: A matrix for the assessment of welfare and cumulative suffering in experimental animals. *Alternatives to Laboratory Animals*, **38**, 205–212. doi: 10.1177/026119291003800304.

Honess, P.E., Johnson, P.J. and Wolfensohn, S.E. (2004) A study of behavioural responses of non-human primates to air transport and re-housing. *Laboratory Animals*, **38**, 119–132. doi: 10.1258/002367704322968795.

Honess, P.E. and Marin, C.M. (2006a) Behavioural and physiological aspects of stress and aggression in nonhuman primates. *Neuroscience & Biobehavioural Reviews*, **30**, 390–412. doi: 10.1016/j.neubiorev.2005.04.003.

Honess, P.E. and Marin, C.M. (2006b) Enrichment and aggression in primates. *Neuroscience & Biobehavioural Reviews*, **30**, 413–436. doi: 10.1016/j.neubiorev.2005.05.002.

Joly, M., Micheletta, J., De Marco, A. et al. (2017) Comparing physical and social cognitive skills in macaque species with different degrees of social tolerance. *Proceedings of the Royal Society B: Biological Sciences*, **284**. doi: 10.1098/rspb.2016.2738.

Joseph, B.E., Wilson, D.W., Henrickson, R.V. et al. (1984) Treatment of pulmonary acariasis in rhesus macaques with ivermectin. *Laboratory Animal Science*, **34**, 360–364.

Justice, W.S.M., O'Brien, M.F., Szyszka, O. et al. (2017) Adaptation of the animal welfare assessment grid (AWAG) for monitoring animal welfare in zoological collections. *Veterinary Records*, **181**, 143. doi: 10.1136/vr.104309.

Kilkenny, C., Browne, W.J., Cuthill, I.C. et al. (2010) Improving bioscience research reporting: the ARRIVE guidelines for reporting animal research. *PLoS Biology*, **8**, e1000412. doi: 10.1371/journal.pbio.1000412.

Kinter, L. and Johnson, D.K. (1998) Remote monitoring of experimental endpoints in animal using radiotelemetry and bioimpedance technologies. In: *International Conference on Humane Endpoints (HEP) in Animal Experiments for Biomedical Research*. Eds Hendriksen,

C.F.M. and Morton, D.B. Zeist. Royal Society of Medicine Press, The Netherlands.

Kondova, I. (2021) The non-human primate as unique model to understand the pathogenesis of human endometriosis.pp 291-300. In: Nonhuman Primate Models in Preclinical Research: Disease Models. Eds. H. Chen and J. Langermans, Nova Science Publishers. ISBN 978-1-53619-931-4.

Krebs, J.R., Davies, N.B. and Parr, J. (1993) *An Introduction to Behavioural Ecology*, 3rd edn. Blackwell Scientific Publications, Cambridge, MA, US.

Kroeker, R., Bellanca, R.U., Lee, G.H. et al. (2014) Alopecia in three macaque species housed in a laboratory environment. *American Journal of Primatology*, **76**, 325–334. doi: 10.1002/ajp.22236.

Kumar, V., Raj, A. and Kumar, P. (2011) Pregnancy diagnosis by laparoscopy in free range rhesus macaques (*Macaca mulatta*). *Open Veterinary Journal*, **1**, 32–34.

Laffins, M.M., Mellal, N., Almlie, C.L. et al. (2017) Evaluation of infrared thermometry in cynomolgus macaques (*Macaca fascicularis*). *Journal of the American Association for Laboratory Animal Science*, **56**, 84–89.

Lewis, S.M., Hotchkiss, C.E. and Ullrey, D.E. (2005) *The Laboratory Primate*. Eds Wolfe-Coote, S. Elsevier Academic Press.

Liddie, S., Goody, R.J., Valles, R. et al. (2010) Clinical chemistry and hematology values in a Caribbean population of African green monkeys. *Journal of Medical Primatology*, **39**, 389–398. doi: 10.1111/j.1600-0684.2010.00422.x.

Liddie, S., Okamoto, H., Gromada, J. et al. (2019) Characterization of glucose-stimulated insulin release protocols in African green monkeys (*Chlorocebus aethiops*). *Journal of Medical Primatology*, **48**, 10–21. doi: 10.1111/jmp.12374.

Lindburg, D.G. (1971) The rhesus monkey in North India: An ecological and behavioral study. In: *Primate Behavior: Developments in Field and Laboratory Research*. Rosenblum, L.A., Academic Press, London.

Lindburg, D.G. (1991) Ecological requirements of macaques. *Laboratory Animal Science*, **41**, 315–22.

Liu, Z., Cai, Y., Wang, Y. et al. (2018) Cloning of macaque monkeys by somatic cell nuclear transfer. *Cell*, **172**, 881–887 e7. doi: 10.1016/j.cell.2018.01.020.

Liu, Z., Li, X., Zhang, J.T. et al. (2016) Autism-like behaviours and germline transmission in transgenic monkeys overexpressing MeCP2. *Nature*, **530**, 98–102. doi: 10.1038/nature16533.

Ljungberg, T. and Westlund, K. (2000) Impaired reconciliation in rhesus macaques with a history of early weaning and disturbed socialization. *Primates*, **41**, 79–88. doi: 10.1007/BF02557463.

Lubbe, A., Hetem, R.S., McFarland, R. et al. (2014) Thermoregulatory plasticity in free-ranging vervet monkeys, *Chlorocebus pygerythrus*. *Journal of Comparative Physiology B*, **184**, 799–809. doi: 10.1007/s00360-014-0835-y.

Lutz, C.K., Coleman, K., Worlein, J.M. et al. (2016) Factors influencing alopecia and hair cortisol in rhesus macaques (*Macaca mulatta*). *Journal of Medical Primatolology*, **45**, 180–188. doi: 10.1111/jmp.12220.

Lutz, C.K., Menard, M.T., Rosenberg, K. et al. (2019) Alopecia in rhesus macaques (*Macaca mulatta*): Association with pregnancy and chronic stress. *Journal of Medical Primatolology*, **48**, 251–256. doi: 10.1111/jmp.12419.

Lutz, C.K. and Novak, M.A. (2005) Environmental enrichment for nonhuman primates: Theory and application. *ILAR Journal*, **46**, 178–191. doi: 10.1093/ilar.46.2.178.

Lyashchenko, K.P., Greenwald, R., Esfandiari, J. et al. (2007) PrimaTB STAT-PAK assay, a novel, rapid lateral-flow test for tuberculosis in nonhuman primates. *Clinical and Vaccine Immunology*, **14**, 1158–1164. doi: 10.1128/CVI.00230-07.

Ma, Y., Li, J., Wang, G. et al. (2016) Efficient production of cynomolgus monkeys with a toolbox of enhanced assisted reproductive technologies. *Scientific Reports*, **6**, 25888. doi: 10.1038/srep25888.

Majolo, B., de Bartoli Vizioli, A. and Schino, G. (2008) Costs and benefits of group living in primates: group size effects on behaviour and demography. *Animal Behaviour*, **76**, 1235–1247.

Mason, S., Premereur, E., Pelekanos, V. et al. (2019) Effective chair training methods for neuroscience research involving rhesus macaques (*Macaca mulatta*). *Journal of Neuroscience Methods*, **317**, 82–93. doi: 10.1016/j.jneumeth.2019.02.001.

Matheson, M.D. and Bernstein, I.S. (2000) Grooming, social bonding, and agonistic aiding in rhesus monkeys. *American Journal of Primatology*, **51**, 177–186. doi: 10.1002/1098-2345(200007)51:3<177: AID-AJP2>3.0.CO;2-K.

Mattison, J.A., Ottinger, M.A., Powell, D. et al. (2007) Endometriosis: clinical monitoring and treatment procedures in rhesus monkeys. *Journal of Medical Primatology*, **36**, 391–398. doi: 10.1111/j.1600-0684.2006.00208.x.

Matz-Rensing, K., Hartmann, T., Wendel, G.M. et al. (2015) Outbreak of tuberculosis in a colony of rhesus monkeys (*Macaca mulatta*) after possible indirect contact with a human TB patient. *Journal of Comparative Pathology*, **153**, 81–91. doi: 10.1016/j.jcpa.2015.05.006.

McDonald, M.M., Agnew, M.K., Asa, C.S. et al. (2021) Melengestrol acetate contraceptive implant use in colobus monkeys (*Colobus guereza*): Patterns through time and differences in reproductive potential and live births. *Zoo Biology*, **40**, 124–134. doi: 10.1002/zoo.21581.

McMillan, J.L., Bloomsmith, M.A. and Prescott, M.J. (2017) An international survey of approaches to chair restraint of nonhuman primates. *Comparative Medicine*, **67**, 442–451.

Moran, S., Chi, T., Prucha, M.S. et al. (2015) Germline transmission in transgenic Huntington's disease monkeys. *Theriogenology*, **84**, 277–285. doi: 10.1016/j.theriogenology.2015.03.016.

Muñoz-Fontela, C., Widerspick, L. and Albrecht, R.A. (2022) Advances and gaps in SARS-CoV-2 infection models. *Plos Pathogens*, **18**, e1010161. doi: 10.1371/journal.ppat.1010161.

Mutch, L.A.K., Klinker, S.T., Janecek, J.J. et al. (2018) Long-term management of vascular access ports in nonhuman primates used in preclinical efficacy and tolerability studies. *Journal of Investigative Surgery*, **13**, 1–12.

NC3R (2017) *NC3Rs Guidelines: Non-Human Primate Accommodation, Care and Use*. London.

Nishimoto-Kakiuchi, A., Netsu, S., Okabayashi, S. et al. (2018) Spontaneous endometriosis in cynomolgus monkeys as a clinically relevant experimental model. *Human Reproduction*, **33**, 1228–1236. doi: 10.1093/humrep/dey095.

Novak, M.A., Hamel, A.F., Kelly, B.J. et al. (2013) Stress, the HPA axis, and nonhuman primate well-being: A review. *Applied Animal Behaviour Science*, **143**, 135–149. doi: 10.1016/j.applanim.2012.10.012.

Novak, M.A., Menard, M.T., El-Mallah, S.N. et al. (2017) Assessing significant (>30%) alopecia as a possible biomarker for stress in captive rhesus monkeys (*Macaca mulatta*). *American Journal of Primatology*, **79**, 1–8. doi: 10.1002/ajp.22547.

Novak, M.A. and Meyer, J.S. (2009) Alopecia: possible causes and treatments, particularly in captive nonhuman primates. *Comparative Medicine*, **59**, 18–26.

NRC (2003a) *Nutrient Requirements of Nonhuman Primates Second Revised Edition*. National Academies Press, Washington D.C.

NRC (2003b) Occupational Health and Safety in the Care and Use of Nonhuman Primates. National Academies Press, Washington D.C.

Overduin-de Vries, A. M., Bakker, F. A., Spruijt, B. M. et al. (2016) Male long-tailed macaques (*Macaca fascicularis*) understand the target of facial threat. *American Journal of Primatology*, **78**, 720–730. doi: 10.1002/ajp.22536.

Owen, D.G. (1992) *Parasites of Laboratory Animals. Laboratory Animal Handbooks No. 12*, Royal Society of Medicine Services Limited, London, UK.

Panarella, M.L. and Bimes, R.S. (2010) A naturally occurring outbreak of tuberculosis in a group of imported cynomolgus monkeys

(*Macaca fascicularis*). *Journal of the American Association for Laboratory Animal Science*, **49**, 221–225.

Pond, C.L., Newcomer, C.E. and Anver, M.R. (1982) Acute gastric dilatation in nonhuman primates: review and case studies. *Veterinary Pathology Suppl* (19 Suppl. **7**), 126–133.

Prescott, M.J. (2016) Online resources for improving the care and use of non-human primates in research. *Primate Biology*, **3**, 33–40.

Prescott, M.J., Nixon, M.E., Farningham, D.A.H. et al. (2012) Laboratory macaques: when to wean? *Applied Animal Behaviour Science*, **137**, 194–207.

Ralph, C.R. and Tilbrook, A.J. (2016) INVITED REVIEW: The usefulness of measuring glucocorticoids for assessing animal welfare. *Journal of Animal Science*, **94**, 457–470. doi: 10.2527/jas.2015-9645.

Ravindran, R., Krishnan, V.V., Dhawan, R. et al. (2014) Plasma antibody profiles in non-human primate tuberculosis. *Journal of Medical Primatolology*, **43**, 59–71. doi: 10.1111/jmp.12097.

Rehmann, P., Gröne, A., Gottstein, B. et al. (2005) Detection of Echinococcus multilocularis infection in a colony of cynomolgus monkeys (*Macaca Fascicularis*) using serology and ultrasonography. *Journal of Veterinary Diagnostic Investigation*, **7**, 183–186. doi:10.1177/104063870501700215

Reinhardt, V. (2003) Working with rather than against macaques during blood collection. *Journal of Applied Animal Welfare Science*, **6**, 189–197. doi: 10.1207/S15327604JAWS0603_04.

Reinhardt, V., Liss, C. and Stevens, C. (1995) Restraint methods of laboratory non-human primates: A critical review. *Animal Welfare*, **4**, 221–238.

Rennie, A.E. and Buchanan-Smith, H.M. (2006) Refinement of the use of non-human primates in scientific research. Part III: refinement of procedures *Animal Welfare*, **15**, 239–261.

Rhoads, M.K., Goleva, S.B., Beierwaltes, W.H. et al. (2017) Renal vascular and glomerular pathologies associated with spontaneous hypertension in the nonhuman primate *Chlorocebus aethiops sabaeus*. *The American Journal of Physiology-Regulatory, Integrative and Comparative Physiology*, **313**, R211–R218. doi: 10.1152/ajpregu.00026.2017.

Rockx, B., Kuiken, T., Herfst, S. et al. (2020) Comparative pathogenesis of COVID-19, MERS, and SARS in a nonhuman primate model. *Science*, **368**, 1012–1015. doi:10.1126/science.abb7314.

Roder, E.L. and Timmermans, P.J. (2002) Housing and care of monkeys and apes in laboratories: adaptations allowing essential species-specific behaviour. *Laboratory Animals*, **36**, 221–242. doi: 10.1258/002367702320162360.

Rogers, J., Raveendran, M., Harris, R.A. et al. (2019) The comparative genomics and complex population history of Papio baboons. *Scientific Advances*, **5**, eaau6947. doi: 10.1126/sciadv.aau6947.

Rox, A., van Vliet, A.H., Sterck, E.H.M. et al. (2019) Factors determining male introduction success and long-term stability in captive rhesus macaques. *PLoS One*, **14**, e0219972. doi: 10.1371/journal.pone.0219972.

Rox, A., van Vliet, A.H., Langermans, J.A.M. et al. (2021) A stepwise male introduction procedure to prevent inbreeding in naturalistic macaque breeding groups. *Animals*, **11**, 545, doi: 10.3390/ani11020545

Sauceda, R. and Schmidt, M.G. (2000) Refining macaque handling and restraint techniques. *Laboratory Animals*, **29**, 47–49.

Schapiro, S.J., Bloomsmith, M.A. and Laule, G.E. (2003) Positive reinforcement training as a technique to alter nonhuman primate behavior: Quantitative assessments of effectiveness. *Journal of Applied Animal Welfare Science*, **6**, 175–187. doi: 10.1207/S15327604JAWS0603_03.

Scheer (2017) Final Opinion on 'The need for non-human primates in biomedical research, production and testing of products and devices (update 2017).

Schuurman, H.J. and Smith, H.T. (2005) Reference values for clinical chemistry and clinical hematology parameters in cynomolgus monkeys. *Xenotransplantation*, **12**, 72–75. doi: 10.1111/j.1399-3089.2004.00186.x.

Schuurman, H.J., Smith, H.T. and Cozzi, E. (2004) Reference values for clinical chemistry and clinical hematology parameters in baboons. *Xenotransplantation*, **11**, 511–516. doi: 10.1111/j.1399-3089.2004.00171.x.

Settlage, D.S. and Hendrickx, A.G. (1974) Electroejaculation technique in *Macaca mulatta* (rhesus monkeys). *Fertility and Sterility*, **25**, 157–159.

Short, C.E. and Bufalari, A. (1999) Propofol anesthesia. *Veterinary Clinics of North America: Small Animal Practice*, **29**, 747–778. doi: 10.1016/s0195-5616(99)50059-4.

Skoura, E., Zumla, A. and Bomanji, J. (2015) Imaging in tuberculosis. *International Journal of Infectious Diseases*, **32**, 87–93. doi: 10.1016/j.ijid.2014.12.007.

Staup, M., Aoyagi, G., Bayless, T. et al. (2016) Characterization of metabolic status in nonhuman primates with the intravenous glucose tolerance test. *Journal of Visualized Experiments*. doi: 10.3791/52895.

Sterck, E.H.M., Zijlmans, D.G.M., de Vries, H. et al. (2019) Determining overweight and underweight with a new weight-for-height index in captive group-housed macaques. *American Journal of Primatology*, **81**, e22996. doi: 10.1002/ajp.22996.

Stoelting, R.K. and Miller, R.D. (2000) Intravenous anesthetics. In: *Basics of Anesthesia*, 4th edn, Eds Miller, R.D. and Stoelting, R.K., pp. 58–69. Churchill Livingstone.

Thomsen, R. (2014) Non-invasive collection and analysis of semen in wild macaques. *Primates*, **55**, 231–237. doi: 10.1007/s10329-013-0393-z.

Turner, P.V., Brabb, T., Pekow, C. et al. (2011) Administration of substances to laboratory animals: routes of administration and factors to consider. *Journal of the American Association for Laboratory Animal Science*, **50**, 600–613.

The European Parliament Council of the European Union (2010) Directive 2010/63/EU of the European Parliament and of the Council of 22 September 2010 on the protection of animals used for scientific purposes. See https://eur-lex.europa.eu/legal-content/EN/TXT/?uri=celex%3A32010L0063

Vernes, M.K. and Louwerse, A.L. (2010) *BPRC's Enrichment Manual for Macaques and Marmosets*. Biomedical Primate Research Centre, Rijswijk, The Netherlands. ISBN: 978-90-812355-2-5

Vervenne, R.A., Jones, S.L., van Soolingen, D. et al. (2004) TB diagnosis in non-human primates: comparison of two interferon-gamma assays and the skin test for identification of *Mycobacterium tuberculosis* infection. *Veterinary Immunology and Immunopathology*, **100**, 61–71. doi: 10.1016/j.vetimm.2004.03.003.

Vierboom M.P., Jonker M., Tak P.P. et al. (2007) Preclinical models of arthritic disease in non-human primates. *Drug Discovery Today*, **12**, 327–335. doi: 10.1016/j.drudis.2007.02.012. Epub 2007 Mar 8. PMID: 17395093.

Wagner, J.E., Kavanagh, K., Ward, G.M. et al. (2006) Old world non-human primate models of type 2 diabetes mellitus. *ILAR Journal*, **47**, 259–71. doi: 10.1093/ilar.47.3.259.

Wallace, P.Y., Asa, C.S., Agnew, M. et al. (2016). A review of population control methods in captive-housed primates. *Animal Welfare*, **25**, 7–20. doi.org/10.7120/09627286.25.1.007

Wergard, E.M., Temrin, H., Forkman, B. et al. (2015) Training pair-housed rhesus macaques (*Macaca mulatta*) using a combination of negative and positive reinforcement. *Behavioural Processes*, **113**, 51–59. doi: 10.1016/j.beproc.2014.12.008.

Westlund, K. (2015) Training laboratory primates – benefits and techniques. *Primate Biology*, **2**, 119–132.

Wickham, L.A., Kulick, A.A., Gichuru, L. et al. (2011). Transurethral bladder catheterization of male rhesus macaques: a refinement of approach. *Journal of Medical Primatology*, **40**, 342–350. doi: 10.1111/j.1600-0684.2011.00494.x.

Wilkinson, A.C., Harris, L.D., Saviolakis, G.A. et al. (1999) Cushing's syndrome with concurrent diabetes mellitus in a rhesus monkey. *Contemporary Topics in Laboratory Animal Science*, **38**, 62–66.

Williams-Fritze, M.J., Smith, P.C., Zelterman, D. *et al.* (2011) Fructosamine reference ranges in rhesus macaques (*Macaca mulatta*). *Journal of the American Association for Laboratory Animal Science*, **50**, 462–465.

Willy, M.E., Woodward, R.A., Thornton, V.B. *et al.* (1999) Management of a measles outbreak among Old World nonhuman primates. *Laboratory Animal Science*, **49**, 42–48.

Willyard, C. (2016) New models: Gene-editing boom means changing landscape for primate work. *Nature Medicine*, **22**, 1200–1202. doi: 10.1038/nm1116-1200.

Wolfe-Coote, S. (2005) *The Laboratory Primate*. Elsevier Academic Press, London, UK.

Wolfensohn, S. and Honess, P. (2005) *Handbook of Primate Husbandry and Welfare*. Blackwell Publishing Ltd., Oxford.

Wolfensohn, S. and Peters, A. (2005) Refinement of neuroscience procedures using nonhuman primates. *Animal Technology and Welfare*, **4**, 49–50.

Wolfensohn, S.E. (1997) Brief review of scientific studies of the welfare implications of transporting primates. *Laboratory Animals*, **31**, 303–305. doi: 10.1258/002367797780596167.

Birds

40 The domestic fowl

Ian J.H. Duncan

Biological overview

Origins

The domestic fowl is derived from the junglefowl, probably mainly from the Burmese red junglefowl (*Gallus gallus spadiceous*, Bonnaterre), but possibly with contributions from the other three junglefowl species (Siegel *et al*. 1992). The junglefowl is a ground-dwelling, gallinaceous bird with territorial males looking after small harems of from 2 to 10 females with their offspring. Junglefowl are considered graminivorous, feeding on leafy material, seeds and grains, but, as with many gallinaceous species, the young chicks require a higher quality diet than this and feed on insects and other invertebrates for the first few weeks of life. Junglefowl are extremely timid and secretive and therefore difficult to study in the wild. They can fly reasonably well and roost in trees at night and occasionally through the day. Otherwise, they spend most of their time on the ground and tend to run from frightening stimuli (Collias & Collias 1967).

Domestic fowl have probably been domesticated for about 5,000 years but early archaeological records are scant. Two features of their early history are of note. The first is that it seems likely the original relationship between human beings and the progenitors of chickens was a predator-prey one. The usual reaction of prey species to predators is a fearful one and the evidence suggests that domestication has not removed this completely (Duncan 1990). The second is that during much of their domestication, chickens were selected for fighting ability, not for their egg or meat producing capabilities (Wood-Gush 1959), and this probably accounts for the aggressiveness of some modern strains.

Lifespan

Domestic fowl have a lifespan of 5–8 years. Commercially, egg-laying hens are kept for only one or two laying years, because egg production declines rather rapidly after this. There is also a trend to extend the laying period to 70 or 80 weeks rather than the traditional 52 weeks. This has led to a stronger focus on resilience and longevity in the breeding of laying hens (Bain *et al*. 2016). Breeding birds of egg-laying strains are also kept for one or two years. Breeding stock for broilers are kept for less than a full laying year because fertility declines so quickly that it is not worthwhile keeping them longer. Broilers themselves, of course, are killed at ages ranging from 32 to 70 days depending on their genetic strain and what final product is required. In general, broilers fed *ad libitum* should not be kept longer beyond their normal production period, as this results in health problems and increased mortality.

The unnaturally short lives of commercial chickens should not necessarily set the pattern for laboratories. Chickens can live healthy lives for at least 4–6 years, and, if possible, this should be made use of.

Social organisation

The basic social unit of junglefowl consists of about 4 to 12 females accompanied by a dominant male and their sub-adult offspring. Dominant males establish and defend territories (Collias *et al*. 1966). From the scant information that is available, it appears that domestic fowl which have gone feral have a very similar organisation (McBride *et al*. 1969; Wood-Gush *et al*. 1978). When in a group, domestic fowl form a social hierarchy. Males and females do not generally interact agonistically although males tend to dominate females passively. Male and female hierarchies are separate. Once formed, the social hierarchy is fairly stable with little social friction. On the other hand, mixing strangers together leads to a lot of fighting.

Under commercial or laboratory conditions, domestic fowl are fairly adaptable. In order to control disease transmission, they are normally kept in single-age groups and this is not a problem for them. Newly hatched chicks are precocial and develop normally without contact with their dam. They are

The UFAW Handbook on the Care and Management of Laboratory and Other Research Animals, Ninth Edition.
Edited by Huw Golledge and Claire Richardson.
© 2024 John Wiley & Sons Ltd. Published 2024 by John Wiley & Sons Ltd.

also able to adapt easily to being kept in single- or mixed-sex groups. As males approach sexual maturity, they may become very aggressive to each other. This is generally not a problem if they are in mixed-sex groups and the sex ratio is kept at 10 or more females per male. However, in all-male groups, the aggression may lead to injury, and it may be necessary to house males individually. In general, domestic fowl will adapt to the range of group sizes normally found in a laboratory, i.e. from 3–4 to several hundred. Aggression tends not to be a major issue in large flocks of laying hens, because of a different mechanism of deciding who is dominant over who in those large flocks. Whereas in small groups, comb size, reflecting testosterone levels, generally determines dominance, in large flocks, body size seems to take precedence (Pagel & Dawkins 1997).

Breeds, strains and genetics

Chickens kept for commercial purposes can generally be divided into three main types, two of which are kept for eggs and one for meat production. Egg-laying strains have been heavily selected for high egg numbers, large egg size and low body weight. Strains kept for meat production have been heavily selected for rapid growth rate, feed conversion efficiency and breast muscle mass In Europe and North America, white-egg-laying strains are derived from the White Leghorn breed whereas brown-egg-laying strains are derived from a variety of breeds but usually include some Light Sussex and Rhode Island Red or Rhode Island White blood. Elsewhere in the world, there may be incorporation of local genetic material such as the Australorp breed in Australia. Meat producing strains (usually referred to as 'broilers') are derived from many different breeds including Cornish and White Rock. Primary Breeding Companies keep selected inbred lines which produce grand-parent, parent and eventually three- or four-way cross hybrid chicks which are sold on the commercial market. This method exploits hybrid vigour and gives an extremely productive and uniform final product, the hybrid chicken. This structure in the poultry industry also separates breeding from commercial production which provides good biological security. It also, of course, provides great genetic security to the primary breeding companies, since the result of breeding commercial stock would be genetic segregation and re-combination and a whole mixture of genotypes of little value.

Reproduction

Reproductive function in domestic fowl is at least partly controlled by day-length. Commercially, egg-laying strains and breeders are kept under short-day conditions (often 8 h light and 16 h dark (8L : 16D) or 10 h light and 14 h dark (10L : 14D)) until they are about 16 weeks of age in the case of laying strains and 20–22 weeks of age in the case of broiler breeders. They are then photo-stimulated by increasing day-length by about 1 h per week to 20–22 weeks (in the case of laying strains) to 14 or 15L : 10 or 9D. Thereafter, day-length usually remains constant. There are various modifications that can be made (see, for example, Lewis & Morris 2006), but this basic lighting programme works well. For ease of management, males and females of the same age are usually used, although it would be possible to successfully photo-stimulate males earlier.

When hens of laying strains are photo-stimulated in week 16, the first egg is usually laid in week 18, the birds reach 5% production in week 20 and peak production, which should be well over 90% (90 eggs per 100 birds per day), is reached in weeks 26–28. There is then a gradual decline in egg production until, at week 72 or 74, the birds should be laying at about 70% (Lewis & Morris 2006). Commercially, day-length is often gradually increased through the laying year but there is no good evidence that this actually stimulates more production. A long day of only 14 or 15 h (in contrast to a very long day of 16 or 18 h) may have more welfare advantages for the hens, in that it provides them with plenty of rest and they do not have an exceptionally long day to fill with activities. With broiler breeders, egg production is delayed by 2–3 weeks and is lower.

It should be remembered that birds differ from mammals in that the male is the homogametic sex carrying two similar sex chromosomes designated ZZ, with females being heterogametic and designated ZW. The fowl has some useful sex-linked traits such as silver (S) and gold (s) down-colour, and slow (K) and fast (k) feathering. These traits enable chicks to be sexed easily at hatching.

Behaviour

The behaviour of the domestic fowl has been well-studied and reported (see, for example, Wood-Gush 1971; Duncan 1980; Appleby et al. 2004; Nicol 2015). Chickens spend a considerable part of the day foraging for food. This is true even if food is provided in a very concentrated and highly nutritious form so that they can consume their requirements in a short time; they still spend many hours pecking, probing and flicking with their beaks and scratching with their feet. A good husbandry system should allow this foraging behaviour to occur unimpeded. Chickens can adapt their drinking behaviour to different sources of water such as troughs, cups or nipples. However, if they have learned to obtain water from one source, they may not recognise it if it is offered from another source.

Other maintenance behaviour includes preening and other activities associated with feather care. Domestic fowl do not bathe in water, but show dustbathing behaviour which functions to rid the feathers of excess lipids. However, this behaviour is not triggered by a build-up of lipids on the feathers but by a combination of other external factors (Duncan et al. 1998). Sleeping and resting are normally done in a perching position but domestic fowl seem able to adapt to flat-footed resting and sleeping.

As mentioned previously, chickens are highly social animals. They also tend to synchronise their activities and do things together as a flock. It is therefore important that the facilities provided allow them to do this. The only activity in which chickens will take turns, is drinking at a limited water source. All these social activities, both agonistic and associative, are organised by a rich repertoire of visual and vocal signals.

Domestic chicks are precocial when they hatch. Although the mother hen would normally be responsible for showing chicks sources of food and water, they are quite able to learn to feed and drink on their own when food and water are obvious. The one function they cannot manage well is thermoregulation; young chicks, therefore, have to be kept in a warm environment for the first few weeks of life, and this is described in some detail later.

Mating behaviour is preceded by elaborate courtship with the male being the initiator and main actor (Wood-Gush 1956). Once inseminated, the hen remains fertile for about 14 days although fertility drops quickly after 7 days. Nesting behaviour is complex and involves both nest site selection and nest building and may occupy 60–90 minutes every time an egg is laid (Duncan & Kite 1989). Extensive evidence suggests that the performance of this behaviour is very important to the hen (Follensbee et al. 1992; Cooper & Appleby 1996; Cronin et al. 2012).

One other behaviour pattern requires special mention, and that is feather pecking and cannibalism which can be a problem in some strains of laying fowl. Outbreaks of feather pecking and cannibalism can occur at any time in a chicken's life but the common times are from 6 to 12 weeks and at point-of-lay. This behaviour has nothing to do with aggression; it is probably some form of foraging behaviour directed at other birds' feathers rather than a potential food source (Blokhuis & Arkes 1984; Blokhuis 1986). Feather pecking behaviour varies substantially between strains of domestic fowl; it has been shown to be a heritable trait (Kjaer & Sørensen 1997) which can be selected against (Kjaer & Hocking 2004). Group selection methods have been shown to be very effective in reducing the incidence of feather pecking within a few generations (Muir & Cheng 2004; Ellen et al. 2008) and at least some of the major breeding companies are reported to be using this technique to reduce feather pecking in their commercial strains while maintaining good productivity (Lay et al. 2011).

However, many other factors may contribute to an outbreak of feather pecking including large group size, wire floor housing, and bright lighting (Kjaer & Vestergaard 1999; Gilani et al. 2013). It has also been shown that the incidence of feather pecking can be reduced by the use of dark brooders during the early rearing phase (Gilani et al. 2012). Dietary modifications, including giving supplementary roughage, can also decrease the likelihood of feather pecking outbreaks (Kalmendal & Wall 2012).

The most effective way to reduce the effects of feather pecking is to beak-trim the birds. However, there is strong evidence that the traditional method of using a hot blade to cut and cauterise the end of the beak causes both acute and chronic pain and therefore reduces the welfare of the birds substantially (Duncan et al. 1989; Gentle et al. 1990). If the strain has a bad reputation for feather pecking, then a better solution is to have the chicks precision-trimmed at the hatchery using infra-red techniques – a procedure which is less traumatic than physically trimming the beaks when the birds are older (Gentle et al. 1997). There also appears to be a link between fearfulness and feather pecking, and fearfulness can be reduced by changing inspection routines and by playing a radio with human voices in the house (de Haas et al. 2014). However, whenever possible, strains with low tendencies to feather peck should be chosen. As stated in the preceding text, many of the primary breeding companies are developing such strains and, if feasible, these should be used (Lay et al. 2011).

Standard biological data

Body weights for various strains of domestic fowl are shown in Table 40.1. Growth rate depends on the strain of chicken being used. The primary breeding companies produce 'Management Guides' with growth curves for each of their hybrids. As an example, females of a light hybrid strain should weigh around 450, 900 and 1,350 g at 6, 12 and 18 weeks of age. If reproductive fitness is important for the research being undertaken, then it is essential that chickens reach the correct weight for age as they are growing. There is usually no problem with light hybrids which can be fed *ad libitum*. Medium hybrids have a slight tendency to gain weight too rapidly, and so growth rate must be checked regularly during the rearing period. Moderate food rationing of the whole group can easily correct any tendency for the birds to gain too much weight. Broiler breeders, on the other hand, have enormous appetites and have to be very severely food restricted in order to be reproductively fit later in life. This has been recognised as a big animal welfare problem in the poultry industry for a considerable time (Mench 1993) with no signs of improvement more recently (e.g. Hocking 2009; Savory 2010). There is no easy solution; the short-term welfare of broiler breeding fowl must be reduced by keeping them on severe food restriction so that they suffer from extreme hunger every day, or they suffer later in life from diseases of excessive weight gain including abnormalities of limb bone development (leg weakness) and obesity. For this reason, laboratories should avoid using broiler breeding fowl if at all possible. Of course, this may not be possible if the birds are being used as a model in obesity or pathological bone growth studies. There are lines of dwarf broiler parent stock available which do not have to be food restricted (or not as severely restricted) as normal broiler parent stock and it may be possible for laboratories to use these lines.

Chickens have a core temperature of about 41.5 °C (Yahav 2015). Like many avian species, they have good control over blood flow to the lower, unfeathered part of the leg

Table 40.1 Average body weights of various types of domestic fowl.

Type of bird	Average weight
Light[1] hybrid adult females	1.3–1.8 kg
Light[1] hybrid adult males	2.0–2.6 kg
Medium[1] hybrid adult females	1.5–2.2 kg
Medium[1] hybrid adult males	3.0–3.6 kg
Female broilers at 42 days	1.9 kg
Male broilers at 42 days	2.2 kg
Broiler breeder adult females	3.0 kg
Broiler breeder adult males	4.0 kg

[1] 'Light' and 'Medium' refer to light and medium body weight birds, the two common types of fowl kept for table egg production.
[2] These weights refer to birds which are food-restricted according to the management guidelines.

and the feet and can use this mechanism to conserve or dissipate heat. The resting heart rate of adult fowl is about 230 beats/min and this increases to about 280–320 beats/min in active but undisturbed birds. When frightened, the heart rate can rise to 460 beats/min (range 380–460) (Duncan 1981).

Uses in research

The domestic fowl, (*Gallus gallus domesticus*), continues to be a popular laboratory animal. It is small and comparatively cheap and easy to maintain. It also has several biological features that make it the species of choice for several avenues of research. For example, there is still great interest in immune function in chickens. B lymphocytes were first described in chickens, the 'B' referring to the bursa of Fabricius. The chicken is also often preferred for classical studies in developmental biology. It lost ground to the mouse some years ago when mouse genetics surged ahead, but the convenience of having the embryo on hand outside the mother has meant that many laboratories have continued to work with chick embryos. The chicken is also favoured for certain oncological studies probably because the avian leucosis viruses are among the better-characterised tumour-forming viruses. The chick embryo is also used fairly widely in general virus research and toxicology studies. Of course, in addition to being used as models for other species and for some general biological principles, chickens are also used in agricultural laboratories specialising in chickens.

Sources of supply

Laboratories using domestic fowl can buy day-old chicks from commercial hatcheries each time more birds are required. A commercial type can be selected to suit the requirements of the particular lines of research. Moreover, the sex of bird required can be specified. However, it should be remembered that choosing to work with only one sex will lead to 50% of chicks being killed after hatching. This should be considered when submitting a research application to the ethical committee. This strategy, of purchasing day-old chicks from a hatchery, will result in a dependable source of uniform birds. Over the short term, it will also result in birds with a very similar genetic make-up. However, the primary breeding companies are constantly striving for improvement, and, every few years, introduce new hybrids and discontinue old ones. If genetic similarity is important for the research over an extended period, then a different strategy should be adopted. Many countries have specialised non-commercial lines of poultry available. These may be research lines maintained by other laboratories, or pure breeds maintained by local fanciers. Information on these sources can usually be obtained from Government Agricultural Departments/Ministries, University Animal Science Departments or Poultry Research Institutes/Centres. Pure breeds may be of interest because they carry particular genes such as the gene for polydactyly carried by the Silkie breed. Another solution is to maintain breeding stock, but this tends to be expensive. The minimum number of breeding birds required to avoid inbreeding problems is about 20 males and 20 females in each generation. This assumes that all 40 birds will contribute to the next generation, which implies the use of artificial insemination. It should be remembered that if the research involves chick embryos, then the source of the eggs is very important. For example, certain research projects might require background information on the disease status and vaccination programme of the parent flock; such information may or may not be available for fertile eggs purchased from a commercial hatchery.

Laboratory management and breeding

Housing

Any well-designed laboratory animal house can be used for chickens. There is advantage in having rooms of sufficient size such that commercial poultry equipment can be used. This would include a ceiling height of 2.5 m. Large rooms also allow for flexibility in the configuration of penning or caging. The surfaces of rooms should be of some impervious material that can be thoroughly cleaned and disinfected. There are various plastic laminates available which, although expensive, serve this purpose extremely well and these should cover the walls and ceiling. The floors of rooms should slope to drains and be of sealed concrete. If possible, all electrical fittings should be sealed so that each room can be pressure-washed. Some system for the removal of manure should be incorporated. As a rough guide, 100 light hybrid laying hens produce about 12 kg manure per day. Also, local authority rules and regulations governing the disposal of waste water should be carefully observed. It may be necessary to provide a large settling tank within the building to remove the bulk of the solids. Ideally, advice from an architect and sewage engineer, who are familiar with local by-laws, should be sought during the design phase of the building. These people should also be consulted if an existing building is being converted to hold chickens.

Lighting

The lights in each room should be fitted with a timer and dimmer so that the length and level of illumination can be controlled automatically. Incandescent lights have the advantage of being cheap and easy to dim, but there are now much more efficient alternatives. Fluorescent lights, although more efficient, are more difficult to dim. Light-emitting diodes (LEDs) are becoming very popular. They have the advantage of being extremely efficient, small and light-weight and are available to emit a variety of wave-lengths. Trials under commercial conditions showed that laying flocks kept under LED lighting had very similar hen-day egg production, egg weight, feed use and mortality rate as flocks under fluorescent lighting (Long et al. 2016). It has also been shown that pullets and laying hens do not have a strong aversion to LED lights although they show a slight preference for fluorescent lighting when given a choice (Liu et al. 2017).

No matter the light source, domestic fowl in laboratories should generally be housed at higher light levels than those used commercially which will allow for easy inspection. It may also be possible to enrich the birds' environment by providing natural light through windows or skylights or by allowing them access to a veranda. General information on lighting is given by Lewis and Morris (2006).

Environmental provisions

General advice on environmental requirements can be found in the report on birds by the Joint Working Group on Refinement (JWGR 2001). The ventilation system should have sufficient capacity to cope with the local climatic conditions and the maximum numbers of birds held in each room. The main purpose of a ventilating system is to remove excess heat and water vapour from the building. It is unlikely that bird density in a laboratory setting will ever be so high as to constitute an over-heating problem, but it should be noted that a light hybrid, medium hybrid and broiler breeding hen produce about 42, 48 and 59 kiloJoules (kJ) of heat per hour. With regard to water production, 100 light hybrid laying hens at normal room temperature produce 11.4 kg respiratory water per day and 8.8 kg faecal water per day, giving a total of 20.2 kg water per day. The ventilation system has to remove much of this water and the efficiency of the system will depend on the relative humidity of the air at the time. The usual formula for calculating fan capacity is to allow 0.17 m^3 air per bird per min. If the laboratory is located in an area where summer temperatures of over 30 °C are common, then an air-conditioning system should be installed.

It is essential that the whole building is fitted with an alarm system which will give warning if there is a power failure to any room. The building should have an emergency generator which switches in automatically in the event of a power failure and, in addition, an alarm system which will notify a responsible person that there is an emergency. Systems are available whereby the alarm will call or text a series of telephone numbers.

Pens or cages?

Probably the first important decision to be made is whether birds can be kept on the floor or if they must be housed in some form of cage. The nature of the research will probably determine which route must be followed. In general, birds should not be kept cages unless there is an overriding scientific reason to do so. However, the fact that a cage environment separates the bird from its faeces, means that cages are more hygienic although more restrictive. There may also be many good scientific reasons for deciding on cages, such as projects requiring faecal collection or if the nature of the research precludes medication with a coccidiostat. Conventional battery cages were banned for commercial use in the European Union (EU) from January 2012; Canada and New Zealand are currently phasing out commercial cages. However, even when birds are not kept in cages, higher welfare standards are required for experimental animals. For example, Directive 2010/63/EU (2010) of the European Parliament on the protection of animals used for scientific purposes has emphasised the principles of replacement, reduction and refinement. This Directive also recommends enriched environments for animals under experiment, including domestic fowl, the need for frequent inspections and early end-points in experiments such that suffering is reduced to a minimum. This Directive also provides minimum enclosure dimensions and space allowances for birds that are substantially greater than for birds being kept commercially. For example, the Directive recommends that a bird weighing 600–1,200 g should be kept in an enclosure of at least 2 m^2 and have space of at least 0.09 m^2.

It may also be possible to brood the chicks and rear the young stock on the floor, while keeping the adult stock in cages. It may even be possible to keep all stock on the floor and move birds into cages for the duration of an experiment. However, it should be realised that if birds have been kept in a relatively enriched environment and are then moved to the more impoverished environment of a cage, they will probably experience frustration, show evidence of this in their behaviour (Duncan 1970) and this in turn may have an effect on the variables being recorded in the experiment. Of course, there are not the same financial constraints on the keeping of birds in a laboratory. So, for example, it may be perfectly feasible to keep laboratory hens in a small floor pen on litter and maintain hygiene by cleaning the pen out each week which would be totally unacceptable financially in commercial practice.

For many research projects, it may be possible to use commercial penning or cages with their furnishings. In other cases, for example in nutritional studies into trace elements, specialised equipment, made of stainless steel or special plastics, may be required.

Information on feeding and drinking equipment is given in the following text.

Brooding phase

Information on optimal environmental conditions for particular strains at different ages is available from breeding companies.

Chicks may be brooded on the floor or in tier brooders. They are not able to regulate their body temperature very well for the first few weeks of life and require warmth. It is usually best to raise the temperature of the room in which chicks are being brooded to say, 24–26 °C, and to provide some supplemental heat.

If brooded on the floor, the extra heat is most easily provided by a suspended electrical heater. More powerful commercial brooders operated by natural gas and other fuels are available if large numbers of chicks are being brooded. For a laboratory, electrical brooders are probably more convenient. It is recommended that dull emitter heaters are used rather than heating lamps since this means that the lighting and heating programmes can be controlled independently. The heater should be suspended above the floor of the pen with some means of adjusting the height, since this is how temperature is controlled. The heater should be switched on 24 h before the chicks are due. A thermometer can be used to check the temperature before the chicks arrive. It should be about 32 °C 15 cm outside the brooder canopy or reflector and 5 cm above the floor. However, the main guide to brooder temperature should be the chicks themselves. When they are placed, they should arrange themselves in a ring below where the brooder is radiating heat. If they huddle directly below the brooder, then they are cold and the brooder should be lowered. If they are spread out as far from the brooder as possible, then they are hot and the brooder should be raised. Dull emitter heaters are capable of brooding a few hundred chicks. Supplemental heat is gradually reduced through the brooding period by raising the height of the brooder.

For the first few days, chicks are usually not allowed access to the whole pen, but are confined to a smaller area, about 1.5 m in diameter, under the brooder using a brooder guard. This is simply a temporary construction made out of a roll of corrugated cardboard, perhaps 30–40 cm high with the ends clipped together to make a circle. It is scrapped after a few days.

Some form of litter with good insulating and absorbing properties should be placed on the floor to a depth of about 3–5 cm. Wood shavings are common, but many other materials can be used. If wood shavings are used, they should be from untreated wood.

Water can be provided in various ways. Chick founts, with a large glass or plastic jar inverted in a plastic or metal dish, are common (see Figure 40.1). Automatic drinking nipples, cups and bells also work well. A bell drinker is a plastic bell-shaped container suspended from the ceiling and supplied with water via a flexible water line from above. Water flows over the outside of the bell and is held in an upturned rim. When a set amount of water is in the rim, the weight of the water operates a stop valve in the supply line. As the birds drink the water, the weight decreases and the valve opens allowing water to flow again (see Figure 40.2). There is some advantage to using nipples since they often have a drop of water hanging from the nipple and this attracts chicks which have a natural tendency to peck at

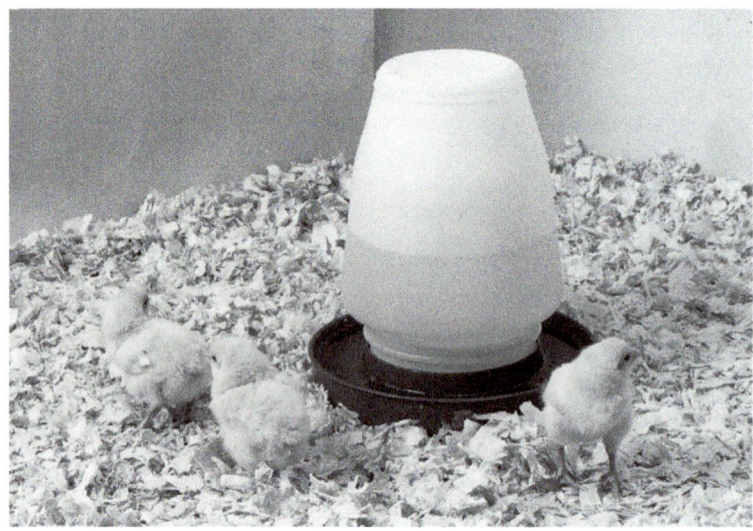

Figure 40.1 A chick fount suitable for supplying chicks with water for the first few weeks of life.

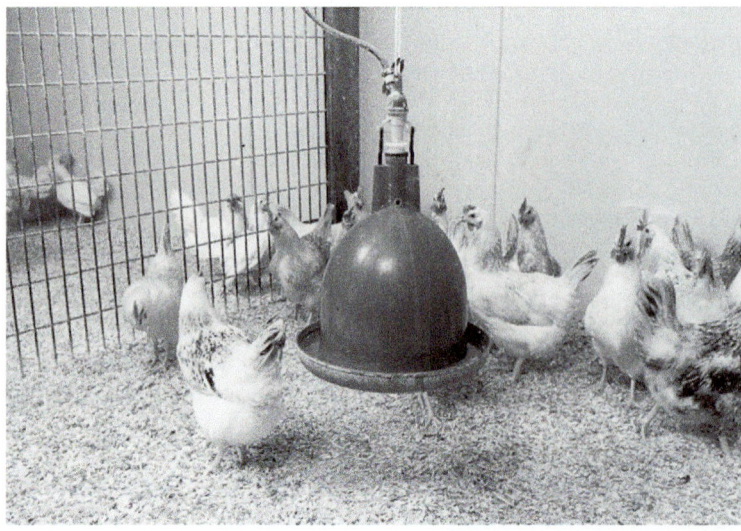

Figure 40.2 A drinking bell suitable for supplying water to all growing and adult birds on the floor.

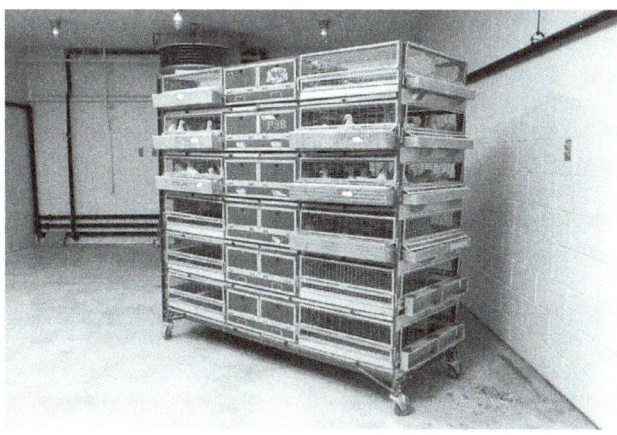

Figure 40.3 A tier brooder.

bright shiny objects. Allow 1.5 cm/chick of water trough access, 1.3 cm/chick if pans or bells are used, 4 automatic cups/100 chicks, or 8 automatic nipples/100 chicks. There should be a daily inspection of all drinkers to ensure there is an unimpeded supply of water.

There are also a variety of feeders available in metal and plastic. Allow 5 cm/chick of trough access or 4 cm/chick if round pans are used. In addition, some extra food should be provided on 'scratch trays' for the first few days. Cardboard trays used for egg storage are ideal for this purpose.

Tier brooders are cages for groups of chicks. Each cage is commonly divided into an enclosed section which is heated electrically with the heat being controlled by a thermostat, and a more open section which allows for inspection. Food and water are supplied from troughs running round the outside of the cage (see Figure 40.3). Tier brooders save space and are often on wheels so they can easily be moved between rooms. The thermostat should be adjusted to provide a temperature of about 32 °C in the enclosed section of the brooder.

As with all neonates, rest and sleep are extremely important for chicks (Malleau *et al.* 2007). Therefore, chicks should be given at least 8 h of darkness every 24 h. When the lights are on, the level of illumination should be fairly high (40 lux) for the first 3–5 days. After this, birds should go on to a lifetime lighting programme. For laying hens and all breeding birds, this will generally mean that, from about 5 days until they are photo-stimulated, they will be kept on a short day, perhaps 8L : 16D. Broilers should be given at least 8 h of darkness every 24 h. Commercially, chickens are kept under very dim light. However, since they are very visual animals, it is suggested that, in a laboratory setting, the level of illumination should be much brighter than this, at least 20 lux.

Rearing phase

After about 4 weeks, young birds generally do not require supplemental heat if they are housed in a room in which the temperature remains above 18 °C. For laying and breeding stock, the phase that follows brooding until they reach sexual maturity at 19–24 weeks is considered the rearing phase. For broilers, the rearing phase covers the period until they are killed at 5–8 weeks. During the rearing phase the optimum room temperature is about 20 °C, but growing birds can easily cope with a range of 18–26 °C. Birds can be reared on the floor or in cages. Once again, the nature of the research will determine which husbandry method is selected, but if at all possible, birds should be reared on the floor. If they are destined to become breeding stock, breeding naturally, then they should be reared on the floor.

Birds should be given plenty of space. If they are being reared in cages, each bird will require a minimum of about 600 cm^2 as they approach sexual maturity, so this capacity should be available. They can be kept at a higher density when they are young, and then be split into smaller groups at a lower density as they grow. If they are reared on the floor on litter, the space required as they approach maturity is about 5 birds/m^2. However, they can be kept more densely than this when young and sub-divided as they grow. Local regulations on bird density should be checked and these should take priority if they allow more space than suggested here.

There are many different kinds of commercial feeders available for floor rearing. Allow 9 cm/bird of trough access or 4 cm/bird if large diameter (120 cm) tube feeders are used. Of course, if any type of food restriction is going to be practised, then these allowances must be greatly increased to 15 cm/bird for troughs and 8 cm/bird for tube feeders, to ensure that all the birds can very easily feed at once. For cage-reared birds, towards the end of the rearing period, allow 9–10 cm/bird of trough space.

Water can be provided by means of troughs, bells, automatic cups or nipples, with cups and nipples being more hygienic. Allow 2.5 cm/bird of water trough access, 2.0 cm/bird of bell access, 9 automatic cups/100 birds, or 12 automatic nipples/100 birds. Birds should be monitored closely if the type of drinker is changed between phases. For example, chicks that have been brooded with nipple drinkers may not recognise water when it is presented in a trough or bell drinker. There should be a daily inspection of all drinkers to ensure there is an unimpeded supply of water. Drinking troughs require frequent cleaning. Bells and cups also require cleaning but less frequently than troughs. Water lines should be checked and flushed regularly since dirt can build up quickly when the house temperature is high.

Since domestic fowl learn to perch at an early age, and since, if given the opportunity, they rest in a perching posture and are strongly motivated to do so (Olsson & Keeling 2002), it is recommended that perches be provided from at least 1 week of age. These should be round, or round with a flattened top, of about 25 mm in diameter for younger birds, and made of reasonably hard wood or plastic. As laying stock birds approach adulthood, the perches should be exchanged for ones with a diameter of about 36 mm (Tauson & Abrahamsson 1994). It is recommended that perches be provided at different heights, one at 5–10 cm above the floor, and at least one other at about 30 cm above the floor. Allow about 30 cm perch length per bird at each level so that the birds can perch communally. Broiler strains also start to perch at 7–10 days of age but stop perching by 20 days, possibly because intensive breeding for large breasts has resulted in their centre of gravity being moved forward making it difficult for them to balance on a perch.

Adult phase

Birds should be moved to their adult quarters at about 16 weeks of age so that they can settle down before the first egg is produced. The optimum temperature for adult chickens is 20–21 °C but the range 16–26 °C is satisfactory. Below 16 °C birds will eat considerably more food to keep warm, and above 27 °C hens may not eat enough to maintain a high level of egg production. At 28–29 °C, they begin to encounter heat stress problems.

It is the housing of adult chickens that raises the most animal welfare concerns. The traditional battery cage, although a hygienic and profitable husbandry system, is much less than ideal from a welfare point of view. Conventional battery cages have been banned in the EU from January 2012 and are in the process of being phased out in Canada and New Zealand. Standards of care in a laboratory should be higher than those in commercial conditions. Laboratories should, therefore, make every attempt to find an alternative, more welfare-friendly husbandry system than cages for keeping adult chickens.

If some type of conventional cage is essential for the research, then it must be of the best possible design. Tauson (1980, 1985) describes how design features of conventional cages may be modified to improve welfare. If some form of conventional cage in a special material such as stainless steel or plastic is necessary, then the cages may have to be built to order. Once again, the modifications suggested by Tauson (1980, 1985) should be incorporated into the design, including an absence of V-shaped spaces where birds can be trapped, a floor slope of no more than 8°, and an appropriate distance that the bird has to stretch to the bottom of the food trough. Cage height should be at least 40 cm throughout the cage. If possible, birds should be kept in small groups of 3 or 4 with 800 cm^2 floor space per bird or at least 600 cm^2 if the birds are small. If birds must be kept in single-bird cages, these should allow about 1,200 cm^2 floor space per bird. If birds are kept in pairs, each cage should have at least 1,800 cm^2 floor space. The minimum feeding space should be 12 cm per bird. In multi-bird cages, birds retain better plumage condition if there are solid rather than wire mesh divisions between cages.

Conventional cages, even those with all the improvements described above, are not suitable for males. It will not generally be possible to keep more than one male to a cage because of the risk of fighting and injury. Cages for males should be 60 cm in height and a space allowance of about 2,500 cm^2 is recommended. Since there are no eggs to roll away, the floor should be level.

The simplest and most hygienic method of supplying water to cages is by means of nipples or cups. One nipple or cup per cage of 3–4 birds is sufficient. However, since chickens do not compete over water, a better configuration is to locate nipples or cups at cage junctions so that 2 or 4 cages can share the facility. This means that birds in each cage will have access to more than one water outlet. There should be a daily inspection of all drinkers to ensure there is an unimpeded supply of water. Drinking cups also require periodic cleaning.

If the type of research being conducted by the laboratory allows alternatives to cages, then there are many systems to choose from. The past 20 years has seen a burgeoning of alternative commercial systems (see, for example, Appleby *et al.* 2004; Lay *et al.* 2011; Rodenburg *et al.* 2012; Friere & Cowling 2013) and a laboratory could easily adopt one of these, either in its commercial form or as a modified scaled-down version. There are two main types of system, one based on floor-housing and the other on modified cages. A good housing system should include the following essential features:

1. The birds should be in reasonably small groups. There is no hard evidence on what the upper threshold might be, above which welfare is reduced. It is likely that a group size of 15–20 is ideal although there is some evidence that social problems are more common with an intermediate flock size of around 30 birds than with a large flock size (Keeling *et al.* 2003). Maintaining birds in appropriately sized groups should not be a problem for most laboratories. Within the group, each bird should have 800 cm^2 of space. Since, in many of these systems, more use is made of vertical space, and birds may 'share' floor space by being at different levels, it is sometimes difficult to make this calculation. As a general rule, laboratories should be generous with space allowances.
2. The birds should be able to feed at the same time; this means that at least 10 cm feed trough space per bird is required, slightly less than this if food is provided from a round pan.
3. Birds should have access to water at all times. Any of the previously described drinkers is suitable. Allow about one cup for 12 hens or one nipple for 8 hens.
4. Hens should have access to a suitable nesting place. Single- or pair-housed birds should each have access to a nestbox, with a ratio of at least one nestbox per two birds provided in larger groups. Communal nestboxes also seem to work quite well. The nest should be secluded but not necessarily dark. It should allow the hen to express the various nest-building motor patterns. Loose nesting material is not essential but a round cup-shaped nest is preferred (Duncan & Kite 1989). It is possible to collect eggs automatically from a nest of this type. If individual nestboxes are used, then allow one nestbox for five hens.
5. Perches should be available for roosting at night and for resting through the day. The best perch designed so far (a perfect perch has not yet been designed) is of reasonably hard wood, circular in profile, 36 mm in diameter and flattened on the top and bottom giving a vertical cross section of 31 mm (Tauson & Abrahamsson 1994). Perches with a mushroom-shaped cross section also work well. Plastic perches tend to be slippier than wooden perches but do give some protection against red mite (*Dermanyssus gallinae*) infestation. If perches are provided at different levels, there should be sufficient length of perch to allow all the birds in a group to perch at the same level. This will require about 15 cm of perch per bird. It should be pointed out that, although on balance, the provision of perches increases welfare, they do have some costs. Perches increase the incidence of bumble foot (an inflammatory infection of the foot pad) and

keel bone deformations, compared with birds kept without perches. On the other hand, perches decrease the incidence of toe pad hyperkeratosis when they are added to conventional battery cages (Tauson & Abrahamsson 1994).

The best alternative systems, whether based on floor-housing or cage-housing, incorporate all these features. The following features are not equally available in the two types of system.

6. It is much easier to provide opportunities for foraging in floor-based housing systems. Since foraging normally occupies a great deal of time, it is probably very important to the chicken. It is not impossible to allow hens in cage-based environments to forage, but it takes some ingenuity and stamina on the part of the caretaker. For example, some type of fresh green material, such as a cabbage or piece of cabbage or net filled with clover could be hung in the cage. Alfalfa hay hung in a net also makes a good foraging substrate. Hanging foraging material in a net means that the hygiene associated with a mesh floor is maintained. However, the labour involved in such a scheme would be considerable and if foraging material is not provided after the chickens have become used the routine, there is then a grave risk of the chickens starting to feather peck. Therefore, if foraging behaviour is considered essential, a floor-based system should be selected.

7. Dustbathing behaviour can be encouraged in cage-based systems by the provision of sandboxes. However, there have been problems associated with these, notably hens laying eggs in the sandboxes, probably because the design was not ideal. On the other hand, dusty locations quickly develop in the litter of floor-based systems, and these are used for dustbathing.

There are so many housing systems available that it is impossible to describe each. Many commercial cage manufacturers are now marketing modified and enriched cages which maintain the hygienic nature if the traditional cage but provide secluded nests, perches and occasionally dust-baths and surfaces to which forage can be added. Fowl are highly motivated to perform 'comfort behaviour' such as wing flapping, feather ruffling and leg stretching, which help to maintain strong leg bones. Modified cages should therefore be large enough to permit all of these behaviour patterns to occur whenever possible. There is one activity that modified cages do not allow full expression to and that is foraging behaviour. Some designs of modified cages incorporate a solid section of floor on which food is regularly scattered. Since foraging behaviour is a social activity, this design works best in larger cages where several hens can engage in the activity simultaneously. Although having a solid floor section within the cage meets some of the birds' foraging needs, it also allows access to any faeces that may be dropped there and so reduces hygiene. Similarly with dust-baths; they allow expression of an important behavioural activity, but they also reduce hygiene. An advantage of a modified cage husbandry system is that the cages can be tiered to save space, and feeding, drinking and egg collection can be automated. They also provide a fairly high standard of hygiene.

Care of aged animals

Occasionally, it may be necessary for laboratories to keep birds beyond their normal commercial lifespan, perhaps because they carry important and rare traits or because the laboratory is interested in the ageing process. In many cases, a deterioration in quality of life with ageing may be gradual and almost imperceptible. It is therefore essential that in these cases, the birds should be observed frequently and carefully by a knowledgeable attendant to ensure that their quality of life is acceptable. Decisions on when states of suffering outweigh states of pleasure are extremely difficult to make but such decisions should always favour ending suffering by euthanasia.

Hygiene

It is essential that newly hatched chicks go into a clean environment. In a laboratory, the best way to achieve this is to copy commercial husbandry and operate an 'all-in, all-out' system. Of course, in a laboratory, 'all-in, all-out' will apply to individual rooms and not to the whole establishment. When each room becomes empty of birds, the room and all the equipment in it, should be thoroughly cleaned and disinfected. If individual rooms can be hermetically sealed, then they should also be fumigated at this time. There may be some advantage in rotating disinfectants and in allowing rooms to stand empty for some days after disinfection. All the equipment in the room should be cleaned and disinfected at the same time as the room is being treated.

It is also good practice to have disinfectant foot baths outside each room so that diseases are not spread inadvertently by the animal care staff. Of course, if the laboratory is dealing with diseases, then much more stringent precautions will have to be taken such as specialist protective clothing and apparatus (a different set for each room or unit), and showering into and out of each room or unit.

Identification and sexing

Small, numbered, metal or plastic wing-tags can be used to give day-old chicks a unique, lifetime identification. There is evidence that plastic wing-tags are superior to metal ones in that they have less deleterious effect on welfare and physiology (Dennis et al. 2008). A special tool is used to clip the tags through the wing-web on the front edge of the wing taking care not to pierce any muscle tissue.

Commercial breeding companies often arrange their day-old chicks to be auto-sexed. Use is made of certain genes carried on the sex chromosomes, such as silver down-colour, barring or fast-feathering. In the case of silver down-colour, for example, cocks (the homogametic sex) which are homozygous recessive for the trait (and gold) are mated with females which are hemizygous dominant (and silver). This results in male progeny in which the males are all heterozygous (and silver) and the females are all hemizygous (and gold). Fast-feathering, controlled by a single gene, is often used to sex broiler chicks. In this case, breeding is arranged such that female chicks are fast-feathering with their emerging primary wing feathers longer than their wing covert feathers. Male chicks, on the other hand are slow-feathering with their primary wing feathers shorter or the same length as their wing coverts. If breeding companies cannot arrange for auto-sexing, then they use vent-sexing in which highly trained personnel are able to sex the chicks using differences in genital papillae.

It is thus simple for a laboratory to buy day-old chicks of the required sex but not so easy to arrange auto-sexing or vent-sexing within the laboratory. If birds of a certain sex are required, the solution may be to rear all the chicks until feather differences become obvious. These differences can usually be identified at a few weeks of age.

Natural breeding

Domestic fowl will breed easily if kept in floor pens. If the experimental procedures dictate that the breeding birds should be kept in cages, then it is advisable to use artificial insemination, since cage breeding is never very successful. Birds are usually photo-stimulated to bring them into breeding condition at around 17–21 weeks of age (a few weeks later for feed restricted, meat-type birds). Rapid growth and reddening of the comb is characteristic of birds coming into breeding condition. In hens, the vent becomes moist and red a few days before the first egg is due and the pubic bones separate from about one finger-width to about three finger-widths.

A sex ratio of about 1 male to 10 females usually works well. Eggs laid 2 days after the sexes are mixed should be fertile. If the laboratory is practising some form of pedigreed mating system, then it should be remembered that hens remain fertile for 7–10 days after one successful copulation. Fertility then drops quite quickly and few fertile eggs should be produced 15 days after the sexes are separated.

Fertile eggs should be collected often in order to get them into ideal storage conditions as quickly as possible. They should be stored, blunt end up, in egg-trays, in an egg storage room designed for the purpose, with a temperature of about 16–18 °C and a relative humidity of 75%. Fertile eggs may be stored for 1 week, but hatchability will decrease after longer storage times.

It is best to warm hatching eggs at room temperature (20–22 °C) for 4–6 hours before setting them in the incubator.

The incubation period for domestic fowl is 21 days. Optimal incubation conditions are a temperature of 37.5–37.7 °C and a relative humidity of 60% for the first 19 days and a temperature of 36.1–37.2 °C and a relative humidity of 75% for the final two days. This is normally achieved by moving the trays from the setter to the hatcher on day 19 of incubation; if the chicks are to be pedigreed, the hatcher must have individual boxes for each egg/chick. The eggs must be turned regularly (commercially they are turned every hour) during the first 19 days.

It has been suggested that eggs should not be exposed to light during the last week of incubation since this increases feather pecking behaviour in the first 3 weeks after hatching (Riedstra & Groothuis 2004). On the other hand, it has been shown that substantial light stimulation during incubation (12 h per day throughout incubation) can be beneficial for welfare in terms of reducing stress and fear responses during the rearing period (Archer & Mench 2014).

If incubation is going to be carried out regularly in a laboratory, then papers which cover the topic such as Hulet (2007), Fasenko (2007) and Decuypere & Bruggeman (2007) should be consulted.

Artificial insemination

Artificial insemination may be necessary because, for example, of a scientific requirement for individually housed hens, or when natural mating results in low fertility, or if specific pedigreed matings are required. The technique is straightforward. For best results, males should be housed individually, otherwise homosexual mating may deplete semen yields. Males can be photo-stimulated to produce semen at a fairly young age but it is normal to do this at about 18 weeks for laying-type males and 20 weeks for meat-type males. They will then start to produce semen at about 20 weeks and 22 weeks, respectively, and collection of semen should start at that time. The procedure for semen collection is well-described by Etches (1996) but requires a highly skilled technician for best results. The male is held with his feet at right angles to his body, and his belly and back is stroked towards the tail with quick firm strokes. This stimulates erection of the phallic folds. When stimulated, the hand massaging the back is then transferred to the cloacal area with the thumb and index finger located on the lateral aspects of the cloaca and slightly anterior to the vent. Gentle pressure can then be used to expel semen from the ductus deferens. The flow of semen can then be collected by aspiration into a collecting ampoule. Care should be taken to collect semen only and avoid urates and faeces. Males should be handled gently and consistently. They become accustomed to being milked by the same operator and changes of personnel should be avoided if possible. A collecting schedule of three times per week (Mondays, Wednesdays and Fridays) will yield good volumes (0.15–0.35 ml) of semen. Etches (1996) recommends collecting the semen into semen diluent at 15 °C, evaluating the semen for sperm density and quality, then arranging the rate of dilution such that each hen gets a standard insemination volume of 0.05 ml containing 100 million sperm cells.

Females can be inseminated as soon as they are in lay and it is better to inseminate later in the day when there is not a hard-shelled egg in the shell gland. The hen is held in the palm of the left hand facing left with the thighs held by the thumb and index finger. Gentle pressure is then exerted in a posterior direction with the left hand as the tail is pressed in an anterior direction with the right hand. This everts the hen's cloaca. A second person then inserts the inseminating pipette into the oviduct to a depth of about 3 cm. The first person releases the pressure on the body cavity allowing the cloaca to return to its natural position and the second person inseminates and withdraws the pipette. Inseminating hens every 5 days will usually maintain a high fertility rate.

Inspection of birds

All birds in a laboratory should be inspected at least twice a day, first thing in the morning and again later in the day. The inspection should be carried out by personnel who are familiar with the healthy appearance and normal behaviour of various classes of domestic fowl. It is good laboratory practice to have check sheets in every bird room on which any departure from normal appearance or behaviour can be recorded. These check sheets should list individual bird numbers in each pen so that any observations or treatments can be recorded at the individual level. Of course, if birds are subjected to any experimental treatment that might jeopardise their welfare, then inspections should be more frequent than this. During routine inspections of the birds, equipment such as feeders and drinkers should be checked. This is also a good opportunity to monitor and record environmental variables such as temperature and ventilation.

Feeding

Commercial poultry rations are formulated to very high standards and laboratories can have confidence in buying these. Complete balanced rations are usually fed, either as a dry mash, pellets or crumbles, which are partially ground-up pellets. The steam and pressure used in pelleting increases the digestibility of a ration so that weight-for-weight, pellets and crumbles are slightly more nutritious than the same ration in mash form. It is advantageous to feed chicks crumbles; the particle size of crumbles is very attractive to chicks and ensures that they ingest plenty of food in the first few days. In the rearing and adult stages, it is usual to choose a mash ration if over-consumption is a problem or if it is necessary to occupy the birds with feeding through a large part of the day and essential if feather pecking is likely to be a problem. (Birds take longer to eat the same quantity of mash compared with pellets or crumbles). If high consumption and quick growth are necessary, or if under-consumption is a problem, then pellets or crumbles should be fed.

The energy in poultry diets normally comes from a cereal, often maize, wheat or barley or a mixture of these, sometimes boosted with soy oil, or a mix of vegetable and animal fat. The protein comes from a source of vegetable protein such as soybean meal supplemented with individual synthetic amino acids. To this is added a pre-mix containing minerals, vitamins and possibly some additives such as an antioxidant, a coccidiostat, xanthophylls to give yolk colour, etc.

Different ages and types of bird have different nutritional requirements which means that, in a laboratory that houses chickens of a range of ages and types, several rations have to be fed. The specifications for the most commonly fed chicken rations are shown in Tables 40.2–40.8.

It should be noted that if hens are producing fertile eggs for hatching, then it is usual to increase the nutrient density of the diet slightly. In addition, special attention is paid to minerals, vitamins and essential amino acids in breeder diets. It is normal for the males in a breeder flock to receive the same ration as the hens. However, they should receive less calcium (< 1.0%). If artificial insemination is being practised and the males are separate from the females, this can be arranged. It can also occur in broiler breeder flocks in which the sexes are fed separately.

It is usual to include a coccidiostat in the rations of young birds being kept on the floor. Rations containing fat should

Table 40.2 Chick starter diet specifications for egg-type strains (from day-old to week 5). The quality of the protein must be high and this can be verified by checking the levels of certain amino acids which should be present at least at the level shown.

Metabolisable energy (ME) (MegaJoules/kilogram)	12.13
Protein (%)	18–20
Arginine (%)	1.0
Lysine (%)	0.9
Methionine (%)	0.4
Tryptophan (%)	0.18
Fibre (%) (upper limit)	3–4
Calcium (%)	1.0
Phosphorus (%)	0.45
Plus a good vitamin and mineral supplement at the recommended level	

Table 40.3 Grower diet specifications for egg-type strains (from week 5 to week 16/17).

Metabolisable energy (ME) (MegaJoules/kilogram)	11.71
Protein (%)	14
Calcium (%)	0.8
Phosphorus (%)	0.4
Plus a good vitamin and mineral supplement at the recommended level	

Table 40.4 Two-phase grower diet specifications for egg-type strains.

	Week 5–11	Week 12–16/17
Metabolisable energy (ME) (MegaJoules/kilogram)	11.92	11.50
Protein (%)	15	13
Calcium (%)	0.8	0.8
Phosphorus (%)	0.4	0.4
Plus a good vitamin and mineral supplement at the recommended level		

Table 40.5 Layer diet specifications for egg-type strains.

Metabolisable energy (ME) (MegaJoules/kilogram)	11.50
Protein (%)	16
Calcium (%)	3.5
Phosphorus (%)	0.4
Plus a good vitamin and mineral supplement at the recommended level	

also have an antioxidant, such as ethoxyquin, to prevent the fat going rancid.

More information on poultry nutrition can be obtained from Leeson & Summers (2000).

If commercial poultry rations are not available, then there are other possibilities which, although not ideal, will provide the essential nutrients. However, if standardised commercial rations are not available, then consider whether it is worthwhile performing research that may not be replicable.

Table 40.6 Breeder diet specifications for egg-type strains.

Metabolisable energy (ME) (MegaJoules/kilogram)	11.71
Protein (%)	17
Calcium (%)	3.7
Phosphorus (%)	0.44
Plus a good vitamin and mineral supplement at the recommended level	

Table 40.7 Three-phase broiler diet specifications.

	Starter (days 1–24)	Grower (days 25–35)	Finisher (days 36–42)
Metabolisable energy (ME) (MegaJoules/kilogram)	12.75	13.18	13.38
Protein (%)	22	20	18
Calcium (%)	1.0	0.95	0.95
Phosphorus (%)	0.42	0.4	0.4
Plus a good vitamin and mineral supplement at the recommended level			

Table 40.8 Broiler breeder diet specifications.

Metabolisable energy (ME) (MegaJoules/kilogram)	12.13
Protein (%)	16.5
Calcium (%)	3.7
Phosphorus (%)	0.45
Plus a good vitamin and mineral supplement at the recommended level	

It should be remembered that birds are very good at balancing their own diet if provided with a variety of ingredients (Dove 1935). Therefore, they could be given a selection of locally available seeds and grains. The local ingredients should be checked against tables of nutrient composition (in any good nutrition textbook) to ensure that they are likely to provide sufficient energy and protein. Leeson and Summers (2000) provide tables of ingredient constraints showing the maximum amount of various ingredients that should be included in diets for different classes of domestic fowl. If soluble vitamins and minerals are available, they could be supplied in the water to supplement local rations. Again, if the birds are laying hens, then some form of supplemental calcium will be required. Also, if whole grains are being fed, then the birds should have access to some form of insoluble grit which is needed to grind the grains in the gizzard.

Laboratory procedures

Handling

As pointed out previously, many strains of domestic fowl have retained their ancestral fear of human beings. They should therefore be handled gently but firmly in order that fear responses are not exacerbated. There is little problem with very young chicks, since fear responses to human beings only develop over the first few days after hatching. There may be some advantage for laboratory managers to habituate birds to human beings and to handling early in life. There is evidence that early handling reduces fearful responses to human beings later (Hughes & Black 1976; Jones & Faure 1981) although some particularly flighty strains may not show much improvement (Murphy & Duncan 1978). Birds should be caught using both hands to pin the bird's wings against its sides. When held firmly like this, birds usually settle down very quickly, and they can be transported over short distances, say between a pen and an examination table within a room. For transporting between rooms, a carrying crate is recommended. Disposable, cardboard, carrying boxes are ideal for this purpose.

If birds are difficult to catch because they show excessive avoidance behaviour, dimming the lights usually helps.

Restraint and blood sampling

Birds may be restrained on their backs, say for examination, with one hand gripping both legs firmly, leaving the other hand free for manipulation. Blood samples are usually drawn from the brachial (wing) vein close to where it passes over the ulna and radius just distal to the joint with the humerus. The easiest method is for one person to restrain the bird on its side using one hand to hold both legs with the other hand over the breast pinning the lower wing to the bird's side. The person taking the sample can then use one hand to extend the other wing. The axillary feathers should be removed from the site or pushed to the side. Whether the needle is inserted into the vein towards or away from the heart is a matter of personal preference. The following sizes of needles are recommended for blood sampling: 0.7 mm × 15 mm long needle (25 G) for 0–2 week old chicks, 0.7 mm × 19 mm (21 G) for 2–6 week old chicks, 0.8 mm × 38 mm (20 G) for 6–18 week old birds, and 0.9 mm × 38 mm for adults.

Monitoring physiological variables

The fact that restraint is an extremely stressful procedure for domestic fowl means that obtaining undisturbed physiological data can be a challenge. Birds are also very intolerant of leads or catheters running from the skin surface. With a great deal of patience, birds can sometimes be habituated to the presence of leads or catheters, but one would then need to question how normal their behaviour was. Birds have extremely flexible necks and can reach almost every part of their bodies with their beaks, which are usually very efficient at removing attachments. The upper neck and head, which cannot be reached by the beak, can be very effectively scratched by the bird's feet. A solution to this problem could be biotelemetry, by which physiological variables are sent from a radio-transmitter on (Duncan et al. 1975) or in the bird (Filshie et al. 1980; Duncan & Filshie 1980) to a receiver some distance away. A bird will habituate to a small device strapped to its back whereas it is very intolerant of attached leads. Once a bird with an implanted device has recovered from anaesthesia, it is free to move about unencumbered. Biotelemetry techniques have improved in the past 30 years and now multichannel devices are available which can transmit up to nine variables simultaneously and even have a two-way capability by which the implanted device can accept commands to perform various tasks within the animal (Axelsson et al. 2007).

Injections and dosing

Intravenous injections are usually given in the brachial vein (see blood sampling in the preceding text). Intramuscular injections are usually given in the muscles of the upper leg. Subcutaneous injections can be given in the neck, the web of the wing or, with the bird restrained on its back, into a patch of loose bare skin at the junction of the breast and leg which makes a very convenient site. It is also possible to arrange *in vivo* microdialysis procedures in poultry (Kops et al. 2014)

Birds can be dosed orally very easily. With the bird restrained in an upright position and the beak held open, pills can be gently pushed to the back of the mouth with a finger. When the head is released, the pill will be swallowed. Liquids can be injected into the crop by way of the oesophagus (taking care to avoid the trachea) by means of a syringe and a flexible plastic tube and with the bird restrained as described above. For best practice, after insertion the correct position of the tube should be confirmed by ensuring it can be felt within the oesophagus.

Anaesthesia and analgesia

Birds are not the easiest class of animals to anaesthetise and those administering anaesthetics to chickens should be properly trained. Specialist texts covering this topic should be consulted, such as Lierz and Korbel (2012) and Lawton (2016).

Chickens should be fasted sufficiently to empty the crop before proceeding with anaesthesia. This will vary from an hour or two with young chicks to overnight for adult birds. It should also be remembered that birds can quickly become hypothermic. Therefore, a warming pad should be used during anaesthesia and some provision should be made to provide heat during recovery, such as a heating lamp over the recovery cage.

With regard to pre-anaesthetics, atropine is generally not used in birds; diazepam (0.5–1.5 mg/kg intramuscularly or intravenously) is the pre-anaesthetic of choice.

Isoflurane is the best anaesthetic agent for chickens. They can be induced in a chamber or by means of a mask with 3–5% isoflurane. They may then be intubated with a non-cuffed endotracheal tube and maintained on 1.0–1.5% isoflurane. Halothane, sevoflurane and methoxyflurane may also be used as anaesthetics but are more likely to produce undesirable side-effects.

For short-term procedures, an injectable mixture of ketamine and xylazine may be used to anaesthetise chickens. The required dosage is about 20 mg/kg ketamine and 2 mg/kg xylazine both given intramuscularly. This anaesthesia may be partially reversed by yohimbine injected intravenously at a rate of 0.2 mg/kg.

There is little information available on analgesics for chickens (see Lawton 2016 for review of local anaesthesia and analgesia in birds). It is thought that butorphanol at a dosage rate of 2.0 mg/kg intramuscularly (Hothersall et al. 2016; Singh et al. 2017) and buprenorphine at a rate of 0.01–0.05 mg/kg intramuscularly have good analgesic effects. Lame broilers will self-medicate with the anti-inflammatory drug carprofen sufficiently to reduce their lameness which suggests that this drug is an effective analgesic for joint pain (Danbury et al. 2000).

Euthanasia

When chickens are to be killed, the method must be humane; that is, it must be painless and must minimise fear and anxiety (see also Chapter 17: Euthanasia and other fates for laboratory animals). It must also be reliable, reproducible, irreversible, simple, safe and rapid (Canadian Council on Animal Care 1993; Close et al. 1996; 1997; Humane Slaughter Association 2001). The recommended method for humanely killing chickens is by overdose of an injectable anaesthetic, such as a barbiturate, given intravenously. Laboratory managers should ensure that a suitably qualified person is readily available to carry out this procedure in emergencies as well as in planned procedures. In an emergency, if barbiturates are available but the carer is inexperienced in intravenous injection, then it can be administered by intracoelomic injection, taking care to avoid the air sacs, at about 1.0–1.5 ml/kg of 20% pentobarbital sodium solution. This causes very little distress, and death occurs quietly after a slightly longer period. In every case after euthanasia by injection, the body should be kept until *rigor mortis* has occurred before disposal of the body. In cases of emergencies when someone with authority to use barbiturates is not available, it is preferable to kill a chicken quickly rather than let it suffer for long, and every effort should be made to use a method of killing that is approved in that country. There are currently two methods available that appear to cause a minimum of suffering viz. manual cervical dislocation and non-penetrating captive bolt.

Manual cervical dislocation requires training on cadavers. In young chicks, the neck may be dislocated by using the thumb to press the neck against the sharp edge of a table or bench. An older bird is held by the legs with the head downwards. The other hand is then placed with the head between the index and second fingers so that the other fingers are under the jaw. By applying pressure downwards with the knuckle of the index finger while simultaneously pulling the jaw upwards, the neck can be dislocated. If cervical dislocation is used, the dislocation should be at as high a level as possible, preferably separating the skull from the vertebral column (C0–C1 vertebral dislocation). This method is only appropriate for smaller birds, that is growing stock and light and medium hybrid hens. Some countries put body weight limits on birds that can be killed by this method (e.g. European Council 2009) and these restrictions should be clearly posted in the laboratory. A supportive glove has been developed to aid manual cervical dislocation. This glove has moveable metal insert fingers designed to fit round the bird's head and aid the twisting motion required to dislocate the bird's neck (Martin et al. 2016). There are other mechanical devices for achieving cervical dislocation but these pose a risk of vertebral crushing with a prolonged death and are not considered humane (Erasmus et al. 2010; Bandara et al. 2019a). The other method of humanely killing birds in the laboratory is by means of a non-penetrating captive bolt that has been specially modified for poultry. A penetrating captive bolt has been shown to be much less effective in killing birds humanely (Martin et al. 2016). There are now several models of non-penetrating captive bolts on the market which have been tested on male and female layer chickens from 10 to 70 weeks of age (Bandara et al. 2019b). These devices are probably not suitable for small birds such as broilers younger that 2–3 weeks or laying stock younger than 10 weeks. Staff should therefore be trained in manual cervical dislocation in order to euthanise smaller birds in emergencies.

Common welfare problems

Disease

Chickens can suffer from a variety of infectious diseases caused by viruses, bacteria, mycoplasma and larger parasitic organisms as well as several metabolic diseases. Birds in a laboratory should be monitored regularly for signs of sickness. Symptoms are usually fairly obvious and would include lethargy, sick bird posture (fluffed feathers, neck withdrawn, eye closure), poor appetite, loss of condition, hens going out of lay, production of malformed eggs, coughing, wheezing, blood in faeces, etc.

It is beyond the scope of this chapter to describe each disease in detail and for more information a standard text should be consulted such as Samour (2016) or Swayne (2017). Neither is this text meant as a diagnostic tool; birds which die or are sick should always be sent to a pathology laboratory for proper diagnosis. What follows is simply a rough guide to the more important diseases. The mode of transmission is given; 'vertical transmission' means that the organism is passed from generation to generation via the egg; 'horizontal transmission' means that the organism is passed from bird to bird by a variety of routes.

Bacterial diseases

There are several *Salmonella* diseases of poultry:

Pullorum disease (Salmonella pullorum)

Symptoms   This is a disease of all poultry and some wild birds with acute white diarrhoea and deaths (up to 50%) in young chicks. If chicks have become infected through the hatching egg, then symptoms, including huddling, can start very early (2nd day). Survivors can be chronically infected with few symptoms. In older birds, there are few symptoms except green-brown diarrhoea.
Transmission   Vertical through the hatching egg (this is the most important).

Horizontal   – in the hatcher, debris and dust from infected eggs
– through the droppings (into feed and water)
– cannibalism, birds eating infected blood and tissues
– birds eating infected eggs
– from infected equipment, e.g. debeakers

Diagnosis   Bacteria are isolated and can be cultured in the laboratory.
Treatment   None is practised. The idea is to eradicate the disease, and this is done by blood-testing breeders for antibodies.
Prevention   Breeders should be blood-tested for the presence of pullorum antibodies and reactors eliminated.

Fowl typhoid (S. gallinarum)

Symptoms   This is a slow spreading disease of all poultry of all ages. Birds show loss of appetite, green diarrhoea, with pale combs and wattles in adults. Mortality can eventually reach 50%.
Diagnosis   Bacteria are isolated and can be cultured in the laboratory.
Transmission   Exactly the same as for Pullorum disease.
Treatment   None is practised and, as for Pullorum, eradication is the answer.
Prevention   Breeders should be blood-tested using an agglutination test.

Paratyphoid e.g. (S. typhimurium, S. montevideo, S. derby)

These are important infections because of the risk of food poisoning to humans.

Symptoms   There are often no symptoms in the birds, sometimes diarrhoea.
Diagnosis   Bacteria are isolated and cultured in laboratory.
Transmission   Spread is mainly horizontal through droppings, equipment and people.
Treatment   This is not a major disease of poultry and treatment is not usually required. However, sulfadimethoxine, furazolidone and tetracycline are all quite effective.
Prevention   Cleaning and disinfection between batches of birds, plus the use of foot baths for personnel, help to reduce the incidence.

A disease as yet un-named (S. enteriditis)

This is very important, not because it causes big losses in poultry, but because the organism infects the ovary and hens lay infected eggs which can cause food poisoning in humans. This disease is now fairly well controlled in most countries through testing and elimination of reactors. There are also vaccines available.

Symptoms   No clear symptoms.
Transmission   Vertical through hatching egg.
Horizontal through egg-eating and possibly through droppings.
Treatment   Recommended not to treat but to eradicate.
Prevention   Breeders should be blood-tested using an agglutination test.

Arizona disease (S. arizonae also known as Arizona hinshawii)

Symptoms Important in turkeys and to a less extent chickens. In young birds there is diarrhoea, listlessness, sometimes nervousness. In older birds there can be paralysis of legs. Mortality can reach 25%.
Transmission Horizontal – in the hatcher (from outside of shell).
– through the droppings (into feed and water).
– from infected equipment.
Treatment Furazolidone is commonly used but eradication is the real answer.
Prevention The organism is very resistant to disinfectants and fumigants (which is why it can be present on the outside of hatching eggs after fumigation). Fumigate at double strength.

Fowl cholera (Pasteurella multocida)

Symptoms In the acute form there are rapid deaths (up to 50%), with 12–18 weeks old being a very susceptible stage. In the chronic form there is swelling of wattles and internal organs can be affected.
Transmission Horizontal, entry by respiratory tract or digestive tract.
Diagnosis Bacteria are isolated and can be cultured in the laboratory.
Treatment Sulfa drugs in drinking water are fairly effective.
Prevention A live vaccine is available and can be given by wing-web but aim for eradication (a blood test is available).

Infectious coryza (Haemophilus paragallinarum)

Symptoms This is a persistent but non-fatal disease of the upper respiratory tract with sneezing, discharge from nostrils and swelling of the face. Organism can only live 5–6 hours outside bird.
Transmission Horizontal through air and drinking water.
Diagnosis Symptoms plus laboratory tests.
Treatment Sulfa drugs are fairly effective.
Prevention Isolation from other poultry, and use all-in, all-out management.

Vibrionic hepatitis (Campylobacter foetus)

Symptoms Birds have pale, withered, scaly combs, show a drop in egg production and watery green diarrhoea. A swollen liver and thickened bile duct are evident at p.m. examination.
Transmission Horizontal through the droppings and so in the feed and on equipment and from room to room on people's feet.
Diagnosis Sick birds should be sent to the pathology laboratory. They will attempt to isolate organism from bile.
Treatment Furazolidone in feed gives quite good results. Injection of streptomycin is also effective.
Prevention Stressed birds seem more susceptible – so avoid stress. Normal sanitary precautions will stop spread.

Coliform infections (Escherichia coli)

Coli Enteritis
Symptoms The organism multiplies and causes lesions in the upper digestive tract. There can be blood in droppings similar to coccidiosis plus listlessness.
Colisepticemia
Symptoms This is often the next stage of coliform infection. The organisms enter the blood stream and infect internal organs.
Air-sac Infection
Symptoms Eventually E. coli reach the air sacs and cause an infection there. The birds cough and wheeze and production falls.
Transmission Mainly horizontal – in the hatcher, infected shells, etc.
– through the droppings (into feed and water).
– from infected dust (into lungs).
– from infected feed.
Diagnosis Bacteria are isolated and cultured in the laboratory.
Treatment Furazolidone and tetracycline can be useful if disease is caught at early stage. Once air sacs are infected, treatment is not effective.
Prevention E.coli infections are a sign of dirty surroundings. So treatment should be accompanied by a clean-up campaign. The usual cleaning, disinfecting and fumigating plus all-in, all-out management will do much to prevent coliform infections.

Omphalitis or navel infection (E. coli, Staphylococcus, Pseudomonas and others)

Symptoms This is a disease of hatching chicks, which seem weak, huddle together, have watery diarrhoea, and an infected open navel. It may be accompanied by 10% mortality.
Transmission Horizontal transmission in hatcher. This disease is *very* infectious.
Diagnosis Send suspect chicks to pathology laboratory for diagnosis. They will identify which organism is responsible.
Treatment No effective treatment. There is little spread of infection once chicks are out of the hatcher.
Prevention The seat of this infection is always the hatcher. If an outbreak occurs, the hatcher must be thoroughly cleaned and fumigated with a fumigant at 3x normal strength. Hatching eggs should be fumigated at 2x strength until infection is eradicated.

Malignant oedema or gangrenous dermatitis (Clostridium septicum)

Symptoms Disease of broilers particularly towards end of the growing period. There is gangrene of muscle and skin so that birds 'fall apart' while still alive. Massive mortality (up to 50%) is common.
Transmission Horizontal.
Diagnosis Fairly obvious but send suspect birds to laboratory for diagnosis. Although *Clostridium septicum* is the

usual organism, *Staphylococcus aureus* can also cause the disease and treatments differ depending on the bacterium that is involved.

Treatment   Penicillin works quite well if the main organism is *Clostridium*. The synthetic penicillin 'Penbritin' is better if *Staphylococcus* is the main organism.

Prevention   This disease can be associated with dirty conditions (but not always). Using litter more than once can increase problem. The disease sometimes appears as a secondary infection after the birds have been weakened by, say, an outbreak of Gumboro disease.

Necrotic enteritis (Clostridium welchii)

Symptoms   This disease is more usually found in broilers. Birds fail to thrive. Mortality commonly reaches 5–10%.

Transmission   Horizontal.

Diagnosis   Small intestine grossly inflamed and distended. Send suspect birds to laboratory for confirmation of diagnosis.

Treatment   Penicillin works quite well.

Prevention   This disease can be associated with dirty conditions (but not always). Thorough disinfection between batches of birds can reduce the incidence.

Mycoplasma diseases

MG (Mycoplasma gallisepticum) or PPLO (pleuropneumonia-like-organism) or CRD (chronic respiratory disease)

Symptoms   This is a respiratory disease affecting the whole respiratory tract particularly the air sacs. Young chicks show sniffling, sneezing and rattling. It is not a killer itself, however, it is often followed by secondary infections particularly with coliforms which make symptoms worse and can lead to 30% mortality. Adult birds have a few symptoms – inactivity, drop in production – but low mortality.

Transmission   Vertical through the hatching egg – this is important.
Horizontal   – through air within a room.
                      – on feet, clothing, feed and equipment between rooms.

Diagnosis   Suspect birds can be diagnosed in a pathology laboratory. There is an agglutination test available.

Treatment   Should only be regarded as a temporary solution. Tylosin is an antibiotic with specific activity against MG.

Prevention   Control can be by vaccination (usually layers) or eradication (usually broilers). Eradication is centred on identifying broiler breeder hens reacting to a blood test, and eliminating them. However, eradication is difficult because MG is *very* infectious.

MS (Mycoplasma synoviae)

Symptoms   Although this is a respiratory disease, the respiratory symptoms are slight and easily missed. What causes the problem is that the organism tends to move to the synovial fluid and the hock and foot pad joints are often affected and become swollen and inflamed. This is mainly a disease of growing birds, particularly 6–14 weeks of age, which become lame and lose their appetites. In older birds, there is a drop in egg production and lameness.

Transmission   Vertical   – through the hatching egg.
Horizontal   – through air within a room.
                      – on feet, clothing, feed and equipment between rooms.

Diagnosis   Suspect birds can be diagnosed in a pathology laboratory. There is an agglutination test available.

Treatment   Oxytetracycline in feed can be useful, but aim for eradication.

Prevention   Eradication by identifying breeder hens reacting to a blood test and eliminating them. Also, hatching eggs can be heat treated to 46 °C before incubation. This kills the organism and only lowers hatchability slightly.

Viral diseases

Infectious bronchitis (IB)

Symptoms   This is a disease of domestic fowl only. In chicks there is wheezing and sneezing and perhaps a nasal discharge. Birds gasp for breath. Typically, it starts very suddenly and spreads very quickly with up to 50% mortality. In a flock, it is likely that all birds will be affected and those that recover will have poor performance in adult life. It is often followed by secondary infections particularly by the coliforms. In adult birds, there are few respiratory symptoms. There is however a huge drop in egg production and a dramatic decrease in egg quality. Soft-shelled, misshapen and wrinkled eggs are very characteristic and albumen quality is poor. Many birds become internal layers.

Transmission   Horizontal   – through air within a room.
                      – on feet, clothing, feed and equipment between rooms.

Diagnosis   Diagnosis is difficult and is often done by eliminating other possibilities. Agglutination tests for antibodies are available.

Treatment   No treatment.

Prevention   There are several vaccines, mostly attenuated, available.
Broilers – at day-old, spray vaccine into mouth or eye (ocular).
Layers – at 2 and 6 weeks give a waterborne or ocular vaccine.
Breeders – at 1, 10 and 30 weeks then every 10–20 weeks during the laying cycle, give a waterborne or ocular vaccine.

Newcastle disease (ND)

Symptoms   A very infectious disease affecting all poultry and some wild birds. There are different forms depending on where in the body the virus strikes. The main symptoms are one of the following:
1. Respiratory difficulty.
2. Nervous disorders ('twisted necks' and 'tumblers').
3. Reduced egg production and quality.

Transmission   Horizontal   – through air within a room.
                      – on feet, clothing, feed and equipment between rooms.

Diagnosis The nervous symptoms give an accurate diagnosis, otherwise it is difficult. Pathology laboratory diagnosis is possible.
Treatment No treatment.
Prevention The usual method is to try to keep completely free from this disease. However, if it gets into the area, then it is wise to vaccinate, since transfer from other sites is very easy. The vaccination programme is complicated – so take advice.

Fowl pox

Symptoms There are two forms of the disease:
1. Dry pox (scabs) on comb, wattles, eyes and earlobes.
2. Wet pox in mouth, trachea, and respiratory tract which eventually cause suffocation. 2 often follows 1.

Transmission Horizontal. The skin must be broken for the virus to enter. This can happen in two ways:
1. Birds pecking each other during fighting.
2. Mosquitos can transmit the disease.

Transmission is therefore usually slow.

Diagnosis The lesions are very symptomatic. If in doubt, a pathology laboratory will take some material from an infected bird and inject it into the face of another bird. If the typical pox develops, then the disease is fowl pox.
Treatment No treatment.
Prevention If fowl pox is a problem, then there are vaccines available. However, vaccines are not used routinely.

Infectious laryngotracheitis (ILT or LT)

Symptoms A very severe respiratory disease usually in chickens over 6 weeks old. The infected birds gasp for breath. There is often haemorrhaging in the respiratory tract and blood can be coughed up. Mortality varies but can reach 30%.
Transmission Horizontal – through air within a room.
– on feet, clothing, feed and equipment between rooms.
Diagnosis Can only be diagnosed in a lab.
Treatment No treatment.
Prevention There is now a very good attenuated vaccine which gives good immunity. Vaccinate at 6 and 16 weeks using ocular route.

Gumboro disease or infectious bursal disease (IBD)

Symptoms Affects chicks aged 20–60 days. Birds are listless, nervous, sleepy, with a whitish diarrhoea which causes them to peck at their vents. Mortality is variable. The problem is that the virus damages the cells in the Bursa responsible for proper working of the immune system. Organism can live several months outside bird – so important to clean and disinfect between batches.
Transmission Horizontal through droppings.
Diagnosis Can only be diagnosed in laboratory.
Treatment No treatment.
Prevention If IBD is a problem in an area, then the usual method is to vaccinate breeders which pass on antibodies in their eggs and this gives protection to the chicks at least for the first part of the vulnerable period.

Avian encephalomyelitis (Epidemic Tremors)

Symptoms Mainly a disease of chicks between 6 and 21 days. They show nervous symptoms including quivering, which is very obvious if the chick is held in the palm of the hand, and paralysis. Many chicks lie on their sides. Mortality is high because chicks cannot get to food or water. Adult birds which become infected show few symptoms but lay infected eggs.
Transmission Vertical – in the hatching egg.
Horizontal – through the droppings.
Treatment No treatment.
Prevention Vaccination of breeders is the answer. Their immunity should be checked regularly as they pass on antibodies to their chicks and this gives good protection.

Marek's disease

Symptoms A tumour-causing virus which is present in most chickens worldwide, but does not always cause tumours. Sometimes tumours enlarge and cause death. The virus can infect the bursa of Fabricius and reduce birds' immunity to other diseases.
Transmission Horizontal. This virus has a unique method of transfer – it lodges in the feather follicles and then gets into the air on skin debris and feather particles. It floats around and is inhaled by other birds. The infected dust and debris can be carried around on feet, clothes, etc.
Diagnosis Tumours are very symptomatic.
Treatment No treatment.
Prevention Several vaccines are available, all derived from herpes virus turkey (HVT).

Avian influenza (Bird Flu)

Symptoms A contagious infection caused by the influenza virus Type 'A', which can affect most bird species, including all poultry species and occasionally some mammalian species. Avian influenza can be classified into two categories, low pathogenic (LPAI) and high pathogenic (HPAI) forms, based on the severity of the illness caused in birds. Avian influenza is a reportable disease. The LPAI form commonly causes only mild symptoms (ruffled feathers, a drop in egg production) and may easily go undetected. The HPAI form spreads very rapidly through poultry flocks, causes disease affecting multiple internal organs, and has a mortality that can approach 100%, often within 48 hours. The great concern is that the H5N1 strain of this virus has been known to infect human beings with a very severe form of influenza with a high mortality rate.
Transmission Horizontal. The main route of transmission is probably as an aerosol, but other routes may be possible.
Diagnosis Laboratory diagnosis is required.
Treatment No treatment.
Prevention No vaccines are available yet for avian influenza.

Parasitic diseases

Other important infectious diseases of chickens are caused by coccidia. These are protozoa that live in the intestinal tract and can cause great damage there. There are several species of coccidia that infect chickens and all belong to the group *Eimeria*. The three most important ones are *E. tenella*, *E. necatrix* and *E. acervulina*. The diseases are generally called 'coccidiosis' no matter which organism is responsible.

Coccidia have a complex life history spent partly in the chicken and partly outside it. Coccidiosis is spread by single-celled bodies known as oocysts. These are passed in the droppings, but are not infectious. They must first go through a process called sporulation, which requires correct conditions of temperature, moisture and air and takes 2–4 days. If the sporulated oocyst is eaten by a chicken, it ends up in the intestines where it multiplies in the gut wall and causes damage. Eventually after 4–7 days, more oocysts are produced and expelled in the droppings and the whole cycle starts again.

The amount of damage is closely related to the number of oocysts present and if only a few are present then little damage is caused. However, if the bird goes on ingesting more and they keep multiplying, very soon there can be millions present – and then the bird has a severe problem. If the numbers build up slowly, then the bird can develop immunity. However, this seldom happens under the artificial conditions found in a laboratory and numbers usually build up very quickly.

Coccidiosis (Eimeria species)

Symptoms Bloody droppings, ruffled feathers, paleness (anaemia due to blood loss) loss of appetite, poor growth, poor production, diarrhoea. The different species of coccidia produce different lesions in different parts of the intestine.

Transmission Through droppings – but of course infected material can be carried on feet, equipment, etc. and so be spread from room to room.

Diagnosis Bloody droppings and characteristic lesions in gut are usually enough for diagnosis. A pathology laboratory can identify the species involved.

Treatment and Prevention There are lots of good coccidiostats available, which can be added to the feed. However, some of them are very specific to some species of coccidia, so it is advisable to get a laboratory identification. Also, coccidia can develop resistance to a particular coccidiostat, so it sometimes helps to rotate coccidiostats from time to time. Birds on the floor will be at biggest risk i.e. most young birds, all broilers, some layer replacements and all breeders.

- A coccidiostat is usually fed to broilers at a rate to completely suppress coccidia since there is no time for broilers to develop immunity.
- With replacement birds (layers and breeders) another strategy is employed. A coccidiostat is fed at full strength for the first 5–6 weeks. It is then gradually withdrawn so that the birds get a very mild coccidiosis. They then slowly develop an immunity and in time the coccidiostat can be withdrawn completely.
- Another approach is to use a so-called 'vaccine'. This is a material which contains a limited number of oocysts and is fed to chicks at about 10–12 days. The idea is that the numbers of oocysts are small and immunity will build up. Obviously a coccidiostat should not be used with this approach.

Warning – Some coccidiostats are *extremely* toxic to other classes of livestock. For example, monensin at normal poultry dosages causes acute heart failure in horses and dogs.

There are some other parasitic diseases of poultry caused by various round and flat worms, but these are unlikely to be a problem in the laboratory. There are also various species of lice that parasitise the skin of domestic fowl, but these are unlikely to be a problem in the laboratory. However, mites can be a serious problem, particularly the common red mite, *Dermanyssus gallinae*. Every effort should be made to keep laboratory facilities free of red mite since an infestation can cause birds extreme distress and major blood loss, and the mite is very difficult to eradicate because of resistance to all permitted arachnicides. Precautions would include an 'all-in, all-out' policy and allowing only hatching eggs or day-old chicks into the facility. If a room does get infected with red mite, it should be left unoccupied by birds for an extended period and the mites will eventually die off.

Metabolic disorders

The implementation of good biological security and the use of vaccines have resulted in control of most of the infectious diseases of chickens. Non-infectious diseases are now of more importance to the poultry industry, and these diseases, usually referred to as 'metabolic disorders', will no doubt be evident in the laboratory, particularly if modern, high-producing strains of chicken are used. The most important ones are sudden death syndrome, ascites, fatty liver and kidney syndrome, and various skeletal disorders in broiler chickens, and liver haemorrhagic syndrome and osteoporosis in laying hens. Most of these disorders have a multifactorial aetiology and are therefore complex. They are mentioned here, simply to warn laboratory managers of their existence. If morbidity due to metabolic disorders is suspected, then more detailed texts such as Leeson *et al.* (1995) or Swayne (2017) should be consulted.

Abnormal behaviour

The occurrence of abnormal behaviour is often a sign that birds are suffering and the laboratory manager should be able to recognise behavioural signs of disease. In addition, some other behavioural symptoms of suffering are fairly easy to recognise. Severe frustration is often characterised by stereotyped back-and-forward pacing and increased aggression (Duncan & Wood-Gush 1971, 1972). Lack of a suitable nesting place is the most likely cause of severe frustration. Severe food restriction often leads to stereotyped pecking at the feeder or some other aspect of the environment (Savory 1989).

Occasionally some strains of chickens in some circumstances will show panic or hysteria. These may be defined as excessive and inappropriate flight-fright reactions, panic having some external trigger and hysteria without an apparent cause (Mills & Faure 1990). Both panic and hysteria seem to have complex aetiologies. However, since they are often associated with large group size, they are unlikely to occur in the laboratory.

Further reading

The primary breeding companies produce 'Management Guides' for each of their hybrids. These set out the management conditions that will optimise the productivity of that particular strain. Laboratories using these hybrids should always ensure that they have the relevant guide. In addition, there are several excellent textbooks on poultry management and husbandry such as Bell and Weaver (2002) which should be used to expand this text. The welfare implications of different commercial husbandry systems are dealt with in some detail by Appleby *et al.* (2004) and Nicol (2015), and these should also be studied.

References

Appleby, M.C., Mench, J.A. and Hughes, B.O. (2004) *Poultry Behaviour and Welfare.* CABI, Wallingford.

Archer, G.S. and Mench, J.A. (2014) Natural incubation patterns and the effects of exposing eggs to light at various times during incubation on post-hatch fear and stress responses in broiler (meat) chickens. *Applied Animal Behaviour Science,* **152,** 44–51.

Axelsson, M., Dang, Q., Pitsillides, K. *et al.* (2007) A novel, fully implantable, multichannel biotelemetry system for measurement of blood flow, pressure, ECG, and temperature. *Journal of Applied Physiology,* **102,** 1220–1228.

Bain, M.M., Nys, Y. and Dunn, I.C. (2016) Increasing persistency in lay and stabilising egg quality in layer laying cycles. What are the challenges? *British Poultry Science,* **57,** 330–335.

Bandara, R.M.A.S., Torrey, S., Turner, P.V. *et al.* (2019a) Efficacy of a novel mechanical cervical dislocation device in comparison to manual cervical dislocation in layer chickens. *Animals,* **9** (in press).

Bandara, R.M.A.S., Torrey, S., Turner, P.V. *et al.* (2019b) Anatomical pathology, behavioural, and physiological responses induced by application of non-penetrating captive bolt devices in layer chickens. *Frontiers in Veterinary Science,* **6,** 1–18.

Bell, D.D. and Weaver, W.D. (Eds) (2002) *Chicken Meat and Egg Production,* 5th edn. Springer, New York.

Blokhuis, H.J. (1986) Feather pecking in poultry: Its relation with ground pecking. *Applied Animal Behaviour Science,* **16,** 63–67.

Blokhuis, H.J. and Arkes, J.G. (1984) Some observations on the development of feather pecking in poultry. *Applied Animal Behaviour Science,* **12,** 145–157.

Canadian Council on Animal Care (1993) Euthanasia. In: *Guide to the Care and Use of Experimental Animals,* Vol. 2. pp. 141–153. CCAC, Ottawa.

Close, B., Banister, K., Baumans, V. *et al.* (1996) Recommendations for euthanasia of experimental animals. Part 1. *Laboratory Animals,* **30,** 293–316.

Close, B., Banister, K., Baumans, V. *et al.* (1997) Recommendations for euthanasia of experimental animals. Part 2. *Laboratory Animals,* **31,** 1–32.

Collias, N.E. and Collias, E.C. (1967) A field study of the Red Junglefowl in North-Central India. *Condor,* **69,** 360–386.

Collias, N.E., Collias, E.C., Hunsaker, D. *et al.* (1966) Locality fixation mobility and social organization within an unconfined population of Red Jungle Fowl. *Animal Behaviour,* **14,** 550–559.

Cooper, J.J. and Appleby, M.C. (1996) Demand for nest boxes in laying hens. *Behaviour Processes,* **36,** 171–182.

Cronin, G.M., Barnett, J.L. and Hemsworth, P.H. (2012) The importance of pre-laying behaviour and nest boxes for laying hen welfare: a review. *Animal Production Science,* **52,** 398–405.

Danbury, T.C., Weeks, C.A., Chambers, J.P. *et al.* (2000) Self-selection of the analgesic drug Carprofen by lame broiler chickens. *Veterinary Record,* **146,** 307–311.

Decuypere, E. and Bruggeman, V. (2007) The endocrine interface of environmental and egg factors affecting chick quality. *Poultry Science,* **86,** 1037–1042.

de Haas, E.N., Bolhuis, J.E., de Jong, I.C. *et al.* (2014) Predicting feather damage in laying hens during the laying period. Is it the past or is it the present? *Applied Animal Behaviour Science,* **160,** 75–85.

Dennis, R.L., Fahey, A.G. and Cheng, H.W. (2008) Different effects of individual identification systems on chicken well-being. *Poultry Science,* **87,** 1052–1057.

Directive 2010/63/EU of the European Parliament (2010) https://eur-lex.europa.eu/legal-content/EN/TXT/?qid=1547424753597&uri=CELEX:32010L0063 (accessed 24 October 2019).

Dove, W.F. (1935) A study of individuality in the nutritive instincts and of the causes and effects of variation in the selection of food. *American Naturalist,* **69,** 469–544.

Duncan, I.J.H. (1970) Frustration in the fowl. In: *Aspects of Poultry Behaviour.* Eds B.N. Freeman and R.F. Gordon, pp. 15–31. British Poultry Science, Edinburgh.

Duncan, I.J.H. (1980) The ethogram of the domesticated hen. In: *The Laying Hen and Its Environment.* Ed. R. Moss, pp. 5–18. Martinus Nijhoff, The Hague.

Duncan, I.J.H. (1981) Telemetry. In: *First European Symposium on Poultry Welfare.* Ed. L.Y. Sørenson, pp. 15–21. Danish Branch of the World's Poultry Science Association, Køge.

Duncan, I.J.H. (1990) Reactions of poultry to human beings. In: *Social Stress in Domestic Animals.* Eds R. Zayan and R. Dantzer, pp. 121–131. Kluwer Academic, Dordrecht.

Duncan, I.J.H. and Filshie, J.H. (1980) The use of radiotelemetry devices to measure temperature and heart-rate in the domestic fowl. In: *A Handbook on Biotelemetry and Radio Tracking.* Eds C.J. Amlaner and D.W. Macdonald, pp. 579–588. Pergamon Press, London.

Duncan, I.J.H., Filshie, J.H. and McGee, I.J. (1975) Radiotelemetry of avian shank temperature using a thin film hybrid microcircuit. *Medical and Biological Engineering,* **13,** 544–550.

Duncan, I.J.H. and Kite, V.G. (1989) Nest site selection and nest building behaviour in domestic fowl. *Animal Behaviour,* **37,** 215–231.

Duncan, I.J.H., Slee, G.S., Seawright, E. *et al.* (1989) Behavioural consequences of partial beak amputation (beak trimming) in poultry. *British Poultry Science,* **30,** 479–488.

Duncan, I.J.H., Widowski, T.M., Malleau, A.E. *et al.* (1998) External factors and causation of dustbathing in domestic hens. *Behavioural Processes,* **43,** 219–228.

Duncan, I.J.H. and Wood-Gush, D.G.M. (1971) Frustration and aggression in the domestic fowl. *Animal Behaviour,* **19,** 500–504.

Duncan, I.J.H. and Wood-Gush, D.G.M. (1972) Thwarting of feeding behaviour in the domestic fowl. *Animal Behaviour,* **20,** 444–451.

Ellen, E.D., Visscher, J., van Arendonk, J.A.M. *et al.* (2008) Survival of laying hens: genetic parameters for direct and associative effects in three purebred layer lines. *Poultry Science,* **87,** 233–239.

Erasmus, M.A., Turner, P.V., Nykamp, S.G. *et al.* (2010) Brain and skull lesions resulting from use of percussive bolt, cervical dislocation by stretching, cervical dislocation by crushing and blunt trauma. *Veterinary Record,* **167,** 850–858.

Etches, R.J. (1996) *Reproduction in Poultry.* CABI, Wallingford, Oxon.

European Council (2009) *European Council Regulation (EC) 1099/2009 of 24 September 2009 on the Protection of Animals at the Time of Killing.*

Fasenko, G.M. (2007) Egg storage and the embryo. *Poultry Science,* **86,** 1020–1024.

Filshie, J.H., Duncan, I.J.H. and Clark, J.S.B. (1980) Radiotelemetry of the avian electrocardiogram. *Medical, Biological and Engineering Computing,* **18,** 633–637.

Follensbee, M.E., Duncan, I.J.H. and Widowski, T.M. (1992) Quantifying nesting motivation of domestic hens. *Journal of Animal Science*, **70**(1), 50 (Abstract).

Friere, R. and Cowling, A. (2013) The welfare of laying hens in conventional cages and alternative systems: first steps towards a quantitative comparison. *Animal Welfare*, **22**, 57–65.

Gentle, M.J., Hughes, B.O., Fox, A. et al. (1997) Behavioural and anatomical consequences of two beak trimming methods in 1- and 10-d-old domestic chicks. *British Poultry Science*, **38**, 453–463.

Gentle, M.J., Waddington, D., Hunter, L.N. et al. (1990) Behavioural evidence for persistent pain following partial beak amputation in chickens. *Applied Animal Behaviour Science*, **27**, 149–157.

Gilani, A.M., Knowles, T.G. and Nicol, C.J. (2012) The effect of dark brooders on feather pecking on commercial farms. *Applied Animal Behaviour Science*, **142**, 42–50.

Gilani, A.M., Knowles, T.G. and Nicol, C.J. (2013) The effect of rearing environment on feather pecking in young and adult laying hens. *Applied Animal Behaviour Science*, **148**, 54–63.

Hocking, P.M. (2009) Feed restriction. In: *Biology of Breeding Poultry*. Ed. P.M. Hocking, pp. 307–330. CABI, Wallingford.

Hothersall, B., Caplen, G., Parker, R.M.A. et al. (2016) Effects of carprofen, meloxicam and butorphanol on broiler chickens' performance in mobility tests. *Animal Welfare*, **25**, 55–67.

Hughes, B.O. and Black, A.J. (1976) The influence of handling on egg production, egg shell quality and avoidance behaviour in hens. *British Poultry Science*, **17**, 135–144.

Hulet, R.M. (2007) Managing incubation: Where are we and why? *Poultry Science*, **86**, 1017–1019.

Humane Slaughter Association (2001) *Practical Slaughter of Poultry. A Guide for Small Producers*. 2nd edn. Humane Slaughter Association, Herts, UK.

JWGR (2001) Laboratory birds: Refinements in husbandry and procedures. Fifth Report of the BVAAWF/FRAME/RSPCA/UFAW Joint Working Group on Refinement. *Laboratory Animals*, **35**(Suppl. 1), S1–S163.

Jones, R.B. and Faure, J.-M. (1981) The effects of regular handling on fear responses in the domestic chick. *Behavioural Processes*, **6**, 135–143.

Kalmendal, R. and Wall, H. (2012) Effects of a high oil and fibre diet and supplementary roughage on performance, injurious pecking and foraging activities in two layer hybrids. *British Poultry Science*, **53**, 153–161.

Keeling, L.J., Estevez, I., Newberry, R.C. et al. (2003) Production-related traits of layers reared in different sized flocks: the concept of problematic intermediate group sizes. *Poultry Science*, **82**, 1393–1396.

Kjaer, J.B. and Hocking, P.M. (2004) The genetics of feather pecking and cannibalism. In: *Welfare of the Laying Hen*. Ed. G.C. Perry, pp. 109–121. CABI, Wallingford.

Kjaer, J.B. and Sørensen, P. (1997) Feather pecking in White Leghorn chickens – a genetic study. *British Poultry Science*, **38**, 333–341.

Kjaer, J.B. and Vestergaard, K.S. (1999) Development of feather pecking in relation to light intensity. *Applied Animal Behaviour Science*, **65**, 243–254.

Kops, M.S., Kjaer, J.B., Güntürkün, O. et al. (2014) Serotonin release in the caudal nidopallium of adult laying hens genetically selected for high and low feather pecking behaviour: An *in vivo* microdialysis study. *Behavioural Brain Research*, **268**, 81–87.

Lawton, M.P.C. (2016) Anaesthesia and analgesia. In: *Avian Medicine*, 3rd edn. Ed. J. Samour, pp. 179–203. Elsevier, St Louis, Missouri.

Lay, D.C., Fulton, R.M., Hester, P.Y. et al. (2011) Hen welfare in different housing systems. *Poultry Science*, **90**, 278–294.

Leeson, S. and Summers, J.D. (2000) *Commercial Poultry Nutrition*, 3rd edn. University Books, Guelph, Canada.

Leeson, S., Diaz, G. and Summers, J.D. (1995) *Poultry Metabolic Disorders and Mycotoxins*. University Books, Guelph, Canada.

Lewis, P. and Morris, T. (2006) *Poultry Lighting: The Theory and Practice*. Northcot, Andover, Hampshire.

Lierz, M. and Korbel, R. (2012) Anesthesia and analgesia in birds. *Journal of Exotic Pet Medicine*, **21**, 44–58.

Liu, K, Xin, H. and Chai, L. (2017) Choice between fluorescent and poultry-specific LED lights by pullets and laying hens. *Transactions of the American Society of Agricultural and Biological Engineers*, **60**, 2185–2195.

Long, H., Zhao, Y., Wang, T. et al. (2016) Effect of light-emitting diode vs. fluorescent lighting on laying hens in aviary hen houses: Part 1 – Operational characteristics of lights and production traits of hens. *Poultry Science*, **95**, 1–11.

Malleau, A.E., Duncan, I.J.H., Widowski, T.M. et al. (2007) The importance of rest in young domestic fowl. *Applied Animal Behaviour Science*, **106**, 52–69.

Martin, J.E., McKeegan, D.E.F., Sparrey, J. et al. (2016) Comparison of novel mechanical dislocation and a modified captive bolt for on-farm killing of poultry on behavioural reflex responses and anatomical pathology. *Animal Welfare*, **25**, 227–241.

McBride, G., Parer, I.P. and Foenander, F. (1969) The social organization and behaviour of the feral domestic fowl. *Animal Behaviour Monographs*, **2**, 125–181.

Mench, J.A. (1993) Problems associated with broiler breeder management. In: *Fourth European Symposium on Poultry Welfare*. Eds C.J. Savory and B.O. Hughes, pp. 195–207. UFAW, Potters Bar, Herts.

Mills, A.D. and Faure, J.-M. (1990) Panic and hysteria in domestic fowl: a review. In: *Social Stress in Domestic Animals*. Eds R. Zayan and R. Dantzer, pp. 248–272. Kluwer, Dordrecht.

Muir, W.M. and Cheng, H.W. (2004) Breeding for productivity and welfare of laying hens. In: *Welfare of the Laying Hen*. Ed. G.C. Perry, pp. 123–138. CABI, Wallingford.

Murphy, L.B. and Duncan, I.J.H. (1978) Attempts to modify the responses of domestic fowl towards human beings. II. The effect of early experience. *Applied Animal Ethology*, **4**, 5–12.

Nicol, C.J. (2015) *The Behavioural Biology of Chickens*. CABI, Wallingford.

Olsson, I.A.S. and Keeling, L.J. (2002) The push-door for measuring motivation in hens: Laying hens are motivated to perch at night. *Animal Welfare*, **11**, 11–19.

Pagel, M. and Dawkins, M.S. (1997) Peck orders and group size in laying hens: 'futures contracts' for non-aggression. *Behavioural Processes*, **40**, 13–25.

Riedstra, B. and Groothuis, T.G.G. (2004) Prenatal light exposure affects early feather-pecking behaviour in the domestic chick. *Animal Behaviour*, **67**, 1037–1042.

Rodenburg, T.B., De Reu, K. and Tuyttens, F.A.M. (2012) Performance, welfare, health and hygiene of laying hens in non-cage systems in comparison with cage systems. In: *Alternative Systems for Poultry – Health, Welfare and Productivity*. Eds V. Sandilands and P. Hocking, pp. 210–224. CABI, Wallingford.

Samour, J. (Ed.) (2016) *Avian Medicine*, 3rd edn. Elsevier, St. Louis, Missouri.

Savory, C.J. (1989) Stereotyped behaviour as a coping strategy in restricted-fed broiler breeder stock. In: *Third European Symposium on Poultry Welfare*. Eds J.-M. Faure and A.D. Mills, pp. 261–264. World's Poultry Science Association, Tours, France.

Savory, C.J. (2010) Nutrition, feeding and drinking behaviour and welfare. In: *The Welfare of Domestic Fowl and other Captive Birds*. Eds I.J.H. Duncan and P. Hawkins, pp. 165–187. Springer, Dordrecht.

Siegel, P.B., Haberfield, A., Mukherjee, T.K. et al. (1992) Jungle fowl - domestic fowl relationships: a use of DNA fingerprinting. *World's Poultry Science Journal*, **48**, 147–155.

Singh, P.M., Johnson, C.B., Gartrell, B. et al. (2017) Analgesic effects of morphine and butorphanol in broiler chickens. *Veterinary Anaesthesia and Analgesia*, **44**, 538–545.

Swayne, D. (Ed.) (2017) *Diseases of Poultry*, 13th edn. Wiley-Blackwell, Ames, Iowa

Tauson, R. (1980) Cages: How could they be improved? In: *The Laying Hen and Its Environment*. Ed. R. Moss, pp. 269–299. Martinus Nijhoff, The Hague.

Tauson, R. (1985) Mortality of laying hens caused by differences in cage design. *Acta Agriculturæ Scandinavica*, **35**, 165–174.

Tauson, R. and Abrahamsson, P. (1994) Foot and skeletal disorders on laying hens. Effects of perch design, hybrid, housing system and stocking density. *Acta Agriculturæ Scandinavica*, Section A, **44**, 110–119.

Wood-Gush, D.G.M. (1956) The agonistic and courtship behaviour of the Brown Leghorn cock. *British Journal of Animal Behaviour*, **4**, 133–142.

Wood-Gush, D.G.M. (1959) A history of the domestic chicken from antiquity to the 19th century. *Poultry Science*, **38**, 321–326.

Wood-Gush, D.G.M. (1971) *The Behaviour of the Domestic Fowl*. Heinemann Educational Books Ltd, London.

Wood-Gush, D.G.M., Duncan, I.J.H. and Savory, C.J. (1978) Observations on the social behaviour of domestic fowl in the wild. *Biology of Behaviour*, **3**, 193–205.

Yahav, S. (2015) Regulation of body temperature, strategies and mechanisms. In: *Sturkie's Avian Physiology*. 6th edn. Ed. Scanes, C.G., pp. 868–905. Academic Press, Amsterdam.

41

The Japanese quail

Rusty Lansford and Kimberly M. Cheng

Biological overview

The Japanese quail (*Coturnix japonica*) belongs to the order Galliformes, family Phasianidae (Chesser et al. 2018), and is a small, chubby, brown-coloured terrestrial migratory bird (Wetherbee 1961). The species is indigenous to East Asia (Latitude 17 °N to 55 °N). Their habitat is in grasslands, croplands, riversides, alpine meadows and grass steppes (Long 1981), and their breeding range extends from northeastern Mongolia through Baikal region to Vitim region of central-eastern Russia, east to Sakhalin Island, and south to Japan, Korea and northeastern China (eastern Shandong). They may also be breeding in Bhutan and Myanmar (del Hoyo et al. 1994). The species' winter range extends from central Japan and central China west through northwestern Thailand and northern Myanmar to northeastern India (Assam), northwestern Bangladesh and Bhutan, with small numbers as far north as Buryatia and Ussuriland (Russia) in mild winters[1]. However, because of climate change and habitat loss, the present-day ranges may be slightly different.

The Japanese quail was previously considered to be a subspecies of the common or European quail, *C. coturnix* (see Crawford 1990). It was given full species status in 1983 (American Ornithologists' Union 1983; Howard & Moore 1984) because no interbreeding has been observed between the common quail and the Japanese quail in areas where the two species are sympatric in Mongolia (Wakasugi 1984). However, more recent crossbreeding experiments between two strains of domestic *C. japonica* and one strain of *C. coturnix* showed that it is easy to obtain the hybrid combinations F1, F2 as well as backcrosses (Derégnaucourt et al. 2002), as confirmed with mtDNA and nuclear DNA analyses (Barilani et al. 2005). Fertility of the hybrid pairs and the hatchability of hundreds of eggs did not differ from those of pure common quail pairs reared under the same conditions. Domesticated Japanese quail from California, USA were introduced in India by Central Avian Research Institute (CARI), Izatnagar, Uttar Pradesh in 1974 (Valavan 2016) that have given rise to several hybrid lines. The Poultry Research Station, Tamil Nadu Veterinary and Animal Sciences University has also released three strains of Japanese quail quails favoured for the taste of their meat and egg-laying traits (Valavan 2016).

The common quail is a popular European game species that is commonly restocked with farm-reared individuals in several European countries, including Greece (Barilani et al. 2005; Tsiompanoudis et al. 2011), Italy (Galli 2003) and The Republic of Serbia, Montenegro, Romania and Spain (Rodriguez-Teijeiro et al. 1993; Puigcerver et al. 2007). It is well-known that common quail are difficult to raise in captivity, whereas Japanese quail are easily bred. The large releases of farmed 'common quail' aroused suspicion that they have been interbred with domestic Japanese quail to increase the captive population. Recent results show that more than 85% of the game farm birds were not just common quail but also had domestic Japanese quail ancestry (Sanchez-Donoso et al. 2012). In some regions, the number of released quails even exceeds the number of wild breeding common quail (Guyomarc'h 2003; Rodriguez-Teijeiro et al. 2005). Introduction of non-native species may cause introgressive hybridisation of maladaptive alleles into native populations. Introgression of domesticated Japanese quail genes in wild common quail populations might affect the phenotypic expression of functional traits, as body size, feather colour, sexual calls and migratory behaviours.

The Japanese quail, which is an Old World quail, should not be confused with the Bobwhite quail (*Colinus virginianus*), a species in the family Odontophoridae (New World quail). Both species have been domesticated and used as food and as research animals.

Japanese quail were originally introduced to North America by the US Fish and Wildlife Service as game birds in 1870, and releases continued into the late 1950s (Standford 1957). Most of the birds released were domestic birds imported from Japan. All stocks released in North America failed to establish and perished within 1 year. However, release attempts in the 1940s on the Hawaiian Islands were successful. Populations survived on Kauai, Molokai, Lanai, Maui and Hawaii (Peterson 1961) and have

---

[1] https://birdsoftheworld.org/bow/species/japqua/cur/introduction (accessed 4 August 2021).

been regularly hunted (Munro 1960). Although the populations originated from released domestic birds, they are now considered wild.

Domestication and origin of domestic and laboratory lines

The first records of domestic quail are from twelfth-century Japan, and it appears that the species was domesticated there during the eleventh century or imported from China in an already domesticated form (Chang *et al.* 2005) at about that time (Howes 1964; Crawford 1990). They were originally kept for their song (Howes 1964), and it has been inferred that lines of quail with particular call types were bred for use in song contests (Taka-Tsukasa 1935; Wakasugi 1984).

Between 1910 and 1941, the Japanese selected quail for increased egg production and by 1940, a thriving industry existed (Howes 1964; Wakasugi 1984). However, all lines of song-type quail and the majority of egg production lines were lost during World War II. Following the war, the quail industry was rebuilt from the few remaining domesticated birds available, possibly with the addition of domesticated lines from Korea, China and Taiwan and quail captured in the wild (Howes 1964; Wakasugi 1984). All present-day laboratory and commercial lines appear to have been derived from this post-war population (Crawford 1990).

General biology

Morphology

The wild-type natal plumage is the same in both sexes (Cheng & Kimura 1990). Chicks have tawny coloured heads with small black patches above the beak. A buff stripe bordered by black stripes runs along the top of the head and there are four dark brown stripes on the back. The back and wings are pale brown (Cheng & Kimura 1990). Juvenile plumage is present at 3–4 weeks of age and full adult plumage is present at about 6 weeks of age. The species is sexually dimorphic in adult plumage (Figure 41.1). In both sexes, body plumage is predominantly brown (Wetherbee 1961; Kawahara 1967, 1973) but it is highly variable in terms of shades of brown and some of the markings on the breast and the throat (Cheng & Kimura 1990). Females have pale-coloured breast feathers which are speckled with dark-coloured spots whereas males have uniform dark rufous breast and cheek feathers. Furthermore, males may develop a white collar while females have cream coloured feathers on the cheeks and do not develop white collars (Urbanski 1984). With domestication came the development of many strains with various plumage colour and pattern (Cheng & Kimura 1990).

Domestic quail reach sexual maturity at 4–5 weeks of age, depending on the lighting schedule. Females enter into full lay at about 6 weeks of age (see also Gerken & Mills 1993). Eggs are variably mottled. The background colour of shells varies from white through to pale brown or blue. The shell colour pigments are porphyrin and biliverdin (Poole 1965). Shell colour, mottling pattern, size and shape vary considerably between females but are consistent for and unique to a given female (Jones *et al.* 1964). Egg weight varies between 8 and 13 g depending on the strain of the bird (see the following text).

Size range and lifespan

Adult wild males and females weigh about 90 and 100 g, respectively (Kawahara 1967), and unselected domestic males and females weigh about 100 and 120 g, respectively. There is considerable variability in body weight between different genetic strains of quail (Gerken & Mills 1993).

The domestic quail is notable for its rapid growth rate (Figure 41.2). Chicks weigh between 8 and 12 g at hatching. They double this weight by 5 days of age and triple it by 8 days of age (Lucotte 1974). By 5–6 weeks of age, birds may weigh 160–250 g depending on sex and strain (Gerken & Mills 1993). Although in the last decade, some commercial meat strains have been bred to achieve above 300 g market weight (Cheng & Nichols 1992).

There appear to be no reports concerning the lifespan of wild quail. Under artificial husbandry conditions, reported

(a) 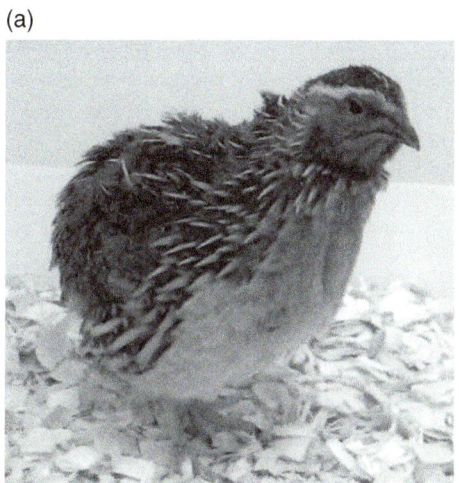   (b)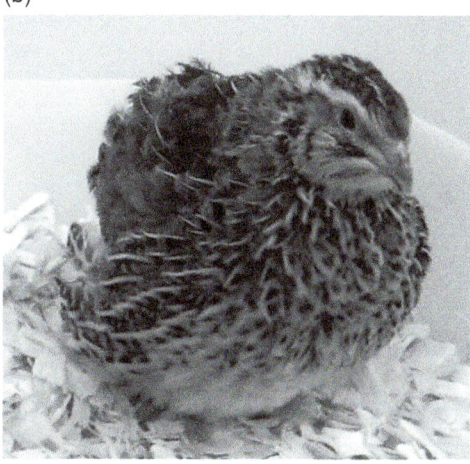

Figure 41.1 Wild-type plumage of male (a) and female (b) adult JQ. Source: Courtesy of David Huss.

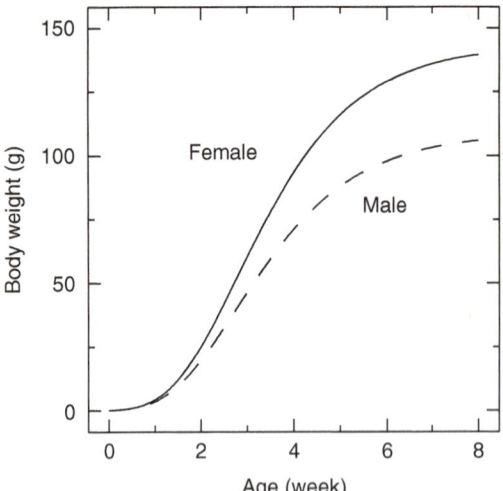

Figure 41.2 Growth curve for male (dashed line) and female (solid line) domestic JQ from hatching to 8 weeks of age. Source: Data from Aggrey (2003).

Table 41.1 Standard biological data for the JQ.

Parameter	Value
Body weight (g)	
1 day	6–8
Adult male	100–130
Adult female	120–160
Organ weight (% body weight)	
Liver	1.95
Heart	0.91
Kidney	0.73
Testes	2.88
Performance and longevity	
Egg weight (g)	9–10
Egg number/100 bird days	80–90
Age at sexual maturity (days)	38–42
Lifespan (months)	24–26
Blood pressure (mmHg)	
Systolic	
Adult male	158.1 ± 4.6[1]
Adult female	156.1 ± 4.7[1]
Diastolic	
Adult male	151.8 ± 4.7[1]
Adult female	146.9 ± 4.2[1]
Heart rate (beats/min)	
Adult male	530.7 ± 17.7[1]
Adult female	489.5 ± 17.1[1]

[1] mean ± se.
Source: Modified from Cooper (1987) and Mills et al. (1999).

lifespan varied depending on breeds, rearing conditions (e.g. continuous lighting) and nutrition factors. In most cases, life was terminated artificially, and the reported lifespan may mean productive lifespan (e.g. see Table 41.1 and Gerken & Mills 1993). Woodard & Abplanalp (1971) reported that males live longer (more than 5 years) than females (less than 4 years). In the authors' laboratory, a male that was kept as a mascot lived for 8 years before being euthanised because of the development of skin tumours.

Social organisation

Studies of social organisation in the wild appear to be limited to those by Taka-Tsukasa (1935), and opportunistic observations have produced conflicting reports (Kawahara 1967; Dement'ev et al. 1967). It has been reported that the birds live in pairs during the breeding season but gather in large flocks during migration and in the winter (Crawford 1990). Observations of feral birds in Hawaii indicate that males are territorial, and mating and nesting takes place within these territories (Schwartz & Schwartz 1949). Members of a pair remain in close proximity before and during the egg-laying period (which implies mate guarding and thus the possibility of extra-pair copulations (McKinney et al. 1983)). Dement'ev et al. (1967) reported that the species is polygamous. Kawahara (1967) noted that males and females live in pairs during the breeding season. On the basis of such evidence and studies of other *Coturnix* species, Kovach (1975) concluded that the mating system is in a transitional state between polygamy and monogamy. However, one of the few studies with captive quail (Orcutt & Orcutt 1976) indicated that males and females formed strong pair bonds, and that males were monogamous and courted only their own female. There is also evidence that quail are able to recognise the calls of a pair-bonded mate (Guyomarc'h 1974). Crowing rate increases in males visually separated from females, and crowing intensity increases with rises in ambient noise levels (Potash 1972, 1975). Crowing patterns of pair-bonded males differ from those of unmated males (Potash 1975). Potash (1975) argued that crowing by males and cricket calls by females serve the function of contact calls when a bonded pair is out of sight of each other. Nichols et al. (1992) studied captive birds in outdoor flight pens and confirmed that males were paired with one female for the whole breeding season. Females also paired with only one male during the breeding season. Nichols (1991) concluded that wild birds are monogamous with some opportunistic forced extra-pair copulations by the male.

Under simulated natural conditions in outdoor flight pens, domestic males are serially monogamous with significantly higher frequencies of extra-pair copulations compared to wild males (Nichols 1991). With higher-density rearing in floor pens or cages, they become promiscuous. Cheng et al. (1989a) observed that the cloacal foam gland in domestic males is much more prominent than that of wild males. Adkins-Regan (1995) suggested that the enlarged foam gland of the domestic males '*hints at a genetically non-monogamous mating system*'.

The common courtship displays performed by wild males include zig-zag dancing, leading, tidbitting, strutting and squatting (Eynon 1968; Nichols 1991). The male initiates sexual behaviour by strutting towards the female. During strutting, the male stretches himself such that his beak, body, head and neck are parallel to the ground, erects his body feathers and walks on his claws and digits with a characteristic stiff-legged gait. Under simulated natural conditions, domestic males also perform these displays but with significantly less frequency and with less specific contexts (Nichols 1991). An indication of female acceptance of the male could be solicitation of copulation by the female. A female would walk in front of her suitor and crouch, inviting the male to mount her

(Nichols 1991). A mated pair also keeps in close vocal contact with each other, giving very quiet calls as they move around together. Under husbandry conditions, the role of the female in courtship and mating appears to be minimal (Kovach 1975). Sefton and Siegel (1973) reported that male courtship displays were rare. The male approaches the female, grabs her head or neck feathers and attempts to mount her without any additional courtship or display behaviour (Farris 1964, 1967; Wilson & Bermant 1972). Cheng (unpublished data) observed mating behaviour of domestic birds using two-male, six-female mating groups in 2.5 × 3.1 m indoor floor pens. Under this situation, a male could dominate the other male and attempt to keep the subordinate male from mating with the females. Often the subordinate male would dash into a group of females and perform zig-zag dancing, and the females responded by scattering in different directions, crouching and hopping up in the air. The subordinate male, and sometimes both males, would start to grab and mount females. During mounting, the male 'grabs' the head or neck feathers of the female, positions himself on the back of the female, spreads his wings and begins treading. The copulatory response sequence results in ejaculation in about half of these cases. While males mount females regardless of the females' receptivity (Lucotte 1974), the type of the female's reaction significantly influenced the latency of the male's grab, mount and cloacal contact responses and also determined the efficiency of the male's copulatory behaviour (Domjan & Nash 1988).

Under husbandry conditions, birds form dominance hierarchies. Although the nature of these hierarchies has not been extensively studied, they appear to be of the peck order type and confer priority of access to resources (Otis 1972; Nol et al. 1996). In group-housed birds, subordinate birds show ambivalent behaviour (Edens et al. 1983). This ambivalent behaviour comprises aspects of both aggressive and submissive behaviour and is an attempt to displace dominant birds from feeders or drinkers. Furthermore, under conditions of deprivation, levels of aggression increase as distance from the food source decreases, and dominance relationships change from a peck order system to a peck dominance system.

Domestic males do not respond well to disruption of established hierarchies. If birds are introduced into established groups, they are likely to be attacked. Attacks are more likely if a stranger is introduced into the home cage of other birds. As a consequence, it is unwise to mix groups of birds or to introduce replacement birds into groups where hierarchies have been established.

Standard biological data

There is a paucity of recent information concerning common physiological parameters in present-day strains of quail. Table 41.1 shows physiological data. Serum chemistry reference values in adult birds including sex-related differences (comparing 16-week-old adult male versus female birds) have been reported in Scholtz et al. (2009). Clinical chemistry data (albumin, total protein, glucose, uric acid, cholesterol, bilirubin, cholinesterase, creatinine, triglycerides, alanine aminotransferase, aspartate aminotransferase and gamma-glutamyl transferase) in blood serum have been reported in Cheng et al. (2010) and Agina et al. (2017).

However, these tables should be considered only a guideline since present-day laboratory and domestic strains may be physiologically different because of selection for other traits, such as body weight or increased egg production (e.g. Alagawany et al. 2014).

Reproduction

Reproduction is strongly dependent on the lighting regimen. Wild birds breed in spring and summer. However, in the laboratory, birds can be maintained in breeding condition all year if they are kept on day lengths of 12 h or more. If birds are kept on short-day lengths (6 h or less), sexual development is delayed or inhibited. Social factors as well as photoperiod influence the onset of sexual maturity. The sound of male vocalisations can speed female sexual development (Guyomarc'h & Guyomarc'h 1984) and males housed with females show faster sexual development than males housed alone (Delville et al. 1984). If birds are transferred from long- to short-day lengths, the gonads regress and reproduction ceases (Sachs 1967). However, some females will lay eggs under short photoperiods or even under continuous darkness (Noble 1972; Stein & Bacon 1976).

If the photoperiod is sufficiently long, sperm production commences at around 4 weeks of age (Mather & Wilson 1964; Ottinger & Brinkley 1978; Ottinger & Brinkley 1979a) and sperm are present in large numbers in the vas deferens and testes by 35 days of age (Ottinger 1978). Males begin crowing at about 2 weeks of age, show cloacal gland development (Cheng et al. 1989b) at about 4 weeks of age and begin mating attempts. Completed copulations may occur only a few days later (Ottinger & Brinkley 1979b).

Male fertility starts to decline as early as 15 weeks of age (Ottinger 1991). Old males have lower fertility than younger males (Woodard & Abplanalp 1967; Ottinger et al. 1983) and males kept on a chronic long-day length photoperiod develop more age-related abnormalities in testes and sperm than males kept on shorter-day length photoperiods (Eroschenko et al. 1977). Advanced age adversely affects sexual behaviour in male quail (see reviews by Ottinger 1983, 1991).

Egg production declines with age (Figure 41.3) and eggs from older females (post-20 weeks) have low hatchability and fertility even though older females are more sexually receptive than younger females (Woodard & Abplanalp 1967). Wild females in their first breeding season display little sexual activity until late in the season and are usually not successful in laying a clutch until their second breeding season (Nichols 1991). Keeping females on chronic long photoperiods shortens their reproductive life presumably because of the physiological demands associated with high egg production.

Breeds, strains and genetics

A wide variety of plumage colour mutants exist (Cheng & Kimura 1990; Butkauskas 2001) and various strains have been selected for physiological and behavioural traits. Details of existing known mutations, gene nomenclature, mutations, physical linkage maps and specific genetic lines can be found in Tsudzuki (2008), Gunnarsson et al. (2007), Mizutani (2002), Cheng and Kimura (1990), Cheng and Nichols (1992), Sato and Lansford (2013) and Somes (1984).

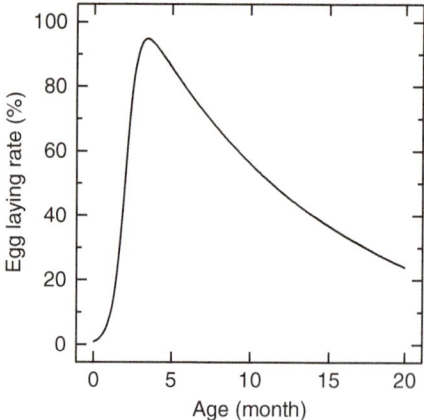

Figure 41.3 Hen-day egg-laying rate as a function of age in domestic JQ. Source: Data from Minvielle et al. (2000).

The karyotype consists of 7 pairs of macrochromosomes (including the sex chromosomes) and 32 pairs of microchromosomes (Shibusawa et al. 2001; Shibusawa et al. 2004). The DNA content per haploid cell is ~1.04 to 1.41 Gb in size (Bachmann et al. 1972; Tiersch & Wachtel 1991; Kawahara-Miki et al. 2013; Wu et al. 2018).

The integrated linkage map has been published by Kayang et al. (2006). Comparative gene mapping of cDNA and genomic DNA clones using fluorescence in situ hybridisation (FISH) revealed that the genetic linkage groups are highly conserved between the chicken and quail; however, the quail differed from the chicken in chromosomes 1, 2 and 8 by pericentric inversion and in chromosome 4 by centromere repositioning (Shibusawa et al. 2001). The first quail draft genome sequence was reported with the N50 contig length of 1.5 kb and then improved and extended by the same group extended the N50 contig length to 32 kb (NCBI BioSample: SAMD00009971) (Kawahara-Miki et al. 2013). Recently, another chromosome level draft genome from a male *Coturnix japonica* individual from an inbred quail line (Cons DD (INRA)) was sequenced at total sequence genome input coverage of ~73 x using an Illumina HiSeq 2500 instrument (NCBI BioSample: SAMN03989050). Long PacBio reads added 20 x coverage to further close gaps in the genome. The assembled male genome Coturnix japonica 2.0 is made up of a total of 2,531 scaffolds (including single contigs with no scaffold association) with an N50 scaffold length of 2.9 Mb (N50 contig length is 511 kb). The assembly sequence size is 0.927 Gb across 33 chromosomes. Coturnix japonica 2.0 has been assigned to more chromosomes and has more annotations with ncRNA, mRNA and pseudogenes predicted than previous versions (Wu et al. 2018). Finally, a total of 16,057 protein-coding genes and 39,075 transcripts were predicted. The annotated Coturnix_japonica_2.0 genome assembly is available at Ensembl[2].

Quail as food animals

Japanese quail have been farmed in many parts of the world. Due to their small body size, fast growth, high rate of egg production and ease of management, they are a practical solution to the problem of animal protein shortage in developing countries and an alternative to chicken in developed countries (Shanaway 1994). Under commercial production systems, quail can be marketed at about 5 weeks of age with an average weight of about 215 g. A feed conversion (feed/gain) ratio of 3.5 is not as efficient as that of broiler chickens (Hoffmann 1990). However, the strength of the quail is in egg production. Domestic hens start egg-laying at about 5–6 weeks of age, eggs are about 10–12 g each, and a hen can produce 280–300 eggs in a year (Minvielle 1998). The feed conversion (feed/egg) ratio of 3.3 makes the quail the champion species in converting feed into eggs (Shanaway 1994). In Japan, birds are mainly kept for egg production. Like the chicken layer operation, birds are kept in cages, quail chicks are vent-sexed at hatch and the males are discarded. In China, males are kept until they are 4–5 weeks old and then sold for meat. Hens are kept for egg production. In the United States and in Europe, birds are used mainly for meat production. Both cage and floor pen systems are used for rearing.

In the past five decades, commercial quail farming has developed in many parts of the world, particularly in Japan, China, Korea, India, Italy, France (Bessei 1977; Minvielle 1998), Spain, Hungary, Poland, Estonia, Russia, Czech Republic, Slovakia (Baumgartner 1993), Saudi Arabia, Southeastern United States, Brazil (Murakami & Ariki 1998) and Chile. US farmers produced ~40 million quail in 2007, which is the most recent available data through the USDA. That was double the number counted in 2002 and ranks the United States fifth in global quail production behind China, Spain, France and Italy. Quail are easing to raise in small spaces, which has made them increasingly popular among backyard farmers.

Quail as laboratory animals

The bird's small size, inexpensive rearing requirements, rapid maturation and adaptability to a wide range of husbandry conditions have made it popular as a laboratory animal for studies of behaviour, development, genetics, growth, endocrinology, nutrition, physiology, pharmacology and toxicology (Padgett & Ivey 1959; Wilson et al. 1959; Reese & Reese 1962; Landsdown et al. 1970). Since quail have been used as a model organism in many research studies, there is an abundance of background information available. Additionally, numerous mutations are known (Cheng & Kimura 1990) and several strains have been developed for use in research (Marks 1978; Shih et al. 1983; Hazard et al. 2005; Minvielle et al. 2007). With the draft genome of the Japanese quail sequenced and assembled (Kawahara-Miki et al. 2013; Wu et al. 2018) and the complete sequence of the mitochondria genome (Nishibori et al. 2001), the species' value as a model animal has been greatly enhanced. There are currently ~150 microsatellite markers identified based on the genome sequences (Kawahara-Miki et al. 2013; Tadano et al. 2014). Another study reported a linkage map with 1735 polymorphic amplified fragment length polymorphisms markers, and

---

[2] http://www.ensembl.org/Coturnix_japonica/Info/Index?db=core;r=3:26260835-26339271 (accessed 4 August 2021)

nine chicken microsatellite markers (Kikuchi *et al.* 2005). Linkage analysis uncovered 578 independent loci. The genome sequence and associated resources will offer essential genetic and genomic reference information, molecular information for making precise primers and nucleic acid probes to use in polymerase chain reaction, multiplexed hybridisation chain reaction-based RNA *in situ* and perturbation reagents including morpholinos, siRNA- and shRNA-based RNA inactivation, and CRISPR-Cas9 targeting approaches (see also Chapter 4: An introduction to laboratory animal genetics).

The Japanese quail is a compelling alternative avian model to the conventional chicken, particularly for researchers who want to generate transgenic birds efficiently (see Bower *et al.* 2011 for a review). This is because the Japanese quail has a shorter generation time compared to chicken (Poynter *et al.* 2009). Moreover, its small body size permits maintenance of transgenic strains by means of small cages with a small modification in an air-conditioned, pathogen-controlled environment of an animal facility (Huss *et al.* 2008). Several tissue-specific fluorescent transgenic lines now exist, which greatly facilitates time-lapse imaging and tissue transplantation (Scott & Lois 2005; Sato *et al.* 2010; Seidl *et al.* 2013; Huss *et al.* 2015; Moreau *et al.* 2018).

The quail has been used extensively as a research model in neuroendocrinology. Since it has prominent and clearly defined sex differences in its behaviour (Ottinger 1989), it has been particularly useful in studies on the endocrine and neural mechanisms that control sexual differentiation and reproductive behaviour (Balthazart & Ball 1998; Balthazart *et al.* 2003; Ball & Balthazart 2004). Gonadotropin-inhibitory hormone, which directly acts on the pituitary to inhibit gonadotropin release, was first discovered in quail (Tsutsui *et al.* 2000). Since much is known about its hormonal regulation of sexual development and behaviour, it is often used as model species for avian toxicology tests (Ottinger *et al.* 2002; Scanes & McNabb 2003) and a key model for examining the effects of endocrine-disrupting chemicals (Halldin *et al.* 1999; Ottinger *et al.* 2001, 2002). Because of the bird's early maturation and short generation time, the bird is best suited for testing transgenerational effects of chemicals (Ottinger *et al.* 2002; Kamata *et al.* 2006). For similar reasons the bird has been a popular model for studying avian genetics (e.g. Minvielle *et al.* 1999; Yang *et al.* 1999; Aggrey 2003; Piao *et al.* 2003; Suda & Okamoto 2003; Kim *et al.* 2007).

The species has been of particular value in studies of photoperiodism and the hormonal control of sexual behaviour (Mills *et al.* 1997). The birds are strongly photoperiodic and have been used to examine how circadian rhythms are entrained in birds as well as the role of melatonin in various physiological processes (Ohta *et al.* 1989; Underwood 1994; Cheng *et al.* 1994; Underwood & Edmonds 1995; Moore & Siopes 2000, 2003; Fu *et al.* 2002; Houdelier *et al.* 2002; Nakahara *et al.* 2003).

Furthermore, quail has many characteristics and behaviour patterns in common with the domestic chicken (*Gallus gallus domesticus*). They have been used to test the nutritive value of various feedstuffs for chickens (e.g., Elangovan *et al.* 2003; Kaya *et al.* 2003), and are increasingly being used as model of that species for studies of applied animal ethology related to animal welfare (Gerken & Petersen 1987; Mills & Faure 1990; Gerken & Mills 1993; Odeh *et al.* 2003).

Although the quail has been, and continues to be, a useful laboratory species, Minvielle (2004) reported that its popularity as a research model, as measured by the number of published papers, had declined between 1992 and 2002. His analysis showed that only 115–120 papers per year were published on the bird in 2001–2002. The authors searched BIOSIS Previews for research papers published between 2003 and 2006 on Japanese quail and found that the number had increased to an average of 154 papers per year. In the 9-year period from 2009 to 2018, there was an average of 164 papers published per year identified by BIOSIS Previews. Minvielle's (2004) reported downward trend seemed to have reversed. However, given the significance of many of the studies outlined above, solely counting the number of published studies on quail may not be a good reflection of their importance as a research model.

Sources of supply (conservation status)

In those countries where quail are farmed for meat or eggs, it may be possible to obtain birds from commercial suppliers. However, one has to be aware that the quality and genetic background of birds from commercial suppliers may vary. This may compromise comparison of results from different experiments or the potential to obtain consistent results from long-term studies. Other sources of supply are laboratories or research stations that maintain breeding populations. In North America, birds of known genetic history and lines selected for particular traits such as atherosclerosis resistance or susceptibility used to be maintained by the Quail Genetic Resource Centre at the University of British Columbia. Because of budgetary problems, the Centre collaborated with the Agassiz Poultry Research Centre (Agriculture and Agri-Food Canada, 6947 #7 Highway, P.O. Box 1000, Agassiz, British Columbia V0M 1A0, Canada) to develop cryopreservation techniques for preserving the quail lines. The fact that *Coturnix* primordial germ cells (PGC), gonadal germ cells (GGC) and gonadal stem cells (GSC) are difficult and expensive to maintain in cell culture has driven the centre to develop a novel cryopreservation technique for testicular and ovarian tissue (Silversides & Liu 2012; Silversides *et al.* 2012; Liu *et al.* 2013; Liu *et al* 2015). Cryopreservation will permit genetically diverse or modified germ cells to be safely stored, reduce the costs and waste of maintaining actively breeding quail lines, preserve genetic diversity in *Coturnix* (Sittmann *et al.* 1966; Kim *et al.* 2007) and potentially endangered avian species, as well as allow for worldwide sharing of genetically modified lines while minimising disease spread issues (Silversides & Liu 2012). Moreover, cryopreservation will avoid all the animal welfare concerns of keeping live breeding populations and shipping live birds.

General husbandry

Different strains of domestic quail differ greatly in their husbandry requirement. The information provided in this section is generic in nature. Researchers working with particular strains of quail may need to modify their husbandry practice accordingly. Management information can usually be obtained from the organisation from which the birds were obtained. Other sources of information include Ottinger and Rattner (1999) and Randall and Bolla (2007).

Housing

Quail can be housed in facilities as diverse as battery cages or outdoor aviaries. The type of housing used will be determined by the nature of the research, statutory requirements, welfare considerations and other factors. Although battery cages have frequently been used, the Joint Working Group on Refinement (JWGR) recommended that, when it is not possible to keep the birds in outdoor aviaries, indoor pens were more suitable than cages, and that if cages have to be used these should be modified to improve the quality of the space they provide (JWGR 2001b). In that report, information on cage sizes used in common practice is also presented together with recommendation for best practice. The European Commission and the RSPCA of England and Wales have provided updated housing guidelines (European Commission 2007; RSPCA 2011) which provide advice on rearing, enrichment and housing. These guidelines also recommend pens rather than cages and that housing systems should allow for the provision of substrate for scratching, pecking and dustbathing, nestboxes and cover whenever possible. In European agricultural research where the housing condition has to be similar to that of commercial farms, the standards laid down by the European Union Directive 98/58/EC and Council Directive 1999/74/EC should be followed (see also Table 41.2). General recommendations adopted under the Council of Europe Convention for The Protection of Farm Animals (ETS No 87) and general and species-specific recommendations under The Protection of Vertebrate Animals used for Experimental and other Scientific Purposes (ETS No 123)[3] should also be consulted. In the UK, in circumstances in which Japanese quail are not defined as domestic poultry under the legislative framework, the housing condition guidelines encompassed within the Wildlife and Countryside Act may have to be followed. In the following sections, the authors provide a description of some commercially available caging systems.

Table 41.2 Space allowances for domestic JQ.

Parameter	Body mass (g)	
	Up to 150	Over 150
Minimum enclosure size (m²)	1.0	1.0
Area per bird: pair-housed (m²)	0.5	0.6
Area per bird: group-housed (m²)	0.10	0.15
Minimum height (cm)	20	30
Minimum length of feeding trough (cm)	4	7

Source: Modified from European Commission (2007); Cheng et al. (2010); RSPCA (2011).

[3]https://www.coe.int/en/web/conventions/full-list/-/conventions/treaty/123 (accessed 4 August 2021)

These are not intended to be descriptions of the ideal as there has been little research in this area, and further research into optimal quail housing is required.

Breeding facilities

Because domestic quail hens do not take to nestboxes readily and eggs laid on the floor are easily soiled and broken, difficult to collect and impossible to pedigree, cages are by far the most practical system for the housing of breeder or layer stock. However, new non-cage housing requirements for farmed poultry has come into effect in Europe in 2012[4]. For keeping breeding birds in floor pens, one has to keep in mind that any aversive events before or during egg formation affect the quality of eggs and offspring phenotypes of quail (Schwabl 1996; Groothuis et al. 2005; Persaud & Galef, Jr. 2005). Even though Buchwalder and Wechsler (1997) have found that quail may use solid-sided nestboxes with a small entrance, no further research has been carried out to facilitate housing breeding quail in floor pens as an alternative to conventional battery cages. It is known that minor differences in housing environment can have significant effects on eggs and offspring. Daily human disturbances have been reported to decrease yolk androgen levels resulting in less reactive offspring (Guesdon et al. 2011). The presence of a shelter seems to help housed quail deal with these disturbances (RSPCA 2011). This transgenerational effect caused by an opportunity to hide could lead to applications in care of laboratory animals, conservation biology and animal welfare.

The quail is a long-day breeder (Wilson & Donham 1988). A lighting regimen of 16–18 h of light and 6–8 h of dark is usually sufficient to maintain a bird in good breeding condition. Less than 10 h of light per day will keep the birds in a non-breeding condition (Robinson et al. 1982)

Brooding facilities

Deep litter floor pens can be used to house birds from hatching to the end of their lives. Deep litter systems can range in size from entire rooms to small boxes mounted on wheels. Heat is provided by lamps, gas burners or radiant heaters suspended above the floor. Wood shavings are the most frequently used floor covering.

Chicks can be kept in wooden boxes until they are 2–3 weeks of age. Typical boxes measure 40 cm × 65 cm × 30 cm (w × d × h). When there is no place to hide, quail will jump upwards with tremendous force in a flight response when startled. If cage height exceeds 30 cm, it will allow the quail to pick up momentum in the flight response which may result in severe head injuries (Gerken & Mills 1993). For this reason, ceilings can be of soft material. However, the soft material should be: (1) non-porous and washable; (2) non-flammable; and (3) not obstruct ventilation. Brooding boxes with soft ceilings are not commercially available. Heat and light can be provided by an infra-red lamp suspended over one end of the box. Temperature directly under the heat source should be 37 °C, allowing the chicks to find their comfort zone as they move towards the other end of the box. The floor of the boxes should be covered with wood shavings or some other form of litter. After 2 weeks, the heat source is no longer needed if the room temperature is maintained

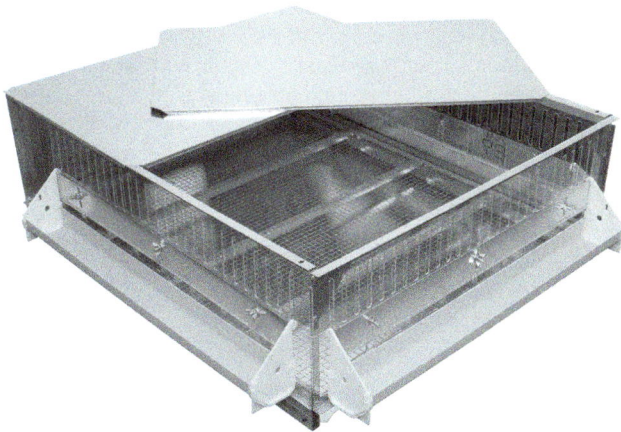

Figure 41.4 Box brooder for JQ chicks. Source: Reproduced with permission of GQF Manufacturing Company.

within the 18–26 °C range. At this age, the juveniles can also be moved to deep litter floor pens.

When justifiable, chicks and juvenile birds may also be kept in commercial battery brooder cages (Figure 41.4). As their name suggests, battery brooder cages are arranged in batteries mounted on metal frames. Heat is provided from radiant heaters which are usually built into the roof of the cage. Light and additional heat can be provided by lamps mounted on the ceiling of the cage. In most commercial brooder cages, the heat source can be controlled by a thermostat. At hatching, quail chicks require an ambient temperature of 37 °C. After 3 days the temperature can be reduced to 35 °C. Thereafter, the temperature can be progressively reduced by 5 °C per week until 25 °C.

Battery brooder cages can be of different sizes but usually measure at least 100 cm × 75 cm × 16–20 cm (w × d × h). Cage roofs are made of solid metal sheeting. Cage sides are made of 1 cm^2 (or smaller) wire mesh or solid metal sheeting. The cage fronts usually serve as hinged doors and are usually made out of vertical wire grill. If trough feeders are attached to the front of the cage, then the space between the bars should be large enough to allow the birds to reach the feeder easily but not so large as to allow chicks to escape. Similar provisions should be made for access to drinkers if these are located outside of the cage. The vertical distance between tiers of cages should be sufficient to allow easy collection and removal of droppings. Obviously, there must be an impervious separation between each tier of cages so as to prevent faeces falling from one level to another. Droppings can be collected on sheets of paper, pull-out trays or moving belts.

Cage floors of 1 cm^2 mesh have been used, which allow for the passage of the droppings from the cage. However, this mesh size is too large to support the feet of chicks under 1 week of age. Therefore, for chicks of less than 1 week of age, the cage floor should be lined with sheets of paper or fine mesh plastic mesh (0.2 cm^2). Some droppings will pass through plastic mesh of this size and with reasonable stocking densities, a single sheet of plastic mesh can be left in place from hatching to about 10 days of age when it is no longer required. Paper sheets, pull-out trays or moving belts should be cleaned before there is excessive accumulation of droppings. In this context, it is important to remember that droppings will not be evenly distributed over the cage floor but will be concentrated in the areas around feeders and drinkers.

Feeders for young chicks must not have high (<2 cm) sides or the birds may not be able to reach the food. Petri dishes make excellent feeders for chicks from hatching to 4 or 5 days of age when food spillage becomes an important problem. From hatching onwards, it is usual to present food in both petri dishes and some other form of feeder so that the chicks are familiar with these other feeders when the petri dishes are removed. In brooder and battery cages, food is usually presented in feeders attached to the front of the cage. These feeders can be simple troughs or more complicated 'back-well feeders'.

The appropriate type of drinker varies with the husbandry system. In small cages and boxes, cage-bird drinkers can be used (one per five birds). When birds are housed in deep litter pens, or boxes, plastic 0.5 l gravity-fed bell drinkers are probably the most appropriate for chicks and sub-adult birds. However, for small chicks it may be advisable to fit drinkers with a grill or rubber ring to reduce the available watering area or some chicks may drown. An alternative solution is to partially fill the drinker with pebbles. Bell drinkers should be placed on wooden sheets to prevent them from becoming clogged with litter. However, this is only a partial solution to clogging and drinkers should be inspected daily and cleaned out when necessary.

Irrespective of the type of housing system used, chicks less than 2 weeks old should be kept under continuous illumination at a minimum of 20 lux light intensity. This is of particular importance when birds are kept in large deep litter pens with a single heat source such as a gas burner. Under such conditions, if a period of darkness occurs, chicks will disperse from beneath the heat source and may die. There is no evidence from corticosterone measurements that quail suffer from being kept under UV-deficient lighting (Smith *et al*. 2005).

Rearing and holding facilities

Juvenile and adult birds can best be housed in deep litter floor pens. They can also be kept in colony or pedigree battery cages that do not have internal sources of heating or lighting (Figure 41.5). Commercial colony cages for adults can often be subdivided into smaller cages for one to three birds.

Floor pens have to be custom-built. They can be of various dimensions depending on the number of birds to be housed and other research requirements. Readers should consult JWGR (2001b) and also see Chapter 40 on domestic fowl.

Like brooder cages, adult cages can be of different sizes. However, commercially available colony cages normally measure 100 cm × 50 cm × 16–20 cm (w × d × h) and pedigree cages suitable for up to three or four birds measure 25 cm × 50 cm × 20 cm (w × d × h).

Pedigree and colony cages usually have roofs made of solid metal sheeting. If the cage roof is not solid metal sheeting but of wire mesh, it is advisable to hang soft, wide plastic strips vertically from the cage roof halfway down the cage for birds to hide behind. This will minimise their flight response and head injuries. The material used for making

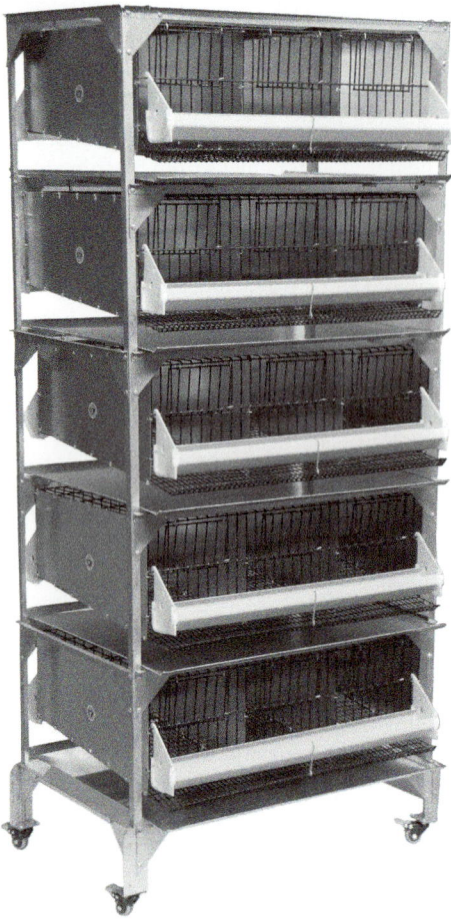

Figure 41.5 Battery breeding cages for adult JQ. Source: Reproduced with permission of GQF Manufacturing Company.

differences in body weight may confound this problem. Lucotte (1974) suggested that stocking densities should be 250 birds/m² during the first week after hatching and 175 birds/m² during the second and third weeks after hatching. However, sex ratio and body weight may require that these estimates be modified (RSPCA 2011). Current recommendations suggest that adult birds should not be kept at stocking densities greater than 40–45 birds/m², thus providing each bird with 225–250 cm² of space (National Research Council (NRC) 1996; National Advisory Committee for Laboratory Animal Research 2004; see also Table 41.2).

In deep litter systems, food can be provided in hoppers which require less maintenance than other feeder types. Quail have high nutritional requirements throughout their lives, particularly during the growing period, so it is important that the feeding space provided is adequate (see Table 41.2). In large deep litter systems, continuous-flow bell drinkers can be used for juvenile and adult birds. These drinkers can be suspended at a height within easy access by the birds but sufficiently high to minimise clogging with litter. Alternatively, cup or nipple drinkers can be installed. Colony cages and pedigree cages are usually equipped with cup or nipple drinkers (one per five birds).

Although juvenile birds readily adapt to changes in drinker type, this is not the case in adult birds. Birds which have been raised with bell drinkers may not recognise nipple or cup drinkers and *vice versa*. Therefore, when birds are transferred from one type of husbandry system to another, it is important to ensure that the animals find the drinkers.

From 3 to 6 weeks of age, birds should be kept under a lighting regimen of 8 h light to 16 h darkness. If this is not the case, females may enter into lay too early, giving rise to reproductive problems (see later in this chapter). Adult birds can be kept on photoperiods of 12–18 h.

these strips should be able to withstand high pressure or steam cleaning without turning brittle. Cages with soft mesh netting roofs are not commercially available but can be custom installed. However, soft mesh netting roofs have the disadvantage that they are flammable, not easily cleaned and disinfected, there is a risk of birds tangling or strangling themselves in a flight response, and they may not easily be used with rack cage systems. Cage sides are made of 1 cm² or smaller wire mesh or solid metal sheeting. Cage floors are made of 1–2 × 1 cm mesh to allow the passage of droppings. The cage floors should be sloping so as to allow eggs to roll out. As for brooder cages, the cage fronts are usually hinged and serve as the cage doors. The cage fronts and backs should be made from wire grill with 2.5 cm spaces between the bars to allow birds to reach food and water easily. Adult cages are mounted on metal frames and arranged in batteries with an impervious separation between tiers. The vertical distance between tiers should be sufficient to allow easy collection and removal of droppings. Again, as for brooder cages, droppings can be collected on sheets of paper, pull-out trays or moving belts.

Domestic quail grow rapidly and reach adult size in 4 weeks. Therefore, stocking densities should be predetermined at hatching or should decrease with the age of the birds, until they reach adult size. Strain, breed and line

Feeding and water

Dietary requirements

Quail chicks have very high requirements for dietary protein and amino acids early in life but these requirements diminish as the birds age. Recommended nutrient levels for growing and breeding birds are shown in Table 41.3. In the case of laying hens, although food intake is low (20–30 g/day), the ratio of egg weight to body is high (approximately 5%) and it is particularly important to ensure a high intake of protein and sulphur amino acids.

Natural and laboratory diets

Wild quail are omnivorous and have a diet composed of small seeds, insects and spiders (Kawahara 1967) and a wide variety of plant materials[4]. Table 41.4 shows the food consumption of birds up to 5 weeks of age. The metabolisable energy value of diets should be in the range of 2600–3200 kcal/kg (Shim & Vohra 1984). In commercial operations where maximising production is a premium, it is usual to

---

[4]https://ec.europa.eu/food/animals/welfare/practice/farm/laying_hens_en (accessed 4 August 2021)

Table 41.3 Nutrient requirements of JQ (NRC 1994). Dietary requirements are on a per kg diet basis, assuming 90% dry matter.

Nutrient	Unit	Diets	
		Starting and growing	Breeding
Metabolisable energy	kcal/kg	2900	2900
Protein and amino acids			
Protein	%	24.0	20.0
Arginine	%	1.25	1.26
Glycine + serine	%	1.15	1.17
Histidine	%	0.36	0.42
Isoleucine	%	0.98	0.90
Leucine	%	1.69	1.42
Lysine	%	1.30	1.00
Methionine	%	0.50	0.45
Methionine + cystine	%	0.75	0.70
Phenylalanine	%	0.96	0.78
Phenylalanine + tyrosine	%	1.80	1.40
Threonine	%	1.02	0.74
Tryptophan	%	0.22	0.19
Valine	%	0.95	0.92
Fat			
Linoleic acid	%	1.0	1.0
Macrominerals			
Calcium	%	0.8	2.5
Chlorine	%	0.14	0.14
Magnesium	mg/kg	300	500
Non-phytate phosphorus	%	0.3	0.35
Potassium	%	0.4	0.4
Sodium	%	0.15	0.15
Trace minerals			
Copper	mg/kg	5	5
Iodine	mg/kg	0.3	0.3
Iron	mg/kg	120	60
Manganese	mg/kg	60	60
Selenium	mg/kg	0.2	0.2
Zinc	mg/kg	25	50
Fat-soluble vitamins			
A	IU/kg	1650	3300
D3	ICU/kg	750	900
E	IU/kg	12	25
K	mg/kg	1	1
Water-soluble vitamins			
B12	mg/kg	0.003	0.003
Biotin	mg/kg	0.3	0.15
Choline	mg/kg	2000	1500
Folacin	mg/kg	1	1
Niacin	mg/kg	40	20
Pantothenic acid	mg/kg	10	15
Pyridoxine	mg/kg	3	3
Riboflavin	mg/kg	4	4
Thiamine	mg/kg	2	2

Table 41.4 Food consumption of sample lines of JQ at different ages.

Age (wk)	Food consumption (g/day)	
	Random-bred line[1]	Commercial meat lines[2]
1		6.8
2	10.2	13.7
3	13.0	15.7
4	17.5	19.8
5		23.5

[1] Data from Farrell et al. (1982).
[2] Data from Güler et al. (2005) and Hyánkova et al. (1997).

provide the birds with 'starter' diets until they are 21 days of age, with 'grower diets' from 3 to 6 weeks of age and 'breeder or layer' diets thereafter. In laboratory operations, the authors found that using a commercial turkey starter diet (26% protein) fortified with extra calcium (2.5%) is satisfactory for feeding quail of all ages. The diet comes in 'crumble' form (crumbled pellets) and has to be ground to a dry mash for feeding newly hatched chicks to 2 weeks old. Thereafter, the diet can be fed as crumbles. Feeding the diet in mesh form will result in high feed spillage and waste. Specially prepared diets for quail may be available from some feed companies. Some commercial game bird diets can also be used for quail. Diet with high wheat content should be avoided, as the feed will become glutinous when moistened and will stick to the toes of the birds and ball up. Advice on quail nutrition in the tropics is available online[5,6].

If the birds are housed in floor pens and are allowed to move freely and express natural behaviour, they will use significantly more energy in their daily activities and that has to be taken into account when formulating the diet (Rutten 2018). It is convenient to use a strong bone and muscle development diet for quail. At 6 weeks post-hatch, when the birds are sexually mature, one can switch to Purina® Game Bird Layena ETTS, which is a complete 16%-protein, high calcium breeder ration formulated to support optimum fertility, embryo development, egg production, strong eggshell and chick vigour in game birds. For nutritional physiology studies, commercial diets may not provide the background consistency of the feed ingredients and the precise level of various nutrients needed. In this situation, a synthetic diet (Table 41.5) may be used.

Water

Clean drinking water must be provided at all times. Water consumption (Table 41.6) increases with age (Farrell et al. 1982; Visser et al. 2000) and is greater in lines selected for increased body mass (Visser et al. 2000). Drinking rates of adults increase as salinity of their drinking water increases,

[5] https://www.hbw.com/species/japanese-quail-coturnix-japonica (accessed 4 August 2021)
[6] http://www.thatquailplace.com/quail/coturn1.htm (accessed 4 August 2021)

Table 41.5 Formula for a synthetic basal diet for laboratory JQ. This diet is used at the UBC Quail Genetic Resource Centre for nutrition research projects.

Ingredient	Amount (g/kg diet)
Soya protein flour (50% protein)	340
Corn starch	400
Limestone	50
Mineral premix	5
Monofos	30
Sucrose	20
Alphacel	70
Vitamin premix	5
D-L methionine	4
Choline chloride	0.8
Tallow	50
Vegetable oil	30

Table 41.6 Water consumption of domestic JQ at different ages.

Age (wk)	Water intake[1] (ml/day)	Water flux[2] (g/day)	
		C strain[3]	P strain[4]
1		18.0	21.0
2	23.3	23.7	30.7
3	26.2	29.7	27.1
4	30.0		
7		40.9	62.1

[1] Farrell et al. (1982).
[2] Visser et al. (2000).
[3] Random-bred line (body mass at 7 wk of age = 184 g).
[4] Rapid growth line (body mass at 7 wk of age = 294 g).

but quail do not tolerate salinities greater than isotonic (150 mM NaCl; Roberts & Hughes 1983).

Environmental provisions

Quail do not readily use conventional nestboxes (see Buchwalder & Wechsler 1997 for a discussion of the improvement of nestbox design and usage) but do use litter for dustbathing. Enriching the environment of chicks by providing coloured objects and other 'toys' reduces fear and aggressive responses in later life (Jones et al. 1991; JWGR 2001b). Providing soft background music and human conversations from radio stations, from poultry farmers' practice and from our own laboratory experience, seems to lessen fear response elicited by humans entering the aviary.

Social grouping

Male quail react vigorously to the presence of unfamiliar males (Selinger & Bermant 1967) and rearing males in pairs and then interchanging pair members leads to an increase in the frequency of aggressive interactions relative to that observed in the original pairs (Edens et al. 1983; Edens 1987). Further, birds that have been left in their 'home' cages are more aggressive than birds that have been transferred to an unfamiliar cage (Edens et al. 1983). Therefore, once groups have been established it is inadvisable to attempt to mix groups or introduce new animals into established groups.

In groups where the male–female ratio is high, misdirected head grabs by males (particularly if the female is not receptive) may result in head wounds and eye damage or loss. Under such circumstances, frequent attempts at mounting may result in wounds and, in extreme cases, the death of the females. Where possible, housing of females in single-sex groups is desirable on welfare grounds. However, this is not the case for males. Breeding birds can be housed in pairs or in trios (one male with two females) (RSPCA 2011). In larger mixed sex groups, the sex ratio should not be more than 1:4. Male homosexual copulation attempts would also be frequent (Wilson & Bermant 1972) and would lead to subordinate males suffering feather loss and injuries similar to those sustained by females.

Sexing

Day-old chicks can be vent-sexed (examination of the cloaca) (Homma et al. 1966) but accuracy is difficult to achieve in practice, except perhaps in Japan where hatcheries hire professional sexers to sex the chicks. However, by the time the chicks are 3–4 weeks old they can be sexed on the basis of plumage colour (Figure 41.1). Researchers working with strains that have plumage colour other than the wild type can identify males at 4 weeks of age by the protruding foam gland above the cloaca (Cheng et al. 1989b).

Recently, molecular approaches are increasingly used to sex chicks and embryos. To determine the host embryo sex, a micromanipulator/microinjection setup can be employed to remove blood/PGCs from the vitelline blood vessel to assay the genome or transcriptome by molecular techniques such as polymerase chain reaction (PCR), reverse transcription PCR (RT-PCR), RNA in situ hybridisation (ISH) or transcriptome sequencing (RNA-seq) for genes that permit sex determination (Griffiths et al. 1996; Jensen et al. 2003; Nagai et al. 2014). For example, HINTW is a robust and reliable marker for female-derived cells (Hori et al. 2000; Nagai et al. 2014) whose expression can be assessed by RT-PCR, RNA in situ hybridisation (ISH), or transcriptome sequencing (RNA-seq). Another method permits extraction of genomic DNA from blood, shell-membrane blood vessels and feathers using Chelex (Jensen et al. 2003). The CHD-1 gene is present on both the W and Z chromosomes (Griffiths et al. 1996; Morinha et al. 2011), but the CHD-1 intron length differs between the two sex chromosomes, resulting in PCR products that separate into two bands for females and a single band for males in most avian species.

Identification

Individual birds can be identified by means of leg bands or wing tags. The use and application of split rings and wing tags is described in JWGR (2001b). Wing bands and tags are readily available from commercial suppliers. Both bands and tags can be placed on birds of any age. However, the banding and tagging of chicks present certain difficulties. Leg bands, which are suitable for small chicks, do not have a diameter sufficient to accommodate the leg of juvenile or adult birds and must be replaced with larger ones when the birds are 1–2 weeks of age. Wing tags can be left in place throughout the life of the birds but only if they are correctly placed in the propatagium (the membrane or fold of skin in front of the humeral and radio-ulnar parts of the wing). However, in chicks the propatagium is very small and there is a risk that some tags will be placed in the muscles of the wing. If this is the case, then the tag will progressively become imbedded in the musculature of the wing as the bird grows. Therefore, birds should be inspected at 1–2 weeks of age and any incorrectly placed tags replaced. #5 Fingerling tags are suitable for quail chicks, and aluminium chick wing bands are suitable for adult quail. Ear tags for mice may also be suitable for the wing tagging of chicks and adults. Transponder microchips could be used as an alternative to leg bands or wing tags. However, these are relatively expensive and do not appear to have been widely used. If birds are housed in floor pens, where they can run around and flap their wings in attempts to fly, the chance of losing a wing tag would be much higher than housing birds in cages. In this situation, the birds should be double tagged with one tag on each wing, to avoid loss of identification (Cheng, personal observations). In pedigree breeding systems, where two or more hens are kept with a male, egg colour, size and shape can be used to identify which of the hens laid them. These parameters vary greatly between individuals but are extremely consistent within individuals over a 3-week period (Lucotte 1974; Cheng, personal observations).

Hygiene

Good hygiene is essential at all stages of husbandry. Incubators and hatchers should be cleaned and disinfected after each use. Rooms, cages, feeders and drinkers must be kept clean and disinfected after each cycle of use. When birds are kept in cages, dropping collectors should be changed or cleaned on a weekly basis. As far as possible, cage floors should be kept free from droppings. In deep litter floor pens, litter should be topped up weekly, with a total clean out and replacement every 2 months. If breeding birds are kept in deep litter floor pens, a cleaning schedule has to be carefully planned because the cleaning procedure will disrupt egg-laying. Where possible, the buildings used to house quail should be emptied periodically and cleaned and disinfected before being used again.

Health monitoring, quarantine and barrier systems

Birds should be carefully inspected at least once daily, and any birds showing signs of sickness or injury should be examined and treated appropriately and any dead birds removed. From hatching to 6 weeks of age, the mortality rate should be less than 5%. During breeding, the mortality rate should be less than 2%. Disease may be indicated by reduced egg output, morbidity and emaciation (see also section on disease). If animals are introduced to existing stock from an external source (this should be avoided if at all possible), it is very important that the source flock is disease free. It is better to bring in fumigated eggs or chicks than adult birds. If chicks or adult birds are brought in from external sources, they should be kept in quarantine for a period of 5–6 weeks. Contact between quail and other birds (particularly, game birds) should be avoided. Access to housing facilities should be restricted to persons who have not been in contact with other birds for 72 h. It is prudent to provide disinfectant footbaths and protective clothing for workers and, for biosecurity reasons, visitors should not be allowed into the husbandry unit. Pest control around housing structures is important and insect screens should be installed to keep flies out.

Transport

It is advisable not to ship quail less than 2 weeks old as they are more sensitive to temperature fluctuation, dehydration and injury. However, if unavoidable, chicks are best transported in commercially available cardboard chick boxes (46 cm × 31 cm × 15 cm) with a floor lining of wood shavings. The boxes should have air holes of a size sufficient to allow adequate ventilation but small enough to prevent the chicks from escaping. When transporting chicks, it is important to ensure that the ambient temperature is suitable (35–30 °C, depending on the age of the chicks) and the time in transit be kept to less than 4 h. Adults should be transported in crates with solid floors and mesh or grill walls and roofs (65 cm × 52 cm × 19 cm for 20 birds). Specially designed crates can be purchased (Figure 41.6). For shipping adults over long distances, it is recommended that a cut open apple be attached to the inside of the crate for birds to peck at to obtain moisture. Time in transit should be limited to less than 8 h unless drinking water can be supplied every 4 h. Information on the transport of laboratory animals is given by Laboratory Animal Science Association (LASA 2005) and IATA[6] (see also Chapter 12: Transportation of laboratory animals).

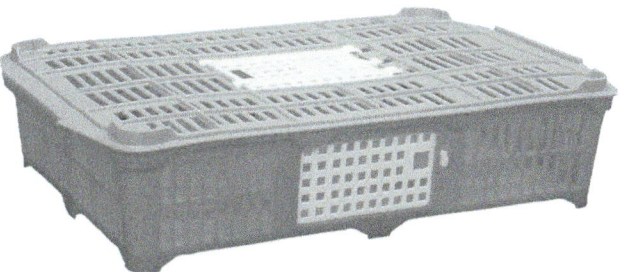

Figure 41.6 Spe[cially designed shipping crate for adult JQ. The crate has openings on the top and the side to facilitate the introduction and removal of birds. Source: Reproduced with permission of KUHL Corporation.

Breeding

Condition of adults

The reproductive status of both male and female quail can be determined from behavioural, hormonal, neuro-anatomical and morphological parameters (for details and references see Mills et al. 1997). However, in practical terms, behavioural and morphological measures are the easiest to apply. Age of sexual maturity can be manipulated by photoperiod. Birds kept under short photoperiod will not become sexually mature. Birds kept under long photoperiod will become sexually mature at 4–5 weeks of age. At sexual maturity, the cloacal diameter of females and the proctodeal (foam) gland of males increase. These anatomical changes and the beginning of sexual behaviour are reliable indicators of sexual maturity.

Breeding systems

The main criteria for the selection of breeding stock are that the birds are in good physical condition and meet the requirements of any selection criteria. However, it should be remembered that quail are extremely susceptible to inbreeding depression. According to Lucotte (1974), the hatchability of eggs falls to near zero after three generations of brother × sister mating. No full-sib mating inbred line has been maintained for more than eight generations (Kim et al. 2007). Therefore, it is important to avoid consanguineous matings. To achieve this in small populations, it is important to maintain pedigree records for breeding stock.

At least three methods exist for the management of breeding birds. Each of these has particular advantages and disadvantages but there is a clear order of preference on both welfare and husbandry grounds.

1. Birds can be housed in small cages containing one male and two or three females. Under such conditions, males do not usually damage the females, the method is not labour intensive and it is possible to pedigree offspring or identify birds which are not reproducing well.
2. Males and females may be kept in individual cages and the males introduced into the cages of the females at intervals of 2–3 days since females are fertile for 3–9 days after a single insemination (Reddish et al. 1996). Males are introduced into the female cages in the morning for a period of 15–30 minutes. This is a sufficiently long period for copulation to take place but short enough to prevent the males from injuring the females. However, this method is extremely labour intensive although it permits one male to be mated to a relatively large number of females.
3. Males and females may be kept together in colony cages containing 5–10 males and 20–40 females. This is not labour intensive, but the males may fight or attempt to copulate with one another, the mating of individual females is irregular and the parents of chicks cannot be identified. This method is probably the least desirable method for the management of breeding birds.

In the authors' laboratory, two males with four females are kept as a unit in a breeding cage and 24 cages (total of 48 males and 96 females) are kept for propagating their random-bred population. They have found this arrangement much more satisfactory than the colony cages.

Artificial insemination (AI)

Techniques for AI of quail have been developed (Wentworth & Mellen 1963; Marks & Lepore 1965; Lepore & Marks 1966), but fertility by AI is highly variable. AI is seldom used in practice because it is difficult to obtain semen that is not contaminated with foam or cloacal products (Buxton & Orcutt 1975). In addition, the volume of semen collected per male is between 3.9 and 6.9 µl (Marks & Lepore 1965) whereas an inseminating dose of 2.5–15 µl is required to achieve acceptable fertility levels. Furthermore, quail lay at the end of the photoperiod (late afternoon). Inseminating the female when there is a hard-shell egg in her oviduct will result in very poor fertility. The best time to inseminate after the egg is laid would be in the dark. For these reasons, reproduction is usually by natural mating rather than by AI.

Germplasm cryopreservation

Cryopreservation permits genetically diverse or modified germ cells to be safely stored, reduce the costs and waste of maintaining actively breeding quail lines. Previous studies have demonstrated that cryopreservation of PGCs is a feasible strategy for the conservation of both male and female germline cells in JQ (Naito et al. 1994; Nakamura et al. 2013; Nandi et al. 2016). Cryopreserved donor-derived germ cells can be thawed and injected into the vitelline blood vessels of stage 15–16 quail embryos. The donor-derived germ cells migrate to and colonise the host embryo's gonadal anlage, thus reconstituting the population of germ cells. The host embryo provides the proper environment for proliferation and maturation of the donor-derived germ cells and facilitate their differentiation into functional eggs and sperm (Trefil et al. 2017).

This approach lets the host's gonad provide the proper growth factor, cellular signals and micro-environment to propagate and maintain the donor-derived germ cells. The collection of genetically valuable embryonic PGC or GGC may not always be feasible. Therefore, routine collection of adult GSC at the time of necropsy could provide a more practical method (Roe et al. 2013), because self-renewing spermatogonial and possibly oogonial stem cells (Jones & Lin 1993) are found throughout the reproductive lifespan of birds. Previous studies have demonstrated that adult chicken and quail gonads contain cells that are capable of migrating and colonising the gonadal ridge following transfer to host chicken embryos at stage 14–17 (Minematsu et al. 2008; Jung et al. 2010; Roe et al. 2013). Likewise, dispersed testicular cells from both prepubertal and adult donors transferred directly into sterilised adult host testes recolonise the seminiferous tubules of the conspecific host, resume spermatogenesis and produce donor-derived offspring (Trefil et al. 2006; Jung et al. 2010). It was recently demonstrated that resumption of spermatogenesis in sterilised adult host chickens occurs following transfer of adult quail spermatogonia (Pereira et al. 2013).

Selective breeding

Traditional animal breeding programmes based on selection on phenotypes to achieve the breeding goal can take many generations and a large population size. With the advances in genome sequencing techniques, genomic-enabled selection is becoming increasingly common in animal breeding. Phenotypes of complex traits can be regressed on thousands of markers concurrently. Applying genomic selection to animal breeding will shorten cycle times, involve smaller number of animals and enable the acceleration of genetic gain (Fulton 2012; Campos et al. 2013).

Incubation of eggs

The nest of the quail, like those of most gallinaceous species, is little more than a simple scrape on the ground with a rim of dry grass or similar material (Kawahara 1967; Nichols 1991). In the wild or in aviaries, quail hens choose to nest in secluded sites within areas containing rough grasses and scattered shrubs (Taka-Tsukasa 1935; Kawahara 1967; Nichols 1991; Schmid & Wechsler 1997). However, little is known about the nesting behaviour of wild birds although it appears that nest-building and incubation are carried out exclusively by the female (Schwartz & Schwartz 1949; Orcutt & Orcutt 1976; Nichols 1991).

In deep litter floor pens, natural incubation of eggs is not practical because quail hens do not readily become broody. Even with nestboxes provided, her nest-building and incubation behaviour is disrupted or not expressed because of close proximity and disturbance from other birds in the pen (Nichols 1991). Eggs can be incubated by bantam hens or pigeons but by far the most practical method is artificial incubation.

Eggs which are intended for incubation should be collected daily. Collection is usually carried out in the morning since most eggs will have been laid at the end of the previous day. Quail eggs have thin and fragile shells, and they therefore should be handled carefully during collection and subsequent manipulations. After collection, the eggs should be stored on cardboard or specially designed polystyrene or foam-rubber trays for quail eggs. Eggs should be stored at 10–15 °C in a well-ventilated room (with a relative humidity of about 40%). Turning stored eggs at regular intervals may help to maintain hatchability. Storage time from collection to setting should be less than 7 days for maximum fertility and should not exceed 14 days since extended storage increases the incidence of embryonic abnormalities (Sittmann et al. 1971). Further, there is a fall in hatchability from 10 days onwards (Kraszewska-Domanska & Pawluczuk 1977). Before setting, eggs should be inspected and any that are dirty, cracked, under- or over-sized, or with shell abnormalities (soft or under or over pigmented) eliminated.

Artificial incubators are of two types – horizontal or vertical. The major difference between these two types of incubators is that horizontal incubators have a single fixed shelf for eggs whereas vertical incubators have several tiers of shelves which can be inclined up to an angle of 45%. Most horizontal incubators are simple in design and can be purchased cheaply. However, they may have low capacity and relatively poor stability of incubation temperature and humidity. More sophisticated horizontal incubators for research use are also available. Vertical incubators have higher capacity and better controlled temperature and humidity than the simple horizontal incubators. Popular models for incubating quail eggs can be obtained from commercial incubator companies.

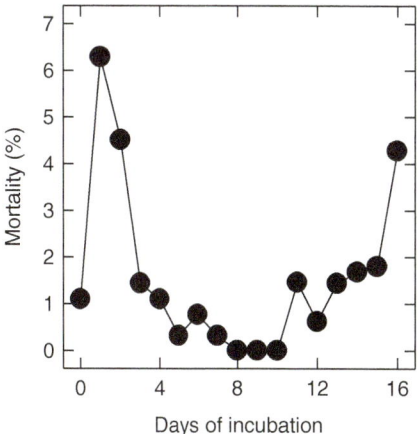

Figure 41.7 Daily embryonic mortality during incubation of JQ eggs. Source: Cheng et al. (2010).

Incubation conditions for quail eggs are similar to those for chicken eggs, but because quail eggs are much smaller than chicken eggs, they are more sensitive to temperature and humidity fluctuations during incubation. In vertical incubators, temperature should be between 37.5 °C and 38 °C. In simple horizontal incubators, where heat loss to the environment tends to be greater than in vertical incubators, the temperature should be set at 39 °C. This higher temperature is used to compensate for the greater temperature fluctuations inherent in these incubators. In both types of incubators, humidity should be 40–50%.

Incubation lasts 16–18 days. Under normal incubation conditions, there are peaks in embryonic mortality during the first 3 days of incubation and during the last 2 days of incubation (Figure 41.7).

Hatching of young

On day 14 of incubation, eggs should be prepared for hatching by transferring them to a hatcher apparatus or arranging them in hatcher trays in the incubator. Eggs should be placed on their sides and should not be turned thereafter. The temperature should be increased to 40 °C and the humidity increased to 70–80%. Eggs hatch between days 16 and 18 of incubation with most chicks hatching on day 17 (Lucotte 1974). However, these values may vary slightly depending on incubation conditions. For example, Wilson et al. (1961) found that the time from setting of eggs to external pipping was about just under 16 days, the time from pipping to hatching about 10 h and the time from hatching to complete drying of the down about 5 h.

Within batches, the time of hatching of quail chicks is synchronised to some degree. This synchronisation of hatching is partially the result of communication between embryos by means of a vocalisation known as clicking which accompanies each air intake (Kovach 1975). Clicking by advanced embryos accelerates hatching in retarded embryos and vice versa (Vince 1966, 1968; Vince & Cheng 1970). Hatchability is therefore better when eggs are put close together in the hatching tray.

Care of young birds

Chicks are nidifugous (precocial) and do not necessarily require parental care post-hatching. Provided that the rearing environment is adequate (see earlier), they have no other specific requirements. In 1974, Lucotte suggested that a mortality rate of 10–15% during the first weeks after hatching should not be considered excessive but with modern management systems it should be considerably less. In the authors' laboratory, quail mortality rate has been below 5% for the last 25 years. The greatest mortality occurs due to 'starve out' on the third and fourth days after hatching when the nutrients from the yolk sack (vitellus) have been depleted and some chicks may fail to adapt to external sources for water and nourishment. It is important to monitor closely at this time.

Care of aged birds

The quail displays a well-defined ageing process (Ottinger et al. 2001; Holmes and Ottinger 2003). Signs of ageing are visible at little over one year of age with evidence of declining function in reproductive, metabolic, neurobiological and behavioural systems (Ottinger & Laoie 2007). The quail exhibit dynamic bone physiology, especially in females because the hollow bones serve as a depot for minerals used in egg production (Ottinger et al. 2001). As a result, ageing females develop bone fragility; they have been well characterised as a model for hormone effects on osteoporosis and the role of vitamin D. They generally live 2–3 years in the wild.

Laboratory procedures

Handling and capture

Quail chicks are very small and must be handled very gently. They should be picked up using only the thumb and forefinger and held in the palm of the hand. When frightened or presented with unfamiliar stimuli, quail frequently injure themselves during the expression of escape behaviour. Therefore, care should be taken to minimise disturbances and staff and visitors should wear clothing with colours familiar to the birds. When birds are caught, they should be held so that their wings are pinned against the body and their legs hang freely. If birds are held by the legs or in such a manner that they can flap their wings, there is a high risk of bone breakage.

Physiological monitoring

Recording of body temperature

Methods for the measurement of body temperature are similar to those used for domestic chickens. The bird can be restrained by holding it facing backwards under your non-dominant arm. Use the arm to lightly hold the wings against your body and slide the hand underneath the legs and gently squeeze them together. Use the other hand to gently insert the thermometer into the cloaca. Yousef et al. (1966) studied the temperature of the hypothalamus, rectum and skin under different environmental conditions. The temperatures observed had the following ranges: hypothalamus 42.7–42.8 °C, rectum 42.0–42.2 °C and skin 39.0–39.8 °C. McNabb and McNabb (1977) describe the measurement of heat transfer across the skin and feather pelts in young birds. Woodard and Mather (1964) have described circadian rhythms in body temperature and Woodard and Wilson (1972) have measured body temperature in relation to oviposition. For further information concerning body temperature, see Wilson (1972).

Collection of blood samples

Blood samples can be taken from the jugular or brachial veins, which clot quickly after the blood sample is taken and prevent from excessive bleeding. Blood can be drawn either from the right or the left veins. The blood volume of quail is approximately 7 ml/100 g body weight (Nirmalan & Robinson 1971) and 0.5 ml blood/100 g body weight can be safely withdrawn. Arora (1979) suggested 0.5 mm diameter (25 G) needles for obtaining blood from the jugular vein and 0.46 mm diameter (26 G) needles for obtaining blood from the brachial vein (see also JWGR 1993). Arora (1979) suggested that for ease of collection, safety and for repeated sampling, the jugular vein was the most suitable site. However, repeated bleeding is not advisable. For a small amount of blood, nicking the brachial vein and immediately collecting the blood with a capillary tube is practical and less invasive. One has to make sure that bleeding has stopped before releasing the bird. The leg veins can be bled as a last resort, but they can be difficult to visualise and should only be done by an experienced bleeder. It is advisable for a novice to first practice bleeding under the supervision of a veterinarian.

Administration of substances

Dosing and injection procedures

The jugular vein is the most suitable site for intravenous injections. Intramuscular injection should be made in the pectoral muscles. Subcutaneous injections should be placed under the skin of the neck. Intra-coelomic injections are sometimes used to administer anaesthetics, but care should be taken not to place the injection into the air sacs.

Liquids can be administered orally by direct intubation of the crop using a standard 12–16 G gavage needle (bulbous tipped 100 mm long) (Ichilcik & Austin 1978). If doses do not need to be precise, it is possible to incorporate compounds into the diet or drinking water.

Although quail are not specifically dealt with, detailed information on the procedures involved in the administration of substances to animals can be found in JWGR (2001a).

Anaesthesia

There has been limited research into appropriate anaesthetics for use in quail but knowledge of the principles of avian anaesthesia have developed considerably in recent years. The report of the JWGR (JWGR 2001b) provides a useful introduction and source of information on anaesthesia and analgesia. Currently, inhalational anaesthesia is the preferred method for anaesthetising birds in many cases. The gas anaesthetic of choice is isoflurane (Carpenter 2000) due to its rapid induction, rapid recovery and minimal myocardial depressant effects. Concentrations have not been set for quail, but the recommended minimum concentration for isoflurane use in birds is 0.5–3%. Although now not often recommended, injectable anaesthetics can be used when inhalation anaesthesia is unavailable (Paul-Murphy and Fialkowshi 2001). However, as many injectable anaesthetics are no longer recommended, a veterinarian should be consulted before they are considered. Paul-Murphy and Fialkowshi (2001) summarise the various injectable drugs and dosages that have been used in birds. Further valuable information on anaesthesia is provided in Chapter 40 on domestic chicken.

Euthanasia

Methods of euthanasia for birds are reviewed in the report of the JWGR (JWGR 2001b) and in the American Veterinary Medical Association (AVMA) Guidelines for the Euthanasia of Animals (AVMA 2013). Each country may have different procedures for euthanising birds, so please check for your own guidelines. The overriding commitment of these guidelines is to provide veterinarians and scientists guidance in relieving pain and suffering of animals that are to be euthanised. In the United States, we typically follow the AVMA Guidelines which details three categories for bird euthanasia: Acceptable Methods, Acceptable with Conditions Methods, and Unacceptable Methods (AVMA 2013; AVMA 2019). Under the category of Acceptable Methods, intravenous injection of an injectable euthanasia agent (i.e., barbiturates) is the quickest and most reliable means of euthanising birds when it can be performed without causing fear or distress (AVMA 2003). A suitable agent for lethal injection is sodium pentobarbital (100 mg/kg administered intraperitoneal). The dose rate for intraperitoneal injection is 6 ml/kg body weight of a 6% solution (Mills et al. 1999). The use of pentobarbital raises legal responsibilities for veterinarians and animal owners to properly dispose of animal remains after death (AVMA 2013). Animal remains containing pentobarbital are potentially poisonous for scavenging wildlife.

Under the AVMA category of Acceptable with Conditions Methods (justified by logistical or scientific basis), quail are usually killed by CO_2 asphyxiation followed by cervical dislocation or lethal injection (AVMA 2013). Quail are placed in an induction chamber that is filled with CO_2 gas (>40%) from a cylinder. Cervical dislocation should be employed as a secondary physical method to ensure death after CO_2. However, it should be noted that, unless the brainstem is destroyed in the process, brain function may persist for some seconds. Incubated eggs may be destroyed by prolonged exposure (>20 minutes) to CO_2, cooling (<4 °C for 4 hours) or freezing (AVMA 2013).

Common welfare problems

Causes of mortality

The highest rates of mortality are usually seen during the first week post-hatching (Löliger & Schubert 1966; Zucker et al. 1967; Lucotte 1974). Careful management (control of temperature, pre-heating of husbandry units and avoidance of draughts) and correct nutrition are important in reducing early mortality. Under proper management, mortality should be less than 5%.

In adult male birds, traumatic injury is the most frequently cited cause of death. Infections of the reproductive organs following prolapse of the uterus, or shell gland, are a common cause of death in adult females (Ernst & Coleman 1966; Löliger & Schubert 1966; Woodard et al. 1973; Nagarajan et al. 1991). Woodard and Abplanalp (1971) estimated that approximately 1% of female birds died from injury or prolapse of the shell gland during each week of their study. However, such mortality can be reduced or prevented by delaying the onset of sexual maturity through manipulation of the photoperiod. The authors found that the frequency of prolapse varied among different strains. If the female can be taken out of egg production (put under a short lighting scheme) when prolapse is first observed, and housed individually to avoid pecking by other birds, the prolapse can generally recover. Prolapses that occur for more than 24 h are difficult to revert.

Other reported causes of mortality in quail include head injuries and emaciation and careful measures should be taken to avoid these. Emaciation appears to occur for a variety of reasons including social competition (Löliger & Schubert 1966; Zucker et al. 1967; Benoff & Rice 1980; Edens et al. 1983) and mechanical difficulties in reaching drinkers and feeders.

Disease

Prophylaxis

Good hygiene and barrier systems which prevent infection from outside sources are the most important aspects of prophylaxis. The implementation of biosecurity measures is critical to prevent the introduction of infectious agents into a quail colony. Such measures include sanitation and quarantine practices, active insect and rodent control programmes, and the inspection of food, water and bedding materials for potential contamination. The introduction of hatching eggs instead of adult birds to the colony reduces the risk of disease transmission from outside source. The health status of the source flock should be carefully evaluated before transfer of eggs or birds. Fumigation of eggs before incubation may help prevent the transmission of diseases from one generation to the next. Ideally, egg incubation and hatching areas are physically separated from the rearing areas, and human traffic always flows from clean to dirty areas. Good ventilation and husbandry (see earlier in this chapter) are important for the prevention of aspergillosis.

Vaccination is not widely practised. With the exception of quail pox vaccine, no vaccines have been developed for quail. However, adult (5-week-old) quail vaccinated against Newcastle disease using chicken vaccines with the strains LaSota, VG-GA, Ulster 2C and B1 conferred 100% protection (Lima *et al*. 2004). Commercial inactivated *Salmonella* vaccines can provide 84% and 90% protection against *Salmonella* Enteritidis (SE) and *Salmonella* Typhimurium (ST) strains, respectively (Mahmoud *et al*. 2016). Chicken vaccine against avian encephalomyelitis (AE) is also effective in adult quail. Many commercially produced feeds contain antibiotics and anticoccidials to prevent diseases and coccidiosis. It is generally advised not to vaccinate quail unless there is a disease outbreak in the area.

Signs of disease

The quail is an extremely disease-resistant species. Although it is susceptible to the majority of diseases found in gallinaceous birds, quail appear to have a much greater resistance to these pathogens than do domestic fowl (Farrow *et al*. 1975). Where disease and excessive mortality do occur, they are frequently a consequence of management failures in high-density production flocks. Many of the symptoms of disease in quail (reduced egg output, morbidity, mortality and emaciation) are common to a wide range of infections. Furthermore, infected birds do not always present obvious clinical symptoms and it is important that specialist help for diagnosis, treatment and control be sought if outbreaks of disease are suspected.

Common diseases

Japanese quail are susceptible to the majority of diseases found in gallinaceous birds. Detailed reviews of diseases affecting quail, along with information on control, prevention and treatment have been published (Barnes 1987; Reed & Jack 2013; Baer *et al*. 2015). A list of some of these diseases is given in Table 41.7.

Infectious diseases

Infectious avian diseases pose a persistent threat to wild and farmed quail populations, along with humans. Similar to other gallinaceous birds, quail are susceptible to a number of avian viral pathogens, most commonly quail bronchitis virus, Newcastle virus, and Eastern Equine Encephalomyelitis (Shivaprasad 2002). Although a brief description of viral pathogens in quail is provided below, the reader can refer to more comprehensive information elsewhere (e.g. Swayne *et al*. 2013).

Viral diseases

Quail bronchitis is an acute, highly contagious and fatal respiratory disease caused by quail bronchitis virus (QBV), a type I avian adenovirus. QBV is highly contagious in

Table 41.7 Natural and experimentally induced diseases of the JQ.

Viral disease	Reference
Quail bronchitis	Mills *et al*. (1999); Reed & Jack (2013)
Newcastle disease	Usman *et al*. (2008); Susta *et al*. (2018)
Eastern Equine Encephalomyelitis	Eleazer *et al*. (1978)
Egg drop syndrome	Mohapatra *et al*. (2014)
Marek's disease	Kenzy and Cho (1969); Cooper *et al*. (2007)
Influenza	Nagarajan *et al*. (2013)
Pox virus	Mills *et al*. (1999); Gülbahar *et al*. (2005)
Avian encephalomyelitis	Hill and Raymond (1962); Sentíes-Cué *et al*. (2016)
Inclusion body hepatitis (adenovirus)	Mills *et al*. (1999)
Lymphoid leucosis	Payne *et al*. (1991)
Reticuloendtheliosis	Theilen *et al*. (1966)
Bacterial diseases	
Pullorum disease (salmonellosis)	Snoeyenbos (1991)
Paratyphoid (salmonellosis)	Mills *et al*. (1999)
Campylobacteriosis	Marumya and Katasube (1988)
Erysipelas	Panigrahy and Hall (1977)
Fowl typhoid	Pomeroy and Nagaraja (1991)
Hexamitiasis	McDougald (1991)
Infectious coryza	Reece *et al*. (1981)
Ulcerative enteritis (quail disease)	Mills *et al*. (1999)
Mycoplasmosis	
(*Mycoplasma gallisepticum*)	Yoder (1991)
(*Mycoplasma synoviae*)	Bencina *et al*. (1987)
Staphylococcosis	Skeeles (1991)
Parasites	
Nematode	Ruff (1991)
coccidiosis	Mohammad (2012); Gesek *et al*. (2014)
Protozoa	
Cryptosporidiosis	Hoerr *et al*. (1986)
Fungal diseases	
Thrush (mycosis of the digestive tract)	Chute (1991)
Aspergillosis	Chaudhary and Sadana (1988)

susceptible flocks, resulting in rapid morbidity and mortality; severe illness is most often observed in chicks less than 6 weeks of age (Reed & Jack 2013). Clinical signs include decreased appetite, ruffled feathers, open-mouth breathing, rales, sneezing, nasal and ocular discharge, and death. Older birds may remain asymptomatic.

Newcastle disease is caused by a single-strand, nonsegmented, negative-sense RNA virus renamed *avian avulavirus* (AAvV) 1. Clinical signs range from subclinical infection to lethargy, ruffled feathers, dyspnoea, torticollis, paralysis and haemorrhagic diarrhoea (Usman *et al*. 2008; Susta *et al*. 2018). Transmission is horizontal via the faecal–oral route or by inhalation of contaminated dust.

Eastern Equine Encephalomyelitis, which quail is susceptible to, is caused by an arbovirus (Alphavirus, family Togaviridae). The virus is typically introduced by mosquitoes and then spreads within a flock via feather picking and cannibalism. Infected birds exhibit depression, tremor, paralysis, torticollis and death. A primary gross finding in a commercial quail flock was duodenal catarrhal enteritis (Eleazer et al. 1978).

Marek's disease, a lymphoproliferative disease caused by a cell-associated herpes virus, is relatively common in commercial flocks of quail (Nagarajan et al. 2013). Transmission occurs through direct contact, and mortality in unvaccinated flocks may range from 10 to 20%. Clinical signs of disease included lethargy, anorexia, weight loss, soft faeces and lime-green urates.

Bacterial diseases

Ulcerative enteritis or 'quail disease' is a fatal enteric disease caused by *Clostridium colinum*, primarily in captive quail but also in several other avian species; genetic susceptibility in quail may vary (Collins et al. 1975). Clinical signs can be acute death with no premonitory signs, diarrhoea, and emaciation. In young quail, 100% mortality can be seen.

Salmonellosis is a major bacterial disease. Quail can be infected with *Salmonella enterica* that cause pullorum disease (*Salmonella pullorum*) and fowl typhoid (*Salmonella gallinarum*). Transmission is both horizontal via the faecal–oral route and vertical via transovarian infection. Japanese quail can harbour multidrug-resistant Salmonella that can be transmitted to humans through consumption of contaminated food or by direct and indirect contact with the carrier birds (Omoshaba et al. 2017). Chicks may present with weakness, decreased appetite, respiratory signs, pale white material on the vent, joint swelling, anaemia and death. Adult birds are subclinical or can exhibit generalised signs of disease, e.g., decreased appetite, diarrhoea, depression, ruffled feathers and decreased egg production.

Campylobacteriosis leads to acute gastroenteritis in quail. It is caused by the gram-negative, microaerophilic bacteria *Campylobacter jejuni* and *C. coli*. Horizontal and vertical transmission are possible. Clinical signs may not be apparent, or diarrhoea can be present.

Naturally occurring infection with *Mycoplasma gallisepticum* and *M. synoviae* has been reported in quail (Murakami et al. 2002; do Nascimento & do Nascimento 1986). Transmission may be horizontal or vertical. Clinical signs of *M. gallisepticum* infection include swelling of the head, nasal discharge, increased lacrimation and decreased egg production. Sinusitis and arthritis have been attributed to *M. synoviae* infection in quail.

Abnormal behaviour

Feather pecking, cannibalism and head-banging (caused by the birds jumping and striking their heads on the cage roof) are the most frequently cited behavioural causes of injury in quail (see Gerken & Mills 1993). Ways to minimise these behaviour patterns have been mentioned in previous sections of this chapter. Females kept in battery cages show pre-laying restlessness similar to that observed in some strains of domestic chickens (Gerken & Mills 1993) and birds of both sexes show vacuum dustbathing behaviour (Gerken 1983). In deep litter floor pens, at higher than recommended stocking densities, and when eggs are not collected daily, egg eating has been observed in some flocks of birds. Stereotyped behaviour can be induced experimentally (Kostal et al. 1992) but its incidence under other conditions is unknown.

Acknowledgements

This chapter is an update of the chapter written by Kimberly Cheng for the previous edition of this book. The authors thank David Huss (University of Southern California) for reviewing an earlier draft of this manuscript. They also thank Cathleen Nichols and Darin Bennett (UBC Quail Genetic Resource Centre) for valuable inputs.

References

Adkins-Regan, E. (1995) Predictors of fertilization in the Japanese quail, *Coturnix japonica*. *Animal Behaviour*, **50**, 1405–1415.

Aggrey, S.E. (2003) Dynamics of relative growth rate in Japanese quail lines divergently selected for growth and their control. *Growth Development and Aging*, **67**, 47–54.

Agina, O.A., Ezema, W.S. and Iwuoha, E.M. (2017) The haematology and serum biochemistry profile of adult Japanese Quail (*Coturnix coturnix japonica*). *Notulae Scientia Biologicae*, **9**, 67–72. DOI: 10.15835/nsb919928.

Alagawany, M., El-Hack, M.E.A., Laudadio, V. et al. (2014) Effect of low-protein diets with crystalline amino acid supplementation on egg production, blood parameters and nitrogen balance in laying Japanese quails. *Avian Biology Research*, **7**, 235–243. doi: https://doi.org/10.3184/175815514X14152945166603 (accessed 31 July 2019).

American Ornithologists' Union (1983) *Check-list of North American Birds*. Allen Press Incorporated, Lawrence, Kansas.

American Veterinary Medical Association (AVMA) (2013) *Guidelines for the Euthanasia of Animals: 2013 Edition*. http://www.avma.org (accessed 10 June 2019).

American Veterinary Medical Association (AVMA) (2019) *Guidelines for the Euthanasia of Animals*. https://www.avma.org/KB/Policies/Pages/Euthanasia-Guidelines.aspx (accessed 15 August 2019).

Arora, K.L. (1979) Blood sampling and intravenous injections in Japanese quail (*Coturnix japonica*). *Laboratory Animal Science*, **29**, 114–118.

Bachmann, K., Harrington, B.A. and Craig, J.P. (1972) Genome size in birds. *Chromosoma*, **37**, 405–416.

Baer, J., Lansford, R. and Cheng, K. (2015). Japanese quail as a laboratory animal model. Chapter 22 In: *Lab Animal Medicine*, 3rd edn. Eds Fox, J.G., Anderson, L.C., Otto, G.M. et al. pp. 1087–1108. San Diego, CA, Academic Press.

Ball, G.F. and Balthazart, J. (2004) Hormonal regulation of brain circuits mediating male sexual behavior in birds. *Physiology and Behavior*, **83**, 329–346.

Balthazart, J., Baillien, M., Charlier, T.D. et al. (2003) The neuroendocrinology of reproductive behavior in Japanese quail. *Domestic Animal Endocrinology*, **25**, 69–82.

Balthazart, J. and Ball, G.F. (1998) New insights into the regulation and function of brain estrogen synthase (aromatase). *Trends in Neurosciences*, **21**, 243–249.

Barilani, M., Derégnaucourt, S., Gallego, S. et al. (2005) Detecting hybridization in wild (*Coturnix c. coturnix*) and domesticated (*Coturnix c. japonica*) quail populations. *Biological Conservation*, **126**, 445–455.

Barnes, H.J. (1987) Veterinary clinics of North America: Small animal practice. *Veterinary Clinics of North America* **17**, 1109–1144. https://doi.org/10.1016/S0195-5616(87)50107-3 (accessed 1 August 2019).

Baumgartner, J. (1993) Japanese quail: genetics, breeding, and production. In: *Proceedings of the 10th International Symposium on Current Problems in Avian Genetics*. Nitra, Slovakia. pp. 11.

Bencina, D.T., Tadina, T. and Dorrer, D. (1987) Mycoplasma species isolated from six avian species. *Avian Pathology*, **16**, 653–664.

Benoff, F.H. and Rice, D.H. (1980) Social dominance and productivity in caged female Japanese quail. *Poultry Science*, **59**, 424–427.

Bessei, W. (1977) Quail breeding in France. *Deutsche Geflugelwirtschaft und Schweineproduktion*, **29**, 4–5.

Bower, D.V., Sato, Y. and Lansford, R. (2011) Dynamic lineage analysis of embryonic morphogenesis using transgenic quail and 4D multispectral imaging. *Genesis* **49**, 619–643. https://doi.org/10.1002/dvg.20754 (accessed 1 August 2019).

Buchwalder, T. and Wechsler, B. (1997) The effect of cover on the behaviour of Japanese quail. *Applied Animal Behaviour Science*, **54**, 335–343.

Butkauskas, D. (2001) *Genetic diversity and reproductive traits of Japanese quail*. PhD dissertation, Institute of Ecology, Lithuania.

Buxton, J.R. and Orcutt, F.S. (1975) Enzymes and electrolytes in the semen of Japanese quail. *Poultry Science*, **54**, 1556–1566.

Campos, de I.C., Hickey, J., Pong-Wong, R. et al. (2013) Whole-genome regression and prediction methods applied to plant and animal breeding. *Genetics*, **193**, 327–345.

Carpenter, N.A. (2000) Anseriform and galliform therapeutics. *Veterinary Clinics of North America*: *Exotic Animal Practice*, **3**, 1–17.

Chang, G.B., Chang, H., Liu, X.P. et al. (2005) Developmental research on the origin and phylogeny of quails. *World's Poultry Science Journal*, **61**, 105–111.

Chaudhary, S.K. and Sadana, J.R. (1988) Experimental aspergillosis in Japanese quails (*Coturnix japonica*). *Mycopathologia* **102**, 179–184.

Cheng, K.M., Hickman, A.R. and Nichols, C.R. (1989b) Role of the proctodeal gland foam of male Japanese quail in natural copulations. *Auk*, **106**, 279–286.

Cheng, K.M. and Kimura, M. (1990) Mutations and major variants in Japanese quail. In: *Developments in Animal and Veterinary Sciences, Vol. 22. Poultry Breeding and Genetics*. Ed. Crawford, R.D., pp. 333–362. Elsevier, Amsterdam.

Cheng, K.M., McIntyre, R.F. and Hickman, A.R. (1989a) Proctodeal gland foam enhances competitive fertilization in domestic Japanese quail. *Auk*, **106**, 287–291.

Cheng, K.M. and Nichols, C.R. (1992) Japanese quail (*Coturnix japonica*): conservation and management of genetic resources in Canada. *Gibier Faune Sauvage*, **9**, 667–676.

Cheng, K.M., Pang, C.S., Wang, Z.P. et al. (1994) A comparison of [125I] iodomelatonin binding sites in testes and brains of heavy meat-type Japanese quail with a random bred strain. *Journal of Heredity*, **85**, 136–139.

Cheng, K.M., Bennett, D.C. and Mills, A.D. (2010) The Japanese Quail. Chapter 42 In: *UFAW Handbook on the Care and Management of Laboratory Animals, 8th Edition*. Eds Hubrecht, R. and Kirkwood, J. pp. 655–673. Blackwell Scientific Publ. London.

Chesser, R.T., Burns, K.J., Cicero, C. et al. (2018). Check-list of North American Birds (online). American Ornithological Society. http://checklist.aou.org/taxa (accessed 7 August 2019).

Chute, H.L. (1991) Thrush (Mycosis of the digestive tract). In: *Diseases of Poultry*. Eds Calnek, B.W., Barnes, H.J., Beard, C.W. et al., pp. 335–337. Wolfe Publications Ltd, London.

Collins, W.M., Hardiman, J.W., Urban, Jr, W.E. et al. (1975) Genetic differences in susceptibility to Ulcerative Enteritis in Japanese quail. *Poultry Science*, **54**, 2051–2054. doi: https://doi.org/10.3382/ps.0542051 (accessed 1 August 2019).

Cooper, D.M. (1987) The Japanese quail. In: *UFAW Handbook on the Care and Management of Laboratory Animals*, 6th edn. Ed. Poole, T.B., pp. 678–686. UFAW, Potters Bar.

Cooper, C. S., Southard, T., Schultz, D. et al. (2007) A case of Marek's disease in Japanese quail (Coturnix japonica)."In Journal of the American Association for Laboratory Animal Science, 46(4), 106–106.

Crawford, R.D. (1990) Origins and history of poultry species. In: *Developments in Animal and Veterinary Sciences, Vol. 22. Poultry Breeding and Genetics*. Ed. Crawford, R.D., pp. 1–41. Elsevier, Amsterdam.

Del Hoyo, J., Elliott, A. and Sargatal, J.(Eds) (1994). *Handbook of the Birds of the World*, Vol. 2. Lynx Edicions, Barcelona, Spain.

Delville, Y., Sulon, J., Hendrick, J.C. et al. (1984) Effect of the presence of females on the pituitary-testicular activity in male Japanese quail (*Coturnix coturnix japonica*). *General Comparative Endocrinology*, **55**, 295–305.

Derégnaucourt, S., Guyomarc'h, J.C. and Aebischer, N.J. (2002) Hybridization between European *Coturnix c. coturnix* and Japanese *Coturnix c. japonica* quail. *Ardea*, **90**, 15–21.

Dement'ev, G.P., Gladkov, N.A., Isakov, Y.A. et al. (1967) In: *Birds of the Soviet Union*. Israel Program for Scientific Translation, Jerusalem.

do Nascimento, M.d.G.F.[1] do Nascimento, E.R. (1986) Infectious sinusitis in *Coturnix* quails in Brazil. *Avian Diseases* **30**, 228–230. doi: 10.2307/1590641

Domjan, M. and Nash, S. (1988) Stimulus control of social behaviour in male Japanese quail, *Coturnix coturnix japonica*. *Animal Behaviour*, **36**, 1006–1015.

Edens, F.W. (1987) Agonistic behaviour and neurochemistry in grouped Japanese quail. *Comparative Biochemistry and Physiology Series A*, **86**, 473–480.

Edens, F.W., Bursian, S.J. and Holladay, S.D. (1983) Grouping in Japanese quail. 1. Agonistic behaviour during feeding. *Poultry Science*, **62**, 1647–1651.

Elangovan, A.V., Verma, S.V.S., Sastry, V.R.B. et al. (2003) Laying performance of Japanese quail fed on different seed meals in diet. *Indian Journal of Animal Nutrition*, **19**, 244–250.

Eleazer, T.H., Blalock, H.G., Warner, J.H., Jr. et al. (1978) Eastern Equine Encephalomyelitis outbreak in *Coturnix* quail. *Avian Diseases*, **22**, 522–525. doi: 10.2307/1589308.

Ernst, R.A. and Coleman, T.H. (1966) The influence of floor space on growth, egg production, fertility and hatchability of *Coturnix coturnix japonica*. *Poultry Science*, **45**, 437–440.

Eroschenko, V.P., Wilson, W.O. and Siopes, T.D. (1977) Function and histology of testes from aged coturnix maintained on different photoperiods. *Journal of Gerontology*, **32**, 279–285.

European Commission (2007) Commission recommendations of 18 June 2007 on guidelines for the accommodation and care of animals used for experimental and other scientific purposes. Annex II to European Council Directive 86/609. See 2007/526/EC. http://eurlex.europa.eu/LexUriServ/site/en/oj/2007/l_197/l_19720070730en00010089.pdf (accessed 13 May 2008).

Eynon, A.E. (1968) *The Agonistic and Sexual Behaviour of Captive Japanese Quail (Coturnix coturnix japonica)*. PhD Thesis, University of Wisconsin.

Farrell, D.J., Atmamihardja, S.I. and Pym, R.A.E. (1982) Calorimetric measurements of the energy and nitrogen metabolism of Japanese quail. *British Poultry Science*, **23**, 375–382.

Farris, H.E. (1964) *Behavioral Development, Social Organization and Conditioning of Courting Behavior in Japanese quail Coturnix coturnix japonica*. PhD dissertation, Michigan State University

Farris, H.E. (1967) Classical conditioning of courting behaviour in the Japanese quail, *Coturnix coturnix japonica*. *Journal of the Experimental Analysis of Behaviour*, **10**, 213–217.

Farrow, W.M., Scmitt, M.W. and Groupe, J. (1975) Responses of isolator – derived Japanese quail and quail cell cultures in selected animal viruses. *Journal of Clinical Microbiology*, **2**, 419–424.

Fu, Z., Inaba, M., Noguchi, T. and Kata, H. (2002) Molecular cloning and circadian regulation of cryptochrome genes in Japanese quail (*Coturnix coturnix japonica*). *Journal of Biological Rhythms*, **17**, 14–27.

Fulton, J.E. (2012) Genomic selection for poultry breeding. *Animal Frontiers*, **2**, 30–36. https://doi.org/10.2527/af.2011-0028 (accessed 1 August 2019)

Galli, L. (2003) *Caratterizzazione genetica di Quaglia Coturnix e rischi d'inquinamento genetico a seguito delle immissioni di soggetti d'allevamento*. PhD Thesis. Genoa: Universita` di Genova.

Gerken, M. (1983). *Untersuchungen zur genetischen Fundierung und Beeinflubarkeit von Verhaltensmerkmalen des Geflügels, durchgeführt in einem Selektionexperiment auf Staubbadedeverhalten bei der japenishcen Wachtel (Coturnix coturnix japonica)* Thesis. Rheinsche Freidrich Wilhelms Universität, Bonn.

Gerken, M. and Mills, A.D. (1993) Welfare of domestic quail. In: *Proceedings of the Fourth European Symposium on Poultry Welfare*. Eds Savory, C.J. and Hughes, B.O., pp. 158–176. UFAW, Potters Bar.

Gerken, M. and Petersen, J. (1987) Bidirectional selection for dust-bathing activity in Japanese quail (*Coturnix coturnix japonica*). *British Poultry Science*, **28**, 23–37.

Gesek, M., Welenc, J., Tylicka, Z. et al. (2014) Pathomorphological changes in the alimentary system of Japanese quails naturally infected with *Eimeria tsunodai*. *Bulletin of Veterinary Institute in Pulawy* **58**, 41–45. doi: 10.2478/bvip-2014-0007

Griffiths, R., Daan, S. and Dijkstra, C. (1996) Sex identification in birds using two CHD genes. *Proceedings in Biological Science*, **263**, 1251–1256.

Groothuis, T.G.G., Müller, W, von Engelhardt, N. et al. (2005) Maternal hormones as a tool to adjust offspring phenotype in avian species. *Neuroscience and Biobehavior* **29**, 329–352.

Guesdon, V., Bertin, A., Houdelier, C. et al. (2011) A place to hide in the home-cage decreases yolk androgen levels and offspring emotional reactivity in Japanese quail. *PLoS One*, **6(9)**, e23941. https://doi.org/10.1371/journal.pone.0023941 (accessed 1 August 2019).

Gülbahar, M.Y., Çabalar, M. and Boynukara, B. (2005) Avipoxvirus infection in quails. *Turkey Journal of Veterinary Animal Science*, **19**, 449–454.

Güler, T., Ertaş, O.N., Çiftçi, M. et al. (2005) The effect of coriander seed (*Coriandrum sativum* L.) as diet ingredient on the performance of Japanese quail. *South African Journal of Animal Science*, **35**, 260–266.

Gunnarsson, U., Hellström, A.R. Tixier-Boichard, M. et al. (2007) Mutations in SLC45A2 cause plumage color variation in chicken and Japanese quail. *Genetics*, **175**, 867–877. doi: 10.1534/genetics.106.063107.

Guyomarc'h, J.C. (2003). Elements for a common quail (*Coturnix c. coturnix*) management plan. *Game and Wildlife Science*, **20**, 1–92.

Guyomarc'h, C. and Guyomarc'h, J.C. (1984) The influence of social factors on the onset of egg production in Japanese quail (*Coturnix coturnix japonica*). *Biology of Behaviour*, **9**, 333–342.

Guyomarc'h, J.C. (1974) *Les vocalisations des Gallinacés – Structure des Sons et des Répertoires. Ontogenèse Motrice et Acquisition de Leur Sémantique (Volumes 1 and 2)*. Thèse de Docteur d'État (Série C, N° d'ordre 198, N° de série 56), Université de Rennes.

Halldin, K., Berg, C., Brandt, I. et al. (1999) Sexual behavior in Japanese quail as a test end pint for endocrine disruption: Effects of in ovo exposure to ethinylestradiol and diethylstilbestrol. *Environmental and Health Perspectives*, **107**, 861–866.

Hazard, D., Couty, M., Faure, J.M. et al. (2005) Relationship between hypothalamic-pituitary-adrenal axis responsiveness and age, sexual maturity status, and sex in Japanese quail selected for long or short duration of tonic immobility. *Poultry Science*, **84**, 1913–1919.

Hill, R.W. and Raymond, R.G. (1962) Apparent natural infection of *Coturnix* hens with the virus of avian encephalomyelitis. Case report. *Avian Diseases*, **6**, 226–227.

Hoerr, F.J., Current, W.L., Haynes, T.B. (1986) Fatal cryptosporidiosis in quail. *Avian Diseases*, **30**, 421–425. doi: 10.2307/1590550.

Hoffmann, E. (1990) *Coturnix Quail*. Cannings, Nova Scotia.

Homma, K., Siopes, T.D., Wilson, W.O. et al. (1966) Identification of sex of day old quail (*Coturnix coturnix japonica*) by cloacal examination. *Poultry Science*, **45**, 469–472.

Hori, T., Asakawa, S., Itoh, Y., et al. (2000) Wpkci, encoding an altered form of PKCI, is conserved widely on the avian W chromosome and expressed in early female embryos: implication of its role in female sex determination. *Molecular Biology Cell*, **11**, 3645–3660. doi:10.1091/mbc.11.10.3645

Houdelier, C., Guyomarc'h, C., Lumineau, S. et al. (2002) Circadian rhythms of oviposition and feeding activity in Japanese quail: effects of cyclic administration of melatonin. *Chronobiology International*, **19**, 1107–1119.

Howard, R. and Moore, A. (1984) *A Complete Checklist of the Birds of the World*, revised edition. Macmillan, London.

Howes, J.R. (1964) Japanese quail as found in Japan. *Quail Quarterly*, **1**, 19–30.

Huss, D., Poynter, G. and Lansford, R. (2008) Japanese quail (*Coturnix japonica*) as a laboratory animal model. *Laboratory Animals (NY)*, **37**, 513–519.

Huss, D., Benazeraf, B., Wallingford, A. et al. (2015) A transgenic quail model that enables dynamic imaging of amniote embryogenesis. *Development*, **142**, 2850–2859.

Hyánkova, L., Dŭdkova, L., Knížetova, H. et al. (1997) Responses in growth, food intake and food conversion efficiency to different dietary protein concentrations in meat-type lines of Japanese quail. *British Poultry Science*, **38**, 564–570.

Ichilcik, R. and Austin, J. (1978) The Japanese quail (*Coturnix coturnix japonica*) as a laboratory animal. *Journal of the South African Veterinary Association*, **49**, 203–207.

Jensen, T., Pernasetti, F.M. and Durrant, B. (2003) Conditions for rapid sex determination in 47 avian species by PCR of genomic DNA from blood, shell-membrane blood vessels, and feathers. *Zoo Biology*, **22**, 561–571.

Joint Working Group on Refinement (1993) Removal of blood from laboratory mammals and birds. First Report of the BVA/FRAME/RSPCA/UFAW Joint Working Group on Refinement. *Laboratory Animals*, **27**, 1–22.

Joint Working Group on Refinement (2001a) Refining procedures for the administration of substances. Report of the BVAAWF/FRAME/RSPCA/UFAW Joint Working Group on Refinement. *Laboratory Animals*, **35**, 1–41.

Joint Working Group on Refinement (2001b) Laboratory birds: refinements in husbandry and procedures. Fifth report of the BVAAWF/FRAME/RSPCA/UFAW Joint Working Group on Refinement. *Laboratory Animals*, **35**, 1–163.

Jones, R.C. and Lin, M. (1993) Spermatogenesis in birds. *Oxford Review of Reproductive Biology*, **15**, 233–264. PMID: 8336978.

Jones, R.B., Mills, A.D. and Faure, J.M. (1991) Genetic and experiential manipulation of fear related behaviour in Japanese quail chicks (*Coturnix coturnix japonica*). *Journal of Comparative Psychology*, **105**, 15–24.

Jones, J.W., Maloney, M.A. and Gilbreath, J.C. (1964) Size, shape and color pattern as criteria for identifying *Coturnix* eggs. *Poultry Science*, **43**, 1292–1294.

Jung, J.G., Lee, Y.M., Kim, J.N. et al. (2010) The reversible developmental unipotency of germ cells in chicken. *Reproduction*, **139**, 113–119.

Kamata, R., Takahashi, S., Shimizu, A. et al. (2006) Avian transgenerational reproductive toxicity test with in ovo exposure. *Archives of Toxicology*, **80**, 846–856.

Kawahara, T. (1967) Wild *Coturnix* quail in Japan. *Quail Quarterly*, **4**, 62–63.

Kawahara, T. (1973) Comparative study of quantitative traits between wild and domestic Japanese quail (*Coturnix coturnix japonica*). *Experimental Animals*, **22**, 139–150.

Kawahara-Miki, R., Sano, S., Nunome, M. et al. (2013) Next-generation sequencing reveals genomic features in the Japanese quail. *Genomics* **101**, 345–353.

Kaya, S., Erdogan, Z. and Erdogan, S. (2003) Effect of different dietary levels of Yucca schidigera powder on the performance, blood parameters and egg yolk cholesterol of laying quails. *Journal of Veterinary Medicine Series A*, **50**, 14–17.

Kayang, B.B., Fillon, V., Inoue-Murayama, M. et al. (2006) Integrated maps in quail (*Coturnix japonica*) confirm the high degree of synteny conservation with chicken (*Gallus gallus*) despite 35 million years of divergence. *BMC Genomics*, **7**, 101–118.

Kenzy, S.G. and Cho, B.R. (1969) Transmission of classical Marek's disease by affected and carrier birds. *Avian Diseases*, **13**, 211–214.

Kikuchi, S., Fujima, D., Sasazaki, S. et al. (2005) Construction of a genetic linkage map of Japanese quail (*Coturnix japonica*) based on AFLP and microsatellite markers. *Animal Genetics* 36, 227–231. https://doi.org/10.1111/j.1365-2052.2005.01295.x (accessed 1 August 2019).

Kim, S.H., Cheng, K.M., Ritland, C. et al. (2007) Inbreeding in Japanese quail estimated by pedigree and microsatellite analyses. *Journal of Heredity*, **98**, 378–381.

Kostal, L., Vyboh, P., Bilcik, B. et al. (1992) Stereotyped pacing in Japanese quail: the role of endogenous opioids. *Journal of Animal Science*, **70**, 24.

Kovach, J.K. (1975) The behaviour of quail. In: *The Behaviour of Domestic Animals*, 3rd edn. Ed. Hafez, E.S.E., pp. 437–453. Bailliere Tindall, London.

Kraszewska-Domanska, B. and Pawluczuk, B. (1977) The effect of periodic warming of stored quail eggs on their hatchability. *British Poultry Science*, **18**, 531–533.

Landsdown, A.B.G., Crees, S.J. and Wilder, R.G. (1970) The Japanese quail: its suitability for embryonic and reproductive investigations. *Journal of the Institute of Animal Technology*, **21**, 71–77.

Laboratory Animal Science Association (2005) Guidance on the transport of laboratory animals. Report of the Transport Working Group established by LASA. *Laboratory Animals*, **39**, 1–39.

Lepore, P.D. and Marks, H.L. (1966) Intravaginal insemination of Japanese quail: Factors influencing the basic technique. *Poultry Science* **45**, 888–891 https://doi.org/10.3382/ps.0450888 (accessed 1 August 2019).

Lima, F.S., Santin, E., Paulillo, A.C. et al. (2004) Evaluation of different programs of Newcastle disease vaccination in Japanese quail (*Coturnix coturnix japonica*). *International Journal of Poultry Science*, **3**, 354–356.

Liu, J., Cheng, K.M. and Silversides, F.G. (2013) Production of live offspring from testicular tissue cryopreserved by vitrification procedures in Japanese quail (*Coturnix japonica*). *Biology of Reproduction* **88**, 1–6.

Liu, J., Cheng, K.M., and Silversides, F.G. (2015) Recovery of fertility from adult ovarian tissue transplanted into week-old Japanese quail chicks. *Reproduction, Fertility and Development* **27**, 281–284.

Löliger, H.C. and Schubert, H.J. (1966) Spontanerkrankungen bei japanischen Wachteln (*Coturnix coturnix japonica*). *Celler Jahrbuch*, **15**, 42–43.

Long, J.L. (1981) *Introduced Birds of the World*. Universe Books, New York.

Lucotte, G. (1974) *Elevage de la caille*. Vigot Frères, Paris.

Mahmoud, H., El-Safty, M. and Hanan, A.A. (2016) Efficacy of commercial inactivated *Salmonella* vaccines in quail. *Benha Veterinary Medical Journal* **31**, 92–95 http://www.bvmj.bu.edu.eg (accessed 28 July 2019).

Marks, H.L. (1978) Long term selection for four-week body weight in Japanese quail under different nutritional environments. *Theoretical and Applied Genetics*, **52**, 105–111.

Marks, H.L. and Lepore, P.D. (1965) A procedure for artificial insemination of Japanese quail. *Poultry Science*, **44**, 1001–1003.

Marumya, S. and Katasube, Y. (1988) Intestinal colonization of Campylobacter jejeuni in young Japanese quails (*Coturnix coturnix japonica*). *Japanese Journal of Veterinary Science*, **50**, 569–572.

Mather, F.B. and Wilson, W.O. (1964) Post-natal testicular development in Japanese quail. *Poultry Science*, **43**, 860–864.

McDougald, L.R. (1991) Other diseases of the intestinal tract. In: *Diseases of Poultry*. Eds Calnek, B.W., Barnes, H.J., Beard, C.W. et al., pp. 804–813. Wolfe Publications Ltd, London.

McKinney, F., Derrickson, S.R. and Mineau, P. (1983) Forced copulation in waterfowl. *Behaviour*, **86**, 250–294.

McNabb, F.M.A. and McNabb, R.A. (1977) Skin and plumage changes during the development of thermoregulatory ability of Japanese quail chicks. *Comparative Biochemistry and Physiology*, **58A**, 163–166.

Mills, A.D. and Faure, J.M. (1990) Diviergierende selektion für soziale motivation und tonische immobilitätswort bei der Japenischen Wachtel (*Coturnix coturnix japonica*). In: Proceedings of the 7th Leipziger Tierzuchtsymposien. Ed. Wussow, J., pp. 87–101. Karl Marx Universisität, Leipzig.

Mills, A.D., Domjan, M., Crawford, L.L. et al. (1997) The behaviour of the Japanese or domestic quail *Coturnix japonica*. *Neuroscience and Biobehavioural Reviews*, **21**, 261–281.

Mills, A.D., Faure, J.M. and Rault, P. (1999) The Japanese quail. In: *UFAW Handbook on the Care and Management of Laboratory Animals*, 7th edn. Ed. Poole, T.B., pp. 697–713. Blackwell Publishing, Oxford.

Minematsu, T., Harumi, T. and Naito, M. (2008) Germ cell-specific expression of GFP gene induced by chicken vasa homologue (Cvh) promoter in early chicken embryos. *Molecular Reproduction and Development*, **75**, 1515–1522.

Minvielle, F. (1998) Genetics and breeding of Japanese quail for production around the world. In: *Proceedings of the 6th World's Poultry Science Association Asian Pacific Poultry Congress*, Nagoya, Japan. pp. 122–127.

Minvielle, F. (2004) The future of Japanese quail for research and production. *World's Poultry Science Journal*, **60**, 500–507.

Minvielle, F., Grossmann, R. and Gourichon, D. (2007) Development and performances of a Japanese quail line homozygous for the diabetes insipidus (di) mutation. *Poultry Science*, **86**, 249–254.

Minvielle, F., Monvoisin, J.-L., Costa, J. et al. (1999) Changes in heterosis under within-line selection or reciprocal recurrent selection: An experiment on early egg production in Japanese quail. *Journal of Animal Breeding and Genetics*, **116**, 363–377.

Minvielle, F., Monvoisin, J.-L., Costa, J. et al. (2000) Long-term egg production and heterosis in quail lines after within-line or reciprocal recurrent selection for high early egg production. *British Poultry Science*, **42**, 150–157.

Mizutani, M. (2002) Establishment of inbred strains of chicken and Japanese quail and their potential as animal models. *Experimental Animals*, **51**, 417–429.

Mohapatra, N., Kataria, J. M., Chakraborty, S. et al. (2014) Egg Drop Syndrome-76 (EDS-76) in Japanese quails (*Coturnix coturnix japonica*): an experimental study revealing pathology, effect on egg production/quality and immune responses. *Pakistan Journal of Biological Science*, **17**, 821–828.

Mohammad, N. (2012). A study on the pathological and diagnosis of *Eimeria* species infection in Japanese quail. *Basrah Journal of Veterinary Research*, **11**, 318–333.

Moore, C.B. and Siopes, T.D. (2000) Effects of lighting conditions and melatonin supplementation on the cellular and humoral immune responses in Japanese quail *Coturnix coturnix japonica*. *General and Comparative Endocrinology*, **119**, 95–104.

Moore, C.B. and Siopes, T.D. (2003) Melatonin enhances cellular and humoral immune responses in the Japanese quail (*Coturnix coturnix japonica*) via an opiatergic mechanism. *General and Comparative Endocrinology*, **131**, 258–263.

Moreau, C., Caldarelli, P., Rocancourt, D. et al. (2018) Timed Collinear Activation of Hox Genes during Gastrulation Controls the Avian Forelimb Position. *Current Biology* **29**, 35–50.e4 https://doi.org/10.1016/j.cub.2018.11.009 (accessed 1 August 2019).

Morinha, F., Carvalho, M., Ferro, A. *et al.* (2011) Molecular sexing and analysis of CHD1-Z and CHD1-W sequence variations in wild common quail (*Coturnix c. coturnix*) and domesticated Japanese quail (*Coturnix c. japonica*). *Journal of Genetics*, **90**, e39–43. https://www.ias.ac.in/article/fulltext/jgen/090/online/e0039-e0043 (accessed 1 August 2019).

Munro, G.C. (1960) *Birds of Hawaii*. Charles E. Tuttle, Rutland, Vermont.

Murakami, A.E. and Ariki, J. (1998) *Produção de Codorna Japonesas*. Jaboticabal, Funep, Brazil.

Murakami, S., Miyama, M., Ogawa, A. *et al.* (2002) Occurrence of conjunctivitis, sinusitis and upper region tracheitis in Japanese quail (*Coturnix coturnix japonica*), possibly caused by Mycoplasma gallisepticum accompanied by Cryptosporidium sp. infection. *Avian Pathology*, **31**, 363–370.

Nagai, H., Sezaki, M., Bertocchini, F., *et al.* (2014) HINTW, a W-Chromosome HINT gene in chick, is expressed ubiquitously and is a robust female cell marker applicable in intraspecific chimera studies. *Genesis*, **52**, 424–430.

Nagarajan, S., Narahari, D., Jayaprasad, I.A. *et al.* (1991) Influence of stocking density and layer age on production traits and egg quality in Japanese quail. *British Poultry Science*, **32**, 243–248.

Nagarajan, K., Thyagarajan, D., Balachandran, C. *et al.* (2013) Incidence of Marek's disease in *Coturnix coturnix japonica* in an organized farm. *Journal Food, Agriculture and Veterinary Sciences*, **3**, 254–257.

Naito, M., Tajima, A., Tagami, T. *et al.* (1994) Preservation of chick primordial germ cells in liquid nitrogen and subsequent production of viable offspring. *Reproduction*, **102**, 321–325. doi: https://doi.org/10.1530/jrf.0.1020321 (accessed 1 August 2019).

Nakamura, Y., Tasai, M., Takeda, K. *et al.* (2013) Production of functional gametes from cryopreserved primordial germ cells of the Japanese quail. *Journal of Reproduction and Development*, **59**, 580–587.

Nakahara, K., Kawan, O.T., Shiota, K. *et al.* (2003) Effects of microinjection of melatonin into various brain regions of Japanese quail on locomotor activity and body temperature. *Neuroscience Letters*, **345**, 117–120.

Nandi, S., Whyte, J., Taylor, L. *et al.* (2016) Cryopreservation of specialized chicken lines using cultured primordial germ cells. *Poultry Science*, **95**, 1905–1911. https://doi.org/10.3382/ps/pew133 (accessed 1 August 2019).

National Advisory Committee for Laboratory Animal Research (2004) *Guidelines on the Care and Use of Animals for Scientific Purposes*. NACLAR, Singapore.

National Research Council (NRC) (1994) *Nutrient Requirements of Poultry*. National Academy Press, Washington, DC.

National Research Council (NRC) (1996) *Guide for the Care and Use of Laboratory Animals*. National Academy Press, Washington, DC.

Nichols, C.R. (1991) *A Comparison of the reproductive and behavioural differences in feral and domestic Japanese quail*. Unpublished MSc Thesis, University of British Columbia.

Nichols, C.R., Robinson, C.A.F. and Cheng, K.M. (1992) Influence of domestication on fecundity and reproductive behaviour in Japanese quail, *Coturnix japonica*. *Gibier Faune Sauvage*, **9**, 743–756.

Nirmalan, G.P. and Robinson, G.A. (1971) Hematology of Japanese quail (*Coturnix coturnix japonica*). *British Poultry Science*, **12**, 475–481.

Nishibori, M., Hayashi, T., Tsudzuki, M. *et al.* (2001) Complete sequence of the Japanese quail (*Coturnix japonica*) mitochondrial genome and its genetic relationship with related species. *Animal Genetics*, **32**, 380–385 https://doi.org/10.1046/j.1365-2052.2001.00795.x (accessed 1 August 2019).

Noble, R. (1972) The effects of estrogen and progesterone on copulation in female quail (*Coturnix coturnix japonica*) housed in continuous dark. *Hormones and Behavior*, **3**, 199–204.

Nol, E., Cheng, K.M. and Nichols, C.R. (1996) Heritability and phenotypic correlations of behaviour and dominance rank of Japanese quail. *Animal Behaviour*, **52**, 813–820.

Odeh, F.M., Cadd, G.G. and Satterlee, D.G. (2003) Genetic characterization of stress responsiveness in Japanese quail. 1. Analyses of line effects and combining abilities by diallel crosses. *Poultry Science*, **82**, 25–30.

Ohta, M., Kadota, C. and Konishi, H. (1989) A role of melatonin in the initial stage of photoperiodism in the Japanese quail. *Biology of Reproduction*, **40**, 935–941.

Omoshaba, E.O., Olufemi, F.O., Ojo, O.E. *et al.* (2017) Multidrug-resistant Salmonellae isolated in Japanese quails reared in Abeokuta, Nigeria. *Tropical Animal Health and Production*, **49**, 1455–1460.

Orcutt, F.S. and Orcutt, A.B. (1976) Nesting and parental behavior in domestic common quail. *Auk*, **93**, 135–141.

Otis, R.E. (1972) *Social organisation in the Japanese quail (Coturnix coturnix japonica): Appetitive and consummatory components*. Unpublished PhD dissertation, Michigan State University.

Ottinger, M.A. (1978) *The relationship of testosterone, sex-related behaviour and morphology during the sexual maturation of the male Japanese quail*. Unpublished PhD dissertation, University of Maryland.

Ottinger, M.A. (1989) Sexual differentiation of neuroendocrine systems and behavior. *Poultry Science*, **68**, 979–989.

Ottinger, M.A. (1983) Sexual behavior and endocrine changes during reproductive maturation and ageing in the avian male. In: *Hormones and Behavior in Higher Vertebrates*. Eds Balthazart, J., Prove, E. and Giles, R., pp. 350–367. Springer-Verlag, Berlin.

Ottinger, M.A. (1991) Neuroendocrine and behavioral determinants of reproductive ageing. *Critical Reviews in Poultry Biology*, **3**, 131–142.

Ottinger, M., Abdelnabi, M., Henry, P. *et al.* (2001) Neuroendocrine and behavioral implications of endocrine disrupting chemicals in quail. *Hormones and Behavior*, **40**, 234–247.

Ottinger, M., Abdelnabi, M., Quin, M. *et al.* (2002) Reproductive consequences of EDCs in birds. What do laboratory effects mean in field species? *Neurotoxicology and Teratology*, **24**, 17–28.

Ottinger, M.A. and Brinkley, H.J. (1978) Testosterone and sex related behavior and morphology: relationship during maturation and in the adult Japanese quail. *Hormones and Behavior*, **11**, 175–182.

Ottinger, M.A. and Brinkley, H.J. (1979a) Testosterone and sex physical characteristics during the maturation of the male Japanese quail. *Biology of Reproduction*, **20**, 905–909.

Ottinger, M.A. and Brinkley, H.J. (1979b) The ontogeny of crowing and copulatory behaviour in Japanese quail (*Coturnix coturnix japonica*). *Behavioural Processes*, **4**, 43–51.

Ottinger, M.A., Duchala, C.S. and Mason, M. (1983) Age-related reproductive decline in the male Japanese quail. *Hormones and Behavior*, **17**, 197–207.

Ottinger, M.A. and Lavoie, E. (2007) Neuroendocrine and immune characteristics of aging in avian species. *Cytogenet Genome Research*, **117**, 352–357. doi: 10.1159/000103198.

Ottinger, M.A. and Rattner, B.A. (1999) Husbandry and care of quail. *Poultry and Avian Reviews*, **10**, 117–120.

Padgett, C.A. and Ivey, W.D. (1959) Coturnix quail as a laboratory research animal. *Science*, **129**, 267–268.

Panigrahy, B. and Hall, C.F. (1977) An outbreak of erysipelas in *Coturnix* quails. *Avian Diseases*, **21**, 708–710.

Paul-Murphy, J. and Fialkowshi, J. (2001) Injectable Anesthesia and Analgesia of Birds. In: *Recent Advances in Veterinary Anesthesia and Analgesia: Companion Animals*. Eds Gleed, R.D. and Ludders, J.W. Electronic publication, International Veterinary Information Service, Ithaca, New York (http://www.ivis.org).

Payne, L.N., Purchase, H.G. and Barnes, H.J. (1991) Lymphoid leukosis. In: *Diseases of Poultry*. Eds Calnek, B.W., Barnes, H.J., Beard, C.W. *et al.*, pp. 386–439. Wolfe Publications Ltd, London.

Persaud, K.N. and Galef, Jr, B.G. (2005) Female Japanese quail (*Coturnix japonica*) mated with males that harassed them are unlikely to lay fertilized eggs. *Journal of Comparative Psychology* **119**, 440–446.

Pereira, R.J., Napolitano, A., Garcia-Pereira, F.L. et al. (2013) Conservation of avian germplasm by xenogeneic transplantation of spermatogonia from sexually mature donors. *Stem Cells Development*, **22**, 735–749.

Peterson, R.T. (1961) *A Field Guide to Western Birds*. Houghton Mifflin Co, Boston.

Piao, J., Shimogiri, T., Maeda, Y. and Okamoto, S. (2003) Analysis of genetic traits by AFLP in the Japanese quail lines selected for large and small body weight. *Japanese Poultry Science*, **40**, J13–J20.

Pomeroy, B.S. and Nagaraja, K.V. (1991) Fowl typhoid. In: *Diseases of Poultry*. Eds Calnek, B.W., Barnes, H.J., Beard, C.W. et al., pp. 87–89. Wolfe Publications Ltd, London.

Poole, H.K. (1965) Spectrophotometric identification of egg shell pigments and time of superficial pigment deposition in the Japanese quail. *Proceedings of the Society for Experimental Biology and Medicine*, **119**, 547–551.

Potash, L.M. (1972) Noise-induced changes in calls of the Japanese quail. *Psychonomic Science*, **26**, 252–254.

Potash, L.M. (1975) An experimental analysis of the use of location calls by Japanese quail, *Coturnix coturnix japonica*. *Behaviour*, **54**, 153–179.

Poynter, G., Huss, D. and Lansford, R. (2009) Japanese quail: an efficient animal model for the production of transgenic avians. *Cold Spring Harbor Protoc*, 2009, pdb emo112. doi:10.1101/pdb.emo112.

Puigcerver, M., Vinyoles, D., and Rodriguez-Teijeiro, J.D. (2007) Does restocking with Japanese quail or hybrids affect native populations of common quail *Coturnix coturnix*? *Biological Conservation* **136**, 628–635. https://doi.org/10.1016/j.biocon.2007.01.007 (accessed 1 August 2019).

Randall, M. and Bolla, G. (2007) Raising Japanese quail. *Primefact* 602. NSW Department of Primary Industries, Australia.

Reddish, J.M., Kirby, J.D. and Anthony, N.B. (1996) Analysis of poultry fertility data. 3. Analysis of the duration of fertility in naturally mating Japanese quail. *Poultry Science*, **75**, 135–139.

Reece, R.L., Barr, D.A. and Owen, A.C. (1981) The isolation of *Haemophilus paragallinarum* from Japanese quail. *Australian Veterinary Journal*, **57**, 350–351.

Reed, W.M. and Jack, S. (2013) *Quail Bronchitis*. Oxford, UK, Wiley-Blackwell.

Reese, E.P. and Reese, T.W. (1962) The quail *Coturnix coturnix* as a laboratory animal. *Journal of the Experimental Analysis of Behaviour*, **5**, 265–270.

Roberts, J.R. and Hughes, M.R. (1983) Glomerular filtration rate and drinking rate in Japanese quail, *Coturnix coturnix japonica*, in response to acclimation to saline water. *Canadian Journal of Zoology*, **61**, 2394–2398.

Robinson, J.E., Follett, B.K. and Dodd, J.M. (1982) Photoperiodism in Japanese quail: the termination of seasonal breeding by photorefractoriness. *Proceedings of Royal Society of London. B.*, **215**. http://doi.org/10.1098/rspb.1982.0030 (accessed 15 August 2019).

Rodriguez-Teijeiro, J., Javie Rodrigo-Rueda, F., Puigcerver, M. et al. (1993) Codornices japonesas en nuestros campos. *Trofeo*, **277**, 48–52.

Roe, M., McDonald, N., Durrant, B., et al. (2013) Xenogeneic transfer of adult Quail (*Coturnix coturnix*) spermatogonial stem cells to embryonic Chicken (*Gallus gallus*) hosts: A model for avian conservation. *Biology of Reproduction*, **129**, 1–7. https://doi.org/10.1095/biolreprod.112.105189

RSPCA (2011) Quail: Good practice for housing and care. In: *Supplementary Resources for Members of Local Ethical Review Processes*, 4th edn, April 2011 www.rspca.org.uk/researchanimals (accessed 20 July 2019).

Ruff, M.D. (1991) Nematodes and Acanthocephalans. In: *Diseases of Poultry*. Eds Calnek, B.W., Barnes, H.J., Beard, C.W. et al., pp. 731–763. Wolfe Publications Ltd, London.

Rutten, P. (2018) Nutrition in cage-free egg layer housing – Diet consideration for alternative layer systems. *Canadian Poultry* December 22–24 http://magazine.canadianpoultrymag.com/publication?i=546297&p=22 (accessed 20 July 2019).

Sachs, B.D. (1967) Photoperiodic control of the cloacal gland of the Japanese quail. *Science*, **157**, 201–203.

Sanchez-Donoso, I., Vila, C., Puigcerver, M. et al. (2012) Are farm-reared quails for game restocking really common quails (*Coturnix coturnix*)?: a genetic approach. *PLoS One*, 7, e39031.

Sato, Y. and Lansford, R. (2013) Transgenesis and imaging in birds, and available transgenic reporter lines. *Development Growth & Differentiation*, **55**, 406–421.

Sato, Y., Poynter, G., Huss, D., et al. (2010) Dynamic analysis of vascular morphogenesis using transgenic quail embryos. *PLoS One*, 5, e12674.

Scanes, C.G. and McNabb, F.M.A. (2003) Avian models for research in toxicology and endocrine disruption. *Avian and Poultry Biology Reviews*, **14**, 21–52.

Schmid, I. and Wechsler, B. (1997) Behaviour of Japanese quail kept in semi-natural aviaries. *Applied Animal Behaviour Science*, **55**, 103–112.

Scholtz, N., Halle, I., Flachowsky, G. et al. (2009) Serum chemistry reference values in adult Japanese quail (*Coturnix coturnix japonica*) including sex-related differences. *Poultry Science*, **88**, 1186–1190.

Schwabl, H. (1996) Environment modifies the testosterone levels of a female bird and its eggs. *Journal of Experimental Zoology* **276**, 157–263.

Schwartz, C.W. and Schwartz, E.R. (1949) *A Reconnaissance of the Game Birds in Hawaii*. Hawaii Board of Commissioners of Agriculture and Forestry, Hilo, Hawaii.

Scott, B. B. and Lois, C. (2005) Generation of tissue-specific transgenic birds with lentiviral vectors. *Proceedings of National Academy of Science U S A*, **102**, 16443–16447.

Sefton, A.E. and Siegel, P.B. (1973) Mating behavior of Japanese quail. *Poultry Science*, **52**, 1001–1007.

Seidl, A. H., Sanchez, J. T., Schecterson, L. et al. (2013) Transgenic quail as a model for research in the avian nervous system: a comparative study of the auditory brainstem. *Journal of Comparative Neurology*, **521**, 5–23.

Selinger, H.E. and Bermant, G. (1967) Hormonal control of aggressive behaviour in Japanese quail (*Coturnix coturnix japonica*). *Behaviour*, **28**, 255–268.

Sentíes-Cué, C.G., Gallardo, R.A., Reimers, N., et al. (2016) Avian encephalomyelitis in layer pullets associated with vaccination. *Avian Diseases*, **60**, 511–515. https://doi.org/10.1637/11306-102115-Case (accessed 1 August 2019).

Shanaway, M.M. (1994) *Quail Production System – A Review*. Food and Agriculture Organization of the United Nations, Rome.

Shibusawa, M., Minai, S., Nishida-Umehara, C., et al. (2001). A comparative cytogenetic study of chromosome homology between chicken and Japanese quail. *Cytogenetics Cell Genetics*, **95**, 103–109.

Shibusawa, M., Nishibori, M., Nishida, C., et al. (2004) Karyotypic evolution in the Galliformes: An examination of the process of karyotypic evolution by comparison of the molecular cytogenetic findings with the molecular phylogeny. *Cytogenetic and Genome Research*, **106**, 111–119. doi: 10.1159/000078570.

Shih, J.C.H., Pullman. E.P. and Kao, K.J. (1983) Genetic selection, general characterization, and histology of atherosclerosis-susceptible and -resistant Japanese quail. *Atherosclerosis*, **49**, 41–53.

Shim, K.F. and Vohra, P.A. (1984). A review of the nutrition of the Japanese quail. *World's Poultry Science Journal*, **40**, 261–274.

Shivaprasad, H.L. (2002) Pathology of Birds – An Overview. *C.L. Davis Foundation Conference on Gross Morbid Anatomy of Animals*. Washington DC.

Silversides, F.G. and Liu, J. (2012) Novel techniques for preserving genetic diversity in poultry germplasm. *Animal Science Reviews* 2012, 207-213 https://www.cabi.org/cabreviews/search/?q=Novel+techniques+for+preserving+genetic+diversity+in+poultry+germplasm.+ (Restricted access).

Silversides, Purdy, P.H., and Blackburn, H.D. (2012) Comparative costs of programmes to conserve chicken genetic variation based on maintaining living populations or storing cryopreserved material. *British Poultry Science* 53, 599-607. http://dx.doi.org/10.1080/00071668.2012.727383 (accessed 1 August 2019).

Sittmann, K., Wilson, W.O. and Mcfarland, L.Z. (1966) Buff and Albino Japanese Quail: Description, Inheritance, and Fitness Traits. *Journal of Heredity*, 57, 119–124. https://doi.org/10.1093/oxfordjournals.jhered.a107487 (accessed 1 August 2019).

Sittmann, K., Abplanalp, H. and Abbott, U.K. (1971) Extended storage of quail, chicken and turkey eggs. 2. Embryonic abnormalities and the inheritance of twinning in quail. *Poultry Science*, 50, 714–722

Skeeles, J.K. (1991) Staphylococcosis. In: *Diseases of Poultry*. Eds Calnek, B.W., Barnes, H.J., Beard, C.W. *et al.*, pp. 293–299. Wolfe Publications Ltd, London.

Smith, E.L., Greenwood, V.J., Goldsmith, A.R. *et al.* (2005) Effect of supplementary ultraviolet lighting on the behaviour and corticosterone levels of Japanese quail chicks. *Animal Welfare*, 14, 103–109.

Snoeyenbos, G.H. (1991) Pullorum disease. In: *Diseases of Poultry*. Eds Calnek, B.W., Barnes, H.J., Beard, C.W. *et al.*, pp. 73–86. Wolfe Publications Ltd, London.

Somes, R.G. (1984) International registry of poultry genetic stocks. *Bulletin of Storrs Agricultural Experimental Station, University of Connecticut*, 469, 1–96.

Standford, J.A. (1957) A Progress Report of coturnix quail investigations in Missouri. Twenty-second North American Wildlife Conference, pp. 316–359.

Stein, G.S. and Bacon, W.L. (1976) Effect of photoperiod upon age and maintenance of sexual development in female *Coturnix coturnix japonica*. *Poultry Science*, 55, 1214–1218.

Suda, Y. and Okamoto, S. (2003) Long term selection for small body weight in Japanese quail II: Changes in reproductive traits from 60 to 65th generations. *Journal of Poultry Science*, 40, 30–38.

Susta, L., Segovia, D., Olivier, T.L., *et al.* (2018) Newcastle Disease Virus Infection in Quail. *Veterinary Pathology*, 55, 682–692.

Swayne, D.E., Glisson, J.R., Mcdougald, L.R., *et al.* (2013) *Diseases of Poultry*. John Wiley & Sons, Inc, New York.

Tadano, R., Nunome, M., Mizutani, M. *et al.* (2014) Cost-effective development of highly polymorphic microsatellite in Japanese quail facilitated by next-generation sequencing. *Animal Genetics*, 45, 881–884.

Taka-Tsukasa, N. (1935) *Coturnix coturnix japonica* Teminick et Schlegel. In: *The Birds of Nippon*, Vol 1. pp. 204–238. Whitherby, London.

Theilen, G.H., Zeigel, R.F. and Twiehaus, M.J. (1966) Biological studies with REV (strain T) that induces reticuloendotheliosis in turkeys, chickens and Japanese quail. *Journal of the National Cancer Institute*, 37, 731–743.

Tiersch, T.R. and Wachtel, S.S. (1991) On the evolution of genome size of birds. *Journal of Heredity*, 82, 363–368. doi: 10.1093/oxfordjournals.jhered.a111105

Trefil P, Aumann D, Koslová A. et al. (2017) Male fertility restored by transplanting primordial germ cells into testes: a new way towards efficient transgenesis in chicken. *Scientific Reports*. 7, 14246. doi: 10.1038/s41598-017-14475-w.

Trefil, P., Micáková, A., Mucksová, J. *et al.* (2006) Restoration of spermatogenesis and male fertility by transplantation of dispersed testicular cells in the chicken. *Biology of Reproduction* 75, 575–581. doi: 10.1095/biolreprod.105.050278

Tsiompanoudis, A.H, Vassilios, J.K. and Bakaloudis, D. (2011) Observations of breeding and wintering European quail *Coturnix coturnix* in northern Greece. *International Journal of Galliformes Conservation*, 2, 38–39.

Tsudzuki, M. (2008) Mutations of Japanese quail (*Coturnix japonica*) and recent advances of molecular genetics for this species. *Poultry Science*, 45, 159–179.

Tsutsui, K., Saigoh, E. and Ukena, K. (2000) A novel avian hypothalamic peptide inhibiting gonadotrophin release. *Biophysical Research Communications*, 275, 661–667.

Urbanski, H.F. (1984) Episodic release of LH in gonadectomized male Japanese quail. *Journal of Endocrinology*, 100, 209–212.

Underwood, H. (1994) The circadian rhythm of thermoregulation in Japanese quail. I. Role of the eyes and pineal. *Journal Comparative Physiology A*, 175, 639–653.

Underwood, H. and Edmonds, K. (1995) The circadian rhythm of thermoregulation in Japanese quail. III. Effects of melatonin administration. *Journal Biological Rhythms*, 10, 284–298.

Usman, B.A., Mani, A.U., El-Yuguda, A.D. *et al.* (2008) The effect of supplemental ascorbic acid on the development of New Castle disease in Japanese quail (*Coturnix coturnix japonica*) exposed to high ambient temperature. *International Journal of Poultry Science*, 7, 328–332.

Valavan, S.E. (2016) Diversified poultry production in India: an overview. *Proceedings of XXV World's Poultry Congress*, 5–9 September 2016, Beijing, China, pp. 297–313.

Vince, M.A. (1966) Artificial acceleration of hatching in quail embryos. *Animal Behaviour*, 14, 389–394.

Vince, M.A. (1968) Retardation as a factor in the synchronization of hatching. *Animal Behaviour*, 16, 332–335.

Vince, M.A. and Cheng, R. (1970) The retardation of hatching in Japanese quail. *Animal Behaviour*, 18, 210–214.

Visser, G.H., Boon, P.E. and Meijer, H.A.J. (2000) Validation of the doubly labelled water method in Japanese quail *Coturnix c. japonica* chicks: is there an effect of growth rate? *Journal of Comparative Physiology*, 170, 365–372.

Wakasugi, N. (1984) Japanese quail. In: *Evolution of Domestic Animals*. Ed. Mason, J.L., pp. 319–321. Longman, London.

Wentworth, B.C. and Mellen, W.J. (1963) Egg production and fertility following various methods of insemination in Japanese quail (*Coturnix coturnix japonica*). *Reproduction*, 6, 215–220. doi: https://doi.org/10.1530/jrf.0.0060215

Wetherbee, D.K. (1961) Investigations in the life history of the common coturnix. *American Midland Naturalist*, 65, 168–186.

Wilson, F.E. and Donham, R.S. (1988) Daylength and control of seasonal reproduction in male birds. In: *Processing of Environmental Information in Vertebrates*. Ed. Stetson, M.H. Proceedings in Life Sciences. Springer, New York, NY.

Wilson, M.I. and Bermant, G. (1972) An analysis of social interactions in Japanese quail, *Coturnix coturnix japonica*. *Animal Behaviour*, 20, 252–258.

Wilson, W.O. (1972) A review of the physiology of *Coturnix* (Japanese) quail. *World's Poultry Science Journal*, 28, 413–423.

Wilson, W.O., Abbott, U.K. and Abplanalp, H. (1959) Developmental and physiological studies with a new pilot animal for poultry – *Coturnix* quail. *Poultry Science*, 38, 1260–1261.

Wilson, W.O., Abbott, U.K. and Abplanalp, H. (1961) Evaluation of *Coturnix* (Japanese quail) as a pilot animal for poultry. *Poultry Science*, 40, 651–657.

Woodard. A.E. and Abplanalp, H. (1967) The effects of mating ratio and age on fertility and hatchability in Japanese quail. *Poultry Science*, 46, 383–388.

Woodard, A.E. and Abplanalp, H. (1971) Longevity and reproduction in Japanese quail maintained under stimulatory lighting. *Poultry Science*, 50, 688–692.

Woodard, A.E., Abplanalp, H., Wilson, W.O. *et al.* (1973) *Japanese Quail Husbandry in the Laboratory*. University of California, Davis, California.

Woodard, A.E. and Mather, F.B. (1964) Effect of photoperiod on the cyclic patterns of body temperature in the quail. *Nature*, **203**, 422–423.

Woodard, A.E. and Wilson, W.O. (1972) Behavioral patterns associated with oviposition in Japanese quail and chickens. *Journal of Interdisciplinary Cycle Research*, **1**, 173–180.

Wu, Y., Zhang, Y., Hou, Z. *et al.* (2018) Population genomic data reveal genes related to important traits of quail. *Gigascience*, **7**, 1–16.

Yang, N., Dunnington, E.A. and Siegel, P.B. (1999) Heterosis following long-term bidirectional selection for mating frequency in male Japanese quail. *Poultry Science*, **78**, 1252–1256.

Yoder, H.W. Jr. (1991) Mycoplasmosis. In: *Diseases of Poultry*. Eds Calnek, B.W., Barnes, H.J., Beard, C.W. *et al.*, pp. 196–212. Wolfe Publications Ltd, London.

Yousef, M.K., McFarland, L.Z. and Wilson, W.O. (1966) Ambient temperature effects on hypothalamic, rectal and skin temperature in coturnix. *Life Sciences*, **5**, 1887–1896.

Zucker, H., Gropp, J., Peh, J. *et al.* (1967) Erfahrungen mit der japanischen Wachtel (*Coturnix coturnix japonica*) als Labortier sowie einige Ergebnisse von Nährstoffbedarfsuntersuchungen. *Tierärztl Umschauft*, **22**, 416–423.

42 The zebra finch

Ruedi G. Nager, Michael J.A. Wilkinson and Graham Law[†]

To the memory of Graham Law, his ingenious creativity, his humour, and his striving to improve the lives of animals and of people who work with animals. He was and will always be an inspiration to us.

Biological overview

Natural history

The zebra finch is a small passerine from the family *Estrildidae* (weaver finches), a group that is found in the Old World tropics and Australasia. All estrildids are similar in structure and habits but vary widely in plumage colour and patterns. However, within the *Estrildidae*, the zebra finch is morphologically, behaviourally and genetically distinct from other species, and forms its own genus *Taeniopygia* set apart from other *Poephila* finches (Christidis 1987).

The Australian zebra finch *Taeniopygia guttata castanotis* (Gould 1837) is widely distributed across the desert and grassland biomes of Australia but is missing from some of the tropical far north and the cool moist south. In Central Australia *T. g. castanotis* is the most common of the weaver finches. It also occurs in the Lesser Sundas and neighbouring islands north of Australia, where they are smaller and form a separate subspecies, the Lesser Sundas zebra finch *T. g. guttata* (Vieillot 1817). There are now also introduced populations in Puerto Rico and Portugal[1]. Zebra finches are sexually dimorphic, the males having a more ornate plumage and a redder bill than females (Figure 42.1). However, in *T. g. guttata* the male has a smaller chest-band and less barring on the throat and upper breast compared with *T. g. castanotis*.

The zebra finch, or at least the subspecies *T. g. castanotis*, is abundant and widespread in the wild. They are opportunistic birds that travel in search of the best resources, occupying arid areas close to accessible surface water allowing for abundant vegetation that provides grass seeds for food and bushes and trees for nesting and roosting; they can also be found in cultivated areas (Zann 1996). Despite their tropical and subtropical distribution, zebra finches tolerate low temperatures, as in the wild they can be exposed to low overnight temperatures (Zann 1996). In the arid areas, zebra finches breed after substantial rains when their food becomes abundant.

Zebra finches are adapted for feeding on a large variety of semi-ripe and ripe grass seeds that are abundant where they live, and they also take dry seeds (Zann 1996). Zebra finches dehusk seeds, and thus prefer seeds of about 1–2.6 mm that are more easily dehusked than smaller seeds (Zann 1996). Zebra finches usually take ripened seeds from the ground, but also take half-ripe seeds from the heads of standing grasses, and this is what they mainly feed to their young. To reach seeds from grass heads they either fly and peck out seeds one at a time, perch on a nearby branch or may even pull the grass head to the ground with their bill or feet. At times, when grass seed is rare, zebra finches may dig into the ground using their bill to randomly search for buried seed (Zann 1996). As their food can be locally abundant, zebra finches are a gregarious species roosting and nesting colonially and foraging in flocks which can help them discover new patches of seed (Zann 1996).

Zebra finches used in research laboratories are derived from *Taeniopygia guttata castanotis*. By the late 1800s, they were frequently bred in captivity in Europe, but large numbers of zebra finches were still being imported from Australia until World War I, and in the 1950s further small numbers of captive-bred birds were imported from Australia (Sossinka 1970). In 1960, the Australian government implemented export bans on all native wildlife. Currently, zebra finches in research laboratories worldwide have presumably been bred for tens of generations without any significant input of wild zebra finches and are genetically clearly distinct from the wild stock (Forstmeier et al. 2007). Captive zebra finches may show alterations in a number of behavioural and other traits as compared to wild zebra finches, including larger body size and delayed female sexual maturity (see later in this chapter) as well as in changes to the structure of distance calls and duration of song phrases (e.g., Sossinka 1970; Slater & Clayton 1991;

[†]Deceased
[1] https://www.iucnredlist.org/species/103818044/104212010 (Accessed 23 June 2022)

The UFAW Handbook on the Care and Management of Laboratory and Other Research Animals, Ninth Edition.
Edited by Huw Golledge and Claire Richardson.
© 2024 John Wiley & Sons Ltd. Published 2024 by John Wiley & Sons Ltd.

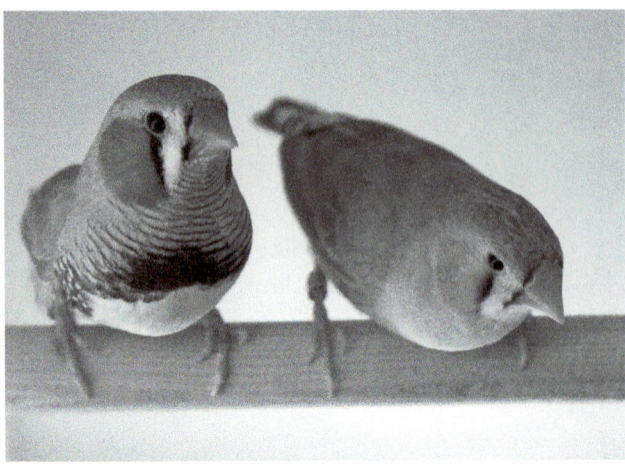

Figure 42.1 Male (left) and female (right) wild-type zebra finches. Females have a grey back, whitish undersides and a white cheek patch bordered by a black stripe. Males are more ornate with reddish brown cheek patches, chestnut brown flanks with white spots and a black-and-white barred chest. Legs are orange in both sexes, but males have a deeper red bill while females' bills are more orange. Source: Photo: G. Law.

Zann 1996). Zebra finches that have been bred in captivity for many generations, however, still respond similarly to a manipulation of their life-history traits compared to wild birds bred in captivity, suggesting that despite significant differentiation between captive and wild populations, the relationship among traits has not changed (Tschirren et al. 2009). There is little information on comparing the physiology of captive and wild birds, but at least the thermal tolerance is still similar between captive-bred and wild zebra finches (Marschall & Prinzinger 1991). Thus, captive birds can adequately represent wild birds for at least studies of life-history evolution. In our view, although care needs to be taken when comparing zebra finches bred in captivity with wild zebra finches – given that the process of domestication has not been robustly studied in captive-bred zebra finches – domestication does not necessarily 'take the wild out of animals' in species that have been maintained in captivity for longer than zebra finches (Wood-Gush & Duncan 1976; Stolba & Wood-Gush 1989; Peplow 2004).

Size range and lifespan

There are morphological differences among different breeding stocks of zebra finches. Among a sample of 18 captive populations, zebra finches in European laboratories were the heaviest (mean body mass: 16.1 g, range 13.7–18.6 g, n = 10 populations), presumably due to selection for large body size by the European aviculturists. Australian captive birds were the lightest (mean: 12.1 g, range 11.9–12.4 g, n = 2), similar in mass to wild birds. North American birds were intermediate in mass (mean: 14.4 g; range 13.7–15.2 g, n = 6; information on body mass from Forstmeier et al. (2007)). Females, but not males, in a captive population had been reported to be skeletally larger than wild birds (Zann 1996). More recent studies on body mass and size of captive populations of zebra finches are lacking.

Zebra finches in the wild are relatively short lived but can reach several years of age in captivity. Their life expectancy is highly variable due to internal and environmental influences. In the wild, about 70% of offspring are lost in the short period between fledging (day 15–20) and nutritional independence (day 35) and only 9% of eggs lead to young surviving to breeding age. Mature free-living birds have an annual mortality of between 72 and 96%, but can occasionally live for up to 5 years, and there is no difference in the survival rates between males and females (Zann 1996). Threats to zebra finch survival in the wild are starvation and predation by snakes, lizards, carnivorous birds and marsupials, but also introduced cats, rats and mice. In captivity, zebra finches still show substantial variation in lifespan with some birds dying at less than 1 year of age while others living for almost 9 years (Heidinger et al. 2012); the oldest bird in captivity on record reached 14.5 years[2]. In captivity, the annual mortality in females has been reported to be higher than in males throughout their lives so that males typically live about 3 years and females about 2 years (Burley 1985). It has not been properly researched whether the longer lifespan of zebra finches in captivity, with its associated wear and tear, negatively affects their welfare.

Social organisation

The zebra finch is a gregarious species forming feeding flocks of a few hundred individuals and nest in colonies ranging from just a few pairs up to 40–50 pairs, but solitary nesting pairs also occur (Zann 1996). Zebra finches can form pair bonds any time during the year when conditions are favourable for breeding and, once paired, develop a strong pair bond during the breeding event (Butterfield 1970). The pair bond is maintained through a series of calls that allow them to recognise and locate their mate (Zann 1996). Only males sing a complex courtship song that they normally learn during the juvenile period between independence from their parents and sexual maturity from any suitable tutor that is available at the time (Eales 1985); females do not sing. Pair bonds don't usually persist beyond the breeding event, presumably due to high mortality rates. In both the wild and in a wild colour-ringed population, even when both pair members have survived to the next breeding event, they have never been observed to re-pair (Zann 1996). No bird has been observed with more than one mate at any one time and only the two parents attend the nest (Zann 1996). Captive zebra finches show mutual mate choice based on plumage colour, song and body condition (Collins & ten Cate 1996; Zann 1996; Jones et al. 2001). As mate choice in the zebra finch is condition-dependent, variation in the susceptibility to rearing conditions and context sensitivity (e.g., where the intensity in competition between males can affect male mating preferences) between sexes and population can lead to differences in mate preferences between populations (Holveck et al. 2011) which warrants further study.

---

[2] http://genomics.senescence.info/species/entry.php?species=Taeniopygia_guttata (Accessed 23 June 2022)

Moreover, female zebra finches can copy mate choice for novel phenotypic traits using public information, further diverging mate preferences between populations (Kniel et al. 2015). Females also may prefer males as mates that are more habituated to captivity (Collins et al. 2008). In the wild, intraspecific brood parasitism is common with 10.9% of offspring and 36% of broods usually containing one or more intraspecific brood parasitic eggs, whereas extra-pair paternity is rare, with 1.7–2.4% of offspring and 5–8% of broods affected (Birkhead et al. 1990; Griffith et al. 2010). In contrast, the levels of extra-pair paternity (15.3–29% of offspring) are higher in captive populations (Burley et al. 1996; Forstmeier et al. 2011; Tschirren et al. 2012; McCowan et al. 2014). This difference between wild and captive population could be due to artificial selection in captivity or to differences in social or environmental factors between the two environments, and possibly because females of the captive population were less choosy, and thus less likely to resist the advances of extra-pair males, than females from the wild population (Rutstein et al. 2007). In summary, zebra finches show mutual mate preference and are only socially – but not genetically – monogamous and the attending parents may not always be the genetic parents of all the young they rear.

Biological data

In captivity, nestlings of zebra finches weigh 0.6–0.9 g at hatching. Over the first 10 days they gain 0.4–0.7 g/day in body mass and about 1 mm/day in tarsus length (Skagen 1988; Martins 2004), but this varies with sex, size of the adult stock birds and food levels (Boag 1987). Typical rectal temperature of healthy captive birds during the day is 41.8 °C (Conover & Messmer 1996) and their thermoneutral zone is around 32 °C (Calder 1964). Haematological values for wild and captive zebra finches are given in Ewenson et al. (2001), with healthy captive zebra finches typically having a heterophil : lymphocyte ratio of 0.17. Captive females kept under thermoneutral conditions have a mean haematocrit of 53.2 % (± standard deviation = 6.6), haemoglobin content of 190.9 ± 20.80 g l^{-1}, red blood cell count of 5.5 ± 0.88 mln μl^{-1} and size of erythrocytes of 57.9 ± 4.21 μm^2; these values are lower in cold acclimated birds (Niedojadlo et al. 2018). Birkhead et al. (2006) give a mean haematocrit of 51.2 (standard deviation = 3.58) for male captive zebra finches, but it is not clear – compared to the female figure above – whether this is a sex or a population difference. Biochemical values for a small sample size of male and female captive zebra finches (n = 10/sex) are given by Patterson and Fee (2015), who reported low albumin and total protein levels for the species. The zebra finch has 40 pairs of chromosomes, but the cells involved in sexual reproduction (germline cells) carry an additional pair of chromosomes (Pigozzi & Solari 1998). These additional chromosomes seem to be widespread in passerines, but absent in non-passerines and may help during sexual reproduction by providing more protein and nutrients for developing sperm and egg cells (Torgasheva et al. 2019).

Reproduction

Zebra finches are opportunistic breeders that breed whenever favourable conditions occur, regardless of time since the last breeding event and photoperiodicity (Zann 1996). In the wild, they typically initiate reproductive behaviour ca. 1–3 months after water becomes available, with young hatching around the time when semi-ripe and ripe seeds – which are more adequate food for nestlings than dry grass seeds – are most abundant (Zann et al. 1995). Thus, zebra finches can respond rapidly to the unpredictable arrival of favourable conditions at any time of year. In order to do so, those inhabiting unpredictable habitat maintain a high level of reproductive readiness (large gonad size and high level of circulating gonadotrophins) and more males show readiness to breed than females (Perfito et al. 2007). Wild zebra finches inhabiting more predictable habitat, where breeding occurs during approximately the same months each year, change their reproductive readiness consistently between the breeding and non-breeding state. When non-breeding birds from the predictable environment were taken into the laboratory they were, however, able to activate their reproductive axis quickly (Perfito et al. 2007). This suggests that there is constant activation of gonads without a refractory period and that the animals can rapidly respond to the presence of favourable breeding conditions, able to breed several times per breeding season (Schielzeth & Bolund 2010). Along with this high reproductive readiness ('hypersexuality') goes an early reproductive maturity in young birds; birds as young as 62–67 days old (median age of birds breeding in the same breeding season in which they hatched: 95 and 92 days for males and females, respectively) have been seen to breed in the wild (Zann 1996). 'Hypersexuality' distinguishes zebra finches from other small passerines and is presumably an adaptation to the unpredictable arid conditions in Australia. However, some aspects of this trait have declined in domesticated zebra finches, with females in captive populations showing a slower sexual development than wild females and laying eggs only as early as 90 days old (Sossinka 1972a).

Zebra finches typically lay a clutch of five white eggs (range two to eight eggs, Zann 1996) that measure about 1.5 × 1 cm, laying one egg each day both in the wild and in captivity. Each egg takes about 4 days of rapid follicle growth before it is laid (Houston et al. 1995). In the wild, parents usually start to incubate on the last or penultimate egg, incubation taking 11–14 days from the day the last egg has been laid and hatching thus occurring over 24–48 h. In captivity, parents start incubation earlier during laying and clutches hatch more asynchronously than in the wild (Gilby et al. 2013). The same shift to an earlier start of incubation is also seen in wild free-living birds brought into captivity, which shows a high level of intraspecific plasticity in incubation behaviour and suggests that the captive environment is likely the main factor behind this behavioural flexibility (Gilby et al. 2013). Both sexes incubate, although only the female has a brood patch, and the sexes differ in incubation temperature and the way they regulate it (Hill et al. 2014). Zebra finches are altricial and the chicks depend on their parents for food and warmth. Young are fed by both sexes, with parents transferring seeds from their crop to the chick's crop. Chicks that have not been fed can be spotted as the crop of fed chicks bulges and seeds can be seen through the skin of the crop. Parents may brood their young for the first few days and can feed their chicks several times during one nest attention bout; therefore, the number of nest visits can be an inaccurate measure of parental feeding effort (Gilby et al. 2011). Young zebra finches fledge about 17–18 days after hatching and feed themselves when ca. 35 days old, but during that time they are still socially dependent on their parents. The young become socially independent between 36 and 50 days after hatching and their sexually dimorphic plumage is developed during this period.

Normal behaviour

The welfare of animals is typically assessed across three aspects: functionality, affective state and naturalness (Fraser 2008). Hence, knowledge on the normal behaviour of zebra finches in the wild is relevant for considering their welfare in captivity, just as it is for many other captive species. Zann (1996) estimates a daily foraging time of 2–4 h and that about 4 g of seeds is needed for wild zebra finches to meet their daily requirements. In search of food, individual zebra finches can range over an area up to at least 1 km around the nest during breeding and are highly mobile when not breeding, deserting an area when conditions become unfavourable (Zann 1996). The lack of genetic differentiation of populations up to 2000 km apart (Forstmeier et al. 2007) supports the view that populations can range over such large distances. Non-breeding zebra finches often roost in old breeding nests or purpose-built nests (Zann 1996). Another energy-demanding activity is moult, and zebra finches have an unusually slow moult for passerines, possibly another adaptation to their arid habitat; a complete primary moult takes approximately 229–239 days in wild individuals and the regrowth of individual feathers takes 21–26 days (Zann 1985). In captivity, the estimated moult duration (70–100 days) is shorter but exhibits a less rigid moulting sequence. When moult and breeding overlap which occurs in both captive and wild animals, captive birds moult more slowly, and this is more pronounced in females than in males (Echeverry-Galvis & Hau 2012). Thus, both arid conditions in the wild and intense breeding activity in captivity can slow the moult.

Sources and supplies

Many research laboratories maintain their own breeding stocks derived from larger stocks of aviculturists. Compared to wild birds, all captive populations have lost some genetic variability even though still showing a substantial variability at 12 highly polymorphic microsatellite markers, suggesting that they are unlikely to have experienced severe genetic bottlenecks (Forstmeier et al. 2007). There is significant genetic and morphological differentiation among captive populations between Australia, Europe and North America, with further differences between regions, particularly in Europe (Zann 1996; Forstmeier et al. 2007), that might have arisen from differences in sources of wild stock, in climatic conditions, and in show standards for size, and from specific breeding programmes focusing on male sexual characteristics (excluding song). Researchers utilising zebra finches are, therefore, not using a genetically uniform stock, and it is essential to give standardised information on the origin of birds used, as recommended in Kilkenny et al. (2010).

There are many colour morphs of zebra finches. The wild type or grey morph is shown in Figure 42.1. The most frequently found colour mutant is fawn which was discovered in wild birds in 1927 (Zann 1996). Aviculturists have bred about 30 main morphs mainly for show competitions and most are mutations of all or particular parts of the plumage[3]. Colour morphs can differ in their morphological and life history traits with potential consequences on fitness in captive birds, although further studies will be required to evaluate fitness effects under natural conditions (Krause et al. 2017). In research laboratories, mainly wild-type and fawn birds are used. The colour mutation fawn is sex-linked, which can be used to sex very young offspring (Birkhead et al. 1989; Kilner 1998). As imprinting on adult plumage colour has a strong effect on mate choice (e.g., Immelmann et al. 1978), its effects may need to be considered in studies on sexual selection and mate selection. If seeking standardisation, one would want to have birds of the same colour morph, but this is difficult to achieve since most colour mutations are recessive and unexpected colour morphs may appear in later generations.

Use in research

The zebra finch is one of the most commonly kept passerines in laboratories (Bateson & Feenders 2010) as it is hardy, easy to keep and one of the most readily bred aviary birds. Zebra finches are inexpensive to buy. They are used in research focusing on the neural basis of song learning, sexual selection, development of sexual preferences and physiological studies such as endocrinology and toxicity testing, but only few studies on animal welfare. The number of publications featuring them reaches over 100 publications per year in recent years.

The fact that the zebra finch genome was the second avian genome to be sequenced to 6× coverage in 2007 made this species attractive for studies including genetic information. The first published zebra finch genome used one male bird from a North American captive breeding population (University of California in Los Angeles, UCLA) that then acted as a catalyst for many subsequent genetic studies on this species.

General husbandry

Species-appropriate husbandry requires a careful selection of environmental conditions that promote desired species-specific behaviours and physiology and prevents abnormal behaviours (Hawkins 2010). The selection of appropriate environmental conditions is typically derived from a good

---

[3] https://ladygouldianfinch.com/features_zmutation.php (Accessed 23 June 2022)

understanding of the species' natural history which, in the case of zebra finches, is well known. Nevertheless, systematic scientific studies evaluating the impact of common husbandry practices (whether or not based on the birds' natural history) on their welfare are, sadly, often lacking; future work is needed to refine guidelines for their husbandry. We base much of the following account on the 'Code of Practice for the Housing and Care of Animals Bred, Supplied or Used for Scientific Purposes'[4].

Enclosure

Enclosures for captive animals need to allow some natural behaviour to be performed (Young 2003) and compatible with the research the animal is used for. In the wild, zebra finches regularly flock in trees and forage on the ground and, therefore, should be given the space to carry out such movements. In the wild, the birds are highly sociable, maintaining close contact to each other and hence, in captivity, they can be maintained at higher densities than many other species (but see below).

There is very little information on the effects of enclosure size on the welfare of zebra finches. The size of the enclosure and the shape and layout of the enclosure's furnishings should be organised so as to maximise space for horizontal flight, as longer cages are associated with fewer abnormal behaviours than shorter cages of the same volume in some captive passerines (Asher et al. 2009; Bateson & Feenders 2010). Moreover, wild-caught starlings kept in smaller cages have been reported to develop more pessimistic cognitive biases – indicative of a negative welfare state – than birds kept in larger cages (Matheson et al. 2008). In a study involving very small numbers of zebra finches, Jacobs et al. (1995) also found reduced activity in a number of behaviours, in pairs kept in cages with an area of 0.11 m² compared to pairs kept in cages with an area of 0.22 m² (N.B. both cage sizes provided less space than currently legally required in European laboratories); so it is possible that small space also detrimentally affects the welfare of captive-bred zebra finches. Perches should be spaced such to enable unimpeded horizontal flights between them. As from 2017, the European Union has implemented regulations requiring minimal space requirements for animals used for scientific purposes (European Union 2010). The minimal space requirements for zebra finches from this EU directive are provided in Table 42.1; different regulations may apply in other parts of the world.

Due to their social nature, zebra finches can be kept in groups, with the best practice stocking densities listed in Table 42.1. Densities higher than the recommended levels can lead to zebra finches producing fewer and poorer-quality offspring (Poot et al. 2012). If, however, accurate information on the offspring's parentage is required, they need to be bred in pairs in separate breeding cages due to the prevalence of intra-specific brood parasitism and extra-pair paternity

Table 42.1 Minimum enclosure dimensions and space allowances for zebra finches as required by the EU Directive 2010/63/EU on the protection of animals used for scientific purposes (European Union 2010).

	Minimum enclosure area (m²)	Minimum height (m)	Minimum number of feeders
Up to 6 birds	1	1	2
7–12 birds	1.5	2	2
13–20 birds	2	2	3
Above 20 birds	+0.05 per each additional bird	2	1 per 6 birds

when breeding in a group (see *Social organisation*). Typically, several breeding pairs are kept in visual and acoustic contact with conspecifics, even though this practice can have detrimental effects (see *Social housing*); the time spent in pairs should be limited to the duration the parents take to raise their offspring to independence (chicks of 35 days of age).

Zebra finches can be housed in standard cages with solid sides on all but the front. It is recommended that cages should be made of an easy-to-clean material to provide a hygienic environment for the birds; cages can be stacked or mounted on wall brackets. Zebra finches can also be kept in aviaries covered with wire mesh of ≤10 mm width or vertical bars not more than 12 mm apart. Aviaries are often indoors. Zebra finches in the wild, however, experience a wide range of environmental conditions and can be exposed to freezing temperatures (Meijer et al. 1996). Thus, they can also be kept outdoors throughout the year, provided they have sufficient protection from wind and rain – such as shrubs – and ideally access to an indoor area with supplemental heating in winter (Joint Working Group on Refinement 2001).

Environmental provisions and enrichments

Typical enrichments provided to passerines include feeding enrichments, ropes or branches of differing diameters, natural floor substrates, water baths and areas of cover (Bateson & Feenders 2010). These can encourage greater use of the space available, performance of natural behaviour patterns and provision of hiding places. In the wild, zebra finches spend a considerable time foraging. As zebra finches normally feed on the ground, seed can be provided on the floor but this, in turn, requires a solid floor and careful consideration of floor covering. Possibilities include paper liner, bark chips, wood shavings, hemp core or sand. A varied substrate gives the advantage of making foraging for spilled seeds more challenging, and increase duration of activity of birds. Bark chips can maintain a hygienic floor litter, but do not work well under the dry conditions usually encountered in laboratory bird rooms. By contrast, hemp core works well under the conditions usually encountered in bird rooms, minimising dust levels for the benefit of the birds and of the staff working with the birds. Seed spillage or intentional scatter feeding on the ground can encourage natural foraging behaviour (Joint Working Group on Refinement 2001). Mixing seeds with husks also increases foraging time and effort, but caution is

[4]https://assets.publishing.service.gov.uk/government/uploads/system/uploads/attachment_data/file/389821/44389_unact_animals_Non-human_primates_Farm_animals_and_Birds.pdf (Accessed 23 June 2022)

warranted when using this feeding method; birds that were provided with mixtures with a husk mass to seed mass ratio of 3 : 1 during their lifetime showed low foraging efficiencies (effectively starving), produced smaller and fewer broods, and had lower survival rates compared to control birds on de-husked seeds (Lemon & Barth 1992; Lemon 1993). However, zebra finches can also pick seeds from heads of standing grass stalks which is a more challenging foraging strategy. This foraging strategy can be simulated in the laboratory by hanging millet sprays from the ceiling of the cage, beyond the reach of a perching bird (Law et al. 2010). Zebra finches readily accept feeding from hanging millet sprays if at the same time the availability of seed on the floor is reduced (Figure 42.2). In order to feed from hanging millet sprays, birds have to fly and hang onto the millet, peck out a seed, and fly back to a perch to dehusk the seed, repeating this operation time and again. The repeated exercise is thought to improve the physical and mental fitness of the birds, as birds had faster flight take-off speeds and improved colour association learning (Law et al. 2010).

When not foraging, wild zebra finches spend much time perching in trees. Perches of a variety of diameters and at different heights should, therefore, be provided. In captivity, where birds have access to perches at varying heights, they most frequently perch high up in the cage and approach the food on the ground by moving to progressively lower perches (pers. obs). Care needs to be taken, however, not to overcrowd the space with perches that would restrict the birds' flight movements. In order to prevent fouling, perches should not be located above food and water dishes placed on the ground. Often doweling rods (ca. 0.5 cm in diameter) fixed to cage walls at both ends are provided as perches but we do not recommend them, as landing on inflexible perches may be detrimental to musculoskeletal health. Sandpaper perch covers should not be used as they can abrade the feet and provide a route for infection. Softer wood or a variety of natural branches (apple, aspen, birch, cactus wood, cherry, elm, maple, mountain ash, pear, pine, poplar and willow) are good alternative perches. Natural branches in a range of diameters (0.5–2 cm), which are often less rigid than artificial perches, allow the muscles of the feet and body involved in balance to be properly exercised and help to keep the claws in good trim. There are commercially available twist perches (perches with a single attachment point) made of plastic or wood that are not of a constant diameter; they give the perch the springiness of a natural branch and sway when the birds land and take off. These perches, as well as commercially available swings designed for zebra finches, help mimic the movement of trees in the wild that causes the birds to exercise a variety of muscles and use the wings for balance with muscle activity being associated with healthier bone and muscle structure (Minor & Lane 1996). Zebra finches like to sit close together and, therefore, perches and swings should be of sufficient length to allow at least two birds to sit on them. We suggest perches be replaced – or cleaned where possible – every 6 weeks to provide a hygienic environment (see *Hygiene* section in the following text).

Zebra finches will use both sand and water baths, sometimes using the bowl communally (Figure 42.3). Access to water baths has been shown to keep the plumage in good condition in several bird species (Brilot et al. 2009) and zebra finches that had their bathing opportunities being removed showed higher basal plasma CORT concentrations (Krause & Ruploh 2016). Baths may only need to be provided for a few hours per day in order to avoid excessive water spillages. Water depth should be around 0.5–1 cm and, if size allows, a flat stone can be placed in the water bath to help prevent the bath tipping over.

Several other enrichments had been suggested for zebra finches. Provision of an optional cover for birds to hide has been suggested, but it can lead to increased fearfulness of the birds over time (Collins et al. 2008). Since zebra finches are

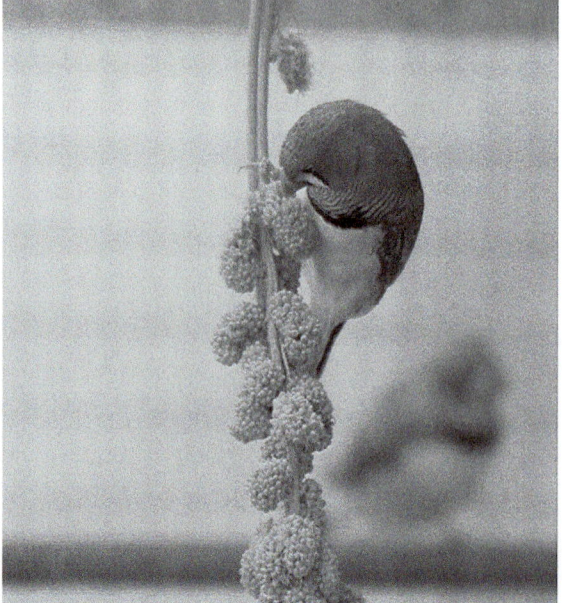

Figure 42.2 Zebra finches feeding on a hanging millet spray. The millet spray is attached to the cage ceiling such that it cannot be reached from a bird sitting on a perch but needs to make a short flight, cling to the swaying millet spray and forage. Source: Photo: G. Law.

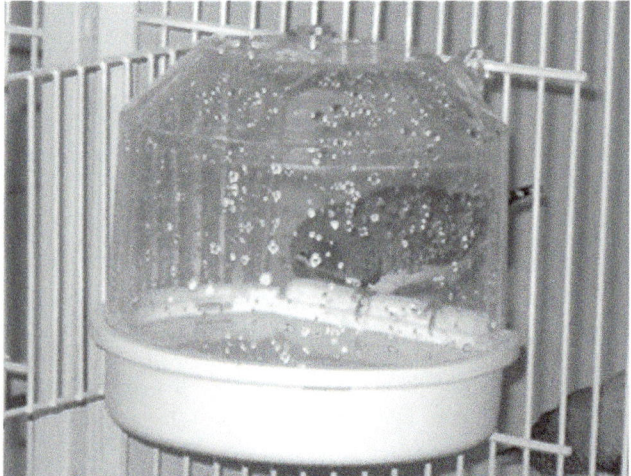

Figure 42.3 Zebra finches entering a water bath. The water bath is attached externally to the cage using one of the opening provided. This allows adding, changing and removing water baths with the least disturbance to the birds. Source: Photo: G. Law.

prolific nest builders and also build roosting nests outside the breeding season, provision of some nest material to non-breeding birds may help provide good sensory stimulation. To increase activity and species-specific nest-building behaviour, nesting material can be attached to the side of the cage, rather than on the ground, and this way the birds have to fly and pull off strands of the material (Law *et al.* 2010). Jacobs *et al.* (1995), using a very small sample size, suggested that simple enrichments such as a larger number of perches, twigs, sand and water baths may result in increased frequency of several desirable behaviours such as vocalisation and singing, and reduced abnormal behaviour, for example, stereotypic hopping. Zebra finches with little opportunity for exercise can become obese (Birkhead *et al.* 2006). Care must be taken, however, to monitor the effects of any enrichments introduced into a laboratory as they can sometimes have unanticipated negative consequences for the birds, as shown by the example of provision of cover to hide (Collins *et al.* 2008).

Feeding and watering

In the wild, zebra finches feed predominantly on a wide variety of grass seeds and supplement their diet with other vegetable matter and insects (Zann 1996). Although captive birds are generally maintained on a diet of foreign finch seed mixes (largely millet and canary seeds), yet their nutritional needs cannot be wholly met by these, and hence a large proportion of bird diseases in captivity have a nutritional basis (Stockdale 2018). Seed-eating passerines – including finches – can selectively pick out oil-based, energy-rich seeds (e.g., rape, sunflower, hemp) and leave out other seeds in a mix, potentially leading to health issues (Stockdale 2018). Therefore, zebra finches need to be offered a balanced diet during their time in the laboratory. Seeds can be provided in feeders mounted on the cage wall or in petri dishes provided on the ground, but the latter method results in a lot of seed spillage. Hanging up millet sprays is another way of providing seeds (see *Environmental provisions and enrichments* section in the preceding text). Because of their high metabolic rate, domesticated zebra finches have a high daily requirement for seed even under standard laboratory conditions (2.3 ± 0.9 g) and this requirement increases when birds are kept below the thermoneutral zone, for instance when kept outdoors (Niedojadlo *et al.* 2018). If birds are kept in social groups, seeds must be provided in several dishes (see Table 42.1) so as to avoid monopolisation of the food by dominant birds at the expense of subordinates. As passerines that have higher body fat are more vulnerable to predation, birds on ad libitum or predictable food will eat less and carry less fat than birds that have less predictable access to food (Cuthill *et al.* 2000), and thus low body fat is not necessarily a sign of poor welfare (Bateson & Feenders 2010).

Zebra finches in captivity are typically provided with dry grass seeds which is what they feed on in the wild during dry periods. However, when coming into the breeding season – when it is wetter – wild birds feed on a greener diet. A greener diet has more readily available nutrients, which benefits both adults and growing chicks. Therefore, during breeding periods, captive birds can also be given some sprouted and soaked seeds. In order to sprout the seeds, normal finch mix can be soaked in clean water, thoroughly rinsed after 24 h and then soaked in water again. After a further 48 h, the seeds are rinsed again, drained thoroughly and placed on paper towels in a flat tray in a warm and dark place. Depending on temperatures, seeds will sprout in 24–36 h and sprouting of over 60% indicates that the seeds are relatively fresh. The sprouted seeds are best offered within the first 36 h after sprouting. Zebra finches also like soaked seeds (soaked for a day in clean water and rinsed), but soaked seeds should be fed immediately as microorganisms can quickly start growing on them.

Zebra finches have a specially adapted muscular gizzard with a tough abrasive keratin-like layer of koilin lining that functions as a gastric mill and mechanically breaks down the food. This is further aided by the birds dehusking seed prior to ingestion. Because of this adaptation, some authors believe zebra finches don't require access to insoluble grit or flint or quartz chips to assist the breakdown of seeds in the gizzard, but this claim is still contested. When these materials have been used as a substitute for soluble calcium, they have been reported to cause digestive disturbances (Taylor 1996). In any case, birds should still be provided with soluble grit (e.g., powdered oyster grit), cuttlefish bone or a proprietary water-soluble calcium supplement to meet the birds' higher calcium requirements during breeding and moulting (Stockdale 2018). Cuttlefish bones, positioned so that the birds have access to the softer side, not only serve as a source of calcium but they have the additional benefit of helping to keep the birds' bill in good trim, avoiding the need to handle birds for beak trimming.

Zebra finches can – once or twice a week – be also offered good-quality greens such as dandelion leaves, freshly cut grass stalks, the darker outer leaves of lettuce, chickweed, spinach, watercress or vegetables (e.g., grated carrots, cucumbers) as well as fruits (e.g., apples, oranges and bananas). It may be necessary to try several vegetables and fruits before deciding what appeals to the individual finches. Greens, vegetables and fruits form an important source of dietary carotenoids that positively influence the bird's health and affect bill coloration (Blount *et al.* 2003a; McGraw *et al.* 2003). They also provide a reasonable level of a few vitamins and minerals, thereby supplementing in some ways what's missing in the seeds (Shepherd 2012). The diet can be further supplemented with insect prey, such as mealworms or cricket nymphs (again one may need to try different insects to see what appeals to the individual finches). This live food, together with other supplements such as commercial egg-based biscuit crumb or minced boiled egg can be occasionally provided as a source of extra protein, especially when breeding. If offered on a regular basis (e.g., once a week), it should be in small amounts and in several separate dishes, so as to prevent birds overeating and causing gastrointestinal disturbances.

As previously mentioned, special attention should be paid to the birds' diet during breeding. Egg formation is a very demanding process both in nutrients and energy requirements. Protein is of paramount importance in egg formation and females use protein stored in muscle tissue to contribute to egg formation. These stores are built up over several weeks prior to breeding. Therefore, females require a protein-enriched diet (e.g., boiled chicken's eggs, commercial protein supplements) from two weeks before breeding. Zebra finches on a protein-rich diet produced larger eggs, larger clutches and had a higher breeding success than birds on a control diet (Selman & Houston 1996). Good sources of calcium (e.g., calcareous grit, cuttlefish bone, fine oyster shell, supplement in drinking water) provided regularly throughout pre-breeding and breeding resulted in eggs with stronger shells compared to females on a calcium-deficient diet (Reynolds 2001). Pre-laying females supplemented with carotenoids mixed into their drinking water and with carotenoid intakes raised to the upper range of that which their normal seed diet provides formed eggs with higher carotenoid content in the yolk resulting in higher hatching and fledging success and in more brightly coloured males compared to offspring from females on a control diet (McGraw et al. 2005). Rearing and conditioning supplements and greens and fruits are a good source for additional carotenoids. The quality of the diet provided during chick rearing can have important consequences on offspring development. Birds receiving a standard seed mixture with a high-protein nestling mixture (approximately 38% protein) had faster growing offspring that attained larger adult size compared to birds on a standard nestling mix that had about 24% protein (Boag 1987). However, effects of rearing diet on offspring development differed between the sexes (Arnold et al. 2007). Growing individuals experiencing a short period of low–quality diet (lower content of protein, total carotenoids, and vitamins A and E) during the nestling period had an altered antioxidant defence system at adulthood (Blount et al. 2003b), and only offspring that continued to have the same dietary treatment throughout development had a better antioxidant defence system when sexually mature (Noguera et al. 2015). Furthermore, nestlings reared on the low–quality diet took longer to initiate egg-laying, and then laid eggs at a slower rate when allowed to breed compared to birds reared on a standard diet (Blount et al. 2006). Compared to birds that were reared on a standard diet of mixed seed supplemented once a week with eggs and germinated seeds, birds whose nestling diet was supplemented with egg and germinated seeds daily, plus fresh greens three times a week, had a higher growth rate and were faster in being trained at associative learning tasks in adulthood (Brust et al. 2014). By comparison, increased compensatory growth rate in response to poor early growth impairs adult cognitive performance (Fisher et al. 2006).

Although zebra finches (provided they are healthy) can survive at least 250 days without water on a diet of dry seed (Cade et al. 1965), this can result in severe bill deformation and poor plumage (Sossinka 1972b). Zebra finches, therefore, should be given access to clean drinking water on a daily basis. Birds would naturally drink from open water surfaces on the ground, but they also easily accept commercially available drinking bottles which help with hygiene. The latter can be mounted externally to the cage, which will also reduce stress to the birds at water changes. When switching from one kind of water container to another, both should be provided for a while so that the birds can get used to the new ones.

Social housing

Zebra finches are social birds during both the breeding and the non-breeding season (Zann 1996). In the wild they roost communally, jostling for a central position, normally the warmest in the roost (Morris 2006). Pair- and group-mates socially interact with each other through intense vocal communication and physical interactions of affiliative (e.g., allopreening, clumping, beak fencing) as well as aggressive (e.g., pecking, chasing, aggressive beak fencing) nature, which are essential to pair-bond establishment and socialisation (Zann 1996; Adkins-Regan 2002). There are legislative requirements for stocking densities of zebra finches used in research in some countries (see Table 42.1 for the European Community). Overcrowding in captivity would be likely to lead to male rivalries that can include aggressive singing and occasionally 'bill fencing' with picked-on birds typically showing feather loss in the head and neck (Poot et al. 2012; Olson et al. 2014). Similar negative effects may occur when kept under skewed sex ratios or inappropriate stocking densities. For example, one study showed how offspring kept at lower stocking densities developed more complex songs than birds kept at high densities (Poot et al. 2012). In another study, offspring reared in larger groups, irrespective of stocking density, secreted a higher glucocorticoid concentration when disturbed, but this effect was only present in females, but not males (Emmerson & Spencer 2018). Males producing directed songs to attract a female have been shown to experience positive reward feedback in the brain, with contrary effects in the case of undirected songs of singly housed males (Huang & Hessler 2008).

Housing individually in cages or soundproof boxes for weeks is commonly used in behavioural neuroscience studies because it facilitates the acquisition of individual data (Olsson et al. 2003). Individual housing represents an impoverished physical and social environment for social animals and can lead to stereotypic behaviours (Garner et al. 2003), can be a potent stressor (Remage-Healey et al. 2003, but see Schweitzer et al. 2014; Crino et al. 2017) and can have moderately detrimental effects on the activity of the brain's limbic region and can modify vocal activity (Elie et al. 2015). Separation from conspecifics by isolating zebra finch males affected their vocal communication and socialisation behaviour even if vocal and visual contacts were maintained (Elie et al. 2015) and resulted in weight loss (Yamahuchi et al. 2017). These results have implications for studies on vocal communication and behavioural neurosciences of individually housed zebra finches, especially in terms of experimental design. If zebra finches need to be housed individually, the time during which they are kept away from others should be minimised (e.g., Joint Working Group on Refinement 2001). The use of mirrors in social birds, as opposed to territorial birds or birds with strict dominance hierarchy where mirrors could result in increased aggression, can mitigate the effects of limited social contact (Henry et al. 2008). There is limited evidence that individually housed zebra finches exposed to mirrors which were occasionally repositioned tended to be less frightened by human disturbance than birds without mirrors (Yamahuchi et al. 2017), but further research is required.

When introducing unfamiliar birds, or regrouping birds, the group needs to be carefully monitored for social compatibility (e.g., unusual weight loss, signs of pecking). If breeding is in groups (i.e., parentage will be uncertain, see *Social organisation* section in the preceding text), care should be taken that an excess of nesting sites is provided, as birds will compete for them and actively and aggressively defend them. Distributing the breeding birds over several smaller aviaries with appropriate stocking densities (see Table 42.1) instead of breeding all together in one large aviary minimises levels of aggression. In 2 : 1 male-biased breeding sex ratios, social instabilities may result in more aggressive behaviours, weight loss, reduced body condition and poorer immune functions, as has been observed in other captive finches (Greives et al. 2007).

In summary, social conditions, group size and density can influence the welfare of zebra finches in laboratories and should be carefully considered.

Identification and sexing

The most common method to individually mark zebra finches is to use split leg rings. If coloured leg rings are required for individual identification, it is important to be aware that the colour of the rings may have profound effects on their social behaviour, mate attractiveness, longevity and offspring sex ratio and development (Burley et al. 1982; Burley 1986, 1988; Swaddle & Cuthill 1994; Cuthill et al. 1997; Arnold et al. 2016); although not all studies have confirmed these effects (see, e.g., Hunt et al. 1997; Rutstein et al. 2004, 2005). In some studies, females preferred males with red leg rings and with symmetrical arrangements of multiple colours and disliked males with green leg rings and with asymmetrical arrangements of multiple colours, and the same colour preferences were found for captive and recently caught wild females. Males most prefer females with black leg rings and least prefer females with light-blue colour rings. Zebra finches do not appear to distinguish between un-ringed birds and those with orange leg rings. Ring colour also affects intra-sexual dominance interactions with red-ringed males being socially dominant over green-ringed males. Hence, it is best to use colours that have less impact on the birds' behaviour and where different colours are unavoidable, to provide a sufficient number of different food sources to avoid dominant birds monopolising the food (Joint Working Group on Refinement 2001). Increasingly, birds are being individually marked with passive integrated transponders (PIT-tags, or microchips), very small glass- or resin-encased devices that respond to an external scanner placed in close proximity and giving an individual recognition and would allow tracking of individual bird's activity and automatically adding to an electronic record of the bird's history. They are cheap and easy to use and can be implanted subcutaneously or can be mounted on a leg ring and may offer an alternative marking method for laboratory birds in the future. There is little known about potential harmful side-effects of PIT-tags on the bird's physiology, anatomy or behaviour but, when implanted, their location can negatively affect the bird's health (Oswald et al. 2018).

The zebra finch is sexually dimorphic and from 2 to 3 months of age the sexes can readily be distinguished on the basis of plumage markings (Figure 42.1) and the fact that only the male sings. In addition, males have a redder beak colour whereas the beak of females is more orange, which may help to determine sex in pure white colour varieties. Before reaching the mature plumage, the sexes may be distinguished by using certain varieties where colour inheritance is sex-linked (Birkhead et al. 1989; Kilner 1998) or by taking a small drop of blood or a feather to use in a molecular sex determination (Griffiths et al. 1996).

Physical environment

In natural environments, temperatures are often highly variable and zebra finches can withstand a wide range of temperatures (Zann 1996). Outside the breeding season, wild zebra finches can experience very cold nights and protect themselves from low temperatures by communal roosting or building non-breeding nests. Birds kept indoors do well when the temperature is maintained between 20 and 25 °C, and extremes are avoided (Joint Working Group on Refinement 2001), but it may be worth considering a slightly reduced overnight temperature – where heating system allows – so as to more closely mimic natural variations in temperature and nocturnal social behaviour (Law et al. 2010). If zebra finches are kept outdoors, the flight areas of the aviaries should be protected from wind and driving rain in the winter months, and suitably shaded areas provided for the summer. Hessian sacking or other garden centre windbreak materials can be used around bird flights to provide protection. Various species of dense shrubs – obviously avoiding poisonous varieties – have been used in aviaries to provide zebra finches with shelter and a secure retreat.

Humidity requirements for captive zebra finches are poorly understood. In the wild, they respond to increased rainfall and humidity – and a corresponding increase in food availability – with breeding activity (Zann et al. 1995). Even under standardised conditions in the laboratory, changes in humidity can trigger nest-building behaviour if suitable nest material is available (Cynx 2001) and seasonal changes in breeding intensity are possibly due to small, uncontrolled variations in humidity (Williamson et al. 2008). Humidity levels between 40 and 80% are typically recommended for breeding birds as low humidity can negatively affect hatching success of eggs, but we have maintained zebra finches in laboratory conditions at ca. 40–55% humidity for many years with no apparent adverse effect (Law et al. 2010). If humidity is too low and there is no automated way of correcting it, it is worth considering the use of a simple source of humidity (e.g., mopping floors with water) to increase ambient humidity.

Zebra finches are diurnal birds and both photoperiod and light quality are important in captive environments. Absolute day length and changes in day length can trigger behavioural and physiological changes. Most zebra finch colonies are kept in light : dark cycles of between 14 : 10 and 12 : 12, with shortening day lengths increasing the probability of breeding (Perfito et al. 2007). At light : dark cycles of 15 : 9, birds showed signs of fatigue (Mak et al. 2015). Under continuous light, mortality increased (Snyder et al. 2013) and impaired spatial and colour association learning (Jha & Kumar 2017), and so checks that light has not been left on accidentally in the birds' dark phase are worth considering. The change from light to dark in the cycle should be gradual, so as to allow birds to find a suitable roost site for the night. Having some dim, background light in the night, equivalent to moon light, may be beneficial for the birds, mimicking natural conditions and reducing fear in case they experience any disturbances during the dark period (Bateson & Feenders 2010; Law et al. 2010). The visual system of zebra finches differs from that of humans in that they perceive light over a larger spectral range – since they can also see in UV – compared to humans – and the UV component of light affects captive zebra finches' mate choice (Bennett et al. 1996). Birds also have a higher flicker fusion frequency than humans (Boström et al. 2016) and perceive television sets, computers and low-frequency fluorescent lights as flickering lights. Both aspects of light quality affect glucocorticoid levels in wild-caught starlings, and light sources that flicker within the starling's range of perception (ca. 30–100 Hz) increased frequency of involuntary muscle spasms (myoclonus) where the bird's entire head would twitch in a rapid and apparently involuntary fashion (Maddocks et al. 2002; Smith et al. 2005a,b; Evans et al. 2012). Although we don't know for certain whether this is also a welfare issue in species with a longer history of captivity, it is likely that zebra finches respond to flickering rate, as their mate choice behaviour is compromised under low frequency flickering rates (ca. 30 Hz, Evans et al. 2006). Therefore, captive zebra finches kept on artificial lighting will most likely benefit from high-frequency (>30 kHz) fluorescent tubes that provide the full natural light spectrum, and other sources of flickering lights should be avoided (Bateson & Feenders 2010). Light levels should be of an appropriate brightness, as bird vision works well in light levels suitable for humans (i.e., around 500 lux). It is also worth considering whether there needs to be an emergency lighting system in case of power failures, as birds will not forage in the dark.

The average temperature, humidity and photoperiod that laboratory zebra finches are exposed to 20.7–22.2 °C, 45.8–48.9% of humidity and a photoperiod of 13.5–13.8 h of day light (Beaulieu 2016; Griffith et al. 2017a). Based on long-term climatic averages for the different Australian biomes, Beaulieu (2016) concluded that the conditions typically encountered in laboratories were unrepresentative of natural conditions. However, Griffith et al. (2017b) argue that temperature, humidity and photoperiod conditions typically used in laboratories are well within the range of conditions seen during the breeding season at typical zebra finch breeding sites. Moreover, Beaulieu (2016) argued that laboratory conditions deviating from average natural conditions were associated with elevated basal glucocorticoid levels indicating that captive zebra finch studies might have been conducted under stressful conditions, although comparing glucocorticoid levels across laboratories and assays is complex, and further cautious studies into this possibility are required (Griffith et al. 2017b).

Adequate air circulation is essential to prevent accumulation of dust and gases (e.g., carbon dioxide, ammonia). In the authors' bird rooms, 13–15 air changes per hour are the norm. This air-changing rate is thought to be adequate for the birds and for the staff working in those rooms, provided sources of dust are minimised by, for example, using a cage litter with low dust emission. Good ventilation should be achieved without causing draughts. Bird house ventilation ducts should be fitted with filters of a suitable size, able to remove fine dust and dander before venting outside. The inevitable build-up of feathers and dust on ventilation ducts can be remedied by regular vacuuming.

Ventilation equipment can – as do other types of equipment – produce noise which needs consideration. Passerine birds have a narrower range of hearing than humans and it is unlikely that they can perceive infra- or ultrasound (Dooling & Therrien 2012). But both acutely and chronically raised noise levels may affect the welfare of the birds and some types of noises (e.g., white noise) are more detrimental than others (Wright et al. 2007). Loud background noise can erode the strong pair bond in zebra finches (Swaddle & Page 2006) and can potentially mask conspecific vocalisation that influences the breeding schedule and clutch size in zebra finch colonies, presumably through social stimulation (Waas et al. 2005). Acoustic enrichment has been little explored in birds, but so far there is some evidence that they respond to playing background natural sounds and music (rock and classic) with increased activity (Robbins & Margulis 2016). It will be worth investigating whether acoustic enrichment is an acceptable method for managing the auditory laboratory environment by masking potentially more stressful sounds such as, for example, chronic loud noise as well as sudden unexpected sounds from ventilation (reviewed in Patterson-Kane & Farnworth 2006). If the decision is taken to play music in bird rooms, the suggestion is to use classical or easy listening music played not above a conversational level (about 60 dB) so as not to interfere with the birds' acoustic communication, and only during the birds' active periods (Patterson-Kane & Farnworth 2006). The potential positive and negative effects of playing music, however, should be carefully monitored for the specific welfare goal after introducing the practice (Kriengwatana et al. 2022).

Hygiene

Hygiene measures in the facility should take account of a variety of factors, such as health status of the birds, proximity to other laboratory animals, potential contact with wildlife, environmental controls and the staff working in the facility. In general, access to the aviary should be restricted to essential staff and protective/dedicated clothing should be donned. The use of masks and other respiratory Personal Protective Equipment (PPE) is particularly important during times of cage/flight cleaning, but some facilities may require their use at all times. Hand-washing facilities within the room facilitate personal and room hygiene, and easy access to running water can also help with daily/weekly husbandry chores (e.g., filling up water fountains).

There should be a plan in place for regular cage/flight/room cleaning and disinfection, based on both animals' and staff wellbeing and the need to control potential build-up of pathogens. Such a plan will depend on factors such as stocking densities, type of caging, type of bedding material, efficiency of heating, ventilation and air conditioning (HVAC) system, health status of animals, risks of entry of adventitious agents.

Facilities may choose to clean and sanitise rooms with water and disinfectants before any new batch of birds arrives and thoroughly decontaminate them (e.g., with hydrogen peroxide vapour) when rooms are empty. Internal bird flights and cages should have the substrates regularly changed; the length of time between changes will depend mostly on the stocking density. Waste substrate and seed from bird cages should, where possible, be vacuumed with low-noise vacuum cleaners fitted with high-efficiency particulate air (HEPA) filters, which help avoid the displacement of fine dust particles into the air. Perches should regularly be removed and washed in disinfectant and then rinsed in fresh water and left to dry before re-use. Cage walls and any cage wire also need periodic cleaning, as do food, water and grit containers. Many of these items will be able to withstand more thorough sterilisation procedures (e.g., VHP) and should be included in the regular plan of periodic decontamination.

Health monitoring, quarantine and barrier systems

A plan for regular health monitoring of birds should be put in place in consultation with veterinary staff and stakeholders. Such a plan will vary depending on the type of facility, the needs and expectations of researchers, regulatory demands, provenance of birds, etc., and will need to include a risk analysis of the potential entry of unwanted pathogens and/or zoonotic agents. In contrast to the case of some of the more common species used in biomedical research, there are no international recommendations for health screening of laboratory zebra finches (nor any other bird species for that matter). Institutions need to formulate their own plans for health screening based, as mentioned before, on local risk analysis and taking advice from veterinarians and other professionals (e.g., occupational health services) considering the health of both birds and humans working in the facility. Zebra finches may be affected by a very wide range of infectious agents (see *Common health and welfare problems* section in the following text) and it is not possible to screen for everything all the time. In addition, the choice of specialised diagnostic laboratories that can handle bird samples is more limited than with other species and – likewise – the range of tests they offer. Hence, careful consideration of what to test for, when and how, is warranted.

There may be sparse information about the health status of birds coming into a facility and, in addition, the stress of transport can lower the animals' natural defences and precipitate disease. Therefore, quarantining new arrivals is a safety policy that has much to recommend it. A dedicated quarantine room, with as much separation from the facility's birds as possible, is best. What this separation entails and what the length of quarantine should be requires a different analysis of risks and discussion with stakeholders. In one survey, many facilities were found to operate a 30-day quarantine period, allowing sufficient time for health screening of new arrivals and/or institution of prophylactic treatments (Patterson & Fee 2015).

All staff should be aware of the normal behaviour of zebra finches and able to recognise when they are ill and need attention (see *Health* section in the following text). Ill or injured individuals may need to be housed individually in a 'hospital cage'. Such a hospital cage should contain a heat source that the bird can move towards or away from and which – ideally – can be regulated. There are commercially available products that offer this feature but, if budgets are tight, an alternative good heat source is a 25 W tungsten bulb with a temperature of about 24 °C. Hospital cages can be located within the same room where the birds are kept, but if there is concern about a contagious disease, it is preferable to keep the hospital cage elsewhere or isolate the sick bird/s in a room with separate air ventilation or appropriate filters so as to protect the stock. Hospital cages should provide a good supply of food in shallow dishes and fresh water in low water bottles placed on or near the floor for easier access.

Breeding

Zebra finches can breed throughout the year in indoor aviaries. However, even under the relatively constant environmental temperature and constant day length of captive breeding facilities, productivity may show seasonal variation with more clutches being produced in summer and autumn (Boruszewska *et al.* 2007; Williamson *et al.* 2008). Captive birds as young as 3 months are physiologically ready to breed, but both age and breeding experience affect reproductive strategies and breeding success in female zebra finches (Williams & Christians 2003; Baran & Adkins-Regan 2014).

To maximise the likelihood of breeding, young birds should be allowed to express mate choice, choosing their own partners from a small mixed-sex group. If particular pairings are required, however, most male/female couples in good condition will breed when placed in the same cage. Pair bond formation between unfamiliar birds can start immediately after introduction, where the male performs a characteristic courtship dance and direct song towards the female and the female carries out an acceptance posture (for more details, see Zann 1996). A sure sign of an established pair bond is when the male and female sit close to and preen each other.

Captive birds need to be provided with suitable nesting sites. Different types of nesting sites are available from wicker baskets and half coconut shells, to re-usable wooden or single-use cardboard nestboxes. Commercially available nestboxes typically have linear dimensions of at least 10 cm and an entrance hole of at least 4 cm diameter. Nestboxes mounted externally to the aviary mesh are convenient since the nest can be checked with minimal disturbance to the breeding birds. Birds need to be provided with suitable nesting material, but not in great excess. Usually, the birds will start to build a nest almost immediately after pairing. Coconut fibre is a good nesting material to build a complex enclosed nest chamber (Figure 42.4), but when offered ready-made nestboxes, birds often build less complex structures. The inside of the nest chamber is lined with some softer material. In captivity, feathers, cotton wool, fine sisal string or moss can be used; it is important to ensure that there is no risk of the birds getting their toes caught in the chosen nesting material. When using nestboxes, birds prefer to sit level with the entrance hole so that, if the entrance is too high up, the bottom of the nestbox can be filled with floor substrate. Provision of nest material should stop once the clutch is complete, as otherwise birds may continue to add nest material over the eggs and lay another clutch on top ('sandwich clutches').

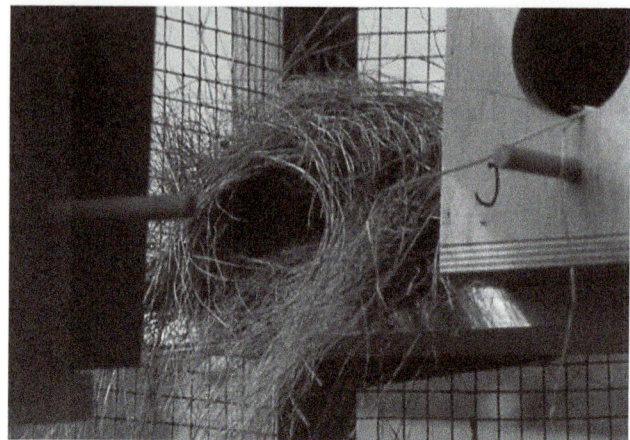

Figure 42.4 Zebra finches build nests when suitable nest support and nest material are available (nest on the left). Similar nests can be built inside nestboxes, which might be more suitable for outdoor aviaries and, when mounted from the outside, minimise disturbance to the breeding birds. Source: Photo: R. Nager.

The onset of breeding can be facilitated by provision of soaked seeds, and greens and/or spraying a fine mist of water over the birds, but these measures are not essential. Also, good nutrition will affect the birds' breeding behaviour (see *Feeding and watering* section in the preceding text). Usually within a week the nest is finished, and the females start laying. In captivity, around the time when the third egg is laid (or even earlier), the birds start sitting on the eggs. This onset of incubation is earlier than in wild birds, resulting in a larger hatching asynchrony than in wild birds (Gilby *et al*. 2013). Both sexes help to incubate the eggs and keep them covered for close to 100% of the time (Gorman & Nager 2003; Gorman *et al*. 2005). At least from the late incubation stage onwards, female zebra finches can recognise their own eggs on the basis of odour (Moskát *et al*. 2016). After approximately 2 weeks of incubation, the eggs will start to hatch. The newly hatched nestlings are blind and only have a few areas of soft down. At hatching, a rearing food (see *Feeding and watering* section in the preceding text) should be provided together with the regular seed mixture. Like most estrildines, zebra finch nestlings are slow developers, and they spend longer in the nest and take longer to reach adult weight than other granivorous species, such as fringillidaes and ploceines (Zann 1996). Both parents feed the nestlings by regurgitating seeds from their crop into the crop of their offspring, albeit the crop of newly hatched nestlings (day 0) is empty as parents only start feeding the next day. Initially, only the right side of the crop is filled and only later, when larger quantities need to be stored, the left side of the crop also fills. Nestling zebra finches are very hardy and 4–5-day-old chicks can endure periods of up to 36 h without being fed and brooded, presumably entering some form of torpor. Nestlings start to make soft begging calls from the third day onwards, feathers start to break through by 6–7 days and eyes open fully by day 10–11. Nestlings can be individually marked using non-toxic pens on the skin and tufts of down, and marks may need to be renewed regularly. From around 8 or 9 days old, nestlings can be ringed with leg rings. To avoid birds leaving the nest prematurely, regular nest checks should be stopped when the birds are about 2 weeks old. When the birds are around 18 days old, they will leave the nest for the first time. Around day 35, the birds will become independent and feed independently, although they will continue to beg for a while longer. Around this time, the bill colour starts to change from black to a lighter colour (which will eventually turn orange or red) and the post-juvenile moult into the adult plumage begins.

For best breeding results, birds should be kept at lower densities than in standard holding accommodation listed in Table 42.1, maintained in an equal sex ratio and provided with an excess of nest sites. When zebra finches breed in groups, both extra-pair paternity and intra-specific brood parasitism can occur (Birkhead *et al*. 1990; Baran & Adkins-Regan 2014). Under good conditions, zebra finches may breed continuously; but it is best not to allow them to produce more than two successive broods before a period of non-breeding. At the end of breeding, the nest should be removed. If two successive clutches are desired, young need to be removed from the parent's cage when independent and housed in their own cage of appropriate size and suitable social environment. If they are left with the parents, they may interrupt the next clutch and the parents may chase off the young birds and pluck their feathers. If a particular behavioural study (e.g., on song learning) requires that young are raised by females alone, it is not necessary to remove the male before day 5, as there is no evidence of young memorising the father's song before that age; a reduction of the brood size may also be advantageous as broods raised by one parent do less well than broods raised by both parents even in captivity (Royle *et al*. 2002). Zebra finches can also be raised from the egg stage onwards by Bengalese finches. However, both interspecific cross-fostering and female-only rearing will affect the behavioural development of the chicks. If pairs fail to feed their chicks at first, particularly first-time breeders, the nestlings can be helped through that period by some hand feeding. Breeding success of zebra finches can vary substantially between laboratories. In a comparative study, only 64% of females that had the opportunity to breed successfully raised at least one fledgling, with hatching failure being the main determinant of breeding success (Griffith *et al*. 2017a). Variation in breeding success between studies can be due to a range of factors (housing, social environment, humidity, temperature, handling, disturbance, diet) and further studies identifying what factors are most influential would help standardise breeding across studies that would allow more generalised conclusions. Mak *et al*. (2015) provide useful further guidelines on how to breed zebra finches in the laboratory.

One of the factors that can explain differences in breeding success between individual pairs is inbreeding. Inbred parents have shown a lower hatching success and inbred females have a lower incubation attentiveness compared to non-inbred females (Pooley *et al*. 2014). Therefore, it is important to keep detailed breeding records and have sufficient accommodation in order to prevent breeding between close relatives, allow the elimination of poor breeders and the efficient rotation of stock used in breeding. Several pedigree software packages are available for this purpose, such as ZooEasy[5] or LaoTzu's Animal Register.

---

[5] https://www.zooeasy.com/ (Accessed 23 June 2022)

Laboratory procedures

Handling

If specific individuals need to be captured and handled on a regular basis, it may be preferable to keep them in small cages where they are more easily and rapidly captured. Although this practice may require an exemption from legally established standard stocking densities – where available – it is less stressful to the individual bird as well as for other birds in the same cage or in other cages in the same room, and might be critically important for studies on stress physiology (Romero & Reed 2005). In large cages, a bird net with padded edges will almost certainly be required for catching birds. Switching off the light can help to catch the bird more quickly in the dark. Once in the hand, birds should be kept with the back inside the palm of the hand, its head between the index and second finger, and the wings gently closed against its sides so that the bird's chest remains free.

Training and habituation for procedures

Acclimating young animals to handling and restraint can reduce fear stress and positively affects the animal's welfare and productivity (Grandin & Shively 2015). Zebra finches are believed not to habituate easily to handling and, compared to many other cage birds, they do not become very tame and are not as inquisitive. Nonetheless, zebra finches will work for food, and can learn to respond to light and colour cues and to discriminate between different songs and sounds. Rewarding zebra finches after disturbance is an effective and simple way to improve their habituation to handling (Collins et al. 2008). Suitable rewards are small pieces of fruit, salad and live insect prey (see Feeding and watering section in the preceding text).

Monitoring methods

Body temperature can be recorded using small temperature probes (<0.5 mm wide) that are carefully inserted into the colorectum via the cloaca. Body temperature can now also be measured using non-invasive methods, like gluing temperature-sensitive radio tags to the birds' skin or using infrared thermal imaging (McCafferty et al. 2015). The new methodology has already been used for assessing a bird's stress response and body condition (Herborn et al. 2015; Jerem et al. 2018) without the need to handle the bird and/or obtain a blood sample. If blood for haematological, hormonal or biochemical analyses is required, it can be collected from three sites: right jugular vein, ulnar/basilar vein and the medial metatarsal vein. As these are all superficial veins, they can be accessed using a sterile needle or lancet and anaesthesia is not normally necessary, with the possible exception of the jugular vein (Chitty 2018). Blood collection should only be carried out by trained and experienced staff. Bleeding can be stopped by pressure from a swab. The vein, in particular the jugular vein, may be more easily recognisable in a well exercised bird with small fat deposits, in turn reducing the duration the bird needs to be handled. The quantity of blood that can be safely collected from healthy individuals is limited to 10% of the circulating blood volume (which is about 0.1 ml for a 16 g zebra finch) and less if the same bird is re-sampled in less than 3–4 weeks (maximum of 1% of circulating blood volume or 0.01 ml for a 16 g zebra finch per 24 h) (Morton et al. 1993). Collection of faeces and urine is easily accomplished by temporarily placing a non-contaminating material (e.g., kitchen roll) over the normal cage's substrate. There are non-destructive methods for collecting a sample of the crop content (Zann & Straw 1984; Chitty 2018), skin and feathers (Chitty 2018) and of semen (Pellatt & Birkhead 1994).

Administration of substances

Some drugs can be mixed with food or drinking water. However, since zebra finches usually remove the husk of the seeds before ingesting them, it is unlikely that they would ingest any drugs on the outside of the seed, unless de-husked seed is used. These oral methods can be useful for administering substances to a large number of birds, but do not permit accurate control of dosage. Suitably sized crop tubes can be used for individual birds, which allows for more accurate dosing. Crop capacity in birds may be estimated at around 30–50 ml/kg (Montesinos 2018).

Injections in small passerines like the zebra finch are difficult and hazardous. Subcutaneous and intramuscular injections can generally be given with a 27 G needle and a 1 ml insulin syringe, but great caution is necessary. A small amount of alcohol is normally used to prepare the site before injection. When the needle is removed, a dry cotton-tipped applicator is placed over the site to apply gentle pressure and stop any bleeding. Subcutaneous injections can be administered at a variety of sites (e.g., inguinal, interscapular, axillary) although the precrural fold is preferable, while intramuscular injections are typically given in pectoral muscles (Montesinos 2018). Intracoelomic injections in zebra finches are possible but great care should be taken in order to avoid damaging air sacs or other internal organs; the midline of the lower third of the body has been recommended (Patterson & Fee 2015). If intraosseous administration is required, the use of a 27–30G needle in the distal ulna or the tibiotarsus is a possibility (Patterson & Fee 2015; Montesinos 2018).

Anaesthesia and analgesia

General anaesthesia can be achieved using gaseous or injectable anaesthetics. As in other species, gaseous anaesthetics have many advantages over injectable ones and they are generally a safer option in birds. However, they do require specialist equipment for precision delivery and considerable knowledge and skills for safe use in small birds. The most commonly used gaseous anaesthetic agents are isoflurane, sevoflurane and desflurane. The latter two agents provide faster induction and recovery when compared to the former, which – although widely used – is an agent capable of causing profound respiratory depression in birds (Speer 2018). Various injectable anaesthetics may be used in finches.

Combinations of ketamine-xylazine, ketamine-midazolam or ketamine-diazepam are possible, and some of these drugs can also be used on their own (or combined with drugs such as butorphanol) to provide sedation rather than anaesthesia. Similarly, drugs used in other species for provision of analgesia, such as opioids and non-steroidal anti-inflammatory drugs, can be used in passerines but bearing in mind that pain assessment in birds is still in its infancy and that analgesic efficacy has not been critically evaluated in most birds. The reader should refer to specialised textbooks or chapters on avian anaesthesia and analgesia (e.g., Samour 2000; Hawkins & Paul-Murphy 2011; Flecknell 2016; Malik & Valentine 2018; Speer 2018) for drug dosages, methods of delivery and monitoring and other pertinent information.

Euthanasia

There are widely referenced guidelines on euthanasia of many different species for veterinarians who carry out or oversee the humane killing of animals[6]. If zebra finches need to be euthanised, overdose of gaseous or injectable anaesthetics can be used; the latter may be preceded by sedation if appropriate. Because of their small size, injectable euthanasia agents are difficult to administer safely and effectively in them and, therefore, use of gaseous anaesthetics is preferable (Eatwell 2008). Exposure to a rising concentration of carbon dioxide in an enclosed chamber has been used, but the humaneness of this method – as in other species – is controversial. Birds can also be killed by neck dislocation by an experienced person but this method – although currently allowed in European legislation – may not be ideal, as evidence from studies in poultry indicates that it does not always lead to immediate loss of brain function (see review by Martin *et al.* 2019). Decapitation is another physical method currently approved in most European countries and the USA, provided it is carried out competently. Some authors advocate the use of gas anaesthesia immediately prior to using physical methods such as decapitation or cervical dislocation, in order to reduce stress and facilitate the procedure (Patterson & Fee 2018).

Common health and welfare problems

Health

Like any other captive bird, laboratory zebra finches can be affected by a variety of infectious diseases caused by bacteria, viruses, parasites, fungi and yeasts (Dorrestein 1996; Jones & Slater 1999) and – if allowed to grow old – ageing and degenerative and metabolic/nutritional disorders (see Table 42.2). However, few – if any – of these disorders manifest themselves in specific, pathognomonic ways. In addition, finches – like other prey species – can hide signs of ill health even to the skilful observer and yet, given their high metabolic rate, disease can take a rapid course. For these

[6]https://www.avma.org/sites/default/files/2020-01/2020_Euthanasia_Final_1-15-20.pdf (Accessed 23 June 2022)

Table 42.2 Some infectious and non-infectious diseases/conditions of zebra finches.

Disease	Comments
Viral	
Avian pox	Uncommon. Conjunctivitis, blepharitis. Self-limiting but may be fatal. Common in some species. Torticollis, depression, weight loss
Paramyxovirus	Severe pancreatitis on *post-mortem*
Papovavirus	Common in some aviaries. Deaths among nestlings and young birds, developmental abnormalities, beak deformities. Hepatocellular necrosis on histopathology
Bacterial	
Enterobacteriaceae	*E. coli* septiceaemia can be a problem in new shipments (stress-related). *Citrobacter, Salmonella* and *Yersinia* have also been reported
Mycobacteria	Tuberculosis (usually due to atypical *M. avium*) can affect finches, and may be more common than previously suspected
Campylobacter	More common in tropical finches such as the Bengalese. Inactivity, yellow droppings and high mortality among fledglings. Can be treated with appropriate antibiotics
Chlamydophila (Psittacosis)	Rare. Conjunctivitis, debilitation, diarrhoea. May see hepatomegaly on *post-mortem*
Pseudomonas	Usually associated with poor hygiene. Foul-smelling diarrhoea
Fungal	
Gastric yeast	*Macrorhabdus ornithogaster* (formerly, Megabacteria) is commonly found in finches. Not too clear whether it can be a primary pathogen, but it can certainly result in a chronic, debilitating condition. Affected birds are fluffed up, constantly hungry and progressively lose condition
Candida	Associated with poor hygiene and unbalanced diets. Crop candidiasis is seen as a distended, thickened crop with a white covering of the mucosa. Can also cause diarrhoea and moulting problems
Parasitic	
Protozoans	Various coccidian species can affect finches. *Isospora serine* (atoxoplasmosis) causes debilitation, diarrhoea and sometimes neurological signs, but is not very common. Other *Isospora* species (causing diarrhoea and weight loss) are more frequently encountered. Trichomoniasis causes respiratory symptoms, regurgitation and emaciation. *Cochlosoma* is not uncommon in Bengalese finches and can cause problems in other varieties. *Toxoplasma* can also be found in finches
Helminths	Both tapeworms and roundworms can be a problem, but they are rare in well-managed aviaries and tend to be associated with the feeding of live food

Table 42.2 (Continued)

Disease	Comments
Arthropods	*Cnemidocoptes* mites can cause abnormal crusting and deformities on the base of the beak. Air sac mites (*Sternostoma tracheacolum*) can cause respiratory signs but are rare in finches
Metabolic/ Nutritional	In general, malnutrition is a major factor behind multiple conditions affecting various organs and systems, especially skin and feathers, reproduction and respiration. Obesity, for example, can be a common problem in captive birds and lead to serious conditions such as fatty liver, atherosclerosis, pancreatitis, diabetes, xanthoma-formation. Excess protein can lead to gout. Calcium and vitamin D deficiencies can lead to misshapen bones, fractures, tremors, egg retention. Vitamin A deficiency can lead to lethargy, nasal discharge, sneezing, conjunctivitis, rhinoliths. Deficiency of B vitamins may lead to various neurological conditions.
Neoplastic	Many different neoplasms can affect finches, from renal/gonadal adenocarcinomas to lymphosarcomas, from thymomas to localised fibromas and lipomas.
Degenerative	Joint disease can affect old birds, limiting their mobility and reducing welfare
Toxic	Various inhalant toxins can significantly compromise the health of birds, including carbon monoxide, Teflon cookware, hair sprays, glues, paints, smoke and formaldehyde. Plant-based toxins include avocado, yew, oleander and lupine. Pesticides such as organophosphates can also be toxic.
Traumatic	By far the most common of these is aggressive pecking from cage mates, but other traumas encountered in the captive environment include accidental concussions, fractures, limb constrictions.

reasons, the emphasis should be placed on good health surveillance and prevention of potential health problems.

In the laboratory setting, with birds living in fairly stable environments, health problems caused by infectious agents are less likely than when birds live in the wild. However, the introduction of new birds (especially if they originate from private owners or bird fanciers) or if birds are kept outdoors at least some of the time can significantly increase the risk of animals coming into contact with infectious agents. Some of these agents (e.g., atoxoplasmosis, avian pox, pseudotuberculosis) can have devastating effects on naïve populations, resulting in high mortality rates. Vaccines developed for use in birds are rare and when available (e.g., canary pox, polyomavirus) are not licensed in all countries. In addition, staff should be aware that the birds can harbour infectious agents that may affect them (zoonosis) and, therefore, should take appropriate precautions when handling them and their environment, especially if birds are showing clinical signs. Although the important zoonotic agent *Chlamydophila psittaci* (the cause of psittacosis, aka ornithosis) is rare in passerines, it needs to be considered as a potential risk. Other possible zoonotic agents that may affect finches are: Campylobacter spp., Salmonella spp., *Mycobacterium avium*, *Yersinia pseudotuberculosis*, *Pasteurella multocida*, Toxoplasma spp. and the red mite *Dermanyssus gallinae*.

As mentioned in previous sections, emergence of health problems in captive finches can be prevented with a few simple measures. Good hygiene with regular and thorough cleaning of enclosures and their furniture is important, and so is the practice of quarantining all newcomers for an appropriate length of time. Birds need a balanced diet together with a good and stimulating environment (see the section *Environmental provisions and enrichments* in the preceding text) that tries to meet their physiological and behavioural requirements. Overcrowding and possible sources of stress such as bullying, the near presence of predators, sudden unfamiliar noises or extremes of temperature should be avoided. In general, it is best to place ill birds in a hospital cage (see *Health monitoring, quarantine and barrier systems* section in the preceding text) and to seek prompt veterinary attention, especially if a contagious disease is suspected.

Readers may refer to in-depth reviews such as Rosskopf and Woerpel (1996), Tully *et al.* (2000), Chitty and Lierz (2008) or Chitty and Monks (2018) for further information on epidemiology, diagnosis, treatment and prevention of diseases in birds.

Behaviour

Inadequate husbandry and/or environmental conditions can result in behavioural problems in laboratory zebra finches. As captive zebra finches are still physiologically and behaviourally similar to wild zebra finches, experiencing an unnatural state has the potential to negatively affect the animal's welfare (Hawkins 2010; Yates 2018). If an animal's physiological and behavioural needs cannot be met, and form and frequency of natural behaviours is expressed differently than in the natural environment, it can develop various abnormal behaviours including repetitive stereotypies (spot picking and route tracing), self-injurious behaviour and mis-directed social behaviours (van Hoek & ten Cate 1998). Lack of data on the importance of natural behaviour patterns to the captive animal and how they can be reliably satisfied in captivity make this a particularly challenging problem. Typical issues encountered in captive environments are poor enclosure design, insufficient space, incompatible social groups, lack of adequate enrichment and inappropriate handling or care. The most common abnormal behaviours seen in captive birds are spot pecking (repeatedly touching a specific spot on the body or in the environment with tip or side of bill) and route tracing (stereotyped jumping from perch to perch) (van Hoek & ten Cate 1998; Garner *et al.* 2003). Aiming to satisfy zebra finches' physical and behavioural needs in the captive situation will allow them to display a broader range of natural behaviours and avoid the development of abnormal ones. If abnormal behaviours are observed, this can be an indication of poor welfare and should be rectified promptly by a thorough revision of the animals' captive environment (including enrichment and social interactions) and their opportunities for performing species-specific behaviours. Care needs to be taken when observing the birds, as their behaviour may change in the presence of an observer, because they are unsettled by it, or afraid or simply interested (Hawkins 2010). Hence, birds should be observed from an appropriate distance or without being seen by them. Getting to know what is normal for the species and even the individual will require significant interest and time investment, but it is essential if one is to detect some of the more subtle behavioural deviations from normality.

Another problematic behaviour in zebra finches is pecking, resulting in feather loss. In zebra finches, this is rarely due to self-directed feather-plucking (Sung 2010), but mostly related to bullying and pecking by cage-mates. There are a range of factors that can trigger this aberrant behaviour including the establishment of dominance hierarchies (for instance, when the social group composition is changed), overcrowding, and lack of appropriate environmental stimulation (Sung 2010; Patterson & Fee 2015). A behaviour indicating good welfare in other species, namely social play, has not been described in finches (Diamond & Bond 2003). Identifying behaviours of zebra finches that are indicators of positive experiences would be of great benefit for a better assessment of their welfare. Given that zebra finches are songbirds and song is one of their characteristic behaviours, its study may be a tool for monitoring their welfare under captive conditions (Yamahachi *et al.* 2017); however, much of our current understanding comes from individually housed birds and, therefore, caution is needed when applying that knowledge.

References

Adkins-Regan, E. (2002). Development of sexual partner preference in the zebra finch: a socially monogamous, pair-bonding animal. *Archives of Sexual Behavior*, **31**, 27–33.

Arnold, K.E., Blount, J.D., Metcalfe, N.B. *et al.* (2007). Sex-specific differences in compensation for poor neonatal nutrition in the zebra finch *Taeniopygia guttata. Journal of Avian Biology*, **38**, 356–366.

Arnold, K. E., Gilbert, L., Gorman, H. E. *et al.* (2016). Paternal attractiveness and the effects of differential allocation of parental investment. *Animal Behaviour*, **113**, 69–78.

Asher, L., Davies, G.T.O., Bertenshaw, C.E. *et al.* (2009). The effects of cage volume and cage shape on the condition and behaviour of captive European starlings (*Sturnus vulgaris*). *Applied Animal Behaviour Science*, **116**, 286–294.

Baran, N.M. and Adkins-Regan, E. (2014). Breeding experience, alternative reproductive strategies and reproductive success in a captive colony of zebra finches (*Taeniopygia guttata*). *PLoS One*, **9**, e89808.

Bateson, M. and Feenders, G. (2010). The use of passerine bird species in laboratory research: implications of basic biology for husbandry and welfare. *Institute for Laboratory Animal Research*, **51**, 394–408.

Beaulieu, M. (2016). A bird in the house: the challenge of being ecologically relevant in captivity. *Frontiers in Ecology & Evolution*, **4**, 141.

Bennett, A.T.D., Cuthill, I.C., Partridge, J.C. and Maier, E.J. (1996). Ultraviolet vision and mate choice in zebra finches. *Nature*, **380**, 433–435.

Birkhead, T.R., Hunter, F.M. and Pellatt, J.E. (1989). Sperm competition in the zebra finch, *Taeniopygia guttata. Animal Behaviour*, **38**, 935–950.

Birkhead, T.R., Burke, T., Zann, R.A. *et al.* (1990). Extra-pair paternity and intra-specific brood parasitism in wild zebra finches *Taeniopygia guttata*, revealed by DNA fingerprinting. *Behavioural Ecology and Sociobiology*, **27**, 315–324.

Birkhead, T.R., Pellatt, E.J., Matthews, I.M. *et al.* (2006). Genic capture and the genetic basis of sexually selected traits in the zebra finch. *Evolution*, **60**, 2389–2398.

Blount, J.D., Metcalfe, N.B., Birkhead, T.R. *et al.* (2003a) Carotenoid manipulation of immune function and sexual attractiveness in zebra finches. *Science*, **300**, 125–127.

Blount, J.D., Metcalfe, N.B., Arnold, K.E. *et al.* (2003b). The effect of pre-breeding diet on reproductive output in zebra finches. *Proceedings of the Royal Society of London Series B-Biological Sciences*, **263**, 1585–1588.

Blount, J.D., Metcalfe, N.B., Arnold, K.E. *et al.* (2006). Effects of neonatal nutrition and adult reproduction in a passerine bird. *Ibis*, **148**, 509–514.

Boag, P. (1987). Effects of nestling diet on growth and adult size of Zebra Finches (*Poephila guttata*). *Auk*, **104**, 155–166.

Boruszewska, K., Witkowski, A. and Jaszczak, K. (2007). Selected growth and development traits of the Zebra Finch (*Poephila guttata*) nestlings in amateur breeding. *Animal Science Papers and Reports*, **25**, 97–110.

Boström, J.E., Dimitrova. M., Canton, C. *et al.* (2016). Ultra-rapid vision in birds. *PLoS ONE*, **11**, e0151099.

Brilot, B., Asher, L. and Bateson, M. (2009). Water bathing alters the speed-accuracy trade-off of escape flights in European starlings. *Animal Behaviour*, **78**, 801–807.

Brust, V., Krüger, O., Naguib, M. and Krause, E.T. (2014). Lifelong consequences of early nutritional conditions on learning performance in zebra finches (*Taeniopygia guttata*). *Behavioural Processes*, **103**, 320–326.

Burley, N. (1985). Leg-band colour and mortality patterns of captive breeding populations of zebra finches. *Auk*, **102**, 647–651.

Burley, N. (1986) Comparison of band colour preferences of two species of estrildid finches. *Animal Behaviour*, **34**, 1732–1741.

Burley, N. (1988). Wild zebra finches have band-colour preferences. *Animal Behaviour*, **36**, 1235–1237.

Burley, N., Krantzberg, G. and Radman, P. (1982). Influence of colour banding on the conspecific preferences of zebra finches. *Animal Behaviour*, **30**, 444–455.

Burley, N.T, Parker, P.G. and Lundy, K. (1996). Sexual selection and extrapair fertilization in a socially monogamous passerine, the zebra finch (*Taeniopygia guttata*) *Behavioral Ecology*, **7**, 218–226.

Butterfield, P.A. (1970). The pair bond in the zebra finch. In: *Social Behaviour in Birds and Mammals*. Ed. Cook, J.H., pp. 149–278. Academic Press, London.

Cade, T.J., Tobin, C.A. and Gold, A. (1965) Water economy and metabolism of two Estrildine finches. *Physiological Zoology*, **38**, 9–33

Calder, W.A. (1964). Gaseous metabolism and water relations of the zebra finch, *Taeniopygia castanotis. Physiological Zoology*, **37**, 400–413.

Chitty, J. (2018). Sample taking and basic clinical pathology. In: *BSAVA Manual of Avian Practice*. Eds Chitty J. and Monks D., pp. 215–231. BSAVA Publications, Gloucester, UK.

Chitty, J. and Lierz, M. (2008). *BSAVA Manual of Raptors, Pigeons and Passerine Birds*. Blackwell Publishing, Oxford.

Chitty, J. and Monks, D. (2018). *BSAVA Manual of Avian Practice*. BSAVA Publications, Gloucester, UK.

Christidis, L. (1987). Phylogeny and systematics of estrildine finches and their relationship to other seed-eating passerines. *Emu*, **87**, 119–123.

Collins, S.A. and ten Cate, C. (1996). Does beak colour affect female preference in zebra finches? *Animal Behaviour*, **52**, 105–112.

Collins, S.A., Archer, J.A. and Barnard, C.J. (2008). Welfare and mate choice in zebra finches: effects of handling regime and presence of cover. *Animal Welfare*, **17**, 11–17.

Conover, M.R. and Messmer, T.A. (1996) Consequences for captive Zebra Finches of consuming tall Fescue seeds infected with the endophytic fungus *Acremonium coenophialum*. *Auk*, **113**, 492–495.

Crino, O.L., Buchanan, K.L., Fanson, B.G. et al. (2017). Divorce in the socially monogamous zebra finch: Hormonal mechanisms and reproductive consequences. *Hormones and Behaviour*, **87**, 155–163.

Cuthill, I.C., Hunt, S., Cleary, C. et al. (1997). Colour bands, dominance, and body mass regulation in male zebra finches (*Taeniopygia guttata*). *Proceedings of the Royal Society of London Series B – Biological Sciences*, **264**, 1093–1099.

Cuthill, I.C., Maddocks, S.A., Weal, C.V. and Jones, E.K.M. (2000). Body mass regulation in response to changes in feeding predictability and overnight energy expenditure. *Behavioral Ecology*, **11**, 189–195.

Cynx, J. (2001). Effects of humidity on reproductive behaviour in male and female zebra finches (*Taeniopygia guttata*). *Journal of Comparative Psychology*, **115**, 196–200.

Diamond, J. and Bond, A.B. (2003). A comparative analysis of social play in birds. *Behaviour*, **140**, 1091–1115.

Dooling, R.J. and Therrien, S.C. (2012). Hearing in birds: what changes from air to water. *Advances in Experimental Medicine and Biology*, **730**, 7–82.

Dorrestein, G.M. (1996). Medicine and surgery of canaries and finches. In: *Diseases of Cage and Aviary Birds*, 3rd edn. Eds Rosskopf, W.J. and Woerpel, R.W., pp. 915–927. William and Wilkins, Baltimore.

Eales, L.A. (1985). Song learning in zebra finches: some effects of song model availability on what is learnt and when. *Animal Behaviour*, **33**, 1293–1300.

Eatwell, K. (2018). Passerine birds: investigation of flock mortality/morbidity. In: *BSVA Manual of Raptors, Pigeons and Passerine Birds*. Eds Chitty, J. and Lierz, M., pp. 370–376. BSVA, Gloucester UK.

Echeverry-Galvis, M.A. and Hau, M. (2012). Molt-breeding overlap alters molt dynamics and behaviour in zebra finches, *Taeniopygia guttata castanotis*. *Journal of Experimental Biology*, **215**, 1957–1964.

Elie, J.E., Soula, H.A., Trouvé, C. et al. (2015). Housing conditions and sacrifice protocol affect neural activity and vocal behavior in a songbird species, the zebra finch (*Taeniopygia guttata*). *Comptes Rendus Biologies*, **338**, 825–837.

Emmerson, M.G. and Spencer, K.A. (2018). Group housing during adolescence has long-term effects on the adult stress response in female, but not male, zebra finches (*Taeniopygia guttata*). *General and Comparative Endocrinology*, **256**, 71–79.

European Union (2010). Directive 2010/63/EU of the European Parliament and of the Council of 22 September 2010 on the protection of animals used for scientific purposes. *Official Journal of the European Union*, **276**, 33–79.

Evans, J.E., Cuthill, I.C. and Bennett, A.T.D. (2006). The effect of flicker from fluorescent lights on mate choice in captive birds. *Animal Behaviour*, **72**, 393–400.

Evans, J.E., Smith, E.L., Bennett, A.T.D. et al. (2012). Short-term physiological and behavioural effects of high- versus low-frequency fluorescent light on captive birds. *Animal Behaviour*, **83**, 25–33.

Ewenson, E.L., Zann, R.A. and Flannery, G.R. (2001). Body condition and immune response in wild zebra finches: effects of capture, confinement and captive-rearing. *Naturwissenschaften*, **88**, 391–394.

Fisher, M.O., Nager, R.G. and Monaghan, P. (2006). Compensatory growth impairs adult cognitive performance. *PLoS Biology*, **4**, e251.

Flecknell, P. (2016). Anaesthesia of common laboratory animal species: special considerations. Other species: birds. In: *Laboratory Animal Anaesthesia*, pp. 249–252. Elsevier, San Diego, California, USA.

Fraser, D. (2008). *Understanding Animal Welfare: The Science in its Cultural Context*. Blackwell-Wiley, Oxford.

Forstmeier, W., Segelbacher, G., Mueller, J.C. et al. (2007). Genetic variation and differentiation in captive and wild zebra finches (*Taeniopygia guttata*). *Molecular Ecology*, **16**, 4039–4050.

Forstmeier, W., Martin, K., Bolund, E. et al. (2011). Female extrapair mating behavior can evolve via indirect selection on males. *Proceedings of the National Academy of Sciences, U.S.A.*, **108**, 10608–10613.

Garner, J.P., Mason, G.J. and Smith, R. (2003) Stereotypic route-tracing in experimentally caged songbirds correlates with general behaviour distribution. *Animal Behaviour*, **66**, 711–727.

Gilby, A.J., Mainwaring, M.C. and Griffith, S.C. (2011). Parental care in wild and captive zebra finches: measuring food delivery to quantify parental effort. *Animal Behaviour*, **81**, 289–295.

Gilby, A.J., Mainwaring, M.C. and Griffith, S.C. (2013). Incubation behaviour and hatching synchrony differ in wild and captive populations of the zebra finch. *Animal Behaviour*, **85**, 1329–1334.

Gorman, H.E. and Nager, R.G. (2003). State-dependent incubation behaviour in the zebra finch. *Animal Behaviour*, **65**, 745–754.

Gorman, H.E., Arnold, K.E. and Nager, R.G. (2005). Incubation effort in relation to male attractiveness in zebra finches (*Taeniopygia guttata*). *Journal of Avian Biology*, **36**, 413–420.

Grandin, T, and Shivley, C. (2015). How Farm animals react and perceive stressful situations such as handling, restraint, and transport. *Animals*, **5**, 1233–1251.

Greives, T.J., Casto, J.M. and Ketterson, E.D. (2007). Relative abundance of males to females affects behaviour, condition and immune function in a captive population of dark-eyed juncos *Junco hyemalis*. *Journal of Avian Biology*, **38**, 255–260.

Griffith, S.C., Crino, O.L., Andrew, S.C. et al. (2017a). Variation in reproductive success across captive populations: Methodological differences, potential biases and opportunities. *Ethology*, **123**, 1–29.

Griffith, S.C., Crino, O.L. and Andrew, S.C. (2017b). Commentary: a bird in the house: the challenge of being ecologically relevant in captivity. *Frontiers in Ecology & Evolution*, **5**, 21.

Griffiths, R., Daan, S. and Dijkstra, C. (1996). Sex identification in birds using two CHD genes. *Proceedings of the Royal Society of London Series B – Biological Sciences*, **263**, 1251–1256.

Griffith, S.C., Holleley, C.E., Mariette, M.M. et al. (2010) Low level of extrapair parentage in wild zebra finches. *Animal Behaviour*, **79**, 261–264.

Hawkins, P. (2010). The welfare implications of having captive wild and domestic birds. In: *The Welfare of the Domestic Fowl and Other Captive Birds*. Eds Duncan, I.J.H. and Hawkins, P., pp. 53–102. Springer Publications, New York.

Hawkins, M.G. and Paul-Murphy, J. (2011). Avian analgesia. *Veterinary Clinics of North America: Exotic Animal Practice*, **14**, 61–80.

Heidinger, B.J., Blount, J.D., Boner, W. et al. (2012). Telomere length in early life predicts lifespan. *Proceedings of the National Academy of Sciences USA*, **109**, 1743–1748.

Henry, L., Le Cars, K., Mathelier, M. et al. (2008). The use of a mirror as a "social substitute" in laboratory birds. *Comptes Rendus Biologies*, **331**, 526–531

Herborn, K., Graves, J.L., Jerem, P. et al. (2015). Skin temperature reveals the intensity of acute stress. *Physiology and Behaviour*, **152**, 225–230.

Hill, D.L., Lindström, J., McCafferty, D.J. and Nager, R.G. (2014). Female but not male zebra finches adjust heat output in response to increased incubation demand. *Journal of Experimental Biology*, **217**, 1326–1332.

Holveck, M-J., Geberzahn, N. and Riebel, K. (2011). An experimental test of condition-dependent male and female mate choice in zebra finches. *PLoS ONE*, **6**, e23974.

Houston, D.C., Donnan, D. and Jones, P.J. (1995). The source of nutrients required for egg production in zebra finches *Poephila guttata*. *Journal of Zoology*, **235**, 469–483.

Huang, Y-C. and Hessler, N.A. (2008). Social Modulation during songbird courtship potentiates midbrain dopaminergic neurons. *PLoS ONE*, **3**, e3281.

Hunt, S., Cuthill, I.C., Swaddle, J.P. et al. (1997). Ultraviolet vision and band-colour preferences in female zebra finches, *Taeniopygia guttata*. *Animal Behaviour*, **54**, 1383–1392.

Immelmann, K., Kalberlah, H.-H., Rausch, P. et al. (1978). Sexuelle Prägung als möglicher Faktor innerartlicher Isolation beim Zebrafinken. *Journal für Ornithologie*, **119**, 197–212.

Jacobs, H., Smith, N., Smith, P. et al. (1995). Zebra finch behaviour and effect of modest enrichment of standard cages. *Animal Welfare*, **4**, 3–9.

Jerem, P., Jenni-Eiermann, S., Herborn, K. et al. (2018). Eye region surface temperature reflects both energy reserves and circulating glucocorticoids in a wild bird. *Scientific Reports*, **8**, 1907.

Jones, A.E. and Slater, P.J.B. (1999). The zebra finch. In: *The UFAW Handbook on the Care and Management of Laboratory Animals*, 7th edn. Ed. Poole, T.B., pp. 722–730. UFAW, Potters Bar.

Jones, K.M., Monaghan, P., and Nager, R.G. (2001). Male mate choice and female fecundity in zebra finches. *Animal Behaviour*, **62**, 1021–1026.

Joint Working Group on Refinement (2001). Laboratory birds: refinements in husbandry and procedures. Fifth Report of the BVAAWF/FRAME/RSPCA/UFAW Joint Working Group on Refinement. *Laboratory Animals*, **35**(Suppl. 1), S1–S163.

Jha, N.A, and Kumar, V. (2017). Effect of no-night light environment on behaviour, learning performance and personality in zebra finches. *Animal Behaviour*, **132**, 29–47.

Kilkenny, C., Browne, W.J., Cuthill, I.C. et al. (2010). Improving bioscience research reporting: the ARRIVE Guidelines for reporting animal research. *PLoS Biology*, **8**, e1000412.

Kilner, R. (1998). Primary and secondary sex ratio manipulation by zebra finches. *Animal Behaviour*, **56**, 155–164.

Kniel, N., Dürler, C., Hecht, I. et al. (2015). Novel mate preference through mate-choice copying in zebra finches: sexes differ. *Behavioral Ecology*, **26**, 647–655.

Krause, T. and Ruploh, T. (2016). Captive domesticated zebra finches (*Taeniopygia guttata*) have increased plasma corticosterone concentrations in the absence of bathing water. *Applied Animal Behaviour Science*, **182**, 80–85.

Krause, E.T., Krüger, O. and Hoffman, J.I. (2017). The influence of inherited plumage colour morph on morphometric traits and breeding investment in zebra finches (*Taeniopygia guttata*). *PLoS ONE*, **12**, e0188582.

Kriengwatana, B.P., Mott, R. and ten Cate, C. (2022). Music for animal welfare: A critical review & conceptual framework. *Applied Animal Behaviour Science*, **251**, 105641.

Law, G., Nager, R.G., Laurie, J. et al. (2010). Aspects of the design of a new birdhouse at the University of Glasgow's Faculty of Biomedical and Life Sciences. *Animal Technology and Welfare*, **9**, 25–30.

Lemon, W.C. (1993). The energetics of lifetime reproductive success in the zebra finch *Taeniopygia guttata*. *Physiological Zoology*, **66**, 946–963.

Lemon, W.C. and Barth, R.H. (1992). The effects of feeding rate on reproductive success in the zebra finch, *Taeniopygia guttata*. *Animal Behaviour*, **44**, 851–857.

Maddocks, S.A., Goldsmith, A.R. and Cuthill, I.C. (2002) Behavioural and physiological effects of absence of ultraviolet wavelengths on European starlings *Sturnus vulgaris*. *Journal of Avian Biology*, **33**, 103–106.

Mak, S-S., Wrabel, A., Nagai, H. et al. (2015). Zebra finch as a developmental model. *Genesis*, **53**, 669–677.

Malik, A. and Valentine, A. (2018). Pain in birds: a review for veterinary nurses. *Veterinary Nursing Journal*, **33**, 11–25.

Marschall, U. and Prinzinger, R. (1991). Vergleichende Ökophysiologie von fünf Prachtfinkenarten (Estrildidae). *Journal für Ornithologie*. **3**, 319–323.

Martin, J.E., Sandilands, V., Sparrey, J. et al. (2019). Welfare assessment of novel on-farm killing methods for poultry. *PLoS ONE*, **14**, e0212872.

Martins, T.L.F. (2004). Sex-specific growth rates in zebra finch nestlings: a possible mechanism for sex ratio adjustment. *Behavioral Ecology*, **15**, 174–180.

Matheson, S.M., Asher, L. and Bateson, M. (2008). Larger, enriched cages are associated with "optimistic" response biases in captive European starlings (*Sturnus vulgaris*). *Applied Animal Behaviour Sciences*, **109**, 374–383.

McCafferty, D.J., Gallon, S. and Nord, A. (2015). Challenges of measuring body temperatures of free-ranging birds and mammals. *Animal Biotelemetry*, **3**, 33.

McCowan, L.S.C., Rollins, L.A. and Griffith, S.C. (2014). Personality in captivity: more exploratory males reproduce better in an aviary population. *Behavioural Processes*, **107**, 150–157.

McGraw, K.J., Gregory, A.J., Parker, R.S. et al. (2003). Diet, plasma carotenoids, and sexual coloration in zebra finch (*Taeniopygia guttata*). *Auk*, **120**, 400–410.

McGraw, K.J., Adkins-Regan, E. and Parker, R.S. (2005). Maternally derived carotenoid pigments affect offspring survival, sex ratio, and sexual attractiveness in a colourful songbird. *Naturwissenschaften*, **92**, 375–380.

Meijer, T., Rozman, J., Schulte, M. et al. (1996) New findings in body mass regulation in zebra finches (*Taeniopygia guttata*) in response to photoperiod and temperature. *Journal of Zoology*, **240**, 717–734.

Minor, M.A. and Lane, N.E. (1996). Recreational exercise in arthritis. *Rheumatic Disease Clinics*, **22**, 563–578.

Montesinos, A. (2018). Basic Techniques. In: *BSAVA Manual of Avian Practice*. Eds Chitty J. and Monks D., pp. 215–231; BSAVA Publications, Gloucester, UK.

Morris, D. (2006). *Watching: Encounters with Humans and Other Animals*. MAX, London.

Morton, D.B., Abbot, D., Barclay, R. et al. (1993). Removal of blood from laboratory mammals and birds. *Laboratory Animals*, **27**, 1–22.

Moskát, C., Golüke, S., Dörrenberg, S. et al. (2016). Female zebra finches smell their eggs. *PLoS One*, **11**, e0155513.

Niedojadlo, J., Bury, A., Cichoń, M. et al. (2018). Lower haematocrit, haemoglobin and red blood cell number in zebra finches acclimated to cold compared to thermoneutral temperature. *Journal of Avian Biology*, e01596.

Noguera, J.C., Monaghan, P. and Metcalfe, N.B. (2015). Interactive effects of early and later nutritional conditions on the adult antioxidant defence system in zebra finches. *Journal of Experimental Biology*, **218**, 2211–2217.

Olson, C.R., Wirthlin, M., Lovell, P.V. and Mello, C.V. (2014). Proper care, husbandry, and breeding guidelines for the zebra finch, *Taeniopygia guttata*. *Cold Spring Harbor Protocols*, **2014**, 1243–1248.

Olsson, I.A.S., Nevison, C.M. Patterson-Kane, E.G. et al. (2003). Understanding behaviour: the relevance of ethological approaches in laboratory animal science, *Applied Animal Behavioural Sciences*, **81**, 245–264.

Oswald, K.N., Evlambiou, A.A., Ribeiro, Â.M. and Smit, B. (2018). Tag location and risk assessment for passive integrated transponder-tagging passerines. *Ibis*, **160**, 453–457.

Patterson, M.M. and Fee, M.S. (2015). Zebra Finches in biomedical research. In: *Laboratory Animal Medicine*. Eds Anderson, L., Otto, G., Pritchett-Corning, K. and Whary, M. pp. 1109–1130; Elsevier, San Diego, California, USA.

Patterson-Kane, E.G. and Farnworth, M.J. (2006). Noise exposure, music, and animals in the laboratory: a commentary based

Pellatt, E.J. and Birkhead, T.R. (1994). Ejaculate size in zebra finches *Taeniopygia guttata* and a method for obtaining ejaculates from passerine birds. *Ibis*, **136**, 97–106.

Peplow, M. (2004). Lab rats go wild in Oxfordshire. *Nature*, https://doi.org/10.1038/news040202-2

Perfito, N., Zann, R.A., Bentley, G.E. et al. (2007). Opportunism at work: habitat predictability affects reproductive readiness in free-living zebra finches. *Functional Ecology*, **21**, 291–301.

Pigozzi, M.I. and Solari, A.J. (1998). Germ cell restriction and regular transmission of an accessory chromosome that mimics a sex body in the zebra finch, *Taeniopygia guttata*. *Chromosome Research*, **6**, 105–113.

Pooley, E.L., Kennedy, M.W. and Nager, R.G. (2014). Maternal inbreeding reduces parental care in the zebra finch, *Taeniopygia guttata*. *Animal Behaviour*, **97**, 153–163.

Poot, H., ter Maat A., Trost, L. et al. (2012). Behavioural and physiological effects of population density on domestic zebra finches (*Taeniopygia guttata*) held in aviaries. *Physiology and Behaviour*, **105**, 821–828.

Remage-Healey, L., Adkins-Regan, E. and Romero, L.M. (2003). Behavioral and adrenocortical responses to mate separation and reunion in the zebra finch. *Hormones and Behaviour*, **43**, 108–114.

Reynolds, S.J. (2001). The effects of low dietary calcium during egg-laying on eggshell formation and skeletal calcium reserves in the zebra finch *Taeniopygia guttata*. *Ibis*, **143**, 205–215.

Robbins, L. and Margulis, S.W. (2016). Music for the birds: effects of auditory enrichment on captive bird species. *Zoo Biology*, **35**, 29–34.

Romero, L.M. and Reed, J.M. (2005). Collecting baseline corticosterone samples in the field: is under 3 min good enough? *Comparative Biochemistry and Physiology* A, **140**, 73–79.

Rosskopf, W.J. and Woerpel, R.W. (1996). *Diseases of Cage and Aviary Birds*, 3rd edn. William and Wilkins, Baltimore.

Royle, N.J., Hartley, I.R. and Parker, G.A. (2002). Sexual conflict reduces offspring fitness in zebra finches. *Nature*, **416**, 733–736.

Rutstein, A.N., Gilbert, L., Slater, P.J.B. et al. (2004). Mate attractiveness and primary resource allocation in the zebra finch. *Animal Behaviour*, **68**, 1087–1094.

Rutstein, A.N., Gorman, H.E., Arnold, K.E. et al. (2005). Sex allocation in response to paternal attractiveness in the zebra finch. *Behavioral Ecology*, **16**, 763–769.

Rutstein, A.N., Brazill-Boast, J. and Griffith, S.C. (2007). Evaluating mate choice in the zebra finch. *Animal Behaviour*, **74**, 1277–1284.

Samour, J. (2000). *Avian Medicine*. Mosby, London.

Schielzeth, H. and Bolund, E. (2010). Patterns of conspecific brood parasitism in zebra finches. *Animal Behaviour*, **79**, 1329–1337

Schweitzer, C., Schwabl, H., Baran, N.M. and Adkins-Regan, E. (2014). Pair disruption in female zebra finches: consequences for offspring phenotype and sensitivity to a social stressor. *Animal Behaviour*, **90**, 195–204.

Selman, R.G. and Houston, D.C. (1996). The effect of pre-breeding diet on reproductive output in zebra finches. *Proceedings of the Royal Society of London Series B – Biological Sciences*, **263**, 1585–1588.

Shepherd, M. (2012). Australian grassfinches in aviculture. In: *Grassfinches in Australia*. Eds Forshaw, J.M and Shepherd, M., pp. 11–34. CSIRO Publishing, Victoria, Australia

Skagen, S.K. (1988). Asynchronous hatching and food limitation: a test of Lack's hypothesis. *Auk*, **105**, 78–88.

Slater, P.J.B. and Clayton, N.S. (1991). Domestication and song learning in zebra finches *Taeniopygia guttata*. *Emu*, **91**, 126–128.

Smith, E.L., Greenwood, V.J., Goldsmith, A.R. and Cuthill, I.C. (2005a) Effect of repetitive visual stimuli on behaviour and plasma corticosterone of European starlings. *Animal Biology*, **55**, 245–258

Smith, E.L., Evans, J.E. and Parraga, C.A. (2005b) Myoclonus induced by cathode ray tube screens and low-frequency lighting in the European starling (*Sturnus vulgaris*). *Veterinary Record*, **157**, 148–150

Snyder, J.M., Molk, D.M. and Treuting, P.M. (2013). Increased mortality in a colony of zebra finches exposed to continuous light. *Journal of the American Association for Laboratory Animal Science*, **52**, 301–307.

Sossinka, R. (1970). Domestikationserscheinungen beim Zebrafinken *Taeniopygia guttata castanotis* (Gould). *Zoologisches Jahrbuch Systematik*, **97**, 455–524.

Sossinka, R. (1972a). Besonderheiten in der sexuellen Entwicklung des Zebrafinken *Taeniopygia guttata castanotis* (Gould). *Journal für Ornithologie*, **113**, 29–36.

Sossinka, R. (1972b). Langfristiges Durstvermögen wilder und domestizierter Zebrafinken (*Taeniopygia guttata castanotis* Gould). *Journal für Ornithologie*, **113**, 418–426.

Speer, B.L. (2018). Basic anaesthesia. In: *BSAVA Manual of Avian Practice*. Eds Chitty J. and Monks D., pp. 215–231; BSAVA Publications, Gloucester, UK.

Stockdale, B. (2018). Nutrition. In: *BSAVA Manual of Avian Practice*. Eds Chitty, J. and Monks, D., pp. 80–97. BSAVA Publications, Gloucester, UK.

Stolba, A. and Wood-Gush, D.G.M. (1989). The behaviour of pigs in a semi-natural environment. *Animal Production*, **48**, 419–425.

Sung, W. (2010). Passerines. In: *Behaviour of Exotic Pets*, 1st edn. Ed. Tynes, V.V., pp. 12–20. John Wiley & Sons Ltd, Chichester, UK.

Swaddle, J.P. and Cuthill, I.C. (1994). Preferences for symmetric males by female zebra finches. *Nature*, **367**, 165–166.

Swaddle, J.P. and Page, L.C. (2006). High levels of environmental noise erode pair preferences in zebra finches: implications for noise pollution. *Animal Behaviour*, **74**, 363–368.

Taylor, E.J. (1996). An evaluation of the importance of insoluble versus soluble grit in the diet of canaries. *Journal of Avian Medicine and Surgery*, **10**, 248–251.

Torgasheva, A.A., Malinovskaya, L.P., Zadesenets, K.S. et al. (2019). Germline-restricted chromosome (GRC) is widespread among songbirds. *Proceedings of the National Academy of Science*, U.S.A., In Press.

Tschirren, B., Rutstein, A.N., Postma, E. et al. (2009) Short- and long-term consequences of early developmental conditions: a case study on wild and domesticated zebra finches. *Journal of Evolutionary Biology*, **22**, 387–395.

Tschirren, B., Postma, E., Rutstein, A.N. and Griffith S.C. (2012). When mothers make sons sexy: maternal effects contribute to the increased sexual attractiveness of extra-pair offspring. *Proceedings of the Royal Society of London Series B – Biological Sciences*, **279**, 1233–1240.

Tully, T.N., Lawton, M.P.C. and Dorrestein, G.M. (2000). *Avian Medicine*. Butterworth-Heinemann, Oxford.

Van Hoek, C.S. and ten Cate, C. (1998) Abnormal behaviour in caged birds kept at pets. *Journal of Applied Animal Welfare Science*, **1**, 51–64.

Waas, J.R., Colgan, P.W. and Boag, P.T. (2005). Playback of colony sound alters the breeding schedule and clutch size in zebra finch (*Taeniopygia guttata*) colonies. *Proceedings of the Royal Society of London Series B – Biological Sciences*, **272**, 383–388.

Williams, T.D. and Christians, J.K. (2003). Experimental dissociation of the effects of diet, age and breeding experience on primary reproductive effort in zebra finches *Taeniopygia guttata*. *Journal of Avian Biology*, **34**, 379–386.

Williamson, K., Gilbert, L., Rutstein, A.N. *et al.* (2008). Within-year differences in reproductive investment in laboratory zebra finches (*Taeniopygia guttata*), an opportunistically breeding bird. *Naturwissenschaften*, **95**, 1143–1148.

Wood-Gush, D.G.M. and Duncan, I.J.H. (1976). Observations on domestic fowl in the wild. *Applied Animal Ethology*, **2**, 255–260.

Wright, A.J., Aguilar, S.N., Baldwin, A.L. *et al.* (2007). Anthropogenic noise as a stressor in animals: a multidisciplinary review. *International Journal of Comparative Psychology*, **20**, 250–273.

Yamahachi, H., Zai, A., Tachibana, R. *et al.* (2017) Welfare of zebra finches used in research. *BioRxiv*, https://doi.org/10.1101/154567

Yates, J. (2018). Naturalness and animal welfare. *Animals*, **8**, 53.

Young, R.L. (2003). *Environmental Enrichment for Captive Animals*. Blackwell Publishing, Oxford.

Zann, R.A. (1985). Slow continuous wing-moult of zebra finches *Poephila guttata* from southeast Australia. *Ibis*, **127**, 184–196.

Zann, R.A. (1996). *The Zebra Finch. A Synthesis of Field and Laboratory Studies*. Oxford University Press, Oxford.

Zann, R.A., Morton, S.R., Jones, K.R. *et al.* (1995). The timing of breeding by zebra finches in relation to rainfall in central Australia. *Emu*, **95**, 208–222.

Zann, R.A. and Straw, B. (1984). A non-destructive method to determine the diet of seed-eating birds. *Emu*, **84**, 40–41.

43

Pigeons and doves

Stephen E.G. Lea, Anthony McGregor, Mark Haselgrove and Catriona M.E. Ryan

Biological overview

General biology

Doves and pigeons make up the order Columbiformes, including over 300 extant species of bird. There is no scientific distinction between the terms 'dove' and 'pigeon'. However, in practice 'dove' is more often used for smaller species, such as the various species of turtle doves and collared doves, and 'pigeon' for larger species, such as the wood pigeon and the crowned pigeons. Some species are known by both names, including the domestic pigeon or rock dove, *Columba livia*.

Over 300 extant species are recognised within Columbiformes. Molecular taxonomy does not support the traditional separation of the family Columbidae (pigeons and doves) from the extinct Raphidae (dodos and solitaires), but no alternative family-level classification has yet been proposed (Pereira et al. 2007; Soares et al. 2016). According to these authors, either two (Soares *et al.*) or three (Pereira *et al.*) major clades are supported by the molecular data: on both accounts, a single major clade, comprising species from both Old and New Worlds, includes both the species usually found in laboratories, the domestic pigeon and the Barbary dove *Streptopelia risoria*.

Columbiform species can be found on every continent except Antarctica, and in most habitats except the driest deserts and icebound terrain. Extant species range in size from around 15 cm in length (beak-tip to tail-tip), for example, the plain-breasted ground dove, *Columbina minuta*, to nearly 75 cm in the case of the Victoria crowned pigeon, (*Goura victoria*) (Gibbs et al. 2001). Their diet consists mostly of fruit or seeds, depending on the species; some species mainly take vegetation (e.g., the common wood pigeon, *Columba palumbus*). Many will eat some small invertebrates along with their usual diet, and a handful take substantial proportions of invertebrates or even reptiles (e.g., the atoll fruit dove, *Ptilinopus coralensis*). So far as is known, all show biparental care, in which both sexes incubate eggs and provision young, including by producing 'crop milk' (described in the following text under Reproduction). In addition, unlike almost all other birds, almost all Columbiform species drink water by sucking it up, using the tongue as a straw, without lifting their heads (see Wickler 1961, for some exceptions).

Despite the large number of species in the order Columbiformes, only two are widely used for research purposes. Both are domestic forms. These are the domestic pigeon (*Columba livia*) and the Barbary dove (*Streptopelia risoria*). In this chapter, we therefore focus on these two species, and basic biological data for them are provided in Table 43.1 (below). Following common usage both in everyday speech and in the non-zoological literature, in the remainder of this chapter these two species will be referred to simply as 'pigeons' (or 'domestic pigeons') and 'doves' (or 'Barbary doves'), respectively; where any other species is intended, it will be identified by its full common and systematic names. Basic information about other species of pigeons and doves can be found in Winkler et al. (2020) and Gibbs *et al.* (2001).

In the case of the pigeon, a distinction needs to be made between three forms: wild, domestic and feral. The wild form is known as the rock dove or rock pigeon. It is native to the coasts of Europe and North Africa, and both coastal and inland regions of southern and western Asia, and is still found in its original habitat. However, it was first domesticated about 5000 years ago (Johnston 1992), and a great variety of different breeds have been bred for different purposes, including meat production, homing and show. All of these are referred to as 'domestic pigeons'. As a result of escapes from captivity and subsequent dispersion, feral pigeons are now found worldwide, though usually in association with humans (Johnston & Janiga 1995). Research birds may be of varieties bred for show, meat (e.g., White Carneau) or homing and racing purposes; neither wild nor feral birds should normally be used, as is discussed further below. Some pigeons carry genes characteristic of the speckled pigeon (*Columba guinea*), probably because of past artificial hybridisation (Vickrey et al. 2018).

In the case of the Barbary dove, no truly wild form exists. It is usually treated as the species *Streptopelia risoria*, though

Table 43.1 Standard biological data (Based on del Hoyo et al. 2019, Powell 1983, Rautenberg 1983, Schleucher & Withers 2002, Calder, 1968 and authors' experience).

	Body weight	Body temperature (cloacal)	Resting respiration rate
Pigeon *Columbia livia*	Wild type 180–360 g; domestics may range up to 1000 g	39.7 °C (range 39–42 °C)	28.3 breaths/min (range 25–30)
Dove *Streptopelia risoria*	130–180 g	41.7 °C	40–42/min

this designation is not accepted in strict taxonomic usage. It is most probably a domesticated variety of the African collared dove (*S. roseogrisea*), or possibly the Eurasian collared dove (*S. decaocto*) (Baptista et al. 2021); it hybridises freely with either. Like pigeons, doves have a long history of domestication, going back at least 3000 years judging from literary references (e.g., in the Hebrew bible, where doves and pigeons are mentioned separately as sacrificial animals). Feral Barbary doves are found, but they do not breed freely in the wild, and are not as common or as widespread as feral pigeons.

There is little sexual dimorphism in appearance between the sexes in either pigeons or Barbary doves; although males are typically 3%–10% heavier, there is great overlap in the weight distributions between the sexes (Johnston & Janiga 1995, p. 18). Behavioural differences are more marked, and these are discussed further in the following text. Individual pigeons have been recorded as living for 35 years in captivity (Carey & Judge 2002), and individual Barbary doves for 12 (e.g., Terrón et al. 2005). The wild-type African collared dove (*Streptopelia roseogrisea*) is slightly smaller than the Barbary dove and is confined to Northern Africa, south of the Sahara, and western-central and southwestern Arabia, occurring in acacia thorn scrub. The collared dove (*Streptopelia decaocto*), which has spread across the north-west of Europe into Britain, is occasionally used as a laboratory bird. It is slightly larger than a Barbary dove and with darker colouration. The courtship and incubation behaviour are very similar to those of the Barbary dove.

Social organisation

Feral pigeons are colonial breeders and often feed together in large numbers (Cramp 1986; Johnston & Janiga 1995), though these are more aggregations caused by local relative food abundance than organised flocks. Aggressive competition for food and partners is often observed where they occur in high densities (Murton et al. 1974). Although the feral pigeon is socially monogamous, frequent pair copulation and intense mate guarding by males suggest a degree of sperm competition (Lovell-Mansbridge 1995). However, when male partners are experimentally removed, females showed no tendency to approach other males or to engage in extra-pair copulations (Lovell-Mansbridge & Birkhead 1998); similarly, when sex ratios are male biased, the frequency of extra-pair copulations does not increase (Marchesan 2002), though breeding success may be reduced because of egg damage (Jankowiak et al. 2018). Higher levels of aggression from cuckolded males may have selected against extra-pair copulations. For example, pair bond structure in females paired with aggressive males is poorer, leading to delayed breeding in these pairs (Erickson & Zenone 1978), which subsequently affects reproductive fitness. Alternatively, Trivers (1972) suggested that one cost of cuckoldry is the withdrawal of parental care by the male. In pigeons and doves, where biparental care is important not only in provisioning young, but also in producing crop milk, the cost of extra-pair copulations for the female is potentially high.

Reproduction

Many aspects of reproductive behaviour and endocrinology have been studied in the Barbary dove. Systematic study of pigeon reproduction has been less intensive, though pigeon fanciers have collected a good deal of practical knowledge.

Courtship and pair bonding

All species of Columbidae seem to form strong pair bonds and show biparental care, and this is certainly true both of the common pigeon and the Barbary dove. Males expend considerable time, energy and physical resources on their offspring, participating in both the incubation of the eggs and in feeding the offspring. This resource-provisioning by the male is mediated by the synchrony of breeding behaviour in male–female pairs, since reproduction is successful only when the male's physical condition is synchronised with egg-laying. Courtship patterns in doves and pigeons perform a number of functions, such as identification of sex and reproductive condition of females, and the synchronisation of the physical condition of the pair (Lehrman 1965; Lovari & Hutchison 1975).

Courtship behaviour in pigeons has been described by Fabricius and Jansson (1963), and in doves by Craig (1909) (for a summary, see Cheng 1979). The initial aggressive courtship by the male consists of chasing, with the body horizontal, and a kah-call, and may alternate with bowing (in doves) or head nodding (in pigeons). In doves, the male will lift his head, inflate the crop and coo as the head is lowered towards the floor. The feet are stamped between bow–coos. In pigeons, depending on the breed, the beak can nearly touch the ground or the breast, and in some types, crests may be fanned out or the tail fanned. The pupil of the eye contracts in both doves and pigeons showing the iris. If the male meets another male, the encounter may result in wing-boxing. However, if opposite sexes meet, the female will alternate between retreating from and approaching the male, and this leads to nesting activity, attempted mating and full copulation 1–2 days after pairing. Courtship in male pigeons has been shown to be elicited by facial features of the female (Patton et al. 2010), but its progress is dependent on both partners showing the appropriate responses to each other (Ware et al. 2017). Females respond to multiple dimensions of the stimuli provided by the male (Partan et al. 2005). In the male Barbary dove, courtship has been shown to be characterised by a transition from initial testosterone-driven aggressive interactions (chasing, bowing and kah-calls) to oestrogen-dependent nest-orientated behaviour (nest display and cooing), and changes in hormonal states accompany these behaviours (Fusani 2008). Since the male dove has no oestrogen circulating in the plasma, testosterone is converted to oestrogen by the enzyme aromatase in the preoptic area and hypothalamus (Hutchison 1991). These general hormonal processes are thought to be widespread in birds, though their triggering is mediated by ecological differences between species (Ball & Balthazart 2004), and thus almost certainly apply to pigeons in some form.

Nest building, ovulation and incubation

Most species of dove and pigeon build rudimentary nests consisting of a few twigs with grass or hay collected by the male and placed in the nest by the female. The female Barbary dove increases wing-flipping (vibration of the wings) when sitting on the nest 4–5 days before egg-laying (Craig 1909). This behaviour in turn stimulates the male to bring nesting material to the female. The time course of the transitions in male courtship behaviour has retarding or accelerating effects on the female's ovarian development. Persistent aggressive courtship patterns by the male are associated with a delay in egg-laying and nest soliciting in the female. However, provisioning of nesting material by the male accelerates the female's ovulation.

In both pigeons and doves, females lay two eggs. The first egg is usually laid in the afternoon, with incubation occurring immediately afterwards. Incubation behaviour is performed by both sexes, although the male usually incubates in the later morning and through the afternoon (Craig 1909), a pattern that is seen also in other related species of dove (e.g., Biricik et al. 1993). Ovulation involves the hormone prolactin, but in the Barbary dove at least, progesterone mediates the initiation of incubation behaviour and egg-laying in the female. During incubation, prolactin levels in both parents increase, and the milk cells lining the crop begin to proliferate to form crop milk, a cheesy, protein-rich suspension which is regurgitated into the beaks of the young; the cellular mechanism of its production is quite similar to that of mammalian milk. So far as is known, this mechanism is found in all species of Columbidae and is unique to them, though an analogous mechanism exists in flamingos and emperor penguins. Young pigeons and doves are fed on crop milk from the first hour of hatching. The crop milk becomes mixed with seeds as the young get older.

Breeds and supply

Barbary doves are available as caged birds throughout the world. They have been bred in a variety of plumage colours, of which the commonest is a pure white; however, the body form and plumage does not vary much between breeds. In contrast, there are over 350 breeds of domesticated pigeon, with great morphological diversity between them, and within each breed there may be a number of colours and markings (Domyan & Shapiro 2017). Pigeon fanciers recognise four main colours: red, black, blue and brown, though white birds are also commonly bred; however, these do not map simply into the genetic variations, as Domyan and Shapiro explain. There are also many plumage types, including fantails, feathered feet and head crests; the genetics of feathered feet have been explored in detail (Domyan et al. 2016). 'Croppers' have the ability to inflate the crop, while 'tumblers and rollers' tumble and roll while in full flight. In our experience, varieties highly bred for particular characteristics are more prone to abnormal behaviour, particularly stereotyped pecking at the environment or plumage, behaviour which is known to be under some degree of genetic control in chickens (Rodenburg & Koene 2003) and may well be in other birds. Accordingly, care should be used when selecting a strain for use in the laboratory. There are genetic linkages between some of the commoner plumage variations to both physiological and behavioural differences (see Leiss & Haag-Wackernagel 1999). Of the four major plumage pattern types (T-check, checker, bar and barless), barless varieties are more likely to have genetic visual deficiencies (Vickrey et al. 2018). Birds bred for exaggerated characteristics such as short beaks or extra-long feathers should be avoided, since they are likely to suffer inherently poor welfare (Savas et al. 2007; Stucki et al. 2008); even fantails and feathered-leg varieties, though not as extreme as many fancy breeds, tend to have broken and soiled feathers under aviary conditions and require extra care in husbandry.

Pigeons and doves are rarely available from specialist laboratory animal suppliers. In some countries, pigeons can be obtained from firms breeding them for the meat trade, but in others this is not possible. Barbary doves and some strains of pigeons are available from bird dealers supplying the pet and fancy trade. A useful source of domestic pigeons is pigeon racers or other fanciers, who discard birds that do not meet their particular standards, which may be irrelevant to laboratory use; however, if the birds are to have free flight, they should not have been allowed to fly free from a previous home, as they may well return there, especially if they are from homing parentage. As both pigeons and doves are domesticated species, there is no need to obtain free-living birds, and this should be avoided, because obtaining pigeons from the wild may import diseases into the laboratory; it is in any case contrary to regulations in many countries, unless wild birds are the specific object of the study. Regardless of origin, birds newly arrived in the laboratory should be immediately inspected for signs of injury, illness or parasites (feather lice are almost inevitable with some sources), and then quarantined for at least two weeks, as well as being deloused.

Uses in the laboratory

The pigeon is the standard avian model organism when comparison between mammals and other phyla are made in physiology, anatomy and brain–behaviour interactions; it has a similar status to the rat or mouse in laboratory studies. Pigeons have been used extensively in visual physiological research (e.g., Medina & Reiner 2000; Karten 2015). Particularly important in some of these studies is the strong lateralisation of brain function that occurs in birds (e.g., Rogers 1996; Ocklenburgh & Güntürkün 2017).

The other major laboratory use for pigeons as a model organism is in experimental psychology in studying visual discrimination, cognition and learning. Pavlovian and instrumental conditioning tasks in conditioning chambers are used extensively with pigeons in experimental psychology (e.g., Cook 2001; Haselgrove et al. 2005; McGregor et al. 2006).

In addition, there has been much investigation of an ability that may be specific to the domestic (homing) pigeon (*Columba livia*): the remarkable ability to return to its loft from unfamiliar sites. The sensory basis and mechanisms of this ability have been studied extensively over the past 50 years (for recent reviews, see Mehlhorn & Rehkamper 2009; Beason & Wiltschko 2015; Bingman 2018). The pigeon is known to use olfaction, magnetic fields and the position of the sun in the sky for long-range homing (Wiltschko & Wiltschko 2013, 2017; Guilford & Taylor 2014). Less well-studied are the mechanisms behind homing in the birds' familiar area. Visual landmarks are thought to be important, and how the pigeon learns and uses information about landmarks is becoming clearer (for review, see Guilford & Biro 2014).

The major laboratory use of doves has been in studies of reproduction, and in particular the interactions of reproductive hormones and behaviour. The reproductive behaviour of doves has been studied in detail, though investigations still continue (e.g., Burns-Cusato et al. 2021; Mitoyen et al. 2021). The endocrine basis of these behaviours has been studied since the 1950s, for example, studies of the androgen-metabolising brain enzymes, the aromatase system (e.g., Hutchison et al. 1986) which forms oestrogen in brain neurones. The control of prolactin secretion and its role in maintaining incubation behaviour and crop milk production is also being extensively studied in the Barbary dove (e.g., Buntin & Buntin 2014). Doves have also been used in studies of immunoreactivity and the role of Gonadotropin-releasing hormone (GnRH) and in particular the way in which its synthesis in the brain is elicited by the social stimuli of courtship (e.g., Mantei et al. 2008).

Laboratory management and breeding

General husbandry

The following recommendations are based on the legal codes covering the European Union (e.g., European Union 2010) and their implementation in the United Kingdom (e.g., Home Office 2014), on reports from animal welfare charities (e.g., Hawkins et al. 2001), and on the authors' personal experience. Further information may be found in Chitty (2018), Chitty and Lierz (2008) and Hawkins (2000).

Housing

Aviaries
Wherever possible, pigeons and doves should be housed in an aviary large enough to permit flight. In temperate conditions, both pigeons and doves will thrive in either indoor or outdoor aviaries. Many of the fittings required for aviaries can be obtained from suppliers to pigeon fanciers. All aviaries should be fitted with perches divided up so that there is one section for each bird ('pigeonholes'); sections should be of 20 cm for doves, 30 cm for pigeons. Longer perches (either shelves or rods) on which the birds can display courtship should also be provided, though they will often be monopolised by a few individuals. Aviaries should offer both the quantity and quality of space to allow the bird to engage in a range of behaviours including flight. Hawkins et al. (2001) recommend (7 m × 3 m × 3 m high) or tunnel aviaries (20 m × 7 m × 3.5 m high). Outdoor aviaries normally consist of two sections, a loft or shed and a wire mesh flight cage, with a window connecting the two; the window can be closed off to allow maintenance, or in extreme weather. It is not necessary to use a purpose-built pigeon loft, but whatever shed is used must be draught-proof but ventilated. If necessary, a supplementary heater may be used. The floors of indoor aviaries, and the sheds of outdoor aviaries, should be covered with suitable bedding to absorb faeces, and this should be replaced regularly. In any indoor housing of pigeons and doves, there is a build-up of white 'dust' (keratinised scales) from the birds' feathers and skin. Wiping with a damp cloth removes this dust, and this should be done at least once a week. In addition, it is essential to have frequent air changes – fans bringing fresh air into the laboratory, and extraction fans to clear laboratories of dust. Outdoor aviaries for doves can be placed on an earth floor, which should be dug over from time to time; aviaries of pigeons require a concrete or other impermeable base, and should be hosed down regularly. Security against predators such as cats and foxes is critical, and smaller predators such as sparrowhawks (*Accipiter nisus*) and weasels (*Mustela nivalis*) have been known to attack birds through the aviary wire, necessitating a double layer of mesh. Everything possible should be done to exclude rats and mice; ensuring grain is not left scattered in or around the aviary will make it less likely that they will be encouraged.

In circumstances where occasional losses of birds can be tolerated, pigeons can be allowed to fly out from outdoor aviaries. A port giving access to the outside should be fitted high on a wall of the flight cage, and should be equipped with no-return bars that can be lowered to ensure that the birds are shut in at night. This kind of housing may be necessary when researching homing, for example. Ideally, there should be no nearby population of wild pigeons from which loft pigeons could acquire diseases and parasites, but given the ubiquity of feral pigeons in urban settings this is unlikely to be achieved absolutely. Accordingly, birds brought into the main colony from such a free-flight situation should be treated like new arrivals in terms of inspection and quarantine. Predators, especially peregrine falcons (*Falco peregrinus*) may render losses from allowing free flight unsupportable, if a resident raptor learns that the aviary offers easy prey. Birds acquired as discards from racing lofts should not be allowed on free flight, as they may return to their previous homes, souring relations with a supplier, and incurring an extra infection risk. A free-flight loft will occasionally attract lost racing birds, and these should be offered back to their owners through the national racing organisation (in the UK, the Royal Pigeon Racing Association). Researchers proposing to set up a free-flight loft should, where possible, get advice from pigeon racers with local experience.

Cages

Pigeons housed either individually, or in pairs in small cages, are often unable to extend their wings fully. Such cages are therefore not appropriate for long-term housing. The European Union (2010) has updated and reaffirmed guidelines on minimum standards of housing that include the housing of pigeons; more detailed advice can be found in an earlier document (Commission of the European Communities 2007). The European Union (2010) recommends long, narrow pens (2 m × 1 m even for a single bird), as these permit short flights. From 2017, it is a legal requirement in the UK that pigeons should be kept in cages no smaller than 2 m^2 (Home Office 2014, Table 2-9-6). Cages should be cleaned at least once a week. Whenever pigeons or doves are kept in cages, they should be given daily access to a room in which exercise flights can be conducted during the morning and/or late afternoon.

When housing pigeons or doves indoors, whether in cages or aviaries, temperatures should be held between 15 ° and 25 °C. Rooms must be well-ventilated. Wolfensohn and Lloyd (2003) recommend at least 10 air changes per hour, although the UK Home Office (2014) recommends 15–20, with the proviso that the ventilation system should not cause the birds to become chilled. Ventilation systems need complete cleaning at least every three years to remove build-up of dust and feathers, and filters need regular inspection and replacement.

Environmental provision and enrichment

Whether pigeons are kept in aviaries or cages, steps should be taken to enrich the captive environment so that they can maximise the expression of more natural behaviours.

Nesting facilities, nesting material and perches are necessary in aviaries, or when birds are paired in cages; further details are given in the following text. In aviaries, a flat tray with clean water for bathing will be used frequently by both sexes. Most pigeons will take the opportunity to bathe in a fine mist of warm water, which can be sprayed at individual birds with a commercial plant sprayer, though the birds should always have the opportunity to escape the spray. Since pigeons are sensitive to ultra-violet light, if birds are caged indoors, it seems advisable to use lighting that emits some UV, such as so-called 'daylight' fluorescent lighting, or, if LED lighting is used, to supplement it with UV emitters; welfare effects of having UV in lighting have not been demonstrated in pigeons, but in chickens and ducks it seems to reduce fear and stress (House et al. 2020; Sobotik et al. 2020). Adding an artificial dawn and dusk lighting (gradual increase and decrease of brightness over a half hour period) similarly seems desirable although welfare benefits have not been demonstrated. As would be expected for a high-latitude species (see Dawson et al. 2001), sexual activity and breeding behaviour in pigeons is sensitive to photoperiod: in the authors' experience, 14 hours of light daily will reliably induce and breeding behaviour; 14 hours of darkness will suppress it. Birds housed in cages may benefit from the provision of toys such as bells and mirrors that can be hung from the cage by chains, though the authors' experience is that pigeons do not pay as much attention to these as some other birds. Before placing any object in a cage or aviary, it should be examined carefully for small parts that might become detached and be ingested.

Social grouping

Doves and pigeons can be maintained as single-sex colonies, but usually the sexes are mixed to prevent excessive aggression. It is advisable to monitor groups closely when first acquired to ensure that birds do not bully or injure others. If housed in pairs, males should not be caged together as they may fight. If birds are housed in individual cages, they should if possible be within sight and hearing of other birds so that some social behaviour can continue. There is a circadian rhythm in bird activity, with more calling and feeding in the morning than the afternoon.

Laboratory feeding and dietary requirements

Food can be provided either in covered bowls or in hoppers attached to the side of the cage or aviary. Suitable bowls can be obtained from suppliers to the fancy. Open bowls should not be used: they result in much food wastage since birds defecate with them, and females may attempt to nest in them. Since some birds consume preferred foods selectively, it is essential that feeders are replenished each day with fresh food. Foraging can be encouraged by scattering seed upon the floor, although not all scattered food will be eaten and there is an obvious risk of contamination with faeces especially if stocking density is high. In addition, hand feeding provides an excellent method to habituate the birds to contact with humans, which is desirable if the birds are to be handled regularly.

Domestic pigeons and many doves are omnivorous (Hawkins et al. 2001; Scullion & Scullion 2010). Consequently, vegetable proteins alone will not provide sufficient nutrients and amino acids for these birds. Thus, a supplement such as turkey starter crumbs or chick-rearing meal should be given. Grains commonly fed to pigeons are kaffir corn, maple peas, hemp, maize, vetch, millet, wheat, oats and barley. Some green food, chick-rearing meal, shell, grit and salt are usually given. Kaffir corn, wheat, maize, millet, finely ground oyster shells and starter turkey crumbs can be fed to doves. Turkey crumbs typically contain vitamins A, D3 and E supplements, ash, methionine, copper (II) sulphate and lasalocid sodium. Starter turkey crumbs are not ideal for pigeons because of their high protein content, but if they are not used, vitamin supplements are required. Adult pigeons require approximately 15–30 g of food per day, and pigeons which have only limited exercise should not be fed *ad libitum* otherwise they tend to become overweight. Provided that body condition is monitored by regular weighing, pigeons can be fed once daily, and should not be given more food than they will promptly clear.

Minerals and vitamins play an important role in bone growth and eggshell formation, and are an essential supplement. Calcium and phosphorus are required in relatively large quantities and can be given as crushed shells, for example, crushed oyster shell, or as powdered or liquid supplements added to the water (although it may be hard to meet daily requirements in this way). Vitamin supplements should also be given, as sufficient vitamins do not occur in cereals and legumes: birds kept indoors need additional vitamin D_3 (or exposure to ultra-violet light), and young birds may need additional vitamin A, especially if it is difficult to include in their diet sources of carotene such as green vegetables and yellow seeds such as maize. Insoluble grit plays a key role in the digestive process of the pigeon and dove as it is stored in the gizzard and used to grind and break down seeds and other fibrous matter before chemical digestion. Suitable mineral and shell materials can be obtained from suppliers to pigeon fanciers.

Water

Fresh water should be provided daily. To prevent the birds fouling the water, the containers should either be covered or mounted on the outside of the cage or aviary. Some birds do not drink when first caged individually. This problem can be avoided by provided the water in see-through reservoirs. Birds which still refrain from drinking can be encouraged to do so by gently immersing their beaks in the water.

Identification and sexing

Individual birds can be identified for life if ringed before they are five days old with closed, numbered rings, which cannot be removed once the bird's toes are fully grown. Coloured split plastic rings can be put in place at any time, though they will occasionally be lost, so additional means of identification (e.g., a careful description of plumage variations, and a photograph) should be used when birds are group-housed. If research involves having the birds on free flight, the laboratory should affiliate to the national racing pigeon organisation (Lang 2010, p. 114ff, gives a list of these), so that their standard rings can be used when birds are bred in the laboratory. If birds ringed in this way get lost and enter fanciers' lofts, they will be returned. Leg-rings with PIT tags attached are available for use in monitoring birds' movements and behaviour. Permanent marking can also be achieved using subcutaneous PIT tags, normally injected under the loose skin at the back of the neck, though not being visible these will not help if birds are lost outside the laboratory.

Although the males of some strains of pigeon have distinctive colouring (e.g., red chequers, mealies and silvers, which show black flecking), in general, the plumage of the male and female pigeon or dove will have the same form throughout the lifespan of the bird, making sexing a difficult task. In the domestic pigeon, the eyes of the young male are more widely spaced than in the female. In adults, the male may be more heavily built than the female and the head rounder with larger ceres than the female who will tend to have a slighter build and a flatter head. Domestic pigeons can also be sexed by their behaviour. Males strut, bob up and down and emit a double 'coo', while females emit only a single coo. In addition, males turn 360° circles, fan out their tails and drag them along the floor while courting a female. At about a year old, once doves and pigeons are sexually mature, the sex of the birds can be determined using observations of courtship behaviour. Each bird is placed in a cage with a known sexually active male. If the unsexed bird is female, it will retreat from the sexually active male and, usually after 5 minutes, the known sexually active male will display nest soliciting and the female will approach the male. If the unsexed bird is a male, aggressive courtship behaviour (chasing, bowing, pecking, kah-calls and wing-boxing) will be displayed. However, it is important to note that identification of sex by either observation of behaviour or external anatomy requires considerable experience before any of these criteria can be used with any degree of accuracy, and even then, they should not be regarded as an entirely accurate method of sex identification. For example, if sex ratios are very uneven, pigeons (especially, females) may form same-sex pairs and show some of the behaviours characteristic of the opposite sex (Jankowiak et al. 2018). More reliable methods of sexing doves and pigeons before the birds are sexually mature include DNA sexing by commercial laboratories (using a blood sample or tissue from a growing feather), or by visually examining the gonads by laparoscopy under general anaesthesia.

Transport and quarantine

Transport of non-human vertebrates within Europe must comply with EU regulations (European Council 2005): for the UK implementation of these (as of 2012), see the Department for Environment, Food and Rural affairs and Home Office code of practice (Home Office 2014). Information on the transport of laboratory animals has been provided by Laboratory Animal Science Association (2005). The Live Animals Regulations (International Air Transport Association 2019) provide comprehensive and regularly updated information concerning international regulations for air transportation of animals. See also Chapter 12: Transportation of laboratory animals.

Providing there is adequate ventilation, pigeons and doves may be transported for short distances in wicker baskets or in cardboard boxes. It is not advisable to give them water continuously as the plumage may become damaged. After a journey of 1–2 h, birds should be given food and water. Upon arrival in the laboratory, it is recommended that incoming birds should be health checked by a vet and any treatments and disease control procedures necessary should be undertaken (e.g., to control internal and external parasites).

Breeding

Condition of adults

A 14 h light/10 h dark regime induces sexual activity in adult male and female doves and pigeons. If, however, artificial light is not used to induce sexual activity, it is best to pair the birds in February or March in northern latitudes. To reduce aggression in the male, it is advisable to introduce the female to a male who has already established a perching and nesting site. Doves and pigeons can form pair bonds and mate for life; therefore, separating breeding pairs may cause distress. However, if the birds are kept in an aviary, breeding can be unsuccessful due to competition for the females from intruder males. Placing pairs in separate cages prevents this interference and allows the behaviour of the pair to be monitored. When the birds are sexually active and behaviourally compatible, egg-laying should occur about 10–12 days after pairing. However, if no eggs are laid within

20 days, then the birds should be paired with different partners. If pairs are compatible, about three to four broods are produced on normal day length during the reproductive season, which is until the end of September in northern latitudes. Maintained on artificial light, pairs will produce young at about 2-monthly intervals for 1–2 years. However, pigeons should be allowed to rest and should not be bred all year round. In particular, they should be allowed to moult normally in the autumn. To avoid separating mates, breeding is usually controlled by adjusting day length, or removing eggs as soon as they are laid.

Nesting, incubation and hatching

When birds are paired, nesting material (straw and twigs), as well as earthenware nesting bowls or papier maché nest pans, should be provided. Filling the nesting bowl with sand or newspaper prevents cracking of the eggs. The male sits on the eggs for shorter periods than the female, usually in the afternoon. Earthenware pans should be disinfected between broods. In the dove, hatching occurs 14 days after the beginning of the incubation period; in pigeons, hatching occurs after 17 or 18 days of incubating.

The young

Young pigeons are called squabs. When first hatched, they are incapable of locomotion, and they do not leave the nest for the first 8–10 days. Both the male and female produce crop milk to feed the young for approximately 10–12 days after hatching. The crop milk, as mentioned earlier, becomes mixed with seeds as the young get older. The parents then continue to feed the squabs grain, until fledging occurs at between 21 and 24 days, and they are able to fly from about 35 days of age. Squabs must be able to grip the substrate with their feet to prevent 'splay leg'. Birds that hatch with splayed legs, or develop them, will never walk, and must be humanely killed. It is usual to leave the parents with the young for the first month, when they can be caged. If permanent identification rings are used (e.g., those supplied by pigeon racing federations), they need to be fitted before the squabs are 7 days old. Young birds should not be allowed to breed until they are at least 36 weeks old.

Reproductive problems

Egg binding (the failure of an egg that has entered the oviduct to be laid) may be caused by soft-shelled or broken eggs, or by infection or malformation of the oviduct. There are multiple possible causes of soft shell, including vitamin D_3 deficiency, infection, and old age, but the commonest cause is deficiency of calcium in the diet. During breeding, pigeons and doves have a particularly high requirement for calcium, which should be freely available, for example, in the form of crushed oyster shell. Females that continually lay soft-shelled eggs should not be used for breeding. Egg binding can be very serious, and signs may include depression, droopy wings, abdominal straining and weakness or paralysis of one or both legs. A hard swelling can usually be felt in the lower abdomen. A lukewarm bath may help the egg pass.

Laboratory procedures

Handling

Pigeons and doves can easily lose feathers if they are improperly handled. To avoid this, quickly grasp the bird from behind around its body and wings (Figure 43.1a). An inexperienced handler may have to use both hands at first, but with

(a)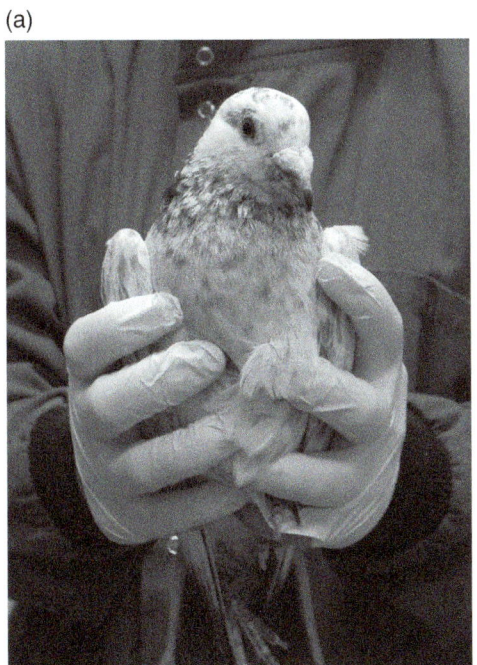

(b)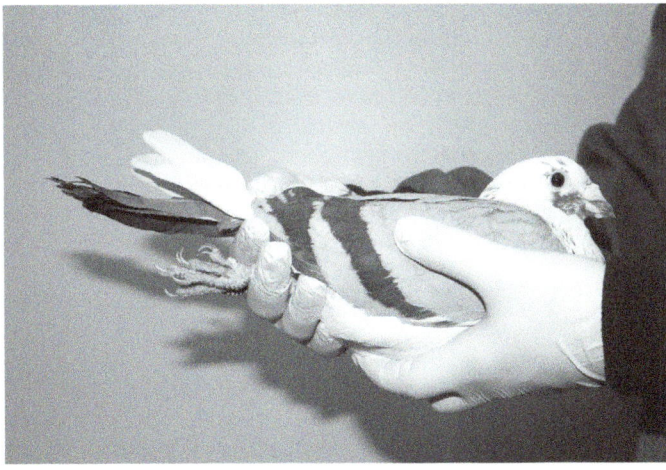

Figure 43.1 (a) An experimenter handling an adult pigeon, using two hands. (b) Holding a smaller bird, giving the handler more freedom.

practice, an adult pigeon or dove can be both caught and held with one hand, leaving the other hand free to open wings, check feather condition, etc. (Figure 43.1b). Avoid pointing the cloaca towards the person, as the bird may defecate, particularly if it is not yet habituated to humans. Pigeons housed in an aviary or in large groups can be caught with a net, and dimming the lights can ease capture. However, if the birds are accustomed to hand feeding, pigeons and doves will fly to the hand. A number of pigeons can be transported a short distance (such as between an aviary/holding room and a nearby laboratory) at the same time by gently placing them headfirst into individual plastic measuring jugs. The pigeon will typically remain in the jug without attempting to escape or showing obvious signs of distress. Similar jugs, or cloth bags, are used to restrain pigeons during weighing. The procedure does not induce tonic immobility, and care is needed to avoid escapes when removing the bird from the restraint, especially if it is not used to being handled.

Behavioural training

Pigeons are frequently used in experiments designed to investigate the psychology of learning and cognition, and behavioural training is also required as a precursor to experiments in psychopharmacology and neuropsychology. Aviary housed birds are normally caged for at least half an hour before testing, to allow them to settle; if cages are baited with a little food, most birds will fly into them without requiring catching. For the tests, the bird is placed into a dark, or dimly illuminated chamber in which visual or (less frequently) auditory stimuli are presented, along with food reward. Before training begins, there is usually a period during which the bird settles. It is good practice for such chambers to be fitted with video cameras so that the bird's behaviour can be monitored and action taken if the equipment malfunctions.

A less stressful procedure for housing, weighing and testing pigeons in the laboratory has been described by Huber (1994; see also Huber et al. 2015). The pigeons are, in this case, housed in outdoor aviaries with perches, a pigeon loft for nesting and hatching eggs, water, but no food. They enter the experimental chamber directly from the outdoor aviary through connecting channels to obtain food. After an acclimatisation phase of several days, the birds enter the channels daily. The animals are weighed automatically on a scale in the floor at the rear of the chamber.

Body temperature

Temperature may be taken by inserting, to a depth of not more than 2 cm, a cloacal thermometer, or thermistor into the cloaca. The mean body temperature of Barbary doves is 41.7 °C, and that of pigeons 39.7 °C, and these averages are typical across a wide range of Columbidae (Schleucher & Withers 2002), though of course there will be some individual variation.

Collection of blood samples

In adult birds, blood samples may be collected from the ulnar, basilica or brachial veins, which run parallel to the external aspect of the humerus, on the underside of the wing; for an illustration, see Scullion and Scullion (2010). It is not necessary to pluck the feathers. The jugular vein, commonly used in other birds, is not suitable in pigeons because there is no apterium (featherless area) allowing access to it. Puncture immediately above the elbow joint is not recommended, as haemostasis can be difficult to achieve at this site. Application of pressure with the thumb at the proximal humerus can help to raise the vein, making it clearly visible. Once the route of the vein is located, feathers can be parted by lightly wiping the injection area with cotton wool soaked in surgical spirit. The blood volume in birds in general is approximately 7 ml/100 g body weight. For a single sample, 0.5 ml/100 g of body weight can be drawn safely (see also Morton et al. 1993).

Administration of substances

As with the collection of blood, it is not necessary to pluck the feathers when administering substances by injection. Lightly wiping the injection site with surgical spirit and parting the feathers will provide sufficient access to the skin.

Oral administration

Solid or liquid oral preparations are best administered in the drinking water or in the feed. However, oral gavage may be necessary for unpalatable substances, or under conditions in which a precise dose is necessary. Take care to avoid the trachea when inserting a tube or substance into the oesophagus. The trachea in the pigeon is located behind the tongue and should be identified before carrying out the procedure. Catheters to be inserted into the oesophagus should be lubricated to avoid damage to either the oesophagus or the pharynx. This procedure requires two people, and firm but gentle restraint of the bird. Morton et al. (2001) recommend a maximum oral dosing volume of 10 ml/kg.

Subcutaneous injection

The most common site for subcutaneous injection is under the loose skin in the back of the neck. The maximum dose is 2–5 ml/kg (Morton et al. 2001).

Intravenous injection

Frequently used sites include the ulnar and medial metatarsal veins. As will the collection of blood, the jugular route is less convenient because of the absence of an apterium. One should aim to use the smallest gauge needle possible for injecting pigeons and doves intravenously. Morton et al. (2001) recommend that the injected volume be no more than 5 ml/kg. It is essential to ensure that the bird is adequately restrained.

Intramuscular injection

Intramuscular injections can be given into the pectoral muscles. Intramuscular injections are painful and can affect mobility. They can also result in death of living tissue (necrosis), it is therefore preferable to administer substances subcutaneously, wherever possible. Intramuscular administration of large volumes should be divided between different injection sites, and the total dose should not exceed 0.05 ml/kg (Morton et al. 2001). Care must be exercised so as to not inject into blood vessels. This can be achieved by refraining from inserting the needle too deeply and, prior to depressing the plunger, withdrawing it slightly to check for signs of blood.

Intraperitoneal injection

Substances should not normally be administered to pigeons or doves by intraperitoneal injection as the substance can easily enter the air sacs and disrupt their function. Further guidance and recommendations of the administration of substances to birds can be found in Harrison and Harrison (1986), Richie et al. (1994), Morton, Jennings et al. (2001), Hawkins et al. (2001), Scullion and Scullion (2010), and Speer (2016).

Anaesthesia

Detailed advice on anaesthesia in birds including pigeons is given by Heatley (2008), and that source should be consulted for further details.

The inhalant anaesthetic, isoflurane, has become the preferred agent for both short and long anaesthesia due to its reliability and the rapid recovery from its effects, which are now well understood (e.g., Botman, Dugdale et al. 2016). Sevoflurane is emerging as a possibly preferable alternative (for review, see Botman, Gabriel et al. 2016).

Prior to anaesthesia, the pigeon must be fasted for at least 2–6 h (depending on weight) to empty its crop and minimise regurgitation. Ophthalmic ointment should be applied to the eyes to prevent the drying of the corneas. Induction of anaesthesia can be achieved with either a face mask, or an induction chamber at 4% isoflurane, and 1–2 l/min total flow. Once induction has occurred, anaesthesia should be maintained using endotracheal intubation. Air exchange is very efficient in birds, and the depth of anaesthesia can change rapidly when using gas inhalants. However, maintenance anaesthesia may be set initially at 2–3% isoflurane and 1–2 l/min flow. Responses should be monitored to maintain a light-to-medium depth of anaesthesia, and concentration of isoflurane adjusted accordingly. The relationships between responsivity and the depth of anaesthesia were reported by Abou-Madi (2001), and a selection of these are shown in Table 43.2. Birds lose heat rapidly during anaesthesia and a heated blanket may not provide sufficient thermal support to prevent a decrease in body temperature; for a comparison of different anaesthetic systems from this point of view, see Boedeker et al. (2005). A heat lamp may be employed during surgery, but care must be taken not to overheat the bird. Body temperature should be monitored with a rectal thermometer.

Wolfensohn and Lloyd (2003) state the importance of flushing with oxygen at the end of anaesthesia to prevent reabsorption of anaesthetic. Warmth and subcutaneous fluids should be provided during recovery from anaesthesia. The wings can be controlled during recovery by wrapping the bird in a towel, taking care not to restrict breathing. The bird should be monitored during recovery in a dark, or dimly lit, quiet area. A smooth recovery can be produced by administering analgesics immediately after surgery, but they can also be administered preoperatively for a smoother induction. Indications of pain in birds can include agitation and restlessness, loss of weight, appetite and variations in the preening of a painful site. Opioids (e.g., butorphanol, 0.5–4 mg/kg intra-muscularly) and non-steroidal anti-inflammatory drugs (e.g., carprofen, 1–4 mg/kg or meloxicam, 0.1–0.5 mg/kg, subcutaneously or by mouth) can be administered as post-operative analgesics (dosages as recommended by Hawkins 2006 and Heatley 2008).

Disposal

It is not always necessary, either legally or practically, for animals that have completed experimental protocols to be killed (Franco 2016). In the particular case of pigeons and doves, which are long-lived, it is common practice to use them repeatedly in many experiments. If the experiments do not cause pain, distress or lasting harm, and if the birds are lodged in good quality aviaries between uses, there is no reason not to do this, though the approval of regulatory authorities should always be obtained. Where resources permit, birds for which no further use is envisaged may be retired to an aviary, perhaps on free flight, so long as their health and quality of life remains good, and the situation offers positive welfare (Rault et al. 2020). However, although wild pigeons and doves may occur in the vicinity of research facilities, laboratory birds must not be simply released to the wild when no longer required, even if they have not undergone any experimental procedures; they are likely to suffer poor welfare unless they have a home loft to return to. If the birds can no longer be maintained in a laboratory colony, therefore, they should be killed. Detailed guidance on methods of killing is included in American Veterinary Medical Association (2020), though the acceptability of particular methods under national legislation should always be confirmed. Several methods of killing birds up to a weight of 1 kg (unlikely to be exceeded except perhaps in the largest specimens of meat breeds of pigeons) are permitted in the United Kingdom under Schedule 1 to the Animals (Scientific Procedures) Act 1986, as amended (Animals in Science Committee 2013), as being consistent with EU regulations. These are:

Anaesthetic overdose

Overdose of an anaesthetic using a route and an anaesthetic agent appropriate for the size and species of animal. Injectable agents such as sodium pentobarbital can be administered

Table 43.2 Levels of anaesthesia (after Abou-Madi 2001).

Response	Light anaesthesia	Medium anaesthesia	Deep anaesthesia
Voluntary blinking	Slow or absent	Slow or absent	Absent
Muscle relaxation	Moderate–good	Good	Absent
Breathing pattern	Rapid and deep	Slow, deep, regular	Slow, shallow
Palpebral reflex[a]	Present or slow	Slow, intermittent	Absent
Pedal reflex[b]	Present or slow	Slow, intermittent	Absent

[a] The palpebral reflex can be elicited by running the finger along the eyelashes.
[b] The pedal reflex can be elicited by squeezing the toes between the thumb and forefinger.

intravenously into the medial metatarsal vein to bring about death (150 mg/kg). Injection may also be given intrahepatically, with the injection site under the sternum along the ventral midline. However, intracoelomic injection should be avoided because the crystallisation of barbiturate drugs may cause pain and distress to the animal, and in general intraorgan routes should only be used in anaesthetised animals because of the risk that they may be painful. Cousquer and Parsons (2007) provide excellent details on locating the medial metatarsal vein and other advice on euthanasia.

CO_2

Exposure to carbon dioxide gas in a rising concentration. The applicability of this method to birds has been controversial because exposure to the gas can result in distress in some animals (Hawkins et al. 2001). It has been argued that argon is a better alternative gas, because unlike carbon dioxide it is not acidic and therefore not an irritant; we have not found any comparative studies involving pigeons or doves, but studies on poultry have not shown a clear advantage of either gas (e.g., McKeegan et al. 2006; Gerritzen et al. 2013).

Cervical dislocation

Dislocation (wringing) of the neck, with the prior use of a sedative or anaesthetic in the case of birds over 250 g, i.e. most pigeons.

Additional methods

Under European Union law and derived national regulations, concussion, decapitation and electrical stunning are also permitted, though these are rarely used.

Whatever method is used, death must be confirmed before disposal of the carcase, for example, by waiting for the onset of rigor mortis; acceptable methods are listed in Animals in Science Committee (2013). Where anaesthetic methods are used, it is common to follow them by cervical dislocation as a confirmatory step. Some methods must only be performed by an appropriately qualified person. Pigeons are long-lived and often used in small numbers, for procedures that may last over several years, so laboratory personnel may not have to perform euthanasia very often; in these conditions, it is better to have all euthanasia done by a veterinary surgeon.

Common welfare problems

Health and disease

Prevention of disease

All birds arriving in a laboratory colony should be immediately inspected for ectoparasites and signs of illness, and in any case quarantined from the main flock for at least a week. In outdoor aviaries or lofts, primary prophylaxis may be aided if wild birds such as sparrows, feral pigeons and wild doves are prevented from entering aviaries. If possible, wild birds should be discouraged from perching on top of aviaries; this is difficult in practice, though the use of solid rather than mesh roofs will limit the problem. Ensuring that food is not spilled around the aviary will reduce the presence of wild birds. Transmission of endoparasites occurs where there is poor hygiene, overcrowding and warm, moist conditions.

Therefore, as secondary prophylactic measures, keep drinking water clean and remove faeces weekly, so as to break the life cycles of these parasites. Suspended aviaries with mesh floors will reduce the problem substantially, but if these are used, pigeons, by nature cliff-dwelling rather than tree-perching birds, should be provided with ledges for perching, and these must then be kept clean.

Health monitoring and signs of disease

Hygiene is of prime importance since infections can spread rapidly from one bird to another. Clinical signs of disease are not always obvious. Daily careful inspection by a person who knows the birds well is a vital precaution in spotting problems early. Birds may initially be examined in the cage or on a perch; a useful additional method of monitoring the health of birds is to keep regular records of the weights of individual birds. In addition to the warning given by loss of weight, daily weighing by a person who knows the bird well gives a further opportunity for anything unusual to be noticed. Redrobe (2002) lists criteria for monitoring health in the perching bird: can it perch? Are its feathers ruffled? Is it alert and responsive? Is its respiration normal? Is there feather loss, or a change in quality of feathers, beak and nails? Is the bird standing with equal weight on both legs and are the wings held at equal lengths? The authors would also recommend observation for changes in faeces. Abnormalities in any of these factors may indicate problems with the bird's health, and certainly indicate poor welfare. Unfortunately, there is currently no equivalent for birds of the 'grimace scale' that can be used to assess welfare in rodents.

Feeding is another good time for health monitoring. If hand feeding, the opportunity may be taken to inspect the feathers which, in a healthy bird, should feel silky to the touch. Redrobe (2002, p. 171) lists common clinical conditions that may be detected when the animal is being handled.

Later signs of illness include the bird remaining in a moribund state on the perch or floor of the aviary, crouched with feathers fluffed out and head down. Birds in this state will not respond to a loud noise such as clapped hands.

More specific information on the diseases most likely to occur in captive pigeons and doves, their diagnosis, and appropriate treatments follows. A particularly good source of information on disease and pathologies in pigeons is Cousquer and Parsons (2007). Other sources include Alkharigy et al. (2018), Marlier and Vindevogel (2006), Nepote (1999), Scullion and Scullion (2010), Rupiper (1998a, 1998b) and Tudor (1991), and general books on avian medicine such as Chitty and Lierz (2008) and Speer (2016). Books for pigeon fanciers, for example, Brown (2015) and Lang (2010), also provide useful non-technical descriptions of symptoms and treatments.

Diseases of pigeons and doves

Endoparasitic infections

The following may occur in pigeons:

1. *Trichomonas gallinae* is a flagellated protozoan which causes trichomoniasis, variously known as 'canker', 'diphtheria' or, particularly in falconry, 'frounce' (note, however, that 'diphtheria' is also used as a term for the

viral disease pigeon pox, described in the following text). Much information about trichomoniasis and its effects in pigeons can be found in the early review by Stabler (1954), and in the recent review of trichomonads in birds by Amin et al. (2014). The domestic pigeon is considered the primary host of *T. gallinae*, although it also occurs naturally in a wide variety of species (e.g., Quillfeldt et al. 2018), especially birds of prey that feed on pigeons. Infection is spread from parents to squabs during feeding, and through contamination of the drinking water. There are thought to be more than 20 strains of *T. gallinae*, varying in virulence, which infect domestic pigeons. The immune response associated with the disease produces yellow round lesions on the epithelium of the mouth, oesophagus and crop, with accompanying diarrhoea and loss of appetite (Narcisi et al. 1991; Gerhold 2016). However, as Frank (2004) points out, with breeders and racers at least, the widespread use of medicines such as metronidazole (antibiotics that are also antiprotozoals) in the 1970s and 1980s led to the near eradication of *T. gallinae* strains that produce these symptoms, making the disease harder to detect. The routine prophylactic treatment of racing birds with nitroimidazoles may also be encouraging the emergence of resistant strains (Rouffaer et al. 2014). In addition, milder strains of *T. gallinae* are thought to enhance immunity against more virulent strains, again making detection of *T. gallinae* infection by presence of symptoms more difficult. However, in the most virulent strain (Jones' Barn), death occurs in almost 96% of infected non-immune birds, through the necrosis of liver and other internal organs (Stabler 1954). Therefore, if infection is suspected treatment is necessary. Infection may be confirmed by a swab taken from the crop lining, and the contents inspected under magnification or by PCR analysis (Gerhold et al. 2008). According to Gerhold (2016), successful treatments include carnidazole (10 mg/kg body wt), metronidazole (60 mg/kg body wt) and dimetridazole (50 mg/kg body wt, PO; or in the drinking water at 0.05% for 5–6 days). Others have questioned the efficacy of nitroimidazole class drugs in eradicating *T. gallinae* from pigeons (e.g. Munoz et al. 1998), while others have called for higher doses for nitroimidazoles for effective treatment (Franssen & Lumeij 1992). Cousquer and Parsons (2007) point out that carnidazole (Spartrix: Harkers) is the only licensed nitroimidazole available in the UK. Tabari et al. (2017) have reported some evidence that an alkaloid extract from the wild rue *Peganum harmala* (commonly used in Middle Eastern folk medicine) might provide a natural alternative.

2. Nematodes, in particular the roundworm *Ascaridia columbae* and the hairworms *Capillaria columbae* and *C. longicollis*, may infect the duodenum and upper part of the small intestine. *A. columbae* average about 2–6 cm in length and 1 mm in thickness, and reproducing worms are generally detectable by visible ova in the faeces. In severe infections, the gut wall may be thinned and transparent, and may occasionally rupture. *Capillaria* species are smaller, at around 2.5 cm in length and much more slender than *A. columbae*. Ova in the faeces may only be detected with microscopy. In both infections, birds are likely to lose weight chronically, develop diarrhoea and suffer a general loss of condition. For both roundworms and hairworms, Walker (2015a) recommends treatment with an avermectin such as Ivermectin ('Ivomec') or Moxidectin at a strength of 10 mg of active drug per litre of drinking water; the actual dose must be calculated by taking into account the extent to which the preparation supplied is already diluted. Fenbendazole can also be used (e.g., Tanveer et al. 2011), though it can have high toxicity in pigeons as in other birds (Howard et al. 2002).

3. Coccidia are a widespread and important group of protozoa, causing the problematic coccidiosis condition in poultry, sheep, dogs, cattle and rabbits. Coccidiosis is most commonly caused by parasites of the genus *Eimeria*. Species in this genus are unusual in having a high degree of host-specificity. Krautwald-Junghanns et al. (2009) review the position for pigeons, in which *Eimeria labbeana* and *E. columbarum* are most common, and affect pigeons at 3–4 months of age most severely. Many birds have a low level of the disease, but affected birds have a greenish diarrhoea, and become emaciated. Diagnosis is through the number of oocysts present in the faeces and is necessary to distinguish the symptoms from those of salmonellosis, trichomoniasis, worm infestation and gut infection. Drug treatments available include amprolium, sulfonamides, clazuril and toltrazuril; Krautwald-Junghanns et al. recommend toltrazuril, with a dosage of 20 mg/kg administered in drinking water for two days.

Ectoparasites

Ectoparasites, such as ticks, mites and lice, may result in feather loss, anaemia and the stunted growth of squabs. Therefore, affected birds should be inspected for the causal organisms.

Some species of lice such as the long feather louse, *Columbicola columbae*, and coccyx louse, *Campanulotes bidentatus*, are common and may cause irritation and damage to the feathers, but feed only from feather dust after attaching themselves to the feather shaft. Very small feather mites such as *Falculifer rostratus* may cause irritation if present in large numbers. If anaemia accompanies skin irritation, then the red mite, *Dermanyssus gallinae*, may be suspected. It should be noted that these mites do not breed on the birds but in cracks and crevices from which they emerge at night. Moxidectin, used for worm infestations, has the advantage of killing any blood-sucking mite. The cage or aviary should be sprayed at the same time as treatment to the bird. Bromocyclen in the form of a dusting powder may be used as a general treatment for most lice and mites. An alternative is a synthetic pyrethroid such as permethrin, sprayed directly on to the bird at 10–20 ml/l of water.

Bacterial and viral diseases

Below is a non-exhaustive list of diseases that may occur in pigeons. Cousquer and Parsons (2007), Chitty and Lierz (2008) and Santos et al. (2020) discuss a wider range of less common diseases.

1. Salmonellosis, also known as paratyphoid, is usually caused by *Salmonella typhimurium* and is the most common bacterial infection of pigeons (the species *S. gallinarum*, which causes fowl typhoid in poultry, is rarely if ever detected in pigeons or doves). *S. typhimurium* organisms can be transmitted in the faeces, crop milk or infected eggs. Clinical signs of infection are extremely variable. Young pigeons often show stunted growth, are underweight and listless, and are affected by diarrhoea. Affected adults may lose weight and develop diarrhoea and swelling of the joints. Swelling and necrosis of the inner eye, known as panophthalmitis, may occur. Isolation and identification of the *Salmonella* microorganisms, usually from faeces or blood, is the only certain means of identifying presence of the disease. In the UK, positive tests for *Salmonella* must be reported, according to orders made under the Animal Health Act (UK Parliament 1981/2015), to the Animal and Plant Health Agency (APHA). Because *Salmonella* is a zoonosis, the risk of a pigeon infecting humans should not be underestimated and strict hygiene measures are essential in handling infected birds. Cousquer and Parsons (2007) recommend that the most severely affected birds be culled and the remainder treated with an antimicrobial, to be determined by culture and sensitivity tests, for 10–14 days.

2. *Chlamydia psittaci*, for a period known as *Chlamydophila psittaci*, is an intracellular bacterium that causes ornithosis in pigeons and respiratory psittacosis in humans; for review, see Balsamo *et al.* (2017). In pigeons, it can be associated with other diseases such as trichomoniasis, pox and herpes virus infections. Symptoms in birds can include lethargy, anorexia, ruffled feathers, conjunctivitis, ocular or nasal discharge or other clinical signs consistent with upper respiratory disease, diarrhoea and signs of liver disease such as excretion of green to yellow-green urates, weight loss and egg infection, and may only appear if the animals are under stress. Humans that have come into contact with infected birds may show influenza-like symptoms such as an abrupt onset of fever, chills, headache, malaise and myalgia that may indicate psittacosis, which may develop into pneumonia. Therefore, if human and pigeon symptoms coincide ornithosis may be suspected. Infection is spread through inhalation or ingestion of nasal discharges or through faeces. The currently favoured treatment is doxycycline or a chlortetracycline-medicated feed, and should be carried out under veterinary supervision (see Baldrey 2020). If antibiotics are not available, or ineffective, the birds should be killed because asymptomatic and treated birds may be carriers, it may be necessary to cull the entire colony. Thorough disinfection of the aviary and cages should be carried out before restocking.

3. Newcastle disease, caused by variants of the avian paramyxovirus 1 (APMV-1 or *Avulavirus* 1), is rare in pigeons. However, there is a strain of APMV-1 which occurs in pigeons, called pigeon paramyxovirus type 1 (PPMV-1); for review, see Pestka *et al.* (2014). Esperón *et al.* (2014) detected PPMV-1 in 44% of a sample of feral pigeons, but not all strains are associated with any clinical signs. Virulent strains of PPMV-1 cause respiratory (e.g., clearly audible breathing sounds and sneezing) and neural symptoms (e.g., by lack of coordination, twitching and paralysis of the legs), and in some cases bloody or watery diarrhoea. The infection spreads rapidly through captive flocks. In the UK, occurrences of APMV-1 and Newcastle disease must be reported, under regulations made under the Animal Health Act (UK Parliament 1981/2015), to the Animal and Plant Health Authority. Amendments to the Act in 2002 and under the Avian Influenza and Newcastle Disease (England and Wales) Order (2003) extended previous powers to protect the public from outbreaks of Newcastle disease in poultry. There is no currently accepted treatment for PPMV-1, though Stenzel *et al.* (2014) have reported some improvement in an experimental use of the antiviral agent methisoprinol. Inactivated and live vaccines are now freely available for use under veterinary supervision and are effective if properly used, although only healthy pigeons should be vaccinated. Infected birds must be culled.

4. Pigeon pox, sometimes referred to as 'diphtheria', is common especially in young birds. The incubation period is usually 1 week. Squabs are infected by their parents. Mosquitoes and other blood-sucking parasites may also play a role in transmission. Therefore, prevention may be facilitated by a clean cage or aviary. Swellings develop on unfeathered areas of the body, particularly around the eyes, beak and legs. Affected birds lose weight and a few young birds may die following spread of the virus to the mouth and throat. Removal of scabs or swellings is not recommended because this is likely to spread infection by releasing viral particles. An infected pigeon is not dangerous to humans. Avian pox viruses are generally quite specific to particular host species (Weli *et al.* 2004), but pigeon pox or closely related forms have been reported in several species of dove and also wood pigeons (*Columba palumbus*) (e.g., Adams *et al.* 2005; Pawar *et al.* 2011), so it may be that all columbids are susceptible to it. There is no treatment, and with care, birds will recover. Vaccines are available and effective, and vaccination is recommended in previously infected populations (Walker 2015b).

5. Avian influenza (AI) received high media coverage when the zoonotic nature of the deadly H5N1 strain was discovered in Hong Kong in 1997. On that occasion, six people died from contact with infected chickens. However, it has been widely reported that should the H5N1 strain mutate to allow transmission between humans then a pandemic, killing millions, would be likely (Webster & Walker 2003), a possibility that may be taken more seriously in the aftermath of the COVID-19 pandemic. H5N1 is only one strain of many that vary in their pathogenicity. Low pathogenic AI infection does not always produce clinical symptoms. However, in the UK, AI is a notifiable disease under the Animal Health Act (1981) and associated amendments, and must be reported to a local DEFRA Animal Health Office if suspected. In birds, clinical signs include respiratory illness, swollen head and loss of appetite. In poultry, high pathogenic AI causes

multiple organ failure, rapid death within 48 h, and spreads through a population very quickly. The disease is spread though contact or faeces, and is not airborne. It had been thought that pigeons did not carry viruses of the H5 type, such as H5N1, but it is now clear that they do (e.g., Elgendy *et al.* 2016; Hassan *et al.* 2018; Tolba *et al.* 2018). AI has a high mutation rate, and the situation for pigeons may change very quickly. The best recommendation is to keep laboratory pigeons under cover and out of contact with wild birds.

6. Mycobacteriosis, caused by a range of mycobacteria, is a common disease in companion birds, including pigeons and doves (see review by Tell *et al.* 2001). Because it is a zoonosis, culling is frequently recommended if it is detected; however, based on an experiment with ring doves, Saggese *et al.* (2014) have argued that a multidrug treatment may be effective.

Nutritional deficiencies

Birds that are not foraging naturally are susceptible to nutritional deficiencies, which they would correct by food choices if living in the wild (Walker 2015c). As noted in the section on feeding and diet in the preceding text, vitamin deficiencies may occur in caged doves and pigeons. Symptoms of vitamin A deficiency include 'rattling' respiratory sounds, resulting from degeneration of mucous membranes in the mouth, and eye infections. Affected birds will lose weight and may move in an uncoordinated way. Birds should be given an oral preparation of vitamin A immediately, and the vitamin supplementation regime should be reviewed.

Signs of poor welfare

The signs of disease listed in the preceding text, such as loss of weight, poor feather condition, lack of response and general changes from the bird's usual stance and behaviour, are all also signs of poor welfare. They are most likely to be detected by someone who is familiar with the individual birds, so consistency in husbandry is important to the bird's welfare as well as very probably reducing their stress. Other indications of poor welfare include foot problems (which may indicate inappropriate flooring or floor covering, or a lack of suitable perches), aggression in group-housed birds (which may indicate overcrowding, or an unsuitable sex ratio), and stereotyped behaviours such as pecking at the cage walls or the bird's own plumage. There is some evidence that cognitive stimulation, including that provided by participating in behavioural experiments, can ameliorate stereotyping (Millar 2013). Birds showing stereotyping should be kept under careful observation; if there is the possibility of moving them to a free-flight aviary, this may reduce the behaviour.

Risks to humans

Health and hygiene

Handlers should wear appropriate protective clothing at all times, to avoid potential health risks from handling birds. The authors recommend the use of a laboratory coat at all times. Cuts and grazes should be covered, and hands and arms washed thoroughly with disinfectant after handling. When handling birds of unknown health status (e.g., wild birds or recent arrivals in the colony, or birds that appear to be sick), disposable examination gloves and a face mask should be worn. Anyone spending substantial time in a colony room or aviary (e.g., for cleaning or extended observation) should always wear a face mask. Handlers should be aware of the zoonotic potential of the pigeon diseases described in the preceding text, and if they need to consult a health professional for any symptoms that could be related to the birds, they should inform the practitioner that they have been in contact with them.

Allergies

Humans can develop pigeon-breeder's lung disease or bird fancier's lung, a form of hypersensitivity pneumonitis caused by inhalation of antigens of pigeon or dove origin (see Quirce *et al.* 2016). This disease is characterised by a diffuse inflammation of the lower respiratory tract. T-lymphocytes recognise a wide range of proteins from pigeons and can induce T-cell proliferation. Feather mites are also a source of allergens for pigeon handlers (see Colloff *et al.* 1997; McSharry *et al.* 2000), with allergic rhinitis (hay fever) being the most common reaction. Dry skin may also occur. Anyone working regularly with pigeons or doves should be kept under observation by their institutional occupational health department, and in particular annual spirometry should be conducted.

Acknowledgements

The authors would like to thank Jemma Dopson and Guillem Esber for providing the photographs for Figure 43.1, and Dr Nigel Taylor for advice.

References

Abou-Madi, N. (2001) Avian anesthesia. *Veterinary Clinics of North America: Exotic Animal Practice*, **4**, 147–167.

Adams, C.J., Feldman, S.H., & Sleeman, J.M. (2005) Phylogenetic analysis of avian poxviruses among free-ranging birds of Virginia. *Avian Diseases*, **49(4)**, 601–605. Doi:10.1637/7369-041805R.1

Alkharigy, F.A., El Naas, A.S. and El Maghrbi, A.A. (2018) Survey of parasites in domestic pigeons (*Columba livia*) in Tripoli, Libya. *Open Veterinary Journal*, **8(4)**, 360–366. Doi:10.4314/ovj.v8i4.2

American Veterinary Medical Association (2020). *AVMA Guidelines for the Euthanasia of Animals: 2020 Edition*. Schaumburg, IL: Author.

Amin, A., Bilic, I., Liebhart, D. and Hess, M. (2014) Trichomonads in birds: A review. *Parasitology*, **141(6)**, 733–747. Doi:10.1017/S0031182013002096

Animals in Science Committee (2013) Consolidated version of the Animals (Scientific Procedures) Act 1986. https://www.gov.uk/government/uploads/system/uploads/attachment_data/file/619140/ConsolidatedASPA1Jan2013.pdf

Baldrey, V. (2020). Guide to using antibiotics in pet birds. *In Practice*, **42**, 394–404. Doi:10.1136/inp.m3092

Ball, G.F. and Balthazart, J. (2004) Hormonal regulation of brain circuits mediating male sexual behavior in birds. *Physiology & Behavior*, **83(2)**, 329–346. Doi:10.1016/j.physbeh.2004.08.020

Balsamo, G., Maxted, A.M., Midla, J.W. et al. (2017) Compendium of measures to control *Chlamydia psittaci* infection among humans (psittacosis) and pet birds (avian chlamydiosis), 2017. *Journal of Avian Medicine and Surgery*, **31**(3), 262–282.

Baptista, L.F., Trail, P.W., Horblit, H.M. et al. (2021) Ring-necked Dove (*Streptopelia capicola*). In: *Cornell Lab of Ornithology Birds of the World*. Eds del Hoyo, J., Elliott, A., Sargatal, J. et al. Ithaca, NY, USA. https://birdsoftheworld.org/bow/species/rindov/cur/introduction.

Beason, R.C. and Wiltschko, W. (2015) Cues indicating location in pigeon navigation. *Journal of Comparative Physiology A – Neuroethology Sensory Neural and Behavioral Physiology*, **201**(10), 961–967. Doi:10.1007/s00359-015-1027-2

Bingman, V.P. (2018) Requiem for a heavyweight: can anything more be learned from homing pigeons about the sensory and spatial-representational basis of avian navigation? *Journal of Experimental Biology*, **221**. Doi:10.1242/jeb.163089

Biricik, M., Kiliç, A. and Sahin, R. (1993) Brutablösung bei freilebenden Palmtauben (*Streptopelia senegalensis*) / The relief at the nest in free-living laughing dove (*Streptopelia senegalensis*) during incubation. *Journal für Ornithologie*, **134**(3), 348–351. Doi:10.1007/BF01640432

Boedeker, N.C., Carpenter, J.W. and Mason, D.E. (2005) Comparison of body temperatures of pigeons (*Columba livia*) anesthetized by three different anesthetic delivery systems. *Journal of Avian Medicine and Surgery*, **19**(1), 1–6. Doi:10.1647/2002-026

Botman, J., Dugdale, A., Gabriel, F. and Vandeweerd, J-M. (2016) Cardiorespiratory parameters in the awake pigeon and during anaesthesia with isoflurane. *Veterinary Anaesthesia and Analgesia*, **43**, 63–71.

Botman, J., Gabriel, F., Dugdale, A.H.A. and Vandeweerd, J.M. (2016) Anaesthesia with sevoflurane in pigeons: minimal anaesthetic concentration (MAC) determination and investigation of cardiorespiratory variables at 1 MAC. *Veterinary Record*, **178**(22), 560. Doi:10.1136/vr.103654

Brown, L. (2015). *Doves as Pets*. NRB Publishing, Las Vegas NV.

Buntin, J.D. and Buntin, L. (2014) Increased STAT5 signaling in the ring dove brain in response to prolactin administration and spontaneous elevations in prolactin during the breeding cycle. *General and Comparative Endocrinology*, **200**, 1–9. Doi:10.1016/j.ygcen.2014.02.006

Burns-Cusato, M., Rieskamp, J., Nagy, M. et al. (2021). A role for endogenous opiates in incubation behavior in ring neck doves (*Streptopelia risoria*). *Behavioural Brain Research*, **399**, 113052. Doi:10.1016/j.bbr.2020.113052

Calder, W.A. (1968) Respiratory and heart rates of birds at rest. *Condor*, **70**(4), 358–365. Doi:10.2307/1365930

Carey, J.R. and Judge, D.S. (2002) *Monographs on Population Aging*. Odense University Press, Odense. https://www.demogr.mpg.de/longevityrecords/

Cheng, M.-F. (1979) Progress and prospects in ring dove research: A personal view. *Advances in the Study of Animal Behavior*, **9**, 97–129. Doi:10.1016/S0065-3454(08)60034-0

Chitty, J. (2018) Pigeons (*Columba livia*). In: *Companion Animal Care and Welfare: The UFAW Companion Animal Handbook*. Ed. Yeates, J. doi:10.1002/9781119333708.ch17

Chitty, J. and Lierz, M. (Eds) (2008). *BSAVA Manual of Raptors, Pigeons and Passerine Birds*. Chichester: Wiley.

Colloff, M.J., Merrett, T.G., Merrett, J. et al. (1997) Feather mites are potentially an important source of allergens for pigeon and budgerigar keepers. *Clinical and Experimental Allergy*, **27**(1), 60–67. Doi:10.1111/j.1365-2222.1997.tb00673.x

Commission of the European Communities (2007) Commission Recommendation of 18 June 2007 on guidelines for the accommodation and care of animals used for experimental and other scientific purposes. *Official Journal of the European Union*, **L197(EN)**, 1–89. http://data.europa.eu/eli/reco/2007/526/oj

Cook, R.G. (2001) *Avian Visual Cognition*. Comparative Cognition Society, Medford MA. http://www.pigeon.psy.tufts.edu/avc/

Cousquer, G. and Parsons, D. (2007) Veterinary care of the racing pigeon. *BMJ In Practice*, **29**(6), 344–355. Doi:10.1136/inpract.29.6.344

Craig, W. (1909) The expressions of emotion in the pigeons, I. The blond ring-dove (*Turtur risorius*). *Journal of Comparative Neurology*, **19**, 29–82. Doi:10.1002/cne.920190103

Cramp, S. (1986) *Handbook of the Birds of Europe, the Middle East and North Africa. The Birds of the Western Palearctic, Vol. IV*. Oxford University Press, Oxford.

Dawson, A., King, V. M., Bentley, G. E., and Ball, G. F. (2001). Photoperiodic control of seasonality in birds. Journal of Biological Rhythms, **16**, 365–380.

Domyan, E.T. and Shapiro, M.D. (2017). Pigeonetics takes flight: Evolution, development, and genetics of intraspecific variation. *Developmental Biology*, **427**, 241–250. Doi:10.1016/j.ydbio.2016.11.008

Domyan, E.T., Kronenberg, Z., Infante, C.R. et al. (2016). Molecular shifts in limb identity underlie development of feathered feet in two domestic avian species. *Elife*, **5**, e12115. Doi:10.7554/eLife.12115

Elgendy, E.M., Watanabe, Y., Daidoji, T. et al. (2016) Genetic characterization of highly pathogenic avian influenza H5N1 viruses isolated from naturally infected pigeons in Egypt. *Virus Genes*, **52**(6), 867–871. Doi:10.1007/s11262-016-1369-z

Erickson, C.J. and Zenone, P.G. (1978) Aggressive courtship as a means of avoiding cuckoldry. *Animal Behaviour*, **26**(1), 307–308. Doi:10.1016/0003-3472(78)90036-2

Esperón, F., Vazquez, B., Sanchez, A. et al. (2014) Seroprevalence of paramyxoviruses in synanthropic and semi-free-range birds. *Avian Diseases*, **58**(2), 306–308. Doi:10.1637/10689-101113-ResNote.1

European Council (2005) Council Regulation (EC) No 1/2005 of 22 December 2004 on the protection of animals during transport... *Official Journal of the European Union*, **48**(L3), 1–44.

European Union (2010) Directive 2010/63/EU of the European Parliament and of the Council. *Official Journal of the European Union*, L276/33. https://eur-lex.europa.eu/legal-content/EN/TXT/PDF/?uri=CELEX:32010L0063&from=EN

Fabricius, E. and Jansson, A.-M. (1963) Laboratory observations on the reproductive behaviour of the pigeon (*Columba livia*) during the pre-incubation phase of the breeding cycle. *Animal Behaviour*, **11**, 534–547.

Franco, N.H. (2016) Killing of animals in science – is it always inevitable? In: *Food Futures: Ethics, Science and Culture*. Eds Olsson, A.S., Araújo, S.M. and Vieira, M.F., pp. 499–504. Wageningen Academic Publishers, Wageningen. Doi:10.3920/978-90-8686-834-6

Frank, K.H. (2004) Canker! Alberta Classic website, downloaded 28 June 2019. http://www.albertaclassic.net/Trichomonas/Trichomonas.php

Franssen, F.F. and Lumeij, J.T. (1992) in vitro nitroimidazole resistance of *Trichomonas gallinae* and successful therapy with an increased dosage of ronidazole in racing pigeons (*Columba livia domestica*). *Journal of Veterinary Pharmacology and Therapeutics*, **15**, 409–415.

Fusani, L. (2008) Testosterone control of male courtship in birds. *Hormones and Behavior*, **54**(2), 227–233. Doi:10.1016/j.yhbeh.2008.04.004

Gerhold, R.W., Yabsley, M.J., Smith, A.J. et al. (2008). Molecular characterization of the trichomonas gallinae morphologic complex in the United States. *Journal of Parasitology*, **94**, 1335–1341. Doi:10.1645/GE-1585.1

Gerhold, R.W. (2016) Overview of trichomonosis. In: *MSD Veterinary Manual, 11th edn.* Eds Allen, D.G., Carter, K.K., Constable, P.D. et al. Merck & Co., Inc., Kenilworth NJ. https://www.msdvetmanual.com/poultry/trichomonosis/overview-of-trichomonosis

Gerritzen, M.A., Reimert, H.G.M., Lourens, A. et al. (2013) Killing wild geese with carbon dioxide or a mixture of carbon dioxide and argon. *Animal Welfare*, **22**(1), 5–12. Doi:10.7120/09627286.22.1.005

Gibbs, D., Barnes, E. and Cox, J. (2001) *Pigeons and Doves: A Guide to the Pigeons and Doves of the World*. Pica, Crowborough UK.

Guilford, T. and Biro, D. (2014) Route following and the pigeon's familiar area map. *Journal of Experimental Biology*, **217**(2), 169–179. Doi:10.1242/jeb.092908

Guilford, T. and Taylor, G.K. (2014) The sun compass revisited. *Animal Behaviour*, **97**, 135–143. Doi:10.1016/j.anbehav.2014.09.005

Harrison, G.J. and Harrison, L. (1986) *Clinical Avian Medicine and Surgery*. Saunders, Philadelphia.

Haselgrove, M., George, D.N. and Pearce, J.M. (2005) The discrimination of structure: III. Representation of spatial relationships. *Journal of Experimental Psychology: Animal Behavior Processes*, **31**, 433–448.

Hassan, M.M., Hoque, M.A., Ujvari, B. and Klaassen, M. (2018) Live bird markets in Bangladesh as a potentially important source for Avian Influenza Virus transmission. *Preventive Veterinary Medicine*, **156**, 22–27. Doi:10.1016/j.prevetmed.2018.05.003

Hawkins, M.G. (2006). The use of analgesics in birds, reptiles, and small exotic mammals. *Journal of Exotic Pet Medicine*, **15**, 177–192. Doi:10.1053/j.jepm.2006.06.004

Hawkins, P. (2000) Refinements in laboratory bird husbandry. *Progress in the Reduction, Refinement and Replacement of Animal Experimentation*, **31(A & B)**, 1313–1318.

Hawkins, P., Morton, D.B., Cameron, D. et al. (2001) Laboratory birds: Refinements in husbandry and procedures. *Laboratory Animals*, **35(S1)**, 1–163.

Heatley, J.J. (2008). Anaesthesia and analgesia. In *BSAVA Manual of Raptors, Pigeons and Passerine Birds*. Eds Chitty, J. and Lierz, M., pp. 97–113. Gloucester, UK: British Small Animal Veterinary Association.

Home Office (2014) *Code of Practice for the Housing and Care of Animals Bred, Supplied or Used for Scientific Purposes*. HMSO, London. https://www.gov.uk/government/uploads/system/uploads/attachment_data/file/388895/COPAnimalsFullPrint.pdf

House, G.M., Sobotik, E.B., Nelson, J.R. and Archer, G.S. (2020). Effects of ultraviolet light supplementation on Pekin duck production, behavior, and welfare. *Animals*, **10**. Doi:10.3390/ani10050833

Howard, L.L., Papendick, R., Stalis, I.H., et al. (2002). Fenbendazole and albendazole toxicity in pigeons and doves. *Journal of Avian Medicine and Surgery*, **16**, 203–210. doi:10.1647/1082-6742(2002)016[0203:FAATIP]2.0.CO;2

Huber, L. (1994) Amelioration of laboratory conditions for pigeons (*Columba livia*). *Animal Welfare*, **3**(4), 321–324.

Huber, L., Heise, N., Zeman, C. and Palmers, C. (2015) The ALDB box: Automatic testing of cognitive performance in groups of aviary-housed pigeons. *Behavior Research Methods*, **47**(1), 162–171. Doi:10.3758/s13428-014-0462-2

Hutchison, J.B., Steimer, T.J. and Hutchison, R.E. (1986). Formation of behaviorally active estrogen in the dove brain – induction of preoptic aromatase by intracranial testosterone. *Neuroendocrinology*, **43**, 416–427. Doi:10.1159/000124558

Hutchison, J.B. (1991) How does the environment influence the behavioural action of hormones? In: *The Development and Integration of Behaviour: Essays in Honour of Robert Hinde*. Ed. Bateson, P., pp. 149–170. Cambridge University Press, Cambridge.

International Air Transport Association (2019) *Live Animals Regulations*, 45th edn. Author, Montréal. https://www.iata.org/publications/store/Pages/live-animals-regulations.aspx

Jankowiak, L., Tryjanowski, P., Hetmanski, T. and Skórka, P. (2018) Experimentally evoked same-sex sexual behaviour in pigeons: better to be in a female-female pair than alone. *Scientific Reports*, **8**. Doi:10.1038/s41598-018-20128-3

Johnston, R.F. (1992) Evolution in the rock dove: skeletal morphology. *Auk*, **109**(3), 530–542.

Johnston, R.F. and Janiga, M. (1995) *Feral pigeons*. Oxford University Press, Karachi.

Karten, H.J. (2015) Vertebrate brains and evolutionary connectomics: on the origins of the mammalian 'neocortex'. *Philosophical Transactions of the Royal Society, B: Biological Sciences*, **370**, 20150060. Doi:10.1098/rstb.2015.0060

Krautwald-Junghanns, M.E., Zebisch, R. and Schmidt, V. (2009) Relevance and treatment of coccidiosis in domestic pigeons (*Columba livia* forma *domestica*) with particular emphasis on toltrazuril. *Journal of Avian Medicine and Surgery*, **23**(1), 1–5.

Laboratory Animal Science Association (2005) Guidance on the transport of laboratory animals: Report of the Transport Working Group established by LASA. *Laboratory Animals*, **39**, 1–39.

Lang, E. (2010) *Pigeon Passion*. IMB Publishing, Barking, UK.

Lehrman, D.S. (1965) Interaction between internal and external environments in the regulation of the reproductive cycle of the ring dove. In: *Sex and Behavior*. Ed. Beach, F.A., pp. 55–380. Wiley, New York.

Leiss, A. and Haag-Wackernagel, D.H. (1999) Plumage polymorphism of the feral pigeon (*Columba livia*). *Journal of Ornithology*, **140**(3), 341–353. Doi:10.1007/BF01651031

Lovari, S. and Hutchison, J.B. (1975) Behavioural transitions in the reproductive cycle of barbary doves (*Streptopelia risoria*). *Behaviour*, **53**, 126–150.

Lovell-Mansbridge, C. (1995) Sperm competition in the feral pigeon, *Columba livia*. Unpublished PhD thesis, University of Sheffield.

Lovell-Mansbridge, C. and Birkhead, T.R. (1998) Do female pigeons trade pair copulations for protection? *Animal Behaviour*, **56**, 235–241.

Mantei, K.E., Ramakrishnan, S., Sharp, P.J. and Buntin, J.D. (2008) Courtship interactions stimulate rapid changes in GnRH synthesis in male ring doves. *Hormones and Behavior*, **54**(5), 669–675. Doi:10.1016/j.yhbeh.2008.07.005

Marchesan, M. (2002) Operational sex ratio and breeding strategies in the feral pigeon *Columba livia*. *Ardea*, **90**(2), 249–257.

Marlier, D. and Vindevogel, H. (2006) Viral infections in pigeons. *Veterinary Journal*, **172**(1), 40–51. Doi:10.1016/j.tvjl.2005.02.026

McGregor, A., Saggerson, A., Pearce, J. and Heyes, C. (2006) Blind imitation in pigeons, *Columba livia*. *Animal Behaviour*, **72**, 287–296. Doi:10.1016/j.anbehav.2005.10.026

McKeegan, D.E.F., McIntyre, J., Demmers, T.G.M. et al. (2006) Behavioural responses of broiler chickens during acute exposure to gaseous stimulation. *Applied Animal Behaviour Science*, **99**(3–4), 271–286. Doi:10.1016/j.applanim.2005.11.002

McSharry, C., Anderson, K. and Boyd, G. (2000) A review of antigen diversity causing lung disease among pigeon breeders. *Clinical and Experimental Allergy*, **30**(9), 1221–1229.

Medina, L. and Reiner, A. (2000) Do birds possess homologues of mammalian primary visual, somatosensory and motor cortices? *Trends in Neurosciences*, **23**(1), 1–12. Doi:10.1016/S0166-2236(99)01486-1

Mehlhorn, J. and Rehkamper, G. (2009) Neurobiology of the homing pigeon: A review. *Naturwissenschaften*, **96**(9), 1011–1025. Doi:10.1007/s00114-009-0560-7

Millar, L.N. (2013) Improving captive animal welfare through the application of cognitive enrichment. Unpublished PhD dissertation, University of Exeter.

Mitoyen, C., Quigley, C., Boehly, T. and Fusani, L. (2021). Female behaviour is differentially associated with specific components of multimodal courtship in ring doves. *Animal Behaviour*, **173**, 21–39. Doi:10.1016/j.anbehav.2020.12.014

Morton, D.B., Abbot, D., Barclay, R. et al. (1993) Removal of blood from laboratory mammals and birds. *Laboratory Animals*, **27**, 1–22.

Morton, D.B., Jennings, M., Buckwell, A. et al. (2001) Refining procedures for the administration of substances. *Laboratory Animals*, **35**, 1–41.

Munoz, E., Castella, J. and Gutierrez, J.F. (1998) in vivo and in vitro sensitivity of *Trichomonas gallinae* to some nitroimidazole drugs. *Veterinary Parasitology*, **78**(4), 239–246. Doi:10.1016/S0304-4017(98)00164-2

Murton, R.K., Thearle, R.J.P. and Coombs, C.F.B. (1974) Ecological studies of the feral pigeon *Columba livia* var III Reproduction and plumage polymorphism. *Journal of Applied Ecology*, **122**, 841–854.

Narcisi, M., Sevoian, M. and Honigberg, B.M. (1991) Pathologic changes in pigeons infected with a virulent *Trichomonas gallinae* strain (Eiberg). *Avian Diseases*, **35**, 55–61.

Nepote, K. (1999) Pigeons as laboratory animals. *Poultry and Avian Biology Reviews*, **10**, 109–115.

Ocklenburg, S. and Güntürkün, O. (2017) *The Lateralized Brain: The Neuroscience and Evolution of Hemispheric Asymmetries*. Academic Press, London.

Partan, S., Yelda, S., Price, V. and Shimizu, T. (2005) Female pigeons, *Columba livia*, respond to multisensory audio/video playbacks of male courtship behaviour. *Animal Behaviour*, **70(4)**, 957–966. Doi:10.1016/j.anbehav.2005.03.002

Patton, T.B., Szafranski, G. and Shimizu, T. (2010) Male pigeons react differentially to altered facial features of female pigeons. *Behaviour*, **147(5–6)**, 757–773. Doi:10.1163/000579510X491090

Pawar, R.M., Bhushan, S.S., Poornachandar, A. et al. (2011) Avian pox infection in different wild birds in India. *European Journal of Wildlife Research*, **57(4)**, 785–793. Doi:10.1007/s10344-010-0488-4

Pereira, S.L., Johnson, K.P., Clayton, D.H. and Baker, A.J. (2007) Mitochondrial and nuclear DNA sequences support a cretaceous origin of Columbiformes and a dispersal-driven radiation in the Paleogene. *Systematic Biology*, **56(4)**, 656–672. Doi:10.1080/10635150701549672

Pestka, D., Stenzel, T. and Koncicki, A. (2014) Occurrence, characteristics and control of pigeon paramyxovirus type 1 in pigeons. *Polish Journal of Veterinary Sciences*, **17(2)**, 379–384. Doi:10.2478/pjvs-2014-0056

Powell, F.L. (1983). Respiration. In: *Physiology and Behaviour of the Pigeon*. Ed. Abs, M., pp. 73–95. London: Academic Press.

Quillfeldt, P., Schumm, Y.R., Marek, C. et al. (2018) Prevalence and genotyping of *Trichomonas* infections in wild birds in central Germany. *Plos One*, **13(8)**, e0200798. Doi:10.1371/journal.pone.0200798

Quirce, S., Vandenplas, O., Campo, P. et al. (2016) Occupational hypersensitivity pneumonitis: an EAACI position paper. *Allergy*, **71**, 765–779. Doi:10.1111/all.12866

Rault, J.L., Hintze, S., Camerlink, I. and Yee, J.R. (2020). Positive welfare and the like: Distinct views and a proposed framework. *Frontiers in Veterinary Science*, **7**. Doi:10.3389/fvets.2020.00370

Rautenberg, W. (1983). Thermoregulation. In M. Abs (Eds.), *Physiology and behaviour of the pigeon*, pp. 131–148. London: Academic Press.

Redrobe, S. (2002) Pigeons. In: *Manual of Exotic Pets, 4th edn*. Eds Meredith, A. and Redrobe, S., pp. 168–178. British Small Animal Veterinary Association, Gloucester.

Richie, B.W., Harrison, G.J., and Harrison, L.R. (1994) *Avian Medicine: Principles and Applications*. Wingers Publishing Inc, Lake Worth FL

Rodenburg, T.B. and Koene, P. (2003). Comparison of individual and social feather pecking tests in two lines of laying hens at ten different ages. *Applied Animal Behaviour Science*, **81**, 133–148. Doi:10.1016/S0168-1591(02)00275-7

Rogers, L. (1996) Behavioral, structural and neurochemical asymmetries in the avian brain: A model system for studying visual development and processing. *Neuroscience and Biobehavioral Reviews*, **20(3)**, 487–503. Doi:10.1016/0149-7634(95)00024-0

Rouffaer, L.O., Adriaensen, C., De Boeck, C. et al. (2014) Racing pigeons: A reservoir for nitro-imidazole-resistant *Trichomonas gallinae*. *Journal of Parasitology*, **100(3)**, 360–363. Doi:10.1645/13-359.1

Rupiper, D.J. (1998a) Diseases that affect race performance of homing pigeon. Part I: Husbandry, diagnostic strategies, and viral diseases. *Journal of Avian Medicine and Surgery*, **12**, 70–77.

Rupiper, D.J. (1998b) Diseases that affect race performance of homing pigeons. Part II: Bacterial, fungal, and parasitic diseases. *Journal of Avian Medicine and Surgery*, **12**, 138–148.

Saggese, M.D., Tizard, I., Gray, P. and Phalen, D.N. (2014) Evaluation of multidrug therapy with azithromycin, rifampin, and ethambutol for the treatment of *Mycobacterium avium* subsp. *avium* in Ringneck Doves (*Streptopelia risoria*): An uncontrolled clinical study. *Journal of Avian Medicine and Surgery*, **28(4)**, 280–289. Doi:10.1647/2012-067R1

Santos, H.M., Tsai, C.Y., Catulin, G.E.M. et al. (2020). Common bacterial, viral, and parasitic diseases in pigeons (*Columba livia*): A review of diagnostic and treatment strategies. *Veterinary Microbiology*, **247**. Doi:10.1016/j.vetmic.2020.108779

Savas, T., Konyali, C., Das, G. and Yurtman, I.Y. (2007) Effect of beak length on feed intake in pigeons (*Columba livia* f. *domestica*). *Animal Welfare*, **16(1)**, 77–83.

Schleucher, E. and Withers, P.C. (2002) Metabolic and thermal physiology of pigeons and doves. *Physiological and Biochemical Zoology*, **75(5)**, 439–450. Doi:10.1086/342803

Scullion, F. and Scullion, G. (2010). Homing pigeons. In: *BSAVA Manual of Exotic Pets, 5th edn*. Eds. Meredith, A. and Johnson-Delaney, C., pp. 188–199. Gloucester, UK: British Small Animal Veterinary Association.

Soares, A.E.R., Novak, B.J., Haile, J. et al. (2016). Complete mitochondrial genomes of living and extinct pigeons revise the timing of the columbiform radiation. *BMC Evolutionary Biology*, **16**. Doi:10.1186/s12862-016-0800-3

Sobotik, E.B., Nelson, J.R. and Archer, G.S. (2020). How does ultraviolet light affect layer production, fear, and stress. *Applied Animal Behaviour Science*, **223**, 104926. Doi:10.1016/j.applanim.2019.104926

Speer, B.L. (2016) *Current Therapy in Avian Medicine and Surgery*. Elsevier, St Louis MO.

Stabler, R.M. (1954) *Trichomonas gallinae*: A review. *Experimental Parasitology*, **3(4)**, 368–402. Doi:10.1016/0014-4894(54)90035-1

Stenzel, T., Tykalowski, B., Smialek, M. et al. (2014) Influence of methisoprinol on the course of an experimental infection with PPMV-1 in pigeons. *Medycyna Weterynaryjna – Veterinary Medicine, Science and Practice*, **70(4)**, 219–223.

Stucki, F., Bartels, T. and Steiger, A. (2008) Zur Beurteilung von Tierschutzaspekten bei Extremzuchten von Rassekaninchen, Rassegeflügel und Rassetauben [Assessment of animal welfare aspects in extreme breeds of rabbits, poultry and pigeons]. *Schweizer Archiv für Tierheilkunde*, **150(5)**, 227–234. Doi:10.1024/0036-7281.150.5.227

Tabari, M.A., Youssefi, M.R. and Moghadamnia, A.A. (2017) Antitrichomonal activity of Peganum harmala alkaloid extract against trichomoniasis in pigeon (*Columba livia domestica*). *British Poultry Science*, **58(3)**, 236–241. Doi:10.1080/00071668.2017.1280725

Tanveer, M.K., Kamran, A., Abbas, M. et al. (2011). Prevalence and chemo-therapeutical investigations of gastrointestinal nematodes in domestic pigeons in Lahore, Pakistan. *Tropical Biomedicine*, **28**, 102–110.

Tell, L.A., Woods, L. and Cromie, R.L. (2001) Mycobacteriosis in birds. *Revue Scientifique et Technique: Office International des Epizooties*, **20(1)**, 180–203. Doi:10.20506/rst.20.1.1273

Terrón, M.P., Paredes, S.D., Barriga, C. et al. (2005) Melatonin, lipid peroxidation, and age in heterophils from the ring dove (*Streptopelia risoria*). *Free Radical Research*, **39(6)**, 613–619. Doi:10.1080/10715760500097831

Tolba, H.M.N., Abou Elez, R.M.M., Elsohaby, I. and Ahmed, H.A. (2018) Molecular identification of avian influenza virus subtypes H5N1 and H9N2 in birds from farms and live bird markets and in respiratory patients. *PeerJ*, **6**, e5473. Doi:10.7717/PeerJ.5473

Trivers, R.L. (1972) Parental investment and sexual selection. In B. Campbell (Ed.), *Sexual Selection and the Descent of Man 1871–1971*, pp. 136–179. Heinemann, London

Tudor, D.C. (1991) *Pigeon Health and Disease*. Iowa State University Press, Ames, IA.

United Kingdom Parliament (2015) *Animal Health Act 1981, As Amended*. HMSO, London. https://www.legislation.gov.uk/ukpga/1981/22

Vickrey, A.I., Bruders, R., Kronenberg, Z. *et al*. (2018) Introgression of regulatory alleles and a missense coding mutation drive plumage pattern diversity in the rock pigeon. *eLife*, **7**, e34803. Doi:10.7554/eLife.34803

Walker, C. (2015a) Parasite control. Australian Pigeon Company website, downloaded 2019-06-27. http://www.auspigeonco.com.au/Articles/Parasite_control.html

Walker, C. (2015b) Pigeon pox vaccination. Australian Pigeon Company website, downloaded 2019-06-27. http://www.auspigeonco.com.au/Articles/pigeonpox.html

Walker, C. (2015c) Vitamin supplements. Australian Pigeon Company website, downloaded 2019-06-27. http://www.auspigeonco.com.au/Articles/vitamin_Supp.html

Ware, E.L.R., Saunders, D.R. and Troje, N.F. (2017) Social interactivity in pigeon courtship behavior. *Current Zoology*, **63(1)**, 85–95. Doi:10.1093/cz/zow066

Webster, R.G. and Walker, E.J. (2003) Influenza: The world is teetering on the edge of a pandemic that could kill a large fraction of the human population. *American Scientist*, **91(2)**, 122–129.

Weli, S.C., Traavik, T., Tryland, M. *et al*. (2004) Analysis and comparison of the 4b core protein gene of avipoxviruses from wild birds: Evidence for interspecies spatial phylogenetic variation. *Archives of Virology*, **149(10)**, 2035–2046. Doi:10.1007/s00705-004-0357-0

Wickler, W. (1961). Über die Stammesgeschichte und den taxonomischen Wert einiger Verhaltensweisen der Vögel. *Zeitschrift für Tierpsychologie*, **18**, 320–342. doi:10.1111/j.1439-0310.1961.tb00423.x

Winkler, D.W., Billerman, S.M. and Lovette, I.J. (2020). Columbidae: Pigeons and doves. In Cornell Lab of Ornithology Birds of the World. https://birdsoftheworld.org/bow/species/columb2/cur/introduction

Wiltschko, R. and Wiltschko, W. (2013) The magnetite-based receptors in the beak of birds and their role in avian navigation. *Journal of Comparative Physiology A: Neuroethology Sensory Neural and Behavioral Physiology*, **199(2)**, 89–98. Doi:10.1007/s00359-012-0769-3

Wiltschko, R. and Wiltschko, W. (2017) Considerations on the role of olfactory input in avian navigation. *Journal of Experimental Biology*, **220(23)**, 4347–4350. doi:10.1242/jeb.168302.

Wolfensohn, S. and Lloyd, M. (2003) *Handbook of Laboratory Animal Management and Welfare*. Blackwell, Oxford.

44 The European starling

Melissa Bateson

Biological overview

General biology

The European starling (*Sturnus vulgaris* L.), henceforth the starling, is a medium-sized songbird with a length of ~22 cm and wingspan of ~40 cm, belonging to the family Sturnidae, sub-order Oscines, order Passeriformes. The starling is an opportunistic and adaptable species, currently found on all of the Earth's continents other than Antarctica. Starlings are common in urban areas and farms, due to their adaptations to foraging on short grass and nesting in cavities provided by buildings. The species is native to most of temperate Europe and western Asia. Northeastern European populations migrate in autumn, with some birds over-wintering in Iberia and Africa. The UK has a resident breeding population and also receives winter migrants from Eastern Europe. Starlings were introduced to Australia (late 1800s), New Zealand (1862), North America (1891), South Africa (1890) and there are recent reports of starlings in South America (Palacio *et al.* 2016). Feare's (1984) monograph on the starling remains an excellent review of the natural history of the species.

Size range and lifespan

Statistics on the body mass of healthy, wild-caught starlings are shown in Table 44.1. Newly hatched chicks weigh around 6.4 g. Juvenile starlings are skeletally fully grown as assessed by tarsus length at the time of fledging. Males are typically slightly skeletally larger than females and adult skeletal size can also be affected by the feeding schedule received by chicks post-hatch, with bird reared under harsher conditions reaching smaller adult size (Nettle *et al.* 2017). Skeletally larger birds are typically also heavier, but body condition (body mass for a given skeletal size) also varies both between and within individuals depending on a number of factors. Males typically have slightly higher body condition than females (Dunn *et al.* 2018a). Early-life feeding schedules can induce enduring differences in body condition, with birds subjected to harsher conditions having either lower or higher condition depending on the treatment (Andrews *et al.* 2015; Dunn *et al.* 2018a). Further factors known to induce more short-term variation in body mass are described in the section on monitoring in the following text.

The annual mortality rate for free-living adult starlings (i.e. at least 1 year of age) is around 55% (Feare 1984). However, mortality should be much lower in captivity where birds are protected from starvation, hypothermia, predation and disease. At Newcastle University, for hand-reared birds kept indoors, we have recorded annual mortality rates of <5%, with no evidence for an increase in mortality with increasing age for birds up to six years of age. Starlings senesce slowly; the mortality rate doubling time for starlings has been calculated at 8 years (cf. 0.3 years for *Mus musculus*) and the maximum recorded longevity for a free-living starling is 22.9 years (Tacutu *et al.* 2013). There are anecdotal reports of captive pet starlings living to over 19 years.

Social organisation

Starlings do not have a strong social structure, but are gregarious throughout the year, forming larger and denser feeding flocks in winter. They form communal roosts in winter that can comprise many thousands of birds. Dominance hierarchies are established in captive flocks, with males dominant to females and adults to juveniles (Bedford *et al.* 2017). Birds may jockey to defend preferred perching positions or feeding sites, and fighting involving grappling with feet and bill stabbing can occasionally occur, but fight-related injuries are rare. During the breeding season, birds will defend a territory immediately around the nest site, with males chasing away other males. Pair bonding does not occur until the weeks immediately before laying. Starlings are primarily monogamous, but polygamous mating systems have also been reported. Both sexes feed the young (Wright & Cuthill 1990).

Reproduction

Starlings are sexually mature at one year of age. The changes in physiology and behaviour preceding breeding are induced by the increased day length in spring in interaction

---

The UFAW Handbook on the Care and Management of Laboratory and Other Research Animals, Ninth Edition.
Edited by Huw Golledge and Claire Richardson.
© 2024 John Wiley & Sons Ltd. Published 2024 by John Wiley & Sons Ltd.

Table 44.1 Body mass in healthy, wild-caught starlings[1]. All masses in g.

Statistic	Male	Female	All
Mean	82.80	78.52	80.62
Standard deviation	6.43	6.37	6.75
Range containing 95%	69.37–95.40	65.96–92.00	67.00–94.00
Range containing 99%	63.00–99.68	60.00–98.94	61.00–99.10

[1] Based on data obtained from the British Trust for Ornithology records extracted on 21/03/2019. Statistics are based on data from 6434 male birds and 6665 females.

Table 44.2 Reproductive data for starlings.

Variable	Mean ± sd	Range
Clutch size (number of eggs)	4.60 ± 0.94	2–9
Incubation (days)	12.38 ± 1.61	10–16
Fledging (days)	20.50 ± 3.25	15–26

with other environmental cues including availability of nest sites and nesting materials (Carbeck et al. 2018). Starlings are usually colonial breeders with nests as little as 1 m apart. They nest in cavities and will readily adopt appropriate nestboxes provided in areas where they are already breeding. Males typically place green plant material in completed nests prior to breeding. The function of this behaviour is unclear and may involve pharmacological effects on nest parasites, female birds and/or nestlings. (Dubiec et al. 2013). In England, first clutches are initiated between early April and late May and second clutches are common. Eggs are pale blue or white-spotted and 30 × 21 mm and weigh ~7 g. Eggs hatch asynchronously, with the last egg often hatching up to 24 h after the others resulting in a runt chick. Basic reproductive data are shown in Table 44.2. Chicks grow fast, reaching their adult weight within two weeks of hatching (Nettle, Monaghan et al. 2015).

Starlings go through a complete moult once each year, following breeding, with juveniles moulting their distinct grey-brown, spotless, plumage at the same time. New feathers are tipped with white or buff giving a spotted appearance that is less apparent by the following breeding season as the pale feather tips wear off.

Normal behaviour

Free-living starlings are probably best known for their spectacular aerial murmurations, which peak in the winter months, but these will not be seen in captivity. Starlings are adapted for terrestrial foraging with powerful legs for walking and a strong, pointed bill for probing into the substrate to locate soil invertebrates. Probing behaviour involves the bird pushing its closed bill into the soil, opening its bill to create a hole while rotating its eyes forwards to gain binocular vision of the contents of the hole (Figure 44.1). Starlings are often seen foraging on the ground both in the wild and in captivity. Hawking of flying insects has also been observed. Starlings are attracted to fruit such as apples, cherries and grapes and are common pests of vineyards and orchards. They will also eat animal feed such as pig pellets and are common around farms. Starlings have relatively long and pointed wings adapted for fast flight across open country. Starlings can be tame and approachable in gardens, but are generally more wary in rural areas. Hand-reared birds can be extremely tame and remain less scared of humans in laboratory conditions (Feenders & Bateson 2011a). Starlings are highly vocal, with both sexes singing, except in the breeding season when only the males sing. They have a complex song, incorporating mimicry, and are open-ended learners extending their repertoire throughout life.

Sources

The vast majority of starlings used in laboratory research are caught from the wild either as adults or juveniles (Asher & Bateson 2008). A number of methods can be used to catch starlings. Walk-in traps and funnel traps can be very successful, especially if live decoy birds are used. However, the ethical and legal considerations of the latter strategy need to be carefully considered. Mist nets and baited, spring-loaded whoosh nets can also be used successfully. The advantage of whoosh netting is that a large number of birds can be caught simultaneously. Adult birds can easily be captured roosting in nestboxes prior to the start of the breeding season. The advantage of catching juvenile birds is that they are of known age and may adapt better to captivity. However, they

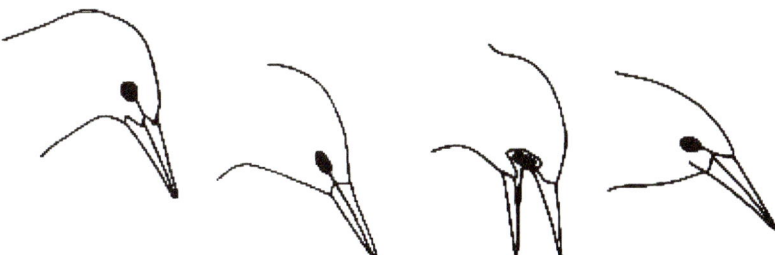

Figure 44.1 Distinctive probing behaviour of a starling. From left to right, the bird searches for indication of a prey item; lowers its head pushing its closed bill into the soil; it opens its bill to create a hole while rotating its eyes forwards; then raises its head to complete the movement. *Source:* Reproduced from *The Starling* by Feare (1984), by permission of Oxford University Press (www.oup.com).

also typically have higher parasite loads and are more prone to developing symptoms of avian pox following capture.

Hand raising chicks is extremely time-consuming, but can be achieved successfully provided chicks are at least 4 days old at the time they are taken from the nest (e.g. Nettle et al. 2017). Hand raising chicks of less than 4 days is reported to be unsuccessful.

Starlings will attempt to breed if housed in mixed-sex aviaries with nestboxes, exhibiting the full range of natural reproductive behaviour including singing, copulation, solicitations, nest construction, laying and incubation (see Calisi et al. 2011). However, the chicks usually die soon after hatching due to the lack of appropriate food (but see Meaden 1993). A solution to this problem is to use a large portable aviary that can be moved around natural pasture during the night so that a constant supply of fresh invertebrates is always available to the birds.

Conservation status

The International Union for the Conservation of Nature and Natural Resources places the starling globally in the category of Least Concern. However, the number of starlings has fallen rapidly in the UK since the early 1980s (Robinson et al. 2005), leading to upgrading of the species' UK conservation listing to Red (>50% population decline). Starlings are rated as SPEC category 3 (declining) in Europe. In the UK, starlings are protected under the Wildlife and Countryside Act 1981, which makes it illegal to intentionally kill, injure or take a starling, or to take, damage or destroy an active nest or its contents. In England, a licence is required from Natural England to disturb, catch or hold starlings. In the USA and Canada, starlings are not protected under wildlife conservation laws due to their status as both an introduced species and agricultural pest. Thus, it is important to check national laws prior to catching wild birds or interfering with their nests.

Use in research

Benefits

Starlings are the most commonly used non-domesticated passerine bird species in laboratory research (Asher & Bateson 2008; Bateson & Feenders 2010). The popularity of the species can be explained by a number of factors. Starlings are widely geographically distributed, locally abundant and relatively easy to catch. Their colonial breeding and readiness to adopt nest boxes make the species ideal if easy access to eggs or chicks in wild populations is required. Furthermore, breeding starlings are very resilient to nest disturbance and tolerate daily nest box visits involving temporary removal of chicks for cross-fostering, weighing, blood sampling or other procedures (Wright & Cuthill 1990; Nettle et al. 2016).

In the laboratory, starlings are robust, settling fast in captivity and usually remaining in good health. Their gregarious nature allows group housing at relatively high densities. They have simple husbandry and dietary requirements. For many experimental purposes, starlings are an ideal size, being large enough for a variety of procedures (e.g. repeated blood sampling (e.g. Gott et al. 2018) and implantation of body temperature loggers (e.g. Dawson 2017)), but small enough to allow behaviour such as flight performance to be studied in captivity (e.g. Brilot et al. 2009; O'Hagan et al. 2015). The starling's voracious appetite and omnivorous diet makes the species ideal for studies of foraging behaviour. Being naturally inquisitive, starlings are easy to train on behavioural tasks; and key-pecking for food can be established quickly using autoshaping procedures (e.g. Feenders & Bateson 2013). These features make starlings ideal for studies of learning, memory and decision making (Bateson, Brilot et al. 2015; Nettle Andrews et al. 2015). Starlings can readily be brought into breeding condition by manipulation of day length, and will sing, choose mates and initiate breeding in captivity (e.g. Buchanan et al. 2003). The life history and telomere dynamics of starlings arguably makes the species a better model for some aspects of human ageing than more conventional laboratory rodent species (Nettle et al. 2017). A three-dimensional digital atlas of the starling brain, which can be used to determine the stereotactic location of identified neural structures, is now available (De Groof et al. 2016). The starling genome has been sequenced and annotated and a de novo assembly of the liver transcriptome is available (Richardson et al. 2017).

Types of research

Starlings are currently used in many areas of pure and applied biological research (reviewed by Asher & Bateson 2008). A search of the Scopus database for articles published over the 5-year period between 2014 and 2018, containing either 'European starling' or 'Sturnus vulgaris' within the title, abstract or keywords, yielded ~23 articles/year reporting studies of captive starlings. This figure does not include field studies on free-living birds (often nest-box populations) that also involve shorter-term handling and scientific procedures, for which the current chapter may also be relevant.

The majority of recent work on starlings is concerned with understanding their behaviour and the cognitive, neural and physiological mechanisms underlying it. Starlings have been an important model in the behavioural ecology of foraging and decision making (Barnett et al. 2014; Bloxham et al. 2014; Smith et al. 2014; van Berkel et al. 2018). They have also been studied in relation to the role played by vision in foraging and anti-predator responses (Butler & Fernández-Juricic 2014; Qadri et al. 2014; Qadri & Cook 2015; Butler et al. 2018). Starlings can be trained to fly in wind tunnels and have been used in studies of avian flight (Stalnov et al. 2015; Gurka et al. 2016; Schulz et al. 2016). Their complex song has made starlings important subjects for studying the neuroethology of hearing, song learning and song production (DeVries et al. 2015; Rouse et al. 2015; Alger et al. 2016; Bregman et al. 2016; Aronowitz et al. 2017; Feenders et al. 2017; Hahn et al. 2017). They have also been used to understand the neuroendocrine control of reproduction and the stress response (Calisi et al. 2016; Fischer et al. 2016; de Bruijn et al. 2017; Riters et al. 2017; Carbeck et al. 2018; Spool et al. 2019). Starlings have recently become an interesting new model for studies of cellular ageing (Nettle et al. 2017; Gott et al. 2018) and the study of life-history trade-offs (Casagrande et al. 2015; Pinxten et al. 2017). The abundance of starlings in urban areas and their tendency to feed at sewage treatment plants has led to the species becoming a popular model in ecotoxicology and specifically understanding the effects of environmental pollutants on cognition and behaviour (Carlson et al. 2014; Zahara et al. 2015; North et al. 2017; Whitlock et al. 2018). Starlings' status as a pest on farms, around airports and in towns has led to their use in research aimed at developing methods for deterring them (Werner et al. 2014; Mahjoub et al. 2015). Finally, the use of starlings in laboratory experiments has led to a recent increase in research specifically addressing the laboratory welfare of this species (Matheson et al. 2008; Feenders & Bateson 2011a; Jayne et al. 2013; George et al. 2014; Bateson, Emmerson et al. 2015).

General husbandry

Enclosures

Free-living starlings are estimated to travel up to 20 km a day between feeding and roosting sites (Feare 1984), meaning that most captive environments are very unnatural in terms of the amount of space they allow. Despite this, captive starlings can be maintained successfully in relatively small cages with the median cage volume revealed by a review of current practice being just 0.42 m^3 (Asher & Bateson 2008). Starlings can also be housed in indoor aviaries or rooms. It is possible to house 20–30 birds in a 2–3 m^2 room with paper or wood chips on the floor. Capture from indoor rooms is easy with the lights turned off. Group housing in large, outdoor aviaries comes closest to the natural situation and is likely to be preferable for welfare. Advantages include natural light, reduced feather damage, greater space for flight and lower maintenance (meaning less disturbance by human caretakers). Disadvantages of large outdoor aviaries are that individuals are less easy to inspect and capture and environmental conditions are harder to control (although the latter is more likely to be a scientific than welfare problem). Where birds have to be kept in smaller cages for scientific reasons (e.g. the need for individual monitoring or frequent capture), a minimum space requirement of 1 m^3 for a singly housed bird has been recommended by the Joint Working Group on Refinement (Hawkins 2001). Long-shaped cages that allow for flight are preferable to squarer or taller cages (Asher, Davies et al. 2009). Small cages (e.g. ~0.15 m^3) can elicit abnormal behaviour, such as somersaulting stereotypies, and have been shown to be associated with the development of pessimistic cognitive biases potentially indicative of a more anxious or depressed state (Matheson et al. 2008; Brilot et al. 2010; Feenders & Bateson 2011b). Small cages with a volume ≤ 0.15 m^3 should therefore be avoided if possible and should not be used for long periods of time. In small cages (0.34 × 0.38 × 0.45 m), crowding (of up to six birds) has been shown to be a source of acute stress in starlings evidenced by decreased preening and increased agonistic behaviour and heart rate (Nephew & Romero 2003). High stocking densities in small cages should be avoided.

Environmental provisions and enrichments

Outdoor aviaries should include an area for roosting that is protected from the weather. Nest boxes should not routinely be provided in mixed-sex aviaries, because they are likely to provoke aggressive nest defence and may encourage unsuccessful breeding attempts. If nestboxes are required for breeding, they should have internal dimensions approximately 13 cm wide, 17 cm deep and 36 cm tall with a 4.5 cm diameter round entrance hole near the top, and should be mounted at least 2.5 m off the ground. Aviaries and cages should be equipped with adequate perches for all birds so as to reduce competition. Plenty of perches at a variety of heights should be provided; birds will tend to spend most of their time on the highest perch available. In aviaries, it is advantageous to have some moving perches (e.g. ropes) since this will help maintain agility. Perches of varying thicknesses and textures (natural branches are ideal) will help maintain healthy claws and feet and provide a variety of substrates for bill-wiping (Witter & Cuthill 1992). Perches should not be located directly over food and water dishes to avoid fouling.

Protective foliage cover in the form of evergreen trees or branches is likely to reduce perceived predation risk in starlings and may be important in reducing anxiety and encouraging birds to use other available enrichment.

Bathing is probably important for feather and skin maintenance and appears to be a strong behavioural need in starlings (Brilot et al. 2009). Starlings deprived of bathing water show increased signs of predation-related anxiety (Brilot & Bateson 2012). Starlings will attempt to bathe in their drinking water unless suitable baths are provided. Trays of bathing water at least 20 cm in diameter and not more than 3 cm deep should be provided, and will need to be replaced daily due to fouling.

Starlings will choose to work for food by searching for it in a substrate such as sand even if the same food is freely available (Inglis & Ferguson 1986; Bean et al. 1999). This so-called contra-freeloading behaviour may suggest a need to perform natural foraging behaviour (Kacelnik 1982), which can be met in captivity by providing a substrate for starlings to probe. Ideally, the entire floor of the enclosure should be covered with a substrate such as bark chippings, but if this is not possible, trays of sand, bark chips or turf should be provided that are large enough. At Newcastle University, we have developed a probing box for starlings (Figure 44.2).

Provision of environmental enrichment for starlings, that must be housed within a small cage for scientific reasons, is associated with fewer abnormal behaviour patterns and more optimistic cognitive biases indicative of a more positive affective state (Bateson & Matheson 2007; Matheson et al. 2008; George et al. 2014). Thus, provision of enrichments may partially offset the negative welfare consequences of

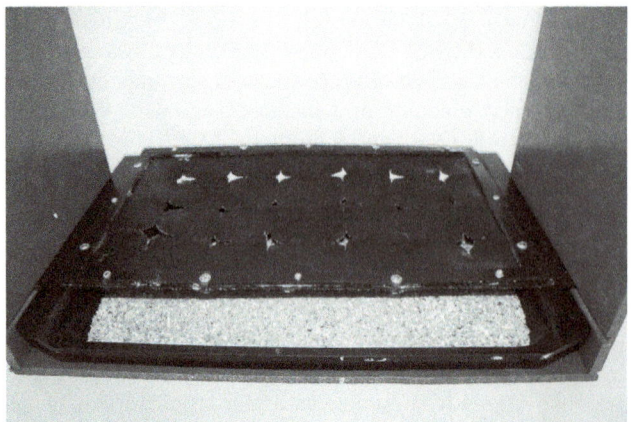

Figure 44.2 The probing box comprises a shallow tray of sand in which mealworms can be dispersed covered by a pierced rubber sheet through which the birds can probe (here shown partially displaced in order to reveal the sand tray). Live mealworms are distributed in the tray of sand daily. The sand facilitates maintenance of the birds' bills while the rubber sheet can be easily cleaned and prevents the birds from fouling the sand.

housing in small cages. Starlings will pay the cost of having to travel through a heavily weighted door to access a cage equipped with a turf probing tray or protective cover, demonstrating the value they attach to these two enrichments (Asher, Kirkden et al. 2009). When birds are group-housed, enrichment items should be large enough not to allow aggressive defence by a single bird (Gill 1995).

Feeding/watering

Starlings are omnivores eating both animal (predominantly insects and their larvae, but also other non-insect invertebrates) and plant material at all times of year (soft fruits in autumn and seeds and cereals in autumn and winter). In captivity, starlings can be kept indefinitely on commercial poultry (chick or turkey) or game bird starter crumbs or dry cat or dog food, provided the animal protein content is around 30% and the fat content around 10%. This diet should be provided *ad libitum* and can be supplemented with live or dried invertebrates (e.g. mealworms or commercial insect-based mixes designed for insectivorous birds) and low-sucrose fruit such as apple pieces, cherries and grapes; the Sturnidae are unable to digest sucrose and high sucrose fruit should be avoided (Martínez del Rio 1990). Live invertebrate prey can be placed in the probing substrate to encourage natural foraging behaviour. Insoluble grit does not appear to be required by starlings. Drinking water should be available at all times, and should be changed at least once a day. Use of gravity dispensers for both food and water will help to reduce fouling. An adequate number of feeders and water bottles should be provided to reduce aggressive interactions in aviaries.

Starling chicks can be hand-reared on soaked dried cat food with a high chicken content and apple puree supplemented with vitamins and calcium blended to a paste-like consistency (Feenders & Bateson 2011a). If accurate quantification of feeding is required, this diet can be liquidised and dispensed directly into the birds' mouths with a repeating pipette (Nettle et al. 2017). Feeding to satiation 10 times per day is sufficient to ensure normal growth in chicks from four days post-hatch. It is not necessary to give chicks fed on the above diet any additional water. Newly hatched chicks will readily beg to humans, but between 10 and 14 days post-hatch they imprint on their parents and stop begging to humans making hand-rearing much more difficult. Thus, chicks for hand-rearing should be taken from the wild between 4 and 10 days post-hatch, ideally before their eyes have opened (around day 6). Although starlings fledge at ~21 days post-hatch, they still rely on their parents for feeding after fledging. Hand-reared birds will need to continue to be hand fed, initially several times a day, for another 7–10 days post-fledging until they are feeding independently. As hand feeding is gradually withdrawn, careful monitoring is required to ensure juvenile birds are getting sufficient food.

Social housing

Captive starlings prefer to be in proximity to conspecifics, and can be housed at relatively high densities as long as adequate roosting perches and food dishes are provided so that all birds can use these simultaneously (Boogert et al. 2006). Groups of 4–12 birds are recommended. It is better to keep several birds together in a larger cage, even if this is at a reduced space per bird. The value that starlings attach to social contact is demonstrated by the fact that isolated birds will forgo foraging in order to be close to a group of conspecifics (Vasquez & Kacelnik 2000).

It is feasible to house starlings individually for scientific purposes, but, if possible, auditory and visual contact with other birds should be maintained. Isolated starlings will work to see still pictures of conspecifics, suggesting that images of starlings are reinforcing (Perret et al. 2015). This research suggests that photographs of starlings could provide a form of environmental enrichment for isolated birds.

Identification and sexing

Starlings can be individually identified with leg rings (bands) of either plastic, rubber or aluminium. Ring size 'C' (diameter 4.3 mm, weight 0.14 g) is usually appropriate for a starling. Split plastic rings and rubber rings are fitted with the tool provided with them, whereas metal rings will require specialist ringing pliers. Rings should be large enough to move freely on the starling's leg but not too large to fall over its foot. Rings are available printed with numbers and also in a range of colours to aid identification of birds without the need for catching. More than one ring can be accommodated on each leg if a large range of colour combinations is required. A microchip can be mounted on a leg ring to allow non-invasive automated identification of a bird when it is in the proximity of a microchip reader. This technology can be used to facilitate automated remote weighing of birds or automated recording of feeder visits in both individually and group-housed birds. Chicks cannot be ringed before ~7 days post-hatch and are most easily identified by marking

Table 44.3 Sexually dimorphic features in starlings.

Variable	Male	Female	Accuracy in juveniles?*
Colour of base of bill	Grey–blue	Salmon pink	100%, but only in the breeding season (when males have yellow bills)
Lightness of iris colour relative to dark chocolate brown pupil	Either dim ring, visible with careful observation or so dark as to be indistinguishable from pupil	Either much lighter with a highly distinct ring or lighter with a clear ring	98% classified correctly using this feature alone
Throat and chest feather length	Mostly long and thin	Range from 50% long and thin, 50% short and wide to mostly short and wide	93–94%
Throat and chest feather tip shape	Range from 50% round, 50% V-shaped to mostly V-shaped	Mostly rounded	81–89%
Mass	Heavier: ≥78 g	Lighter: <78 g	70–72%
Tarsus length	Longer: ≥29.3 mm	Shorter: <29.3 mm	65–67%
Speckling (density of pale feather tips)	Fewer to no spots	More spots	Not a useful trait in juveniles

* Figures are taken from an analysis in Smith, Cuthill et al. (2005).

the top of the head with non-toxic paint; such marks will need to be renewed every couple of days.

Starlings are sexually dimorphic and can be accurately sexed from external features alone (see Table 44.3). Juveniles can be more difficult to sex based on plumage; however, 98% can be correctly classified based on iris colour alone (Smith, Cuthill et al. 2005). Molecular sexing can be performed on DNA from a drop of blood or a mouth swab.

Physical environment

Keeping any bird species in captivity requires careful attention to the physical environmental conditions selected. Starlings originate in temperate areas and have evolved to time their annual cycle of reproduction to coincide with seasonal fluctuations in climate and food supply. Therefore, the physiological state and behaviour of starlings are sensitive to environmental cues including temperature and photoperiod. Choosing the correct physical environment is important not only to optimise welfare, but also to achieve the desired scientific objectives (Bateson & Feenders 2010).

Temperature and humidity

Starlings can withstand a wide range of temperatures and humidity as evidenced by their geographic distribution, and will thrive in outdoor aviaries (in the UK climate) provided that some shelter is available. Inside, it is typical to maintain laboratory temperatures at 14–20 °C; however, deviations from this range are unlikely to cause problems. Starlings have been shown to mount an acute stress response to a rapid 3 °C drop in ambient temperature (De Bruijn & Romero 2011). However, repeated exposure to weather-related stressors (including a rapid 3 °C drop in ambient temperature) does not appear to cause common symptoms of chronic stress (de Bruijn et al. 2017). Ambient temperature is known to affect foraging decisions and fat storage (Cuthill et al. 2000; Bateson 2002; Chatelain et al. 2013).

There is no information on the humidity requirements of starlings or the effects of changes in humidity. Provision of water baths (recommended) allows birds the option to increase the humidity in the micro-climate around their body. Exposing starlings to a short bout of artificial rain has been shown to induce an acute stress response (De Bruijn & Romero 2013).

Photoperiod

Photoperiod is extremely important in starlings because, like other temperate-zone species, they use the annual change in day length to control the seasonal onset of breeding and moult (Nicholls et al. 1988; Dawson 2007). Photorefractoriness is the stage of the annual cycle in which the reproductive system is inactive and the gonads are regressed. This state is present in juvenile birds and in adults it is caused by exposure to long days following the breeding season. The short days of winter render birds photosensitive, such that when days lengthen in spring, the neuroendocrine changes leading to gonadal maturation and breeding are stimulated. Thus, exposure to long days has opposite effects on the physiology and behaviour of birds depending on their experience. The threshold day length necessary to induce photorefractoriness in starlings is higher than that required to induce reproductive development. As a consequence, starlings can be maintained in reproductive condition for very long periods (possibly indefinitely) on a regime of 11 L: 13 D. Prolonged exposure (>30 days) to long days (> 12 hours light) results in a photorefractoriness, gonadal regression and finally moult. In starlings held on 13 L: 11 D, the gonads will remain regressed indefinitely and birds will never come into breeding condition.

To maintain a natural seasonal cycle in starlings housed indoors, it is necessary to alter the light schedule on a weekly basis to keep step with the natural day length outside. The welfare consequences of altering the natural seasonal cycle are unknown. If birds are kept indoors for long periods, then it is advisable to expose them to a sequence of short and long days to stimulate an annual moult and thus maintain feather condition. Moult duration can be reduced from 119 days for birds held on constant long days of 18 L : 6 D to 92 days by gradually reducing the period of daylight by 1 h/week from 18 L : 6 D to 12 L : 12 D; however, this acceleration is bought at the expense of reduced final feather quality (Dawson 2004). Following a period of long days, photosensitivity in starlings can be reinstated by a period of 25–35 days of 8 L : 16 D (Goldsmith & Nicholls 1984).

For birds housed indoors, either the daily transition between light and dark should be gradual in order to allow birds to find a roosting site for the night, or a dim nightlight should be provided.

Quality of light

Like humans, birds rely heavily on their visual sense. However, the frequency at which a flickering light source is perceived as continuous is believed to be higher in birds than in humans (>100 Hz vs. 50–60 Hz, respectively), leading to concern that starlings may be able to perceive the flicker from conventional low-frequency fluorescent lights (100 Hz in Europe and 120 Hz in the USA) and cathode ray tube monitors. In preference tests, starlings prefer high-frequency (>30 kHz) over low-frequency (100 Hz) lighting, indicating that they can detect a difference (Greenwood et al. 2004). Myoclonus (involuntary muscle twitching) is induced in starlings exposed to fluorescent lighting and cathode ray tube monitors flickering below 150 Hz (Smith & Evans 2005). Birds are less active and have higher basal corticosterone levels under low-frequency lighting, suggesting that they may find it more stressful (Smith, Greenwood et al. 2005). Starlings also show changes in mate choice in low- and high-frequency lighting, becoming less consistent in the preferences in low-frequency conditions (Evans et al. 2006). It is therefore recommended that, if natural light is not available, rooms are lit with high-frequency fluorescent lights (>150 Hz).

Most birds, including starlings, have an additional retinal cone type tuned to UV wavelengths meaning that if they are housed in laboratories without UV light, they may be deprived of visual information usually available to them in the outside world. There is some evidence to suggest that starlings may prefer a light environment containing UV (Greenwood et al. 2002), and that being housed in a UV-deficient light environment causes higher basal corticosterone levels and changes in behaviour (Maddocks et al. 2002). Lack of UV light may also be involved in the development of hyperkeratosis (see the following text). It is therefore recommended that starlings are housed in rooms with full-spectrum lighting. Specialist UV lamps marketed for parrots can be used in starling aviaries.

Noise

Birds perceive sounds in a different frequency range from humans and laboratory rodents. Whereas humans hear well in the range of 0.2–8 kHz, passerines have a narrower range, hearing best in the range of 1–5 kHz (Heffner 1998). There is no evidence that passerines can perceive infra- or ultrasound, so sources of such sound are not a welfare concern for starlings. However, raised noise levels are likely to be stressful and cause changes in both physiology and behaviour (Rich & Romero 2005).

Hygiene

The main disadvantage of starlings as an experimental animal is the large quantities of droppings (faeces and urates) they produce. The floor covering needs to be replaced daily in smaller cages, but in larger aviaries less frequent cleaning is necessary. Cleaning can be stressful for birds, particularly those in cages, but stress can be reduced if husbandry is conducted as quietly as possible, ideally by a familiar person, at a similar time each day (Rich & Romero 2005). It may also help if birds are provided with high perches and/or cover to which they can retreat during husbandry.

Starlings can carry zoonotic pathogens and therefore pose an infection risk. One analysis of bacteria present in free-living starling droppings showed that most did not belong to the specific types most often found in humans, suggesting that starlings are unlikely to present a major source of infection for humans (Gautsch et al. 2000). However, avian influenza (AI), which can be fatal in humans, can occur in wild starlings. Starlings show only mild symptoms of AI and recover quickly (Perkins & Swayne 2003; Ellis et al. 2021), meaning that infection could be missed. Some laboratories routinely screen incoming starlings for common pathogens including *Salmonella*, *Yersinia* and coccidia.

Recently acquired starlings should be kept isolated from existing laboratory stock for at least 2 weeks to establish as far as possible that birds are free from infectious diseases and to allow screening for zoonoses and treatment for parasites (see the following text). During AI outbreaks in wild birds, incoming birds should be quarantined for 4 weeks, during which human contact is limited to essential husbandry and biosecurity measures are enhanced.

Care of aged animals

Starlings can be maintained in captivity for many years without obvious signs of senescence. Starlings' claws and bills are adapted for walking and probing in soil and can become overgrown in captivity where they are not naturally abraded. Provision of rough wooden or sandpaper-covered perches and probing substrates (see Figure 44.2) can help (Cuthill et al. 1992), but usually birds will need to be caught and their bills and claws trimmed with nail clippers every few months. Overgrowth of the upper mandible will result in feeding and preening problems. It is important to check regularly that leg rings have not become too tight as a result of hyperkeratosis-related thickening of leg scales. In starlings kept for over a year indoors, the most significant problem that we have encountered at Newcastle University is development of hyperkeratosis (see section in the following text on common health and welfare problems).

Laboratory procedures

Handling

Capture by hand is possible in smaller cages. Since birds will not fly in the dark, it is often easier to turn off the room lights and use a small torch to locate birds. In larger cages or

The European starling

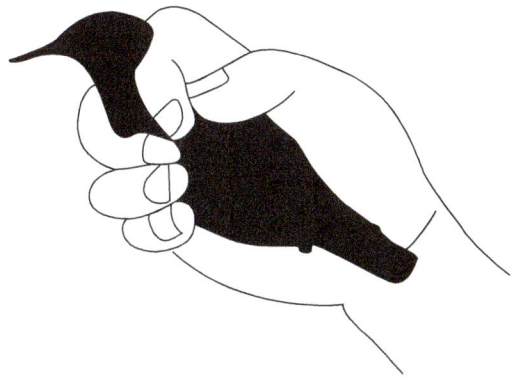

Figure 44.3 A recommended way to hold a starling: the bird's head is held between the index and middle finger with its back in the palm of the hand. The ring finger, little finger and thumb rest across the bird's closed wings to prevent them from flapping.

outdoor aviaries, a net (with padded edges) will be necessary. Birds will usually fly towards the light, and an indoor aviary can easily be emptied by turning off the lights and allowing the birds to fly into an adjacent lit room. Starlings can be trained to enter a small transport cage by reinforcing this behaviour with a preferred treat such as mealworms. Cotton drawstring bags are ideal for transporting starlings over short distances. A recommended procedure for holding a starling is shown in Figure 44.3.

Training procedures

Captive starlings can be rapidly habituated to familiar humans if human visits are associated with beneficial consequences such as provision of mealworms or water baths. It is not unusual for well-habituated birds to take mealworms directly from humans. However, if birds are to be released to the wild, consideration should be given as to the possible adverse consequences of extensive habituation to humans.

Starlings can be easily trained to perform responses including hopping on perches, flying through mazes, probing holes through paper, going through push-doors, pecking lids off wells/dishes, and pecking illuminated keys or touchscreens. Pecking illuminated keys for food reward can be trained using standard autoshaping procedures (Bateson & Kacelnik 1995; Feenders & Bateson 2013). Other behaviour patterns such as hopping between perches or using their feet to remove the stopper from a food container will need to be trained by gradual shaping with positive reinforcement.

Starlings learn to work for preferred treats such as live mealworms with minimal or no prior food deprivation (Bloxham et al. 2014). However, if birds are being reinforced with their normal diet or operant pellets, it may be necessary to restrict their food intake by removing *ad libitum* food for a period of time immediately prior to the training session. Since birds do not eat during the night, it often works well to remove *ad libitum* food at the end of the day and start the daily training session first thing the following morning when birds are hungry; birds can then be fed *ad libitum* following the training session for the remainder of the day (e.g. Dunn et al. 2018b). This method is recommended as being safer and easier to implement than attempting to maintain birds at a percentage of their free-feeding mass, because it does not rely on the establishment of a stable baseline mass, which can be problematic in starlings (see section on weighing below). Body mass should be monitored regularly in birds that are food restricted.

Monitoring methods

Weighing

Birds can be weighed manually by catching and placing in a cloth bag or plastic decapitation cone (see Figure 44.4a). If regular monitoring of body mass is necessary (e.g. for birds that are food restricted), it is desirable to find a weighing method that does not require catching. Starlings can be

(a)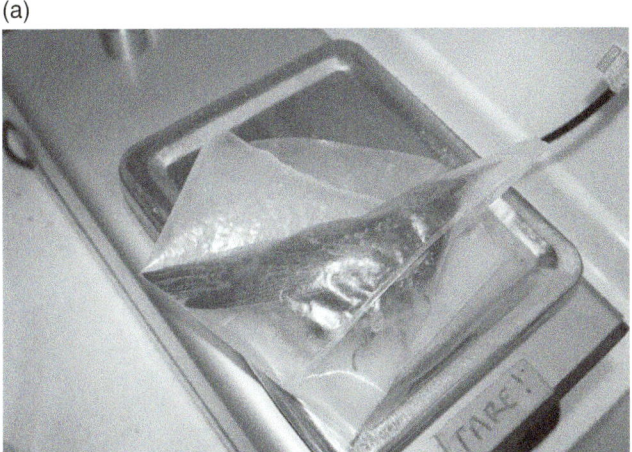

(b)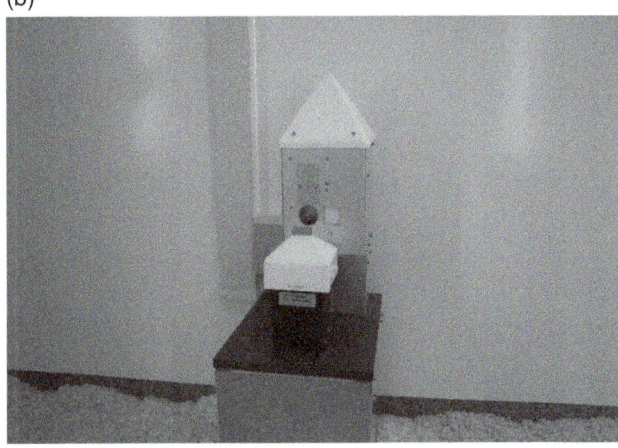

Figure 44.4 Methods for weighing starlings. (a) Using a decapitation cone to weigh a starling on standard electronic balance. (b) The system developed at Newcastle University that allows microchipped starlings to weigh themselves every time they forage from an operant feeding station. The short wooden perch is designed to accommodate a single starling and sits on an electronic balance equipped with a microchip reader. The bird can feed from a hopper located behind the circular aperture on the feeding station (see Bateson et al. 2021).

trained to come to a balance in their cage for mealworms. The balance can either be connected to a computer or read directly (a video camera or binoculars can be used for this in the case of shy birds). Another potentially less labour-intensive option is fit a balance to a regularly used perch within the home cage/aviary. A balance can be combined with a microchip reader in order to allow group-housed birds equipped with microchips to be weighed regularly without catching (see Figure 44.4b; Bateson et al. 2021).

It is important to be aware that individual birds can vary substantially in mass. Starlings show a daily cycle of body mass, increasing their mass between dawn and dusk and losing mass over night when they do not forage; a bird can lose up to 10 g on a long winter night (Tait 1973). Mass also varies with season; birds can be as much as 15 g heavier in winter than summer. Other factors known to influence body condition include predictability of food (birds on unpredictable feeding schedules are heavier: Cuthill et al. 2000; Witter et al. 1995), dominance status (dominant birds are lighter: Witter & Swaddle 1995), housing conditions (captive birds are lighter in individual cages than in aviaries: Dunn et al. 2018a) and moult (birds can become very light during moult). In studies where mass is important, birds should be weighed at the same time of day (preferably before it is light in the morning when the gut is empty).

Body temperature

Body temperature can be measured using a cloacal probe or by placing a fast-responding thermocouple thermometer under the wing against the bare skin. Starlings are homoeothermic with normal body temperature described as 39–40 °C (Feare 1984). The thermoneutral zone—the range of ambient temperatures over which feather insulation alone can maintain body temperature—is approximately 15–40 °C (Feare 1984). If frequent temperature measurements are required, this can be accomplished by surgically implanting a small temperature logger (e.g. one model available is 17 × 6 mm and weights 1 g) sub-dermally on the nape of the neck (Dawson 2017). Such loggers will later need to be removed in order to download the data.

Heart rate

Heart rate of caged starlings has to be measured continuously with a nearby external receiver using small heart rate transmitters (20 × 10 × 10 mm, 4 g) surgically implanted in the inter-scapular space or the abdominal cavity (Nephew & Romero 2003; De Bruijn & Romero 2013). Birds were reported to be able to fly and behave normally following recovery from surgery. In the latter study, baseline heart rates of ~330–380 bpm were recorded for singly caged birds, with heart rates rising to ~540 bpm when five intruder birds were introduced into the cage.

Blood sampling

In adult starlings, blood samples are most easily taken from the brachial (alar) vein. The metatarsal vein can also be used, but this is harder to locate quickly if rapid sampling is required. Use of the jugular vein is not recommended due to the risks of accidentally puncturing the nearby carotid artery. With some practice holding and positioning birds, it is straightforward for a single person to collect blood from either the right or left brachial or metatarsal veins unassisted (see Figures 44.5a and 44.5b). For right-handers puncturing the vein with the right hand, the easiest vein to access is the left brachial vein. Use of alcohol for site preparation is not recommended, because it causes cooling, and the consequent vasoconstriction can make the vein hard to locate, but water (applied with wet cotton wool) can be used to temporarily damp down downy feathers around the sampling site. No feather plucking should be necessary to expose the brachial or metatarsal veins. The vein is punctured with a sterile 25G (orange) needle, and the resulting drop or pool of blood collected with one or more microcapillary tubes (usually, 75 μl tubes are convenient). Once the sample has been collected, light pressure should be applied to the puncture site with a cotton wool ball to staunch any further bleeding. In the case of the brachial vein, it is usually possible to place the cotton wool under the bird's wing and hold the bird as in Figure 44.3 for a few minutes. Usually, bleeding stops very quickly, but occasionally light pressure will need to be

(a)

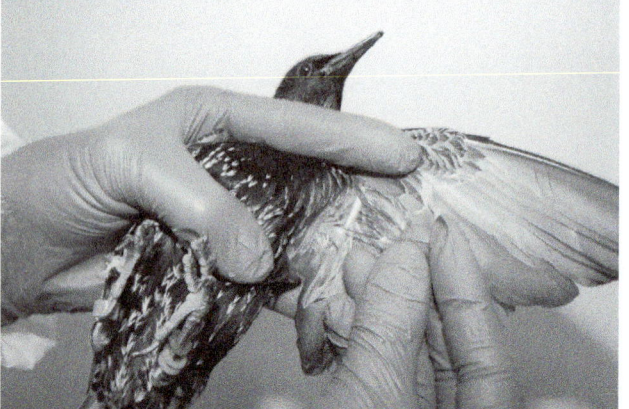

(b)

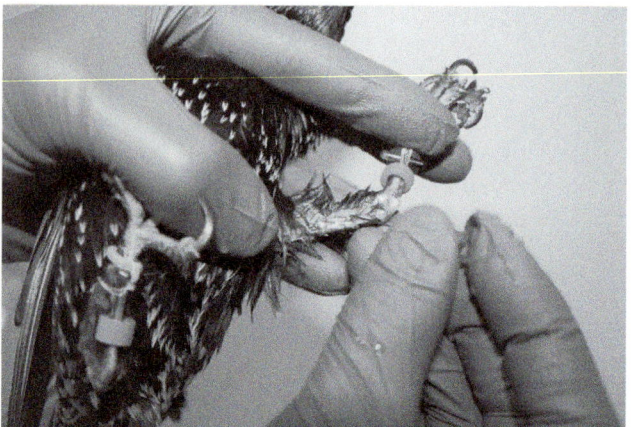

Figure 44.5 Holding a starling for blood sampling. (a) Left brachial vein and (b) Left metatarsal vein.

applied for several minutes. The bird should be held until bleeding has completely ceased.

In newly hatched chicks (1–4 days), the feet and legs are better developed than the wings and blood is therefore most easily taken from the metatarsal vein. Due to lack of plumage, no water is required to expose the vein and it can easily be seen in good light. Measures must be taken to keep chicks warm while they are out of the nest. Chemical heating pads can be used to create a warm transport container for chicks and researchers handling chicks should ensure that their hands are warm.

Whatever the age of the bird, as small a volume of blood as possible should be taken. Following standard guidance, not more than 10% of the blood volume should be taken at one time and less than 15% of the blood volume should be taken in any 30-day period (Wolfensohn & Lloyd 2008). A starling can be assumed to have a total of 70 µl of blood per g body weight. Thus, a maximum of 70 µl can be taken at any one time from a 10 g nestling and 490 µl from a 70 g adult. These limits should be applied conservatively to allow for the fact that it is not always possible to stop bleeding as soon as the required sample has been collected. Repeatedly puncturing the same vein within a 48-hour period is not recommended so, if a single puncture yields insufficient blood, another vein should be used to complete the sample. Occasionally, puncturing a vein will result in the formation of a haematoma. If this occurs, attempts to withdraw blood from that vein should be abandoned and another vein selected. Following the above guidelines, we have never observed any ill effects of blood sampling in starling chicks (from 2 days post-hatch) or adults.

Administration of substances

For substances that can be administered by mouth, feeding birds with injected mealworms should be considered as a non-invasive approach. Mealworms can be carefully injected, via the mouthparts with a hypodermic needle (e.g. Barnett et al. 2007).

The easiest injection site for intramuscular injections on a starling is the pectoral muscle (the largest muscle in the body), but care should be taken, especially if repeated injections are required, because damage to this muscle can cause impairment of flight. Subcutaneous injections in starlings can be made into the inguinal leg fold (e.g. Kelm-Nelson et al. 2012). Intraperitoneal injections in starlings should be avoided due to the risk of injecting into air sacs. Subcutaneous silastic implants have been used to deliver chronically raised levels of hormones such as testosterone (e.g. Spool et al. 2019).

Anaesthesia and analgesia

Invasive procedures should always be accompanied by appropriate anaesthesia and analgesia. A range of different anaesthetic protocols using both injectable and inhaled agents have been described in starlings. Starlings should be food deprived for ~1 hour prior to anaesthesia (Lierz & Korbel 2012).

Inhaled anaesthetics are preferable because they are more controllable and can be delivered non-invasively, in oxygen, via a face mask, avoiding the need for painful injections. Starlings have been successfully anaesthetised for 2–3 hours with isoflurane used at 2–5% for induction and 1.5–3% for maintenance (e.g. Bee & Klump 2004).

Birds anaesthetised with ketamine only can become very excitable during recovery, risking injury. Therefore, ketamine should always be used in combination with an alpha-2-agonist. The following protocols have been described in starlings. For minor surgery (implantation of a heart rate transmitter), birds have been anaesthetised using ketamine (30 mg/kg) and xylazine (10 mg/kg) injected into the pectoral muscle (De Bruijn & Romero 2011). For fMRI, birds have been anaesthetised with 0.4 ml of a mixture containing 0.5 ml of ketamine (50 mg/ml) and 10 ml of medetomidine (1 mg/ml) injected into the pectoral muscle. In the latter protocol, anaesthesia was maintained at a constant depth by continuously infusing the mixture at a rate of 0.10 ml/h through a catheter positioned in the pectoral muscle (De Groof et al. 2017). Urethane is commonly used in acute neurophysiological experiments on starlings due to its minimal effects on physiological variables and the fact that a single injection (7 ml/kg) provides immobility for several hours (Kozlov & Gentner 2016). Urethane is controversial due to its toxicity and its use is not appropriate when recovery is required.

Birds are extremely susceptible to hypothermia, and it is advisable to control the bird's temperature during anaesthesia (e.g. by using a heated pad) and to monitor body temperature with a cloacal probe. Body temperature in starlings should be maintained at 41.5 ± 0.5 °C (De Groof et al. 2017). To monitor depth of anaesthesia during procedures, respiration rate and amplitude can be constantly measured with a small pneumatic sensor positioned under the bird (De Groof et al. 2017). The different stages of avian anaesthesia are described by Lierz and Korbel (2012). During recovery from anaesthesia, birds should be carefully monitored until they can perch normally. Recovery should take place in a quiet, warm (~25 °C), dimly lit environment.

If a procedure or injury involves tissue damage and/or there are changes in the bird's posture, temperament or normal behaviour (e.g. decline in feeding or activity), it should be assumed that the bird could be experiencing pain. Pain, or likely pain, in birds should be treated as it would be in mammals (Machin 2005). The anaesthetics ketamine and medetomidine both additionally have analgesic properties in other species and thus may provide some analgesia following anaesthesia in starlings. Unfortunately, there is very little information available on analgesia in starlings specifically. Since the effects of drugs can vary widely between avian species (Lierz & Korbel 2012), the use of drugs not previously given to starlings should be approached with caution and doses may need adjustment. Opioids are used to treat chronic and acute pain in mammals. There is some evidence that subcutaneous injection of opioid drugs affects the latency of starlings to withdraw their feet from hot water, suggesting that opioids might be effective analgesics in this species. However, the dose of fentanyl used (0.25 mg/kg) did not produce significant analgesia compared to a water control (Kelm-Nelson et al. 2012). The opioid butorphanol (1.0 mg/kg) has been shown to produce analgesia in African grey parrots (Paul-Murphy et al. 1999), but there is no record of its use in starlings. Nonsteroidal anti-inflammatory drugs (NSAIDs) are used to treat inflammatory and chronic pain. Carprofen and meloxicam are the NSAIDs of choice in birds (Lierz & Korbel 2012), but their use has not been reported in starlings. Ketoprofen has been used to treat post-surgical pain in starlings at a dose of 10 mg/kg (De Bruijn & Romero 2011), but there are no data on whether this dose is effective in this species. Use of local anaesthetics is not recommended in birds (Lierz & Korbel 2012).

Euthanasia

A range of different procedures can be used for euthanasia of starlings, the most common being concussion and cervical dislocation by striking the head on a hard surface followed by cervical dislocation or decapitation. This has the advantage of being quick, but requires confidence on the part of the handler. A widely used refinement involves inducing the bird with an inhaled anaesthetic such as isoflurane prior to decapitation. The best alternative is injection with sodium pentobarbital. The injection should ideally be intrahepatic, with the injection site under the sternum along the ventral midline.

Alternatives to euthanasia should be considered where possible for starlings captured from the wild as juveniles or adults. Release to the wild may be an option, but there are several considerations (ASAB 2018). First, it is important to determine whether release is permitted by local legislation. In England, it is common practice (and indeed sometimes a requirement of licensing bodies such as Natural England) to release wild-caught starlings following research. If release is legally possible, the researcher should assess whether it might be injurious both to the released animal and to existing populations in the area. Ideally, birds should be given a period (e.g. 2 weeks) in a large, outdoor aviary to re-acclimatise to outdoor conditions if they have been inside and to build up and exercise their flight muscles prior to release. The release site should be either near the site of original capture, or at another location frequented by wild starlings. Hand-reared birds should not be released to the wild, because they are likely to lack the necessary experience to survive.

Common health and welfare problems

Starlings are generally extremely robust and suffer few health and welfare problems in captivity. Here, we present the most common health problems reported in a questionnaire sent to researchers in both Europe and North America with extensive experience keeping starlings in the laboratory.

Injuries

Captive starlings often seem to acquire minor cuts and abrasions on the gripping surface of their feet. Signs of such injuries include traces of blood on perches or cage paper and birds perching on one leg. Birds with foot injuries should be caught, examined and monitored carefully, but these injuries usually resolve within a few days without the need for specific treatment. Foot problems can be caused by a build-up of dirt on the birds' feet. This problem is simply resolved by providing a water bath. Feather damage, especially to the primaries and tail, is common in birds housed in wire mesh cages. Although this is unsightly, it is unlikely to be a welfare problem unless birds are about to be released, in which case it could affect flight performance. Feather damage can be prevented by housing birds in smooth walled cages.

Dietary-related health problems

Hyperkeratosis characterised by raised overgrown scales on feet and legs, overgrown beak and nails and poor feather condition is common in captive starlings. In extreme cases, scales become irritating to the birds and cause problems with their leg rings. The cause of hyperkeratosis is currently unclear, and a number of possible factors have been discussed, including insufficient protein in the diet, lack of access to natural daylight and lack of bathing water. Many poultry diets and softbill diets designed for fruit-eating Mynahs contain insufficient protein for starlings (see Feeding/watering section for details). Our experience based on attempts to manage the condition at Newcastle University is that provision of sufficient dietary protein and baths are not sufficient to prevent hyperkeratosis and that lighting is likely to be critical. If starlings are kept inside, then manipulating the day length to initiate a moult and provision of UV lighting (specialist bulbs designed for parrots are available) may help reduce hyperkeratosis. There is some anecdotal evidence that hyperkeratosis is at least partially reversible in starlings.

Parasites and infectious diseases

Parasites and infectious diseases are not thought to be a major cause of mortality in free-living starling populations (Feare 1984), and captive starlings rarely have disease problems if husbandry is good. However, the species is host to a wide range of parasites with infection rates in free-living birds being higher in juveniles than adults and peaking in the summer. It is good practice to quarantine incoming birds and treat them for parasites.

Ectoparasites include feather lice, ticks and mites. These can be vectors of disease in addition to producing clinical signs of anaemia, feather loss and skin lesions. Ectoparasites can be treated with ivermectin applied topically to the back of the neck. Starlings are recorded hosts of many endoparasites including nematodes, trematodes, cestodes and acanthocephalans. The gapeworm (*Syngamus trachea*) is a long red nematode that attaches to the trachea of birds. The worms cause bleeding in the throat and can block the trachea. Starlings infected with gapeworm can often be heard coughing. Nematode worms in starlings can be treated with the following drugs: fenbendazole (by addition to feed), flubendazole (by addition to feed), ivermectin (by mouth or applied to skin) and levamisole (by addition to drinking water).

Avian pox is a viral disease that produces wart-like lesions on the bird's head, particularly around the eyes and the base of the bill. Badly affected birds may need to be euthanised, but most usually recover without treatment. It is common for birds to develop the disease shortly after capture from the wild. Juvenile starlings seem particularly susceptible to pox, but survivors appear to become immune, and captive adults rarely develop the disease.

Aspergillosis is a common fungal infection of starlings causing clinical signs ranging from mild debility to sudden death. It is usually secondary to immunosuppression from chronic stress or other primary diseases, and can also occur in the presence of high concentrations of the fungus in the environment. Clinical diagnosis of aspergillosis is difficult, and prognosis is poor.

Signs of poor welfare

Dawkins (2006) suggests that animal welfare can be assessed by focusing on just two questions: 'are the animals healthy?' and 'do they have what they want?'. If the answer to either or both of these questions is negative, then welfare is likely to be suboptimal. Acute poor health is relatively easy to recognise in starlings. A starling that is unwell or in pain will typically be lethargic, perching with a hunched posture and its feathers puffed up. The wings may droop and the eyes may be partially closed (Figure 44.6). Any bird exhibiting these signs should be caught immediately, weighed and subjected to a thorough physical examination. Chronic ill health and/or maintenance in an environment that does not provide for starlings' behavioural needs are likely to be reflected in more subtle changes in plumage, body weight and behaviour. Sustained weight loss in the absence of any environmental changes that might induce strategic weight regulation (see the section in the preceding text on weighing) is a cause for concern. The development of abnormal behaviour patterns such as stereotypies is usually associated with inadequate housing. The most frequently reported abnormal behaviour pattern exhibited by caged starlings is the somersaulting or flipping stereotypy (although incidences of stereotypy are relatively low compared with other captive birds). This appears to be most common in birds housed in small barren cages, and can be reduced by adding enrichment to the cage or returning victims to a larger aviary. Somersaulting appears to be restricted to birds caught from the wild as adults and may originate from a greater escape motivation in these individuals (Feenders & Bateson 2011b). At Newcastle University we have not observed somersaulting in hand-reared starlings.

There is evidence that singing is rewarding in starlings and thus should be associated with a positive affective state (Riters 2011; Kelm-Nelson *et al.* 2012). Presence of song could therefore be a good indicator of positive welfare in captive starlings.

Acknowledgements

I would like to thank the following individuals: Lucy Asher (Newcastle University) for her contributions to the previous version of this chapter; Kathy Murphy (Newcastle University), Heidi Lehmann (Massey University, New Zealand), Lauren Riters (University of Wisconsin) and Annemie Van Der Linden (University of Antwerp) for advice on avian anaesthesia and analgesia.

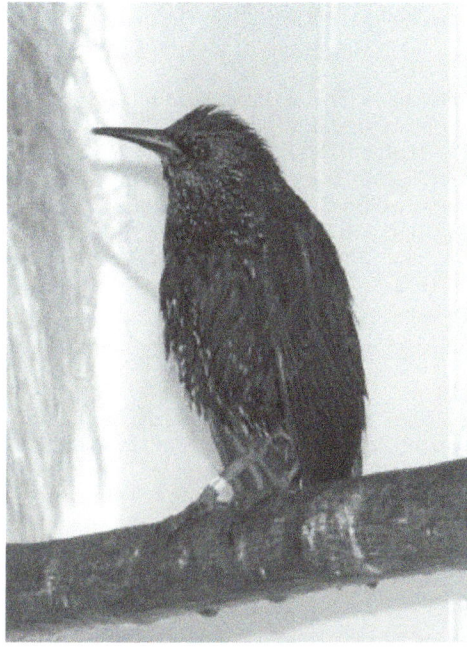

Figure 44.6 A starling in poor health. Note the drooping wings and poor feather condition. This bird has mild hyperkeratosis: note the heavy, overgrown bill and thickened leg scales.

References

Alger, S.J., Larget, B.R. and Riters, L.V. (2016) A novel statistical method for behaviour sequence analysis and its application to birdsong. *Animal Behaviour*, **116**, 181–193. doi: 10.1016/j.anbehav.2016.04.001.

Andrews, C. *et al.* (2015) Early-life adversity increases foraging and information gathering in European starlings, *Sturnus vulgaris*. *Animal Behaviour*, **109**, 123–132. doi: 10.1016/j.anbehav.2015.08.009.

Aronowitz, J.V., Newman, K.L. and McDermott, C.R. (2017) Estradiol modulates hemispheric lateralization of auditory evoked neural activity in male European starlings (*Sturnus vulgaris*). *The Journal of Neuroscience*, **37**(33), 7800–7802. doi: 10.1523/jneurosci.1414-17.2017.

ASAB (2018) Guidelines for the treatment of animals in behavioural research and teaching. *Animal Behaviour*, **135**, I–X. doi: 10.1016/j.anbehav.2017.10.001.

Asher, L. *et al.* (2009) The effects of cage volume and cage shape on the condition and behaviour of captive European starlings (*Sturnus vulgaris*). *Applied Animal Behaviour Science*, **116**(2–4), 286–294.

Asher, L. and Bateson, M. (2008) Use and husbandry of captive European starlings (*Sturnus vulgaris*) in scientific research: a review of current practice. *Laboratory Animals*, **42**(2), 1–16. doi: 10.1258/la.2007.007006.

Asher, L., Kirkden, R.D. and Bateson, M. (2009) An empirical investigation of two assumptions of motivation testing in captive starlings (*Sturnus vulgaris*): do animals have an energy budget to "spend"? and does cost reduce demand?. *Applied Animal Behaviour Science*, **118**(3–4), 152–160.

Barnett, C.A., Bateson, M. and Rowe, C. (2007) State-dependent decision making: educated predators strategically trade off the costs and benefits of consuming aposematic prey. *Behavioral Ecology*, **18**(4), 645–651. doi: 10.1093/beheco/arm027.

Barnett, C.A., Bateson, M. and Rowe, C. (2014) Better the devil you know: avian predators find variation in prey toxicity aversive. *Biology Letters*, **10**(11), 20140533. doi: http://dx.doi.org/10.1098/rsbl.2014.0533.

Bateson, M. (2002) Context-dependent foraging choices in risk-sensitive starlings. *Animal Behaviour*, **64**, 251–260.

Bateson, M., Brilot, B.O. et al. (2015) Developmental telomere attrition predicts impulsive decision-making in adult starlings. *Proceedings of the Royal Society B: Biological Sciences*, **282**, 20142140. doi: 10.1098/rspb.2014.2140.

Bateson, M., Emmerson, M. et al. (2015) Opposite effects of early-life competition and developmental telomere attrition on cognitive biases in juvenile European starlings. *PLoS One*, **10**(7), e0132602. doi: 10.1371/journal.pone.0132602.

Bateson, M. and Feenders, G. (2010) The use of passerine bird species in laboratory research: implications of basic biology for husbandry and welfare. *ILAR journal*, **51**(4), 394–408.

Bateson, M. and Kacelnik, A. (1995) Preferences for fixed and variable food sources: variability in amount and delay. *Journal of the Experimental Analysis of Behavior*, **63**(3), 313–329. doi: 10.1901/jeab.1995.63-313.

Bateson, M. and Matheson, S.M. (2007) Performance on a categorisation task suggests that removal of environmental enrichment induces "pessimism" in captive European starlings (*Sturnus vulgaris*). *Animal Welfare*, **16**(S), 33–36.

Bateson, M., Andrews, C., Dunn, J., et al. (2021). Food insecurity increases energetic efficiency, not food consumption: an exploratory study in European starlings. *PeerJ*, **9**, p.e11541.

Bedford, T. et al. (2017) Effects of early life adversity and sex on dominance in European starlings. *Animal Behaviour*, **128**. doi: 10.1016/j.anbehav.2017.03.026.

van Berkel, M. et al. (2018) Can starlings use a reliable cue of future food deprivation to adaptively modify foraging and fat reserves?. *Animal Behaviour*, **142**, 147–155. doi: 10.5281/zenodo.1193788.

Bloxham, L. et al. (2014) The memory of hunger: developmental plasticity of dietary selectivity in the European starling, Sturnus vulgaris. *Animal Behaviour*, **91**, 33–40. doi: 10.1016/j.anbehav.2014.02.025.

Boogert, N.J., Reader, S.M. and Laland, K.N. (2006) The relation between social rank, neophobia and individual learning in starlings. *Animal Behaviour*, **72**(6), 1229–1239. doi: 10.1016/j.anbehav.2006.02.021.

Bregman, M.R., Patel, A.D. and Gentner, T.Q. (2016) Songbirds use spectral shape, not pitch, for sound pattern recognition. *Proceedings of the National Academy of Sciences*, **113**(6), 1666–1671. doi: 10.1073/pnas.1515380113.

Brilot, B.O., Asher, L. and Bateson, M. (2009) Water bathing alters the speed–accuracy trade-off of escape flights in European starlings. *Animal Behaviour*, **78**(4), 801–807. doi: 10.1016/j.anbehav.2009.07.022.

Brilot, B.O., Asher, L. and Bateson, M. (2010) Stereotyping starlings are more "pessimistic". *Animal cognition*, **13**(5), 721–31. doi: 10.1007/s10071-010-0323-z.

Brilot, B.O. and Bateson, M. (2012) Water bathing alters threat perception in starlings. *Biology Letters*, **8**(3), 379–381. doi: 10.1098/rsbl.2011.1200.

de Bruijn, R., Reed, J.M. and Romero, L.M. (2017) Chronic repeated exposure to weather-related stimuli elicits few symptoms of chronic stress in captive molting and non-molting European starlings (*Sturnus vulgaris*). *Journal of Experimental Zoology Part A: Ecological and Integrative Physiology*, **327**(8), 493–503. doi: 10.1002/jez.2134.

De Bruijn, R. and Romero, L.M. (2011) Behavioral and physiological responses of wild-caught European starlings (Sturnus vulgaris) to a minor, rapid change in ambient temperature. *Comparative Biochemistry and Physiology – A Molecular and Integrative Physiology*, **160**(2), 260–266. doi: 10.1016/j.cbpa.2011.06.011.

De Bruijn, R. and Romero, L.M. (2013) Artificial rain and cold wind act as stressors to captive molting and non-molting European starlings (*Sturnus vulgaris*). *Comparative Biochemistry and Physiology – A Molecular and Integrative Physiology*, **164**(3), 512–519. doi: 10.1016/j.cbpa.2012.12.017.

Buchanan, K.L. et al. (2003) Song as an honest signal of past developmental stress in the European starling (*Sturnus vulgaris*). *Proceedings of the Royal Society B: Biological Sciences*, **270**, 1149–1156. doi: 10.1016/S0018-506X(03)00124-7.

Butler, S.R. and Fernández-Juricic, E. (2014) European starlings recognize the location of robotic conspecific attention. *Biology Letters*, **10**(10). doi: 10.1098/rsbl.2014.0665.

Butler, S.R., Templeton, J.J. and Fernández-Juricic, E. (2018) How do birds look at their world? A novel avian visual fixation strategy. *Behavioral Ecology and Sociobiology*, **72**(3). doi: 10.1007/s00265-018-2455-0.

Calisi, R.M. et al. (2011) Social and breeding status are associated with the expression of GnIH. *Genes, Brain and Behavior*, **10**(5), 557–564. doi: 10.1111/j.1601-183X.2011.00693.x.

Calisi, R.M. et al. (2016) Patterns of hypothalamic GnIH change over the reproductive period in starlings and rats. *General and Comparative Endocrinology*, **237**, 140–146. doi: 10.1016/j.ygcen.2016.08.015.

Carbeck, K.M. et al. (2018) Environmental cues and dietary antioxidants affect breeding behavior and testosterone of male European starlings (*Sturnus vulgaris*). *Hormones and Behavior*, **103**, 36–44. doi: 10.1016/j.yhbeh.2018.05.020.

Carlson, J.R., Cristol, D. and Swaddle, J.P. (2014) Dietary mercury exposure causes decreased escape takeoff flight performance and increased molt rate in European starlings (*Sturnus vulgaris*). *Ecotoxicology*, **23**(8), 1464–1473. doi: 10.1007/s10646-014-1288-5.

Casagrande, S. et al. (2015) Birds receiving extra carotenoids keep singing during the sickness phase induced by inflammation. *Behavioral Ecology and Sociobiology*, **69**(6), 1029–1037. doi: 10.1007/s00265-015-1916-y.

Chatelain, M., Halpin, C.G. and Rowe, C. (2013) Ambient temperature influences birds' decisions to eat toxic prey. *Animal Behaviour*, **86**(4), 733–740. doi: 10.1016/j.anbehav.2013.07.007.

Cuthill, I.C. et al. (2000) Body mass regulation in response to changes in feeding predictability and overnight energy expenditure. *Behavioral Ecology*, **11**(2), 189–195.

Cuthill, I., Witter, M. and Clarke, L. (1992) The function of bill-wiping. *Animal Behaviour*, **43**(1), 103–115. doi: 10.1016/S0003-3472(05)80076-4.

Dawkins, M.S. (2006) A user's guide to animal welfare science. *Trends in Ecology & Evolution*, **21**(2), 77–82. doi: 10.1016/j.tree.2005.10.017.

Dawson, A. (2004) The effects of delaying the start of moult on the duration of moult, primary feather growth rates and feather mass in common starlings Sturnus vulgaris. *Ibis*, **146**(3), 493–500. doi: 10.1111/j.1474-919x.2004.00290.x.

Dawson, A. (2007) Seasonality in a temperate zone bird can be entrained by near equatorial photoperiods. *Proceedings of the Royal Society B: Biological Sciences*, **274**(1610), 721–725. doi: 10.1098/rspb.2006.0067.

Dawson, A. (2017) Daily cycles in body temperature in a songbird change with photoperiod and are weakly circadian. *Journal of Biological Rhythms*, **32**(2), 177–183. doi: 10.1177/0748730417691206.

DeVries, M.S. et al. (2015) Differential relationships between D1 and D2 dopamine receptor expression in the medial preoptic nucleus and sexually-motivated song in male European starlings (*Sturnus vulgaris*). *Neuroscience*, **301**, 289–297. doi: 10.1016/j.neuroscience.2015.06.011.

Dubiec, A., Góźdź, I. and Mazgajski, T. D. (2013) Green plant material in avian nests. *Avian Biology Research*, **6**(2), 133–146. doi: 10.3184/175815513X13615363233558.

Dunn, J. et al. (2018a) Early-life begging effort reduces adult body mass but strengthens behavioural defence of the rate of energy intake in European starlings. *Royal Society Open Science*, **5**(5). doi: 10.1098/rsos.171918.

Dunn, J. et al. (2018b) 'Evaluating the cyclic ratio schedule as an assay of feeding behaviour in the European starling (*Sturnus vulgaris*)', *PLoS One*, **13**(10), 1–15. doi: 10.1371/journal.pone.0206363.

Ellis, J.W., Root, J.J., McCurdy, L.M., et al. (2021) Avian influenza A virus susceptibility, infection, transmission, and antibody kinetics in European starlings. *PLoS Pathogens*, **17**(8), p.e1009879.

Evans, J.E., Cuthill, I.C. and Bennett, A.T.D. (2006) The effect of flicker from fluorescent lights on mate choice in captive birds. *Animal Behaviour*, **72**(2), 393–400. doi: 10.1016/j.anbehav.2005.10.031.

Feare, C. (1984) *The Starling*. Oxford: Oxford University Press.

Feenders, G. et al. (2017) Temporal ventriloquism effect in european starlings: Evidence for two parallel processing pathways. *Behavioral Neuroscience*, **131**(4), 337–347. doi: 10.1037/bne0000200.

Feenders, G. and Bateson, M. (2011a) Hand-rearing reduces fear of humans in European starlings, *Sturnus vulgaris*. *PloS One*, **6**(2), p. e17466. doi: 10.1371/journal.pone.0017466.

Feenders, G. and Bateson, M. (2011b) The development of stereotypic behavior in caged European starlings, *Sturnus vulgaris*. *Developmental psychobiology*, **54**(8), 773–784. doi: 10.1002/dev.20623.

Feenders, G. and Bateson, M. (2013) Hand rearing affects emotional responses but not basic cognitive performance in European starlings. *Animal Behaviour*, **86**(1), 127–138. doi: 10.1016/j.anbehav.2013.05.002.

Fischer, C.P., Franco, L.A. and Romero, L.M. (2016) Are novel objects perceived as stressful? The effect of novelty on heart rate. *Physiology and Behavior*, **161**, 7–14. doi: 10.1016/j.physbeh.2016.04.014.

Gautsch, S., Odermatt, P. and Burnens, A.P. (2000) The role of starlings (Sturnus vulgaris) in the epidemiology of potentially human bacterial pathogens. *Schweizer Archiv fur Tierheilkunde*, **142**, 165–172 (in German).

George, I. et al. (2014) Assessing video presentations as environmental enrichment for laboratory birds. *PLoS One*, **9**(5), e96949. doi: 10.1371/journal.pone.0096949.

Gill, E.L. (1995) Environmental enrichment for captive starlings. *Animal Technology*, **45**, 89–93.

Goldsmith, A.R. and Nicholls, T.J. (1984) Prolactin is associated with the development of photorefractoriness in intact, castrated, and testosterone-implanted starlings. *General and Comparative Endocrinology*, **54**(2), 247–255. doi: 10.1016/0016-6480(84)90178-3.

Gott, A. et al. (2018) Chronological age, biological age, and individual variation in the stress response in the European starling: a follow-up study. *PeerJ*, 1–19. doi: 10.7717/peerj.5842.

Greenwood, V.J. et al. (2002) Do European starlings prefer light environments containing UV?. *Animal Behaviour*, **64**(6), 923–928. doi: 10.1006/anbe.2002.1977.

Greenwood, V.J. et al. (2004) Does the flicker frequency of fluorescent lighting affect the welfare of captive European starlings?. *Applied Animal Behaviour Science*, **86**(1–2), 145–159. doi: 10.1016/j.applanim.2003.11.008.

De Groof, G. et al. (2016) A three-dimensional digital atlas of the starling brain. *Brain Structure and Function*, **221**(4), 1899–1909. doi: 10.1007/s00429-015-1011-1.

De Groof, G. et al. (2017) Topography and lateralized effect of acute aromatase inhibition on auditory processing in a seasonal songbird. *The Journal of Neuroscience*, **37**(16), 4243–4254. doi: 10.1523/jneurosci.1961-16.2017.

Gurka, R. et al. (2016) Flow pattern similarities in the near wake of three bird species suggest a common role for unsteady aerodynamic effects in lift generation. *Interface Focus*, **7**(1), 20160090. doi: 10.1098/rsfs.2016.0090.

Hahn, A.H. et al. (2017) Song-associated reward correlates with endocannabinoid-related gene expression in male European starlings (*Sturnus vulgaris*). *Neuroscience*, **346**, 255–266. doi: 10.1016/j.neuroscience.2017.01.028.

Hawkins, P. (2001) Laboratory birds: Refinements in husbandry and procedures. Fifth Report of the BVAAWF/FRAME/RSPCA/UFAW Joint Working Group on Refinement. *Laboratory Animals*, **35**(Suppl.), S1–S163.

Heffner, H.E. (1998) Auditory awareness. *Applied Animal Behaviour Science*, **57**(3–4), 259–268. doi: 10.1016/S0168-1591(98)00101-4.

Jayne, K., Feenders, G. and Bateson, M. (2013) Effects of developmental history on the behavioural responses of European starlings (*Sturnus vulgaris*) to laboratory husbandry. *Animal Welfare*, **22**(1), 67–78. doi: 10.7120/09627286.22.1.067.

Kacelnik, A. (1982) Information primacy or preference for familiar foraging techniques? A critique of Inglis & Ferguson. *Animal Behaviour*, **35**, 925–926.

Kelm-Nelson, C.A., Stevenson, S.A. and Riters, L.V. (2012) Context-dependent links between song production and opioid-mediated analgesia in male European starlings (*Sturnus vulgaris*). *PLoS One*, **7**(10). doi: 10.1371/journal.pone.0046721.

Kozlov, A.S. and Gentner, T.Q. (2016) Central auditory neurons have composite receptive fields. *Proceedings of the National Academy of Sciences*, **113**(5), 1441–1446. doi: 10.1073/pnas.1506903113.

Lierz, M. and Korbel, R. (2012) Anesthesia and analgesia in birds. *Journal of Exotic Pet Medicine*, **21**(1), 44–58. doi: 10.1053/j.jepm.2011.11.008.

Machin, K.L. (2005) Avian analgesia. *Seminars in Avian and Exotic Pet Medicine*, **14**, 236–242. doi: 10.1016/j.cvex.2010.09.011.

Maddocks, S.A., Goldsmith, A.R. and Cuthill, I.C. (2002) Behavioural and physiological effects of absence of ultraviolet wavelengths on European starlings *Sturnus vulgaris*. *Journal of Avian Biology*, **33**(1), 103–106.

Mahjoub, G., Hinders, M.K. and Swaddle, J.P. (2015) Using a "sonic net" to deter pest bird species: Excluding European starlings from food sources by disrupting their acoustic communication. *Wildlife Society Bulletin*, **39**(2), 326–333. doi: 10.1002/wsb.529.

Martínez del Rio, C. (1990) Dietary, phylogenetic, and ecological correlates of intestinal sucrase and maltase activity in birds. *Physiological Zoology*, **63**, 987–1011.

Matheson, S.M., Asher, L. and Bateson, M. (2008) Larger, enriched cages are associated with "optimistic" response biases in captive European starlings (*Sturnus vulgaris*). *Applied Animal Behaviour Science*, **109**(2–4), 374–383. doi: 10.1016/j.applanim.2007.03.007.

Meaden, F. (1993) *Keeping British Birds: An Avicultural Guide to European Species*. Blandford, London.

Nephew, B.C. and Romero, L.M. (2003) Behavioral, physiological, and endocrine responses of starlings to acute increases in density. *Hormones and Behavior*, **44**(3), 222–232. doi: 10.1016/j.yhbeh.2003.06.002.

Nettle, D., Monaghan, P. et al. (2015) An experimental demonstration that early-life competitive disadvantage accelerates telomere loss. *Proceedings of the Royal Society B: Biological Sciences*, **282**(1798), 20141610. doi: 10.1098/rspb.2014.1610.

Nettle, D., Andrews, C.P.C.P. et al. (2015) Developmental and familial predictors of adult cognitive traits in the European starling. *Animal Behaviour*, **107**, 239–248. doi: 10.1016/j.anbehav.2015.07.002.

Nettle, D. et al. (2016) Brood size moderates associations between body size, telomere length and immune development in European starling nestlings. *Ecology and Evolution*, **6**, 1–11. doi: 10.1002/ece3.2551.

Nettle, D. et al. (2017) Early-life adversity accelerates cellular ageing and affects adult inflammation: experimental evidence from the

European starling. *Scientific Reports*, **7**, 40794. doi: 10.1038/srep40794.

Nicholls, T.J., Goldsmith, A.R. and Dawson, A. (1988) Photorefractoriness in birds and comparison with mammals. *Physiological Reviews*, **68(1)**, 133–176. doi: 10.1152/physrev.1988.68.1.133.

North, M.A., Rodriguez-Estival, J. and Smits, J.E.G. (2017) Biomarker sensitivity to vehicle exhaust in experimentally exposed European starlings. *Environmental Science and Technology*, **51(22)**, 13427–13435. doi: 10.1021/acs.est.7b03836.

O'Hagan, D. et al. (2015) Early life disadvantage strengthens flight performance trade-offs in European starlings, *Sturnus vulgaris*. *Animal Behaviour*, **102**, 141–148. doi: 10.1016/j.anbehav.2015.01.016.

Palacio, F.X., Maragliano, R.E. and Montalti, D. (2016) Functional role of the invasive European Starling, *Sturnus vulgaris*, in Argentina. *Emu*, **116(4)**, 387–393. doi: 10.1071/MU16021.

Paul-Murphy, J.R., Brunson, D.B. and Miletic, V. (1999) Analgesic effects of butorphanol and buprenorphine in conscious African grey parrots (*Psittacus erithacus erithacus* and *Psittacus erithacus timneh*). *American Journal of Veterinary Research*, **60**, 1218–1221.

Perkins, L.E.L. and Swayne, D.E. (2003) Varied pathogenicity of a Hong Kong-origin H5N1 avian influenza virus in four passerine species and budgerigars. *Veterinary paThology*, **40(1)**, 14–24.

Perret, A. et al. (2015) Social visual contact, a primary "drive" for social animals?. *Animal Cognition*, **18(3)**, 657–666. doi: 10.1007/s10071-015-0834-8.

Pinxten, R. et al. (2017) Experimental inhibition of a key cellular antioxidant affects vocal communication. *Functional Ecology*, **31(5)**, 1101–1110. doi: 10.1111/1365-2435.12825.

Qadri, M.A.J. and Cook, R.G. (2015) The perception of Glass patterns by starlings (*Sturnus vulgaris*). *Psychonomic Bulletin and Review*, **22(3)**, 687–693. doi: 10.3758/s13423-014-0709-z.

Qadri, M.A.J., Romero, L.M. and Cook, R.G. (2014) Shape from shading in starlings (*Sturnus vulgaris*). *Journal of Comparative Psychology*, **128(4)**, 343–356. doi: 10.1037/a0036848.

Rich, E.L. and Romero, L.M. (2005) Exposure to chronic stress downregulates corticosterone responses to acute stressors. *American Journal of Physiology-Regulatory Integrative and Comparative Physiology*, **288(6)**, R1628–R1636.

Richardson, M.F., Sherwin, W.B. and Rollins, L.A. (2017) De novo assembly of the liver transcriptome of the European Starling, *Sturnus vulgaris*. *Journal of Genomics*, **5**, 54–57. doi: 10.7150/jgen.19504.

Riters, L.V. (2011) Pleasure seeking and birdsong. *Neuroscience and Biobehavioral Reviews*, **35(9)**, 1837–1845. doi: 10.1016/j.neubiorev.2010.12.017.

Riters, L.V., Cordes, M.A. and Stevenson, S.A. (2017) Prodynorphin and kappa opioid receptor mRNA expression in the brain relates to social status and behavior in male European starlings. *Behavioural Brain Research*, **320**, 37–47. doi: 10.1016/j.bbr.2016.11.050.

Robinson, R.A., Siriwardena, G.M. and Crick, H.Q.P. (2005) Status and population trends of starling *Sturnus vulgaris* in Great Britain. *Bird Study*, **52(3)**, 252–260. doi: 10.1080/00063650509461398.

Rouse, M.L. et al. (2015) Reproductive state modulates testosterone-induced singing in adult female European starlings (*Sturnus vulgaris*). *Hormones and Behavior*, **72**, 78–87. doi: 10.1016/j.yhbeh.2015.04.022.

Schulz, D. et al. (2016) Flying starlings, PET and the evolution of volant dinosaurs. *Current Biology*, **26(7)**, R265–R267. doi: 10.1016/j.cub.2016.02.025.

Smith, E.L. et al. (2005) Effect of repetitive visual stimuli on behaviour and plasma corticosterone of European starlings. *Animal Biology*, **55(3)**, 245–258. doi: 10.1163/1570756054472827.

Smith, E.L. et al. (2005) Sexing starlings *Sturnus vulgaris* using iris colour. *Ringing & Migration*, **22(4)**, 193–197. doi: 10.1080/03078698.2005.9674332.

Smith, E.L. and Evans, J.E. (2005) Myoclonus induced by cathode ray tube screens and low-frequency lighting in the European starling (*Sturnus vulgaris*). *Veterinary Record*, **157**, 148–150.

Smith, K.E., Halpin, C.G. and Rowe, C. (2014) Body size matters for aposematic prey during predator aversion learning. *Behavioural Processes*, **109(PB)**, 173–179. doi: 10.1016/j.beproc.2014.09.026.

Spool, J.A. et al. (2019) Co-localization of mu-opioid and dopamine D1 receptors in the medial preoptic area and bed nucleus of the stria terminalis across seasonal states in male European starlings. *Hormones and Behavior*, **107**, 1–10. doi: 10.1016/j.yhbeh.2018.11.003.

Stalnov, O. et al. (2015) On the estimation of time dependent lift of a European starling (*Sturnus vulgaris*) during flapping flight. *PLoS One*, **10(9)**, 1–21. doi: 10.1371/journal.pone.0134582.

Tacutu, R. et al. (2013) Human ageing genomic resources: integrated databases and tools for the biology and genetics of ageing. *Nucleic Acids Research*, **41(D1)**, 1027–1033. doi: 10.1093/nar/gks1155.

Tait, M.J. (1973) Winter food and feeding requirements of the starling. *Bird Study*, **20**, 226–236.

Vasquez, R.A. and Kacelnik, A. (2000) Foraging rate versus sociality in the starling *Sturnus vulgaris*. *Proceedings of the Royal Society B*, **267**, 157–164.

Werner, S.J. et al. (2014) European starling feeding activity on repellent treated crops and pellets. *Crop Protection*, **63**, 76–82. doi: 10.1016/j.cropro.2014.05.001.

Whitlock, S.E. et al. (2018) Environmentally relevant exposure to an antidepressant alters courtship behaviours in a songbird. *Chemosphere*, **211**, 17–24. doi: 10.1016/j.chemosphere.2018.07.074.

Witter, M.S. and Swaddle, J.P. (1995) Dominance, competition, and energetic reserves in the European starling, *Sturnus vulgaris*. *Behavioral Ecology*, **6(3)**, 343–348. doi: 10.1093/beheco/6.3.343.

Witter, M.S., Swaddle, J.P. and Cuthill, I.C. (1995) Periodic food availability and strategic regulation of body mass in the European Starling, *Sturnus vulgaris*. *Functional Ecology*, **9(4)**, 568–574. doi: 10.2307/2390146.

Wolfensohn, S. and Lloyd, M. (2008) *Handbook of Laboratory Animal Management and Welfare*. 3rd edn. Oxford University Press, Oxford.

Wright, J. and Cuthill, I. (1990) Biparental care: manipulation of partner contribution and brood size in the starling, *Sturnus vulgaris*. *Behavioral Ecology*, **1(2)**, 116–124.

Zahara, A.R.D. et al. (2015) Latent cognitive effects from low-level polychlorinated biphenyl exposure in juvenile European starlings (*Sturnus vulgaris*). *Environmental Toxicology and Chemistry*, **34(11)**, 2513–2522. doi: 10.1002/etc.3084.

45 Corvids

Rachael Miller, Martina Schiestl and Nicola S. Clayton

Biological overview

General biology

The family Corvidae comprises of 123 bird species across 21 genera in the order Passeriformes, and includes crows, ravens, magpies and jays (Clayton & Emery 2007; Del Hoyo et al. 2015). Corvids are found across the world, with some species occupying broad ranges, for instance, being found across Europe (e.g. rook *Corvus frugilegus*, carrion crow *Corvus corone*) and Asia (e.g. Azure-winged magpie *Cyanopica cyanus*, Western jackdaw *Coloeus monedula*, Eurasian jay *Garrulus glandarius*), North America (e.g. Clark's nutcracker *Nucifraga columbiana*, Pinyon jay *Gymnorhinus cyanocephalus*, Blue jay *Cyanocitta cristata*, American crow *Corvus brachyrhynchos*) and Australia (e.g. Australian raven *Corvus coronoides*), while other species are island endemics (e.g. Hawaiian crow or 'Alalā *Corvus hawaiiensis*, New Caledonian crow *Corvus moneduloides*, Mariana crow *Corvus kubaryi*) (Madge & Burn 1994). Corvids utilise almost all terrestrial habitats, including open agricultural areas, woodlands, forests, coastal regions, mountains and many species are also found in urban and suburban settings, like parks and gardens (Madge & Burn 1994; Del Hoyo et al. 2015).

Size range and life span

Corvids are medium to large passerines, that vary in colour from mainly black or blue coloured plumage, some with white or grey areas, or brightly coloured (Madge & Burn 1994). The sexes are generally similar in colour and size, though in some species, the males are larger and heavier (e.g. in ravens and crows). They range in size and weight from 40 g and 20 cm in the dwarf jay (*Cyanolyca nanus*) to over 1400 g and 65 cm in the common raven (*Corvus corax*) and thick-billed raven (*Corvus crassirostris*) (Beaman & Madge 2010; Del Hoyo et al. 2015). Corvids can be relatively long-lived and some species/individuals may live over 20 years. It is possible to estimate the age-class in several corvid species (in first calendar year, second calendar year or adults), such as in ravens and crows, by checking the colouration inside the mouth (Svensson 1992; Madge & Burn 1994) (Figure 45.1).

Social organisation

As with most birds, corvids are monogamous comprising primarily of bonded pairs, which mate for life, and remain together throughout the year (Clayton & Emery 2007). Corvid sociality varies across species – and sometimes between populations – with all species living in either pairs or groups (none are naturally solitary), which should be reflected in their laboratory housing (Table 45.1). For example, rooks and jackdaws will forage, roost and breed in social groups throughout the year, while Eurasian jays typically live in territorial pairs. Some species, like New Caledonian crows and 'Alalā crows, live in family groups. Age influences sociality in some species, like common ravens and carrion crows, with younger birds coming together to forage, roost and find pair partners (Clayton & Emery 2007). Season also influences social organisation, with birds coming together in groups outside of the breeding season, though living in territorial pairs during breeding season (Clayton & Emery 2007).

In order to establish pairs for pair housing from a group situation (e.g. from a group of juvenile or sub-adult ravens or jays), observations of social interactions – both affiliative (i.e. positive) and agonistic (i.e. negative) interactions – can be used to identify which individuals are likely to respond well to be paired together as adults and/or in breeding season (see Normal behaviour section). For instance, Eurasian jays will share food directly with pair partners in the run-up to breeding season, which can be a reliable indicator of a pair bond forming. This approach provides individuals with the opportunity to form pairs naturally, i.e. to select their own partners. If pairs need to be set up outside of a group setting, for instance, if two adult birds are sourced separately, care must be taken during the introduction and interactions between the birds monitored closely for signs of aggression. Ideally, new individuals may be initially housed with visual access though no physical access to one another in order to monitor behavioural responses to one another, before being placed in

---

The UFAW Handbook on the Care and Management of Laboratory and Other Research Animals, Ninth Edition.
Edited by Huw Golledge and Claire Richardson.
© 2024 John Wiley & Sons Ltd. Published 2024 by John Wiley & Sons Ltd.

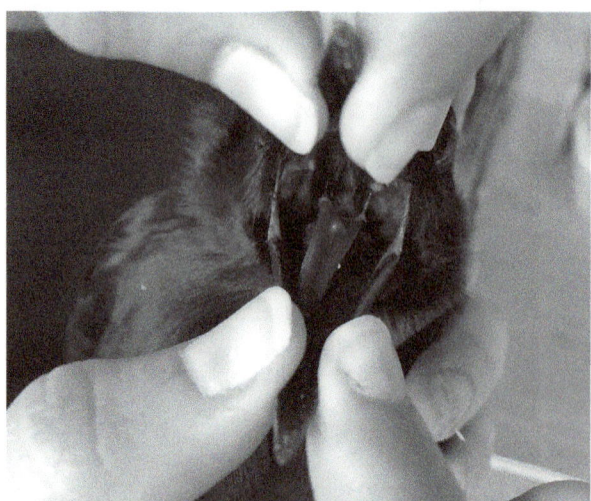
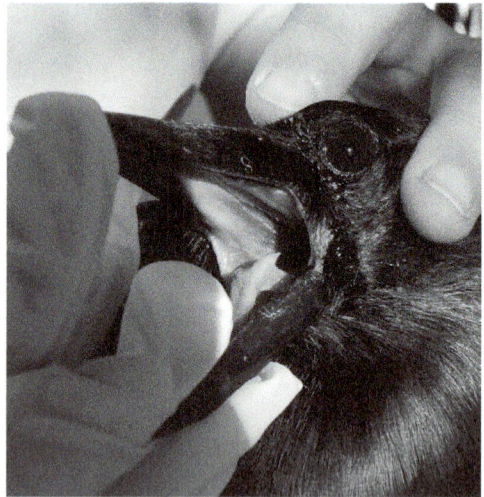

Figure 45.1 Example of New Caledonian crow beak coloration for aging estimates. Left picture of an adult bird, with completely black inside the mouth and right picture of a juvenile crow, with pink inside the oral cavity. Source: Martina Schiestl (2017).

Table 45.1 Housing for corvid species typically used in laboratory research.

Species	Social organisation (Clayton & Emery 2007)	Appropriate lab housing
Eurasian jay (*Garrulus glandarius*)	Territorial pairs in adulthood	Pair housing during the breeding season; possible to hold in a group outside of the breeding season
Common raven (*Corvus corax*)	Territorial pairs in adulthood	Pair housing for adult birds; possible to hold in a group as juveniles and sub-adults
Carrion crow (*Corvus corone*)	Territorial pairs in adulthood, generally not cooperative breeders except in one Spanish population	Pair housing for adult birds; possible to hold in a group as juveniles and sub-adults
New Caledonian crow (*Corvus moneduloides*)	Family groups	Pairs or family groups
'Alalā (*Corvus hawaiiensis*)	Family groups	Pairs or family groups
Rooks (*Corvus frugilegus*)	Colonial pairs, mixed sex, mixed age flocks	Pair or group housing. Can be housed in mixed-species aviaries with jackdaws – require adequate space and opportunities for pairs to defend micro territories within the colony
Jackdaws (*Coloeus monedula*)	Colonial pairs, mixed sex, mixed age flocks	Pair or group housing. As above with rooks
Azure-winged magpie (*Cyanopica cyanus*)	Cooperative breeders – family and social groups	Pair or group housing
Red-billed chough (*Pyrrhocorax pyrrhocorax*)	Colonial pairs, forage in flocks	Pair or group housing
Clark's nutcracker (*Nucifraga columbiana*)	Territorial pairs	Pair housing
Pinyon jay (*Gymnorhinus cyanocephalus*)	Colonial, cooperative breeding	Pair or group housing
Blue jay (*Cyanocitta cristata*)	Territorial pairs	Pair housing
Californian scrub-jay (*Aphelocoma californica*)	Territorial pairs in adulthood	Pair housing; possible to hold in a group as juveniles and sub-adults
Florida scrub-jay (*Aphelocoma coerulescens*)	Colonial, cooperative breeding	Pair or group housing

the same aviary. Single housing should be avoided wherever possible, unless required specifically for other scientific or welfare purposes, such as illness, and if necessary, then visual access to conspecifics should ideally be provided.

Reproduction

Corvid nests are typically constructed from sticks in an open cup shape, lined with grass and other soft materials, and located in trees, shrubs or on ledges, including cliff edges in ravens and choughs (Del Hoyo *et al*. 2015), and artificial structures, like telegraph poles in other species. Pairs tend to build nests together; the female undertakes incubation and the male often feeds the female during incubation (Del Hoyo *et al*. 2015). Corvids lay between 1 and 9 light blueish-green eggs, though on average from 2 to 4, in one or two clutches per season (Holyoak 1967; Fox 2003). Some species are cooperative breeders, and so helpers are permitted to assist in rearing nestlings. In some species, like carrion crows and common ravens, fledglings and juveniles will stay with the parents for several months before leaving to join non-breeder flocks. In European corvids, breeding season typically runs from March to June (Holyoak 1967). Incubation ranges across species, from 16 to 22 days (Fox 2003). The nestling period varies between species, for instance, from 12 days in Florida scrub-jays (*Aphelocoma coerulescens*) to up to 45 days in pied crows (*Corvus albus*) (Del Hoyo et al. 2015). Fledging typically occurs around 38 days for ravens, 34 days for crows and 27 days for magpies (Whitmore & Marzluff 1998).

Normal behaviour (wild and captive)

Corvids engage in both social affiliative (i.e. positive) interactions and agonistic (i.e. negative) interactions with other birds. They engage in affiliative pair bonding behaviours, like aerobatic displays, food sharing, mutual preening (preening another bird's body) and bill twining (bill holding) (Clayton & Emery 2007). Other affiliative behaviours may include touching another bird, contact sitting (sitting beside another bird), feeding or playing close to another bird and sharing food or objects (Fraser & Bugnyar 2010). Agonistic behaviours may include stealing food (either directly from another bird or by recovering the cache of another bird), displacement (approaching another bird so the other retreats), pecking, chasing or physically attacking and in some cases injuring other birds (Clayton & Emery 2007). Some species will also support their affiliates in fights, and reconcile after aggressive conflicts with valuable partners (Seed et al. 2007; Fraser & Bugnyar 2011; Sima et al. 2018).

They use a range of species-specific vocalisations and displays. For example, they use vocalisations to communicate about food (e.g. food-associated calls that ravens give when food is difficult to access (Heinrich 1988), and begging calls from chicks). They also use calls to communicate about threats (e.g. alarm or mobbing, for instance, in response to a predator) or to indicate submissiveness while interacting with more dominant conspecifics. They also use calls to inform others about their location (e.g. long-distance calls) and in courtship (Kroodsma 1985). The number of different calls uttered varies between species, but in the limited species studied varies from 14 to 80 calls, with ravens emitting the largest number of calls documented (Del Hoyo et al. 2015). Ravens respond differently to the calls of familiar and unfamiliar individuals, and even discriminate between familiar birds based on their relationship with those individuals from up to 3 years ago (Boeckle & Bugnyar 2012). As songbirds, corvids will also sing, for instance, see work on the whispering song of the magpie (Birkhead 2010). Corvids also produce loud and quiet calls so presumably the function of song is for mate choice rather than territoriality in this family of birds, in contrast, for example with great tits that sing to defend territories (Krebs et al. 1978). They can also mimic a variety of sounds (Goodwin 1976). Displays tend to involve erecting head and/or body feathers and can be utilised during courtship as well as agonistic displays (Gwinner 1964).

Like other birds, they spend a good proportion of their daylight hours foraging for food (Miller et al. 2014). When it is dark, they tend to roost on branches off of the ground.

Other normal behaviours include auto-preening (preening one's own body), wiping the beak on another surface, scratching oneself, stretching and manipulating or playing with food or objects. Corvids may also 'sun-bathe' by positioning themselves in the sunlight and sometimes stretching out a wing/leg. Adult corvids will go through a full-annual moult, which mainly takes place post-breeding season, though in some species, starts while birds are still feeding their young (Madge & Burn 1994; Del Hoyo et al. 2015). At this time, as moulting can be very energy consuming, it is particularly important to ensure that any unnecessary stress is avoided. It may also be sensible to provide additional supplements at this time, such as 'Avipro Avian Probiotic' in the water, to help boost the immunity of the birds.

Most corvid species engage in some level of caching behaviour, i.e. hiding food or non-food items for later recovery. Note that not all corvid species cache – one notable example is the jackdaw, which has implications for how they forage and remember, and should be kept in mind when designing enrichment (Clayton & Krebs 1994). Object play may contribute to caching development and learning about social relations with conspecifics, particularly in young birds (Clayton et al 1994; Bugnyar & Kotrschal 2002; Bugnyar et al. 2007). Caching behaviour has been utilised in a number of cognitive experiments to explore corvid understanding of the perspectives of others and memory (Bugnyar & Heinrich 2005; Dally et al. 2006; Clayton et al. 2007; Grodzinski & Clayton 2010). Most species are also quite neophobic, i.e. aversive to novel stimuli (Greenberg & Mettke-Hofmann 2001), with levels of neophobia varying between species, individuals and age groups (Heinrich 1999; Miller et al. 2015). As mentioned in the Social organisation section and elaborated further in the Social housing section, corvids can be quite territorial, varying across species and typically most prominent during breeding season.

Sources/supply/conservation status

The International Union for Conservation of Nature (IUCN) has classified 77.9% of corvid species as least concern status, though some species have decreasing populations, such as rooks, Siberian jay (*Perisoreus infaustus*), white-winged magpie (*Urocissa whiteheadi*) and grey jay (*Perisoreus canadensis*). The remaining corvid species are classified as near threatened, vulnerable, endangered or critically endangered, including the Florida scrub-jay, Pinyon jay, Mariana crow, Yellow-billed magpie (*Pica nutalli*), Amami jay (*Garrulus lidthi*) and Flores crow (*Corvus florensis*) (Del Hoyo et al. 2015). The 'Alalā crow is classified as extinct in the wild, though efforts are being made for a species reintroduction (Madge & Burn 1994; Del Hoyo et al. 2015).

In the UK, all corvid species – ravens, carrion/ hooded crows, jackdaws, Eurasian jays, Eurasian magpies (*Pica pica*), red-billed choughs and rooks – are protected under the Wildlife and Countryside Act 1981 and the Wildlife (Northern Ireland) Order 1985 making it illegal to intentionally take, injure or kill these birds, or their eggs/active nests. However, the UK government does issue general licences allowing certain corvid species to be killed or taken by authorised persons using permitted, legal methods in order to conserve other species, preserve public health (including air safety) or prevent substantial damage to crops or livestock.

In many countries, to obtain corvids from the wild for research purposes, an appropriate national licence or permission is required. For instance, in the UK, this is a Natural England Licence or Scottish Natural Heritage Licence (Cambridge 2014) and in the USA, you need both a federal and a state permit. It is possible that some corvid species, namely those that are not classified as threatened, may be sourced via zoological collections, while adhering to national legislation and procedures, including quarantine. Threatened corvid species are likely to be protected through Convention on International Trade in Endangered Species (CITES) legislation. It may also be an option to bolster laboratory samples through breeding within labs or transferring birds between labs, following the national guidelines. We discuss breeding in captivity in the Breeding section.

Use in research

The interest in using corvids for research has drastically increased in recent years (Figure 45.2), primarily within the research areas of: zoology, behavioural sciences, ecology, psychology, biomedicine and evolutionary biology, with a smaller number of studies in other topics, like veterinary science, neurosciences and conservation (Web of Knowledge 2018). For example, in 2008, there were 18 papers within the fields of behaviour and cognition using corvids, comprising 170 individuals in total (Bateson & Feenders 2010) (note that some may include repeated samples). Non-invasive cognitive/behavioural research has indicated that corvids often perform comparably to primates, including young children, in cognitive tasks in both the social and physical domains, like social learning, cooperation, planning for the future, reasoning about cause and effect, and taking into account the perspective of others (see reviews in Emery & Clayton 2004; Seed *et al*. 2009). In the UK, many behavioural, developmental and cognitive studies are classified as non-regulated procedures by the Home Office, if they do not require any invasive procedures (Cambridge 2014).

We note that there is very little published research on the welfare of corvids in laboratory settings at present (though see Samour 2016). However, many of the general husbandry procedures from other more commonly held captive bird species apply similarly to corvids (Hawkins *et al*. 2001). We present this information in the following sections, with reference to published research on corvids and other bird species. We also draw on our own experience of working professionally with various corvid species, including Eurasian jay, carrion crow, common raven, rook, California scrub-jay, azure-winged magpie and New Caledonian crow, in both captive and field settings, including laboratories and zoos, in the UK, Austria, United States, New Zealand and New Caledonia. Furthermore, we wish to advocate and fully support the study of corvid welfare in future.

To our knowledge, there are approximately 15–20 corvid species used in laboratory-based research worldwide (see Table 45.1 for species examples), though this is increasing all the time. Furthermore, there are 24 species of interest to the Corvid interest group in the Association of Zoos and Aquariums for management in zoological collections. These include species held for research, rehab or education: magpie jay (*Calocitta sp.*), pied crow, Guam/ Mariana crow, common crow, common raven, Chihuahuan raven (*Corvus cryptoleucus*), fish crow (*Corvus ossifragus*), scrub-jay, blue jay and black-billed magpie (*Pica hudsonia*) (Fox 2003).

General husbandry

Enclosures

As far as possible, corvids should be provided with species-specific social housing, as discussed in Social organisation section (see Table 45.1), and with an abundance of space and complexity, given their renowned intelligence and territoriality (Emery & Clayton 2004; Clayton & Emery 2007). If the birds must be held in smaller aviaries, then training and enrichment should be a priority. The safest housing option is in single-species enclosures (Fox 2003). The one exception to this is the housing of rooks and jackdaws together, as these two species are often seen foraging together in the wild and roosting together (Jolles *et al*. 2013). Like most other bird species, corvids require space for foraging, flight and outside enclosure access for natural light and weather.

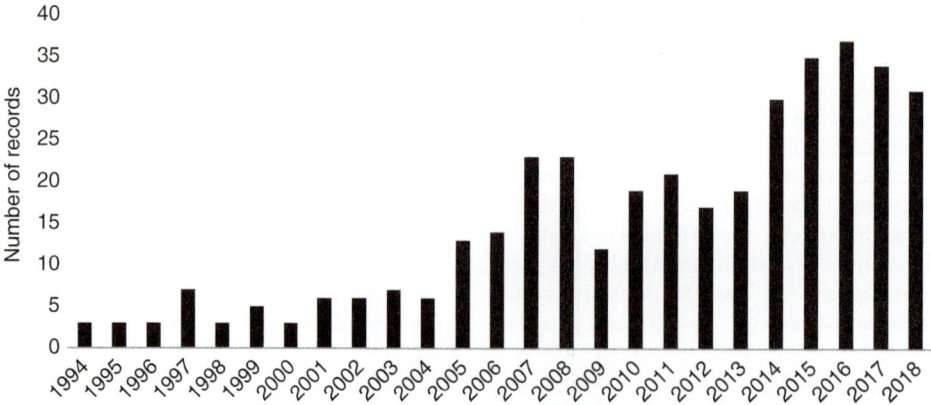

Figure 45.2   Number of records with 'corvid' in topic per year (Web of Knowledge 2018).

Natural behaviours including foraging, caching (where applicable), roosting and social interactions should be promoted. It is preferable to provide access to heated housing for colder months, particularly for species being held in countries outside of their natural range – though few species need to be shut inside overnight in winter as most corvids are hardy species. They need adequate shelter from the elements and from humans/conspecifics if required, and sufficient perching and shelving at different heights in a variety of sizes (length and diameter) and textures (e.g. smooth vs coarse). For species that will also spend time on the ground, rocks and logs can be provided. Coarse sand or small stones are ideal substrates as they allow the birds to dig and cache, while providing drainage and facilitating cleaning (Fox 2003).

Housing must be secure to prevent escape or predator access. It is critical to have a safety cage, i.e. double-door entry system, in place at the entrance to the aviary, and an enclosed space (e.g. a room/corridor) for entering inside testing compartments, to ensure that staff can enter and leave safely without the birds escaping or being trapped in the door. It is beneficial to ensure that nets and other required equipment for catching a bird are on hand, should they manage to enter the safety cage or another area they are not supposed to be. Wire mesh in outside enclosures should be checked regularly for holes and mended as required. To observe birds without disturbing them or influencing their behaviour, hides (e.g. a shed with 1-way glass) may be used. Corvid aviaries may be constructed from wooden or metal frame with wire mesh with the mesh size applicable for the species. For example, at University of Cambridge, the internal mesh size used for Eurasian jays and rooks is 2.6×8 cm (indoor) and 3×1.5 cm (outside). It is possible to use netting for the roof, providing regular checks for any developing holes are done.

There are not currently minimum enclosure requirements specified for corvids; therefore, at present, those stipulated for other bird species (Hawkins *et al.* 2001), like chickens (*Gallus gallus domesticus*) and pigeons (e.g. *Columba livia domestica*), should be followed, though we highlight that these are minimum requirements rather than optimal ones (Cambridge 2014). Hence efforts should be made to exceed these minimum space allocations. The critical point is allowing room for flight; hence, the enclosure height and volume is most important. This allows exercise and also enables birds to escape close contact with humans without injuring themselves. Birds should have unlimited access to these flight areas unless confinement is justified on scientific, husbandry or welfare grounds.

As examples, we present the laboratory housing currently in place for Eurasian jays and rooks at the University of Cambridge in the UK (Figure 45.3) and common raven at the University of Vienna in Austria (Figure 45.4). At Cambridge University, the Eurasian jays are held in species-specific groups outside of breeding season with a large outdoor aviary (3 m height × 5 × 20) and smaller aviaries attached to them (3 m height × 1 × 6), which have access to indoor testing compartments (3 m height × 1 × 2). The birds have access to the indoor compartments outside of testing, which provide heated housing. During breeding season and post-breeding season moult, the jays are separated in pairs and held temporarily in the smaller aviaries to prevent aggression between pairs. They are then re-introduced into the group for the remainder of the year. The jays therefore have a large flight space, a variety of perching, options for shelter and foraging/caching opportunities. The rooks are held together throughout the year, as per their natural species history. We note that, in the past, rooks and jackdaws were traditionally held together in the same aviary (the same one currently used just for rooks), as these species are often found together naturally in the wild (Jolles *et al.* 2013).

At Vienna University, the ravens have an all-year outdoor aviary complex (total size ~680 m^2), with sheltered areas where they are protected from rain/snow and sun. They are housed either in pairs or social groups, depending on age. Every pair/group has access to a large main aviary and adjoining visually isolated experimental compartment (~20 m^2 per compartment), to which they have access at all times. The compartments are separated via sliding doors.

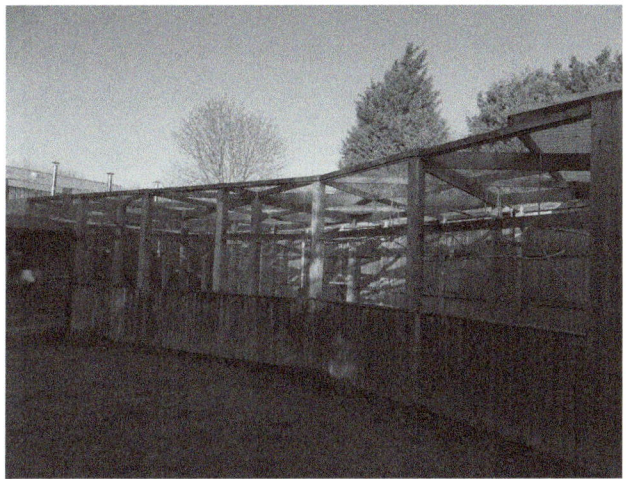 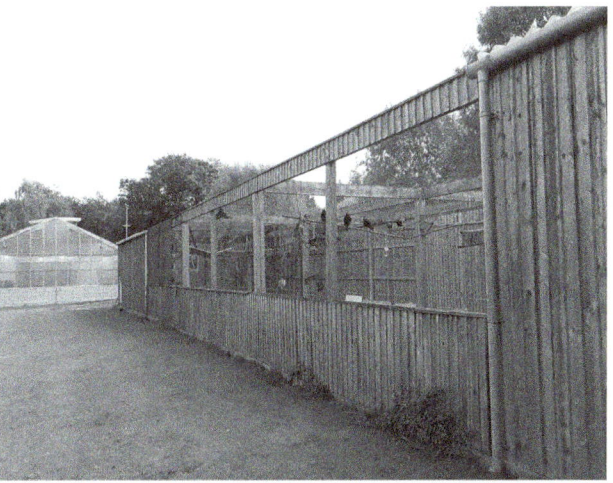

Figure 45.3 Left: Example of Eurasian jay outside aviary; right: Example of rook outside aviary: large outside aviaries with numerous smaller attached aviaries which access internal housing/testing compartments, University of Cambridge. Sources: left: Rachael Miller (2018); right: Anna Frohnwieser (2017).

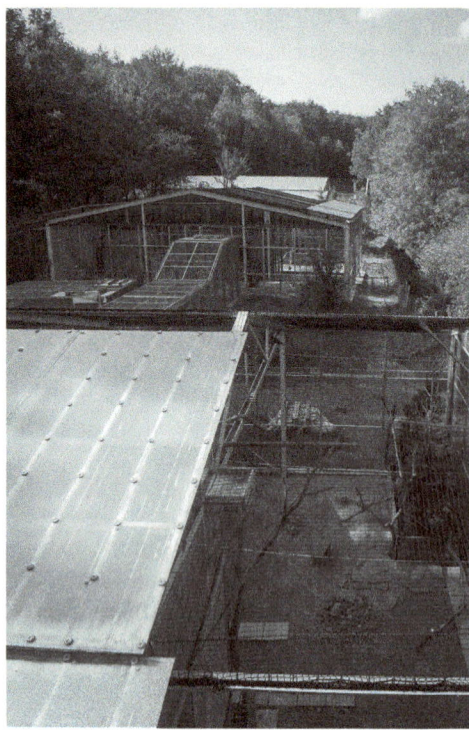

Figure 45.4 Example of common raven all year outdoor aviary complex: large aviary with numerous connected compartments, separated via sliding doors and access to visually isolated experimental compartments, University of Vienna. Source: Alexandru Munteanu (2018).

Breeding pairs have access to nesting areas and nesting material and all niches are furnished with cameras to be able to observe the process from a distance. The compartments are furnished with a variety of branches, bathing possibilities and different substrates that allow the birds to cache. The whole complex is connected via runways, so the ravens can be easily moved around, without having to catch them (Massen et al. 2014).

Feeding and watering

Corvids are typically generalist and omnivorous in diet, and like many other passerines, will eat a variety of fruits (like berries), insects, grains, nuts, seeds and eggs/meat (like small mammals, chicks of other species and carrion) (Fox 2003; Bateson & Feenders 2010). Laboratory diets may contain formulated soaked dog/cat food pellets or formulated bird food (e.g. an insectivorous mix), and should also offer a similar variety of fresh components, like fruit, vegetables, seeds, nuts and meat/eggs/insects, as far as possible. Other than eggs, dairy items (e.g. cheese, yogurt) and bread should be limited. For example, for the Eurasian jay facilities at University of Cambridge, UK, the main diet composes primarily of soaked cat biscuits, cooked egg, mixed wild bird seeds and nuts, fruit (e.g. pear, apple, berries, grapes) and vegetables (e.g. potato, broccoli, squash, courgette, green beans) with grit for digestion and vitamin supplement ('Nutrobal' 3 × per week, cuttlefish). Note that the nuts and insects are often reserved for testing/training, as they are likely to be highly preferred food items. During breeding season, Avipro is added to the soaked cat biscuits.

Food should be presented in dishes or scattered on clean platforms, with the number of dishes/platforms accounting for the number of birds present to prevent aggression over food sources. For instance, one dish per bird/pair in a pair housing situation, or one dish for approximately every three birds in a group housing situation. The daily diet should be presented off-the-ground whenever possible, to minimise attracting and/or contamination from rodents. The amount of food provided can be determined by monitoring the consumption and weighing left-over food. It may need to be changed seasonally, such as being increased in breeding season.

Some food items used for enrichment, however, may be presented on the ground as part of a 'scatter-feed' or in a foraging tray, such as insects (enrichment discussed further in next section). Animal care staff should be vigilant for signs of rodents (e.g. faeces), and take action to control rodent presence if required. Food should be supplemented with vitamins (e.g. MVS 30, Nutrobal). Cuttlefish bone should be provided – grated over food and/or placed within reach of perches, especially during the breeding season when calcium levels may be low, particularly in egg-laying females. All corvid species require access to clean drinking water, available on an ad-lib basis. Corvids will also bathe regularly; therefore, providing shallow baths with daily-refreshed water, is recommended.

Environmental provisions and enrichment

Enrichment can aid in alleviating boredom and/or abnormal behaviours in captive animals (King 1993; Nicol 1995), and can be food based, sensory, physical and cognitive (de Azevedo et al. 2007). For food-based enrichment, whole deceased chicks or mice can be provided (e.g. ravens, crows), peanuts and acorns (e.g. Eurasian jays), or whole or large pieces of fruit or vegetable, like melon, papaya, mango, corn on the cob or halved coconuts speared on perches/wire (for most species). Live insects like mealworms, wax moth larvae, crickets, cockroaches and locusts, or dog treats (e.g. 'Frolic') can be reserved for testing/training and/or enrichment. Food 'treats' can be presented as a scatter-feed, in a foraging tray (e.g. with sand or bark pieces, on the ground, platform or suspended) and hidden in tubes, bottles, cardboard containers and pet toys to encourage natural foraging behaviours. It may also be frozen within ice, or be scattered into the water (though only if it won't contaminate drinking water). As most corvid species cache, i.e. hide food for later, this behaviour can be promoted by providing a range of potential caching locations, like varied substrates on the ground or in foraging trays.

For physical enrichment, as mentioned in the previous section, corvids like to bathe, so opportunities for doing so in water and in sand should be provided. Perches should be variable in diameter (natural sticks are best as they vary in size and textures, as opposed to wooden dowels), with several perching options located across the aviary, while still allowing space for free-flight. Thick rope can also be used for a variable perch. Corvids tend to like opportunities to peck into wood; therefore, old natural logs (once cleaned with disinfectant) or wooden parrot chew toys can be provided. These items could also have holes drilled into them for hiding treats. Corvids also like to dig; therefore, providing a variety of substrates (e.g. bark, straw, sand), is beneficial. Re-branching (i.e. replacing old branches) can help to enrich the physical environment. A water sprinkler may be provided for hot days – though ensuring the birds can avoid it if they prefer. Species-appropriate nestboxes and nesting material can promote natural breeding behaviour, even in cases where breeding is not desired (so e.g. eggs can be removed/replaced/pipped).

Sensory enrichment may include incorporating olfactory stimuli (e.g. herbs/spices like banana extract, perfume) or visual stimuli (e.g. mirror). Cognitive enrichment may be a regular occurrence for lab corvids, depending on the nature of the research they are involved in, and is likely to be stimulating for the birds. In cases where the birds are not held for the purposes of cognitive/behavioural testing, the corvids could still benefit from being presented with simple problem-solving tasks. For example, nuts/insects hidden inside an opaque plastic bottle without a lid, requiring the animal to manipulate the bottle to cause the food to fall out, or food in a transparent tube, requiring the animal to use a pre-placed stick to push/pull the food out. Some pet toys also provide opportunities for problem solving to find hidden food. Furthermore, some aspects of training, particularly when using positive reinforcement, may be enriching for the animals (Laule & Desmond 1998; Westlund 2014). Training for health monitoring, e.g. weight, or testing purposes, like moving animals between cages, can also reduce the stress that would otherwise be associated with handling (Laule & Desmond 1998). We elaborate further on these points in the Training for procedures section.

Most corvid species are quite neophobic, as highlighted in the Normal behaviour section; therefore, any new items should be presented gradually and the behavioural responses of the birds to these items noted and responded to in future enrichment. For instance, if the birds respond very fearfully to a new item being placed inside their aviary, this item could be introduced more gradually by initially placing it in view but outside of the aviary to allow the birds to familiarise with it, before attempting to place it inside the aviary once more. If the birds continue to respond fearfully, this stimulus should potentially be removed and no longer used as an enrichment option. Where possible, it is sensible to try to vary the enrichment provided on a regular basis to prevent the birds from losing interest in it. Some species will spend some time on the ground (like ravens) while others tend to remain primarily at height (like Eurasian jays), and this should be taken into account when providing enrichment.

Finally, it is critical that any enrichment items presented to the animals are safe and do not put them at risk. It is usually sensible to ensure that any new items are approved by the animal care manager/team prior to use, and carefully monitored while initially present in the aviary. It is also important to ensure that enrichment food is balanced with the daily diet, particularly for high-fat/protein items, like nuts/meat.

Social housing

Corvids are social and should be housed in pairs or groups, depending on species, age and season. We have covered this topic in the Social organisation section (and in Table 45.1). If it is essential for birds to be housed singly, for example due to experimental constraints, then it should be time limited. If they need to be held singly on a longer-term basis, such as due to aggression received by conspecific(s), then the birds should be held with visual and acoustic access to conspecifics. In the UK, single housing requires a Home Office Project Licence.

As with other birds housed socially, care must be taken to observe for signs of aggression between individuals, which is particularly likely for some of the less social corvid species in the approach to and during breeding season, including Eurasian jays, ravens and carrion crows. Even if pairs are physically separated, but in adjacent compartments, if the barrier is mesh, it is likely that additional covering (e.g. matting, plastic sheeting) over the mesh will be required to prevent the birds from attacking one another through the mesh. Signs of aggression to look out for may include reluctance for an individual to approach food in the presence of others, listening out for aggression-related vocalisations, any physical injuries on the birds or feather plucking, or any evidence of such in the aviary (e.g. blood, excessive amounts of dropped feathers, or broken feathers). Some corvids will attack a group member if they are injured or unwell; therefore, this individual may need to be temporarily removed from the group while they heal. Some corvid species, like ravens, show strict dominance hierarchies with groups that will influence access to resources, including food, perches and mates. It can be helpful to monitor dominance interactions through behavioural observations as these can help in identifying individuals of lower rank that may be more likely to receive aggression from conspecifics and/or limited access to resources.

Identification and sexing

It is essential to be able to individually identify corvids for research and welfare purposes. There are several means of enabling identification of individual corvids – most are applicable to all corvid species. Metal and/or plastic leg rings with identifying colours and/or letters/numbers can be used (De Beer et al. 2001). With plastic rings, applying superglue to the ring to aid in closing it is often necessary. In some bird species, like zebra finches (Taeniopygia guttata), the colour of rings has been found to influence social behaviour, including mate choice, longevity and offspring sex ratio (Burley et al. 1982) in some though not all studies (Hunt et al. 1997). To our knowledge, whether there is any influence of colour rings on corvid behaviour is yet to be tested. Wing tags can also be used to aid in identification, though, unlike leg rings, are invasive to apply. Note that depending on the material used to attach wing tags, birds may be able to remove them. As with marking any bird, care should be taken to use the correct size of ring or tag per species, applied by an experienced person or under the supervision of one, and visually checked regularly to ensure no issues arise (like toes being caught in rings or rings being discarded by the bird).

For captive corvids, it can be helpful to take individual photographs which can then be used for identifying through plumage markings in some species. Typically, this method is more difficult to learn, as in many corvid species, individuals physically look very similar to one another. Therefore, it may be best used as a back-up or additional means of identifying, and alongside individual behavioural differences. It is also possible to dye or temporarily mark feathers or toenails to aid in identification. For example, temporarily applying a small dot of tip-ex to the toenails of hatchlings can aid in identification until the chicks are large enough to receive their leg ring.

Recent advances in animal tracking have enabled the use of satellite tracking of wild birds, including some corvids like New Caledonian crows and common ravens (Rutz & Hays 2009; Loretto et al. 2016). Small transmitters are attached to a harness strapped to the bird's body and their movements can then be tracked. This has been particularly useful in wild birds. In the wild and captivity, Passive Integrated Transponder (PIT) tags can be used to monitor the movement, relations between individuals and apparatus access to specific individuals, such as in great tits (*Parus major*) (Aplin et al. 2013).

Sexing corvids is most reliably achieved through blood or feather sexing DNA analysis.

In some species, sex can also be determined through external biometrics as size differences exist between sexes, though note that there is often size overlap between sexes, particularly in juveniles. Fletcher and Foster (2010) found 85–93% accuracy in sexing larger males and smaller females. For example, wing length is longer in male carrion crows, rooks and jackdaws than female conspecifics (Fletcher & Foster 2010).

Physical environment

Excessive noise or vibration can negatively influence bird behaviour. A dawn-dusk lighting regime (e.g. 8:16 for indoor housing only or 12:12 day/night cycle where outside housing is also available) and good ventilation are important for indoor housing. In starlings, recent research suggested that full-spectrum lights for inside housing, including UV, are important to prevent hyperkeratosis (Bateson & Asher 2010), though it is not currently known whether this is also applicable for corvids. Presently, to our knowledge, most corvids held for scientific purposes have access to outside housing; therefore, the type of indoor light sources may be less critical than other lab species housed entirely indoors. Note that birds will not feed in very low light intensity (Cambridge 2014). The minimum UK Home Office requirements for bird indoor housing are: temperature of 16–23 °C, humidity of 30–80% and air changes of 8–12/hour (Cambridge 2014). Outdoor housing should provide suitable wind and rain cover, and shade from the sun.

Hygiene

It is important to note that birds can potentially carry zoonotic diseases i.e. diseases that are transmissible to humans, like salmonellosis and chlamydiosis, and staff may develop allergies to feather dust (Cambridge 2014). Therefore, care should be taken when working with these birds or handing them. For example, protective clothing including face masks, glasses and footwear/ shoe covers may need to be worn. Staff should routinely wash hands after contact with birds or their enclosures, or wear disposable gloves. Some corvids are capable of causing injury to humans, through bites, pecks or scratches, so gloves may be worn during handling (Cambridge 2014). If possible, it is also beneficial to use a towel/breathable bag to restrain a bird, as this reduces likelihood of being pecked/scratched, and sometimes gloves can reduce the sensitivity of the fingers so are not ideal when more intricate procedures are required during handling, like taking blood or ringing.

Enclosures should be cleaned thoroughly on a regular basis using appropriate disinfectants and any build-up of faeces or old food should be removed daily. This includes cleaning of substrates/flooring, perches and walls. It is recommended to use vinegar or other approved cleaning substances rather than bleach as a general disinfectant, as bleach can cause long-term damage to the birds if handled incorrectly. As highlighted in earlier sections, year-round bathing opportunities are important for maintaining healthy plumage and to enable the birds to maintain their personal hygiene. The bath should be deep enough so the birds can fully emerge themselves in it (Whitworth et al. 2007). Clearly ensuring diseases and infections are prevented and treated is critical for the welfare of the birds, staff and the research.

Quarantine, barrier systems and transportation

New arrivals or sick birds should be isolated from others until deemed safe for (re-) introduction to the other birds. For example, until clear faecal sample results are obtained, with faecal samples typically screened for both bacteriology (e.g. chlamydia, salmonella, campylobacter – which are zoonotic diseases) and parasitology (usually around 28 days for quarantined birds). For sick birds, dimmed lighting and an available heat source should be used. Barrier systems should be in place for humans going between isolation and general holding, including, as applicable, foot baths or shoe covers, changing clothes/jackets/plastic suits, wearing gloves, etc. For any deaths where the cause is unknown, post-mortem examinations should be conducted to ascertain the cause of death.

Corvids can be transported in wooden or plastic boxes, like secure cat carriers with breathing holes, of an adequate size for the species. The carrier should be lined, for instance, with newspaper or plastic matting. Most animals prefer to travel in dimmed light/darkness as it calms them. Small amounts of food (not meat) and/or water may be provided, though is usually only necessary for longer journeys. It is helpful to be able to add/remove food and water dishes through small hatches for longer journeys rather than opening the main carrier door and risking an escape. This also enables food and water to be provided at specific time points rather than leaving it in the carrier for the entire journey (which could lead to spilled or spoiled food).

Breeding

At the start of breeding season, it can be beneficial to increase enrichment, particularly in offering live food, i.e. insects. Corvids should be provided with nesting material, including sticks of varying width and length, plus softer materials, like grass, in early breeding season. If breeding is to be promoted, the birds should be provided with nest location options, preferably at a height and distance from care staff. Nest baskets, boxes and platforms, depending on species, may be provided. For the best breeding results, and successful pair housing of adults, it is best to allow individuals to select their own partner, where possible. Even if the intention is not to allow successful breeding, it can be important to let captive birds 'go through the motions' of building nests and laying eggs, even when those eggs are then removed/replaced or pipped to prevent the eggs from hatching. Care should be taken when approaching the nest, as some species/individuals may be highly aggressive towards humans; therefore, protective clothing, like lab glasses and a helmet, may be necessary. Note that in some countries, including the UK, there are regulations governing the euthanasia of embryos (see Euthanasia section).

With regard to artificial incubation, temperature and humidity is typically 37.5 or 38 °C and around 31–69% relative humidity, varying per species (Whitmore & Marzluff 1998). Once the eggs start to pip, they should be placed in a hatcher at 35 °C and 73% relative humidity, and after hatching, into a brooder at 35 °C, though adjusted in response to chick behaviour (shivering vs. panting) (Whitmore & Marzluff 1998). In common ravens, American crows and black-billed magpies, chicks fed large amounts of food grew faster and were healthier than those fed smaller amounts, or less regularly. However, no captive feeding regime enabled the chicks to grow as quickly as wild-reared birds. Survival 3 months post-release was positively correlated with feeding frequency (Whitmore & Marzluff 1998). When hand-rearing corvids, researchers often wish to habituate the birds to humans and start training for welfare and research early to ensure they are comfortable working with humans later on. Where possible, it may be beneficial to introduce the birds to humans in general (i.e. both sexes, varying hair colours, heights, etc.), rather than just specific humans involved in hand-rearing, during the rearing and juvenile period. It is also important to provide early exposure to conspecifics to ensure that these individuals behave as naturally as possible (critical particularly for cognitive testing) and are not over-attached to a human carer to the detriment of their interactions with their own species (Fox 2003).

Laboratory procedures

Handling

Handling can be very stressful for animals, including corvids, and should be avoided unless necessary. For instance, for veterinary checks, enclosure moves and in case of injury or illness. Where possible, rather than or at least prior to catching and handling, injured or sick birds should be observed closely while in the enclosure (Cambridge 2014). Corvids should be caught using bird nets with padded edges, and secure size-appropriate pet carriers can be used for secure transport. Ideally, the birds should be encouraged into a small space for catching to ensure the catching process is as quick and efficient as possible. While in the hand, the bird should be held securely, by an experienced person, for example, using the one-handed 'ringer's hold' (Figure 45.5). The bird's body is supported by the thumb, ring and little fingers, with the head restrained by the index and middle fingers (Sutherland et al. 2004; Whitworth et al. 2007). For larger corvid species, like crows and ravens, the two-handed grip may be used, with the hands placed either side of the bird so its wings are held against the body, with thumbs placed on the bird's backbone and fingers curled around the breast and abdomen and legs tucked up underneath the body (Whitworth et al. 2007) (Figure 45.5). Sometimes, it is helpful to use a combination of these two techniques for handling larger corvids, depending on the purpose for handling. For example, the ringer's hold may be used while taking head measurements if the body is

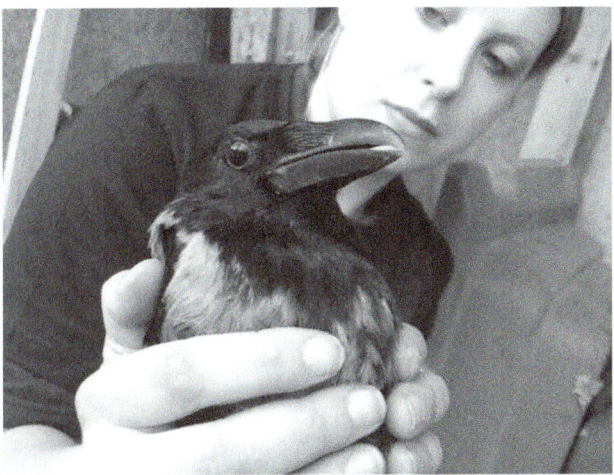
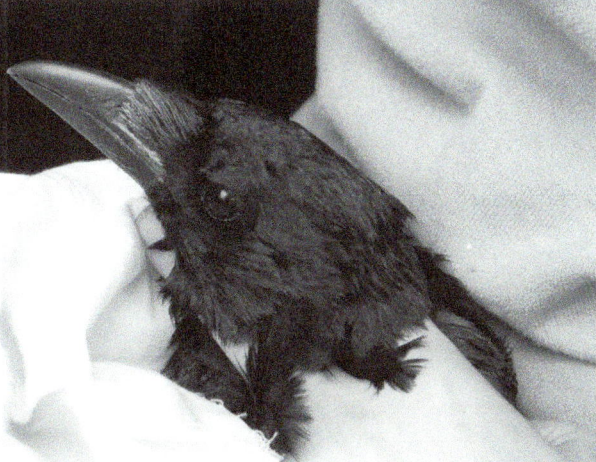

Figure 45.5 Example of crow handling: left photo: two-handed grip; Right photo: ringer's grip. Source: Gavin Harrison (2011).

secured within a material bag. The proper amount of restraint should be used, with the bird held firmly to prevent struggling or injury to the handler, but without restricting its respiration or heart function. Gasping is a clear sign that the pressure should be reduced (Whitworth et al. 2007). Birds should never be grabbed by the wings/ legs or tail if they escape during handling, but netted or cornered and covered with a material bag or towel before the hold is regained (Whitworth et al. 2007). During handling, it is beneficial to cover the bird's head with breathable material/hood and/or to place them inside a breathable material (e.g. cotton) bag or towel. This helps the bird to remain calm during the process and limits potential injuries to handlers.

Training and habituation for procedures

Corvids are well-suited for training, as they are quick learners, reward-motivated and often highly adaptable to human presence and environmental pressure (Fox 2003). Training using positive reinforcement techniques, such as those described in detail for husbandry training of marabou storks (*Leptoptilos crumenifer*) (Miller & King 2013) and other bird species (Heidenreich 2004), can be an extremely efficient and stress-minimised means of monitoring health and moving birds for research testing. For example, training can be used for taking weights by encouraging a bird to stand briefly on a perch attached to a set of scales, or allowing brief touching of feet or body to closely monitor condition or assess injuries, in return for small rewards (e.g. mealworms, nuts, dog biscuits). It is possible to train birds to provide faecal samples in specified locations (much like you might train a cat to use a litter tray or a dog to wait to defecate outside), and, in some cases, even to allow blood to be taken without physically catching the bird. Training can also be used for introducing birds to one another in a gradual manner, which can be helpful particularly in aggressive species (Miller & King 2013). Rather than catching birds for testing, birds can be trained to enter testing areas/compartments voluntarily, which ensures they are more relaxed for these procedures and therefore more likely to produce natural behaviours and engage in cognitive tasks. Training has even been used in other species, like dogs and primates (Nieder 2005), to enable eye-tracking and brain scans – which could potentially be utilised for corvids too. See also Chapter 15: The use of positive reinforcement training techniques to enhance the care and welfare of laboratory and research animals.

Some corvid species and individuals are highly neophobic (Greenberg & Mettke-Hofmann 2001), which should be considered during training and when introducing new areas, items and/or persons. Most species, including rooks, jackdaws, ravens and carrion crows, need sufficient time to adapt to changes in their environment. They may show stress reactions initially; therefore, a gradual introduction via a trusted person can be helpful. In a research set up, it is suggested to have the experimental compartment(s) as part of the 'home' aviary, so the birds can roam around the complex by themselves as much as they need outside of testing times. Therefore, during testing times when birds may be temporarily separated from the group, they are more likely to be comfortable enough to participate in testing. Where possible, aviaries and/or test areas should be located in areas where there is reduced disturbance by passing people, particularly during critical test trials.

Monitoring methods

Captive corvids should be monitored on a daily basis, with each bird visually checked to ensure they are well and behaving normally. The birds may for instance be checked during feeds, when (depending on the location of the food dishes) they are likely to come close to a human, or during testing. Weights can be monitored regularly without handling the birds by training them to stand on scales (see Training section) for a small food reward. If the scales are left inside the aviary, the birds are able to slowly get used to them and over time see them as normal part of the environment, thereby reducing neophobic behaviour towards the scale. Weight monitoring is likely to be particularly important in case of dietary and seasonal changes, as some corvid species react with gain/loss of weight during different seasons and the food supply may have to be adjusted accordingly.

It may be advisable to hold an annual health check of all birds, where each bird is caught and physically checked more closely, including eyes, nails, body condition. Nails or bills may need to be trimmed – though adequate environmental provisions should negate this need, such as ensuring the birds have access to perches of varying sizes and materials, and items that they can peck.

When necessary, blood samples can be collected from the alar or brachial wing vein, or in larger species, the jugular vein in a similar manner to other bird species (Cambridge 2014; Samour 2016). Faecal samples can be collected from the floor of the aviary, for instance, by placing down clean sheeting beneath favoured perches and collecting after a set period of time. Depending on the social housing, these may be grouped or individual/pairs samples by aviary. If a bird is restrained already, then a cloacal swab can be used for a faecal smear. These faecal samples can then be analysed for bacteriology and/or parasitology as required. The regularity of faecal monitoring may vary between collections depending on factors like funding for covering these costs. For example, at University of Cambridge and the University of Vienna, the corvid faecal samples are checked on a monthly basis. Treatment if required, and following veterinary advice, can then be administered individually upon positive results, thereby, where possible, limiting potential negative impact of regular long-term treatment on the birds' health and/or resistance against treatment courses.

Administration of substances

Where possible, it is recommended to administer substances without having to catch the bird, as handling can be an added stressor for sick birds. For non-invasive administration, substances can be given orally, i.e. pes os (PO), by mixing it into the normal diet and/or in the water, or via a syringe directly into the mouth. Corvids are generally quite good at detecting hidden medicine (especially if it has a bad/strong taste), so it is advisable to use larger amounts of food than the regular diet to hide it, or to use preferred treats, like hiding it inside an insect, like a locust or wax moth larva. If the birds can taste the medication and are repelled by it, it can become increasingly difficult to routinely administer it. Therefore, another strategy for non-invasive medication is to train the birds using positive reinforcement to take medicine PO voluntarily in return for a reward.

The parenteral route is the invasive method of drug administration via subcutaneous (SC), intramuscular (IM) or intravenous (IV) injections. IM injections are inserted into the pectoral or thigh muscles, and it is recommended to alternate sites whenever possible, as they can induce muscle trauma. SC injections are inserted into the inguinal web, interscapular area or axillary region right under the skin and are the preferred method for injecting larger substance volumes, such as to administer fluids. IV injections are mainly used during critical care treatment as a very rapid therapeutic level is achieved via this route (Samour 2016).

Anaesthesia and analgesia

As local anaesthesia can lead to high stress levels in birds, full anaesthesia is usually the recommended method (Samour 2016). Here, it is important to first check that the crop is empty or deprive the bird of food for 1–2 hours beforehand. This is particularly important in smaller bird species, in order to avoid regurgitation and hypoglycaemia during the procedure (Samour 2016). Prevention of heat loss is important via a heat source, insulation and minimum of feather removal and applied water/alcohol when preparing the skin (Cambridge 2014). During anaesthesia procedures, the bird should be closely monitored including their reflexes, respiration, heart rate and temperature (Cambridge 2014). Following the procedure, the bird should be kept in a quiet, darkened, padded box while recovering.

The two gaseous agents most routinely used in practice are Isoflurane and Sevoflurane. The second one is part of the next generation of gaseous anaesthetic agents as it has a lower blood gas partition coefficient than isoflurane (0.69), therefore giving a shorter recovery time than isoflurane. The gaseous agent of choice, plus oxygen as a carrier gas, can be easily administered by using a face mask, which helps reduce potentially more stressful procedures like injection and handling. To put on the face mask, it is best to use a towel to restrain the bird (Samour 2016). Inhalation anaesthetics are often preferable to injectable ones, as there is easier control of anaesthetic depth and improved oxygenation due to using oxygen concurrently. For injectable anaesthetics, the weight of the bird should be obtained to determine the correct drug dosage (Cambridge 2014).

It is important to note that isoflurane anaesthesia does not provide postoperative analgesia, i.e. pain relief (Dohoo 1990). Note that there are no analgesics with a veterinary licence for corvids. The most commonly used pain relief drug is Meloxicam ('Metacam'), which is an nonsteroidal anti-inflammatory analgesic, with a dose of 0.1 mg/kg SC or PO (Paul-Murphy & Ludders 2001). Signs of pain in birds are often obscure and subtle. Therefore, behavioural changes must be looked out for, including sitting on the floor instead of a perch, squatting, fluffed up feathers, drooping of wings/head, fast moving eye lids and/or reduced appetite (Hawkins & Paul-Murphy 2011). Note that behavioural changes do not manifest equally over all individuals and/or species. Hence, the presence of trained staff and regular observation intervals is very important (Speer 2015).

Euthanasia

If it is necessary to euthanise a bird, it is important to choose a humane method that will lead to a quick state of unconsciousness with the minimum of pain and fear. If the body is to be used for scientific research, then this should also be considered before euthanising the bird. Euthanasia should only be performed by veterinarians or other professionally trained personnel. It should be handled respectfully and professionally. Once a bird has been euthanised, the death should be confirmed – for instance, through dislocation of the neck, destruction of the brain, exsanguination or confirming rigour mortis onset (Cambridge 2014).

The following is a list of approved euthanasia methods for birds (Orosz 2006; Cambridge 2014; Speer 2015):

1. Pentobarbital euthanasia via a route other than intravenously. Can only be used when the bird is already under anaesthesia via isoflurane or sevoflurane. Pentobarbital should not be administered IM as it can be painful. In our experience, this is the most refined method.
2. Overdose of inhaled anaesthetics using a route and agent appropriate for the size and species of the animal. Can be used for all birds.
3. Exposure to carbon dioxide in a rising concentration: appropriate rate of application is important so that the increase in carbon dioxide is rapid enough to have a short time to the loss of posture and consciousness, but slow enough that there is reduced aversion or reaction to the gas. Can be used for birds up to 1.5 kg.
4. Dislocation of the neck. Can be used for birds up to 3 kg.
5. Concussion of the brain by striking the cranium. Can be used for birds to up 250 g.

Methods for foetal, larval and embryonic forms:

1. Before 50% of incubation length is complete, eggs can be euthanised by the above-mentioned methods 1–3, via refrigeration (under 4 °C for 4 hours), disruption of membranes or maceration in apparatus approved under appropriate slaughter legislation.
2. Once 50% of incubation length is complete, euthanasia can be conducted via the above methods 1–5, plus decapitation up to weight of 50 g, as studies suggest that the neural tube of the bird embryo is already formed at this stage.

Common welfare problems

Health

Corvids are typically quite hardy species. However, many diseases that are a concern for other bird species are also a concern for corvids, including a variety of parasites.

Transmission of parasites from adult to young individuals may be one of the reasons that young are affected routinely in the nest, e.g. gapeworm (*Syngamus trachea*) (Żuchowska 1987; Samour 2016). The following are some parasites that need constant monitoring and/or treatment (Żuchowska 1987; Berto *et al.* 2011; Samour 2016):

- *Coccidiosis*: single celled protozoa, which cause diarrhoea (with/without blood), weight loss, depression and the bird may stop eating. Birds may also be carriers without showing any signs of illness.
- *Capillariosis*: a round worm species. Most clinical signs in young birds include weight loss, diarrhoea, regurgitation, anaemia and oral necrotic plaques.
- *Cestoda*: a helminth species. As this parasite competes for food with the host, it does not cause serious health problems unless the bird is immune-deficient or the parasite numbers grow excessively. Clinical signs are diarrhoea (from severely damaged intestine walls), malnourishment and weight loss.
- *Syngamosis*: a gapeworm species, which causes laboured breathing. Infected birds stretch out their necks, open their mouths and gasp for air. Other clinical signs include: coughing, weakness and shaking of the head.

Rickets can affect corvids and is characterised by defective bone formation in young birds. It is caused by malnutrition during the nestling phase and results mainly from a vitamin D or phosphorus deficiency (Thompson 2007). Rickets leads to bone deformations, resulting in the birds suffering from deformed beak and legs. Treatment for early-stage rickets can be provided via parenteral administration of vitamin D as well as ultraviolet light. To avoid rickets, an adequate balanced diet and access to ultraviolet light during development is important (Cousquer *et al.* 2007; Stieger-Vanegas *et al.* 2013).

Viral diseases can also occur in corvids. One example is avian influenza, which is spread all over the world and occurs in multiple bird species (Swayne & Halvoson 2008). Transmission occurs via respiratory tract and faeces, with an incubation period from several hours to 3 days. Testing is done either via a direct antigen test or polymerase chain reaction (PCR) on oropharyngeal or cloacal swabs. It is caused by orthomyxovirus with three antigenically distinct types: A, B and C, with B and C only occurring in humans (Speer 2015). If avian influenza is confirmed in poultry or other captive birds in the UK, then various control measures would come into effect on the premises and the surrounding areas in accordance with the Avian Influenza of Avian Origin in Mammals (England) (No 2) Order 2006 (Cambridge 2014). Vaccination is a possible preventative measure; however, the performance of many vaccines and the vaccination schedule in non-poultry species is not well-defined. Therefore, vaccination may provide no more additional protection of outdoor caged birds than adequate biosecurity (Speer 2015).

Common injuries in corvids include injured toes and/or claws, usually causing the individual to limp for a short period of time. In general, corvids are good at dealing with small injuries. Therefore, provided there is not excessive bleeding or an open wound, it is usually recommended to just observe their general behaviour (i.e. food intake, movement, social interactions) and to check for swelling in the injured area to deduce whether additional action is required. After a day or two, the bird should move around normally. In case of larger wounds, a veterinary assessment will be necessary. To avoid further injuries to the individual, transportation in a small, dark box with a towel or other soft matting is advised. If birds are bandaged or require further daily treatments, the bird should be kept in a box inside or next to his social partner/group so as to avoid add further stress due to social isolation. As corvids are intelligent and quick learners (Emery & Clayton 2004), setting up a routine for care is helpful to help limit the general stress level. For example, after arriving in the morning, immediately changing the bandage and/or administration of medication, cleaning the box and then giving the bird either the normal food or a reward. This way, the birds can learn quickly that nothing further is likely to happen to them for the remainder of the day and so may be more relaxed (M. Schiestl, personal communication 2019).

Before catching a bird, it is usually recommended to use non-invasive visual assessment -checking for visible wounds, general appearance, behaviour, weight, food intake, collect and test faecal sample – to identify whether a bird is injured and/or sick. This approach is recommended because handling and restraint can be highly stressful for birds, and may also impact on some health indicator parameters, including respiratory and heart rate. If the bird is found to be wounded or unwell, only then it is recommended to catch the bird for a close-up appraisement by a veterinarian. If the bird is handled, it can also be checked over to assess the skin and feather condition, look for bald patches, swelling or bleeding, or a general loss of condition. These factors may indicate bacterial or parasitic infections, feather plucking or other injuries (Cambridge 2014; Speer 2015).

Behaviour and abnormal behaviour

In order to assess a bird's welfare, including their behavioural and mental state, it is important to have sufficient information about their natural behavioural repertoire and/or experience to be able to judge it accordingly. This is particularly important for new personnel/staff, who we recommend take time to observe the birds for a period of time and become acquainted with the common behaviours shown in a pair/group. We cover normal corvid behaviours in the Biological overview section. Abnormal behaviour is usually defined as changed frequency, intensity or latency of normal behaviours, common for class, sex and age, which does not have any adaptive value for survival and fitness of the individual bird. The signs of abnormal behaviours can be subtle, such as change in body posture, feather condition, fast/slow moving eyelids, faster/slower breathing and unresponsiveness. Therefore, as mentioned before, it is important that personnel/staff are trained to be able to interpret the behaviour correctly and act accordingly (Samour 2016).

Signs of poor welfare

Signs of poor welfare that could indicate a disease or injury include: changes to an individual's appearance (murky feathers, fluffed feathers, unusual crouching position, fast moving eyelids), posture, temperament, appetite, respiration or locomotory skills, and/or the presence of any unusual bodily fluids in the enclosure, like blood, diarrhoea or mucus (Cambridge 2014; Speer 2015). For example, lack of interest in food or severe weight loss can often be a late warning signal for poor health in birds (Samour 2016). Signs of acute distress include gasping, laboured or open-mouthed breathing (Samour 2016). Note that signs of pain can vary by species and/or individual differences within species, for instance, some species may show increased vocalisations and strong avoidance reactions to painful situations, while others may become quiet and unresponsive (Cambridge 2014). Further signs of poor welfare include birds being obese/malnourished, a bare environment, lack of social stimulation and the inability to perform natural behaviours (e.g. caching in caching corvid species is severely limited if the birds are living in an aviary with a concrete floor). Additionally, stereotypic behaviours can be a sign of poor welfare as they can result from suboptimal environmental conditions, such as lack of opportunity to interact with conspecifics or objects, or insufficient holding/flight space (Bateson & Feenders 2010). These are typically behaviours that are repetitive, invariant and serve no clear goal or function (Cambridge 2014; Speer 2015). Examples may include excessive feather plucking and pacing. Stereotyping is easier to prevent than to cure, however, addressing issues with the environment, increasing enrichment and training can aid in reducing stereotyping if it starts (Bateson & Feenders 2010). It is therefore critical to be aware of what is normal behaviour for each species and individual under care. Communication between animal care staff and researchers is also important to ensure information between everyone is exchanged properly.

Acknowledgements

We thank Megan Lambert for comments on this chapter. This work was funded by the European Research Council under the European Union's Seventh Framework Programme (FP7/2007-2013)/ERC Grant Agreement No. 3399933, awarded to Nicola S. Clayton (funding Rachael Miller, Nicola S. Clayton).

References

Web of Knowledge. (2018) Retrieved from the World Wide Web: Webofknowledge.com
Aplin, L.M., Farine, D., Morand-Ferron, J. et al. (2013) Individual personalities predict social behaviour in wild networks of great tits (*Parus major*). *Ecology Letters*, **16**, 1365–1372.
Bateson, M. and Asher, L. (2010) The European starling. In: *The UFAW Handbook on the Care and Management of Laboratory and Other Research Animals*, 8th edn. Eds Hubrecht, R. and Kirkwood, J. Wiley-Blackwell, Bognor Regis.
Bateson, M. and Feenders, G. (2010) The use of passerine bird species in laboratory research: implications of basic biology for husbandry and welfare. *ILAR Journal*, **51**, 394–408.
Beaman, M. and Madge, S. (2010) *The Handbook of Bird Identification: For Europe and the Western Palearctic*. A&C Black, London.
Berto, B.P., Flausino, W., McIntosh, D. et al. (2011) Coccidia of new world passerine birds (Aves: Passeriformes): a review of Eimeria Schneider, 1875 and Isospora Schneider, 1881 (Apicomplexa: Eimeriidae). *Systematic Parasitology*, **80**, 159.
Birkhead, T. (2010) *The Magpies: The Ecology and Behaviour of Black-Billed and Yellow-Billed Magpies*. A&C Black, London.
Boeckle, M. and Bugnyar, T. (2012) Long-term memory for affiliates in ravens. *Current Biology*, **22**, 801–806.
Bugnyar, T. and Heinrich, B. (2005) Ravens, *Corvus corax*, differentiate between knowledgeable and ignorant competitors. *Proceedings of the Royal Society B: Biological Sciences*, **272**, 1641–1646.
Bugnyar, T. and Kotrschal, K. (2002) Observational learning and the raiding of food caches in ravens, *Corvus corax*: is it 'tactical' deception? *Animal Behaviour*, **64**, 185–195.
Bugnyar, T., Schwab, C., Schloegl, C. et al. (2007) Ravens judge competitors through experience with play caching. *Current Biology*, **17**, 1804–1808.
Burley, N., Krantzberg, G. and Radman, P. (1982) Influence of colour-banding on the conspecific preferences of zebra finches. *Animal Behaviour*, **30**, 444–455.
Cambridge, U.O. (2014) University Biomedical Services Home Office Personal Licence course (Avian) notes. Summarises information based on Home Office Legislation and the EU Directives on the Protection of Animals Used for Scientific Purposes.
Clayton, N.S., Dally, J.M. and Emery, N.J. (2007) Social cognition by food-caching corvids. The western scrub-jay as a natural psychologist. *Philosophical Transactions of the Royal Society B: Biological Sciences*, **362**, 507–522.
Clayton, N.S. and Emery, N.J. (2007) The social life of corvids. *Current Biology*, **17**, R652–R656.
Clayton, N.S., Griffiths, D. and Bennett, A. (1994) Storage of stones by jays *Garrulus glandarius*. *Ibis*, **136**, 331–334.
Clayton, N.S. and Krebs, J.R. (1994) One-trial associative memory: comparison of food-storing and nonstoring species of birds. *Animal Learning & Behavior*, **22**, 366–372.
Cousquer, G., Dankoski, E. and Patterson-Kane, J. (2007) Metabolic bone disease in wild collared doves (*Streptopelia decaocto*). *Veterinary Record*, **160**, 78–84.
Dally, J.M., Emery, N.J. and Clayton, N.S. (2006) Food-caching western scrub-jays keep track of who was watching when. *Science*, **312**, 1662–1665.
de Azevedo, C.S., Cipreste, C.F. and Young, R.J. (2007) Environmental enrichment: a GAP analysis. *Applied Animal Behaviour Science*, **102**, 329–343.
De Beer, S., Lockwood, G., Raijmakers, J. et al. (2001) SAFRING bird ringing manual. *ADU Guide*, **5**, 104.
Del Hoyo, J., Elliott, A., Sargatal, J. et al. (2015) *Handbook of the Birds of the World Alive*. Lynx Edicions, Barcelona.
Dohoo, S.E. (1990) Isoflurane as an inhalational anesthetic agent in clinical practice. *The Canadian Veterinary Journal*, **31**, 847.
Emery, N.J. and Clayton, N.S. (2004) The mentality of crows: convergent evolution of intelligence in corvids and apes. *Science*, **306**, 1903–1907.
Fletcher, K. and Foster, R. (2010) Use of external biometrics to sex carrion crow *Corvus corone*, Rook *C. frugilegus* and Western Jackdaw *C. monedula* in Northern England. *Ringing & Migration*, **25**, 47–51.
Fox, T. (2003) Corvids: Husbandry and Management. A brief review, originally presented at the AZA 2003 Eastern Regional. Association of Zoos and Aquariums Eastern Regional.
Fraser, O.N. and Bugnyar, T. (2010) The quality of social relationships in ravens. *Animal Behaviour*, **79**, 927–933.
Fraser, O.N. and Bugnyar, T. (2011) Ravens reconcile after aggressive conflicts with valuable partners. *PLoS One*, **6**, e18118.
Goodwin, D. (1976) *Crows of the World*. Cornell University Press, London.
Greenberg, R. and Mettke-Hofmann, C. (2001) Ecological aspects of neophobia and neophilia in birds. In: *Current Ornithology*, pp. 119–178. Springer, New York.

Grodzinski, U. and Clayton, N.S. (2010) Problems faced by food-caching corvids and the evolution of cognitive solutions. *Philosophical Transactions of the Royal Society B: Biological Sciences*, **365**, 977–987.

Gwinner, V.E. (1964) Untersuchungen uber das Ausdrucks-und Sozialverhalten des Kolkraben (*Corvus corax* L.). *Zeitschrift für Tierpsychologie*.

Hawkins, M.G. and Paul-Murphy, J. (2011) Avian analgesia. *Veterinary Clinics: Exotic Animal Practice*, **14**, 61–80.

Hawkins, P., Morton, D., Cameron, D. et al. (2001) Laboratory birds: refinements in husbandry and procedures. *Laboratory Animals*, **35**, 1–163.

Heidenreich, B. (2004) Training birds for husbandry and medical behavior to reduce or eliminate stress. Association of Avian Veterinarians Conference.

Heinrich, B. (1988) Winter foraging at carcasses by three sympatric corvids, with emphasis on recruitment by the raven, *Corvus corax*. *Behavioral Ecology and Sociobiology*, **23**, 141–156.

Heinrich, B. (1999) *Mind of the Raven*. Cliff Street Books, New York.

Holyoak, D. (1967) Breeding biology of the Corvidae. *Bird Study*, **14**, 153–168.

Hunt, S., Cuthill, I.C., Swaddle, J.P. and Bennett, A.T. (1997) Ultraviolet vision and band-colour preferences in female zebra finches, *Taeniopygia guttata*. *Animal Behaviour*, **54**, 1383–1392.

Jolles, J.W., King, A.J., Manica, A. and Thornton, A. (2013) Heterogeneous structure in mixed-species corvid flocks in flight. *Animal Behaviour*, **85**, 743–750.

King, C.E. (1993) Environmental enrichment: is it for the birds? *Zoo Biology*, **12**, 509–512.

Krebs, J., Ashcroft, R. and Webber, M. (1978) Song repertoires and territory defence in the great tit. *Nature*, **271**, 539.

Kroodsma, D.E. (1985) Voices of the New World Jays, Crows, and Their Allies. Family Corvidae. *The Auk: Ornithological Advances*, **102**, 433.

Laule, G. and Desmond, T. (1998) Positive reinforcement training as an enrichment strategy. DC: Smithsonian Institution. CiteseerX.

Loretto, M.-C., Schuster, R. and Bugnyar, T. (2016) GPS tracking of non-breeding ravens reveals the importance of anthropogenic food sources during their dispersal in the Eastern Alps. *Current zoology*, **62**, 337–344.

Madge, S. and Burn, H. (1994) *Crows and Jays: A Guide to the Crows, Jays and Magpies of the World*. A&C Black, London.

Massen, J.J., Pašukonis, A., Schmidt, J. and Bugnyar, T. (2014) Ravens notice dominance reversals among conspecifics within and outside their social group. *Nature Communications*, **5**, 3679.

Miller, R., Bugnyar, T., Pölzl, K. and Schwab, C. (2015) Differences in exploration behaviour in common ravens and carrion crows during development and across social context. *Behavioral Ecology and Sociobiology*, **69**, 1209–1220.

Miller, R. and King, C. (2013) Husbandry training, using positive reinforcement techniques, for Marabou stork *Leptoptilos crumeniferus* at Edinburgh Zoo. *International Zoo Yearbook*, **47**, 171–180.

Miller, R., Schiestl, M., Whiten, A. et al. (2014) Tolerance and social facilitation in the foraging behaviour of free-ranging crows (*Corvus corone corone*; *C. c. cornix*). *Ethology*, **120**, 1248–1255.

Nicol, C. (1995) Environmental enrichment for birds. *Environmental Enrichment Information Resources for Laboratory Animals 1965–1995*, 1–3.

Nieder, A. (2005) Counting on neurons: the neurobiology of numerical competence. *Nature Reviews Neuroscience*, **6**, 177.

Orosz, S. (2006) Guidelines for euthanasia of nondomestic animals. American Association of Zoo Veterinarians.

Paul-Murphy, J. and Ludders, J.W. (2001) Avian analgesia. *Veterinary Clinics of North America: Exotic Animal Practice*, **4**, 35–45.

Rutz, C. and Hays, G.C. (2009) New frontiers in biologging science. *Biology Letters*, **5**, 289–292.

Samour, J. (2016) *Avian Medicine*. Mosby International Ltd, Missouri.

Seed, A.M., Clayton, N.S. and Emery, N.J. (2007) Postconflict third-party affiliation in rooks, *Corvus frugilegus*. *Current Biology*, **17**, 152–158.

Seed, A.M., Emery, N.J. and Clayton, N.S. (2009) Intelligence in corvids and apes: a case of convergent evolution? *Ethology*, **115**, 401–420.

Sima, M.J., Matzinger, T., Bugnyar, T. and Pika, S. (2018) Reconciliation and third-party affiliation in carrion crows. *Ethology*, **124**, 33–44.

Speer, B. (2015) *Current Therapy in Avian Medicine and Surgery*. Elsevier Health Sciences, Missouri.

Stieger-Vanegas, S., Garret, R., McKenzie, E. and Löhr, C. (2013) Vertebral fractures in two alpaca crias with rickets syndrome. *Australian Veterinary Journal*, **91**, 437–440.

Sutherland, W.J., Newton, I. and Green, R. (2004) *Bird Ecology and Conservation: A Handbook of Techniques*. Oxford University Press, Oxford.

Svensson, L. (1992) *Identification Guide to European Passerines*. British Trust of Ornithology, Stockholm.

Swayne, D.H. and Halvoson, D.A. (2008) Influenza. In: *Diseases of Poultry*. Ed. Saif, Y.F., pp. 620–636. Blackwell Publishing, Ames, IA.

Thompson, K. (2007) Bones and joints. In: *Jubb, Kennedy and Palmer's Pathology of Domestic Animals*, pp. 1–184. Elsevier, Philadelphia.

Westlund, K. (2014) Training is enrichment – and beyond. *Applied Animal Behaviour Science*, **152**, 1–6.

Whitmore, K.D. and Marzluff, J.M. (1998) Hand-rearing corvids for reintroduction: importance of feeding regime, nestling growth, and dominance. *The Journal of Wildlife Management*, 1460–1479.

Whitworth, D., Newman, S., Mundkur, T. and Harris, P. (2007) *Wild Birds and Avian Influenza: An Introduction to Applied Field Research and Disease Sampling Techniques*, Food & Agriculture Org.

Żuchowska, E. (1987) Role of synanthropic corvid birds (Corvidae) in the transmission of parasites to zoo birds. *Wiadomości Parazytologiczne*, **33**, 193–198.

Reptiles and Amphibia

46 Terrestrial reptiles: lizards, snakes and tortoises

John E. Cooper

Introduction

There are approximately 11,000 extant species of reptiles (class Reptilia). Number of species and nomenclature follow the Reptile Database[1]. The majority of reptiles are lizards and snakes (order Squamata). More than 40 species in the order Testudines that can be regarded as terrestrial – called 'tortoises' in Europe, Australasia and elsewhere but in North America usually referred to (with marine and freshwater aquatic chelonians) as 'turtles'. There are just over 20 species of crocodiles, alligators, caimans and their allies (order Crocodylia), and the unique lizard-like tuatara (order Rhynchocephalia), neither of which is dealt with in this chapter.

Much has been published over the years, in various languages, concerning the husbandry and captive care of reptiles. General information about the biology, restraint and treatment of reptiles can be found in various earlier texts. For instance, useful, succinct, summaries for lizards are provided by Schumacher (2003), for snakes by Mitchell (2003) and for chelonians by Raphael (2003). This chapter does not attempt to provide details of the husbandry of individual species. Instead, it outlines and explains the general biological principles underlying successful reptile husbandry.

Many of the requirements of reptiles, and the husbandry techniques appropriate for successfully maintaining them in captivity, are significantly different from those of mammals or birds. With a few exceptions (see, e.g. Thorogood & Whimster 1979; Wisniewski 1992), relatively little has been published specifically on the laboratory management of terrestrial reptiles: therefore, it is often necessary (and wise) to extrapolate from the experiences of those who successfully keep and breed these species in private collections or in zoos. While some of the accounts tend to be anecdotal, others are based on sound observation and study – see, e.g., Divers (1995), Frye (1993), Harling (1993, 1994), Langerwerf (1990, 1991), Rose (1992), Sheriff (1988), Sweeney (1993) and Townson (1994). A useful overview of laboratory management of reptiles is the chapter by O'Rourke et al. (2019).

[1] www.reptile-database.org (Accessed 25 May 2022)

Biological overview

Anatomy

Reptiles are vertebrate animals that show considerable variation in morphology, especially modifications to limbs, vertebral column, and pectoral and pelvic girdles (Davis 1981). There are snakes with vestiges of hindlimbs and lizards that are legless; an example of the latter are members of the family Scincidae (Schumacher 2003). Some indication of the complexity of structures in the cephalic region of squamate reptiles (snakes and lizards) is given in Figure 46.1. The integument of all reptiles is particularly important in terms of biology and health and is, therefore, discussed in detail in the next section.

The integument

In almost all reptile species, the outer layer of the skin, the epidermis, is thickened (see Figure 46.1) and highly keratinised to form plate-like scales (Figures 46.2 and 46.3), which in places overlap one another (imbrication). The surface of the epidermis is lost periodically, a process known as ecdysis or sloughing, and is replaced by growth of new cells from deeper layers. In snakes, the entire skin is shed, usually in one piece, including the keratinous 'spectacle', which covers the eye. Changes in the spectacle, characterised by an opacity or translucency, are a sign that sloughing is imminent. In many lizards, the skin is lost in small portions, the process taking place more or less simultaneously over the entire surface of the body. Some species, such as *Abronia* species shed their skins whole. In other reptiles, the process tends to be piecemeal.

Sloughing (shedding) is an important physiological event (Maderson 1965). When reptiles are kept in laboratories, it is important that detailed records of sloughing are maintained as a change in frequency, or a failure of/difficulty in shedding (dysecdysis), may indicate ill-health. It is good practice to retain shed skins, in a sealed plastic bag, so that they can be examined in the laboratory as part of routine health monitoring (see section on health) (Figure 46.4).

The UFAW Handbook on the Care and Management of Laboratory and Other Research Animals, Ninth Edition.
Edited by Huw Golledge and Claire Richardson.
© 2024 John Wiley & Sons Ltd. Published 2024 by John Wiley & Sons Ltd.

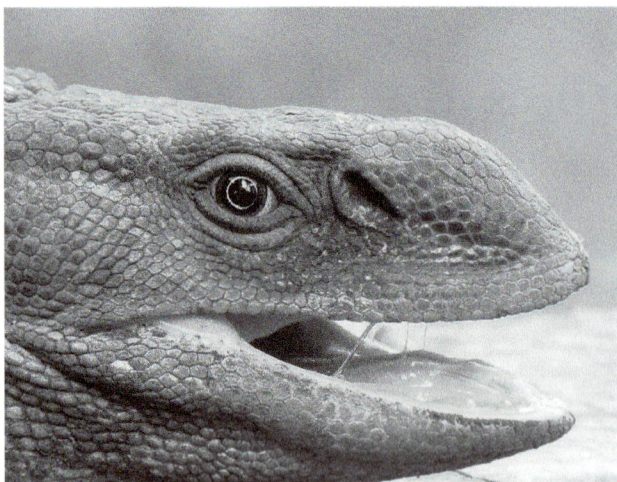

Figure 46.1 Head of a monitor lizard (*Varanus* sp.), illustrating the detailed scalation. The animal has a clear, shiny, eye, usually indicative of health.

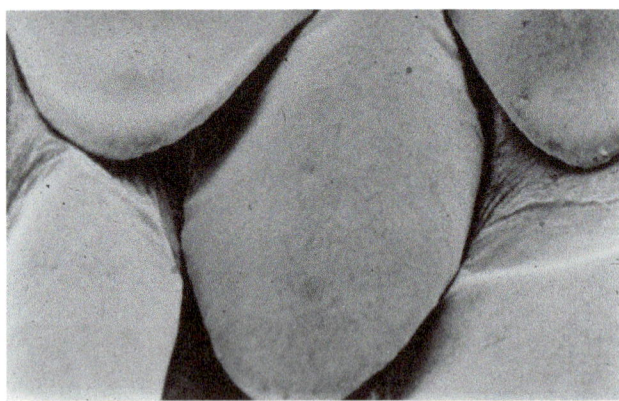

Figure 46.2 A low-power scanning electron microscope view of the skin of a skink (*Leiolopisma telfairii*), showing the overlapping scales.

The 'shell' of terrestrial chelonians consists in most cases of bone, sometimes of cartilage, that is covered with connective tissue and highly keratinised stratified squamous epithelium. It is well-innervated and sensitive to trauma and painful stimuli. The care of, and veterinary attention to, chelonians can be specialised (McArthur *et al.* 2004).

Ectothermy and behavioural thermoregulation

The conventional wisdom has been that, apart from rare exceptions, such as brooding pythons, reptiles cannot control their body temperature by internal means. As ectothermic animals, reptiles rely on external sources to maintain a preferred body temperature (PBT)/preferred optimal temperature zone (POTZ) (see below for terminology) and this in turn allows for optimal biological function. There is, however, some evidence indicating that certain species (black rat snake, *Elaphe obsoleta obsoleta* (now named '*Pantherophis obsoletus*'); corn snake, *Elaphe guttata* (*Pantherophis guttatus*); Eastern box turtle, *Terrapene carolina*) were able to regulate their body temperatures independently of their environment (Raske *et al.* 2012).

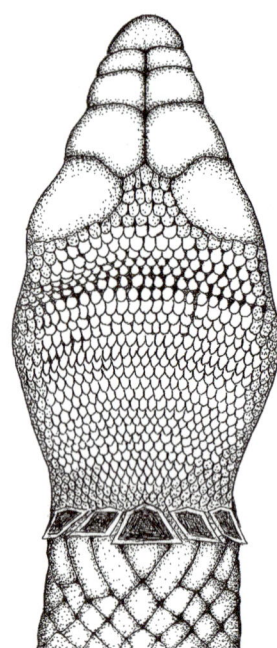

Figure 46.3 Line drawing of *Lacerta viridis* head (drawn courtesy of the Edward Elkan Reference Collection).

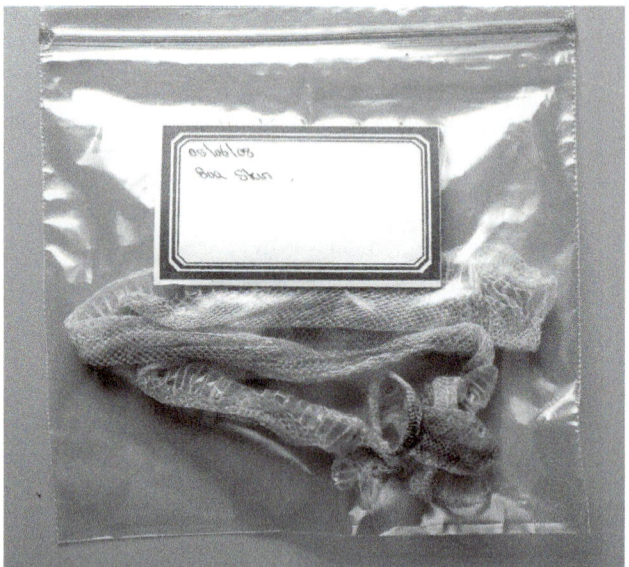

Figure 46.4 A sloughed (shed) skin from a boa constrictor. Regular and complete sloughing is usually a sign of good health in snakes. Under laboratory conditions, the sloughing cycle should be monitored and shed skins carefully preserved, in sealed plastic bags, so that they can be examined for parasites and evidence of disease (photo: Richard Spence).

Notwithstanding this interesting work, the generality that reptiles are ectotherms means that the temperature(s) within their cage or enclosure can have profound effects on the animals' health and welfare – this and other environmental features are usually dictated by the keeper of the animal. The amount of heat produced by reptiles is small and because they have no insulation (hair or feathers) it can be rapidly lost. Without some external source of heat, the body temperature

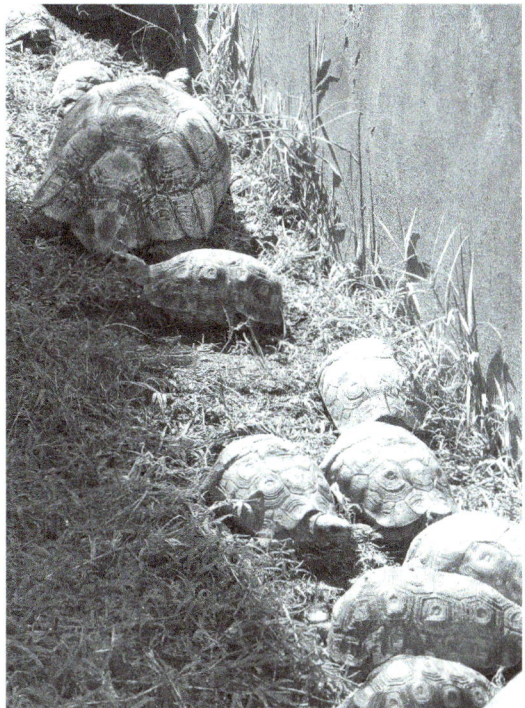

Figure 46.5 A mixed group of leopard (*Stigmochelys pardalis*) and hinge-back (*Kinixys belliana*) tortoises in an outdoor pen. This sort of management is popular in the tropics because it is inexpensive and provides natural sunlight (note how the tortoises are thermoregulating in the sunlit area). It offers environmental enrichment but may predispose animals to damage and predation.

of a reptile will approximate to its immediate surroundings. Many species of reptiles adjust their behaviour to take advantage of external heat sources, usually either direct sunlight or sun-warmed substrates such as rocks, sand or (less frequently) water (Figure 46.5). Typically, a reptile will lie in the sun ('basking') until its body temperature rises to a threshold level ('upper thermoregulatory set point') at which metabolic rate is optimal and it will begin to perform other kinds of behaviour such as searching for food, courtship and mating and defensive aggression (Schieffelin & Queiroz 1991).

It can be important in research, both in the laboratory and the field, to be able to measure the body temperatures of reptiles. A non-invasive method, using an infrared temperature gun, was described for chelonians by Cerreta et al. (2018).

Basking often involves flattening and positioning the body so that the maximum surface area is exposed to solar radiation. When the animal stops basking, these postures are no longer maintained. If it remains in the sun, it may nevertheless drop in temperature because the rate of heat gain has been reduced. If it moves into the shade, for example while feeding, it will cool. In both cases, a second threshold temperature ('lower thermoregulatory set point') will be reached, and the animal will seek sunlight and resume basking. In small lizards, the rates of heat loss and heat gain are rapid, and as they move from sun to shade and back again, they are often called 'shuttling heliotherms'. This method of maintaining a relatively high body temperature by basking to gain heat (and in very hot environments, actively seeking to cool by spending long periods in the shade or panting) is termed 'behavioural thermoregulation'. It is a key to understanding many aspects of reptile biology, including how best to provide suitable conditions in captivity.

The actual threshold temperatures (Firth & Turner 1982) vary from species to species, and sometimes among individuals of the same species, depending upon various factors (Huey 1982). The mean temperatures recorded in active animals (mean activity temperature (MAT); Pough & Gans 1982) will thus fluctuate. More than 500 species of reptiles for which MATs or similar thermoregulatory data are available were listed in Avery (1982), Meek and Avery (1988) and Peterson et al. (1993). Another term used by herpetologists is 'preferred optimum temperature zone' (POTZ) or 'preferred optimum temperature range' (POTR) and published data are available on the POTZ for numerous species of reptile, some of which may be kept in laboratories. Different heat sources can influence the behaviour of captive reptiles (Thomas et al. 2019).

It is vital under laboratory conditions to ensure that the temperature of different areas in the reptile's environment is properly monitored and recorded. Maximum and minimum thermometers are the basic tools but digital thermography is increasingly being used (Fleming et al. 2003). Thermostats are an important item in any reptile house and should be pulse-proportional so as to regulate energy flow to the heat source. Pulse proportional stats are only used with lightless heat sources. Dimming is required for heating lamps; pulse proportional stats will blow the lamp quickly.

Behavioural interactions

A useful and topical review of the normal (natural) behaviour of reptiles is provided by Durso and Maerz (2019). Some specific considerations are discussed below.

Many species of reptile are territorial, and when group-housed they may form dominance hierarchies. In nature, animals with low status can usually flee to alternative locations. This option is not available in a small cage, and low-status individuals may be subject to chronic stress (see later) and sustain physical injury. They may be excluded from basking, feeding or retreat sites, and as a consequence fail to thrive. It follows that great care must be exercised if potentially territorial reptiles are kept together in cages. There are, however, measures that can be taken to reduce agonistic interactions. Enriching the environment by increasing complexity and installing refugia (see later) can ensure that individuals encounter one another less frequently, and may actually reduce territory size in some species, e.g. *Anolis aeneus* (Eason & Stamps 1991). Providing multiple basking and feeding sites and non-communal retreats may also minimise aggression.

Special senses

Some reptiles have colour vision and a few can sense the near ultraviolet (UV) (Fleishman et al. 1993). All chelonians and many lizards have a parietal/pineal eye/gland situated at the top of the head which is connected to the pineal organ. This has a lens and a retina, but because it lies beneath the scales, cannot form an image. It responds to the wavelength and intensity of light and seems to be concerned with rhythmic behaviour, seasonal reproductive cycles and thermoregulation.

All terrestrial reptiles can respond to vibrations (an important consideration in the positioning of cages as proximity to electrical and other equipment may have adverse effects), and many can hear. Few reptiles vocalise, an exception being some species of gecko. Even the sounds made by copulating tortoises may serve as communication (Galeotti *et al.* 2005).

There are other aspects of reptile senses that differ from those in mammals. Direct olfaction is generally not well-developed (there is current interest in this subject in respect of chelonians), but lizards and snakes have forked tongues, the tips of which can be inserted into the paired organs of Jacobson at the top of the palate. This provides a kind of 'touch–smell' sense, and enables the animals to obtain detailed information about the immediate environment and to make extensive use of communication by pheromones. Such communication is often important in mediating social behaviour (Mason 1992; Alberts *et al.* 1994a) and physiology (Alberts *et al.* 1994b). The 'touch–smell' sense may also enable reptiles to detect the presence of other species, including potential predators and possible prey. Discrimination using this sense can be subtle. Many snakes can use chemical cues to follow the 'trails' of prey, and this is particularly important for those species that track envenomated victims until they die – so-called 'strike-induced chemosensory searching'. Some pythons and certain other snakes have small pits on the side of the head that are sensitive to infrared radiation, and enable them to sense the presence of warm-blooded prey.

Lights and heaters in a captive reptile's cage serve to simulate what the animal encounters in the wild but the subject is far more complex than just copying nature, as succeeding text will demonstrate. An important initial point that should be made is that electrical equipment must be correctly installed and used and properly monitored – to protect the animals and staff alike.

UV radiation is important to most species of reptile and will be discussed in more detail later. It can influence social behaviour (Fleishman *et al.* 1993). There is evidence, for example, that secretions from the femoral glands of some desert iguanas and certain lacertids selectively absorb long-wave UV radiation; deposits from these glands left in the environment will be very obvious to another individual (Alberts 1989; Alberts *et al.* 1994a). Chin glands in certain chelonians may play a similar role (Alberts *et al.* 1994b).

Size and lifespan

Adult reptiles range in size from lizards that measure 40 mm or less in length and weigh less than 1 g, to snakes that are more than 6 m in length (e.g. *Python reticulatus*, *Eunectes murinus*). The largest lizards are *Varanus* spp., which may reach 3 m in length, and have a body mass of over 150 kg.

In general, smaller reptiles live for shorter periods than do larger ones. Small lizards characteristically have a maximum longevity of 10 years; larger lizards may live for more than 30 years. Pythons and boas can also survive for more than three decades, but the potential longevity of most other snakes is not known. Small species of tortoise have a life-expectancy of 20 years; larger species more than 100. Reptiles are likely to survive longer in captivity than they would in the wild (Roitberg & Smirina 2006).

Hibernation and aestivation

Some species of reptile hibernate, others will undergo periods of aestivation when environmental conditions are hot, dry and adverse.

The physiology of hibernation (brumation) is complex and some examples draw attention to the remarkable resilience of certain reptile species to hypoxia (Jackson 2002).

There is much published advice on how best to prepare reptiles, mainly tortoises, for hibernation (see, e.g., McArthur *et al.* 2004). Under laboratory conditions, however, these and other species are usually kept awake during the cold months, by maintaining them at a higher temperature (see, e.g., Arbour *et al.* 2007).

Sex determination and reproduction

Most reptile species (all chelonians and crocodilians, most lizards and some snakes) lay eggs. Some lizards and certain snakes, particularly but not exclusively those that inhabit cold climates (e.g. the European common lizard, *Zootoca vivipara*) or high altitudes where incubation of eggs may be retarded (e.g. certain Central African chameleons) produce live young. In such taxa, the eggs are retained in the oviducts until the young are ready for independent existence. Reptiles that produce live young are usually termed 'viviparous' or 'live-bearing' but the word 'ovoviviparous' is sometimes also used.

Fertilisation in reptiles is internal, and may follow elaborate courtship behaviour (Hernandez-Divers 2001). Male lizards and snakes have two intromittent organs, the hemipenes: chelonians have one hemipenis (phallus).

Some species of reptiles are sexually dimorphic, showing distinct colour, markings, size or anatomical features such as the presence of femoral pores in certain lizards (Schumacher 2003).

Distinguishing the sex of monomorphic species or (of almost all) juvenile reptiles can be difficult but various methods can be used. In snakes, scale counts often help (male snakes usually have a longer tail, with more subcaudal scales, than do females) and even a sloughed skin can be used to determine this (Cooper & Cooper 2007) (Figure 46.4).

'Cloacal probing', using a slender, blunt object of suitable size, is the most frequently employed technique for the sexing of snakes and the larger lizards. If the probe cannot be advanced when gently directed caudally from the cloaca, the animal is female. In males, the probe will enter a sulcus which contains an invaginated hemipenis (Frye 1991). Probing is used routinely by herpetologists but the technique needs to be properly learned if damage to animals is to be prevented. Probing is best taught using a freshly dead reptile.

As discussed in more detail in the section on reproduction, sex determination in some species, such as sea turtles, is temperature-dependent (Ewert *et al.* 1994), and this has to be borne in mind when incubating eggs under laboratory conditions. Egg-laying female reptiles usually bury their eggs in soil or sand. Eggs of most species are oval or round in shape and are surrounded by a shell, which may be hard as a result of impregnation with calcium salts, or soft and leathery. In nature, the site at which the eggs are laid is important. Protection from predators is necessary but the temperature will affect the rate of development and, in some species, the sex of the offspring. Relative humidity is also relevant. If it is too low, the eggs will dehydrate; if too high, they will drown or become infected by fungi or bacteria (see later).

Laboratory management

General

The Council of Europe provided recommendations for minimum housing standards for reptiles used in research (Council of Europe 2006). In the USA, Reinhardt & Kreger (2002) provided information about the laboratory housing of reptiles as did the Canadian Council on Animal Care (CCAC) in their various guidelines.

Some reptiles can be kept satisfactorily in large aquaria, wooden cages with a glass panel or open-topped wooden or fibreglass containers. Certain species appear to require such cages to be only very simply furnished in order to thrive – a *'clinical habitat'* (Varga 2019) that lends itself well to laboratory research. Others need more specialised accommodation, and may thrive better if the internal construction and 'furnishing' of the cage bear some relationship to their normal environment – a *'naturalistic habitat'* (Varga 2019). Thus, sand-burrowing lizards (e.g. *Chalcides ocellatus*) remain in far better condition if they have sand in which to burrow, as do arboreal species (e.g. most *Anolis* lizards) when provided with branches on which they can climb.

Species that are 'sit-and-wait' predators (e.g. many species of snakes and geckos), and herbivorous reptiles, usually need little space. Some species, such as most lizards in the families Lacertidae and Teiidae, will be restricted by smaller cages. In these, they often spend much of their time trying to get out, possibly suggesting that a motivation to range is being thwarted. This has been linked with poor welfare in mammals (Clubb & Mason 2003). The immediate action should be to provide such species with more space but scientific data on the significance of escape-like behaviour in reptiles are scant.

Reptiles are adept at escaping from cages and enclosures. Many species climb or burrow and, by flattening their bodies, can squeeze through small holes or cracks.

Handling and restraint

Competent handling and restraint are as important for reptiles as they are for other species of laboratory animals. Training of staff is highly desirable and in some countries such as the UK, may be mandatory before appropriate licences are issued. See also Chapter 14: Attaining competence in the care of animals used in research. Inexperienced research workers can learn much from herpetologists.

Smaller lizards and snakes can usually be rested, or restrained gently, on the hand for routine inspection or movement from one cage to another. Many species of snake will support themselves if allowed to move from hand to hand. When restraint of snakes and lizards is necessary, they should be grasped firmly behind the head while supporting the body. Support is particularly important for snakes and legless lizards which become injured or stressed if they are allowed to 'dangle'. The handling of venomous snakes is referred to later. Care must be taken with lizards to ensure that the tail is not grasped or pinned, since certain species can spontaneously shed it (autotomy) (Bellairs & Bryant 1985). Some geckos not only shed their tails extremely readily but their skin may easily tear away from the underlying tissue.

Large lizards, such as iguanas and monitors, have a powerful, possibly toxic (see later), bite and can also inflict damage with their tail and claws. It is a wise precaution to use leather gloves when handling them.

Chelonians can usually be handled by grasping the 'shell' (carapace and plastron) and land tortoises, in contrast to many species of terrapin and turtle, rarely bite. Restraint of tortoises in order to carry out procedures is less easy. It may be possible to grasp the animal's head but sometimes light anaesthesia is required to facilitate this and other investigative techniques.

Training and habituation of captive reptiles can facilitate handling and thereby minimise stress to both animal and personnel (see later).

Species used in the laboratory

Table 46.1 lists some of the species of reptile that are used widely for research. Most of them can now be obtained as captive-bred animals. A very few species of captive-bred terrestrial reptile are produced commercially specifically for research purposes – *Anolis carolinensis*, for example.

Whenever possible, reptiles for research should be captive-bred and obtained from reliable sources. In many parts of the world, however, wild-caught reptiles are routinely used in studies. Animals may sometimes need specifically to be taken from the wild – for example, because the research is concerned with free-living reptiles – for example, reintroduction or translocation conservation projects.

It is essential to adhere to relevant legislation. Even common and widespread species of reptile may be covered by national laws, requiring (for example) a licence to take them from the wild or to retain them in captivity.

The UK is one of many countries that have such legislation. The Wildlife and Countryside Act 1981 and other legislation may require a licence to authorise the taking or keeping of reptiles. A Dangerous Wild Animals Act 1976 licence may be necessary to keep venomous snakes and lizards. Regulations implementing the Convention (CITES) apply to the movement between countries of reptiles listed on the Appendices to the Convention. Permits are required for the import and export of live and dead specimens and their derivatives, including blood samples and tissues for DNA analysis.

The Animal Welfare Acts in the UK (see below) apply to all captive reptiles, imposing a duty of care to provide for their welfare needs and providing provisions to prevent unnecessary suffering. Reptiles used in scientific research are subject to the Animals (Scientific Procedures) Act 1986.

Terrestrial reptiles: lizards, snakes and tortoises

Table 46.1 Some terrestrial reptile species that are frequently kept in laboratories.

Scientific name	Common English name	Studies for which the species is commonly used	Reference
Lizards			
Anolis carolinensis	American (green) anole	A wide range of physiological topics, especially neuroethology and colour change	Harling (1994), O'Rourke et al. (2019)
Anolis sagrei	Brown anole		
Chalcides ocellatus	Eyed or ocellated skink	A wide range of physiological topics	Wisniewski (1992)
Chamaeleo spp.	Chameleons	Colour change, sensorimotor coordination of eyes and tongue	Townson (1994)
Eublepharis macularius	Leopard gecko	Skin grafts, temperature-dependent sex determination	Thorogood & Whimster (1979), Wisniewski (1992)
Gekko gecko	Tokay gecko	Eye and brain	Wisniewski (1992)
Iguana iguana	Common or green iguana	Metabolism and physiology	Frye (1993), Divers (1995)
Podarcis muralis and *P. sicula* (and other small lacertid lizards)	European wall lizards	Neurotransmitters, physiology of endogenous rhythms, endocrinology	Langerwerf (1990, 1991), Harling (1993) Townson (1994)
Pogona spp.	Bearded dragons	Endocrinology	Sheriff (1988)
Tiliqua spp.	Blue-tongued skinks	A wide range of physiological topics	Rose (1992), Townson (1994)
Various species	Various species	Studies of biological rhythms and seasonal cycles	Underwood (1992), cited by O'Rourke et al. (2019)
Various species	Various species	Control mechanisms for reproductive cycles and comparative endocrinology	Moore & Lindsey (1992), cited by O'Rourke et al. (2019)
Various species	Various species	Neuroethology	Crews & Gans (1992), cited by O'Rourke et al. (2019)
Various species	Various species	Regenerative processes	Bellairs & Bryant (1985), cited by O'Rourke et al. (2019)
Aspidoscelis spp.	Whiptail lizards	Parthenogenesis and other reproductive strategies	O'Rourke et al. (2019)
Snakes			
Elaphe (*Pantherophis*) spp.	Corn and rat snakes	A wide range of physiological topics	Bartlett (1993)
Lampropeltis spp.	King snakes	A wide range of physiological topics	Edwards (1991)
Thamnophis spp.	Garter snakes	Various; especially muscle physiology, reproductive endocrinology, physiology of hibernation	Sweeney (1993)
Tortoises			
Terrapene Carolina	Carolina box turtle	Sensory physiology	
Testudo graeca and *T. hermanni*	European tortoises	Physiology of the pineal and associated organs	Jackson (1991), British Chelonia Group (undated)
Trachemys scripta elegans	Red-eared sliders	Physiology and infectious disease research	O'Rourke et al. (2019)
Various species	Various species	Research on *Salmonella* and other bacterial pathogens	Arbour et al. (2007).

The Good Practice Guidelines[2] are produced for private keepers but applicable in no small part to reptiles in captivity.

These Good Practice Guidelines are designed to provide keepers of reptiles and amphibians with the steps needed to ensure the needs of their animal(s) are met, as required by Section 9 of the Animal Welfare Act 2006, Section 24 of the Animal Health and Welfare (Scotland) Act 2006 or Section 9 of the Welfare of Animals Act (Northern Ireland) 2011.

The uses of reptiles in research

Reptiles and other ectothermic vertebrates have played a significant part in scientific research. Cooper (1977) reviewed the role of such species and stressed that they can serve as useful models for studies on the origin and aetiology of human diseases.

It is important to remember that reptiles are kept for research and study in many parts of the world. In some countries, they do not receive legal protection once they are held in captivity. Nor – often because of cultural or religious convictions – is welfare always accepted as an essential precept when reptiles are managed in laboratories. Researchers are sometimes encouraged to do experimental work on reptiles (or amphibians) because such animals are readily and inexpensively acquired and apparently not demanding in terms of housing and feeding. As a result, reptiles may be inadequately managed, making research results questionable. There is, therefore, always a need to consider the care and management (the title of this volume) of all laboratory reptiles, not just those in countries and jurisdictions where standards are already high.

Reptiles are used for biomedical research, for teaching students and for simple, non-invasive, studies on nutrition, growth or reproduction (O'Rourke et al. 2019). Examples are given in Table 46.1.

---

[2] http://data.parliament.uk/DepositedPapers/Files/DEP2015-0315/Good_Practice_Guidelines_For_the_Welfare_of_Privately_Kept_Reptiles.pdf (Accessed 25 May 2022)

Tortoises have long been used in studies of sensory physiology, work that led to a better understanding of pain in these animals (Rosenberg 1972) and contributing substantially to more humane methods for euthanasia (Cooper *et al*. 1984; UFAW/World Society for the Protection of Animals (WSPA) 1989; WSPA 1994).

One use of reptiles has attracted generally high standards of management throughout the world because of the importance of the end-product – venom. Snakebite is classified as a 'Neglected Tropical Disease (NTD)'. It kills over 95,000 people each year and leaves thousands more with permanent physical disabilities.

Traditional laboratory conditions are the order of the day in many venom research establishments in the 'western' world – for example, the Alistair Reid Venom Research Unit at the Liverpool School of Tropical Medicine in England. However, especially in the tropics, where snakes can often be obtained (caught) locally and then easily and inexpensively maintained, venom collection may take place '*in situ*' in open-air or simply constructed enclosures. Often these reptiles serve two purposes, in that they can also be displayed to the public.

Three examples from Kenya, where the author has worked, illustrate the different approaches. The Nairobi Snake Park has for over half a century been part of the National Museums of Kenya. Snakes are kept primarily for display, but some are also 'milked' for their venom. Bio-Ken, on the Kenya Coast, founded by the late James and Sanda Ashe, in contrast, has its own small laboratory, carries out research on venom and hosts biannual snakebite seminars attended by experts from many countries. The third example is the recently established Kenya Snakebite Research and Intervention Centre (KSRIC) which is based at the Institute of Primate Research (IPR) near Nairobi. KSRIC boasts a modern 'Herpetarium' (Figure 46.6), where snakes are kept for venom production and research. The snakes are housed in temperature- and light-controlled rooms, with shelves of labelled plastic box cages, each containing a water dish and an upturned cut-out bowl as a refuge. Every day staff, always working in pairs (Figure 46.7), check each snake's weight and skin condition, look for any evidence of parasites and monitor behaviour. While KSRIC is of necessity primarily orientated towards to venom and

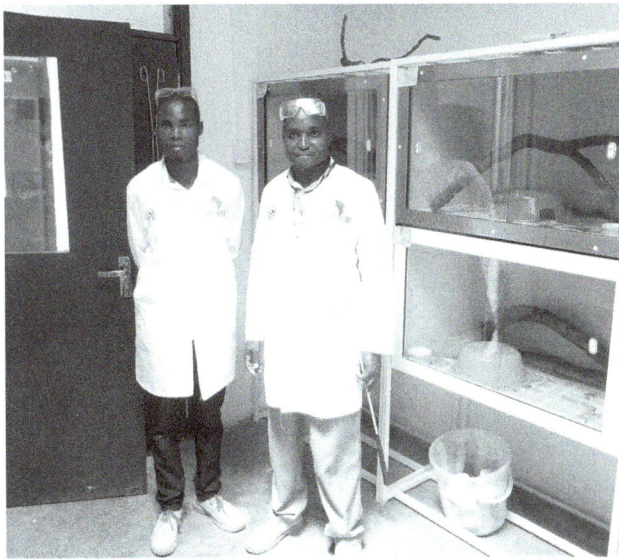

Figure 46.7 Staff at the Kenya Snakebite Research and Intervention Centre (KSRIC) always work in pairs.

biomedical research, the focus as far as staff are concerned is unwaveringly on the importance of keeping and tending reptiles humanely.

It must not be forgotten that far more research is performed on free-living reptiles than on those kept in captivity. Field studies may include capture, identification, marking, weighing and measuring, implantation of transponders or other devices, sample collection (Hernandez-Divers *et al*. 2004a) and surgical procedures. The principles of safe and humane fieldwork have been detailed in guidelines produced by various bodies and the challenges and responsibilities presented by such activities discussed by, for example, Cooper (2013a,b). Legal and ethical considerations of working in the field were explained in considerable detail by Cooper M.E. (2013).

The importance of using non-invasive or minimally invasive techniques in reptile research cannot be over-estimated. It serves both to promote the welfare of the study animals and to minimise stress that may adversely affect results. The principles of minimally invasive procedures in reptiles were included in the paper by Cooper (1998).

All reptiles deserve the highest level of care. An important prerequisite is an understanding of the natural history and biology of the species. For some, there may be extensive published information – *Iguana iguana*, for example (Jacobson 2003). For others, data may be sparse or largely anecdotal.

Temperature and thermoregulation

An understanding of the principles of thermoregulation is essential to those keeping reptiles in captivity, perhaps particularly so when the animals are being managed for research purposes where control of environmental parameters is important.

Knowledge of the natural history of the species is, as always, an important prerequisite. Many nocturnal geckos and lizards and snakes from the leaf litter or lower levels of

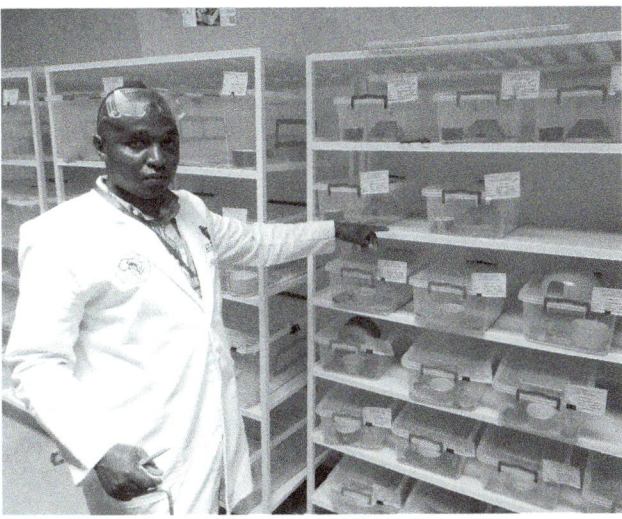

Figure 46.6 The senior herpetologist at the Kenya Snakebite Research and Intervention Centre (KSRIC) points out a labelled plastic box cage.

tropical rain forests do not routinely thermoregulate. Ideally, they require air temperatures that equate with their natural environments. However, during the day some species warm themselves by (for example) pressing themselves on to the warm rock under which they live and then use the heat obtained to help sustain them at night.

Most species of reptile do, however, need to thermoregulate and this can be accommodated under laboratory conditions by providing a diversity of substrate temperatures, using heating pads, lamps or other sources of surface warmth. All electrical devices must be properly fitted and carefully monitored, to protect both animals and personnel. Bulbs, for example, should be positioned so that the animal can approach close enough to be able to warm readily, but not so near that it will burn itself (Divers & Stahl 2019) either from the infrared radiation itself or from a substrate that has been heated by the radiation. Care must be taken that laboratory cages do not become too hot. There must be areas that are sufficiently cool to enable the reptiles to lose heat as well as to gain it. This can often be achieved by placing the bulb(s) at one end of the cage. The heat should not be switched on for too long; 8–10 h per day is ideal for most species. The longer there is heat provided, the more protracted the period for which the reptile maintains its activity temperature and the greater its metabolic expenditure. Various papers, mainly relating to studies on captive and free-living European common lizards (*Zootoca vivipara*), have described research relevant to the care of this and possibly other species under laboratory conditions (Avery 1984, 1994). Avery (1984) suggested that relatively short daily exposure to radiant heat minimises the risk of respiratory disease caused by the bacterium *Aeromonas*, while Guillette *et al.* (1995) postulated that the daily period for which radiant heat is available may affect the immune system. The air temperature when the heating bulb is switched off may be allowed to vary: this corresponds to the situation in all but the most stable of tropical climates. There is often a tendency to keep the background temperature too high and this may be deleterious for species from desert or montane environments, where high solar radiation during the day can be followed by cool nights. Successful captive husbandry and breeding in environments in which temperatures were carefully controlled and monitored was reported in relation to the Malagasy panther chameleon, *Furcifer pardalis* (Ferguson 1994). Similar data are required for other species and those who keep reptiles under laboratory conditions are in a particularly strong position to carry out the necessary studies.

Light

Natural light (in which the greatest energy is in the blue part of the spectrum) often appears to result in better survival, growth and reproduction of reptiles than does artificial light (which usually peaks in the yellow), although the reasons for this are not fully understood. There is some evidence that the duration of the daily photoperiod may be an important factor, controlling reproductive cycles in many species (Avery 1994), and this must be taken into account by those wishing to breed reptiles in captivity. The value of natural (solar) lighting must never be overlooked. In many reptile collections in the tropics, including some used for research purposes (see later), sunlight is the only source of UVB-b and the animals appear to fare very well.

Ultraviolet radiation

In recent years, much has been published – and even more discussed – concerning the provision of ultraviolet heat and light for captive reptiles. Probably, the most up-to-date and authoritative publication on the topic is the chapter by Baines and Cusack in the multi-author tome 'Reptile and Amphibian Medicine and Surgery' (Divers & Stahl 2019). Baines and Cusack point out that, in nature, sunlight interacts with features of a reptile's environment, creating a microhabitat with superimposed gradients of heat, light and ultraviolet (UV) radiation; the result may range from full sun to full shade. They go on to explain that by self-regulating their exposure to solar radiation, reptiles are able to use these gradients for thermoregulation and, in some cases, for UV photoregulation. Deviations from the optimal range can serve as stressors and adversely affect a reptile's health.

Baines and Cusack go on to emphasise the difficulties that characterise the provision of suitable 'photo-microhabitat' for captive reptiles. This is largely because of the paucity of field studies that report the daily light and UV exposure of free-living reptiles. Thus, while in the wild natural sunlight varies (its spectrum and radiance are influenced by the height of the sun in the sky, by the amount of cloud cover, and by the degree of shading from environmental factors) in captivity a lamp is either on or off, and its spectrum and radiance vary little, if at all.

In 2004, a far-sighted group of reptile keepers in the UK, Frances Baines, Andy Beveridge, Rachel Hitch and Rob Lane, started to study scientifically the use of UV lighting in reptile husbandry. Their work, combined with those of others, was called the UV Tool Project and led in 2005 to the launch of the website[3] on 26 July 2005 and the Reptile and Amphibian Working Group UV-TOOL – UV Guide UK (Baines *et al.* 2016).

In 2010, Ferguson and colleagues published records of daily UV exposure of 15 species of free-living reptile that had been monitored using the UV Index (UVI), measured with a Solarmeter 6.5 UV Index meter (Ferguson *et al.* 2010). Ferguson *et al.* observed that, based on their daily sun exposure, the 15 species could be assigned places in one of four microhabitats or 'zones'; subsequently designated the 'Ferguson Zones'.

In 2012, the British and Irish Association of Zoos and Aquaria (BIAZA), working with private herpetologists, specialist reptile keepers and zoological collections, allocated Ferguson Zones to 254 species of reptile and amphibian and suggested appropriate UV lighting options for these animals in captivity. These recommendations were published in the free access online Journal of Zoo and Aquarium Research.

Important contributions towards a better understanding of lighting for reptiles have also been made by John Courteney-Smith who has made much of his material

---

[3] http://www.uvguide.co.uk/ (Accessed 25 May 2022)

available to reptile keepers[4]. Courteney-Smith points out that, historically, advice for reptiles was simply to buy a 5% UVB lamp for forest animals and a 10% lamp for desert animals. No real thought was given to the unique adaptations of the species and their basking behaviour or the distance between the lamp and the animal. The Arcadia Reptile Light Guide[5] seeks to rectify this by enabling reptile keepers to make an informed choice of lighting for their charges.

Space does not permit detailed description here of how best to provide artificial lighting and heating for reptiles in laboratories but the scientist or technician who keeps such animals for research should read the chapter by Baines and Cusack (2019) and other reliable literature[6,7]. It should be noted that Baines and Cusack stress that, although artificial lighting cannot totally replicate natural sunlight it can, when used properly, make a substantial contribution to raising standards of reptile husbandry.

Relative humidity (RH)

Only limited data are available on the humidity requirements of reptiles: much of the available information is based on observational and anecdotal evidence. Laboratory environments often have drier air than do the microhabitats of free-living reptiles. This may prove deleterious – even to desert species, which spend much of their lives in humid burrows. The RH in rooms housing reptiles, or in individual cages, can be increased in many ways. Spraying with water from a mist nozzle is effective but labour-intensive. One very simple measure is to furnish cages with living plants; transpiration will raise the RH. High humidity zones can be created within the cage by the use of 'humidity boxes' or, on a larger scale, by installing dripper systems or waterfalls.

Various diseases of the skin, scales and the carapace and plastron (chelonians) may be induced or exacerbated by too high or too low humidity. In particular, Gram-negative bacteria such as *Aeromonas* and *Pseudomonas* and certain fungi are likely to multiply excessively under damp conditions.

Ventilation and air changes

Optimum ventilation for laboratory reptiles can be difficult to achieve. Too little ventilation results in inadequate diffusion of oxygen into, and carbon dioxide out of, a cage and can also increase humidity, leading to condensation. Too much ventilation, on the other hand, can make it difficult to control the temperature and keep the RH high. The optimum ventilation for a particular cage design must sometimes be determined by trial and error; there is increasingly a tendency to specify the number of air changes in order to conform with research protocols and, ostensibly, to promote health and welfare. These are not necessarily the most appropriate for a given species (Cooper & Williams 1995).

Environmental enrichment

The welfare of a captive reptile is likely to be enhanced if its accommodation is appropriate to the species (Varga 2019). However, despite some advances in our understanding of environmental requirements in recent years, there remains a need for more properly designed research.

This is an area that has attracted considerable attention in recent years. Guidance and resources are available, especially online, but the methods of enrichment advocated are not always backed up with scientific evidence.

Notwithstanding the points above, many species of terrestrial reptiles can be maintained, apparently successfully, in relatively plain cages and such containment seems to satisfy their behavioural requirements. As discussed earlier, however, some taxa thrive better in cages or enclosures that mimic the natural environment (Figure 46.5).

There are species of reptile that clearly benefit from environmental enrichment. When, for example, small European lacertid lizards are kept in plain unfurnished cages, they tend to spend long periods motionless, often basking at length beneath the bulb that is provided for thermoregulation. Creating an area of spatial diversity, even simply by adding a number of wooden blocks, results in a dramatic change in behaviour. The lizards then bask for only relatively short periods, interspersing this with periods of movement (presumably looking for food) among the blocks, behaviour that is much closer to that seen in the field (Avery 1994).

Training and habituation

Training and habituation are increasingly part of good management of reptiles (Skurski *et al.* 2019). It can facilitate the performance of procedures and will reduce risks to staff. For example, lizards can be taught to feed at the same location each day. Snakes can learn by association and some species, e.g., iguanas, recognise cause and effect relationships. Habituation has been studied in some reptiles (Xavier *et al.* 2006) but needs further research.

The importance of 'good stockmanship' cannot be overemphasised. Those who tend captive reptiles, especially technicians, should exhibit an empathy with their charges and, preferably, have personal experience of herpetology.

Refugia (hiding places)

Most species of reptiles, like almost all metazoan animals, have periods of the day when they are active. When they are not active, they seek some kind of refuge – in burrows, under rocks or in crevices, high in trees or among dense vegetation (many terrestrial chelonians). Failure to provide a refuge for captive reptiles may be stressful (Hernandez-Divers 2001).

Physiological measures of stress were initially investigated some years ago (Kreger & Mench 1993; Guillette *et al.* 1995)

---

[4] https://chameleonacademy.com/member/john-courteney-smith-mrsb/ (Accessed 25 August 2022)
[5] https://www.arcadiareptile.com/lighting/guide/ (Accessed 25 May 2022)
[6] http://www.uvguide.co.uk/files/BIAZA-UVTool-introduction.pdf (Accessed 25 May 2022)
[7] http://www.reptilesmagazine.com/Reptile-Health/Habitats-Care/Reptile-Lighting-Information/ (Accessed 25 May 2022)

followed by studies on behavioural means of detecting and possibly measuring stress in diverse species of reptile (Greenberg 1995; Warwick *et al.* 1995). This issue was also discussed by Warwick *et al.* (2013) but that paper has been challenged in some quarters. There is at present little clear-cut evidence that the methods described contribute substantially to welfare of reptiles in laboratories.

It is conventional wisdom that captive reptiles should be provided with a refuge that mimics places where they would hide in nature. Given a choice, snakes prefer an opaque refuge to one with transparent walls, although the latter are more convenient from the standpoint of the reptile-keeper (Chiszar *et al.* 1987). It is best not to disturb individuals in the refuge. For similar reasons, as a general rule, it is preferable not to alter the internal arrangements of a cage once an individual has become familiar with it, especially under laboratory conditions where standardisation of procedures is so important. This is because many reptiles learn the immediate topography of their enclosure and can become stressed when it alters (Chiszar *et al.* 1995). On the other hand, many herpetologists and veterinarians would argue that a novel environment can encourage chemosensory behaviour and thereby promote welfare. The relationships between refugia and other elements of cage design are important.

Hygiene

It is usually a basic tenet of captive management of animals that cages should be cleaned regularly in order to minimise build-up of parasites or other pathogens. This can be particularly important where infections might compromise research. Hygiene is also important to reduce the risk of spread of zoonotic infections. However, there are indications that cage-cleaning for certain reptiles should not be too frequent. Some of the chemicals in faeces can act as pheromones and may be used for communication. Some snakes, for example, thrive less well in clean cages than in cages containing some faeces and leaving a small amount of faecal material in a cage every time it is cleaned reduces the incidence of escape behaviour (Chiszar *et al.* 1980). In contrast, certain species of gecko avoid contact with their own faeces, probably to minimise exposure to parasites (Brown *et al.* 1998).

Disinfection of cages should be preceded by thorough cleaning. The choice of a disinfectant is important. Some can be toxic, especially to small reptiles. Disinfectants have different modes of action. Under circumstances where quality disinfectants are unavailable or prohibitively expensive, hot water is an easy and cheap alternative, preferably followed by drying in the sun or in a hot-air oven.

There is evidence for some mammalian species that irregular husbandry can be a stressor. While there are few equivalent unequivocal data for reptiles, consideration should be given to regular cleaning routines.

Diet and feeding

Reptiles as a class eat a variety of foods though many species have narrow food preferences. Lizards are predominantly carnivorous (a few species are herbivorous), and snakes are almost entirely carnivorous. Chelonians vary: as a general rule, terrestrial species (land tortoises) are primarily vegetarian while freshwater aquatic species (terrapins) are carnivorous. Rendle and Calvert (2019) provide a very useful review of the nutritional needs of captive reptiles and Brown *et al.* (2019) of the features of the gastro-intestinal system.

Reptiles have relatively low metabolic rates and high net food-conversion efficiencies. Over-feeding is often as much of a problem as underfeeding, and can lead to a range of pathological conditions (see later). Small and medium-sized lizards, and most chelonians, need feeding daily. Large lizards and many snakes should be fed less frequently: some large snakes probably feed in nature less than once per week or once per month. The essential requirements are a regime and diet that will ensure the maintenance of bodyweight in non-breeding adults, and normal growth by juveniles. Many reptiles cease feeding spontaneously from time to time, especially just prior to skin-shedding.

In nature, most vertebrate prey is taken alive. The question of whether it is acceptable to feed living mammalian or avian prey to snakes and large lizards in captivity raises important ethical and sometimes legal issues (Cooper, M.E. 2019; Cooper *et al.* 2019). Many large reptiles will feed on dead animals; others quickly learn to do so. It is the animal that persistently refuses to feed on anything but living prey which creates a dilemma. Some authorities take the view that feeding living prey may be acceptable as a last resort (if the predator would otherwise starve to death) but that the prey animal should be removed from the cage immediately if the predator takes no interest in it, in the interests of both predator and prey. In the UK, the offering of live prey is not, *per se*, illegal but it may provide grounds for a criminal action.

Live vertebrates should not be used as food and even invertebrates should be used in a way that is sensitive to the fact that they too are living animals – see later. There are many methods to simulate the movement of non-living prey: these include placing them in a Petri dish on an automatic shaker, or employing tongs to shake the prey, or dragging the food item around the vivarium so as to create a scent trail for the snake/lizard to follow.

Some snakes refuse to feed in captivity. They can be force-fed (Cooper & Jackson 1981), often now referred to as 'assisted feeding', but it is preferable to try to coax them to feed spontaneously first. One technique, often successful with pythons and boas, is to condition them always to feed in the same place, which may be marked with scent of potential prey from time to time to reinforce the association. Other ruses include hiding the food in a tube or another unexpected location.

In some jurisdictions, live feeding (using vertebrate animals) is either illegal or discouraged by codes of practice. When dead animals are used as food, they should be killed humanely – for instance, using a Schedule-1 method following the (UK) Animals (Scientific Procedures) Act 1986 (ASPA) – see later – or according to the American (US) AVMA Guidelines.

Most authorities concur that the diets of reptiles should be as varied as possible, as this helps to reduce nutritional disorders that are so commonly encountered in captivity (Frye 1991, 1994, 1996; Rendle 2019; Boyer & Scott 2019). This injunction applies to herbivorous as well as insectivorous or carnivorous species. Because tortoises, iguanas and other herbivorous reptiles feed with apparent relish on soft leaves and fruits, it is sometimes not appreciated that their diets in nature are usually very varied, and often include insects, molluscs and other invertebrates which may be swallowed deliberately or accidentally and usefully contribute to the animal's nutrient intake.

Insectivorous reptiles will often take only living prey. Invertebrates can be purchased from dealers who breed the animals for the pet trade or propagated within the laboratory animal facility. It is important to ensure that such animals are from a reliable source and health checks on them may be advisable as they can be a source of infection.

Although legal constraints do not usually apply, there are ethical issues relating to the feeding of live invertebrates to reptiles and other animals (see earlier). Cooper and Williams (2014) debated this predicament in their paper on the feeding of live food to 'exotic' animals. They pointed out that over the past two decades, concerns regarding the health and welfare of invertebrates have grown, discussion and studies on whether invertebrates 'suffer' pain have become prevalent, and, in its wake, some limited analysis and discussion of the ethical considerations of using these animals as live prey.

Crickets such as by *Gryllus assimilis* and *Gryllus bimaculatus* are popular food items. Any not eaten within a few hours should be removed as they are nocturnal and may nibble the appendages of lizards if allowed to remain in the cage and increase the risk of autoinfection with parasites.

Mealworms are larvae of the beetle *Tenebrio molitor* and are easy to breed, although this is subject to high standards of management, including hygiene. So-called 'giant mealworms' are suitable for larger species of reptile. Mealworms should not form a major part of the diet, however, because they contain far too high a concentration of phosphorus ions relative to calcium ions. Sooner or later, reptiles fed a diet of mealworms succumb to disorders caused by mineral imbalance (Frye 1991, 1996). Many reptile keepers 'preload' or 'gutload' mealworms and other invertebrates with calcium, and sometimes other minerals, vitamins and plant material, by adjusting their diet immediately prior to using them as food. Finke *et al.* (2005) evaluated four dry commercial gut-loading products for improving the calcium content of crickets.

Invertebrate prey can also be dusted externally with minerals to increase dietary intake but care must be taken to ensure that the invertebrate is ingested quickly as some species, especially crickets, quickly groom and remove the dust.

An increasingly large range of dietary supplements is available commercially, some formulated specifically for reptiles. They all contain vitamin D and calcium; some are very finely ground, so that the particles adhere readily to the cuticle of invertebrate prey. Almost all captive reptiles need dietary supplementation: the only possible exceptions are those kept in large, open outdoor enclosures, with exposure to natural sunlight and a varied diet. In some studies and locations (e.g. the tropics), it may be acceptable to allow the reptiles to eat insects that have flown into the enclosure from outside.

Many reptiles are susceptible in captivity to mineral deficiencies or imbalances. These may result from a faulty diet or from insufficient exposure to appropriate ultraviolet radiation. There are four main reasons why problems associated with calcium arise so commonly:

1. Inadequate calcium in the diet.
2. Calcium: phosphorus ratio is too low.
3. A dietary deficiency of vitamin D_3.
4. Inadequate exposure to UV radiation, which in many species is necessary for dermal synthesis of cholecalciferol, the metabolic precursor of vitamin D. It is important to note that it is UV-b light in the range 290–320 nm that is of prime importance in converting vitamin D. The amount of UV-b that is available to the reptile can be measured using an appropriate meter. All of terrestrial UV is important, including UV-a which probably not only provides more vitamin D, but also regulates and recycles D3 production.[8]

These mineral deficiencies or imbalances can give rise to various skeletal disorders (Frye 1991), referred to by many by the generic, rather imprecise, name *'metabolic bone diseases'*. The term MBD includes nutritional secondary hyperparathyroidism (NSHP), renal secondary hyperparathyroidism (RSHP), fibrous osteodystrophy (Figure 46.8), osteomalacia, osteoporosis and osteopetrosis. Clinical signs can include impaired weight-bearing and locomotion, tetany, paralysis, prolapses and retarded growth.

In chelonians, abnormalities of the carapace, characterised by doming of scutes, is generally referred to as 'pyramidal shell growth (PSG)'. PSG is commonly seen in captive tortoises but can be a normal morphological feature of some species, such as Indian star tortoises (*Geochelone elegans*) and some tent tortoise species (*Psammobates* spp.). As indicated above, PSG primarily affects the carapace, especially the central vertebral scutes, producing a knobby pyramidal shape rather than an evenly rounded smooth carapace. There is

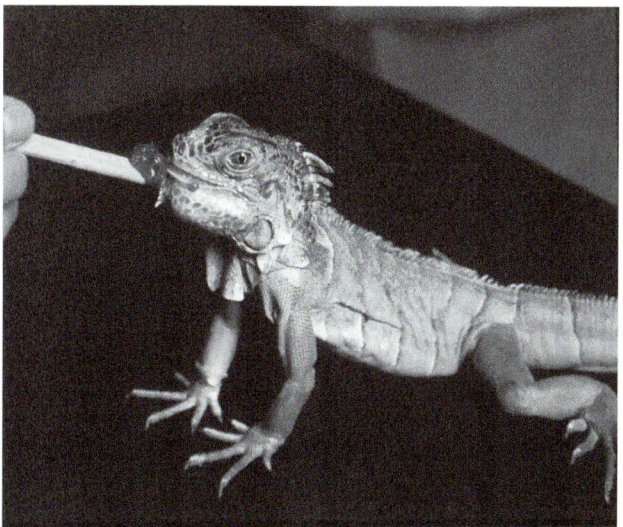

Figure 46.8 A green iguana (*Iguana iguana*) with metabolic bone disease. The swelling of the lower jaw is a sign of fibrous osteodystrophy. A balanced diet will usually prevent the development of this condition under laboratory conditions.

---

[8] https://youtu.be/L83RApPPri8 (Accessed 25 August 2022)

thicker bone underlying the annuli of the scutes and, with pronounced PSG, the vertebral column may separate from the dorsally domed dermal bone.

PSG has long been considered indicative of an osteodystrophy associated with an inadequate calcium-phosphorus balance and a high protein intake. Recent work, however, suggests that the condition may be complex (Boyer & Scott 2019).

One of the few scientific studies on PSG was in African spurred tortoises (*Centrochelys sulcata*), reared under different RH conditions ('dry' 24–58%, 'mid' 31–75%, and 'humid' 45–99) and different protein intake (14%, 19%, and 31% DM), and Ca:P ratios of greater than 3.7:1.21 The study showed a trend for greater pyramiding under drier conditions. The least pyramiding was found in the experimental group (environmental humidity of 45%–99%) and the most pyramiding in the group with 24%–58% environmental humidity; the two groups had identical dietary protein intake (19% DM). The authors concluded that if PSG was to be kept to a minimum, hiding areas with relatively high humidity should be provided. It was speculated that, during humid seasons, there is a concurrent increase in growth of plants of higher nutritional value. Conversely, during dry seasons, nutritional quality decreases and growth slows. Many tortoises naturally seek humid refuges in burrows or under foliage at soil level. Therefore, it is argued, providing in captivity a dry environment with constant rich nutrition is unnatural and may contribute to PSG.

Another study, on African spurred tortoises and leopard tortoises, found that increased heat exposure at night leads to increased growth rate and a significant increase ($P < 0.05$) in the prevalence of PSG. RH values and diet quality were the same in treatment and control groups (that received no nocturnal heat). The authors suggested that unnatural growth rate may lead to deposition of material between keratin scutes at a greater rate than the bone shell can spread, leading to conical upgrowth of carapacial scutes.

Both these studies point out that increased growth rates lead to more PSG. It seems probable that the condition is multifactorial but is largely independent of dietary calcium and phosphorus.

There is no treatment for PSG. Shell deformities are permanent, and only new shell growth can be corrected. The prevalence of the condition can be reduced with better nutrition, such as more hay, grasses and commercial tortoise diets, humid retreats for growing tortoises, and by slowing growth rate with an ambient drop in temperature at night. Concurrent anorexia or nutritional secondary hyperparathyroidism can complicate treatment and prognosis.

Osteodystrophic disorders ('metabolic bone diseases', MBD) are more relevant to laboratory reptiles than PSG because MBD can affect any species. Again, there is much published information, some of it (especially on the internet) anecdotal and not evidence-based. Useful data are to be found in a number of places in the book by Divers and Stahl (2019). John Courteney-Smith, referred to earlier, has developed the Earth Pro Recovery programme for confirmed MBD reptiles.[9] The programme, which has been tested on a range of species, is tailored to dietary needs and takes account of the animals' age, sex and bodyweight.

Various vitamin deficiencies are recognised or suspected in captive reptiles. Hypovitaminosis A was the first to be properly described and documented. In chelonians, it can produce characteristic ocular lesions. Other effects may include retarded healing of wounds and predisposition to infectious diseases (Cooper *et al.* 1980). Studies have been carried out on the vitamin A requirements of some species – chameleons, for example (Abate *et al.* 2003).

It is not only a deficiency of vitamin A that can cause disease in captive reptiles. Hypervitaminosis A may result from excessive administration resulting in skin lesions.

How much to feed laboratory reptiles is an important consideration (see earlier). Condition scores play a crucial part in monitoring nutritional status (see later).

Underfeeding will result in weight loss, 'poverty lines' and weakness. However, such findings can also be the result of providing an adequate but unsuitable diet, or because a reptile is unwell and unable to feed, or is unwilling to do so on account of stressors, including territorial or other aggression. Too low an ambient temperature or other adverse environmental factors may also be a cause of decreased feeding behaviour and food intake.

Over-feeding of captive reptiles can result in a range of pathological changes, including hepatic lipidosis (Divers & Cooper 2000). Some information on food intake of captive snakes in relation to body weight is provided by Kirkwood and Gili (1994).

Laboratory reptiles should always be provided with water. Dehydration can rapidly prove fatal in reptiles, in part because it leads to renal damage and the development of visceral gout (Figure 46.9). Some species will use water for bathing as well as for drinking. Snakes may immerse themselves in water when sloughing is imminent. How water is presented is important. Some lizards and chelonians will drown if they fall into a water container from which they are unable to escape. Chameleons will not usually drink from a water bowl: they should be provided with water in the form of drops on foliage, using a spray.

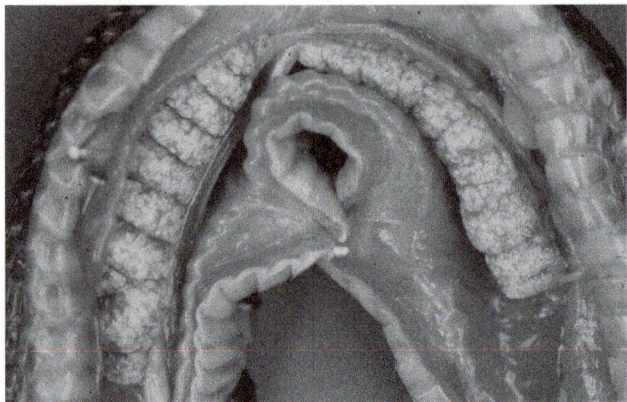

Figure 46.9 *Post-mortem* appearance of a Jamaican boa (*Epicrates subflavus*). The kidneys are white as a result of deposition of urates (visceral gout), possibly because of dehydration.

---

[9] https://www.arcadiareptile.com/earthpro/feeding-programme/ (Accessed 25 May 2022)

Identification and marking

The marking for identification of captive reptiles is important both for scientific and legal reasons (Cooper & Cooper 2007). It has long been recognised that many individual reptiles can be identified by a combination of their size, colour, pattern and, in certain lizards, the state of the tail (since this may have been broken off in the past, and be at various stages of regrowth). It is possible to build up databases of sets of pictures of individuals – e.g., of the plastral markings of tortoises.

When individual reptiles cannot be recognised visually, it is necessary to mark them. Methods for snakes were reviewed by Lang (1992). Clipping ventral scales is simple and effective, but the animal must usually be handled in order to see the marks. Implanted transponder tags, commonly termed 'microchips', are routinely used in zoos and in the pet trade in many countries and may be a legal requirement for certain species as part of enforcing legislation – e.g., for tortoises that are traded in the European Union under EC Regulations 338/97 and 865/2006 (Cooper & Cooper 2007). Transponders are also regularly used in field studies (Germano & Williams 1993). There are correct and incorrect methods of implanting microchips, most dictated by factors such as practicability and welfare, some by legal regulations. A useful review insofar as reptiles are concerned is to be found at the website of the British Veterinary Zoological Society[10].

Welfare and welfare assessment

As a general rule, the application of the Five Freedoms will do much to promote the welfare of captive reptiles (Rayment-Dyble 2019). As with all species that are kept in the laboratory, the assessment of welfare of reptiles is of great importance. Over 30 years ago, guidelines for the recognition of pain, distress and discomfort in laboratory mammals were first formulated in the UK (Morton & Griffiths 1985). Little comparable advice appears to have been devised for laboratory reptiles, although general criteria/guidelines for recognising pain, distress and discomfort were developed by WSPA (1994) and Warwick et al. (1995). More recently, Warwick et al. (1995) published a paper about abnormal behaviour in reptiles, including signs of 'captivity-stress, injury and disease' (sic), and suggested that greater awareness of such issues might help veterinarians and reptile keepers.

'Welfare audit' is increasingly being used to assess the well-being of zoo animals, including reptiles, and many British zoological collections use a welfare evaluation form for this purpose. Aspects that are assessed include environmental parameters such as UV light (with reference to the Ferguson zone – see earlier), light intensity (lux) and temperature; and behavioural implications such as opportunities for basking, whether there is space appropriate to the species' size and activity pattern, and the depth and constitution of substrate and whether it allows for normal behaviour and/or egg laying (Baines 2017).

Some reptile behaviour is considered to be associated with stressors and stress (Hernandez-Divers 2001; Warwick et al. 2019). Stereotypy, for example, is well-recognised in captivity: it has received little scientific attention in reptiles in contrast to the situation in domesticated mammals and birds (Mason & Rushen 2006).

There are limited data on the physiological effects of handling and restraining some species of reptile (e.g. Kreger & Mench 1993). Chelonians readily defaecate when handled or contained and, indeed, these 'stress faeces' (Josseaume 2002) are used in some research studies.

A useful review of early thinking concerning stress in reptiles was provided by Denardo (2006), and Hernandez-Divers (2001) provided a very useful introduction to reptile ethology, including examples of normal and abnormal behaviour patterns. Interactions between stress and other aspects of reptile metabolism were discussed by Guillette et al. (1995).

Reproduction

General considerations

Breeding reptiles in captivity demands care and attention to detail, and is usually time-consuming (Wright & Raiti 2019). Many species require either a natural seasonal regime of temperature and photoperiod (and occasionally also rainfall), or artificial regimes that mimic seasonality (Chiszar et al. 1994). Most temperate species require the 'priming' effects of cool-induced hibernation or quiescence in order to promote breeding, e.g., *Zootoca vivipara* (Gavaud 1991). Social behaviour often has a modulating effect on the development of reproductive condition, for example in *Anolis* lizards. Successful reproduction may depend on the correct social context (Hernandez-Divers 2001). In the leopard gecko (*Eublepharis macularius*), for example, females will lay only if sexually mature males are present. In the American anole (*Anolis carolinensis*), courtship displays by males facilitate ovarian growth in females, whereas aggressive interactions, which may occur if more than one male is present, may inhibit ovarian development (Crews et al. 1994).

Most reptiles are oviparous. Under laboratory conditions, the eggs should be removed immediately after laying, because they need a carefully controlled environment for successful development. In addition, the hatchlings may be eaten by the adults. Gecko eggs, however, should not be removed, because they are laid in such a way that they adhere to hard surfaces such as rocks or the walls of a cage. They can be protected by taping a small plastic container over them until they hatch. Temperature, substrate, substrate moisture and RH of the surrounding atmosphere are particularly important. reptile eggs should not be moved or turned during incubation.

Role of temperature

All reptile species have an optimum temperature for incubation of their eggs. This is usually lower than the mean activity temperatures maintained by adults. Eggs incubated at

---

[10] http://bvzs.org.uk (Accessed 25 May 2022)

Table 46.2 Lizards, terrestrial chelonians and crocodilians that have unequivocally been shown to have temperature-dependent sex determination (TSD). There are many other species which are likely to have TSD. Most reptile species have not been studied in sufficient detail to know whether their sex determination is genetic, environmental or temperature-dependent. The data in this table are mostly from Ewert et al. (1994), Lang and Andrews (1994) and Viets et al. (1994).

Lizards	Agama agama, A. caucasia
	Dipsosaurus dorsalis
	Eublepharis macularius
	Gekko japonicas
	Hemitheconyx caudicinctus
	Tarentola boettgeri
	Phelsuma madagascariensis
Chelonians (terrestrial species)	Testudo graeca, T. hermanni Terrapene ornate
Crocodilians	Alligator mississippiensis, A. sinensis
	Caiman crocodilus
	Crocodylus palustris, C. johnstoni, C. moreletii, C. niloticus, C. porosus, C. siamensis
	Gavialis gangeticus
	Paleosuchus trigonatus

temperatures that lie outside the optimum have lower levels of hatching success, and may be associated with developmental abnormalities (see later).

There are many species of reptiles in which the sex of an embryo depends not on sex chromosomes but on the temperature during the early stages of incubation (Table 46.2).

Three general patterns are seen (Lance 1994):

1. Higher temperatures produce males, lower temperatures produce females; this applies in many species of lizards and in alligators.
2. The opposite effect: higher temperatures produce females; lower temperatures produce males e.g. in many chelonians.
3. Intermediate temperatures produce males, higher and lower temperatures produce females. This occurs in the leopard gecko (*Eublepharis macularius*), the snapping turtle (*Chelydra serpentina*) and some crocodiles.

In most of the species that show temperature-dependent sex determination (TSD), the transition from production of one sex to production of the other takes place within a comparatively narrow range of temperatures (intersexes are rare). In American alligators (*Alligator mississippiensis*), however, intermediate temperatures result in the production of a mixture of males and females. The actual temperatures that are important for producing changes in the sex ratio vary from species to species, and sometimes geographically within a species. Fluctuating temperatures may produce different results from constant temperatures. Table 46.2 lists lizard species shown to exhibit TSD. Because of the complexity of responses, no attempt has been made to provide crucial temperatures. The implications of TSD for the breeding of those reptile species in which it occurs are profound; in management programmes for sea turtles, sexing by endoscopy is increasingly being used to ensure an even mix of sexes when juvenile animals are returned to the sea.

Substrate

The eggs of many reptiles may be incubated on damp tissue paper, *Sphagnum* moss, peat, sand, polystyrene foam or other substrates. The medium most frequently used, however, is vermiculite. Made primarily for insulating buildings, vermiculite is cheap, relatively non-toxic and absorbent; it contains sufficient air-filled spaces among the granules that diffusion of air can readily take place. Whatever medium is employed, it should be used only once. There has been much discussion about the extent to which eggs should be buried in the substrate. Packard and Phillips (1994) recommended that eggs of species with flexible shells should be half-buried; those with rigid shells should be placed in small depressions at the surface of the medium.

Health and diseases

The aim in captivity is to provide reptiles with good welfare, of which physical health is a vital component. Under laboratory conditions, it is particularly important to establish health profiles for the animals so as to help ensure consistency of research results, to detect early signs of disease and to promote welfare (see later). The diagnosis and treatment of reptile diseases are primarily the remit of the veterinarian, preferably one with experience of reptile medicine and surgery (Frye 1994). A useful table of differential diagnoses is to be found in an Appendix to the BSAVA Manual of Reptiles (Girling & Raiti 2019). The prevention and management of many diseases of reptiles are predicated by good husbandry.

The animal technician and research worker, who are familiar with the behaviour and natural history of the species, have an important part to play in disease prevention and in health monitoring.

Health monitoring

Health monitoring involves the regular and routine investigation of live reptiles, *post-mortem* examination of any animals that die or have to be culled, and laboratory studies on samples from live reptiles, dead reptiles and their environment. Relatively little has been published on the health monitoring of laboratory reptiles but methods used for lizards, snakes, chelonians and other species in zoological collections and conservation programmes (Woodford 2001) can be usefully adapted. Cooper (1989) wrote specifically about the health monitoring of laboratory reptiles and amphibians and stressed the importance of using minimally-invasive methods whenever wild animals are involved (Cooper 1998).

The exclusion of infectious disease is facilitated by the use of quarantine, whereby incoming reptiles are kept separately prior to their introduction to the colony. During this period, the animals should be screened for pathogens and, if possible, health monitored. Subsequently, as in other fields of laboratory animal science, there is a need to maintain the reptiles' status by having efficient barrier systems, with rules to which all staff adhere.

An essential aspect of monitoring the health and, to a certain extent, the welfare of captive reptiles is the assessment of body condition. This is not always easy or straightforward; for example, some reptiles go through normal, cyclical, periods of fat deposition or loss. Essentially, however, body condition scoring (BCS) implies that laboratory reptiles are weighed and measured on a regular basis. How these data are processed may depend on the species: formulae are available for Mediterranean tortoises (e.g. Jackson 1991; Hailey 2000; Willemser & Hailey 2002).

Newer books do not necessarily supersede older works. Often the latter contain sound, basic information which can be of great value to research workers and animal technicians. Scientific literature about reptile diseases goes back to the seminal work of Reichenbach-Klinke and Elkan (1965): although now over 40 years old, their book remains a useful guide to some aspects, especially parasite identification. In subsequent decades, texts such as those by Cooper and Jackson (1981) and Frye (1991) provided herpetologists, including those working in laboratories, with relevant information from the growing field of medical and surgical treatment, leading to the current authoritative texts by Girling and Raiti (2019) and Divers and Stahl (2019). It is important to remember that not all relevant texts are in English. For example, excellent sources of information on lizards, snakes and tortoises are the relevant chapters in the German work *Krankheiten der Heimtiere* (Gabrisch & Zwart 2015).

The effects of captivity on health

Captivity imposes physical, behavioural and physiological constraints on reptiles. Confinement in a relatively small space, often in close contact with others of the same species, can precipitate infectious or non-infectious disease and compromise welfare (Arena & Warwick 1995). So can stressors associated with, for example, the absence of somewhere for the reptile(s) to hide – see later (refugia). These are important ethical, often legal, considerations when reptiles are kept in laboratories. Examples of health problems that are due to, or exacerbated by, captivity are given later, under Non-infectious diseases.

The effect of captivity and of regular 'milking' of venomous snakes attracted interest in the 1970s when the author was working in East Africa. Strong evidence emerged that such stressors (especially when coupled with trauma) could cause, or predispose to, infections affecting the buccal cavity and the skin and lead to bacterial septicaemia (Cooper & Nares 1971; Cooper 1973; Cooper & Leakey 1976;).

The influence of temperature on health

The immune responses of reptiles, both humoral (production of antibodies) and cellular, are temperature-dependent and, therefore, less effective at lower temperatures (Guillette *et al*. 1995). Some species respond to bacterial (and perhaps other) infections, or the introduction of bacterial pyrogens, by spontaneously seeking higher body temperatures the

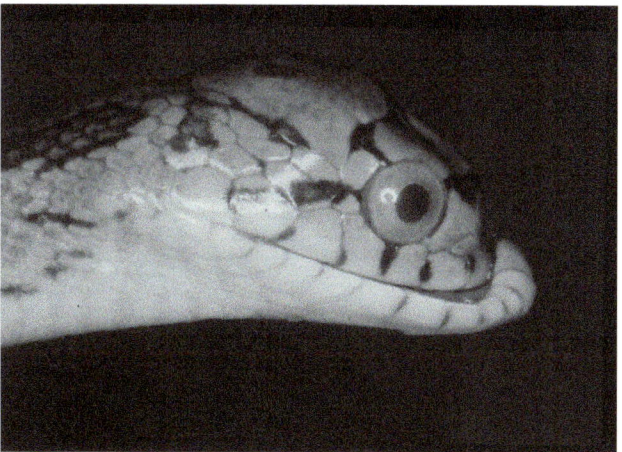

Figure 46.10 A developmental abnormality, an undershot jaw and hydrocephalus, in a captive-bred king snake (*Lampropeltis* sp.). Such anomalies can have a genetic aetiology, often associated with inbreeding, or follow temperature fluctuations during incubation.

so-called '*behavioural fever*' (Ramos *et al*. 1993). For these reasons, many authorities suggest that sick reptiles undergoing treatment should be kept warm or assisted in doing so by providing a temperature gradient and given the opportunity to maintain high body temperatures by basking for longer periods than usual (Frye 1991).

As mentioned elsewhere, adverse or fluctuating temperatures can affect the survival and health of neonatal reptiles. An increased prevalence of developmental abnormalities may be indicative of such a situation (Figure 46.10).

Cerreta *et al*. (2018) described methods of body temperature assessment in *Chelonoidis chathamensis*.

Non-infectious diseases

Reptiles kept in the laboratory are particularly prone to non-infectious disease, largely because they are confined in captivity and, therefore, more likely to encounter physical insults. The latter include trauma (physical damage to rostrum (Figure 46.11) or limbs, often associated with cage design or insensitive management), electrocution (from poorly maintained electrical circuits), burns (from proximity to badly positioned bulbs or heaters) and drowning (deep water containers from which lizards and chelonians, is particular, cannot escape). Non-infectious insults can readily lead to infectious disease – for example, a wound may become infected with bacteria.

One of the most common problems encountered in captive reptiles is damage to the rostrum, caused by the animals colliding with the walls of the cage or enclosure, especially when they are trying to escape (a behaviour that can develop into a stereotypy). Attempts to reduce the incidence of such lesions include giving individuals as large a cage as is practicable, providing refugia (see the preceding text) and avoiding disturbance and stress whenever possible. Painting or otherwise marking vertical glass surfaces so that they are opaque can also sometimes reduce the incidence of collisions. Some materials are particularly damaging, e.g., wire mesh, which should

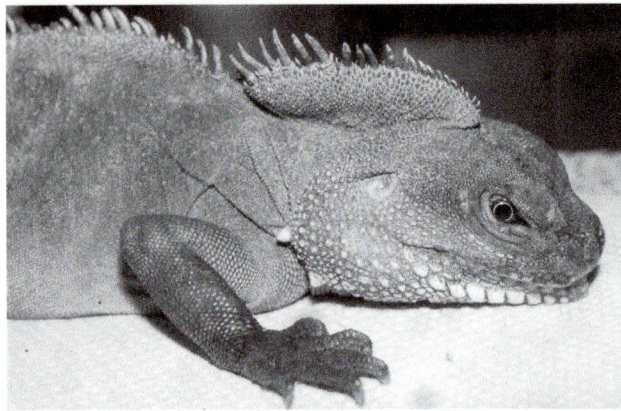

Figure 46.11 Chronic damage to the rostrum of a water dragon (*Physignathus* sp.) due to repeated rubbing on the glass sides of its cage.

be screened with protective partitions made from other materials. Treatment is by cleaning the wound (Frye 1991) followed by standard medication and prevention of further trauma. Burns, usually caused by an animal being able to get to close to the hot surface of a bulb or heating pad, can also be treated (Divers & Stahl 2019). In lizards and snakes, which shed their skins regularly, the area of the burn can become a site of incomplete ecdysis and a focus for infection.

Chelonians in captivity often have overgrowth of the highly keratinised edges to the mouth. This is usually because the diet is softer than that in the wild but underlying disease (possibly including hepatic dysfunction) may play a part. Treatment is initially by burring the beak to restore normal anatomy. Prevention includes ensuring that the diet is as varied as possible and contains harder material, such as fibrous plants. Overgrowth of the claws, also caused by insufficient abrasion, may occur in chelonians and large lizards.

Snakes in captivity often fail to slough properly (dysecdysis – see earlier). There can be many reasons for this, including poor health, malnutrition, dehydration and endocrine imbalances caused by failure to provide the correct photothermal stimuli that cue seasonal cycles of reproduction and activity (Avery 1994). A dysecdytic snake can be helped to shed by soaking for about an hour in warm water.

Other non-infectious diseases include poisoning, genetic/congenital/developmental abnormalities and metabolic disorders associated with old age and/or dietary imbalances. Poisoning can result from overdosage of medical agents, prolonged exposure to toxins (e.g. insecticidal preparations) or ingestion of toxic material in the food. Developmental abnormalities may be present at birth (congenital) or appear later in life. They may or may not have an underlying genetic basis. Environmental factors may play a part in producing some abnormalities, especially during incubation of eggs. All such anomalies should be investigated and documented and specimens retained for study (Bellairs 1981; Cooper et al. 1998).

Infectious diseases

Many infectious agents can cause morbidity (ill-health) or mortality (death) in captive reptiles. While some organisms appear to be frank pathogens, many others are opportunists that take advance of an injured or immunocompromised animal. Host–parasite relations are still poorly understood in reptiles but knowledge of these is often the key to the prevention or control of infectious disease. Experimental work on reptiles is yielding useful information about inflammatory and other responses in reptiles (Tucunduva et al. 2001).

Bacteria

Numerous pathological conditions in captive reptiles are caused by bacteria (Wellehan and Divers 2019a).

The particular role of Gram-negative species such as *Aeromonas* and *Pseudomonas* was recognised many years ago (Cooper & Jackson 1981). Pneumonia, often coupled with a septicaemia, is one such example. Necrotic stomatitis ('mouth rot') is another; it is not a single disease entity, but a syndrome that was originally considered to be caused by a wide range of bacteria (Cooper & Sainsbury 1994) but which may also be due to viruses, including herpesviruses and ranaviruses (Gray and Chinchar 2015). Necrotic dermatitis ('scale rot') shows a similar pattern, as does 'shell rot' in chelonians. 'Blister disease' of snakes and lizards, characterised by fluid-filled vesicles on the skin, is often a result of a non-infectious factor, adverse humidity: the lesions can quickly become secondarily infected by bacteria.

Subcutaneous abscesses are often seen in lizards and snakes and are usually due to bacteria (Figure 46.12). The pus of reptiles is semi-solid, often laid down over several weeks in concentric layers, and needs to be removed surgically.

Salmonella is of particular importance under laboratory conditions because of the zoonotic risk (see later). The genus consists of over 2400 serotypes, a number of which (some termed 'Arizona' – *S. enterica arizonae*) may be isolated from captive reptiles, including those kept for research purposes, and may cause pathological lesions and clinical signs of disease (Cambre et al. 1980; Onderka & Finlayson 1985; Gene & Loeschner 2002).

Many other bacteria may cause disease in captive reptiles (Cooper 1999) including *Neisseria* species, especially *N. iguanae* (Plowman et al. 1987; Barrett et al. 1994) and *Mycobacterium* species (Soldati et al. 2004). *Devriesea agamarum* can be the

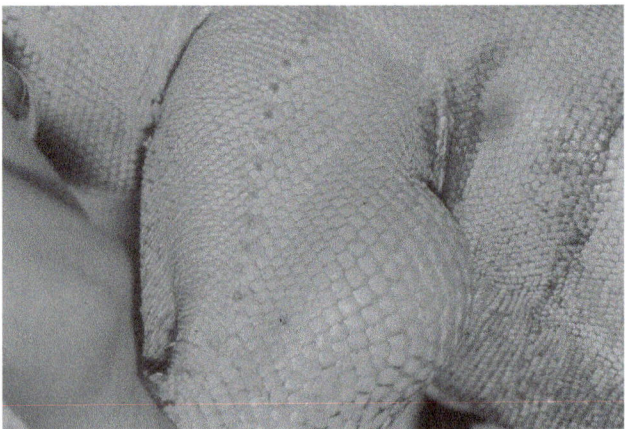

Figure 46.12 A subcutaneous abscess in the hindlimb of a green iguana. The pus in such a case is likely to be semi-solid and needs to be removed surgically. This is a male animal and the row of femoral pores is very apparent.

cause of skin lesions (cheilitis) in *Uromastyx* spp. and others (Hellebuyck *et al.* 2009).

Any breach in the skin may permit the ingress of bacteria which can then cause a localised infection, such as an abscess or cellulitis, possibly followed by bacteraemia and septicaemia, often with fatal results (Cooper 1999).

Most bacterial diseases may be treated with standard antibiotics following sensitivity testing and appropriate palliation (Knotek 2019; Carpenter 2012; Divers & Stahl 2019). Reliable pharmacokinetic data are available on a number of antibacterial agents such as enrofloxacin (Young *et al.* 1997). Antibiotics should only be administered to laboratory reptiles following appropriate sensitivity tests and, whenever possible (in view of concerns about antimicrobial resistance, AMR) preference given to other ways of combating bacteria – for instance, the treatment of external lesions using hypochlorous acid (*Vetericyn Plus*, Petlife International Ltd). The eggs of reptiles may be infected with and may spread bacterial and other diseases. The *post-mortem* examination of reptile eggs was detailed by Cooper (2019).

Mycoplasmata (mycoplasmas) can be the cause of upper respiratory tract disease in tortoises (Jacobson *et al.* 2014).

Fungi

Austwick and Keymer (1981) provided a useful earlier review of mycotic infections of reptiles. Later reports augmenting the earlier work included those by Nichols *et al.* (1999) and Bertelsen *et al.* (2005). Current thinking is summarised by Wellehan and Divers (2019b).

Nannizziopsis and *Paranannizziopsis* spp. are causes of dermatitis and systemic disease, especially *Nannizziopsis guarroi* (e.g. Sigler *et al.* 2013). *Ophidiomyces ophiodiicola* is a significant, apparently emerging disease, cause of fungal disease in snakes. In addition to occurring in a wide range of taxa in captivity, it causes death in free-living vipers in North America and has been found in free-living snakes in Europe (e.g. Lorch *et al.* 2016; Franklinos *et al.* 2017).

Mycotic infections need to be diagnosed early, using a variety of clinical and laboratory techniques (Wellehan & Divers 2019b).

Viruses

The importance of viral infections in reptiles began to be appreciated nearly 40 years ago (Clark & Lunger 1981). Since then great advances have been made, with a range of viruses recognised as causes of disease in various parts of the world (Just *et al.* 2001; Marschang 2011). A number of these are potentially important in the laboratory maintenance of terrestrial reptiles:

- paramyxoviruses, genus *Ferlavirus*, primarily in snakes but also in lizards and chelonians (Jacobson *et al.* 2001; Hyndman *et al.* 2013). Paramyxovirus infection in caiman lizards (Dracaena guianensis). Transmitted via aerosol as well as direct contact. Especially important in viperids; severe outbreaks can occur in laboratories where vipers are kept for venom collection – the first description was in a laboratory with a large viper collection in Switzerland (Foelsch & Leloup 1976). Associated with respiratory and (less commonly) neurological disease. Diagnosis is by polymerase chain reaction (PCR) detection of viral RNA. The highest virus loads are to be found in the lungs. Tracheal washes can be tested in live animals and can be combined with investigation of oral/cloacal swabs. Serology is also possible (haemagglutination inhibition) but reactivity depends on many factors – time post infection, immune system of the host, genotype with which the animal was infected, virus type used for testing. Persistent infections have been suspected but not proven.
- herpesviruses, in lizards, snakes and chelonians (Jacobson 2007). These are most important in chelonians. Various genotypes. Herpesviruses are the cause of diphtheroid-necrotising stomatitis in many tortoise species and fibropapillomatosis in sea turtles (see, for example, Cooper & Seebaransingh 2008).

There are sporadic reports of herpesviruses, in squamates. Diagnosis is by PCR detection using material from lesions.

- adenoviruses in lizards (Julian & Durham 1982; Wellehan *et al.* 2004). Very common in squamate reptiles. Various genotypes, all belonging to the genus *Atadenovirus*. Especially common in bearded dragons (*Pogona vitticeps*). Associated with gastro-intestinal disease, CNS signs, respiratory disease and liver lesions, but also found in clinically healthy animals. Possible factor in multifactorial disease processes, possibly particularly important in juveniles. Also found in chelonians; more genetically diverse viruses, 'testadenoviruses' are believed to have co-evolved with chelonians – infection is not always associated with disease (Doszpoly *et al.* 2013). The genus *Siadenovirus* was associated with a severe disease outbreak and high mortality in a mixed species group following illegal import into the USA (Rivera *et al.* 2009). The genus *Atadenovirus* was detected in a *Testudo graeca* with stomatitis and oesophagitis (Garcia-Morante *et al.* 2016). Diagnosis is by PCR using cloacal swabs or samples from liver or intestine.
- ranaviruses in tortoises, occasionally lizards and snakes (Duffus *et al.* 2015). Associated mostly with vasculitis and haemorrhage, hepatic necrosis, upper digestive tract disease, respiratory disease in chelonians, skin lesions and haemorrhage in lizards. The same viruses can be transmitted between amphibians and reptiles – sometimes fish. Diagnosis is by PCR; tissues are more sensitive than swabs (e.g. liver, tail clips). Blood can also be tested.
- reoviruses of various reptiles, mostly squamates (e.g. Marschang *et al.* 2002, Marschang 2019). Associated most often with upper respiratory and upper digestive tract disease, also with pneumonia and CNS signs. Described in outbreaks with mixed infections. Diagnosis is mostly by PCR on oral and cloacal swabs and tissues.
- Reptarenaviruses (Chang and Jacobson 2010; Stenglein *et al.* 2012; Hetzel *et al.* 2013; Chang *et al.* 2016; Stenglein *et al.* 2017). These viruses are the cause of inclusion body disease (IBD) in boas and pythons, which is very widespread throughout the world. Very genetically diverse viruses that produce intra-cytoplasmic inclusions, made up of viral protein, in a wide variety of cells. Clinical

signs very varied; often involve the CNS, but also skin, respiratory and digestive tracts. Lymhoproliferative disorders. Boas are commonly infected with many inclusions throughout the body; the boas may remain clinically healthy for extended periods of time. Pythons show fewer inclusions, often only in neurons; they tend to develop severe disease quickly. IBD is considered a progressive disease. Diagnosis is by detection of typical inclusions in cells (e.g. in liver (biopsies), oesophageal tonsils, blood or buffy coat smears). Diagnosis can be difficult in pythons – inclusions are often only in the CNS. PCR can be used for virus detection (oesophageal swabs, whole blood, tissues, CNS in pythons).

- Nidoviruses. Order *Nidovirales*, subfamily *Serpetovirinae* (Stenglein et al. 2014; Hoon-Hanks et al. 2018; O'Dea et al. 2018; Zhang et al. 2019). Cause severe respiratory disease in pythons. Very common in captive pythons, especially certain species. Similar viruses have been found in *Tiliqua* spp. in Australia, and similar viruses have been associated with severe die-off of Bellinger River turtles (*Myuchelys georgesi*) in Australia. Diagnosis is by PCR.

Captive reptiles can be screened serologically for certain viruses – for example, ferlaviruses and some herpesviruses of chelonians (testudinid herpesvirus 1 and 3, the types most commonly found in Mediterranean tortoises (Marschang 2019)). Serology can provide information on whether an animal has been in contact with an antigen or one that cross-reacts with it, but does not necessarily provide information on whether the reptile remains infected. In the case of herpesviruses, which cause latent infections, an animal with antibodies should be considered to be persistently infected. Virus detection is most commonly performed by PCR, which should be considered an important part of excluding infectious disease from laboratory colonies of snakes, lizards and chelonians.

Many viruses can be involved in multifactorial disease processes. Treatment of viral infection in reptiles is generally difficult and relies mostly on supportive therapy. Reptiles that survive infection and become clinically healthy will often remain carriers. Quarantine, hygiene and regular testing are important. The general rule in laboratory animal work should be to exclude such pathogens by obtaining reptiles from 'clean' captive-bred sources and by quarantining and screening incoming stock.

Protozoa

Keymer (1981) provided an excellent seminal review of protozoa of reptiles, and Barnard and Upton (1994) produced a practical *'veterinary guide'* to many of these species. The most up-to-date information is probably the chapter by Wellehan and Walden (2019). Some intestinal protozoa are beneficial – for example, ciliates that aid digestion in tortoises and large herbivorous lizards (Troyer 1982).

Haematozoa (blood-borne protozoa), haemoparasites, are not uncommonly seen in terrestrial reptiles, both in wild (free-living) and captive animals. In a number of cases, their classification remains uncertain, as does the understanding of their significance (Davies & Johnston 2000; Wellehan & Walden 2019)). The presence of haematozoa in blood smears should be noted during routine health monitoring. Smears should be examined on two occasions, at least 14 days apart, during any quarantine period.

Entamoeba invadens has a direct life cycle, with cysts being passed in faeces. Meerovitch (1958, 1961) elucidated the life stages of this protozoon. She concluded that the parasite is usually a commensal in chelonians, where it ingests plant polysaccharides. In snakes, *E. invadens* proves pathogenic because they are carnivorous and, in the absence of plant ingesta, the *Entamoeba* obtains its polysaccharide requirements from intestinal mucosal secretions, rendering the gut wall susceptible to invasion. It follows that, in laboratories, herbivorous and carnivorous/omnivorous reptiles should not be kept together and strict hygiene must be practised when moving from one reptile species to another.

The coccidian parasite *Cryptosporidium* is increasingly a problem in reptile collections – e.g., in leopard geckos (Deming et al. 2008) – and is difficult to treat. It can be zoonotic.

Helminths and pentastomids

All of the major groups of parasitic worms are found in reptiles. Tapeworms (Cestoda) and flukes (Trematoda) are not usually a major problem in captive reptile husbandry, especially in the laboratory, as they require the appropriate intermediate host as part of their life cycle. The same is true of pentastomids which, although worm-like in appearance, are in fact highly modified arthropods. The life cycles of pentastomids are complex, and, depending on the species of parasite, a reptile may be a definitive or an intermediate host. Most infections of reptiles with pentastomes are asymptomatic.

In comparison, many species of nematodes have direct life cycles and these worms can increase rapidly under suitable conditions. A range of clinical signs and pathological lesions may be seen in infected reptiles. Treatment of the affected animal must be coupled with hygiene and other measures in order to prevent re-infection. Parasitic worms are readily treated with various anthelmintics but care must always be taken as adverse sequelae sometimes result. Ivermectin can be toxic to chelonians (Frye 1991) and should be employed with appropriate caution in all reptile species. Treatment during quarantine, coupled with microscopical examination of faeces, will help to limit and control nematode infestations in laboratory reptiles.

Ticks and mites

Ticks and other ectoparasites of reptiles can be pathogenic in their own right, causing local or systemic disease, or they may transmit other organisms (Burridge 2001). Ticks (Figure 46.13) can be removed with forceps, but care must be taken that the mouthparts do not remain because they may become a focus for infection with bacteria and other pathogens. Certain acaricides, such as permethrins, are effective in control but, as with all treatment under laboratory conditions, may be contra-indicated in reptiles that are part of an experimental procedure.

Mites, especially the 'snake mite', *Ophionyssus natricis*, can be the cause of ill-health or death in laboratory reptiles. Parasitic mites feed on blood, and can transmit viruses,

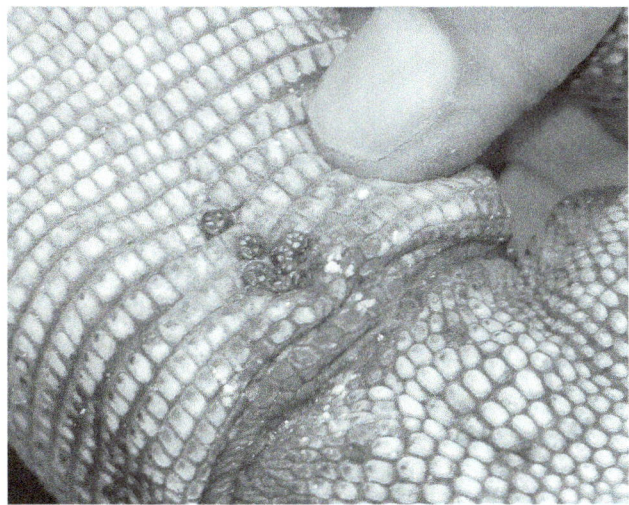

Figure 46.13 Cloacal region of a monitor lizard, showing the presence of tightly attached *Amblyomma* ticks.

spirochaetes, rickettsiae, bacteria and protozoa. The parasites and their eggs can survive in crevices in the environment for long periods.

Fipronil wipes can be used, with care, to kill mites or ivermectin can be administered topically or by injection. Large reptiles can be treated with proprietary (dog and cat) flea sprays (Frye 1991) Under laboratory conditions, where the use of drugs that have a systemic effect may be contraindicated, mites can be killed by painting the reptile with vegetable oil, which is then blotted off (Espinosa *et al.* 1998) or trapped with sticky tape and removed. An alternative approach may be to biological control, making use of predatory acarines that feed on *Ophionyssus natricis* (Schilliger *et al.* 2013; Mendyk 2015).

Routine treatment and quarantine of incoming animals will help to prevent the introduction of mites to a laboratory animal facility. Scrupulous attention to hygiene is then necessary to prevent treated animals from becoming re-infected. Davies and Knotek (2019) discussed therapeutics and medication of reptiles.

Health and physiological monitoring

Standard veterinary procedures for reptiles are applicable to those that are kept for research. Imaging is practicable using radiography, ultrasonography, magnetic resonance imaging (MRI) and computed tomography (CT) scanning (Raiti 2019).

Collection of samples and laboratory investigations

Samples may need to be taken from reptiles for research purposes, for health monitoring or for diagnostic purposes. Samples can be of many types. Some, such as faeces, can be collected without handling the reptile, while others, such as blood, will necessitate invasive techniques. The most appropriate methods will depend on many factors, including the temperament, size and anatomy of the reptile. Veterinary texts provide useful guidance (see, for example, Divers & Stahl 2019).

Blood sampling can be an important part of research procedures involving reptiles. It is also a useful adjunct to health monitoring. Specific papers relating to laboratory work are available – e.g., on blood sampling of lizards (Brown 2007) – while other texts refer more to pet, zoo and wild animals. Sampling sites depend upon the species and the requirements but include withdrawing blood from a vein (jugular, caudal/coccygeal, brachial, abdominal or subcarapacial), heart orbital sinus or via a toe-nail clip. However, in order to perfect techniques specific training is necessary, preferably under the supervision of an experienced veterinarian.

Whole blood is the best material for routine haematology. All anticoagulants can affect cell morphology and staining characteristics. Although lithium heparin is commonly used (see the following text), EDTA is preferable for leucocyte counts and morphology in lizards and snakes but EDTA can cause haemolysis in chelonians. Lithium heparin, however, allows for the examination of (a) whole blood for haematology (complete blood count, packed cell volume [PCV], total solids), and (b) plasma for biochemical tests – all from the same sample.

The amount of blood and frequency of sampling are important considerations in experimental work where regular bleeding may be part of the research protocol. In some countries, quantity and frequency may be stipulated in regulations designed to promote welfare. Where this is not the case, a general rule is not, on any one occasion, to remove a sample of blood that is more than 1% of the body weight of the animal. The author's personal guideline for repeat bleeding is to restrict the volume to 0.7% (i.e. 7 ml of blood per kilogram body weight) and to take this amount from the reptile no more frequently than once a week.

Reference values for blood are available for some species and often include both haematological and biochemical figures (see, for example, Heatley and Russell 2019). There is a need nevertheless to expand these databases and those scientists and laboratory animal veterinarians who take blood samples from reptiles for other purposes should, whenever possible, also prepare smears and carry out haematological and biochemical analyses. Such information is not just of scientific importance: it can also enhance health monitoring and assist in the assessment of welfare.

Laboratory investigation of samples taken from reptiles are covered by a number of authors, for example, bacteriology by Cooper (1999), haematology by Heatley and Russell (2019) and cytology by Camus and Yeuroukis (2019).

Methods of treatment

Terrestrial reptiles may need to be treated with medicinal agents either as part of an experiment or for health reasons. Supportive care is always important and useful information is to be found in texts directed at veterinary nurses/technicians (Cooper *et al.* 2003; McBride & Hernandez-Divers 2004; Mitchell 2004). Emergency and critical care have been covered by a number of authors, e.g., of chelonians by Norton (2005). Techniques for dosing and injection procedures are described in various publications (e.g. Knotek 2019 and Divers & Stahl 2019). The dose and the frequency of administration of some agents may need to be based on allometric scaling.

Telemetry

Telemetry is a well-established procedure in field studies on reptiles and both invasive and non-invasive techniques for attaching a transmitter can be adapted to laboratory research (e.g. Ferrell et al. 2005).

Surgical procedures

Both experimental and therapeutic surgery may be carried out on laboratory reptiles. These do not differ significantly from those employed in veterinary practice (Divers 2019). Under laboratory conditions, it is particularly important to minimise invasive techniques. Endoscopy, for example, can be used very successfully in reptiles as first demonstrated nearly 30 years ago and often reduces the need to perform traumatic, painful or stressful procedures (Brearley et al. 1991; Hernandez-Divers et al. 2004b).

Anaesthesia and analgesia

Anaesthestic methods for reptiles have advanced dramatically in recent years and much has been published in both books and journals (Bertelsen 2019). Awareness of the susceptibility of reptiles to painful stimuli has prompted studies on analgesia (Greenacre et al. 2005). This information is of great relevance to the use of reptiles in research where procedures may be performed that may cause pain.

Euthanasia

Laboratory reptiles may need to be killed at the end of an experiment, or on welfare grounds because of injury, disease or old age. Some nations may have local regulations regarding acceptable techniques. Euthanasia of terrestrial reptiles presents special problems (UFAW/WSPA 1989; Cooper 2019), on account of the low metabolic rates of many and the ability of some species to tolerate hypoxia for long periods (Jackson 2002). Useful resumés of methods of euthanasia for reptiles are given by Cooper (2019).

Decapitation and cervical dislocation are no longer standard methods, because of concerns that the animal may continue to be aware of painful stimuli for a period after the process. Nevertheless, in the UK, Schedule I of the Animals (Scientific Procedures) Act 1986 continues to permit the use of decapitation so long as it is followed immediately by physical destruction of the brain. Freezing is also no longer advocated by most authorities, again on welfare grounds. The exception is dropping small reptiles (of 1 cm maximum diameter) into liquid nitrogen. Other methods that are now considered unacceptable include drowning, overdose of anaesthetic agents by certain routes and use of neuromuscular blockers.

The currently preferred techniques, where practicable, are an overdose of either an appropriate volatile agent, such as isoflurane, or of a barbiturate given by injection (Cooper 2019).

It is important for legal as well as for welfare reasons to be able to determine correctly if a euthanised animal is indeed dead (Cooper et al. 2019).

Zoonoses and other health hazards

Any laboratory animal can present a hazard to those who work with or tend it. The dangers may be infectious, physical or toxic. Pathogenic bacteria that may be transmitted from reptiles to humans include *Salmonella*, *Leptospira*, *Mycobacterium* and *Cryptosporidium* (Johnson-Delaney and Gal 2019).

Salmonella is always considered a particular hazard, although it is not easy to quantify the dangers, partly because so many serotypes or strains may be involved (Burnham et al. 1998).

Under laboratory conditions, it is important to draw up proper risk assessments (see next section). A useful summary of precautions, including reference to the BVZS Guidelines, was provided by Redrobe (2002). Handling animals using appropriate techniques (see Handling and restraint) will lessen the likelihood of physical injury.

A number of species of snake and two species of lizard have traditionally been considered venomous. However, research on monitor lizards and iguanids indicates that other species have saliva which may cause tissue damage (in addition to infection) if the animal bites (Fry et al. 2006). It is important, therefore, to be aware of the identity of any snake or lizard that is to be kept in the laboratory. If in doubt, advice should be sought and full precautions put into place.

Details of techniques for keeping and handling venomous squamates are not included here: useful guidelines are provided by Boyer (2019) and Johnson (2019). These animals should be managed only by trained personnel and a proper risk assessment carried out. Venomous species should be handled with appropriate equipment, such as tongs or a snake-hook (Locke 2008). In order to restrain venomous snakes for radiography or injection, they may be induced to enter a rigid transparent plastic tube (Locke 2008), of a diameter equivalent to that of the snake. Once the snake is inside, the ends can be closed with bungs. For injection, tubes have small holes drilled at appropriate points so that a needle can be inserted. This technique should not be used for narrow-bodied venomous species such as kraits or mambas, as these may succeed in turning around within the tube.

Other legal considerations

The importance of adhering to relevant legislation when keeping reptiles was emphasised earlier. Reference should be made to Cooper, M.E. (2019) and Cooper et al. (2019).

In many countries, reptiles are covered by laws that regulate the use of animals in research. Other statutes may also be relevant, including those concerning conservation of endangered species, welfare, dangerous wild animals and zoonoses. Where there is no legislation controlling the maintenance and use of terrestrial reptiles for research, it is wise to use and follow established codes of practice. Sometimes, specific guidelines are available, for example, those produced for field research on reptiles in Canada (Canadian Council on Animal Care (CCAC) 2003) and the USA (ASIH/HL/SSAR 1987); if this is not the case or the guidelines are inappropriate, the researchers (in collaboration with others) should formulate and use their own.

Conclusion

Understanding of the needs of captive reptiles, including those kept in laboratories, has advanced considerably in the past 10 years. However, an awareness of the sentience of reptiles is not new. In his book *The Natural History and Antiquities of Selborne* ('The Natural History of Selborne' first published in 1789), the English parson and naturalist Gilbert White wrote '. ….the most abject reptile and torpid of beings distinguishes the hand that feeds it, and is touched, with the feelings of gratitude'.

Acknowledgements

I am grateful to Roger Avery, my former teacher, for permitting me to base some of this chapter on his original text in a previous edition and to David Alderton, once one of my students and now a colleague and much-valued advisor, for helpful guidance on the contents.

Rachel Marschang, John Courteney-Smith and Matthew Rendle kindly commented on an early draft and provided helpful comments. Chris Mitchell provided valuable advice regarding welfare assessment in zoos and drew my attention to the BIAZA welfare auditing toolkit. My wife, Margaret E. Cooper, checked the sections on legislation and risk assessment.

Over the years, I have learnt much about the management of venomous snakes from friends and colleagues in East Africa and elsewhere, among them Jonathan Leakey, Jackson Iha, Stephen Spawls, Geofrey Kepha, Paul Rowley, Edouard Crittenden and David Warrell.

The editor and anonymous referees made helpful comments. I am indebted to them all.

References

Abate, A.L., Coke, R., Ferfuson, G. *et al*. (2003). Chameleons and vitamin A. *Journal of Herpetological Medicine and Surgery*, **13**, 23–31.

Alberts, A.C. (1989). Ultraviolet visual sensitivity in desert iguanas: implications for pheromone detection. *Animal Behaviour*, **38**, 129–137.

Alberts, A.C., Jackintell, L.A. and Phillips, J.A. (1994a). Effects of chemical and visual exposure to adults on growth hormones, and behaviour of juvenile green iguanas. *Physiology and Behaviour*, **55**, 987–992.

Alberts, A.C., Rostal, D.C. and Lance, V.A. (1994b). Studies on the chemistry and social significance of chin gland secretions in the desert tortoise, *Gopherus agassizii*. *Herpetological Monographs*, **8**, 116–124.

Arbour, E.K., Chacra, N.A., Gali-Mouhtaseb, H. *et al*. (2007). Performance, bacterial shedding and microbial drug resistance in two tortoise species. *Veterinary Record*, **161**, 62–65.

Arena, P.C. and Warwick, C. (1995). Miscellaneous factors affecting health and welfare. In: *Health and Welfare of Captive Reptiles*. Eds Warwick, C., Frye, F.L. and Murphy, J.B., pp. 263–283. Chapman and Hall, London.

ASIH/HL/SSAR (1987). *Guidelines for Use of Live Amphibians and Reptiles in Field Research*. USA. http://iacuc.ucsd.edu/PDF_References/ASIH-HL-SSAR%20Guidelines%20for%20Use%20of%20Live%20Amphibians%20and%20Reptiles.htm (Accessed 03 January 2009).

Austwick, P.K.C. and Keymer, I.F. (1981). Fungi and actinomycetes. In: *Diseases of the Reptilia*. Eds Cooper, J.E. and Jackson, O.F., pp. 193–231. Academic Press, London.

Avery, R.A. (1982). Field studies of body temperatures and thermoregulation. In: *Biology of the Reptilia 12. Physiology C. Physiological Ecology*. Eds Gans C. and Pough F.H., pp. 93–166. Academic Press, London.

Avery, R.A. (1984). Physiological aspects of lizard growth: the role of thermoregulation. *Symposia of the Zoological Society of London*, **52**, 407–424.

Avery, R.A. (1994). The effects of temperature on captive amphibians and reptiles. In: *Captive Management and Conservation of Amphibians and Reptiles*. Eds Murphy, J.B., Adler, K. and Collins, J.T., pp. 47–51. Society for the Study of Amphibians and Reptiles, Ithaca, New York.

Baines, F.M. (2017). UV or not UV? An in-depth look at UV light and its proper use with reptiles. In: *Reptiles* magazine, Jan-Feb 2017 16-25. Available online at http://www.reptilesmagazine.com/An-In-Depth-Look-At-UV-Light-And-Its-Proper-Use-With-Reptiles/

Baines, F.M. and Brames, H. (2010). Preventive reptile medicine and reptile lighting. In: *Proc. ARAV 1st Int Conference on Reptile and Amphibian Medicine*, Munich. Eds Öfner, S. and Weinzierl, F., pp. 3–13. March 4–7, 2010. Verlag Dr. Hut, 80538 München, Germany.

Baines, F., Chattell, J., Dale, J. *et al*. (2016). How much UV-B does my reptile need? The UV-Tool, a guide to the selection of UV lighting for reptiles and amphibians in captivity. *Journal of Zoo and Aquarium Research*, **4**(1), 42–63. Available online at: http://www.jzar.org/jzar/article/view/150

Baines, F.M. and Cusack, L. (2019). Environmental Lighting. (2019). In: *Mader's Reptile and Amphibian Medicine and Surgery*. Eds Divers, S.J. and Stahl, S.J., pp. 131–138. Elsevier, St. Louis, Missouri, USA.

Barnard, S.M. and Upton, S.J. (1994). *A Veterinary Guide to the Parasites of Reptiles, Vol 1: Protozoa*. Krieger, Florida.

Barrett, S.J., Schlater, L.K., Montali, R.J. *et al*. (1994). A new species of *Neisseria* from iguanid lizards, *Neisseria iguanae* sp. nov. *Letters in Applied Microbiology*, **18**, 200–202.

Bartlett, R.D. (1993). Comments on the *obsoleta*-complex rat snakes of Florida (with mention of three extralimital forms). *Tropical Fish Hobbyist*, **41**, 120–137.

Bellairs, A.d'A. (1981). Congenital and developmental diseases. In: *Diseases of the Reptilia*. Eds Cooper, J.E. and Jackson, O.F., pp. 469–485. Academic Press, London.

Bellairs, A. d'A and Bryant, S.V. (1985). Autotomy and regeneration in reptiles. In: *Biology of the Reptilia, Development B, volume 15*. Eds Gans, C. and Billett, F., pp. 301–410. John Wiley & Sons, New York.

Bertelsen, M.F. (2019). Anaesthesia and analgesia. In: *BSAVA Manual of Reptiles*, 3rd edn.. Eds Girling, S.J. and Raiti, D., pp. 200–209. British Small Animal Veterinary Association, Gloucester

Bertelsen, M.F., Crawshaw, G.J., Sigler, L. *et al*. (2005). Fatal cutaneous mycosis in tentacled snakes (*Erpeton tentaculatum*) caused by the *Chrysosporium* anamorph of *Nannizziopsis vriesii*. *Journal of Zoo and Wildlife Medicine*, **36**, 82–87.

Boyer, D.M. (2019). Special considerations for venomous reptiles. In: *BSAVA Manual of Reptiles*, 3rd edn. Eds Girling, S.J. and Raiti, D., pp. 482–487. British Small Animal Veterinary Association, Gloucester.

Boyer, T.H. and Scott, P.W. (2019). Nutritional Diseases In: *Mader's Reptile and Amphibian Medicine and Surgery*. Eds Divers S.J. and Stahl, S.J., pp. 932–950. Elsevier, St. Louis, Missouri, USA.

Burnham, B.R., Atchley, D.H., De Fusco, R.P. et al. (1998). Prevalence of fecal shedding of *Salmonella* organisms among captive green iguanas and potential public health implications. *Journal of the American Veterinary Medical Association*, **214**, 48–50.

Brearley, M.J., Cooper, J.E. and Sullivan, M. (1991). *Colour Atlas of Small Animal Endoscopy*. Mosby, London.

British Chelonia Group (undated) *Care Sheet: Mediterranean Tortoises Testudo graeca and T. hermanni*. British Chelonia Group, Chippenham. http://www.britishcheloniagroup.org.uk (Accessed 26 January 2009).

Brown, C. (2007). Blood sample collection in lizards. *Lab Animal Europe*, **36**, 23–24.

Brown, S.G., Gomes, F. and Miles, F.L. (1998). Faeces avoidance behaviour in unisexual and bisexual geckos. *Herpetological Journal*, **8**, 169–172.

Brown, S.J.L, Naylor, A.D, Machin, R.A. and Pellett, S. (2019). Gastrointestinal system. In: *BSAVA Manual of Reptiles*, 3rd edn. Eds Girling, S.J. and Raiti, D., pp. 284–308. British Small Animal Veterinary Association, Gloucester.

Burridge, M.J. (2001). Ticks (Acari: Ixodidae) spread by the international trade in reptiles and their potential roles in dissemination of diseases. *Bulletin of Entomological Research*, **91**, 3–23.

Cambre, R.C., Green, D.E., Smith, E.E. et al. (1980). Salmonellosis and Arizonosis in the reptile collection at the National Zoological Park. *Journal of the American Veterinary Medical Association*, **177**, 800–803.

Camus, M.S. and Yeuroukis, C.K. (2019). Cytology. In: *Mader's Reptile and Amphibian Medicine and Surgery*. Eds Divers, S.J. and Stahl, S.J., pp. 361–364. Elsevier, St. Louis, Missouri, USA.

Canadian Council on Animal Care (2003). *Guidelines on the Care and Use of Wildlife*. CCAC, Ottawa.

Carpenter, J.W. (2012). *Exotic Animal Formulary*, 4th edn. Elsevier Saunders, Philadelphia.

Cerreta, A.J., Lewbart, G.A., Diaz, R. et al. (2018). *Chelonoidis chathamensis*. Methods of body temperature assessment. *Herpetological Review*, **49**(4), 696–697.

Chang, L.W. and Jacobson, E.R. (2010). Inclusion body disease, a worldwide infectious disease of boid snakes: a review. *Journal of Exotic Pet Medicine*, **19**(3), 216–225.

Chang, L.W., Fu, D., Stenglein, M.D. et al. (2016). Detection and prevalence of boid inclusion body disease in collections of boas and pythons using immunological assays. *The Veterinary Journal*, **218**, 13–18.

Chiszar, D., Radcliffe, C.W., Boyer, T. et al. (1987). Cover-seeking behaviour in red spitting cobras (*Naja mossambica pallida*): effects of tactile cues and darkness. *Zoo Biology*, **6**, 161–167.

Chiszar, D., Smith, H.M. and Carpenter, C.C. (1994). An ethological approach to reproductive success in reptiles. In: *Captive Management and Conservation of Amphibians and Reptiles*. Eds Murphy, J.B., Adler, K. and Collins, J.T., pp. 147–173. Society for the Study of Amphibians and Reptiles, Ithaca, New York

Chiszar, D., Tomlinson, W.T., Smith, H.M. et al. (1995). Behavioural consequences of husbandry manipulations: indicators of arousal, quiescence and environmental awareness. In: *Health and Welfare of Captive Reptiles*. Eds Warwick, C., Frye, F.L. and Murphy, J.B., pp. 186–204. Chapman and Hall, London.

Chiszar, D., Wellborn, S., Wand, M.A. et al. (1980). Investigatory behaviour in snakes. II. Cage cleaning and the induction of defecation in snakes. *Animal Learning and Behaviour*, **8**, 505–510.

Clark, H.F. and Lunger, P.D. (1981). Viruses. In: *Diseases of the Reptilia*. Eds Cooper, J.E. and Jackson, O.F., pp. 136–164. Academic Press, London.

Clubb, R. and Mason, G. (2003). Captivity effects on wide-ranging carnivores. *Nature*, **425**, 473–474.

Cooper, J.E. (1973). Veterinary aspects of recently captured snakes. *British Journal of Herpetology*, **5**(11), 368–374.

Cooper, J.E. (1977). Diseases of lower vertebrates and biomedical research. *Laboratory Animals*, **11**, 119–123.

Cooper, J.E. (1989). Health monitoring and quality control of reptiles and amphibians kept for biomedical research. *Proceedings of the Third International Colloquium on the Pathology of Reptiles and Amphibians*, Florida, pp. 4–7.

Cooper, J.E. (1998). Minimally invasive health monitoring of wildlife. *Animal Welfare*, **7**, 35–44.

Cooper, J.E. (1999). Reptilian microbiology. In: *Laboratory Medicine. Avian and Exotic Pets*. Ed. Fudge, A.M., pp. 223–227. Saunders, Philadelphia.

Cooper, J.E. (2013a). What is fieldwork? In Field Techniques in Exotic Animal Medicine. *Journal of Exotic and Pet Medicine*, **22**(1), 7–16.

Cooper, J.E. (2013b). Editor. Field Techniques in Exotic Animal Medicine. *Journal of Exotic and Pet Medicine*, **22**(1).

Cooper, J.E. (2019). Euthanasia and *post-mortem* examination. In: *BSAVA Manual of Reptiles*, 3rd edn. Eds Girling, S.J. and Raiti, D., pp. 240–256. British Small Animal Veterinary Association, Gloucester.

Cooper, J.E. and Cooper, M.E. (2007). *Introduction to Veterinary and Comparative Forensic Medicine*. Blackwell Publishing, Oxford.

Cooper, J.E., Dutton, C.J. and Allchurch, A.F. (1998). Reference collections: their importance and relevance to modern zoo management and conservation biology. *Dodo*, **34**, 159–166.

Cooper, J.E., Dutton, C.J. and Belle, J. (2003). Exotic pets and wildlife. In: *Jones's Animal Nursing*. Eds Lane, D.R. and Cooper, B., pp. 265–308. Elsevier, Oxford.

Cooper, J.E., Ewbank, R. and Rosenberg, M.E. (1984). Euthanasia of tortoises. *Veterinary Record*, **115**, 635.

Cooper, J.E. and Jackson, O.F. (Eds) (1981). *Diseases of the Reptilia*. Academic Press, London.

Cooper, J.E. and Leakey, J.H.E. (1976). A septicaemic disease of East African snakes associated with enterobacteriaceae. *Transactions of the Royal Society of Tropical Medicine and Hygiene*, **70**, 80–84.

Cooper, J.E., McClelland, M.H. and Needham, J.R. (1980). An eye infection in laboratory lizards associated with an *Aeromonas* sp. *Laboratory Animals*, **14**, 149–151.

Cooper, J.E., Merck, M. and Cooper, M. E (2019). Forensics. In: *Mader's Reptile and Amphibian Medicine and Surgery*. Eds Divers, S.J. and Stahl, S.J., pp 1464–1475. Elsevier, St. Louis, Missouri, USA.

Cooper, J.E. and Nares, P. (1971). Clinical and *post-mortem* examination of snakes at the Nairobi Snake Park. *East African Wildlife Journal*, **9**, 166–170.

Cooper, J.E. and Sainsbury, A.W. (1994). Review: oral diseases of reptiles. *Herpetological Journal*, **4**, 117–125.

Cooper, J.E. and Seebaransingh, R. (2008). Fibropapillomatosis in a green turtle (*Chelonia mydas*) from Trinidad. *West Indian Veterinary Journal*, **8**, 77–80.

Cooper, J.E. and Williams, D.L. (1995). Veterinary perspectives and techniques in husbandry and research. In: *Health and Welfare of Captive Reptiles*. Eds Warwick, C., Frye, F.L. and Murphy, J.B., pp. 98–111. Chapman and Hall, London.

Cooper, J.E. and Williams, D.L. (2014). The feeding of live food to exotic pets: issues of welfare and ethics. *Journal of Exotic Pet Medicine*, **23**(**2014**), 244–249.

Cooper, M.E. (2013). Legal and ethical considerations of working in the field. *Journal of Exotic Pet Medicine*, **22**(1), 17–33.

Cooper, M.E. (2019). Laws and Regulations—International. In: *Mader's Reptile and Amphibian Medicine and Surgery*. Eds Divers, S.J. and Stahl, S.J., pp. 1447–1452. Elsevier, St. Louis, Missouri, USA.

Council of Europe (2006). Multilateral Consultation of Parties to the European Convention for the Protection of Vertebrate Animals used for Experimental and other Scientific Purposes (ETS 123)

Appendix A. *Cons 123 (2006) 3*. Available from URL: http://www.coe.int/t/e/legal_affairs/legal_co-operation/biological_safety,_use_of_animals/laboratory_animals/2006/Cons123(2006)3AppendixA_en.pdf (Accessed 31 July 2008).

Crews, D., Bergeron, J.M., Bull, J.J. et al. (1994). Temperature-dependent sex determination in reptiles: proximal mechanisms, ultimate outcomes, and practical applications. *Developmental Genetics*, **15**, 297–312.

Crews, D. and Gans, C. (1992). The interaction of hormones, brain and behavior: an emerging discipline in herpetology. In: *Biology of the Reptilia 18. Physiology E*. Eds Gans C. and Crews D., pp. 1–23. Chicago University Press, Chicago.

Davies, A.J. and Johnston, M.R.L. (2000). The biology of some intraerythrocytic parasites of fishes, amphibia and reptiles. *Advances in Parasitology*, **45**, 1–107.

Davies, R. and Knotek, S. (2019). Therapeutics and medication. In: *BSAVA Manual of Reptiles*, 3rd edn. Eds Girling, S.J. and Raiti, D., pp. 176–199. British Small Animal Veterinary Association, Gloucester.

Davis, P.M.C. (1981). Anatomy and physiology. In: *Diseases of the Reptilia*. Eds Cooper, J.E. and Jackson, O.F., pp. 9–73. Academic Press, London.

Deming, C., Greiner, E. and Uhl, E.W. (2008). Prevalence of *Cryptosporidium* infection and characteristics of oocyst shedding in a breeding colony of leopard geckos. (*Eublepharis macularius*). *Journal of Zoo and Wildlife Medicine*, **39**, 600–607.

Denardo, D. (2006). Stress in captive reptiles. In: *Reptile Medicine and Surgery*, 2nd edn. Ed. Mader, D.R., pp. 119–123. Saunders Elsevier, St. Louis, Missouri.

Divers, S.J. (1995). The green iguana (*Iguana iguana*): a guide to successful captive management. *British Herpetological Society Bulletin*, **51**, 7–26.

Divers, S.J. (2019). Surgery: principles and techniques. In: *BSAVA Manual of Reptiles*, 3rd edn. Eds Girling, S.J. and Raiti, D., pp. 210–239 British Small Animal Veterinary Association, Gloucester.

Divers, S.J. and Cooper, J.E. (2000). Reptile hepatic lipidosis. *Seminars in Avian and Exotic Pet Medicine*, **9**, 153–164.

Divers, S.J. and Stahl, S. (Eds) (2019). *Mader's Reptile and Amphibian Medicine and Surgery*, 3rd edn. Elsevier St. Louis, Missouri.

Doszpoly, A., Wellehan, J.F. Jr, Childress, A.L. et al. (2013). Partial characterization of a new adenovirus lineage discovered in testudinoid turtles. *Infection, Genetics and Evolution*, **17**, 106–112.

Duffus, A.L.J., Waltzek, T.B., Stöhr, A.C. et al. (2019). Natural behavior. In: *Mader's Reptile and Amphibian Medicine and Surgery*. Eds Divers, S.J. and Stahl, S.J., pp. 90–99. Elsevier, St. Louis, Missouri, USA.

Eason, P.K. and Stamps, J.A. (1991). The effect of visibility on territory size and shape. *Behavioural Ecology*, **3**, 166–172.

Edwards, J. (1991) It's just the beginning – my experience with Florida kingsnakes. *Snake Breeder*, **8**, 3–4.

Espinosa, R.E., Tracey, C.R. and Tracey, C.R. (1998). A safe single-application procedures for eradicating mites on reptiles. *Herpetological Review*, **29**, 35–36.

Ewert, M.A., Jackson, D.R. and Nelson, C.E. (1994). Patterns of temperature-dependent sex determination in turtles. *Journal of Experimental Zoology*, **270**, 3–15.

Ferguson, G.W. (1994). Old World chameleons in captivity: growth, maturity and reproduction of Malagasy *Chamaeleo pardalis*. In: *Captive Management and Conservation of Amphibians and Reptiles*. Eds Murphy, J.B., Adler, K. and Collins, J.T., pp. 323–331. Society for the Study of Amphibians and Reptiles, Ithaca, New York.

Ferguson, G., Brinker, A., Gehrmann, W. et al. (2010). Voluntary exposure of some Western-Hemisphere snake and lizard species to ultraviolet-B (UVB) radiation in the field: How much UVB should a lizard or snake receive in captivity? *Zoo Biology*, **29(3)**, 317–334.

Ferrell, S.T., Marlar, A.B., Alberts, A.C. et al. (2005). Surgical technique for permanent intracoelomic radiotransmitter placement in anegada iguanas (*Cyclura pinguis*). *Journal of Zoo and Wildlife Medicine*, **36**, 712–715.

Finke, M.D., Dunham, S.U. and Kwabi, C.A. (2005). Evaluation of four dry commercial gut loading products for improving the calcium content of crickets, *Acheta domesticus*. *Journal of Herpetological Medicine and Surgery*, **15**, 7–12.

Firth, B.T. and Turner, J.S. (1982). Sensory, neuronal and hormonal aspects of thermoregulation. In: *Biology of the Reptilia 12. Physiology C. Physiological Ecology*. Eds Gans, C. and Pough, F.M., pp. 213–274. Academic Press, London.

Fleishman, L.J., Loew, E.R. and Leal, M. (1993). Ultraviolet vision in lizards. *Nature*, **365**, 397.

Fleming, G.J., Isaza, R., Spire, M.F. et al. (2003). The use of digital thermography for environmental evaluation of reptile enclosures. *Journal of Herpetological Medicine and Surgery*, **13**, 38–42.

Foelsch, D.W. and Leloup, P. (1976). Fatale endemische Infektion in einem Serpentarium. *Tieraerztl Praxis*, **4**, 527–536.

Franklinos, L.H.V., Lorch, J.M., Bohuski, E. et al. (2017). Emerging fungal pathogen Ophidiomyces ophiodiicola in wild European snakes. *Scientific Reports*, **7(1)**, 3844.

Fry, B.G., Vidal, N., Norman, J.A. et al. (2006). Early evolution of the venom system in lizards and snakes. *Nature*, **439**, 584–588.

Frye, F.L. (1991). *Biomedical and Surgical Aspects of Captive Reptile Husbandry*. Krieger, Florida.

Frye, F.L. (1993). *Iguanas: A Guide to their Biology and Captive Care*. Krieger, Florida.

Frye, F.L. (1994). *Reptile Clinician's Handbook*. Krieger, Florida.

Frye, F.L. (1996). *A Practical Guide for Feeding Captive Reptiles*, 2nd edn. Krieger, Florida.

Gabrisch, K. and Zwart, P. (2015) *Krankheiten der Heimtiere*. Schlütersche, Hannover.

Gal, J., Dobos-Kovacs, M. and Sos, E. (2003). Nodular dermatitis of emerald swift (*Sceloporus malachiticus*) kept in captivity. *Magyar Allatorvosok Lapja*, **125**, 44–48.

Galeotti, P., Sacchi, R., Fasola, M. et al. (2005). Do mounting vocalizations in tortoises have a communication function? A comparative analysis. *Herpetological Journal*, **15**, 61–71.

Garcia-Morante, B., Pénzes, J.J., Costa, T. et al. (2016). Hyperplastic stomatitis and esophagitis in a tortoise (*Testudo graeca*) associated with an adenovirus infection. *Journal of Veterinary Diagnostic Investigation*, **28(5)**, 579–583.

Gavaud, J. (1991). Role of cryophase temperature and therophase duration in thermoperiodic regulation of the testicular cycle in the lizard *Lacerta vivipara*. *Journal of Experimental Zoology*, **260**, 239–246.

Germano, D.J., and Williams, D.F. (1993). Field evaluation of using passive integrated transponder (PIT) tags to permanently mark lizards. *Herpetological Review*, **24**, 54–56.

Girling, S.J. and Raiti, P. (Eds) (2019). *BSAVA Manual of Reptiles*, 3rd edn. British Small Animal Veterinary Association, Gloucester.

Gray, M.J. and Chinchar, V.G. (Eds) *Ranaviruses: Lethal Pathogens of Ectothermic Vertebrates*, pp. 9–58. Springer Open.

Greenacre, C., Paul-Murphy, J., Sladky, K.K. et al. (2005). Reptile and amphibian analgesia. *Journal of Herpetological Medicine and Surgery*, **15**, 24–29.

Greenberg, N. (1995). Ethologically informed design in husbandry and research. In: *Health and Welfare of Captive Reptiles*. Eds Warwick, C., Frye, F.L. and Murphy, J.B., pp. 239–262. Chapman and Hall, London.

Guillette, L.J., Cree, A. and Rooney, A.A. (1995). Biology of stress: interactions with reproduction, immunology and intermediary metabolism. In: *Health and Welfare of Captive Reptiles*. Eds Warwick, C., Frye, F.L. and Murphy, J.B., pp. 32–81. Chapman and Hall, London.

Hailey, A. (2000). Assessing body mass condition in the tortoise, *Testudo hermanni*. *Herpetological Journal*, **10**, 57–61.

Harling, R. (1993). Successfully keeping and breeding *Podarcis pityusensis* in indoor vivaria. *British Herpetological Society Bulletin*, **44**, 38–40.

Harling, R. (1994). The successful keeping and breeding of *Anolis carolinesis*. *British Herpetological Review*, **27**, 71–72.

Heatley, J.J. and Russell, K.E. (2019). Hematology. In: *Mader's Reptile and Amphibian Medicine and Surgery*. Eds Divers, S.J. and Stahl, S.J., pp. 301–318. Elsevier, St. Louis, Missouri, USA.

Hellebuyck, T., Martel, A., Chiers, K. et al. (2009). *Devriesea agamarum* causes dermatitis in bearded dragons (*Pogona vitticeps*). *Veterinary Microbiology*, **134**(3-4), 267–271.

Hetzel, U., Sironen, T., Laurinmäki, P. et al. (2013). Isolation, identification, and characterization of novel arenaviruses, the etiological agents of boid inclusion body disease. *Journal of Virology* 87, 10918–10935.

Hernandez-Divers, S.J. (2001). Clinical aspects of reptile behavior. *Veterinary Clinics of North America Exotic Animal Practice*, **4**, 599–612.

Hernandez-Divers, S.J., Cooper, J.E. and Cooke, S.W. (2004a). Diagnostic techniques and sample collection in reptiles. *Compendium on Continuing Education of the Practicing Veterinarian*, **26**, 470–483.

Hernandez-Divers, S.J., Stahls, Hernandez-Divers, S.M. et al. (2004b). Coelomic endoscopy of the green iguana (*Iguana iguana*). *Journal of Herpetological Medicine and Surgery*, **14**, 10–18.

Hoon-Hanks, L.L., Layton, M.L., Ossiboff, R.J. et al. (2018). Respiratory disease in ball pythons (*Python regius*) experimentally infected with ball python nidovirus. *Virology*, **517**, 77–87.

Huey, R.B. (1982). Temperature, physiology and ecology of reptiles. In: *Biology of the Reptilia 12. Physiology C Physiological Ecology*. Eds Gans, C. and Pough, F.H., pp. 25–91. Academic Press, London.

Hyndman, T.H., Shilton, C.M. and Marschang, R.E. (2013). Paramyxoviruses in reptiles: a review. *Veterinary Microbiology*, **165**(3-4), 200–213.

Jackson, O.F. (1991). Reptiles. Part 1. Chelonians. In: *Manual of Exotic Pets*. Eds Beynon, P.H. and Cooper, J.E., pp. 221–243. British Small Animal Veterinary Association, Cheltenham.

Jackson, D.C. (2002). Hibernating without oxygen: physiological adaptations of the painted turtle, *Chrysemys picta*. *Journal of Physiology*, **543**, 731–737.

Jacobson, E.R. (2003). *Biology, Husbandry and Medicine of the Green Iguana*. Krieger, Melbourne, Florida.

Jacobson, E.R. (2007). *Infectious Diseases and Pathology of Reptiles*. Taylor and Francis, New York.

Jacobson, E.R., Brown, M.B., Wendland, L.D. et al. (2014). Mycoplasmosis and upper respiratory tract disease of tortoises: A review and update. *The Veterinary Journal*, **201**, 257–264.

Jacobson, E.R., Origgi, F., Pessier, A.P. et al. (2001). Paramyxovirus infection in caiman lizards (*Dracaena guianensis*). *Journal of Veterinary Diagnostic Investigation*, **13**, 143–151.

Johnson, R. (2019). Venomous species. In: *Mader's Reptile and Amphibian Medicine and Surgery*. Eds Divers, S.J. and Stahl, S.J., pp. 162–167. Elsevier, St. Louis, Missouri, USA.

Johnson-Delaney, C.A. and Gal, J. (2019). Reptile zoonoses and threats to public health. In: *Mader's Reptile and Amphibian Medicine and Surgery*. Eds Divers, S.J. and Stahl, S.J., pp. 1359–1365. Elsevier, St. Louis, Missouri, USA.

Josseaume, B. (2002). Faecal collector for field studies of digestive responses in forest tortoises. *Herpetological Journal*, **12**, 169–172.

Julian, A.F. and Durham, P.J.K. (1982). Adenoviral hepatitis in a female bearded dragon (*Amphibolurus barbatus*). *New Zealand Veterinary Journal*, **30**, 59–60.

Just, F., Essbauer, S., Ahne, W. et al. (2001). Occurrence of an invertebrate iridescent-like virus (Iridoviridae) in reptiles. *Journal of Veterinary Medicine. Series B*, **48**, 685–694.

Keymer, I.F. (1981). Protozoa. In: *Diseases of the Reptilia*. Eds Cooper, J.E. and Jackson, O.F., pp. 235–290. Academic Press, London.

Kirkwood, J.K. and Gili, C. (1994) Food consumption in relation to bodymass in some snakes in captivity. *Research in Veterinary Science*, **57**, 35–38.

Kreger, M.D. and Mench, J.A. (1993). Physiological and behavioral effects of handling and restraint in the ball python (*Python regius*) and the blue-tongued skink (*Tiliqua scincoides*). *Applied Animal Behaviour Science*, **38**, 323–336.

Lance, V.A. (1994). Environmental sex determination in reptiles: pattern and process. *Journal of Experimental Zoology*, **270**, 1–127.

Lang, M. (1992). A review of techniques for marking snakes. *Smithsonian Herpetological Information Service*, **90**, 1–19.

Lang, J.W. and Andrews, H.V. (1994). Temperature-dependent sex determination in crocodilians. *Journal of Experimental Zoology*, **270**, 28–44.

Langerwerf, B.A.W.A. (1990). The successful breeding of lizards from temperate regions. In: *Care and Breeding of Captive Reptiles*. Eds Townson, S., Millichamp, N.J., Lucas, D.G.D. et al., pp. 20–35. British Herpetological Society, London.

Langerwerf, B.A.W.A. (1991). A large scale lizard breeding facility in Alabama. *British Herpetological Society Bulletin*, **36**, 43–46.

Locke, B. (2008). Venomous snake restraint and handling. *Journal of Exotic Pet Medicine*, **17**, 273–284.

Lorch, J.M., Knowles, S., Lankton, J.S. et al. (2016). Snake fungal disease: an emerging threat to wild snakes. *Philosophical Transactions of the Royal Society of London B Biological Sciences*, **5**, 371(1709).

Maderson, P.F.A. (1965). Histological changes in the epidermis of snakes during the sloughing cycle. *Journal of Zoology, London*, **146**, 98–113.

Marschang, R.E (2011). Viruses infection reptiles. *Viruses*, **3**(11), 2087–2126.

Marschang, R.E. (2019). Virology. In: *Mader's Reptile and Amphibian Medicine and Surgery*. Eds Divers, S.J. and Stahl, S.J., pp. 247–269. Elsevier, St. Louis, Missouri, USA.

Marschang, R.E., Donahoe, S., Manvell, R. et al. (2002). Paramyxovirus and reovirus infections in wild-caught Mexican lizards (*Xenosaurus* and *Abronia* spp.). *Journal of Zoo and Wildlife Medicine*, **33**, 317–321.

Mason, R.T. (1992). Reptilian pheromones. In: *Biology of the Reptilia 18. Physiology E Hormones, Brain and Behavior*. Eds Gans, C. and Crews, D., pp. 114–128. Chicago University Press, Chicago.

Mason, G. and Rushen, J. (2006). *Stereotypic Animal Behaviour: Fundamentals and Applications to Welfare*, 2nd edn. CAB International, Wallingford.

McArthur, S.D., Wilkinson, R.J. and Meyer, J. (2004). *Medicine and Surgery of Tortoises and Turtles*. Blackwell Publishing, Oxford.

McBride, M. and Hernandez-Divers, S.J. (2004). Nursing care of lizards. *Veterinary Clinics of North American Exotic Animal Practice*, **7**, 375–396.

Meek, R. and Avery, R.A. (1988). Thermoregulation in chelonians. *Herpetological Journal*, **1**, 253–259.

Meerovitch, E. (1958). Some biological requirements on host–parasite relations of *Entamoeba invadens*. *Canadian Journal of Zoology*, **36**, 513–523.

Meerovitch, E. (1961). Infectivity and pathogenicity of polyxenic and monoxenic *Entamoeba invadens* to snakes kept at normal and high temperatures and natural history of reptile amoebiasis. *Journal of Parasitology*, **47**, 791–794.

Mendyk, R.W. (2015). Preliminary notes on the use of the predatory soil mite *Stratiolaelaps scimitus* (Acari: Laelapidae) as a biological control agent for acariasis in lizards. *Journal of Herpetological Medicine and Surgery*, **25**(1-2), 24–27.

Mitchell, M. (2003). Ophidia (snakes). In: *Zoo and Wild Animal Medicine*, 5th edn. Eds Fowler, M.E. and Miller, R.E., pp. 82–93. Saunders, St Louis.

Mitchell, M.A. (2004). Snake care and husbandry. *Veterinary Clinics of North America Exotic Animal Practice*, **7**, 42–446.

Moore, M.C. and Lindsey, J. (1992). The physiological basis of behavior in male reptiles. In: *Biology of the Reptilia 18. Physiology E*. Eds Gans C. and Crews D., pp. 70–113. Chicago University Press, Chicago.

Morton, D.B. and Griffiths, P.H. (1985). Guidelines on the recognition of pain, distress and discomfort in experimental animals and an hypothesis for assessment. *Veterinary Record*, **116**, 431–436.

Nichols, D.K., Weyant, R.S., Lamirande, E.W. et al. (1999). Fatal mycotic dermatitis in captive brown tree snakes (*Boiga irregularis*). *Journal of Zoo and Wildlife Medicine*, **30**, 111–118.

Norton, T.M. (2005). Chelonian emergency and critical care. *Seminars in Avian and Exotic Pet Medicine*, **14**, 106–130.

O'Dea, M.A., Jackson, B., Jackson, C. et al. (2016) Discovery and partial genomic characterisation of a novel Nidovirus associated with respiratory disease in wild shingleback lizards (*Tiliqua rugosa*). *PLoS One*, **11**(11), e0165209.

Onderka, D.K. and Finlayson, M.C. (1985). Salmonellae and salmonellosis in captive reptiles. *Canadian Journal of Comparative Medicine*, **49**, 268–270.

O'Rourke, D.P., Nowlan, P. and Retnam, L. (2019). Laboratory Management and Medicine. In: *Mader's Reptile and Amphibian Medicine and Surgery*. Eds Divers, S.J. and Stahl, S.J., pp. 1414–1420. Elsevier, St. Louis, Missouri, USA.

Packard, G.C. and Phillips, J.A. (1994). The importance of the physical environment for the incubation of reptile eggs. In: *Captive Management and Conservation of Amphibians and Reptiles*. Eds Murphy, J.B., Adler, K. and Collins, J.T., pp. 195–208. Society for the Study of Amphibians and Reptiles, Ithaca, New York.

Peterson, C.R., Gibson, A.R. and Dorcas, M.E. (1993). Snake thermal ecology: the causes and consequences of body-temperature variation. In: *Snakes: Ecology and Behavior*. Eds Seigel, R.A. and Collins, J.T., pp. 241–314. McGraw-Hill, New York.

Plowman, C.A., Montali, R.J. Phillips, L.G. et al. (1987). Septicemia and chronic abscesses in iguanas (*Cyclura cornuta* and *Iguana iguana*) associated with a *Neisseria* species. *Journal of Zoo Animal Medicine*, **18**, 86–93.

Pough, F.H. and Gans, C. (1982). The vocabulary of reptilian thermoregulation. In: *Biology of the Reptilia 12. Physiology C Physiological Ecology*. Eds Gans, C. and Crews, D., pp. 17–23. Academic Press, London.

Raiti, P. (2019). Non-invasive imaging. In: *BSAVA Manual of Reptiles*, 3rd edn. Eds Girling, S.J. and Raiti, D., pp. 134–159. British Small Animal Veterinary Association, Gloucester.

Ramos, A.B., Don, M.T. and Muchlinski, A.E. (1993). The effect of bacteria infection on mean selected body temperature in the common agama, *Agama agama*: a dose-response study. *Comparative Biochemistry and Physiology A*, **105**, 479–484.

Raphael, B.L. (2003). Chelonians (turtles, tortoises). In: *Zoo and Wild Animal Medicine*, 5th edn. Eds Fowler, M.E. and Miller, R.E., pp. 48–58. Saunders, St Louis.

Raske, M., Lewbart, G., Dombrowski, D. et al. (2012). Body temperatures of selected amphibian and reptile species. *Journal of Zoo and Wildlife Medicine*, **43**(3), 517–521.

Rayment-Dyble, L. (2019). Reptile pet trade and welfare. In: *BSAVA Manual of Reptiles*, 3rd edn. Eds Girling, S.J. and Raiti, D., pp. 26–35. British Small Animal Veterinary Association, Gloucester.

Redrobe, S. (2002). Reptiles and disease – keeping the risks to a minimum. *Journal of Small Animal Practice*, **43**, 471–472.

Reichenbach-Klinke, H. and Elkan, E. (1965). *The Principal Diseases of Lower Vertebrates*. Academic Press, London.

Reiner, A.J. (1992). Neuropeptides in the nervous system. In: *Biology of the Reptilia 17. Neurology C*. Eds Gans, C. and Ulinski, P.S., pp. 587–739. Chicago University Press, Chicago.

Reinhardt, V. and Kreger, M.D. (2002). Laboratory housing of reptiles and amphibians. In: *Comfortable Quarters for Laboratory Animals*. Ed Reinhardt, V. Animal Welfare Institute.

Rendle, M. (2019). Nutrition. In: *BSAVA Manual of Reptiles*, 3rd edn. Eds Girling, S.J. and Raiti, D., pp. 49–69. British Small Animal Veterinary Association, Gloucester.

Rendle, M. and Calvert, I. (2019). Nutritional problems. In: *BSAVA Manual of Reptiles*, 3rd edn. Eds Girling, S.J. and Raiti, D., pp. 365–396. British Small Animal Veterinary Association, Gloucester.

Rivera, S., Wellehan, J.F. Jr., McManamon, R. et al. (2009). Systemic adenovirus infection in Sulawesi tortoises (*Indotestudo forstenii*) caused by a novel siadenovirus. *Journal of Veterinary Diagnostic Investigation* **21**(4), 415–426.

Roitberg, E.S. and Smirina, E.M. (2006). Age, body size and growth of *Lacerta agilis boemica* and *L. strigata*: a comparative study of two closely related lizard species based on skeleton-chronology. *Herpetological Journal*, **16**, 133–148.

Rose, T.A. (1992). Husbandry and successful breeding of the New Guinea blue-tongued skink. *Association for the Study of Reptiles and Amphibians Monograph*, **2**, 22–28.

Rosenberg, M.E. (1972). Excitation and inhibition of motorneurones in the tortoise. *Journal of Physiology*, **221**, 715–730.

Sheriff, D. (1988). The inland bearded dragon, *Pogona vitticeps*, and its maintenance and breeding in captivity. *Royal Zoological Society of Scotland Annual Report*, **76**, 49–55.

Schieffelin, C.D. and de Queiroz, A. (1991). Temperature and defense in the common garter snake: warm snakes are more aggressive than cold snakes. *Herpetologica*, **47**, 230–237.

Schilliger, L.H., Morel, D., Bonwitt, J.H. and Marquis, O. (2013). *Cheyletus eruditus* (Taurrus): an effective candidate for the biological control of the snake mite (*Ophionyssus natricis*). *Journal of Zoo and Wildlife Medicine*, **44**(3), 654–659.

Schumacher, J. (2003). Lacertilia (lizards, skinks, geckos) and amphisbaenids (worm lizards). In: *Zoo and Wild Animal Medicine*, 5th edn. Eds Fowler, M.E. and Miller, R.E., pp. 73–81. Saunders, St Louis, Missouri

Skurski, M.L, Fleming, G.J., Daneault, A. and Pye, G.W. (2019). Behavioral training and enrichment of reptiles In: *Mader's Reptile and Amphibian Medicine and Surgery*. Eds Divers S.J. and Stahl, S.J., pp. 100–104. Elsevier, St. Louis, Missouri, USA.

Soldati, G., Lu, Z.H., Vaughan, L. et al. (2004). Detection of Mycobacteria and Chlamydiae in granulomatous inflammation of reptiles: a retrospective study. *Veterinary Pathology*, **41**, 388–397.

Stenglein, M.D., Sanders, C., Kistler, A.L. et al. (2012). Identification, characterization, and in vitro culture of highly divergent arenaviruses from boa constrictors and annulated tree boas: candidate etiological agents for snake inclusion body disease. *MBio*, **3**, e00180-12.

Stenglein, M.D., Jacobson, E.R., Wozniak, E.J. et al. (2014). Ball python nidovirus: a candidate etiologic agent for severe respiratory disease in *Python regius*. *MBio*, **5**, e01484-14.

Stenglein, M.D., Sanchez-Migallon, Guzman, D., Garcia, V.E. et al. (2017). Differential disease susceptibilities in experimentally Reptarenavirus-Infected boa constrictors and ball pythons. *Journal of Virology*, **91**, e00451-17.

Sweeney, R. (1993). *Garter Snakes: Their Natural History and Care in Captivity*. Blandford, London.

Thomas, O., Kane, D. and Michaels, C.J. (2019). Effects of different heat sources on the behaviour of blue tree monitors (*Varanus macraei*). *The Herpetological Bulletin*, **149**, 41–43.

Thorogood, J. and Whimster, I.W. (1979). The maintenance and breeding of the leopard gecko, *Eublepharis macularius*, as a laboratory animal. *International Zoo Yearbook*, **19**, 74–78.

Townson, S. (1994). *Breeding Reptiles and Amphibians*. British Herpetological Society, London.

Troyer, K. (1982). Transfer of fermentative microbes between generations of a herbivorous lizard. *Science*, **216**, 540–542.

Tucunduva, M., Borelli, P. and Silva, J.R.M.C. (2001). Experimental study of induced inflammation in the Brazilian boa (*Boa constrictor constrictor*). *Journal of Comparative Pathology*, **125**, 174–181.

UFAW/WSPA (1989). *Euthanasia of Amphibians and Reptiles*. Report of a Joint UFAW/WSPA Working Party UFAW, Potters Bar/WSPA, London.

Underwood, H. (1992). Endogenous rhythms. In: *Biology of the Reptilia 18. Physiology E*. Eds Gans C. and Crews D., pp. 229–297. Chicago University Press, Chicago.

Varga, M. (2019). Captive maintenance. In: *BSAVA Manual of Reptiles*, 3rd edn. Eds Girling, S.J. and Raiti, D., pp. 36–48. British Small Animal Veterinary Association, Gloucester.

Viets, B.E., Ewert, M.A., Talent, L.G. et al. (1994). Sex-determining mechanisms in squamate reptiles. *Journal of Experimental Zoology*, **270**, 45–56.

Warwick, C., Frye, F.L. and Murphy, J.B. (1995). *Health and Welfare of Captive Reptiles*. Chapman and Hall, London.

Warwick, C., Arena, P, Lindley, S. et al. (2013). Assessing reptile welfare using behavioural criteria. *In Practice*, **35**(3), 123–131.

Wellehan, J.F.X., and Divers (2019a). Bacteriology. In: *Mader's Reptile and Amphibian Medicine and Surgery*. Eds Divers, S.J., Stahl, S.J., pp. 235–246. Elsevier, St. Louis, Missouri, USA.

Wellehan, J.F.X., and Divers (2019b). Mycology. Divers SJ, Stahl SJ Eds *Mader's Reptile and Amphibian Medicine and Surgery*. Elsevier, St. Louis, Missouri, USA. Pp. 270–280.

Wellehan, J. and Walden, H.D.S. (2019). Parasitology (Including Hemoparasites). In: *Mader's Reptile and Amphibian Medicine and Surgery*. Eds Divers, S.J. and Stahl, S.J., pp. 281–300. Elsevier, St. Louis, Missouri, USA.

Wellehan, J.F.X., Johnson, A.J., Harrach, B. et al. (2004). Detection and analysis of six lizard adenoviruses by consensus primer PCR provides further evidence of a reptilian origin for the atadenoviruses. *Journal of Virology*, **78**, 13366–13369.

Willemser, R.E. and Hailey, A. (2002). Body mass condition in Greek tortoises: regional and interspecific variation. *Herpetological Journal*, **12**, 105–114.

Wisniewski, P.J. (1992). Maintenance and breeding of some lizards from arid areas under laboratory conditions. *Association for the Study of Reptiles and Amphibians Monograph*, **2**, 49–53.

Woodford, M.H. (2001). *Quarantine and Health Screening Protocols for Wildlife prior to Translocating and Release into the Wild*. OIE, Paris.

Wright, K.M. and Raiti, D (2019). Breeding and neonatal care. In: *BSAVA Manual of Reptiles*, 3rd edn. Eds Girling, S.J. and Raiti, D., pp. 70–88. British Small Animal Veterinary Association, Gloucester.

WSPA (1994). *Pain Assessment and Euthanasia of Ectotherms*. Scientific Advisory Panel Report 09/90, revised 02/94. World Society for the Protection of Animals, London.

Xavier, G., Winne, C. and Fedewa, L. (2006). Ontogeny of anti-predator behavioural habituation in cottonmouths. *Ethology*, **112**, 608–615.

Young, L.A., Schumacher, J., Papich, M.G. and Jacobson, E.R. (1997). Disposition of enrofloxacin and its metabolite ciprofloxacin after intramuscular injection in juvenile Burmese pythons (*Python molurus bivittatus*). *Journal of Zoo and Wildlife Medicine*, **28**, 71–79.

Zhang, J., Finlaison, D.S., Frost, M.J. et al. (2018). Identification of a novel nidovirus as a potential cause of large scale mortalities in the endangered Bellinger River snapping turtle (*Myuchelys georgesi*). *PLoS One*, **13**(10), e0205209.

Other sources of information

Herpetological societies exist in many countries of the world. Most publish newsletters, members' information sheets, journals or bulletins, often in different languages and many have their own websites.

The British Chelonia Group produces *Care Sheets* relating to most of the species of terrestrial chelonians likely to be found in captivity. These are obtainable from the British Chelonian Group[11].

Journals published in English (and, where appropriate, the associations that publish them) that are of particular relevance to the care and use of reptiles include the *Herpetological Journal* (British Herpetological Society), *Applied Herpetology*, *Copeia* (American Society of Ichthyologists and Herpetologists), *Herpetological Review* (American Society of Ichthyologists and Herpetologists) and *Journal of Herpetological Medicine and Surgery* (Association of Amphibian and Reptilian Veterinarians (ARAV)).

There are numerous websites that provide advice on the care of reptiles in captivity. Some but not all of the information given is sound. Some websites refer to legislation that affects the keeping and use of reptiles.

---

[11] http://www.britishcheloniagroup.org.uk/

47 An amphibian 'laboratory model', *Xenopus*

Richard Tinsley

Biological overview

As their name suggests, amphibians are adapted to life in two environments: in water and on land. They evolved from fish, and their descendants gave rise to the reptiles, birds and mammals. While they have characteristics typical of all tetrapod vertebrates (including the pentadactyl limb), they also have specialisations that are unique among tetrapods (including use of the skin as a respiratory surface). The life history of amphibians is also exceptional because development (ontogeny) recapitulates evolution (phylogeny): the tadpole is fish-like and transforms into a fundamentally terrestrial tetrapod juvenile. This metamorphosis is unique among vertebrates: the juvenile stage is redesigned and reconstructed from the components that made up the larva.

Amphibians arose in the late Devonian period, 380–360 million years ago (mya), and radiated in the Carboniferous, Permian and Triassic leading to great diversity and a worldwide distribution during a period of around 120 million years. However, all these lines became extinct and present-day amphibians, the Lissamphibia, appear first in the Triassic and diversify in the Jurassic. There is no overlap in the fossil record between the extinct groups that represented 'The Age of the Amphibians' and the ancestors of modern taxa. The precise origins of present-day amphibians are uncertain; their earliest fossils are morphologically similar to modern representatives. Thus, the Pipidae (the family including *Xenopus*) has fossils in the Cretaceous (125 mya) resembling current species. The major diversification of anurans is relatively recent with genera such as *Bufo* appearing in the Paleocene (60 mya) and *Rana* in the Eocene (50 mya). This evolution is roughly contemporaneous with that of the mammals.

There are three orders of lissamphibians. Apoda (alternatively called Caecilia or Gymnophiona) comprise about 213 species. Urodela (alternatively called Caudata) – newts and salamanders – comprise about 737 species. Anura (or Salientia or Batrachia) – frogs and toads – have about 7140 species (Stuart *et al.* 2008; Amphibiaweb 2019). They are easily distinguished: apodans have no limbs or limb girdles and are worm-like, burrowing in tropical soils; urodeles have a long tail and limbs more or less equal in length; anurans have a very short vertebral column, no tail, and hindlimbs typically longer than forelimbs, adapted for jumping.

The skin of amphibians acts as a respiratory surface (in addition, in most species, to the lungs and buccal cavity). It is delicate, kept moist by extensive mucus secretion, highly permeable and well supplied with blood vessels. Water can be absorbed rapidly through the skin but most amphibians on land lose water by continuous evaporation. The kidneys cannot concentrate urine to conserve water; nitrogenous wastes are eliminated primarily as urea (or ammonia) in very dilute urine. These features preclude measures to restrict water loss and most amphibians are confined to damp environments. The urinary bladder serves as an important water store: this water can be resorbed into the body during dehydration (a process impossible in higher tetrapods).

Skin pigmentation has an important role in defence, providing either camouflage or, conversely, warning coloration to deter predators. Skin secretions include highly toxic compounds and also a great diversity of peptides that have antimicrobial properties.

Amphibians are ectothermic, with body temperature dependent on the external environment, but they regulate temperature both behaviourally and by evaporative cooling. At very low temperatures, amphibians enter a state of torpor: they seek refuges, their metabolic rate slows and food intake stops.

Most but not all amphibians return to water to breed. The larval (tadpole) stage has a wide range of food types including vegetation, microscopic particles and aquatic prey. After metamorphosis, most amphibians are carnivorous, feeding primarily on small invertebrates. With some exceptions, prey capture occurs on land involving terrestrial and aerial targets for which vision is the predominant sense: movement triggers a feeding response. There is typically no overlap in food types (and hence competition) between tadpoles (in water) and juveniles and adults (on land).

Over the past 30 years, there have been worldwide reports of declining amphibian populations – at least 43% of the world's species declining and about one-third (32%) classified as threatened. Habitat loss represents the greatest threat, followed by pollution. Disease caused by the chytrid fungus *Batrachochytrium dendrobatidis* and *Ranavirus* has been responsible for dramatic population declines. In addition, many species are declining for unknown reasons (Stuart *et al.* 2008; IUCN 2019).

The use of amphibians in research

Amphibians have a long history of use in research. Major advances in fundamental knowledge of physiology and biochemistry were first made on amphibians, with studies subsequently including embryology and endocrinology, genetics and immunology. Over the past 50 years, *Xenopus laevis* has been one of the most intensively used of all 'laboratory animals' (alongside the mouse and chick) in developmental, cell and molecular biology (Gurdon 1996) (although Zebrafish now have greater use). *Xenopus tropicalis* was the first vertebrate to be cloned and the first amphibian to have its genome sequenced. Other recent interest has focused on amphibian skin peptides for their antibiotic properties and applications in anti-cancer treatment.

European Directive 2010/63, together with wildlife legislation in member countries, has created a major change in research use of amphibians. Laboratory work on animals caught in the natural environment is no longer permitted (with very few exceptions) and is restricted to animals specifically bred for research, supplied by recognized establishments. The need for this change was highlighted in Tinsley (2010).

Amphibians are maintained in the laboratory to meet a series of needs.

1. A reference collection for a species, including captive breeding programmes. Animals may be originally wild-caught (including those rescued from threatened habitats) or derived from captive breeding, and are maintained for conservation, research and education. Typically, the appropriate husbandry is that employed in zoos and conservation institutions aiming for long-term survival and reproduction in near-natural conditions.
2. For research on the animals themselves including: behaviour, sensory perception, physiology, response to infection. Such research requires animals in an optimum state with respect to 'whole body' condition, energy and other reserves, and natural reactions to environmental stimuli. Time scales for maintenance may relate to the period of a research project rather than 'long-term'.
3. For research involving products of the animals (especially eggs). Here, the requirement for performance is among the most demanding. The quality of eggs required for molecular and developmental biology may gradually become unsatisfactory even from animals apparently in good health. The timescale for maintenance of individual animals may involve repeated use (e.g., oöcyte removals) but is terminated when performance deteriorates.

These different uses may also be distinguished in terms of increasing scale, from relatively small numbers for [1] to many hundreds for [3] requiring a 'rolling population' available for use on demand.

General considerations for the husbandry of amphibians

Given the range of species kept for different purposes and with very different needs, it is not possible to provide detailed guidance for all. This section outlines some general points but more detailed information can be found in AmphibianArk (2019). Ideally, all purposes should be met by maintenance in one set of conditions known to ensure optimum physiological state, life span and well-being for a species. In practice, these conditions have often not been established empirically.

Some husbandry handbooks that address the needs of mesic amphibians (including *Rana*, *Bufo*, *Triturus* species) recommend a solid substrate (glass, plastic, metal, ceramic tiles) and a continuous flow of water, designed to wash away faecal material. These conditions are optimal for observation, but not for well-being. Provision of live prey (crickets, mealworms, etc.) may be ineffective if these become trapped in water and die. Light levels are often too high, and frogs may huddle together creating a risk of skin damage from urination. Laboratory aquarium design and size must avoid circumstances where natural escape responses will result in collision with tank walls, etc.

For many urodeles, caecilians and 'amphibious' anurans, maintained at relatively small scale for conservation, research and education ([1] in the preceding text), it is most effective to reproduce environmental conditions closely matching natural habitats. Despite their ecological diversity, most amphibians occur in habitats providing cover, concealment from predators, relatively high humidity, and protection from dehydration and major temperature fluctuations. Most activity is nocturnal, corresponding with greatest availability of terrestrial invertebrate prey. Populations are often established near water bodies and a common startle response by a frog on land is to leap into water. These characteristics should guide the provision of laboratory accommodation. Depending on species, maintenance conditions should provide choice between areas with water and 'land'; the choice of substrate (including damp sterilised soil, seedling compost or other specialised media) depends on the species, humidity/pH and hygiene requirements. The surface layer should be replaced, generally at weekly intervals. Active live food is needed to stimulate recognition but choice of food type should take account of behaviour: for instance, urodeles typically react slowly to prey organisms whereas anurans respond with a rapid 'snap'. Refuges provide concealment and increased humidity (in 'caves', under vegetation, etc.), but conditions must allow for inspection to check well-being.

While semi-natural conditions represent the best approach to maintenance of mesic amphibians, the previous edition of this Handbook (Tinsley 2010a) included an unusual example of an anuran adapted to xeric conditions. The purpose of this was to show that successful husbandry procedures can be devised even for species with highly specialised requirements but these rely on detailed knowledge of ecology, physiology and behaviour 'in the wild'. The aim was also to show that husbandry may require an unorthodox approach but the principles may be adapted for other amphibians (see also Michaels *et al.* 2014). Spadefoot toads, *Scaphiopus couchii*, occur in the southwestern deserts of North America. They escape the most arid conditions buried below the desert surface for over 10 months each year; during this, they do not feed but rely on stored energy reserves. Emergence is triggered by torrential summer rainfall; the toads spawn in newly formed ponds and then feed intensively on desert invertebrates, typically on a maximum of 20 nights each year, before returning to hibernation as drought increases. One of the challenges for laboratory maintenance is to ensure that feeding for a few weeks provides reserves for the following 11 months (details in Tocque et al. 1995, Tinsley 1999). Toads cannot be fed simply by providing live prey (crickets, mealworms) on the soil surface during darkness: they remain buried. However, they adapt readily to being removed gently from the soil, isolated in bare aquarium tanks and given prey in daylight: they respond immediately, despite unnatural conditions, feed to satiation within an hour and can then be returned to soil.

Procedures involving individual maintenance allow detailed records of body weight gain, food intake, etc. (with uneaten prey items weighed and subtracted from the weight initially offered). Tocque et al. (1995) showed that body weight increased in proportion to weight of food ingested. Toads given 24 meals could eat a total weight of food equivalent to twice their original body weight, increasing in weight by around 100%. The nutritional quality of food significantly influenced body weight gain and fat body accumulation: toads amassed large fat reserves (up to 14% of their body weight) when fed with lipid-rich mealworms compared with those fed crickets (fat bodies up to 10% toad body weight). However, while ensuring energetic needs for hibernation, a lipid-rich diet does not achieve good growth (including bone formation). For this, crickets should be fed on a high-protein diet and dusted with mineral and vitamin supplements. These procedures can be useful for other anuran species. Thus, feeding animals individually avoids within-group competition and provides records of food intake and body weight change; in turn, knowledge of individual weight gain gives assurance of adequate energy reserves for performance in research (Figure 47.1).

A case study for detailed review: the husbandry of *Xenopus* species

The major focus of this chapter on the husbandry of *Xenopus* reflects an exceptional need in laboratory animal welfare. For most laboratory animals, there are standardised procedures for maintenance, specifying preferred accommodation, temperature, diet, etc. These are recognised as ensuring optimum conditions for growth, development and well-being. By contrast, while *Xenopus* is one of the most intensively used laboratory animals, there is no consensus on how it should be maintained and there have been no experimentally proven tests to guide protocols. This deficiency has been highlighted repeatedly in the literature. Major and Wassersug (1998) surveyed husbandry practices in 'Xenopus laboratories' and found wide variation and little agreement in methods employed. They emphasised the pressing need for experimental evidence to support decisions. Twenty-five years later, this need still exists and represents a major anomaly in laboratory animal welfare.

The following sections review current knowledge relevant to laboratory maintenance of *Xenopus*. For some key protocols, published recommendations are contradictory (e.g., whether *Xenopus* should be maintained in aquaria with or without refuges, in hard or soft water, in recirculating systems or static tanks). The few attempts to test alternative regimes have flaws in design, measurement and/or statistical analysis (see the following text). Therefore, an approach has been taken here to provide *discussion* of potential effects of a series of factors influencing welfare. For some published accounts, the evidence is examined critically so that readers can judge the basis for conclusions.

Without proven experimental evidence for husbandry recommendations, the present review is inevitably phrased as 'in the view of the present author'. The strength of this approach relies on fieldwork observations on the ecology and behaviour of *Xenopus* in east, west and southern Africa and on introduced populations in Europe and the USA. These observations (during over 50 years) are also supported by experience of maintaining a dozen species of *Xenopus* in the laboratory (Figure 47.2).

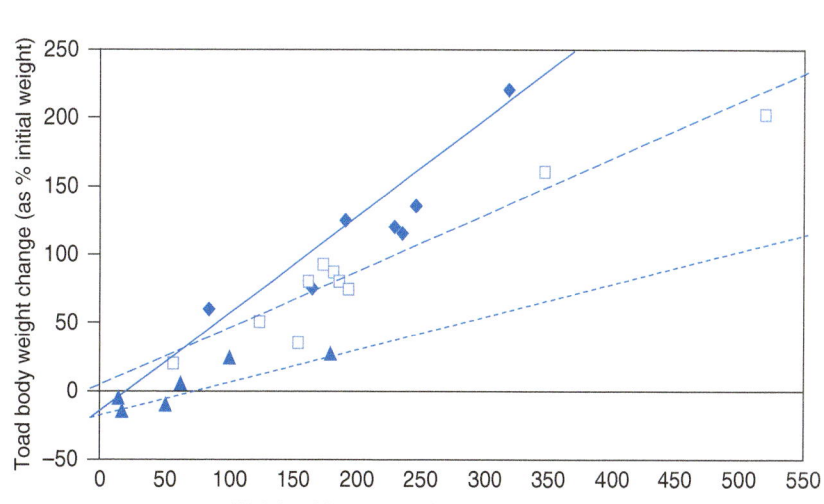

Figure 47.1 Laboratory experimental data showing the exceptional capacity of *Scaphiopus couchii* to convert food intake into body growth (and hence energy reserves). Toads (n = 6–9 for each data point) were fed individually *ad libitum*, given 28 meals in 56 days at 25° C, with crickets (solid diamonds), mealworms (open squares) or woodlice (solid triangles). Food sources significantly influenced body weight increase and efficiency of fat body accumulation: woodlice represent an inferior food diet with almost no growth or fat storage; greatest body weight increase with crickets and mealworms includes lipid that enables survival through dormancy for over 1 year without further feeding. Source: Adapted from Tocque et al. (1995), which provides full details of procedures.

Biological overview

Diversity, biogeography

Xenopus species in sub-Saharan Africa occur in still waters of swamps, ponds and streams and in man-made habitats including dams, flooded pits, ditches and wells. They are less common or absent from rivers or lakes, especially those with well-established fish communities. In general, *Xenopus* species prefer cloudy water and areas of vegetation where they are hidden from aerial predators once below the surface. They are cryptic and nocturnal. Information on ecology is reviewed by Tinsley *et al.* (1996).

Xenopus is described in the literature as a frog or a toad, but these popular terms do not have strict scientific relevance, and *Xenopus* is actually distant from both 'divisions'. Although the use of a genus name alone is not accepted scientifically, the name *Xenopus* will be used as an informal designation in this account for the species of *Xenopus* and *Silurana*.

There are currently 29 species of Xenopus (Evans *et al.* 2015). These are of major genetic and evolutionary interest because they form a polyploid series with two lineages: one with chromosome numbers of 20 and 40 (*Silurana*), the other with 36, 72 and 108 chromosomes (*Xenopus*). Some authors considered this distinction justifies a separate genus, *Silurana*, but recent assessment recognises the common origin of these lineages and *Silurana* now has the rank of subgenus (Evans *et al.* 2015). *Xenopus* (*Silurana*) *tropicalis* is extensively used in laboratory research as the only diploid species (2n=20), with a shorter generation time; all other species with higher ploidy levels evolved through allopolyploidisation (Evans *et al.* 2015). The innovative work of Ben Evans, McMaster University, has provided meticulous interpretation of molecular genetic relationships, demonstrating remarkable reticulated evolution generated principally by multiple rounds of interspecies hybridization (Furman *et al.* 2018).

There are broad distinctions between the species groups based on geographical distribution and habitat type, but it is difficult to determine niche separation at a fine scale: in some areas up to four species occur in the same ponds. However, the two species most commonly employed in research, *laevis* and *tropicalis*, are ecologically distinct. *Xenopus laevis* is a generalist savannah species distributed from the Cape to Sudan, but typically occupying cooler areas in each region. There is significant evolutionary divergence within the species *X. laevis* from South Africa. The form occurring in the winter rainfall area of the western Cape is distinct from that in the summer rainfall area further north (Measey & Channing 2003). Fortunately, this should not cause confusion for existing research findings because worldwide export of *X. laevis* has mostly been from the Cape.

Xenopus tropicalis is limited to lowland tropical forest in West Africa, from Nigeria to Senegal. It is not found outside the forest canopy. This suggests a strict requirement for shade but perhaps also for relative uniformity of conditions including temperature (where ponds are not exposed to fluctuations in sunshine). Water temperature in natural habitats is typically around 25 °C (Tinsley *et al.* 1996). *Xenopus tropicalis* is not simply a warmer-water version of *X. laevis*: there are striking differences in behaviour and environmental preferences (obvious to laboratory workers who maintain both), but there is little detailed field information.

Ecology

Information on the ecology of *X. laevis* is necessary to appreciate the thermal limits of this 'laboratory amphibian'. At the Cape, South Africa, *X. laevis* experiences a Mediterranean climate with temperatures below 10 °C in winter and above 25 °C in summer. Records from introduced northern hemisphere

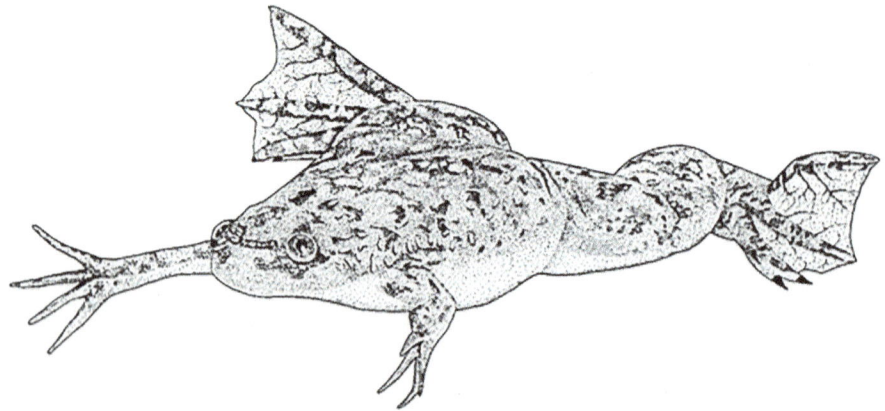

Figure 47.2 *Xenopus laevis*, illustrating the flattened, streamlined body with limbs splayed laterally; powerful leg muscles and webbed feet enable rapid swimming; the innermost 3 digits carry black claws (2 are visible in this view). The forelimbs are directed forward, not involved in supporting the body, with a principal role in sweeping food into the mouth. The eyes are directed upwards, the nostrils are near the tip of the snout, there is no visible eardrum. 'Stitches' around the eyes and along the flanks represent the lateral line system, sensitive to movement, vibrations and pressure changes (and hence precise location of unseen prey). Mature females are pear-shaped, males are slimmer with parallel flanks; body length (snout – vent length) is typically 90–130 mm in adult females, about 25% less in males; body weight of large females is 100–150 g. The sexes are distinguished by size but also by the presence of cloacal labia in females and dark gloves on the fore arms of males in breeding condition. The dorsal skin is camouflaged with irregular mottled patterns of olive, brown and greenish-grey; expansion and contraction of melanophores enables darkening and lightening of the body to match background colour. The venter is predominantly creamy-white.
Source: From Tinsley and Kobel (1996): cover drawing by Timothy Colborn, University of Bristol.

populations show tolerance of wider extremes. In eastern USA, animals overwinter beneath ice in frozen ponds; in Arizona, X. laevis occurs in ponds whose summer temperatures reach 30 °C (close to the thermal maximum). In addition to longer-term seasonal variations in temperature, Xenopus naturally experience short-term fluctuations between pond areas exposed to sun and in deep shade. Temperature records in ponds inhabited by introduced X. laevis in the UK show an annual cycle between 4 and 24 °C, and short-term changes (especially in spring and autumn) of up to 8 °C over a few days. In these UK populations, X. laevis experience temperatures below 10 °C for over 6 months (October to March) (Tinsley et al. 2011), but still show fast growth rates, excellent condition and successful breeding. Experience from the author's laboratory shows that X. laevis can acclimatise to long-term maintenance (up to 2 years) at 10 and 15 °C and can be maintained in the shorter term at 5 °C.

Xenopus laevis is normally very robust, with potential to survive more than 20 years in the laboratory. Successive recaptures of individually marked *X. laevis* in an introduced population in Wales show that lifespan can also exceed 20 years in the wild (Tinsley et al. 2012). Long-term laboratory experience has shown that *Xenopus* can spawn successfully after 15 years captivity.

Much of the diet comprises small invertebrates but *Xenopus* may also feed communally exploiting larger prey items including carrion. As a scavenger, *Xenopus* differs from most amphibians where, if there is no movement, a potential food item is not recognised. Both tadpoles and post-metamorphs of *Xenopus* feed in the same environment but there is no overlap in diet since the tadpoles are filter-feeders. However, juvenile and adult *Xenopus* may feed on tadpoles. This habit allows efficient exploitation of energy sources: tadpoles feed on phytoplankton which gains energy directly from sunlight, and adults trap this source of nutrients by cannibalism.

Xenopus laevis has been released into the wild and established self-maintaining populations outside Africa (Tinsley & McCoid 1996). The current list of locations includes Europe (France, Portugal, Italy), North America (many areas but most abundantly in California), South America (Chile), Ascension Island, China and Japan. Introduced populations occurred in the UK for over 50 years but are now extinct (Tinsley et al. 2015b). Many localities have a Mediterranean climate equivalent to that at the Cape, but the diversity of habitat conditions confirms the adaptability of *X. laevis*. This adaptability has contributed to its success as a 'model organism' in laboratory research.

Sensory perception, behaviour and communication

Perception of the environment employs the lateral line system, sight, touch, chemoreception/olfaction and hearing (Elepfandt 1996a,b). In contrast to terrestrial anurans, *Xenopus* retains the lateral line system after metamorphosis. These sense organs detect pressure changes and vibrations enabling accurate location of movements (including prey). The orientation of the eyes gives binocular vision of the area on and above the water surface: submerged *Xenopus* can respond to and precisely locate objects (prey, for instance) a few centimetres above the water. Touch is important to find food in turbid water: stroking the insides of the forelimbs and digits elicits a feeding response. *Xenopus* has two distinct classes of olfactory receptors, one specialised for detecting odours in water (related to receptors in fish), the other for detecting airborne odours (related to those in mammals).

There have been few studies of *Xenopus* behaviour in the wild especially because typical habitats have cloudy water. Valuable insight has come from direct observations at clear water sites. Baird (1983) observed that air-breathing is synchronised within groups of *X. laevis*, controlled socially by stimuli from others in the group. Ringeis et al. (2017) described a wealth of complex interactions at night in which male *X. laevis* establish territories underwater and defend the borders against other males; they show complex social behaviour, dominant/subordinate hierarchy, spatial cognition, complex learning and long-term memory (Elepfandt 1996a,b). Communication is dominated by vocal signalling using a highly specialised mechanism to create underwater sounds (Kwong-Brown et al. 2019) and an auditory system modified for reception (Elepfandt 1996b). Both sexes have an extensive vocal repertoire based on clicks, used in male–female, female–male and male–male communication. The male advertisement call is a continuous trilling made by the larynx without any visible movement.

The laboratory worker is generally unaware of any of this complex social organisation when *Xenopus* are housed in relatively small rectangular aquaria.

Laboratory maintenance of *Xenopus*

Current recommendations for care of *Xenopus* are based on:

a. Personal descriptions by researchers of systems in their own laboratories, with the rationale 'this works for us'. These accounts benefit from first-hand experience, but there is often little comparison with alternative regimes or justification for choices adopted.
b. Accounts that describe problems with specific aspects of *Xenopus* maintenance or performance, followed by explanation of changes made to previous protocols in order to resolve difficulties. This approach may be helpful for workers experiencing similar circumstances but there is typically no data analysis or assurance that the changes implemented were actually responsible for the improvement.
c. Attempts to test quantitatively the effect of specific environmental factors or maintenance protocols on *Xenopus* condition (growth rates, behaviour, oöcyte quality). Typically, these are tests of single factors within an environment where the effects of co-occurring factors are unknown. Interpretation is strongly dependent on appropriate statistical analysis.
d. Use of standardised automated systems for maintenance, with environmental design (tanks), water characteristics (water chemistry, methods of water change, etc.) determined by commercial manufacturers. Rationale for design may be influenced by the technology employed for tropical fish (especially, Zebrafish). Basic parameters for space, water depth, etc. generally follow European and national

guidelines. The scientific basis for these decisions (by governments, manufacturers, etc.) is generally not made explicit (or is unknown). Some laboratories report problems with achieving research needs (oöcyte quality) after the switch from previous systems.

A review of the literature indicates that practices (from all four approaches) are often accepted uncritically: indeed, with so little evidence, there may be no basis for judgement. The design of improved welfare procedures based on quantitative experimental studies presents some significant challenges.

A. There is typically marked variation in growth rates, maturation times and condition of *Xenopus* within groups maintained in experimental trials (e.g., Hilken *et al.* 1995). These differences are pronounced even for individuals belonging to the same subgroup maintained with the same husbandry (Tinsley 2010a). Genetic effects may have confounded some published trials, but variability may also be influenced by competition and stress.
B. The value of experiments is dependent on sound design, including controls, standardisation of environmental factors, and comprehensive statistical analysis of data (see also Chapter 3: The design of animal experiments).
C. Experiments must take account of interactions involving behavioural responses within groups of *Xenopus*: complex behaviour involving long-term memory, learning, habituation and hierarchy may confound simple trial comparisons.
D. Monitoring and evaluation of trials must consider subtle effects that husbandry protocols may have on *Xenopus* condition, perhaps operating at a subclinical level over several years before becoming symptomatic (see the following text regarding oöcyte quality).

Alternative approaches to laboratory provision

The European Directive 2010/63 now limits laboratory research to *Xenopus* supplied by recognized breeding establishments and this is also the case, by choice for many large '*Xenopus* laboratories' worldwide. Outside Europe, however, research on *X. laevis* exported from South Africa may continue. These are caught as adults, after at least 3 years in natural habitats, and laboratory conditions are often totally at variance with their previous experience. Nocturnal animals accustomed to the security of cloudy water are likely to experience stress in high-density populations in clear, shallow water, illuminated from all sides (and even below), with frequent disturbance and exposure to predation.

Semi-natural environments

For long-term maintenance of reference collections of *Xenopus* species, it is best to attempt simulation of environmental conditions reflecting the habitats of *Xenopus* in the wild. Without detailed information on long-term effects of specific parameters, it seems sensible to provide a relatively large-scale environment, especially for big active species such as *X. laevis*. Most other species in the genus are smaller and aquarium dimensions can be reduced. Suitable conditions can be created with an aquarium with thick glass walls, darkened on three sides but with the front panel clear for inspection, a dark base, and light coming primarily from above. *Xenopus* in such aquaria do not appear to react to minor movements lateral to the tank. Water depth should be at least 50 cm (ideally, deeper for adult *X. laevis*). A three-dimensional environment can be created with leafy plants (plastic foliage is easier to 'maintain' at low light levels and to wash/sterilise). There should be at least a partial covering at the water surface. Where there is good illumination, including daylight, this surface covering can be provided by natural growth of duckweed (*Lemna* spp.) or by floating synthetic material (resembling lily pads). These conditions allow *Xenopus* to reach the surface while hidden from direct exposure. The water should be still, without appreciable circulation; aeration is unnecessary and should be avoided since a stream of aerator bubbles may be 'deafening' to *Xenopus*. Other services, including water pumps, must not produce vibrations. Rounded gravel is an effective substrate in which sections of drain pipes or plant pots are partially embedded as refuges. A stable environment with good water quality can be achieved if the bottom gravel supports a culture of bacteria that de-nitrify metabolic wastes.

To maintain equilibrium in water quality, animals must not be over-fed (avoiding breakdown of uneaten food in the gravel). This management works well with 'chunky' food items (bovine heart, meal worms, etc.) that are ingested intact, without creating debris. It is impractical with pellet-type food which disintegrates if not eaten quickly. Food input requires judgement (noting the amount of food eaten within 30–60 min). Animals fed to satiation with one or a few meals each week will maintain optimum physiological condition (with good gonad and fat body development). The complexity of setting up 'semi-natural' habitats is offset by ease of maintenance: the frequency of water changes can be judged from water clarity and accumulation of anoxic sediment in the gravel. With good management, water changes may be every few months (sooner if algal blooms occur in sunlight). Water changes require removal of animals to temporary holding tanks while the aquarium is emptied and cleaned. The gravel should be thoroughly washed and re-introduced together with some of the original sediment from which de-nitrifying bacteria can re-establish.

Detailed observations of *Xenopus* in 'semi-natural' environments can give valuable insight into behaviour. In this author's experience, if *Xenopus* (particularly, the smaller species) are provided with an island, they will spend much time out of water, especially at night. It is not known whether this meets important physiological needs. Perhaps *X. laevis* is regarded as exclusively aquatic in the laboratory only because animals are not provided with any alternative.

This approach works well for small populations of rare species, especially those sensitive to disturbance (Purpose [1] in the preceding text), but most laboratories require replicated systems for larger populations (Purposes [2] and [3]).

Large-scale maintenance systems

Requirements for aquarium provision, including housing systems, nutrition and water quality, are considered in detail by Green (2010). Most approaches focus principally on controlling variations in the aquatic environment influenced by feeding, waste removal and water chemistry. Requirements are met by three alternative designs: aquaria containing static water which is completely replaced at intervals (so-called 'fill and dump'); flow-through systems that replace water continuously, with trickle input balanced by drainage to waste; re-circulating systems with filtration and sterilisation of recycled water and automatic control of physical and chemical characteristics.

The choice between systems is influenced by space, water supply and cost. Static systems are low cost in terms of equipment but expensive in terms of maintenance (technician time). Recirculating systems have high set-up costs for equipment but are time-efficient for maintenance.

The design of large-scale accommodation involves a series of unexplored assumptions about welfare; thus, for efficiency of cleaning, aquaria routinely have a hard, bare substrate (a plastic or glass tank bottom) but this contrasts starkly with the soft mud typical in natural habitats. As already noted, basic procedures achieving optimum environmental conditions for *Xenopus* have not yet been established. The following sections review the key parameters in *Xenopus* husbandry.

Environmental conditions

Aquarium rooms should be maintained in relatively dim illumination (not 'office' or 'domestic' lighting). Summer photoperiod at the Cape (for *X. laevis*) is around 14 h light: 10 h dark, but *X. tropicalis* in equatorial latitudes would naturally experience around 12 h L: 12 h D. The day: night change in the laboratory should involve gradual transition in light levels, not an 'on–off' switch. Tanks with darkened sides and a black base help provide appropriate seclusion; tests for corticosterone production have shown that stress levels are reduced in *Xenopus* maintained on a black background compared with white (Holmes *et al*. 2016).

Xenopus can jump more than their own body length above the water surface, so tanks should have secure lids with air holes. Animals should not be able to reach the lid as this may result in nasal trauma. Some commercially available modular systems for *Xenopus* have lids only about 5 cm above the water surface. Counter-intuitively, laboratory-raised animals in these circumstances do not typically show nasal damage: perhaps they become conditioned to the spatial limitations of their 'habitats', inhibiting natural behaviour. *Xenopus* raised from metamorphosis in such systems may adapt well and not experience stress; animals raised in large open tanks (or caught in the wild) may find such restrictions stressful.

Water depth

Spatial dimensions of aquarium tanks – water depth and tank area – should represent an important factor in the laboratory environment of *Xenopus* (as for most active predators in captivity). However, water depths in most laboratory regimes contrast strikingly with conditions in natural habitats.

The survey by Major and Wassersug (1998) showed that different laboratories employed water depths ranging from 5 to 25 cm without rationale for choices. Body size has a major effect on suitability and it must be assumed that most data relate to adult *X. laevis* (typically, 90–130 mm SVL for full-grown females). Water depth has generally received little attention in overviews of *Xenopus* husbandry or it has been dismissed as unimportant. Major and Wassersug concluded that depth may not be a crucial factor in laboratory husbandry, citing observations by Tinsley *et al.* (1996) that *X. laevis* may be found at various water depths in the wild. However, occurrence does not equate with preference nor with successful long-term establishment and reproduction.

The few attempts in the literature to test effects of water depth have significant flaws in design or analysis. Hilken *et al.* (1994) carried out preference tests with *X. laevis* maintained on a sloping tank base giving water depths from 15 to 25 cm. Most individuals were reported to prefer deeper water. Their body weight range was 13–50 g (length was not given) so size differences within the group were considerable. These preference data may have been confounded by competition since Hilken *et al.* noted that 'smaller frogs were forced into the more shallow areas'. Hilken *et al.* (1995) measured growth of *X. laevis* maintained for 8 months in water depths of 5, 10 and 20 cm and found no significant differences in length (SVL) or weight. However, the experimental design created other major changes besides depth: tank volumes with increasing depth were 1.6, 3.1 and 6.2 l, respectively, with corresponding effects on density, potentially confounding the analysis. Sample sizes were small and did not take account of sex.

Observations on behaviour 'in the wild' and in 'semi-natural' aquaria provide an alternative perspective. In natural habitats, *Xenopus* rarely remain at the water surface, potentially exposed to aerial predators, except when concealed by surface vegetation. Characteristically, shallow clear water is avoided. Where there is no vegetation, visits to the surface to breathe are extremely rapid (< 1 sec) and groups of animals in the same area may break the surface simultaneously and disappear within seconds (Baird 1983 and personal observations), reducing vulnerability to predators. In habitats with surface vegetation, *Xenopus* may spend long periods 'hanging' from the water surface with only the snout tip and nostrils protruding and the body and legs extended vertically below. In this attitude, they are not visible from above but, if there is a threat or disturbance, they can propel themselves rapidly downwards with a backward contraction of the body assisted by the sliding pelvis and powerful thrusts of the webbed feet.

The observation that *Xenopus* frequently adopts a posture in aquaria with its nose tip at the surface has led to the suggestion that maximum water depth should allow animals to stand on the tank bottom and reach the surface without effort. This interpretation is probably anthropocentric. In deep aquaria, hanging from the surface appears to be 'effortless', achieved for long periods without swimming movements since *Xenopus* use the air in their lungs adjust buoyancy.

Following the assumption that animals prefer to stand on the tank bottom, *minimum* water depth would be equated approximately with snout-vent length plus extended hind limb length. These two measurements are almost equal in X. *laevis* so, by this criterion, water depth for large adult females would be at least 20 cm, up to about 25 cm. Few accounts of laboratory practices meet this condition: some specify less (or much less) than SVL alone (e.g., 5–10 cm by Dawson et al. 1992). Animals in the growth experiments of Hilken et al. (1995) had mean SVL 68 mm maintained in water 5 cm deep. A few accounts cite water depth just above SVL (e.g., 15 cm by Brown & Nixon 2004) but without allowing for leg length. The most recent European Directive (2010/63) relates water depth for 'aquatic anurans' (presumably, *Xenopus*, as specified in previous Directives on this subject) to a series of body sizes with each depth closely matching or just less than SVL. Thus, for body length 6–9 cm, minimum water depth should be 8 cm; for length 9–12, depth 10 cm; for length >12, depth 12.5 cm.

In water depths too shallow for the 'stand on the bottom' criterion (less than SVL plus leg length), *Xenopus* that are disturbed cannot perform the rapid downward escape reflex, hitting the tank base as they contract backwards. This restriction is even greater in depths equal to or less than SVL (without leg length): attempts to escape downwards lead to frantic swimming in all directions. With these shallow depths, animals can rest with nostrils exposed only by maintaining an oblique angle to the surface. In this attitude, they make frequent adjustments to their position as their feet slide on the tank bottom. Alternatively, they may float horizontally on the surface with head and inflated lungs exposed above the water surface. This position is never found in natural habitats (e.g., Baird 1983).

These observations suggest that *Xenopus* in natural habitats might experience stress in two respects in clear shallow water: exposure to predation from above and inability to escape below. These twin factors would explain the avoidance of shallow water in the wild, yet these are inherent in many laboratory aquarium systems.

In widely used modular recirculating systems for *Xenopus*, water depth is 'taken care of' by the size of tanks supplied by manufacturers. In a selection of current designs, water depths are 10, 13.5 and 15 cm. Depending on body lengths, this range conforms to European Commission recommendations. However, in the view of the present author, tanks with these water depths may be appropriate for smaller species, including X. *tropicalis*, and for juvenile X. *laevis* but are very considerably too shallow for adult female X. *laevis*.

Several early studies (e.g., Landgrebe 1939) showed that adverse conditions, including shallow water and overcrowding, lead to ovary regression. Severe restrictions in space and depth cause overt pathology and a poor response to hormone-induced ovulation. Conditions that are improved but still not optimal – where ill-effects are not obvious – may have subclinical effects on subtle measures of well-being. For this reason, the present author advocates that water depth for adult female X. *laevis* should be not less than 30 cm (i.e. about 50% greater than SVL plus extended leg length) and, for largest individuals, preferably 40–50 cm. Carefully designed experiments are required to test potential effects on oöcyte quality and duration of reproductive success.

Tank area and population density

Guidance from observations 'in the wild' is less informative for this parameter: little is known of factors influencing within-population interactions. Field studies by Ringeis et al. (2017) provided detailed insight into behaviour (principally, mating interactions) in X. *laevis* in a pond with clear water. Inevitably, in a single population such as this, density is influenced by previous immigration/emigration, breeding and predation within the confines of the habitat rather than indicating preference. For laboratory populations in Europe, Directive (2010/63) relates minimum surface area to numbers of animals, e.g., 600 cm^2 for 'aquatic anurans' with 9–12 cm SVL and 150 cm^2 for each additional animal.

Most assessments of density in the husbandry literature are based on water volume per animal but do not specify the 3-dimensional parameters of basal area of aquaria and water depth. Typically, there is little comparative information on numbers of individuals per tank or body sizes. Densities vary widely: Major and Wassersug's (1998) survey of then-current practices reported water volumes ranging from 0.5 to 20 (mean 5) l per *Xenopus*. Specific recommendations include 2 l/animal by The National Academy of Sciences and 12 l/animal by The Council of Europe in 2006 and European Commission in 2007 (see Tinsley 2010a). Among accounts by authors of their own facilities, Wu and Gerhart (1991) reported a density of 2000–3000 large 'fully adult' X. *laevis* in a tank of 800 l (i.e. average 0.27–0.4 l/animal). Hilken et al. (1995) tested effects of density on growth rates in mixed sex groups of X. *laevis* in either 8.6 or 14 l of water/animal (volumes greater than in most other reports). After 9 months, animals at the lower density were significantly heavier and longer (SVL) than at higher density. This could provide rare evidence for a clear-cut effect of aquarium design on growth. However, analysis may have been confounded by considerable variation in body sizes and other limitations noted in the preceding text; so, interpretation is uncertain, emphasizing – again – that rigorous experiments with appropriate sample size and statistical analysis are urgently needed.

Very fast growth rates of juvenile X. *laevis* can be achieved at relatively high density (1.5–2 l/animal at 40–50 mm SVL) if feeding is intensive. This outcome may not necessarily indicate good practice; instead, it may parallel the fast growth characteristics of intensively reared animals in agriculture and aquaculture. The body growth of these animals will change the parameters of space, density and relative water depth during maintenance: sub-adults with 50 mm SVL may have adequate space in 1.5 l of water/animal but experience progressive deterioration in habitat suitability as their SVL increases to 120 mm.

Feeding

There is relatively little discussion in the literature about optimum diets for *Xenopus* species. A range of alternative diets appears to satisfy nutritional requirements although there have been no quantitative tests. Commercially formulated composite diets include regulated quantities of proteins, fats, carbohydrates, minerals, trace elements, etc.; these are similar to or the same as those designed and tested for intensive rearing of fish. Some authors support a diet of organ meat (including bovine heart muscle) (see Tinsley 2010a). In some vertebrates, such diets may lead to deficiency diseases. The studies on *Scaphiopus* (in the preceding text) emphasized the need to boost the nutritional value of prey organisms with protein and vitamin supplements before feeding to the toads. Small, solid pieces of meat have the advantage of less debris during feeding, especially in 'semi-natural' aquaria. Other diets are reviewed by Reed (2005). Live food such as *Tubifex* carries risks of infection.

Some accounts of *X. laevis* maintenance emphasise the presumed benefits of a so-called 'feeding frenzy'. Certainly, animals that are stimulated to feed simultaneously avoid the outcome where those reacting slowly may miss a meal. This also accords with circumstances in nature where one *Xenopus* finding a food source may trigger searching behaviour by others in the vicinity. A 'frenzy' can be advantageous when an item is too big for one individual to ingest alone: a group of *Xenopus* can quickly shred large-bodied prey or carrion by repeated scratching with sharp hindfoot claws. However, this author is not convinced that this behaviour is an advantage in the laboratory. When two or more individuals attempt to ingest the same food item, violent struggles, kicking with the claws and biting are potentially damaging. Pieces of food (e.g., cubes of meat) should be small enough to be swallowed quickly, avoiding simultaneous 'capture' by other individuals. In practice, *X. laevis* become conditioned to a regular feeding routine and all individuals may respond together when food is given, so a 'frenzy' may not improve intake.

Different authorities advocate feeding *X. laevis* at a variety of frequencies. Young post-metamorphs require frequent feeding: gut size limits food intake per meal and significant gaps between meals may reduce growth. Fastest development to maturity is achieved with daily feeding. However, full-grown adults can maintain excellent condition and develop ripe ovaries with one or two (large) meals per week. The key to this regimen is that all individuals in a tank should be fed to satiation avoiding competitive effects that might induce differences in growth rate and size. Satiation can be achieved by providing sufficient food so that a surplus always remains uneaten after a meal. Otherwise there can be no assurance that some individuals are not under-fed (or unfed). A meal appropriate to each population can be added to the aquarium, which is then inspected about an hour later; if all food has been eaten, more can be added until just a few items remain. The slight excess can be removed at the end of the day, avoiding fouling of the water. This process of matching food supply to need is more difficult with a pellet-type diet where uneaten food disintegrates relatively quickly and an excess leads to greater water fouling.

Feeding regimes that impose a short time limit on food availability should be avoided. For instance, feeding by groups of *X. laevis* was limited to 10 min by Kaplan (1993) and 5 min by Delpire et al. (2011) before removal of the 'excess' by net. This practice favours animals more dominant and aggressive in the within-group hierarchy. Body size variation will increase if some individuals consistently feed well and others badly at each meal. The disruption of netting uneaten food early during feeding may create alarm and regurgitation and animals may experience stress as they continue searching for food after removal (including attacking each other).

Water changes

Feeding (frequency and food type), aquarium water volume and population density all affect water quality. Approaches to maintaining quality represent the major management concern in '*Xenopus* laboratories' influencing equipment and workload (hence financial costs) and ultimately animal welfare and suitability for research.

Individual aquaria with static water are simple systems for maintenance, typically involving draining and replacing the tank water at regular intervals (every few days or once per week). This 'fill-and-dump' routine creates a cycle of changes in water quality between feeding and cleaning; deterioration in water quality (including increasing ammonia levels and accumulation of debris from feeding and faecal output) is determined by the intervals between water changes and, in turn, frequency of feeding. Feeding with commercial formulations (pellets) produces earlier deterioration in water quality (especially from disintegration of uneaten pellets), so more frequent water changes may be necessary.

For *X. laevis* maintained in static systems, there are two approaches to the feeding/water change sequence. Where animals are fed once or twice weekly and the water is also changed once or twice, some lab regimens advocate feeding on the day before the water change. Alternatively, the water change is carried out first and the animals are fed immediately afterwards. In the first case, animals feed in water containing accumulated waste from the previous week (faeces, shed skin and other debris) and then experience major disturbance from the water change after food intake, potentially provoking regurgitation. In the second case, maximum pollution (lowest water quality) occurs in the period preceding feeding but water change at this point ensures that food ingestion takes place in clean water, avoiding re-ingestion of faeces, etc. In practice, *X. laevis* readily become conditioned to the change-then-feed sequence and begin to search for food immediately after transfer to clean water. Thus, the meal is eaten more efficiently, with less debris, and animals are undisturbed (for several days) after food intake, so digestion avoids disruption from water changes.

Animals must be transferred to water at the same temperature. The smoothest changes are achieved by direct transfer of animals from one tank to a duplicate, limiting disturbance to the moment of transfer. For a series of tank changes, the just-vacated tank can then be cleaned out, refilled and used to receive animals from the next tank to be changed, and so on. An alternative approach is to transfer animals to a temporary 'holding' tank; the original container is washed, re-filled and the same animals are returned to it. Animals and tanks always remain together, reducing risks of spread of infection, but this method increases disturbance during temporary holding.

Xenopus may be moved between tanks by net (with mesh size avoiding transfer of debris); they should not be picked up in groups in a net such that they fall on top of each other. For experienced laboratory workers, it is often least disruptive to transfer animals gently by hand. Using naked hands (without gloves) provides a check on condition: roughening of *Xenopus* skin and decrease in slipperiness (reduced mucus secretion) give early warning of poor health (see section on Welfare). However, disposable gloves should be worn where there are concerns about zoonotic infections (see Safety considerations in the following text).

Tanks should be washed thoroughly between water changes, removing biofilm and growths of algae, but should never be cleaned with bleach or abrasive materials – the roughened surface may be more easily colonised by microorganisms. Maintenance protocols for water changes should incorporate common sense hygiene measures. Nets, holding containers, cleaning cloths, etc. should be washed thoroughly (ideally with hot water) between uses. Most pathogens affecting *X. laevis* have no resistant stages and do not survive complete drying (the capillarid skin nematode is an exception). So, equipment should be dried thoroughly between uses (with aquaria propped upside-down to drain completely). Containers (including plastic aquaria) must not be stacked with moisture trapped inside.

An alternative approach to this 'fill-and-dump' protocol involves draining the water from static tanks while the animals remain *in situ* and refilling with clean water without moving the occupants. Some laboratories have timer-controlled draining followed by an automatic refill. In the view of this writer, these procedures raise major welfare concerns. Rapid decrease in water depth and temporary exposure of animals out of water is highly stressful. *Xenopus* experiencing these conditions show great alarm as the water level falls, scrambling over each other when exposed. The torrent of water produced during refilling creates further panic and shock. Effects on stress behaviour can be seen if water is siphoned out of a 'semi-natural' aquarium housing an otherwise-undisturbed population of *Xenopus*; it is also evident on a larger scale in ponds 'in the wild' when water is pumped out (e.g., as supplies for irrigation). In both cases, there is frenzied agitation with animals jumping at the surface (up tank walls or pond banks) as the water level falls.

To meet the needs of water quality, some '*Xenopus* systems' employ a flow-through of fresh water with replaced water passing to drain. The exchange may be gradual and continuous or periodic with timer-controlled operation. This approach depends on abundant water provision but is vulnerable to fluctuations in supply water chemistry.

In each of these approaches, if water changes result in incomplete removal of tank water there are significant risks of infection. Thus, partial water changes in static tanks (sometimes with 50% of water replaced at each change), drainage of tanks while the *Xenopus* are left *in situ* and flow-through systems dependent on slow input of replacement water are all undesirable because complete removal of sediment is impossible: pathogen infective stages may persist and re-infect the group (see section on Parasites).

For the most intensive use of *Xenopus*, the large scale of accommodation makes the various labour-intensive methods impractical. Increasingly, '*Xenopus* laboratories' are adopting automated or semi-automated systems in which racks of aquaria are maintained with comprehensive environmental control (including temperature and water chemistry), and with water quality regulated by continuous recirculation and filtration. With purpose-built recirculation systems, water changes are achieved with continuous removal and replacement, avoiding cyclical variation in water quality: typically, 10% of the water is replaced each day and passed through biological, mechanical and charcoal filters before UV sterilisation. Refuges and other enrichment may interfere with water flow routes so tanks should be removed and cleaned regularly. At the time of writing (2019), there are innovative developments in tank design involving automatic removal of debris from the tank bottom (by suction or partial draining); this reduces the disturbance (and workload) of netting uneaten food and improves water quality. Mechanical and electrical equipment (including pumps, filters) must not generate vibrations transmitted to *Xenopus* within aquaria; these services should be located remotely from racks of tanks.

Temperature

Xenopus laevis can adapt to a wide range of temperatures, but laboratory studies show that there are complex behavioural, physiological and immunological interactions accompanying temperature change. Maintenance at different temperatures must take account of rate of change, allowing time for physiological adjustments. Green *et al.* (2003) attributed deaths of laboratory-maintained *X. laevis* to thermal shock following direct transfer from 16 to 23 °C. There are no established data for rates of change that are tolerated. Changes of about 5 °C over 2–5 days accord with conditions experienced naturally, but, for greater changes, animals should acclimate at intermediate temperatures. *Xenopus* should not be transferred directly between tanks of water at different temperatures; animals should be moved in water at their original temperature to new conditions where this water then warms or cools gradually. Alternatively, with thermostatically controlled heater/chiller units, settings should be changed by only about 2 °C per day.

Immune function in *Xenopus* (as in other ectotherm vertebrates) is temperature-dependent (Robert & Ohta 2009). Immune responses of *X. laevis* are most effective above 20 °C; *X. laevis* are progressively immunosuppressed below about 18 °C. Recommendations in the literature for maintenance at lower temperatures (including 15 or 16 °C) may predispose to pathogenic infection. At low temperatures (including 10 °C), *X. laevis* will not tolerate frequent disturbance. Thus, long-term maintenance at low temperatures is best achieved in stable aquaria with water changes at several month intervals (see the preceding text).) Food supply should be inversely proportional to temperature, corresponding with metabolic needs. *Xenopus laevis* may remain in good condition in long-term maintenance at 25 °C but require increased food supply to fuel higher metabolic rate and frequent water changes to remove waste products. *Xenopus tropicalis* is less tolerant of temperature change and indirect evidence of pathogenic infections in laboratory populations suggests that immunosuppression may be significant below about 20 °C.

Hence, *X. laevis* will adapt to temperatures throughout the range 15–25 °C, but on either side of the central band of about 18–22 °C animals will be more vulnerable to co-occurring stress. Hilken *et al.* (1995) found no significant differences in growth of *X. laevis* maintained at 19, 22 or 24 °C. However, this result is counter to biological principles: metabolic rate may differ by 50% with a 5 °C change. As noted earlier, these results may have limitations reflecting methodology and analysis.

Water chemistry

Green (2010) provides a comprehensive overview of water quality (including filtration, water chemistry, alkalinity, conductivity, pH). Godfrey and Sanders (2004) recommended maintenance in hard water based on their experience where poor oöcyte quality in soft water was followed by a change to hard water and subsequent improvement. For observations such as these, over a period of years, it is difficult to exclude other co-occurring factors. This highlights the need for specifically designed controlled quantitative trials (as in other aspects of *Xenopus* husbandry).

There is an unresolved debate concerning alternative water supplies provided by potable tap water or RO water (purified by reverse osmosis reconstituted with salts). It might be expected that domestic supplies intended as drinking water should meet the needs of *X. laevis*, but supply pipes must not contaminate the water with metals such as copper and lead which have serious effects on oöcyte quality. Water must be dechlorinated (most simply by allowing it to stand for 12–24 h); where water supplies are treated with chloramines these can be removed with commercial aquarium agents containing sodium thiosulphate.

Environmental enrichment

It is intuitive that environmental enrichment based on natural habitats should improve well-being in the laboratory (see also Chapter 10: Enrichment: Animal welfare and scientific validity). In their survey of laboratory practices, Major and Wassersug (1998) reported a 50 : 50 split in cover or no cover among *Xenopus* facilities. Only 20% provided 'local refuges' (pots, tubes, stones, etc.). In the past 20 years, there has been greater impetus to provide enrichment routinely. This trend has been welcome even though the published assessments are contradictory.

Hilken *et al*. (1995) recorded growth in two groups (each 4 males, 4 females) with or without refuges. After 7 months, body weight (but not length) was significantly greater in the group without refuges and these animals were reported to be less shy, reacting to disturbance with less panic. However, the methodology had the same limitations as other tests in these investigations (see the preceding text).

Brown and Nixon (2004) conducted preference tests with various forms of enrichment, recording that enriched areas with opaque tubes were preferred. They observed behaviours opposite to those reported by Hilken *et al*. (1995): animals with enrichment were more active and reacted to disturbance with less panic than those in barren aquaria. Oöcyte quality and quantity were assessed after 4–8 months: Brown and Nixon reported that both measures were 'consistently improved' in enriched compared with non-enriched environments, but differences were not statistically significant (quantity, $p=0.2$; quality, $p=0.1$). Food consumption and body weights were not recorded but the authors reported that 'all *X. laevis* appeared to consume the same amount of food and no obvious body weight gains or losses were seen'. Clearly, these data are not sufficient for sound conclusions.

The wider literature refers to two forms of cover: first, a refuge creating local seclusion into which one or a few individuals can retreat to 'safety' (i.e. as if from predators in the water), and second, a partial or complete covering over the tank surface (i.e. as if restricting exposure to aerial predators). It might be predicted that both are important in reducing stress: observations on the behaviour of *Xenopus* in laboratory aquaria (especially with semi-natural conditions) provide a valuable guide. Several authors, together with personal observations, suggest that *Xenopus* prefer to have contact between their dorsal surface and the inside of the refuge (Hilken *et al*. 1994; Brown & Nixon 2004; Archard 2012) and may squeeze into narrow spaces between enrichment items and the tank sides or base. Individuals frequently locate themselves in the opening of the refuge adopting a 'ready to feed' attitude with forelimbs outstretched (Figure 47.4). This behaviour gives the impression of an apparently natural response to environmental conditions. However, it would not be surprising if *Xenopus* provided with secure refuges might show stress behaviour in open spaces between refuges. This would accord with exposure in clear, shallow water, and would concur with the findings of Hilken *et al*. (1994, 1995) that *Xenopus* provided with refuges remained shy and were slow to emerge and feed. In these circumstances, exposure could be reduced by a cover over the entire aquarium provided by a tinted lid.

Refuges in the form of pipes and flowerpots must be sufficiently heavy that they cannot be moved or upturned by the movements of startled *Xenopus*. The numbers and sizes of refuges should be sufficient to accommodate all individuals to avoid aggressive interactions and competition. Torreilles and Green (2007) reported how refuges could reduce bite wounds in large *X. laevis* populations (see the following text).

Refuges must allow for periodic inspection to ensure health but reducing stress with refuges would be negated if animals must be evicted from hiding places to check well-being. Translucent red or blue tubes appear to provide equally effective refuges as opaque black or grey tubes, enabling inspection without disturbance.

Breeding

Reproductive processes and procedures

Spawning by *X. laevis* in South African habitats is triggered by recent rainfall, a rise in water levels and a fall in water temperature after previous temperatures around 20 °C. This would have the selective advantage that heavy rain washes sediments into ponds, enriching nutrient status and promoting algal blooms that provide a food supply for tadpoles (Tinsley *et al*. 1996). Although spawning appears to be optimal at 20 °C, fieldwork on introduced populations in Wales demonstrates that *X. laevis* can spawn and complete development through metamorphosis at 15 °C. Males in mating condition develop black nuptial gloves on the inner surface of the arms to grip the female; in receptive females, the cloacal labia become pink. Amplexus is inguinal (around the waist).

One of the major advantages of *Xenopus* for laboratory research derives from the ease with which breeding can be induced at any time of year. In South Africa and other areas with cool winter temperatures, age at sexual maturity is generally 2 years for males and 3 years for females. In favourable conditions in the laboratory (and 'in the wild' in California with temperatures at least 20 °C for most of the year), X. laevis can reach maturity at about 6 months post-metamorphosis (8 months from the egg stage) (Tinsley & Kobel 1996).

Spawning of X. laevis can occur spontaneously in the laboratory at around 20–22 °C but is usually induced by injection of human chorionic gonadotrophin (hCG). Females should have been well fed for 1–3 months and should be plump and pear shaped, reflecting an enlarged ovary. Nuptial gloves can be induced by isolating males for a week before spawning. Typically, two injections are given 48 h apart: a primer to bring animals into mating condition and a final dose to stimulate spawning. Male and female are kept separate after priming and put together after the final injection. Doses are related to body size but, for adult X. laevis, the primer may be 50 IU for males and 100 IU for females, with final doses 100 IU and 300 IU, respectively. The tank in which spawning occurs should have a platform of plastic (not wire) netting through which eggs can settle avoiding risk of being eaten by the parents.

To prevent damage to spawn, adults should be removed from tanks and eggs left *in situ* until they hatch. Larvae break free after about 48 h (at 22 °C) and attach to a vertical surface until remaining yolk is absorbed. The tadpoles are filter-feeders, sieving microscopic particles from water while hovering head-down at an angle of 45° with the tip of the tail flickering continuously. In the wild, tadpoles of X. laevis form large schools, all orientated in the same direction and swimming in unison. Under natural conditions, body length (head to tail tip) typically exceeds 90 mm with a highly muscular tail, but in the laboratory maximum body size is considerably less. This size difference might suggest that typical laboratory conditions for rearing tadpoles are sub-optimal.

Tadpoles are fed diets with particle size appropriate for the gill filtering apparatus. These include finely powdered plant material (nettle powder, algae), commercial fish food, finely ground pellets intended for adult X. laevis, and milk (which produces a droplet suspension of suitable size for filtration). Feeding frequency should allow the suspension to be cleared between meals. The amount of food required increases with development; material that settles to the tank bottom can support an infusorial culture that adds to the food supply. Large aquaria may become relatively stable with water changes at intervals of a few weeks but, with intensive feeding, once-weekly changes may be required. Water quality can be maintained with gentle aeration but X. laevis tadpoles also breathe air, visiting the surface about every 30 min in normoxic water.

Oviposition induced by hormonal stimulation typically results in deposition of eggs *en masse* – often several thousand eggs – on the bottom of a container. Under natural conditions, the mode of egg deposition differs: the mating pair swim slowly throughout oviposition, eggs are released singly or in small groups and are stuck to vegetation, stones and vertical surfaces. This ensures that eggs develop above anoxic mud and benthic predators. It is possible that rapid, massive deposition of eggs in the laboratory results from over-stimulation of the reproductive tract by high hormone dosage, but it is not known whether this affects egg quality. Observations of spontaneous spawnings in semi-natural aquaria with water depth 50 cm show that the amplexed pair undertake extensive coordinated movements resulting in trails of eggs adhering to the tank sides up to the water surface. In laboratory stimulation of egg deposition, *Xenopus* are typically housed in shallow water in a container only about 50% larger than the female; there is no possibility of swimming during egg release. It remains to be investigated whether spatial restrictions on natural behaviour during induced oviposition might have a significant stress effect and whether this might influence egg quality.

Reproductive output: oöcyte quality

Problems reported in the literature are at three levels. First, a failure of egg production by X. laevis recently brought into the laboratory (from 'the wild' and commercial suppliers) for which the contributing factors include temperature, food supply and natural seasonal cycles. Second, variation during laboratory maintenance involving a temporary reduction in egg quality followed by recovery. Third, a history of laboratory performance in which females have good oöcyte production for 2–3 years, followed by gradual deterioration until animals are considered 'not fit for purpose' (and are usually culled).

Failures with recently arrived animals were more common with X. laevis exported from South Africa. At the Cape (the source of most supplies), X. laevis breeds from early spring to mid/late summer, typically September to February. Females may spawn up to three times during this period, so some adults brought into laboratories for oöcyte 'harvesting' have gravid ovaries prepared for ovulation while others have depleted ovaries following recent natural spawning. These animals may be accustomed to natural water temperatures close to those experienced in laboratories (i.e. around 20 °C). By contrast, adult X. laevis collected during April–July (late autumn/winter at the Cape) may be taken from water at low temperatures (around 10 °C), unprepared for immediate spawning, and transfer to laboratory temperatures represents a shock. The equivalent natural cycle involving an anovulatory period in winter has been observed in introduced populations in San Francisco (Farrell *et al.* 2007). These natural seasonal cycles may explain part of the variation in physiological state of X. laevis immediately after importation. Use of lab-raised X. laevis in research should eliminate these problems.

Some laboratories report temporary failures of oöcyte production in established X. laevis colonies. These may occur over a few months and have been linked with seasonal effects, but deterioration and recovery have occurred in laboratories isolated from variations in temperature and photoperiod. Contributing factors are unexplained.

For laboratories (outside Europe) that use wild-caught imports, X. laevis should have a period of intensive feeding at optimum temperatures for 2–3 months between arrival and first use. Intensive feeding is also essential between successive spawnings to ensure regrowth of ovaries. Husbandry procedures must ensure that all females feed to satiation at each meal, avoiding the possibility that feeding by some individuals in a group is compromised by competition and dominance hierarchies.

Regarding temperature for oviposition by *X. laevis*, most laboratories employ the range 19–23 °C in agreement with conditions in the wild. Accumulation of ripe oöcytes may begin in early spring (in Cape habitats) at about 16 °C; this explains reports that good quality eggs may be harvested at temperatures lower than those optimal for spawning.

Identifying the longer-term problems of permanent deterioration in egg quality is more difficult. Green (2002) reviewed factors affecting oögenesis, emphasising the importance of temperature and food supply (as in the preceding text) and also age of the female. In the laboratory, female *X. laevis* may contain up to 1000 mature oocytes after sexual maturity. At 2–3 years, both lab-raised and wild females are highly productive, capable of laying 3 or 4 clutches/year, each with more than 20,000 eggs (Tinsley & McCoid 1996). This productivity continues in older females (aged 4.5–15 years) in the wild but may decline in lab-raised *Xenopus* when 3–4 years old. Significantly, the first spawnings of lab-raised *X. laevis* and the first spawnings of wild-caught *X. laevis* in the laboratory produce good quality eggs, but there is subsequent deterioration of both. This suggests that it is duration of laboratory maintenance, and hence some deficiency in laboratory environment and/or husbandry procedures that influences deterioration in oöcyte quality rather than female age. Green (2002) considered a series of other factors that might affect egg quality including bacterial and fungal infections of eggs after harvesting. Elsner *et al.* (2000) identified particular problems with oöcytes obtained surgically using clean but not aseptic techniques which resulted in antibiotic-resistant infections; quality was restored with antiseptic surgery and enhanced antibiotic treatment.

There have been few attempts to test husbandry practices quantitatively against oöcyte quantity and quality. Delpire *et al.* (2011) compared the functional activity of a membrane co-transporter in eggs from *X. laevis* maintained in static tanks or a recirculating system. Oöcytes from females in static tanks were reported to be consistently superior. Unfortunately, interpretation was confounded by differences including water chemistry and temperature, tank dimensions, water depth and amount and frequency of feeding, so it cannot be used to generate recommendations.

Laboratory procedures

Handling

The slippery skin of *X. laevis* makes capture by predators – and laboratory handling – difficult. The powerful hindlimbs and sharp claws may deter inexperienced handlers who must be neither too tentative nor too rough. The hand is positioned palm down above the animal in water so its head is facing the handler's wrist; the index finger is moved between the animal's hindlimbs and flexed forward beneath its abdomen; the thumb and remaining fingers are closed around the animal's flanks. The animal can then be lifted above the water surface with its body held gently but firmly against the palm of the hand and its legs hanging between thumb and forefinger on one side and forefinger and middle finger on the other. In this position, the animal is unable to bring its hindlimbs forward to push itself away or scratch the handler. Small agile individuals are best caught with two hands enclosing the animal in cupped palms. Temporary immobilisation can be achieved by holding the wet animal in soft paper towelling which can be discarded after a single use. *Xenopus* typically become calm when they experience light pressure on their dorsal surface and their eyes are covered.

Latex and nitrile gloves cause high mortality in amphibian tadpoles including *X. laevis* and unwashed vinyl gloves are also toxic (Cashins *et al.* 2008). There is currently no evidence for negative effects on juveniles or adults but lethality in tadpoles suggests the need for caution. Hand creams that might irritate amphibian skin must not be used.

In addition to the characteristic mucus skin secretions of *X. laevis* (present at all times), animals stressed by rough handling may discharge a milky exudate from the body surface. This is highly toxic, intended to deter predators and has an acrid odour. Secretions coalesce to form glutinous strands that are difficult to remove from surfaces. This exudate is toxic to the animals themselves. *Xenopus* that acquire a covering of thick white secretion become paralysed and die within about 10 min. The effects spread to others in the same tank. If recognised quickly, the symptoms can be prevented by transferring affected animals to clean water and gently removing the glutinous secretion with a succession of pieces of paper towel. Production of the exudates stops when animals are calmed and they can recover in several changes of clean water, but all containers, surfaces, etc. must be thoroughly washed to remove chemical traces that might affect other *Xenopus* or handlers. This extreme defence reaction may be encountered in *X. laevis* recently caught in the wild, but is rare in animals habituated to laboratory conditions. Most disastrously, it may occur during transport if animals are crowded and/or subjected to unfavourable conditions.

Administration of substances

For injection (e.g., hormone stimulation of spawning), *X. laevis* can be held securely by the extended hindlimbs if these are gripped together in soft paper towelling just posterior to the pelvis. There must be no possibility that one or both legs can be brought forward, allowing the animal to push itself free. The abdomen and anterior of the animal can then be rested on the bench surface (on damp paper towel) with hindlimbs immobilized: in this position, an injection can be given without risk of movement that could lead to injury. Gonadotrophic and other hormones are typically introduced into the dorsal lymph sac; fluid in this large subdermal space is quickly transported into the general circulation and around the body. It is most efficient to introduce the hypodermic needle very superficially (almost horizontally) through the skin of the dorsal thigh and forwards through the septum separating the lymph spaces of upper leg and back. Injected fluid can then be expelled into the dorsal lymph sac with reduced risks of leakage and entry of infection.

The needle should meet only fine superficial capillaries so there should be no bleeding or bruising.

Monitoring methods

For measurement of weight and length (e.g., to record growth rates), it is least stressful to weigh animals in a container of water on a top pan balance. Differences of a few grams between successive weights of the same animal are not significant since these may result from presence or absence of urine in the bladder and from gut contents. In *Xenopus*, measurement of body length (typically, the distance from the tip of the nose to the cloaca, i.e. snout–vent length, SVL, or more strictly to the tip of the urostyle, SUL) is prone to errors created by the sliding pelvis. The forward-directed iliac processes of the pelvic girdle articulate with the sacral vertebrae by means of a sliding joint (resembling the sliding seat of some rowing boats). This adaptation, enabling an individual to shorten or lengthen its spine by up to 15%, is effective in rapid escape movements and also burrowing in mud. Accurate SVL data require *Xenopus* to be measured in a relaxed 'standard' position (without the legs being contracted up to the body, reducing length, nor extended too fully, increasing length). With practice, this can be done in a few seconds with animals transferred quickly from water to damp paper towel on a flat surface. A flexible transparent ruler is most efficient; callipers should be avoided because of risk of injury if the animal moves suddenly. It is difficult to reduce variation between successive measurements of the same individual to <2 mm; therefore, differences of 1 or 2 mm in a series of length measurements cannot be considered significant. Even with this error margin, valuable data on growth and condition can be compiled. Reliability is improved if the same investigator makes successive measurements, standardizing the method of holding the animal and the degree of contraction or extension.

Identification and marking techniques

Removal of digits for individual identification is not acceptable and, in *Xenopus*, cut toes re-grow. PIT tags (passive integrated transponders) or microchips introduced beneath the skin produce a unique signal that can be read with a portable scanner. However, the process of inserting the tag (ca. 5 mm long, 1 mm diameter) seems questionable on welfare grounds. Needle injectors work effectively on the thick skin of mammals where the point of insertion in elastic tissues closes as the needle is withdrawn. However, in amphibians, including *X. laevis* with relatively inelastic skin, the perforation can remain open risking infection and sometimes loss of the tag. Visible Implanted Elastomers (VIE tags), using combinations of coloured spots beneath the skin, require multiple injection sites (and hence potential pathogen entry) and VIE may have poor visibility in the heavily pigmented skin of *Xenopus*.

In many amphibians, the skin is too delicate to tolerate dye injection or branding but *Xenopus* is unusual in having relatively tough skin. Reed (2005) and Green (2010) considered branding ineffective but this author's field studies, based on populations of several thousand *X. laevis*, have confirmed the value of dye marks and brands (e.g., Tinsley et al. 2012, 2015b). Introduction of dye (typically, alcian blue) with a pressure injector produces discrete spots that remained visible for over 20 years (in long-lived *X. laevis* in the wild). Freeze-branding using metal numbers and letters also produces dark, easily read figures on the white belly skin that are permanent (again >15 years in natural populations) and have never been found to cause skin damage or infection (details in Tinsley et al. 2015a, Supplementary Information). Methods involving the numbering of individuals may be valuable for large populations or for long-term laboratory maintenance of animals that may be moved between different treatments. However, for aquaria holding small groups of animals, it is simpler and quicker to base individual identification on photographs of the dorsal skin patterns of the occupants in each tank (attached to the tank or record book). These pigmentation patterns remain constant in *Xenopus* even when background colour changes. They can be analysed with digital imaging and machine vision techniques to produce a single hexadecimal digit characterizing individuals (see Tinsley 2010a).

Anaesthesia/analgesia

MS222 (tricaine methane sulphonate) is the most effective anaesthetic, administered by immersion of animals in a 0.05–0.10% solution. MS222 forms an acidic solution in water and should be buffered to pH7 with sodium bicarbonate. Adult *X. laevis* left in MS222 for about 10 min after loss of reflexes will take 20–30 min to recover when transferred to clean, preferably flowing, water (but times vary with body size and temperature). During anaesthesia and recovery, animals should be propped with nostrils above the water surface and, if out of water, should be kept wet with damp tissue. Alternatives including Benzocaine are reviewed by Smith et al. (2018). There is an urgent need for information on analgesics effective with *Xenopus*, particularly for surgical removal of oöcytes. Some alternative agents are considered by Green (2010) and Smith et al. (2018) and references, but there is limited information on drug doses and their safety margins; potential effects on oöcyte quality are unknown.

Euthanasia

Among several alternative methods (Reed 2005), an overdose of MS222 (generally, 2–3 g/l of water, buffered to ph7) is most effective and humane (Archard & Goldsmith 2010). After unconsciousness, time to death is variable (more than 1 h) but animals should then be double-pithed to destroy brain and spinal cord tissue. Where perfusion might wash out MS222, barbiturate overdose (injected into the dorsal lymph sac) may be recommended.

Transport

It is predictable that an animal with a secretive lifestyle would be distressed by transport and re-housing (see also Chapter 12: Transportation of Laboratory Animals). Problems include exposure to unfavourable environmental conditions (especially, heat, poor water quality, restricted access to air), stress from overcrowding, and physical damage from movement within containers. Holmes et al. (2018) assayed waterborne corticosterone levels as an indicator of stress and found that release rates increased in transported animals, remaining elevated for the following 7 days.

Xenopus laevis are sometimes transported with minimal water in insulated boxes packed with damp moss or sponge. The light packaging reduces cost but the method risks stress and injury. Although *X. laevis* tolerates emersion from water in a damp environment, they continue to excrete ammonia that can cause skin burns. Without water, animals are more vulnerable to temperature fluctuations; containers must not be exposed to sun during transport.

From personal experience, it seems better to transport *Xenopus* in clean water deep enough to cover all individuals. Water has the disadvantage that it transmits vibrations, but sterile sponge reduces waves and provides a more stable covering for submerged animals. Polystyrene boxes that are waterproof (lined with polythene sheeting) provide insulation, but air holes must not become blocked. In relatively shallow boxes, *Xenopus* may jump and hit their heads, incurring injuries ('red nose' symptoms) and subsequent bacterial infection: the rough surface of polystyrene should be padded with a lining of sponge. Animals should not be fed for 3–4 days before travelling to reduce fouling of water. For transport over shorter distances between laboratories, animals can be carried in relatively deep water (around 30 cm) in tall containers (with lids above jumping height), at a time of day avoiding high temperatures.

Safety considerations

There are no records of transfer of infection from *Xenopus* species to humans. However, some bacterial infections are the same as or closely related to human pathogens so there is, potentially, a zoonotic risk. Common sense hygiene measures should be adopted when handling *Xenopus* and aquarium water. The use of gloves is recommended (these reduce sensitivity in handling, missing information on the animal's condition from its skin texture, but this should be weighed against protection for the handler). *Mycobacteria*, including *M. chelonae* and *M. marinum*, are important concerns for anyone immunosuppressed; specialist medical advice should be obtained. Treatment for these infections in humans is difficult; *M. chelonae* is resistant to most antibiotics and to some disinfectants. Although each of the reports of lethal outbreaks in laboratory *Xenopus* emphasized that no human cases occurred among staff (see section on Health and disease, in the following text), it would be prudent for immunosuppressed individuals to avoid contact with aquaria and aquatic organisms altogether.

Skin secretions of *Xenopus* species are toxic. Workers handling *X. laevis* must avoid transfer of mucus to their eyes (if irritated, eyes should be washed with copious amounts of water). The defensive response of *Xenopus* to extreme physical stress, involving discharge of milky exudate from the body surface, potentially represents a greater concern for laboratory workers (see section on Handling, in the preceding text). Warning signs include the acrid odour, white glue-like strands and rapid deaths of affected *Xenopus*. Accounts of the natural history of *X. laevis* in South Africa describe the deaths of animals (including dogs) that have bitten *Xenopus*. Since *Xenopus* can recover if quickly washed with clean water (see the preceding text), the same remedy should be appropriate for humans. All contaminated laboratory surfaces must also be thoroughly washed.

Workers with *Xenopus* should avoid inhalation and skin contact with MS222 (see the preceding text); gloves should be worn; solutions should be prepared under a fume hood and kept covered.

Common Welfare Problems

Gas bubble disease affects *Xenopus* exposed to water supersaturated with gases, especially nitrogen. Supersaturation arises when air is drawn into water pumped under pressure to supply aquarium systems. Gas bubbles accumulate in the vascular system leading to haemorrhages in foot webbing and limbs. Tsai et al. (2017) reported deaths following exposure for <1 hour; recovery of surviving *Xenopus* appeared complete after 2 weeks but, although individuals were apparently in good condition, oöcyte quantity and quality were still reduced 6 months later (after which these animals were culled).

The sensitivity of *X. laevis* to noise and severe vibrations transmitted through water has been documented in animals exposed to building construction work (Felt et al. 2012). During a 30 min exposure, symptoms included buoyancy problems, inability to submerge, skin sloughing and stomach eversion resulting in airway obstruction and death. Effects were attributed to over-stimulation of hair cells in the lateral line system.

Bite wounds (and cannibalism) may be associated with aggression and the 'feeding frenzy'. Torreilles and Green (2007) described how introduction of refuges in crowded populations of *X. laevis* reduced the incidence of bite wounds from 5% annually in tanks without enrichment to about 0.5% after addition of sections of pipe. While this case confirms the value of refuges, it also illustrates conditions promoting aggression which should not occur in laboratory maintenance. In addition to the relatively high density (150 animals in 300 l of water), groups of *Xenopus* were removed each month and replaced with different individuals. This practice may constantly challenge the social hierarchy and increase aggression within a colony (Chum et al. 2013).

Thermal shock leading to death has been reported among *X. laevis* experiencing a sudden temperature change of only 2–5 °C (Green et al. 2003; Green 2010). However, the report actually involved a change from 16 to 23 °C (deaths caused by the 2–5 °C change related to other anuran species).

Stress

The development of sensitive assays for corticosterone has provided insight into the responses of *Xenopus* to stress. Archard and Goldsmith (2010) tested effects of various euthanasia methods on circulating plasma corticosterone levels. Apart from the primary findings (that the highest MS222 concentration tested, buffered to pH7, caused least stress), the study produced the significant result that the order of removal of *X. laevis*, taken in sequence from tanks containing groups of animals, was positively related to corticosterone levels. This could be associated with repeated disturbance of remaining animals as the next-in-turn is taken from the holding tank. It might also reflect stress induced by increasing awareness of the progressive removal (capture) of co-habitants (i.e. that alarm is contagious). This alarm response may resemble the agitation shown by groups of *Xenopus* when water levels are suddenly reduced (see the preceding text).

Measurement of corticosterone has been refined in non-invasive studies where release rates have been assayed in water containing *Xenopus*. Holmes *et al*. (2016) recorded increased stress in *Xenopus* housed in tanks with a white background compared with those on a black background (in agreement with the preference tests of Hilken *et al*. (1994) and others). Additionally, increased atypical behaviour was recorded in the white background group. Holmes *et al*. (2018) reported equivalent effects with elevated corticosterone in water following transportation and re-housing (see the preceding text).

Care of aged animals

Laboratories supporting mass maintenance of *Xenopus* 'egg producers' are unlikely to justify the upkeep of females once the quality and quantity of eggs has declined. For others with less intensive maintenance, the concept of 'aged' is more flexible. *Xenopus* species can reproduce successfully aged 15 years and survival in the wild and the laboratory may exceed 20 years (see the preceding text). While still healthy, these can meet conservation needs for captive breeding or can be 'retired' as pets for *Xenopus* enthusiasts.

Health and disease

The older literature describes a range of pathological conditions affecting *Xenopus* including degenerative diseases, neoplasms and microbial infections (considered from a medical perspective by Dr Edward Elkan and others). These conditions are rare and illustrate three related principles (Tinsley 1995). First, *X. laevis* may carry some pathogens without symptomatic disease until there is a physiological check caused by malnutrition, temperature change or other environmental stress. Until this point, the condition may apparently be controlled, becoming overtly pathogenic only following the additional precipitating factor. Second, once disease has become established, pathogenesis may develop to an extreme degree before *X. laevis* exhibits obvious ill-effects. Commonly, in tuberculosis of the lungs, liver or gut, a considerable part of the organ may become non-functional before illness and death occur. Reichenbach-Klinke and Elkan (1965) observed that such *'crippling injuries and disease would have killed warm-blooded animals at a much earlier stage'*. Third, in overcrowded conditions of laboratory maintenance, one animal may develop severe disease (tuberculosis, for instance) and die, while others in the same aquarium remain unaffected. These observations suggest immune defences are normally highly effective in controlling disease.

For skin damage including minor infections, natural immunity is often the best means of recovery (without antibiotics). In the writer's experience, affected *Xenopus* should be maintained in isolation in darkened aquaria and undisturbed surroundings. They should be transferred to clean water daily, so that skin healing is not hampered by elevated ammonia or bacterial populations. Feeding should be restricted to food taken immediately by the animal, with uneaten food removed to prevent contamination. Where this natural recovery is effective, improvement is visible over about a week, with progressive reduction in areas of damaged skin until completely healed. If there is deterioration, antibiotic treatment may be required (under direction from a vet). With severe pathology and visible distress, recovery is often unlikely and outbreaks are best managed by early culling. Strict hygiene is essential (especially with nets, tanks and tank-cleaning materials).

Microbial infections

Ranaviruses are associated with amphibian disease outbreaks worldwide and have been recorded in laboratory populations and commercial supplies of *X. laevis*. Adult *X. laevis* are resistant to FV3, clearing infection within a few weeks, but the virus can then remain quiescent in apparently healthy hosts (Robert *et al*. 2007). This covert infection can cause acute systemic disease when host immunity is compromised and is transmissible to others including tadpoles in which it is lethal. Laboratory populations of *Xenopus* – as potential asymptomatic carriers of *Ranavirus* – therefore constitute a risk for wider dissemination into the environment (see Biosecurity in the following text).

A comprehensive review of microbial infections of *X. laevis* by Green (2010) includes diagnosis, clinical aspects and drugs used in treatment: this and more recent references should be consulted for detailed information. A familiar condition (for all amphibians) is the skin infection 'red leg', often attributable to secondary infection following injury, stress or another primary infection. Agents implicated include *Aeromonas hydrophila*, *Pseudomonas* spp. and *Staphylococcus* spp. causing epidermal bleeding progressing to severe generalized sepsis. *Chryseobacterium* (*Flavobacterium*) spp. cause fatal septicaemia and are significant because of their resistance to antibiotics, chlorine and chloramines. Most bacterial infections associated with high mortality in laboratory epidemics are ubiquitous in aquatic environments and are opportunistic pathogens in the laboratory. There is typically no treatment and culling is recommended to reduce risks of further spread. Other agents causing mortality in laboratory *Xenopus* populations include *Chlamydia pneumoniae*, *Cryptosporidium* spp., and nontuberculous mycobacteria including *Mycobacterium chelonae*, *M. xenopi*, *M. liflandii*, *M. marinum* and an *M. ulcerans*-like infection (Green *et al*. 2000; Trott *et al*. 2004; Fremont-Rahl *et al*. 2011; and others). Infection may be transmitted vertically through oöcytes or sperm, remaining subclinical until triggered by stress including low temperatures and handling during oöcyte collection (see Fremont-Rahl et al. 2011). Some of these mycobacteria are potentially zoonotic (see sections on Safety in the preceding text, and Biosecurity in the following text).

Devastating epidemics among *X. tropicalis* may be linked to the higher water temperatures employed in husbandry (favouring faster bacterial multiplication) or, perhaps, to greater stress experienced by this tropical forest species in the laboratory environment.

Fungal infections

The chytrid fungus, *Batrachochytrium dendrobatidis* (*Bd*), occurs in most wild and laboratory populations of *X. laevis*. Infection causes epidermal damage but in wild populations this appears normally to be relatively minor. Lethal infections have been recorded in lab populations, especially of *X. tropicalis*. Control of laboratory epidemics relies on culling and comprehensive disinfection of equipment with antifungal chemicals. In a survey of *Bd* based on RT-PCR assays, nearly 90% of UK laboratories carried infection (Tinsley et al. 2015a). Field and lab evidence from introduced *X. laevis* in the UK shows that data on infection levels are strongly influenced by environmental factors. Heavy infections in two UK laboratories accompanied stress: low temperature in one and infection with *Pseudocapillaroides xenopodis* (see Parasites section) in the other. Tests on *X. laevis* in UK field populations showed prevalence twice as high in April (84% after 6 months at <10 °C) than in July (43% after 3 months at ≥15 °C). Parallel experiments with lab-raised *X. laevis* recorded 100% prevalence at 10 °C but only 3% at 20 °C. During repeat testing of lab-maintained populations, most individuals were *Bd*-negative even when they shared aquaria with *Bd*-positive animals (Table 47.1). Field studies showed no *Bd* infection in UK native amphibian species associated with the populations of *X. laevis* and no evidence of declining numbers, even where the introduced and native species had shared habitats for 50 years. This 'neutral' outcome in the UK could be specific to the environmental conditions, or the *Bd* lineages introduced with the *X. laevis*, or the native species 'at risk' in the UK. In other world regions where *X. laevis* has been introduced, this 'silent carrier' may be responsible for spread to susceptible amphibian species in the wild. Within laboratories, *Bd* in *Xenopus* represents a major threat to other co-housed amphibian species: in one such cross-infection 'spill-over', the Mallorcan Midwife Toad, *Alytes muletensis*, acquired *Bd* from infected *Xenopus gilli*, both maintained in species recovery programmes in the same facility (Tinsley et al. 2015a) (see Biosecurity in the following text).

Saprolegnia spp. are typically associated with fish but can cause secondary skin infections in amphibians including *Xenopus*. These fungi have an impact on laboratory research where *Xenopus* oöcytes become infected *in vitro*.

Parasites

Xenopus species carry a richer assemblage of parasites than most other anurans – over 25 genera from seven invertebrate groups infecting almost every organ of the body. This spectrum reflects a dual 'inheritance': some parasites are characteristic of groups found in anurans, reflecting a common evolutionary origin, and some are related to parasites of fish, reflecting an ecological origin through shared diet, habitats, etc. All have ancient evolutionary relationships (not recent transfers), and almost all are strictly host-specific to *Xenopus* so are not a hazard for other amphibians. References to these parasites are listed in Tinsley (1995, 1996) and Jackson & Tinsley (2001) with further details in Tinsley (2010b) (Figure 47.3).

In countries where wild-caught *Xenopus* are used in research, parasite infections may transmit within pre-existing laboratory populations and compromise welfare, physiological function and research use. The natural parasite fauna of *Xenopus* should not be encountered in European institutions. If these parasites are discovered, then the source of infection would raise serious concerns.

Potential for transmission depends on life cycle characteristics. Parasites with indirect life cycles that require specific intermediate hosts (including snails and insects) should not be able to transmit in laboratories and so, if present at capture, will gradually decline. Thus, although potentially worrying to non-specialists, expulsion of gut parasites, including tapeworms (*Cephalochlamys namaquensis*), nematodes (*Camallanus* and *Batrachocamallanus* species) and several species of digenean flukes (Figure 47.3d,e,g), has no implications for spread (but indicates the possibility of more worms within the consignment of *Xenopus*). Parasites with indirect life cycles employing *Xenopus* species as intermediate hosts also cannot transmit within lab populations; these include *Tylodelphylus xenopodis* (pericardium) (Figure 47.3h) and encysted metacercariae (eyelids and lateral line organs). Because they complete their life cycles in predators of *Xenopus* (typically, birds), pathological effects in delicate organs may impair behaviour or stamina, predisposing to capture by final hosts (reviewed by Tinsley 1996).

Parasites with direct life cycles (a single host species) have the potential to increase in numbers and spread from host to host. One nematode parasite of *X. laevis*, *Pseudocapillaroides xenopodis*, is notorious for devastating epidemics in laboratory populations. Affected hosts develop roughened skin, become anorexic, emaciated and die. Lethal infections have occurred in *X. laevis* a year after importation from South Africa, so laboratory populations may include individuals carrying pre-existing asymptomatic infection. A thymus-dependent immune response protects against development of disease; overt symptoms may follow immunosuppression including reduction in water temperature (Tinsley 1995). Infection can be treated with anthelmintic drugs, including thiabendazole and ivermectin. The eggs are highly resistant and can spread between aquaria on nets, etc.

Three other parasites have direct life cycles with the potential to transmit within lab populations: two monogeneans (*Protopolystoma xenopodis* and *Gyrdicotylus gallieni*) and an acarine mite (*Xenopacarus africanus*) (Figure 47.3b,c,a). For all three, primary infection can trigger an immune response that eliminates the parasites (Tinsley 1996). In laboratories where different populations of *X. laevis* are maintained separately from one another, infection would eventually die out. However, if new imports of *X. laevis* or successive

Table 47.1 *Batrachochytrium dendrobatidis* in laboratory populations of adult *Xenopus laevis*: changes in detectable infection with time. Records of *Bd* infection were determined by RT-PCR assay using TaqMan probes. Animals, all originating from the same stock at the European *Xenopus* Resource Centre, were allocated to 8 tanks each with 4 animals of a single sex and monitored over 19 weeks at 18.5 °C. Solid blocks indicate the periods of maintenance when individuals tested positive for *Bd* at the start of the respective time intervals; for all other blocks, tests for *Bd* were negative.

Chytrid was present in the overall population but only 9 of 352 tests (2.6%) were positive over the 19 weeks of observation. All animals in 4 of the groups (tanks) were *Bd* negative over the complete sequence of 11 tests. In each of 2 tanks, 1 animal showed a single positive test. Only 2 animals showed repeat infections: in #23, the episodes were separated by 10 weeks without detectable infection; in #16, the second episode continued as 3 successive positive results in the final 7 weeks of sampling; with this exception, all other positive tests were followed on the next screening by a negative result. In all groups except one (tank D), the positive infection was restricted to a single individual, without any detectable occurrence in the other animals in the same tank. In 4 of the weeks, the tests indicated that all animals were free of detectable infection; in 6 of the weeks when infection was detected, only a single host was *Bd*-positive (prevalence 3%). This low prevalence is consistent with published field surveys but the repeat testing showed that the specific individuals involved fluctuated with time. Source: Adapted from Tinsley (2015a).

Tank/Animal		Weeks 1	3	5	6	7	8	10	11	12	13	19
A (females)	1											
	2				■	■						
	3											
	4											
B (females)	5											
	6											■
	7											
	8											
C (females)	9											
	10											
	11											
	12											
D (females)	13										■	
	14											
	15											
	16			■						■	■	■
E (males)	17											
	18											
	19											
	20											
F (males)	21											
	22											
	23	■							■			
	24											
G (males)	25											
	26											
	27											
	28											
H (males)	29											
	30											
	31											
	32											

generations of laboratory-produced animals are mixed with previously established populations, the naïve individuals provide a chain of susceptible hosts allowing infection to persist for long periods (even for years). In the recent past, *X. africanus*, has been a consistent 'passenger' with consignments of *X. laevis* from a major supplier, evidently transmitted within stock facilities before dispatch.

One of the most important of these parasites for low-level chronic pathology is *Protopolystoma xenopodis*. Adults in the urinary bladder produce eggs that pass out with the urine, develop for about 3 weeks in sediment and release larvae that invade the next host via the cloaca. Juvenile worms develop in the kidneys for 2–3 months before migrating to the bladder and beginning egg production.

Burdens of *P. xenopodis* in the urinary bladder are strictly regulated (reviewed by Tinsley 2004). Despite continuous transmission in the wild, numbers of adult worms remain low (mean <2 adults/host). So, although these parasites feed on blood, there is an effective limit on blood loss. However, juvenile infections in the kidneys are potentially more serious. Most worms are killed by an immune response within about a month post-infection; however, repeated invasion by infective stages may produce a 'rolling' population of parasites responsible for continual pathology including tissue

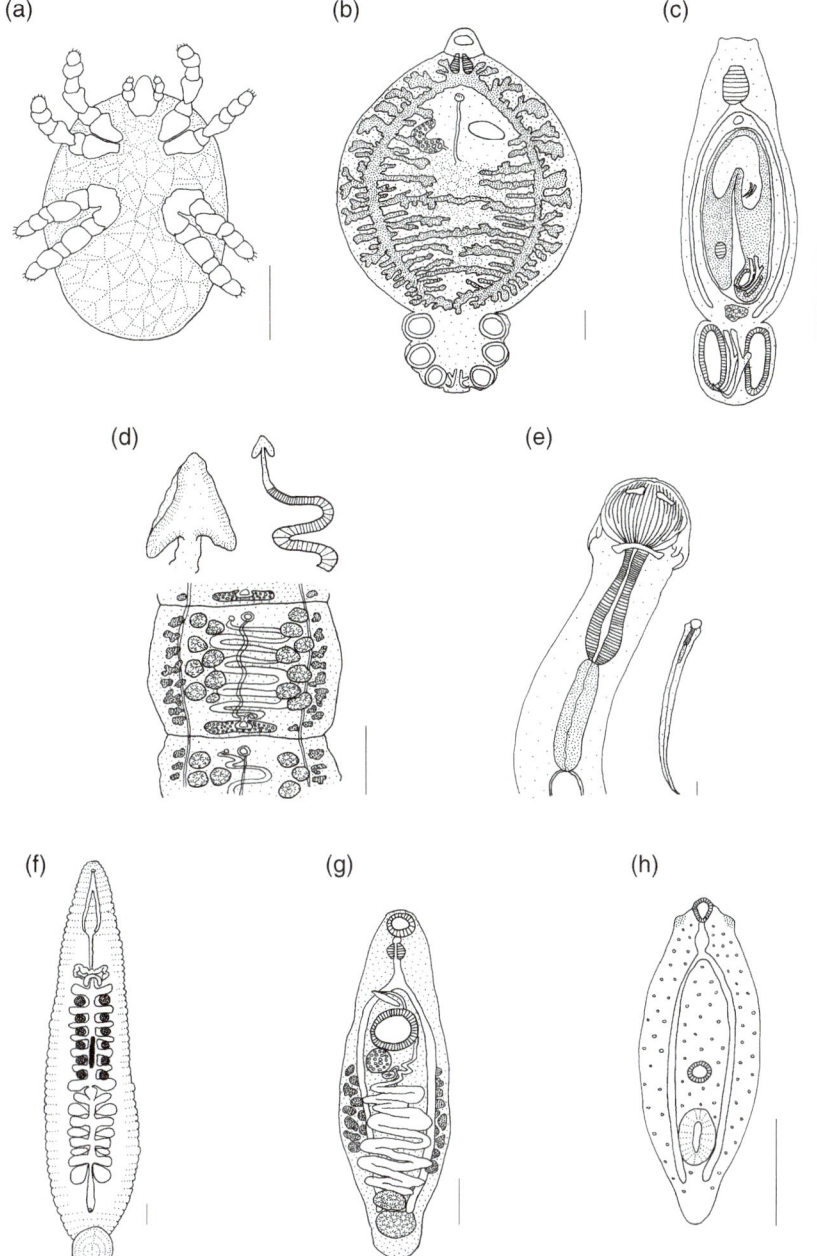

Figure 47.3 Selected parasites of *Xenopus laevis* showing morphological features enabling diagnosis of laboratory infections. (a) *Xenopacarus africanus* (acarine mite; nasal and eustachian passages). Reproduction occurs within the host and heavy infections may accumulate in laboratory *Xenopus* populations. Larval stages are white; digestion of host blood produces black pigmentation as the mites develop. (b) *Protopolystoma xenopodis* (monogenean platyhelminth; urinary bladder and kidneys): blood-feeding flukes with a direct life cycle; infections can transmit during laboratory maintenance if sediment accumulates in aquaria (see text). (c) *Gyrdicotylus gallieni* (monogenean platyhelminth; oral cavity). An offspring develops to maturity within the uterus of the parent worm and may, in turn, contain a further embryo in its uterus. Progeny emerge directly at the site of infection producing rapid increase in parasite numbers; host-to-host transfer of worms occurs by contact. (d) *Cephalochlamys namaquensis* (tapeworm, intestine): infections can be detected when mature segments are passed in water; arrowhead-shaped scolices may also be expelled following host stress or hormone treatment. (e) Several species of camallanid nematodes attach by a chitinized buccal capsule to the wall of the oesophagus, stomach and intestine. As in the tapeworm (d), life cycles require a copepod intermediate host and transmission does not normally occur in laboratory maintenance. (f) *Marsupiobdella africana* (leech; external skin): this species is unique among leeches in brooding up to 50 offspring in a ventral pouch; when developed, the young emerge through a mid-ventral pore and attach to *Xenopus*, feeding on blood from epidermal capillaries. (g) *Oligolecithus elianae* (digenean platyhelminth; intestine). This and 3 other species of digeneans occurring in the stomach, intestine, gall bladder and rectum have complex life cycles with a snail intermediate host; they do not transmit in laboratory populations of *Xenopus*. (h) *Tylodelphylus xenopodis* (digenean platyhelminth; pericardial cavity): larvae may be detected only at host dissection; worms released from the pericardial membranes sometimes occur on the surface of the ovaries. Infections result from skin penetration by larvae from snail intermediate hosts in natural habitats. Related trematodes, all requiring transfer to a predator of *Xenopus* to complete their life cycles, occur in the body cavity, lateral line system and eyelids. There is no laboratory transmission but infections may represent a confounding factor in laboratory procedures. The pathogenic nematode, *Pseudocapillaroides xenopodis*, is not shown; fine thread-like worms may be found in teased fragments of skin examined as fresh, wet preparations under the microscope; eggs hatch within epidermal tunnels created by adult worms; parasite burdens accumulate in individual hosts and transmit by contamination. For references to parasite infections, see text. All scale bars = 250 μm.

damage, blood-feeding and stimulation of inflammatory and other anti-parasitic responses.

This life cycle can be controlled in the laboratory when parasite eggs are removed before they complete development. Minimum time to hatching is 26 days at 20 °C (but only 18 days at 25 °C) (Tinsley et al. 2011). With static tank maintenance, weekly water changes provide a wide safety margin preventing re-infection (assuming aquaria are emptied, rinsed and refilled with a complete change of clean water). With husbandry procedures involving partial water changes, infective larvae may develop in the tank sediment, re-infect the occupants and initiate pathogenic disease. The situation with recirculating systems is unexplored but will depend on frequency of tank cleaning alongside the flow-through water exchange. With a water replacement rate of 10% per day, eggs should be removed – on average – within 10 days, but the risks of autoinfection are increased where sediment accumulates around enrichment items that impede water flow. Tanks should be disconnected and thoroughly cleaned at least every 2 weeks.

Quarantine

New arrivals of *Xenopus* must be kept separate from existing laboratory populations. This is essential not only to prevent introduction of new infections but also to avoid adding naïve hosts that could maintain an asymptomatic infection already present in the laboratory. However, while quarantine is essential, the previous sections show that it cannot completely prevent disease introductions. Several of the highly pathogenic parasite infections can occur in lab-maintained animals for over a year without symptoms and then create epidemics (including *Pseudocapillaroides xenopodis*). Infections of adult *Protopolystoma xenopodis* can be detected by recovery of eggs passed in water (see Tinsley 2004) but developing worms may remain undetected in the kidneys for up to a year (Tinsley et al. 2012). Table 47.1 shows that chytrid fungus may be undetected by RT-PCR assays for over 3 months and subsequently test positive. Infections may be kept in check by effective immune responses, but the potential remains for severe disease when immunity is compromised by stress and other factors. Quarantine is also ineffective in identifying parasites employing *Xenopus* as intermediate hosts (including *T. xenopodis* in the pericardium); heavy parasite burdens may remain viable but undetected for several years.

The objective of quarantine is also defeated in infections with *Ranavirus* and several bacterial agents, especially the mycobacteria which may remain latent until immune control is compromised. The possibility of vertical transmission of mycobacteria via oöcytes or sperm raises major concerns; outbreaks among lab-bred animals may originate from previous generations of wild-caught parents (see section on Health and disease in the preceding text).

Biosecurity

Although quarantine does not protect against introduction of infection, scrupulous laboratory hygiene is essential to limit transfer within facilities. Maintenance of groups of *Xenopus* in separate tanks provides some restriction on spread of infection, enabling outbreaks to be contained. Prevention of infection in recirculating systems depends on effectiveness of in-line sterilization of recycled water. There are special risks of introduction of bacteria pathogenic for *Xenopus* where the agents are free-living in origin, carried in water supplies. Different species of *Xenopus* must be isolated from one another to prevent disease transfer; other 'non-amphibian' taxa may represent carriers of *Mycobacteria* spp. transmissible to *Xenopus* including Zebrafish (a potential source of epidemics in *X. laevis* even when spatially separated within animal facilities). While strict hygiene precautions are essential to prevent disease within laboratories (considered in the preceding text in the sections on Water changes, Safety, and the various groups of infectious agents), equivalent measures must control against transfer into the external environment. Routine protocols should include the use of footwear (or coverings) restricted to designated areas, and sterilization of floors and other surfaces with agents such as Virkon. The other major route for potential dissemination of laboratory infections into the external environment is via drainage water. The possibility of environmental contamination by *Bd* can be prevented by heating effluent water to 60 °C or treatment with disinfectants before discharge.

Signs of poor welfare

In response to unfavourable conditions or poor health, *X. laevis* may adopt a 'hunched' posture with fore- and hindlimbs held close to the body and head depressed. Skin texture is an important indicator of well-being: it should have a glossy appearance and slippery feel (reflecting effective mucus production), but in ill-health may feel relatively rough and 'dry'. In healthy animals, the process of moulting involves separation of large sheets of outer keratinised skin which are typically pushed into the mouth with the forelimbs and eaten. When animals are unhealthy or stressed, the outer skin is shed into the water in small fragments. In chronic ill-health, there may be pinpoint haemorrhages visible on the white skin of the belly and legs.

The presence of bite marks on the limbs indicates aggression; this can be alleviated by reducing density, introducing more refuges and avoiding addition of new animals into established tank populations.

Floating and an inability to submerge is symptomatic of several pathological conditions. Accumulation of fluid in the dorsal lymph sac may indicate failure of the lymph hearts near the base of the spine. Damaged noses may indicate shallow water depth, an inappropriate tank cover or disturbed behaviour reflecting stress.

Poor welfare and stress may be evident from the tank water when it becomes cloudy with small fragments of shed skin. *Xenopus* with very different body sizes should not be maintained together.

Concluding remarks

Use of amphibians as 'laboratory animals' in research and teaching was formerly motivated by the belief that populations in the wild (especially of frogs) are an abundant, easily

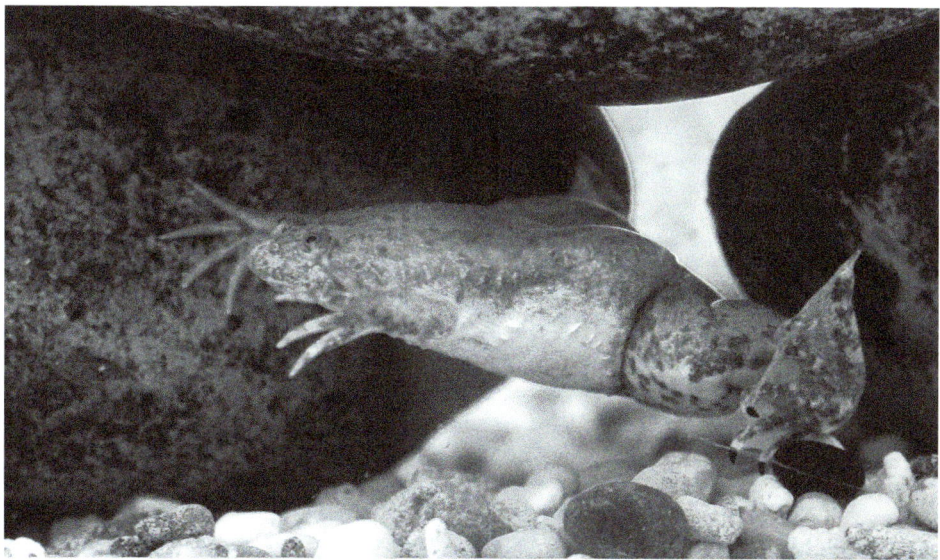

Figure 47.4 *Xenopus victorianus*: adult female in a 'semi-natural' aquarium illustrating the distinctive posture of animals maintained in good environmental conditions with optimum welfare. This individual occupies the entrance to a refuge (in this case, a 'cave' which is backlit to enhance the photograph but, in practice, would have a black background to increase seclusion); forelimbs are outstretched in readiness to capture prey (including, in nature, organisms that may drift or swim past in the water column or that land on the water surface above); hindfoot webbing is expanded and leg muscles flexed to enable rapid movement. The prominent bulges on the posterior dorsum are created by the large inflated lungs in the body cavity allowing submergence for up to about 1 h; in nature, rapid intake of air at the surface (<1 sec) is synchronized and socially controlled within groups of *Xenopus* but breathing behaviour may be disrupted in laboratory maintenance. The alert, responsive disposition of this individual contrasts with body attitudes typical of poor welfare (see text). Source: Tinsley, R.C. (2010b) / with permission from CABI.

caught, relatively inexpensive source of live vertebrate material for practical exercises. However, in almost all cases now, large-scale capture of frogs is not sustainable, physiological condition is often poor (especially because of inappropriate maintenance) and large-scale use cannot be justified. This conclusion is inescapable on the grounds of conservation, ethics, welfare and cost, but use of amphibians is also unacceptable scientifically where reliability of results may be compromised by poor condition or stamina. However, laboratory use of *X. laevis* differs in important respects. Populations in natural habitats are abundant and there are no major conservation concerns. Most importantly, supplies to many major laboratories worldwide are now provided by specialized breeding establishments. Indeed, European Directive 2010/63 makes this obligatory in member countries.

While it is essential to improve conditions for all amphibians in laboratory research (Brod *et al.* 2019), most of this account has focused on *Xenopus* because of the anomaly that this is one of the most intensively used laboratory animals internationally – as a 'model organism' – but laboratory conditions compromise the most demanding research, and there are no overall standardized procedures based on experimentally proven evidence for optimum husbandry.

Given the lack of quantitative validation for maintenance protocols, this chapter has adopted the approach of relating observations 'in the wild' to interpreting the requirements for improved laboratory welfare. The discussion still leads to the conclusion that well-designed controlled experiments are essential to resolve uncertainties. However, as a focus for those future studies, a general principle from this review is

that effects potentially compromising physiological condition (including oögenesis) are likely to be subtle and long-term. This is prompted in part by the finding that reproductive performance (egg quality) may be satisfactory during short-term maintenance of *X. laevis* but declines after about 3 years. This short effective 'life span' contrasts with outcomes 'in the wild' (and in semi-natural lab maintenance) where females can spawn prolifically for 15 years or more. So, the challenge is to identify and exclude suboptimal laboratory conditions that have negative effects over (or after) several years.

Some of the case studies for *X. laevis* (in the preceding text) show long-term ill-effects after initial recovery from setbacks. Thus, *Xenopus* that had apparently recovered after gas bubble disease still had impaired oöcyte production 6 months later. This could suggest that poor reproductive performance in later life could have its origins in previous stress.

Some of the more obviously unfavourable conditions in the laboratory environment have (or should have) now been improved, such as the provision of refuges and dark substrates, but others considered in this chapter remain. In this author's assessment, the most important candidate for major improvement – rarely considered in the literature – is living space, especially water depth. All comparisons with conditions in natural habitats and observations of behaviour in aquaria suggest that water depth is far too low in laboratory husbandry. The physical and behavioural stress induced by shallow water could contribute to chronic low-level debilitation whose effects accumulate over time to affect reproductive performance. Some water change procedures incorporate sudden reductions in water depth including complete drainage of tank water while the animals remain *in situ*. For an aquatic animal with abilities for complex monitoring of its environment (see the preceding text), sudden disappearance of its habitat and exposure out of water could represent a significant shock. In this writer's opinion, laboratory procedures that repeatedly impose such obvious distress should be reconsidered.

Looking to the future, the need for rigorous quantitative trials of alternative husbandry protocols (as emphasized throughout this chapter) remains urgent. Among other measures, the trials must use the criterion most critical for research – oöcyte quality. There is also a need for greater knowledge of the behaviour and sensory perception of *Xenopus* to increase understanding of responses to environmental conditions in laboratory maintenance. Finally, it should be emphasized that the key to high standards of welfare lies with laboratory personnel with a natural sympathy for living amphibians, able to recognize behaviour patterns and other indicators of good health and absence of stress. This understanding is best achieved with a thorough knowledge of the 'natural history' of the species and the patience for careful first-hand observation.

Acknowledgements

Research on *Xenopus* has been supported by grants from the Biotechnology and Biological Sciences Research Council, including BB/C506272/1 and BB/D523051/1. I am grateful to many people who discussed *Xenopus* facilities and shared their experiences, including Sir John Gurdon, Matt Guille, Rue Jones-Green, Mollie Millington, Jean-Philippe Mocho, Clare Sims, Nicola Watts and Stephen Woodley; special thanks also to Heather Tinsley.

References

AmphibianArk (2019). http://www.amphibianark.org/husbandry-documents/?wpfb_cat=3#wpfb-cat-3 (Accessed 12 September 2019).

Amphibiaweb (2019). http://amphibiaweb.org (Accessed 12 September 2019).

Archard, G.A. and Goldsmith, A.R. (2010). Euthanasia methods, corticosterone and haematocrit levels in *Xenopus laevis*: evidence for differences in stress? *Animal Welfare*, **19**, 85–92.

Archard, G.A. (2012). Effect of enrichment on the behaviour and growth of juvenile *Xenopus laevis*. *Applied Animal Behaviour Science*, **139**, 264–270.

Baird, T.A. (1983). Influence of social and predatory stimuli on the air-breathing behavior of the African clawed frog, *Xenopus laevis*. *Copeia*, **1983**, 411–420.

Brown, M.J. and Nixon, R.M. (2004). Enrichment for a captive environment – the *Xenopus laevis*. *Animal Technology and Welfare*, **3**, 87–95.

Brod, S., Brookes, L. and Garner, T.W.J. (2019). Discussing the future of amphibians in research. *Lab Animal*, **48**, 16–18.

Cashins, S.D., Alford, R.A. and Skerratt, L.F. (2008). Lethal effect of latex, nitrile, and vinyl gloves on tadpoles. *Herpetological Review*, **39**, 298–301.

Chum, H., Felt, S., Garner, J. et al. (2013). Biology, behavior, and environmental enrichment for the captive African clawed frog (*Xenopus* spp). *Applied Animal Behaviour Science*, **143**, 150–156.

Dawson, D.A., Schultz, T.W. and Shroeder, E.C. (1992). Laboratory care and breeding of the African clawed frog. *Frog Care*, 31–36.

Delpire, E., Gagnon, K.B., Ledford, J.J. et al. (2011). Housing and husbandry of *Xenopus laevis* affect the quality of oocytes for heterologous expression studies. *Journal of the American Association for Laboratory Animal Science*, **50**, 46–53.

Directive 2010/63/EU of the European Parliament and of the Council. https://eur-lex.europa.eu/legal-content/EN/TXT/?uri=CELEX:32010L0063 (Accessed 2 February 2019).

Elepfandt, A. (1996a). Sensory perception and the lateral line system in the clawed frog, *Xenopus*. In: *The Biology of Xenopus*. Eds Tinsley, R.C. and Kobel, H.R., pp. 97–120. The Zoological Society of London, Clarendon Press, Oxford.

Elepfandt, A. (1996b). Underwater acoustics and hearing in the clawed frog, *Xenopus*. In: *The Biology of Xenopus*. Eds Tinsley, R.C. and Kobel, H.R., pp. 177–193. The Zoological Society of London, Clarendon Press, Oxford.

Elsner, H.-A., Hönck, H.-H., Willmann, F. et al. (2000). Poor quality of oocytes from *Xenopus laevis* used in laboratory experiments: prevention by use of antiseptic surgical technique and antibiotic supplementation. *Comparative Medicine*, **50**, 206–211.

Evans, B.J., Carter, T.F., Greenbaum, E. et al. (2015). Genetics, morphology, advertisement calls and historical records distinguish six new polyploid species of African clawed frog (*Xenopus*, Pipidae) from West and Central Africa. *PLOS ONE* | DOI:10.1371/journal.pone.0142823

Farrell, K., Bouley, D. and Green, S. (2007). Seasonal oogenesis in feral South African clawed frogs (*Xenopus laevis*). *Proceedings Association of Reptilian and Amphibian Veterinarians*, 129–130.

Felt, S.A., Cowan, A.M., Luong, R. et al. (2012). Mortality and morbidity in African clawed frogs (*Xenopus laevis*) associated with construction noise and vibrations. *Journal of the American Association for Laboratory Animal Science*, **51**, 253–256.

Fremont-Rahl, J.J., Ek, C., Williamson, P.L.C. et al. (2011). *Mycobacterium liflandii* outbreak in a research colony of *Xenopus* (*Silurana*) *tropicalis* frogs. *Veterinary Parasitology*, **48**, 856–867.

Furman, B.L.S., Dang, U.J., Evans, B.J. et al. (2018). Divergent subgenome evolution after allopolyploidization in African clawed frogs (*Xenopus*). *Journal of Evolutionary Biology*, **31**, 1945–1958.

Godfrey, E.W. and Sanders, G.E. (2004). Effect of water hardness on oocyte quality and embryo development in the African clawed frog (*Xenopus laevis*). *Comparative Medicine*, **54**, 170–175.

Green, S.L. (2002). Factors affecting oogenesis in the South African clawed frog (*Xenopus laevis*). *Comparative Medicine*, **52**, 307–312.

Green, S.L. (2010). *The Laboratory Xenopus sp*. CRC Press, Boca Raton.

Green, S.L., Lifland, B.D., Bouley, D.M. et al. (2000). Disease attributed to *Mycobacterium chelonae* in South African clawed frogs (*Xenopus laevis*). *Comparative Medicine*, **50**, 675–679.

Green, S.L., Moorhead, R.C. and Bouley, D.M. (2003). Thermal shock in a colony of South African clawed frogs (*Xenopus laevis*). *Veterinary Record*, **152**, 336–337.

Gurdon, J.B. (1996). Introductory comments: *Xenopus* as a laboratory animal. In: *The Biology of Xenopus*. Eds Tinsley, R.C. and Kobel, H.R., pp. 3–8. The Zoological Society of London, Clarendon Press, Oxford.

Hilken, G., Willman, F., Dimigen, J. et al. (1994). Preference of *Xenopus laevis* for different housing conditions. *Scandanavian Journal of Laboratory Animal Science*, **21**, 71–80.

Hilken, G., Dimigen, J. and Iglauer, F. (1995). Growth of *Xenopus laevis* under different laboratory rearing conditions. *Laboratory Animals*, **29**, 152–162.

Holmes, A.M., Emmans, C.J., Jones, N. et al. (2016). Impact of tank background on the welfare of the African clawed frog, *Xenopus laevis* (Daudin). *Applied Animal Behaviour Science*, **185**, 131–136.

Holmes, A.M., Emmans, C.J., Coleman, R. et al. (2018). Effects of transportation, transport medium and re-housing on *Xenopus laevis* (Daudin). *General and Comparative Endocrinology*, **266**, 21–28.

IUCN (2019). The Red List of Threatened species. Version 2019-2. http://www.iucnredlist.org. (Accessed 12 September 2019).

Jackson, J.A. and Tinsley, R.C. (2001). Host-specificity and distribution of cephalochlamydid cestodes: correlation with allopolyploid evolution of pipid anuran hosts. *Journal of Zoology*, **254**, 405–419.

Kaplan, M.L. (1993). An enriched environment for the African clawed frog (*Xenopus laevis*). *Lab Animal*, **22**, 25–28.

Kwong-Brown, U., Tobias, M.L., Elias, D.O. *et al*. (2019). The return to water in ancestral *Xenopus* was accompanied by a novel mechanism for producing and shaping vocal signals. *eLife*, **8**, e39946

Landgrebe, F.W. (1939). The maintenance of reproductive activity in *Xenopus laevis* for pregnancy diagnosis. *Journal of Experimental Biology*, **16**, 89–95.

Major, N. and Wassersug, R.J. (1998). Survey of current techniques in the care and maintenance of the African clawed frog (*Xenopus laevis*). *Contemporary Topics*, **37**, 57–60.

Measey, G.J. and Channing, A. (2003). Phylogeography of the genus *Xenopus* in southern Africa. *Amphibia-Reptilia*, **24**, 321–330.

Michaels, C.J., Gini, B.F. and Preziosi, R.F. (2014). The importance of natural history and species-specific approaches in amphibian ex-situ conservation. *Herpetological Journal*, **24**, 135–145.

Reed, B.T. (2005). *Guidance on the Housing and Care of the African Clawed Frog Xenopus laevis*. Research Animals Department, RSPCA, Horsham

Reichenbach-Klinke, H. and Elkan, E. (1965). *The Principal Diseases of Lower Vertebrates*. Book II Diseases of Amphibians. T.F.H. Publications, New Jersey.

Ringeis, A., Krumscheid, B., Bishop, J. *et al*. (2017). Acoustic communication and reproductive behaviour in the aquatic frog *Xenopus laevis* (Pipidae), a field study. *African Journal of Herpetology*, **66**, 122–146.

Robert, J., Abramowitz, L., Gantress, J. and Morales, H.D. (2007). *Xenopus laevis*: a possible vector of ranavirus infection? *Journal of Wildlife Diseases*, **43**, 645–652.

Robert, J. and Ohta, Y. (2009). Comparative and developmental study of the immune system in *Xenopus*. *Developmental Dynamics*, **238**, 1249–1270.

Smith, B.D., Vail, K.J., Carroll, G.L. *et al*. (2018). Comparison of etomidate, benzocaine, and MS222 anesthesia with and without subsequent flunixin meglumine analgesia in African clawed frogs (*Xenopus laevis*). *Journal of the American Association for Laboratory Animal Science*, **57**, 202–209.

Stuart, S.N., Hoffmann, M., Chanson, J.S. *et al*. (2008). *Threatened Amphibians of the World*. Lynx Edicions, Barcelona, Spain; IUCN, Gland, Switzerland; and Conservation International, Arlington.

Tinsley, R.C. (1995). Parasitic disease in amphibians: control by the regulation of worm burdens. *Parasitology*, **111**, S153–S178.

Tinsley, R.C. (1996). Parasites of *Xenopus*. In: *The Biology of Xenopus*. Eds Tinsley, R.C. and Kobel, H.R., pp. 233–261. The Zoological Society of London, Clarendon Press, Oxford.

Tinsley, R.C. (1999). Parasite adaptation to extreme conditions in a desert environment. *Parasitology*, **119**, S31–S56.

Tinsley, R.C. (2004). Platyhelminth parasite reproduction: some general principles derived from monogeneans. *Canadian Journal of Zoology*, **82**, 270–291.

Tinsley, R.C. (2010a). Amphibians, with special reference to *Xenopus*. In: *The UFAW Handbook on the Care and Management of Laboratory and other Research Animals*, 8th edn. Eds. Hubrecht, R. and Kirkwood, J., pp. 741–760. Wiley-Blackwell, Oxford.

Tinsley, R.C. (2010b). *Xenopus*. In: *The Encyclopaedia of Applied Animal Behaviour and Welfare*. Eds. Mills, D.S. *et al*. CAB International, Wallingford.

Tinsley, R.C. and Kobel H.R. (1996). *The Biology of Xenopus*. The Zoological Society of London, Clarendon Press, Oxford.

Tinsley, R.C. and McCoid, M.J. (1996). Feral populations of *Xenopus* outside Africa. In: *The Biology of Xenopus*. Eds Tinsley, R.C. and Kobel, H.R., pp. 81–94. The Zoological Society of London, Clarendon Press, Oxford.

Tinsley, R.C., Loumont, C. and Kobel, H.R. (1996). Geographical distribution and ecology. In: *The Biology of Xenopus*. Eds Tinsley, R.C. and Kobel, H.R., pp. 35–59. The Zoological Society of London, Clarendon Press, Oxford.

Tinsley, R.C., Coxhead, P.G., Stott, L.C. *et al*. (2015a). Chytrid fungus infections in laboratory and introduced *Xenopus laevis* populations: assessing the risks for UK native amphibians. *Biological Conservation*, **184**, 380–388.

Tinsley, R.C., Stott, L.C., Viney, M.E. *et al*. (2015b). Extinction of an introduced warm-climate alien species, *Xenopus laevis*, by extreme weather events. *Biological Invasions*, **17**, 3183–3195.

Tinsley, R.C., Stott, L.C., York, J.E. *et al*. (2012). Acquired immunity protects against helminth infection in a natural host population: long-term field and laboratory evidence. *International Journal for Parasitology*, **42**, 931–938.

Tinsley, R.C., York, J.E., Everard, A.L.E. *et al*. (2011). Environmental constraints influencing survival of an African parasite in a north temperate habitat: effects of temperature on egg development. *Parasitology*, **138**, 1029–1038.

Tocque, K., Tinsley, R.C. and Lamb, T. (1995). Ecological constraints on feeding and growth of *Scaphiopus couchii*. *Herpetological Journal*, **5**, 257–265.

Torreilles, S.L. and Green, S.L. (2007). Refuge cover decreases the incidence of bite wounds in laboratory South African clawed frogs (*Xenopus laevis*). *Journal of the American Association for Laboratory Animal Science*, **46**, 33–36.

Trott, K., Stacey, B.A., Lifland, B.D. *et al*. (2004). Characterization of a *Mycobacterium ulcerans*-like infection in a colony of African tropical clawed frogs (*Xenopus tropicalis*). *Comparative Medicine*, **54**, 309–317.

Tsai, J.Y., Felt, S.A., Bouley, D.M. *et al*. (2017). Acute and chronic outcomes of gas-bubble disease in a colony of African clawed frogs (*Xenopus laevis*). *Comparative Medicine*, **67**, 4–10.

Wu, M. and Gerhart, J. (1991). Raising *Xenopus* in the laboratory. *Methods in Cell Biology*, **36**, 3–18.

Fish

48 Fishes

Sonia Rey Planellas and Carlos Garcia de Leaniz

Introduction: Fish, the most diverse vertebrate taxon

The single most distinguishing feature of fish is perhaps their sheer diversity. With over 33,000 known species (Froese & Pauly 2019), fish harbour more diversity than all the other vertebrates put together. Fish are present in all continents, in all waters, and occupy virtually every aquatic niche. They live in waters with temperatures that range from −2 °C to 40 °C and salinities that range from less than 0.5 g/kg in freshwater to up to 130 g/kg (four times full seawater) in the case of some euryhaline species inhabiting extreme coastal and arid environments (Kültz 2015). Some species like the mangrove killifish (*Kryptolebias marmoratus*), the mudskippers (family Oxudercidae) and the walking catfish (*Clarias batrachus*) are amphibious in nature and can remain out of the water for relatively long periods thanks to specialised skin cells and various adaptations that let them breathe air.

Fish range in size from 8 mm in length when mature in the case of the Cyprinid *Paedocypris progenetica* (the smallest known vertebrate (Kottelat *et al.* 2006)) to over 12 metres (the whale shark *Rhincodon typus* (Colman 1997)) and their life span ranges from 2 months for the sign eviota, *Eviota sigillata*, a small coral reef fish with the shortest lifespan of any vertebrate (Depczynski & Bellwood 2005), to 112 years for the bigmouth buffalo (*Ictiobus cyprinellus*), a freshwater Cypriniforme native to North America (Lackmann *et al.* 2019) or even 392 years (Nielsen *et al.* 2016) for the Greenland shark (*Somniosus microcephalus*).

Some species are live bearers like the guppy (*Poecilia reticulata*) and give birth to a few fully developed fry while others like the sunfish (*Mola mola*) can release in excess of 300 million eggs at a time (Froese & Pauly 2019). Unique among vertebrates, the mangrove killifish can produce hermaphrodites and self-fertilise, producing offspring that are genetically identical to their parents (Consuegra *et al.* 2013), while the Amazon molly (*Poecilia formosa*) reproduces through gynogenesis which results in only females (Schartl *et al.* 1995). One species, the African turquoise killifish (*Nothobranchius furzeri*), has become the animal model of choice for studying the process of ageing, as its embryos can pause development (diapause) for years, longer than the animal's average lifespan of only four to six months (Harel *et al.* 2015).

What is a fish?

Their sheer diversity makes it difficult to define with precision what a fish is; there is no universally accepted common definition of 'fish'. Fish have been defined as a 'a cold-blooded animal that lives in water, breathes with gills, and usually has fins and scales'[1] as 'cold-blooded vertebrates provided with gills throughout life, and whose limbs, if present, are modified into fins'[2], but also as 'aquatic, craniate, gill-bearing animals that lack limbs with digits'[3]. In an earlier version of this chapter, Turnbull and Berrill (2010) defined fish as 'aquatic vertebrates that rely, at least in part, on gills for respiration in the adult form'.

The vast majority of fishes are bony fishes (Class Osteichthyes, 96%), with skeletons composed of true bone tissue, as opposed to cartilage (Class Chondrichthyes including sharks, skates and rays, 4%), and the Agnathans (<1%), which are primitive jawless fish that include the lampreys and hagfishes. Among the bony fishes, the largest family is the Cyprinids (carps, goldfish, zebrafish) which, with c. 3,000 species and 370 genera, is also the largest family of vertebrates, followed by the Cichlids (>1,650 species described, and possibly 2,000–3,000 additional species yet to be described) which include the Tilapiine tribe that encompasses the tilapias, one of the most important farmed fish species worldwide. So, in many ways, to understand what a fish is, and what their needs are, one must consider the Cyprinids (like the goldfish) and the Cichlids (like the tilapias) first.

---

[1] https://www.merriam-webster.com/dictionary/fish [English Language Learners Definition of fish] (Accessed September 20, 2021)
[2] https://www.oed.com/ (Accessed July 27, 2021)
[3] https://en.wikipedia.org/wiki/Fish (Accessed July 27, 2021)

Fish in research

The use of fish in research has grown exponentially during the last twenty years, amounting to tens of millions of fish annually. In the USA alone, around 3.5–7 million fish are used for research each year, roughly 7% of all experimental animals (The American Anti-Vivisection Society 2021). This includes fish model species, such as the zebrafish (see Chapter 49: Zebrafish), but also species increasingly being used for aquaculture, one of the fastest growing food industries. Indeed, the need to domesticate and diversify more species for the aquaculture industry is one of the reasons behind the increasing use of fish in research, particularly in areas related to fish farming such as nutrition, reproduction, genetics, health, physiology and welfare. The number of scientific publications on fish welfare alone has increased more than twentyfold since 2010 (Figure 48.1).

In the UK, a total of 375,532 fish were used in regulated animal research procedures during 2020, of which 83% were zebrafish and 17% were other fish (UK Home Office 2021). Fish were the second most commonly used animals in experimental procedures (13%), second only to mice (72%) (UK Home Office 2021). The majority (67%) of research using fish in the UK during 2020 involved the nervous system and animal behaviour (UK Home Office 2021). In the EU, 1.2 million fish were used for regulated research during 2017 (13% of the total number of animals used) (Abbott 2020), 41% of which were zebrafish and 59% were other fish species (European Commision 2020). Although the identity of fish species other than zebrafish is not provided, these likely include Atlantic salmon (*Salmo salar*), rainbow trout (*Oncorhynchus mykiss*), European sea bass (*Dicentrarchus labrax*), gilthead sea bream (*Sparus aurata*), Nile tilapia (*Oreochromis niloticus*), goldfish (*Carassius auratus*), three-spined stickleback (*Gasterosteus aculeatus*) and the guppy (*Poecilia reticulata*), as these are the species most commonly used in fish research (Table 48.1).

Bibliographic analysis (Figure 48.2) indicates that different fish species are used in different areas of research, the observed distribution being markedly different from what one would expect if species choice followed a uniform distribution. For example, goldfish is mostly used in physiology and studies of adaptation; guppies and sticklebacks for behavioural and evolutionary work; salmon and trout for ecological and aquaculture studies; cleaner fish, sea bream, sea bass and tilapia for aquaculture-related studies; tilapia and trout for nutrition; while zebrafish is mostly used for research into disease, evolution, biomedicine, physiology and toxicology. The results also indicate that despite the continued increase in the number of fish used for scientific purposes, research on fish welfare is still modest compared to other research areas, and that sea bass is the only species where research effort on welfare slightly exceeds the expected value from a uniform distribution.

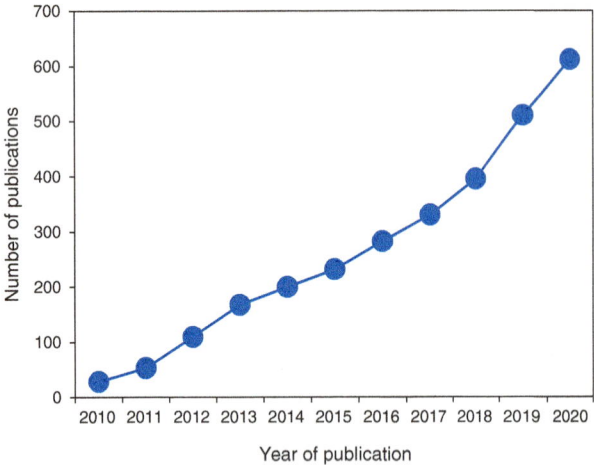

Figure 48.1 Cumulative number of scientific publications with the term 'fish welfare' in the title, the keywords or in the main body of text in articles published during the last 10 years. Source: Web of Science, all databases from 2010–2020.

Table 48.1 Fish species cited in 345 publications with the term 'fish welfare' in the title, the keywords or in the main body of text in articles published during the last 10 years (2009–2020) appearing in two or more articles. A further 95 species were cited in only one publication and are not presented here.

Common name	Scientific name	No. of publications	%
Atlantic salmon	*Salmo salar*	139	19.50
Rainbow trout	*Oncorhynchus mykiss*	72	10.10
European sea bass	*Dicentrarchus labrax*	46	6.45
Gilthead sea bream	*Sparus aurata*	32	4.49
Zebrafish	*Danio rerio*	30	4.21
Atlantic cod	*Gadus morhua*	29	4.07
Nile tilapia	*Oreochromis niloticus*	23	3.23
Common carp	*Cyprinus carpio*	20	2.81
Turbot	*Psetta maxima*	15	2.10
African mud catfish	*Clarias gariepinus*	13	1.82
Senegalese sole	*Solea senegalensis*	13	1.82
European eel	*Anguilla anguilla*	9	1.26
Mozambique tilapia	*Oreochromis mossambicus*	9	1.26
Arctic char	*Salvelinus alpinus*	8	1.12
Goldfish	*Carassius auratus*	7	0.98
South American catfish	*Rhamdia quelen*	7	0.98
Brown trout	*Salmo trutta*	7	0.98
Three-spined stickleback	*Gasterosteus aculeatus*	5	0.70

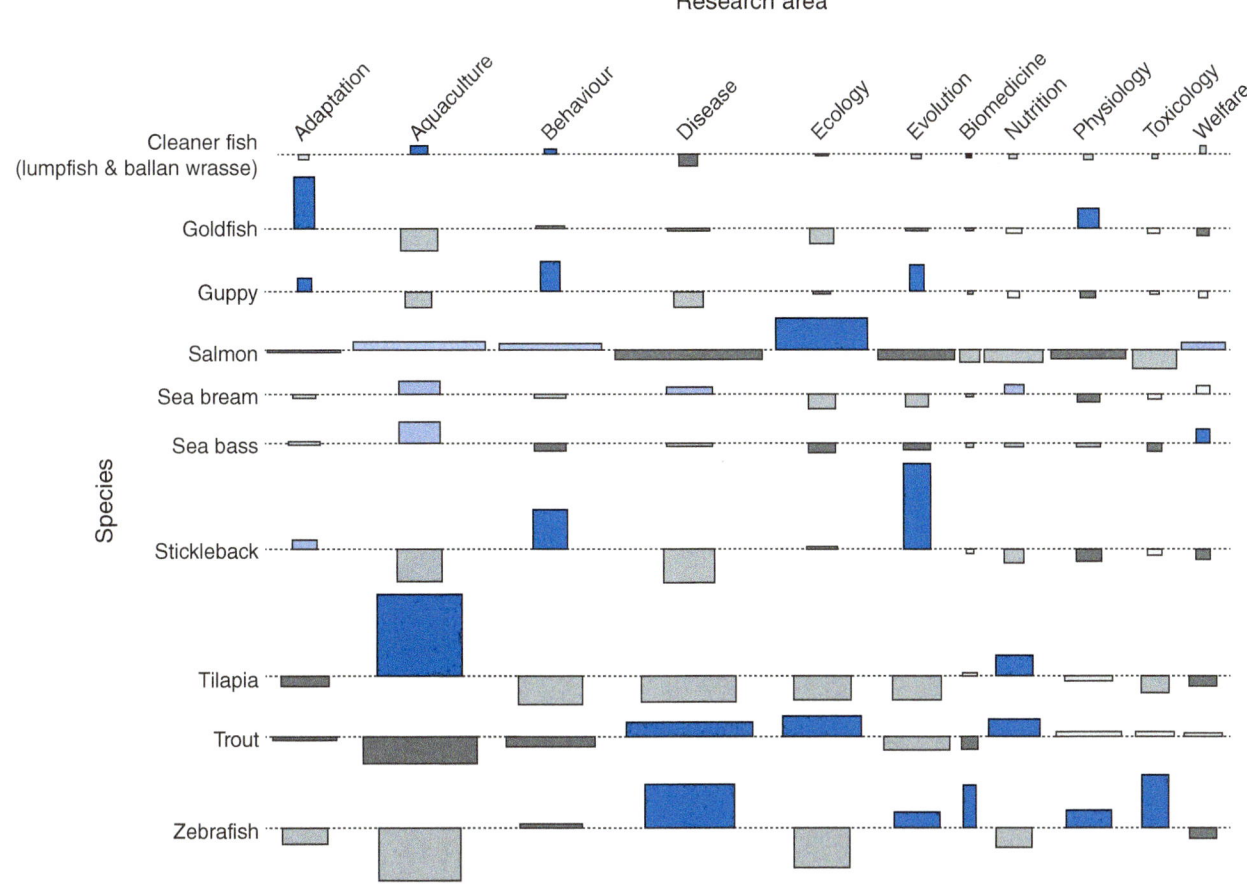

Figure 48.2 Association plots showing the use of different fish species in different areas of research based on 12,696 papers retrieved from Google Scholar with the common name of the species and the research area in the title as search strings. The area of each box is proportional to the difference in observed and expected frequencies. Dark blue boxes indicate positive associations above the random expectation and grey boxes negative associations. The results indicate that different species are used in different contexts and research areas (Likelihood Ratio = 4367.2, df = 90, P< 0.001).

Implementing the Three Rs in fish research

The high diversity and plasticity of fish has important consequences for research design (covered in Chapter 3: The design of animal experiments) and also for implementing the Three Rs (covered in Chapter 2: The Three Rs). Imprecise or biased results can be generated due to uncontrolled sources of variation, and this is particularly true for fish research where studies may involve hundreds or even thousands of individuals, sourced from the wild or other very heterogenous sources (farms, pet shops, etc.), and typically housed across multiple tanks or aquaria.

Most teleost fish have a duplicated genome (Taylor et al. 2003) and this contributes to their extreme diversity and plasticity (Volff 2005) and generates additional sources of variation among otherwise similar individuals. Thus, to increase the precision and statistical power of fish studies (and reduce the number of fish required for research), the effects of plasticity, genetic variation and housing conditions need to be taken explicitly into account. For example, subtle differences in light intensity, temperature or noise may exist between otherwise identical tanks and these can generate individual differences in physiology or behaviour (Wysocki et al. 2007). How fish are handled or anaesthetised can also generate unwanted variation (Thompson et al. 2016), and some fish may change their behaviour by eavesdropping on their neighbours which may violate the assumption of statistical independence (Fernandes Silva et al. 2019) and may require that tanks are visually isolated from one another. Likewise, alarm cues, free cortisol and other steroid hormones can accumulate in recirculation systems commonly used in fish research (Mota et al. 2014, 2017) and this can potentially influence the behaviour and physiology of experimental fish sharing the same (recirculated) water (Martins et al. 2009). Lack of standardisation in housing conditions can lead to variation in the fish microbiota (Vatsos 2017) that can affect the results of experiments and reduce reproducibility.

In order to implement the Three Rs, 'nuisance variables' need to be measured so that they can be treated as covariates (Meyvis & Van Osselaer 2017), and tank effects need to be explicitly incorporated into data analysis (Thorson & Minto 2015), perhaps using generalised linear mixed modelling (Venables & Dichmont 2004; Bolker et al. 2009). An alternative to increase statistical power and reduce sample size would be to use reactive fish with low cortisol response levels that adapt well to captivity (Vindas et al. 2017; Champneys et al. 2018), so that noise caused by family or tank effects is reduced.

Genetic variation can also reduce statistical power to detect treatment effects (Festing & Altman 2002). To overcome this, researchers tend to employ relatively large sample sizes, but this limits efforts to fully implement the Principle of Reduction. Traditionally, a larger number of fish was used for experimental purposes than other vertebrates on the grounds that mortality during the larval and juvenile stages is typically much higher in fish than in other vertebrate taxa. Fish are often sold by weight, not by numbers, and this – for a long time – also reflected how they were viewed as experimental animals. However, a high early life stage mortality is no longer justification for using a large number of experimental fish. An alternative to large samples is the use of isogenic lines with reduced genetic variation (Franěk et al. 2020), although these are seldom completely homozygous (Guryev et al. 2006) and may result in loss of fitness and severe birth defects (Shinya & Sakai 2011) which have welfare implications and renders them unsuitable for some areas of research. Other approaches include using naturally inbred species like the mangrove killifish (Consuegra et al. 2013), mono-sex lines if available (e.g. Nile tilapia, rainbow trout) and rearing fish communally in common garden experiments to reduce tank effects. *A priori* screening for stress-coping styles can reduce the variability of gene expression studies too (Mackenzie et al. 2009).

In the case of biomedical or translational research, fish need to fulfil several additional criteria: they must have similar response to those of humans (face validity), the mechanisms underlying behavioural variation must be similar to that found in humans (constructive validity), and the promoter (e.g. drugs) should have the same effects in the animal model as it does in humans (Denayer et al. 2014; Ferreira et al. 2020). Finally, while replacement is difficult in most areas of fish research, it is not impossible. For example, Kazlauskaite et al. (2021) have developed an *in vitro* simulator of the Atlantic salmon gastrointestinal tract to study the influence of the gut microbiome on fish nutrition. *In silico* studies are also widely used to study the dynamics of fish swimming and shoaling, therefore, dispensing with the need to use live fish (Mwaffo et al. 2017). Increasingly, animal models are being replaced by robotics, *in vitro* techniques, and other approaches whenever possible (see also Chapter 2: The Three Rs) in order to reduce animal numbers used in experimentation and refine methods to minimise welfare costs. The same considerations of the Three Rs apply to fish as to any other vertebrate (NORECOPA 2016).

Husbandry overview and welfare requirements of main fish species used in research

General guidelines for maintaining fish for research have been provided by Clark et al. (1997), DeTolla et al. (1995), American Fisheries Society (2014), Canadian Council on Animal Care (2005) and Sneddon and Wolfenden (2019) among others. There are also many excellent guides for maintaining ornamental (aquarium) fish that provide a wealth of information applicable to the care of laboratory fish (Hawkins 1981; Gay 2005; Gay 2009; Alderton 2019).

However, an appreciation of fish diversity is important for animal technicians, veterinarians and researchers responsible for the health and welfare of fish used in research because, in the case of fish, clearly one size does not fit all. The welfare needs and husbandry requirements of most species of fish are not known.

Below we provide an overview of the husbandry and welfare requirements of the main species used in fish research (see also d'Angelo & de Girolamo 2021). In addition to the species listed in Table 48.1, we have also included information on two species of facultative cleaner fish, the lumpfish (*Cyclopterus lumpus*) and the ballan wrasse (*Labrus bergylta*) which are increasingly being used for research into sea lice control in salmon farming (Powell et al. 2018b; Treasurer 2018a).

The huge diversity of fish species used in research Smith (2013) makes it difficult to provide general husbandry guidelines, as these will not always be appropriate (Johansen et al. 2006). We have selected instead 10 species which are representative of the most commonly used fish in research, based on the number of experimental procedures in the UK (UK Home Office 2021) and the number of publications using scientometrical analysis (de Castilhos Ghisi & de Oliveira 2016), and discussed their specific requirements. Many of the species we discuss are used in aquaculture research, including Atlantic salmon, rainbow trout, sea bass, sea bream and tilapia, as well as two species of cleaner fish (lumpfish and ballan wrasse) used in salmon farming. Other species such as goldfish, guppies and three-spined stickleback are held in captivity and used in behavioural, ecological, toxicological and evolutionary studies. Zebrafish husbandry is not included here as it is covered in Chapter 49. Many other fish species are being used as experimental models for human disease (Schartl 2014) but there is limited guidance on their specific husbandry and welfare requirements. A similar situation occurs with research into ornamental fish, a growing industry (Leal et al. 2016; Evers et al. 2019) for which there are few specific welfare guidelines, but for which we discuss the requirements of the goldfish as a case example, as it has similar needs as the koi carp.

According to EU Directive 2010/63/EU on the protection of animals used for scientific purposes, the following environmental parameters should be monitored for fish used in research: dissolved oxygen, nitrogen compounds, pH, salinity, temperature, lighting, noise, stocking density and water volume. An indicative range of optimal parameters and key husbandry traits for the most common fish species used in research, excluding zebrafish, is given in Table 48.2 and Table 48.3, respectively. Please note that although salinity, light, noise and volume are specifically mentioned in the Directive, they are either not monitored routinely (e.g. noise) or standards are lacking. An image for each of the main fish species used in research can be seen in Figure 48.3.

Goldfish

The goldfish (*Carassius auratus*) is a ray-finned fish belonging to the family Cyprinidae (Carps and minnows). Although native to central Asia, China and Japan, the species has now been introduced into more than 60 countries throughout the world and many feral populations have established (Casal 2006). The species is easily reared in the laboratory

Table 48.2 Indicative range of optimal water parameters for fish described in the text.

Species	O_2 (mg/l)	Temp (°C)	pH	Free ammonia (NH_3, mg/L)	Reference
Goldfish (Carassius auratus)	>5	20–24	6.0–8.0	<0.0500	Froese and Pauly (2019) Watson et al. (2004)
Guppy (Poecilia reticulata)	>4	18–28	7.0–8.0	<0.2000	Wedemeyer (1996)) Mills (1999) Andrews (2002) Froese and Pauly (2019)
Three-spined stickleback (Gasterosteus aculeatus)	>5	4–13.5	7.4–8.3	<0.0001	Froese and Pauly (2019) Schluter (2021) Bakker and Mundwiler (2021)
Tilapia (general) (Oreochromis sp.)	3–8	25–30	6.5–9.0	<0.2400	Stickney (1993) Ross (2000) Hussain (2004)
Rainbow trout (Oncorhynchus mykiss)	>6.5	4–20	7.0–8.0	<0.0125	McLarney (1998) RSPCA (2020) MacIntyre et al. (2008) Noble et al. (2020)
Atlantic salmon (Salmo salar)	>6.5	4–17	6.0–8.0	<0.0125	Froese and Pauly (2019) Noble et al. (2018) RSPCA (2018)
Other Salmonids (general)	>6.5	>0–20	6.0–9.0	<0.0125	Bromage and Shepherd (1992) Noble et al. (2018)
Lumpfish (Cyclopterus lumpus)	>7.3	7–16	7.3–8.5	<0.0050	Garcia de Leaniz et al. (2022) Treasurer et al. (2018a)
Ballan wrasse (Labrus bergylta)	>7	8–16	7.4–8.2	<0.1000	Treasurer et al. (2018a) RSPCA (2018)
Gilthead Sea bream (Sparus aurata)	6–9	12–21	7–8	<0.1000	Froese and Pauly (2019)
Sea bass (Dicentrarchus labrax)	6–9	14–20	7.9–8.2	<0.5000	Pillay and Kutty (2005)

and is an important animal research model, particularly for studies of cognition, memory and adaptation (Lushchak et al. 2001; Rodríguez et al. 2002; Portavella et al. 2004; Roesner et al. 2008) as seen in Figure 48.2.

It has been estimated that over 81 million goldfish were sold in the USA during 2013 (National Agricultural Statistics Service 2019) and that up to 589 million freshwater fish were imported into the UK in 1987–1989, the most common of which were goldfish, although precise numbers are unknown (Maceda-Veiga et al. 2013). Goldfish are traded in over 100 countries and there are more than 300 varieties obtained by selective breeding (Bristol Aquarists' Society 2020), but the most common single tail goldfish used in research are the 'common', 'feeder' and 'comet' varieties (Smartt 2008; Bristol Aquarists' Society 2020).

In the wild goldfish are found in eutrophic, slow flowing and well vegetated freshwater habitats within a wide range of temperatures (0–35 °C) (Watson et al. 2004). The species is omnivorous and will readily feed on commercial dry food in the laboratory; it can easily live in excess of 10 years in captivity where it prefers to live in groups of 5 or more individuals (Froese & Pauly 2019), although few fish will be used for that long in experiments.

Goldfish are very hardy and tolerate relatively low dissolved oxygen and are easily bred in the laboratory. The female will lay adhesive eggs that attach to submerged vegetation during the breeding season, multiple spawnings being the norm which are triggered by a drop in water temperature. Eggs will hatch within 2–9 days post-fertilisation, depending on water temperature, and fry will start feeding 2–3 days after hatching (Watson et al. 2004). Goldfish are social and very inquisitive and prefer to be reared in slow flowing waters with a pH between 6 and 8 (Table 48.3) and temperature between 20 and 24 °C (although they will tolerate 8–30 °C (RSPCA 2019)). They are very voracious, so appropriate filtration is required with weekly water replacements of 10–25% of water volume to maintain water quality and periodic water quality checks. The minimum recommended aquarium size is 100 cm in length and a capacity of more than 50 L, or 4 times the adult body size (RSPCA 2019). More detailed information on the rearing of goldfish can be found in Anders and Ostrow (1986); Smartt (2008); RSPCA (2019); Bristol Aquarists' Society (2020).

Guppy

The guppy (Poecilia reticulata) is a live-bearing, ray-finned teleost belonging to the family Poeciliidae (Poeciliids). The species (also called 'rainbow fish') is characterised by its bright colours that have made it one of the most common freshwater fishes for the aquarium, and also one widely used for research, particularly for studies of adaptation, behaviour and evolution (Magurran 2005), as seen in Figure 48.2. The guppy is a tropical species naturally found in the Northern Hemisphere between 2 and 14 °N of latitude, in densely vegetated streams with temperatures ranging from 18 to 28 °C, with an optimum of 23–24 °C. The guppy has been introduced widely for mosquito control (Froese & Pauly 2019) and feral populations now exist in many parts of the world (Lindholm et al. 2005; El-Sabaawi et al. 2016; Leduc et al. 2021).

Table 48.3 Key husbandry traits of different fish species used in laboratory research.

Husbandry trait	Goldfish	Guppy	Three-spined stickleback	Nile tilapia	Rainbow trout	Atlantic salmon	Lumpfish	Ballan wrasse	Gilthead sea bream	Sea bass	Zebrafish
Typical life span in the laboratory (yr)	3–5	1–2	1–2	1–2	1–2	<1	<1	1–2	2–3	2–3	1–2
Ease to breed lines in the laboratory	Easy	Easy	Easy	Easy	Moderate	Not possible	Not possible	Difficult	Difficult	Difficult	Easy
Aggression	Low	Low	High*	High*	Moderate	High	Moderate	Moderate	Low	Low	Low
Hardiness	High	High	High	High	Moderate	Low	High	Moderate	Low	Low	High
Fecundity (egg or embryo/kg)	63,000	189,000	9,000	73	2,200	2,000	55,000	160,000	1,200,000	638,000	444,000
Typical 1st year length (cm)	13	3	4	18	10	8	12	8	21	22	5
Ease to feed in the laboratory	Easy	Easy	Easy	Easy	Easy	Easy	Moderate	Moderate	Difficult	Moderate	Easy
Trophic level§	2.4	3.0	3.3	2.0	3.8	4.1	3.7	3.2	3.2	3.6	3.1
Domestication	High	High	Low	High	Moderate	Moderate	Low	Low	Low	Low	High
Min. aquarium size (cm)	100	60	60	210	—	—	—	—	—	—	50
Indicative density in laboratory (g/L)	0.5	0.6	1.2	14	12	12	20	5	20	12	0.5
Sexual dimorphism	Yes	Yes	Yes	Yes	Yes	Yes	Yes	Yes	Yes	Yes	Yes
Cannibalism	Common	Common	Common	Common	Rare	Rare	Common	Rare	Rare	Common	Rare

* During breeding;
§ trophic level: the position in the trophic chain, a measure that considers both the diet composition and the trophs of the food items with primary producers and detritus having a TL of 1 and top fish predators a TL of 4 and above (Froese & Pauly 2019).

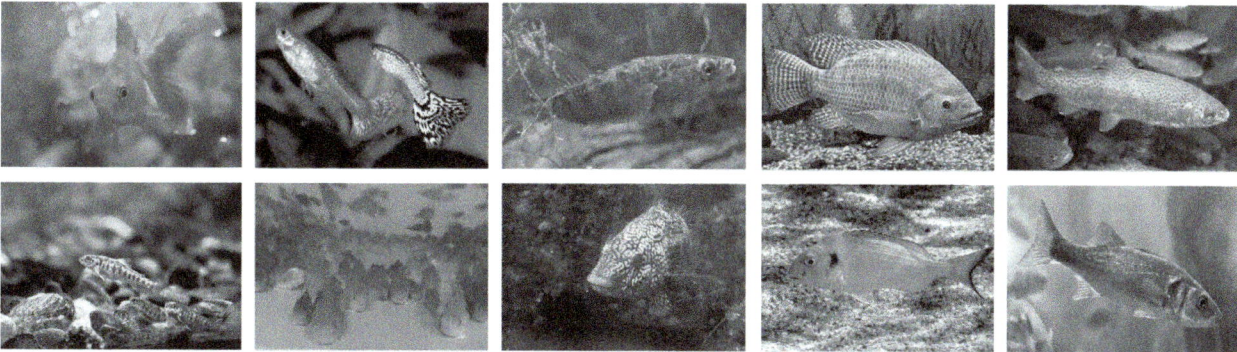

Figure 48.3 Images for each of the main fish species used in research. From left to right and top to bottom: goldfish *(Carassius auratus)*, guppy *(Poecilia reticulata)*, three-spined stickleback *(Gasterosteus aculeatus)*, Nile tilapia *(Oreochromis niloticus)*, rainbow trout *(Oncorhynchus mykiss)*, Atlantic salmon *(Salmo salar)*, lumpfish *(Cyclopterus lumpus)*, ballan wrasse *(Labrus bergylta)*, gilthead sea bream *(Sparus aurata)* and European sea bass *(Dicentrarchus labrax)*. *Source:* Unknown Author/licensed under CC BY-SA.

Guppies are very easy to breed in captivity, and as they reach maturity after only 2–3 months, their short life cycle makes them ideal for evolutionary and genetic studies. The species has also been widely used in ecotoxicology and LC50 data exist for 30 different compounds (Froese & Pauly 2019). Many different varieties have been produced for the aquarium trade (Fernando & Phang 1985; Nakajima & Taniguchi 2001; Khoo *et al.* 2002).

In the wild, the diet of the guppy consists of zooplankton, small insects and detritus, giving it a trophic level of 2.8–3.2 (Froese & Pauly 2019), but they readily feed on commercial dry diets in the laboratory.

The anal fin of male guppies has been transformed into a gonopodium that is used as a copulatory organ for internal fertilisation. Females can store sperm for later fertilisation and may produce 20–40 live young every four weeks (Froese & Pauly 2019). Guppies do not display parental care and cannibalism is common, although this can vary considerably between populations (Nilsson *et al.* 2011), as does shoaling behaviour (Magurran & Seghers 1990).

The minimum recommended aquarium size for keeping guppies is 60 cm in length, and being a shoaling species, 5 or more individuals should be housed together (Froese and Pauly 2019) at a density of ~0.6 g/L (Table 48.3). A good account of the use of guppies in research is provided by Magurran (2005), particularly in relation to evolutionary studies. Detailed information on the rearing of guppies can be found in Mozart (1998) and Ohlyan *et al.* (2011).

Three-spined stickleback

The three-spined stickleback (*Gasterosteus aculeatus*) is a small, ray-finned fish belonging to the family Gasterosteidae. Most stickleback populations complete their life cycle entirely in freshwater but there are anadromous populations that move to brackish water to feed and return to freshwater to spawn (Froese & Pauly 2019). Sticklebacks are benthopelagic and can be found in waters up to 100 m deep but usually inhabit much shallower regions, typically heavily vegetated areas with a mud or sandy substrate (Froese & Pauly 2019). They are subtropical, inhabiting waters with temperatures ranging from 4 to 20 °C. The main water quality requirements and husbandry traits are given in Tables 48.2–48.3.

The three-spined stickleback is an important animal model for behavioural and evolutionary research (see Figure 48.2; Huntingford & Ruiz-Gomez 2009; Norton & Gutiérrez 2019). Niko Tinbergen, one of the founders of ethology, based much of his seminal work on this species because they are common in the wild, are easy to rear in the laboratory and provide interesting questions for research (Huntingford & Ruiz-Gomez 2009). The biology of the species is described in Ostlund-Nilsson *et al.* (2006).

Three-spined sticklebacks typically live 1–2 years in captivity, where they reach ~5 cm in length. Their trunk and caudal peduncle are covered with bony scutes, that along with 3–4 sharp dorsal spines, offer protection against predators. Adult three-spined sticklebacks are carnivorous (trophic level = 3.3–3.4) and feed mostly on worms, crustaceans, insects and small fishes in the wild (Froese & Pauly 2019). Cannibalism, of both eggs and fry, is relatively common (Foster *et al.* 1988; Smith & Reay 1991; Mehlis *et al.* 2009).

During the breeding season, the breast region of the males turns bright red or orange and they become highly territorial. The male constructs a nest with plant material that is glued together with a special protein produced in the kidney. The female is then encouraged to enter the nest and deposit her eggs, which are fertilised by the male who will then guard and keep them aerated until hatching. Males chase away other males and non-gravid females, but may allow another gravid female and fertilise their eggs in the same nest (Ostlund-Nilsson *et al.* 2006). Nest construction is repeatable and its quality and complexity are thought to be used by the female to assess male fitness (Rushbrook *et al.* 2008).

The species is relatively easy to rear in the laboratory. The minimum aquarium size is 60 cm (>50 L) and the indicative density in captivity is 1.2 g/L with partial water exchanges (10% volume) every week. The following practical breeding guidance is provided by Brown (2016): Males and females are separated and fed a high-protein diet during the breeding season. Adequate nesting material, like cotton fibres and similar, need to be provided in the aquarium for the male to build the nest. After the nest is built, the female is introduced, but removed after laying her eggs, leaving the male to fan and tend the nest. When the larvae hatch, the male is removed to prevent cannibalism, and the larvae are fed initially on infusorians (including microalgae, amoeba, rotifers,

Paramecium and other ciliates) which can be easily cultured in the laboratory as described in Sharpe (2020), Das *et al.* (2012) and Mukai *et al.* (2016). As the fish grow, they can be fed on aquarium fish food, including dried bloodworms, *Tubifex*, shrimp and frozen *Daphnia*. They can also take flake fish food.

Nile tilapia

The Nile tilapia (*Oreochromis niloticus*) is a ray-finned, tropical freshwater fish of the family Cichlidae (Cichlids). It is a benthopelagic species that lives in shallow waters within a temperature range of 14–33 °C (Froese & Pauly 2019). Native to Africa (Nile basin, Senegal, Gambia, Volta, Niger, Benue (Nigeria) and Chad), it has been widely introduced elsewhere too (Casal 2006). After the Cyprinids, Cichlids are the second largest vertebrate family. The Tilapiine cichlid tribe includes ~100 species that inhabit mainly freshwater habitats, including shallow streams, ponds, rivers and lakes. Some species can also survive in brackish water.

Nile tilapia is one of the most important aquaculture species worldwide, having been hailed as the 'aquatic chicken' (Little 1998; Coward & Little 2001) and also as 'the most important food fish on the planet' (Fitzsimmons *et al.* 2011). The species has been extensively used for aquaculture and nutrition research (Figure 48.1) and is considered to be the first farmed fish, with many commercial strains (FAO 2005; El-Sayed 2020). However, it is also one of the most invasive fishes (Lowe *et al.* 2000), its expansion being limited only by cold temperatures. An overview of the biology and culture of Nile tilapia is given in FAO (2005) and El-Sayed (2020), and its rearing alongside other species (polyculture) is reviewed in Wang and Lu (2016). The water quality requirements and husbandry traits are given in Tables 48.2–48.3.

Nile tilapia are mainly diurnal and can live up to 10 years and reach over 5 kg, although their typical life span in the laboratory is much shorter. They grow fast in captivity and can reach 18 cm at the end of the first year. They are omnivorous grazers and filter feeders which will feed on phytoplankton, periphyton, aquatic plants, small invertebrates, benthic fauna and detritus in the wild. Their trophic level is consequently low (TL = 2.0; Froese & Pauly 2019).

Sexual maturity is reached after 3–6 months and spawning takes place when temperatures reach ~20–24 °C and the fish weigh ~30 g (Froese & Pauly 2019). At this point, the male digs a pit in a sandy or gravely substrate that serves as a spawning nest to which the female is attracted to spawn via elaborate courtship displayed by the male. Nile tilapia are maternal mouthbrooders and after the eggs are fertilised, the female will incubate the eggs in her mouth and brood the fry until the yolk sac is absorbed, typically 1–2 weeks after fertilisation (FAO 2005). Males are highly territorial during the breeding season and will guard the nest and fertilise a succession of females. As with other fish species, males that invest more in nest building tend to attract the highest number of females (Mendonça & Gonçalves-de-Freitas 2008). In captivity, 3 females are normally housed together for every male to reduce competition. Females may spawn every 4 weeks and brood up to 200 eggs at any given time (Froese & Pauly 2019), although they generally brood fewer than 30 eggs, depending on body size.

For laboratory rearing, three methods of reproduction can be used: manual stripping of gametes and artificial fertilisation using the dry method, collection of fertilised eggs from the female's mouth, or collection of free-swimming fry after these have been brooded by the female. Eggs can be incubated in upwelling jars or in hatching baskets suspended from troughs. For larval rearing, temperature is increased to 28 °C and yolk sac reabsorption takes 5–10 days (FAO 2005). As males grow significantly faster than females, production of mono-sex all male tilapia is desirable in commercial aquaculture, this being achieved directly by sex reversal of the fry via administration of methyltestosterone in the feed (Hiott & Phelps 1993; FAO 2005), or indirectly through the use of YY male broodstock obtained via oestrogen feminisation of the parents, the so-called 'GMT technology' (Beardmore *et al.* 2001). A short 4 °C increase in water temperature 10–30 days post-fertilisation has also been used to increase the proportion of males (Nivelle *et al.* 2019).

In commercial recirculation facilities, Nile tilapia can be reared at densities as high as 60–120 g/L (FAO 2005) but a lower density has been recommended for maintaining high welfare (~34 g/L; Zaki *et al.* 2020). On the other hand, too low densities (<6 g/L) can increase aggression and chronic stress (Champneys *et al.* 2018), resulting in higher disease susceptibility (Ellison *et al.* 2018; Rodriguez-Barreto *et al.* 2019; Ellison *et al.* 2020). An optimal density of 6 individuals/m² has been recommended for outdoor enclosures (Bhujel 2000), and an indicative density of ~14 g/L for a typical fish rearing laboratory facility can be recommended (Champneys *et al.* 2018). However, as there is an interaction between density and social stress, it is difficult to determine optimal densities across all contexts and this requires further attention (Gonçalves-de-Freitas *et al.* 2019).

Rearing Nile tilapia in the laboratory is not difficult as the species is very sturdy, tolerates a wide range of conditions and readily accepts pelleted food which can be administered using on-demand feeders, which tend to reduce competition and waste (Benhaïm *et al.* 2017). Tilapia fry can be sourced from many suppliers and are easy to transport and there are now guidelines for assessing and improving their welfare (Neto & Giaquinto 2020; Pedrazzani *et al.* 2020) which facilitate their use as laboratory fish. The main challenges for maintaining an experimental population in the laboratory reflect the need to grade and thin the fish regularly as they can outgrow tanks quickly, and to manage the sex reversal process if all male fish are desired.

Rainbow trout

The rainbow trout (*Oncorhynchus mykiss*) is a ray-finned fish belonging to the family Salmonidae (Salmonids) native to the Pacific basins of North America but widely introduced to many countries (Casal 2006), where it has become invasive (Lowe *et al.* 2000; Garcia de Leaniz *et al.* 2010). There are several strains that reflect a history of domestication, going back to the 1950s (Cowx 2005). The species is used extensively in research, particularly in relation to disease, ecology and nutrition (Figure 48.2).

A good overview of the behaviour and ecology of rainbow trout (and other Pacific salmonids) is given by Quinn (2005). Welfare guidelines for the species have been published by

Noble et al. (2020). There is an extensive literature on the artificial rearing of rainbow trout, which is broadly similar to the rearing of other salmonids and is well-described in Pennell and Barton (1996), Willoughby (1999) and Woynarovich et al. (2011). An account of the global expansion of the species is provided by Halverson (2010) and a summary of impacts can be found in Hardy (2018), while the main conservation issues are discussed in Lichatowich (2001). The water quality requirements and main husbandry traits for the species are given in Tables 48.2–48.3.

Rainbow trout can live entirely in freshwater rivers or lakes, or migrate to sea to feed in the case of anadromous populations (called 'steelhead') before returning to freshwater to spawn. They are benthopelagic and inhabit the upper 200 m of the water column with temperatures ranging from 10 to 24 °C. They feed on macro-invertebrates of aquatic and terrestrial origin and can become piscivorous when they reach 15–20 cm in length (Monnet et al. 2020), at which point they may migrate to a lake, estuary or the sea. They have a trophic level of 3.8 (Froese & Pauly 2019) and will establish social hierarchies around feeding territories.

Sexual maturation occurs after 2 years in males and 3 years in females, with spawning taking place from November to May in its natural range, although strains have been developed that spawn at any time of year using temperature and photoperiod manipulation. Like other salmonids, artificial fertilisation in rainbow trout is easily achieved using the dry method: the eggs are stripped from the female by abdominal massage and fertilised with the sperm of one or more males before water is added to activate the sperm. In the wild, the female uses her powerful tail to dig a pit in a gravely substrate called a 'redd' and deposit her eggs, which are rapidly fertilised by one or more males and then covered by subsequent tail beats by the female. A female may dig more than one redd during the spawning season and mate with multiple males. The eggs will develop in the redds and the alevins will emerge from the gravel when their yolk sac is nearly reabsorbed, and disperse typically downstream in search of a suitable feeding territory. The eggs of rainbow trout are large (3–6 mm) and in captivity they are generally incubated in vertical incubators (either upwelling or downwelling) or in hatching trays or boxes suspended from raceways or troughs (Willoughby 1999; Woynarovich et al. 2011).

Rainbow trout should not be kept in rectangular glass aquaria as they require ample space, strong water flow and plenty of cool, well-oxygenated water. Instead, juveniles can be reared in troughs or in circular tanks connected to an appropriately sized Recirculation Aquaculture Systems (RAS). The main challenges for laboratory rearing are the need to maintain cold temperatures during the summer that will typically require a chiller, and the tendency for trout to leap out of the water which will require closely fitted lids on the tanks. Eggs can be sourced from many commercial farm suppliers, are easily incubated in the laboratory and juveniles can be kept for several months in tanks without much difficulty as they easily feed on pellets. However, keeping rainbow trout to maturity, breeding them and maintaining an experimental line will require a larger recirculation infrastructure with a capacity of at least 5,000 L and tanks with a volume of ~1,200 L or more.

Atlantic salmon

Like rainbow trout, the Atlantic salmon (*Salmo salar*) is a ray-finned fish belonging to the family Salmonidae. Atlantic salmon are native to both sides of the North Atlantic but have also been widely introduced to the southern hemisphere for aquaculture purposes (Garcia de Leaniz et al. 2010), notably to Chile which is the largest salmon producer after Norway. The species is used extensively in fish research, particularly in ecology (Figure 48.2). Most populations of Atlantic salmon are anadromous and migrate to sea as 'smolts' after 1–3 years in freshwater, but land-locked (potadromous) populations that reside entirely in freshwater also exist on both sides of the North Atlantic (Mills 1989).

The literature on Atlantic salmon is very extensive. Overviews of the biology and ecology of the species are given in Mills (1989); Shearer (1992); Jonsson and Jonsson (2011) and Hendry and Cragg-Hine (2003). Atlantic salmon are structured into locally adapted populations maintained by homing (Garcia de Leaniz et al. 2007a; Garcia de Leaniz et al. 2007b), which has implications for exploitation (Hindar et al. 2007) and management (Verspoor et al. 2007), but also for research as populations can differ widely in fitness-related traits (Garcia de Leaniz et al. 2007b). Practical guidance on artificial rearing is provided by Jones (2004), and welfare guidelines for the species are given in Noble et al. (2018). Tables 48.2–48.3 provide information on the water quality requirements and main husbandry traits for the species.

The reproduction and juvenile stages of Atlantic salmon are very similar to those of rainbow trout described in the preceding text. Atlantic salmon feed mostly on aquatic insects and crustaceans in freshwater and on fish and crustaceans at sea (Shearer 1992; Jonsson & Jonsson 2011). The species has a trophic level of 4.1 (Froese & Pauly 2019). Juveniles are territorial and will defend feeding stations in running waters, but territoriality is replaced by scramble competition in rearing tanks and in sea cages, where rearing densities are much higher than in wild. Grading is necessary in captivity to prevent the development of a bimodal size distribution (Storebakken & Austreng 1987; Skilbrei 1991) as this can compromise welfare (Cubitt et al. 2008). At sea, Atlantic salmon are commonly found in the upper (210 m) water column, where water temperatures range between 2 °C and 9 °C (Froese & Pauly 2019), although in sea cages they grow best within the 6–16 °C range (Jones 2004).

The challenges for rearing Atlantic salmon in the laboratory are similar to those of rainbow trout: they need strong flows and cool, well-oxygenated water and are unsuitable to be kept in aquaria. Vertical incubators and shallow, horizontal troughs (fitted with artificial substrate) can be used for egg development and rearing of alevins and fry, but deeper GRP circular tanks of at least 1,200 L capacity connected to a properly sized RAS (5,000 L or more) are needed for longer rearing. Having a good water temperature control system Is essential to keep Atlantic salmon indoors as buildings tend to become too warm for the species during the summer. As for rainbow trout, eggs can be sourced from commercial hatcheries or from wild parents (where this is allowed) and transported easily into the laboratory where they can be reared for several months on artificial aquafeeds. However, keeping Atlantic salmon in the laboratory for longer than a few months is not advisable, as some individuals may smolt on the spring of their first year (after they reach ~10–12 cm/100 g) and would need to be transferred to much larger sea water tanks.

Lumpfish

The Atlantic lumpfish or lumpsucker (*Cyclopterus lumpus*, L.) is a ray-finned fish belonging to the Order Scorpaeniformes and the family Cyclopteridae. Its scientific name, *Cyclopterus lumpus*, makes reference to its ventral suction disc or sucker (from the Greek *kyklos* = circle and *pteryx*, *pterygium* = fin) that lumpfish use to attach to suitable surfaces, and which along with their round tadpole-like shape (*lumpus*), absence of scales and swim bladder, and presence of tubercles, are the most distinguishing features of the species. The main sources on information on the biology of the species are Davenport (1985) and more recently Powell *et al.* (2018a).

Lumpfish are benthopelagic (Froese & Pauly 2019) with a wide boreal distribution in both sides of the North Atlantic. The species is found over a wide depth range (0–860 m), although it is most commonly found within 50–150 m from the surface (Stein 1986). Lumpfish have become very popular as cleaner fish to control sea lice infestations in salmon farming, and their use in aquaculture research has increased accordingly (Figure 48.2). However, being a new species to aquaculture, their husbandry and welfare requirements are not as well-known as those of other species and there is therefore a need for practical guidance. The main welfare issues for lumpfish are related to habitat preferences, feeding, provision of shelters, health and disease management, and artificial reproduction (Powell *et al.* 2018b; Eliasen *et al.* 2020; Gutierrez Rabadan *et al.* 2021; García de Leaniz *et al.* 2021; Rey *et al.* 2021).

The diet of lumpfish is very varied and includes planktonic organisms, small crustaceans, ctenophores and polychaetes, but also seagrass, insects, small fish and fish eggs (Davenport 1985). Newly hatched larvae initially feed on surface plankton, switching to small crustaceans, larger amphipods and decapods as they grow in size (Powell *et al.* 2018a). In captivity, lumpfish are fed on enriched *Artemia* nauplii during the first 2–3 weeks after hatching and then weaned onto commercial diets. They aggregate in large clumps when young, attached to a suitable surface with their suction discs, but become progressively more pelagic and solitary as they grow (Powell *et al.* 2018a). In the laboratory, tanks should be provided with structures where lumpfish can attach, dark colours being best as lumpfish tend to avoid pale structures.

Keeping lumpfish until maturation in the laboratory is not difficult but getting them to reproduce is challenging; as their life cycle has not yet been closed in captivity (Powell *et al.*, 2018b), it is not possible to maintain experimental lines in the laboratory. Cannibalism is relatively common among larvae (Powell *et al.* 2018a) but its impact can be reduced by frequent grading. Typically, one should ensure that the largest individuals in a tank never reach a size twice as large as that of the smallest ones. This means that fish that have hatched at markedly different times should not be pooled and reared together as this might exacerbate any initial size differences. The species can switch between two different foraging strategies, actively swimming for food or clinging and waiting, depending on prey availability and metabolic rate (Killen *et al.* 2007). The incidence of lumpfish with deformed suckers can be high and varies between families. Lumpfish with severely deformed suckers cannot cling to the substrate and tend to spend too much energy swimming which may lead to emaciation and death. Therefore, the advice is to screen and humanely kill severely deformed lumpfish at the earliest opportunity (Garcia de Leaniz *et al.* 2021).

The typical length after their first year is around 12 cm and although densities of up to 60 g/L are used in commercial hatcheries, densities in the laboratory are probably best kept at around 20 g/L. The main difficulties in the laboratory is to keep the water temperature low (~10 °C) and this will normally require the use of appropriate chillers, particularly during the summer months. Lumpfish need *Artemia* for start feeding, and will wean onto commercial dry feed readily, although a high incidence of cataracts has sometimes been reported in fish fed commercial diets compared to wild lumpfish (Imsland *et al.* 2018; Imsland *et al.* 2019; Paradis *et al.* 2019). The water quality requirements and main husbandry traits for the species are shown in Tables 48.2–48.3.

Ballan wrasse

The ballan wrasse is a ray-finned marine Perciform fish belonging to the family Labridae that is usually found in the upper (30 m) surface layer of the Eastern North Atlantic, from Norway to Morocco (Froese & Pauly 2019). The young use the intertidal areas and move to the littoral zone as they grow, being commonly associated with rocks and seaweed. Ballan wrasse are all females when they hatch and become males after 4–14 years (Froese & Pauly 2019).

After lumpfish, ballan wrasse (*Labrus bergylta*) is the main species used for research on the use of cleaner fish in aquaculture (Powell *et al.* 2018b; Treasurer 2018b). The main sources of information on ballan wrasse biology and husbandry are Helland *et al.* (2014), Treasurer (2018a) and Noble *et al.* (2019). As with lumpfish, broodstock are typically caught from the wild as availability of farmed wrasse is limited. Broodstock can be kept in 1.5 m diameter tanks with low light and are provided with artificial kelp as enrichment. To encourage spawning in captivity, sex ratios typically consist of 4–10 females at a stocking density of 5–12 g/L (Helland *et al.* 2014). Males can become aggressive when the number of females is low.

Larvae are typically fed on rotifers 4–5 days after hatching and then on *Artemia* 25–30 days post-hatch, lasting for 20–70 days depending on temperature, after which they are weaned onto dry feed (Helland *et al.* 2014). Ballan wrasse will grow to ~8 cm after their first year and although higher densities are used in commercial hatcheries, densities in the laboratory are probably best kept at around 5–15 g/L (Lein & Helland 2014; Noble *et al.* 2019).

The main husbandry traits and water quality requirements are given in Tables 48.2–48.3. Maintaining ballan wrasse for research in the laboratory is constrained by the need to have cultures of rotifers and *Artemia* for initial feeding and, as with lumpfish, to maintain low temperatures (in this case, below 16 °C) with the use of chillers during the summer. Other rearing challenges include 'clumping' behaviour (i.e. dense aggregations) seen among larvae which appears to be a response to stress and can promote fin erosion; clumping can be reduced by reducing disturbances (including reducing light levels and noise) and increasing water flow (Skiftesvik *et al.* 2014).

Gilthead sea bream

The gilthead sea bream (*Sparus aurata*) is a ray-finned fish belonging to the family Sparidae (Porgies) which has become increasingly important as an aquaculture species since the 1990s (Colloca & Cerasi 2005), particularly in Greece, Turkey and Spain.

Gilthead sea bream are benthopelagic, being associated with seagrass beds, rocky and sandy habitats typically up to 30 m deep. They are distributed in subtropical waters (16–20 °C) between 15 and 62 °N of latitude (Froese & Pauly 2019). They are sedentary and may form loose aggregations. In the wild, their diet consists of molluscs, crustaceans and fish, but they also feed occasionally on seaweed (Colloca & Cerasi 2005). The species has a trophic level of 2.8–3.7 (Froese & Pauly 2019). Most gilthead sea bream are males when they hatch and become females during their second or third year, although in captivity the extent and timing of sex reversal varies depending on social structure and hormone levels (Colloca & Cerasi 2005).

Spawning in captivity can be controlled by manipulating the photoperiod and the water temperature, and also by stimulation of the ovaries with injection of Gonadotrophin-releasing hormone agonists (GnRHa). Females can lay up to 80,000 eggs every day during the spawning season that can last up to 4 months (Colloca & Cerasi 2005).

Gilthead sea bream larvae are fed on enriched rotifers for 3–4 days, and are then supplemented with enriched *Artemia* for 10 additional days until complete metamorphosis takes place, normally 32–35 days post-hatch (Colloca & Cerasi 2005). Microalgae are used during larviculture to create "green wate" conditions which have proved beneficial for the development of larvae (Papandroulakis *et al*. 2001). The use of substrate has also shown to be beneficial as a form of structural enrichment in captivity (Batzina & Karakatsouli 2012). Frequent feeding (every 2 hrs for 12 hrs) at 18 °C and 35–37% salinity are required during the initial stages (Colloca & Cerasi 2005) which may be difficult to achieve in the laboratory. A high incidence of skeletal deformities has been observed among larvae in some intensive systems but this can be reduced by lowering densities and by increasing tank volume (Prestinicola *et al*. 2013). Densities up to 20 g/L had no effect on welfare in captivity (Araújo-Luna *et al*. 2018).

The water quality requirements and main husbandry traits are given in Tables 48.2–48.3. Moretti *et al*. (1999) provide extensive guidance on hatchery production. As with many other marine species, the rearing of gilthead sea bream in the laboratory is constrained by the availability of broodstock and the need to set up cultures of rotifers and *Artemia* for initial feeding. The species is also very sensitive to cold temperatures and frequent grading is necessary to reduce competition and the onset of large size differences (Moretti *et al*. 1999).

European sea bass

The European sea bass (*Dicentrarchus labrax*) is a ray-finned fish belonging to the family Moronidae. The species occupies a very wide niche with respect to salinity (3–37%) and water temperature (8–24 °C) (Froese & Pauly 2019). Sea bass are demersal and are typically found in the littoral zone, in the upper 100 m of the water column. Like sea bream, the culture of sea bass has increased exponentially since the 1990s, particularly in Mediterranean countries, Greece and Turkey being the largest producers. European sea bass were the second marine fish farmed commercially in Europe, after Atlantic salmon, and is currently the most important fish cultured in the Mediterranean (Bagni 2005). Sea bass are an important species for research in aquaculture, but also into welfare (Figure 48.2), as it is a high cortisol response species and its stress response is well-known (Fanouraki *et al*. 2011; Samaras *et al*. 2016). The main sources of information on the general biology of the species is Pickett and Pawson (1994), and more recently Vázquez and Muñoz-Cueto (2014). The main husbandry requirements are presented in Tables 48.2–48.3, and guidance on methods for hatchery production is given in Moretti *et al*. (1999).

Sea bass can grow very fast under the right conditions, and can reach 22 cm at the end of their first year and mature at 32 cm (Froese & Pauly 2019), when they are 2–4 years old. They will aggregate in groups during the breeding season, spawning taking place once a year in coastal shallow waters and near estuaries, usually between January and June, depending on populations. Young sea bass feed initially on zooplankton and then progressively shift to worms, crustaceans and fish larvae, with adults being piscivorous. The species has a trophic level of 3.5–3.8 (Froese & Pauly 2019).

The sex ratio during artificial breeding is kept at 2 males per female, which are housed together and allowed to batch spawn in suitable tanks (Bagni 2005). Control of maturation is facilitated by intramuscular injection of human chorionic gonadotropin (Bagni 2005), and out-of-season gametogenesis can also be achieved by manipulating the temperature and photoperiod. The eggs of sea bass typically develop in 3 days and the 3 mm larvae reabsorb the yolk sac in 7–10 days, taking ~75 days from hatching to metamorphose into 1.5–2.5 g juveniles (Bagni 2005). Larvae are fed enriched rotifers and *Artemia* during first feeding (Moretti *et al*. 1999).

Sea bass will form loose schools when they are young, becoming more solitary as they grow. Being euryhaline, sea bass can be reared in the laboratory under a wide range of temperatures and salinities, but have a high cortisol response and are easily stressed (Samaras *et al*. 2016). As for other marine species, the biggest challenges for rearing sea bass in the laboratory lie in the need to culture live prey for the larval stages, the high frequency of feeding required (every 10–15 minutes for juveniles (Bagni 2005)) which makes husbandry labour intensive, and the need for a marine recirculation aquaculture system with good filtration and a life support system. Frequent grading is necessary to reduce excessive size heterogeneity as this can lead to aggression and cannibalism (Moretti *et al*. 1999). Nevertheless, being a common farmed species, juveniles can be sourced from commercial hatchery suppliers which will dispense with the need to rear the more challenging larval stages.

Fish welfare

The number of papers on fish welfare has increased substantially over the last 10 years (Figure 48.1) and welfare monitoring has now become a normal requirement for field and laboratory work, as well as in aquaculture production systems (Johansen *et al*. 2006; Kiessling *et al*. 2012; Sloman *et al*. 2019). Maintaining high welfare is important for animal research because fish raised under good welfare conditions tend to perform better and are more likely to produce repeatable results than those in poor welfare.

Studies on fish preferences and coping styles (such as those generated by COPEWELL https://cordis.europa.eu/project/id/265957 and other programs) have made it possible to quantify the behavioural and physiological needs of fish better, and to gain insights into the underlying mechanisms (Huntingford *et al.* 2006; Martins *et al.* 2012; Castanheira *et al.* 2015). There are undoubtedly still lots of questions to be resolved, but a better understanding of the sensory world of fish and their cognitive abilities (Saraiva *et al.* 2018) is central to improvement of fish welfare (Figure 48.4). In this sense, the use of zebrafish (*Danio rerio*) as an animal research model has improved understanding of fish behaviour in general and resulted in better methods of monitoring fish welfare (see Chapter 49: Zebrafish). Zebrafish studies are beginning to unravel the neural mechanisms associated with the ability to cope with stress, anxiety and fear, paving the way for better control of fish welfare (Kalueff *et al.* 2013; Stewart *et al.* 2014).

Fish are now regarded as sentient animals and have the same level of protection as terrestrial vertebrates (Canadian Council on Animal Care 2005; Farm Animal Welfare Council 2014; Jenkins *et al.* 2014; NORECOPA 2016). In Europe, for example, fish are protected from the time that they are capable of independent feeding on the assumption that they can experience pain, suffering and distress.

There is a considerable body of work indicating the capacity of fish and other aquatic organisms, like cephalopods and decapods, to suffer and feel pain (Sneddon 2015; Brown & Dorey 2019) and this has changed the way legislators are protecting them.

Main welfare issues in fish

Fish held under laboratory conditions may face several welfare issues, most commonly those related to husbandry, handling and transport. Other welfare issues may arise due to the experimental procedures themselves, the definition of humane end-points and the method used for euthanasia.

Handling and transport are covered in the next sections, along with other activities that can also compromise welfare as part of experimental procedures, including the administration of substances, experimental set-ups and changes in diet. We finish by briefly discussing the concept of positive welfare, in contrast to the more common emphasis on monitoring poor welfare.

How to measure welfare in fish?

This is the one of the most difficult issues that arises when there are potential welfare problems with fish. Welfare indicators (or Operational Welfare Indicators: OWIs) exist for only a few species of fish such as the Atlantic salmon (Noble *et al.* 2018), the rainbow trout (Noble *et al.* 2020) or the lumpfish (Garcia de Leaniz *et al.* 2021; Gutierrez Rabadan *et al.* 2021). Welfare indicators can be classified into direct (animal based), when they measure attributes of the fish themselves, or indirect (environment based) when they assess the environment the fish live in (Noble *et al.* 2020). Direct, animal-based welfare indicators tend to be invasive or require handling and can be further subdivided into OWIs – which can be measured in a commercial setting – and Laboratory Based Welfare Indicators (LABWIs) which require access to laboratory facilities. Good (operational) welfare indicators

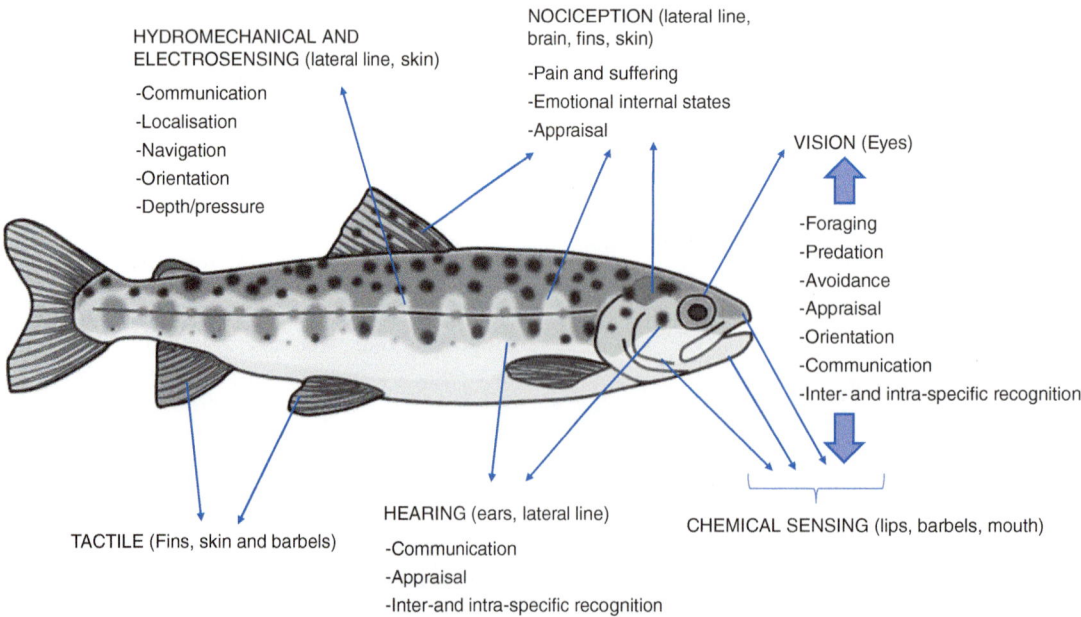

Figure 48.4 The sensory world of fish. Source: Adapted from Saraiva *et al.* (2018). Domestication and Welfare in Farmed Fish; doi: 10.5772/intechopen.77251. Source: Fish drawing courtesy of Dr Peter E. Jones, CSAR, Swansea University.

should be informative, easy to measure and non-invasive, or minimally invasive. They should be repeatable (Gutierrez Rabadan *et al.* 2021), usually following a scoring system (by training laboratory or farm staff) and integrated into routine husbandry procedures. The measurements must be relevant to the welfare of the species, and ideally be non-lethal. Intuitively, the most straightforward welfare indicators might be a record of mortalities and signs of ill health, and this is implemented in laboratories as a daily routine check. Removing any mortalities and sending regular samples for analysis is also essential for good husbandry (Johansen *et al.* 2006). However, recording mortalities alone will not improve welfare, as when mortalities occur welfare has already been compromised and may be too late to take remedial actions. Simple pathological investigations such as skin scrapes and eye dabs can be done on anaesthetised fish to investigate the presence of parasites. Gill biopsies and tissue samples on mortalities can also be explored for pathological signs of disease and parasitism (Sneddon & Wolfenden 2019).

Better welfare indicators include monitoring various physiological parameters (including growth and blood parameters), monitoring environmental parameters (but for this the species requirements need to be known) and assessing changes in behaviour to detect signs of sickness, pain or distress (including activity levels, position in the tank or cage, feeding response). Some fish welfare indicators are individual based (e.g. skin damage, deformities, blood parameters), while others refer to the group (e.g. shoaling behaviour, mortality, feeding behaviour), and yet others relate to the environment (oxygen levels, temperature, etc.), as shown in Table 48.4. New and emerging technologies to assess fish welfare have been developed recently and reviewed on a just published manuscript by Barreto and colleagues (Barreto *et al.* 2021).

However, an integrated welfare assessment should be implemented and designed specifically for each fish species and each rearing system and ideally measure different welfare aspects (Toni *et al.* 2019). For some farmed fish, like Atlantic salmon, what constitutes good welfare is fairly well-known (Noble *et al.* 2018) but for most species this is not so clear. A 'welfare assessment toolbox' based on some general guidelines can be designed for each species used for experimental purposes and incorporated into the normal husbandry protocols (see Figure 48.5).

Table 48.4 Examples of individual- and group-based indicators used to assess fish welfare for different fish species (from Rey *et al.* 2019).

Individual-Based Welfare Indicators	**Physical Health**	Mortalities
		Opercula and/or gill damage
		Colour changes (e.g. eye darkening, pale gills, skin colour)
		Fin damage
		Gill health index (Parasites/Amoebic gill disease (AGD))
		Snout damage
		Deformities
		Parasite infection
		Skin damage and appearance: lesions/abrasions/injuries/
		Scale loss and haemorrhage (Skin Index)
		Bacterial load
		Body condition (hepatosomatic index, Fulton condition index)
		Standard growth rates (SGR)
	Physiology	Blood parameters (lactate, glucose, cortisol)
		Ventilation rate
		Muscle pH
		Immune parameters
		Smoltification state
		Heart rate
Group-Based Welfare Indicators	**Behaviour**	Crowd intensity (scale 1–5 in RSPCA)
		Feeding and anticipatory behaviours and recovery time after stress
		Social interactions
		Spatial distribution (vertical and horizontal)
		Abnormal (e.g. lethargy, isolation)/Normal behaviours
		Spiralling, gulping sickness behaviours
		Reaction to carers
		Activity (swimming behaviour, leaping)
	Environment	Water quality (pH, oxygen, ammonia, nitrites and nitrates)
		Temperature, turbidity
		Water flow rates and current speed
		Light
		Kairomones and steroids in the water
		Salinity
		Stocking density
		Scales in water
		Enclosure design/substrate access

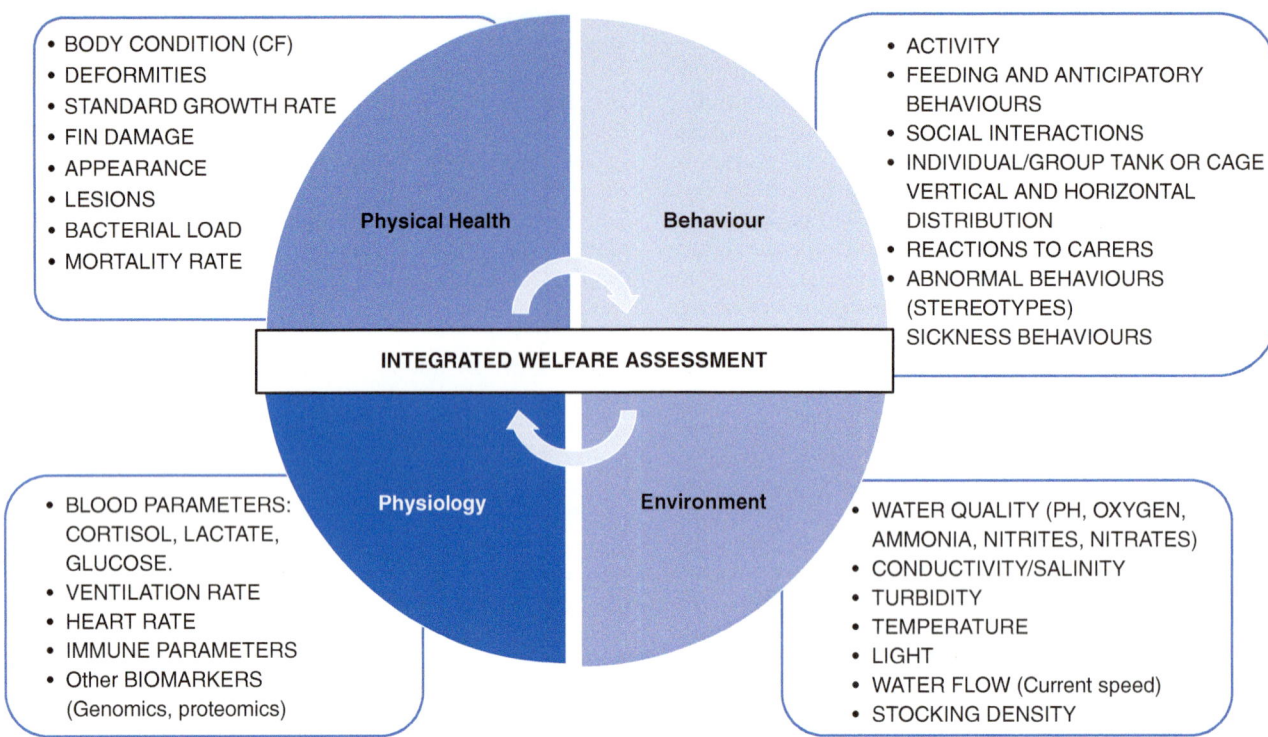

Figure 48.5 An integrated fish welfare assessment should include measurements on physical health, behaviour, physiology and the physical environment of the fish.

Fish differ widely in the range of optimal environmental conditions and husbandry requirements, including minimum tank size, stocking densities, diet, vulnerability to disease, hardiness, adaptation to captivity and response to stress, but detailed information has only been compiled for a few species (Tables 48.2–48.3). This means that for work on most other species, researchers must obtain information from the literature and data repositories (such as FishBase[4] (Froese & Pauly 2019 and FishEthoGroup[5])) and build on their experience and adopt a precautionary approach (e.g., on water quality), noting that conditions that are optimal for growth are normally also optimal for survival.

In addition to water quality, other parameters to consider are environmental noise, light conditions, temperature and photoperiod: the latter can affect the fish circadian rhythms positively or negatively and must be tailored to each species. For example, Nile tilapia appears to prefer a yellow background and blue light (Volpato and Barreto 2001; Luchiari et al. 2006) while the availability of a temperature gradient is important for many species. Most times, these parameters are not considered because of poor knowledge or because they are difficult to measure or maintain in the laboratory despite mounting evidence of their influence on fish welfare (Villamizar et al. 2012; Boltana et al. 2013; Rey et al. 2015a; Rey et al. 2015b).

A Qualitative Behavioural Assessment (QBA) based on animal body language is available for farmed terrestrial animals that makes it possible to quantify the behaviour of individuals as well as that of the group based on a Visual Analogue Scale (VAS) scoring system (Rutherford et al. 2012). QBA has been developed and validated recently for fish (Jarvis et al. 2021) and studies are underway to test their use in farmed fish under different rearing systems. QBA could also be used for fish in research settings. A similar tool to QBA has also recently been developed and validated for farmed fish, and this promises to be a powerful OWI for fish under laboratory conditions (Ellis 2020). Paradigms such as the successive negative contrast (SNC) used in rats could be translated into fish research as a behavioural OWI (Ellis et al. 2020).

Underwater cameras are increasingly being used for routine visual monitoring of laboratory (Ellis et al. 2019) and recent advances in the use of sensors and optical technology (Parra et al. 2018), Artificial Intelligence (Føre et al. 2018) and machine learning (Saberioon et al. 2017; Valletta et al. 2017) are facilitating the assessment of fish behaviour and welfare addressing the needs for Precision Fish Farming (O'Donncha et al. 2021). Powerful tracking software (such as Ethovision, or free programs such as IDtracker, Ctrax, DeepLabCut, Tracktor, Zebtrack, Biotracker and plugins for ImageJ) are available for tracking zebrafish and other small fish under controlled environments, while biosensors (such as BioSort[6]) can use face recognition to monitor individual fish under commercial conditions. Sonar and camera systems have also been used to monitor feeding behaviour, estimate biomass and assess behavioural responses to environmental stressors and these could be incorporated into operational welfare indicators (Pautsina et al. 2015; Schraml et al. 2020; Bekkozhayeva et al. 2021; O'Donncha et al. 2021).

---

[4] https://www.fishbase.de/ (Accessed July 27, 2021)
[5] http://www.apc.gov.uk/reference/apc_supplementary_review_schedule_1.pdf
[6] https://www.biosort.no/?lang=en (Accessed September 27, 2021)

Signs of poor welfare and humane end-points in fish

Fish welfare indicators should be clear enough to give reliable warnings of poor welfare. Indicators of poor welfare can be detected at the individual level, including abnormal behaviours such as thigmotaxis, freezing or lethargy, extreme physiological values, external physical damage and abnormalities such as deformities, loss of scales or fin damage among others. At the group level, fish can display changes in swimming activity patterns, shoaling behaviour, aggression and feeding responses (Table 48.4). Changes in the position of fish in the water column can also reveal a stress response or a deviation from normal conditions (Sneddon 2009; Martins et al. 2012; Millot et al. 2014; Sneddon et al. 2014; Sneddon 2019).

Stress can be a reliable indicator of poor welfare, but it is often difficult to measure, and requires handling and blood extraction in the case of physiological parameters, like plasma cortisol, lactate or glucose (Ellis et al. 2012), although cortisol can now also be detected non-invasively in the skin mucus, faeces and also in the water (Ellis et al. 2013; Sadoul & Geffroy 2019; Uren Webster et al. 2020).

Despite the fact that fish are legally afforded the same level of protection as terrestrial vertebrates, guidelines for the use of fish in research are often more permissive or vague than those for birds or mammals. This is particularly evident in relation to humane end-points and systems for scoring severity (Hawkins et al. 2011). Although some countries have specific guidelines for choosing appropriate end-points for fish (Canadian Council on Animal Care 2005; Sneddon 2009), in most cases each laboratory refers to their animal care and welfare manager or veterinarian to decide on suitable end-points for fish under their care in accordance with a legislation that is notoriously vague.

Mitigation measures and positive welfare: the use of enrichment in fish research

According to Shepherdson (1989) the aim of environmental enrichment in zoos and aquaria is to *'provide an environment in which animals behave as closely as possible to their wild counterparts'*. Short- and long-term abnormal behaviours such as increased aggression or stereotypies (persistent repetition of a specific behaviour) can be mitigated using enrichment in captivity (Swaisgood & Shepherdson 2006; Näslund & Johnsson 2016) as this has been shown to promote more natural behaviours (Roberts et al. 2011; Roberts et al. 2014; Stringwell et al. 2014; Jones et al. 2021); see also Chapter 10: Environmental enrichment: animal welfare and scientific validity. Enrichment can take many forms: sensorial, physical, dietary, social and occupational (Näslund & Johnsson 2016), but some forms work better than others for different fish (Williams et al. 2009). For example, structural enrichment seems to work well for many fish as it adds novel features, as well as places to hide, forage and interact, and this is thought to have positive effects on fish welfare. The addition of novel objects to the typical barren artificial environment can make fish more resilient but it can also generate short-term neophobia (Champneys et al. 2018). Other potential problems with enrichment may arise due to competition for enriched sites that can lead to aggression or exclusion of some individuals. For this reason, structural enrichment needs to be applied in a way that ensures that all animals benefit from the novel features. Problems may also arise when enriched habitats become more difficult to clean or interfere with the provision of food or normal husbandry, or when non-inert materials are used that can leach toxic chemicals or contaminate tissue. Such problems can often be solved by different means – for example, vegetation and substrate heterogeneity can be simulated by the use of pictures and textured backgrounds in glass aquaria[7].

Some fish can experience chronic social stress because of aggression, territoriality, dominance and the formation of social hierarchies and these can be mitigated by grading, as individuals of similar sizes are less likely to engage in agonistic interactions. However, this cannot be completely eliminated, and it will also depend on the social structure and life cycle of the species. For example, lumpfish (*Cyclopterus lumpus*) can be very aggressive, and their growth varies a lot under farm conditions, but aggression can be greatly reduced by grading and by using structural enrichment that increases the surface available for clinging. In this case, a combination of grading and enrichment can help mitigate an undesirable behaviour that can lead to fin damage and poor welfare (Turner 2016; Rey et al. 2021).

Laboratory procedures

Administration of substances

There are three main routes of substance administration to fish: in the food, by injection and by immersion. Regardless of the route, the administration of substances should always be conducted under veterinary advice and supervision and requires appropriate training of staff administering them.

Oral administration

Substances can be added directly to the food – for example, immunostimulants, antibiotics or vaccines can be delivered mixed or incorporated into the fish food (Shaalan et al. 2016). They should be properly mixed or coated with the food to avoid leaching prior to consumption. Research into the benefits of prebiotics and probiotics in fish farming has increased much in recent years (Dawood et al. 2018), but it is important to remember that this also needs to meet welfare standards, to ensure that the welfare of fish is not being compromised. Growth, swimming activity, behaviour and other welfare indicators should be monitored, and experiments terminated if mortalities increase or significant welfare issues are detected. The administration of antibiotics and vaccines should always follow veterinary advice as their use may be regulated by national legislation.

---

[7]https://aquariumblueprints.com/do-you-need-a-background-for-your-fish-tank/ (Accessed September 27, 2021)

Injection and cannulation

The administration of substances by injection or cannulation requires that fish are anaesthetised or sedated first (see anaesthesia section in the following text). Three types of injection can be used for substance administration in fish: Intraperitoneal (IP) or intracoelomic, intramuscular (IM) and intravenous (IV; Figure 48.6). IP injections are applied to the peritoneal area, in the body cavity, typically at the base of the pelvic fin. The tip of the needle is inserted under a scale and is pushed through the abdominal wall into the body cavity and then directed parallel to the ventral surface. IM injections are usually applied into the large dorsal muscle area of the fish, close to the dorsal fin. They can also be administered into the pectoral muscle, at the base of the pectoral fin. IV injections are usually applied to the caudal venous sinuses of the fish, through the ventral side of the caudal peduncle; IV injections are less common and are mainly used in large fish and for specific purposes. Not all fish have the same body plan, and the specific sites of injection may differ between species, but the preceding are the most common ones.

Bath immersion

As with other routes of administration, delivery of substances via immersion should be carried out under the supervision of a veterinary surgeon, who will advise on dosage and duration. Indicative doses can normally be calculated from drug instructions, but treatment of some pathologies and parasites may require specific medicines and a detailed diagnosis. During bath treatments, fish normally have to be handled and moved between tanks or containers. This might cause stress and aversive responses should be monitored. Good aeration and careful monitoring will typically be required to ensure water quality is maintained, particularly if baths last for some time.

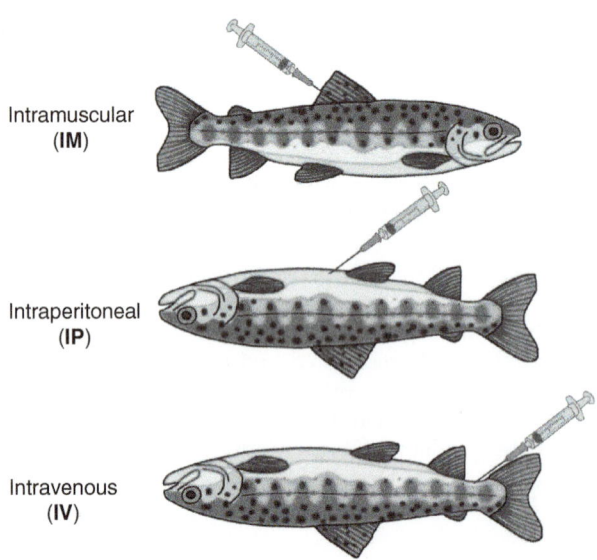

Figure 48.6 The three most common types of injection in fish. The precise location of needle insertion depends on body plan and may differ slightly from the locations shown here for brown trout. Source: Drawing courtesy of Dr Peter E. Jones, CSAR, Swansea University.

Anaesthesia and analgesia

The use of anaesthetics and analgesics for fish is licensed in many countries and only products approved by the relevant Food and Drug administration can legally be used when fish are used for food. Not all substances can be used in all species (Readman et al. 2017) – for example, some anaesthetics can have adverse effects on some species but not in others (Martins et al. 2018; Pounder et al. 2018).

Anaesthetics are substances that induce insensitivity to pain or (in the case of sedatives) leave animals sedated or unconscious if used as general anaesthetics. Because fish are considered to be sentient animals, they need to be anaesthetised before carrying any scientific procedure that can result in significant pain or distress. Most fish become very stressed when they are removed out of the water, and handling and restraint should typically be conducted under sedation. Several anaesthetics are commonly used for fish, the most common ones being MS222 (tricaine methane sulphonate, sold under the trade name Finquel[8]), benzocaine, clove oil, and 2-phenoxy-ethanol (Coyle et al. 2004; Saint-Erne 2015; Priborsky & Velisek 2018). Other agents such as metomidate or quinaldine are less commonly used. Anaesthetics are usually delivered as a bath, and diluted (buffered) in acetone, water or ethanol prior to use. Larger fish can be anaesthetised by injection and can operated on out of the water if their gills are kept irrigated with anaesthetic dosed water using a pump with temperature control to create a small recirculation system (Hawkins 1981).

It is recommended that prior to anaesthesia, for experimental procedures fish fasted for a minimum of 6 h (or longer for species with a high metabolic rate or at warm temperatures) in order to reduce basal metabolic rate and oxygen consumption. Due to the variability in the responses of different fish to anaesthetics, published doses should be used with care as they are only indicative (NORECOPA 2016). Correct anaesthesia of fish should result in rapid induction and quick recovery, as well as in immobilisation and analgesia during the procedure. The concentrations and times depend on fish species, body size and the objective of the anaesthesia: sedation, deep sleep or euthanasia. It can also vary depending on water temperature and pH. Proper aeration, consideration of maximum loading densities and monitoring of water quality are essential. Water should preferably come from the holding tank or aquatic system where the animals are held. The correct duration of the procedure can be assessed using behavioural observations (ataxia or random swimming, loss of righting reflex and response to stimuli like pinching the base of the tail), respiratory rate and gill colour (pink to light red are correct).

Analgesics are drugs designed to reduce or relieve pain without causing loss of consciousness. Analgesics have been tested in zebrafish, and to lesser extent in sticklebacks, carp and trout (Sneddon 2012). However, they probably work well in other fish species, even those distantly related to model species. The main analgesics used to reduce pain and discomfort are opioid agents (morphine, butorphanol and buprenorphine), non-steroidal anti-inflammatory drugs

---

[8] https://www.drugs.com/vet/finquel-ms-222-tricaine-methanesulfonate.html (Accessed July 27, 2021)

(ketoprofen and carprofen) and local anaesthetics such as lidocaine (Sneddon 2012). These can reduce the stress response to different experimental procedures such as fin clipping (Deakin et al. 2019).

More detailed information on the use of anaesthetics and analgesics in fish can be found in Ross and Ross (2009), Readman et al. (2013), NORECOPA (2016) and Schroeder et al. (2021)

Handling

Fish vary in their ability to withstand handling, but capture and handling are undoubtedly stressful (Mazeaud et al. 1977; Billard et al. 1981; Pickering 1981; Pickering et al. 1982; Barton & Iwama 1991; Wendelaar Bonga 1997; Cook et al. 2015). Proper handling is not only important for the health and welfare of fish, but can also improve statistical power and experimental precision by reducing an unwanted source of variation (Pottinger & Calder 1995).

Fish skin is very different from that of terrestrial animals. The epithelium is relatively thin, unstratified and consists of live cells with no keratinisation. The surface layer has a complex pattern, which is species-specific, and has a large surface area that helps to retain a superficial layer of mucus that harbours a distinctive skin microbiome than varies among fish species (Legrand et al. 2020), but also among individuals and populations (Uren Webster et al. 2018). The skin has numerous free nerve endings that may act as nociceptors (pain receptors) and respond to mechanical pressure less than 0.1 g; thus, rough handling has the potential to be painful (Sneddon 2019). Specialised cells in the epidermis produce mucus that is continually sloughed off. The scales are contained within pockets of dermis extending up into the epidermis, and therefore removal of scale creates a wound spreading into the vascular tissue. Thus, the loss of a scale is not equivalent to losing hair or the ends of claws. Most fish – including salmonids – have delicate skins. Physical handling must be kept to a minimum and any abrasive or dry surfaces must be avoided, fish should only come in contact with soft, non-abrasive wet surfaces. This means that nets should be soft, knotless and submerged in the water prior to handling. Mesh size should be small enough to avoid parts of the fish protruding through the nets as this can cause damage and have a negative welfare effect. Fish should be handled with wet hands or with wet gloves and kept moist at all times, as even brief periods of air exposure can be highly stressful to most species (Sloman et al. 2001; Lankford et al. 2006). Fish skin can desiccate very rapidly in warm conditions with rapid airflow, and can freeze quickly when the temperature is below freezing.

Capturing fish from a tank can be difficult and stressful to the fish and can also cause injuries; this is especially true in the case of larger fish and when fish are housed in large tanks, or the tanks have objects or structures. Capturing fish with a hand net is a skill that requires practice and inexperienced people can spend a lot of time chasing a fish, which can be very stressful and potentially damaging. Corralling fish with two hand nets can facilitate capture, while passive handling – where fish enter the net voluntarily – can also be encouraged in some species.

Many fish can be weighed in a tared container filled with water, and this is probably preferably to weighing the fish out of the water. There are numerous references in the literature that advocate blotting the fish dry prior to weighing to reduce experimental error, but it is doubtful this is justifiable. Blotting is damaging to the fish, and the small amount of water removed is probably less than the content of the gut and the water in the mouth and the opercular cavity. If groups of fish are weighed in a net, their total weight should not be too heavy, or fish at the bottom risk suffering injury from crushing. The type of net used to move fish can also impact on fish welfare, knotless and rubber nets being preferred (Powell 2021).

Occasionally, fish may have to be held in temporary containers, such as when administering an anaesthetic. While adequate aeration in such vessels is essential, excessive aeration can disturb the fish and even damage them. The need for anaesthesia when handling fish is dependent on the species of fish and its previous experiences. Some fish may be easily handled with little or no signs of distress or attempts to escape – for example, some flatfish may be handled quite easily, even out of water, providing their eyes are covered. Others, for example, salmonids, may be severely stressed by even the gentlest of handlings. Once again, the necessity for anaesthesia requires an assessment based on familiarity with the fish.

Transportation

Wherever possible, fish should be transported in water even for very short periods of time (<1 minute). Many commercial farms now use fish pumps rather than nets to move fish. Oxygen levels must be maintained during transport, and stocking densities kept to a level that will not result in loss of water quality over the trip duration. Typical densities used for commercial fish transport range from 40 to 150 kg/m^3 for trout (Noble et al. 2020; RSPCA 2020), and ~ 40 kg/m^3 for lumpfish (personal observation). Commercial fish transporters recommend that the fish should not be disturbed during transport unless absolutely necessary. Therefore, there should be a remote method of monitoring dissolved oxygen, and water should not be exchanged during under normal circumstances. On a small scale, fish can be transported in sealed plastic bags. Usually two bags, one within the other, would be used to reduce the risk of breaking, especially with fish with spiny fin rays such as tilapia or many species of catfish. The inner bag should be one-third filled with water from the tank the fish are kept in (provided that is of high quality) and the remainder of the bag filled with oxygen. The neck of the bag can be twisted and bent over before being firmly tied with cable ties or a strong elastic band. For the transport of small fish, the corners of the bag may be tied off to provide a rounded rather than pointed corner to avoid fish becoming trapped and suffering from hypoxia.

Temperature fluctuations should be kept to a minimum during transport. For this, bags may be packed in insulating polystyrene boxes surrounded by ice packs (in the case of cold-water species) and should not be transported during periods of high temperatures. For larger groups of fish, insulated transportation tanks are used. In this case, fish should be starved for at least 6 h in the case of small fish (<400 g) and for 48 h in the case of larger fish (>400 g) as this reduces metabolic rate and oxygen consumption.

On arrival at the destination, fish should be acclimatised to the new environment. Acclimatisation is necessary not only to equilibrate the water temperature but also other water quality parameters such as pH. Even the most adaptable species have a limited capacity to adapt rapidly, and therefore every effort should be made to ensure that conditions during transport and arrival are as similar as possible. In some cases, this may require that the water is adjusted slowly over a period of several days to reduce any rapid changes following transportation – for example, in pH or salinity. Under normal circumstances, the bags should be floated on the new water until temperature has equilibrated (30–60 minutes). Either during this time or subsequently, some of the recipient water should be mixed with that in the bag to avoid any rapid changes in water chemistry. Acclimatising fish on arrival is always a compromise. Fish should not be confined for longer than necessary and, if they have already endured a long trip, it may be necessary to aerate the bag during the acclimatisation period. In some circumstances, when water quality has deteriorated to dangerous levels (as it may happen if some fish have died during transport), then the need for acclimatisation may be secondary to the urgent need for clean water. Under such circumstances, the surviving fish should be separated from the dead ones and placed in clean water with a similar temperature as soon as possible.

Fish should be closely monitored after transport for signs of ill health since moving fish can result in disruption of the social structure and result in social stress, aggression and injuries (Adams *et al.* 1998).

The International Air Transport Association's Live Animals Regulations (LAR) Manual 2021, contains details of transporting fish and is available from the IATA website[9]. See also Chapter 12: Transportation of laboratory animals.

Training and habituation during procedures

Disturbance can result in poor welfare, but it can also interact with other aspects of the environment – for example, with stocking density (Turnbull *et al.* 2005). In some circumstances, occasional disturbances can be more detrimental to fish than chronic exposure to mild disturbance (Adams *et al.* 2007). Some species can be trained to use self-feeding (i.e. on-demand) feeders (Alanärä & Brännäs 1996) and can use visual cues to anticipate feeding (Stien *et al.* 2007), which can reduce scramble competition and improve welfare. Some species have even been trained to approach zookeepers and allow them to conduct health checks (*pers comm*. From Epcot Center, Orlando, USA). In Norway, the Three Rs Working Group suggested that it may be possible to reduce some of the negative impacts of experimental procedures by training fish to associate a food reward when they enter the net (Hawkins *et al.* 2011).

Monitoring and sampling methods

Health monitoring

Most current guidelines for monitoring fish health refer to quarantine protocols for new fish arriving at a research facility. A distinction is usually made depending on the origin of the fish (from the wild or from other facilities), the species and the type of facility, but there is a need for better, harmonised criteria. Ensuring experimental fish are in good health is paramount for research since the health of fish can have a more significant effect on the outcome of the study than the experimental treatment itself.

New arrivals can bring parasites and infectious pathogens into the rearing system and cause disease outbreaks, while some pathogens can be endemic in cultured and wild populations of fish, such as *Mycobacterium* spp. infections in zebrafish and *Flavobacterium psychrophilum* in trout. Therefore, health management is much more than just keeping infections out of a fish facility. It concerns all aspects of the construction and management of the system and should be a central consideration when establishing any fish holding facility. Strategies designed to avoid introducing new diseases, and to control them if they occur are essential.

Health monitoring comprises the detection of problems (surveillance) as well as their identification (diagnosis). Wherever possible, protocols for monitoring health and welfare should be species-specific; it is often not appropriate to provide generic guidelines covering all species of fish (Johansen *et al.* 2006). Microscopy of skin scrapes, eye dabs and gill biopsies can be useful in identifying signs of infection or parasitism (Sneddon & Wolfenden 2019).

Blood plasma samples and haematocrit counts can provide useful insights into general health status; however, most blood parameters are highly variable and this can make it difficult to reach a conclusion (Johansen *et al.* 2006). Despite a scarcity of publications, the volume of blood in fish is estimated to be 2–5% of body weight and CCAC guidelines[10] recommend that no more than 1 ml of blood should be extracted per kilogram of body weight in live fish (Hawkins *et al.* 2011). Such blood volume is high compared to mammals (where only up to 10% of circulating blood volume is recommended to be drawn in a single bleed). Fish should be sedated during blood sampling to reduce stress and avoid diverting blood from the spleen to the rest of the body caused by the 'fight or flight' stress response. A recent review (Lawrence *et al.* 2020) provides best practices for blood sampling in fish, and suggests that blood volumes should be within 0.1%–10% of fish mass, although this is merely indicative as the volume of blood that can be extracted from live fish without causing harm is species and context dependent.

Tissue samplings are also common, and samples can be processed for histopathology or extracted for PCR analysis (mainly for pathogen identification). Those are common husbandry and health monitoring procedures for research facilities that have specific standard operational protocols (SOPs) depending on the fish species.

---

[9] https://www.iata.org/en/publications/store/live-animals-regulations/ (Accessed July 27. 2021)

[10] https://www.ccac.ca/Documents/Standards/Guidelines/Fish.pdf (Accessed July 27, 2021)

Sampling for genetic background

The most common techniques for obtaining tissue samples for fish genetic analysis (including parentage assignment) are fin clipping and skin swabbing. Fin clipping is the removal of all or part of a fin, usually to identify an individual or a population. It can be used to identify fish for monitoring purposes or also to identify their genetic background (via DNA extraction and genotyping). It can be a stressful (and probably painful) event and a source of infection if not done under good hygienic conditions. The removal of even a small amount of fin can have an adverse effect on the swimming ability of fish (Horak 1969; Dietrich & Cunjak 2006), although this is not always the case and may depend on species and fish size (Gjerde & Refstie 1988). Using anaesthetics and analgesics is recommended, but standard procedures are only available for zebrafish[11]. A less intrusive alternative to fin clipping is skin swabbing (Breacker et al. 2017; Tilley et al. 2020), and this does not require the use of anaesthesia or analgesia.

Physiological and reproductive status

Physiological monitoring of stress, reproductive status, and immunocompetence is common in fish research, and can also be used to monitor welfare and health. Most physiological parameters are monitored by extracting blood or by analysing other tissue samples. They are mostly invasive techniques that sometimes require euthanasia. Tissue samples can be used for biochemical analysis, histopathology or molecular biology. Stress indicators commonly used are levels of cortisol, lactate and glucose in blood plasma, and monoamines, dopamine, catecholamines and noradrenaline in brain and blood plasma (Schreck et al. 2016). For monitoring of reproductive status, changes in behaviour, colouration, body shape and chemical cues (reproductive pheromones) can be used. Ultrasound and endoscopy can also be used under anaesthesia (Wildhaber et al. 2005; Bryan et al. 2007), and hormonal changes related to reproduction can be assessed by analysis of steroids and gonadotropins in blood plasma (Zohar 2021). The gene expression of reproductive hormones and their receptors can be examined in brain (for GnRHs) and pituitary samples (for LH).

The large diversity of fish makes it hard to evaluate their reproductive state and there is a huge variability in development of the gonads and the physiological parameters associated with reproduction. Mechanisms of sex determination and differentiation are highly variable in fish and may differ between genera or even between species, and are under genetic and environmental control, depending on temperature, light, photoperiod and social context (Devlin & Nagahama 2002; Baroiller et al. 2009; Sandra & Norma 2010).

High diversity also poses problems for sampling the immune status of fish. The immune response varies considerably between species, and also within species, depending on context and genetic background, and there is a conspicuous lack of harmonised, common markers for the cellular and molecular components of the immune system (Tort et al. 2003;

Randelli et al. 2008). To evaluate the immune status of fish, both the cellular and the molecular level can be explored. Blood serum can be analysed for molecules involved in the immune response. These may include antimicrobial (AMPs) and antiviral peptides, enzymes (lysozyme, caspases, proteases), transferrin, complement, prostaglandins (PGE2), reactive oxygen intermediates (ROIs), cyclooxygenase-2 (COX-2), cytokines, chemokines and lectins, as well as toll like receptors (TLRs). Many immune biomarkers can also be studied at the transcriptome level such as the complement system, Mx genes and inflammation markers, cytokines and interleukins (Randelli et al. 2008). In addition to blood, other tissues can be used to examine the immune response in fish, including the head kidney, liver and spleen (Yuan et al. 2008; Millán et al. 2011; Pardo et al. 2012).

Behaviour

Video analysis software can be used to track the location of fish in a tank, their position in the water column, as well as their swimming activity and related behaviours, including swimming speed, distance covered, acceleration, number of turns, laterality, or time spent freezing. Many different software packages are available including free programs (Franco-Restrepo et al. 2019) and proprietary ones (Noldus, Viewpoint). Passive integrated transponder (PIT tags) can be used to identify individuals and determine their location (Acolas et al. 2007), but these have limited application in laboratory studies outside large tanks or flumes. PIT tags can also be used for behavioural studies (feeding response and group behaviour) and for individual or group behavioural selection tests (e.g., risk taking in groups). Acoustic telemetry can be a good tool for monitoring fish in sea cages and this is especially useful for aquaculture research (Muñoz et al. 2020). Tagging of animals should be done humanely with the use of anaesthesia and post-operative analgesia should be considered (Sloman et al. 2019). Fish identification, marking and tagging is a rapidly evolving field and recent reviews are provided by Axelsson et al. (2020) and Sandford et al. (2020).

Euthanasia

There is a general lack information on humane end-points for fish (Johansen et al. 2006; Sneddon 2009). LD50 testing is no longer allowed on mammals, but it is still used in fish (Braunbeck et al. 2005). Euthanasia requires an appropriate humane killing method, and any handling or restraint should have as few adverse effects on the animals (see Chapter 17: Euthanasia and other fates for laboratory animals). Most of the information relating to the humane killing of fish is in the context of slaughter of farmed fish (Robb & Kestin 2002; Van De Vis et al. 2003; Lines & Kestin 2005) but specific guidance on the best methods for euthanising fish in research is generally lacking (but see Neiffer & Stamper (2009)).

The two techniques recommended in the UK for humane killing of adult fish used in research are concussion and destruction of the brain prior to regaining of consciousness, and overdose of a suitable anaesthetic. In other jurisdictions, other techniques can also be used. For example, electrical stunning is permissible in Europe under 20210/63/EU and

---

[11]https://iacuc.ucsf.edu/sites/g/files/tkssra751/f/wysiwyg/STD%20PROCEDURE%20-%20Aquatic%20-%20Fin%20Clipping%20of%20Zebrafish.pdf (Accessed July 27, 2021)

in the USA, immersion in carbon dioxide saturated water or ethanol are also viable options (American Veterinary Medical Association 2020).

However, even while an overdose of anaesthetic is considered a humane method for killing fish (but note that the choice of anaesthetic may be species-specific), it also requires that death is confirmed or assured by a second method. This can be through confirmation of permanent cessation of the circulation, destruction of the brain, dislocation of the neck, exsanguination (i.e. fatal blood loss), the onset of *rigor mortis* or instantaneous destruction of the body in a macerator. The choice of method to confirm or assure death will depend on any subsequent sample collection – for example if brain tissue is required, it will not be appropriate to destroy the brain to assure death.

Some problems may arise with the euthanasia of heavily armoured fish, as it may be difficult to effectively concuss them, or with species that differ widely in their susceptibility to anaesthesia, for example, with air breathers. In these cases, the dose of anaesthetic might need to be increased to reduce time to death, while avoiding any irritant or aversive effect of the anaesthetic. Euthanising large numbers of fish, or very small fish, can also be a problem since concussion may not be feasible and following anaesthetic overdose it may be difficult to confirm death in a short period of time. Large fish can also pose a problem since capture and restraint prior to killing may be difficult and stressful to the fish. Adding anaesthetic to the water where the fish are kept may avoid handling stress, but this may not always be possible if only some individuals need to be euthanised, or the tanks or aquaria are connected to a shared recirculation system.

Other methods of euthanasia that are used in some places include maceration, chilling (which raises welfare concerns) and electrical stunning[5]. Electrical stunning is widely used in trout farming (Lines & Kestin 2005) and is also permissible in the EU, but it has not yet been recommended in the UK as a valid technique for killing fish used in research.

Acknowledgements

Revised and updated from Chapter 49 by James F. Turnbull and Iain Berrill in *The UFAW Handbook on The Care and Management of Laboratory and Other Research Animals, 8e*. We are grateful to Tim Ellis, Huw Golledge and an anonymous referee for their valuable comments and insights.

References

Abbott, A. (2020). Animal-research data show effects of EU's tough regulations. *Nature*, **12 February 2020**, 1–3.

Acolas, M.-L., Roussel, J.-M., Lebel, J.M. and Baglinière, J.-L. (2007) Laboratory experiment on survival, growth and tag retention following PIT injection into the body cavity of juvenile brown trout (*Salmo trutta*). *Fisheries Research*, **86**, 280–284.

Adams, C., Turnbull, J., Bell, A. *et al.* (2007) Multiple determinants of welfare in farmed fish: stocking density, disturbance, and aggression in Atlantic salmon (*Salmo salar*). *Canadian Journal of Fisheries and Aquatic Sciences*, **64**, 336–344.

Adams, C.E., Huntingford, F.A., Turnbull, J.F. and Beattie, C. (1998) Alternative competitive strategies and the cost of food acquisition in juvenile Atlantic salmon (*Salmo salar*). *Aquaculture*, **167**, 17–26.

Alanärä, A. and Brännäs, E. (1996) Dominance in demand-feeding behaviour in Arctic charr and rainbow trout: The effect of stocking density. *Journal of Fish Biology*, **48**, 242–254.

Alderton, D. (2019) *Encyclopedia of Aquarium and Pond Fish*. Dorling Kindersley Ltd., Attleborough, Norfolk.

American Fisheries Society (2014) *Guidelines for the Use of Fishes in Research*. p. 104. American Fisheries Society, Bethesda, Maryland.

American Veterinary Medical Association (2020) *AVMA Guidelines for the Euthanasia of Animals: 2020 Edition*. p. 121. Schaumburg, IL, USA: American Veterinary Medical Association.

Anders, J. and Ostrow, M. (1986) Goldfish in research: use and maintenance. *Laboratory Animals*, 33–41.

Andrews, C. (Ed.) (2002) *The Interpet Guide to Fish Breeding*. Interpet Publishing, Surrey.

Araújo-Luna, R., Ribeiro, L., Bergheim, A. and Pousão-Ferreira, P. (2018) The impact of different rearing condition on gilthead seabream welfare: Dissolved oxygen levels and stocking densities. *Aquaculture Research*, **49**, 3845–3855.

Axelsson, M., Peterson, E., Gräns, A. and Ljung, P.E. (2020) Fish identification, Marking and Tagging Methods. The Swedish 3Rs Center, Swedish Board of Agriculture, pp. 38.

Bagni, M. (2005) Sea bass. In: *Cultured Aquatic Species Information Programme*. Rome [online]: FAO.

Bakker, T.C.M. and Mundwiler, B. (2021) Nest-site selection in a fish species with paternal care. *Hydrobiologia*, **848**, 641–650.

Baroiller, J.-F., D'Cotta, H. and Saillant, E. (2009) Environmental effects on fish sex determination and differentiation. *Sexual Development*, **3**, 118–135.

Barreto, M.O., Rey Planellas, S., Yang, Y. *et al.* (2021) Emerging indicators of fish welfare in aquaculture. *Reviews in Aquaculture* n/a.

Barton, B. and Iwama, G. (1991) Physiological changes in fish from stress in Aquaculture with emphasis on the response and effects of corticosteroids. *Annual Review of Fish Diseases*, **44**, 3–26.

Batzina, A. and Karakatsouli, N. (2012) The presence of substrate as a means of environmental enrichment in intensively reared gilthead seabream Sparus aurata: growth and behavioral effects. *Aquaculture*, **370**, 54–60.

Beardmore, J., Mair, G. and Lewis, R. (2001) Monosex male production in finfish as exemplified by tilapia: applications, problems, and prospects. *Aquaculture*, **197**, 283–301.

Bekkozhayeva, D., Saberioon, M. and Císař, P. (2021) Automatic individual non-invasive photo-identification of fish (Sumatra barb *Puntigrus tetrazona*) using visible patterns on a body. *Aquaculture International*.

Benhaïm, D., Akian, D.D., Ramos, M. *et al.* (2017) Self-feeding behaviour and personality traits in tilapia: A comparative study between Oreochromis niloticus and Sarotherodon melanotheron. *Applied Animal Behaviour Science*, **187**, 85–92.

Bhujel, R.C. (2000) A review of strategies for the management of Nile tilapia (*Oreochromis niloticus*) broodfish in seed production systems, especially hapa-based systems. *Aquaculture*, **181**, 37–59.

Billard, R., Bry, C. and Gillet, C. (1981) *Stress, Environment and Reproduction in Teleost Fish*. Academic Press, Bristol.

Bolker, B.M., Brooks, M.E., Clark, C.J. *et al.* (2009) Generalized linear mixed models: a practical guide for ecology and evolution. *Trends in Ecology & Evolution* **24**, 127–135.

Boltana, S., Rey, S., Roher, N. *et al.* (2013) Behavioural fever is a synergic signal amplifying the innate immune response. *Proceedings of the Royal Society B: Biological Sciences*, **280**, 20131381.

Braunbeck, T., Böttcher, M., Hollert, H. *et al.* (2005). Towards an alternative for the acute fish LC50 test in chemical assessment: the fish embryo toxicity test goes multi-species-an update. *ALTEX-Alternatives to Animal Experimentation*, **22**, 87–102.

Breacker, C., Barber, I., Norton, W.H.J. *et al.* (2017). A low-cost method of skin swabbing for the collection of DNA Samples from small laboratory fish. *Zebrafish*, **14**, 35–41.

Bristol Aquarists' Society (2020). Goldfish. http://www.bristol-aquarists.org.uk/

Bromage, N. and Shepherd, J. (1992). Fish, their requirements and site evaluation. In: *Intensive Fish Farming*, Eds Shepherd, J. and Bromage, N., pp. 17–49. Blackwell Publishing, Oxford.

Brown, C. (2016) Does anybody have experience with breeding three-spined stickleback in aquarium? ResearchGate.

Brown, C. and Dorey, C. (2019) Pain and emotion in fishes – fish welfare implications for fisheries and aquaculture. *Animal Studies Journal*, **8**, 175–201.

Bryan, B.J., Wildhaber, M., Papoulias, D. et al. (2007) Estimation of gonad volume, fecundity, and reproductive stage of shovelnose sturgeon using sonography and endoscopy with application to the endangered pallid sturgeon. *Journal of Applied Ichthyology*, **23**, 411–419.

Canadian Council on Animal Care (2005) Guidelines on the care and use of fish in research, teaching and testing. In: *Canadian Council on Animal Care*, p. 94.

Casal, C. (2006) Global Documentation of fish introductions: The growing crisis and recommendations for action. *Biological Invasions*, **8**, 3–11.

Castanheira, M., Conceição, L., Millot, S. et al. (2015) Coping styles in farmed fish: Consequences for aquaculture. *Reviews in Aquaculture*, **9**, 23.

Champneys, T., Castaldo, G., Consuegra, S. and Garcia de Leaniz, C. (2018) Density-dependent changes in neophobia and stress-coping styles in the world's oldest farmed fish. *Royal Society Open Science*, **5**, 181473.

Clark, J.D., Gebhart, G.F., Gonder, J.C., Keeling, M.E. and Kohn, D.F. (1997). The 1996 guide for the care and use of laboratory animals. *ILAR Journal*, **38**, 41–48.

Colloca, F. and Cerasi, S.I. (2005) *Sparus aurata*. In: *Cultured Aquatic Species Information Programme*. Rome: FAO Fisheries Division [online].

Colman, J.G. (1997) A review of the biology and ecology of the whale shark. *Journal of Fish Biology*, **51**, 1219–1234.

Consuegra, S., Ellison, A., Allainguillaume, J. et al. (2013) Balancing selection and the maintenance of MHC supertype variation in a selfing vertebrate. *Proceedings of the Royal Society B: Biological Sciences*, **280**.

Cook, K.V., Lennox, R.J., Hinch, S.G. and Cooke, S.J. (2015) FISH Out of WATER: How Much Air is Too Much? *Fisheries*, **40**, 452–461.

Coward, K. and Little, D. (2001) Culture of the 'aquatic chicken': present concerns and future prospects. *Biologist (London, England)*, **48**, 12–16.

Cowx, I.G. (2005) *Oncorhynchus mykiss*. In: *Cultured Aquatic Species Information Programme*. Rome [online]: FAO Fisheries Division.

Coyle, S.D., Durborow, R.M. and Tidwell, J.H. (2004) *Anesthetics in Aquaculture*: Southern Regional Aquaculture Center Stoneville.

Cubitt, K.F., Winberg, S., Huntingford, F.A. et al. (2008) Social hierarchies, growth and brain serotonin metabolism in Atlantic salmon (*Salmo salar*) kept under commercial rearing conditions. *Physiology & Behavior*, **94**, 529–535.

Das, P., Mandal, S.C., Bhagabati, S. et al. (2012) Important live food organisms and their role in aquaculture. *Frontiers in Aquaculture*, **5**, 69–86.

Davenport, J. (1985) *Synopsis of biological data on the lumpsucker, Cyclopterus lumpus (Linnaeus, 1758)*: Food & Agriculture Org.

Dawood, M.A., Koshio, S. and Esteban, M.Á. (2018) Beneficial roles of feed additives as immunostimulants in aquaculture: A review. *Reviews in Aquaculture*, **10**, 950–974.

d'Angelo, L. and de Girolamo, P. (Eds) (2021) *Laboratory Fish in Biomedical Research. Biology, Husbandry and Research Applications for Zebrafish, Medaka, Killifish, Cavefish, Stickleback, Goldfish and Danionella translucida*. Academic Press, London.

Deakin, A.G., Buckley, J., AlZu'bi, H.S. et al. (2019) Automated monitoring of behaviour in zebrafish after invasive procedures. *Scientific Reports*, **9**, 1–13.

de Castilhos Ghisi, N. and de Oliveira, E.C. (2016) Fish welfare: The state of science by scientometrical analysis. *Acta Scientiarum. Biological Sciences*, **38**, 253–261.

Denayer, T., Stöhr, T. and Van Roy, M. (2014) Animal models in translational medicine: Validation and prediction. *New Horizons in Translational Medicine*, **2**, 5–11.

Depczynski, M. and Bellwood, D.R. (2005) Shortest recorded vertebrate lifespan found in a coral reef fish. *Current Biology*, **15**, R288–R289.

DeTolla, L.J., Srinivas, S., Whitaker, B.R. et al. (1995) Guidelines for the Care and Use of Fish in Research. *ILAR Journal*, **37**, 159–173.

Devlin, R.H. and Nagahama, Y. (2002) Sex determination and sex differentiation in fish: An overview of genetic, physiological, and environmental influences. *Aquaculture*, **208**, 191–364.

Dietrich, J.P. and Cunjak, R.A. (2006) Evaluation of the impacts of Carlin tags, fin clips, and Panjet tattoos on juvenile Atlantic salmon. *North American Journal of Fisheries Management*, **26**, 163–169.

El-Sabaawi, R.W., Frauendorf, T.C., Marques, P.S. et al. (2016) Biodiversity and ecosystem risks arising from using guppies to control mosquitoes. *Biology Letters*, **12**, 20160590.

El-Sayed, A.-F.M. (2020) *Tilapia Culture*. Academic Press, Oxford.

Eliasen, K., Patursson, E.J., McAdam, B.J. et al. (2020) Liver colour scoring index, carotenoids and lipid content assessment as a proxy for lumpfish (*Cyclopterus lumpus* L.) health and welfare condition. *Scientific Reports*, **10**, 8927.

Ellis, T., Yildiz, H.Y., López-Olmeda, J. et al. (2012) Cortisol and finfish welfare. *Fish Physiology and Biochemistry*, **38**, 163–188.

Ellis, T., Sanders, M. and Scott, A. (2013) Non-invasive monitoring of steroids in fishes. *Veterinary Medicine Austria*, **100**, 255–269.

Ellis, T., Rimmer, G.S.E., Parker, S.J. et al. (2019) In-tank underwater cameras can refine monitoring of laboratory fish. *Animal Welfare*, **28**, 191–203.

Ellis, S.L., Riemer, S., Thompson, H. and Burman, O.H. (2020) Assessing the external validity of successive negative contrast–implications for animal welfare. *Journal of Applied Animal Welfare Science*, **23**, 54–61.

Ellis, M.A. (2020) Fin damage in juvenile Atlantic salmon: Farm and experimental, causes and consequences (PhD). The University of Stirling, Stirling, UK.

Ellison, A.R., Uren Webster, T.M., Rey, O. et al. (2018) Transcriptomic response to parasite infection in Nile tilapia (*Oreochromis niloticus*) depends on rearing density. *BMC Genomics*, **19**, 723.

Ellison, A.R., Uren Webster, T.M., Rodriguez-Barreto, D. et al. (2020) Comparative transcriptomics reveal conserved impacts of rearing density on immune response of two important aquaculture species. *Fish Shellfish Immunology*, **104**, 192–201.

European Commission (2020) Report on the Statistics on the Use of Animals for Scientific Purposes in the Member States of the European Union in 2015–2017, p. 20.

Evers, H.G., Pinnegar, J.K. and Taylor, M.I. (2019) Where are they all from? – sources and sustainability in the ornamental freshwater fish trade. *Journal of Fish Biology*, **94**, 909–916.

Fanouraki, E., Mylonas, C., Papandroulakis, N. and Pavlidis, M. (2011) Species specificity in the magnitude and duration of the acute stress response in Mediterranean marine fish in culture. *General and Comparative Endocrinology*, **173**, 313–322.

FAO (2005) *Oreochromis niloticus*. In: *Cultured Aquatic Species Information Programme*. Rome [online]: FAO Fisheries and Aquaculture Department.

Farm Animal Welfare Council (2014) Opinion on the Welfare of Farmed Finfish. p. 16.

Fernandes Silva, P., Garcia de Leaniz, C. and Luchiari, A.C. (2019) Fear contagion in zebrafish: A behaviour affected by familiarity. *Animal Behaviour*, **153**, 95–103.

Fernando, A. and Phang, V. (1985) Culture of the guppy, Poecilia reticulata, in Singapore. *Aquaculture*, **51**, 49–63.

Ferreira, G.S., Veening-Griffioen, D.H., Boon, W.P. et al. (2020) Levelling the translational gap for animal to human efficacy data. *Animals*, **10**, 1199.

Festing, M.F. and Altman, D.G. (2002) Guidelines for the design and statistical analysis of experiments using laboratory animals. *ILAR Journal*, **43**, 244–258.

Fitzsimmons, K., Martinez-Garcia, R. and Gonzalez-Alanis, P. (2011) Why tilapia is becoming the most important food fish on the planet. In: *Better Science, Better Fish, Better Life. Proceedings of the Ninth International Symposium on Tilapia in Aquaculture*, Eds Liping, L. and Fitzsimmons, K., pp. 9–19. Shanghai Ocean University, Shanghai, China: AquaFish Collaborative Research Support Program.

Føre, M., Frank, K., Norton, T. et al. (2018) Precision fish farming: A new framework to improve production in aquaculture. *Biosystems Engineering*, **173**, 176–193.

Foster, S., Garcia, V. and Town, M. (1988) Cannibalism as the cause of an ontogenetic shift in habitat use by fry of the threespine stickleback. *Oecologia*, **74**, 577–585.

Franco-Restrepo, J.E., Forero, D.A. and Vargas, R.A. (2019). A review of freely available, open-source software for the automated analysis of the behavior of adult zebrafish. *Zebrafish*, **16**, 223–232.

Franěk, R., Baloch, A.R., Kašpar, V. et al. (2020) Isogenic lines in fish – a critical review. *Reviews in Aquaculture*, **12**, 1412–1434.

Froese, R. and Pauly, D. (2019) FishBase World Wide Web electronic publication.

Garcia de Leaniz, C., Gutierrez Rabadan, C., Barrento, S.I. et al. (2022) Addressing the welfare needs of farmed lumpfish: knowledge gaps, challenges and solutions. *Reviews in Aquaculture* **14**, 139–155.

Garcia de Leaniz, C., Fleming, I.A., Einum, S. et al. (2007a) Local adaptation. In: *The Atlantic Salmon: Genetics, Conservation and Management*, Eds Verspoor, E., Stradmeyer, L. and Nielsen, J., pp. 200–239. Blackwell, Oxford.

Garcia de Leaniz, C., Fleming, I.A., Einum, S. et al. (2007b) A critical review of adaptive genetic variation in Atlantic salmon: implications for conservation. *Biological Reviews*, **82**, 173–211.

Garcia de Leaniz, C., Gajardo, G. and Consuegra, S. (2010) From best to pest: Changing perspectives on the impact of exotic salmonids in the southern hemisphere. *Systematics and Biodiversity*, **8**, 447–459.

Gay, J. (2005) *The Perfect Aquarium: The Complete Guide to Setting Up and Maintaining an Aquarium*. Hamlyn, UK.

Gay, J. (2009) *Aquarium Manual: The Complete Step-by-step Guide to Keeping Fish*. J H Haynes & Co Ltd., 192 pages.

Gjerde, B. and Refstie, T. (1988) The effect of fin-clipping on growth rate, survival and sexual maturity of rainbow trout. *Aquaculture*, **73**, 383–389.

Gonçalves-de-Freitas, E., Bolognesi, M.C., Gauy, A.C.d.S. et al. (2019) Social behavior and welfare in Nile tilapia. *Fishes*, **4**, 23.

Guryev, V., Koudijs, M.J., Berezikov, E. et al. (2006) Genetic variation in the zebrafish. *Genome Research*, **16**, 491–497.

Gutierrez Rabadan, C., Spreadbury, C., Consuegra, S. and Garcia de Leaniz, C. (2021) Development, validation and testing of an Operational Welfare Score Index for farmed lumpfish *Cyclopterus lumpus* L. *Aquaculture*, **531**, 735777.

Halverson, A. (2010) *An entirely Synthetic Fish: How Rainbow Trout Beguiled America and Overran the World*. Yale University Press, London.

Hardy, R. (2018) Invasive Species Compendium. CABI.

Harel, I., Benayoun, B.A., Machado, B. et al. (2015) A platform for rapid exploration of aging and diseases in a naturally short-lived vertebrate. *Cell*, **160**, 1013–1026.

Hawkins, A.D. (Ed.) (1981) *Aquarium Systems*. Academic Press, London.

Hawkins, P., Dennison, N., Goodman, G. et al. (2011) Guidance on the severity classification of scientific procedures involving fish: report of a Working Group appointed by the Norwegian Consensus-Platform for the Replacement, Reduction and Refinement of animal experiments (Norecopa). *Laboratory Animals*, **45**, 219–224.

Helland, S., Dahle, S., Hough, C. and Borthen, J. (2014) Production of ballan wrasse (*Labrus bergylta*). Science and Practice. p. 136. The Norwegian Seafood Research Fund (FHF).

Hendry, K. and Cragg-Hine, D. (2003) Ecology of the Atlantic Salmon. In: *Conserving Natura 2000 Rivers Ecology Series*, p. 36. English Nature, Peterborough, UK.

Hindar, K., Garcia de Leaniz, C., Koljonen, M.-L. et al. (2007) Fisheries exploitation. In: *The Atlantic Salmon: Genetics, Conservation and Management*, Eds Verspoor, E., Stradmeyer, L. and Nielsen, J., pp. 306–330. Blackwell, Oxford.

Hiott, A.E. and Phelps, R.P. (1993) Effects of initial age and size on sex reversal of *Oreochromis niloticus* fry using methyltestosterone. *Aquaculture*, **112**, 301–308.

Horak, D.L. (1969) The effect of fin removal on stamina of hatchery-reared rainbow trout. *The Progressive Fish-Culturist*, **31**, 217–220.

Huntingford, F.A., Adams, C., Braithwaite, V.A. et al. (2006) Current issues in fish welfare. *Journal of Fish Biology*, **68**, 332–372.

Huntingford, F.A. and Ruiz-Gomez, M.L. (2009) Three-spined sticklebacks *Gasterosteus aculeatus* as a model for exploring behavioural biology. *Journal of Fish Biology*, **75**, 1943–1976.

Hussain, M.G. (2004) *Farming of tilapia: Breeding Plans, Mass Seed Production and Aquaculture Techniques*. Momin Offset Press, Dhaka.

Imsland, A.K.D., Reynolds, P., Jonassen, T.M. et al. (2019) Comparison of diet composition, feeding, growth and health of lumpfish (*Cyclopterus lumpus* L.) fed either feed blocks or pelleted commercial feed. *Aquaculture Research*, **50**, 1952–1963.

Imsland, A.K.D., Reynolds, P., Jonassen, T.M. et al. (2018) Effects of three commercial diets on growth, cataract development and histopathology of lumpfish (*Cyclopterus lumpus* L.). *Aquaculture Research*, **49**, 3131–3141.

Jenkins, J.A., Bart, H.L., Bowker, J.D. et al. (2014) Guidelines for use of fishes in research – revised and expanded, 2014. *Fisheries*, **39**, 415–416.

Jarvis, S., Ellis, M.A., Turnbull, J.F. et al. (2021) Qualitative behavioral assessment in juvenile farmed Atlantic salmon (*Salmo salar*): Potential for on-farm welfare assessment. *Frontiers in Veterinary Science*, **8**.

Johansen, R., Needham, J.R., Colquhoun, D.J. et al. (2006) Guidelines for health and welfare monitoring of fish used in research. *Laboratory Animals*, **40**, 323–340.

Jones, M. (2004) *Salmo salar*. In: *Cultured Aquatic Species Information Programme*. Rome [online]: FAO Fisheries Division.

Jones, N.A.R., Webster, M.M. and Salvanes, A.G.V. (2021) Physical enrichment research for captive fish: Time to focus on the DETAILS. *Journal of Fish Biology* n/a.

Jonsson, B. and Jonsson, N. (2011) *Ecology of Atlantic Salmon and Brown Trout: Habitat as a Template for Life Histories*. Springer Science & Business Media.

Kalueff, A.V., Gebhardt, M., Stewart, A.M. et al. (2013) Towards a comprehensive catalog of zebrafish behavior 1.0 and beyond. *Zebrafish*, **10**, 70–86.

Kazlauskaite, R., Cheaib, B., Heys, C. et al. (2021) SalmoSim: The development of a three-compartment in vitro simulator of the Atlantic Salmon GI tract and associated microbial communities.

Khoo, G., Lim, K.F., Gan, D.K. et al. (2002) Genetic diversity within and among feral populations and domesticated strains of the guppy (*Poecilia reticulata*) in Singapore. *Marine Biotechnology*, **4**, 367–378.

Kiessling, A., van de Vis, H., Flik, G. and Mackenzie, S. (2012) Welfare of farmed fish in present and future production systems. *Fish Physiology and Biochemistry*, **38**, 1–3.

Killen, S.S., Brown, J.A. and Gamperl, A.K. (2007) The effect of prey density on foraging mode selection in juvenile lumpfish: balancing food intake with the metabolic cost of foraging. *Journal of Animal Ecology*, **76**, 814–825.

Kottelat, M., Britz, R., Hui, T.H. and Witte, K.-E. (2006) *Paedocypris*, a new genus of Southeast Asian cyprinid fish with a remarkable sexual dimorphism, comprises the world's smallest vertebrate. *Proceedings of the Royal Society B: Biological Sciences*, **273**, 895–899.

Kültz, D. (2015) Physiological mechanisms used by fish to cope with salinity stress. *Journal of Experimental Biology*, **218**, 1907–1914.

Lackmann, A.R., Andrews, A.H., Butler, M.G. et al. (2019) Bigmouth Buffalo *Ictiobus cyprinellus* sets freshwater teleost record as improved age analysis reveals centenarian longevity. *Communications Biology*, **2**, 197.

Lankford, S., Adams, B., Adams, T. and Cech, J. Jr. (2006) Using specific antisera to neutralize ACTH in sturgeon: A method for manipulating the interrenal response during stress. *General and Comparative Endocrinology*, **147**, 384–390.

Lawrence, M.J., Raby, G.D., Teffer, A.K. et al. (2020) Best practices for non-lethal blood sampling of fish via the caudal vasculature. *Journal of Fish Biology*, **97**, 4–15.

Leal, M.C., Vaz, M.C.M., Puga, J. et al. (2016) Marine ornamental fish imports in the European Union: an economic perspective. *Fish and Fisheries*, **17**, 459–468.

Leduc, A.O., Thomas, S.A., Bassar, R.D. et al. (2021) The experimental range extension of guppies (*Poecilia reticulata*) influences the metabolic activity of tropical streams. *Oecologia*, 1–17.

Legrand, T.P., Wynne, J.W., Weyrich, L.S. and Oxley, A.P. (2020) A microbial sea of possibilities: current knowledge and prospects for an improved understanding of the fish microbiome. *Reviews in Aquaculture*, **12**, 1101–1134.

Lein, I. and Helland, S. (2014) Establishment of ballan wrasse broodstock. In: *Production of Ballan Wrasse (Labrus bergylta). Science and Practice*, Eds Helland, S., Dahle, S., Hough, C. and Borthen, J., pp. 10–13. The Norwegian Seafood Research Fund, Oslo.

Lichatowich, J. (2001) *Salmon without Rivers: A History of the Pacific Salmon Crisis*. Island Press, Washington DC.

Lindholm, A.K., Breden, F., Alexander, H.J. et al. (2005) Invasion success and genetic diversity of introduced populations of guppies *Poecilia reticulata* in Australia. *Molecular Ecology*, **14**, 3671–3682.

Lines, J. and Kestin, S. (2005) Electric stunning of trout: Power reduction using a two-stage stun. *Aquacultural Engineering*, **32**, 483–491.

Little, D. (1998) Options in the development of the aquatic chicken. *Fish Farmer*, **7**, 35–37.

Lowe, S., Browne, M., Boudjelas, S. and De Poorter, M. (2000) 100 of the World's Worst Invasive Alien Species A selection from the Global Invasive Species Database p. 12: Invasive Species Specialist Group (ISSG), World Conservation Union (IUCN).

Luchiari, A.C., do Amaral Duarte, C.R., de Morais Freire, F.A. and Nissinen, K. (2006) Hierarchical status and colour preference in Nile tilapia (*Oreochromis niloticus*). *Journal of Ethology*, **25**, 169–175.

Lushchak, V.I., Lushchak, L.P., Mota, A.A. and Hermes-Lima, M. (2001) Oxidative stress and antioxidant defenses in goldfish *Carassius auratus* during anoxia and reoxygenation. *American Journal of Physiology-Regulatory, Integrative and Comparative Physiology*, **280**, R100–R107.

Maceda-Veiga, A., Escribano-Alacid, J., de Sostoa, A. and García-Berthou, E. (2013) The aquarium trade as a potential source of fish introductions in southwestern Europe. *Biological Invasions*, **15**, 2707–2716.

MacIntyre, C.M., Ellis, T., North, B.P. and Turnbull, J.F. (2008) The influences of water quality on the welfare of farmed rainbow trout: a review. In: *Fish Welfare*, Ed. Branson, E., pp. 150–184. Blackwell Publishing, Oxford.

MacKenzie, S., Ribas, L., Pilarczyk, M. et al. (2009) Screening for coping style increases the power of gene expression studies. *PLoS One*, **4(4)**, e5314. doi:10.1371/journal.pone.0005314

Magurran, A. and Seghers, B. (1990) Population differences in the schooling behaviour of newborn guppies, *Poecilia reticulata*. *Ethology*, **84**, 334–342.

Magurran, A.E. (2005) *Evolutionary Ecology: The Trinidadian Guppy*. Oxford University Press, Oxford.

Martins, C.I., Galhardo, L., Noble, C. et al. (2012) Behavioural indicators of welfare in farmed fish. *Fish Physiology and Biochemistry*, **38**, 17–41.

Martins, C.I., Ochola, D., Ende, S.S. et al. (2009) Is growth retardation present in Nile tilapia *Oreochromis niloticus* cultured in low water exchange recirculating aquaculture systems? *Aquaculture*, **298**, 43–50.

Martins, T., Valentim, A., Pereira, N. and Antunes, L.M. (2018) Anaesthetics and analgesics used in adult fish for research: A review. *Laboratory Animals*, **53**, 325–341.

Mazeaud, M.M., Mazeaud, F. and Donaldson, E.M. (1977) Primary and secondary effects of stress in fish: Some new data with a general review. *Transactions of the American Fisheries Society*, **106**, 201–212.

McLarney, W.O. (1998) *Freshwater Aquaculture: A Handbook for Small Scale Fish Culture in North America*. Vancouver, British Columbia: Hartley & Marks Publishers.

Mehlis, M., Bakker, T.C. and Frommen, J.G. (2009) Nutritional benefits of filial cannibalism in three-spined sticklebacks (*Gasterosteus aculeatus*). *Naturwissenschaften*, **96**, 399–403.

Mendonça, F.Z. and Gonçalves-de-Freitas, E. (2008) Nest deprivation and mating success in Nile tilapia (Teleostei: Cichlidae). *Revista Brasileira de Zoologia*, **25**, 413–418.

Meyvis, T. and Van Osselaer, S.M.J. (2017) Increasing the power of your study by increasing the effect size. *Journal of Consumer Research*, **44**, 1157–1173.

Millán, A., Gómez-Tato, A., Pardo, B.G. et al. (2011) Gene expression profiles of the spleen, liver, and head kidney in turbot (*Scophthalmus maximus*) along the infection process with *Aeromonas salmonicida* using an immune-enriched oligo-microarray. *Marine Biotechnology*, **13**, 1099–1114.

Millot, S., Cerqueira, M., Castanheira, M.F. et al. (2014) Use of conditioned place preference/avoidance tests to assess affective states in fish. *Applied Animal Behaviour Science*, **154**, 104–111.

Mills, D. (1989) *Ecology and Management of Atlantic salmon*. Springer Science & Business Media, London.

Mills, D. (Ed.) (1999) *The Interpet Bumper Guide to Tropical Aquarium Fishes*. Interpet Publishing, Surrey.

Monnet, G., Rosenfeld, J.S. and Richards, J.G. (2020) Adaptive differentiation of growth, energetics and behaviour between piscivore and insectivore juvenile rainbow trout along the Pace-of-Life continuum. *Journal of Animal Ecology*, **89**, 2717–2732.

Moretti, A., Pedini Fernandez-Criado, M., Cittolin, G. and Guidastri, R. (1999) *Manual on Hatchery Production of Seabass and Gilthead Seabream*. p. 205. Food and Agriculture Organization of the United Nations, Rome.

Mota, V.C., Martins, C.I., Eding, E.H. et al. (2014) Steroids accumulate in the rearing water of commercial recirculating aquaculture systems. *Aquacultural Engineering*, **62**, 9–16.

Mota, V.C., Martins, C.I., Eding, E.H. et al. (2017) Water cortisol and testosterone in Nile tilapia (*Oreochromis niloticus*) recirculating aquaculture systems. *Aquaculture*, **468**, 255–261.

Mozart, H. (1998) *Guppies. Keeping and Breeding Them in Captivity*. Chelsea House Publications, Neptune City, NJ.

Mukai, Y., Sani, M., Mohammad-Noor, N. and Kadowaki, S. (2016) Effective method to culture infusoria, a highly potential starter feed for marine finfish larvae. *International Journal of Fisheries and Aquatic Studies*, **4**, 124–127.

Muñoz, L., Aspillaga, E., Palmer, M. et al. (2020) Acoustic telemetry: A tool to monitor fish swimming behavior in sea-cage aquaculture. *Frontiers in Marine Science*, **7**, 1–12.

Mwaffo, V., Butail, S. and Porfiri, M. (2017) In-silico experiments of zebrafish behaviour: Modeling swimming in three dimensions. *Scientific Reports*, **7**, 1–18.

Nakajima, M. and Taniguchi, N. (2001) Genetics of the guppy as a model for experiment in aquaculture. *Genetica*, **111**, 279–289.

Näslund, J. and Johnsson, J.I. (2016) Environmental enrichment for fish in captive environments: Effects of physical structures and substrates. *Fish and Fisheries*, **17**, 1–30.

National Agricultural Statistics Service (2019) 2018 Census of Aquaculture. United States Department of Agriculture.

Neiffer, D.L. and Stamper, M.A. (2009) Fish sedation, anesthesia, analgesia, and euthanasia: Considerations, methods, and types of drugs. *ILAR Journal*, **50**, 343–360.

Neto, J.F. and Giaquinto, P.C. (2020). Environmental enrichment techniques and tryptophan supplementation used to improve the quality of life and animal welfare of Nile tilapia. *Aquaculture Reports*, **17**, 100354.

Nielsen, J., Hedeholm, R.B., Heinemeier, J. *et al.* (2016) Eye lens radiocarbon reveals centuries of longevity in the Greenland shark (*Somniosus microcephalus*). *Science*, **353**, 702–704.

Nilsson, K., Lundbäck, S., Postavnicheva-Harri, A. and Persson, L. (2011) Guppy populations differ in cannibalistic degree and adaptation to structural environments. *Oecologia*, **167**, 391–400.

Nivelle, R., Gennotte, V., Kalala, E.J.K. *et al.* (2019) Temperature preference of Nile tilapia (*Oreochromis niloticus*) juveniles induces spontaneous sex reversal. *PLoS One*, **14**, e0212504.

Noble, C., Gismervik, K., Iversen, M.H. *et al.* (Eds) (2018) *Welfare Indicators for Farmed Atlantic Salmon: Tools for Assessing Fish Welfare*. Nofima.

Noble, C., Gismervik, K., Iversen, M.H. *et al.* (Eds) (2020) *Welfare Indicators for Farmed Rainbow Trout: Tools for Assessing Fish Welfare*. Nofima.

Noble, C., Iversen, M.H., Lein, I. *et al.* (2019) An introduction to Operational and Laboratory based Welfare Indicators for ballan wrasse (*Labrus bergylta*). In: *RENSVEL OWI FACT SHEET SERIES*, p. 43: FHF.

NORECOPA (2016) Fish as research animals.

Norton, W.H. and Gutiérrez, H.C. (2019) The three-spined stickleback as a model for behavioural neuroscience. *PLoS One*, **14**, e0213320.

O'Donncha, F., Stockwell, C.L., Planellas, S.R. *et al.* (2021). Data driven insight into fish behaviour and their use for precision aquaculture. *Frontiers in Animal Science*, **30**. 10.3389/fanim.2021.695054.

Ohlyan, S., Sihag, R.C. and Yadava, N.K. (2011) Efficacy of different aquarium designs fabricated for the breeding of the guppy. *Journal of Nature Science and Sustainable Technology*, **5**, 243.

Ostlund-Nilsson, S., Mayer, I. and Huntingford, F.A. (2006) *Biology of the Three-Spined Stickleback*. CRC Press, Boca Raton, FL.

Papandroulakis, N., Divanach, P., Anastasiadis, P. and Kentouri, M. (2001) The pseudo-green water technique for intensive rearing of sea bream (*Sparus aurata*) larvae. *Aquaculture International*, **9**, 205–216.

Paradis, H., Ahmad, R., McDonald, J. *et al.* (2019) Ocular tissue changes associated with anterior segment opacity in lumpfish (*Cyclopterus lumpus* L) eye. *Journal of Fish Diseases*, **42**, 1401–1408.

Pardo, B.G., Millán, A., Gómez-Tato, A. *et al.* (2012) Gene expression profiles of spleen, liver, and head kidney in turbot (Scophthalmus maximus) along the infection process with *Philasterides dicentrarchi* using an immune-enriched oligo-microarray. *Marine Biotechnology*, **14**, 570–582.

Parra, L., García, L., Sendra, S. and Lloret, J. (2018) The use of sensors for monitoring the feeding process and adjusting the feed supply velocity in fish farms. *Journal of Sensors*, **2018**.

Pautsina, A., Císař, P., Štys, D. *et al.* (2015) Infrared reflection system for indoor 3D tracking of fish. *Aquacultural Engineering*, **69**, 7–17.

Pedrazzani, A.S., Quintiliano, M.H., Bolfe, F. *et al.* (2020) Tilapia on-farm welfare assessment protocol for semi-intensive production systems. *Frontiers in Veterinary Science*, **7**, 991.

Pennell, W. and Barton, B.A. (1996). *Principles of Salmonid Culture*. Elsevier, Amsterdam.

Pickering, A. (Ed.) (1981) *Stress and Fish*. Academic Press, London.

Pickering, A., Pottinger, T. and Christie, P. (1982) Recovery of the brown trout, *Salmo trutta* L., from acute handling stress: a time-course study. *Journal of Fish Biology*, **20**, 229–244.

Pickett, G.D. and Pawson, M.G. (1994) *Sea Bass: Biology, Exploitation and Conservation*. Springer Science & Business Media, Berlin.

Pillay, T.V.R. and Kutty, M.N. (2005) *Aquaculture: Principles and Practises*. Blackwell Publishing, Oxford.

Portavella, M., Torres, B. and Salas, C. (2004) Avoidance response in goldfish: emotional and temporal involvement of medial and lateral telencephalic pallium. *Journal of Neuroscience*, **24**, 2335–2342.

Pottinger, T. and Calder, G. (1995) Physiological stress in fish during toxicological procedures: a potentially confounding factor. *Environmental Toxicology and Water Quality*, **10**, 135–146.

Pounder, K.C., Mitchell, J.L., Thomson, J.S. *et al.* (2018) Physiological and behavioural evaluation of common anaesthesia practices in the rainbow trout. *Applied Animal Behaviour Science*, **199**, 94–102.

Powell, A. (2021) Rubber net mesh reduces scale loss during routine handling of farmed Atlantic salmon (*Salmo salar*). *Animal Welfare*, **30**, 19–24.

Powell, A., Pooley, C., Scolamacchia, M. and Garcia de Leaniz, C. (2018a) Review of lumpfish biology In: *Cleaner Fish Biology and Aquaculture Applications*, Ed. Treasurer, J.W., pp. 98–121. 5M Publishing Ltd., Sheffield.

Powell, A., Treasurer, J.W., Pooley, C.L. *et al.* (2018b) Use of lumpfish for sea-lice control in salmon farming: challenges and opportunities. *Reviews in Aquaculture*, **10**, 683–702.

Prestinicola, L., Boglione, C., Makridis, P. *et al.* (2013) Environmental conditioning of skeletal anomalies typology and frequency in gilthead seabream (*Sparus aurata* L., 1758) juveniles. *PLoS One*, **8**, e55736.

Priborsky, J. and Velisek, J. (2018) A review of three commonly used fish anesthetics. *Reviews in Fisheries Science & Aquaculture*, **26**, 417–442.

Quinn, T.P. (2005) *The Behavior and Ecology of Pacific Salmon and Trout*. University of Washington Press, Seattle.

Randelli, E., Buonocore, F. and Scapigliati, G. (2008) Cell markers and determinants in fish immunology. *Fish and Shellfish Immunology*, **25**, 326–340.

Readman, G.D., Owen, S.F., Knowles, T.G. and Murrell, J.C. (2017) Species specific anaesthetics for fish anaesthesia and euthanasia. *Scientific Reports*, **7**, 7102.

Readman, G.D., Owen, S.F., Murrell, J.C. and Knowles, T.G. (2013) Do fish perceive anaesthetics as aversive? *PLoS One*, **8**, e73773.

Rey, S., Digka, N. and MacKenzie, S. (2015a). Animal personality relates to thermal preference in wild-type zebrafish, *Danio rerio*. *Zebrafish*, **12**, 243–249.

Rey, S., Huntingford, F.A., Boltana, S. *et al.* (2015b) Fish can show emotional fever: Stress-induced hyperthermia in zebrafish. *Proceedings of the Royal Society B: Biological Sciences*, **282**, 20152266.

Rey, S., Little, D.C. and Ellis, M.A. (2019) Farmed fish welfare practices: Salmon farming as a case study. Retrieved from https://www.aquaculturealliance.org/wp-content/uploads/2020/05/FarmedFishWelfarePractices_26_May_2020.pdf

Rey, S., Treasurer, J., Pattillo, C. and McAdam, B.J. (2021) Using model selection to choose a size-based condition index that is consistent with operational welfare indicators. *Journal of Fish Biology* n/a.

Robb, D. and Kestin, S. (2002) Methods used to kill fish: Field observations and literature reviewed. *Animal Welfare*, **11**, 269–282.

Roberts, L., Taylor, J. and Garcia de Leaniz, C. (2011) Environmental enrichment reduces maladaptive risk-taking behavior in salmon reared for conservation. *Biological Conservation*, **144**, 1972–1979.

Roberts, L.J., Taylor, J., Gough, P.J. *et al.* (2014). Silver spoons in the rough: can environmental enrichment improve survival of hatchery Atlantic salmon *Salmo salar* in the wild? *Journal of Fish Biology*, **85**, 1972–1991.

Rodriguez-Barreto, D., Rey, O., Uren-Webster, T.M. *et al.* (2019) Transcriptomic response to aquaculture intensification in Nile tilapia. *Evolutionary Applications*, **12**, 1757–1771.

Rodríguez, F., López, J.C., Vargas, J.P. *et al.* (2002) Conservation of spatial memory function in the pallial forebrain of reptiles and ray-finned fishes. *Journal of Neuroscience*, **22**, 2894–2903.

Roesner, A., Mitz, S.A., Hankeln, T. and Burmester, T. (2008) Globins and hypoxia adaptation in the goldfish, *Carassius auratus*. *The FEBS Journal*, **275**, 3633–3643.

Ross, L.G. (2000) Environmental physiology and energetics. In: *Tilapias: Biology and Exploitation*, Eds Beveridge, M.C. and McAndrew, B.J., pp. 89–128. Springer, Dordrecht.

Ross, L.G. and Ross, B. (2009) *Anaesthetic and Sedative Techniques for Aquatic Animals*. John Wiley & Sons, Oxford.

RSPCA (2018) RSPCA Standards for Farmed Atlantic Salmon. p. 89. Horsham, UK Royal Society for the Prevention of Cruelty to Animals.

RSPCA (2019) How should I keep and care for my goldfish? In: *RSPCA Knowledgebase*.

RSPCA (2020) RSPCA Standards for Farmed Rainbow Trout. p. 51. Horsham, UK: Royal Society for the Prevention of Cruelty to Animals.

Rushbrook, B., Dingemanse, N.J. and Barber, I. (2008) Repeatability in nest construction by male three-spined sticklebacks. *Animal Behaviour*, **75**, 547–553.

Rutherford, K.M., Donald, R.D., Lawrence, A.B. and Wemelsfelder, F. (2012). Qualitative behavioural assessment of emotionality in pigs. *Applied Animal Behaviour Science*, **139**, 218–224.

Saberioon, M., Gholizadeh, A., Císař, P. et al. (2017) Application of machine vision systems in aquaculture with emphasis on fish: State-of-the-art and key issues. *Reviews in Aquaculture*, **9**, 369–387.

Sadoul, B. and Geffroy, B. (2019) Measuring cortisol, the major stress hormone in fishes. *Journal of Fish Biology*, **94**, 540–555.

Saint-Erne, N. (2015) Anesthesiology in fish. In: *40th World Small Animal Veterinary Association Congress, Bangkok, Thailand, 15–18 May, 2015. Proceedings book*, pp. 353–355: World Small Animal Veterinary Association.

Samaras, A., Papandroulakis, N., Costari, M. and Pavlidis, M. (2016) Stress and metabolic indicators in a relatively high (European sea bass, *Dicentrarchus labrax*) and a low (meagre, *Argyrosomus regius*) cortisol responsive species, in different water temperatures. *Aquaculture Research*, **47**, 3501–3515.

Sandford, M., Castillo, G. and Hung, T.C. (2020) A review of fish identification methods applied on small fish. *Reviews in Aquaculture*, **12**, 542–554.

Sandra, G.-E. and Norma, M.-M. (2010) Sexual determination and differentiation in teleost fish. *Reviews in Fish Biology and Fisheries*, **20**, 101–121.

Saraiva, J.L., Castanheira, M.F., Arechavala-López, P. et al. (2018) Domestication and welfare in farmed fish. In: *Animal Domestication*. IntechOpen.

Schartl, M. (2014) Beyond the zebrafish: Diverse fish species for modeling human disease. *DMM Disease Models and Mechanisms*, **7**, 181–192.

Schartl, M., Wilde, B., Schlupp, I. and Parzefall, J. (1995) Evolutionary origin of a parthenoform, the Amazon molly *Poecilia formosa*, on the basis of a molecular genealogy. *Evolution*, **49**, 827–835.

Schluter, D. (2021). How to raise stickleback. In: *Schluter Lab*. Vancouver, BC.

Schraml, R., Hofbauer, H., Jalilian, E. et al. (2020) Towards fish individuality-based aquaculture. *IEEE Transactions on Industrial Informatics*, **17**, 1–1.

Schreck, C.B., Tort, L., Farrell, A.P. and Brauner, C.J. (2016) *Biology of Stress in Fish*. Academic Press, London.

Schroeder, P., Lloyd, R., McKimm, R. et al. (2021) Anaesthesia of laboratory, aquaculture and ornamental fish: *Proceedings of the first LASA-FVS Symposium. Laboratory Animals*, **55**, 317–328.

Shaalan, M., Saleh, M., El-Mahdy, M. and El-Matbouli, M. (2016) Recent progress in applications of nanoparticles in fish medicine: a review. *Nanomedicine: Nanotechnology, Biology and Medicine*, **12**, 701–710.

Sharpe, S. (2020) How to Culture Your Own Infusoria at Home. Infusoria as Fish Food. The Spruce Pets.

Shearer, W.M. (1992) *The Atlantic Salmon: Natural History, Exploitation and Future Management*. Fishing News Books

Shepherdson, D. (1989) Review of environmental enrichment in zoos. *Ratel*, **16**, 35–40.

Shinya, M. and Sakai, N. (2011) Generation of highly homogeneous strains of zebrafish through full sib-pair mating. *G3: Genes| Genomes| Genetics*, **1**, 377–386.

Skiftesvik, A.B., Durif, C. and Bjelland, R. (2014) Understanding and remediating clumping behaviour. In: *Production of ballan wrasse (Labrus bergylta). Science and Practice*, Eds Helland, S., Dahle, S., Hough, C. and Borthen, J., pp. 70–71. The Norwegian Seafood Research Fund (FHF).

Skilbrei, O.T. (1991) Importance of threshold length and photoperiod for the development of bimodal length–frequency distribution in Atlantic salmon (*Salmo salar*). *Canadian Journal of Fisheries and Aquatic Sciences*, **48**, 2163–2172.

Sloman, K., Taylor, A., Metcalfe, N. and Gilmour, K. (2001) Stress from air emersion fails to alter chloride cell numbers in the gills of rainbow trout. *Journal of Fish Biology*, **59**, 186–190.

Sloman, K.A., Bouyoucos, I.A., Brooks, E.J. and Sneddon, L.U. (2019). Ethical considerations in fish research. *Journal of Fish Biology*, **94**, 556–577.

Smartt, J. (2008) *Goldfish Varieties and Genetics: Handbook for Breeders*: John Wiley & Sons, New York.

Smith, C. and Reay, P. (1991) Cannibalism in teleost fish. *Reviews in Fish Biology and Fisheries*, **1**, 41–64.

Smith, S.A. (2013) Welfare of Laboratory Fishes. *Laboratory Animal Welfare*, 301–311.

Sneddon, L.U. (2009) Pain perception in fish: Indicators and endpoints. In: *ILAR Journal*, pp. 338–342.

Sneddon, L.U. (2012) Clinical Anesthesia and Analgesia in Fish. *Journal of Exotic Pet Medicine*, **21**, 32–43.

Sneddon, L.U. (2015) Pain in aquatic animals. *Journal of Experimental Biology*, **218**, 967–976.

Sneddon, L.U. (2019) Evolution of nociception and pain: evidence from fish models. *Philosophical Transactions of the Royal Society B: Biological Sciences*, **374**, 20190290.

Sneddon, L.U., Elwood, R.W., Adamo, S.A. and Leach, M.C. (2014) Defining and assessing animal pain. *Animal Behaviour*, **97**, 201–212.

Sneddon, L.U. and Wolfenden, D.C.C. (2019) Ornamental Fish (Actinopterygii). In: *UFAW Companion Animal Handbook*, Ed. Yeates, J., pp. 440–466. Wiley Blackwell.

Stein, D.L. (1986). Cyclopteridae. In: *Fishes of the North-Eastern Atlantic and the Mediterranean*. Eds Whitehead, P.J.P., Bauchot, M.-L., Hureau, J.-C. et al., pp. 1269–1274. UNESCO, Paris.

Stewart, A.M., Braubach, O., Spitsbergen, J. et al. (2014) Zebrafish models for translational neuroscience research: From tank to bedside. *Trends in Neurosciences*, **37**, 264–278.

Stickney, R.R. (1993) Tilapia. In *Culture of Nonsalmonid Freshwater Fishes*, Ed. Stickney, R.R., pp. 81–115. CRC Press, Boca Raton.

Stien, L.H., Bratland, S., Austevoll, I. et al. (2007) A video analysis procedure for assessing vertical fish distribution in aquaculture tanks. *Aquacultural Engineering*, **37**, 115–124.

Storebakken, T. and Austreng, E. (1987) Ration level for salmonids: I. Growth, survival, body composition, and feed conversion in Atlantic salmon fry and fingerlings. *Aquaculture*, **60**, 189–206.

Stringwell, R., Lock, A., Stutchbury, C.J. et al. (2014) Maladaptation and phenotypic mismatch in hatchery-reared Atlantic salmon *Salmo salar* released in the wild. *Journal of Fish Biology*, **85**, 1927–1945.

Swaisgood, R. and Shepherdson, D. (2006) Environmental enrichment as a strategy for mitigating stereotypies in zoo animals: A literature review and meta-analysis. *Stereotypic Animal Behaviour: Fundamentals and Applications to Welfare: Second Edition*, pp. 256–285.

Taylor, J.S., Braasch, I., Frickey, T. et al. (2003) Genome duplication, a trait shared by 22,000 species of ray-finned fish. *Genome Research* **13**, 382–390.

The American Anti-Vivisection Society (2021) Animals in Science. Which Animals are Used: Fish.

Thompson, R.R.J., Paul, E.S., Radford, A.N. et al. (2016) Routine handling methods affect behaviour of three-spined sticklebacks in a novel test of anxiety. *Behavioural Brain Research*, **306**, 26–35.

Thorson, J.T. and Minto, C. (2015). Mixed effects: A unifying framework for statistical modelling in fisheries biology. *ICES Journal of Marine Science*, **72**, 1245–1256.

Tilley, C.A., Carreno Gutierrez, H., Sebire, M. et al. (2020) Skin swabbing is a refined technique to collect DNA from model fish species. *Scientific Reports*, **10**, 18212.

Toni, M., Manciocco, A., Angiulli, E. et al. (2019) Assessing fish welfare in research and aquaculture, with a focus on European directives. *Animal*, **13**, 161–170.

Tort, L., Balasch, J. and Mackenzie, S. (2003) Fish immune system. A crossroads between innate and adaptive responses. *Inmunologia*, **22**, 277–286.

Treasurer, J. (Ed.) (2018a) *Cleaner Fish Biology and Aquaculture Applications*. 5M Publishing, Sheffield.

Treasurer, J. (2018b) *An Introduction to Sea Lice and the Rise of Cleaner Fish*. Sheffield: 5m Publishing ltd.

Turner, J. (2016) Video tracking of behaviour and tank distribution of lumpfish (*Cyclopterus lumpus*) related to fin damage to develop operational welfare indicators. (*MSc. Thesis*). The University of Stirling, Stirling.

Turnbull, J., Bell, A., Adams, C. et al. (2005) Stocking density and welfare of cage farmed Atlantic salmon: Application of a multivariate analysis. *Aquaculture* **243**, 121–132.

Turnbull, J.F. and Berrill, I.K. (2010) Fish. In: *The UFAW Handbook on the Care and Management of Laboratory and Other Research Animals*, Eds. Hubrecht, R.C. and Kirkwood, J. Blackwell, Chichester.

UK Home Office (2021) *Annual Statistics of Scientific Procedures on Living Animals Great Britain 2020*. p 30.

Uren Webster, T.M., Consuegra, S., Hitchings, M. and Garcia de Leaniz, C. (2018) Interpopulation variation in the Atlantic Salmon microbiome reflects environmental and genetic diversity. *Applied and Environmental Microbiology*, **84**, e00691-18.

Uren Webster, T.M., Rodriguez-Barreto, D., Consuegra, S. and Garcia de Leaniz, C. (2020). Cortisol-Related Signatures of Stress in the Fish Microbiome. *Frontiers in Microbiology*, **11**, 1621.

Valletta, J.J., Torney, C., Kings, M. et al. (2017) Applications of machine learning in animal behaviour studies. *Animal Behaviour*, **124**, 203–220.

Van De Vis, H., Kestin, S., Robb, D. et al. (2003) Is humane slaughter of fish possible for industry? *Aquaculture Research*, **34**, 211–220.

Vatsos, I. (2017) Standardizing the microbiota of fish used in research. *Laboratory Animals*, **51**, 353–364.

Vázquez, F.J.S. and Muñoz-Cueto, J.A. (2014) *Biology of European Sea Bass*. CRC Press, Boca Raton, FL.

Venables, W.N. and Dichmont, C.M. (2004) GLMs, GAMs and GLMMs: an overview of theory for applications in fisheries research. *Fisheries Research*, **70**, 319–337.

Verspoor, E., Garcia de Leaniz, C. and McGinnity, P. (2007) Genetics and Habitat Management. In: *The Atlantic Salmon: Genetics, Conservation and Management*, Eds Verspoor, E., Stradmeyer, L. and Nielsen, J., pp. 410–434. Oxford: Blackwell.

Villamizar, N., Ribas, L., Piferrer, F. et al. (2012) Impact of daily thermocycles on hatching rhythms, larval performance and sex differentiation of zebrafish. *PLoS One*, **7**, e52153.

Vindas, M.A., Gorissen, M., Höglund, E. et al. (2017) How do individuals cope with stress? Behavioural, physiological and neuronal differences between proactive and reactive coping styles in fish. *Journal of Experimental Biology*, **220**, 1524–1532.

Volff, J. (2005). Genome evolution and biodiversity in teleost fish. *Heredity*, **94**, 280–294.

Volpato, G.L. and Barreto, R.E. (2001) Environmental blue light prevents stress in the fish Nile tilapia. *Brazilian Journal of Medical and Biological Research*, **34**, 1041–1045.

Wang, M. and Lu, M. (2016) Tilapia polyculture: A global review. *Aquaculture Research*, **47**, 2363–2374.

Watson, C.A., Hill, A.V.S. and Pouder, D.B. (2004) Species profile: Koi and Goldfish. In *SRAC Publications*, p. 6.

Wedemeyer, G. (1996) *Physiology of Fish in Intensive Culture Systems*. Springer Science & Business Media, London.

Wendelaar Bonga, S.E. (1997). The stress response in fish. *Physiological Reviews*, **77**, 591–625.

Wildhaber, M., Papoulias, D., DeLonay, A. et al. (2005) Gender identification of shovelnose sturgeon using ultrasonic and endoscopic imagery and the application of the method to the pallid sturgeon. *Journal of Fish Biology*, **67**, 114–132.

Williams, T., Readman, G. and Owen, S. (2009) Key issues concerning environmental enrichment for laboratory-held fish species. *Laboratory Animals*, **43**, 107–120.

Willoughby, S. (1999) *Manual of Salmonid Farming*. Blackwell Science Ltd, Chichester.

Woynarovich, A., Hoitsy, G. and Moth-Poulsen, T. (2011) Small-scale rainbow trout farming. In: *FAO Fisheries and Aquaculture Technical Paper*, p. 92. Rome: FAO.

Wysocki, L.E., Davidson III, J.W., Smith, M.E. et al. (2007) Effects of aquaculture production noise on hearing, growth, and disease resistance of rainbow trout *Oncorhynchus mykiss*. *Aquaculture*, **272**, 687–697.

Yuan, C., Pan, X., Gong, Y. et al. (2008) Effects of Astragalus polysaccharides (APS) on the expression of immune response genes in head kidney, gill and spleen of the common carp, *Cyprinus carpio* L. *International Immunopharmacology*, **8**, 51–58.

Zaki, M.A.A., Alabssawy, A.N., Nour, A.E.-A.M. et al. (2020) The impact of stocking density and dietary carbon sources on the growth, oxidative status and stress markers of Nile tilapia (*Oreochromis niloticus*) reared under biofloc conditions. *Aquaculture Reports*, **16**, 100282.

Zohar, Y. (2021) Fish reproductive biology – Reflecting on five decades of fundamental and translational research. *General and Comparative Endocrinology*, **300**, 113544.

49 Zebrafish

Carole Wilson

Introduction

Nowadays, many research institutions and academia boast the zebrafish (*Danio rerio*) among their complement of animal models. This small tropical fish from South Asia has seen a dramatic rise in its use as a research model during the last thirty years (Figure 49.1). Along with other species, including *salmon*, *trout* and other smaller species including *killifish*, fish are the second most used animal group in research after mice in the UK, and are currently classified by genus rather than individual species. In 2019, 16% of all licensed scientific procedures in the UK were performed on fish, and they accounted for 12% of all breeding of animals with genetic modifications (UK Home Office 2020a). Chapter 48: Fishes contains information on the more general use of fish in research.

Zebrafish are of interest to the biomedical research community because they are vertebrates that share approximately 70% commonality with human genes and some 82% in common with human disease-causing genes (Howe et al. 2013). In addition to their small size and robustness, zebrafish are highly fecund. This, coupled with the fact their transparent embryos are externally fertilised and develop very rapidly outside the body, makes them excellent candidates for research. In general, they are largely viewed as a very cost-effective model that is easy to work with. However, while their husbandry requirements are often assumed to be relatively simple and commonly known, the broadness of husbandry and welfare guidelines for them suggests otherwise (Nevalainen et al. 2002).

Zebrafish were historically kept in laboratories by research staff in relatively simple setups, but as the model system has grown in popularity, scale and sophistication, so too has the complexity of their housing, husbandry and welfare needs. The scientific value of zebrafish has expanded greatly beyond the production of wild-type fish embryos - encompassing chemical screens, the production of transgenic fish and, more recently, the introduction of gene editing, including clustered regularly interspaced short palindromic repeats (CRISPR) technologies (Hwang et al. 2013). Thus making ideas and scientific disciplines open up that were only imagined a few years ago.

Biological overview

General biology

Zebrafish, first described in the 1800s (Clark K.J; Ekker 2013), are a small tropical freshwater teleost, although many of their natural environments may also be described as temperate. Their taxonomy classification is in the order Cypriniformes, family Cyprinidae, subfamily Danioninae and genus *Danio*. There are approximately 2,400 other members of the cyprinid family, which included carp, barbs, and goldfish, all of which are toothless in the mouth but retain pharyngeal teeth. Fusiform in shape, as adult between 20 and 40 mm from the snout to the caudal peduncle. They are so named for the characteristic horizontal striping pattern on each side of the body. They have three unpaired fins and two sets of paired fins, as well as two sets of barbels (Harper and Lawrence 2011).

In the wild, they are distributed across much of South Asia, including India, Bangladesh, Pakistan and Nepal (Sundin et al. 2019). They appear to prefer areas with overhanging vegetation and, while they inhabit various waters, they are generally found inhabiting slow flowing shallow pools and slow to moderate flowing rivers, often with mud and silt bottoms (Parichy 2015). They tolerate a wide variety of water conditions, including pH and salinity, as well as differences in water turbidity (Engeszer et al. 2007; Spence et al. 2008; Suriyampola et al. 2016). An omnivorous species, they feed on a wide range of diets, such as zooplankton, small insects, algae and other plant materials (Spence et al. 2008). Many other fish species share these environments including related species such as *Dario dario* and *Danio meghalayensis*, as well as species such as knifefish, needlefish and catfish, which are likely to prey on zebrafish (Engeszer, Patterson, et al. 2007).

Zebrafish are ectothermic, regulating body temperature according to environmental conditions and temperature. They are seasonal breeders in the wild and an 'r' selected species – free spawning with the ability to lay up to several hundreds of eggs per clutch. The embryos develop very rapidly with no parental care and become capable of free feeding after five days post fertilisation (dpf) under a standard

---

The UFAW Handbook on the Care and Management of Laboratory and Other Research Animals, Ninth Edition.
Edited by Huw Golledge and Claire Richardson.
© 2024 John Wiley & Sons Ltd. Published 2024 by John Wiley & Sons Ltd.

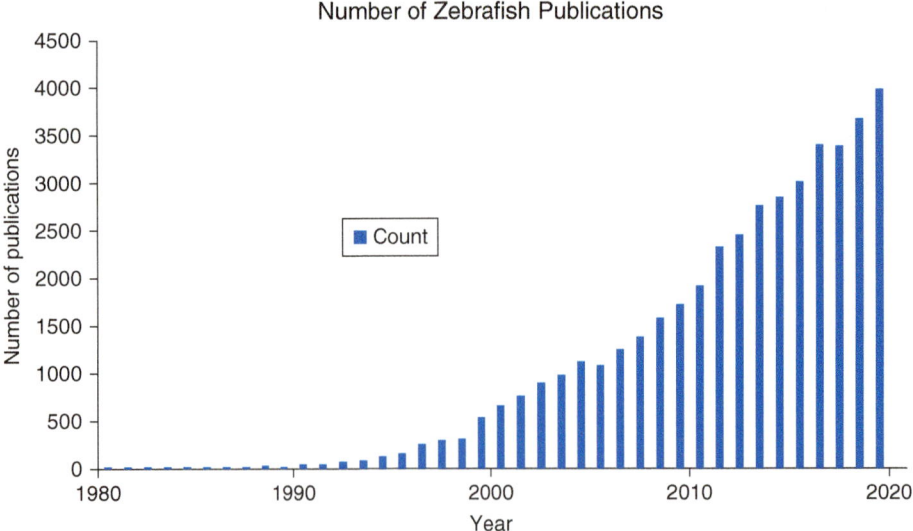

Figure 49.1 Cumulative number of scientific publications citing zebrafish as the animal model, from a search of PubMed using search terms all zebrafish and /or *danio rerio* and /or *brachydanio*. Source: Karen Dunford

laboratory temperature of 28.5°C (Kimmel *et al.* 1995). Developmental rate will be affected by environmental temperatures: cooler water will slow development and warmer water speed development, although it should not be assumed that all features will develop equally under different temperatures (Kimmel *et al.* 1995).

Laboratory zebrafish have undergone a process of domestication; wild zebrafish are much more genetically diverse than those lines which can be found in the laboratory, which are now genetically distinct from any wild-type population (Whiteley *et al.* 2011). The two main lines of laboratory fish are TU, originally created from a pet shop population in Germany, and AB, originating similarly in the USA. TU and AB each appear to have a common ancestor which, although they are distinct, lacks a sex determining locus at the tip of chromosome 4 (Wilson *et al.* 2014). Much of the genetic variation has been lost from most laboratory lines, probably a consequence of bottlenecking and genetic drift, but also because of different breeding strategies between institutions, to the point where different lines have now evolved into distinct sub-lines (Suurvali *et al.* 2020).

Size and life span

Zebrafish are small cyprinids, approximately 20–40 mm in length, although they will vary in size according to both the conditions they are kept in and, to an extent, the genetic line (Meyer *et al.* 2013). Even individual fish kept under the same standard conditions will vary in size (Singleman and Holtzman 2014). Zebrafish from outdoor farms in Florida generally exceed the size of any zebrafish kept under standard laboratory conditions (author's personal observation).

The rate of growth will vary given individual laboratory conditions, including environmental conditions and the impact of nutrition. However, for example, under the standard condition of 28°C, at 24 hours larval fish will measure approximately 1.9 mm long, rising to 3.7 mm by day three (Kimmel *et al.* 1995). At the beginning of the juvenile period, fish will be approximately 10.9–11.7 mm (Parichy *et al.* 2009), and will attain adult size at 25 mm at approximately 90 days. One study showed that skeletal length at death increased with age suggesting indeterminate growth (Gerhard *et al.* 2002).

Although there have been anecdotal reports of zebrafish being kept for up to four years in captivity, this is not a common practice. It is recommended that 18 months should be the maximum life span of a zebrafish held in a breeding programme (UK Home Office; 2020b). After this time, it is usual to see reduced fertility and fecundity and fish becoming more susceptible to illness (Wilson & Dunford 2015). In the wild, zebrafish are thought to be seasonal and so are unlikely to live more than a year, especially given the instability of their environments.

Zebrafish development

Development in zebrafish occurs very rapidly in the initial embryonic stages (Figure 49.2), and developmental stages up to 120 hours post fertilisation (hpf) are very temperature dependent. These described are held at 28.5°C (Kimmel *et al.* 1995) (Table 49.1). General development of zebrafish is highly impacted by a wide variety of environmental factors including, but not exclusively, water temperature (Kimmel *et al.* 1995), water quality and stocking density (Singleman and Holtzman 2014), lighting conditions (Villamizar *et al.* 2014) and, in later stages, nutritional factors and dietary regimes (Watts *et al.* 2012; Perera & Yufera 2016; Lawrence *et al.* 2012).

Reproduction

In the wild, zebrafish usually spawn seasonally, but under laboratory conditions they can spawn all year round. When sexual maturity is reached, they are highly fecund and fertile. Females are capable of spawning every 2–3 days and laying in excess of 200 eggs in each clutch. Ovulation and spawning are dependent on the presence of males and the eggs produced are fertilised externally, with no parental care. Courtship behaviour is induced by female pheromones in response to male olfactory cues – the release of steroid glucuronide (Vandenhurk and Lambert 1983). Photoperiod and first daylight induces spawning in fish (Tsang *et al.* 2017).

Mating behaviour is displayed as males circling females and trying to lead them to spawning sites and, in part, is controlled by aggression in courtship behaviours – dominance patterns in both male and female – and it is linked to fish size. Larger males and females tend to be dominant, and when similar sized fish are together, they show less

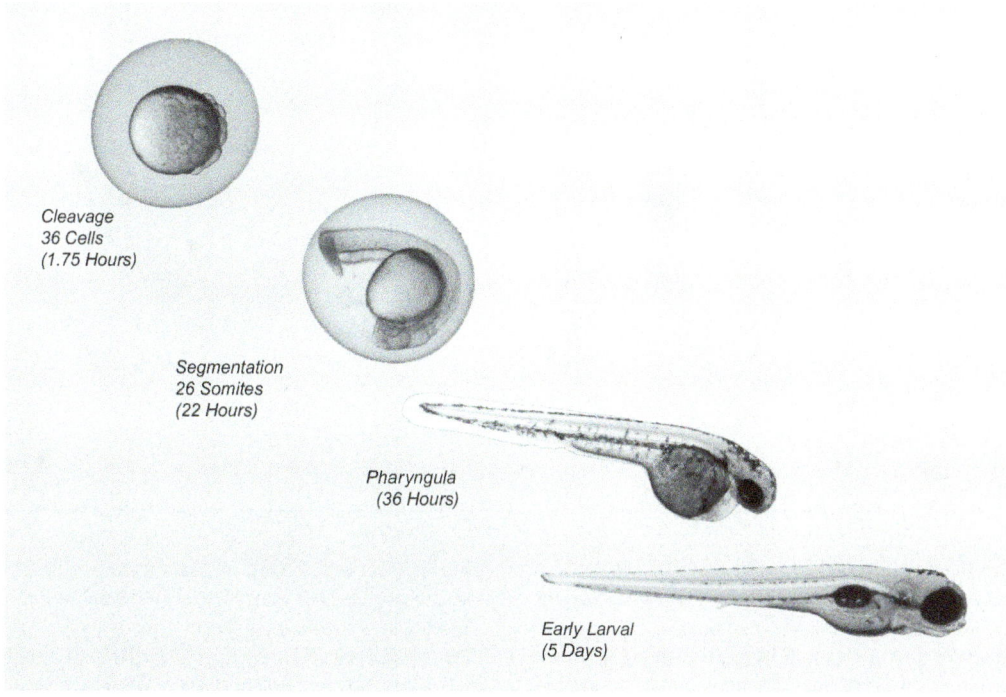

Figure 49.2 Brief pictorial diagram of four of the developmental stages, as described in Table 49.1.

Table 49.1 Brief description of the stages of zebrafish development.

Period	Development	Time at period (post fertilisation)	References
Zygotic	1 cell over a large yolk, which can sustain the developing embryo for at least 96 hours before any exogenous feeding needs to occur	0–0.75 hours post fertilisation	(Kimmel et al. 1995) (Wilson 2012)
Cleavage	2–64 cell Cell division begins to occur	0.75–2.25 hours post fertilisation	
Blastula	64–1000 cell After 3 hours, asynchronous cell division begins – leading into 30% epiboly	1000 cell occurs at approximately 2.25–5 hours post fertilisation	
Gastrulation	Ends in formation of the tail bud at approximately 10 hours post fertilisation.	Approximately 5–10 hours post fertilisation	
Segmentation	Begins with first somite furrow and ends in formation of 26 somites Spontaneous muscular twitching at 20 somites Start of formation of lens and otic vesicle	10–24 hours post fertilisation	
Pharyngula	Beginning of period – • Formation of blood cells on yolk • Heartbeat • Beginning of pigmentation At end of this period – • Body begins to straighten • Fin development begins	24–48 hours post fertilisation	
Hatching	Larval fish leaves the chorion Rapid organ development Ends in protruding mouth stage at 72 hours	48–72 hours post fertilisation	

(Continued)

Table 49.1 (Continued)

Period	Development	Time at period (post fertilisation)	References
Early larval	72 hours – swim bladder inflates Early feeding behaviour begins	3–approximately 13 dpf	(Guerrera et al. 2015)
	Mouth develops	3 dpf	(Lee et al. 2018)
	Gut develops a hollow tube	3–5 dpf	(Wilson 2012)
	Digestive tract opens, digestive enzymes secreted	3–7 dpf	
	Body Length 3.7–4 mm	5 dpf	
	Yolk sac completely depleted and reabsorbed. Exogenous feeding begins	7 dpf	
	Sexual differentiation begins (all fry beginning as female)	8 dpf	
	Body length 4.5–8 mm	10 dpf	
Metamorphosis	Ends when full adult pigmentation and fin complement are complete	15–20 dpf	(Parichy 2003) (Wilson 2012)
Juvenile	Follows metamorphosis	Approximately 30–90 dpf	(Wilson 2012)
Adult	Achieved at sexual maturity Fully developed gonads Potentially indeterminate growth	In laboratory: 2–3 months old or 25 mm or over	(Engeszer, Alberici da Barbiano, et al. 2007) (Gerhard et al. 2002) (Spence et al. 2008) (Wilson 2012)

aggression towards one another (Paull *et al.* 2010). Enriched sites are preferred for spawning – shallow, vegetated areas with good water circulation (Spence, Ashton, and Smith 2007). In a laboratory setting, fish will spawn in bare tanks (personal observation), but there is evidence that environmental enrichment, plastic grass and leaves increases the number of eggs laid (Wafer *et al.* 2016). In the wild, mating appears to happen frequently between individual males and females separate from the shoal (Hutter *et al.* 2010). In the laboratory and where possible, group mating appears to happen more frequently, and this may be tied to high stocking density in the tanks, lack of the ability for sexual selection and altered mating tactics (Hutter *et al.* 2010).

Social organisation

Zebrafish are a shoaling species, a behaviour which recognisably begins at 14–15 dpf (Facciol and Gerlai 2020). In the wild, they often form small shoals of 5–20 (Pritchard *et al.* 2001), but in faster flowing water they can form shoals of up to 300 individuals, with males preferring to associate with larger groups of females (Suriyampola *et al.* 2016). Shoaling behaviour influences mate choice and recognition, and mates are often chosen from the same shoal (Engeszer, Ryan, and Parichy 2004). Other work shows that fish will preferentially associate with fish displaying the same pigment patterns as those they first shoaled with (Spence *et al.* 2008). Dominance hierarchies form in both male and female groups; in a laboratory setting, these appear to be largely based on body size. Males of similar size will be less aggressive to one another. Dominant females will choose both the best spawning sites and larger bodied males, who are likely to be dominant (Paull *et al.* 2010). They also have been shown to secrete pheromones that suppress subordinate females (Gerlach 2006), which may have little effect in wild habitats when fish can vacate an area but are perhaps more relevant in a captive situation.

In a laboratory setting, zebrafish are usually kept in groups, with the numbers of fish depending on the age of the fish and the tank size. Often these fish are derived from a single clutch and represent the same genetic line (personal observation). There is some debate about the most appropriate stocking density. Crowding does appear to increase stress in adult fish, dependent on tank size, acclimation time to the tank and feeding regimes (Ramsay *et al.* 2006) and crowding in bare tanks also appears to increase aggression in females and decrease levels of fecundity (Carfagnini *et al.* 2009). Five adult fish per litre has been suggested (Matthews, Trevarrow, and Matthews 2002), or four to ten fish per litre (Alestrom *et al.* 2020) to maintain water quality. Although exposing young fish (six weeks post fertilisation) to overcrowding induces stress (Fontana *et al.* 2021), recommendations for numbers of larval fish are higher than adult fish – suggestions ranging between 100 per 35 mL for embryos and 250 per litre for 5–10 dpf (Alestrom *et al.* 2020) to more conservative estimates of 40–50 fish per litre for the early larval period (Matthews *et al.* 2002; Harper & Lawrence 2011).

Sources

Zebrafish are the only fish species on Schedule 2 in the UK and on Annex 1 in the European Directive 2010/63/EU. This means tighter control is required of the sources from which laboratory zebrafish originate. The source must be one where the fish have been purpose-bred for use in scientific research. If zebrafish are to be taken from the wild or another non-purpose-bred source, it needs to be stated, authorised and justified in a project licence. Therefore, zebrafish cannot be sourced from anywhere other than designated establishments of breeding and supply or other reputable sources from outside of the UK.

There are no commercial sources of laboratory zebrafish as there are with research mice. There are, however, two academic resource centres established. The first, Zebrafish International Resource Centre (ZIRC)[1] was established in Oregon over 20 years ago, now funded by the National Institutes of Health (NIH). The second is the European Zebrafish Resource Centre (EZRC)[2], based in the Karlsruhe Institute of Technology in Germany, established in 2012, and initially funded by the Klaus Tschira Foundation and EU ZF-HEALTH project. Other sources include the Chinese Zebrafish Resource Centre (CZRC)[3], Sinnhuber Aquatic Research Laboratory (SARL)[4], collaborators or some of the bigger institutions, but many genetically modified fish are created in house.

Whatever the source, it is common for fish to be classified as intellectual property, usually requiring material transfer agreements (MTAs) between the collaborating institutions to be executed prior to exchange.

Transport

Before any transportation of zebrafish can take place, all the proper legislative permissions must be in place (see Chapter 8: Legislation and oversight of the conduct of research using animals: a global overview; and Chapter 12: Transportation of laboratory animals). In the UK, if obtaining zebrafish from outside the country, then authorisation to import is required from the Fish Health Inspectorate[5]. Other regions and countries will have differing legislation.

Transportation of adult zebrafish is similar to that of many other small fish. They need to be shipped in plastic bags, and taped at the edges to stop fish becoming trapped in them. The bags are typically filled with one-third of water and two-thirds of either air or oxygen enriched air (depending on the numbers of fish held within the bags and their age and size) as covered in International Air Transport Association (IATA) regulations (IATA 2021), and are often placed inside another similarly sized bag to reduce the risk of water loss due to breakage. These bags are then placed into a polystyrene box with a cardboard wrapper for transport.

The rules that surround the transport of embryonic forms are less clear – embryos and recently hatched forms would not benefit from transport in polythene bags due to their size and general fragility. These life stages are normally transported in rigid containers such as conical tubes and culture vessels, but, as a general principle, should be transported in such containers and under conditions with particular regard to space, temperature and oxygen levels.

Other transportation considerations will be the same as those that exist for all other fish species and other vertebrates, and include such things as transporting as quickly as possible and causing the animals as little stress as possible (OATA 2020)[6]. These factors are also covered in Chapter 48: Fishes.

Uses in research

Zebrafish have become a very popular vertebrate model over a wide range of biological scientific disciplines, more than any other fish species.

The first uses of zebrafish and embryos were as models for fisheries and toxicological research (Laale 1977), but it has flourished as a model in the last 40 years after George Streisinger pioneered their use to study features and organisation of vertebrate development in 1972 at the University of Oregon (Grunwald and Eisen 2002).

Christiane Nüsslein-Volhard, who had been working on large-scale genetic screening of *Drosophila*, realised the potential of zebrafish as a system that might allow substantial genetic screening in a vertebrate model and was responsible for the creation of the large-scale screen in Tubingen (Nusslein-Volhard 2012). The Nüsslein-Volhard and Wieschaus screening strategy was to focus on mutations with clearly defined phenotypes that allowed identification of genes that have a unique role in a specific developmental process (Ingham 1997) including embryogenesis, behaviour, physiology, health and disease. Simultaneously, another large-scale screen was set up by Marc Fishman and Wolfgang Driever in the USA and between the two screens approximately 4,000 embryonic lethal mutant phenotypes were discovered (Grunwald and Eisen 2002).

From this point, the model expanded into many other scientific disciplines and gained further momentum, enabled by two technological breakthroughs – the completion of its genome sequencing in 2002 at the Sanger Centre (Howe et al. 2013) and the development and application of genome-editing technologies (Gaj, Gersbach, and Barbas 2013), now dominated by CRISPR-cas9 (see also Chapter 4: An introduction to laboratory animal genetics).

Although zebrafish have many physiological differences from humans, they do share many similarities including homologous organ and tissue function, as well as orthologs with many highly conserved functional regions. These traits have led to them becoming prominent models for disease and drug discovery. Because of their small size, transparency that facilitates the visualising of phenotypes and ease of array in 96 well plates, embryos are becoming widely used in small-molecule screens (MacRae and Peterson 2015). These screens can be roughly divided into four types – morphological, therapeutic, pathway and behavioural. Morphological screens use compounds to create anatomical differences and patterning deviations from normal development (Teixido et al. 2019). Therapeutic screens identify small molecules that can ameliorate disease phenotypes, examples of which include enhancers of cardiovascular development, function and regeneration (Tu and Chi 2012; X.-X.I. Zeng 2018). Pathway screens look at the ability of a compound to interact with a specific cellular pathway, while behavioural screens have a wide variety of

---

[1] https://zebrafish.org/home/guide.php (Accessed June 14, 2022)
[2] https://www.ezrc.kit.edu/ (Accessed June 14, 2022)
[3] http://en.zfish.cn/ (Accessed June 14, 2022)
[4] https://ehsc.oregonstate.edu/SARLfeature (Accessed June 14, 2022)
[5] https://www.gov.uk/guidance/import-or-export-live-fish-and-shellfish (Accessed June 16, 2022)

[6] https://ornamentalfish.org/wp-content/uploads/Transport-code-final.pdf (Accessed June 16, 2022)

purposes, such as social preference testing (Ogi et al. 2021) and neuropsychiatric drug targets (Williams and Hong 2016).

In addition to the work that is carried out on embryonic and larval forms, research is also carried out on adult fish. Zebrafish have tissue regenerative abilities that have made them a model of interest to study tissue regeneration in general, including fins and hearts (Gemberling et al. 2013) and more specifically, spinal and heart injury; for example, cryoinjury, which is a surgically induced lesion, is used to damage the heart of adult fish (Chablais and Jazwinska 2012). Control of regeneration appears to be organ specific and not all tissues can regenerate (Marques, Lupi, and Mercader 2019). Development of similar cancer phenotypes in humans and zebrafish has led to genetically modified fish used for tumour modelling and visualisation (Hason and Bartunek 2019), as well as the creation of zebrafish models for personalised medicine (Baxendale, van Eeden, and Wilkinson 2017). Zebrafish may also be used for ageing studies as they can mimic ageing in humans; for example, they show spinal curvature as an age-related phenotype generated by muscle abnormalities (Gerhard et al. 2002).

General husbandry

Zebrafish welfare

Interest in zebrafish welfare has grown substantially since the 1970s. However, because they are naturally robust and can thrive across an extensive range of environments (Spence et al. 2008; Suriyampola et al. 2016), specific guidelines for their well-being are difficult to find and very broad in their nature when they are available (Alestrom et al. 2020). It is generally accepted that there is still much to understand about true zebrafish husbandry and welfare and many of their basic requirements are still not known (Strahle et al. 2012; Lidster et al. 2017; Graham et al. 2018).

The perception of zebrafish as a very inexpensive and easy model to keep and preconceived ideas surrounding sentience have hindered the development and realisation of many of their optimal welfare and husbandry requirements. This has resulted in the establishment of a wide range of different husbandry and welfare practices across institutions worldwide. A survey conducted in 2017 (Lidster et al. 2017) showed disparity in many husbandry practices including, but not limited to: stocking density, diet, feeding frequency, as well as diversity in environmental enrichment. Husbandry technology has become slightly more uniform in some areas when welfare needs have become clearer, but still in many areas husbandry practice remains very diverse.

An example of this is evident in feeding and nutritional practices. Over the last few years, considerably more information has become available on this subject. There are a number of studies that evaluate fish performance on different diets (Siccardi et al. 2009; Watts et al. 2016). These and other studies examine how nutritional components of diets – proteins, carbohydrates, fats and vitamins, minerals and other micronutrients, as well as the volume and times of feeding a day – influence fish growth, survival, body condition and reproductive capacity. Despite considerable published information addressing the dietary needs of zebrafish and advice on ways of feeding, different practices prevail through all life stages, and these are not well-standardised. This may reflect differences in resources, such as the size of facility, technical help and expertise available, legislative needs, as well as different beliefs and reliance upon anecdotal evidence. But it is clear that zebrafish are affected by these differences in husbandry practices, and in the case of feeding, this can be witnessed by different growth rates published (Siccardi et al. 2009; Lawrence et al. 2012; Fowler et al. 2019; Fowler et al. 2021).

That said, there are a few practices that are generally adhered to; for example, it is generally agreed that zebrafish should be kept in a water temperature of around 28.5°C (Westerfield 2007), varying by +/− 0.5°C for larval forms under 120 hpf, which also is the standard for development tables (Kimmel et al. 1995). The deviation around 28.5°C for older life stages is wider, 24–29°C, as suggested by FELASA guidelines (Alestrom et al. 2020), although in the wild, it is known they survive at much wider temperature conditions – from 6°C to over 38°C (Spence et al. 2008).

Physical environment

Most zebrafish facilities use some kind of recirculating aquatic system (RAS), comprising of three parts – racking, tanks and water filtration. These are usually compatible with scientific requirements and do not have the large water requirements of a flow through system. These systems can be fairly simple: an individual rack with a few tanks on it or very complex, with many racks supporting complex arrangements of small polycarbonate tanks linked together with a shared filtration plant (Figure 49.3a and b).

The racking provides support for the tanks and is usually a stainless-steel structure divided in shelves. It also incorporates the pipework to feed water to the tanks and gravity drains dirty water to the water filtration plant.

Polycarbonate tanks come in a variety of volumes usually between 0.75 and 10 L, all used for different purposes, from isolation and growing larval stages to the larger tanks designed to hold large numbers of adult stock fish. These tanks are usually comprised of three or four parts – the tank itself, a lid, a baffle and a siphon, which slots into the back of the tank and controls water flow through the tank by pushing water coming into the tank towards the bottom of the tank and then exiting behind the baffle. This design facilitates good flow of water around the tank and moves solid wastes out into the filtration system (Figure 49.4).

The source of water is very important and will be dependent on where the institution is situated. Many institutions use reverse osmosis (RO) to treat incoming water, and then add back in desirable salts and minerals to replace those removed through the purification process.

Water filtration in zebrafish aquaria usually comprise of four main components – mechanical, biological and chemical filtration and water disinfection. Mechanical filtration removes solids. Nitrifying bacteria in biological filtration breaks down components of the nitrogen cycle: ammonia into nitrite and then further to nitrate. Chemical filtration, such as activated carbon removes colourants and odours and finally, water disinfection is achieved by ultraviolet light.

Hygiene practices and biosecurity measures will be determined, to some extent, by the size and resources of individual

(a) 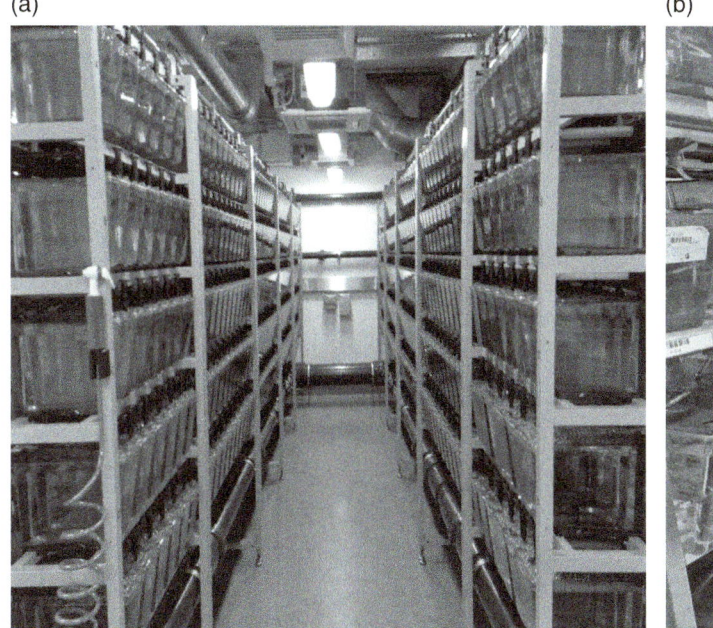 (b)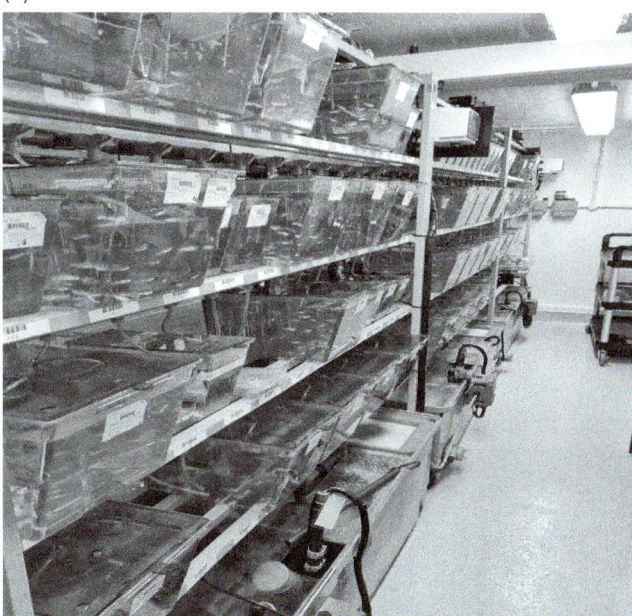

Figure 49.3a and b Common tank and racking arrangements for zebrafish. Different systems but still performing the same function. (a) Without under racking sump arrangement, water will flow back to water filtration plant (not shown). (b) With under racking sump arrangement, usually contains bio-filtration, whish water passes across back to water filtration plant (not shown). Picture: Paul Barwood

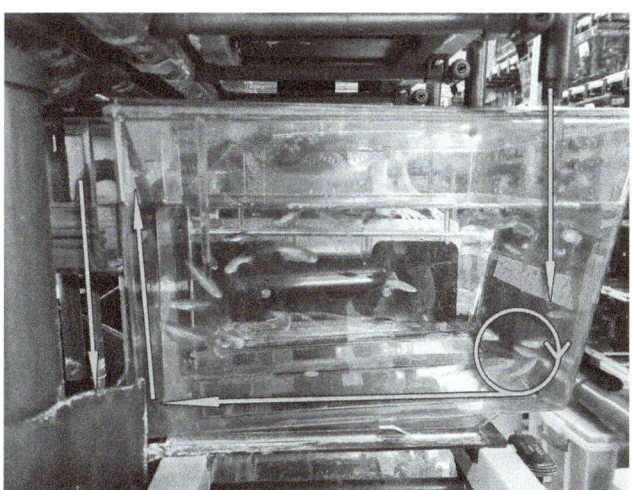

Figure 49.4 The arrowed line indicates flow of water through the tank, entering through the front of the tank and exiting through the back of the tank. Note: These tanks rely, to an extent, on the water flow rate to create good water circulation. Source: Karen Dunford

institutions. In larger facilities, it can be considered good practice to implement a flow of traffic – staff visit the cleanest rooms or areas first and quarantine rooms or other areas which contain fish with a lower or unknown health status last. At a minimum, quarantine areas need to be considered for adult and larval forms arriving from sources with either unknown health status or with a known pathogen status undesirable to the incoming facility. Although it is increasingly common to receive health screening information from the exporting institutions, it is wise to keep those animals separate from the main colony, given that there are not yet standards for reporting.

Equipment must be kept clean – an area for cleaning must be present so items such as tanks, nets (Garcia and Sanders 2011; Collymore, Porelli, et al. 2014) and other related paraphernalia can be washed and then undergo either disinfection or sterilisation. It is harder to clean the system itself; most have pipework is fairly inaccessible and, therefore, difficult to clean and consideration has to be given to biological filtration, as this cannot be subject to either disinfection or sterilisation.

Until recently, many zebrafish facilities were not seen to employ vigorous use of personal protective equipment (PPE), which is considered standard in rodent facilities. It was not unusual to see staff in everyday clothing in fish facilities, but this is becoming less common nowadays (author's personal observation). Several recommendations of PPE have been made: the use of lab coats, dedicated footwear, overshoes or footbaths and gloves (Borges *et al*. 2016; Canadian Council on Animal Care, 2020), which serve to protect staff from zoonotic diseases, such as *Mycobacterium marinum*.

It is now widely recognised that good hygiene can prevent and slow the spread of disease and that these practices should be linked to a robust health monitoring programme to inhibit the spread of pathogens. To this end, the last few years have seen the development of Specific Pathogen Free (SPF) programmes for zebrafish, which raise the standards of hygiene and actively seek to exclude specific diseases from programmes. These are not commonly applied, but are certainly far beyond the standards of hygiene often present in zebrafish programmes of 10 to 15 years ago (Kent *et al*. 2011; Barton *et al*. 2016).

For further information on physical environment for laboratory zebrafish, Lawrence and Mason give a broad overview of water production and treatment, as well as tanks and racking (Lawrence and Mason 2012). *The Laboratory Zebrafish* (Harper and Lawrence 2011) covers all aspects of aquatic systems extensively, while recent innovations are discussed in *Laboratory Fish in Biomedical Research* (Newell & Brocca 2021).

Environmental parameters

Water quality is a suite of environmental parameters which require consideration. The primary factors should be temperature, pH, conductivity, dissolved oxygen and compounds of the nitrogen cycle. Compounds such as chlorines and other chemicals found in source water are detrimental to the health of zebrafish (Alestrom *et al.* 2020) and should be avoided; other contaminants, such as copper, can be found in fittings as well as source water (Harper and Lawrence 2011) and also require removal. There are other compounds found in water that are less well-understood but may have more subtle effects on research and should be considered, as they can affect both health and behaviour, as well as experimental outcomes. These include compounds such as calcium (Metz *et al.* 2014), pheromones (Diaz-Verdugo *et al.* 2019), cortisol (Pavlidis *et al.* 2013), levels of detritus and build-up of potentially pathogenic biofilms (Chang, Lewis, and Whipps 2019).

Often 14 light:10 dark photoperiods are maintained in zebrafish facilities, with the option of a dawn and dusk period (Alestrom *et al.* 2020), which is normal in a mammalian unit (author observation), but unlike some other fish species, zebrafish show no preference for shade (Jones *et al.* 2019). An all light or all dark environment has a detrimental effect on larval fish development (Villamizar *et al.* 2014) and attention should also be paid to other light sources; for example, fire signs within the fish rooms, as these can also affect breeding patterns if not regulated carefully (Adatto, Krug, and Zon 2016).

Room temperature should be considered. Water temperature is usually kept around 28.5 °C for reproduction and development (Kimmel *et al.* 1995), with a broader range for fish maintenance. In the UK, this is usually achieved by heating the water in the aquatic system itself – however, this might be supplemented by heating the room but with care regarding an acceptable room temperature for staff.

Environmental parameters are summarised in Table 49.2 and further general guidance, including environmental parameters, can be found in CCAC guidelines: Zebrafish and other small, warm-water laboratory fish ('CCAC guidelines: Zebrafish and other small, warm water laboraoty fish' 2020), as well as FELASA guidelines (Alestrom *et al.* 2020).

Table 49.2 Summary of suggestions for the basic environmental parameters desirable for zebrafish.

Environmental parameters for zebrafish			
	Parameter	*Notes*	*References*
Temperature	28.5 °C – for development 24–29°C	Have temperature tolerances 6.7–41.7°C	(Lawrence 2007) (Varga 2011)
pH	7–8	Can tolerate 6–8.5	(Lawrence 2007) (Varga 2011) (Castranova *et al.* 2011)
Conductivity	Usual range 500–700 µS	Can be highly variable 150–1700 µS	(Varga 2011)
Dissolved oxygen	7.8 mg/L	Similar to oxygen saturation	(Lawrence 2007)
Hardness	75–200 mg/L	Should be at least 75 mg/L	(Lawrence 2007) (Varga 2011)
Ammonia	0	Should not rise above <0.1 mg/L	(Lawrence 2007) (Varga 2011) (Castranova *et al.* 2011)
Nitrite	0	Should not rise above <1 mg/L	(Lawrence 2007) (Varga 2011) (Castranova *et al.* 2011)
Nitrates	<25 mg/L	Can tolerate 1000 mg/L – but this is undesirable, can be removed by water changes	(Lawrence 2007)
Photoperiod Light:Dark	14:10	Is sometimes set at 12:12	(Lawrence 2007) (Westerfield 2007)
Lux	54–354 lux at water surface	Not yet well-defined	(Lawrence 2007)
Stocking density	5–10/L juvenile/adults <50/L fry	Five fish per litre	(Castranova *et al.* 2011) (Lawrence 2011) (Pavlidis *et al.* 2013) (Varga 2011)

Environmental enrichment

Briefly, environmental enrichment improves the quality of life of the animals and allows species-specific behaviours (see Chapter 10 – Enrichment: animal welfare and scientific validity). This is a more controversial subject than for most mammalian species as these already have a substantial body of evidence demonstrating the benefits of environmental enrichment. In zebrafish facilities, barren tanks are currently the most usual set up, due in part to the numbers of tanks. In terms of structural enrichment, there is evidence to both support and not support its use – placing plastic plants in a tank can improve breeding (Wafer et al. 2016) and lower aggression (Carfagnini et al. 2009), but other studies have shown this to increase aggression (Woodward et al. 2019). The use of plastic plants/objects in tanks may also affect scientific outcomes – plastics leaching into the water can alter gene regulation and change immune responses (Limonta et al. 2019), but also encourage brain cell proliferation and can be seen as a positive for zebrafish welfare (von Krogh et al. 2010). Using submerged plants, a ruin-like plastic object and gravel in the bottom for 21–28 days (Marcon et al. 2018) showed zebrafish with reduced vulnerability to stress and its biochemical impact compared with a standard environment. Also, learning rate is enhanced in larval fish grown in an enriched environment than those grown in a bare tank (Spence and Smith 2008). Validated environmental enrichment should be the default option for zebrafish, and if it is not used, researchers should show it is detrimental to their work. There is a movement towards the use of images of gravel placed underneath tanks as a form of non-invasive enrichment, which has a positive welfare benefit while not having any of the negatives associated with structural enrichment in the tank (Schroeder et al. 2014). Another study showed preference of zebrafish for structured environments (clay pot and plants), but behavioural diversity was the same in the empty compartment of the tank (Kistler et al. 2011).

All fish show preference for structural enrichment, including plastic plants and gravel images in the bottom of tanks over bare tanks, but this varies according to social grouping. Group-housed fish show less dominant and aggressive behaviour overall and will use plastic plants and gravel substrates as enrichment. When housed as a pair, dominant fish tend to choose an enriched environment, while subordinate fish will spend time in unenriched, bare sides of tanks (Schroeder et al. 2014). Care must be taken to create compatible groups – mismatched sized fish can create heightened aggression and fish raised in structurally rich environments can also grow at different rates and that variance in size can also elevate aggression (Spence, Magurran, and Smith 2011). The practice of singularly housing zebrafish is discouraged by the Home Office, but there is evidence that if kept in single tanks by themselves, they may benefit from being allowed to see other fish around them (Schroeder et al. 2014) and potentially from some forms of structural enrichment (Collymore, Tolwani, and Rasmussen 2015).

Other forms of enrichment can be considered, such as occupational enrichment – providing water flow within the tank to provide an opportunity for exercise (DePasqual et al. 2019). Nutritional enrichment is commonly used by giving the zebrafish live food. In larval forms, the use of live food, including *Paramecium*, elicits a hunting response (Lau et al. 2019). It is also common for facilities to use the addition of live food, including *Artemia* as both a food stuff and as enrichment as it stimulates prey-capture behaviour (Alestrom et al. 2020).

Health monitoring

Health monitoring in zebrafish facilities should be considered in terms of supporting both rigorous husbandry and hygiene regimens (Martins, Monteiro, et al. 2016), and in so doing reducing and limiting the effect of both non-pathogenic and pathogenic disease on animal welfare and scientific reproducibility of results. This should begin tankside with daily observation of the fish, which is a legal requirement both under UK and European legislation, and can often be done while feeding. It is important to develop a system that allows for a more standardised way of checking and monitoring fish; however, there is currently no universally approved approach for this. The phenotype of a fish is starting point for this and any animals showing signs that are inconsistent with the normal or expected phenotype should be considered either for closer monitoring, removal from the system or potential treatment. For example, fish should be considered for removal if they are anorexic, showing abnormal swimming, curvature of the spine or changes in body colour; these conditions are linked both to disease but also old age, so should be closely monitored if connected to an ageing project. There are different ways to do this, including the development of traffic light systems and body condition scoring indices (Wilson 2013; Clark et al. 2018) these help determine the seriousness of the phenotype, many of which require instant removal from the system and are indicators of potential pathogens (Sanders et al. 2020).

The second stage of health monitoring is to create a programme that examines the pathogenic circumstance of the facility; this ordinarily would include a sentinel screen and perhaps some or all of the following – polymer chain reaction (PCR), culture or histological (where appropriate), examination of detritus and biofilms from tanks and sumps, water and sick fish removed from the system.

How a sentinel screening is approached will depend on individual circumstances. Often fish can be set up in a sentinel tank that is supplied with water drawn from the sump waste. Sometimes sentinels can be either side of the water treatment/filtration plant of the system (pre- and post-filtration) but it can be argued that sentinels directly after water treatment are monitoring the effectiveness of filtration rather than identifying pathogens. How often, how many and how old sentinels are when they are used for assessment will depend on the size of the facility, how it is being used, the degree of statistical confidence required (Marancik et al. 2020) and often financial constraints (Collymore, Crim, and Lieggi 2016). For example, if previous screening shows a facility to be clear of a certain disease, the screening interval between testing for that pathogen could be increased. Similarly, if imported fish come in with no indication of health status and are being held in a quarantine area, then an increase in health screening may be warranted. In the case of small numbers of fish, for example those being held in a quarantine area, it may not be feasible to hold dedicated sentinel fish. Rather, it might be more appropriate to use sick or older fish from the colony and employ other ways of health monitoring, including embryos, detritus and biofilms (Mocho et al. 2017). Table 49.3 lists some of the most commonly screened for pathogens in zebrafish, as well as some non-pathogenic disease.

Feeding

The nutritional needs of zebrafish are still largely unknown (Lawrence 2007; Ulloa et al. 2011; Watts et al. 2012). This has led to very varied feeding practices across institutions, with no standardised practice.

There is general agreement about the importance of dietary proteins for the promotion of growth and reproduction – although different sources of protein can influence body mass in terms of both lean and fat composition (Smith et al. 2013).

Lipids are also essential to fulfil both energy requirements. Essential fatty acids (EFAs) are required for normal development and to absorb fat soluble vitamins. Polyunsaturated fatty

Table 49.3 Summary of some of the most common pathogenic and non-pathogenic disease affecting zebrafish and the tank-side clinical signs that may accompany them.

Pathogens affecting zebrafish			
Pathogen	Clinical signs	Observations	References
Mycobacterium chelonae	May present as subclinical Low-level chronic disease Dermal lesions and ulceration	Opportunist species Fairly ubiquitous Found in many facilities Found in biofilms TU line may be more susceptible than other lines Can be present and transmitted through live food	(Whipps et al. 2012) (Chang et al. 2019) (Whipps et al. 2008)
Mycobacterium haemophilum	High levels of chronic disease and mortality Overt emaciation Overt lethargy Chronic and diffuse inflammation Raised scales/dropsy Ulcers/haemorrhage	Suboptimal environmental conditions exacerbate infection Found in biofilms	(Whipps et al. 2012) (Whipps et al. 2007) (Racz et al. 2019)
Mycobacterium marinum	High levels of chronic disease and high mortality Raised scales/swollen abdomen Reddened gills Overt emaciation Overt lethargy, reduced swimming Chronic and diffuse inflammation Ulcers	Zoonotic affecting fish and staff. Suboptimal environmental conditions exacerbate infection Found in biofilms	(Mason et al. 2016) (Whipps et al. 2012) (Astrofsky et al. 2000) (Swaim et al. 2006)
Other mycobacterium species M. peregrinum M. abscessus M. fortuitum	Low level of chronic disease Clinical signs – as above	Also found in biofilms May cause disease when challenged experimentally	(Whipps et al. 2012) (Astrofsky et al. 2000)
Pseudoloma neurophilia microsporidium	Often subclinical Probable increased mortality and lower fecundity Causes emaciation and skeletal deformities.	Prevalent in conventional zebrafish facilities Both horizontally and vertically transmission Difficult to detect in analysis of detritus, biofilms and water. Males more heavily parasitised than females	(Kent, Harper, and Wolf 2012) (Spagnoli et al. 2015) (Sanders et al. 2013) (Kent et al. 2018)
Pseudocapillaria tomentosa Nematode	Subclinical through to high mortality Expressed outwardly as emaciation	Eggs can be seen in detritus Males more heavily parasitised than females Intestinal parasite	(Kent et al. 2002) (Kent et al. 2018) (Kent et al. 2012)

Table 49.3 (Continued)

Pathogen	Clinical signs	Observations	References
Pathogens affecting zebrafish			
Edwardsiella ictaluri Bacteria	High and acute mortality Haemorrhage in skin, opercula, and base of fins and abdomen Behavioural change	Originally thought to be specific to catfish species	(Hawke et al. 2013) (Kent et al. 2020)
Flavobacterium columnare Bacteria	Clinical or subclinical infection Severe gill disease Tail/Fin rot Necrosis of tissues		Health Monitoring for your zebrafish colonies[7] (von Gersdorff Jorgensen 2016)
Ichthyophthirius multifiliis Protozoan parasite (Also known as Ich or White Spot)	Affects skin and gills Increased mucus and laboured breathing To a lesser extent infects nasal and buccal cavities		(von Gersdorff Jorgensen 2016)
ISKNV (infectious spleen and kidney necrosis virus)	Lethargy Loss of appetite Abnormal swimming Swollen abdomen	Can cross species barrier – so need for high biosecurity	(Bermudez et al. 2018)
Non-pathogenic disease – water quality			
Poor water quality Metal toxicities Ammonia and nitrate toxicity	Gill lesions Laboured breathing Decreased growth Mortality	Can occur in new systems or overcrowded systems	(Kent et al. 2020) (Pullium et al. 1999)
Gas bubble disease (gas super saturation)	Gas bubbles appear in skin and/or gills	Caused by gas super saturation conditions in water, then gas being released from solution and super saturate fish's bodily fluids with gas resulting in bubbles in the tissues	(Kent et al. 2020) Water Quality Problems[8]

acids (PUFAs) must be provided in the diet as they cannot be synthesised by zebrafish, but they can convert them into highly unsaturated fatty acids (HUFAs), of which eicosapentaenoic (20:5n-3:EPA), docosahexaenoic (22:6n-3:DHA) and arachidonic acids (20:4n-6:AA) (Harper and Lawrence 2011) are an important requirement for normal growth, egg production and fertilisation success (Watts et al. 2012). It has been shown that different ratios of the fatty n3 and n6 acids have different effects on zebrafish, including body composition and spawning, with a ratio of 5:1 n6 to n3 being optimal for embryo viability (Fowler, Dennis-Cornelius, et al. 2020).

Although it has been stated zebrafish have no dietary requirement for carbohydrate (Harper and Lawrence 2011), at levels of under 5%, growth rates may be affected, along with body composition and condition (Fowler, Williams, et al. 2020) and its inclusion in the diet may improve resistance to hypoxia stress (Ma et al. 2020).

Vitamins are received through the diet – vitamin C is highly soluble and needs to be delivered in an insoluble form or from a live diet. Also water soluble, vitamin B complex is involved in growth and the absence of B7 (biotin) lowers survival rates, growth rates and weight gain (Fowler, Williams, et al. 2020). Vitamins A, D, E and K are fat soluble. Vitamin A is involved in vision and fin development. D has a role in hormonal control affecting bone growth and maintenance (Fowler, Williams, et al. 2020). Vitamin E has a role, protecting against oxidation stress (Fowler, Williams, et al. 2020) and also impacts the function of vitamin C, so deficiencies in E can lead to skeletal muscle degeneration and mobility issues (Lebold et al. 2013).

Minerals are also important for physiological function and these can be received either through diet or through the aquatic environment (Harper and Lawrence 2011). Calcium, phosphorus and magnesium are absorbed through the water and diet (Harper & Lawrence 2011; Fowler, Williams, et al. 2020) and are involved in bone, skin and scale formation. Other trace minerals are also taken up through diet, for example manganese, zinc and selenium (Fowler, Williams, et al. 2020), which are also required for biological function (Harper and Lawrence 2011).

Another feeding consideration is particle size – larval and juvenile fish require a particle size that reflects their smaller gape size. A 5 dpf larval fish has a mouth width of 180–200 μm and a 15 dpf larval fish has a mouth width of 290–320 μm (Onal and Langdon 2016). This must be reflected in the particle size of food offered. Both live foods, *Paramecium* and rotifer (salt water *Brachionus plicatilis* or fresh water *Brachionus calyciflorus*), are small, ranging 150–260 μm making them suitable

---

[7] https://www.idexxbioresearch.com/hubfs/Zebrafish_Booklet.pdf (Accessed 16 June 2022)
[8] https://zebrafish.org/wiki/health/disease_manual/water_quality_problems (Accessed 16 June 2022)

for first feeds, but *Artemia*, at first hatch, are approximately 475–500 μm and are best suited to older larval stages and juvenile to adult fish. Commercial diets of different particle size are also fed to all life stages, but one study showed that at first feed larval fish preferred 21–45 μm capsules and 15 dpf larvae preferred capsules in the 47–75 μm size range – smaller than the maximum they can ingest (Onal and Langdon 2016).

Historically, commercial diets for ornamental fish (Creaser 1934) have formed the diet of laboratory zebrafish. More recently, diets formulated for aqua-cultural fish species (Fowler et al. 2019) have also become more readily available. These diets usually have a high protein content of around 60%, promoting rapid growth for both juvenile and larval forms; this is often seen as a requirement for fish involved in intensive breeding programmes, which, although often aspired to, may not be the best for fecundity and fertility (Monteiro et al. 2018). The particle sizes are available in preference sizes for both larval and adult fish. Most of these diets also contain a lipid content of around 15%, another source of energy, as well as EFAs. Some of these diets are microencapsulated, enhancing the feed ability to retain water soluble nutrients (Harper and Lawrence 2011). Commercially, available foods are not currently available for different stages of growth, so these diets are the same for all life stages, but presented in different particle sizes.

It is common for adult fish to be fed two to three times a day, sometimes more if they are being fed by automatic feeders, although it has also been suggested that adult fish will function well-being fed 5% of body weight once a day (Lawrence et al. 2012). The amount of food fed varies from facility to facility – some feeding as a percentage of body weight, some feeding to a perceived satiation point.

Care of larval and juvenile fish

Unlike mammals and some fish species, zebrafish offer no parental care, so in a laboratory environment this must be provided by technical/research staff. Fertilisation takes place outside of the body and the embryos must be removed from adult fish to avoid cannibalism. For the first seven days of life, an embryo feeds endogenously on the yolk sac, its sole source of nutrition for the first four days of life; a larval fish is not sufficiently well-developed to begin exogenous feeding until the gut tube is formed, the mouth and anus are both open and the gas bladder has been inflated (see the biological data section for more information on larval development). It is normal during this period to keep the embryos in water in Petri dishes or some other small container so that the water can be easily changed/refreshed, and development can be monitored. The water can either be system water – drawn off of the main aquaria – filtered system water, reconstituted fish water or an embryo medium. The number of embryos kept in a dish is variable, from 50 to 250 (see social organisation for more information). After 3–4 dpf (largely temperature dependent), swim bladder inflation should have occurred (Wilson 2012) and the embryo should be well-developed enough to begin exogenous feeding (Kaushik, Georga, and Koumoundouros 2011); the normal procedure is to provide food after 5 dpf (Table 49.1).

The majority of facilities feed a combination of both live and dry diets at this stage. Live diets encourage hunting behaviour and are linked to higher survival rates and brain circuitry development (Avitan et al. 2020). Although zebrafish can be raised on either a live or formulated diet, evidence suggests that larval fish have lower survival and growth rates when exclusively fed on a formulated diet (Goolish, Okutake, and Lesure 1999). For more information related to type of feeding of young zebrafish stages, please see the Feeding section of this chapter.

It is important that there is enough food within the water that pre-metamorphic fish find food easily and do not have to expend excessive energy trying to find food. This can create a water quality problem: in static or very slow dripping water, larval fish do not foul the water as adults would, but feeding can. Even though it is known that early stage larval fish can tolerate higher levels of ammonia (Best et al. 2010), efforts should be made to ensure that water volume, flow and quality are balanced. The challenge is to maintain a readily accessible food source without compromising the water quality. Siphoning waste from tanks is one way to deal with this (Norton et al. 2019).

Perhaps one of the most important aspects of larval rearing is to make gradual changes to each stage of management – this is critical as large changes in any aspect of husbandry acts as a stressor for the younger stages of growth and can lower survival rates (Wilson 2012). For example, it is important to change diets slowly, adding in new, larger particle diets, while gradually phasing out smaller particle sizes and increasing the amounts of feed presented; similarly, flow rates should also be gradually increased, each change being dependent on the size of the fish and stage of their development.

Breeding All colony management and successful breeding strategies are dependent on two primary elements: breeding behaviour of the fish and the purpose of breeding itself. There are reports that optimal breeding of zebrafish should be done once every ten days (Nasiadka and Clark 2012); however, good results can be achieved by setting up fish twice a week (unpublished research, UCL). Spawning the fish too often can decrease the quality and quantity of eggs produced but infrequent spawning will cause the eggs to be reabsorbed or plugs of necrotic cells may form and block the oviduct, causing a condition colloquially known as being 'egg bound' (Nasiadka and Clark 2012). The health status of the fish will always influence spawning and reproductive success, so mating unhealthy fish is unlikely to have a good outcome.

In addition to unhealthy fish, over- and under-spawning problems exist around decreased fertility and viability associated with inbreeding depression, and the need to maintain some level of hybrid vigour (Monson and Sadler 2010). It is important to maintain heterozygosity within wild-type lines to keep producing large clutches of eggs. Wild-type lines of zebrafish are not isogenic and should not have lost heterozygosity as defines an inbred strain (such as a mouse strain) but may come from an institutionally closed colony, which may affect scientific reproducibility (Crim and Lawrence 2021) and lead to institutional variation between lines of wild-type fish. Although it is important to maintain genetic variability, wild-type lines lack the genetic variation of wild zebrafish (Coe et al. 2009).

Breeding protocols are varied across facilities and are dependent on the type of work taking place. The most common types of crosses are pair and group crossing (Nasiadka and Clark 2012). Group crossings are used primarily to maintain genetic diversity – as more than two individuals will have contributed to the offspring, and for this reason they are often used for line propagation (Nasiadka and Clark 2012). There are several other ways to achieve this: combining embryos from spawning of smaller groups, round robin breeding scheme[9] and the creation of hybrid lines (Nasiadka & Clark 2012), as well as constant refreshment of wild-type lines from external sources. Pair crosses often have other applications: identification of carriers of recessive mutations (Nasiadka & Clark 2012) or fish carrying targeted transgenes (Tsang *et al.* 2017), for example.

Sex ratios are also important. One study found female-biased ratios increased egg production compared to an equal sex bias (Rahmann *et al.* 2021); however, many facilities use sex ratios of either two females to three males or one female to two males. This may be suboptimal due to male aggression, so a reversal of these ratios may be more desirable (Tsang *et al.* 2017). Another study also reported heightened male aggression in sex ratios in which males outnumbered females, resulting in a reduction of eggs produced (Ruhl *et al.* 2009).

The equipment used for breeding can be very diverse and include large and small tanks holding the fish in static water (Castranova and Wang 2020) and mass spawning systems (Adatto *et al.* 2011) which hold 38–380 L of water and can be used for the rapid collection of thousands of eggs staged at the same point in development (Castranova and Wang 2020).

Very small tanks (0.8–1 L) should be avoided (Tsang *et al.* 2017); however, they are frequently used for a variety of purposes – for genotyping and pair spawning, for example. Care should be taken when employing this breeding strategy as water quality can quickly deteriorate, especially if set up overnight (author, unpublished work). Small tanks with static water in volume under 200 mL can decrease egg production (Tsang *et al.* 2017).

Fish can also be bred in their home tanks on an aquatic system – often as a solid bottom container with a mesh screen top – which can be placed towards the water column allowing fish to spawn in shallow water (Castranova and Wang 2020). Whatever method and tank are employed for breeding, the eggs must be physically separated from the adult fish otherwise they will be eaten.

Other extrinsic factors will also influence successful breeding, including, but not limited to, water quality and enrichment – fish have been shown to prefer gravel to no substrate (Schroeder et al. 2014; Spence, Ashton, and Smith 2007), which also suggests that marbles and other similar substrates in tanks may increase number of eggs laid. Breeding is also heavily influenced by light levels, light cycle and light spectrum. All of these may affect spawning, hatching of eggs, larval development, growth and behaviour (Villamizar *et al.* 2014; Tsang *et al.* 2017). A gradual 30-minute light change mimicking dawn and dusk, with a light cycle of 14 hours light:10 hours dark is usually recommended (Tsang *et al.* 2017). Intrinsic aspects of laboratory zebrafish relevant to breeding are also discussed under biological data, and reproduction within this chapter.

Sexing Sex differentiation occurs between 20 and 25 dpf; from 8 dpf, gonad development begins, but at this time all fry develop as female. At approximately 20–25 dpf, a transition begins – when ovary development stops in male fish and testis development begins (Kossack and Draper 2019).

As adult and sexually mature fish, males are usually more streamlined and bullet shaped than females, which are usually rounder in the body[10] sometimes exhibiting a more swollen belly and are slightly larger and heavier (Georga and Koumoundouros 2010). In some lines, it can be possible to tell the sexes apart by colouration; males appear more yellow while females can appear more silver and duller in colour, but this may also be influenced by dietary carotenoids. Courtship behaviour can also give clues to the sex of a fish – males can be observed chasing females (Paull *et al.* 2008). Usually, the clearest way of identification is that females also have a prominent papilla (sometimes referred to as an 'egg flap') which covers the urogenital opening (see Figure 49.5a). This is not present in males, who display prominent breeding tubercle clusters in the pectoral fins (McMillan *et al.* 2015) (see Figure 49.5b).

Individual identification

It is not uncommon to keep zebrafish in their hundreds, if not thousands, so they are normally not identified as individuals. Identification is harder to achieve than in most mammalian species for several reasons. Colonies can be separated into small numbers of fish in tanks, but these numbers are still usually far higher than the numbers of mice kept in a cage. They are also capable of regenerating most tissues, so marking them in an equivalent way to ear notching in mice, for example fin clipping, is not an option. Other ways of identification have been suggested, such as natural pigment patterns (Delcourt *et al.* 2018), which are likely to have limited use if all the fish housed together are of the same line and with very similar pigmentation (author's own observation).

Tags can also be used for individual identification – passive integrated transponders (PIT tags) (Delcourt *et al.* 2018). This means of identification is not without disadvantage; zebrafish are very small and to insert a PIT tag so it does not interfere with the fish's ability to swim or disrupt internal organs is a very skilled job, as well as being perceived as expensive, and so is very uncommon. Another potential identification method is injected dyes for short-term tagging and identification (Cheung, Chatterjee, and Gerlai 2014), which would work for small groups of fish. Visible implant elastomer (VIE) can have good results and be relatively long lasting for identifying individual fish (Hohn and Petrie-Hanson 2013), but others report the colours of the elastomer influence social preferences (Frommen *et al.* 2015), and could be problematic in that way. A novel refined protocol to implement VIE has recently been published with positive results (Racz *et al.* 2021). From personal experience, the success of this type of tagging will be dependent on the skill and experience of the person performing the procedure.

---

[9] Round robin breeding explained at https://zfin.org/ZDB-GENO-960809-7 (Accessed 16 June 2022)

[10] https://sciencing.com/tell-male-female-zebrafish-apart-5954254.html (Accessed June 21, 2022)

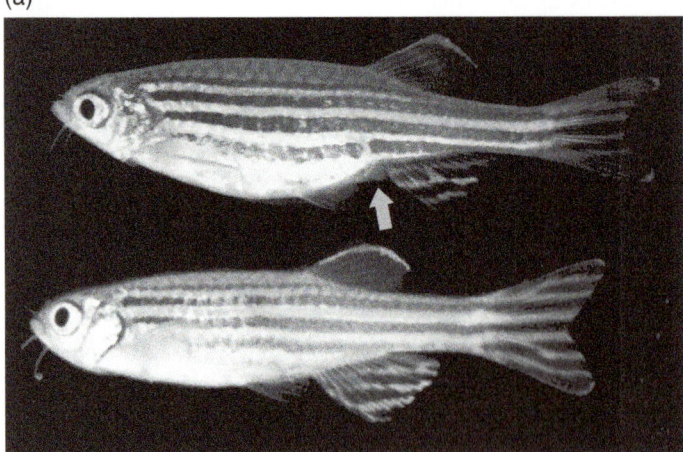
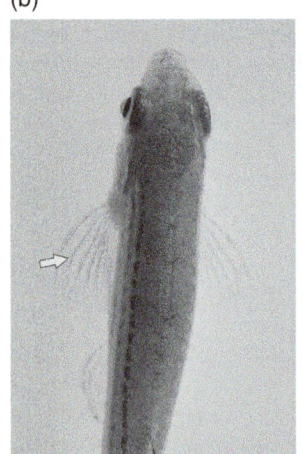
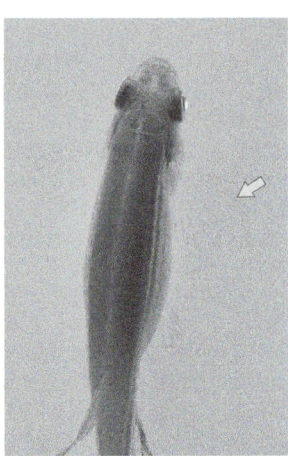

Figure 49.5a and b (a) The female above arrow shows the prominent papilla and slightly rounder in the body, male below, slightly more bullet shaped. (b) The male on the left-hand side shows the prominent breeding tubercle clusters, the arrow pointing to one of them, not present in the female on the right-hand side, as shown by the arrow showing the absence.

Laboratory procedures

Handling

The majority of adult handling is by netting. As good general practice, no fish should be chased around a tank with a net, and exposure to the air should occur for the shortest possible amount of time. Poor netting technique can be very stressful for fish and excessive exposure to air during this procedure results in elevated levels of stress, but the process of domestication and selection appears to mean laboratory zebrafish recover from it relatively well (Ramsay et al. 2009). Adult zebrafish should be anaesthetised if they are removed from water for anything other than brief netting and tank transfer. If they are manipulated for reasons such as cardiac injury, they must be anaesthetised and inverted on a sponge with a groove cut into it to hold them in place. Care should be taken when touching an adult zebrafish as, unlike mammalian species, they do not have a skin layer comprised of keratin; instead their scales are made from bone with a mucus layer above them, which can be damaged, leaving the fish susceptible to infection (Aman et al. 2018).

Training/habituation for procedures

This is not a generally used technique for adult fish. However, there are some examples of training fish to go to a certain area – for example, to avoid an electric shock (Xu et al. 2007) or to receive a reward (Pilehvar, Town, and Blust 2020), indicating that zebrafish can be trained. Also, before behavioural testing, adult zebrafish can be placed in the apparatus to habituate to the environment. The process of habituation in adult zebrafish is also described for the novel tank test when the animals spend more time in the top of the tank over time, as they learn that the top of the tank is also safe (Wong et al. 2010). Habituation is also widely used in behavioural tests on larvae, where an animal will stop responding to a repetitive stimulus – for example, rapid transition from daylight to complete darkness causes a larval fish to show a startle response by swimming very fast in a particular pattern, but repeated exposure to complete darkness will result in larval zebrafish decreasing that activity (Randlett et al. 2019). The stimuli can be visual, acoustic or touch related (Lopez-Schier 2019; Roberts et al. 2019).

Blood collection

Until fairly recently, most zebrafish blood collection was usually lethal. In the last few years, methods to take repeated blood samples have been developed and used for various reasons including diet induced obesity, glucose metabolism and haematological studies. This sampling is performed by inserting a heparinised capillary needle into the dorsal aorta, located posterior to the anus and ventral to the spine. The amount of blood that can be collected is related to body mass and that is estimated as a volume that is 2–3.8% of body weight. A single collection should not exceed 5 µl of blood and repeated collections should not exceed 2 µl per week or 2–5 µl every two weeks (Zang et al. 2015).

Administration of substances

In embryonic and larval forms, administration is typically carried out by substances added to the water, but this is typically ineffective in adult zebrafish. The use of oral gavage for adult zebrafish will produce more precise results – both in terms of amount and timing of substance administered (Dang et al. 2016). It is helpful to use fish of similar size to ensure the tubing required is of a similar size. No more than 5µl of substance should be administered, and the procedure should take no more than 45 seconds per fish. Improvements on original gavage techniques have been accomplished, including the use of more flexible tubing (Collymore, Rasmussen, and Tolwani 2013).

Injection

In a similar way to oral gavage, intraperitoneal injection has the advantage of giving a known dose of a substance to an adult fish (Kinkel *et al.* 2010). Other injection sites include intramuscular and intravenous and are covered in Chapter 48: Fishes.

Genotyping

There are several ways of collecting biological materials for the purpose of genotyping zebrafish. The least invasive method would be via visual inspection of an embryonic or larval phenotype – usually an examination of offspring from heterozygous parents which do not show a phenotype but which would be present in 25% homozygous offspring. This kind of screening is most usually used for testing zebrafish created from forward genetic screening and, as such, the gene would be unknown. This can be a time-consuming process and may not always be accurate.

Fin clipping is currently the most common way of genotyping in the UK and is covered in a pre-written Home Office protocol describing breeding[11]. The fish must be anesthetised before a small part of the adult caudal fin is removed for analysis. The percentage of the fin removed is likely to depend on the size of the fin but the least amount possible to achieve analysis: some suggestions are 0.25 cm of the fin (De Lombaert *et al.* 2017), 40% (Deakin *et al.* 2019) and half way between the end of the scales and the tip of the caudal fin[12]. Some protocols in the UK describe 10% as a further refinement (authors own observation).

As a potentially painful procedure (Deakin *et al.* 2019), there has been significant work undertaken to refine and present alternatives, including fin clipping of larval forms as young as 3 dpf, which involves removal of a small section of the tip of caudal fin, causing blastema formation at the site of the wound and normal fin regeneration follows (Wilkinson *et al.* 2013). This allows genotyping of fish before they become legally protected at 5 dpf in the UK, but requires more technical skill than fin clipping an adult. Another method is the Zebrafish Embryonic Genotyper (ZEG), which oscillates and shakes embryos, sloughing off enough cells to be collected for PCR (Lambert *et al.* 2018). This is less invasive, and also eliminates the need to grow embryos to adulthood for genotyping.

More recently, skin swabbing (Tilley *et al.* 2020), adapted from work done in other fish species, including blue green sunfish, Atlantic cod and stickleback (Breacker *et al.* 2017), has attracted attention as both an alternative and a refinement to fin clipping. Buccal swabbing, a procedure that was also developed in other fish species, has also been investigated (Lawton 2017).

Anaesthesia/analgesia

The most common way to administer either anaesthetics or analgesia is to add them to the water. When zebrafish are subjected to surgeries, it should be presumed that both anaesthesia and analgesia are provided. Likely, the most commonly used anaesthetic is tricaine methansulfonate (MS-222) (Readman *et al.* 2013). This compound is generally available in a powdered form that must be buffered (for freshwater fish) and dissolved in water. MS-222 can be used on all life stages of fish. It initially causes the fish to move rapidly and have increased ventilation before losing both the righting mechanism and body movement (Matthews and Varga 2012). The addition of MS-222 to water lowers pH and so the water needs to be buffered to 7 with either TRIS, sodium hydroxide or sodium bicarbonate to avoid this and prevent it from causing acidosis (Harper and Lawrence 2011). Other adverse side effects include increased stress responses, bleeding from the gills – possibly as a result of increased blood pressure or vasoconstriction (Deebani *et al.* 2019) – and decreased heart rate as a result of its muscle relaxant qualities. There is some suggestion that repeated usage of MS-222 may lead to slower recovery times and alteration of other parameters – a dynamic that should be taken into account when calculating dosage volumes (Matthews & Varga 2012; Owen & Kelsh 2021). Given the wide range of adverse effects, its use as a recommended anaesthetic for zebrafish should be revised (Readman *et al.* 2013).

Another widely used anaesthetic is 2-Phenoxyethanol (2-PE). Unlike MS222, 2-PE comes in an oily liquid form and, although it is widely used in aquaculture, its mechanism of action is poorly understood. It is also difficult to control the depth of anaesthesia (author's own observation, (Owen and Kelsh 2021).

Other anaesthetics have been used in zebrafish, including metomidate hydrochloride, which may only be suitable for procedures where only immobilisation is required (Collymore, Tolwani, *et al.* 2014). This is also true of etomidate (Martins, Valentim, *et al.* 2016). Isoflurane cannot be recommended for use as a single agent as it is difficult to dose and appears to induce stress in adult fish (Collymore, Tolwani, *et al.* 2014). However, it may be more promising for long-term anaesthesia when combined with other agents such as MS-222 (Lockwood et al. 2017; Huang *et al.* 2010). Combinations of propofol and lidocaine appear less adverse than MS-222 (Valentim *et al.* 2016). Other anaesthetics include clove oil – of which eugenol is the active component, which induces good anaesthesia but may promote delayed recovery times (Martins, Valentim, *et al.* 2016) – and benzocaine, the method of action of which is less defined for zebrafish, but is structurally similar to MS-222, suggesting similarities between the two (Wynd *et al.* 2017). Comparisons of different anaesthetics have shown that many cause aversive behaviours in zebrafish, including MS-222 and 2-PE, but etomidate does not elicit the same response (Readman *et al.* 2017). These studies suggest that there is still much work to be done with regard to the refinement and understanding of anaesthesia in zebrafish. This uncertainty is reflected in the broad range of dosage rates (Table 49.4a and b) that have to be adapted for each procedure and life stage.

---

[11]Standard Genetically altered zebrafish protocols pgs 11 – 28 https://assets.publishing.service.gov.uk/government/uploads/system/uploads/attachment_data/file/1086446/Genetically_Altered_Zebrafish_Protocols.pdf (Assessed 11 November 2022)

[12]https://zfin.atlassian.net/wiki/spaces/prot/pages/356155929/Fin+Amputations(Assessed 11 November 2022)

Table 49.4a Summary of single anaesthetics suitable for zebrafish and suggested dosages.

Single anaesthetics used for zebrafish				
Anaesthetics used for zebrafish	Published dosages (recovery)	Recommended dosage for recovery	Published dosages (euthanasia)	References
MS-222	164 mg/L 100 mg/L 150 mg/L 200 mg/L	164 mg/L	200–300 mg/L 0.168 mg/mL (prior to liquid nitrogen immersion) >300–900 mg/L (fry) 250 mg/L 400 mg/L	(Matthews and Varga 2012) (Martins, Valentim, et al. 2016) (Readman et al. 2013) (Collymore, Tolwani, et al. 2014) (Lockwood et al. 2017) (Wynd et al. 2017) (Strykowski and Schech 2015) (Wilson et al. 2009) (Collymore, Banks et al. 2016) (Davis et al. 2015) (Thurman, Rasmussen, and Prestia 2019) (Ferreira, Olsson, and Valentim 2018)
2-Phenoxyethanol Clove oil (active ingredient eugenol)	0.3 mL/L 55 mg/L 55–140 mg/L	0.3 mL/L 55 mg/L	50 mg/L	(Readman et al. 2013) (Collymore, Tolwani, et al. 2014) (Martins, Valentim, et al. 2016) (Davis et al. 2015) (Ferreira, Olsson, and Valentim 2018)
Eugenol	60–100 ppm 60–100 µg/L	60–100 µg/mL	>1500 µL (fry)	(Strykowski and Schech 2015) (Grush, Noakes, and Moccia 2004) (Matthews and Varga 2012) (Readman et al. 2013)
Isoeugenol Benzocaine	20 mg/L 100 mg/L	20 mg/L 100 mg/L	250 mg/L	(Wynd et al. 2017) (Readman et al. 2013) (Wynd et al. 2017) (Thurman et al. 2019)
Lidocaine (mixed)	325 mg/L 100 mg/L (unmixed)	325 mg/L 100 mg/L (unmixed)	400 mg/L >350 mg/L	(Readman et al. 2013) (Ferreira, Olsson, and Valentim 2018) (Collymore, Tolwani, et al. 2014) (Collymore Banks et al. 2016)
Etomidate	2 mg/L	2 mg/L	6 mg/L	(Martins, Valentim, et al. 2016) (Readman et al. 2013) (Ferreira, Olsson, and Valentim 2018)
Metomidate hydrochloride	10 mg/L stock 13.5 mg/L	10 mg/L stock 13.5 mg/L		(Collymore, Tolwani, et al. 2014)
Propofol	1.25 mg/L 2.5 mg/L	1.25 µg/L 2.5 mg/L	40 mg/L for 20 mins 120 mg/L for 10 mins	(Martins, Valentim, et al. 2016) (Chu et al. 2020) (Valentim et al. 2016)

Table 49.4b Summary of combined anaesthetics suitable for zebrafish and suggested dosages.

Combination anaesthetics	Published dosages (recovery)	Published dosages (euthanasia)	References
Etomidate + lidocaine Propofol + lidocaine	0.2 µg/L + 100 µg/L 1.25 µg/mL + 100 µg/mL 2.5 mg/L + 50 mg/L	20 mg/L + 100 mg/L	(Martins, Valentim, et al. 2016) (Martins, Valentim, et al. 2016) (Valentim et al. 2016) (Ferreira, Olsson, and Valentim 2018)
Ketamine + metedomidine MS222 + isoflurane	100 µg/mL + 1.25 µg/mL 65 + 65 ppm		(Martins, Valentim, et al. 2016) (Huang et al. 2010)

Analgesia in zebrafish is an important area of interest in zebrafish research, given that fish exhibit behavioural changes similar to pain responses of higher vertebrates (Sneddon 2003). A good candidate appears to be lidocaine, a local anaesthetic agent that blocks sodium channels and reduces stress levels, as shown by decreased fin wafting after a fin clipping procedure accompanied by decreased cortisol levels (Schroeder and Sneddon 2017). Although lidocaine is an anaesthetic, the dosage required for full anaesthesia can result in high mortality and so has a narrow safety margin (Collymore, Tolwani, et al. 2014), making it a better choice for analgesia as no side effects have been observed (Sneddon 2012). Morphine, an opioid, is another likely analgesia candidate, especially for regeneration studies when lidocaine may interfere and delay fin regeneration (Lelek et al. 2020). Opioids may also have adverse effects such as respiratory depression (Ohnesorge, Heinl, and Lewejohann 2021). Non-steroidal anti-inflammatory drugs (NSAIDs) also appear to have analgesic properties in zebrafish. More research is required as they appear to be beneficial only in adults and inflammatory pain. A summary of selected analgesia agents and suggested dosages for zebrafish appears in Table 49.5.

Euthanasia

Successful euthanasia will depend on the age of the fish – in both adult and larval forms of zebrafish – and will have to follow regional legislative practice. In the UK, Schedule 1 of the Animals (Scientific Procedures) Act 1986[13] (ASPA) lists appropriate methods of killing animals, only one of which is practical for zebrafish – overdose of an anaesthetic using a route and anaesthetic agent appropriate for the size and species of animal. For zebrafish, this will usually involve an overdose of anaesthetic, for which there is no consensus of opinion as to which is the most humane (von Krogh et al. 2021). This is followed by a confirmation of death – of which there are a few practical options – destruction of the brain, rigour mortis and instantaneous destruction of the body in a macerator are the most likely, as other confirmation methods are impractical for zebrafish. Larval forms over the age of 5 dpf should be treated in the same way, with protected stages up to at least 14 dpf high doses of anaesthetic appear to be more effective (Strykowski and Schech 2015). In the UK, embryonic and larval forms under 5 dpf are not protected under ASPA, but are also much more resistant to overdose of anaesthetic (Strykowski and Schech 2015). This allows the use of more practical methods of euthanasia, such as rapid chilling and addition of bleach to tank water, which is more effective (Matthews & Varga 2012; Strykowski & Schech 2015).

Outside of the UK, other methods of euthanasia are acceptable, for example hypothermic shock or rapid chilling in water temperatures of 0–4 °C (Matthews and Varga 2012) can be used for all ages of zebrafish and is approved by the American Veterinary Association (AVMA guidelines)[14]. While this is an ineffective method of euthanasia for larger bodied and/or cold water species, it has been successful in several studies using zebrafish (Wilson et al. 2009; Matthews & Varga 2012; Strykowski & Schech 2015; Wallace et al. 2018).

Severity classification and humane endpoints

Severity classification and humane endpoints in zebrafish welfare are currently less well-defined than in mammalian species. Both still remain problematic and difficult to define, as they are unable to show facial expressions or vocalise (Sneddon 2011). Lacking facial muscles excludes grimace scales (Sotocinal et al. 2011; Miller & Leach 2015; George et al. 2019) used for assessing pain in mammals and cannot be applied to zebrafish, as they lack the facial muscles to give clues to pain.

Behavioural responses to pain are similar to those of higher vertebrates, suggesting fish in general do feel pain (Sneddon 2003) and perhaps suggest ways in which humane endpoints can be defined. Behavioural responses in prey animals can be subtle – healthy zebrafish swim constantly, using all of the water column, whereas zebrafish after a painful treatment increase their use of the bottom of the tank and reduce swimming activity (Deakin et al. 2019). Automated behavioural monitoring to determine pain is being developed, which may be very useful to determine pain after an invasive procedure (Deakin et al. 2019), but currently, this may be perceived as too cost prohibitive to be applied to large fish in a system.

Table 49.5 Summary of analgesic agents for use with zebrafish and suggested dosages.

Analgesia in zebrafish		
Analgesic agent	Published dosage	References
Lidocaine	1 mg/kg	(Sneddon 2012)
	2–5 mg/L	(Martins, Valentim, et al. 2016)
		(Schroeder 2016)
Morphine	3 µL (intramuscular)	(Taylor et al. 2017)
	48 mg/L (larvae)	(Taylor et al. 2017)
		(Lopez-Luna et al. 2017a)
		(Lopez-Luna et al. 2017b)
Buprenorphine	0.1 mg/L	(Steenbergen and Bardine 2014)
	0.2 mg/L	
	0.5 mg/L	(Steenbergen 2018)
		(Schroeder and Sneddon 2017)
Acetylsalicylic acid	1 mg/L (more studies necessary)	(Schroeder and Sneddon 2017)
Diclofenac	40 mg/kg (injected intraperitoneal)	(Costa et al. 2019)
Indomethacin	0.2 mg/L	(Magalhaes et al. 2017)

---

[13] Schedule 1, Standard Methods of Humane Killing, Page 27 – 28, https://assets.publishing.service.gov.uk/government/uploads/system/uploads/attachment_data/file/619140/ConsolidatedASPA1Jan2013.pdf (Accessed 21 June, 2022)

[14] AVMA Guidelines for the euthanasia of Animals: 2020 edition. https://www.avma.org/sites/default/files/2020-01/2020-Euthanasia-Final-1-17-20.pdf (Accessed June 21, 2022)

Overt signs of ill health can also be used to determine both severity limits and humane endpoints, and attempts have been made to standardise health terms (Goodwin et al. 2016) as well as the use of body condition scoring (Wilson et al. 2013; Clark et al. 2018). This has been the approach in the UK; the Home Office has provided protocols to be used in project licences for both the standard breeding of genetically altered zebrafish, as well as guidance on how to use them[15]. It is expected that the majority of this work would fall under a mild severity limit, including both fin clipping and cryopreservation work. The stated humane endpoints under this protocol include culling fish that show signs of suffering greater than minor or transient, or compromise their health or well-being, for example: abnormal growth, swimming, feeding and behaving abnormally. For those fish with a moderate severity limit, it is expected that the applicant should state the adverse effects – for example, effects from genetic alteration.

The classification of moderate severity in the UK and Europe are procedures that are likely to cause short-term moderate pain, suffering or distress, and procedures that are likely to cause moderate impairment of the well-being or general condition of the animal[16]. Suggestions for monitoring this are easily detectable disturbance of an animal's normal state, which may be difficult to ascertain in zebrafish but may be aided body condition scoring and standardised reference terms (author's own observation). Procedures, such as cardiac injury, which are more invasive, carried out on older animals and cause tissue damage (Gonzalez-Rosa, Burns, and Burns 2017) are classified as moderate.

Severe severity levels are discouraged in general and are not frequently applied in zebrafish, partly due to their small size and the prevalence of use of embryos before 5 dpf when they are not protected by law in the UK and Europe. However, in some toxicological studies, death can be considered an endpoint and this would be classified as a severe severity, as may some genetic line modifications (Hawkins et al. 2011).

Research into pain and suffering still remains a fairly recent area of study, but it can be assumed that anaesthesia and analgesia should be provided in response to tissue damage (Sneddon 2009). Both humane endpoints and severity limits can also be judged by clinical signs – for example respiration rates, food consumption and swimming behaviours (Hawkins et al. 2011) – but what must also be considered are environmental and husbandry stressors. This can include sex, sex ratios, tank size and stocking densities (Buenhombre et al. 2021).

Welfare problems

Many welfare problems associated with zebrafish and their husbandry are common to all fish species and are discussed in Chapter 48. Much is derived from our lack of understanding of the species and fish in general. As ectothermic poikilotherms, their intrinsic needs are more directly connected to their extrinsic requirements than a mammalian species, so the smallest of differences in the environment can affect zebrafish, in turn having effects on their husbandry and welfare in ways we do not fully understand. Although there are more guidelines for zebrafish husbandry and welfare, compared to many other fish species, they are still very broad and not particularly descriptive, which has led to inconsistent interpretation and a lack of standardisation in welfare methodology. This can lead to a wide range of welfare problems including low survival rates at embryonic and juvenile stages, pathogen load and disease related issues, water quality and nutritional issues, as well as variability in wild-type lines.

Culturally, we appear guilty of a dissociation with fish in general and do not appear to share the same empathy with zebrafish as we do with mammalian models. This sentiment is echoed in legislation; ASPA 1986 asks that project licence holders should involve animals with the lowest capacity to feel pain, suffering, distress or lasting harm (HomeOffice 2020) and this is often interpreted to include zebrafish. This also seems to be supported by the belief of some that fish do not feel pain; Rose et al. suggests this was because of fish lacking brain structures such as the cerebral cortex, which is only present in mammalian species (Rose et al. 2014). However, these beliefs are now being challenged by a body of work that shows that fish do feel pain, with much of the evidence coming from studies done directly with zebrafish (Sneddon 2009, 2015). Unlike many other fish species, the scientific purposes for which zebrafish are used have often led to them being housed in multi-species units. When this is the case, primary care may be delivered by people who, because they are more familiar with mammalian species, may find it difficult to adapt to working with a species that is so unfamiliar and living in an environment that is difficult to relate to.

Our lack of understanding of the model coupled with lack of standardisation of husbandry and welfare can have a potential impact on scientific outcomes and reproducibility of results, as well as negatively affecting the welfare of the fish. Improving education on the species and having more robust guidelines and greater communication across the stakeholders will do much to further and improve the husbandry and welfare needs of the zebrafish.

References

Adatto, I., Lawrence, C., Thompson, M. and Zon, L.I. (2011). A new system for the rapid collection of large numbers of developmentally staged zebrafish embryos. *PLoS One*, **6**.

Adatto, I., Krug, L. and Zon, L.I. (2016). The red light district and its effects on zebrafish reproduction. *Zebrafish*, **13**, 226–229.

Alestrom, P., D'Angelo, L., Midtlyng, P.J. et al. (2020). Zebrafish: Housing and husbandry recommendations. *Laboratory Animals*. **54**, 213–224.

Aman, A.J., Fulbright, A.N. and Parichy, D.M. (2018). Wnt/beta-catenin regulates an ancient signaling network during zebrafish scale development. *Elife*, **7**.

Astrofsky, K.M., Schrenzel, M.D., Bullis, R.A. et al. (2000). Diagnosis and management of atypical Mycobacterium spp. infections in established laboratory zebrafish (Brachydanio rerio) facilities. *Comparative Medicine*, **50**, 666–672.

---

[15]https://assets.publishing.service.gov.uk/government/uploads/system/uploads/attachment_data/file/785930/Standard_GA_zebrafish_breeding_protocols_FINAL.pdf (Accessed June 21, 2022).

[16]https://assets.publishing.service.gov.uk/government/uploads/system/uploads/attachment_data/file/276014/NotesActualSeverityReporting.pdf (Accessed June 21, 2022)

Avitan, L., Pujic, Z., Molter, J. et al. (2020). Behavioral signatures of a developing neural code. *Current Biology*, **30**, 3352–3363.

Barton, C.L., Johnson, E.W. and Tanguay. R.L. (2016). Facility design and health management program at the Sinnhuber Aquatic Research Laboratory. *Zebrafish*, **13**, S39–S43.

Baxendale, S., van Eeden, F. and Wilkinson, R. (2017). The Power of zebrafish in personalised medicine. *Personalised Medicine: Lessons from Neurodegeneration to Cancer*, **1007**, 179–197.

Bermudez, R., Losada, A.P., de Azevedo, A.M. et al. (2018). First description of a natural infection with spleen and kidney necrosis virus in zebrafish. *Journal of Fish Diseases*, **4**(8), 1283–1294.

Best, J., Adatto, I., Cockington, J., et al. (2010). A novel method for rearing first-feeding larval zebrafish: Polyculture with Type L saltwater rotifers (Brachionus plicatilis). *Zebrafish*, **7**, 289–295.

Borges, A.C., Pereira, N., Franco, M. et al. (2016). Implementation of a Zebrafish Health Program in a research facility: A 4-year retrospective study. *Zebrafish*, **13**, S115–S26.

Breacker, C., Barber, I., Norton, W.H.J. et al. (2017). A low-cost method of skin swabbing for the collection of DNA samples from small laboratory fish. *Zebrafish*, **14**, 35–41.

Buenhombre, J., Daza-Cardona, E.A., Sousa, P. and Gouveia, A. (2021). Different influences of anxiety models, environmental enrichment, standard conditions and intraspecies variation (sex, personality and strain) on stress and quality of life in adult and juvenile zebrafish: A systematic review. *Neuroscience and Biobehavioral Reviews*, **131**, 765–791.

Canadian Council on Animal Care. (2020). *CCAC Guidelines: Zebrafish and Other Small, Warm Water Laboratory Fish*. ISBN 978-0-919087-84-2

Carfagnini, A.G., Rodd, F.H., Jeffers, K.B. and Bruce, A.E.E. (2009). The effects of habitat complexity on aggression and fecundity in zebrafish (Danio rerio). *Environmental Biology of Fishes*, **86**, 403–409.

Castranova, D., Lawton, A., Lawrence, C. et al. (2011). The effect of stocking densities on reproductive performance in laboratory zebrafish (Danio rerio). *Zebrafish*, **8**, 141–146.

Castranova, D. and Wang, C.M. (2020). Zebrafish breeding and colony management. *Zebrafish in Biomedical Research: Biology, Husbandry, Diseases, and Research Applications*, pp. 357–364.

Chablais, F. and Jazwinska, A. (2012). Induction of myocardial infarction in adult zebrafish using cryoinjury. *Jove-Journal of Visualized Experiments*, (62), 3666. doi: 10.3791/3666

Chang, C.T., Benedict, S. and Whipps, C.M. (2019). Transmission of Mycobacterium chelonae and Mycobacterium marinum in laboratory zebrafish through live feeds. *Journal of Fish Diseases*, **42**, 1425–1431.

Chang, C.T., Lewis, J. and Whipps, C.M. (2019). Source or sink: Examining the role of biofilms in transmission of Mycobacterium spp. in laboratory zebrafish. *Zebrafish*, **16**, 197–206.

Cheung, E., Chatterjee, D. and Gerlai, R. (2014). Subcutaneous dye injection for marking and identification of individual adult zebrafish (Danio rerio) in behavioral studies. *Behavior Research Methods*, **46**, 619–624.

Chu, D.K., Jampachaisri, K. and Pacharinsak, C. (2020). High dose propofol effectively euthanizes zebrafish (Danio rerio). *Thai Journal of Veterinary Medicine*, **50**, 13–16.

Clark, K.J. and Ekker, S.C. (2013). Zebrafish. *Brenner's Encyclopedia of Genetics*, 2nd edn., pp. 396–398. Elsevier: San Diego.

Clark, T.S., Pandolfo, L.M., Marshall, C.M., et al. (2018). Body condition scoring for adult zebrafish (Danio rerio), *Journal of the American Association for Laboratory Animal Science*, **57**, 698–702.

Coe, T.S., Hamilton, P.B., Griffiths, A.M., et al. (2009). Genetic variation in strains of zebrafish (Danio rerio) and the implications for ecotoxicology studies, *Ecotoxicology*, **18**, 144–150.

Collymore, C., Banks, E.K. and Turner, P.V. (2016). Lidocaine hydrochloride compared with MS222 for the euthanasia of zebrafish (Danio rerio), *Journal of the American Association for Laboratory Animal Science*, **55**, 816–820.

Collymore, C., Crim, M.J. and Lieggi, C. (2016). Recommendations for health monitoring and reporting for zebrafish research facilities, *Zebrafish*, **13**, S138–S148.

Collymore, C., Porelli, G., Lieggi, C. and Lipman, N.S. (2014). Evaluation of 5 cleaning and disinfection methods for nets used to collect zebrafish (Danio rerio). *Journal of the American Association for Laboratory Animal Science*, **53**, 657–660.

Collymore, C., Rasmussen, S. and Tolwani, R.J. (2013). Gavaging adult zebrafish. *Jove-Journal of Visualized Experiments*, (78), 5069.

Collymore, C., Tolwani, A., Lieggi, C. and Rasmussen, S. (2014). Efficacy and safety of 5 anesthetics in adult zebrafish (Danio rerio). *Journal of the American Association for Laboratory Animal Science*, **53**, 198–203.

Collymore, C., Tolwani, R.J. and Rasmussen, S. (2015). The behavioral effects of single housing and environmental enrichment on adult zebrafish (Danio rerio). *Journal of the American Association for Laboratory Animal Science*, **54**, 280–285.

Costa, F.V., Rosa, L.V., Quadros, V.A., et al. (2019). Understanding nociception-related phenotypes in adult zebrafish: Behavioral and pharmacological characterization using a new acetic acid model. *Behavioural Brain Research*, **359**, 570–578.

Creaser. (1934). The technic of handling the zebra fish (Brachydanio rerio) for the production of eggs which are favorable for embryological research and are available at any specified time throughout the year. *Copeia*, **1934**, 159–161.

Crim, M.J. and Lawrence, C. (2021). A fish is not a mouse: understanding differences in background genetics is critical for reproducibility. *Lab Animal*, **50**, 19–25.

Dang, M., Henderson, R.E., Garraway, L.A. and Zon, L.I. (2016). Long-term drug administration in the adult zebrafish using oral gavage for cancer preclinical studies. *Disease Models & Mechanisms*, **9**, 811–820.

Davis, D.J., Klug, J., Hankins, M., et al. (2015). Effects of clove oil as a euthanasia agent on blood collection efficiency and serum cortisol levels in Danio rerio. *Journal of the American Association for Laboratory Animal Science*, **54**, 564–567.

De Lombaert, M.C.M., Rick, E.L., Krugner-Higby, L.A. and Wolman, M.A. (2017). Behavioral characteristics of adult zebrafish (Danio rerio) after MS222 anesthesia for fin excision. *Journal of the American Association for Laboratory Animal Science*, **56**, 377–381.

Deakin, A.G., Buckley, J., AlZu'bi, H.S. et al. (2019). Automated monitoring of behaviour in zebrafish after invasive procedures. *Scientific Reports*, **9**.

Deebani, A., Iyer, N., Raman, R. and Jagadeeswaran, P. (2019). Effect of MS222 on Hemostasis in Zebrafish. *Journal of the American Association for Laboratory Animal Science*, **58**, 390–396.

Delcourt, J., Ovidio, M., Denoel, M., et al. (2018). Individual identification and marking techniques for zebrafish. *Reviews in Fish Biology and Fisheries*, **28**, 839–864.

DePasqual, C., Fettrow, S., Sturgill, J. and Braithwaite, V.A. (2019). The impact of flow and physical enrichment on preferences in zebrafish. *Applied Animal Behaviour Science*, **215**, 77–81.

Diaz-Verdugo, C., Sun, G.J., Fawcett, C.H., et al. (2019). Mating suppresses alarm response in zebrafish. *Current Biology*, **29**, 2541–2546.

Engeszer, R.E., Alberici da Barbiano, L., Ryan, M.J. and Parichy, D.M. (2007). Timing and plasticity of shoaling behaviour in the zebrafish, Danio rerio. *Animal Behaviour*, **74**, 1269–1275.

Engeszer, R.E., Patterson, L.B., Rao, A.A. and Parichy, D.M. (2007). Zebrafish in the wild: A review of natural history and new notes from the field. *Zebrafish*, **4**, 21–U126.

Engeszer, R.E., Ryan, M.J. and Parichy, D.M. (2004). Learned social preference in zebrafish. *Current Biology*, **14**, 881–884.

Facciol, A. and Gerlai, R. (2020). Zebrafish shoaling, its behavioral and neurobiological mechanisms, and its alteration by embryonic alcohol exposure: A review. *Frontiers in Behavioral Neuroscience*, **14**.

Ferreira, J.M., Olsson, A.S. and Valentim, A.M. (2018). Adult zebrafish euthanasia: Efficacy of anaesthesia overdose versus rapid cooling. *PeerJ Preprints*, **2018**, 12–17.

Fontana, B.D., Gibbon, A.J., Cleal, M., et al. (2021). Moderate early life stress improves adult zebrafish (Danio rerio) working memory but does not affect social and anxiety-like responses. *Developmental Psychobiology*, **63**, 54–64.

Fowler, L.A., Dennis-Cornelius, L.N., Dawson, J.A. et al. (2020). Both dietary ratio of n-6 to n-3 fatty acids and total dietary lipid are positively associated with adiposity and reproductive health in zebrafish. *Current Developments in Nutrition*, **4**.

Fowler, L.A., Powers, A.D., Williams, M.B., et al. (2021). The effects of dietary saturated fat source on weight gain and adiposity are influenced by both sex and total dietary lipid intake in zebrafish. *PLoS One*, **16**.

Fowler, L.A., Williams, M.B., D'Abramo, L.R. and Watts, S.A. (2020). Zebrafish nutrition-moving forward. *Zebrafish in Biomedical Research: Biology, Husbandry, Diseases, and Research Applications*, 379–401.

Fowler, L.A., Williams, M.B., Dennis-Cornelius, L.N., et al. (2019). Influence of Commercial and laboratory diets on growth, body composition, and reproduction in the zebrafish Danio rerio. *Zebrafish*, **16**, 508–521.

Frommen, J.G., Hanak, S., Schmidl, C.A. and Thunken, T. (2015). Visible Implant Elastomer tagging influences social preferences of zebrafish (Danio rerio). *Behaviour*, **152**, 1769–1781.

Gaj, T., Gersbach, C.A. and Barbas, C.F. (2013). ZFN, TALEN, and CRISPR/Cas-based methods for genome engineering. *Trends in Biotechnology*, **31**, 397–405.

Garcia, R.L. and Sanders, G.E. (2011). Efficacy of cleaning and disinfection procedures in a zebrafish (Danio rerio) facility. *Journal of the American Association for Laboratory Animal Science*, **50**, 895–900.

Gemberling, M., Bailey, T.J., Hyde, D.R. and Poss, K.D. (2013). The zebrafish as a model for complex tissue regeneration. *Trends in Genetics*, **29**, 611–620.

Georga, I. and Koumoundouros, G. (2010). Thermally induced plasticity of body shape in adult zebrafish Danio rerio (Hamilton, 1822). *Journal of Morphology*, **271**, 1319–1327.

George, R.P., Howarth, G.S. and Whittaker, A.L. (2019). Use of the rat grimace scale to evaluate visceral pain in a model of chemotherapy-induced mucositis. *Animals*, **9**.

Gerhard, G.S., Kauffman, E.J., Wang, X., et al. (2002) Life spans and senescent phenotypes in two strains of Zebrafish (Danio rerio). *Experimental Gerontology*, **37**, 1055–1068.

Gerlach, G. (2006). Pheromonal regulation of reproductive success in female zebrafish: female suppression and male enhancement. *Animal Behaviour*, **72**, 1119–1124.

Gonzalez-Rosa, J.M., Burns, C.E. and Burns, C.G. (2017). Zebrafish heart regeneration: 15 years of discoveries. *Regeneration*, **4**, 105–123.

Goodwin, N., Karp, N.A., Blackledge, S., et al. (2016). Standardized welfare terms for the zebrafish community. *Zebrafish*, **13**, S164–S168.

Goolish, E.M., Okutake, K. and Lesure, S. (1999). Growth and survivorship of larval zebrafish Danio rerio on processed diets. *North American Journal of Aquaculture*, **61**, 189–198.

Graham, C., von Keyserlingk, M.A.G. and Franks, B. (2018). Zebrafish welfare: Natural history, social motivation and behaviour. *Applied Animal Behaviour Science*, **200**, 13–22.

Grunwald, D.J. and Eisen, J.S. (2002). Timeline – Headwaters of the zebrafish emergence of a new model vertebrate. *Nature Reviews Genetics*, **3**, 717–724.

Grush, J., Noakes, D.L.G. and Moccia, R.D. (2004). The efficacy of clove oil as an anaesthetic for the zebrafish, Danio rerio (Hamilton). *Zebrafish*, **1**, 46–53.

Guerrera, M.C., De Pasquale, F., Muglia, U. and Caruso, G. (2015). Digestive enzymatic activity during ontogenetic development in zebrafish (Danio rerio). *Journal of Experimental Zoology Part B-Molecular and Developmental Evolution*, **324**, 699–706.

Harper, C. and Lawrence, C. (2011). *The Laboratory Zebrafish*. CRC Press, Taylor and Francis Group: San Diego.

Hason, M. and Bartunek, P. (2019). Zebrafish models of cancer-new insights on modeling human cancer in a non-mammalian vertebrate. *Genes*, **10**.

Hawke, J.P., Kent, M., Rogge, M., et al. (2013). Edwardsiellosis caused by Edwardsiella ictaluri in laboratory populations of zebrafish Danio rerio. *Journal of Aquatic Animal Health*, **25**, 171–183.

Hawkins, P., Dennison, N., Goodman, G., et al. (2011). Guidance on the severity classification of scientific procedures involving fish: report of a Working Group appointed by the Norwegian Consensus-Platform for the Replacement, Reduction and Refinement of animal experiments (Norecopa). *Laboratory Animals*, **45**, 219–224.

Hohn, C. and Petrie-Hanson, L. (2013). Evaluation of visible implant elastomer tags in zebrafish (Danio rerio). *Biology Open*, **2**, 1397–1401.

Howe, K., Clark, M.D., Torroja, C.F.J., et al. (2013). The zebrafish reference genome sequence and its relationship to the human genome. *Nature*, **496**, 498–503.

Huang, W.C., Hsieh, Y.S., Chen, I.H., et al. (2010). Combined use of MS-222 (Tricaine) and isoflurane extends anesthesia time and minimizes cardiac rhythm side effects in adult zebrafish. *Zebrafish*, **7**, 297–304.

Hutter, S., Penn, D.J., Magee, S. and Zala, S.M. (2010). Reproductive behaviour of wild zebrafish (Danio rerio) in large tanks. *Behaviour*, **147**, 641–660.

Hwang, W.Y., Fu, Y.F., Reyon, D., et al. (2013). Efficient genome editing in zebrafish using a CRISPR-Cas system. *Nature Biotechnology*, **31**, 227–229.

IATA. (2021). *Live Animals Regulations (LAR)* (International Air Transport Association).

Ingham, P.W. (1997). Zebrafish genetics and its implications for understanding vertebrate development. *Human Molecular Genetics*, **6**, 1755–1760.

Jones, N.A.R., Spence, R., Jones, F.A.M. and Spence-Jones, H.C. (2019). Shade as enrichment: Testing preferences for shelter in two model fish species. *Journal of Fish Biology*, **95**, 1161–1165.

Kaushik, S., Georga, I. and Koumoundouros, G. (2011). Growth and body composition of zebrafish (Danio rerio) larvae fed a compound feed from first feeding onward: Toward implications on nutrient requirements. *Zebrafish*, **8**, 87–95.

Kent, M.L., Bishop-Stewart, J.K., Matthews, J.L. and Spitsbergen, J.M. (2002). Pseudocapillaria tomentosa, a nematode pathogen, and associated neoplasms of zebrafish (Danio rerio) kept in research colonies. *Comparative Medicine*, **52**, 354–358.

Kent, M.L., Buchner, C., Watral, V.G. et al. (2011). Development and maintenance of a specific pathogen-free (SPF) zebrafish research facility for Pseudoloma neurophilia. *Diseases of Aquatic Organisms*, **95**, 73–79.

Kent, M.L., Gaulke, C.A., Watral, V. and Sharpton, T.J. (2018). Pseudocapillaria tomentosa in laboratory zebrafish Danio rerio: Patterns of infection and dose response. *Diseases of Aquatic Organisms*, **131**, 121–131.

Kent, M.L., Harper, C. and Wolf, J.C. (2012). Documented and potential research impacts of subclinical diseases in zebrafish. *Ilar Journal*, **53**, 126–134.

Kent, M.L., Sanders, J.L., Spagnoli, S. et al. (2020). Review of diseases and health management in zebrafish Danio rerio (Hamilton 1822) in research facilities. *Journal of Fish Diseases*, **43**, 637–650.

Kimmel, C.B., Ballard, W.W., Kimmel, S.R. et al. (1995). Stages of embryonic-development of the zebrafish. *Developmental Dynamics*, **203**, 253–310.

Kinkel, M.D., Eames, S.C., Philipson, L.H. and Prince, V.E. (2010). Intraperitoneal injection into adult zebrafish. *Journal of Visualized Experiments: JoVE*. DOI: 10.3791/2126 [Online publication.]

Kistler, C., Hegglin, D., Wurbel, H. and Konig, B. (2011). Preference for structured environment in zebrafish (Danio rerio) and checker barbs (Puntius oligolepis). *Applied Animal Behaviour Science*, **135**, 318–327.

Kossack, M.E. and Draper, B.W. (2019). Genetic regulation of sex determination and maintenance in zebrafish (Danio rerio). *Sex Determination in Vertebrates*, **134**, 119–149.

Laale, H.W. (1977). Biology and use of zebrafish, brachydanio-rerio in fisheries research – literature-review. *Journal of Fish Biology*, **10**, 121–173.

Lambert, C.J., Freshner, B.C., Chung, A. et al. (2018). An automated system for rapid cellular extraction from live zebrafish embryos and larvae: Development and application to genotyping. *PLoS One*, **13**.

Lau, J.Y.N., Bianco, I.H. and Severi, K.E. (2019). Cellular-level understanding of supraspinal control: what can be learned from zebrafish?. *Current Opinion in Physiology*, **8**.

Lawrence, C. (2007). The husbandry of zebrafish (Danio rerio): A review. *Aquaculture*, **269**, 1–20.

Lawrence, C. (2011). Advances in zebrafish husbandry and management, Chapter 23 in H.W. Detrich, M. Westerfield and L.I. Zon (Eds.), *Methods in Cell Biology*, Vol. 2, 429–451, Elsevier: San Diego.

Lawrence, C., Best, J., James, A. and Maloney, K. (2012). The effects of feeding frequency on growth and reproduction in zebrafish (Danio rerio). *Aquaculture*, **368**, 103–108.

Lawrence, C. and Mason, T. (2012). Zebrafish housing systems: A review of basic operating principles and considerations for design and functionality. *Ilar Journal*, **53**, 179–191.

Lawton, S. (2017). Do Buccal swabs from Zebrafish give enough of a sample of DNA to be used as a viable non-invasive method of genotyping?. *Animal Technology and Welfare*, **16**, 155–164.

Lebold, K.M., Lohr, C.V., Barton, C.L. et al. (2013). Chronic vitamin E deficiency promotes vitamin C deficiency in zebrafish leading to degenerative myopathy and impaired swimming behavior. *Comparative Biochemistry and Physiology C-Toxicology & Pharmacology*, **157**, 382–389.

Lee, S.L.J., Horsfield, J.A., Black, M.A. et al. (2018). Identification of sex differences in zebrafish (Danio rerio) brains during early sexual differentiation and masculinization using 17 alpha-methyltestoterone. *Biology of Reproduction*, **99**, 446–460.

Lelek, S., Simões, M.G., Hu, B. et al. (2020). Morphine alleviates pain after heart cryoinjury in zebrafish without impeding regeneration. *bioRxiv [Preprint]*.

Lidster, K., Readman, G.D., Prescott, M.J. and Owen, S.F. (2017a). International survey on the use and welfare of zebrafish Danio rerio in research. *Journal of Fish Biology*, **90**, 1891–1905.

Limonta, G., Mancia, A., Benkhalqui, A. et al. (2019). Microplastics induce transcriptional changes, immune response and behavioral alterations in adult zebrafish. *Scientific Reports*, **9**.

Lockwood, N., Parker, J., Wilson, C. and Frankel, P. (2017). Optimal anesthetic regime for motionless three-dimensional image acquisition during longitudinal studies of adult nonpigmented zebrafish. *Zebrafish*, **14**, 133–139.

Lopez-Luna, J., Al-Jubouri, Q., Al-Nuaimy, W. and Sneddon, L.U. (2017a). Impact of analgesic drugs on the behavioural responses of larval zebrafish to potentially noxious temperatures. *Applied Animal Behaviour Science*, **188**, 97–105.

Lopez-Luna, J., Al-Jubouri, Q., Al-Nuaimy, W. and Sneddon, L.U. (2017b). Reduction in activity by noxious chemical stimulation is ameliorated by immersion in analgesic drugs in zebrafish. *Journal of Experimental Biology*, **220**, 1451–1458.

Lopez-Schier, H. (2019). Neuroplasticity in the acoustic startle reflex in larval zebrafish. *Current Opinion in Neurobiology*, **54**, 134–139.

Ma, Q., Hu, C.T., Yue, J.J.Y. et al. (2020). High-carbohydrate diet promotes the adaptation to acute hypoxia in zebrafish. *Fish Physiology and Biochemistry*, **46**, 665–679.

MacRae, C.A. and Peterson, R.T. (2015) Zebrafish as tools for drug discovery. *Nature Reviews Drug Discovery*, **14**, 721–731.

Magalhaes, F.E.A., de Sousa, C.A.P.B., Santos, S.A.A.R. et al. (2017). Adult zebrafish (Danio rerio): An alternative behavioral model of formalin-induced nociception. *Zebrafish*, **14**, 422–429.

Marancik, D., Collins, J., Afema, J. and Lawrence, C. (2020). Exploring the advantages and limitations of sampling methods commonly used in research facilities for zebrafish health inspections. *Laboratory Animals*, **54**, 373–385.

Marcon, M., Mocelin, R., Benvenutti, R. et al. (2018). Environmental enrichment modulates the response to chronic stress in zebrafish. *Journal of Experimental Biology*, **221**.

Marques, I.J., Lupi, E. and Mercader, N. (2019). Model systems for regeneration: Zebrafish. *Development*, **146**.

Martins, S., Monteiro, J.F., Vito, M. et al. (2016). Toward an integrated zebrafish health management program supporting cancer and neuroscience research. *Zebrafish*, **13**, S47–S55.

Martins, T., Valentim, A.M., Pereira, N. and Antunes, L.M. (2016). Anaesthesia and analgesia in laboratory adult zebrafish: A question of refinement. *Laboratory Animals*, **50**, 476–488.

Mason, T., Snell, K., Mittge, E. et al. (2016). Strategies to mitigate a Mycobacterium marinum outbreak in a zebrafish research facility. *Zebrafish*, **13**, S77–S87.

Matthews, M., Trevarrow, B. and Matthews, J. (2002). A virtual tour of the Guide for zebrafish users. *Lab Animal*, **31**, 34–40.

Matthews, M. and Varga, Z.M. (2012). Anesthesia and Euthanasia in zebrafish. *Ilar Journal*, **53**, 192–204.

McMillan, S.C., Geraudie, J. and Akimenko, M.A. (2015). Pectoral fin breeding tubercle clusters: A method to determine zebrafish sex. *Zebrafish*, **12**, 121–123.

Metz, J.R., Leeuwis, R.H.J., Zethof, J. and Flik, G. (2014). Zebrafish (Danio rerio) in calcium-poor water mobilise calcium and phosphorus from scales. *Journal of Applied Ichthyology*, **30**, 671–677.

Meyer, B.M., Froehlich, J.M., Galt, N.J. and Biga, P.R. (2013). Inbred strains of zebrafish exhibit variation in growth performance and myostatin expression following fasting. *Comparative Biochemistry and Physiology a-Molecular & Integrative Physiology*, **164**, 1–9.

Miller, A.L. and Leach, M.C. (2015). Using the mouse grimace scale to assess pain associated with routine ear notching and the effect of analgesia in laboratory mice. *Laboratory Animals*, **49**, 117–120.

Mocho, J.P., Martin, D.J., Millington, M.E. and Torres, Y.S. (2017). Environmental screening of Aeromonas hydrophila, Mycobacterium spp., and Pseudocapillaria tomentosa in zebrafish systems. *Jove-Journal of Visualized Experiments*, (130), 55306. doi: 10.3791/55306

Monson, C.A. and Sadler, K.C. (2010). Inbreeding depression and outbreeding depression are evident in wild-type zebrafish lines. *Zebrafish*, **7**, 189–197.

Monteiro, J.F., Martins, S., Farias, M. et al. (2018). The impact of two different cold-extruded feeds and feeding regimens on zebrafish survival, growth and reproductive performance. *Journal of Developmental Biology*, **6**.

Nasiadka, A. and Clark, M.D. (2012). Zebrafish breeding in the laboratory environment. *Ilar Journal*, 53, 161–168.

Nevalainen, T., Blom, H.J.M., Guaitani, A. et al. (2002). FELASA recommendations for the accreditation of laboratory animal science education and training – Report of the Federation of European Laboratory Animal Science Associations Working Group on Accreditation of Laboratory Animal Science Education and Training. *Laboratory Animals*, **36**, 373–377.

Newell, B. and Brocca, M. (2021). Chapter 2, Housing and maintenance of zebrafish, new technologies in laboratory aquatic systems and considerations for facility design. In: *Laboratory Fish in Biomedical Research*, Eds Paolo de Girolamo and Livia d'Angelo. Science Direct.

Norton, A., Franse, K.F., Daw, T. et al. (2019). Larval rearing methods for small-scale production of healthy zebrafish. *Eastern Biologist*, **2019**, 33–46.

Nüsslein-Volhard, C. (2012). The zebrafish issue of Development. *Development*, **139**, 4099–5103.

OATA. (2020). Code for the transport of ornamental fish general principles. https://ornamentalfish.org/wp-content/uploads/Transport-code-final.pdf. Accessed 25 Oct 2020.

Ogi, A., Licitra, R., Naef, V. et al. (2021). Social preference tests in zebrafish: A systematic review. *Frontiers in Veterinary Science*, **7**.

Ohnesorge, N., Heinl, C. and Lewejohann, L. (2021). Current methods to investigate nociception and pain in zebrafish. *Frontiers in Neuroscience*, **15**.

Onal, U. and Langdon, C. (2016). Diet size preference of zebrafish (Danio rerio) larvae fed on cross-linked protein-walled capsules. *Zebrafish*, **13**, 556–562.

Owen, J.P. and Kelsh, R.N. (2021). A suitable anaesthetic protocol for metamorphic zebrafish. *PLoS One*, **16**.

Parichy, D.M. (2003). Pigment patterns: fish in stripes and spots. *Current Biology*, **13**, R947–R50.

Parichy, D.M. (2015). Advancing biology through a deeper understanding of zebrafish ecology and evolution. *Elife*, **4**.

Parichy, D.M., Elizondo, M.R., Mills, M.G. et al. (2009). Normal table of postembryonic zebrafish development: Staging by externally visible anatomy of the living fish. *Developmental Dynamics*, **238**, 2975–3015.

Paull, G.C., Filby, A.L., Giddins, H.G. et al. (2010). Dominance hierarchies in zebrafish (Danio rerio) and their relationship with reproductive success. *Zebrafish*, **7**, 109–117.

Paull, G.C., Van Look, K.J.W., Santos, E.M. et al. (2008). Variability in measures of reproductive success in laboratory-kept colonies of zebrafish and implications for studies addressing population-level effects of environmental chemicals. *Aquatic Toxicology*, **87**, 115–126.

Pavlidis, M., Digka, N., Theodoridi, A. et al. (2013). Husbandry of zebrafish, Danio Rerio, and the cortisol stress response. *Zebrafish*, **10**, 524–531.

Perera, E. and Yufera, M. (2016). Soybean meal and soy protein concentrate in early diet elicit different nutritional programming effects on juvenile zebrafish. *Zebrafish*, **13**, 61–69.

Pilehvar, A., Town, R.M. and Blust, R. (2020). The effect of copper on behaviour, memory, and associative learning ability of zebrafish (Danio rerio). *Ecotoxicology and Environmental Safety*, **188**.

Pritchard, V.L., Lawrence, J., Butlin, R.K. and Krause, J. (2001). Shoal choice in zebrafish, Danio rerio: the influence of shoal size and activity. *Animal Behaviour*, **62**, 1085–1088.

Pullium, J.K., Dillehay, D.L. and Webb, S. (1999). High mortality in zebrafish (Danio rerio). *Contemporary Topics in Laboratory Animal Science*, **38**, 80–83.

Racz, A., Allan, B., Dwyer, T. et al. (2021). Identification of individual zebrafish (Danio rerio): A refined protocol for VIE tagging whilst considering animal welfare and the principles of the 3Rs'. *Animals*, **11**.

Racz, A., Dwyer, T. and Killen, S.S. (2019). Overview of a disease outbreak and introduction of a step-by-step protocol for the eradication of mycobacterium haemophilum in a zebrafish system. *Zebrafish*, **16**, 77–86.

Rahmann, U.O., Jaman, A., Shajahan, M. and Islam, M.S. (2021). Impact of sex ratio on the spawning success of zebrafish in the laboratory settings. *Progressive Agriculture*, **32**, 78–83.

Ramsay, J.M., Feist, G.W., Varga, Z.M. et al. (2006). Whole-body cortisol is an indicator of crowding stress in adult zebrafish, Danio rerio. *Aquaculture*, **258**, 565–574.

Ramsay, J.M., Feist, G.W., Varga, Z.M. et al. (2009). Whole-body cortisol response of zebrafish to acute net handling stress. *Aquaculture*, **297**, 157–162.

Randlett, O., Haesemeyer, M., Forkin, G. et al. (2019). Distributed plasticity drives visual habituation learning in larval zebrafish. *Current Biology*, **29**, 1337-45 e4.

Readman, G.D., Owen, S.F., Knowles, T.G. and Murrell, J.C. (2017). Species specific anaesthetics for fish anaesthesia and euthanasia. *Scientific Reports*, **7**.

Readman, G.D., Owen, S.F., Murrell, J.C. and Knowles, T.G. (2013). Do fish perceive anaesthetics as aversive?. *PLoS One*, **8**.

Roberts, A.C., Chornak, J., Alzagatiti, J.B. et al. (2019). Rapid habituation of a touch-induced escape response in Zebrafish (Danio rerio) Larvae. *PLoS One*, **14**.

Rose, J.D., Arlinghaus, R., Cooke, S.J. et al. (2014). Can fish really feel pain?. *Fish and Fisheries*, **15**, 97–133.

Ruhl, N., McRobert, S.P. and Currie, W.J.S. (2009). Shoaling preferences and the effects of sex ratio on spawning and aggression in small laboratory populations of zebrafish (Danio rerio). *Lab Animal*, **38**, 264–269.

Sanders, J.L., Monteiro, J.F., Martins, S. et al. (2020). The impact of pseudoloma neurophilia infection on body condition of zebrafish. *Zebrafish*, **17**, 139–146.

Sanders, J.L., Watral, V., Clarkson, K. and Kent, M.L. (2013). Verification of intraovum transmission of a microsporidium of vertebrates: Pseudoloma neurophilia infecting the Zebrafish, Danio rerio. *PLoS One*, **8**, e76064.

Schroeder, P., Jones, S., Young, I.S. and Sneddon, L.U. (2014). What do zebrafish want? Impact of social grouping, dominance and gender on preference for enrichment. *Laboratory Animals*, **48**, 328–337.

Schroeder, P. (2016). Exploring suitable analgesics in zebrafish – a combined approach. In: *13th FELASA Congress*, 32. Brussels, Belgium.

Schroeder, P.G. and Sneddon, L.U. (2017). Exploring the efficacy of immersion analgesics in zebrafish using an integrative approach. *Applied Animal Behaviour Science*, **187**, 93–102.

Siccardi, A.J., Garris, H.W., Jones, W.T. et al. (2009). Growth and survival of zebrafish (Danio rerio) fed different commercial and laboratory diets. *Zebrafish*, **6**, 275–280.

Singleman, C. and Holtzman, N.G. (2014). Growth and maturation in the zebrafish, Danio Rerio: A staging tool for teaching and research. *Zebrafish*, **11**, 396–406.

Smith, D.L., Barry, R.J., Powell, M.L. et al. (2013). Dietary protein source influence on body size and composition in growing zebrafish. *Zebrafish*, **10**, 439–446.

Sneddon, L.U. (2003). The evidence for pain in fish: The use of morphine as an analgesic. *Applied Animal Behaviour Science*, **83**, 153–162.

Sneddon, L.U. (2009). Pain perception in fish: Indicators and endpoints. *Ilar Journal*, **50**, 338–342.

Sneddon, L.U. (2011). Pain perception in fish evidence and implications for the use of fish. *Journal of Consciousness Studies*, **18**, 209–229.

Sneddon, L.U. (2012). Clinical anesthesia and analgesia in fish. *Journal of Exotic Pet Medicine*, 21, 32–43.

Sneddon, L.U. (2015). Pain in aquatic animals. *Journal of Experimental Biology*, **218**, 967–976.

Sotocinal, S.G., Sorge, R.E., Zaloum, A. et al. (2011). The Rat Grimace Scale: A partially automated method for quantifying pain in the laboratory rat via facial expressions. *Molecular Pain*, **7**.

Spagnoli, S.T., Xue, L., Murray, K.N. et al. (2015). Pseudoloma neurophilia: a retrospective and descriptive study of nervous system and muscle infections, with new implications for pathogenesis and behavioral phenotypes. *Zebrafish*, **12**, 189–201.

Spence, R., Gerlach, G., Lawrence, C. and Smith, C. (2008). The behaviour and ecology of the zebrafish, Danio rerio. *Biological Reviews*, **83**, 13–34.

Spence, R., Ashton, R. and Smith, C. (2007). Oviposition decisions are mediated by spawning site quality in wild and domesticated zebrafish, Danio rerio'. *Behaviour*, **144**, 953–966.

Spence, R., Magurran, A.E. and Smith, C. (2011). Spatial cognition in zebrafish: The role of strain and rearing environment. *Animal Cognition*, **14**, 607–612.

Spence, R. and Smith, C. (2008). Innate and learned colour preference in the zebrafish, Danio rerio. *Ethology*, **114**, 582–588.

Steenbergen, P.J. (2018). Response of zebrafish larvae to mild electrical stimuli: A 96-well setup for behavioural screening. *Journal of Neuroscience Methods*, **301**, 52–61.

Steenbergen, P.J. and Bardine, N. (2014). Antinociceptive effects of buprenorphine in zebrafish larvae: An alternative for rodent models to study pain and nociception?. *Applied Animal Behaviour Science*, **152**, 92–99.

Strahle, U., Scholz, S., Geisler, R. et al. (2012). Zebrafish embryos as an alternative to animal experiments-A commentary on the definition of the onset of protected life stages in animal welfare regulations. *Reproductive Toxicology*, **33**, 128–132.

Strykowski, J.L. and Schech, J.M. (2015). Effectiveness of recommended euthanasia methods in larval zebrafish (Danio rerio). *Journal of the American Association for Laboratory Animal Science*, **54**, 81–84.

Sundin, J., Morgan, R., Finnoen, M.H. et al. (2019). On the observation of wild zebrafish (Danio rerio) in India. *Zebrafish*, **16**, 546–553.

Suriyampola, P.S., Shelton, D.S., Shukla, R. et al. (2016). Zebrafish social behavior in the Wild. *Zebrafish*, **13**, 1–8.

Suurvali, J., Whiteley, A.R., Zheng, Y.C. et al. (2020). The laboratory domestication of zebrafish: From diverse populations to inbred substrains. *Molecular Biology and Evolution*, **37**, 1056–1069.

Swaim, L.E., Connolly, L.E., Volkman, H.E. et al. (2006). Mycobacterium marinum infection of adult zebrafish causes caseating granulomatous tuberculosis and is moderated by adaptive immunity. *Infection and Immunity*, **74**, 6108–6117.

Taylor, J.C., Dewberry, L.S., Totsch, S.K. et al. (2017). A novel zebrafish-based model of nociception. *Physiology & Behavior*, **174**, 83–88.

Teixido, E., Kiessling, T.R., Krupp, E. et al. (2019). Automated morphological feature assessment for zebrafish embryo developmental toxicity screens. *Toxicological Sciences*, **167**, 438–449.

Thurman, C.E., Rasmussen, S. and Prestia, K.A. (2019). Effect of 3 euthanasia methods on serum yield and serum cortisol concentration in zebrafish (Danio rerio). *Journal of the American Association for Laboratory Animal Science*, **58**, 823–828.

Tilley, C.A., Gutierrez, H.C., Sebire, M. et al. (2020). Skin swabbing is a refined technique to collect DNA from model fish species. *Scientific Reports*, **10**.

Tsang, B., Zahid, H., Ansari, R. et al. (2017). Breeding Zebrafish: A review of different methods and a discussion on standardization. *Zebrafish*, **14**, 561–573.

Tu, S. and Chi, N.C. (2012). Zebrafish models in cardiac development and congenital heart birth defects. *Differentiation*, **84**.

UK Home Office. (2020a). *Annual Statistics of Scientific Procedures on Living Animals, Great Britain 2019*. In UK Home Office (Ed.) (Her Majesty's Stationery Office: ISBN 978-1-5286-2042-0).

UK Home Office. (2020b). Project licence: standard conditions, Home Office. Accessed 21.10.2020.

Ulloa, P.E., Iturra, P., Neira, R. and Araneda, C. (2011). Zebrafish as a model organism for nutrition and growth: Towards comparative studies of nutritional genomics applied to aquacultured fishes. *Reviews in Fish Biology and Fisheries*, **21**, 649–666.

Valentim, A.M., Felix, L.M., Carvalho, L. et al. (2016). A new anaesthetic protocol for adult zebrafish (Danio rerio): Propofol combined with Lidocaine. *PLoS One*, **11**.

Vandenhurk, R. and Lambert, J.G.D. (1983). Ovarian-steroid glucuronides function as sex-pheromones for male Zebrafish, Brachydanio-Rerio. *Canadian Journal of Zoology-Revue Canadienne De Zoologie*, **61**, 2381–2387.

Varga, Z.M. (2011). Aquaculture and husbandry at the Zebrafish International Resource Center. *Zebrafish: Genetics, Genomics and Informatics*, 3rd edn, **104**, 453–478.

Villamizar, N., Vera, L.M., Foulkes, N.S. and Sanchez-Vazquez, F.J. (2014). Effect of lighting conditions on zebrafish growth and development. *Zebrafish*, **11**, 173–181.

von Gersdorff Jorgensen, L. (2016). The dynamics of neutrophils in zebrafish (Danio rerio) during infection with the parasite Ichthyophthirius multifiliis. *Fish Shellfish Immunol*, **55**, 159–164.

von Krogh, K., Higgins, J., Torres, Y.S. and Mocho, J.P. (2021). Screening of anaesthetics in adult zebrafish (Danio rerio) for the induction of euthanasia by overdose. *Biology-Basel*, **10**.

von Krogh, K., Sorensen, C., Nilsson, G.E. and Overli, O. (2010). Forebrain cell proliferation, behavior, and physiology of zebrafish, Danio rerio, kept in enriched or barren environments. *Physiology & Behavior*, **101**, 32–39.

Wafer, L.N., Jensen, V.B., Whitney, J.C., et al. (2016). Effects of environmental enrichment on the fertility and fecundity of zebrafish (Danio rerio). *Journal of the American Association for Laboratory Animal Science*, **55**, 291–294.

Wallace, C.K., Bright, L.A., Marx, J.O., et al. (2018). Effectiveness of rapid cooling as a method of euthanasia for young zebrafish (Danio rerio). *Journal of the American Association for Laboratory Animal Science*, **57**, 58–63.

Watts, S.A., Lawrence, C., Powell, M. and D'Abramo, L.R. (2016). The vital relationship between nutrition and health in zebrafish. *Zebrafish*, **13**, S72–S76.

Watts, S.A., Powell, M. and D'Abramo, L.R. (2012). Fundamental approaches to the study of zebrafish nutrition. *Ilar Journal*, **53**, 144–160.

Westerfield, M. (2007). *The zebrafish Book: A Guide for the Laboratory Use of Zebrafish*. University of Oregon Press, Eugene.

Whipps, C.M., Dougan, S.T. and Kent, M.L. (2007). Mycobacterium haemophilum infections of zebrafish (Danio rerio) in research facilities. *Fems Microbiology Letters*, **270**, 21–26.

Whipps, C.M., Lieggi, C. and Wagner, R. (2012). Mycobacteriosis in zebrafish colonies. *Ilar Journal*, **53**, 95–105.

Whipps, C.M., Matthews, J.L. and Kent, M.L. (2008). Distribution and genetic characterization of Mycobacterium chelonae in laboratory zebrafish Danio rerio. *Diseases of Aquatic Organisms*, **82**, 45–54.

Whiteley, A.R., Bhat, A., Martins, E.P., et al. (2011). Population genomics of wild and laboratory zebrafish (Danio rerio). *Molecular Ecology*, **20**, 4259–4276.

Wilkinson, R.N., Elworthy, S., Ingham, P.W. and van Eeden, F.J.M. (2013). A method for high-throughput PCR-based genotyping of larval zebrafish tail biopsies. *Biotechniques*, **55**, 314–316.

Williams, C.H. and Hong, C.C. (2016). Zebrafish small molecule screens: Taking the phenotypic plunge. *Computational and Structural Biotechnology Journal*, **14**, 350–356.

Wilson, C. and Dunford, K. (2015). Implementation of an integrated zebrafish health management program at the UCL fish facility. In https://static1.squarespace.com/static/58065fb61b631b37ff3ce66a/t/5c52dee7b8a045df091dd44f/1548934893670/LASA+Winter+Meeting+2015.pdf: UCL.

Wilson, C., Dunford, K., Nichols, C., Callaway, H. and Hakkesteeg, J. (2013). Body condition scoring for laboratory zebrafish. *Animal Technology and Welfare*, **12**, 7.

Wilson, C. (2012). Aspects of larval rearing. *Ilar Journal*, **53**, 169–178.

Wilson, C.A., High, S.K., McCluskey, B.M., et al. (2014). Wild sex in zebrafish: Loss of the natural sex determinant in domesticated strains. *Genetics*, **198**, 1291–1308.

Wilson, J.M., Bunte, R.M. and Carty, A.J. (2009). Evaluation of rapid cooling and tricaine methanesulfonate (MS222) as methods of euthanasia in zebrafish (Danio rerio). *Journal of the American Association for Laboratory Animal Science*, **48**, 785–789.

Wong, K., Elegante, M., Bartels, B., et al. (2010). Analyzing habituation responses to novelty in zebrafish (Danio rerio). *Behavioural Brain Research*, **208**, 450–457.

Woodward, M.A., Winder, L.A. and Watt, P. (2019). Enrichment increases aggression in zebrafish. *Fishes*, **4**, 22.

Wynd, B.M., Watson, C.J., Patil, K., Sanders, G.E. and Kwon, R.Y. (2017). A dynamic anesthesia system for long-term imaging in adult zebrafish. *Zebrafish*, **14**, 1–7.

Xu, X.J., Scott-Scheiern, T., Kempker, L. and Simons, K. (2007). Active avoidance conditioning in zebrafish (Danio rerio). *Neurobiology of Learning and Memory*, **87**, 72–77.

Zang, L.Q., Shimada, Y., Nishimura, Y., et al. (2015). Repeated blood collection for blood tests in adult zebrafish. *Jove-Journal of Visualized Experiments*, (102), e53272. doi: 10.3791/53272.

Zeng, X-XI and Zhong, T.P. (2017). Zebrafish. In: *Encyclopedia of Cardiovascular Research and Medicine*. Eds R.S. Vasan and D.B. Sawyer. Elsevier, Amsterdam.

Cephalopoda

50 Cephalopoda

Meghan Holst, Ryan B. Howard and Robyn J. Crook

Foreword

This chapter is an updated and revised version of the previous Cephalopoda chapter in the UFAW handbook, written originally by Peter Boyle for the 7th edition in 1999, and updated by Bernd Budelmann for the 8th in 2010. In the years since the original chapter and its update were published, research into cephalopod mariculture, husbandry and welfare has experienced somewhat of an explosion, with hundreds of new papers appearing in the literature on these topics. Because there are now a number of excellent and recent references on cephalopod phylogeny, anatomy and physiology, in this latest iteration we have streamlined some of the original content on cephalopod physiology and behaviour, and included expanded sections on welfare, housing, enrichment and procedures that reflect updated and expanded knowledge in these areas. In the past ten years, there has also been considerable expansion in the number of species available for use in research labs, and it is not possible to provide comprehensive information on the specific needs for each species. We have instead attempted to provide information that should be widely applicable to those most common species (for example, *Octopus vulgaris, O. bimaculoides, Abdopus spp., Sepia officinalis, S. bandensis, Doryteuthis pealei, Euprymna scolopes*; see for example Figure 50.1), with emphasis on aspects of welfare and husbandry that are particularly important for cephalopods and that differ most significantly from the standard needs of other aquatic species.

Biological overview

General biology

Phylogeny

Cephalopods appear in the fossil record about 530 mya, having evolved from a monoplacophoran-like mollusc through conversion of their external shell into a buoyancy apparatus (Kröger *et al.* 2011). Today, the classes Nautiloidea and Coleoidea contain the roughly 800 described, extant species of cephalopods today.

Nautiluses, of the subclass Nautiloidea, are often referred to as 'living fossils' due to their early diversification and primitive appearance. They are easily recognisable among cephalopods as the only ectocochleate group, or lineage that retained their external shells. Though fossil evidence suggests nautiluses were once prolific in the oceans there are now only two accepted genera, Allonautilus and nautilus (Ward & Saunders 1997).

Coleoidea appeared more recently in the Devonian, and includes all extant cuttlefish, squid, and octopuses. Coleoidea contains two superorders: Decapodiformes and Octopodiformes. Decapodiformes refers to the 10 appendages present in cuttlefish and squid, which all have 8 arms and 2 tentacles. The five orders that comprise Decapodiformes are Spirulida (ram's horn squid), Sepiida (cuttlefish), Myopsida ('closed eye' or inshore squids), Oegopsida ('open eye' or pelagic squid) and Sepiolida (bobtail squids). Octopodiformes likewise refers to the eight limbs present in species of octopuses. There are two orders, Octopoda and Vampyromorpha (Strugnell *et al.* 2005; Strugnell & Nishiguchi 2007). The main order of octopuses that receives attention for their laboratory uses is Octopoda. Most decapods found in research laboratories belong to either Sepiolida or Sepiida, which are highly amenable to culture from eggs, or Myopsida, which are invariably wild-caught. Sepiida, the cuttlefish, are also used extensively and are popular laboratory animals due to their relative ease of culture from eggs.

Anatomy

Cephalopods share certain basic features of their body organisation with the gastropods, bivalves and other molluscs. The typical molluscan shell originally present in the cephalopods is greatly reduced or lost in the modern forms, as it is in some other molluscan lines, such as many marine gastropods and the terrestrial slugs. The radula, a ribbon of chitinous teeth which functions in gastropods and chitons as a versatile feeding organ for rasping or scraping, is one of the most characteristic molluscan features. It is present,

---

The UFAW Handbook on the Care and Management of Laboratory and Other Research Animals, Ninth Edition.
Edited by Huw Golledge and Claire Richardson.
© 2024 John Wiley & Sons Ltd. Published 2024 by John Wiley & Sons Ltd.

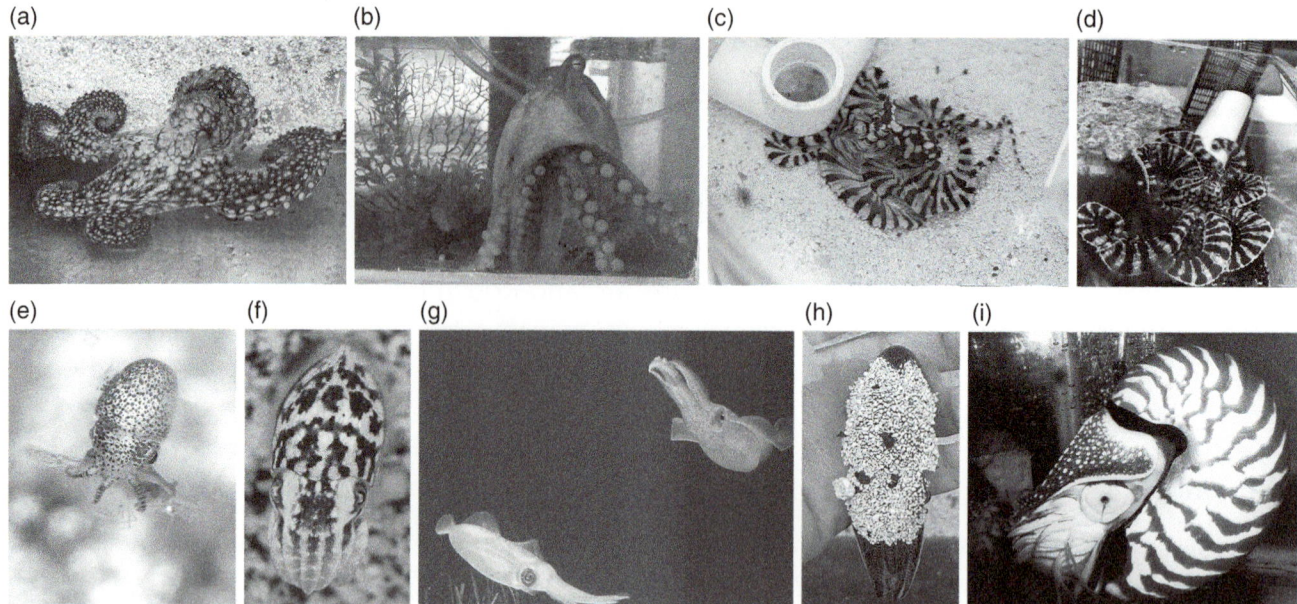

Figure 50.1 Representatives of common species used in research laboratories and found in public aquaria. (a) *Abdopus aculeatus*. (b) *Octopus bimaculoides*. (c) *Wunderpus photogenicus*. (d) *Thaumoctopus mimicus*. (e) *Euprymna scolopes*. (f) *Sepia bandensis*. (g) *Sepioteuthis sepioidea*. (h) *Euprymna berryi*. (i) *Nautilus pompilius*. Source: Images: Robyn Crook, except B., courtesy of Lisa Abbo.

too, in all cephalopods, although its role in feeding may be subsidiary to other structures. From here, the anatomical differences among cephalopod species grow quickly, so the general anatomy of Nautiloids and Coleoids will be handled separately.

Nautiloids are the only extant cephalopods with external shells, which are divided into a series of chambers by calcareous septa or partitions. The last and largest chamber is occupied by the body, which allows the head to retract into the heavily calcified shell and protects the animal from predatory attacks. When retracted, modified tentacles form a hood that closes the shell's opening (Ward 1987). The 90 or more tentacles (depending on species) are attached to the anterior part of the head and house the buccal mass at their base. The buccal mass, like other coleoids, contains the radula, beak and mandibular muscles. The hyponome (funnel) extends from the shell ventral to the head and is used in propulsion. Nautiluses do not have an ink sac, and there is little external sexual dimorphism.

All coleoids have lost the external shell and its protective functions. Instead, they rely on rapid locomotion, their dynamically camouflaging skin and ink secreting organs as their primary means of defence. Unique to coleoids are their pigment containing organs, chromatophores, which are used to change skin colour (Messenger 2001). Chromatophores may work in conjunction with papillae, hydrostatic muscles that change skin texture (Allen *et al*. 2014), to alter the appearance of the animal (although deep-water species may have absent or greatly reduced chromatophores and papillae, and instead may have photophores and other bioluminescent skin elements for camouflage and signalling (Johnsen *et al*. 1999; Robison *et al*. 2003; Bush *et al*. 2009)). Most coleoids, *Cirrina* and *vampyroteuthidae* excluded, have an ink sac. Key anatomical features are illustrated in Figure 50.2.

Nervous system

The nervous system of cephalopods is among the largest and most complex of all the invertebrates, both in terms of raw number of cells and in the number of different lobes. The brain mass/body mass ratio surpasses that of the primitive or lower vertebrates (Nixon & Young 2003; Hanlon & Messenger 2018). In general, the nervous system consists of a large central brain located between the eyes, along with multiple peripheral ganglia with varying degrees of elaboration within the mantle and arms. While each clade of the coleoid cephalopods shows some specialisations to their nervous systems, their general anatomy and function are similar. The nautiloid nervous system is considerably different, being both smaller and less elaborated than that of the coleoids (Nixon & Young 2003).

Nautiloids

The nautilus brain is a simple ring-like structure that circles the oesophagus (Young 1965). Unlike in coleoids, where the brain is easily accessible for surgical and other manipulations, the nautilus brain is deep in the solid muscle tissue under the hood, and in normal anatomical position is caudal to the uppermost part of the shell. It is, therefore, difficult to access the brain without removing the animal from its shell.

A single supraesophageal cord connects diffuse optic and olfactory lobes located lateral and dorsal on the cord, and relatively few nerves radiate from this part of the CNS. The lateral parts of the brain encompass lobes hypothetically involved in motor control and sensory integration (Young 1965), although these presumptions are based on structural and positional analogy to better studied regions of the coleoid brain, and their actual function in nautilus is unstudied. The suboesophageal cord is divided into an

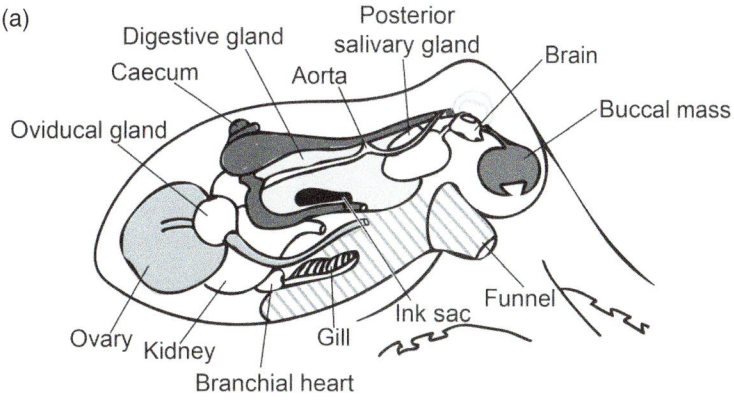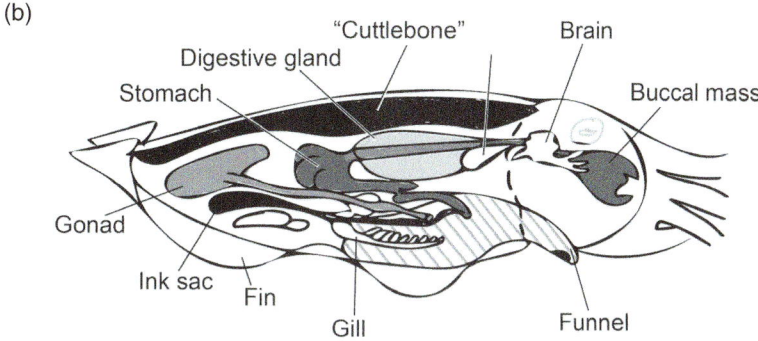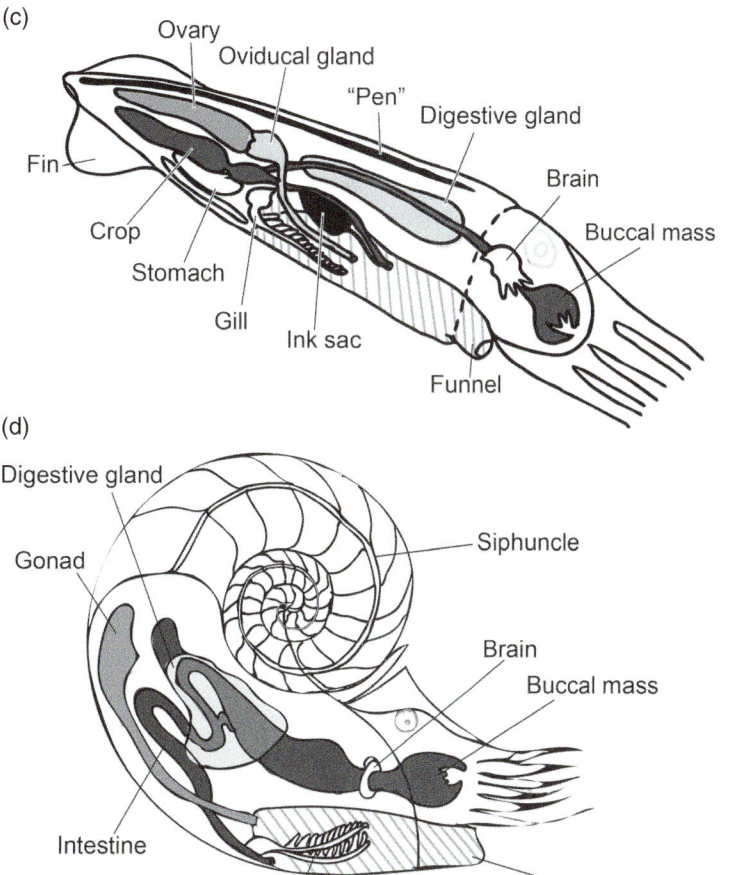

Figure 50.2 Sketch plan of the gross anatomy of the four major groups of cephalopods. (a) Octopus, (b) Cuttlefish, (c) Squid and (d) Nautilus. Source: Modified from the 8th Edition.

anterior and posterior ring, with multiple nerves radiating rostrally and caudally, respectively. Notably absent from the nautiloid brain are defined supraesophageal lobes, which in coleoids govern executive processing and potentially, affective states. However, although structurally these regions appear absent, there are no published records of neurophysiological function of the nautiloid brain, and thus it is impossible to rule out these abilities in nautilus. Notably, several studies have demonstrated learning and memory abilities in nautilus that are equivalent to those of coleoid cephalopods (Crook & Basil 2008a; Crook & Basil 2008b; Crook et al. 2009; Crook & Basil 2013), indicating that the dedicated 'learning and memory' lobes found in the coleoid brain have functional equivalents in the much simpler nautiloid brain. Thus, we caution that although much of the justification for welfare concern in cephalopods is grounded in rationales based on neural complexity of coleoids, nautiloids should be given equal consideration when considering welfare.

Nautiloid sense organs are likewise simpler than those of coleoids. The eye is a simple 'pinhole-camera' type, with no lens or cornea. The pupil opens directly to seawater and the retina contains only photoreceptors, as is the case for all cephalopods (Yamamoto et al. 1965; Gray 1970; Muntz & Raj 1984). The eyes are adapted to low light levels and the pupillary reflex is slow, in the order of minutes (Muntz & Raj 1984; Muntz 2010). The olfactory sense, in contrast to that of vision, is quite well-developed in nautiloids. Each of the tentacles is covered in both contact and distance chemoreceptors, and nautilus are adept at tracking odour plumes over quite long distances (Basil et al. 2000; Basil et al. 2002; Basil et al. 2005). The olfactory lobe is larger, comparatively, than that of coleoids, and presumably this is the primary sensory modality of these deep-water cephalopods (Young 1965).

Coleoids

In coleoids, the brain is greatly expanded compared with nautiloids, with distinct divisions between lobes. For octopus, there are an estimated 500 million neurons, although approximately 2/3 are outside the central brain mass (Young 1963; Nixon & Young 2003). A great deal of information is available on the neuroanatomy of the system and the division of function between the many lobes.

The traditional view of the coleoid brain is that the suboesophageal areas of the brain are concerned with the control of groups of muscles, while the supraesophageal lobes are concerned with higher motor centres and cognitive function (Boycott & Young 1955; Young 1960, 1962; Young & Boycott 1971). However, these functional divisions are likely to be oversimplifications, and the application of novel neurobiological and genetic tools are likely to permit more nuanced understanding of structure/function relationships in the coleoid brain (Shigeno et al. 2008; Shigeno et al. 2010; Shigeno & Ragsdale 2015).

It is certainly true that there are clear divisions of function between various lobes. Groups of muscles known to be controlled from centres in the suboesophageal brain include those of the arms, mantle, head, funnel, fins and chromatophores (Young 1976). Some regions are allocated to receptor information and analysis. Most notable of these are the optic lobes, large ganglionic masses located laterally on each side of the brain and receiving large numbers of small optic nerves (Young 1962). The optic lobes are primarily concerned with processing incoming visual information; however, recent evidence suggests they also play a role in control of body patterning (Liu & Chiao 2017) and memory storage (Sanders 1975; Chrachri & Williamson 2004; Marini et al. 2017). Olfactory lobes are present although much smaller than the very large optic lobes, reflecting the heavy investment in vision as a sensory modality of great importance to coleoids.

In addition to the brain is a series of peripheral ganglionic masses. These are extensive and contain enormous numbers of nerve cells with functions primarily concerned with systems where they are located. For example, there are an estimated 3×10^8 in the nerve cords of the arms alone, and these ganglia govern local movements of the arms and suckers, including complex, co-ordinated movements involved in grasping, prey handling and defensive withdrawal (Matzner 2000; Sumbre et al. 2001; Gutfreund et al. 2006; Hague et al. 2013; Nesher et al. 2014). The main ganglionic masses in a typical octopod are shown in Figure 50.3. Certain movements of the arms (Rowell 1963; Rowell 1966; Matzner 2000; Sumbre et al. 2001; Gutfreund et al. 2006), mantle (Gray 1960) and buccal mass (Boyle 1983) take place in isolation from the central nervous system.

Sense organs

The skin of coleoids, particularly of the suckers and lips, is liberally supplied with receptor cells responsive to tactile and chemical stimuli. Octopuses are responsive to a very light touch on almost any part of the surface, and may be taught to discriminate between objects which differ only in the quality of surface texture (Wells 1959; Wells & Young 1975). Mechanically sensitive cells are known also to be located within the blocks of somatic muscle (Alexandrowicz 1960; Graziadei 1965), and in the skin and superficial tissues in octopuses (Gray 1960; Alupay et al. 2014; Perez et al. 2017), cuttlefishes (Kier & Messenger 1985) and squid (Crook et al. 2013). Mechanonociceptors, neurons tuned specifically to damaging or noxious mechanical stimuli, have also been described in octopus and squid, and presumably are also present in cuttlefish (Crook et al. 2013; Alupay et al. 2014). There is currently no evidence for either thermal or chemical nociceptors in any cephalopod species.

Both contact and distance chemoreceptors are present in cephalopods, and are involved in feeding (Boal & Golden 1999; Anraku et al. 2005; Hanlon & Shashar 2008; van Giesen et al. 2020), detection and recognition or conspecifics (Walderon et al. 2011), and detection of predators (Gilly & Lucero 1992; Fouke & Rhodes 2020). Discrimination between objects can be made on the basis of chemical differences (Wells 1963; Wells & Young 1965; Gutnick et al. 2011).

Cephalopods have large camera-type eyes placed laterally and dorsally. There is a highly refractile spherical lens which focuses light onto a retina of receptive cells (Nautilus operates on the different principle of the 'pinhole' camera.). General accounts of cephalopod behaviour, and experimental studies on prey capture (Chiao et al. 2015; Almansa et al. 2017) confirm the importance of visual input to

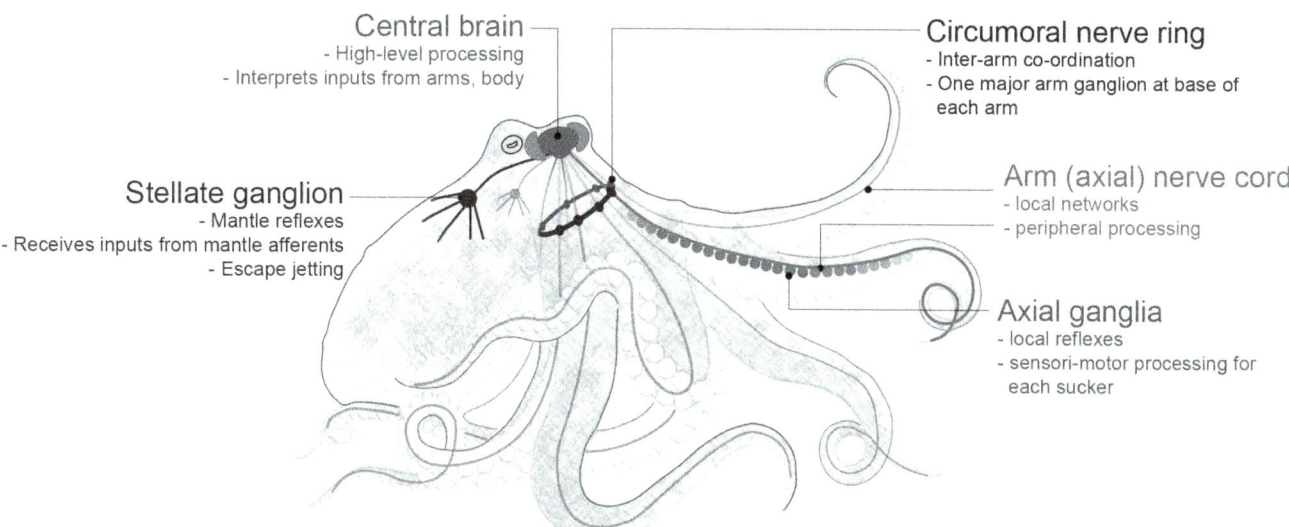

Figure 50.3 Schematic of the principal ganglionic masses of the octopus and their principal functions.

cephalopods. There are also well-known examples of the role played by visual stimuli in sexual recognition by *Sepia* (Hall & Hanlon 2002). Visual acuity is high (Packard 1969), and although still somewhat controversial, most evidence suggests cephalopods are colourblind (Hanlon & Shashar 2008; Chiao et al. 2011). The recent discovery of extra-ocular opsins in the skin of cephalopods (Mäthger et al. 2010; Ramirez & Oakley 2015) and theoretical work on the unique shape of the cephalopod pupil (Stubbs & Stubbs 2016) has only deepened the mystery of how cephalopods achieve their exceptional colour-matching camouflage abilities, as the photopigment found in these receptors has the same spectral sensitivity as in the eye.

Chromatophores and other skin elements

Cephalopods are important laboratory animal models for studies of vision, visual signalling and camouflage. At the centre of such studies is the remarkable dynamic skin colouration achieved by many shallow-water cephalopods, mediated by various elements within the skin. These include chromatophores, iridophores and leucophores, pigmentary and structural elements that determine skin colour (Messenger 2001; Hanlon & Messenger 2018), and papillae, muscular hydrostats that control skin texture (Allen et al. 2014). These elements are under direct neural control (Dubas & Boyle 1985; Saidel & Monsell 1986; Novicki et al. 1990; Wardill et al. 2012; Gonzalez-Bellido et al. 2018), allowing for almost instantaneous changes in colour, reflectance and texture in response to changes in the visual environment (Barbosa et al. 2008; Allen et al. 2009; Chiao et al. 2015). Skin colour, texture and tone are useful outward indicators of animal health. Paralysis of regions of chromatophores can indicate local tissue infection, nerve damage or the onset of senescence (Sanders & Young 1974; Saidel & Monsell 1986; Andrews et al. 2013; Imperadore et al. 2017), where skin quality declines gradually at first and then severely towards the end of life (see senescence, later in this chapter).

Diet, digestion and excretion

Cephalopods are obligate carnivores, and the overwhelming majority are active hunters. Diets of wild cephalopods are comprised primarily of crustaceans, fish and molluscs, which are mostly taken as live prey throughout the cephalopod lifespan. While crustaceans are believed to be the preferred prey of most cephalopod species (Boucaud-Camou & Boucher-Rodoni 1966), and key in sustaining their demanding growth requirements, the reason is still unclear (Iglesias et al. 2014; Villanueva et al. 2014). Additional reports exist of cephalopods eating polychaete worms, hydroids, echinoderms and gelatinous fauna (Hoving & Haddock 2017; Olmos-Pérez et al. 2017). Furthermore, certain species of cephalopods scavenge and eat dead prey, like some deep-sea cephalopods that have elongated filaments, which serve to catch detritus (Hoving & Haddock 2017).

After ingestion, the already fragmented meal enters a rather short digestive tract consisting of a crop in some taxa, then stomach, caecum and intestine. Some digestion takes place within the lumen of the gut, but most digestion and absorption take place in the large digestive gland (Boucaud-Camou & Boucher-Rodoni 1966; Sykes et al. 2017). Entry into the gland of food particles and the egress of excretory material into the gut lumen occur through a pair of short ducts connecting the digestive gland to the caecum. Long strings of pigmented faeces (the residues of the digestive process, usually pink–brown depending on diet composition) bound by mucus, are released from the anus into the exhalent water flow.

Digestive excretion occurs by the release of pigmented material from digestive gland cells into the lumen of the gut (Boucaud-Camou & Boucher-Rodoni 1966). Excretion from the blood system occurs via excretory tissue surrounding the lateral venae cavae (Schipp et al. 1975). The main venous return from the anterior part of the body, the anterior vena cava, divides into two lateral venae cavae before entering the branchial heart of each side. The excretory cells (kidney tissues) are grouped into flocculent masses (renal appendages) sited on fine diverticula of the lateral venae cavae. The urine is formed, probably by ultrafiltration and secretion, into a coelomic pericardial space, from which it drains into the mantle cavity through a short duct and renal papilla. Little is known about the composition and flow of urine.

Reproduction

Cephalopods are gonochoristic (dioecious), and oviparous, and fertilisation is achieved by direct mating. Various reviews of the details of reproduction are available (Arnold & Williams-Arnold 1977; Wells & Wells 1977; Rocha et al. 2001).

Sexual maturity is controlled by secretion of hormones from the optic gland that drive the maturation of ovary and testis (Di Cosmo & Di Cristo 1998; Di Cosmo et al. 2001; Polese et al. 2015), and is generally irreversible once begun. At the onset of sexual maturity, there is an apparently rapid process of gonad growth, yolk secretion and ripening of accessory glandular systems. To some degree, sexual maturity is controlled by body size and water temperature, giving it a seasonal aspect (Martins 1982; Lipiński & Underhill 1995; Hernández-García et al. 2002; Otero et al. 2007).

In the male, ripe sperm are packaged into complicated spermatophores and stored in a special spermatophoric (Needham's) sac until mating occurs. The male transfers sperm to the female by passing ripe spermatophores along a muscular groove in one arm which becomes modified for this function (the hectocotylus, hectocotylised arm) at sexual maturity (Thompson & Voight 2003; Wodinsky 2008; Huffard & Godfrey-Smith 2010; Figure 50.4).

The course of fertilisation after mating varies among different cephalopod types. Sperm may be held by the female in special pouches at the base of the arms or within the mantle cavity (sepioids and squid) (Ikeda et al. 1993; Shaw & Sauer 2004; Hoving et al. 2010; Sato et al. 2010; Bush et al. 2012), or enter the female genital tract and lodge in the oviducal glands (octopus) (Froesch & Marthy 1975; Tosti et al. 2001; Di Cristo & Di Cosmo 2007; Olivares et al. 2017), or even pass into the ovary itself (Eledone) (Boyle & Knobloch 1983; Perez & Haimovici 1991; Boyle & Chevis 1992). These mechanisms allow the possibility of opportunistic matings and sperm storage in cephalopods. The longest interval between mating and egg laying was recorded in Octopus tetricus at 114 days (Joll 1976).

Multiple matings and multiple paternity of broods seems to be the norm for most cephalopod species (Shaw & Boyle 1997; Buresch et al. 2001; Quinteiro et al. 2011; Naud et al. 2016). The sperm storage organs of females may contain spermatophores from many males, but mechanisms of sperm selection and sperm competition are not completely understood (Naud et al. 2005; Squires et al. 2014).

Post-laying care of eggs varies among the different taxa. In octopuses, care of egg masses is obligate for their survival. Females lay eggs either in dens, where they remain to aerate and groom the eggs until they hatch, or hold egg masses in a protective posture in their arms while they rest on the substrate (Boletzky 1998; Rocha et al. 2001; Drazen et al. 2003). Females almost always fast during egg care and die shortly after eggs hatch. Incubation periods for octopuses vary from a typical 1–3 months for shallow-water tropical species, to an astounding 53 months, reported in the deep-sea octopus Graneledone (Robison et al. 2014). Squid and cuttlefish typically lay eggs adhered to the substrate or to sea grasses, where they incubate with no further parental care. Egg masses may be coated in protective biofilms to inhibit the growth of pathogenic bacteria and fungi (Gomathi et al. 2010; Gromek et al. 2016; Kerwin & Nyholm 2017), and they are protected from predators either by being concealed in tight spaces (Boletzky 1998), or laid in such vast aggregations that predation has minimal impact on overall reproductive success (Augustyn 1990; Sauer & Smale 1991; Sauer et al. 1992). Some exceptions to these general rules are known; the

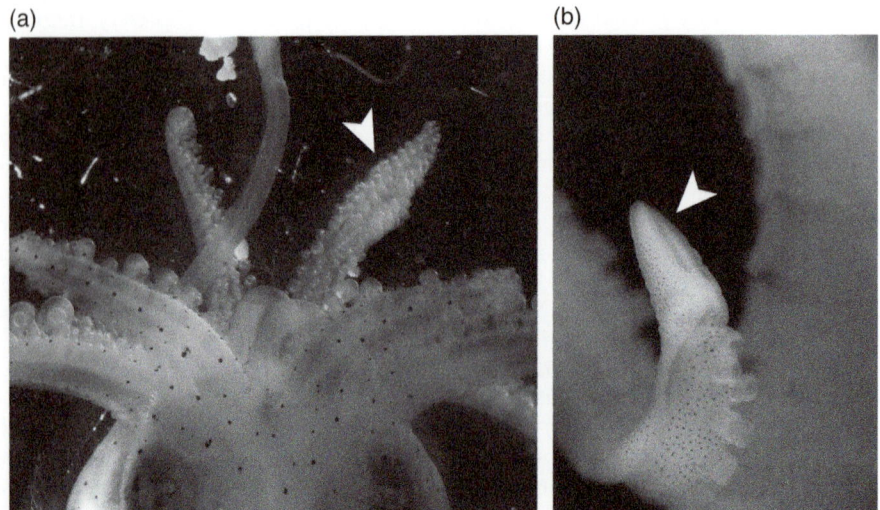

Figure 50.4 Reproductive arm modifications of two male cephalopods. (a) A hectocotylised arm of the sepiolid Euprymna scolopes. Ventral view showing the underside of arm L1 (arrowhead), which is shortened, thickened and displays tightly packed, long-stalked suckers at its tip. This arm is inserted into mantle cavity of the female during mating. (b) The ligula of the tropical pygmy octopus O. bocki. Arm R3 is modified at its tip be bare of suckers. A groove in the skin of the arm provides a channel for the spermatophore to move before it is placed into the female's ˙le cavity by the arm tip.

deep-sea squid, *Gonatus onyx*, for example, broods its eggs by holding them in its arms as it swims (Seibel *et al.* 2005), and the octopus Argonauta secretes a shell-like encasement to protect its eggs until hatching (Finn & Norman 2010). In all cases, there is no post-hatching parental care, and hatchlings are independent, actively swimming hunters from the moment they hatch.

Uses in research

Legislation and regulation

As of the time of writing, at least some cephalopod species and life stages are regulated in nearly all major research nations and all nations within the EU. The notable exception to this rule is the USA, where no invertebrate species is included currently in federal research regulations.

In general, the motivation for inclusion of cephalopods in national or federal regulations governing welfare relates to their relative complexity compared with other invertebrates, and with that, the likely capacity for pain, suffering and distress. There is a clear need for further research work elucidating the capacities of cephalopods for higher cognitive and emotional states relevant to welfare, as far as possible within the existing legal frameworks that now exist for cephalopod research. Additionally, research work that develops refinements to all research-related procedures is imperative and sorely needed at the time of writing.

Different nations and regulatory agencies have different thresholds and definitions for procedures using cephalopods. Readers are urged to refer to their institutional, local and federal agencies for clear indications on what specific activities involving cephalopods are likely to be regulated or require approval. For EU members, detailed information on procedures, endpoint and severity assessments may be found in Fiorito *et al.* 2015 and Cooke *et al.* 2019.

General husbandry

Acquisition, capture and transport of cephalopods

Few research laboratories have access to captive bred stocks of cephalopods, although there are growing efforts, at the time of writing, to develop sustainable cultures of a selection of species for use in research, including cuttlefish, octopuses and sepiolids. However, most research laboratories rely on wild-caught adults or wild-collected eggs. Methods for collection of wild cephalopods vary. Most octopuses and sepiolids are collected by hand. Loliginid squids and deeper water species may be collected by trawl nets, which results in considerable physical trauma and high mortality. *Octopus vulgaris* and other coastal octopuses are often sourced from local fisheries using pot traps, which allows for animals to be captured in good physical condition with minimal stress. Regardless of capture method, a universal drawback of wild-collected specimens is unknown genetic background, age and previous history; for experiments in physiology and behaviour, these sources of variation can be considerable.

Transportation and shipping of cephalopods presents several serious welfare-related concerns. Cephalopods have unusually high metabolic rates and voracious appetites, which results in rapid water fouling. Compounding the rapid degradation of water quality is some cephalopod species' propensity to ink when stressed or jostled; two things that are common during packing and shipping. Ink contains high levels of ammonia (Derby *et al.* 2007; Derby 2014), which is toxic in even very low concentrations.

Minimising water fouling is best done by packing animals for transport in relatively large volumes of water. In general, the bottom 1/3 of a large shipping bag should be filled with water and the top 2/3 either with compressed air or oxygen. Bags should be double or triple layered to avoid punctures from cephalopods chewing through the bags (this is particularly common with nautiluses), and packed within insulated containers with either heat or cold packs, depending on the water temperature. Octopuses should always be packed singly. Squid and cuttlefish may tolerate being packed in pairs if female or immature, but singly is preferable. Cephalopods should not be fed immediately prior to transport as this risks accelerating water fouling (Figure 50.5), but prolonged fasting is also inadvisable due to cephalopods' high metabolic rates.

Upon arrival, acclimation to local water conditions is essential. If animals are to be housed in an 'open' seawater system that is of the same general parameters as those of the capture location, only temperature acclimation is necessary. This can be achieved by floating the shipping bags in the

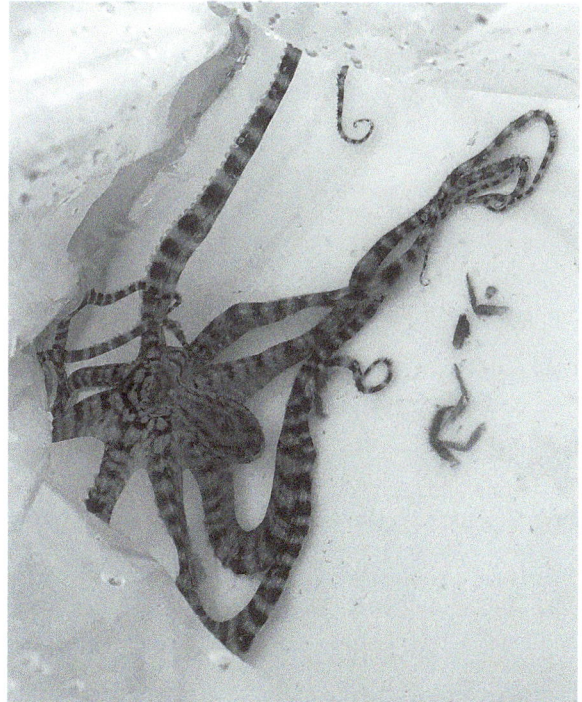

Figure 50.5 An octopus (*Thaumoctopus mimicus*) with crab legs and other detritus in the shipping bag upon arrival. This animal was likely fed shortly before shipping and was carrying uneaten crab parts in the arm crown. Discarded food and faeces contribute to fouling of shipping water. Feeding animals shortly before shipping should be avoided if possible.

tank water to equilibrate the temperature of the shipping water to the tank water, and then animals can be released. In 'closed' or recirculating seawater systems, gradual drip acclimation is recommended, where water from the housing system is mixed progressively into the shipping water, until all the shipping water has been replaced. This process typically takes several hours, depending on the distance between the shipping water and home tank water in terms of pH, salinity, alkalinity and temperature.

During transport, animals consume the oxygen in the transport water and thus indirectly slow the ionisation of ammonium to ammonia. However, if the transport water is over oxygenated, or oxygenated quickly upon acclimation at the destination, oxygen can quickly convert ammonium to ammonia. For this reason, it is important not to over oxygenate the transport water prior to shipment, and acclimation should use air stones with ambient air as opposed to pure oxygen. Air stones may present their own issues as well, as air bubbles can become trapped in the mantle and cause buoyancy dysregulation. Air stones, if used, should be placed in an area inaccessible to the animal, and close to the water surface.

Maintenance, housing and colony management

A standard terminology was adopted by Boletkzy and Hanlon (1983) to describe the various phases of holding cephalopods in captivity.

- *Maintenance*: Holding wild-caught late juvenile or adult stages at the same approximate developmental stage for varying periods of time, with no specific intention of growing them to more advanced stages.
- *Rearing*: Growing a cephalopod over a certain period of time without reaching production of a second generation.
- *Culture*: Growing a cephalopod at least from hatching through the complete life cycle (juvenile and adult stages, sexual maturity, mating and egg laying), to hatching viable young of the first filial (F1) generation.

Although the term culture is also used collectively to refer to the whole process, these aspects of holding cephalopods in the laboratory will be dealt with separately.

Enclosures

Most cephalopods are not communal animals; some species aggregate in the wild and will tolerate group housing, but no cephalopod species is truly social. Some common lab cephalopods, such as *Euprymna spp.* and *Sepia spp.* can be kept together before they become sexually mature, when aggressive interactions between males and male harassment of females impairs welfare (Hanlon *et al.* 1997). Most species of cuttlefish may be held in communal tanks throughout all life stages (Panetta *et al.* 2017), although again, the onset of sexual maturity can result in aggression, which is detrimental to animal welfare. All octopus species that are used commonly in laboratory settings are obligately solitary, and may be stressed by the presence of neighbours (Hanlon & Forsythe 2008). In general, visual isolation is sufficient to minimise stress, with most successful housing arrangements permitting the continuous flow of water among visually isolated enclosures without apparent harm.

Space requirements vary considerably depending on the species and life-stage to be housed. 'Space' here refers to enclosure size, not to total water volume, which almost invariably should be far larger than the individual enclosure volume. Some cephalopods, such as squid and cuttlefish, need housing that is large enough for normal swimming behaviour to occur (including startle and escape jetting) without risking injuries to their skin against enclosure walls. Pelagic squid species are particularly difficult to keep. Even when large enclosures are provided for pelagic species, maintaining them for long periods is considered extremely challenging and is typically only attempted at large marine stations with access to free-flowing seawater and very large tank sizes. Some other squid species exhibit behaviours more tractable to laboratory housing, for example, the bobtail squids (sepiolids) in the genera *Rossia* and *Euprymna* (Hanlon *et al.* 1997). Sepiolids are growing in popularity as laboratory animals, partly because they can be housed in relatively high densities and are more sedentary than the myopsid squids.

Enclosure shape is also of critical importance. For frequently swimming species such as squid and cuttlefish, enclosures with sharp corners should be avoided. Instead, they do best in circular or oval enclosures, particularly as hatchlings and juveniles. Octopuses and other benthic species can more readily utilise enclosures with corners, which are often found in commercially available rack systems. For any octopus enclosure, preventing escapes is vital; many octopuses will attempt to explore above the water surface, and are adept at removing unsecured lids and squeezing through any small space. Tightly fitted lids over enclosures are necessary, or where lids are impractical or not available, porous material glued just above the water surface can prevent sucker adhesion to tank walls, and thus prevent escapes. Artificial turf, Velcro and other porous materials are popular for this purpose, but should be used with care as there have been occasional reports of skin irritation. The vertical extent must be longer than the reach of the arm to be effective.

Likewise outflows to drains and filtration systems must be enclosed; the 'rule of thumb' is that any opening larger than the size of animals' eye can be an escape risk. Wrapping outflows in mesh or filling gaps with well-secured sponge material is usually sufficient to prevent escapes. In addition, any exposed pump impellers or moving parts represent entanglement and injury risks to arms, which can be probed into even the smallest of spaces; these should also be shielded by mesh or placed in non-housing areas of tank systems, such as sumps.

Water quality

In marine systems other than those of single-pass, flow-through design, there are challenges in maintaining good water quality. In closed-loop or recirculating systems, the accumulation of nitrogenous and phosphate waste products must be managed, which requires extensive filtration systems and careful, daily monitoring for abnormal water quality values.

Rates of water 'turnover' (the number of times per hour the full water volume transits a given point, such as a circulation pump or filter) provide a basic indication of how effectively wastes may be removed from the water volume. Turnover rates should vary with the type of animals housed, enclosure size and setup, and total water volume. There is no single rule as to what turnover rate is correct or ideal for a given species, life-stage, enclosure size or temperature, but it should be sufficient to effectively and promptly remove waste, while also supplying appropriate flow for natural behaviours. Inadequate flow can result in the build-up of waste in the housing enclosure and poor oxygenation. Excessive flow may interfere with feeding and other natural behaviours, or cause physical injury from washing against hard surfaces. Careful monitoring of water chemistry parameters, animal behaviour and general physical condition should be employed to identify correct water flow parameters for each system.

While all fish and aquatic invertebrates require good water quality to maintain good welfare status, cephalopods are especially sensitive to water quality outside of healthy parameters. Water quality should be tested regularly and issues correctly promptly. In recirculating systems, the maintenance of biological as well as physical and chemical filtration, is essential for maintaining animal health.

There are many good guides on biofiltration, nutrient cycling and management of organic waste in enclosed seawater systems, so only brief information is given here. A comprehensive overview of system types for cephalopods and water quality parameters is given in Fiorito et al. (2015).

Nitrogenous waste

The nitrogen cycle is a natural phenomenon whereby bacteria consume, and thus remove, nitrogenous waste from its environment. Nitrogenous waste is present in the marine environment as ammonia, ammonium, nitrite and nitrate. Each form of nitrogen becomes less toxic, respectively.

Nitrogenous waste accumulates in fixed water volumes from the decomposition of food, faeces and detritus. Cephalopods are known as being 'messy eaters', discarding non-preferred pieces of prey and producing copious faecal matter. Unless waste produces are removed daily from housing enclosures by siphoning or hand collection, nitrogenous waste can be hard to manage even in a tank with excellent biological filtration. Nitrogenous waste begins in the form of ammonium (NH_4) and ammonia (NH_3). Ammonia is the ionised form and is more toxic than unionised ammonium. Both ammonium and ammonia are present in seawater, and are often referred to as 'total ammonia nitrogen' (TAN). Ammonium is converted to ammonia when pH rises and as oxygen is more readily available. Ammonia (NH_3) converts to nitrite (NO_2) and nitrate (NO_3) as it is oxidised by denitrifying bacteria (Guerdat et al. 2011). Once nitrogenous waste is in the form of nitrate, it is most easily removed by regular water changes.

Cephalopods may tolerate traces of ammonia for extended periods, and can withstand higher levels for short periods (during shipping, for example). However, ideally housing water should be maintained at 0.00 ppm ammonia (Potts 1965; Luke et al. 2014), Concentrations of ammonia outside of the acceptable range indicate the need for an immediate water change, followed by investigation to locate the source of the contamination, often a dead animal or a piece of decaying food that has been missed in daily cleaning. Ammonia levels should drop rapidly if denitrifying bacteria are present in the system and proactive clean-up occurs as soon as a spike in level is detected.

Nitrite (NO_2), while less toxic than ammonia, should also be closely monitored. A healthy system should remain between 0.01 and 0.05 ppm. System water should never reach above 0.1 ppm, and will have negative health implications when left unmitigated (Boyle 1981; Hanlon & Forsythe 1985; Lee et al. 1998). Nitrate (NO_3) is the least toxic form of nitrogenous waste. Even though higher concentrations of nitrate can be tolerated, levels should not exceed 20 ppm. Nitrate levels higher than 20 ppm have been documented to cause distress in cephalopods specifically, and may cause repetitive inking in some species (Hanley et al. 1998; Luke et al. 2014; Fiorito et al. 2015). Nitrate can be consumed by vegetation, if grown in the same water as the housing system, but it most efficiently removed through regular water changes.

pH

Cephalopods will typically do best within a pH range equivalent to that of natural seawater, between 8.0 and 8.3. Values outside of these ranges can be tolerated, but should not reach outside 7.5–8.5. pH values outside of this range will have negative physiological effects on cephalopods even after short exposures; in cephalopods, binding of oxygen to the blood pigment haemocyanin is highly dependent on pH (Lykkeboe et al. 1980; Bridges 1995), and variations in pH outside normal ranges can have rapid negative effects on health. pH varies with salinity and temperature, and is stabilised by water alkalinity. Maintaining adequate levels of alkalinity can be aided by the addition of crushed coral (calcium carbonate) to tank floors, or in mesh bags within sumps or filtration sections. Alternatively, regular testing and buffering of the water is effective to maintain alkalinity levels over 180 mg/L.

Dissolved oxygen

Oxygen saturation in cephalopod housing systems should remain above 90% at all times. Levels are temperature dependent, and most cephalopods can tolerate short-term variations; however, levels below 65% can cause stress, especially when exposed chronically (Lee et al. 1998; Cerezo Valverde & García García 2005). Oxygen levels can be improved by providing adequate enclosure turnover and by adding aerators within the system. Aerators such as air stones should be placed carefully to ensure that water turbulence does not impede the natural swimming behaviour of the animal, and does not embolise the animal by entrapping bubbles within the mantle. Octopuses will play with objects placed in their enclosures (Kuba et al. 2006), which includes air stones, and are thus at risk of air entrapment. Healthy animals seem mostly able to avoid this problem, perhaps because they can clear air by cleaning the mantle cavity with their arms. Cuttlefish and squid, which are unable to reach arms into their mantle cavities, can accumulate trapped air by swimming through bubble clouds. Animals that seem unable to swim downwards from the water surface or who swim in midwater with an elevated caudal mantle should be investigated for trapped air. Gently holding the animal vertically with the head uppermost while submerged should release the air bubbles through the siphon or mantle opening at the neck.

Lighting

Most cephalopods in research laboratories are found naturally in quite shallow water, and thus are adapted to fairly high light levels. However, artificial fluorescent lights can be excessively bright and may show high-frequency flickering, which is likely to stressful to cephalopods especially when inadequate shelter is provided within tank spaces. Lighting should replicate natural photoperiod of a natural light cycle, with 12:12 regimes year-round being appropriate for almost all tropical species. Diurnal variation in light levels contributes to many physiological aspects of cephalopods including feeding, growth and development. Animals should never be exposed to 24-hour light unless it is absolutely necessary for the experiment of interest. Dull red light or moonlight is acceptable during night hours for short periods of observation; however, red light is not 'invisible' to cephalopods as occasionally claimed (Muntz 1986; Hanlon & Messenger 2018). The use of infra-red light to observe natural night-time and within-shelter behaviours is well-tolerated. IR-transparent, black glass is commercially available and can be used to construct housing enclosures and shelters within tanks, allowing complete visibility of animals within enclosures without disturbance from visible light.

Enclosure cleaning

Detritus, faeces and uneaten food should be removed from housing tanks daily to avoid build-up of waste products and poor water quality that may cause physiological stress. Tropical (i.e., warm water) systems are especially sensitive to spikes in ammonia, nitrite and nitrate as warmer temperatures increase the speed of waste decomposition. It is important to ensure waste is removed from the system by moving habitat during enclosure cleans, and fluidising substrate when siphoning. Depending on the species, these cleanings can be quite disruptive; octopuses may need to be removed from their dens, and sand-burying cephalopods such as bobtail and pyjama squids will need to swim during siphoning. Visual disturbance from insertions of hands and arms or cleaning tools can cause startle behaviours such as inking, which if excessive can lead to increased water ammonia levels. For these reasons, cleaning should occur no more than once daily, and less frequently if animals are not feeding (common in the first few days after arrival in the lab, during senescence, or in periods of egg brooding for female octopuses). Occasionally, it may be necessary to completely drain and disinfect housing tanks, or scrub down tanks to remove accumulated algae or other sources or fouling. In such cases, any detergents or chemical cleaners should be washed thoroughly from all parts of the housing system before animals are reintroduced, a process which may take several hours. Tanks should never be cleaned with detergents or other chemicals while animals are housed in the same system.

Filtration

For long-term maintenance in recirculating systems, cephalopods require extensive filtration systems to keep water chemistry within appropriate natural parameters and to manage waste. Filtration is broadly divided into biological, chemical and physical. Biological filtration primarily removes nitrogenous waste, chemical filtration primarily removes other inorganic toxins (chlorine, phosphates and various metals) and physical or mechanical filtration removes suspected particles. In general, cephalopods have similar filtration needs as do other marine species, with the exception of often needing additional removal of protein. Protein skimmers (also called protein fractionators) are this standard for recirculating cephalopod systems, made necessary by the constant discharge of mucus from the skin into the water, the decay of dropped food items, and the need for rapid removal of ink from the water column. Protein skimmers use high water flow rates and intense aeration with microbubbles to create foam in which the waste is trapped and then can be removed from collection cups. Protein skimmers may also remove micronutrients from the water, but these are generally replenished through normal scheduled water changes.

Housing design and enrichment

No cephalopod will prosper in a barren tank. Cephalopods may be stressed by exposure to observers and lack of structure in their housing enclosures. Different species require different types of housing enrichment, but all cephalopods should be provided areas within their enclosure where they can shelter from visual disturbances, and appropriate structure to permit the normal exercise of a range of species-appropriate behaviour (Mather & Anderson 1999; Cooke et al. 2019). For example, benthic cephalopods of different species may prefer very fine substrate, such as the burrowing octopus, *Muusoctopus leioderma*, while others may prefer small pebbles to pull into their dens, such as the red octopus, *Octopus rubescens*. Keeping fine or rocky substrate clean and free from decaying food and other detritus is challenging, as it requires daily removal of visible waste and weekly siphoning that fluidises sand and removes small waste particles that are trapped in the substrate, creating excessive nitrogenous waste. Because highly enriched environments can make non-invasive observations of animal health more difficult, make capture more challenging and potentially more dangerous to the animal, and are harder to keep clean, a balance must be struck between enrichment and practicality.

Benthic animals that do not bury in sand but den in tight crevices will need enclosure furniture that allows them to construct dens. For example, many coastal species of octopus will naturally hide in tight crevices in a reef habitat (Forsythe & Hanlon 1997; Huffard et al. 2005). In an enclosure setup, this can be accomplished by providing PVC pipe, PVC caps, terra cotta plant pots, or rocks of varying sizes and shapes to allow the animal to retreat into a den and pull substrate around it. Many octopus species will hold rocks and shells around them once in a crevice to become completely hidden from predators. Most octopuses will readily occupy offcuts of PVC pipe or small flowerpots, which can be lifted and placed into experimental setups and the animal gently encouraged to move out of the shelter using gently probing. The use of coral rocks with natural holes and crevices should be avoided, as octopuses will inevitably find their way into the smallest of spaces and then be all but impossible to remove when necessary.

Sepiolids and *Sepia* will bury if given sandy substrate of a particle size that can be relatively easily blown by the siphon of the animal. Most cuttlefish will bury if given the opportunity but can be housed on bare tank floors if provided plastic plants or other vertical structures to permit reasonable camouflage and concealment. Sepiolids such as *Euprymna* should be considered obligate buriers, and provided a sand bed of at least one inch depth to allow full concealment during daylight hours. This can be inconvenient for daily health and monitoring inspections, but in general, concealed animals are healthy animals. For benthic and burying animals, enclosures with opaque walls and bottoms are preferable to clear plexiglass (such as is used for housing zebrafish in rack systems).

Pelagic species such as the loliginid squid may be inhibited by tank furnishing like plastic plants, and become trapped in tank corners during normal swimming behaviour. Sandy substrate is useful to encourage resting or sitting behaviour (rather than endless swimming), and tanks should be opaque and covered to block high light and visual disturbance. Loliginid squid can be housed in a tank that is large in surface area but of quite shallow depth (30–60 cm), which allows for their strong horizontal swimming and jetting behaviour. Round or oval tanks, or square tanks with rounded corners, are preferable to tanks with sharp corners in which squid can get trapped during jetting. The overall size of the enclosure should be such that several strong jets in a row can be performed without constraint. Strong water flow and high levels of aeration are necessary when housing squid, but inflows and air stones should be positioned to not interfere with normal swimming behaviour.

Multiple studies have shown that cognitive behaviour is impaired when cephalopods are reared in impoverished environments (Dickel *et al.* 2000; Lee *et al.* 2010; Poirier *et al.* 2005). Regardless of the species, it is critical to research the natural habitat and behaviour and to provide the animal with housing enrichment that stimulates innate behaviour (Figure 50.6). Barren or inappropriate housing conditions will likely cause chronic stress for lab cephalopods, and will affect physiological and behavioural studies and the overall welfare of the lab animal.

Feeding in the laboratory

All cephalopods are carnivores, and nearly all, including all common laboratory species, are active hunters. As such, provision of live prey is ideal. Some species can be trained in the juvenile period to take dead or prepared food items, but this can require considerable effort from lab personnel. In general, octopuses are relatively easy to transition to non-live prey, whereas cuttlefish require quite extensive training. Sepiolids and myopsid squid, the other groups used commonly in laboratories, are very unlikely to take inanimate prey even with extensive training efforts. Nautilus, in particular, takes dead food and probably is a regular scavenger in the field (Saunders & Ward 2010). Figure 50.7 illustrates laboratory feeding in some species.

Despite a few exceptions, for most practical purposes, keeping and growing live cephalopods will entail regular supplies of live prey of suitable species.

Most juvenile and adult octopuses will eat almost any type of crustacean of appropriate size (crabs, shrimps, squat lobsters, etc.). Many species, for example *Octopus vulgaris*, *O. bimaculatus* and *E. dofleini*, will also readily take a variety of gastropod or bivalve molluscs. Adult squid and cuttlefish will catch fish and pelagic crustacea such as euphausids. Ideally, a choice of prey from the species range likely to be available in the natural habitat and of a size readily tackled by the cephalopod should be supplied. The ideal size relative to the body size of the cephalopod varies by taxon; octopuses are certainly capable of killing crustacea of their own size, but as a general guide, suitable prey organisms would be not more than about 10% of the mass of the octopus. In contrast, the small sepiolids will tackle shrimp prey at least as long as themselves and sometimes much larger. Juvenile *Euprmyna scolopes* prefer mysid shrimp larger than their own body size and will consume several per day (Hanlon *et al.* 1997).

Like many marine invertebrates, octopuses can survive without food for periods of at least several weeks, but feeding rates of healthy, growing cephalopods are high. For cool temperate, warm water and tropical species, daily rates of food intakes for octopods range from 1 to 10% of body weight, and up to 15% of body weight for some squid (O'Dor & Wells 1987). Flesh retrieval from crabs is around 50% of the gross body weight. Therefore, to fuel even a 5% feeding rate for a 500 g octopus, at least 50 g of crab will have to be supplied daily. Except where measured levels of food intake are required, food should be supplied ad libitum. Live food supply on this scale places significant demands on collections made in the field, or from commercial supply at high expense.

Growth

High food intakes, coupled with exceptional rates of gross food conversion efficiency, result in very high growth rates. Growth conversion efficiency (that is the growth increment expressed as a percentage of the food intake over the same period) ranges normally between 40% and 60% on a wet-weight basis, or even higher for octopods, and somewhat lower for squid, 25–40% (O'Dor & Wells 1987; Lee 1995; Koueta & Boucaud-Camou 2001). This means that for even a relatively slow-growing species such as *Eledone cirrhosa*, 100 g of crab meat ingested results in 40 g of octopus growth (Boyle & Knobloch 1982; Boyle *et al.* 1982).

Various mathematical expressions have been used to describe cephalopod growth (Forsythe & Van Heukelem 1987). Growth in laboratory-held octopuses generally follows two phases: an early phase, best described by an exponential relationship, during which most of the adult size is achieved, followed by a much slower logarithmic growth phase. During

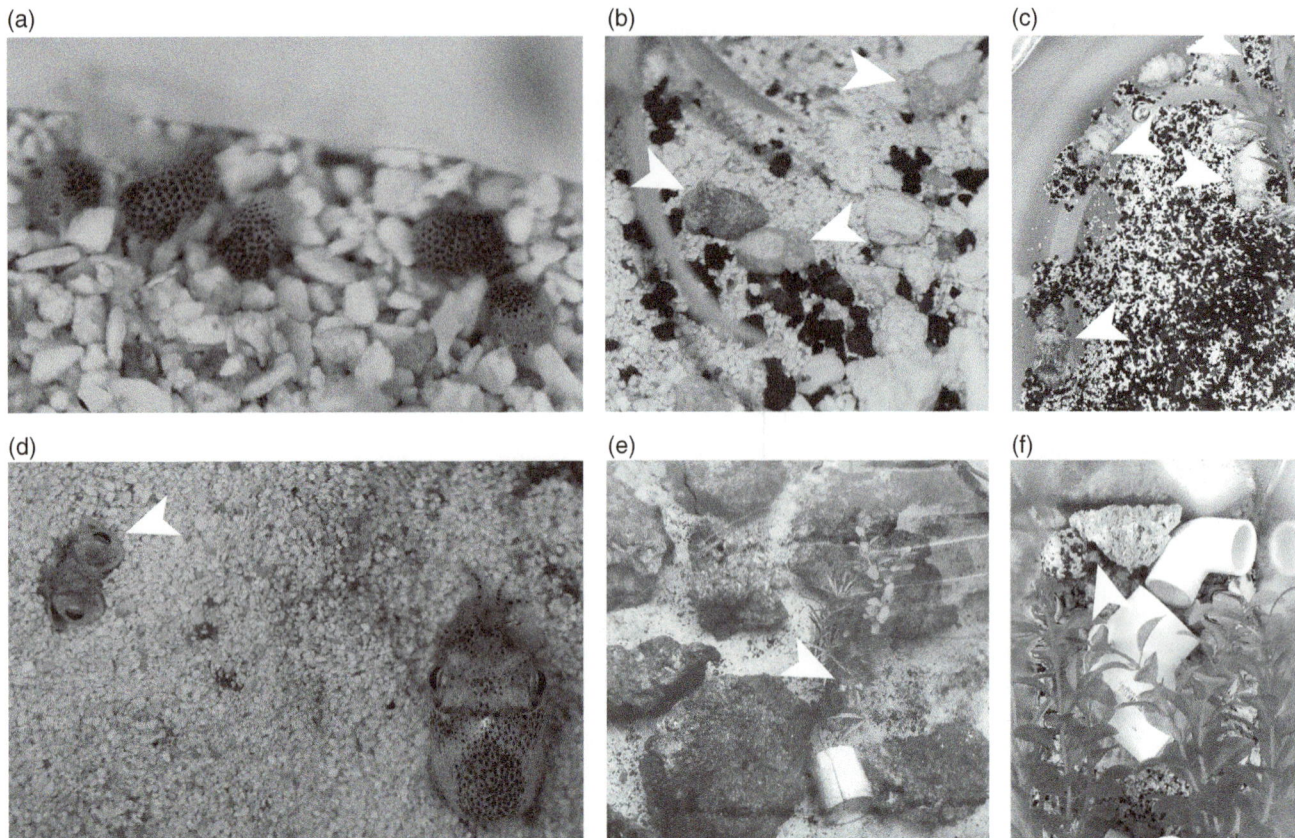

Figure 50.6 Examples of species-appropriate housing enrichments. (a) newly hatched *Euprymna* scolopes settle among grains of sand in their enclosure. (b) Newly hatched *Sepia bandensis* (arrowheads) camouflage among a mix of rocks, sand and pebbles. Artificial vegetation provides additional structure. (c) Juvenile *S. bandensis* in a shallow 'grow-out' tub with the same contents as in B. As animals grow the sand is used for partial burying and permits normal expression of camouflage behaviour. (d) Adult *E. scolopes* bury completely in sand if it is sufficiently deep. Here two females are visible hunting for food. (e) An adult *S. Bandensis* (arrowhead) swims in complex habitat tank, containing sand, rocks, plants and other structures. This is ideal for normal expression of breeding behaviour but would not be appropriate for animals needing to be caught for experimental procedures regularly. (f) An *Octopus bocki* (arrowhead) shelters in a den made from shells and rocks within a complex housing enclosure. Housing enrichment should balance the needs of the animal against practical needs of experimenters to view, capture and manage the animal.

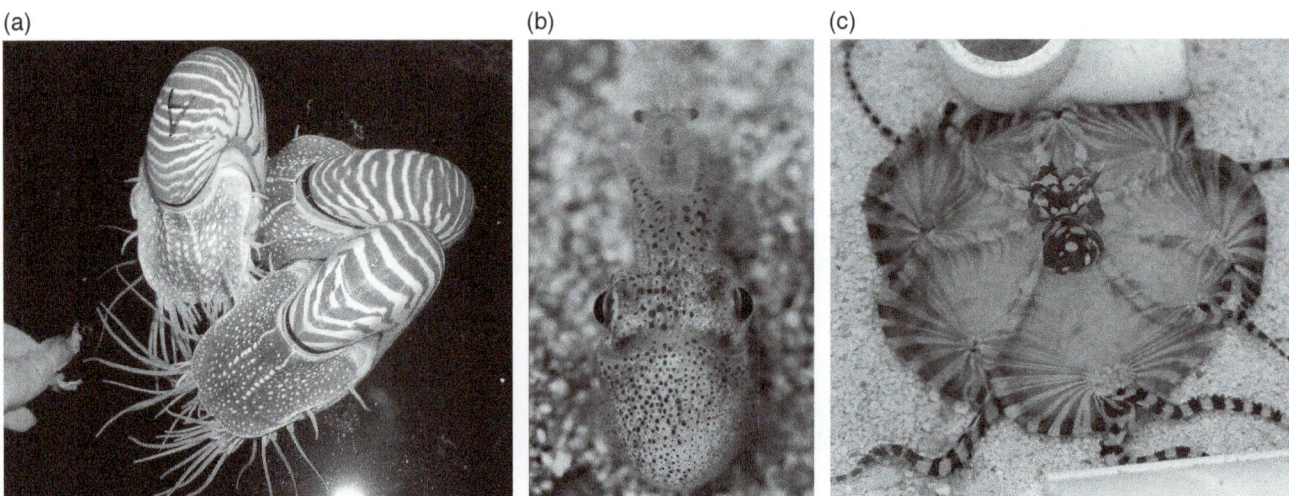

Figure 50.7 Feeding in the laboratory. Some species will readily accept dead or frozen food. Other species require live prey throughout their lifespans. (a) These nautilus are fed on frozen fish heads. (b) A juvenile *E. scolopes* consuming a live grass shrimp. (c) An octopus (*Wunderpus photogenicus*) displaying arm-web enveloping of a live crab.

the early part of the first phase, maximum instantaneous growth rates (the percentage increase in body weight per day) range from 4 and 8%. Animals nearing their adult size are more likely to be growing at 1–2% per day or less (Joll 1977; Wells & Clarke 1996; Koueta et al. 2000; Domingues et al. 2005).

Where field data are available, growth rates are correspondingly high (Hanlon et al. 1983; Boyle 1990), leading most authors to believe that the aquarium growth performance is not abnormal. There are, however, wide differences between individuals, and many animals brought in from the field will not begin to feed as readily or grow as fast.

Captive breeding and colony management

The culture and breeding of cephalopods in laboratory conditions is not widely undertaken, although recent efforts to close lifecycles of commonly used research species have been quite successful (Iglesias et al. 2004; Berger 2011; Grasse 2014; Vidal et al. 2014). Obtaining cephalopods for research from sources other than wild collection is desirable, and in some cases is required unless an exception is granted (see 2010/63/EU and Fiorito et al. 2015). There is also growing interest in cephalopods as developmental biology and genetically modifiable models, with many species being cultured for such experiments.

The availability of captive bred research specimens is still extremely limited, and most breeding is done within individual laboratories, with reared animals used 'in house' and not sold or provided to other research institutions.

There are many examples of cephalopods raised in captivity from eggs brought in from the field or laid in the aquarium (Figure 50.8), but successful breeding through multiple generations requires either especially favourable conditions of open seawater circulation or considerable effort to maintain high-quality closed circulation systems, along with

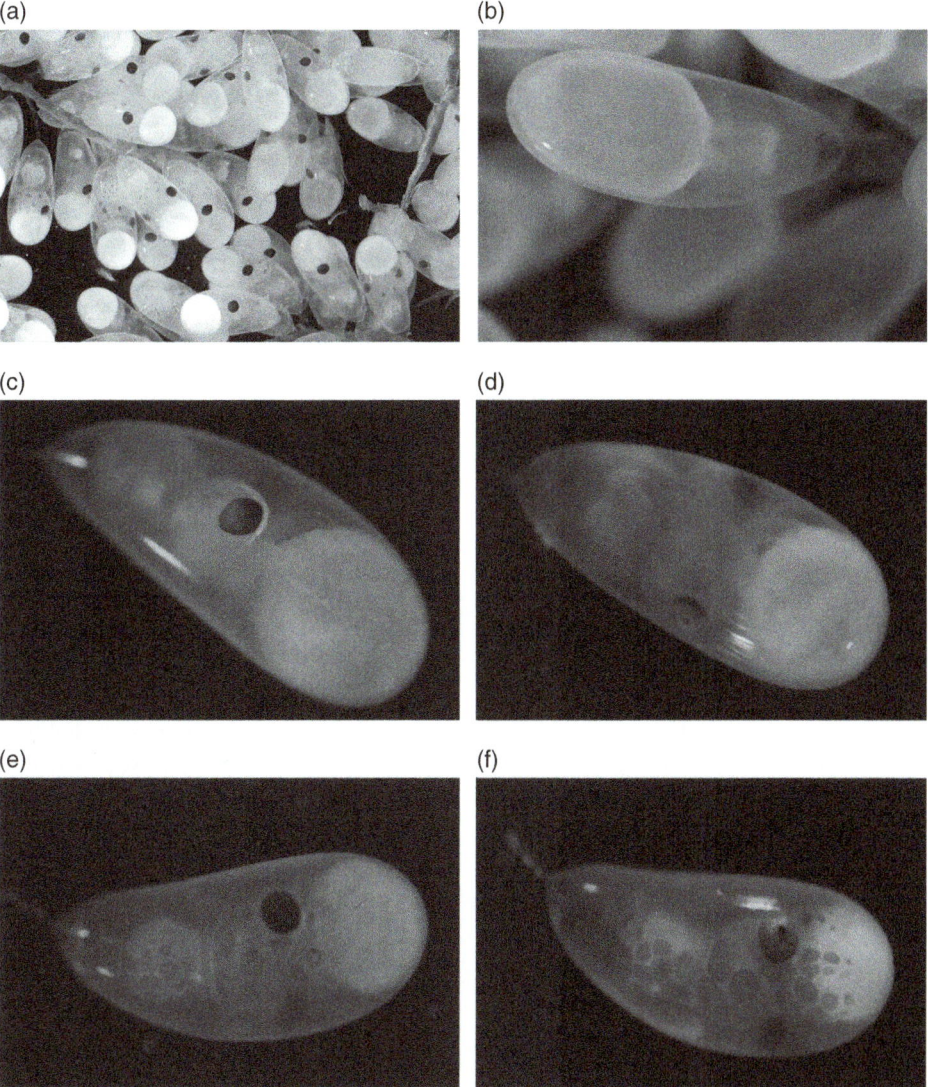

Figure 50.8 Octopuses are growing in popularity in developmental biology and genetic manipulation, due to their large numbers of eggs, amenability to manipulation and transparent egg capsule. A developmental sequence of an unidentified tropical octopus. (a) Eggs laid in strings against a tank wall. (b,c,d) As the embryo develops, the eyes become pigmented and chromatophores develop and become active. (e and f). As hatching nears, the yolk diminishes.

dedicated and highly experienced husbandry staff (Grasse 2014). Hatchling cephalopods often require very specialised housing in kreisel-type tanks to keep them in contact with food items and away from tank edges (Higgins et al. 2012; Vijai et al. 2015). In either case, apart from the practical difficulties of housing and handling small hatchling animals, the main problem is the supply of sufficient live food of suitable type and size. While on-growing using prepared or pelleted diets has been attempted successfully in octopus (Lee et al. 1991; Domingues et al. 2007; Rosas et al. 2007; Quintana et al. 2008; Butler-Struben et al. 2018) and cuttlefish (Hanlon et al. 1991; Castro et al. 1993; Domingues et al. 2005), successful culture of hatchling paralarvae on anything other than copious volumes of highly specific live foods, often carefully supplemented or 'gut loaded' with additional nutrition (Villanueva 1994; Domingues et al. 2001; Ikeda et al. 2005; Seixas et al. 2010) has thus far proved impossible.

Sexing

Males and females may be distinguished externally by the presence of modifications to the arm of the mature male used for sperm transfer during mating. In octopods, it is the third right arm (counting from the dorsal midline) which becomes thickened; a fold in the skin along the arm develops and the tip usually becomes modified and hook-like (Wells 1978; Thompson & Voight 2003). In myopsid squid, it is the fourth (ventral) left or right (Smith et al. 1987; Zecchini et al. 1996; Sabirov et al. 2012), and in sepiolids, it is the first left or right (Moynihan 1983; Nabhitabhata et al. 2005). Observation of the hectocotylised arm in sepiolid squid and octopus is the primary means of sexing adult animals. In loliginid squid and cuttlefish, the hectocotylus is harder to observe directly, and sexing is instead done by observation of the white testis in males and the pink accessory nidamental gland in females, both visible through the mantle musculature (Hanlon et al. 1999). In cuttlefish, sexing is based primarily on behaviours and body patterning (see Montague et al. 2021 for helpful figures).

Mating

Pairing captive cephalopods for mating needs to be managed carefully to prevent stress, fighting, possible physical injury or, rarely, cannibalism. Even in species where group housing is well-tolerated, mating can involve aggressive behaviours among rival males (Huffard et al. 2010; Cummins et al. 2011), and towards females. In general, mating occurs at night and the typical practice is to place a single male into the female enclosure at dusk, and remove the male the next morning. Most cephalopods engage in some sort of courtship behaviour where the male signals to the female with specialised chromatophore patterns and body postures (Arnold 1990; Hanlon et al. 1994; Huffard 2007). Mating occurs after the female reciprocates interest with chromatophore patterns and postures of her own. The usual approach is for the male hectocotylus to be inserted into the mantle cavity of the female. Peristaltic and 'pumping' movements of the male arm transfer spermatophores to the female.

Not all species engage in visual courtship behaviours that result in females choosing their mates; for example, males of the *Euprymna* genus show no obvious courtship behaviour, and instead pursue and grapple females into the mating position, holding the female restrained during spermatophore transfer (Hanlon et al. 1997; Franklin et al. 2014).

Mating in cephalopods is always one to one, although each individual may perform a series of matings with different partner, resulting in multiple paternity in egg clutches (Shaw & Boyle 1997; Van Camp et al. 2004; Bo et al. 2016). Underwater video observations show that while single male and female pairs are formed at mating, small 'sneaker males' may successfully fertilise the same female during the egg-laying process (Hall & Hanlon 2002; Iwata et al. 2011).

Female cephalopods have various methods of holding sperm transferred from the male, in buccal membranes or within the mantle cavity. In *Octopus vulgaris*, the sperm enters the oviducts and lodges in the oviducal glands (Tosti et al. 2001; Wodinsky 2008), while in *Eledone cirrhosa* spermatangia (ruptured spermatophores) travel all the way into the ovary (Boyle & Knobloch 1983). Fertilisation is then truly internal, and its timing is essentially determined by the female.

In oegopsid squid, spermatophores may be held in the buccal membrane of the female (*Todarodes*) (Takahama et al. 1991; Ikeda et al. 1993), attached to the base of the gills (*Illex*) (Villanueva et al. 2011) or even pushed into cuts in the mantle and neck musculature, presumably by the male during copulation (Hoving et al. 2010). Mating in the different taxa takes place in a number of positions; often from a distance with minimal contact in octopus (Mather 1998; Huffard 2007; Huffard & Godfrey-Smith 2010), in a 'head to head' position in cuttlefish (Hall & Hanlon 2002; Montague et al. 2021), with the male grasping the female from beneath around the neck in sepiolids (Franklin et al. 2014), and with the male swimming below, or inverted above, in sepioid squid (Chichery 1985; Jantzen & Havenhand 2002). In culture conditions, sufficient space and habitat complexity should be provided during mating attempts to allow for the natural performance of mating behaviour, and for reasonable shelter opportunities for either of the sexes to avoid harassment and aggression during or after courtship.

Egg laying

Many cephalopod species will lay viable eggs in aquarium conditions. Often this occurs when gravid females close to egg laying are brought in from the field, but a number of species, mostly those with large eggs (Hanlon & Forsythe 1985), have successfully laid eggs after long-term rearing, having stored sperm from mating encounters prior to capture. There is not clear agreement on how early in life a female may be mated and store viable sperm, but reports of fertilised eggs laid after multiple months in isolation suggest that mating may occur quite early in the juvenile stage in octopuses.

Sepioids lay small numbers (25–1000) of large eggs (1–10 mm in diameter) usually within a period of a few weeks. They are individually deposited, firmly fixed to a hard substrate, each enclosed in a tough sheath, which considerably increases the size of each egg. Octopods may also lay large eggs, ranging in size from about 2 mm in length (*Octopus vulgaris*) up to 12–15 mm (*O. bimaculoides*, *O. briareus*, *Eledone moschata*, *Bathypolypus spp.*) or even larger in some Antarctic species (Daly 1996). Estimates for total fecundity in octopods range from minima of 25–50 (*O. joubini, O. australis*) to well over 100,000 (*O. vulgaris, O. tetricus, O. cyanea*). The eggs are in strings, attached usually in the protection of rocks or an overhang. Egg laying is completed in less than a day or may take several weeks. Females of many species are known then to brood the egg mass, blowing sea water over it, keeping the eggs clear of epigrowths and protecting them against predators. This behaviour usually continues until hatching of the juveniles is completed. Myopsid squid (*Loligo*) also lay benthic egg masses in the form of a cluster of finger-like capsules, each containing perhaps 100 eggs, and no further maternal care is provided. These are commonly retrieved from spawning grounds by trawlers, but may also be laid in the aquarium (Hanlon *et al.* 1989). Oegopsid squid, in contrast, lay large, diffuse egg masses, neutrally buoyant in the water column, and consequently their eggs are rarely available for culture (but see Balch *et al.* 1985).

Egg masses to be cultured need gentle circulation of clean aerated seawater. Commonly used methods to achieve this include suspending the egg masses in water from threads across the tank, or in containers such as net bags or floating plastic strainers. Egg masses deposited on hard surfaces, such as those of sepiolids and *Sepia*, can be gently scraped away and placed in mesh baskets or in egg 'tumblers' (upright tubes using an airlift to provide gentle, constant movement of eggs and water; see examples in Grasse (2014)). Direct agitation from stirrers or aeration bubbles should be avoided, and low light levels should be maintained. Eggs should not be disturbed once the hatching date approaches as unexpected mechanical stimuli can result in premature hatching (usually indicated by the presence of a large external yolk sac held in the arm crown), and these premature emergers have very poor survival (von Boletzky 2004). Water quality for egg incubation should be maintained carefully, as eggs are vulnerable to predation from microfauna such as copepods, and may also be infected by pathogenic bacteria (Figure 50.9). Eggs and egg masses showing signs of infection should be removed promptly from the incubation chamber and disposed of.

Hatchlings

Development time in the egg depends on species and temperature, and ranges from fewer than 10 to over 100 days. Once the embryo approaches maturity, a natural tranquiliser in the perivitelline fluid acts to prevent premature hatching (Marthy *et al.* 1976; Weischer & Marthy 1983), although excessive mechanical or visual agitation can lead to premature emergence. At hatching, the developed embryo actively breaks out of the enclosing egg coats using a special hatching gland and the organ of Hoyle, a sharp spine-like structure on the caudal mantle, which is resorbed shortly after hatching (Segawa *et al.* 1988; Guerra *et al.* 2001; Lee *et al.* 2009).

Hatchlings can be collected from incubation tanks or the main enclosure using a transfer pipette or turkey-baster, making sure there is not excessive force applied during the aspiration. For species with hatchlings that bury immediately in substrate (such as *Euprymna berryi*), gentle puffing of the sand to encourage hatchlings to swim up into the water column allows aspiration without the risk of abrasion by sand grains during movement. Larger hatchlings of octopuses can be moved in small beakers or other vessels. Collection in nets and exposure to air should be avoided completely.

Hatchling rearing enclosures should be isolated from adults and other potential predators, and should be not overly large to encourage frequent encounters between hatchlings and their live prey. Shallow (~10–20 cm) tubs are ideal for cuttlefish and sepiolids, and gentle circular water movement encourages hunting behaviour. Strong flow, or flow patterns that trap hatchlings against the edges of enclosures or wash

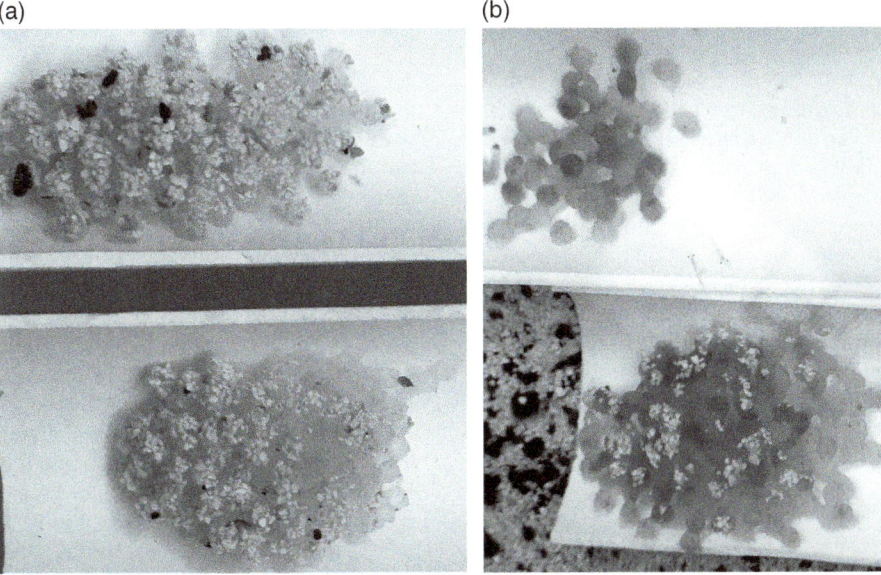

Figure 50.9 (a) A healthy clutch of *E. scolopes* eggs in the early stages of incubation. Eggs are laid on halves of PVC pipe and covered with sand by the female. (b) A bacterial infection has overtaken two clutches of eggs in the later stages of incubation, killing the embryos. Eggs of any cephalopod species that show signs of infection or infestation should be removed promptly and their enclosure removed and disinfected. Quarantine of eggs that were kept in the same water volume may be necessary.

them against the substrate are likely to lead to high mortality. Aeration using air stones placed into the rearing tubs at very low bubbling rates is acceptable, although care should be taken to ensure that bubbles are not causing excessive agitation. Inflow and outflow pipes should be screened, and may need to be isolated further for species with weak swimming abilities that may become trapped on outflow screens. Whether to use substrate, and of what type, depends somewhat on the species; cuttlefish can be reared in bare-bottom tanks, but sepiolids such as *Euprymna* do best with a shallow layer of fine sand that allows the small hatchling to bury during daylight hours. Somewhat lower light levels that are acceptable for adults during the day are ideal for hatchlings, and dull red light or very low white light (similar to light levels on a clear, starry night) are ideal for night-time hours. Many cephalopod hatchlings exhibit a diel vertical migration pattern which facilitates night-time hunting of planktonic prey that rises towards the surface at night (Moynihan 1983; Anderson & Mather 1996; Zeidberg & Hamner 2002). Total darkness (such as would occur in an enclosed room with no windows and all lights out) should be avoided; if windows or skylights are not present in the culturing facility, very dull artificial light should be provided at night to facilitate hunting behaviour that relies on the hatchling viewing the shadow of prey items against light from overhead.

Cephalopod hatchlings are active immediately upon hatching, first feeding on the remains of the yolk provision for the egg. After a period of half a day to about a week (depending on species and temperature), they will begin to feed on live food. At this point, a variety of appropriately small crustacean food must be supplied, such as newly hatched artemia, copepods, mysids, shrimps and newly metamorphosed crabs (Villanueva 1994; Iglesias & Fuentes 2014; Panetta et al. 2017), depending on species preference but also largely on local availability; some trial and error is expected for culture efforts located outside the natural habitat of the cephalopod species being reared. If food items available are not those likely to be consumed in the wild, special attention should be paid to ensuring a correct balance of nutrients. This is often achieved by supplementing the diet of intended food organisms, such as rotifers, artemia and mysid shrimps (Koueta et al. 2002; Villanueva et al. 2004; Seixas et al. 2010; Navarro et al. 2014). Various fatty-acid and vitamin supplements can be fed or introduced into the housing water for food animals, or the food animals can be bathed in such solutions shortly prior to feeding to cephalopod hatchlings.

Some facilities report that hatchling survival is best if food is limited in the first 24 hours after hatching, perhaps to avoid hatchlings becoming habituated to prey movement before yolk sac depletion drives hunger cues that initiate hunting behaviour. Thereafter, food should be supplied liberally, although the ideal prey/hatchling ratio depends on multiple factors including species, enclosure size, prey type and hatchling age.

Care of aged animals

Nearly all cephalopod species enter a period of senescence after reaching sexual maturity. Length of senescent periods varies considerably, from a few days in very short-lived species, such as the Hawaiian bobtail squid, *Euprymna scolopes* (Hanlon et al. 1997), up to a year or longer in the giant Pacific octopus, *Enteroctopus dofleini* (Anderson et al. 2002). In semelparous cephalopods, the period of senescence is defined by the onset of the reproductive stage, to eventual death from terminal decline of the nervous system and other tissues, leaving the animal vulnerable to predation and infection (Anderson et al. 2002; Pascual et al. 2010; Fiorito et al. 2015; Roumbedakis & Guerra 2019).

While all cephalopods likely experience similar symptoms of senescence, most literature focuses on octopus and cuttlefish species. Although senescence also occurs in squids, there is little formal description of how the process may or may not differ among the various orders. Senescence is most often described in species that are displayed by public aquaria or common in research laboratories culturing through multiple generations, such as the giant Pacific octopus, *Enteroctopus dofleini* (Anderson et al. 2002) and the common European cuttlefish, *Sepia officinalis* (Chichery & Chichery 1992a; Chichery & Chichery 1992b; Forsythe et al. 1994; Halm et al. 2000).

Senescence almost always includes anorexia, skin deterioration without signs of healing, sinking of the eyes, stereotypic uncoordinated movement, apathetic behaviours, abnormal morphology and sometimes autophagy (Higham 1957; Bradley 1974; Budelmann 1998; Anderson et al. 2002). If infection is acquired during the senescent stage, animals generally do not respond to treatment, suggesting that the normal immune response (Castellanos-Martínez & Gestal 2013) declines during senescence (Anderson et al. 2002). Behaviour is often unpredictable, becoming repetitive and stereotypic, and cognitive performance declines (Chichery & Chichery 1992a). Early symptoms of senescence may parallel signs of disease, stress or illness; this presents a husbandry challenge when the age of wild-caught specimens is unknown.

Senescence is induced through reproductive hormones regulated by the optic gland, and is influenced by environmental factors such as light and temperature (Wodinsky 1977; Anderson et al. 2002; Wang & Ragsdale 2018). Once cephalopods enter senescence, the symptoms and terminal decline are irreversible. The only exception to this has been through experimental removal of the optic gland, where brooding anorexic females of *Octopus hummelinki* began feeding again, and lived up to 9 months post gamete deposition (Wodinsky 1977). In some species, the onset of senescence can be delayed by reducing water temperatures towards physiological minimums and carefully limiting food intake, which slows growth and thus extends lifespan.

In the wild, mature female octopuses will find a secluded habitat or den to lay their eggs and depending on the species, will tend them until they hatch. Females fast the entire time they are brooding eggs, metabolising their own muscle tissue for fuel (O'Dor & Wells 1978), which results in significant weight loss. This is also seen in captive specimens even when food is readily available to the animal; at the Seattle Aquarium, mean percent weight loss for brooding *E. dofleini* was 49.5% (Anderson et al. 2002). In cephalopods without maternal egg care such as cuttlefish and squid, females decline rapidly after egg laying, which may occur in a single event or spaced over several days or weeks.

Male reproductive maturity is marked by behavioural onset of mate-seeking, and in some species, greatly increased male-male aggression (Cummins et al. 2011; Shashar & Hanlon 2013). While males typically show external signs of senescence after mating, some captive animals without the chance to mate may drop spermatophores onto enclosure floors in early senescence, or may display senescent behaviours before depositing sperm.

Captive cephalopods often experience delayed or extended senescence as they may not have the opportunity to mate and do not have natural predators. Given that senescent animals may persist in captive conditions with significantly compromised health, decline and signs of poor welfare should be monitored closely by lab personnel. Decisions on when and if to euthanise moribund animals in terminal decline are not standard. There are differing opinions on whether senescence, as a 'natural process', should be allowed to conclude in the natural death of the animal, or whether humane euthanasia at the point where the animal is unable to right itself or shows increasingly severe skin lesioning, is preferable (Holst & Miller-Morgan 2020). Certainly, if similarly extensive skin lesions as those that characterise late-stage senescence were to occur in younger, otherwise healthy animals, immediate treatment or euthanasia would be considered necessary to protect welfare. The willingness to allow senescent animals to endure extensive tissue degradation is grounded in the belief that the peripheral sensory system and the central brain likely degenerate in parallel with the external body surface, rendering the aged animal insensible to its multiple injuries. However, this assumption has never been tested, and as such we urge caution when considering welfare evaluations for senescent animals. Concluding when clinical signs of decline may compromise the animals' welfare can be difficult, but tools provided by Fiorito et al. (2015) and Holst and Miller-Morgan (2019) can aid in making appropriate decisions about euthanasia of aged animals.

While declines in behavioural performance have been demonstrated in ageing animals (Chichery & Chichery 1992a; Chichery & Chichery 1992b; Anderson et al. 2002; Holst & Miller-Morgan 2020), it is unclear how senescence may change other aspects of behaviour and physiology, which should be taken into account during experiments. If possible, avoiding the use of senescent animals in procedures is desirable; given that their performance is likely to be unpredictable, the use of senescent animals may result in the need for increased sample sizes, and the broad applicability of findings made from animals in poor health is likely to be limited. This is of course complicated by the issue of wild collection as the source of most laboratory octopus and squid. Hand-collection of octopuses from the wild, a common method for small tropical species particularly, may inadvertently target senescent animals given that senescence is associated with increased wandering behaviour. The likely over-representation of senescent octopuses in laboratories may be partly responsible for octopus' reputation as being particularly difficult animals to keep healthy; even the most experienced aquarists cannot prolong the life of a terminally reproductive cephalopod.

Laboratory procedures

Handling and health monitoring

Handling cephalopods is usually necessary for health inspections, movement of animals between enclosures, during behavioural experimental procedures and for performing invasive procedures.

Cephalopod skin is delicate and is easily damaged by nets and other restraints. The mucus layer that is secreted by the skin offers some protection from abrasion, but extreme care is necessary to avoid causing injury during handling procedures, particularly for squid, whose skin is the thinnest and most injury-prone among the coleoids. Physical handling should be minimised as any contact with abrasive or dry surfaces is detrimental and undoubtedly highly stressful (Hanlon 1990; Walsh et al. 2002).

Capture of animals from holding tanks may be done with fine-gauge, knotless nets, immersed into the water and moved with slow, steady movements beneath the animal, then gently lifted to bring the animal close to the surface. Once contained in the net, the animal should be transferred while still submerged to a bucket or other smooth-walled container for movement out of the holding tank. Direct exposure to air should be completely avoided for squid and cuttlefish. Nets should be disinfected regularly. Octopuses, particularly those that naturally inhabit the inter-tidal region, can withstand brief air exposure during handling and movement. Capture of free-swimming cephalopods from holding tanks is a skill that requires some practice and familiarity with the animals' behaviour. Fast and aggressive movements of nets and personnel during capture will result in panicked animals that ink and collide with walls and other physical structures, causing problems with water quality and general health.

Squid and cuttlefish can be weighed in a fixed, known volume of seawater and the water weight subtracted. Octopuses, which are generally more tolerant of brief periods out of water, can be weighed by placing them directly onto a scale, but blotting the surface of the skin dry is not advised, as it disrupts the mucus layer and risks abrading the skin. Some very large octopuses, such as the giant Pacific octopus, *Enteroctopus dofleini*, may be weighed in a net that is lifted briefly out of the water, but this procedure is usually preceded by extensive reward training where the animal is trained to move by itself into and out of the net, minimising stress from being actively captured by handlers.

Handling during health monitoring and more invasive procedures may necessitate sedation, particularly for some species of squid. Cuttlefishes and octopuses are relatively easily habituated to gentle handling, as are the sepiolid squids; however, the loliginid squids are difficult to habituate and tend to be flighty and unpredictable in laboratory conditions (Hanlon 1990). Very light sedation using a low concentration of ethanol in seawater (0.5–1.0% v/v), or a dilute mix of seawater and magnesium salt (1:4 or 1:3 ratio of 300 mM $MgCl_2$:SW), should be sufficient to facilitate brief episodes of handling typical of what would be required for normal health monitoring (physical inspection of the mantle cavity, weighing, injections, etc.), or very brief veterinary or experimental procedures (injection, tissue biopsy, etc.)

(Mooney et al. 2010; Gleadall 2013). For handling procedures that are prolonged, a combination of sedation and habituation is ideal. Blood draws, for example, are normally done under light general anaesthetic (Collins & Nyholm 2010). For such procedures, a period of habituation to capture, handling and movement in and out of the home tank should reduce stress and minimise complications that can occur during sedation and immobilisation.

Non-invasive health monitoring is desirable given cephalopods' delicate skin and aversions to being handled. However, accurate health indicators are difficult to obtain for group-housed animals because identifying individuals is challenging, particularly for larger school groups of squid. Octopuses, while being easy to identify individually due to their solitary housing requirements, are difficult to inspect in sufficient detail without coaxing them from their shelters. For day-to-day monitoring, determining that animal is displaying appropriate, species-specific schooling or sheltering behaviour and not showing any obvious signs of injury, is more than likely sufficient given the drawbacks of disturbing animals for the sake of gaining more information about their welfare in the absence of indications for concern. The use of non-invasive behavioural assays of feeding motivation is popular for establishing normal health prior to use in experimental procedures, and is likely also a useful indicator of good welfare status (Cooke & Tonkins 2015; Tonkins et al. 2015). Additional non-invasive metrics of health welfare may include assessment of skin colouration and texture, swimming behaviour and buoyancy, reaction to visual stimuli, and normal use of arms and tentacles (see Fiorito et al. 2015 for detailed descriptions).

From a safety standpoint, handling also carries risks for laboratory personnel, most commonly of being bitten. All cephalopods will attempt to bite when defending themselves from being grasped either by a human hand or a predator, and there are numerous reports of divers being bitten by curious or defensive cephalopods in the wild (McMichael 1964; Snow 1970; Zeidberg & Robison 2007; Tennesen 2015). The beak is sharp, and the buccal musculature is surprisingly strong, even in small animals. Most typical laboratory species are rather small and their bites, although painful, do not cut through skin, but larger octopuses and nautiluses have sufficient strength to inflict skin-penetrating bites. Detaching a biting cephalopod is difficult, as the bite is usually accompanied by tight grasping of the hand with the suckers. Bites often occur when the animal is being handled out of water and most cephalopods will release their grasp if placed back into water and allowed to escape to a shelter. If a bite penetrates the skin, the area should be washed thoroughly with very hot water (Atkinson et al. 2006; Loten et al. 2006) and monitored for swelling and signs of infection, which can be serious (Campanelli et al. 2008; Aigner et al. 2011). Nearly all cephalopods have some sort of salivary toxin used to immobilise invertebrate prey, but some species are highly venomous to vertebrates (the blue-ringed octopus species complex, the flamboyant cuttlefish and potentially other species such as the pyjama squid) and these species must be housed and handled with extreme care (McMichael 1964; Sheumack et al. 1978; Sheumack et al. 1984; Ruder et al. 2013).

Surgery

Surgical procedures in cephalopods fall into two main categories: veterinary need and experimental research. The latter category contains the vast majority of published reports of surgical procedures from which animals recovered (see Fiorito et al. 2015 for review), with only a handful of accounts of surgical treatment of illness or injury (Harms et al. 2006). Surgical techniques should be generally similar to those used in other aquatic animals such as fish, although there are some additional factors to consider when undertaking surgery on cephalopods.

While a sterile environment and equipment is ideal, in practice it is unlikely that sterile seawater and general anaesthetic solutions are readily available or available in sufficient quantities for surgery except on very small specimens. Incision sites are usually not scrubbed prior to procedures, as there is little known about the efficacy of different scrub liquids nor of their potentially deleterious effects on skin integrity. The use of antibiotic drugs, either topical or systemically applied, as a prophylactic measure against infection of surgical sites is likewise unstudied in cephalopods, and there are no reports of antibiotic use after survival surgery in published literature. Certainly, naturally occurring wounds can become infected (see 'Infections' section, later in this chapter), so careful monitoring of surgical sites after surgery should be standard. Signs of infection are likely to include degradation or necrosis of skin around the surgical site, or raised and discoloured areas. Whole-animal signs of infection are loss of appetite, changed behaviour, lethargy and death.

Different methods of closure of incisions in cephalopod skin has been reported in a number of studies. The use of sutures of different types is common, as is the use of tissue glue (Chichery & Chanelet 1976; Chichery & Chanelet 1978; Andrews & Tansey 1981; Harms et al. 2006; Shomrat et al. 2008). While there are anecdotal reports of octopuses using their fine manipulation skills to remove sutures placed in their skin, it is not clear whether this could be alleviated by using a different type of suture thread or by using discontinuous sutures.

Post-surgical analgesia is not routinely given in cephalopods. Not only are there no validated drugs available that can be given either locally or systematically for analgesia after surgical procedures, but there is also no consensus on how to evaluate animals for signs of pain and distress or for their alleviation in the presence of drugs. The need for dedicated studies of effects of common analgesic drugs is cephalopods is needed urgently at the time of writing. The most suitable option for post-surgical analgesia currently is the application of local anaesthetic at the time of surgery, which prevents nociceptive sensitisation both at the surgical site and more generally across the body surface (Crook et al. 2013). Both lidocaine and magnesium chloride solution are effective local anaesthetics (Butler-Struben et al. 2018); however, because magnesium chloride causes local muscle relaxation it may lead to uncontrolled bleeding if injected at the site of incisions. For this reason, veterinary preparations of lidocaine or the other '-caine' anaesthetics (which are often formulated with a vasoconstrictor such as adrenaline) are preferable for use at surgical sites.

Anaesthesia and analgesia

The implementation of Directive 2010/63/EU/, with its requirement for humane and effective anaesthesia of cephalopods subject to invasive procedures, has highlighted the relative dearth of knowledge of effective anaesthesia of cephalopods. Although there have been numerous studies published which describe some form of 'general anaesthesia' in cephalopod subjects, anaesthesia has traditionally been evaluated via effects on motor output only, which has led to considerable disagreement about whether typically used chemical agents are true anaesthetics, paralytics or both (Messenger et al. 1985; Mooney et al. 2010; Gleadall 2013; Polese et al. 2014; Fiorito et al. 2015). In addition, there has been minimal investigation of efficacy of commonly used local anaesthetic agents, which may be useful for minor procedures.

Immersion is the only currently validated method for general anaesthetic in cephalopods; immersion may be considered equivalent to inhalant anaesthesia for terrestrial species, as the presumptive primary mode of action is exchange across the respiratory membrane surface. Successful general anaesthesia by injection has not been reported.

Historically, the preferred anaesthetic for cephalopods was immersion in urethane, which resulted in reliable and readily reversible immobility, allowing for handling and surgical procedures (Andrews & Tansey 1981; Gleadall 2013); however, its now-recognised carcinogenic effects have removed it from use as a general anaesthetic for cephalopods. Instead, researchers have relied on either solutions of magnesium chloride salt or ethanol in seawater to anaesthetise animals for procedures, but only recently have these two substances been demonstrated to have 'true' anaesthetic effects; that is, they achieve complete but reversible blockade of sensation, as well as immobilisation and loss of organised neural output from the CNS (Butler-Struben et al. 2018).

Octopuses and cuttlefish may be readily and reversibly anaesthetised by transfer to a container of sea water containing either general anaesthetic solution. Depth of anaesthesia is controlled only by concentration and the period of immersion.

For magnesium chloride, a solution of 330 mM $MgCl_2.6H_2O$ mixed into distilled, fresh water may then be mixed with seawater at either a 1:3, 1:2 or 1:1 ratio, depending on the species and the individual; it is recommended to start with the lowest concentration (1:3), then increase the concentration of the magnesium chloride mix after 5–10 minutes if the animal is not showing signs of sedation. The appropriate dose also depends somewhat on the procedure being attempted; for basic handling, external examination or brief injections, a low dose that achieves mild sedation (i.e., the animal is quiescent but still shows some signs of responsiveness to handling) should be sufficient. Higher doses are necessary for more invasive procedures. At doses up to 1:1, respiratory arrest should not occur even when an animal is deeply anaesthetised; although respiration might slow considerably, it should recover spontaneously when the solution is changed to normal seawater without the need for mantle massage or other experimenter interventions. An important caveat to the use of magnesium chloride for potentially painful procedures is that there is a considerable period (up to 15 minutes in some cases) where the animal is behaviourally unresponsive to stimulation but sensation is not yet blocked (Butler-Struben et al. 2018); it is thus necessary to wait at least this long after the animal loses peripheral reflex responses to noxious stimulation, such as skin pinch, before proceeding with surgical procedures. This same effect occurs in reverse upon recovery.

Ethanol may also be used at doses of 1–2% in seawater. Progressively increasing the concentration can avoid behavioural signs of distress reported in some studies; a starting dose of 0.5%, increased every 5–10 minutes until the animal shows signs of sedation is recommended to avoid this complication. Unlike magnesium chloride solutions, there is minimal lag time between behavioural signs of anaesthesia and cessation of sensory neuron signal to the central brain, making ethanol generally a better choice where direct monitoring of the nervous system is not possible. Ethanol also produces less suppression of respiration and has considerably faster induction and recovery times, making for shorter procedure durations overall (Butler-Struben et al. 2018). It is important to note that cooling in chilled seawater is not an effective anaesthetic, although it may be useful as an adjuvant to other methods, as suggested by Fiorito et al. (2015). However, this is likely to be appropriate only for temperate species. Chilling tropical species below their natural thermal limit is likely to cause stress and increase mortality.

Visible signs of general anaesthesia are the progressive loss of activity, loss of righting reflex and paling of the skin (Figure 50.10). Cessation of breathing, previously considered a sign of 'complete' anaesthesia, is both undesirable and unnecessary, and should it occur, immediate perfusion of the mantle with clean seawater should begin, along with manual respiration (rhythmic squeezing of the mantle by hand) until ventilation is spontaneous and the animal shows signs of recovery.

Local and regional anaesthetics have been used with good success in several studies (Andrews et al. 1981; Crook et al. 2014; Fiorito et al. 2015; Butler-Struben et al. 2018). Injectable anaesthetics can be used to infiltrate skin and muscle prior to incisions, and are ideally used in conjunction with general sedation or anaesthesia for more invasive procedures. Lidocaine (0.5%) and magnesium chloride (isotonic, or 330 mM) produced complete blockade of afferent nerve signal for at least 30 minutes after injection into the mantle of cuttlefish and octopus (Butler-Struben et al. 2018), and produced no long-term ill-effects on sensation or chromatophore function at 24 hours after injection. Both substances cause local relaxation of chromatophores in the infiltrated area, providing a useful visual indication of the margins of the anaesthetised region.

The use of anaesthetics in cephalopods remains at a relatively primitive stage. Little is known of the central effects of these compounds and the parameters of adjustment of anaesthetic type or concentration to cephalopod species and body size. At the time of writing, only these two anaesthetic substances have been validated (i.e., they have been shown to inhibit sensory processing, not only motor function), and this validation is currently limited to small, tropical species. Future studies focusing on larger species, temperate species and other drugs are needed, and we expect that they will follow within the next several years as the need for better anaesthetics is recognised.

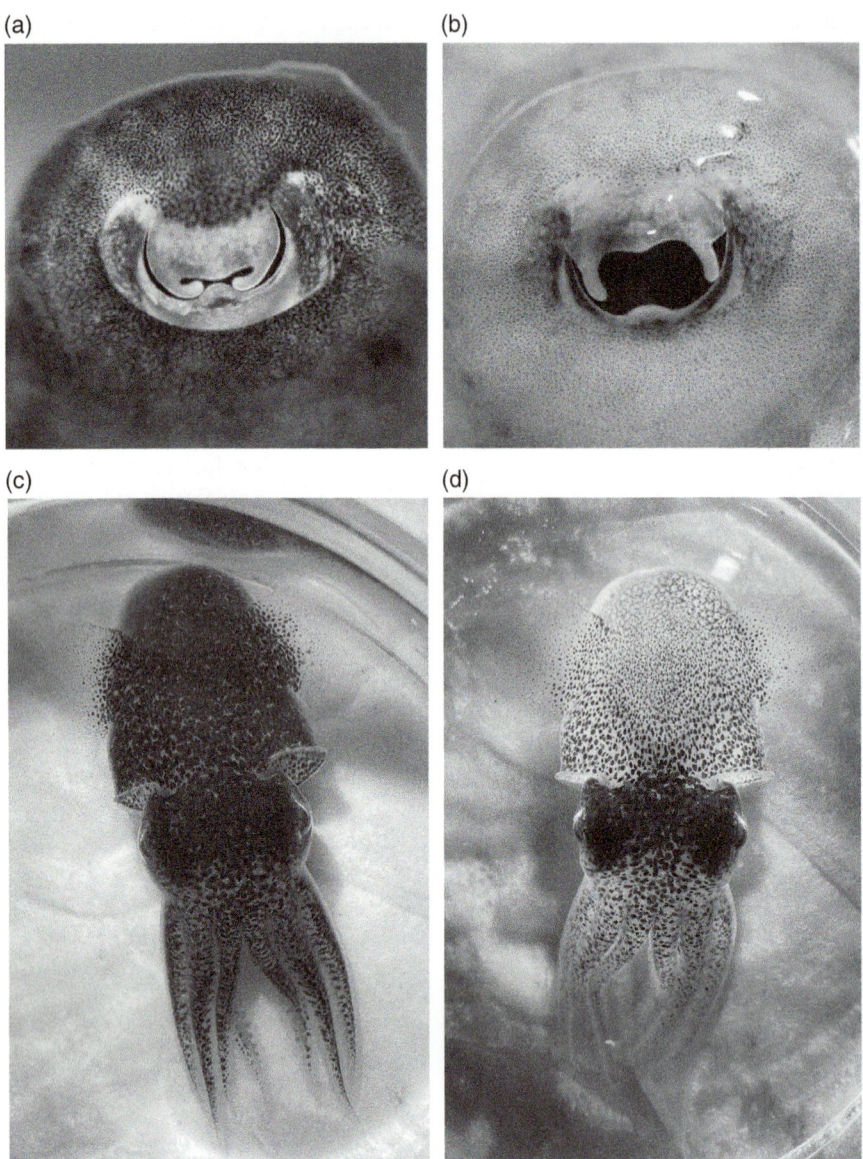

Figure 50.10 Signs of general anaesthesia in two species of cephalopod. (a and b) As anaesthesia induction progresses, the pupil of *Sepia bandensis* begins to relax and expand, and the pupillary light reflex is lost. (c and d). Progressive relaxation of chromatophores in the sepiolid *Euprymna berryi*. As anaesthesia plane deepens, the animal becomes progressively paler. The chromatophores across the top of the head are often the last to relax. This animal is sedated but not yet completely anaesthetised.

Euthanasia

Humane methods of killing cephalopods remain poorly studied. In most cases, the simplest and most effective primary method is terminal anaesthesia, typically via a high dose of ethanol in seawater (2–3%, introduced progressively), or isotonic (330 mM) $MgCl_2$ solution. With either substance, respiration should cease completely within 5–10 minutes (often much faster for tropical species). However, respiratory arrest and cardiac arrest may not occur simultaneously. If the heart is still beating, even without respiratory movements of the mantle, oxygenated haemolymph is still delivered to tissues, and the possibility that the animal is still conscious and sensate cannot be discounted. Where cardiac activity cannot be measured directly, waiting 10–15 minutes after the cessation of breathing movements should ensure that the brain is non-functional (Butler-Struben et al. 2018).

Secondary methods (also termed 'completion of killing' or 'confirmation of death') vary depending on intended use of tissues. If the CNS is not required, complete destruction of the brain is a quick and effective method of ensuring death. Using a scalpel or razorblade, a midline cut is made through the head between the eyes. There is no need to expose the brain for this procedure; the overlying skin and cartilage-like cranium is sliced through easily. Four to six additional longitudinal cuts should be made through the brain and optic lobes to ensure complete tissue destruction. As the brain is sliced, there may be reflex movement of the arms or chromatophores of the head, but there should be no co-ordinated movements of multiple arms, nor directed movement towards the area of sliced skin. Other methods of confirmation of death are rapid freezing, gill clipping, aortic transection or perfusion through the aorta or ocular sinus cavity with a fixative such as paraformaldehyde.

Killing cephalopods without anaesthesia should only be attempted if the need for unadulterated tissue is justified, and in countries where cephalopods are included in vertebrate animal protections, justification and formal approval is likely needed. If a purely physical method is used, this should only be done by trained and experienced personnel. The most common method for octopuses is decerebration, using the same technique as described above but without initial anaesthesia. Placing the animal upright on a smooth surface allows the arms and suckers to adhere, stabilising the animal and reducing interference by the arms as the first cut is made through the brain. Ideally, the procedure should be completed within 30 seconds to minimise distress.

Common welfare problems

Health and diseases

Parasitism, infections and other diseases

Cephalopods carry a wide variety of parasites and symbionts (Castellanos-Martínez & Gestal 2013; Roumbedakis et al. 2018) which include viruses, bacteria, fungi, sporozoans, ciliates, dicyemids (mesozoa), monogeneans, digeneans, cestodes, acanthocephalans, nematodes, polychaetes, hirudineans, branchiurans, copepods and isopods.

Although there are many reports of parasites found in both wild and captive cephalopods, and in a range of tissue types, there are relatively few detailed investigations of their potentially pathological effects on cephalopod health (Pascual et al. 1996; Gestal et al. 2002; Castellanos-Pascual et al. 2010; Martínez et al. 2014; Roumbedakis et al. 2018; Pascual et al. 2019), and likewise there are few, if any, recent studies on how parasite infection may most effectively be treated (Barord et al. 2012; Sykes & Gestal 2014). Approaches for removing external parasites on fish often involve immersion dips of either low-salinity water, formalin or other drug solution (for example, Fajer-Ávila et al. 2003; Katharios et al. 2006; Ohno et al. 2009); given the delicate skin of cephalopods and the low tolerance of salinity changes in most species (Hendrix et al. 1981; Nabhitabhata et al. 2001; Şen 2005), these approaches are likely to be counterproductive. Most reports of metazoan parasites come from naturally infected, wild-collected cephalopods, and as such, evaluation of their potentially deleterious effects is challenging. Heavy parasite loads are likely, as they are in any host species, to affect growth and vigour (Pascual et al. 2019), but whether there is any net benefit to attempting to remove naturally acquired parasites from wild-collected laboratory cephalopods is not clear.

Bacterial infections in captive cephalopods are relatively common, particularly as consequences of skin lesions caused by physical injury (Hanlon et al. 1983; Hanlon & Forsythe 1990; Oestmann et al. 1997 Gestal et al. 1998; Farto et al. 2003; Farto et al. 2019). Vibriosis is reported as particularly common (Ford et al. 1986), with multiple species of these Gram-negative bacteria found in skin lesions and internal organs in various cephalopod species (Sykes & Gestal 2014). Treatment with either oral or injected antibiotics is effective in some cases, but it is necessary to recognise signs of infection early if treatment is to be successful; in many cases, unless there are clear external signs of infection (Hanlon et al. 1984) there are few other validated indicators of infection prior to the animal declining irreversibly. Fungal infections have been reported occasionally in captive cephalopods (Figure 50.11) but detailed reports of genera involved, symptoms, ill-effects and treatments are scarcer still (Jones & O'Dor 1983; Hanlon & Forsythe 1985; Hanlon 1990; Polglase et al. 2009; Sykes & Gestal 2014; Polglase 2019), with only one detailed case report of surgical excision of skin eruptions and systemic treatment with antifungal drugs, which ultimately proved unsuccessful, perhaps due to insufficient treatment duration or secondary bacterial infection (Harms et al. 2006). Fungal fruiting bodies have been recorded emerging from the skin of two infected, senescent adult squid, but because the individuals were already showing declining health, no treatment or further identification of the fungus was attempted, and instead the animals were euthanised. Given the relatively few case reports of fungal infections from mature or senescent cephalopods, it appears that fungal pathogens have low virulence in otherwise healthy animals, and may be opportunistic invaders of otherwise compromised hosts.

Preventing the spread of pathogens in research aquaria is achieved primarily by maintaining good water quality and good husbandry; appropriate biological, chemical and mechanical filtration is essential both for removing pathogens and their nutrients from the water, and avoiding chronic stress that renders cephalopods vulnerable to opportunistic infections. Additionally, ultraviolet filtration is useful in removing micro-organisms from the water column, but flow rate and light cycles may need to be adjusted based on changing bioloads or in response to suspected outbreaks. Quarantine of new animals and any showing signs of illness is essential, as is proactive treatment of suspected infection. The use of prophylactic antibiotic agents after surgeries is not yet commonplace for cephalopods, and the efficacy of such approaches, along with efficacy of treatments for incidental infections, requires further study.

Injuries

Cephalopods in captive conditions are prone to injuries (Figure 50.12). Their delicate skin, propensity to startle easily and their very forceful swimming movements make them particularly vulnerable to injuries from collisions with enclosure walls. Additionally, group-housed species can inflict injuries on one another during aggressive encounters during mating, and inadvertently during competition for food items. Wild-caught cephalopods may enter laboratory settings carrying significant injuries acquired during the collection process. Cuts and abrasions of the skin inflicted by nets or rough handling are a frequent cause of mortality, especially in squids, usually within a few days of capture (Summers & McMahon 1974; Summers et al. 1974; Chabala et al. 1986; Hanlon 1990). For cephalopods that suffer mild, survivable abrasions or bruising, recovery may be possible

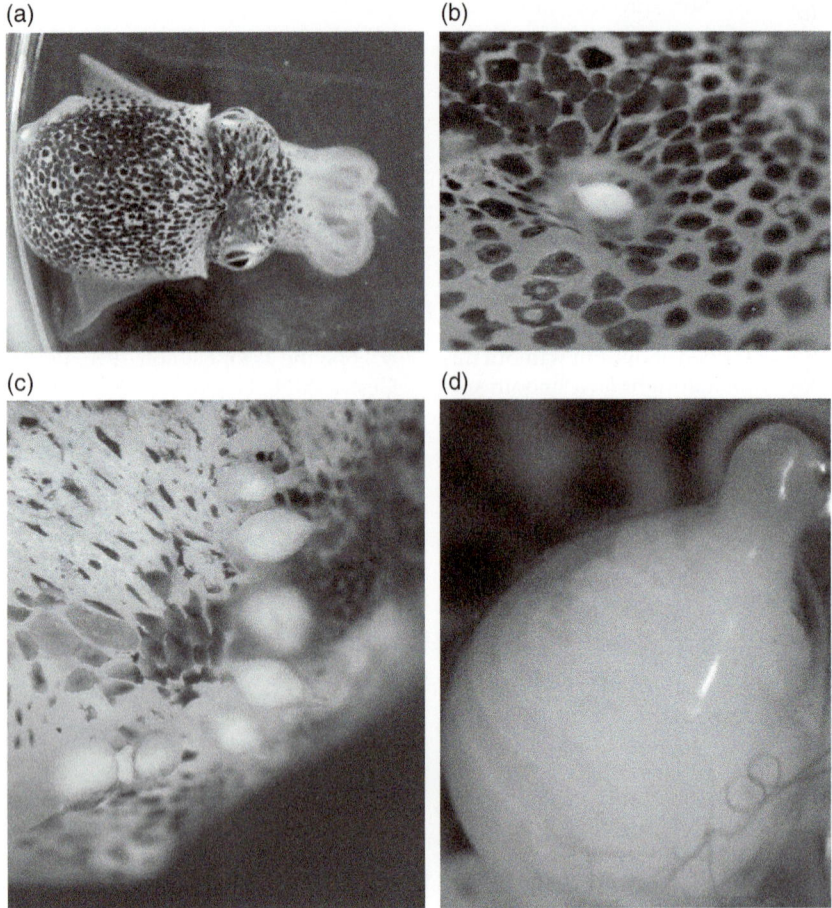

Figure 50.11 Opportunistic fungal infection in two senescent females of *Euprymna scolopes*. (a) Fungal growth is visible beneath the skin on the caudal mantle. (b) A closeup of the infected area in A. (c and d) A different animal, photographed post-euthanasia. Fungal fruiting bodies have erupted through the skin. (d) A closeup of C. The species of fungus was not identified, and did not spread to other healthy animals in the colony.

with excellent husbandry, provision of ample live food, minimal disturbance and excellent water quality.

Some octopus species will autotomise arms when handled during collection (Alupay 2013), which can affect behaviour dramatically (Alupay et al. 2014). Wild-caught animals may also carry existing injuries from failed predation attempts in various stages of healing when they are collected. There is little evidence to suggest that treatment with antibiotics or other drugs in the period immediately after collection is useful. In general, allowing a lengthy period of days to weeks of acclimation time after capture is likely to provide the best outcome. For animals that appear to decline further after capture (indicated by development of skin lesions or extensions of existing lesions, loss of appetite and abnormal behaviour), euthanasia may be the best course of action.

Injuries acquired once within laboratory or aquarium settings are most commonly derived from collisions with physical structures in the environment. Lesions of skin on the posterior mantle are common in octopus, cuttlefish and squid alike, and will typically enlarge further unless the source of the injury is remedied. If a change of physical environment is not possible, reducing disturbance from external may be sufficient to reduce startle behaviours that ing into enclosure walls. Group housing of cuttlefish and squid, particularly when groups are of mixed sex, can also promote aggressive encounters. Once sexually mature, males will bite, grapple and pursue other males, resulting in injuries from the beak, sucker hooks and from collisions. Close monitoring of interactions among animals is necessary when animals approach a size or age when sexual maturity is near, and separation of males into solitary housing is the only effective strategy for preventing these types of injuries. In general, groups of females are less prone to aggressive interactions, but still may injure each other in competition for food items.

Cannibalism and autophagy

Many cephalopod species, particularly octopus and squid, have been reported to be cannibalistic in the wild (Sauer & Smale 1991; Rasero et al. 1996; Ibánez & Keyl 2010; Hernández-Urcera et al. 2014) and will attack and kill conspecifics if kept in the same enclosure. For cephalopods that can be kept communally, small animals may be killed and eaten by larger ones, but the incidence of this behaviour depends very much on the size range of animals held together, the stocking density and provision of adequate food and places of shelter (Hanlon et al. 1983; Hanlon & Forsythe 1985). In the field, the

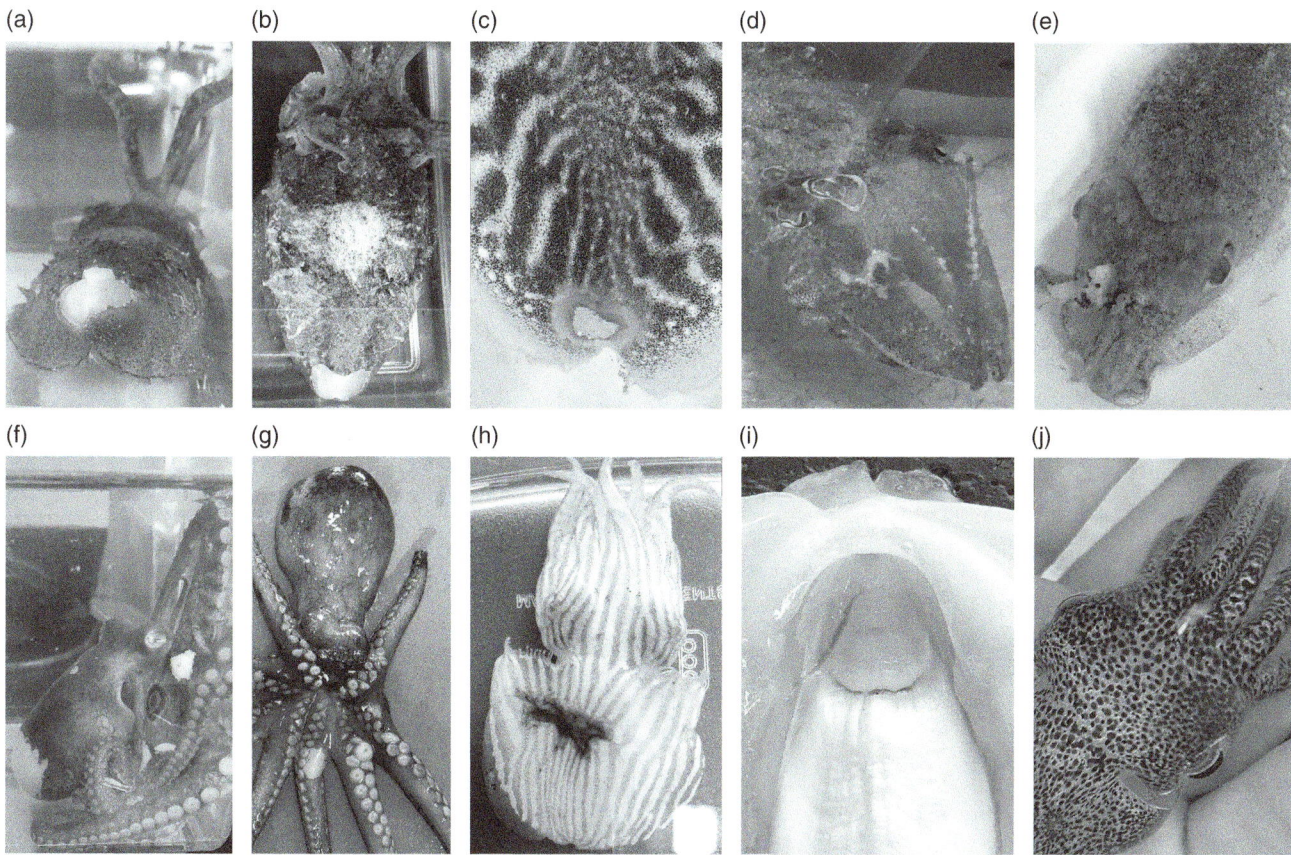

Figure 50.12 Examples of injuries affecting various laboratory cephalopods. (a and b). *Sepia officinalis* showing ulceration of the caudal tip of the mantle, usually caused by colliding with tank walls. (c) A similar lesion showing spreading infection around the wound margins. (d) This *S. officinalis* is showing several wounds from agonistic encounters. The circular scar on the head is a characteristic bite wound. (e) *S. officinalis* with a facial laceration. (f) A senescent female *Octopus bimaculoides* showing ulceration of the caudal mantle and arms. (g) A second example of senescence-associated skin ulceration in *O. bimaculoides*. This animal also shows evidence or autotomy on arm L1 (arrowhead). (h) *Sepiolida lineolata (pyjama squid)* with a large abrasion on the dorsal mantle. (i) *S. officinalis* with a fractured cuttlebone and large hematoma over the caudal mantle, presumably from a forceful collision with the tank wall. (j) Female *E. berryi* with a spermatophore embedded in the skin of the arm crown. Source: All images courtesy of Lisa Abbo, Staff Scientist and veterinarian, Marine Biological Laboratory, Woods Hole, MA, USA, except J. – R Crook.

diet of many cephalopods includes smaller representatives of their own species (Nixon 1987). In certain squids, e.g., *Illex illecebrosus*, it appears that during long migratory journeys the smaller members of the shoal form a normal and major component of diet for the larger animals (Santos & Haimovici 1997), thus cannibalism in laboratory settings is not necessarily indicative of undue stress or abnormal physiology, but rather is a normal aspect of behaviour in many species (that nonetheless should be ameliorated as much as possible). Some cephalopods may be cannibalistic during mating (Anderson *et al*. 2002; Hanlon & Forsythe 2008). If attempting to breed cephalopods in the laboratory, it is usually best to move a male into a female enclosure overnight, then separate the pair the next morning; while this method does not guarantee either successful mating or complete prevention of attacks, it seems to greatly reduce the risks to breeding animals (see section 'mating').

Autophagy, the deliberate consumption of the animal's own body, is known to occur in cephalopods, and is usually an indicator of extreme stress or illness (Reimschuessel & Stoskopf 1990). Autophagy in cephalopods may be a mechanism to remove a damaged area of tissue. After arm autotomy, octopuses engage in extended grooming behaviour of holding the arm stump in the beak (Alupay *et al*. 2014), but whether this involves consumption of some remaining tissue is not known. Dysesthesia is a relatively common cause of self-mutilation in laboratory rodents (Christensen *et al*. 1996; Kohn *et al*. 2007), and it has been proposed as a similar cause of autophagy in octopuses (Reimschuessel & Stoskopf 1990).

There have also been observations of autophagy occurring during senescence and disease (Anderson *et al*. 2002), and even as a contagion spreading between cephalopods sharing the same system (Budelmann 1998). Autophagy can progress quickly and cause death within a matter of hours or days. Reports of autophagy indicate that the behaviour is difficult to interrupt once it begins, and if autophagy is observed, euthanasia is highly recommended for individuals that will not cease the behaviour. Euthanasia is also recommended if it occurs at more than one location on the animal. If there are several cephalopods that share the same system, autophagic animals should be removed to reduce the risk of autophagy in the entire population.

Conclusions

Although there has been enormous progress made on cephalopod welfare, husbandry and culture since the last iteration of the UFAW handbook in 2010, compared to the extent of information and wealth of detail available for laboratory vertebrates, the cephalopods remain poorly served. In the past 10–15 years, the clade has enjoyed something of a resurgence of popularity as research animals, spurred largely by the publication of the octopus genome (Albertin et al. 2015) and recent breakthroughs in husbandry (Dan et al. 2018). As a result of the implementation of Directive 2010/63/EU (Smith et al. 2013; Fiorito et al. 2015), there is now an ongoing and urgent need to develop, validate and standardise best practices and their legislation across research laboratories not only in the European Union, but throughout the world. We anticipate that in the coming years, improved procedures for capture and transport, captive breeding and research methods will be developed, greatly improving both the welfare of captive cephalopods and the quality, reliability and repeatability of research studies in which they are used.

References

Aigner, B.A., Ollert, M., Seifert, F., et al. (2011). *Pseudomonas oryzihabitans* cutaneous ulceration from octopus vulgaris bite: a case report and review of the literature. *Arch. Dermatol.* **147**, 963–966.

Albertin, C.B., Simakov, O., Mitros, T., et al. (2015). The octopus genome and the evolution of cephalopod neural and morphological novelties. *Nature* **524**, 220–224.

Alexandrowicz, J. (1960). A muscle receptor organ in *Eledone cirrhosa*. *J. Mar. Biol. Assoc. UK* **39**, 419–431.

Allen, J.J., Mäthger, L.M., Barbosa, A. and Hanlon, R.T. (2009). Cuttlefish use visual cues to control three-dimensional skin papillae for camouflage. *J. Comp. Physiol. A* **195**, 547–555.

Allen, J.J., Bell, G.R.R., Kuzirian, A.M., et al. (2014). Comparative morphology of changeable skin papillae in octopus and cuttlefish. *J. Morphol.* **275**, 371–90.

Almansa, E., Rocha, F.J., Roura, A., et al. (2017). Cephalopods as predators: a short journey among behavioral flexibilities, adaptions, and feeding habits. *Front. Physiol.* | www.frontiersin.org **1**, 598.

Alupay, J.S. (2013). Characterization of arm autotomy in the Octopus, *Abdopus aculeatus* (d'Orbigny, 1834).

Alupay, J.S., Hadjisolomou, S.P. and Crook, R.J. (2014). Arm injury produces long-term behavioral and neural hypersensitivity in octopus. *Neurosci. Lett.* **558**, 137–142.

Anderson, R.C. and Mather, J.A. (1996). Escape responses of *Euprymna scolopes* Berry, 1911 (Cephalopoda: Sepiolidae). *J. Molluscan Stud.* **62**, 543–545.

Anderson, R.C., Wood, J.B. and Byrne, R.A. (2002). Octopus senescence: the beginning of the end. *J. Appl. Anim. Welf. Sci.* **5**, 275–283.

Andrews, P.L.R. and Tansey, E.M. (1981). The effects of some anaesthetic agents in *Octopus vulgaris*. *Comp. Biochem. Physiol. Part C, Comp.* **70**, 241–247.

Andrews, P.L.R., Messenger, J.B. and Tansey, E.M. (1981). Colour changes in cephalopods after neurotransmitter injection into the cephalic aorta. *Proc. R. Soc. London – Biol. Sci.* **213**, 93–99.

Andrews, P.L.R., Darmaillacq, A.-S., Dennison, N., et al. (2013). The identification and management of pain, suffering and distress in cephalopods, including anaesthesia, analgesia and humane killing. *J. Exp. Mar. Biol. Ecol.* **447**, 46–64.

Anraku, K., Archdale, M.V., Hatanaka, K. and Marui, T. (2005). Chemical stimuli and feeding behavior in Octopus, *Octopus vulgaris*. *Phuket Mar. Biol. Cent.* **66**, 221–227.

Arnold, J. (1990). Squid mating behavior. In: *Squid as Experimental Animals*. Eds. Adelman, W.J., Jr., Arnold, J.M., and Gilbert, D.L. Plenum Press, New York.

Arnold, J. and Williams-Arnold, L. (1977). Cephalopoda: decapoda. In: *Reproduction of Marine Invertebrates, Volume IV Molluscs: Gastropods and Cephalopods*. Eds. Giese, A. and Pearse, J.S., pp. 243–290. Academic Press, New York.

Atkinson, P.R.T., Boyle, A., Hartin, D. and McAuley, D. (2006). Is hot water immersion an effective treatment for marine envenomation? *Emerg. Med. J.* **23**, 503–508.

Augustyn, C.J. (1990). Biological studies on the chokker squid *Loligo vulgaris reynaudii* (cephalopoda; myopsida) on spawning grounds off the south-east coast of South Africa. *South African J. Mar. Sci.* **9**, 11–26.

Balch, N., O'Dor, R. and Helm, P. (1985). Laboratory rearing of rhynchoteuthions of the ommastrephid squid *Illex illecebrosus* (Mollusca: Cephalopoda). *Vie milieu* **35**, 243–246.

Barbosa, A., Mäthger, L.M., Buresch, K.C., et al. (2008). Cuttlefish camouflage: the effects of substrate contrast and size in evoking uniform, mottle or disruptive body patterns. *Vision Res.* **48**, 1242–1253.

Barord, G.J., Ju, C. and Basil, J.A. (2012). First report of a successful treatment of a mucodegenerative disease in the Chambered Nautilus (*Nautilus pompilius*). *J. Zoo Wildl. Med.* **43**, 636–639.

Basil, J.A., Hanlon, R.T., Sheikh, S.I. and Atema, J. (2000). Three-dimensional odor tracking by *Nautilus pompilius*. *J. Exp. Biol.* **203**, 1409–1414.

Basil, J.A., Lazenby, G.B., Nakanuku, L. and Hanlon, R.T. (2002). Female nautilus are attracted to male conspecific odor. *Bull. Mar. Sci.* **70**, 217–225.

Basil, J., Bahctinova, I., Kuroiwa, K., et al. (2005). The function of the rhinophore and the tentacles of *Nautilus pompilius* L. (Cephalopoda, Nautiloidea) in orientation to odor. *Mar. Freshw. Behav. Physiol.* **38**, 209–221.

Berger, E. (2011). Aquaculture of Octopus species: present status, problems and perspectives. *Plymouth Student Sci.* **4**, 384–399.

Bo, Q.K., Zheng, X.D., Gao, X.L. and Li, Q. (2016). Multiple paternity in the common long-armed octopus *minor* (Sasaki, 1920) (Cephalopoda: Octopoda) as revealed by microsatellite DNA analysis. *Mar. Ecol.* **37**, 1073–1078.

Boal, J.G. and Golden, D.K. (1999). Distance chemoreception in the common cuttlefish, *Sepia officinalis* (Mollusca, Cephalopoda). *J. Exp. Mar. Biol. Ecol.* **235**, 307–317.

Boletzky, S.V. (1998). Cephalopod eggs and egg masses. *Oceanography Mar. Biol. An Annu. Rev.* 36, 341–371.

Boletzky, S.V. and Hanlon, R.T. (1983). A review of the laboratory maintenance, rearing and culture of cephalopod mollusks. *Memoirs of the National Museum Victoria*, No. 44.

Boucaud-Camou, E. and Boucher-Rodoni, R. (1966). Feeding and digestion in cephalopods. In: *Physiology of Mollusca*. Eds. Saleuddin, A. and Wilbur, K., pp. 97–124. Academic Press, London.

Boycott, B.B. and Young, J.Z. (1955). A memory system in *Octopus vulgaris* Lamarck. *Proc. R. Soc. London. Ser. B, Biol. Sci.* 449–480.

Boyle, P.R. (1981). Methods for the aquarium maintenance of the common octopus of British waters, *Eledone cirrhosa*. *Lab. Anim.* **15**, 327–331.

Boyle, P.R. (1983). *Cephalopod Life Cycles*. Academic Press, UK.

Boyle, P.R. (1990). Cephalopod biology in the fisheries context. *Fish. Res.* **8**, 303–321.

Boyle, P.R. and Chevis, D. (1992). Egg development in the octopus *Eledone cirrhosa*. *J. Zool.* **227**, 623–638.

Boyle, P.R. and Knobloch, D. (1982). On Growth of the Octopus *Eledone Cirrhosa*. *J. Mar. Biol. Assoc. United Kingdom* **62**, 277–296.

Boyle, P.R. and Knobloch, D. (1983). The female reproductive cycle of the octopus, *Eledone cirrhosa*. *J. Mar. Biol. Assoc. United Kingdom* **63**, 71–83.

Boyle, P.R., Knobloch, D. and Gaillard, J. (1982). Sexual maturation in the octopus *Eledone cirrhosa* Lamarck. *Proc. 7th Int. Malacol. Congr. 31 – Sept. 7,1980*, **22**, 189–196.

Bradley, E.A. (1974). Some observations of *Octopus joubini* reared in an inland aquarium. *J. Zool.* **173**, 355–368.

Bridges, C.R. (1995). Bohr and Root Effects in Cephalopod Haemocyanins – Paradox or Pressure in *Sepia officinalis*? *Mar. Freshw. Behav. Physiol.* **25**, 121–130.

Budelmann, B.U. (1998). Autophagy in Octopus. *South African J. Mar. Sci.* **20**, 101–108.

Buresch, K.M., Hanlon, R.T., Maxwell, M.R. and Ring, S. (2001). Microsatellite DNA markers indicate a high frequency of multiple paternity within individual field-collected egg capsules of the squid *Loligo pealeii*. *Mar. Ecol. Prog. Ser.* **210**, 161–165.

Bush, S.L., Robison, B.H. and Caldwell, R.L. (2009). Behaving in the dark: locomotor, chromatic, postural, and bioluminescent behaviors of the deep-sea squid *Octopoteuthis deletron* Young 1972. *Biol. Bull.* **216**, 7–22.

Bush, S.L., Hoving, H.J.T., Huffard, C.L., et al. (2012). Brooding and sperm storage by the deep-sea squid *Bathyteuthis berryi* (Cephalopoda: Decapodiformes). *J. Mar. Biol. Assoc. United Kingdom* **92**, 1629–1636.

Butler-Struben, H.M., Brophy, S.M., Johnson, N.A. and Crook, R.J. (2018). in vivo recording of neural and behavioral correlates of anesthesia induction, reversal, and euthanasia in cephalopod molluscs. *Front. Physiol.* **9**.

Campanelli, A., Sanchez-Politta, S. and Saurat, J.H. (2008). Cutaneous ulceration after an octopus bite: infection due to *Vibrio alginolyticus*, an emerging pathogen. *Ann. Dermatol. Venereol.* **135**, 225–227.

Castellanos-Martínez, S. and Gestal, C. (2013). Pathogens and immune response of cephalopods. *J. Exp. Mar. Biol. Ecol.* **447**, 14–22.

Castellanos-Martínez, S., Diz, A.P., Álvarez-Chaver, P. and Gestal, C. (2014). Proteomic characterization of the hemolymph of *Octopus vulgaris* infected by the protozoan parasite *Aggregata octopiana*. *J. Proteomics* **105**, 151–163.

Castro, B.G., Paul DiMarco, F., DeRusha, R.H. and Lee, P.G. (1993). The effects of surimi and pelleted diets on the laboratory survival, growth, and feeding rate of the cuttlefish *Sepia officinalis* L. *J. Exp. Mar. Biol. Ecol.* **170**, 241–252.

Cerezo Valverde, J. and García, B. (2005). Suitable dissolved oxygen levels for common octopus (*Octopus vulgaris cuvier*, 1797) at different weights and temperatures: analysis of respiratory behaviour. *Aquaculture* **244**, 303–314.

Chabala, L.D., Morello, R.S., Busath, D., et al. (1986). Capture, transport, and maintenance of live squid (*Loligo pealei*) for electrophysiological studies. *Pflugers Arch. Eur. J. Physiol.* **407**, 105–108.

Chiao, C.-C., Kenneth Wickiser, J., Allen, J.J., et al. (2011). Hyperspectral imaging of cuttlefish camouflage indicates good color match in the eyes of fish predators. *PNAS* **108**.

Chiao, C.-C., Chubb, C. and Hanlon, R.T. (2015). A review of visual perception mechanisms that regulate rapid adaptive camouflage in cuttlefish. *J. Comp. Physiol. A. Neuroethol. Sens. Neural. Behav. Physiol.* **201**, 933–945.

Chichery, R. (1985). The behavior and natural history of the Caribbean reef squid *Sepioteuthis sepioidea*. *Behav. Processes* **10**, 328–329.

Chichery, R. and Chanelet, J. (1976). Motor and behavioural responses obtained by stimulation with chronic electrodes of the optic lobe of *Sepia officinalis*. *Brain Res.* **105**, 525–532.

Chichery, R. and Chanelet, J. (1978). Motor responses obtained by stimulation of the peduncle lobe of *Sepia officinalis* in chronic experiments. *Brain Res.* **150**, 188–193.

Chichery, R. and Chichery, M.P. (1992a). Learning performances and aging in cuttlefish (*Sepia officinalis*). *Exp. Gerontol.* **27**, 233–239.

Chichery, M.P. and Chichery, R. (1992b). Behavioural and neurohistological changes in aging Sepia. *Brain Res.* **574**, 77–84.

Chrachri, A. and Williamson, R. (2004). Cholinergic and glutamatergic spontaneous and evoked excitatory postsynaptic currents in optic lobe neurons of cuttlefish, Sepia officinalis. *Brain Res.* **1020**, 178–187.

Christensen, M.D., Everhart, A.W., Pickelman, J.T. and Hulsebosch, C.E. (1996). Mechanical and thermal allodynia in chronic central pain following spinal cord injury. *Pain* **68**, 97–107.

Collins, A.J. and Nyholm, S.V. (2010). Obtaining hemocytes from the Hawaiian bobtail squid Euprymna scolopes and observing their adherence to symbiotic and non-symbiotic bacteria. *J. Vis. Exp.*, (36), 1714.

Cooke, G.M. and Tonkins, B.M. (2015). Behavioural indicators of welfare exhibited by the common European cuttlefish (Sepia officinalis). *J. Zoo Aquarium Res.* **3**, 157–162.

Cooke, G.M., Tonkins, B.M. and Mather, J.A. (2019). Care and enrichment for captive cephalopods. In: *The Welfare of Invertebrate Animals*. Eds. Carere, C. and Mather, J., pp. 179–208. Springer, Cham.

Crook, R.J. and Basil, J.A. (2008a). A role for nautilus in studies of the evolution of brain and behavior. *Commun. Integr. Biol.* **1**, 18–19.

Crook, R. and Basil, J. (2008b). A biphasic memory curve in the chambered nautilus, Nautilus pompilius L. (Cephalopoda: Nautiloidea). *J. Exp. Biol.* **211**, 1992–1998.

Crook, R.J. and Basil, J.A. (2013). Flexible spatial orientation and navigational strategies in chambered nautilus. *Ethology* **119**, 77–85.

Crook, R.J., Hanlon, R.T. and Basil, J.A. (2009). Memory of visual and topographical features suggests spatial learning in nautilus (Nautilus pompilius L.). *J. Comp. Psychol.* **123**, 264–274.

Crook, R.J., Hanlon, R.T. and Walters, E.T. (2013). Squid have nociceptors that display widespread long-term sensitization and spontaneous activity after bodily injury. *J. Neurosci.* **33**, 10021–10026.

Crook, R.J., Dickson, K., Hanlon, R.T. and Walters, E.T. (2014). Nociceptive sensitization reduces predation risk. *Curr. Biol.* **24**, 1121–1125.

Cummins, S.F., Boal, J.G., Buresch, K.C., et al. (2011). Extreme aggression in male squid induced by a β-MSP-like pheromone. *Curr. Biol.* **21**, 322–327.

Daly, H. (1996). Ecology of the Antarctic octopus Pareledone from the Scotia Sea. Doctoral dissertation, University of Aberdeen.

Dan, S., Iwasaki, H., Takasugi, A., et al. (2018). An upwelling system for culturing common octopus paralarvae and its combined effect with supplying natural zooplankton on paralarval survival and growth. *Aquaculture* **495**, 98–105.

Derby, C.D. (2014). Cephalopod ink: production, chemistry, functions and applications. *Mar. Drugs* **12**, 2700–2730.

Derby, C.D., Kicklighter, C.E., Johnson, P.M. and Zhang, X. (2007). Chemical composition of inks of diverse marine molluscs suggests convergent chemical defenses. *J. Chem. Ecol.* **33**, 1105–1113.

Di Cosmo, A. and Di Cristo, C. (1998). Neuropeptidergic control of the optic gland of Octopus vulgaris: FMRF- amide and GnRH immunoreactivity. *J. Comp. Neurol.* **398**, 1–12.

Di Cosmo, A., Di Cristo, C. and Paolucci, M. (2001). Sex steroid hormone fluctuations and morphological changes of the reproductive system of the female of Octopus vulgaris throughout the annual cycle. *J. Exp. Zool.* **289**, 33–47.

Di Cristo, C. and Di Cosmo, A. (2007). Neuropeptidergic control of Octopus oviducal gland. *Peptides* **28**, 163–168.

Dickel, L., Boal, J.G. and Budelmann, B.U. (2000). The effect of early experience on learning and memory in cuttlefish. *Dev. Psychobiol.* **36**, 101–110.

Domingues, P.M., Sykes, A. and Andrade, J.P. (2001). The use of Artemia sp. Or mysids as food source for hatchlings of the cuttlefish (Sepia officinalis L.); effects on growth and survival throughout the life cycle. *Aquac. Int.* **9**, 319–331.

Domingues, P.M., Dimarco, F.P., Andrade, J.P. and Lee, P.G. (2005). Effect of artificial diets on growth, survival and condition of adult cuttlefish, Sepia officinalis Linnaeus, 1758. *Aquac. Int.* **13**, 423–440.

Domingues, P.M., López, N., Muñoz, J.A., et al. (2007). Effects of a dry pelleted diet on growth and survival of the Yucatan octopus, *Octopus maya*. *Aquac. Nutr.* **13**, 273–280.

Drazen, J.C., Goffredi, S.K., Schlining, B. and Stakes, D.S. (2003). Aggregations of egg-brooding deep-sea fish and cephalopods on the Gorda escarpment: a reproductive hot spot. *Biol. Bull.* **205**, 1–7.

Dubas, F. and Boyle, P. (1985). Chromatophore motor units in *Eledone cirrhosa* (Cephalopoda: Octopoda). *J. Exp. Biol.* **431**, 415–431.

Fajer-Ávila, E.J., Abdo-de la Parra, I., Aguilar-Zarate, G., et al. (2003). Toxicity of formalin to bullseye puffer fish (*Sphoeroides annulatus* Jenyns, 1843) and its effectiveness to control ectoparasites. *Aquaculture* **223**, 41–50.

Farto, R., Armada, S.P., Montes, M., et al. (2003). Vibrio lentus associated with diseased wild octopus (*Octopus vulgaris*). *J. Invertebr. Pathol.* **83**, 149–156.

Farto, R., Fichi, G., Gestal, C., et al. (2019). Bacteria-Affecting Cephalopods. In *Handbook of Pathogens and Diseases in Cephalopods*, pp. 127–142. Cham, Springer International Publishing.

Finn, J.K. and Norman, M.D. (2010). The argonaut shell: gas-mediated buoyancy control in a pelagic octopus. In: *Proceedings of the Royal Society B: Biological Sciences*, pp. 2967–2971. The Royal Society.

Fiorito, G., Affuso, A., Basil, J., et al. (2015). Guidelines for the Care and Welfare of Cephalopods in Research –A consensus based on an initiative by CephRes, FELASA and the Boyd Group. *Lab. Anim.* **49**, 1–90.

Ford, L.A., Alexander, S.K., Cooper, K.M. and Hanlon, R.T. (1986). Bacterial populations of normal and ulcerated mantle tissue of the squid, Lolliguncula brevis. *J. Invertebr. Pathol.* **48**, 13–26.

Forsythe, J.W. and Hanlon, R.T. (1997). Foraging and associated behavior by Octopus cyanea Gray, 1849 on a coral atoll, French Polynesia. *J. Exp. Mar. Biol. Ecol.* **209**, 15–31.

Forsythe, J.W. and van Heukelem, W.F. (1987). Growth. In: *Cephalopod Life Cycles, Vol. II*. Ed. Boyle, P.R., pp. 135–155. Academic Press, London.

Cooke, G.M., Tonkins, B.M. and Mather, J.A. (2019). Care and enrichment for captive cephalopods. In: *The Welfare of Invertebrate Animals*. Eds. Carere, C. and Mather, J., pp. 179–208. Springer, Cham.

Forsythe, J.W., DeRusha, R.H. and Hanlon, R.T. (1994). Growth, reproduction and life span of Sepia officinalis (Cephalopoda: Mollusca) cultured through seven consecutive generations. *J. Zool.* **233**, 175–192.

Fouke, K.E. and Rhodes, H.J. (2020). Electrophysiological and motor responses to chemosensory stimuli in isolated cephalopod arms. *Biol. Bull.* **238**, 1–11.

Franklin, A.M., Squires, Z.E. and Stuart-Fox, D. (2014). Does predation risk affect mating behavior? An experimental test in dumpling squid (Euprymna tasmanica). *PloS One* **9**, e115027.

Froesch, D. and Marthy, H.J. (1975). The structure and function of the oviducal gland in octopods (Cephalopoda). *Proc. R. Soc. London – Biol. Sci.* **188**, 95–101.

Gestal, C., Abollo, E. and Pascual, S. (1998). Rickettsiales-like organisms in the gills of reared Octopus vulgaris (Mollusca, Cephalopoda). *Bull. Eur. Assoc. Fish Pathol.* **18**, 13–14.

Gestal, C., Páez de la Cadena, M. and Pascual, S. (2002). Malabsorption syndrome observed in the common octopus vulgaris infected with Aggregata octopiana (Protista: Apicomplexa). *Dis. Aquat. Organ.* **51**, 61–65.

Gilly, W.F. and Lucero, M.T. (1992). Behavioral responses to chemical stimulation of the olfactory organ in the squid Loligo opalescens. *J. Exp. Biol.* **162**, 209–229.

Gleadall, I.G. (2013). The effects of prospective anaesthetic substances on cephalopods: summary of original data and a brief review of studies over the last two decades. *Clin. Psychol. Rev.* **33**, 23–30.

Gomathi, P., Nair, J.R. and Sherief, P.M. (2010). Antibacterial activity in the accessory nidamental gland extracts of the Indian squid, Loligo duvauceli Orbigny. *Indian J. Mar. Sci.* **39**, 100–104.

Gonzalez-Bellido, P.T., Scaros, A.T., Hanlon, R.T. and Wardill, T.J. (2018). Neural Control of Dynamic 3-Dimensional Skin Papillae for Cuttlefish Camouflage. *iScience* **1**, 24–34.

Grasse, B. (2014). The biological characteristics, life cycle, and system design for the flamboyant and Paintpot Cuttlefish, Metasepia sp., cultured through multiple generations. *Drum Croak.* **45**, 58–71.

Gray, J.A.B. (1960). Mechanically excitable receptor units in the mantle of the octopus and their connexions. *J. Physiol.* **153**, 573–582.

Gray, E.G. (1970). A note on synaptic structure of the retina of Octopus vulgaris. *J. Cell Sci.* **7**, 203–215.

Graziadei, P. (1965). Muscle receptors in cephalopods. *Proc. R. Soc. London. Ser. B. Biol. Sci.* **161**, 392–402.

Gromek, S.M., Suria, A.M., Fullmer, M.S., et al. (2016). Leisingera sp. JC1, a bacterial isolate from Hawaiian bobtail squid eggs, produces indigoidine and differentially inhibits vibrios. *Front. Microbiol.* **7**.

Guerdat, T.C., Losordo, T.M., Classen, J.J., et al. (2011). Evaluating the effects of organic carbon on biological filtration performance in a large scale recirculating aquaculture system. *Aquac. Eng.* **44**, 10–18.

Guerra, A., Rocha, F., González, A.F. and Bückle, L.F. (2001). Embryonic stages of the Patagonian squid Loligo gahi (Mollusca: Cephalopoda). *Veliger* **44**, 109–115.

Gutfreund, Y., Matzner, H., Flash, T. and Hochner, B. (2006). Patterns of motor activity in the isolated nerve cord of the octopus arm. *Biol. Bull.* **211**, 212–222.

Gutnick, T., Byrne, R.A., Hochner, B. and Kuba, M. (2011). Octopus vulgaris uses visual information to determine the location of its arm. *Curr. Biol.* **21**, 460–462.

Hague, T., Florini, M. and Andrews, P.L.R. (2013). Preliminary in vitro functional evidence for reflex responses to noxious stimuli in the arms of Octopus vulgaris. *J. Exp. Mar. Biol. Ecol.* **447**, 100–105.

Hall, K.C. and Hanlon, R.T. (2002). Principal features of the mating system of a large spawning aggregation of the giant Australian cuttlefish Sepia apama (Mollusca: Cephalopoda). *Mar. Biol.* **140**, 533–545.

Halm, M.P., Agin, V., Chichery, M.P. and Chichery, R. (2000). Effect of aging on manipulative behavior in the cuttlefish, Sepia. *Physiol. Behav.* **68**, 543–547.

Hanley, J.S., Shashar, N., Smolowitz, R., et al. (1998). Modified laboratory culture techniques for the European cuttlefish Sepia officinalis. In: *Biological Bulletin*, pp. 223–225.

Hanlon, R.T. (1990). Maintenance, rearing and culture of teuthoid and sepioid squids. In: *Squid as Experimental Animals*, pp. 35–62. Boston, MA: Plenum Press, New York, NY.

Hanlon, R.T. and Forsythe, J.W. (1985). Advances in the laboratory culture of octopuses for biomedical research. *Lab. Anim. Sci.* **35**, 33.

Hanlon, R.T. and Forsythe, J.W. (1990). Diseases caused by microorganisms. In: *Diseases of Mollusca: Cephalopoda*. Ed. Kinnie, O., pp. 23–46. Hamburg, Biologische Anstalt Helgoland.

Hanlon, R.T. and Forsythe, J.W. (2008). Sexual cannibalism by Octopus cyanea on a Pacific coral reef. *Mar. Freshw. Behav. Physiol.* **41**, 19–28.

Hanlon, R. and Messenger, J. (2018). *Cephalopod Behaviour*. Cambridge University Press, Cambridge.

Hanlon, R.T. and Shashar, N. (2008). Aspects of the sensory ecology of cephalopods. In: *Sensory Processing in Aquatic Environments*, pp. 266–282. New York, NY, Springer New York.

Hanlon, R.T., Hixon, R.F. and Hulet, W.H. (1983). Survival, growth, and behavior of the loliginid squids Lologi plei, Loligo pealei, and Lolliguncula brevis (Mollusca: Cephalopoda) in closed sea water systems. *Biol. Bull.* 637–685.

Hanlon, R.T., Forsythe, J.W., Cooper, K.M., *et al.* (1984). Fatal penetrating skin ulcers in laboratory-reared octopuses. *J. Invertebr. Pathol.* **44**, 67–83.

Hanlon, R.T., Yank, W.T., Turk, P.E., *et al.* (1989). Laboratory culture and estimated life span of the Eastern Atlantic squid, Loligo forbesi Steenstrup, 1856 (Mollusca: Cephalopoda). *Aquac. Res.* **20**, 15–34.

Hanlon, R.T., Turk, P.E. and Lee, P.G. (1991). Squid and cuttlefish mariculture: an updated perspective. *J. Cephalop. Biol.* **2**, 31–40.

Hanlon, R.T., Smale, M.J. and Sauer, W.H.H. (1994). An ethogram of body patterning behavior in the squid Loligo vulgaris reynaudii on spawning grounds in South Africa. *Biol. Bull.* **187**, 363–372.

Hanlon, R.T., Claes, M.F., Ashcraft, S.E. and Dunlap, P.V. (1997). Laboratory culture of the Sepiolid Squid Euprymna scolopes: a model system for bacteria-animal symbiosis. *Biol. Bull.* **192**, 364–374.

Hanlon, R.T., Maxwell, M.R., Shashar, N., *et al.* (1999). An ethogram of body patterning behavior in the biomedically and commercially valuable squid *Loligo pealei* off Cape Cod, Massachusetts. *Biol. Bull.* **197**, 49–62.

Harms, C.A., Lewbart, G.A., McAlarney, R., *et al.* (2006). Surgical excision of myotic (Cladosprorium sp.) granulomas from the mantle of a cuttlefish (Sepia officinalis). *J. Zoo Wildl. Med.* **37**, 524–530.

Hendrix, J.P., Hulet, W.H. and Greenberg, M.J. (1981). Salinity tolerance and the responses to hypoosmotic stress of the bay squid Lolliguncula brevis, a euryhaline cephalopod mollusc. *Comp. Biochem. Physiol. – Part A Physiol.* **69**, 641–648.

Hernández-García, V., Hernández-López, J.L. and Castro-Hdez, J.J. (2002). On the reproduction of Octopus vulgaris off the coast of the Canary Islands. *Fish. Res.* **57**, 197–203.

Hernández-Urcera, J., Garci, M.E., Roura, Á., *et al.* (2014). Cannibalistic behavior of octopus (octopus vulgaris) in the wild. *J. Comp. Psychol.* **128**, 427–430.

Higgins, F.A., Bates, A.E. and Lamare, M.D. (2012). Heat tolerance, behavioural temperature selection and temperature-dependent respiration in larval Octopus huttoni. *J. Therm. Biol.* **37**, 83–88.

Higham, T.F. (1957). Nature note: autophagy in octopods. Hesiod vindicated. *Classical Rev.* **7**, 16–17.

Holst, M. and Miller-Morgan, T. (2020). The use of a species specific health and welfare assessment tool to monitor health, stress and welfare of the giant Pacific octopus, Enterocotpus dofleini. *J. Appl. Anim. Welf. Sci.*, **24**(3), 272–291.

Hoving, H.J.T. and Haddock, S.H.D. (2017). The giant deep-sea octopus Haliphron atlanticus forages on gelatinous fauna. *Sci. Rep.* **7**.

Hoving, H.J.T., Lipinski, M.R., Videler, J.J. and Bolstad, K.S.R. (2010). Sperm storage and mating in the deep-sea squid Taningia danae Joubin, 1931 (Oegopsida: Octopoteuthidae). *Mar. Biol.* **157**, 393–400.

Huffard, C.L. (2007). Ethogram of Abdopus aculeatus (d'Orbigny, 1834) (Cephalopoda: Octopodidae): can behavioural characters inform octopodid taxonomy and systematics? *J. Molluscan Stud.* **73**, 185–193.

Huffard, C.L. and Godfrey-Smith, P. (2010). Field observations of mating in Octopus tetricus Gould, 1852 and Amphioctopus marginatus (Taki, 1964) (Cephalopoda: Octopodidae). *Molluscan Res.* **30**, 81–86.

Huffard, C.L., Boneka, F. and Full, R.J. (2005). Underwater bipedal locomotion by octopuses in disguise. *Science* **307**, 1927.

Huffard, C.L., Caldwell, R.L. and Boneka, F. (2010). Male-male and male-female aggression may influence mating associations in wild octopuses (Abdopus aculeatus). *J. Comp. Psychol.* **124**, 38.

Ibánez, C. and Keyl, F. (2010). Cannibalism in cephalopods. *Rev. Fish Biol. Fish.*, **20**(1), 123–136.

Iglesias, J. and Fuentes, L. (2014). Octopus vulgaris. Paralarval Culture. In: *Cephalopod Culture*, pp. 427–450. Dordrecht, Springer Netherlands.

Iglesias, J., Otero, J.J., Moxica, C., Fuentes, L. and Sánchez, F.J. (2004). The completed life cycle of the octopus (Octopus vulgaris, Cuvier) under culture conditions: paralarval rearing using Artemia and zoeae, and first data on juvenile growth up to 8 months of age. *Aquac. Int.* **12**, 481–487.

Iglesias, J., Villanueva, R. and Fuentes, L. (2014). *Cephalopod Culture*. Eds. Iglesias, J., Fuentes, L., and Villanueva, R. Springer, Dordrecht.

Ikeda, Y., Sakurai, Y. and Shimazakj, K. (1993). Fertilizing capacity of squid (Todarodes pacificus) spermatozoa collected from various sperm storage sites, with special reference to the role of gelatinous substance from oviducal gland in fertilization and embryonic development. *Invertebr. Reprod. Dev.* **23**, 39–44.

Ikeda, Y., Sakurazawa, I., Ito, K., *et al.* (2005). Rearing of squid hatchlings, Heterololigo bleekeri (Keferstein 1866) up to 2 months in a closed seawater system. *Aquac. Res.* **36**, 409–412.

Imperadore, P., Shah, S.B., Makarenkova, H.P. and Fiorito, G. (2017). Nerve degeneration and regeneration in the cephalopod mollusc Octopus vulgaris: the case of the pallial nerve. *Sci. Rep.* **7**.

Iwata, Y., Shaw, P., Fujiwara, E., *et al.* (2011). Why small males have big sperm: dimorphic squid sperm linked to alternative mating behaviours. *BMC Evol. Biol.* **11**, 236.

Jantzen, T.M. and Havenhand, J.N. (2002). Preliminary field observations of mating and spawning in the squid Sepioteuthis australis. *Bull. Mar. Sci.*, **71**(2), 1073–1080.

Johnsen, S., Balser, E. J., Fisher, E.C. and Widder, E.A. (1999). Bioluminescence in the Deep-Sea Cirrate Octopod Stauroteuthis syrtensis Verrill (Mollusca: Cephalopoda). *Biol. Bull.* **197**, 26–39.

Joll, L.M. (1976). Mating, egg-laying and hatching of Octopus tetricus (Mollusca: Cephalopoda) in the laboratory. *Mar. Biol.* **36**, 327–333.

Joll, L.M. (1977). Growth and Food Intake of Octopus Tetricus (Mollusca: Cephalopoda) in Aquaria. *Mar. Freshw. Res.* **28**, 45–56.

Jones, G.M. and O'Dor, R.K. (1983). Ultrastructural observations on a thraustochytrid fungus parasitic in the gills of squid (Illex illecebrosus LeSueur). *J. Parasitol.* **69**, 903.

Katharios, P., Papandroulakis, N. and Divanach, P. (2006). Treatment of Microcotyle sp. (Monogenea) on the gills of cage-cultured red porgy, Pagrus pagrus following baths with formalin and mebendazole. *Aquaculture* **251**, 167–171.

Kerwin, A.H. and Nyholm, S.V. (2017). Symbiotic bacteria associated with a bobtail squid reproductive system are detectable in the environment, and stable in the host and developing eggs. *Environ. Microbiol.* **19**, 1463–1475.

Kier, W.M. and Messenger, J.B. (1985). Mechanoreceptors in the fins of the cuttlefish, *Sepia officinalis*. *J. Exp. Biol.* **119**, 369–373.

Kohn, D.F., Martin, T.E., Foley, P.L., *et al.* (2007). Guidelines for the assessment and management of pain in rodents and rabbits. *J. Am. Assoc. Lab. Anim. Sci.* **46**, 97–108.

Koueta, N. and Boucaud-Camou, E. (2001). Basic growth relations in experimental rearing of early juvenile cuttlefish Sepia officinalis L. (Mollusca: Cephalopoda). *J. Exp. Mar. Biol. Ecol.* **265**, 75–87.

Koueta, N., Castro, B.G. and Boucaud-Camou, E. (2000). Biochemical indices for instantaneous growth estimation in young cephalopod Sepia officinalis L. *ICES J. Mar. Sci.* **57**, 1–7.

Koueta, N., Boucaud-Camou, E. and Noel, B. (2002). Effect of enriched natural diet on survival and growth of juvenile cuttlefish Sepia officinalis L. *Aquaculture* **203**, 293–310.

Kuba, M.J., Byrne, R.A., Meisel, D.V. and Mather, J.A. (2006). When do octopuses play? Effects of repeated testing, object type, age, and food deprivation on object play in Octopus vulgaris. *J. Comp. Psychol.* **120**, 184–190.

Lee, P.G. (1995). Nutrition of cephalopods: fueling the system. *Mar. Freshw. Behav. Physiol.* **25**, 35–51.

Lee, Y.-H., Yan, H.Y. and Chiao, C.-C. (2010). Visual contrast modulates maturation of camouflage body patterning in cuttlefish (Sepia pharaonis). *J. Comp. Psychol.* **124**(3), 261–270.

Lee, Y., Yan, H.Y. and Chiao, C.-C. (2012). Effects of early visual experience on the background preference in juvenile cuttlefish Sepia pharaonis. *Biol. Lett.*, **8**(5), 740–743.

Lee, P.G., Forsythe, J.W., Di Marco, F.P., et al. (1991). Initial palatability and growth trials on pelleted diets for cephalopods. *Bull. Mar. Sci.* **49**, 362–372.

Lee, P., Turk, P., Forsythe, J., et al. (1998). Cephalopod culture: physiological, behavioral and environmental requirements. *Aquac. Sci.* **46**, 417–422.

Lee, P.N., Callaerts, P. and de Couet, H.G. (2009). The embryonic development of the Hawaiian bobtail squid (Euprymna scolopes). *Cold Spring Harb. Protoc.* 2009, pdb.ip77.

Lipiński, M.R. and Underhill, L.G. (1995). Sexual maturation in squid: quantum or continuum? *South African J. Mar. Sci.* **15**, 207–223.

Liu, T.-H. and Chiao, C.-C. (2017). Mosaic organization of body pattern control in the optic lobe of squids. *J. Neurosci.* **37**, 768–780.

Loten, C., Stokes, B., Worsley, D., et al. (2006). A randomised controlled trial of hot water (45° C) immersion versus ice packs for pain relief in bluebottle stings. *Med. J. Aust.* **184**, 329–333.

Luke, D., Cohen, J. and Aquatic Invertebrate Taxon Advisory Group (2014). *Giant Pacific Octopus (Enteroctopus dofleini) Care Manual*. Aquatic Invertebrate Taxon Advisory Group (AZA).

Lykkeboe, G., Brix, O. and Johansen, K. (1980). Oxygen-linked CO_2 binding independent of pH in cephalopod blood. *Nature* **287**, 330–331.

Marini, G., De Sio, F., Ponte, G. and Fiorito, G. (2017). Behavioral analysis of learning and memory in cephalopods (Chapter 1.24). In: *Learning and Memory: A Comprehensive Reference*, Ed. Bryne, J.H., pp. 441–462. Academic Press, Oxford, UK.

Marthy, H.J., Hauser, R. and Scholl, A. (1976). Natural tranquilliser in cephalopod eggs. *Nature* **261**, 496–497.

Martins, H.R. (1982). Biological studies of the exploited stock of loligo forbesi (Mollusca: Cephalopoda) in the azores. *J. Mar. Biol. Assoc. United Kingdom* **62**, 799–808.

Mather, J.A. (1998). How Do Octopuses Use Their Arms? *J. Comp. Psychol.* **112**, 306–316.

Mather, J. and Anderson, R. (1999). Exploration, play and habituation in octopuses (Octopus dofleini). *J. Comp. Psychol.* **113**(3), 333.

Mäthger, L.M., Roberts, S.B. and Hanlon, R.T. (2010). Evidence for distributed light sensing in the skin of cuttlefish, *Sepia officinalis*. *Biol. Lett.* **6**, 600–603.

Matzner, H. (2000). Neuromuscular system of the flexible arm of the Octopus: physiological characterization. *J. Neurophysiol.* **83**, 1315–1328.

McMichael, D.F. (1964). The identity of the venomous octopus responsible for a fatal bite at Darwin, northern territory. *J. Malacol. Soc. Aust.* **1**, 23–24.

Messenger, J.B. (2001). Cephalopod chromatophores: neurobiology and natural history. *Biol. Rev.* **76**, 473–528.

Messenger, J.B., Nixon, M. and Ryan, K.P. (1985). Magnesium chloride as an anaesthetic for cephalopods. *Comp. Biochem. Physiol. Part C Comp. Pharmacol.* **82**, 203–205.

Montague, T.G., Rieth, I.J. and Axel, R. (2021). Embryonic development of the camouflaging dwarf cuttlefish, *Sepia bandensis*. *Dev. Dyn.* Dvdy.375.

Mooney, T.A., Lee, W.-J. and Hanlon, R.T. (2010). Long-duration anesthetization of squid (Doryteuthis pealeii). *Mar. Freshw. Behav. Physiol.* **43**, 297–303.

Moynihan, M. (1983). Notes on the behavior of Euprymna scolopes (Cephalopoda: Sepiolidae). *Behaviour* **85**, 25–41.

Muntz, W.R.A. (1986). Short communications: the spectral sensitivity of Nautilus Pompilius. *J. Exp. Biol.* **126**, 513–517.

Muntz, W.R.A. (2010). Visual behavior and visual sensitivity of Nautilus pompilius. In: *Nautilus*, pp. 231–244. Springer, Dordrecht.

Muntz, W.R.A. and Raj, U. (1984). On the visual system of Nautilus Pompilius. *J. Exp. Biol.* **109**, 253–263.

Nabhitabhata, J., Asawangkune, P., Amornjaruchit, S. and Promboom, P. (2001). Tolerance of eggs and Hatchlings of neritic cephalopods to salinity changes. *Phuket Mar. Biol. Cent. Spec. Publ.* **25**, 91–99.

Nabhitabhata, J., Nilaphat, P., Promboon, P. and Jaroongpattananon, C. (2005). Life Cycle of Cultured Bobtail Squid, Euprymna hyllebergi. *Phuket Mar. Biol. Cent. Res. Bull.* **66**, 351–365.

Naud, M.-J.J., Shaw, P.W., Hanlon, R.T. and Havenhand, J.N. (2005). Evidence for biased use of sperm sources in wild female giant cuttlefish (Sepia apama). *Proc. R. Soc. B Biol. Sci.* **272**, 1047–1051.

Naud, M.-J.J., Sauer, W.H.H., McKeown, N.J., et al. (2016). Multiple mating, paternity and complex fertilisation patterns in the chokka squid Loligo reynaudii. *PloS One* **11**, e0146995.

Navarro, J.C., Monroig, Ó. And Sykes, A.V. (2014). Nutrition as a key factor for cephalopod aquaculture. In: *Cephalopod Culture*, pp. 77–95. Dordrecht, Springer Netherlands.

Nesher, N., Levy, G., Grasso, F.W. and Hochner, B. (2014). Self-recognition mechanism between skin and suckers prevents octopus arms from interfering with each other. *Curr. Biol.* **24**, 1271–1275.

Nixon, M. (1987). Cephalopod diets. In: *Cephalopod Life Cycles. Comparative Reviews*. Ed. Boyle, P.R., pp. 201–219. Academic Press, London.

Nixon, M. and Young, J.Z. (2003). *The Brains and Lives of Cephalopods*. Oxford University Press, Oxford, UK.

Novicki, A., Budelmann, B.U. and Hanlon, R.T. (1990). Brain pathways of the chromatophore system in the squid *Lolliguncula brevis*. *Brain Res.* **519**, 315–323.

O'Dor, R.K. and Wells, M.J. (1978). Reproduction versus somatic growth: hormonal control in Octopus vulgaris. *J. Exp. Biol.* **77**, 15–31.

O'Dor, R.K. and Wells, M.J. (1987). Energy and nutrient flow in cephalopods. In: *Cephalopod Life Cycles, Vol. II*, Ed. Boyle, P.R., pp. 109–133. Academic Press, London.

Oestmann, D.J., Scimeca, J.M., Forsythe, J., et al. (1997). Special considerations for keeping cephalopods in laboratory facilities. *J. Am. Assoc. Lab. Anim. Sci.* **36**, 89–93.

Ohno, Y., Kawano, F. and Hirazawa, N. (2009). The effect of oral antibiotic treatment and freshwater bath treatment on susceptibility to Neobenedenia girellae (Monogenea) infection of amberjack (Seriola dumerili) and yellowtail (S. quinqueradiata) hosts. *Aquaculture* **292**, 248–251.

Olivares, A., Avila-Poveda, O.H., Leyton, V., et al. (2017). Oviducal glands throughout the gonad development stages: a case study of Octopus mimus (cephalopoda). *Molluscan Res.* **37**, 229–241.

Olmos-Pérez, L., Roura, Á., Pierce, G.J., et al. (2017). Diet composition and variability of wild Octopus vulgaris and Alloteuthis media (Cephalopoda) Paralarvae: a metagenomic approach. *Front. Physiol.* **8**.

Otero, J., González, Á.F., Sieiro, M.P. and Guerra, Á. (2007). Reproductive cycle and energy allocation of Octopus vulgaris in Galician waters, NE Atlantic. *Fish. Res.* **85**, 122–129.

Packard, A. (1969). Visual acuity and eye growth in octopus vulgaris (Lamarck). *Monit. Zool. Ital. – Ital. J. Zool.* **3**, 19–32.

Panetta, D., Solomon, M., Buresch, K. and Hanlon, R.T. (2017). Small-scale rearing of cuttlefish (Sepia officinalis) for research purposes. *Mar. Freshw. Behav. Physiol.* **50**, 115–124.

Pascual, S., Gestal, C., Estévez, J.M., et al. (1996). Parasites in commercially-exploited cephalopods (Mollusca, Cephalopoda) in Spain: an updated perspective. *Aquaculture* **142**, 1–10.

Pascual, S., González, A.F. and Guerra, A. (2010). Coccidiosis during octopus senescence: preparing for parasite outbreak. *Fish. Res.* **106**, 160–162.

Pascual, S., Abollo, E., Mladineo, I. and Gestal, C. (2019). Metazoa and related diseases. In *Handbook of Pathogens and Diseases in Cephalopods*, pp. 169–179. Cham, Springer International Publishing.

Perez, J.A.A. and Haimovici, M. (1991). Sexual maturation and reproductive cycle of Eledone massyae, Voss 1964 (Cephalopoda: Octopodidae) in Southern Brazil. *Bull. Mar. Sci.* **49**, 270–279.

Perez, P.V., Butler-Struben, H.M. and Crook, R.J. (2017). The selective serotonin reuptake inhibitor fluoxetine increases spontaneous afferent firing, but not mechanonociceptive sensitization, in octopus. *Invertebr. Neurosci.* **17**, 10.

Poirier, R., Chichery, R. and Dickel, L. (2005). Early experience and postembryonic maturation of body patterns in cuttlefish (Sepia officinalis). *J. Comp. Psychol.* **119**, 230–237.

Polese, G., Winlow, W. and Di Cosmo, A. (2014). Dose-dependent effects of the clinical anesthetic isoflurane on octopus vulgaris: a contribution to cephalopod welfare. *J. Aquat. Anim. Health* **26**, 285–294.

Polese, G., Bertapelle, C. and Di Cosmo, A. (2015). Role of olfaction in Octopus vulgaris reproduction. *Gen. Comp. Endocrinol.* **210**, 55–62.

Polglase, J.L. (2019). Cephalopod diseases caused by fungi and Labyrinthulomycetes. In: *Handbook of Pathogens and Diseases in Cephalopods*, pp. 113–122. Cham, Springer International Publishing.

Polglase, J.L., Bullock, A.M. and Roberts, R.J. (2009). Wound healing and the haemocyte response in the skin of the Lesser octopus Eledone cirrhosa (Mollusca: Cephalopoda). *J. Zool.* **201**, 185–204.

Potts, W. (1965). Ammonia Excretion in Octopus dofleini. *Comp. Biochem. Physiol.* **14**, 339–355.

Quintana, D., Domingues, P. and García, S. (2008). Effect of two artificial wet diets agglutinated with gelatin on feed and growth performance of common octopus (Octopus vulgaris) sub-adults. *Aquaculture* **280**, 161–164.

Quinteiro, J., Baibai, T., Oukhattar, L., *et al.* (2011). Multiple paternity in the common octopus vulgaris (Cuvier, 1797), as revealed by microsatellite DNA analysis. *Molluscan Res.* **31**, 15–20.

Ramirez, D.M. and Oakley, T.H. (2015). Eye-independent, light-activated chromatophore expansion (LACE) and expression of phototransduction genes in the skin of Octopus bimaculoides. *J. Exp. Biol.* **218**, 1513–1520.

Rasero, M., Gonzalez, A.F., Castro, B.G. and Guerra, A. (1996). Predatory relationships of two sympatric squid, Todaropsis eblanae and Illex coindetii (Cephalopoda: Ommastrephidae) in Galician waters. *J. Mar. Biol. Assoc. United Kingdom* **76**, 73–87.

Reimschuessel, R. and Stoskopf, M.K. (1990). Octopus automutilation syndrome. *J. Invertebr. Pathol.* **55**, 394–400.

Robison, B.H., Reisenbichler, K.R., Hunt, J.C. and Haddock, S.H.D. (2003). Light production by the arm tips of the deep-sea cephalopod Vampyroteuthis infernalis. *Biol. Bull.* **205**, 102–109.

Robison, B., Seibel, B. and Drazen, J. (2014). Deep-sea octopus (Graneledone boreopacifica) conducts the longest-known egg-brooding period of any animal. *PloS One* **9**, e103437.

Rocha, F., Guerra, A. and González, A.F. (2001). A review of reproductive strategies in cephalopods. *Biol. Rev. Camb. Philos. Soc.* **76**, 291–304.

Rosas, C., Cuzon, G., Pascual, C., *et al.* (2007). Energy balance of Octopus maya fed crab or an artificial diet. *Mar. Biol.* **152**, 371–381.

Roumbedakis, K. and Guerra, Á. (2019). Cephalopod senescence and parasitology. In: *Handbook of Pathogens and Diseases in Cephalopods*, pp. 207–211. Cham, Springer International Publishing.

Roumbedakis, K., Drábková, M., Tyml, T. and Di Cristo, C. (2018). A perspective around cephalopods and their parasites, and suggestions on how to increase knowledge in the field. *Front. Physiol.* **9**, 1573.

Rowell, C.H.F. (1963). Excitatory and inhibitory pathways in the arm of octopus. *J. Exp. Biol.* **40**, 257–270.

Rowell, C.H.F. (1966). Activity of interneurones in the arm of Octopus in response to tactile stimulation. *J. Exp. Biol.* **44**, 589–605.

Ruder, T., Sunagar, K., Undheim, E.A.B., *et al.* (2013). Molecular phylogeny and evolution of the proteins encoded by coleoid (cuttlefish, octopus, and squid) posterior venom glands. *J. Mol. Evol.* **76**, 192–204.

Sabirov, R.M., Golikov, A.V., Nigmatullin, C.M. and Lubin, P.A. (2012). Structure of the reproductive system and hectocotylus in males of lesser flying squid Todaropsis eblanae (Cephalopoda: Ommastrephidae). *J. Nat. Hist.* **46**, 1761–1778.

Saidel, W.M. and Monsell, E.M. (1986). Organization of the motor neuron components of the pallial nerve in octopus. *Brain Res.* **374**, 30–36.

Sanders, G.D. (1975). The cephalopods. *Invertebr. Learn.* **3**, 1–101.

Sanders, G.D. and Young, J.Z. (1974). Reappearance of specific colour patterns after nerve regeneration in Octopus. *Proceeding R. Soc. London B, Biol. Sci.* **186**, 1–11.

Santos, R.A. and Haimovici, M. (1997). Food and feeding of the short-finned squid Illex argentinus (Cephalopoda: Ommastrephidae) off southern Brazil. *Fish. Res.* **33**, 139–147.

Sato, N., Kasugai, T., Ikeda, Y. and Munehara, H. (2010). Structure of the seminal receptacle and sperm storage in the Japanese pygmy squid. *J. Zool.* **282**, 151–156.

Sauer, W.H.H. and Smale, M.J. (1991). Predation patterns on the inshore spawning grounds of the squid Loligo vulgaris reynaudii (Cephalopoda: Loliginidae) off the south-eastern Cape, South Africa. *South African J. Mar. Sci.* **11**, 513–523.

Sauer, W.H.H.H., Smale, M.J. and Lipinski, M.R. (1992). The location of spawning grounds, spawning and schooling behaviour of the squid Loligo vulgaris reynaudii (Cephalopoda: Myopsida) off the Eastern Cape Coast, South Africa. *Mar. Biol.* **114**, 97–107.

Saunders, W.B. and Ward, P.D. (2010). Ecology, distribution, and population characteristics of Nautilus. In: *Nautilus: Topics in Geobiology, Vol. 6*, pp. 137–162. Springer, Dordrecht.

Schipp, R., von Boletzky, S. and Doell, G. (1975). Ultrastructural and cytochemical investigations on the renal appendages and their concrements in dibranchiate cephalopods (Mollusea, Cephalopoda). *Zeitschrift für Morphol. Der Tiere* **81**, 279–304.

Segawa, S., Yang, W., Marthy, H. and Hanlon, R.T. (1988). Illustrated embryonic stages of the eastern Atlantic squid Loligo forbesi. *The Veliger* **30**, 230–243.

Seibel, B.A., Robison, B.H. and Haddock, S.H.D. (2005). Post-spawning egg care by a squid. *Nature* **438**, 929.

Seixas, P., Otero, A., Valente, L.M.P., Dias, J. and Rey-Méndez, M. (2010). Growth and fatty acid composition of Octopus vulgaris paralarvae fed with enriched Artemia or co-fed with an inert diet. *Aquac. Int.* **18**, 1121–1135.

Şen, H. (2005). Incubation off European Squid (*Loligo vulgaris* Lamarck, 1798) eggs at different salinities. *Aquac. Res.* **36**, 876–881.

Shashar, N. and Hanlon, R.T. (2013). Spawning behavior dynamics at communal egg beds in the squid Doryteuthis (Loligo) pealeii. *J. Exp. Mar. Biol. Ecol.* **447**, 65–74.

Shaw, P.W. and Boyle, P.R. (1997). Multiple paternity within the brood of single females of *Loligo forbesi* (Cephalopoda: Loliginidae), demonstrated with microsatellite DNA markers. *Mar. Ecol. Prog. Ser.* **160**, 279–282.

Shaw, P.W. and Sauer, W.H.H. (2004). Multiple paternity and complex fertilisation dynamics in the squid *Loligo vulgaris reynaudii*. *Mar. Ecol. Prog. Ser.* **270**, 173–179.

Sheumack, D.D., Howden, M.E.H., Spence, I. and Quinn, R.J. (1978). Maculotoxin: a neurotoxin from the venom glands of the octopus Hapalochlaena maculosa identified as tetrodotoxin. *Science (80-.).* **199**, 188–189.

Sheumack, D.D., Howden, M.E.H. and Spence, I. (1984). Occurrence of a tetrodotoxin-like compound in the eggs of the venomous blue-ringed octopus (*Hapalochlaena maculosa*). *Toxicon* **22**, 811–812.

Shigeno, S. and Ragsdale, C.W. (2015). The gyri of the octopus vertical lobe have distinct neurochemical identities. *J. Comp. Neurol.* **523**, Spc1–Spc1.

Shigeno, S., Sasaki, T., Moritaki, T., *et al.* (2008). Evolution of the cephalopod head complex by assembly of multiple molluscan body parts: evidence from Nautilus embryonic development. *J. Morphol.* **269**, 1–17.

Shigeno, S., Takenori, S. and Boletzky, S. von (2010). The origins of cephalopod body plans: a geometrical and developmental basis for the evolution of vertebrate-like organ systems. In *Cephalopods – Present and Past*, Tokai University Press, Tokyo, pp. 23–34.

Shomrat, T., Zarrella, I., Fiorito, G. and Hochner, B. (2008). The octopus vertical lobe modulates short-term learning rate and uses LTP to acquire long-term memory. *Curr. Biol.* **18**, 337–342.

Smith, P.J., Mattlin, R.H., Roeleveld, M.A. and Okutani, T. (1987). Arrow squids of the genus nototodarus in New Zealand waters: systematics, biology, and fisheries. *New Zeal. J. Mar. Freshw. Res.* **21**, 315–326.

Smith, J.A., Andrews, P.L.R., Hawkins, P., et al. (2013). Cephalopod research and EU Directive 2010/63/EU: requirements, impacts and ethical review. *J. Exp. Mar. Biol. Ecol.* **447**, 31–45.

Snow, C.D. (1970). Two accounts of the northern octopus *dofleini*, biting scuba divers. *Res. Reports fish commission Oregon* **2**, 103.

Squires, Z.Z.E., Wong, B.B.B.M., Norman, M.D.M. and Stuart-Fox, D. (2014). Multiple paternity but no evidence of biased sperm use in female dumpling squid *Euprymna tasmanica*. *Mar. Ecol. Prog. Ser.* **511**, 93–103.

Strugnell, J. and Nishiguchi, M.K. (2007). Molecular phylogeny of coleoid cephalopods (Mollusca: Cephalopoda) inferred from three mitochondrial and six nuclear loci: a comparison of alignment, implied alignment and analysis methods. *J. Molluscan Stud.* **73**, 399–410.

Strugnell, J., Norman, M., Jackson, J., Drummond, A.J. and Cooper, A. (2005). Molecular phylogeny of coleoid cephalopods (Mollusca: Cephalopoda) using a multigene approach; the effect of data partitioning on resolving phylogenies in a Bayesian framework. *Mol. Phylogenet. Evol.* **37**, 426–441.

Stubbs, A.L. and Stubbs, C.W. (2016). Spectral discrimination in color blind animals via chromatic aberration and pupil shape. *Proc. Natl. Acad. Sci. U. S. A.* **113**, 8206–8211.

Sumbre, G., Gutfreund, Y., Fiorito, G., et al. (2001). Control of Octopus arm extension by a peripheral motor program. *Science (80-.)*. **5536**, 1845–1848.

Summers, W.C. and McMahon, J.J. (1974). Studies on the maintenance of adult squid (*Loligo pealei*). I. Factorial survey. *Biol. Bull.* **146**, 279–290.

Summers, W.C., McMahon, J.J. and Ruppert, G.N.P.A. (1974). Studies on the maintenance of adult squid (*Loligo peali*). II. Empirical extensions. *Biol. Bull.* **146**, 291–301.

Sykes, A.V. and Gestal, C. (2014). Welfare and diseases under culture conditions. In *Cephalopod Culture*, pp. 97–112. Dordrecht, Springer Netherlands.

Sykes, A.V., Almansa, E., Cooke, G.M., et al. (2017). The digestive tract of cephalopods: a neglected topic of relevance to animal welfare in the laboratory and aquaculture. *Front. Physiol.* **8**.

Takahama, H., Kinoshita, T., Sato, M. and Sasaki, F. (1991). Fine structure of the spermatophores and their ejaculated forms, sperm reservoirs, of the Japanese common squid, *Todarodes pacificus*. *J. Morphol.* **207**, 241–251.

Tennesen, M. (2015). March of the Red Devil. *New Sci.* **227**, 32–35.

Thompson, J.T. and Voight, J.R. (2003). Erectile tissue in an invertebrate animal: the Octopus copulatory organ. *J. Zool.* **261**, 101–108.

Tonkins, B.M., Tyers, A.M. and Cooke, G.M. (2015). Cuttlefish in captivity: an investigation into housing and husbandry for improving welfare. *Appl. Anim. Behav. Sci.* **168**, 77–83.

Tosti, E., di Cosmo, A., Cuomo, A., et al. (2001). Progesterone induces activation in Octopus vulgaris spermatozoa. *Mol. Reprod. Dev.* **59**, 97–105.

Van Camp, L.M., Donnellan, S.C., Dyer, A.R. and Fairweather, P.G. (2004). Multiple paternity in field- and captive-laid egg strands of *Sepioteuthis australis* (Cephalopoda: Loliginidae). *Mar. Freshw. Res.* **55**, 819–823.

Van Giesen, L., Kilian, P.B., Allard, C.A.H. and Bellono, N.W. (2020). Molecular basis of chemotactile sensation in octopus. *Cell* **183**, 594–604.e14.

Vidal, E.A.G., Villanueva, R., Andrade, J.P., et al. (2014). Cephalopod culture: current status of main biological models and research priorities. In: *Advances in Marine Biology*, pp. 1–98.

Vijai, D., Sakai, M., Wakabayashi, T., et al. (2015). Effects of temperature on embryonic development and paralarval behavior of the neon flying squid *Ommastrephes bartramii*. *Mar. Ecol. Prog. Ser.* **529**, 145–158.

Villanueva, R. (1994). Decapod crab zoeae as food for rearing cephalopod paralarvae. *Aquaculture* **128**, 143–152.

Villanueva, R., Riba, J., Ruíz-Capillas, C., et al. (2004). Amino acid composition of early stages of cephalopods and effect of amino acid dietary treatments on Octopus vulgaris paralarvae. *Aquaculture* **242**, 455–478.

Villanueva, R., Quintana, D., Petroni, G. and Bozzano, A. (2011). Factors influencing the embryonic development and hatchling size of the oceanic squid *Illex coindetii* following in vitro fertilization. *J. Exp. Mar. Biol. Ecol.* **407**, 54–62.

Villanueva, R., Sykes, A.V., Vidal, E.A.G., et al. (2014). Current status and future challenges in cephalopod culture. In: *Cephalopod Culture*, pp. 479–489. Dordrecht, Springer Netherlands.

Von Boletzky, S. (2004). A brief survey of cephalopod culture techniques. *Aquaculture* **2**, 229–240.

Walderon, M.D., Nolt, K.J., Haas, R.E., et al. (2011). Distance chemoreception and the detection of conspecifics in Octopus bimaculoides. *J. Molluscan Stud.* **77**, 309–311.

Walsh, L.S., Turk, P.E., Forsythe, J.W. and Lee, P.G. (2002). Mariculture of the loliginid squid Sepioteuthis lessoniana through seven successive generations. *Aquaculture* **212**, 245–262.

Wang, Z.Y. and Ragsdale, C.W. (2018). Multiple optic gland signaling pathways implicated in octopus maternal behaviors and death. *J. Exp. Biol.* **221**.

Ward, P.D. (1987). *The Natural History of Nautilus*. Allen & Unwin, Sydney.

Ward, P.D. and Saunders, W.B. (1997). Allonautilus: a new genus of living nautiloid cephalopod and its bearing on phylogeny of the Nautilida. *J. Paleontol.* 1054–1064.

Wardill, T.J., Gonzalez-Bellido, P.T., Crook, R.J. and Hanlon, R.T. (2012). Neural control of tuneable skin iridescence in squid. *Proc. Biol. Sci.* **279**, 4243–52.

Weischer, M.-L. and Marthy, H.-J. (1983). Chemical and physiological properties of the natural tranquilliser in the cephalopod eggs. *Mar. Behav. Physiol.* **9**, 131–138.

Wells, M.J. (1959). A touch-learning centre in Octopus. *J. Exp. Biol.* **36**, 590–612.

Wells, M.J. (1963). Taste by touch: some experiments with Octopus. *J. Exp. Biol.* **40**, 187–193.

Wells, M.J. (1978). *Octopus. Physiology and Behaviour of an Advanced Invertebrate*. Chapman and Hall, London.

Wells, M.J. and Clarke, A. (1996). Energetics: the costs of living and reproducing for an individual cephalopod. *Philos. Trans. R. Soc. B Biol. Sci.* **351**, 1083–1104.

Wells, M. and Wells, J. (1977). Cephalopoda: Octopoda. In: *Reproduction of Marine Invertebrates, Molluscs: Gastropods and Cephalopods*. Ed. Giese, A., pp. 291–330. Academic Press, New York.

Wells, M.J. and Young, J.Z. (1965). Split-brain preparations and touch learning in the octopus. *J. Exp. Biol.* **43**, 565–579.

Wells, M.J. and Young, J.Z. (1975). The subfrontal lobe and touch learning in the octopus. *Brain Res.* **92**, 103–121.

Wodinsky, J. (1977). Hormonal inhibition of feeding and death in Octopus: control by optic gland secretion. *Science (80-.)*. **198**, 948–951.

Wodinsky, J. (2008). Reversal and transfer of spermatophores by Octopus vulgaris and O. hummelincki. *Mar. Biol.* **155**, 91–103.

Yamamoto, T., Tasaki, K., Sugawara, Y. and Tonosaki, A. (1965). Fine structure of the octopus retina. *J. Cell Biol.* **25**, 345–359.

Young, J.Z. (1960). The failures of discrimination learning following the removal of the vertical lobes in Octopus. *Proc. R. Soc. London. Ser. B. Biol. Sci.* **153**, 18–46.

Young, J.Z. (1962). The optic lobes of Octopus vulgaris. *Philos. Trans. R. Soc. Lond. B. Biol. Sci.* 19–58.

Young, J.Z. (1963). The number and sizes of nerve cells in Octopus. *Proc. Zool. Soc. London* 229–254.

Young, J.Z. (1965). The central nervous system of Nautilus. *Philos. Trans. R. Soc. Lond. B. Biol. Sci.* 1–25.

Young, J.Z. (1976). The nervous system of Loligo. II. Suboesophageal centres. *Philos. Trans. R. Soc. Lond. B. Biol. Sci.* 101–167.

Young, J.Z. and Boycott, B.B. (1971). *The Anatomy of the Nervous System of Octopus vulgaris*. Clarendon Press, Oxford.

Zecchini, F., Vecchione, M. and Roper, C.F.E. (1996). A quantitative comparison of hectocotylus morphology between Mediterranean and western Atlantic populations of the squid *Illex coindetii* (Mollusca: Cephalopoda: Oegopsida: Ommastrephidae). *Proc. Biol. Soc. Washingt.* **109**, 591–599.

Zeidberg, L.D. and Hamner, W.M. (2002). Distribution of squid paralarvae, *Loligo opalescens* (Cephalopoda: Myopsida), in the Southern California Bight in the three years following the 1997–1998 El Niño. *Mar. Biol.* **141**, 111–122.

Zeidberg, L.D. and Robison, B.H. (2007). Invasive range expansion by the Humboldt squid, *Dosidicus gigas*, in the eastern North Pacific. *Proc. Natl. Acad. Sci. U. S. A.* **104**, 12948–12950.

Decapoda

51 Decapod crustaceans

Robert W. Elwood and Ray W. Ingle

Introduction

The order Decapoda includes shrimps, prawns, crayfish, lobsters, true crabs and hermit crabs. Many species are used in the food industry, either captured from wild or reared in aquaculture. Some may be reared in their early stages and then released to supplement wild stocks. Most are a convenient size for keeping in captivity and many are not too difficult to maintain. Some are used as pets. At present, there are few legal constraints on collecting, importing or captive breeding, although with the recognition that some crabs and crayfish are invasive that is likely to change. There are also risks of introducing diseases to native populations or captive stocks. A detailed source to the literature on care and management of captive decapods is given by Ingle (1995) and discussions of the possibility that they might experience pain and thus might suffer from poor treatment is given by Elwood (2012).

Decapod Biology

Structure

Decapods are segmented, typically with five segments forming the head, eight forming the thorax and six forming the abdomen, and each segment typically bears a pair of appendages. The head has the antennules, antennae, mandibles, first and second maxillae. They also have a carapace enclosing the thorax and gills, moveable stalked eyes, the flagellum of each antennule is divided (biramous), a broad flat exopod (scaphocerite) is on the antenna, the first three pairs of thoracic appendages (maxillipeds) are modified for feeding and the following five pairs (pereiopods or walking legs) are developed for walking. In some groups, notably hermit crabs, the size of the 4th and 5th pereiopods is reduced and may be vestigial (McLaughlin1982). The first and/or second pairs of pereiopods usually bear claws (chelipeds), which in some species are large, powerful and often asymmetrically developed. The third walking legs may also be chelae but these pincers are typically small. The abdomen usually has five pairs of pleopods (swimmerets) and the final appendages are the typically flattened uropods, but again there may be modification and/or loss of the abdominal appendages, especially in hermit crabs. The crayfish is a typical example and shown in Figure 51.1 to show the appendages and main body parts. The classification of decapods and aspects of their biology that need to be known for successful maintenance in captivity are briefly described.

Classification and identification

Various classifications have been proposed for decapods. The one given in Table 51.1 shows the taxonomic positions of the genera and species mentioned in the text.

Many species are maintained in captivity for research and the aquarium trade. Correct identification is important when assessing requirements of decapods held in captivity and literature of specialised works for identifying decapods is given by Ingle (1995). Life histories vary, particularly those of the two suborders, and it is necessary to know something about these before captive rearing is attempted. Vernacular names, where these are known, are given for all decapods mentioned and in the tabulated classification in Table 51.1. Note that the terms 'prawn' and 'shrimp' are widely used but have no specific attributes in the scientific classification. Indeed, small and large individuals within a single species may be called shrimp and prawns, respectively.

Moulting (ecdysis)

Decapods typically have a hardened exoskeleton that prevents normal growth. Increased body size is only achieved by shedding the exoskeleton, a process known as *ecdysis* or *moulting*. This allows the newly formed soft shell beneath to expand and then harden. The short period of actual ecdysis has profound effects on normal life style and preparing for and recovering from moulting have considerable impacts on behaviour.

The UFAW Handbook on the Care and Management of Laboratory and Other Research Animals, Ninth Edition.
Edited by Huw Golledge and Claire Richardson.
© 2024 John Wiley & Sons Ltd. Published 2024 by John Wiley & Sons Ltd.

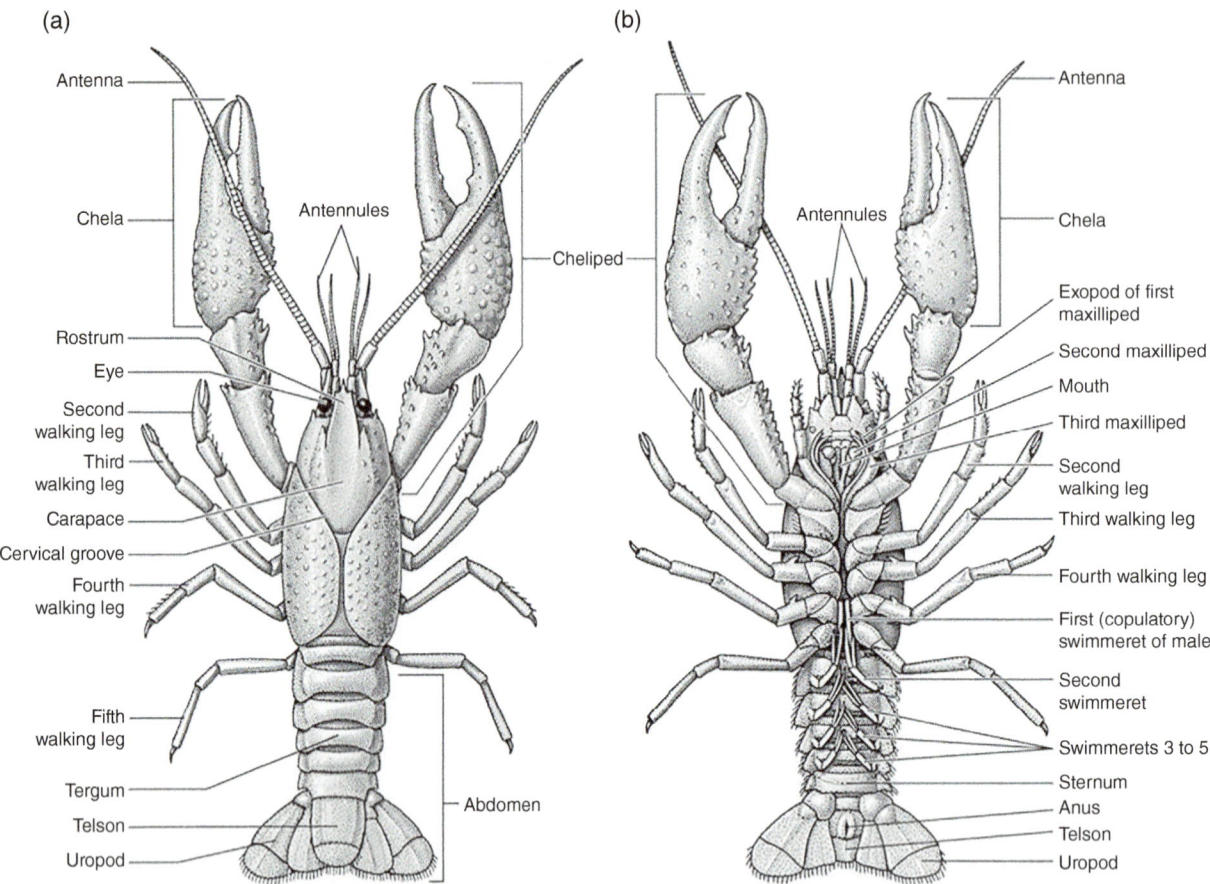

Figure 51.1 External structure of a male crayfish: (a) dorsal aspect; (b) ventral aspect. The walking legs are also called *pereiopods*, and the swimmerets are also known as *pleopods*. The first pleopod in males is hardened and used in copulation. Source: The McGraw Hill Companies slide 9 from chapter 19: Aquatic Mandibulates. Accessed from: https://slideplayer.com/slide/7632032/

Moulting frequently occurs at night. In clawed lobsters, *Homarus*, regions of the carapace, especially the thoraco-abdominal membrane and the cephalothoracic wall above the pereiopods, are weakened forming 'fracture planes' by withdrawing minerals from the old exoskeleton (Aiken 1980). Water is ingested and absorbed into the body tissues. This increases hydrostatic pressure, which causes the carapace to lift and distend the thoraco-abdominal membrane. During this passive phase, the lobster is usually quiescent and may become stressed if disturbed, and crayfish may exhibit anxiety-like states during moult and take fewer risks (Bacqué-Cazenave *et al.* 2019).

The lobster rolls onto its side, the thoraco-abdominal membrane splits transversely, the carapace hinges forward and the anterior appendages are withdrawn, followed by withdrawal of the abdomen. Lubrication of limbs by a moulting fluid assists withdrawal. The upper meral region of the larger cheliped is also softened prior to moulting and the propodal muscles are temporarily reduced in size by dehydration to allow easier extraction of the limb. Nevertheless, losses of the larger claw and other limbs may occur and may lead to death during or after ecdysis. In crab-like decapods, pre-ecdysial fractures occur along the carapace epimeral suture. Shedding the old shell can take from as little as three minutes for crawfishes *Panulirus*, twenty minutes for clawed-lobsters *Homarus*, to one to three hours for shore crabs *Carcinus*. The exoskeleton is very soft immediately after ecdysis. It hardens within a few hours for prawns but may take from three to sixteen days for the shore crab *Carcinus*.

In clawed lobsters and freshwater crayfish, some of the calcium withdrawn from the exoskeleton is stored as paired lens-shaped concretions of approximately 8–10 mm diameter termed 'gastroliths'. These are located on the mid-cardiac walls of the alimentary canal and are shed into the cardiac chamber during moulting where they are broken up by the cardiac teeth (gastric mill) and dissolved. The calcium liberated is reabsorbed by the hepatopancreas, deposited in the exoskeleton via the haemolymph (blood) and used for recalcifying the tips of limbs and mouthparts to enable feeding. In clawed lobsters, *Homarus*, most of the old moulted exoskeleton is then eaten so that additional minerals are recovered. In shore crabs *Carcinus*, at least half the calcium used for hardening the exoskeleton is taken up from the surrounding sea water.

There are two main types of moulting cycle. First, anecdysis is a seasonal moult, and the intermoult period is prolonged. It is typical for freshwater cambarid crayfish, crawfish, some true (brachyuran) crabs such as fiddler crabs (*Uca*) and some spider crabs, for example, the thorn-back

Table 51.1 Classification of those decapods commonly maintained in captivity.

Order Decapoda
Suborder Dendrobranchiata
Superfamily Penaeoidea
Family Penaeidae (penaeid shrimps or prawns): *Penaeus (Penaeus) monodon* Fabricius, 1798 (Giant Tiger Prawn); *Penaeus (Marsupenaeus) japonicus* Bate, 1888 (Kuruma Prawn)

Suborder Pleocyemata
Infraorder Stenopodidea
Family Stenopodidae: *Stenopus hispidus* (Olivier, 1811) (Banded or Coral Shrimp)

Infraorder Caridea (caridean shrimps or prawns)
Superfamily Atyoidea
Family Atyidae (atyid shrimps or prawns)
Superfamily Palaemonoidea
Family Hymenoceridae: *Hymenocera picta* Dana, 1852 (Harlequin or Clown Shrimp). Family Palaemonidae (palaemonid and periclimenid shrimps or prawns): *Macrobrachium australiense* Holthuis, 1950; *Macrobrachium rosenbergii* (de Man, 1879) (Freshwater Giant Prawn); *Palaemon adspersus* Rathke, 1837 (Baltic Prawn); *Palaemon serratus* (Pennant, 1777) (Common Prawn); *Palaemonetes varians* (Leach, 1814) (Atlantic Ditch Prawn); *Periclimenes (Periclimenes) pedersoni* Chace, 1958 (Pederson's Cleaning Shrimp)
Superfamily Alpheoidea
Family Alpheidae (alpheid shrimps or prawns): *Lysmata amboinensis* (de Man, 1888) (Red-back Cleaner Shrimp)
Superfamily Pandaloidea
Family Pandalidae (pandalid shrimps or prawns): *Pandalus borealis* Kroyer, 1838 (Northern Shrimp); *Pandalus montagui* Leach, 1814 (Pink Shrimp)
Superfamily Crangonoidea
Family Crangonidae (crangonid shrimps or prawns): *Crangon crangon* (Linnaeus, 1758) (Brown Shrimp)

Infraorder Astacidea
Superfamily Nephropoidea (clawed lobsters)
Family Nephropidae: *Enoplometopus* species (reef lobsters); *Homarus americanus* H. Milne Edwards, 1837 (American Clawed Lobster); *Homarus gammarus* (Linnaeus, 1758) (European Clawed Lobster); *Nephrops norvegicus* (Linnaeus, 1758) (Norway Lobster)
Superfamily Astacoidea: (northern hemisphere freshwater crayfish)
Family Astacidae (astacid crayfish): *Astacus astacus* (Linnaeus, 1758) (Noble Crayfish); *Astacus leptodactylus* Eschscholtz, 1823 (Long-clawed Crayfish); *Austropotamobius pallipes* (Lereboullet, 1858) (White-clawed Crayfish); *Pacifastacus (Pacifastacus) leniusculus leniusculus* (Dana, 1852) (Signal Crayfish). Family Cambaridae (cambarid crayfish): *Procambarus (Scapulicambarus) clarkii* (Girard, 1852) (Red Swamp Crayfish)
Superfamily Parastacoidea (southern hemisphere freshwater crayfish)
Family Parastacidae (parastacid crayfish): *Cherax destructor* Clark, 1936 (Yabby)

Infraorder Thalassinidea: (thalassinid mud shrimps or lobsters)
Superfamily Thalassinoidea
Family Callianassidae: *Callianassa* and *Upogebia* species
Infraorder Palinura
Superfamily Palinuroidea
Family Palinuridae (crawfish or spiny lobsters): *Palinurus elephas* (Fabricius, 1787) (European Crawfish/Spiny Lobster); *Panulirus* species

Infraorder Anomura
Superfamily Paguroidea
Family Coenobitidae (coenobite crabs, includes semi-terrestrial hermit crabs): *Birgus latro* (Linnaeus, 1758) (Robber Crab); *Coenobita* species (land hermit crabs). Family Paguridae (marine hermit crabs): *Pagurus bernhardus* (Linnaeus, 1758) (Soldier Hermit Crab). Family Lithodidae (stone or false crabs): *Paralithodes camtschaticus* (Tilesius, 1815) (King Stone Crab)
Superfamily Galatheoidea
Family Galatheidae (squat lobsters): *Pleuroncodes monodon* (H. Milne Edwards, 1837) (Red Squat Lobster); *Galathea* species. Family Porcellanidae (porcelain crabs): *Petrolisthes* and *Porcellana*

(*Continued*)

Table 51.1 (Continued)

Infraorder Brachyura (true crabs)
Section Dromiacea
Superfamily Dromioidea
Family Dromiidae (sponge crabs): *Dromia personata* (Linnaeus, 1758) (Linnaeus's Sponge Crab)
Section Oxyrhyncha (spider crabs)
Superfamily Majoidea
Family Majidae: *Inachus dorsettensis* (Pennant, 1777) (Scorpion Spider Crab); *Libinia emarginata* Leach, 1815 (Common Spider Crab); *Macropodia rostrata* (Linnaeus, 1761) (Long-legged Spider Crab); *Maja squinado* (Herbst, 1788) (Thorn-back Spider Crab); *Mithrax spinosissimus* (Lamarck, 1818) (Lazy Crab); *Stenorhynchus seticornis* (Herbst, 1788) (Arrow Crab)
Section Oxystomata
Superfamily Dorippoidea
Family Dorippidae: (sharp-mouth or face crabs): *Medorippe* species
Superfamily Leucosioidea
Family Calappidae (calappid or box crabs): *Calappa* species
Section Cancridea
Superfamily Cancroidea
Family Cancridae (cancrid crabs): *Cancer pagurus* (Linnaeus, 1758) (European Edible Crab). Family Corystidae: *Corystes cassivelaunus* (Pennant, 1777) (Long-armed Crab)
Section Brachyrhyncha
Superfamily Portunoidea (portunid crabs, includes swimming crabs)
Family Portunidae: *Carcinus aestuarii* Nardo, 1847 (Mediterranean Shore Crab); *Carcinus maenas* (Linnaeus, 1758) (North Atlantic Shore Crab); *Necora puber* (Linnaeus, 1767) (Velvet Swimming Crab); *Portunus* species
Superfamily Xanthoidea
Family Goneplacidae (goneplacid or angular crabs). Family Xanthidae (xanthid crabs): *Rhithropanopeus harrisii* (Gould, 1841) (Dwarf Crab); *Trapezia* species; *Xantho* species
Superfamily Grapsidoidea
Family Gecarcinucidae (gecarcoidean crabs, includes land crabs): *Cardisoma guanhumi* Latreille, 1803 (Great Land Crab); Gecarcoidea and *Gecarcinus* species (land crabs). Family Grapsidae: *Geosesarma* and *Sesarma* (sesarmid or mangrove crabs); *Grapsus* and *Pachygrapsus* (grapsid or rock crabs)
Superfamily Pinnotheroidea
Family Pinnotheridae (pinnotherid or pea crabs): *Pinnotheres pisum* (Linnaeus, 1767) (European or Linnaeus's Pea Crab)
Superfamily Potamoidea (potamonid or freshwater crabs)
Family Potamautidae: Potamonautes. Family Potamidae. Potamon. Family Pseudothelphusidae Pseudothelphusa
Superfamily Ocypodoidea
Family Ocypodidae (ocypodid crabs, includes racing and fiddler crabs): *Uca (Australuca) bellator signatus* (Hess, 1865); *Uca (Leptuca) lactea* (de Haan, 1835)
Superfamily Hapalocarcinoidea
Family Hapalocarcinidae (hapalocarcinid or coral crabs)

spider crab, *Maja squinado*. Second, diecdysis occurs throughout the year and is typical for many pleocyemate prawns and some brachyuran crabs. For these, the intermoult period is of relatively short duration. However, temperature can influence these two patterns of ecdysis. Shore crabs *Carcinus*, for example, remain in the diecdysial state during summer but may revert to an overwinter anecdysial condition. For some, particularly spider crabs (oxyrhynchs), further moults may never occur beyond the one to puberty, and other brachyuran crabs may eventually reach a state in which further moulting and growth ceases. Crabs that grow to an exceptionally large size, such as the European edible crab *Cancer pagurus*, perhaps continue to moult throughout their entire lives.

Captive environments may not provide all the conditions required for successful moulting. 'Moulting death' sometimes occurs in which the claws, walking legs or abdomen cannot be extracted from the old shell, or the new shell fails to harden and may become contorted.

Hormones

Hormones control numerous functions in decapods and levels of hormones may change during larval development, and within a developmental stage (Chang 2001). Ecdysteroids, for example, play a key role in the moult cycle and decapods have low levels of these during the postmoult and intermoult periods but a marked increase occurs in early premoult, which then declines by the time ecdysis occurs. Crustacean Hyperglycaemic Hormone (CHH) regulates haemolymph glucose levels and is released in times of stress. CHH also changes during the moult cycle, being relatively low during postmoult and intermoult but increases during the premoult (Chang 2001), at a time thought to be stressful (Bacqué-Cazenave *et al*. 2019). CHH is also released when the animal is injured (Patterson *et al*. 2007) or subject to potentially painful stimuli such as electric shock (Elwood & Adams 2015). CHH is also involved in the regulation of onset of vitellogenesis and thereby reproduction (Swetha *et al*. 2011).

These and other hormones are stored within the eye-stalks of decapods and ablation of the eye-stalks has marked effects. Unilateral or bilateral ablation has been used in many experimental studies, but they are used most in commercial cultivation of several species of prawn and shrimp (Taylor *et al*. 2004). Captive conditions often inhibit females from developing mature ovaries, and even if a given species develops ovaries and spawns in captivity, eyestalk ablation may increase egg production.

Behaviour

Rhythms

Many activities of decapods are rhythmic, controlled internally by hormones and influenced externally by tidal, lunar and seasonal cycles. These endogenous rhythms may persist in captivity for several weeks but gradually become out of phase with the free-living populations. Imposed rhythm entrainment should be taken into consideration when assessing laboratory requirements for experimental studies, particularly on behaviour (Naylor 1988).

Feeding

A greater variety of food is often available for free-living decapods than for those held in captivity. The diet of many appears to be unspecialised, but there is a general tendency towards either herbivorous or carnivorous traits and a few species may be true omnivores. The shape of the cheliped dactyl and propodus of brachyuran crabs provides an indication of feeding preferences. Many spider crabs (oxyrhynchs), some xanthid and rock crabs (grapsids) are essentially herbivores. The tips of their chelipeds are spoon-shaped and used to scrape or pick algal growths from surfaces. Cancrid, portunid and calappid crabs are typical carnivores. Many prey upon molluscs by chipping away the shell and consuming the soft parts. The chelipeds of these species are shaped as powerful pincers. Portunid crabs swim after their prey and are particularly cannibalistic. Omnivorous decapods are represented by astacoidean crayfish, some sesarmid, grapsid, ocypodid, gecarcoidean, potamonid crabs and coenobite hermit crabs. Some spider crabs are opportunistic omnivores and ingest the small amphipod crustaceans trapped among the algae, which they also consume.

Aggression

Decapods frequently show agonistic behaviour towards conspecifics and have been the subjects of numerous studies on resource partitioning (e.g. burrows, space, mates, food) and contest resolution (Arnott & Elwood 2008, 2009). Some contests do not proceed further than displays but many become escalated with physical contact that may involve grappling, holding and crushing of appendages or, in the case of hermit crabs, vigorous rapping of the shells together (Briffa & Elwood 2000). These fights are energetically demanding (Briffa & Elwood 2005) and injurious, and attempts should be made to minimise fights when decapods are kept in captivity. Also, in hermit crabs, one individual may attack another in order to take its shell. If evicted, the loser would normally get the winner's shell, but in large groups the loser might be disturbed while it is naked and lose contact with the winner's old shell. The crab may then remain naked and could be subject to cannibalism. Further, recently moulted decapods may be particularly prone to injury by conspecifics and hence be less successful in contests for resources.

There are several ways by which fights, or the adverse consequences of fights can be reduced. First is to reduce the number of animals per holding tank/enclosure. If there is only one animal, it cannot fight, but even with a few animals there may be few contests because the animals may learn from encounters and not fight those opponents again (Gherardi & Atema 2005). Second, if there are plenty of shelters competition for those will be reduced. Further, decapods may spend most of the time within individual shelters and thus avoid contact with each other. Reducing aggression might be achieved with the addition of seaweed to containers holding shore crabs or by providing plenty of empty shells to hermit crabs. Third, claws may be bound, so they cannot be used to grasp and crush opponents, this being a common practice in the lobster industry. However, the impact of binding claws on the welfare of animals needs to be assessed and it is not recommended for animals used in research.

Cannibalism

We have noted that moulting has inherent risks of detached appendages or incomplete ecdysis leading to death, and that newly moulted animals may be less successful in contests. They may also be unable to defend themselves and are prone to cannibalism. This is a natural phenomenon but is a major problem in aquaculture because it has marked negative consequences for survival during larval culture, nursery culture and growing out to adult stages (Romano & Zeng 2017). Because of this, the problem has received much study aimed at reducing cannibalism and these studies are useful in protecting animals held for research. The key findings are that cannibalism is decreased by (a) reducing stocking density, (b) increasing habitat complexity and availability of shelters, (c) reducing size heterogeneity and (d) providing suitable foods. Further, there may be sex differences in cannibalism, with a higher cannibalism by males. Another method proposed to reduce cannibalism is to manipulate specific neurotransmitters known to influence aggression. This might be achieved on a small scale by injection of either the neurotransmitter or antagonists and by feed containing either high or low levels of amino acid precursors.

Habitat choice

Decapods often need different conditions at successive stages of development. This is obvious when the lifestyles of pelagic larvae are compared with requirements of later benthic stages. However, environmental differences may not be obvious for other species. For example, some penaeid prawns are migratory; they spawn offshore but the larvae and early post-larvae migrate into less saline coastal water, later returning to the offshore waters to complete development. Juveniles of some freshwater *Macrobrachium* prawns spend part of their lives in brackish or saline water.

Methods they use for concealment also must be recognised. Many decapods avoid predation by burying themselves or burrowing diurnally and foraging nocturnally. Penaeid and crangonid prawns burrow into sand or sandy mud by displacing the substrate with strong water currents created by rapidly beating the pleopods. Many cancrid, portunid and calappid crabs burrow backwards into substrates. Some clawed lobster, thalassinid mud lobsters and crabs construct semi-permanent burrows. Mud lobster tunnels often extend vertically and horizontally for considerable distances. Goneplacid and particularly ocypodid crabs consolidate their burrows by methodically excavating and dumping substrates near or around the opening. Some spider crabs (*Inachus*, *Macropodia* and *Stenorhynchus*) use their chelipeds to remove pieces of weed or sessile animals (sponges etc.) from substrates and fasten these to hook-shaped setae on limbs and body surfaces producing an effective camouflage. Sometimes these acquired organisms are eaten thus ensuring a readily available food source (Crane 1975; Warner 1977; Lancaster 1988; Holdich & Lowery 1988).

Reproduction

Decapods may mate and spawn in captivity, and this is preceded by a change in behaviour. The male freshwater prawn *Macrobrachium australiense*, for example, excavates a depression in the aquarium substrate where copulation occurs. Some 20 hours after mating the female adopts a hunched stance and extrudes her eggs that become attached to setae on the pleopods. Male clawed lobsters and freshwater crayfish use the chelipeds for turning the female onto her back in order to extrude spermatophores onto her sternum. Mated females of many shrimps, lobsters and crayfish can be recognised by the white concretions of spermatophores on their sterna. Extensive grooming by the female of her pleopod setae is an indication that spawning will soon occur. Female clawed lobsters mate shortly after moulting while the exoskeleton is still soft. Male hermit crab may hold the gastropod shell occupied by a female for some hours or days prior to copulation and intruder males may fight to take over the guarding position, and hence the mating opportunity (Yasuda et al. 2011). Mate guarding is also typical for portunid and cancrid crabs in which the male carries the female beneath him for a few days before she moults and may even assist with shedding of her old exoskeleton. Copulation occurs immediately after the moult and can last for several hours. The male may not release the female until her exoskeleton has partially hardened. However, precopulatory moults do not occur in many decapods such as penaeid prawns, some hermit crabs, some xanthid crabs and most semi-terrestrial crabs.

Use in research

Research on decapods is diverse and publications may fit broad topics such as environmental science, physiology, anatomy/morphology, life sciences/biomedicine and fisheries. Studies may also be described as nutrition/dietetics, developmental biology, genetic/heredity, behavioural sciences, biodiversity/conservation, reproduction, endocrinology, toxicology, neuroscience and evolutionary biology. Many studies may investigate more than one of these areas. A substantial proportion involve field collections and specimens may have a procedure at that time and/or be killed or transported alive to the laboratory. The techniques employed in the studies are as diverse as the topics. The final section of this chapter considers potential welfare problems that might occur and ways that they may be minimised.

Management of decapods in captivity

Water quality

Most decapods live in either saline or freshwater habitats, although a few species will move into brackish water (shore crabs *Carcinus*) or need low salinities for part of their lives (some freshwater prawns, *Macrobrachium*). A limited number (semi-terrestrial hermit crabs and brachyuran land crabs) can survive with access to only very small quantities of water.

For aquatic species, an understanding of water quality management is important for successful long-term maintenance (Kinne 1976). The control of ammonia, nitrites and to a lesser degree nitrates, is important for successful maintenance of decapods (Romano & Zeng 2013). Between 60 and 80% of total nitrogenous products resulting from protein breakdown is liberated as ammonia. Ideally, levels of total ammonia should not exceed 0.10 mg/l in closed systems, but in practice this level is not easy to maintain for long periods. In newly established systems, and when the mass of decapods is increased in holding tanks, ammonia levels should be checked daily. For measurements of total ammonia levels (NH3-N, NH4-N), colorimetric methods are more accurate than colour chart test kits.

Nitrite is less harmful to decapods than ammonia; however, levels in both sea and freshwater should not exceed 0.10–0.20 mg/l. Levels exceeding 75–100 mg/l cause moulting difficulties and in general it is advisable to keep concentrations below about 20 mg/l by partial water changes. Nitrate, being less toxic, has received less study than has the effects of ammonia and nitrite (Romano & Zeng 2013).

Calcium is an important ion when evaluating water quality for freshwater decapods but there is usually enough calcium in sea water for marine decapods. During moulting, approximately 90% of calcareous material is lost from the exoskeleton. This is replaced from stored calcium (gastroliths) in some but extracted from the water by others. The shore crab *Carcinus maenas*, for example, obtains half of the calcium required for calcifying the exoskeleton from sea water. Thin exoskeletons are often an indication of calcium deficiency. For marine decapods, hardness levels should not fall below about dH7 (100 + mg/l) and for freshwater forms, a total hardness of dH3–6 (50–100 mg/l) is recommended. Calcium-based salts can be added to increase water hardness when necessary but regular partial water changes will usually maintain normal hardness values.

The effect of pH changes on decapods is not well-understood. In practice, pH is affected by carbon dioxide excreted by decapods and by filter bacteria. Lowering pH increases respiration and an increase from just pH7 to pH8 can cause a tenfold rise in un-ionised ammonia in sea water. For marine decapods, a pH range of 8.0–8.3 and for freshwater forms between 7.1 and 7.8 should be maintained. Commercially available chemical buffers can be added to water to increase pH values should this fall to below those given above, but partial water changes will also restore values.

Oxygen is only moderately soluble in water and decreases as salinity and temperature rise. Levels are reduced also by bacterial decomposition of uneaten food and by requirements of filter bacteria. Oxygen use by decapods is temperature related but, in general, marine decapods have lower oxygen uptakes than freshwater forms. Decapods from deep waters are less efficient at adapting to low oxygen levels than intertidal and freshwater forms. Oxygen requirements may be higher at times of moulting. The lowest critical threshold is about 2 mg/l, but oxygen levels should be maintained near to saturation by aeration and/or water circulation, not only in the water itself but also in substrates in which prawns and some crabs bury themselves. At 25 °C, saturation in sea water is about 4.8 mg/l and in freshwater 8.2 mg/l.

Carbon dioxide is highly soluble in both fresh and sea water. In holding vessels, significant rises in carbon dioxide are usually the result of respiratory metabolism but increases can occur also if there is a decline in pH and when bicarbonates break down into carbon dioxide and water. It is rarely necessary to measure carbon dioxide levels in holding waters. Circulating the water by vigorous aeration easily removes carbon dioxide via the water/air interface.

Rising temperature increases decapod metabolism, lowers oxygen concentrations in the body, and increases levels of ammonia and carbon dioxide. Decreases in temperature slow down metabolism to a point where some species cease to feed, and it also affects biological efficiency of filters because bacterial populations in these may take time to become acclimatised to temperature changes. In general, offshore and deep-water decapods that experience only gradual seasonal changes have a more limited temperature tolerance than intertidal and terrestrial forms. Rapid temperature changes cause stress and sometimes death by affecting enzyme producing systems. Most temperate water decapods can acclimatise to temperatures between 7 and 15 °C and tropical species to a range between 20 and 25 °C, but it is always useful to know the seasonal fluctuations experienced in the natural environment. Latitudinal temperature differences are important. The pink shrimp *Pandalus montagui*, for example, collected from its southernmost range in waters of 15 °C, will tolerate temperatures as high as 17 °C in captivity but prawns living further north in waters of 7 °C will not survive above 11 °C. Exceptionally, some intertidal decapods can become acclimatised to quite high temperatures. The temperate common prawn *Palaemon serratus* has been reared successfully in water temperatures as high as 30 °C and the intertidal fiddler crabs *Uca (A) bellator signatus* and *Uca (L) lactea* can withstand gradual rises in temperature to as high as 42 °C. However, most decapods are least stressed when they are kept within the temperature ranges encountered in their natural habitats and to which their metabolism is adapted.

Systems for keeping decapods

Small to medium sized decapods that are exclusively aquatic can be kept in the types of aquarium systems designed for fish. Large aquatic and semi-aquatic decapods, including those that may need to be individually housed, are best kept in a system of the type illustrated in Figure 51.2a with recirculating water. The large holding tank (ht) can accommodate many individual vessels as shown, to hold small decapods. It can also be used by itself to house a few large forms, but then a standpipe must be fitted to the outlet to maintain water at a suitable level. The wood or fibreglass lid (ld) can be hinged longitudinally and glass or Perspex® observation windows fitted; these can be covered with coloured transparent film to reduce light intensity. This unit incorporates a settlement tank (st) that reduces the amount of coarse suspended matter reaching the filter media. Suitable baffles (rb) installed in this tank slow down water circulation and promotes effective settlement of suspended particles. When it is necessary to flush out bottom sludge, the pump circulating the water is switched off, the baffles are raised slightly, and the swing

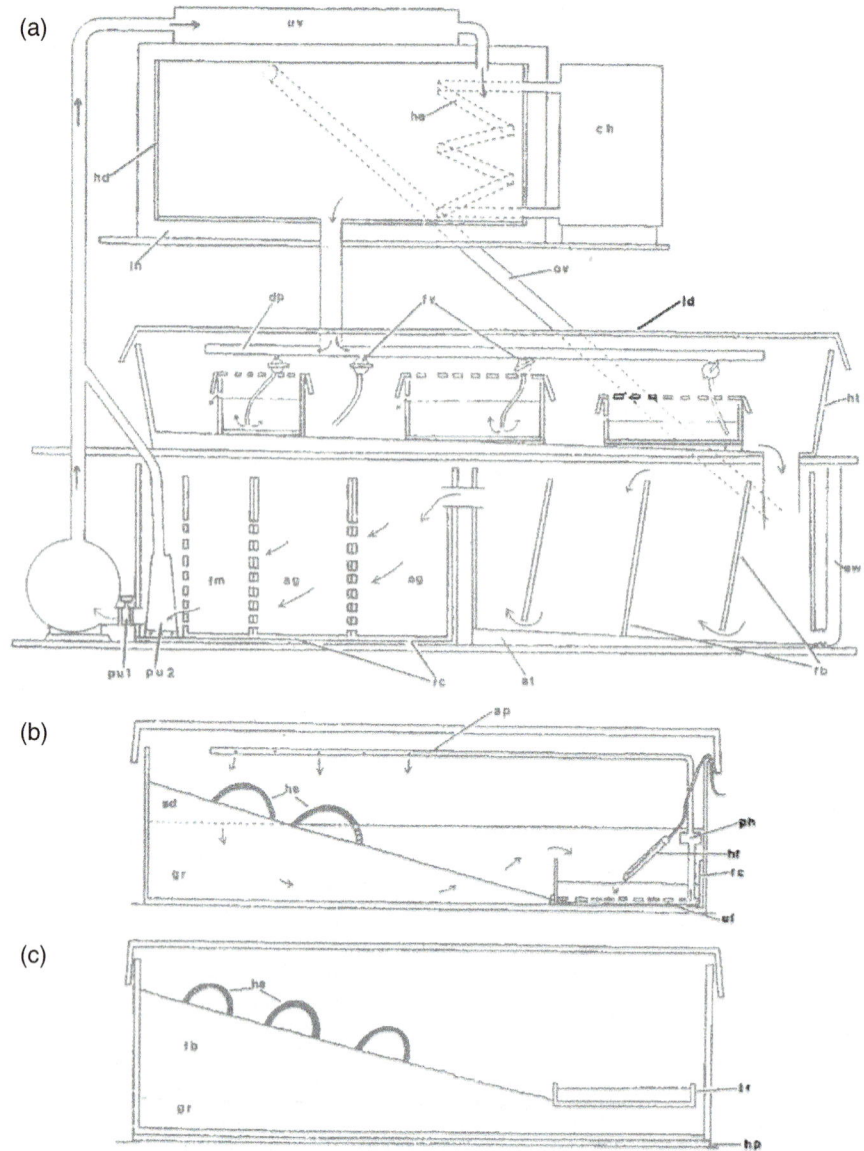

Figure 51.2 Schematic figures of modules for holding decapods in captivity; (a) multiple holding system; (b) module for maintaining intertidal species; (c) module for maintaining semi-terrestrial crabs. **ag** aggregate filter media; **ch** cooler/heater unit; **dp** distribution pipe; **fb** forest bark; **fm** foam filter media; **fv** flow control valves; **gr** gravel; **hd** header tank; **he** heat exchange coil; **hp** heater pad; **hr** heater/thermostat; **hs** hides; **ht** holding tank; **in** insulation jacket; **ld** lid; **ov** overflow; **ph** power head; **pu1** external pump or **pu2** submersible pump; **rb** removable baffle unit; **rc** removable vessels containing filter media; **sd** sand; **sp** spray-bar; **st** settlement tank; **sw** swing-arm standpipe; **tr** heavy tray; **uf** undergravel filter; **uv** ultra-violet unit.

arm standpipe (sw) is lowered. Alternatively, the sludge can be siphoned or pumped from the settlement tank. Filter brushes can be used in place of baffles but during removal for cleaning much of the sediment trapped on brush hairs usually becomes detached and re-suspended in the water and this must be allowed to settle before sludge removal. Water from the settlement tank flows through the filter media contained in perforated canisters (rc) or mesh bags that are easily removed for flushing if they become too clogged to allow adequate water flow through the system. Filter media consist of gravel or plastic aggregate (ag) and cellular foam (fm). Either an external (pu1) or submersible (pu2) pump can be used to circulate water. Both must have couplings to allow easy replacement and standby pumps should always be at hand. For sea-water systems, external pumps with plastic magnetic coupled impellers are preferable. It is important that the capacity of the settlement tank is greater than that of the header tank so that it does not overfill should the pump fail. Alternatively, a solenoid operated cut-off valve can be incorporated in the header tank outlet pipe.

Individual vessels within the large holding tank may be commercially available Perspex® boxes or specially made glass aquaria constructed with silicone adhesive. Lids are essential and must be secured to prevent animals escaping. The ability of decapods to get out of enclosures can be very surprising. Water outlets from these boxes should consist of numerous perforations because crabs often sit over and block single exits. It is advisable to maintain an air space between the lid and water surface. For those intertidal crabs known to frequently leave the water, hides can be provided, such as clay flowerpots, that extend above the water level.

Crabs that normally inhabit intertidal regions, for example, ocypodid crabs, that burrow, and species that spend time out of water, can be housed in the type of module shown in Figure 51.2b. This simulates an average natural habitat but is without tidal movements. The substrate should be taken from, or represent as near as possible, that of the normal habitat. It is not always easy to achieve adequate water circulation through muddy/sand substrates; this is best done with a power head pump (ph). The activities of the inhabitants often stir up the substrate and cause filters to become clogged. Thus, frequent partial water changes may be required, and under gravel filters should be installed in vessels (rc) that can be removed easily for cleaning.

A better system is the tidal apparatus shown in Figure 51.3. This is particularly suitable for keeping ocypodid crabs. The essential components consist of a mesh screen (ms) inserted a short distance from each end of the holding vessel. Water is periodically pumped into the tank through the air/water lift (wt) and from the reservoir (re) placed below the tank level. This water percolates through the substrate (st) and is drained out through the constant level siphon (ls). The air lift pump is regulated by a time switch and, as the inflow is greater than the outflow, the substrate is eventually flooded, simulating a high tide. When the air pump is switched off, the substrate is slowly drained to the siphon level. The substrate is kept biologically active by inoculations of glucose/yeast solutions and artificial light is provided to stimulate photosynthesis.

Semi-terrestrial and terrestrial crabs are best kept in the vivarium-type module shown in Figure 51.2c. In this container, the water is restricted to a receptacle (tr) heavy enough to prevent it from being overturned by the animals. If required, a thermostatically controlled heating pad (hp) is a convenient method for raising the temperature of the container and allow water to condense on the inner surfaces of the module to provide the humidity needed for some crabs. Gravel and forest bark, previously sterilised, are suitable substrates and clay drains or flowerpots make satisfactory hides. An escape proof lid must be fitted.

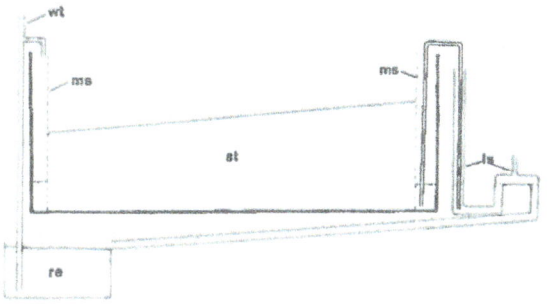

Figure 51.3 A module to simulate tidal conditions. **ls** constant-level siphon; **ms** mesh screens; **re** reservoir; **st** substrate; **wt** water lift. Source: Redrawn from a Figure by Quinn and Fielder (1978)

Special requirements of captive decapods

In their natural habitat many species of penaeid prawns, crangonid shrimps and some crabs habitually burrow into bottom substrates during daylight but emerge during darkness to feed. Many other decapods burrow to lesser degrees and for all decapods the substrate in holding vessels must be of adequate depth. Burrowing could disturb an under-gravel filter, but this can be protected by a mesh placed above the filter. Thalassinid mud lobsters construct branching and often deep burrows in the seabed and when these are held in captivity a substrate depth of at least 0.5 m should be provided. Substrates of these depths sometimes become anaerobic in laboratory conditions causing deterioration of water quality; however, mud lobsters can sometimes be induced to live in plastic pipes as a substitute for their normal burrow.

Rearing in captivity

Rearing equipment

Difficulties may arise when rearing marine decapods because early pelagic larval stages (zoeae) and the later benthic stages (megalopa and post-larvae) require different conditions. Further, mortalities may be high during the transition from a pelagic to benthic mode of life. Some decapods are difficult to rear through all larval stages because, in captivity, females shed their eggs or embryonic development ceases (thalassinid mud lobsters). The newly hatched larvae may be very small (some grapsid crabs) and require special food whereas others have prolonged larval development (crawfish). Freshwater decapods, however, are easier to rear because they are well-developed at hatch and their food requirements are like those of the adults.

Because of the nature of their development, penaeid prawns are best reared in the type of modules shown in Figure 51.4a,b. The fibreglass or polyurethane hatching tank (hv) of 90–900 litres capacity has air lines (al) arranged around the internal circumference; the air-line diffusers extend to the tank bottom. Water is circulated via a primary filter (fl), a pump (pu) and external filter (fu). Female prawns bearing spermatophores are placed into the hatching tank and removed after spawning. The nauplii that hatch from the eggs are siphoned onto a suitable size mesh and transferred to rearing vessels (Figure 51.4b). These are inverted polyurethane carboys or large bottles from which the bases have been removed. The sizes of these vessels depend upon the numbers of larvae being reared, 250 nauplii per litre is suggested. The rearing water is kept in motion by aeration through the air supply tube (ad) inserted into the central neck of the screw cap (cp). This tube also functions as a drain tube for daily water changes. A mesh barrier (mc) prevents larvae from being siphoned out during water changes.

Early larval stages are fed with algae, unconsumed quantities of which are small enough to pass through the mesh barrier during each water change. Later-stage larvae are fed with brine shrimp nauplii, if uneaten these rapidly grow to a size that will not pass through the mesh barrier. These larger nauplii should not be allowed to accumulate in the rearing vessel where they will compete with the prawn larvae for

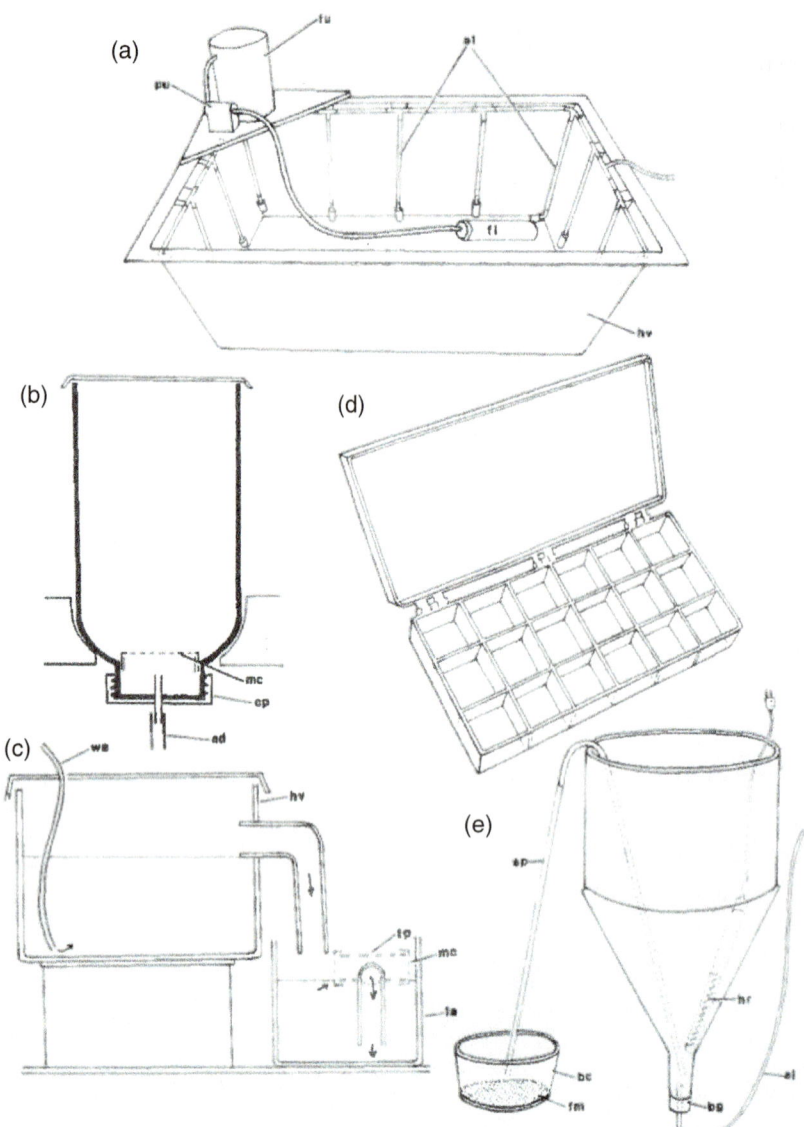

Figure 51.4 Apparatus used for rearing decapods: (a) module for spawning and hatching penaeid prawns (dendrobranchiate decapods); (b) inverted polyurethane bottle or carboy adapted for mass rearing of decapod larvae (the base has been removed and the air supply inserted into the neck region); (c) module for hatching and retaining pleocyemate decapod larvae (caridean shrimps, lobsters and crabs) – females carrying eggs are placed into upper container, hatched larvae are carried over into larval (lower container) trap and retained by the mesh covering both ends of internal horizontal part of T-piece outflow; (d) compartmented transparent Perspex® box – a single larva is placed into each compartment and examined by placing box on a light source; (e) a brine shrimp hatcher constructed from a plastic bin cemented to a large funnel. **ad** tube carrying air supply and also for draining water; **al** air lines; **bc** brine shrimp collector; **bg** rubber bung; **cp** screw cap; **fl** screen filter; **fm** fine mesh; **fu** filter unit; **hr** heater/thermostat; **hv** hatching vessel; **la** larval trap; **mc** mesh collar; **pu** pump; **sp** siphon; **tp** T-piece; **wa** water supply. Source: (a) Drawn from figure 1 photograph by Cook (1967).

oxygen and algal food. Large nauplii are removed by attracting them towards a light source directed at one side of the vessel from where they are then siphoned off. The contents of the rearing module are emptied periodically into a shallow dish and the developmental stages of the prawns assessed. Post-larvae are removed and further reared through later stages in aquaria or in the type of module shown in Figure 51.2a. A suggested stocking density is 10–20 per square metre for post-larvae of 4–5 mm in length.

Females of caridean prawns, clawed lobsters, hermit crabs, crayfish and crabs incubate their eggs attached to the pleopods; this makes it easy to recognise ovigerous specimens. Females with eggs should be housed individually in vessels with aerated water that is partially changed daily. An alternative method is to maintain each female in the type of vessels shown in Figure 51.4c connected to a water flow. When the larvae hatch, they are carried into the larval trap (la). This incorporates a mesh barrier fixed onto each end of a T-piece (tp) inserted into an inside wall of the vessel. Water flow must be regulated at the time of egg hatching to prevent delicate larvae being forced against the retaining mesh and damaged.

Rearing larvae

Newly hatched larvae are removed as soon as possible from either system described above using a wide bore pipette. Various methods for rearing are available: First, compartmental boxes with hinged lids may be used (Figure 51.4d). Each compartment is half filled with water, supplied with food and usually contains a single larva. At 24- or 48-hour intervals, larvae are transferred, via a wide bore pipette, to boxes containing freshly prepared rearing water and food. This method is suitable for studying the progress of individual larvae, particularly when moulted exuviae are needed for morphological or growth studies. Compartmented boxes are also suitable for rearing early post-larval stages of many marine decapods and the young of freshwater crayfish. Later stages can be grown on in aquaria or in the system shown in Figure 51.2a.

Second, larvae can be reared in a mass culture module of the type shown in Figure 51.4b, stocked at about 200 larvae per litre and by the same methods described for rearing penaeid prawns. Larvae with very long spines, such as porcelain crab zoeae, can become entangled with each other (resulting in high mortalities) in mass culture vessels and should be stocked at very low densities and given minimum water circulation.

A third method involves removal of eggs from the female's pleopods and then incubating them in vessels installed on mechanical shakers; the holding water should be changed at intervals. Detached freshwater crayfish eggs have been successfully hatched in units through which water flows at a rate of 75 ml per minute. Fish hatchery 'Zuger jars' also have been used for hatching crayfish eggs. Fungal infection of eggs can be reduced by dipping the eggs daily in a bath of 10–20 ppm of malachite green.

Growing on post-larval forms

When growing-on, adequate shelter should be provided to reduce mortalities at the vulnerable periods of moulting that occur frequently during these early stages of growth. Small plastic tubes are suitable for lobsters and crabs. Post-larval hermit crabs must be given empty gastropod shells of suitable sizes for concealing their soft abdomens.

Foods and feeding

Food for larval decapods

Very small larvae require algae as food until they become large enough to consume brine shrimp nauplii; the latter is universally used as food for rearing marine decapods (Provasoli et al. 1957). For example, two days or so after hatching the nauplii of penaeid prawns moult to the protozoeal stage. These are approximately 1.0 mm in length and filter feed on suspended algal cells – e.g. *Skeletonema, Thalassiosira, Melosira, Nitzschia, Tetraselmis, Isochrysis, Phaeodactylum* and *Cyclotella*. The numbers of cells fed to larvae can vary from 5000 to 70,000 per ml depending upon the algae used. Small quantities of yeast or soycake can be added to these feeds. Approximately nine days after hatching the larvae moult to the mysis stage and algae should be replaced gradually by newly hatched brine shrimp nauplii fed at 2–5 per ml. Alternatively, commercial micro-encapsulated foods can be used. The post-larval stages that appear approximately 12 days after hatching are initially fed with large brine shrimp nauplii, but this diet is gradually replaced with the type of food used to feed juveniles.

By contrast, newly hatched caridean prawns, lobsters and crabs are usually large enough to consume small brine shrimp nauplii, but a few may require algae during very early stages. At the megalopal stage, the food should be gradually changed to the adult diet. Food requirements of the phyllosoma larvae of crawfish are not fully understood. A few have been reared to late larval stages on combinations of algae, brine shrimp nauplii and mussel meat.

Culturing food for larval decapods

Algae

Algae are usually cultured in large conical flasks. Bubbling filtered air or carbon dioxide through the media increases growth rates of some species. The flasks can be placed near a north facing window or very close to one or more fluorescent tubes that have a spectrum near to daylight. Weekly sub-culturing may be necessary when cultures are growing rapidly. Standard bacteriological sterilisation methods should be used for all glassware and during sub-culturing to prevent contamination. Pure strains of algae can be obtained from appropriate culture centres.

Two media are commonly used for culturing the types of algae mentioned above:

Erdschreiber medium stock solution is prepared as follows: (a) For nitrate/phosphate solution, dissolve 20 gm sodium nitrate ($NaNO_3$) and 2 gm sodium hydrogen orthophosphate ($Na_2HPO_4.12H_2O$) in 100 ml distilled water. Autoclave plugged flasks at 104 kPa for 20 minutes and store in a refrigerator. (b) 1000 ml cleared soil extract is prepared by sieving 1 kg of untreated soil added to 1000 ml of tap water and autoclaving at 104 kPa for one hour, cooling and decanting off the cloudy liquid into 150 ml plugged flasks that are boiled to resterilise, then cooled and centrifuged to precipitate the fine clay (or after autoclaving filter decanted liquid through Whatman no. 1 filter paper into plugged flasks and autoclave for 20 minutes); store flasks in a deep freeze until required. (c) Culture water for approximately one litre culture of algae is prepared by autoclaving 1000 m flasks of sea water, allowing these to cool to ambient temperature and then slowly adding to each flask, using a sterilised pipette, 2 ml of (a) and 100 ml of (b). Flame the necks of flasks before and after decanting then inoculate with the algal culture.

Miquel Allen medium stock solution is prepared as follows: (a) 100 gm potassium nitrite (KNO3), 2 gm potassium bromide (KBr), 1 gm potassium iodide (KI), distilled water 1000 ml. (b) 25 gm sodium hydrogen orthophosphate (Na2HPO4.12H2O), 12.5 gm calcium chloride (CaCl2.6H2O), 12.5 ml ferric chloride (FeCl3, 58% w/v sol.), 14.5 ml hydrochloric acid conc. (HCL), 500 ml distilled water. (c) Prepare the culture medium by adding 2 ml of (a) and 1 ml of (b) to 1000 ml of sea water. Heat to 70 °C and maintain at this temperature for 20 minutes, cool and decant off the clear liquid into sterilised flasks and inoculate with the algal culture.

Brine shrimp

The naupliar stages of the brine shrimp (*Artemia salina*) have proved the best food for rearing decapods. Vacuum-packed cans of brine shrimp eggs are available from commercial aquaculture retailers. Cans should be labelled with a guaranteed percentage of 70–95% hatch. Various methods have been described for hatching these eggs (Sorgeloos 1980). A simple device for this purpose is shown in Figure 51.4e. The hatcher is constructed of a large plastic funnel cemented to a plastic barrel the base of which has been removed. Brine shrimp eggs are kept in suspension by strong aeration through the air tube (al) and a light source is provided above the container for at least the first twelve hours of incubation to promote hatching. The water should be maintained at about 25° C and in normal strength sea water or saline solutions made with commercial grades of sodium chloride prepared with fresh water having a pH value of 8–9. Egg densities when hatching should not exceed about 10 g/l. Eggs must be kept in suspension, water oxygen levels maintained near to saturation and with continuous illumination throughout incubation to ensure a good hatch. Nauplii culled within one hour of hatching have maximum nutritive values; unharvested nauplii grow appreciably within 24 hours and may be too large for newly hatched decapod larvae to consume.

Hatched nauplii are collected by switching off the air supply and allowing the nauplii to swim towards a light source directed at a region near the base of the funnel from where they are removed through the siphon (sp) into the collector (bc) and retained on a fine mesh (fm). The inside end of the siphon should be located about 5–10 mm above the bung (bg) and the inside surface of the funnel can be finely scored to promote the adhesion of empty egg capsules as water is slowly siphoned off when collecting the nauplii. All the equipment should be thoroughly cleaned in very hot water and scrubbed to remove bacterial films before using again.

When brine shrimp eggs are hatched, most empty egg capsules will remain separated from the nauplii because the latter are siphoned from the hatcher (Figure 51.4e). However, the egg capsules can be removed from the eggs before hatching by the method described below. Decapsulated eggs can be hatched immediately or stored in saturated brine at −4 °C. There are advantages in using decapsulated eggs. Incubation time is considerably reduced, chemicals used for decapsulation also disinfect the eggs by removing and killing bacteria attached to the capsule surfaces; the risk of bacterial contamination of larval cultures is thus reduced. Less energy is used by brine shrimp nauplii during the hatching process and they emerge with a higher nutritive value. Some decapod larvae will even accept decapsulated eggs as food.

The following method is suitable for decapsulating 10 gm of eggs.

1. Dissolve 5 gm of calcium hypochlorite ($Ca(OCl)_2$) in approximately 1000 ml of freshwater; aerate for ten minutes; stabilise the pH by adding 3 gm of calcium oxide (CaO); continue aeration for a further 10 minutes; store overnight to allow cooling and precipitation; siphon off the supernatant and use this as a decapsulation bath.
2. Hydrate the brine shrimp eggs in sea water for one hour and keep them in suspension by aeration.
3. Transfer the eggs into a stainless steel or nylon mesh cage and suspend this in the decapsulation bath; this should be surrounded with ice to prevent the bath temperature from exceeding 35 °C. Keep the eggs in suspension by aeration and when the egg colour changes from dark brown to orange or white (usually within 5–10 minutes), the mesh cage containing the decapsulated eggs is removed and the eggs washed very thoroughly for at least 10–15 minutes in running fresh water.
4. Place the mesh cage containing the decapsulated eggs into a deactivation bath of 0.10 N hydrochloric acid (HCl) for 3–4 minutes and then wash again very thoroughly in running fresh water.

The rotifer (*Brachionus plicatilis*) is sometimes used for feeding very small decapod larvae. The rotifers are cultured in flasks, maintained at 20–22 °C and fed with algae such as *Dunaliella*, *Chlorella* and yeast (see Liao *et al.* 1983 for culture methods). Populations should be allowed to reach 100 rotifers per ml before feeding to larvae.

Food for adult decapods

Many marine species are easy to maintain on natural foods containing shrimp and fish meal. These foods can be either freshly prepared or purchased as frozen or freeze-dried commercial products. Freshwater crayfish will eat aquatic plants, lettuce and spinach, supplemented with meat or fish. Adult crayfish appear predominantly herbivorous and juveniles carnivorous. Semi-terrestrial coenobite hermit crabs and carcoidean crabs, although omnivores, seem to thrive on diets of leaves and fruit in captivity. Small quantities of soya bean supplement will usually make up any nitrogenous deficits. Brine shrimps, reared to late naupliar or adult stage, are highly nutritious food for juvenile and adult decapods.

Artificially prepared foods are also suitable and are now marketed for commercial shrimp rearing. Prepared food for penaeid prawns can comprise a mixture of 45% shrimp meal, 20% high gluten wheat flour, 18% fish meal 13% corn ground, 8% soybean meal, 5% brewer's yeast and 1% vitamins and minerals. These ingredients must be bound together to prevent immediate disintegration when being manipulated by decapods. In this formula the high gluten wheat flour serves as a binder. Other binding agents are agar, carboxymethyl cellulose, polyvinyl alcohol, gelatin and casein (see Kinne 1976 for method of preparation). For feeding marine portunid crabs, mussel meat (*Mytilus*) and wrack weed (*Fucus*) can be dried, pulverised and added to melted agar, the mixture poured into petri dishes, allowed to solidify and then cut into cubes of an appropriate size for feeding. Deposit feeding crabs such as ocypodids, and suspension feeding haplocarcinid coral crabs will usually need food composed of fine particles unless their substrates are rich in organic material.

Many prawns and crabs characteristically dismember large pieces of food, and some regurgitate food to 'work it over' again. The quantity of food given is a compromise between the amount immediately consumed and that which can be safely left uneaten and not foul the water. The amount of food consumed and assimilated is often high. For example, adult Baltic prawns *Palaemon adspersus* consume an equivalent of 2.2% of their body weight each 24 hours. Further, juvenile clawed lobsters *Homarus* have an assimilation efficiency of 81% when fed a diet of brine shrimps and the common spider crab *Libinia* 90–95% when fed on algae, fish and mussel.

Collecting, handling and transporting decapods

Collecting

Methods for collecting live decapods vary from simply catching them by hand, with nets or with baited hand-held lines, to using elaborate traps and suction devices. The technique used will depend upon the type of habitat and substrate. Semi-terrestrial ocypodid and gecarcoidean land crabs are often easier to collect at night when momentarily stunned by torchlight (Ng 2017). They can also be dug from their burrows or by waiting near the burrow entrance for the crabs to emerge and then cutting off retreat with a spade. Intertidal spider, cancrids, some xanthid and porcelain crabs often remain immobile when they are exposed and are thus easy to capture. Hermit crabs will typically withdraw into their shells and may then fall over, making them easy to see and then capture in intertidal pools. Porcelain crabs cling tightly to rock surfaces, readily shed limbs and should be detached with care. Portunid and grapsid crabs are agile and adept at slipping into inaccessible fissures in rocks. Shallow-water prawns can be collected using hand nets or with a roller push net (Figure 51.5a). SCUBA diving is a good method for collecting decapods in deeper waters. This method allows selective collecting and causes minimum environmental damage, also it may be the least stressful for the animals. Hand collected specimens are placed into plastic bags.

Pelagic decapods, particularly larval stages, can be collected with a tow net. Trawling is often used to collect offshore benthic decapods but only on seabeds that are not extensively rocky. Lightly calcified decapods can be damaged when they become compressed in the cod-end of a trawl as it is brought onto the deck; nevertheless, trawling is often the only method for obtaining deep water decapods. On rocky bottoms, baited traps of commercial design (Figure 51.5b) are effective for collecting lobsters and crabs, and for freshwater crayfish. The bait retainer (br) holds the

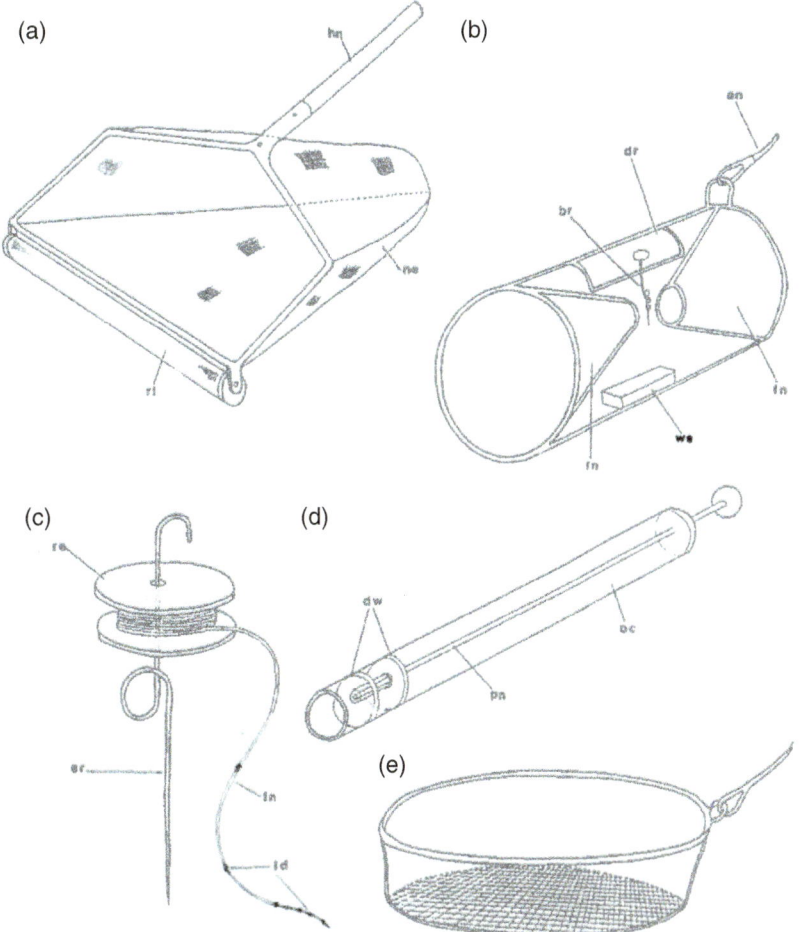

Figure 51.5 Equipment for collecting decapods: (a) roller-type push net; (b) funnel-shaped trap; (c) device for collecting mud lobsters/shrimps; (d) suction gun (e) large plastic sieve. **an** anchor line; **br** bait retainer; **dr** door; **dw** double washer; **fn** funnels; **hn** handle; **ld** small lead shot (substitute); **ln** line; **ne** net bag; **oc** outer Perspex® cylinder; **pn** plunger; **re** line reel; **rl** roller; **sr** securing rod; **we** weight. Source: (a) Drawn from a photograph published by Manning (1975). (b) Drawn from figure 2 of de Vaugelas (1985).

fish, mussel or other meat to which the decapod is attracted through one of the wide-mouth funnels (fn), the inner ends of these are narrowed to reduce escape. A device for extracting mud shrimps from burrows is shown in Figure 51.5c. The fine line (ln), weighted at the end with lead shot substitute and on a reel (re) is secured by a rod (sr) near to the burrow. The weighted end (ld) is lowered into the burrow and left for 2–3 days. This line is ingested by the mud shrimp before being rejected as inedible but becomes entangled in the limbs holding the shrimp as it is carefully dug out of the burrow. A suction gun (Figure 51.5d) is useful for capturing burrowing decapods. The Perspex® cylinder (oc) of the one shown is approximately 1 m in length and 60 mm in diameter. The plunger (pn) has a double neoprene washer (dw) at the lower end and the handle is large enough to be firmly held. The end of the gun is pushed into the burrow mouth and the plunger rapidly withdrawn. The contents of the tube are quickly ejected into a floating sieve (Figure 51.5e) conveniently attached to the operator by a line or held by an assistant. The sand or mud in the sieve is gently washed away to reveal captured decapods. A suction gun can be used when SCUBA diving. The contents are slowly released into an empty plastic bag that is then secured underwater and inspected for captured decapods after returning to the diving vessel.

Apart from nets of appropriate sizes and protective footwear when working on rocky shores, the most useful items for collecting small to medium size decapods are plastic buckets and bowls for sorting catches, and plastic bags that can be secured with strong elastic bands for transporting catches. Captured decapods should be retained with only a small quantity of bagged water to provide a maximum surface area for gaseous exchanges. Bags should be supported in lightweight plastic boxes. If captured decapods have obvious sharp spines, two or more bags, one within the other, should be used. On exposed sunny shores or even on a ship's deck, water within plastic bags can quickly reach temperatures lethal to decapods. If adequate shade is not available, the bags should be submerged in the sea, river or lake until they can be transported to the laboratory. Buckets containing more than one decapod should include weed to provide shelter and reduce agonistic behaviour. Very large decapods need to be transferred immediately into plastic tanks of an appropriate size and provided with aeration if available. They can be also transported successfully in shallow darkened vessels with minimum water and covered with wet cloth on which, if necessary, are placed small bags of ice cubes.

Handling

Small decapods are best handled in a net, taking care not to damage delicate antennae and limbs. Lobsters and crabs should be grasped firmly near the dorso-posterior part of the carapace using the thumb and forefinger and quickly turned ventral side uppermost. In this reversed position, they will often assume a cataleptic state, but it is wise to restrain the abdomen of small lobsters and crayfish with the third and fourth fingers gently pressed against the underside to prevent a 'tail-flip' escape reflex. The powerful chelipeds of some large crabs (robber crab *Birgus* and some land crabs) can cause serious wounds by puncturing skin and even crushing small finger bones.

Transporting decapods

Plastic bags contained in strong boxes can be used. Many intertidal crabs will travel satisfactorily packed only in damp weed and several small crabs can be housed in one bag providing it contains liberal amounts of weed. Decapods collected from offshore waters must be fully immersed and large decapods should be housed individually. A high humidity (90–95%) must be maintained if clawed lobsters and crawfish are transported in damp weed as even slight drying of the gills can cause irreversible damage to these delicate organs resulting in a short captive life. Polystyrene boxes give excellent insulation. Bagged ice cubes can be included if necessary but should not be in direct contact with the specimens.

Collecting restrictions

The survival of many decapod species is now threatened by habitat destruction or by other negative changes in environments. The World Conservation Monitoring Centre, Cambridge, UK collects data on threatened species and habitats. This information is published as the IUCN Red List of Threatened Animals and is periodically updated. It is necessary to know which species are protected and if restrictions exist governing their capture and export from or import to the countries concerned. Although regulations will apply to faunas in designated conservation areas, they may be also applicable to species outside of these regions. For example, in the UK the native, white-clawed crayfish *Austropotamobius pallipes* is legally protected by the Wildlife and Countryside Act of 1986 and it is an offence to take this species from the wild.

Restraining, anaesthetising and killing decapods

Restraining

Decapods are not easy crustaceans to restrain physically. When possible, mild or deep anaesthesia should be used if they must be immobilised. A restraining device for large shrimps comprises a foam-lined trough in which the shrimp is held and then immobilised with 'Velcro' straps fastened across the trough. The chelae of crabs can be immobilised using plastic coated wire tape. Allow the crab to grasp the tape approximately 50 mm from the far end, then quickly wrap the tape around the closed chelae and secure by twisting the ends together. However, the welfare implications of holding the chelae closed for long periods has not yet been assessed and this method should only be employed if other methods are not available.

Anaesthesia and analgesia

Anaesthesia is usually achieved by totally immersing decapods in an appropriate solution of anaesthetic. Xylazine hydrochloride at concentrations of 70 mg/kg body weight induces anaesthesia within 5–6 minutes and maintains this state for approximately 45 minutes (Oswald 1977). Procaine hydrochloride at 25 mg/kg body weight causes anaesthesia within 20–30 seconds, total paralysis within 4 minutes and an unconscious state for 2–3 hours; used at 60 mg/kg recovery takes as long as 10 hours. Halothane used at 0.5% by volume anaesthetises freshwater crayfish within approximately 15 minutes. Tricaine methanesulfonate (MS-222) used at concentrations of 0.3–0.5% for small crabs of 10–14 mm carapace width causes anaesthesia within about 30 minutes, larger crabs of 33–36 mm carapace width require exposures exceeding one hour. *These chemicals must be handled with care and the operator must avoid direct contact with any anaesthetics by wearing suitable protective clothing.* Clove oil (Ghanawi et al. 2019) and eugenol (Li et al. 2018) may also be effective anaesthetics.

Large lobsters or very large crabs are best immobilised by injections into the abdomen of isobutanol (2-methyl-1-propanol). At a concentration of 1.0μ1/10 gm live weight at 15 °C, anaesthesia is induced within 2 minutes and recovery takes about 18 minutes. Injecting this anaesthetic at temperatures of 6–8.5 °C and concentrations of 4.0μ1/10 gm body weight sustains anaesthesia for as long as 184 minutes.

Local anaesthetics have been used to mitigate negative effects of eye-stalk ablation. Various methods of ablation leave different types of wounds and probably induce different levels of stress. Application of local anaesthetics and coagulating agents have been used to reduce the stress, and possible pain from ablation (e.g. Taylor et al. 2004). For example, prawns *Macrobrachium americanum* treated with lignocaine showed less rubbing, flicking and sheltering than those without the anaesthetic following ablation (Diarte-Plata et al. 2012)

Morphine has been suggested to have an analgesic effect on decapods. In the crab, *Chasmagnathus granulatus*, morphine produced a dose-dependent reduction of crab sensitivity to electric shock, and this was reversed by the opioid antagonist, naloxone (Lozada et al. 1988). However, when an experimental test was used that should have resulted in more movement; if there was an analgesic effect, there was no sign of a specific analgesia. Rather, there was a general immobility, and no specific analgesia could be established (Barr & Elwood 2011).

To prevent cannibalism, decapods should never be returned to communal holding vessels until they appear to have fully recovered from the effects of anaesthetics.

Euthanasia

Small decapods, including larvae, can be killed quickly by overdosing with anaesthetics. Methyl (methanol) or ethyl (ethanol) alcohols, or the industrial methylated spirit used for preserving animal tissues, when added slowly to water causes anaesthesia leading to death. Decapods of a medium to large size can be humanely killed by long-lasting anaesthetising (see previous sections), wrapping in a cloth or plastic and placing in a deep freeze. If undamaged tissues are needed for histological studies, the decapod should be anaesthetised and then immersed in the appropriate fixative. For large decapods, this should be injected through the thoraco-abdominal membranes and/or membranes between leg segment to ensure adequate penetration of the fixative into tissues. There may be occasions when the animal should be killed quickly but prior preparation is not possible. In this case, while killing lobsters and crabs an awl may be inserted between the mouthparts and directed upwards at an angle of about 45° rapidly destroying the brain and central nerve mass.

Recent studies have focused on the welfare implications of different methods of killing decapods (Conte et al. 2021). Fregin and Bickmeyer (2016) suggest avoiding the use of cooling, magnesium chloride and carbon dioxide but did recommend slow heating and electrical stunning as methods with high welfare. However, different species may respond differently to electrical stunning with crayfish and shrimp being effectively killed but crabs less so (Weineck et al. 2018).

Diseases of decapods

Invasive organisms

A variety of disease-producing and fouling organisms may cause problems for decapods (Couch 1983; Johnson 1983; Overstreet 1983; Bateman & Stentiford 2017) but the pathogen profile might differ between age classes (Bateman et al. 2011). Some bacterial and fungal infections are serious and may cause rapid death.

Some diseases should be notified to the relevant national authorities (see OIE list of diseases of crustaceans[1]).

Heavy infestations (fouling) by commensals can cause stress and render decapods susceptible to diseases. Poor water quality can produce stress that allows bacteria and fungi, normally present in water, to invade tissues often through the cuticle or membranes damaged during agonistic encounters. These regions are particularly vulnerable at times of moulting. Knowledge of diseases and their treatments for invertebrates is relatively poor when compared with that known for fish. Most of the information available for decapods relates to species that are cultured and commercially farmed (shrimps, lobsters and freshwater crayfish). Clinical symptoms, however, are well-known for commonly occurring diseases such as lobster gaffkaemia, which affects European lobsters, and crayfish plague *Aphanomyces astaci*, the latter being responsible for extinctions of native populations of European crayfish. Here we list the main groups of causative organisms, however, we suggest that The OIE Manual of Diagnostic Tests be consulted for guidance[2].

1. Viruses. Viral infections have been reported from various decapods (Bateman & Stentiford 2017) but few of these pathogens have been formally characterised and classified. However, some have devastating consequences on the global crustacean farming industry. Transmission occurs through viral contaminated water and by cannibalism.
2. Bacteria. These are often opportunistic pathogens, invading tissues of stressed or wounded decapods producing disease symptoms and death, if invasions are not

---

[1] https://www.cefas.co.uk/international-database-on-aquatic-animal-diseases/oie-listed-diseases/ (Accessed 24 March, 2022)
[2] https://www.oie.int/en/what-we-do/standards/codes-and-manuals/aquatic-manual-online-access/ (Accessed March 24, 2022)

suppressed by the host's defence mechanism or by treatment (for bacteria in crabs, see Wang 2011). Damage caused by infections may be either to the exoskeleton by chitin destroying (chitinoclastic) species, to the gills by filamentous forms, or to the haemocoele and muscle tissues by various septicaemia-causing species. Infections can interfere with moulting. Bacterial infections of haemocoelic tissues hinder the clotting efficiency of haemolymph, cause reductions in numbers of circulating haemocytes and local necrosis of gills, muscles and antennal glands. The progress of many infections is usually temperature dependent.

  Chitinoclastic bacteria causing shell disease (rust disease or black spot) easily gain entrance through damaged epicuticle and this layer can be degraded also by lipolytic (fat degrading) bacteria present in poor quality water, particularly when suspended sewerage sludge is present. Various chitinolytic or chitinoclastic bacteria produce the enzyme chitinase that is capable of degrading carapace chitin (Wang 2011). Lesions are obvious and become progressively deeper during later stages allowing entry of opportunistic bacteria and fungi. Shell disease often causes high mortalities when lobsters are crowded into holding tanks especially when gills become badly damaged.

  Early clinical symptoms are not always obvious in bacterial infections causing septicaemic conditions, but advanced stages of infection are often marked by prolonged lethargy and stiffened, trembling limbs. Rickettsiae is usually visible using light microscopy and by staining tissues with specific stains. Rickettsia has been described for shore crabs *Carcinus aestuarii* and *C. maenas* (Eddy et al. 2007) and causes death when experimentally transmitted to healthy crabs.

  Muscle tissues of prawns become opaque, gills may turn black (melanised) and body colouration becomes abnormal. Not all strains of a pathogen are necessarily virulent as is the case for the gram-positive coccus (*Aerococcus*) that causes clawed lobster gaffkaemia disease, but the lobster's defence mechanisms are not effective against virulent strains. *Aerococcus* has been isolated from several species of crabs and may occur also in penaeid prawns; these decapods could be reservoirs of infections if they form part of the lobster's diet (Davies & Wootton 2017).

3. Fungi. Aquatic fungi may be opportunistic pathogens that normally live as saprophytes, and many appear to be normal epibionts. Fungi causing burnt spot disease, signified by red to black regions on the cuticle, may be chitinoclastic and partially parasitic. Crayfish plague that is caused by the water mould (*Aphanomycetes astaci*) may be exclusively parasitic. Infected crayfish are disoriented and the limbs droop when crayfish are removed from water. *Fusarium* infections cause blackening of gills, and the carapace is heavily melanised when decapods are infected with the *Haliphthoros* fungus.

4. Ellobiopsids. These are a group of hyphae-like producing organisms whose taxonomic affinities are uncertain. They have a bulb-shaped branching structure located within the host's tissue from which protrude external finger-like processes. How they affect their host is not known and their prevalence in decapods uncertain.

5. Protozoans. Many species of protozoans infect decapods (Stentiford 2008). They range from opportunistic invaders to true parasites. The amoeba *Paramoeba perniciosa* enters tissues through external lesions, particularly if these are developed during moulting. The amoebae invade the haemolymph and chiefly non-epithelial tissues causing lysis; in advanced infections, the tissues are filled with the amoebae. Infected decapods become lethargic, and the ventral surfaces turn grey. Species of ciliophorans of the genus *Anophrys* infect tissues and haemolymph feeding upon the haemocytes and haemolymph causing death by anaemia. Many ciliophorans are ectocommensals. *Lagenophrys* occurs on the gills of crabs and *Cothurnia* on freshwater crayfish, excessive numbers can cause asphyxiation. Some, such as *Synophrya*, can become endoparasitic. Some protozoans infecting decapods live as intracellular parasites and have complex life histories. *Urosporidium crescens*, for example, is a hyperparasite of digenean trematodes (see 6b in the following text) turning them black. Decapod tissues have a speckled appearance (pepper disease) when numbers of infected metacercariae of these trematodes are present. Many of the microsporidian protozoans that infect decapods are particularly pathogenic (Stentiford et al. 2012). Muscle opacity is often a symptom of such infections.

6. Metazoans. Decapods are hosts to a considerable number of metazoans (reviewed primarily for crabs by Stentiford 2008). When present on body surfaces in large numbers, they are considered as fouling organisms. Some derive benefit from shelter and a supply of food and do not appear to affect their host. Others are true parasites occurring as larval stages in body tissues utilising decapods as intermediate hosts in their life cycle (digenean flukes). The major metazoans associated with decapods are briefly reviewed below.

    a. Branchiobdellids. These are leech-like commensal/parasitic oligochaete annelid worms, which attach by suckers to gills of freshwater crayfish, marine shrimps and crabs. They may damage these delicate organs.

    b. Digenean trematodes (flukes). Cercariae (an infective larva) damage decapod gills by coating or penetrating the surfaces. Cercariae develop into metacercariae that become imbedded in the host tissue, grow and damage organs. Decapods may be infected when newly captured but show no obvious symptoms other than melanisation of infected regions. Even heavy infections may not adversely affect decapods although metabolism may be altered and render them susceptible to bacterial and fungal infections, or predation in communal holding vessels.

    c. Nemerteans (ribbon worms). Juveniles of the nemertean *Carcinonemertes carcinophila* occur on the gills of true crabs and secrete a mucous capsule that causes gill lamellae to stick together. After the female crab has spawned, the juvenile worms migrate to the egg mass and feed upon eggs and developing larvae. The worm's faeces and the yolk released from damaged eggs induce secondary infections and encourage epibionts. Nemerteans may also be found in juvenile crabs.

d. Nematodes (roundworms). Many species infect decapods, the majority occur as juvenile stages, affecting the host to varying degrees.
e. Crustaceans. Several crustaceans parasitise decapods. The degenerate adult stage of the cirripede rhizocephalans (*Sacculina*), related to barnacles, occurs as a conspicuous sac between abdomen and thoracic sterna of crabs and affects behaviour and reproduction of the host. Isopods of the sub-order Epicaridea inhabit the branchial cavities of prawns, lobsters and their allies. In prawns, their presence is often indicated by a blister-like swelling of the carapace branchial region. The parasites feed on haemolymph and affect maturation and respiration of the host. A related group, the entoniscid isopods, cause deterioration of the ovaries. Early stages of infection are sometimes denoted by a brownish pigment beneath the host's abdominal membranes. Small crabs can die from entoniscid infections.

Prevention and treatment

Measures can be taken to reduce the risk of diseases developing in captive held decapods. Avoid introducing damaged animals into healthy stocks and do not overcrowd as this usually raises agonistic levels. Maintain good water quality and minimise water-borne bacterial populations by u.v. water treatment. Ensure adequate oxygen levels and prevent extremes of temperatures in holding vessels. Legally approved antibiotics of appropriate strengths added to holding water are sometimes used to control general bacterial problems and antibiotics can be incorporated in food to treat specific infections *when the causative agents have been identified*. One mg/per kg body weight of Vancomycin protects lobsters against gaffkaemia infections for at least 15 days. Antibacterial agents such as oxolinic acid, nitrofurazone (Furacin) and the nifurpirinol (Furanace = Prefuran), also the fungicide/protozoacide malachite green are all suitable agents for treating some ectoparasites. *Fusarium* fungal infections can be controlled with a 6.3 ppm solution of malachite green and killed with a 6.2 ppm solution of dichloroisocyanurate. Furanace is effective for treating *Haliphthoros* fungal infections. Ectoparasites on semi-terrestrial crabs sometimes can be reduced by lowering the humidity to dry the shell, even a 2–4-hour bath in 1.5–2.5% of hydrochloric acid has been used to remove these parasites. Buquinolate has been used to treat protozoan microsporan infections.

A licence many be required to legally obtain and use antibiotics and restrictions may govern the use of other chemicals for treating decapod diseases. The reader must consult the appropriate regulations of his or her country before purchasing or using these agents.

Welfare problems in decapods

There is little legal protection for the welfare of decapods, largely because of a belief that these animals respond to noxious stimuli purely by reflex responses that do not require central processing. Thus, it is argued that they do not experience pain (Sherwin 2001). However, several studies have shown that the responses are more than mere reflexes and are generally consistent with the idea of pain (Sneddon et al. 2014). For example, prawns and crabs brushed with acetic acid on antennae, eyes or mouth parts show prolonged rubbing of the specific treated area (Barr et al. 2008; Elwood et al. 2017) but that rubbing is reduced if a local anaesthetic is applied (Barr et al. 2008). Shore crabs learn to avoid a shelter after two trials if it is coupled with electric shock and, instead, use one in which no shock is experienced (Magee & Elwood 2013). Further, hermit crabs trade-off shock avoidance with the need to avoid predators (Magee & Elwood 2016) and to keep a high-quality shell (Appel & Elwood 2009a; Elwood & Appel 2009), indicating central decision-making. Hermit crabs shocked within their shell show a high motivation to get a new shell for many hours after the experience (Appel & Elwood 2009b; Elwood & Appel 2009). Crayfish show anxiety-like behaviour after shock and become risk averse, but this is eliminated by injection of an anti-anxiolytic drug (Fossat et al. 2014, 2015). Electric shock also causes a physiological stress response that is independent of the behavioural response in crabs (Elwood & Adams 2015) and the stress response is also seen in crabs that have had one claw removed in a manner that causes damage at the joint but not when autotomy is induced (Patterson et al. 2007).

It is important to be clear, however, that these observations of non-reflex responses, coupled with physiological change, do not prove pain because that is not possible for any species. They do, however, disprove the notion that crustaceans show only reflexes without central processing and thus the observations are consistent with pain experience. The precautionary principle has been applied to vertebrates and the evidence for that move is not too dissimilar to that described in the preceding text (Birch 2017). However, there has been a reluctance to accept that evidence and offer protection for decapods (Diggles 2019). This stance is clearly illogical, and decapods should be given the benefit of doubt and thus should be treated in ways that maintain good welfare (Birch 2017). Although there has been a recent growth in organisations and jurisdictions that promote or require humane treatment for decapods (Rowe 2018), the latter remains rare. One notable exception is the recent recognition of decapods being sentient by the UK parliament (Crump et al. 2022), however, that provides no specific protection for these animals. However, it should be recognised that scientific advance usually precedes legislative change, often with considerable time between the two but those using animals do not have to wait for legislation. Scientists should carefully evaluate the experimental procedures to be employed and refine these to minimise harm to the subjects. We should also consider experimental design and sample sizes to minimise the numbers of animals subjected to the most harmful procedures. It might be difficult, however, to replace the subjects because most work on decapods is species specific. Whenever possible, science should promote good practice even if that is not currently required by law.

Acknowledgements

We are grateful to authors and publishers for permission to redraw figures from the sources cited and that have been reproduced from Ingle (1995).

References

Aiken, D.E. (1980). Moulting and growth. In: *The Biology and Management of Lobsters*, Vol. 1. Eds Cobb, J.S. and Phillips, B.F., pp. 91–163. Academic Press, London.

Appel, M. and Elwood, R.W. (2009a). Motivational trade-offs and the potential for pain experience in hermit crabs. *Applied Animal Behaviour Science*, **119**, 120–124.

Appel, M. and Elwood, R.W. (2009b). Gender differences, responsiveness and memory of a potentially painful event in hermit crabs. *Animal Behaviour*, **78**, 1373–1379.

Arnott, G. and Elwood, R.W. (2008). Information-gathering and decision-making about resource value in animal contests. *Animal Behaviour*, **76**, 529–542.

Arnott, G. and Elwood, R.W. (2009). Assessment of fighting ability in animal contests. *Animal Behaviour*, **77**, 991–1004.

Bacqué-Cazenave, J., Berthomieu, M., Cattaert, D. et al. (2019). Do arthropods feel anxious during molts? *Journal of Experimental Biology*, **222(2)**, jeb186999.

Barr, S. and Elwood, R.W. (2011). No evidence of morphine analgesia to noxious shock in the shore crab, *Carcinus maenas*. *Behavioural Processes*, **86**, 340–344.

Barr, S., Laming, P.R., Dick, J.T.A. and Elwood, R.W. (2008). Nociception or pain in a decapod crustacean? *Animal Behaviour*, **75**, 745–751.

Bateman, K.S. and Stentiford, G.D. (2017). A taxonomic review of viruses infecting crustaceans with an emphasis on wild hosts. *Journal of Invertebrate Pathology*, **147**, 86–110.

Bateman, K.S., Hicks, R.J. and Stentiford, G.D. (2011). Disease profiles differ between non-fished and fished populations of edible crabs (*Cancer pagurus*) from a major commercial fishery. *ICES Journal of Marine Science*, **68**, 2044–2052.

Birch, J. (2017). Animal sentience and the precautionary principle. *Animal Sentience*, **16(1)**. DOI: 10.51291/2377-7478.1200

Briffa, M. and Elwood, R.W. (2000). The temporal pattern of shell rapping within bouts indicates costly signalling. *Animal Behaviour*, **59**, 159–165.

Briffa, M. and Elwood, R.W. (2005). Rapid change in energetic status in fighting animals: causes and effects of strategic decisions. *Animal Behaviour*, **70**, 119–124.

Chang, E.S. (2001). Crustacean hyperglycemic hormone family: old paradigms and new perspectives. *American Zoologist*, **41**, 380–388.

Conte, F., Voslarova, E., Vecerek, V., Elwood, R., Coluccio, P., Pugliese, M., and Passantino, A. (2021). Humane slaughter of edible decapod crustaceans. *Animals*, **11**(4), 1089.

Cook, A. M. (1967) *FAO Experience Paper 37*, Food and Agriculture Organization of the United Nations.

Couch, J.A. (1983). Diseases caused by Protozoa. In: *The Biology of Crustacea, Vol. 6 Pathobiology*, Ed. Provenzano, A.J., pp. 79–113. New York: Academic Press.

Crane, J. (1975). *Fiddler Crabs of the World*. Ocypodidae: Genus UCA. Princeton University Press, New Jersey.

Crump, A., Browning, H., Schnell, A., Burn, C., and Birch, J. (2022). Sentience in decapod crustaceans: A general framework and review of the evidence. *Animal Sentience* 32(1). DOI: 10.51291/2377-7478.1691.

Davies, C.E. and Wootton, E.C. (2017). Current and emerging diseases of the European lobster (*Homarus gammarus*): a review. *Bulletin of Marine Science*, **94**, 959–978.

De Vaugelas, J. (1985). A new technique for collecting large-sized callianassid mud-shrimp (Decapoda, Thalassinidea). *Crustaceana*, **49**(1), 105–109. http://www.jstor.org/stable/20104071

Diarte-Plata, G., Sainz-Hernández, J.C., Aguiñaga-Cruz, J.A. et al. (2012). Eyestalk ablation procedures to minimise pain in the freshwater prawn *Macrobrachium americanum*. *Applied Animal Behaviour Science*, **140**, 172–178.

Diggles, B.K. (2019). Food for thought: review of some scientific issues related to crustacean welfare. *ICES Journal of Marine Science*, **76**, 66–81.

Eddy, F., Powell, A., Gregory, S. et al. (2007). A novel bacterial disease of the European shore crab, *Carcinus maenas* – molecular pathology and epidemiology. *Microbiology*, **153**, 2839–2849.

Elwood, R.W. (2012). Evidence for pain in decapod crustaceans. *Animal Welfare*, **21**, 23–27.

Elwood, R.W. and Adams, L. (2015). Electric shock causes physiological stress responses in shore crabs, consistent with prediction of pain. *Biology Letters*, **11**. DOI: 10.1098/rsbl.2015.

Elwood, R.W. and Appel, M. (2009). Pain in hermit crabs? *Animal Behaviour*, **77**, 1243–1246.

Elwood, W., Dalton, N. and Riddell, G. (2017). Aversive responses by shore crabs to acetic acid but not to capsaicin. *Behavioural Processes*, **140**, 1–5.

Fossat, P., Bacque-Cazenave, J., De Deurwaerdere, P., Delbecque, J.-P. and Cattaert, D. (2014). Anxiety-like behavior in crayfish is controlled by serotonin. *Science*, 344:1293–1297.

Fossat, P., Bacque-Cazenave, J., De Deurwaerdere, P. et al. (2015). Serotonin, but not dopamine, controls stress response and anxiety-like behavior in crayfish, *Procambarus clarkii*. *Journal of Experimental Biology*, **218**, 2745–2752.

Fregin, T. and Bickmeyer, U. (2016). Electrophysiological investigation of different methods of anesthesia in lobster and crayfish. *PLoS ONE*, **11**, e0162894.

Ghanawi, J., Saoud, G., Zakher, C. et al. (2019). Clove oil as an anaesthetic for Australian redclaw crayfish *Cherax quadricarinatus*. *Aquaculture Research* doi.org/10.1111/are.14319.

Gherardi, F. and Atema, J. (2005). Memory of social partners in hermit crab dominance. *Ethology*, **111**, 271–285.

Holdich, D.M. and Lowery, R.S. (1988). *Freshwater Crayfish Biology, Management and Exploitation*. Croom Helm, London.

Ingle, R.W. (1995). *The UFAW Handbook on The Care & Management of Decapod Crustaceans in Captivity*. Universities Federation for Animal Welfare, Potters Bar.

Johnson, P.T. (1983). Diseases caused by viruses, rickettsiae, bacteria and fungi. In: *The Biology of Crustacea*, Vol. 6. Ed. Provenzano, A.J., pp. 2–78. Academic Press, New York.

Kinne, O. (1976). Cultivation. Part 2 In: *Marine Ecology, Vol. 3 A Comprehensive Integrated Treatise on Life in Oceans and Coastal Waters*. Ed Kinne, O., pp. 1–1293. John Wiley & Sons, Chichester.

Lancaster, I. (1988). *Pagurus bernhardus* (L.) – an introduction to the natural history of hermit crabs. *Field Studies*, **7**, 187–238.

Li, Y., She, Q., Han, Z. et al. (2018). Anaesthetic effects of eugenol on grass shrimp (*Palaemonetes sinensis*) of different sizes at different concentrations and temperatures. *Scientific Reports*, **8**, 11007.

Liao, C., Su, H.M. and Lin, J.H. (1983). Larval food for penaeid prawns. *CRC Handbook of Mariculture, Vol. 1, Crustacean Aquaculture*. Ed. McVey, J.P., pp. 43–69. CRC Press, Florida.

Lozada, M., Romano, A. and Maldonado, H. (1988). Effects of morphine and naloxone on a defensive response of the crab *Chasmagnathus granulatus*. *Pharmacology Biochemistry & Behavior*, **30**, 635–640.

Magee, B. and Elwood, R.W. (2013). Shock avoidance by discrimination learning in the shore crab (*Carcinus maenas*) is consistent with a key criterion for pain. *Journal of Experimental Biology*, **216**, 353–358.

Magee, B. and Elwood, R.W. (2016). Trade-offs between predator avoidance and electric shock avoidance in hermit crabs demonstrate a non-reflexive response to noxious stimuli consistent with prediction of pain. *Behavioural Processes*, **130**, 31–35.

Manning, R. B. (1975). Two methods for collecting decapods in shallow water. *Crustaceana*, **29**(3), 317–319. http://www.jstor.org/stable/20102275.

McLaughlin, P.A. (1982). Comparative morphology of crustacean appendages. In: *The Biology of Crustacea Vol 2*. Ed. Bliss, D.E., pp. 197–256. Academic Press, New York.

Naylor, E. (1988). Rhythmic behaviour of decapod crustacea. *Symposia of the Zoological Society of London*, **59**, 177–199.

Ng, P.K.L. (2017). Collecting and processing freshwater shrimps and crab. *Journal of Crustacean Biology*, **37**, 115–122.

Oswald, R.L. (1977). Immobilization of decapod Crustacea for experimental procedures. *Journal of the Marine Biological Association of the United Kingdom*, **57**, 715–721.

Overstreet, R.M. (1983). Metazoan symbionts. In: *The Biology of Crustacea Vol. 6 Pathobiology*. Ed. Provenzano, A.J., pp. 155–250. Academic Press, New York.

Patterson, L., Dick, J.T.A. and Elwood, R.W. (2007). Physiological stress responses in the edible crab *Cancer pagurus* to the fishery practice of de-clawing. *Marine Biology*, **152**, 265–272.

Provasoli, L., McLaughlin, J.J.A, and Droop, M. (1957). The Development of artificial media for marine algae. *Archives of Microbiology*, **255**, 392–428.

Quinn, R. H., and Fielder, D. R. (1978). A Laboratory beach system for prolonged maintenance of sand crabs, Mictyris Latreille, 1806 and Scopimera De Haan, 1833 (Decapoda, Brachyura). *Crustaceana*, **34**(3), 310–313. http://www.jstor.org/stable/20103286

Romano, N. and Zeng, C. (2013). Toxic effects of ammonia, nitrite, and nitrate to decapod crustaceans: a review on factors influencing their toxicity, physiological consequences, and coping mechanisms. *Reviews in Fisheries Science*, **21**, 1–21.

Romano, N. and Zeng, C. (2017). Cannibalism of decapod crustaceans and implications for their aquaculture: A review of its prevalence, influencing factors, and mitigating methods. *Reviews in Fisheries Science & Aquaculture*, **25**, 42–69.

Rowe, A. (2018). Should scientific research involving decapod crustaceans require ethical review? *Journal of Agricultural and Environmental Ethics*, **31**, 625–634.

Sherwin, C.M. (2001). Can invertebrates suffer? Or how robust is argument-by-analogy? *Animal Welfare*, **10**, S104–S118.

Sneddon, L.U., Elwood, R.W., Adamo, S.A. and Leach, M.C. (2014). Defining and assessing animal pain. *Animal Behaviour*, **97**, 202–212.

Sorgeloos, P. (1980). The use of brine shrimp *Artemia* in aquaculture. In: *Proceedings of the International Symposium on the Brine Shrimp, Artemia salina, Vol. 3, Ecology, Culturing, Use in Aquaculture*. Eds Persoone, G., Sorgeloos, P., Roles, O. and Jaspers E. Universa Press, Wetteren, Belgium, pp. 23–56.

Stentiford, G.D. (2008). Diseases of the European edible crab (*Cancer pagurus*): a review. *ICES J Mar Sc* 65:1578–1592.

Stentiford, G.D., Neil, D.M., Peeler, E.J. et al. (2012). Disease will limit future food supply from the global crustacean fishery and aquaculture sectors. *Journal of Invertebrate Pathology*, **110**, 141–157.

Swetha, C.H., Sainath, S.B., Ramachandra Reddy, P. and Sreenivasula Reddy, P. (2011). Reproductive endocrinology of female crustaceans: perspective and prospective. *Journal of Marine Science: Research & Development*, S:3.

Taylor, J., Vinatea, L., Ozorio, R. et al. (2004). Minimizing the effects of stress during eyestalk ablation of *Litopenaeus vannamei* females with topical anesthetic and a coagulating agent. *Aquaculture*, **233**, 173–179.

Yasuda, C., Suzuki, Y. and Wada, S. (2011). Function of the major cheliped in male–male competition in the hermit crab *Pagurus nigrofascia*. *Marine Biology*, **158**, 2327–2334.

Wang, W. (2011). Bacterial diseases of crabs: a review. *Journal of Invertebrate Pathology*, **106**, 18–26.

Warner, G.F. (1977). *The Biology of Crabs*. Elek (Scientific Books), London.

Weineck, K., Ray, A.J., Fleckenstein, L.J. et al. (2018). Physiological changes as a measure of crustacean welfare under different standardized stunning techniques: cooling and electroshock. *Animals*, **8**, 158.

Index

Note: Page numbers in *italics* refer to figures; those in **bold** to tables or boxes.

AAALAC International 105, 107, 114, 289
Abnormal Toxicity Test 8
'accelerated lambing' systems 618
accelerometers *561*
acclimation 243
acclimatisation, fish 923
accreditation process 107
ACLAM *see* American College of Laboratory Animal Medicine
activity monitoring 560
acute food restriction/deprivation (fasting) 203
acute gastric dilatation 734
ADABs *see* affect-driven attention biases
addressing undesirable behaviour 241–242
ad libitum feeding 202–203, 385–386
   acute food restriction/deprivation (fasting) 203
   calorie or diet restriction 202–203
   food restriction 203–204
   laboratory mice 254
   pair feeding 204–205
   regulation of diet-restriction studies 204
   torpor 203
adults
   cats 554
   condition of 556–557
   decapods 1004–1005
   farm pigs **573**
   female laboratory opossum *303*
   hamsters 422
   horse 649
   Japanese quail *770*
   laboratory mice 344
   pig 579–580
   rat, laboratory 388–389
   tree shrews 332
   Tupaia belangeri **328**
   Xenopus laevis **898**
   zebrafish 937
Adverse Outcome Pathways (AOP) 7
AECs *see* Animal Ethics Committees
affect-driven attention biases (ADABs) 72–73
African green monkeys 723
agar gel diets 194
age 59
ageing animals/aged animals care 251, 311
   cattle 602–603

cephalopoda 974–975
dogs and macaques 263–264
ferrets 510
gerbils 412
guinea pigs 473
laboratory dog 527–528
in mice 254, **255–258**
mouse as model of 252
rabbits, laboratory 493–494
in research 252
for scientific purposes 264–265
zebra finch as 252–253, *261*, 261–263, **262**, *262–263*
zebrafish as 253, 263, *263*
aggressive interactions 312–313, 438
Agreement on International Humane Trapping Standards (AIHTS) 97
AGY *see* Avian Gastric Yeast
AIHTS *see* Agreement on International Humane Trapping Standards
airline executives 188
air transport process 184
ALF *see* Animal Liberation Front
algae 1003
alleles 41–42
allergic respiratory disease 656
Alligator mississippiensis 868
allocoprophagy 461
alopecia scoring **67**, *734*
alternative methods *see* Three Rs
Amblyomma ticks 873
Ambystoma mexicanum 253
amelioration 631
American alligators (*Alligator mississippiensis*) 868
American barn *634*
American College of Laboratory Animal Medicine (ACLAM) 228
American Veterinary Medical Association (AVMA) 394
amphibian 881–902
   husbandry 882–883
   in research 882
amyloidosis 426, 657–658
anaesthesia 16, 75, 91–92
   anaesthetic chamber for *317*
   capuchin monkeys 716

cat, domestic 563
cattle 604
cephalopoda 977, *978*
corvids 849
decapod crustaceans 1006–1007
dog, laboratory 535–537, **536**
ferrets 511–513, **512**
fishes 922–923
fowl, domestic 753
gerbil, laboratory 411
guinea pigs 475–476, **477**
horses 650
inhalation 91–92, *92*
injectable 92
Japanese quail 777
laboratory opossums 316–317
marmosets and tamarins 698–699
for mouse 358–359, **359**
mouse lemurs (*Microcebus* spp.) 672–673
naked mole-rat (NMR) 453–454
old world monkeys (OWM) 729
pigeons and doves 815
pigs and minipigs 588–590
rabbit, laboratory 497–498
rat, laboratory **393**, 393–394, **394**
recovery 92
reptiles, terrestrial 874
of sheep and goats 623
starling 833–834
and stress 86
Syrian hamster 425
tree shrews 335
volatile 274
voles 437
wild boar *92*
Xenopus 894
zebra finch 799–800
zebrafish 947–949, **948**
analgesia 16, 75, 316–318
   cat, domestic 562
   cattle 604
   cephalopoda 977, *978*
   corvids 849
   decapod crustaceans 1006–1007
   dog, laboratory 535–537, **536**
   ferrets 511–513
   fishes 922–923

The UFAW Handbook on the Care and Management of Laboratory and Other Research Animals, Ninth Edition.
Edited by Huw Golledge and Claire Richardson.
© 2024 John Wiley & Sons Ltd. Published 2024 by John Wiley & Sons Ltd.

fowl, domestic 753
gerbil, laboratory 411
guinea pigs 476, **477**
horses 651
laboratory opossums 316–317
marmosets and tamarins 698–699
for mice 358–359, **360**
mouse lemurs (*Microcebus* spp.) 672–673
naked mole-rat (NMR) 453–454
old world monkeys (OWM) 729
pigs and minipigs 588–590
rabbit, laboratory 497–498
rat, laboratory 393–394, **394**
reptiles, terrestrial 874
starling 833–834
tree shrews 335
Xenopus 894
zebra finch 799–800
zebrafish 947–949, **948, 949**
analysis of covariance (ANCOVA) 29, **30**, 37, 198
analysis of variance (ANOVA) 29, 36–37
Anatomy of the Laboratory Mouse, The (Cook) 345
Ancare Enrichment Unit (Model MH16RDRC) 309, *309*
Anglo-Nubian goat breeds 613
Animal and Plant Health Agency (APHA) 98, 184
animal-based research 5
animal care staff
  competence 220–234
    delivering training to 220
    national training schemes 227–228
    and supervisors 220
Animal Ethics Committees (AECs) 116, 284
animal experiments design
  research strategy 23–26
  statistical analysis 36–38
  steps in 27–32
  types of 32–36
  variation 26–27
  see also experimental designs
animal facilities
  acceptance of FRT data 135
  budget 128
  building management system (BMS) 132
  client team 127–129
  commissioning 133
  construction team 132
  cost consultants 128
  design process 129–130
  design team 130–132
  heating, ventilation and air conditioning (HVAC) 132
  legislation 125–126
  overriding requirements 123
  pre-handover demonstration of 133–135
  procurement models 126–127
  project brief for 123–124
  project team 130
  purpose and function 122
  Soft Landings 135–136
  special requirements for 135
  specifications 133
  types 124–125
  User Requirement Specification 128, *128*
  value engineering 128–129
Animal factor 28, 29
Animal Liberation Front (ALF) 188
animal management practices 238
animal room, containments 152–153

animals
  behaviour 31
  marking and identification 13
  and procedure 23–24
  production 10–11
  research facilities *see* animal facilities
  re-use of 10
  transport 13
  welfare 1, 11
  wild-caught 14
Animals (Scientific Procedures) Act (ASPA 1986) 95, 183, 874
Animal Transport Certificate (ATC) 185
Animal & Veterinary Service (AVS) 116
animal welfare 184
Animal Welfare Act (AWA) 97, 117, 394
Animal Welfare Amendment Act (No. 2) 2015 117
animal welfare assessment grid (AWAG) 726
Animal Welfare Body (AWB) 224
animal welfare constraints 272
Animal Welfare Regulations (AWR) 105, 393
AniMatch 11
anophthalmia 353–354
anxiety 50
AOP *see* Adverse Outcome Pathways
APHA *see* Animal and Plant Health Agency
Aphanomyces astaci 1008
appropriate education 221
aquatic species 253, 276
Archemyobia (Nearchemyobia) latipilis 311
architect's responsibility 131
Arizona disease 755
ARRIVE guidelines **24**, 32, 60, 197
artificial burrow systems 449–450
artificial insemination 557
  fowl, domestic 750
  Japanese quail 774
ASAB *see* Association for the Study of Animal Behaviour
Asia, legislation and oversight 113–116
aspergillosis 835
Association for the Study of Animal Behaviour (ASAB) 99
Association's Rules of Accreditation 107
ATC *see* Animal Transport Certificate
Atlantic salmon (*Salmo salar*) 915–916
atrial thrombosis 426
Australia, legislation and oversight 116–117
Australian marsupial species 302
automated in-cage behavioural phenotyping 58
automated systems 74
automutilation 336
autonomic responses 70
autosomes 41
avian avulavirus 778
Avian encephalomyelitis (Epidemic Tremors) 757
Avian Gastric Yeast (AGY) 262
Avian influenza (Bird Flu) 757, 818
avian pox 835
AVMA *see* American Veterinary Medical Association
AWA *see* Animal Welfare Act
AWAG *see* animal welfare assessment grid
AWB *see* Animal Welfare Body
AWR *see* Animal Welfare Regulations

Babesia microti 438
baboons 723
bacterial artificial chromosome (BAC) 304

bacterial diseases 514–515, 779
bacterial infections 426
bacteriophages 50
ballan wrasse 916
bank voles (*Myodes glareolus*) 432, 436, *436*
barbering *67*, 354–355
bar-biting, in rats *71*
barrier integrity 135
BASC *see* British Association for Shooting and Conservation
Batrachochytrium dendrobatidis 882, 897, **898**
BCS *see* body condition score
bedding, guinea pigs 471
begging 461
behaviour/abnormal behaviour 319–320
  cattle 606
  corvids 850
  environmental enrichment on 140–141
  fowl, domestic 758
  horses 631
  laboratory opossums 319–320
  mouse, laboratory 352–353
  mouse lemurs (*Microcebus* spp.) 675
  pigs and minipigs 592
  rat, laboratory 395
  training *see* training/habituation
  and welfare 438–439
behavioural fever 869
behavioural management 364–366
behavioural measures
  affect-driven attention biases (ADABs) 72–73
  anticipatory behaviour 72
  home-cage behaviours **71**
  monitoring routine behaviour 70–71
  stereotypic behaviour 71–72
  vocalisations 72
behavioural testing 15
behavioural thermoregulation 856–857
Beijing Municipality 115
beneficial austerity 209
beneficial enrichment 142
bespoke systems 160–161
best practice 236
binocular vision 570
biocontainment 125, 126, 150, *152*
biological data
  cell, tissue and embryo culture 306
  genetic stocks and strains 304–306
  normal behaviour 304
  reproduction 303–304
  social organisation 303
biological filtration 968
biological replication 31
biomedical research 340
biosecurity 645, 900
biotelemetry 168
BIPs *see* border inspection posts
birds 276
  containment systems 166–167
  inspection of 750–751
biting and kicking, horses 631
blood sampling procedure 15, 318, 425, 453
  gerbil, laboratory 410
  guinea pigs 473–475, *474*
  horses *651*
  pigs and minipigs 584–586, *584–586*
  for voles 436
  zebrafish 946
bloody tears 68
body condition score (BCS) 601, 641

Index

body size effects 198
body weight 68–69
border inspection posts (BIPs) 186
Bordetella bronchiseptica 498, 565
Borrelia burgdorferi 438
box/stall walking 631
brain measures 73
branchiobdellids 1008
breeding 311–313
    behaviour and biology 349–352
    capuchin monkeys 714
    cat, domestic 556–559
    cephalopoda 971–972
    and colony management 362
    corvids 847
    dog, laboratory 528–531
    failure 365
    ferrets 509–510
    gerbil, laboratory 408–410
    harem 362
    horses 645–648
    inbred strains **45**
    Japanese quail 774–776
    laboratory management and 384–395
    marmosets and tamarins 695–696
    naked mole-rat (NMR) 452
    pigeons and doves 812–813
    rabbits, laboratory 494–495
    rat 382–384, 389–390
    sheep and goats 617–620
    Syrian hamster 420–424
    tree shrews 332–334
    voles 434–435
    zebra finch 797–798
brine shrimp (*Artemia salina*) 1004
British Association for Shooting and Conservation (BASC) 99
broad-based phenotyping 55–57
Brown Norway rat 380, 385
Bruce effect 352
BSAVA Manual of Reptiles 868
BSRIA *see* Building Services Research and Information Association
budget 128
building information modelling (BIM), 131
building management system (BMS) 132, 134
Building Services Research and Information Association (BSRIA) 136
buprenorphine 75, 318

Caecilia or Gymnophiona 881
cafeteria-style diets 692
caged rabbits *490*
cage trap *90*, *91*
CALAS *see* Canadian Association for Laboratory Animal Science
Callithrix jacchus 205, 683, *684*, **687**, **688** *see also* marmosets and tamarins
callitrichids species *684*, **685**, 689, 699
calorie/diet restriction 202–203
Campylobacteriosis 779
Campylobacter jejuni 779
Canadian Association for Laboratory Animal Science (CALAS) 227
Canadian Council for Animal Care (CCAC) 99
canine distemper 514
cannibalism 344
captive cephalopods *see* cephalopoda
captive environments 138–139
captive mouse lemurs 666–667

capture of wild animals 90–95
    extreme weather conditions 90
    non-targets 90
    time of day 90
    time of year 90
capturing behaviour 240–241
capuchin monkeys 707–717
    administration of substances 716
    anaesthesia 716
    biological data 708–709
    breeding 714
    care of aged 715
    environmental provisions 710–711
    euthanasia 716
    feeding 714–715
    habitats and feeding habits 708
    handling and training 715
    health 716–717
    physical environment 713
    physiological monitoring 715–716
    quarantine 713
    signs of poor welfare 717
    social grouping 711–713
    social organisation 707–708
    and squirrel monkeys *712*
    uses in research 709–710
carbohydrates 192
carbon dioxide 273–274, 276, 336, 477, 999
Carcinonemertes carcinophila 1008
Carcinus maenas 999
cardiac and pulmonary functions 583–584
cardiomyopathy 516
care-staff associations 227
Cas9 50–51
casting sheep 622
Catarrhini see Old World monkeys
cat, domestic 546–566, *549–550*
    anaesthesia 563
    analgesia 562
    biological data **547**
    breeding 556–559
    dietary requirements 553–554
    disease 563–566
    enrichment 551, *551*, 551–552, **552–553**
    environmental provisions 551–552
    euthanasia 563
    feeding and watering 552–555
    function 551, *551*, **552–553**
    genetics of 546
    group housing 550–551
    handling 559–560
    health monitoring 556
    housing 549–552
    hygiene 555–556
    monitoring methods 560–561
    monitoring welfare 566
    physical environment 555
    reproduction 547–548
    social organisation 547
    training 560
catheterisation 651
cattle
    accommodation 600
    administration of substances 604
    anaesthesia and analgesia 604
    behaviour/abnormal behaviour 606
    biological data for 596–597, **597**
    care of aged animals 602–603
    ectoparasites 605
    enclosures 599–600
    endoparasites 605
    environmental enrichment 600

    euthanasia 604
    eye infection/injury 605
    feeding/watering 600–601
    handling 603
    health (diseases/injuries) 604–606
    health monitoring 602
    hygiene 602
    lameness 605
    lifespan 596
    mastitis 605
    metabolic diseases 605
    mobility 605
    monitoring methods 603
    natural history 596
    physical environment 601
    pneumonia 605–60
    quarantine and biosecurity 602
    reproduction **597**, 597–598
    ringworm 606
    samples collection 603–604
    scours (diarrhoea) 606
    signs of poor welfare 606
    size range 596
    social housing 601
    sources and supply 598
    training/habituation 603
    transportation 598–599
Cattle Health Plan 602
Cavia tschudii 465
C57BL/6J strain 44, *355*, 356
CCAC *see* Canadian Council for Animal Care
Cebus apella **708**
Cebus capucinus 711
Cebus genus 707
cell-specificity 42–43
central dogma of biology, 42
cephalopoda 959–982
    anaesthesia and analgesia 977, *978*
    anatomy 959–962
    breeding and colony management 971–972
    cannibalism and autophagy 980
    capture and transport of 965–966
    care of aged animals 974–975
    chromatophores and skin elements 963
    diet, digestion and excretion 963–964
    dissolved oxygen 967–968
    enclosure cleaning 968
    euthanasia 978–979
    feeding 969
    filtration 968
    handling and health monitoring 975–976
    hatchlings 973–974
    health and diseases 979–981
    housing design and enrichment 968–969
    legislation and regulation 965
    lighting 968
    maintenance, housing and colony management 966
    nitrogenous waste 967
    oxygen saturation in 967
    phylogeny 959
    reproduction *964*, 964–965
    sense organs 962–963
    species of *978*
    water quality 966–968
Cercopithecidae 721
Cercopithecids 721
Cercopithicines 721
cestoda 850
chaff *640*
champing 648

chelonians 870
Chelonoidis chathamensis 869
chemical filtration 968
chemical-induced mutagenesis 47–48
chemical methods 411–412
chemical mutagenesis 47
chemical restraint, in horses 650
chicks 745, *746*, 747
'chisel-toothed digging' 446
chi-squared test 37–38
Chlamydia psittaci 565, 818
Chlamydophila felis 565
Chlamydophila psittaci 818
Chlorocebus 723
chromodacryorrhoea 68, *68*
chromosomes 41
chronic interstitial nephritis 412
chronic lymphocytic enterocolitis (CLE) 699
chronic obstructive pulmonary disease 656
CIDR devices *see* controlled internal drug release devices
CIOMS *see* Council for International Organizations of Medical Sciences
CITES legislation *see* Convention on International Trade in Endangered Species legislation
CLE *see* chronic lymphocytic enterocolitis
client team 127–129
clinical disease 624
cloacal prolapse 319
closed-formula diets 193
Clostridium difficile 159
Clostridium piliforme 412
Clustered Regularly Interspaced Short Palindromic Repeats (CRISPR) 50–51
coccidiosis *(Eimeria species)* 758
Code of Ethical Conduct (CEC) 117
cognitive bias methods 73
cognitive enrichment 845
coleoidea 959
colic 654–655
coliform infections *(Escherichia coli)* 755
colony management 362
  cephalopoda 971–972
commercial breeding 749
commercial diets 944
commercial software 36
commissioning 133
Committee for the Purpose of Control and Supervision of Experiments on Animals (CPCSEA) 115
common raven *(Corvus corax)* 839
communications 296
competence (staff) 220–234
  defined 222
  developing practical skills 226–227
  education and training, purpose of 221–224
  element of Directive 2010/63/EU 228–229
  evaluation 229–232
  legal and ethical considerations 221
  levels of **227**
  national training schemes 227–228
  new employees, orientation of 225–226
  quality schemes 232–233
  reflective and self-directed learning 229
completely randomised design 32, *32*
compliance system 107
computer-aided design (CAD) 131
computer software 32
concept design 129

conditional transgenesis 50
conditioned reinforcer 239
confirmatory experiments 25
congenital cataract 353–354
conjunctivitis 655, *655*
Conservation (Natural Habitats, &c.) Regulations 1994 96
constant-nutrition diets 193
constraints, on killing method 270–272
construction planning 129
construction team 132
constructs 48
construct validity 24
consumer demand 74–75
containment systems
  animal room 152–153
  barrier **154**
  bespoke systems 160–161
  birds 166–167
  checklist for 167
  for ferrets 163–164, *164*
  filter-top cages *158*, 158–159
  flexible film isolators 153–155, *154*
  for guinea pigs 163
  hamsters 162–163
  individually ventilated cage (IVC) 155–158, *157*, **158**
  laminar flow booths 160
  legislative requirements 168
  for mice 161–162
  for nonhuman primates 164–165
  pigs 165
  protective clothing 151–152
  for rabbits 163
  for rats 162
  rigid isolators 155
  ruminants 165–166
  species 161–167
  types 151–161
  ventilated cabinets *159*, 159–160
contingent harms 12–14
continued use 269–270
continuing professional development (CPD) 18, 224, 231–232
continuous monitoring 124
continuous schedule 241
contractor procurement models 126–127
contract/procurement factors 124
control 340–341
control diets 207
  and experimental diets 207
control groups 10, 33
controlled atmosphere killing 273–274
controlled internal drug release (CIDR) devices 617
controls 59
conventional cages *308*
conventional phenotyping 58
Convention on International Trade in Endangered Species (CITES) legislation 98, 841
cooperative feeding 244–245
core design, repeated measures design 36
corvids
  administration of substances 848–849
  anaesthesia and analgesia 849
  behaviour and abnormal behaviour 850
  biology 839
  breeding 847
  enclosures 842–844
  environmental provisions and enrichment 844–845

euthanasia 849
feeding and watering 844
handling *847*, 847–848
health 849–850
hygiene 846
identification and sexing 845–846
life span 839
monitoring methods 848
normal behaviour (wild and captive) 841
physical environment 846
quarantine and barrier systems 846
reproduction 840–841
signs of poor welfare 850–851
size range 839
social housing 845
social organisation 839–840
sources/supply/conservation status 841–842
training and habituation 848
transportation 846
use in research 842
corvid species, housing for **840**
Corynebacterium kutscheri 426
cost consultants 128
Coturnix japonica see Japanese quail
Council for International Organizations of Medical Sciences (CIOMS) 103, **103–104**
Council of Agriculture (COA) 115
Council on Accreditation 107
Countryside and Rights of Way (CRoW) Act 2000 96
CPCSEA *see* Committee for the Purpose of Control and Supervision of Experiments on Animals
CPD *see* continuing professional development
Cre-lox systems 366
crib-biting/wind-sucking 632
Cricetus cricetus 419
cross-over designs 34
CRoW Act 2000 *see* Countryside and Rights of Way Act 2000
cubicles 160
'culture of care' 221
cumulative ammonia 363
cumulative severity 269
cumulative suffering 269
cuniculus 85
Cyclopterus lumpus 910
cynomolgus macaques 721–722
cytoplasm 42
cytotoxicity data 9

Danio meghalayensis 933
Danio rerio see zebrafish
Dario dario 933
data sharing, wild animals 88
dead animals, use of 277
decapod crustaceans
  aggression 997–998
  anaesthesia and analgesia 1006–1007
  behaviour 997–998
  cannibalism 998
  classification and identification 993, **995–996**
  collecting *1005*, 1005–1006
  diseases 1007–1009
  feeding 997
  habitat choice 998
  handling 1006
  hormones 997
  management 998–1009

decapod crustaceans (cont'd)
    modules for holding 1000
    moulting (ecdysis) 993, 997
    rearing in 1001–1003, 1002
    reproduction 998
    restraining 1006
    structure 993
    systems for keeping 999
    transporting 1006
    use in research 998
    welfare problems in 1009
Decapodiformes 959
decision-making process 25–26
'deductive science' 6
delivering training method 224
dental care 642–643
dental disease 264
deoxyribonucleic acid (DNA) 40
    and cell-specificity 42–43
    chromosomes 41
    fragments 48
    genes and alleles 41–42
    gene structure 41
    molecule of inheritance 40
    non-coding 43
    protein-coding 40–41
    protein synthesis 42
    structure of 42
Department of Defense (DoD) 113
dependent variables 27
Dermanyssus gallinae 748, 817
desensitisation 243–244
Design of Experiments (DoE) 35
design process 129–130
    animal experiments *see* animal experiments design
    experimental *see* experimental design
design team 130–132
Destructive Imported Animals Act (1932) 97
detailed design 129
Devriesea agamarum 870
diarrhoea 336, 624, 717
Dictyocaulus arnfieldi 643
Didelphis marsupialis 302
Didelphis virginiana 301, 302
dietary requirements 553–554
diets 191–192
    as basis for irreproducibility 206–209
    and calorie restriction 202
    as enrichment 205
    formula form 193
    hardness 199
    ingredient-based 192–193
    laboratory animal 192
    natural and laboratory 424, 581
    non-nutrients in 208–209
    nutrient levels in 207–208, **208**
    physical form 193–194
    supplementary products 194
    types 192–194
diphtheria 818
direct harms 12, 14–16
directional flow containment systems 161
Directive 2010/63/EU 187, 223, 231, 264, 285, **286**, 598, 977
    competence of 228–229
Dirofilaria immitis 515
discourse model 292
discrete data 37–38
discrimination 9
discriminative ability 23–24

disease-containment strategy 168
diseases
    bacterial 514–515
    cat, domestic 563–566
    cephalopoda 979–981
    clinical 624
    decapod crustaceans 1007–1009
    dog, laboratory 539–541
    fowl, domestic 754–758
    guinea pigs 478–480
    Japanese quail 777–779, **778**
    reptiles, terrestrial 868–873
    see also non-infectious diseases
dispatch method **94**
'disperser males' 446
dissolved oxygen 967–968
diurnal feeding rhythms 200–201
Djungarian Hamster (*Phodopus sungorus*) 203
documentation 184–186
DoD *see* Department of Defense (DoD)
dog, laboratory 518–541
    ageing and management of 263–264
    anaesthesia 535–537, **536**
    analgesics 535–537, **536**
    behavioural problems 538
    care of aged animals 527–528
    diseases of 539–541
    enrichment 522
    environmental provisions 522
    euthanasia 537
    feeding and watering 522–525
    food restriction 203
    handling and training 531–532
    health monitoring 527
    husbandry practices 520
    lighting 527
    methods for restraining 533
    noise 527
    and non-human primates (NHPs) 251
    nutritional requirements of **525**
    physical environment 526–527
    physiological monitoring 532–533
    reproduction 519, **519**
    social housing 525–526
    social organisation 519
    standard biological data in 519, **519**
    transport 521
    ventilation and relative humidity 527
domestication
    guinea pig 466, **466**
    laboratory mouse 341–343
domestic dog (*Canis lupus familiaris*) 518
dopaminergic functioning 73
dosing 14–15
    equipment used 15
    formulations administered 15
    frequency and duration 15
    route of administration 14–15
    volume administered 15
double-stranded DNA repair 51
dozing 459
Dromiciops gliroides 301
'drop method' 274
Drosophila melanogaster 303
dry diets 524
dustbathing behaviour 749
dwarf jay (*Cyanolyca nanus*) 839
dye marking 725

Eastern Equine Encephalomyelitis 779
Ebola 164
echinococcus 732

Echinococcus multilocularis 732
ectoparasites 311, 605
education, purpose of 221–224
effective desensitisation 243
egg bound 944
egg-type strains **751–752**
EHC *see* Export Health Certificate
electronic identification systems 579
embryonic stem (ES) cell 49–50
EMMA *see* European Mouse Mutant Archive
EMPReSS 56
Encephalitozoon cuniculi 499
endocrine disorders 733
endometriosis 733
endoparasites 605
endpoints 269
energy 194–198
engineering *vs.* performance standards 103, 104
enrichment 150, 341
    animal behaviour and 138–140
    and animal safety 143
    and behavioural management 364–366
    cat, domestic 551, *551*, **552–553**
    cephalopoda 968–969
    for chickens in high containment *167*
    diets as 205
    environment *see* environmental enrichment
    environmental provisions and 308–309
    and experiment 144
    in fishes 921
    and human safety 143–144
    mouse, laboratory 360–362
    needed 138–140
    programme 144–145
    proposed 143
    for rats *163*
    validation 144
Entamoeba invadens 872
environmental changes, guinea pigs 472
Environmental Crimes Law 118
environmental disturbance 452
environmental DNA 8
environmental enrichment 13, 137–145
    approaches to 138
    in captive environments 138–139
    cattle 600
    corvids 844–845
    dog, laboratory 522
    domestic cat 551–552
    effect of 140–141
    field-based *636*
    gerbil, laboratory 405–406
    guinea pigs 469–470
    horses 636
    mouse lemurs (*Microcebus* spp.) *667*, *668*
    naked mole-rat (NMR) 450–451
    needed 138–140
    old world monkeys 727
    opportunity 549
    rabbits, laboratory 490–491
    reptiles, terrestrial 863
    sheep and goats 616
    terminology 138
    zebrafish 941
    see also enrichment
environmental factors 58, 254
Environmental Protection Act 1990 97
Environmental Protection Agency (EPA) 113
environmental provisions 450
environment, ferrets 508
EPA *see* Environmental Protection Agency
epidural anaesthesia 590

equine serum gonadotropin (eSG) 316
ERC *see* ethical review committee
Erdschreiber medium 1003
Estrildidae (weaver finches) 787
ethical review
   balancing harm and benefit 289–290
   benefit 286–287
   challenges 291–293
   ethics committees 284
   euthanasia 278
   experimental design 287
   origin of 281–282
   place 284–285
   in practice 291
   public perspectives 283
   reduction 287–289
   refinement 287–289
   replacement 287–289
   3Rs 290–291
   underlying philosophy 282–283
   undertaken 283–284
ethical review committee (ERC) 224
ethics committees 284
   self-assessment checklist for 294–296
N-ethyl-N-nitrosourea (ENU) mutagenesis 48, 55
EU Directive 2010/63/EU *see* Directive 2010/63/EU
EUMODIC *see* European Mouse Disease Clinic
Eumorphia 56
Euprymna scolopes 980
Euprymna spp. 966
Eurasian magpies (*Pica pica*) 841
EU Regulation (1143/2014) 97
European Conditional Mouse Mutagenesis programme (EUCOMM) 56
European ethics committees 284
European hamsters (*Cricetus cricetus*) 419
European Mouse Disease Clinic (EUMODIC) 56
European Mouse Mutant Archive (EMMA) 56
European regulation 183
European sea bass (*Dicentrarchus labrax*) 917
European starling *see* starling
Europe, Council Regulation (EC) No 1/2005 187
Europe, legislation and oversight 108–110
EUROTOX *see* Federation of European Toxicologists & European Societies of Toxicology
euthanasia 268–278
   aquatic species 276
   capuchin monkeys 716
   carbon dioxide for 411
   cat, domestic 563
   cattle 604
   cephalopoda 978–979
   corvids 849
   dead animals, use of 277
   dog, laboratory 537
   ethical committees 278
   foetal forms 276–277
   fowl, domestic 753–754
   gerbil, laboratory 411–412
   horses 654
   humane and scientific endpoints 269
   human factors 277–278
   killing method *see* killing method
   laboratory opossum 318
   marmosets and tamarins 699
   mouse, laboratory 360
   mouse lemurs (*Microcebus* spp.) 673
   naked mole-rat (NMR) 453–454
   neonates 276
   of neonates 412
   non-human primates 276
   old world monkeys (OWM) 729–730
   parenteral anaesthetic overdose 275–276
   physical methods 274–275
   pigs and minipigs 590–591
   rabbit, laboratory 498
   reptiles, terrestrial 874
   sheep and goats 623
   starling 834
   training 277–278
   tree shrews 336
   voles 437
   Xenopus 894
   zebra finch 800
   zebrafish 949
excessive nutrients 195–196
exercise, horses 641
exons 41
Experimental Design Assistant (EDA) **24**
experimental designs 9
   blinding of 32
   choosing 31
   decision-making process 25–26
   ethical review 287
   purpose of 24–25
   randomisation 32
   statistical analysis 32, 36–38
   steps in 27–32
   types of 32–36
experimental modulating factors 289–290
experimental unit 28, 32
   replication of 29–30
experiments
   confirmatory 25
   exploratory 25
   pilot 24–25
   purpose 25
   types of 24–25
   within-animal 25, 28
expert judgement 11
exploratory experiments 25
Export Health Certificate (EHC) 184
extended matching questions (EMQs) 230
external telemetry devices 533
external validity 24, 26, 142
extinction 242
extruded diets 193
ex vivo systems 8
eye infection/injury 605

'face' validity 24
facial expressions 726
facility accommodation factors 124–125
facility reliability test (FRT) 134–135
factorial design **34**, 34–35, **35**
faecal sampling 89, 411
farm animals 237
farm pigs 570–571, *571*, **571, 574, 577**
Fasciola hepatica 643
fates, for animals 268–278
Federation of European Laboratory Animal Science Associations (FELASA) 105, 106, 227, 228, 233, 353, 387
   training scheme 228
Federation of European Toxicologists & European Societies of Toxicology (EUROTOX) 233
feeding/watering 196–198
   ad libitum 202–203
   as basis for irreproducibility 206–209
   cat, domestic 552–555
   cattle 600–601
   cephalopoda 969
   cooperative 244–245
   corvids 844
   decapod crustaceans 997
   delivery systems 197–198
   diurnal rhythms 200–201
   dog, laboratory 522–525
   fowl, domestic 751–752
   gerbil, laboratory 406
   guinea pigs 471
   horses *637*, 637–638
   marmosets and tamarins 692–693
   Monodelphis domestica 309–310
   mouse, laboratory 360–362
   naked mole-rats, 450–451
   pair 204–205
   pigeons and doves 811–812
   pigs and minipigs 581–582
   quality 196–197
   rabbits 200–201, 491
   rat, laboratory 385–386
   sheep and goats 620–621
   starling 828
   Syrian hamster 424
   thirst and need for 196
   tree shrews 329–331
   voles 433
   zebra finch *792*, 793–794
   zebrafish 942–944
feline immunodeficiency virus (FIV) 564
feline infectious peritonitis (FIP) 564–565
feline leukaemia virus (FeLV) 564
feline panleukopenia (FPV) 565
Felis silvestris 546
Felis silvestris catus 546
FeLV *see* feline leukaemia virus
females
   guinea pigs 467
   laboratory opossums 303, 311
   mixed-sex groups 472
   newborn and suckling 433
   Syrian hamster *422*, *422*, *423*
ferrets 506–516
   anaesthesia 511–513, **512**
   analgesics 511–513
   behaviour 507
   biological and breeding data **507**
   care of aged animals 510
   containment systems for 163–164, *164*
   enriched environment *508*
   environment 508
   euthanasia 513
   handling 510, *510*
   husbandry and management 508–510
   jugular venepuncture in *511*
   minor techniques 510–511
   neoplasia in 516
   nutrition 508
   reproduction and breeding 509–510
   ventilated unit for *164*
fidelity 23, 24
field-based environmental enrichment 636
field studies of wildlife 84–99
   best practice guidelines 99
   capture, handling, release 90–95
   legislation appropriate to 95–99
   reasons for 85
   three Rs 87–89
   welfare impacts of 85–87

field vole *(Microtus agrestis)* 432
fight-related injuries 673–674
filter-top cages *158,* 158–159
financial and technical constraints 272
fin clipping 925
FIP *see* feline infectious peritonitis
fipronil wipes 873
fire protection (FP) engineer 131
Fisher's exact test 37–38
fishes 907–926
   acclimatisation 923
   anaesthesia and analgesia 922–923
   Atlantic salmon *(Salmo salar)* 915–916
   ballan wrasse 916
   enrichment in 921
   European sea bass *(Dicentrarchus labrax)* 917
   gilthead sea bream *(Sparus aurata)* 917
   goldfish *(Carassius auratus)* 910–911
   guppy *(Poecilia reticulata)* 911–913
   handling 923
   individual-and group-based indicators **919**
   injection and cannulation 922, *922*
   integrated fish welfare assessment *920*
   lumpsucker *(Cyclopterus lumpus,* L.) 916
   nile tilapia *(Oreochromis niloticus)* 914
   poor welfare and humane end-points 921
   rainbow trout *(Oncorhynchus mykiss)* 914–915
   in research 908–917
   sensory world of *918*
   species **912**
   three-spined stickleback *(Gasterosteus aculeatus)* 913–914
   training and habituation 924–925
   water parameters for **911**
   welfare 908, **908**, 917–921
fitch 506
FIV *see* feline immunodeficiency virus
Five Freedoms *632,* 867
fixed effect 27
fixed formulation 193
flexible film isolators 153–155, *154*
flukes (Trematoda) 872
fluorescent lighting 311, 744
Flynn's Parasites of Laboratory Animals (Baker) 353
foaling 646
foetal forms 276–277
food animals, Japanese quail as 766
food chamber *449*
food, foraging for 200
footprint efficiency 362
foraging behaviour 86
formal scientific validation 19
formal validation process 19
formula types 193
forward genetics approach 47
fowl cholera *(Pasteurella multocida)* 755
fowl, domestic 741–759
   abnormal behaviour 758
   adult phase 748–749
   anaesthesia and analgesia 753
   artificial insemination 750
   behaviour 742–743
   breeds, strains and genetics 742
   brooding phase 745–747
   care of aged animals 749
   diet specifications **751–752**
   disease 754–758
   egg-type strains **751–752**
   environmental provisions 745
   euthanasia 753–754
   feeding 751–752
   handling 752
   housing 744
   hygiene 749
   identification and sexing 749–750
   injections and dosing 753
   lifespan 741
   lighting 744–745
   monitoring physiological variables 752–753
   natural breeding 750
   pens or cages 745
   rearing phase 747
   reproduction 742
   restraint and blood sampling 752
   social organisation 741–742
   sources of supply 744
   standard biological data 743–744
   types of **743**
   uses in research 744
fowl typhoid *(S. gallinarum)* 754
FPV *see* feline panleukopenia
fracture 657
Friedman's test 38
FRT *see* facility reliability test
Fukomys damarensis 443
Furcifer pardalis 862
fur colouration 675

Gallus gallus domesticus see fowl, domestic
Gallus gallus spadiceous 741
gapeworm *(Syngamus trachea)* 850
gas bubble disease 895
gasping 848
gastrointestinal system 654–656
gavage 204
GCP *see* good clinical practice
gels and pastes 194
gene editing 50
gene nomenclature 43
general anaesthesia 16, 393
genes 41–42
genetically modified animals (mice) 40
   animal models 50
   development 54
   laboratory animal genetics 46–50
   phenotyping 54–61
   rise of 352
   welfare of 54–55
genetic drift 44
genetic engineering 48
genetic heterogeneity 26
genetics 43–46, 59, 366
   of domestic cats 546
   and genomics 304, 383–384
   rat, laboratory 382–384
   strains and 327
genetic variation 26–27
genital swabs 651–652
genomics 304
   genetics and 383–384
genotyping 8
gerbil, laboratory
   activity patterns 402
   anaesthesia 411
   analgesia 411
   blood sampling 410
   breeding 408–410
   common welfare problems 412–413
   enclosures 405
   environmental enrichment 405–406
   environmental provisions 405
   euthanasia 411–412
   external features 400–401
   feeding/watering 406
   handling 410
   identification and sexing 407–408
   monitoring methods 410
   physical environment 408
   senses and communication 401–402
   social housing 406–407
   social organisation 402–404
   standard biological data 400
   taxonomy 400
   transportation 408
   uses in research 404–405
German Laboratory 2020 programme 123
germ-free/gnotobiotic animals 153
gestation 724
gilthead sea bream *(Sparus aurata)* 917
gloves wearing 152
GLP *see* Good Laboratory Practice
glucocorticoid analysis methods **69**
glucocorticoids 69
Goeldi's monkey *(Callimico goeldi)* 686
Golden Hamster 419
goldfish *(Carassius auratus)* 910–911
Gonatus onyx 965
good clinical practice (GCP) 633
Good Laboratory Practice (GLP) 113, 145, 208
Göttingen Minipigs **571**
gram-negative species 870
grass cubes *639*
great tits *(Parus major)* 846
green iguana *(Iguana iguana)* 865
grey mouse lemur *(Microcebus murinus)* 662
grinding extruded diet 193
grooming transfer test *66*
ground and powdered diet 193
ground transportation 187
group housing
   cats 550–551
   sheep and goats 614–615
Gryllus assimilis 865
guide RNA molecule (gRNA) 50, *51*
guinea pigs 75, 155, 200, 465–480
   administration techniques 473
   anaesthesia 475–476, **477**
   analgesia 476, **477**
   bedding 471
   biochemical data **479**
   biological data 466–467, **467**
   blood collection 473–475, *474*
   care of aged animals 473
   containment systems for 163
   diseases 478–480, **479**
   domestication 466, **466**
   enclosures and environmental enrichment 469–470
   environmental changes 472
   feeding/watering 471
   female 467
   haematological data **479**
   handling 473, *473*
   health monitoring 472–473, **473**
   high-fibre requirements 194
   identification and sexing 472, *472*
   newborn 466
   reproductive data for **467**
   social housing **471**, 471–472
   social organisation in *468*
   use in research 469
   welfare assessment in 478

Gumboro disease 757
guppy (*Poecilia reticulata*) 911–913

habituation 243
half-suit isolators *155*
halogenated volatile anaesthetics 272
hamster parvovirus (HaPV) 426
hamster polyomavirus 426
hamsters, containment systems 162–163
handling
   animals for humane killing 277
   capuchin monkeys 715
   cattle 603
   cephalopoda 975–976
   corvids *847*, 847–848
   dog, laboratory 531–532
   domestic cat 559–560
   ferrets 510, *510*
   fishes 923
   guinea pigs 473, *473*
   horses *649*, 649–650
   marmosets and tamarins 696–697
   Monodelphis domestica 315–316
   mouse *357*, 357–358
   mouse lemurs (*Microcebus* spp.) 672
   naked mole-rat (NMR) 452, *453*
   pigeons and doves *813*, 813–814
   pigs and minipigs 582–583, *583*
   rabbits, laboratory 495–496
   rat, laboratory *390*, 390–391
   sheep and goats 621–623
   Syrian hamster 424
   transportation 923–924
   tree shrews 334
   voles 435–436
   wild animals 91, *91*, 153
   zebrafish 946
hand rearing 334
hands-on exercises 226
haploid 42
HaPV *see* hamster parvovirus
harem breeding 362
'HARKing' 25
harm–benefit analysis 290
harmonising 8
hay diets 194
hay racks 620
health (diseases/injuries) 454
health monitoring
   basic type of 353
   cat, domestic 556
   cattle 602
   cephalopoda 975–976
   dog, laboratory 527
   gerbil, laboratory 408
   guinea pigs 472–473, **473**
   horses 648–649
   Japanese quail 773
   marmosets and tamarins 694–695
   mouse illnesses 353
   mouse lemurs (*Microcebus* spp.) 672
   naked mole-rat (NMR) 451
   pigeons and doves 816
   and quarantine 311
   rabbits, laboratory 493
   rat, laboratory 386–387, **388**
   reptiles, terrestrial 868–869
   sheep and goats 617
   tree shrews 331
   zebra finch 797
   zebrafish 941–942

'healthy ageing' 252
heating, ventilation and air conditioning (HVAC) 132
Helicobacter mustelae 514
hemosiderosis 699
hepatic cirrhosis 426
herbivores 636
heredity factor 40
herpes B virus infection 716
Heterocephalus glaber see naked mole-rat (NMR)
hibernation 203
high-fidelity fallacy 8–9
high-fidelity system 23
hill breeds, of sheep 614
home-cage monitoring 58, **65**, 71, **71**
Home Office Project Licence 845
homologous recombination 50
homology arms 50
homology-directed repair (HDR) 50
homozygous 44
hoof care, horses 642, *642*
hormones, decapod crustaceans 997
horses
   abnormal behaviour 631
   administration of substances 652–658
   analgesics 651
   behaviour 630–632
   biological data 628–629, **629**
   biosecurity 645
   biting and kicking 631
   blood sampling procedure *651*
   breeding 645–648
   chemical restraint 650
   in containment facility 654
   crib-biting/wind-sucking 632
   dental care 642–643
   environmental enrichment 636
   euthanasia 654
   exercise 641
   faecal sampling 652
   feeding *637*, 637–638
   field shelter 635
   foal behaviour 647–648
   gastrointestinal system 654–656
   general anaesthesia 650
   handling and training *649*, 649–650
   health monitoring and record keeping 648–649
   herd of ponies *629*
   hoof care 642, *642*
   housing **634**, *634*, 634–635
   identification 640
   low-roughage diets in 631
   normal behaviour 630–631
   nutrition 637–640
   optimising air quality in stables 635
   pain and distress 632
   parasites (endoparasites), prevention of 643–644
   physical examination 651
   physiological monitoring 651–652
   reproduction 629–630
   reuse or rehoming 633–634
   roughages 639–640
   skin infections of **657**
   social organisation 628
   transportation 644
   urine sampling 652
   use in research 632–633
   vaccinations 645

   walker machine *641*
   weaving/box (stall) walking 631
   weight monitoring 641, *641*
   wood chewing 631–632
housing 310, 365
   cat, domestic 549–552
   cattle 601
   containments *see* containment systems
   corvids 845
   for corvid species **840**
   dog, laboratory 525–526
   enrichment *see* enrichment
   guinea pigs **471**, 471–472
   horses **634**, *634*, 634–635
   naked mole-rat (NMR) 451
   pigeons and doves 810
   rabbits, laboratory 491–492
   rat, laboratory 385
   special arrangements 150–169
   zebra finch 794–795
HPA system *see* hypothalamic pituitary–adrenocortical system
human/animal relationship 242
humane endpoints 16–17, 269, 413
   planning, implementing and reviewing 17
   in practice 16–17
humane experimental technique 5
   principles of 6
humane killing method 14, 277
human factors 277–278
human genome 40, 41
human hearing, ranges *346*
husbandry programme 264
hydrocephalus 356
hyperlipaemia 658
hyperoestrogenism 515
hypersexuality 789
hypervitaminosis A 866
hypothalamic pituitary– adrenocortical (HPA) system 468, 478
hypothermia 317
hypovitaminosis A 866

IACUC *see* Institutional Animal Care and Use Committee
IAEC *see* Institutional Animal Ethics Committees
IATA Live Animals Board 183
IBD *see* infectious bursal disease
ICLAS *see* International Council for Laboratory Animal Science
idiopathic peripheral vestibular disease 675
ILAR Guidelines 196
immune response 70
IMPC *see* International Mouse Phenotyping Consortium
imperforate vagina 356
IMPReSS *see* International Mouse Phenotyping Resource of Standardised Screens
inbred mouse strains 43–44, *44*, 343, *343*
   breeding **45**
   characteristics of 45
   gene variants in **46**
   of other species 46
   phenotypes between **46**
   selecting an appropriate 46
incandescent lights 744
India, legislation and oversight 115–116
Indian National Science Academy 115
individual housing, cats 549–550

individually ventilated cage (IVC) 155–158, 157, **158,** *162,* 363
infanticide 409, 426
infectious bronchitis (IB) 756
infectious bursal disease (IBD) 757
infectious coryza (*Haemophilus paragallinarum*) 755
infectious diseases 318–319, 778
 reptiles, terrestrial 870–873
infectious laryngotracheitis (ILT or LT) 757
in-foal mares 646
INFRAFRONTIER project 56
infrared thermography 410
ingredient-based diet types 192–193
 natural-ingredient diets 192
 purified diets 192–193
inhalation anaesthesia 91–92, 393, 476, 589–590, 833
inhaled volatile anaesthetics 274
in-house training 225
injectable anaesthesia 92, 589
injection types 587
injuries 85–86, 565
injurious aggression 365
in silico studies, wild animals 87
inspection system 107
Institute of Animal Technology (IAT) 227
Institutional Animal Care and Use Committee (IACUC) 104–106, 224
Institutional Animal Ethics Committees (IAEC) 115
insulinomas 516
integrational transgenesis 48–49, **49**
'intentional' training 236
internal validity 26
international accreditation 107
International Association of Colleges of Laboratory Animal Medicine (IACLAM) 228
International Committee for Standardized Genetic Nomenclature 43
International Council for Laboratory Animal Science (ICLAS) 103, **103–104,** 228
International Culture of Care Network 18
International Guiding Principles for Biomedical Research Involving Animals 103, **103–104**
International Index of Laboratory Animals 383
International Institute for Sustainable Laboratories² (I²SL) 123
International Knockout Mouse Consortium 50
international legislation 99
International Mouse Phenotyping Consortium (IMPC) 45, 56, 57
International Mouse Phenotyping Resource of Standardised Screens (IMPReSS) 56, 57
International Society for Transgenic Technologies 225
intradermal injections 15, 587
intramuscular (IM) injections 587, 588, 621, 653, *653,* 728
intraperitoneal (IP) injections 392, 437, 497, 588
intravenous (IV) injections 391, 437, 588, 621
introns 41
In-Use services 130
invasive non-native species **98**
invasive tissue marking 94
in vitro replacement systems 6, 8

in-vitro techniques 233
InVivoStat power analysis *30,* 31, 37
isoflurane 411
isolators
 flexible film 153–155, *154*
 half-suit 155
 for piglets 166
 potential welfare issues **156**
 rigid 155
 use with poultry *166*
ISO 19650 standard 132
Israeli Animal Welfare Law 118
IVC *see* individually ventilated cage
ivermectin 871
Ixodes trianguliceps 438

jackpot/bonus 241
Jamaican boa *866*
Japanese quail 762–779, *764*
 administration of substances 776
 anaesthesia 777
 artificial insemination 774
 biological data for **764**
 box brooder for 769
 breeding 774–776
 breeds, strains and genetics 765–766
 disease 777–779, **778**
 domestication 763
 eggs 775
 environmental provisions 772
 feeding and water 770–772
 as food animals 766
 food consumption **771**
 handling and capture 776
 health monitoring 773
 housing 768–770
 husbandry 767–768
 hygiene 773
 identification 773
 as laboratory animals 766–767
 morphology 763
 mortality, causes of 777
 mortality during incubation 775
 nutrient requirements **771**
 physiological monitoring 776
 quarantine and barrier systems 773
 reproduction 765
 sexing 772
 size range and lifespan 763–764
 social grouping 772
 social organisation 764–765
 sources of supply 767
 space allowances for **768**
 standard biological data 765
 synthetic basal diet for **772**
 transport 773
 water consumption of **772**
Japan, legislation and oversight 113–114
jills 506
Joint Nature Conservation Committee (JNCC) 99
Joint Working Group on Refinement (JWGR) 768, 777
journey planning 183–186
 air transport 184
 documentation 184–186
 ground transport 183–184
 journey time 186
 points of entry 186
journey time 186
juvenile crow, *840*
JWGR *see* Joint Working Group on Refinement

Kenya Snakebite Research and Intervention Centre (KSRIC) *861*
ketamine 590
ketamine hydrochloride 729
kidney, mouse 344
killing method
 cephalopoda 978
 constraints on 270–272
 ethical committees 278
 human factors 277–278
 laboratory animals 273–274
 rabbit, laboratory 498
 scientific purposes **271**
 selection 272–273
kitten development 558, *558*
Knockout Mouse Project (KOMP) 56
knowing 222
KOMP *see* Knockout Mouse Project
Korean Animal Protection Law 114
Kruskal-Wallis test 38
KSRIC *see* Kenya Snakebite Research and Intervention Centre
Kyoto Wistar 383

laboratory animals
 genetics
  gene nomenclature 43
  genetically altered (GA) 46–50
  genetic drift 44
  inbred line 45
  inbred strains 43–44, 46
  molecular genetics 40–43
  outbred strains 46
  substrains 44–45
 Japanese quail as 766–767
 mouse 340–367
 rabbits 484–500
 rat 379–395, **389**
 transportation *see* transportation, of laboratory animals
 voluntary food intake in 198–202, *199, 200*
'LABORATORY ANIMALS' label 185
Laboratory Based Welfare Indicators (LABWIs) 918
laboratory diets 264, 581
laboratory opossums 301–320
 adult female 303
 behavioural/abnormal behaviour 319–320
 biological data **303**
 bred genetic stocks of **305**
 cell, tissue and embryo culture 306
 developmental biology 306
 developmental stages of 306–307
 female 303, 311
 general husbandry 307–313
 iPSCs of 306
 marsupials 301–302
 partially and fully inbred strains of **305**
 procedures 315–318
 reproductive problems 319–320
Labrus bergylta 910
LABWIs *see* Laboratory Based Welfare Indicators
Laelaps hilaris 438
lameness, in cattle 605
laminar flow booths 160, *160*
laminitis 656–657
LAPS system 276
large factorial designs 35
larval and juvenile fish 944–945
laryngeal mask airway (LMA) 590
Latin America, legislation and oversight 118

Index

Latin square design 33–34, *34*
Lawsonia intracellularis 426
learning 222
LEDs *see* light-emitting diodes
Lee-Boot effect 352
legal constraints 270–272
legislation and oversight 101–118
   harmonisation of guidelines 107–118
   history 102
   institutional and governmental review 106–107
   principles 102–107
   research animal facilities 125–126
Leontocebus fuscicollis 686
Leontopithecus rosalia 686
Leptospira spp. 388
less sentient species, wild animals 87
liability 184
library racking systems 157
licences 98–99
lifelong learning 231–232, *232*
light–dark (LD) cycles 448
light-emitting diodes (LEDs) 744
light intensity 690
liquid diets 193–194
lissamphibians 881
Listeria monocytogenes 674
'LIVE ANIMALS' label *185*
living fossils 959
lizards **868**
Ljungan virus 438
LMA *see* laryngeal mask airway
locomotor activity, circadian pattern of *327*
Long-Evans hooded 383
longevity 202–203
lower critical concentration (LCC) 195, *195*
low-roughage diets, in horses 631
lumpsucker (*Cyclopterus lumpus*, L.) 916
lung pathology 426
Lyme disease 438
lymphocytic choriomeningitis virus (LCMV) 426

Macaca fascicularis 205, **732**
Macaca mulatta 205, 242, **732**
macaques, ageing and management of 263–264
Macrobrachium australiense 998
Macropus eugenii 302
magnitude of reinforcement 241
maintenance, client's facility 134
male
   cephalopods *964*
   mixed-sex groups 472
   Syrian hamster 422
   voles 438
malignant oedema/gangrenous dermatitis (*Clostridium septicum*) 755–756
malocclusion 356
management, of wild animals 85
mangrove killifish (*Kryptolebias marmoratus*) 907
Mann-Whitney test 38
marabou storks (*Leptoptilos crumenifer*) 848
mare
   features of **645**
   stages of **647**
Marek's disease 757, 779
marking, animals
   animals 13
   invasive tissue 94
   natural 94
   physical 94
   of wild animals 93–94
Marmosa robinsoni 302
marmosets and tamarins 164
   administration of substances 698
   anaesthesia/analgesia 698–699
   behavioural indicators 700
   biological data 687, **688**
   biology 683–686
   body mass and lifespan 686–687
   breeding and rearing 695–696
   care of aged animals 695
   euthanasia 699
   external genitalia *694*
   feeding/watering 692–693
   handling 696–697, *697*
   health monitoring 694–695
   identification and sexing 693–694
   indicators of positive welfare 699–700
   management and breeding 690–696
   normal behaviour (wild and captive) 688
   physical environment and hygiene 694
   quarantine and barrier system 694–695
   senses and communication 688–689
   social housing 693
   social organisation and reproduction 687
   sources and supply 689
   training/habituation 697
   transport 694–695
   use in research 689–690
marmoset species 683–686
marsupials
   biology of 301–302
   laboratory 302–303
Martindale-type suit *151*, 152
mastitis 605
mating systems 333
   rat, laboratory 381–382
maturation 431
maturity levels 132
MBD *see* metabolic bone diseases
mechanical, electrical and plumbing (MEP) services 131
meiosis 42
Meloxicam 849
memory 222
MEP services *see* mechanical, electrical and plumbing services
Mesocricetus auratus 419
messenger RNA (mRNA) 42
'metabolically hungry' 191
metabolic bone diseases (MBD) 865, 866
metabolic diseases 605
metric model 292
mice *see* mouse
microbiome 343
Microcebus lehilahytsara 666
Microcebus murinus 662
microchipping 94
microphthalmia 353–354
microsampling 15, 391
Microtus agrestis 430, 432
Microtus montanus 438
Microtus pensylvanicus 430
milk, in gerbils 411
minimal requirements 195
minimising animal harm 287
Ministry of Food and Drug Safety (MFDS) 114
Ministry of Science and Technology (MOST) 114
Miquel Allen medium 1004

MMA syndrome 592
mobility, in cattle 605
molecular biology 48
molecular genetics 40–43
   central dogma of *42*
monitoring methods 334, 452–453
   cat, domestic 560–561
   cattle 603
   corvids 848
   marmosets and tamarins 697–698
   rabbit, laboratory 496–497
   rabbits, laboratory 496–497
   Xenopus 894
   zebra finch 799
Monodelphis domestica 301–303, **304**, *305*, *315*
   brain of 307
   breeding 311–313
   feeding/watering 309–310
   hygiene 311
   identification and sexing 310
   newborn 307
   non-infectious diseases 319
   physical environment 311
   social housing 310
Monodelphis species 301
monogamous pairings 312
Moraxella catarrhalis 498
Morris water maze 362
mortality
   causes of 777
   effects of field studies 86
mosaic 50
MOST *see* Ministry of Science and Technology
moulting (ecdysis) 993, 997
Mouse Genome Informatics resource 44
mouse, laboratory 340–367
   ad-libitum feeding of 254
   administration guidelines for **358**
   ageing in 254, **255–258**
   ageing–related adverse effects in *259–260*
   ambient temperature requirements 345
   anaesthesia 358–359, *359*
   analgesics 358–359, **360**
   basic biology 343–345, **344**
   behaviour 348–352
   blood withdrawal routes for **359**
   breeding behaviour and biology 349–352
   containment systems for 161–162
   control 340–341
   conventional phenotyping 58
   enrichment 360–362, *361*
   euthanasia 268–278, 360
   feeding and watering 360–362
   genetically modified *see* genetically modified animals
   genetics 40–51
   glass tower blocks and tyrannosaurs 362–364
   handling *357*, 357–358
   health and/or welfare problems in **65**
   illnesses 353–356
   infectious agents **354**
   killing methods 273–274
   maintenance behaviour 348
   as model of ageing 252
   mouseness of 341–343
   natural biology and behaviour **65**
   necropsy 360
   positive reinforcement training techniques 236–247
   problem and abnormal behaviour 352–353

mouse, laboratory (cont'd)
　procedures 357–360
　rack of IVCs used to 157
　rat and human hearing ranges 346
　reproductive and developmental values
　　for 349
　sensory world of 345–348
　social behaviour 348–349
　stress 340–341
　surgery 359–360
　transportation 171–188
　vaginal epithelium 350
　voluntary food intake in 198–202
　well-being 340–341
mouse lemurs (*Microcebus* spp.)
　662–675, *663*
　abnormal behaviour 675
　administration of substances 672
　anaesthesia and analgesia 672–673
　biological data 670–672
　body mass 670, *670*, **671**
　body temperature 670–671, *671*
　breeding, 668–670
　diseases and injuries 673–675
　drug application and medical treatment
　　in **673**
　ecology 662–663
　environmental enrichment
　　667, *668*
　euthanasia 673
　handling and health monitoring 672
　housing, food and water 667
　identification 668
　infant development 671–672
　oestrus cycle **669**
　physical environment 667–668
　reproduction 664
　sampling 672
　senses and communication 665
　sociality 664–665
　sources and conservation 665–666
　taxonomy 662
　uses in research 666–667
mouseness, of mouse 341–343
Mouse Phenome Database (MPD) 56
Mouse Phenome Project 56
mouse sense 345–348
　magnetoreception 347–348
　smell and taste 347
　touch 346–347
　vision 345–346
mouthing 648
MPD *see* Mouse Phenome Database
mRNA *see* messenger RNA
MS (Mycoplasma synoviae) 756
multiple choice questions (MCQs) 230
multi-use technique, wild animals 88
Mus musculus 341–342, 382
Mustela eversmanii 506
Mustela nigripes 506
Mustela putorius 506
mutations 43
　in laboratory animals 47–50
　spontaneous 47
mutual grooming 630, *631*
Muusoctopus lieoderma 968
Mycobacterium microti 437
Mycobacterium tuberculosis 732
Mycoplasma spp. 565
mycoplasmata (mycoplasmas) 871
Myo7a gene 47
Myodes glareolus 432

NAEAC *see* National Animal Ethics Advisory
　Committee
naked mole-rat (NMR) 442–455, *443*, *462–464*
　administration of substances 453
　anaesthesia 453–454
　analgesia 453–454
　biology 442–443, 446
　breeding 452
　care of aged animals 451–452
　characteristic features 446
　enclosures/artificial burrow
　　systems 449–450
　environmental enrichment 450–451
　environmental provisions 450
　ethogram for non-vocal behaviours
　　459–461, 459–464
　euthanasia 453–454
　handling and habituation 452, *453*
　hygiene and health monitoring 451
　mating system 446
　monitoring methods 452–453
　natural history 442–443
　normal behaviour 448
　ovarian cycle of *447*
　parturition 462
　reproduction 446–448
　size range and lifespan 443–445
　social housing 451
　social organisation 445–446
　sources/supply/conservation status 449
　striking aspect 448
Nannizziopsis guarroi 871
Nannizziopsis spp. 871
nasopharyngeal swabbing 651, *652*
National Advisory Committee for Laboratory
　Animal Research (NACLAR) 116
National Animal Ethics Advisory Committee
　(NAEAC) 117
National Centre for 3Rs (NC3Rs) 99, 168
National Competent Authorities 230
National Institutes of Health 193
National Permit Committee 118
National Research Council of the United
　States (NRC) 194
National Training Information Service 227
national training schemes 227–228
natural and laboratory diets 424, 581
natural breeding 750
natural food intake patterns 199
　during gestation and lactation 200
　in non-reproducing animals 199
　in reproducing animals 200
natural-ingredients diets 192, 195, **207**, 208
natural markings 94
Nature Conservation (Scotland) Act 2004 96
NC3Rs *see* National Centre for 3Rs
nebulisation 653–654, *654*
necropsy, laboratory mouse 360
necrotic enteritis (Clostridium welchii) 756
necrotic stomatitis 870
negative reinforcement training (NRT) 237,
　237–238
nematodes 817
nemerteans 1008
neonates
　euthanasia of 276, 412
　mortality in male pups 409
　rats 389
neoplasia 261
　in ferrets 516
　in mouse lemurs 674
neoplasms 426

Nervus ischiadicus 475
nested design 31
nestling voles 431
neuro-physiological sensitivity 14
neutering, effects of 559
newborn laboratory opossum 307, *307*
newcastle disease (ND) 756–757, 778, 818
new employees, orientation of 225–226
New Zealand, legislation and oversight 117
New Zealand Veterinary Association 117
New Zealand White (NZW) rabbits 485, 492
nile tilapia (*Oreochromis niloticus*) 914
Nipple drinkers 197
nitrite 999
nitrogen 274
nitrogenous waste 967
noise, starling 830
non-coding DNA 43
nonessential nutrient 195
non-human primates (NHPs) 200, 205, 721
　containment systems for 164–165
　dogs and 251
　euthanasia 276
　food restriction 203
　training 237
　wooden 186
non-infectious diseases 319, 353–356, 479
　anophthalmia/microphthalmia/congenital
　　cataract 353–354
　barbering 354–355
　C57BL/6 mice *355*
　hydrocephalus 356
　imperforate vagina 356
　malocclusion 356
　reptiles, terrestrial 869–870
　ulcerative dermatitis 356
　unexpected genetic effects 356
　vaginal septa 356
　wounding secondary to aggression 356
non-invasive sampling methods 15, 89
non-nutrients, in diets 208–209
non-obese diabetic (NOD) mice 352
'non-parametric' methods 36–38
non-random sampling 36
nonrapid eye movement (NREM) sleep *328*
non-sentient organisms 8
non-steroidal anti-inflammatory drugs
　(NSAIDs) 651, 949
non-target species 87
non-vertebrate species 187
NORINA database 8
North America, legislation and
　oversight 110–113
nucleic acid codons 41
nucleotides 41
nutrients 191
　excessive 195–196
　ferrets 508
　horses 637–640
　levels in diet 207–208, **208**
　during pregnancy 529
　requirements 194–195
　unintended nutrient deficiency 205–206
　and water requirements 194–198
nutritional deficiencies 191, 624

obesity 675, 734
Octopodiformes 959
octopus (*Thaumoctopus mimicus*) 965
Octopus rubescens 968
Octopus vulgaris 84
oesophageal obstruction (choke) 655

Index

oestrous control 531
oestrous cycle 409
OIE *see* World Organisation for Animal Health
old world monkeys (OWM) 721–734
   acute gastric dilatation 734
   administration of substances 728
   alopecia 734
   anaesthesia and analgesia 729
   biological data 721–723, **724**
   endocrine disorders 733
   endometriosis 733
   environment and hygiene 727
   euthanasia 729–730
   handling 727–728
   health 730
   housing, husbandry, and enrichment 726–727
   infectious diseases 730–733
   injuries 730
   intoxications 734
   macaque breeding groups 723–725
   marking 725
   nutrient deficiencies **734**
   nutritional aspects 733–734
   obesity 734
   sampling methods 728–729
   skin and hair abnormalities 733
   transportation 725
   use in research 725
   welfare 730
   welfare assessment 726
olfaction 347
olfactory sense 467
omnivorous species 933
omphalitis/navel infection 755
one-piece full suit *152*
open-formula diets 193
operant conditioning 237
Ophidiomyces ophiodiicola 871
Ophionyssus natricis 872, 873
oral dosing technique 562
organs-on-chips 8
orientation, new employees 225–226
osteoarthritis 528
osteodystrophic disorders 866
outbred strains 46, 390
outcome measures 27
overriding requirements 123
OWM *see* old world monkeys
oxygen 999
oxygen saturation, in cephalopoda 967
oxytetracycline 412

Paedocypris progenetica 907
pain and distress, horses 632
pain assessment 590
pair-and group-housed animals 12
pair feeding 204–205
pairings 312
Palaemon adspersus 1005
Palaemon serratus 999
palatability 201
Pandalus montagui 999
parametric tests 38
Paramoeba perniciosa 1008
paramyxovirus infection 871
Paranannizziopsis spp. 871
parasites (endoparasites) 498–499, 515, 897–900
   prevention of 643–644
parasitic diseases 757–758
parasitic infestations 427

paratyphoid 818
parenteral anaesthetic overdose 275–276
parturition 409, 598, 646–647
Passalurus ambiguus 499
passive integrated transponder (PIT tags) 925
passive restraint *559*
Pasteurella multocida 498
pellet diets 193
pellet hardness effects 201–202
penis prolapse 336
pens/cages 745
People's Republic of China, legislation and oversight 114–115
performance specifications 133
peri-anaesthetic care 535
persistent frustration 606
personal protective equipment (PPE) 151
pheasant, handling of *91*
phenotyping 43, **46**, 54–61
   broad-based 55–57
   challenges 58–60
   genetic modification 54, 55
   hierarchical approach 57
   hypothesis-driven 57–58
   issues with conventional 58
   Mouse Phenome Project 56
   pipeline 57
   systematic 55–57
   welfare of 54–55
physical barriers 150
physical enrichment 13
physical environment
   cat, domestic 555
   cattle 601
   corvids 846
   dog, laboratory 526–527
   gerbil 408
   marmosets and tamarins 694
   rabbits, laboratory 492–493
   starling 829
   zebra finch 795–796
   zebrafish 938–940
physical marking 94
physical methods 274–275, 412
physical punishment 242
Physignathus sp. 870
physiological measures 69
physiological monitoring 391
   capuchin monkeys 715–716
   dog, laboratory 532–533
   horses 651–652
   Japanese quail 776
   pigs and minipigs 583–584
   stress 925
   Syrian hamster 424–425
   voles 436–437
physiological stress response 69
phytoestrogens 208
pigeons and doves 807–819
   administration of substances 814
   allergies 819
   anaesthesia 815, **815**
   behavioural training 814
   biological data 807–808, **808**
   breeding 812–813
   breeds and supply 809
   cages 811
   cervical dislocation 816
   diseases 816–819
   environmental provision and enrichment 811
   feeding and dietary requirements 811–812

   handling *813*, 813–814
   health monitoring 816
   housing 810
   intramuscular injections 814–815
   intraperitoneal injections 815
   intravenous injection 814
   nutritional deficiencies 819
   reproduction 808–809
   social grouping 811
   social organisation 808
   subcutaneous injection 814
   transport and quarantine 812
   uses in laboratory 809–810
   water 812
pigs and minipigs 570–592
   abnormal behaviour 592
   acclimation 582
   administration of substances 587–588
   anaesthesia and analgesia 588–590
   biological data 570
   biopsies 587
   blood sampling 584–586, *584–586*
   breeding 579–581
   breeds, strains and genetics 574, *576*
   cardiac and pulmonary functions 583–584
   categories **575**
   dietary requirements 581–582
   diseases 591–592
   ear tattoo *580*
   environmental provisions 578
   euthanasia 590–591
   faeces 586
   farm and miniature **574, 577**
   feeding 581–582
   handling and restraining 582–583, *583*
   health monitoring 579
   housing 575–577
   identification and sexing 579
   injection *587*, 587–588, **588**
   lifespan 570
   liquids 587
   milk 586
   nutrient requirements of **582**
   oestrous symptoms 573
   physical environment and hygiene 577–578
   physiological monitoring 583–584
   picking up *583*
   presentation of food and water 578–579
   quarantine and barrier systems 579
   reproduction 572–573
   reproductive problems 592
   senses communication and cognition 570–572
   size range 570
   social grouping 578
   social organisation 572
   sources of supply 574–575
   transport 579
   urine 586
   uses in laboratory 575
   water 581
   young 580–581
pigs, containment systems 165
pilot experiments 24–25
pin worm *(Oxyuris equi)* 643
PIT tags *see* passive integrated transponder
Places Other than Licensed Establishments (POLEs) 95–96
plasma corticosterone *380*
Plasmodium simium 716
PLoS Biol **24**
pneumonia 605–60

Index

point of entry (POE) 186
poisonous plant Ragwort *639*
polycarbonate cages 307
polycystic disease 426
polypropylene 307
population dynamics, effects of field studies 86
positive reinforcement training (PRT) 236–247, *237*, 560, 715
  benefits 236, 238–239
  methods 239–241
  negative reinforcement training and 238
  objectives 239
  techniques 240–241
  tools 239–240
positive reinforcers 239
post-surgical analgesia 16
potential welfare issues
  of isolators **156**
  of IVCs **158**
  room as containment barrier **154**
power analysis 29–30
practical skills 226–227
prairie vole 431
precise reinforcement 243
precision 142
'predictive' validity 24
pre-emptive analgesia 16
preference tests 73–74
pregnancy 332
  determination 598
  domestic cat 557
  gerbils 49
  and newborns 714
PREPARE guidelines 18, 20, **24**, 60, 357
prescriptive specifications 133
primary conjunctivitis 655
primary responsibility 224
Principles of Humane Experimental Technique, The (Russell & Burch 1959) 5
problem and abnormal behaviour 352–353
procedural training 13
procurement models 126–127
  advantages and disadvantages **127**
project brief 123–124, 129
  for animal facilities 123–124
'project evaluation' 107
project manager (PM) 130
project procurement strategy 126
project team 130
promoters 42
prophylaxis 564, 591, 777–778
proposed enrichment 143
protective clothing 151–152
protein-coding DNA 40–41
protein fractionators 968
protein skimmers 968
Protopolystoma xenopodis 898, 900
protozoa 850
  reptiles, terrestrial 872
protozoans 1008
Pseudocapillaroides xenopodis 897, 900
pseudo-replication 28, 31
PSG *see* pyramidal shell growth
psychological stress 75
pullorum disease (*Salmonella pullorum*) 754
punishment/negative reinforcement 15–16, 237, 241–242
pup injury 426
purified diets 192–193, 195
'purposeful ageing' of animals 251, 264
pyramidal shell growth (PSG) 865

QBA *see* Qualitative Behavioural Assessment
quail bronchitis 778
Qualitative Behavioural Assessment (QBA) 920
qualitative dependent variables 27
Quality of Life (QoL) 566
quality schemes 232–233
quantitative dependent variables 27
quarantine and barrier systems 331

rabbits, laboratory 484–500
  administration of drugs 497
  anaesthesia/analgesia 497–498
  biological data 485–486
  breeding 494–495
  caged *490*
  cardiovascular and respiratory functions in **485**
  care of aged animals 493–494
  clinical chemistry in **486**
  environmental enrichment 490–491
  euthanasia 498
  feeding/watering 491
  general biology (natural history) 484
  haematology in **485**
  handling 495–496
  health monitoring 493
  killing 498
  monitoring methods 496–497
  normal behaviour 486–487
  physical environment 492–493
  reproduction 486
  in research 487–488
  sexing 492
  size range and lifespan 484
  social housing 491–492
  training/habituation 496, *496*
  welfare problems 498–499
rabbits, wild
  containment systems for 163
  feeding 200–201
  food restriction 203
  and guinea pigs 200
  high-fibre requirements 194
  'muesli' feeds for 205
  social organisation 485
  unintended nutrient deficiency 205
radiation-induced germ-line mutagenesis 47
rainbow trout (*Oncorhynchus mykiss*) 914–915
random effects 28
randomisation 32
randomised block design 33, *33*, 37
RAO *see* recurrent airway obstruction
rasping 642–643
Rat Genome Database (RGD) 383
rationalising 8
rat, laboratory 379–395, **389**
  abnormal behaviour 395
  anaesthesia **393,** 393–394, **394**
  analgesia 393–394, **394**
  biology and history 379–380
  environmental provisions 384–385
  feeding/watering 385–386
  general husbandry 384–385
  handling and training *390*, 390–391
  health monitoring 386–387, **388**
  identification and sexing 386
  mating system and reproduction 381–382
  during nasal administration *392*
  neonates 389
  procedures 390–395
  quarantine and barrier systems 386–387

  reproductive problems 395
  restraining *391*
  sensory systems 380
  size range and lifespan 381
  social housing 385
  social organisation 381
  standard biological data 382
  strains and genetics 382–384
  transportation 388
  well-being in 395
  Wistar rats **382**
rats, wild
  bar-biting in *71*
  chromodacryorrhoea in *68*
  containment systems for 162
  enrichment for *163*
  and human hearing ranges *346*
  natural biology and behaviour of *65*
Rattus norvegicus 380, 382
Rattus rattus 380
read-across approach, wild animals 87–88
rearing 334
recommended allowance 195
record-keeping 694
  horses 648–649
records 231
recurrent airway obstruction (RAO) 656
red tears 68
reduction 9–11, 287–289
  experimental design 9–10
  optimising animal production 10–11
  principles 5, 6
  and refinement 9
  re-use of animals 10
  wild animals 88
reference resources 107
refinement 11–17, 287–289
  assessing animal well-being 11
  contingent harms 12–14
  direct harms 14–16
  observation schedules 12
  principles 5, 6
  scoring systems 11–12
  wild animals 88–89
reflection 229
refugia, terrestrial reptiles 863–864
regression 241
regulations
  of diet-restriction studies 204
  and standards 186–187
regulatory DNA 42–43
regulatory sequences 42
reinforcement
  delivery of 241
  magnitude of 241
  schedules of 241
  selective or differential 241
relative humidity (RH) 863
release or rehoming 270
release, wild animals 94–95
reliability 133–134
remote cameras, wild animals 88–89
renal diseases 675
repeated factor, repeated measures design 36
repeated measures design 35–36
repetition 240
replacement 7–9, 287–289
  high-fidelity fallacy 8–9
  methods 8
  principles 5, 6
  strategies 8
  wild animals 87–88

replicability 142
reproduction
 animals 200
 behaviour 86
 biological data 303–304
 cat, domestic 547–548
 corvids 840–841
 decapod crustaceans 998
 dog, laboratory 519, **519**
 ferrets 509–510
 fowl, domestic 742
 guinea pig **467**
 husbandry systems 548
 Japanese quail 765
 mouse, laboratory **349**
 naked mole-rat (NMR) 446–448
 pigeons and doves 808–809
 pigs and minipigs 572–573
 problems of laboratory opossums 319–320
 rabbit, laboratory 486
 rat, laboratory 381–382, **389**, 395
 reptiles, terrestrial 858–859, 867–868
 starling 824–825
 voles 430–431, 434–435
 zebra finch 789–790
 zebrafish 934–936
reptiles, terrestrial 855–875
 anaesthesia and analgesia 874
 anatomy 855
 bacteria 870–871
 behavioural interactions 857
 diet and feeding 864–866
 ectothermy and behavioural thermoregulation 856–857
 environmental enrichment 863
 euthanasia 874
 handling and restraint 858–859
 health and diseases 868–873
 health monitoring 868–869
 helminths and pentastomids 872
 hibernation and aestivation 858
 hygiene 864
 identification and marking 867
 infectious diseases 870–873
 integument 855–856
 light 862
 non-infectious diseases 869–870
 protozoa 872
 refugia 863–864
 relative humidity 863
 reproduction 867–868
 sex determination and reproduction 858–859
 size and lifespan 858
 special senses 857–858
 species used in laboratory 859–860
 telemetry 874
 temperature and thermoregulation 861–862
 ticks and mites 872–873
 training and habituation 863
 ultraviolet radiation 862–863
 uses of 860–861
 ventilation and air changes 863
 viral infections 871–872
 welfare and welfare assessment 867
 zoonoses and health hazards 874
Republic of Korea 114
research
 ageing animals in 252–253
 animal facilities *see* animal facilities
 ethics review *see* ethical review
 journals 19
 laboratory animals 236–247

 quality 184
 scientific 269
 tree shrews use in 327–329
 wildlife 84–99
 wildlife studies 95–96
research, testing and teaching (RTT) 117
resource equation 29
respiratory protective equipment (RPE) 151
respiratory system, mouse 345
resting herd 630
restraint 13
retrospective assessments 285
reuse/rehoming
 of animal 10, 269
 horses 633–634
reward/positive reinforcement 15–16
rhesus macaques 721–722
Rhincodon typus 907
ribosome 42
rigid isolators 155
ringing 93
ringworm 606
RNA-guided endonucleases (RGEN) 50
rooting 349
rotifer (*Brachionus plicatilis*) 1004
roughages 639–640
routine welfare monitoring 65–69
 body weight 68–69
 cage observations 65
 of physical appearance 66–67, **67**
RPE plus down-draught table 151
rumenal fermentation 609, 610, 623
ruminal contents 604
ruminants, containment systems 165–166
Rus-LASA *see* Russian Association for Laboratory Animal Science
Russian Association for Laboratory Animal Science (Rus-LASA) 118
Russian Federation 118
Russian law 102

safety and environmental constraints 272
Saguinus geoffroyi 686
Saguinus oedipus 686
saliva 561
 samples 93
Salmonella enterica 779
Salmonella typhimurium 818
salmonellosis 779
sampling
 blood 15, 318, 410, 425, 453
 non-invasive 15
 non-random 36
 urine and faecal 411
 of wild animals 92–93
SAM system *see* sympathetic–adrenomedullary system
SANGER-MGP *see* Wellcome Trust Sanger Institute Mouse Genetics Project
Sapajus libidinosus 708
Sapajus spp. 708–710, *709*
Saprolegnia spp. 897
Scandinavian Federation for Laboratory Animal Science (Scand-LAS) 579
Scand-LAS *see* Scandinavian Federation for Laboratory Animal Science
schedules of reinforcement 241
Science Council of Japan (SCJ)
 guidelines 113–114
scientific application of animals 115
scientific constraints 272
scientific endpoints 269

scientific research 269
scientific training 18
scientific validation 19
SCJ guidelines *see* Science Council of Japan guidelines
scours (diarrhoea) 606
SE *see* structural engineer
sebaceous gland carcinomas 412
sedation 650
selective or differential reinforcement 241
self-directed learning 229
self-injurious behaviours (SIB) 239
semi-synthetic diets 192
sensory enrichment 636, 845
sensory systems 380
sensu strictu 342
sentinels 353
Sepia bandensis 970
Sepia officinalis 981
Sepia spp. 966
sepiolids 969
sequential testing, wild animals 88
services engineer 131
severity 290
sexing 59
 corvids 845–846
 domestic cat 555
 gerbil, laboratory 407–408
 guinea pigs 472, *472*
 Japanese quail 772
 marmosets and tamarins 693–694
 pigs and minipigs 579
 rabbits, laboratory 492
 rat, laboratory 386
 reptiles, terrestrial 858–859
 Syrian hamster 421
 voles 433–434
 zebrafish 945
sexual maturity 964
shaping/successive approximation 240
shearing and fleece care 625
shedding, of winter coat *629*
sheep and goats
 ageing and normal life span 625
 anaesthesia of 623
 biological overview 609
 breeding 617–620
 choice of breed 613–614
 common diseases 624–625
 enclosures, pasture and shelters 614
 environmental enrichment 616
 euthanasia 623
 feeding 610, 620–621
 group housing 614–615
 handling 621–623
 health monitoring 617
 identification 616
 individual penning **615**, 615–616, *616*
 injections 621–623
 lumbar spine of *618*
 natural behaviour 609–611
 open-plan barn 615
 perceptual and cognitive abilities 611–613
 quarantine and barrier systems 617
 reproductive behaviour 610–611
 social organisation 609–610
 source of animals 614
 standard biological data 613
 training 621–623
 transport and movement 617
 uses in laboratory 614
 welfare assessment 623

shipping box *314*
SHIRPA protocols 55–57
short-term sedation 716
SHR *see* spontaneous hypertensive rat
signal-to- noise ratio 25
signs of poor welfar 336
Simian Immunodeficiency virus (SIV) 731
Singapore, legislation and oversight 116
single-and two-stage design-and-build models 126–127
single-housing 526
single nucleotide polymorphisms (SNPs) 44
single photon emission computed tomography (SPECT) 334
single-sex groups 433
SIV *see* Simian Immunodeficiency virus
skin infections, of horses 657
skin pigmentation 881
skin swabbing 925
S-labs 123
smart traps 89
Sminthopsis crassicaudata 302
snakes 870
social enrichment 13
social grouping
   capuchin monkeys 711–713
   pigeons and doves 811
social housing *see* housing
socialisation training 244
social isolation and distress 438
social organisation
   capuchin monkeys 707–708
   corvids 839–840
   domestic cat 547
   fowl, domestic 741–742
   gerbil, laboratory 402–404
   in guinea pigs *468*
   horses 628
   pigs and minipigs 572
   rat, laboratory 381
   zebrafish 936
social stratification 468
Soft Landings 135–136
solitary housing 471
Sorex sinuosus 203
South Africa, legislation and oversight 118
South African National Standard (SANS) 118
soybean oil 192
soy isoflavones 208
spatial behaviour 86
species 161–167
   aquatic 276
   mice 161–162
   signs and care for 253–264
   training for 236–237
specifications 133
specific-locus test 48
Specific Pathogen-Free (SPF) 26
SPECT *see* single photon emission computed tomography
spermatogenesis 630
SPF *see* Specific Pathogen-Free
spontaneous activity 201
spontaneous hypertensive rat (SHR) 46, 383
spontaneous mutations 47
spontaneous spongiform brainstem degeneration 675
spontaneous tumours *336*
Sprague-Dawley albino 383
squirrel monkeys *712*
stability 133–134
staff quality 566
staff training 153
stallions 648
Staphylococcus aureus 479
starling 824–835
   anaesthesia and analgesia 833–834
   biology 824
   blood sampling *832*, 832–833
   body mass in **825**
   care of aged animals 830
   conservation status 826
   environmental provisions and enrichments 827–828
   euthanasia 834
   feeding/watering 828
   handling 830–831, *831*
   hygiene 830
   identification and sexing 828–830
   monitoring methods 831–833
   noise 830
   normal behaviour 825
   parasites and infectious diseases 834
   photoperiod 829
   physical environment 829
   probing behaviour of *825*
   reproduction 824–825
   reproductive data for **825**
   sexually dimorphic features in **829**
   size range and lifespan 824
   social organisation 824
   training procedures 831
   use in research 826–827
   weighing *831*
statistical analysis
   experimental designs 32
   types of 36–38
statistical design, wild animals 88
statistical power 29
statistical test 29
stereotypic behaviour 71–72, 139, 320
   voles 438–439
stereotyping 631, 851
stomach, mouse 344
strains 26
   and genetics 327
   rat, laboratory 382–384
Streptococcus equi 645
Streptococcus zooepidemicus 656
stress 340–341, 565–566
   anaesthesia and 86
   effects of 85
   physiological monitoring 925
   Xenopus 895–896
'stress' hormones 70
stressors 603
structural engineer (SE) 131
study design *see* experimental design
sub-contractors 132
subcutaneous (SC) injections 437, 511, 728
substrains 44–45
supplementary products 194
suppliers of building materials 132
surgery 16, 318
   mouse, laboratory 359–360
survival, effects of field studies 86
sympathetic–adrenomedullary (SAM) system 468
synchronisation technique 597
synthetic diets 192
Syrian hamster *420*
   anaesthesia 425
   approaching *424*
   behaviour 419–420
   breeding 420–424
   dimensions and space allowances **421**
   dosing routes for 425–426
   ecology 419
   feeding 424
   female 422, *422*, *423*
   growth curves for *423*
   handling 424
   identification and sexing 421
   lifting *424*
   male *422*
   optimal reproductive life of 423
   physiological monitoring 424–425
   reproductive data for **422**
   scruffing *425*
   taxonomy 419
   uses in laboratory 420
   water 424
systematic phenotyping 55–57
system/equipment failure 134–135

Taeniopygia guttata *see* zebra finch
Taeniopygia guttata castanoti 787
tagging animals 93
tail-cuff method 326
Taiwan, legislation and oversight 115
tamarins 164
tamarin species 686
tamoxifen 201
TAN *see* total ammonia nitrogen
tapetum lucidum 665
tapeworms (Cestoda) 643–644, 872
target 239–240
targeted transgenesis 49–50
tattooing 331
T2DM *see* Type 2 DM
teaching behaviour 240
teat scoring systems 605
technical design 129
technical replication 31
telemetric systems 93, 168, 532–533
temperature 450
temperature-dependent sex determination (TSD) **868**
test sensitivity 142
tetracycline 412
The Air Cargo Tariff and Rules (TACT) 186
thick-billed raven (*Corvus crassirostris*) 839
thoracic compression 276
Three Primary Standards 107
Three Rs (3Rs) 5, 102–107
   definitions 102
   ethical framework of 221
   ethics review 290–291
   in fish research 909–910
   funding bodies 18
   holistic approach to 7
   individual activity 18
   institution activity 18
   international and national efforts 19–20
   origin and evolution 6–7
   principles 102–107
   responsibility for 18–20
   scientific journals 19
   using ageing animals *see* ageing animals
   wildlife studies 87–89
   working definitions 7
   see also reduction; refinement; replacement
three-spined stickleback (*Gasterosteus aculeatus*) 913–914
Three Ss 7
time out 241–242

Tiritrichomonas mobilensis 336
TIVA *see* Total Intravenous Anaesthesia
TMRs *see* total mixed rations
toe tattooing 421
torpor 203
tortoises 855
total ammonia nitrogen (TAN) 967
Total Intravenous Anaesthesia (TIVA) 497
total mixed rations (TMRs) 600
touch, mouse senses 346–347
traditional model 126
training/habituation
   capuchin monkeys 715
   cat, domestic 560
   cattle 603
   corvids 848
   dog, laboratory 531–532
   education and 221–223
   euthanasia 277–278
   FELASA 228
   fishes 924–925
   horses 649–650
   in-house 225
   'intentional' 236
   laboratory animals 245–247
   marmosets and tamarins 697
   of mice to perform 358
   national training schemes 227–228
   nonhuman primates 237
   opportunities 225
   programme 223–224
   programme development 245–247
   rabbits, laboratory 496, *496*
   rat, laboratory 390–391
   reptiles, terrestrial 863
   sheep and goats 621–623
   socialisation 244
   for species 236–237
   tree shrews 334
   zebra finch 799
tranquillisers 183
transfer RNA (tRNA) 42
transgene
   targeted insertion of 49
transgenesis 48
transgenic strains 48
transmissible spongiform encephalopathies (TSEs) 614
transportation, of laboratory animals 13, 314–315
   animal rights movement 187–188
   cattle 598–599
   of cephalopods 965–966
   container design and construction 177–181
   container stocking density 181–182
   corvids 846
   current laws, regulations and standards 186–187
   decapod crustaceans 1006
   dog 521
   environmental provisions during 490
   gerbil, laboratory 408
   handling 923–924
   health and welfare 172–177
   horses 644
   Japanese quail 773
   journey planning 183–186
   marmosets and tamarins 694–695
   old world monkeys (OWM) 725
   pigeons and doves 812
   pigs and minipigs 579

   principles and requirements 171–172
   rat 388
   sheep and goats 617
   stressors during 182–183
   tree shrews 331–332
   voles 435–436
   Xenopus 894–895
   zebrafish 937
'treatment' factor 27
tree shrews 324–337
   administration of substances 334
   anaesthesia 335
   analgesia 335
   biological data 326–327
   breeding 332–334
   common welfare problems 336
   euthanasia 336
   feeding 329–330
   general biology 324–325
   general husbandry 329–334
   handling 334
   hand rearing 334
   health monitoring 331
   identification and sexing 331
   intubation 335
   laboratory procedures 334–336
   mating systems 332
   monitoring methods 334
   Scandentia **325**
   size range and lifespan 325–326
   social organisation 326
   sources of supply 327
   transport 331–332
   use in research 327–329
   water 330–331
Trichuris trichiura 732
trickle cube/hay feeders *636*
trio mating 362
TSD *see* temperature-dependent sex determination
t-test 36–37
tuberculosis 437, 716
tumours 336
Tupaia belangeri 324, *325, 326,* 327
   adult **328**
   housing and rearing 330
   for inhalation anaesthesia *335*
   nesting 332
   newborn 333
   pregnancy 332
Tupaia belangeri chinensis 326
Tupaia glis 326, 327
Tupaia taenia quentini 336
Tupaiidae 326
Tupaiids 333
Tylodelphylus xenopodis 897
Type 2 DM (T2DM) 732
type I (autoimmune) diabetes 352
Tyzzer's disease 412

UBT *see* Usable Buildings Trust
UK, animal research laboratories in 125
ulcerative dermatitis 356
ulcerative enteritis 779
ultraviolet radiation 862–863
understanding 222, 224–225
undesirable penthouse shoebox 362
unexpected genetic effects 356
unintended nutrient deficiency 205–206
United States Department of Agriculture's (USDA) 104
unit of replication 28

Universities Federation for Animal Welfare (UFAW) 5
   mission of 1
upper critical concentration (UCC) 195, *195*
Uracil (U) 42
urine 534
   collection, guinea pig 474–475
   and faecal sampling 411, 561
   Syrian hamster 425
urolithiasis 602
Urosporidium crescens 1008
URS *see* User Requirement Specification
Usable Buildings Trust (UBT) 136
user advisor, role of 127
User Requirement Specification (URS) 128, *128*

vaccinations 778
   horses 645
vacutainer systems 621
vaginal septa 356
vaginal smears 436–437
validation 133–134
   enrichment 144
validity 26, 287, 289
value engineering (VE) 128–129
VAP *see* vascular access port
variability, nuisance source of 33
variable-formula diets 193
variable/intermittent schedule 241
variations 43
vascular access port (VAP) 728–729
vasculitis 675
vasopressin 70
VAS scoring system *see* Visual Analogue Scale scoring system
ventilated cabinets *159*, 159–160
ventilation system 155, 493, 745
verbal commands 648
verification 133
vervet monkeys 723
veterinary care 104–105
vibrionic hepatitis (*Campylobacter foetus*) 755
video analysis software 925
VIE *see* visible implant elastomer
viraemia 731
viral diseases 564–565, 778, 850
visible implant elastomer (VIE) 945
Visual Analogue Scale (VAS) scoring system 920
vitamin A 943
vitamin C 943
vitamin E 943
vitamin E deficiency 424
vivaria 122
volatile anaesthetics 274
voles
   anaesthesia 437
   breeding 434–435
   euthanasia 437
   food and water 433
   general biology 430
   housing 432–433
   identification and sexing 433–434
   infants or pups 431
   laboratory animal 431
   nestling 431
   physical environment 432
   physiological monitoring 436–437
   reproduction 430–431, 434–435
   social grouping 433
   social isolation and distress 438
   sources of supply 431

voles (cont'd)
　　stereotypic behaviour 438–439
　　transport and handling 435–436
　　welfare problems 437–439
voluntary accreditation, of animal care 107
voluntary food intake, in laboratory
　　　animals 198–202, *199*, *200*
　　body size effects 198
　　diurnal feeding rhythms 200–201
　　environmental effects 201
　　foraging for food 200
　　in non-reproducing animals 199
　　palatability and variety effects 201
　　pellet hardness effects 201–202
　　in reproducing animals 200
　　spillage 198–199
voluntary water intake 638

Waardenburg syndrome 516
walker machine, horses *641*
wasting marmoset syndrome 699
Watanabe heritable hyperlipidaemic (WHHL)
　　　rabbits 488
watering *see* feeding/watering
water voles 430
weaning 334, 435, 530
　　age 410
　　and rearing 557–558
weasels (*Mustela nivalis*) 92
weaving/box (stall) walking 631
weighing starling *831*
weight loss 624
weight monitoring, horses 641, *641*
welfare
　　animal 1, 11
　　behaviour and 438–439
　　changes in 70–73
　　contingent harms 12–14
　　costs 12–14
　　direct harms 12, 14–16
　　environmental enrichment on 140–141
　　fish 908, *908*, 917–921
　　importance of 5
　　of laboratory and research animals 236–247
　　legislation 138
　　monitoring systems 166
　　well-being 11
　　wildlife studies 85–87
　　zebrafish 938
welfare assessment 11, 55, 64–76
　　basic principles 64
　　and changes 69–70
　　in guinea pigs 478
　　old world monkeys (OWM) 726
　　reptiles, terrestrial 867
　　routine monitoring 65–69
　　sheep and goats 623
　　toolbox 64, 65, 73
　　zebra finch **262**
　　for zebra finches **262**
welfare audit 867
well-being 340–341
Wellcome Trust Sanger Institute Mouse
　　　Genetics Project (SANGER-MGP) 56
well-fleeced sheep 614
well-functioning ethics review 292
Welsh Mountain pony 633
WHHL rabbits *see* Watanabe heritable
　　　hyperlipidaemic rabbits

white-tailed deer 152
Whitten effect 352
wild animals/mammals
　　being observed by CCTV 164, *164*
　　capuchin monkeys 707–717
　　field studies *see* field studies of wildlife
　　handling 91, *91*, 153
　　management of 85
　　old world monkeys (OWM) 721–734
　　research facilities *see* research animal
　　　　facilities
　　voles 430–439
wild boar
　　anaesthesia of 92
　　using infrared 89
wild-caught animals 14
wild cavy (*Cavia aperea*) *see* guinea pigs
Wildlife and Countryside Act (WCA) 96–97
wildlife research 84
Wild Mammals (Protection) Act 1996 97
wild-type GM mouse 347
Wild-Type Groningen rats 383
wild-type plumage 763
Wistar albino 383
Wistar rats **382**, *385*
within-animal experiments 25, 28
wood chewing 631–632
wooden nonhuman primate *186*
World Organisation for Animal Health (OIE) 103
worming plan 644, *644*
wounding secondary to aggression 356
wounds 657

xanthan gum 193
X chromosomes 41
Xenopus 881–902
　　administration of substances 893–894
　　anaesthesia/analgesia 894
　　biosecurity 900
　　breeding 891–893
　　care of aged animals 896
　　diversity, biogeography 884
　　environmental conditions 887–893
　　environmental enrichment 891
　　euthanasia 894
　　handling 893
　　health and disease 896–900
　　identification and marking
　　　　techniques 894
　　laboratory maintenance 885–887
　　large-scale maintenance systems 887
　　monitoring methods 894
　　safety considerations 895
　　semi-natural environments 886
　　species 883
　　stress 895–896
　　temperature 890
　　transport 894–895
　　water chemistry 891
　　see also Xenopus laevis
Xenopus laevis 253, 881–902
　　behaviour and communication 885
　　ecology 884, 884–885
　　parasites of *899*
　　see also Xenopus
Xenopus tropicalis 253

Y chromosomes 41
Yersinia spp 691, 732

zebra finch 252–253, 262–263, 787–802,
　　788, *798*
　　administration of substances 799
　　ageing-related adverse effects in *261*
　　anaesthesia and analgesia 799–800
　　behaviour 801
　　biological data 789
　　breeding 797–798
　　enclosures 791
　　environmental provisions and
　　　　enrichments 791–793
　　euthanasia 800
　　feeding and watering 792, 793–794
　　handling 799
　　health monitoring 797
　　humidity requirements for 795
　　hygiene 796–797
　　identification and sexing 795
　　infectious and non-infectious
　　　　diseases 800–801
　　monitoring methods 799
　　natural history 787–788
　　normal behaviour 790
　　physical environment 795–796
　　quarantine and barrier systems 797
　　reproduction 789–790
　　size range and lifespan 788
　　social housing 794–795
　　social organisation 788–789
　　sources and supplies 790
　　training and habituation 799
　　use in research 790
　　welfare assessment system for **262**
zebrafish 253, 263, *263*, 933–950
　　administration of substances 946
　　anaesthesia/analgesia 947–949,
　　　　948, **949**
　　as animal model *934*
　　blood collection 946
　　classification and humane
　　　　endpoints 949–950
　　development 934, **935–936**
　　environmental enrichment 941
　　environmental parameters **940**, 940
　　euthanasia 949
　　feeding 942–944
　　general biology 933–934
　　genotyping 947
　　handling 946
　　health monitoring in 941–942
　　injection 947
　　larval and juvenile 944–945
　　pathogenic and non-pathogenic
　　　　disease **942–943**
　　perception 938
　　physical environment 938–940
　　reproduction 934–936
　　sexing 945
　　size and life span 934
　　social organisation 936
　　sources 936–937
　　training/habituation 946
　　transportation 937
　　uses in research 937–938
　　welfare 938
　　welfare problems 950
zinc-finger nucleases (ZFNs) 50
zoonosis 437–438
Zootoca vivipara 862